Diseases of Poultry

TENTH EDITION

Diseases

of

Poultry

TENTH EDITION

Edited by B. W. Calnek
with
H. John Barnes
Charles W. Beard
Larry R. McDougald
Y. M. Saif

Editorial Board for the American
Association of Avian Pathologists

Iowa State University Press   Ames, Iowa, USA

Iowa State University Press
2121 South State Avenue
Ames, IA 50014

Orders: 1-800-862-6657
Office: 1-515-292-0140
Fax: 1-515-292-3348

Tenth edition, 1997

Library of Congress Cataloging-in-Publication Data
Diseases of poultry / edited by B.W. Calnek, with H. John Barnes ... [et al.].—10th ed.
      p.   cm.
   Includes bibliographical references and index.
   ISBN 0-8138-0427-2
   1. Poultry—Diseases. I. Calnek, B. W.
SF995.D69 1997
636.5′0896—dc21   97-2161

Last digit is the print number: 9 8 7 6 5 4 3 2 1

Contents

Contributing Authors

DENNIS J. ALEXANDER. Department of Avian Virology, Central Veterinary Laboratory, New Haw, Addlestone, Surrey KT15 3NB, England

ARTHUR A. ANDERSEN. National Animal Disease Center, P.O. Box 70, Ames, IA 50010

JAMES J. ARENDS. S & J Farms Animal Health Consultants, Willow Spring, NC 27592

LAWRENCE H. ARP. Department of Toxicology and Pathology, Hoffman-La Roche, 340 Kingsland Street, Nutley, NJ 07110

RICHARD E. AUSTIC. Department of Animal Science, New York State College of Agriculture and Life Sciences, Cornell University, Ithaca, NY 14853

TREVOR J. BAGUST. International Projects and Programs Division, University of Melbourne, Parkville, Victoria 3052, Australia

H. JOHN BARNES. College of Veterinary Medicine, North Carolina State University, 4700 Hillsborough, Raleigh, NC 27606

C. BAXTER-JONES. BUTA, P.O. Box 727, Lewisburg, WV 24901

CHARLES W. BEARD. 130 Red Fox Run, Athens, GA 30605

HERMAN A. BERKHOFF. Department of Microbiology, Pathology, and Parasitology, College of Veterinary Medicine, North Carolina State University, 4700 Hillsborough, Raleigh, NC 27606

A. J. BERMUDEZ. Veterinary Medical Diagnostic Laboratory, University of Missouri-Columbia, P.O. Box 6023, Columbia, MO 65205

PETER M. BIGGS. Willows, London Road, St. Ives, Huntingdon, Cambs PE17 4ES, England

PAT J. BLACKALL. Animal Research Institute, Yeerongpilly, Qld 4105, Australia

J. M. BRICKER. Intervet, Inc., 405 State Street, Millsboro, DE 19966

THOMAS P. BROWN. Department of Avian Medicine, College of Veterinary Medicine, University of Georgia, Athens, GA 30602-4875

V. VON BÜLOW. Freie Universität Berlin, Institut für Geflügelkrankheiten, Koserstr. 21, D-14195 Berlin, Germany

B. W. CALNEK. Unit of Avian Medicine, Department of Microbiology and Immunology, College of Veterinary Medicine, Cornell University, Ithaca, NY 14853

DAVID CAVANAGH. Institute for Animal Health, Compton Laboratory, Compton, Newbury, Berkshire RG 20 7NN, England

R. P. CHIN. California Veterinary Diagnostic Laboratory System, Fresno Branch, School of Veterinary Medicine, University of California, Davis, 2789 S. Orange Avenue, Fresno, CA 93725

HAROLD L. CHUTE. 432 Main Street, Orono, ME 04473

WILLIAM L. CURRENT. Infectious Disease Research (MC7R2), Bldg. B98A/2, Mail Drop 0428, Lilly Corporate Center, Indianapolis, IN 46285

JAMES F. DAVIS. Georgia Poultry Laboratory, 4457 Oakwood Road, P.O. Box 20, Oakwood, GA 30566

JOHN E. DOHMS. Department of Animal and Food Sciences, College of Agricultural Sciences, University of Delaware, Newark, DE 19717-1303

C. H. DOMERMUTH. Virginia-Maryland Regional College of Veterinary Medicine, Virginia Tech and State University, Blacksburg, VA 24061

R. DROUAL. California Veterinary Diagnostic Laboratory System, Fresno Branch, School of Veterinary Medicine, University of California, Davis, 2789 S. Orange Avenue, Fresno, CA 93725

J. P. DUCHATEL. Faculty of Veterinary Medicine, University of Liege, Liege, Belgium

B. C. EASTERDAY. School of Veterinary Medicine, University of Wisconsin-Madison, Madison, WI 53706

J. FABRICANT. Unit of Avian Medicine, Department of Microbiology and Immunology, College of Veterinary Medicine, Cornell University, Ithaca, NY 14853

A. M. FADLY. Avian Disease and Oncology Laboratory, USDA Agricultural Research Service, 3606 E. Mount Hope Road, East Lansing, MI 48823

MARTIN D. FICKEN. Pfizer Central Research, P.O. Box 80809, Lincoln, NE 68501

RICHARD K. GAST. Southeast Poultry Research Laboratory, USDA Agricultural Research Service, 934 College Station Road, Athens, GA 30605

G. YAN GHAZIKHANIAN. Nicholas Turkey Breeding Farms, P.O. Box Y, Sonoma, CA 95476

J. R. GLISSON. Department of Avian Medicine, College of Veterinary Medicine, University of Georgia, Athens, GA 30602-4875

MARK A. GOODWIN. Georgia Poultry Laboratory, 4457 Oakwood Road, P.O. Box 20, Oakwood, GA 30566

R. E. GOUGH. Department of Avian Virology, Central Veterinary Laboratory, New Haw, Addlestone, Surrey KT15 3NB, England

JAMES E. GRIMES. Texas Veterinary Medical Diagnostic Laboratory, P.O. Drawer 3040, College Station, TX 77841-3040 (Deceased)

W. B. GROSS. 1509 Lark Lane, Blacksburg, VA 24060

JAMES S. GUY. College of Veterinary Medicine, North Carolina State University, 4700 Hillsborough, Raleigh, NC 27606

SCOTT HAFNER. 252 Ashbrook Drive, Athens, GA 30605

DAVID A. HALVORSON. 301 Veterinary Science, 1971 Commonwealth Avenue, University of Minnesota, St. Paul, MN 55108

C. F. HELMBOLDT. Box 155, Rockport, ME 04856

VIRGINIA S. HINSHAW. University of Wisconsin, School of Veterinary Medicine, 2015 Linden Drive W., Room 3174, Madison, WI 53706

FREDERIC J. HOERR. Veterinary Diagnostic Laboratory, 1001 Wire Road, P.O. Box 2209, Auburn, AL 36831-2209

TADAO IMADA. National Institute of Animal Health, Kannondai, Tsukuba 305, Japan

SHERMAN W. JACK. Mississippi State University, College of Veterinary Medicine, Box 9825, Mississippi State, MS 39762

M. S. JAFFERY. K & N's Poultry Farm, 406 Noor Estate, Sharea Faisal, Karachi, Pakistan

RICHARD J. JULIAN. Department of Pathology, Ontario Veterinary College, University of Guelph, Guelph, Ontario NIG 2W1, Canada

HITOSHI KAWAMURA. Tochigi Laboratory, Gem Corporation, 82-1 Ogura, Imaichi, Tochigi 321-11, Japan

KIRK C. KLASING. Department of Avian Sciences, College of Agricultural and Environmental Sciences, University of California, Davis, CA 95616

S. H. KLEVEN. Department of Avian Medicine, College of Veterinary Medicine, University of Georgia, Athens, GA 30602-4875

LOUIS LEIBOVITZ. 3 Kettle Hole Road, Falmouth, MA 02540

DAVID H. LEY. Department of Food Animal and

Equine Medicine, College of Veterinary Medicine, North Carolina State University, 4700 Hillsborough, Raleigh, NC 27606

R. E. LUGINBUHL. 401 N.W. 130th Avenue, Plantation, FL 33325

PHIL D. LUKERT. Department of Medical Microbiology, College of Veterinary Medicine, University of Georgia, Athens, GA 30602-4875

E. T. MALLINSON. Virginia-Maryland Regional College of Veterinary Medicine, University of Maryland Campus, College Park, MD 20742

MASAKAZU MATSUMOTO. College of Veterinary Medicine, Oregon State University, Corvallis, OR 97331

LARRY R. MCDOUGALD. Department of Poultry Science, University of Georgia, Athens, GA 30602-4875

J. B. MCFERRAN. 19 Knocktern Gardens, Belfast, Northern Ireland BT4 3LZ

M. S. MCNULTY. Department of Agriculture for Northern Ireland, Veterinary Sciences Division, Stormont, Belfast, Northern Ireland BT4 3SD

K. V. NAGARAJA. Avian Disease Research Program, College of Veterinary Medicine, University of Minnesota, St. Paul, MN 55108

SYED A. NAQI. Unit of Avian Medicine, Department of Microbiology and Immunology, College of Veterinary Medicine, Cornell University, Ithaca, NY 14853

R. A. NORTON. Department of Poultry Science, Auburn University, Auburn, AL 36849-5416

N. O. OLSON. Department of Animal and Veterinary Sciences, West Virginia University, Morgantown, WV 26505

L. N. PAYNE. Institute for Animal Health, Compton Laboratory, Compton, Newbury, Berkshire RG20 7NN, England

F. WILLIAM PIERSON. VA-MD Regional College of Veterinary Medicine, Virginia Tech, Blacksburg, VA 24601

B. S. POMEROY. Avian Disease Research Program, College of Veterinary Medicine, University of Minnesota, St. Paul, MN 55108

RODNEY L. REECE. National Registry of Domestic Animal Pathology, Elizabeth Macarthur Agricultural Institute, Private Mail Bag 8, Camden, NSW 2570, Australia

WILLIE M. REED. Animal Health Diagnostic Laboratory, Michigan State University, B646 W. Fee Hall, East Lansing, MI 48824-1316

W. MALCOLM REID. Department of Poultry Science, University of Georgia, Athens, GA 30602-4875 (Deceased)

D. L. REYNOLDS. Veterinary Medical Research Institute, College of Veterinary Medicine, Iowa State University, Ames, IA 50011

JOHN L. RICHARD. Midwest Area National Center for Agricultural Utilization Research, USDA Agricultural Research Service, 1815 N. University Street, Peoria, IL 61604

C. RIDDELL. Western College of Veterinary Medicine, University of Saskatchewan, 52 Campus Drive, Saskatoon, Saskatchewan, Canada S7N 5B4

RICHARD B. RIMLER. National Animal Disease Center, P.O. Box 70, Ames, IA 50010

JOHN K. ROSENBERGER. Department of Animal and Food Sciences, College of Agricultural Sciences, University of Delaware, Newark, DE 19717-1303

M. D. RUFF. USDA, Agricultural Research Service, Beltsville, MD 20705

Y. M. SAIF. Food Animal Health Research Program, OARDC, Ohio State University, 1680 Madison Avenue, Wooster, OH 44691

T. S. SANDHU. Unit of Avian Medicine, College of Veterinary Medicine, Duck Research Laboratory, 217 Old Country Road, Eastport, NY 11941

KAREL A. SCHAT. Unit of Avian Medicine, Department of Microbiology and Immunology, College of Veterinary Medicine, Cornell University, Ithaca, NY 14853

MILTON L. SCOTT. Department of Animal Science, New York State College of Agriculture and Life Sciences, Cornell University, Ithaca, NY 14853

SIMON M. SHANE. School of Veterinary Medicine, Louisiana State University, Baton Rouge, LA 70803

H. L. SHIVAPRASAD. California Veterinary Diagnostic Laboratory System, Fresno Branch, School of Veterinary Medicine, University of California, Davis, 2789 S. Orange Avenue, Fresno, CA 93725

J. KIRK SKEELES. Department of Animal and Poultry Sciences, University of Arkansas, Fayetteville, AR 72701

WILFRED T. SPRINGER. 11921 King Richard Drive, Baton Rouge LA, 70815-6318

DAVID E. SWAYNE. Southeastern Poultry Research Laboratory, USDA Agricultural Research Service, 934 College Station Road, Athens, GA 30605

CHARLES O. THOEN. Department of Microbiology, Immunology, and Preventive Medicine, College of Veterinary Medicine, Iowa State University, Ames, IA 50011

DEOKI N. TRIPATHY. Department of Veterinary Pathobiology, College of Veterinary Medicine, University of Illinois at Urbana-Champaign, Urbana, IL 61801

H. VINDEVOGEL. Faculty of Veterinary Medicine, University of Liege, Bld de Colonster 20/BAT B.42, 4000 Liege, Belgium

DENNIS P. WAGES. College of Veterinary Medicine, North Carolina State University, 4700 Hillsborough, Raleigh, NC 27606

J. E. WILLIAMS. 2103 Kumquat Drive, Edgewater, FL 32141

R. L. WITTER. Avian Disease and Oncology Laboratory, USDA Agricultural Research Service, 3603 E. Mount Hope Road, East Lansing, MI 48823

L. W. WOODS. California Veterinary Diagnostic Laboratory System, Davis Branch, University of California, School of Veterinary Medicine, P.O. Box 1770, W. Health Science Drive, Davis, CA 95617

P. R. WOOLCOCK. California Veterinary Diagnostic Laboratory System, Fresno Branch, School of Veterinary Medicine, University of California, Davis, 2789 S. Orange Avenue, Fresno, CA 93725

PRISCILLA B. WYRICK. Department of Microbiology and Immunology, School of Medicine, University of North Carolina at Chapel Hill, Campus Box 7290, 804 Faculty Laboratory Office Building, Chapel Hill, NC 27599

RICHARD YAMAMOTO. Department of Population Health and Reproduction, School of Veterinary Medicine, University of California, Davis, CA 95616

HARRY W. YODER, JR. 360 Brookwood Drive, Athens, GA 30605

D. V. ZANDER. 18340 160th Avenue N.E., Woodinville, WA 98072

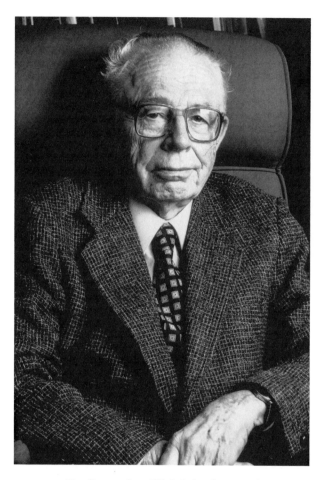

Dedicated to W. Malcolm Reid

Foreword

The revised tenth edition of *Diseases of Poultry* comes six years after the previous edition. Historically, that six-year interval has been appropriate because it allows a buyer of the text five or six years use on the investment, yet revisions are frequent enough to incorporate information on new techniques, research findings, and emerging diseases. The computer has greatly facilitated this revision, as it did the ninth edition, but there is still a great deal of effort expended by the editor and associate editors, as well as a large number of contributing authors, to bring out a new edition.

Expansion of the poultry industry is continuing in all categories and in all areas of the world, fueled by and keeping pace with an increased demand for poultry products. That demand is the result of the desire by many people to consume less animal fat and to enjoy economical but tasty food. The creative products that have been developed by the further-processing industry, and the numerous commercial outlets that have added poultry products to their menus, have obviously had an impact. Some of the former fast-food hamburger outlets now generate a quarter of their sales from breakfast meals featuring eggs. Virtually all of those outlets now include chicken breast fillet sandwiches as an important menu addition. Neither the achievements in new-product development nor the trend for more meals to be consumed outside the home are likely to end in the foreseeable future.

While consumer demand has driven the continuing expansion of the poultry industry, the resulting increased poultry population density and the rearing of different types of incompatible poultry species in close proximity have presented major disease challenges. Researchers and poultry veterinarians have had to effectively deal with the disease aspects of that expansion. Although advances in genetics and nutrition have obviously had a significant positive impact on the poultry industry, the ability to prevent and control disease has been crucial in allowing the poultry production process to function efficiently.

Earlier editions of *Diseases of Poultry* were written and used primarily by poultry veterinarians in the United States. Major changes in the text through the years have accompanied the inclusion of contributions from experts in many highly specialized fields and from many countries of the world. This has made it truly an international text, both in origin and utilization. Because all major diseases of poultry are covered and because of the benefits of a broader and more global perspective, the text has improved over the years.

It is clear that understanding the molecular genetics of causative agents will have a major role in keeping infectious diseases of poultry in check. Fortunately, the specialty of poultry disease research has attracted scientists with training in this discipline. That asset, coupled with the ability of many other researchers who were trained in more conventional approaches to the study of infectious diseases to acquire knowledge and skills in molecular methods, ensures that poultry disease researchers are at the forefront of understanding and controlling infectious diseases.

Immunization innovations include the use of vectored vaccines in which genes coding for protective antigens have been inserted into the genome of nonpathogenic poxviruses or herpesviruses. These will likely receive continued scrutiny and may see extensive use in the next decade. We may also come to rely on protective antigens prepared in vitro by inserting the appropriate genes into baculoviruses, which then produce the antigens in insect cell cultures. Also, protective antigens will likely be "engineered" in the laboratory once the sequence and secondary/tertiary structures are determined. The use of DNA as a vaccine to direct the production of protective antigen within the host is also a likely possibility.

Regardless of how rapid and extensive are the changes in approaches to poultry disease prevention and control, *Diseases of Poultry* will incorporate them with each new edition. These timely revisions provide both the student and professional with a convenient and reliable source of information that has ample references for additional reading. The many editions of *Diseases of Poultry* can most assuredly be added to the list of factors that have led to the continuing expansion and phenomenal success of the poultry industry.

Charles W. Beard

Preface

This edition of *Diseases of Poultry* marks a milestone. It is the fifth edition produced by an editorial committee appointed by the American Association of Avian Pathologists (AAAP), equaling the number edited by H.E. Biester, initially with Louis DeVries, and later with L.H. Schwarte. Four of the five original AAAP committee members have been replaced over the years. H. John Barnes joined the group for the eighth edition, replacing C.F. Helmboldt; for the ninth edition, Charles W. Beard took over for M.S. Hofstad. The present committee has two new members: Larry R. McDougald and Y.M. Saif have replaced W. Malcolm Reid and Harry W. Yoder, Jr., respectively. B.W. Calnek, who became the chief editor after Dr. Hofstad's retirement, remains as the only member from the original AAAP committee.

In the course of the five AAAP-sponsored editions, the number of contributing experts has increased 240% to the present total of 96, 30 of whom are new authors or co-authors. Also, the number of countries from which authors were selected expanded from two to nine, representing four continents. Thus, there has been a strong trend toward broader representation for authorship and a clear recognition that poultry diseases do not respect either borders or continents.

Readers of this edition will find a number of significant changes in addition to the usual updated material in all chapters and subchapters. Staphylococcosis, *Riemerella anatipestifer* (previously *Pasteurella anatipestifer*), and infectious anemia have been expanded to full chapter status, and intestinal spirochetosis and *Mycoplasma iowae* infection have each been accorded subchapter status. On the other hand, some chapters or subchapters have been absorbed, merged, or moved. Erysipelas is now a subchapter in Other Bacterial Diseases; subchapters on nematodes and acanthocephalans, and cestodes and trematodes, are now in a new chapter entitled Internal Parasites; and pseudotuberculosis has been moved from the Pasteurellosis (now called Fowl Cholera) chapter to Other Bacterial Diseases. Parvovirus infection of chickens has been deleted because the condition described is thought to have been the same as infectious anemia. Also, material on the so-called malabsorption syndrome has been removed from the Reovirus Infections chapter (new title, Viral Arthritis) and from the Developmental, Metabolic, and Miscellaneous Disorders chapter. It is discussed separately in a new chapter (see below).

Chapters or subchapters on colibacillosis, paratyphoid infections, and arbovirus infections have been completely revised. A new subchapter entitled Interactions between Nutrition and Infectious Disease has been added to the Nutritional Diseases chapter, and the chapter on viral enteric infections has a new subchapter covering enterovirus infections.

An entirely new chapter (Chap. 37) addresses the problems of a number of emerging diseases and diseases of complex or unknown etiology, many of which were not previously discussed in the book. These include so-called Angara disease, so-called spiking mortality syndromes of chickens and turkeys, multicausal respiratory disease, transmissible viral proventriculitis, hepatic lipidosis, pigeon circovirus infection, Muscovy duck parvovirus infection, gangliosidosis in emus, multicentric histiocytosis, *Ornithobacterium rhinotracheale* infection, enteric disease complex (malabsorption syndrome), squamous cell carcinoma, big liver and spleen disease, fulminating disease of guinea fowl, and hepatitis–plenomegaly syndrome.

This edition also represents an effort to improve the illustrations. Nearly one quarter of the 414 black and white photographs are new, and the number of color plates has more than doubled to 25 (of these, 20 are totally or partially new).

The editorial committee members thank all of the contributors who prepared new material or revised existing material for the production of this edition.

EDITORIAL COMMITTEE
B.W. Calnek, Chairman
H. John Barnes
Charles W. Beard
Larry R. McDougald
Y.M. Saif

Diseases of Poultry

TENTH EDITION

1 Principles of Disease Prevention: Diagnosis and Control

D. V. Zander, A. J. Bermudez, and E. T. Mallinson

INTRODUCTION. This chapter acquaints the reader with basic principles of poultry sanitation and disease prevention and control. It also introduces the student to basic necropsy procedures and provides information on insecticides and disinfectants. For information on specific diagnostic techniques and control measures, the reader is referred to the respective chapters covering specific diseases in this text and to Whiteman and Bickford (49).

This chapter does not cover all the detailed disease control methods or all types of poultry, but attempts only to outline and illustrate some fundamental concepts. Each poultry enterprise is different; therefore, the basic concepts must be applied according to conditions and facilities existing in individual situations. To keep abreast of the flow of research and information, a constant review of current literature and recommendations applicable to specific diseases, special enterprises, and various geographic areas is necessary. Excellent journal sources of current information are *Avian Diseases, Avian Pathology, Poultry Science, Journal of Applied Poultry Research,* and *World's Poultry Science Journal,* and there are many publication and trade journals with special emphasis on particular segments of poultry husbandry, e.g., *Poultry International, International Hatchery Practice, Poultry Digest, Broiler Industry, Egg Industry, Turkey World,* and others including publications in various languages. Standard textbooks on chicken and turkey production, husbandry, and nutrition are other sources of information. A good practical manual on commercial chicken production is North and Bell (32).

HOST–PARASITE RELATIONSHIP. Disease results when normal body functions are impaired, and the degree of impairment determines severity of the disease. Disease may occur from deficiency of a vital nutrient or ingestion of a toxic substance. It may result from injury or physical stress with which the bird cannot cope, or it may be the consequence of harmful action of infectious and parasitic agents.

Some nutritional deficiencies are temporary and reversible when the nutrient is supplied in adequate amounts; others are irreversible. Disease resulting from stress is related to its severity and duration. Injuries such as extreme beak trimming tend to persist for a long time and may be permanent. Diseases caused by infectious and parasitic agents are frequently complex and depend upon characteristics of both host and parasite.

Whether disease results from parasitism depends on number, type, and virulence of the parasite; route of entry to the body; and defense status and capabilities of the host. The latter depends partly on the host's prior disease encounters (e.g., infectious bursal disease, or IBD), nutritional status, and genetic ability to organize resistance mechanisms; environmental stresses; and kind and timing of countermeasures employed (drugs, changes of environment).

Some virulent organisms rapidly overcome the resistance of even the healthiest hosts. Less virulent strains or types cause moderate to severe illness, but most birds respond and return to a state of health. Still other strains or types cause no marked reaction, and the host shows little or no obvious signs of ill health. Some infectious agents may not cause dramatic effects themselves, but predispose the host to more serious infections by other agents. Some microorganisms are not considered pathogenic because they are usually found in and around individuals considered "normal"; it must be recognized, however, that so-called nonpathogenic and low pathogenic organisms can also cause serious losses when the right circumstances exist. Severe physical stresses such as chilling, overheating, water deprivation, starvation, and concurrent infection by other disease agents can reduce the host's ability to resist, and thus may precipitate a disease condition that can be detected (e.g., clinical mycoplasmosis following infectious bronchitis, or clinical salmonellosis in chilled or water-deprived chicks).

Coccidiosis provides a good example of the relationship between the number of invading organisms and the severity of the resulting infection, since the

3

morbidity and mortality of the host species are usually proportional to the number of coccidial oocysts ingested. A similar situation exists for many other infectious diseases. A mild roundworm infection may not be serious, whereas a severe infection can be very detrimental. The titer of a live virus vaccine may be so low that an immunizing infection does not occur following administration. A good reason for removing moribund and dead birds from a flock is to reduce the number of infectious organisms available to penmates. Thorough washing and disinfecting of a building may not render it sterile, but it can reduce the number of infectious organisms to such a low level that they cannot cause disease.

By following sound disease-preventive practices before and after arrival of new flocks; making sure the flock has adequate, properly placed, good quality feed and water; applying judicious and timely vaccines and medications; and providing a less stressful environment, the poultry producer can control the probability of a flock becoming infected, as well as the severity and outcome of an infection.

Influence of Modern Practices. Avian disease specialists must continually seek new knowledge about the nature and control of specific diseases. Meanwhile, persons responsible for production of poultry meat, table- and hatching-eggs, chicks and poults, feed ingredients, and mixed feeds should practice the basic techniques and management principles that will prevent occurrence of disease. They should also provide the physical facilities and quarantine capabilities necessary for control and elimination of diseases that occasionally gain entrance, so that they do not become a continuing problem. Economic losses, sometimes relatively subtle, resulting from disease can mean the difference between success or failure in the poultry business. Those who disregard the basic principles of disease prevention may succeed in times of a favorable market, but do not remain competitive when the margin of profit is very small. A new modern enterprise with many good buildings and labor-saving equipment, but constructed and operated without regard to fundamental disease control and eradication principles, may function free of disease for a few years. All too frequently, a troublesome disease gains entrance and thereafter becomes a constant costly burden because of the extreme cost of depopulation required to eradicate it.

When new farms and buildings are designed and constructed, and production is programmed with the objective of excluding diseases or eradicating them when they gain entry, poultry can be maintained free of most harmful diseases in a practical manner with a minimum of effort. The poultry producer who uses fundamental management practices that prevent disease outbreaks has little need for detailed knowledge of the many infectious diseases affecting poultry.

Facilities need not be new to be adequate. Frequently, old farms can be enlarged and production reprogrammed to exclude or eradicate disease. Many old poultry buildings, hatcheries, and feed mills can be redesigned to favor exclusion, eradication, or control of disease. Strict application of disease-preventive management techniques has enabled producers to maintain specific-pathogen-free chickens on farms of standard design and construction (15).

The trend in all agricultural industries continues toward larger units, fewer farmers, and corporate enterprise. The chicken and turkey industries have been leaders in this trend, which has placed emphasis on efficiency of operation and lower costs of production. Survival in the industry has depended upon continual adoption of newer and more efficient practices. It is sometimes forgotten that efficiency in disease prevention is as important as efficiency in cleaning, feeding, bird handling, and egg processing. The resulting evolution of management systems has altered the emphasis in disease-control practices and will continue to do so; e.g., the shift in housing of egg-laying flocks from floor pens to cages has altered the approach to control of intestinal diseases and parasites and has increased emphasis on control of cannibalism through reduced light intensity and surgical removal of sharp beak tips (beak trimming).

New problems in feed formulation have arisen because certain vitamins and minerals normally found in the litter are not available to caged birds. Windowless, insulated, light- and temperature-controlled poultry houses have reduced environmental stresses from extremes in weather. Chickens in such houses require less feed in cold weather than those without this protection, which necessitates new considerations in feed formulation.

Corporation farming accelerated the move toward integrated control and operation of two or more segments of the industry such as feed manufacturing, breeder flock management, hatchery operation, pullet rearing, broiler and turkey grow-out phases, laying farm production, egg processing, turkey and broiler slaughter and processing, and even retail distribution. Integration of the industry has concentrated under one decision-making body the disease control practices for millions of birds, as well as several phases in the production chain of eggs and meat. Thus, sound health practices and emergency quarantine measures decided upon by one or a few individuals can be quickly and effectively applied to large numbers of birds. Through integration, it has become economically practical to employ veterinarians full time and place responsibility for disease control directly in the hands of specialized avian pathologists. Disease considerations are sometimes reduced to simple cost accounting, whereby the economic loss from a disease and the costs of treating it are weighed against the costs of its eradication and of maintenance of the clean status, before determining the course of action.

Where established management and industry practices allow or contribute to spread and propagation of some disease agent, attempts are frequently made to expose flocks to the disease deliberately at an opportune time. This practice is successful for many viral diseases and has led to widespread use of specially prepared vaccines. The practice is much less successful for bacterial infections and is more likely to perpetuate the disease. Exposure to culturally altered or selected naturally occurring attenuated strains of pasteurella, bordetella, and staphylococci have been used with considerable success in turkey flocks (24). Except for prevalent and highly contagious diseases for which effective vaccines are available, it is usually more economical to keep poultry free of disease than to burden them with it deliberately or by accident, provided the costs of eradication and of maintenance of a free status do not exceed the costs resulting from outbreaks of the disease. Poultry producers with extremely large, compact, multiple-age, egg-laying enterprises find it more economical to expose pullet flocks to some bacterial agents that are endemic on the layer premises to which they may later be moved (*Haemophilus paragallinarum*, *Mycoplasma gallisepticum*) than to attempt the costly adult depopulation necessary to eradicate infections.

The poultry industry can no longer be considered composed of localized businesses limited to certain states or areas. It is characterized by multistate and even multinational companies moving products daily between locations and to various markets. Because of the high cost of scientific poultry breeding, producers throughout the world depend on a few organizations for their highly efficient breeding and production stocks. In the case of turkeys, most of the world's breeding stock originates from one of three locations in North America. For such a system to function smoothly and efficiently, widespread and daily shipments of hatching eggs, poults, chicks, started pullets, and adult fowl across state and national boundaries are essential and necessitate reevaluation of old concepts of health regulations. Specialized avian pathologists have evolved to guide the course of health control measures. Diagnostic facilities, both private and government, are available in major poultry-producing areas of the world. Except where importation and use are restricted by government regulation, high-quality

vaccines and drugs are available wherever poultry is raised commercially. Breeding of poultry on a scientific basis has created strains of uniform quality with a high degree of resistance against diseases for which satisfactory drugs and vaccines are not available. Good quality feed is the rule, not the exception.

Yet disease still takes a heavy toll from all types of poultry enterprise. Those who exercise farm management decisions (caretaker, owner, flock supervisor, corporate manager, money lender) have the power to reduce these losses through management for disease control. They must be made aware of the responsibilities and continually encouraged to develop a philosophy of disease prevention through management and to concentrate on amortized long-term advantages and not just short-term savings.

Cardinal principles of disease prevention and control are the same for the chicken hobbyist, fancy-bird breeder, and game-bird farmer as for the corporation with several million turkeys, broilers, or laying hens. The backyard flock maintained without regard for disease control can perpetuate a disease that constitutes a threat to a large productive industry. On the other hand, since most such flocks are not vaccinated, they may be susceptible to diseases against which large commercial flocks are protected. The greatest hazard to commercial producers that is created by fancy breeds and backyard flocks is the possible perpetuation of diseases that have been eradicated from the industry. Thus, it is a sound principle of disease prevention that no employee of a commercial unit have any contact with poultry, or pet or hobby birds, at home or elsewhere.

Many producers attempt to save money through substitution of cheaper feed ingredients or unproven equipment and housing, or fail to keep equipment operating as the manufacturer recommends. This frequently leads to poor growth or adult performance that is mistakenly attributed to a nonexistent mysterious disease. Considering the capital investment and daily minimum maintenance costs of a flock of chickens, maximum performance (growth, egg production) should be the primary husbandry goal.

With better control over diseases of all kinds, providing optimum bird comfort throughout the house has become a very important management factor in obtaining maximum performance. That is not achieved solely by windowless, insulated, light- and temperature-controlled houses. Such factors as overcrowding, poor beak trimming, uneven temperatures, and uncomfortable air currents on caged birds that cannot move to a more comfortable location also adversely affect performance. Proper orientation of feeders, waterers, and light promotes good performance; slight, seemingly insignificant changes from proven systems can have a pronounced adverse effect on performance of both caged and floor-housed flocks of chickens and other commercial fowl. Poor performance of adults is often traceable to detrimental events that occurred during the rearing period.

Meat birds are bred to grow fast and large, but the flocks kept for breeding must have feed intake restricted to prevent obesity and poor adult performance. Feed restriction must be carefully controlled to prevent aggressive birds from getting most of the available feed. Two systems are widely used: daily restriction and skip-a-day feeding. The former requires special feeding equipment or procedures to ensure that feed is presented to the entire flock simultaneously so that all birds begin eating at the same time. In the skip-a-day system, feed is given in larger quantities on alternate days, permitting the recessive birds to obtain their share even if they have to wait their turn to eat. In either system, special provision must be made in formulating feeds to provide adequate coccidiostat and essential nutrients in the reduced amount consumed.

Poultry and game birds are very cannibalistic under any circumstances. Under most modern systems, beak trimming is a virtual necessity, and special machines have been manufactured for this purpose. Beak trimming is performed on birds of various ages, depending on the husbandry system in use. The extremely dim light used in light-tight poultry houses greatly reduces or prevents cannibalism, but chicks reared under natural or bright light frequently have their beaks trimmed lightly at 1 day of age or a few days after delivery to the brooder. This early mild trimming is not severe enough to be permanent; therefore, beaks of such flocks of breeders or commercial layers are frequently trimmed again before maturity. Some methods and ages of early beak trimming can protect chickens from cannibalism throughout life if other management factors (e.g., light intensity) are favorable.

Biosecurity. *Biosecurity*—safety from transmissible infectious diseases, parasites, and pests— is a term that embodies all of the measures that can or should be taken to prevent viruses, bacteria, fungi, protozoa, parasites, insects, rodents, and wild birds from entering or surviving and infecting or endangering the well-being of the poultry flock.

The reader is referred to a series of eight videotapes illustrating biosecurity measures and the many threats to poultry health that biosecurity is designed to prevent. These were produced by the United States Department of Agriculture (USDA), Animal Plant Health Inspection Service (APHIS), Veterinary Services. Inquire at your state APHIS veterinary office for further information. These professionally filmed tapes are also available from state extension offices and major poultry industry trade associations. They provide graphic biosecurity training for workers, managers, and owners in all types of broiler, layer, turkey, game bird, breeder farm, hatchery, feed mill, transportation, and live-bird market operations.

BIOSECURITY GUIDELINES. Specific disease-prevention guidelines, targeted to different sectors of industry (truckers, service workers, farm owners, catching crews, and others), are often available from university extension specialists. A 14-page booklet, *Biosecurity for Poultry,* published by the Mid-Atlantic States Cooperative Extension Poultry Health and Management Unit, and available from the University of Maryland Extension Service, is an informative example of such cooperatively produced guidelines.

SOURCES OF INFECTION AND PROTECTIVE MEASURES AGAINST THEM.

Infections gain entrance to a flock from various sources. To understand why various preventive practices are recommended, it is important to review briefly the sources and routes of infection.

Humans. Because of their mobility, duties, curiosity, ignorance, indifference, carelessness, or total concentration on current profit margin, humans constitute one of the greatest potential causes of introduction of disease. Rarely is this because they become infected and shed the disease agent, but rather because they track infectious diseases, use contaminated equipment, or manage their flocks in such a way that spread of disease is inevitable.

Most frequently, footwear is suspected as the means of transport of disease, but hands can become contaminated with exudates when lesions and discharges are examined. Clothing can also become contaminated with dust, feathers, and excrement. At least one avian disease pathogen (Newcastle disease virus) has been found to survive for several days on the mucous membrane of the human respiratory tract and has been isolated from sputum (47).

NEIGHBORS. A frequent source of infection is a disease outbreak at a neighboring farm. Disease inspection visits among producers are a common way of spreading disease. If a neighbor's flock is afflicted with a very interesting new disease, discuss it by telephone. It is best to warn neighbors not to visit when a disease is in progress, and by all means do not walk around on a neighbor's farm for any purpose.

CONTRACT WORK CREWS. Much of poultry farm

procedure requires sporadic use of a crew of several workers, e.g., blood testing, beak trimming, vaccinating, inseminating, sexing, weighing, and moving birds from one location to another. The producer or farm manager frequently has difficulty in assembling a crew who are available and knowledgeable about handling poultry. Therefore, crews who service many poultry enterprises are contracted. Such crews travel about the poultry community handling many flocks, and must be regarded as a potential source of infection. Thus, they should take stringent precautions to safeguard the health of every flock with which they work.

VISITORS. Disease outbreaks in a community have been known to follow the path of a careless visitor. If visitors do not enter premises or buildings, they cannot track in diseases.

The source of a new or dreaded disease is often puzzling. World trade and travel are becoming more commonplace. It is not uncommon for a person to leave one farm in the morning and be visiting another farm or place of business in another part of the country or another continent on the same day. Some disease agents can easily survive that time frame. All who travel should be cognizant of this and guard against introduction of disease into their own flocks or onto premises of clients, competitors, friends, or fellow producers when returning from a trip. Protective footwear and clothing are not readily available in all countries and poultry areas. A good preventive measure when returning from a trip is to sanitize shoes and launder all clothing worn on farms.

Recovered Carriers.
Carrier birds are those that have apparently recovered from a clinical infection but still retain the infectious organism in some part of the body. While they appear healthy, the infectious agent continues to multiply in the body and to be eliminated into the environment. Like actively infected flocks, they can perpetuate a disease on a farm and constitute a disease threat to other birds. Many commonly occurring diseases are known to be transmitted by carriers. Carrier birds can be a potential source of disease through the various practices noted below.

MULTIPLE AGES. Multiple ages on a premises constitute a serious disease potential from both actively infected fowl and recovered carriers, particularly if birds of differing ages are closely associated through management practices or proximity. Disease agents that result in chronic infections or recovered carriers are passed by various means, including direct contact, to each new susceptible flock brought onto the premises. Serious drops in production may occur in young laying flocks moved onto laying premises where carrier birds from previous disease outbreaks remain.

STARTED PULLETS. Pullets are frequently reared to or near point-of-lay by a specialized pullet rearer or on a separate premises unit belonging to the laying-farm owner. This practice has become established in the industry for many sound reasons. Pullets can, however, be a potential source for introduction of a disease onto a layer farm if they have been exposed on the pullet farm and, as a result, have become recovered carriers of some disease not existing on the layer farm. Another hazard is assembling mature pullets reared in different geographic areas onto a single layer premises, even an all-in, all-out layer premises. Those reared in one area may have been exposed to and recovered from, but carrying, a disease agent not found in the area where the other pullets were reared.

FORCE-MOLTED HENS. Force-molting of laying hens or breeders is frequently practiced (particularly during times of economic stress) to supply a special market, meet an emergency egg demand, or improve declining shell quality, or because it is deemed economical at the time. One advantage of keeping force-molted hens, rather than rearing new replacement pullets, is that old hens are not apt to suffer a disease that normally occurs during the rearing age. If such flocks are force-molted and held in the same house, there is little danger of disease problems developing. Conversely, a producer who collects spent hens for molting from many poultry farms and mixes them on one premises at one time runs a serious risk, since any of the force-molted groups may be carriers of a disease to which the others are susceptible.

POULTRY SHOW STOCK. Birds exhibited at poultry shows may be exposed to actively infected or symptomless carrier birds of other exhibitors from which they may contract disease. The contact-infected stock may not develop active signs until returned to the owner's farm, where they may then be a source of new infection. Breeders of fancy birds and game birds and youths with poultry projects (4-H, Future Farmers of America) must recognize the extreme hazards of returning birds exhibited in shows and fairs and of introducing partly grown or adult birds for special breeding purposes. A cardinal rule for show stock is that it should never be returned to the owner's farm. If birds must be shown, individuals should be selected that can be sold after the exhibition. If they must be returned, they should be quarantined for several weeks. In some areas, exhibition-type poultry should be vaccinated against some diseases. Check with a local avian pathologist or veterinary diagnostic laboratory.

BREEDING STOCK. Adult stock considered especially desirable for breeding purposes may be symptomless carriers and serve as a source of infection for the breeding farm. It is best to purchase such stock as hatching eggs or day-old chicks and to rear them in an isolated off-farm quarantine area until there is reasonable assurance that they are free of infection.

MIXED SPECIES OF POULTRY. One species that is naturally very resistant to a disease may act as a carrier of that disease for another species that is very susceptible. Some death losses and debilitation from histomoniasis may occur in chickens, but in turkeys the losses can be disastrous. Therefore, even with routine use of drugs to prevent histomoniasis, the two species should never be run together, and turkeys should not be run on a dirt yard or floor that has recently had chickens on it.

Also, a silent (inapparent) mycoplasma infection in chickens may spread to mycoplasma-free turkeys and erupt into a full-blown case of sinusitis and air sac infection. Other diseases may be rather innocuous in one species of fowl, but very serious in another. It is also advisable to keep meat and laying chickens separated, since the same disease may have different economic importance in the two types.

Other Sources

HOSPITAL PEN. Sick birds from several pens collected into one hospital pen or house and later returned to their respective quarters may carry back not only the condition for which they were removed, but one or more diseases contracted while in the hospital area. Therefore, hospital pens are not recommended for routine segregation of sick birds except as a way-station en route to the diagnostic laboratory or crematorium. If and when used for a special purpose (observation, injury, cannibalism), they should be temporary arrangements within the house and should hold birds from only one pen or house.

CULL PEN. Cull pens still exist on some poultry farms. Nonlaying hens are frequently culled from a flock and marketed for meat. Nonproducing hens in good health present no health hazard for humans or poultry. Cull birds in obviously poor health may or may not be afflicted with an infectious disease. The producer should suspect the worst and destroy such birds rather than hold them for slaughter.

BACKYARD AND PET FOWL. Poultry kept as pets or to supply household eggs or meat are just as capable of carrying and transmitting disease as are commercial flocks. Pet barnyard fowl of a rare or interesting nature may also carry disease to commercial poultry. The risk to the invested enterprise is too great to permit such a part-time hobby by a resident owner or employee. Cockfighting is banned in many states, but these game fowl seem to be transported around the country, constituting an effective way to carry disease. Some employees may own or handle these fowl, and thus could introduce a serious disease to the poultry enterprise where they work. Poultry farm and hatchery owners and workers should be especially cautious about contact with imported ornamental pet birds or migratory waterfowl because they can be symptomless carriers of diseases that are highly virulent for domestic poultry.

LIVE-BIRD MARKETS. These are buildings usually in the inner cities in which poultry of all types, ages, and health status are assembled by small buyers to supply a demand for live fowl for those who wish to examine the fowl live prior to slaughter or prefer to kill and dress fowl at home (Fig. 1.1). Such facilities are rarely depopulated, cleaned, and disinfected, and thus are ideal situations for transmission and propagation of poultry diseases. In addition, the hauling equipment and vehicles may not be cleaned and disinfected after each use. Such equipment, hauled throughout the poultry industry areas where a few birds of different types or age are bought at various places, is an excellent means of transmitting diseases. Good managers and owners will keep such buyers and their equipment out of their farms and offices. The live-bird market trade has been strongly associated with the propagation and spread of avian influenza and laryngotracheitis.

Egg-borne Diseases. Egg-borne diseases are transmitted from the infected dam to newly hatched offspring by means of the fertile egg. Some disease agents are carried inside the shell as a result of shedding into the egg prior to addition of the shell and membranes. Others are carried on the shell or penetrate from the shell surface through natural pores after the egg is laid.

The agent may gain entrance to the egg as a result of infection of the ovary and ovarian follicles (transovarian transmission), as a result of contamination of the free ovum in the peritoneal cavity, or by contact in the oviduct. Once the shell and membranes are added, the organism enjoys a protected location where it is not easily destroyed. From there it can later invade the developing embryo, and lesions are frequently observed in tissues and organs of offspring at hatching. Transovarian transmission seems to be limited to only a few of the many diseases that affect poultry and most of these have been eradicated from breeding flocks.

When the freshly laid egg cools from body tem-

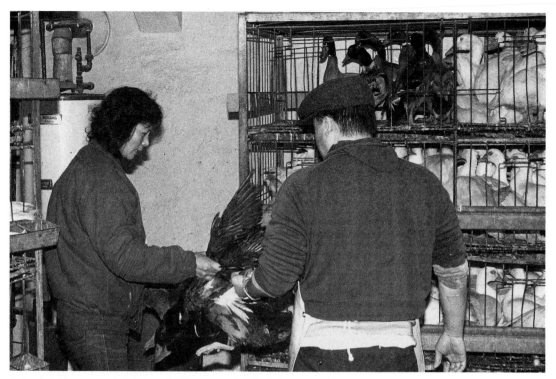

1.1. Urban live-bird markets are rarely depopulated and disinfected. Diseases are readily propagated and transmitted to new birds brought in to replenish the supply. Commercial production managers are sometimes tempted to deal with live-bird markets because of the increased profits afforded by this association. These short-term profits are extremely small compared to the severe losses which can occur if infectious agents of high pathogenicity are introduced into the commercial poultry industry. (Univ Maryland)

perature to nest, room, or cool-room temperature, a pressure differential occurs between the inside of the egg and the atmosphere. Any fluid on the shell surface is drawn inward. Motile bacteria are aided by this pressure differential to penetrate the shell. The primary contamination of this nature is from enteric organisms, particularly salmonellae and coliforms, but other types of bacteria and fungi also may be drawn into the egg. For preventive measures, see Breeder Flock Management and see Management of Hatching Eggs.

Equipment. Diseases and parasites can be carried on equipment. Cleaning equipment and vehicles usually have accumulations of litter and feces that can be a threat to other farms and houses where they may be transported for succeeding assignments. They should be washed free of litter and droppings before use in another farm area.

Mites are frequently found on eggs and can be transported from farm to farm in corrugations of egg cases taken into chicken houses. Wire crates and baskets do not offer these hiding places. Residues of *Salmonella*-contaminated eggs on egg flats may be a potential method of introducing disease. Use of washed and disinfected plastic egg flats and moving of stacked flats of uncased eggs on racks and pallets reduce the hazard of transmission of diseases and parasites among farms.

Fowl pox, infectious bursal disease, and Marek's disease viruses, coccidia, roundworm eggs, and other infectious material can be carried on crates, footwear, and vehicles, particularly on the floor and foot control pedals of a vehicle.

Artificial inseminating equipment, particularly reused inseminating tubes, offer an excellent method of transmitting disease.

Poultry hauling equipment can disseminate infectious material through feathers, feces, blood, exudates, and skin encrustations left in the crates or picked up at the slaughter plant. Hauling equipment should be washed and disinfected after use before being taken to another farm (Fig. 1.2).

Miscellaneous Sources

LABORATORY EXPOSURE. Frequently, a producer, particularly a small flock owner, hobbyist, or

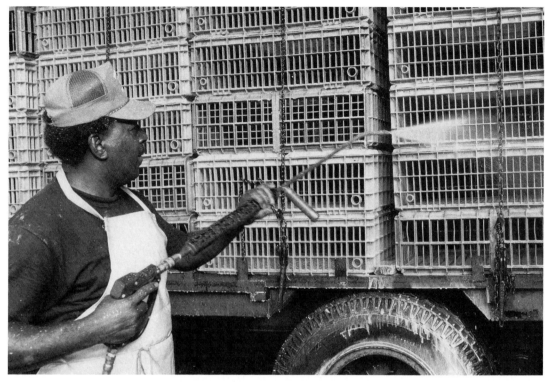

1.2.   Soiled vehicles and equipment can carry disease agents. They should be thoroughly washed and disinfected after each live haul. One gram of chicken manure can contain enough viral particles to infect 1 million birds with avian influenza. (Davidek)

game bird owner, will want to take a bird home after the veterinarian has examined it at the laboratory. While in the receiving area or diagnostic facilities, even for a short time, live poultry have a good opportunity to contact some disease agent. Except under special circumstances (exotic birds, valuable pet) no bird should be returned from the laboratory to the farm, because it could develop disease and be the source of a new infection on the home premises. The bird should either be sacrificed and necropsied or, if a pet, referred to a private clinician.

A disease may be tracked from laboratory surroundings to a farm by careless laboratory or service workers or the producers. Clean and frequently washed and disinfected laboratory areas are the responsibility of the veterinarian. Precautions against tracking disease from the laboratory to the farm are the responsibility of the producer and service worker.

RODENTS.   Rodents contaminate feed and litter with their excrement. They are particularly hazardous to *Salmonella* control, since they are frequently infected with these organisms and can perpetuate the disease on a farm.

HOUSEHOLD PETS.   Dogs and cats, like rodents, are capable of harboring enteric organisms that are infectious to poultry. When these pets are not confined to the household area, but roam continually among the poultry in the pens and yards, they constitute a serious health hazard. Such pets are just as capable of tracking contaminated material on their feet and in their hair as people.

WILD BIRDS.   Wild birds are capable of carrying a variety of diseases and parasites. Some cause illness in the wild birds themselves; for others, the birds act as mechanical carriers. Every effort should be made to prevent their nesting in the poultry area. Imported zoological specimens destined for zoos are not a direct contact threat because the zoos are located in cities, but they should be considered as a potential source of introduction of an exotic disease or parasite. Exotic ornamental pet birds constitute a real hazard because they become widely dispersed and may be purchased by poultry workers. On numerous occasions, exotic birds in or destined for pet stores have been found infected with a virulent exotic form of Newcastle disease virus, which in at least one instance was the source of a serious and costly outbreak in poultry. Stringent entry quarantine requirements to apprehend and destroy infected birds provide a good barrier against introduction and dissemination by carrier birds, but failures can occur (illegal smuggling), and producers should be wary of such personal pets. Domestic pigeons can also be a source of dangerous strains of Newcastle disease virus.

INSECTS. Many insects act as transmitters of disease. Some are intermediate hosts for blood or intestinal parasites; others are mechanical carriers of disease through their biting parts. Still others, because of their feeding habits and hiding places, appear to be reservoirs of disease whereby the infectious agent survives from one flock to the next.

FEED. Some ingredients may contain infectious agents, particularly salmonellae, from contamination at their source or anywhere along the production line or storage areas. Methods are available for sterilizing feed, but they increase cost of the final product. Pelleting, if done properly, is a practical method of greatly reducing contaminants because of the heat generated in the process, but it is not dependable for complete sterilization. Meat meal is the feed ingredient most apt to introduce *Salmonella* spp. This hazard can be avoided by using only vegetable protein ingredients, supplemented as necessary with synthetic amino acids. Such formulations are recommended for breeder rations if pelleting capabilities are not available.

MANAGEMENT FACTORS IN DISEASE PREVENTION.

The more important physical principles of disease prevention include favorable geographic location of the farm in respect to other poultry units, proper location of buildings in relation to each other and to prevailing wind currents, proper design of the building inside and out, and design and positioning of equipment. Long-range planning and programming of the operation, whether large or small, is very important and should consider movement patterns of various vehicles and equipment, work traffic of regular and holiday caretakers and special work crews, feed delivery and storage, and the system for moving eggs and flocks from the farm. An avian pathologist can be helpful in avoiding some common pitfalls, but to avoid high-risk disease situations, consultation should be done when the farm is being designed and the production programmed, rather than after it is developed and serious trouble is evident.

Good disease-prevention practices are perhaps best illustrated as a chain that is only as strong as its weakest link. Many sound principles can be discredited by failure to carry out one or two related ones, which are either overlooked or not considered essential. While it may not always be possible to use all the practices, the more that are followed, the greater the chances of avoiding disease outbreaks.

Isolation. Not all producers follow the same disease control practices. A close neighbor may disregard sound principles and be burdened with diseases until forced out of business by economic pressures. In the meantime, disease agents present on his premises may be blown or carried by various vectors and fomites to adjacent premises; thus, a disease may occasionally gain entrance even on well-managed units. Until a disease has been eradicated, it serves as a reservoir and potential source of infection for future flocks on the same premises and those on adjacent premises. The closer the houses of one premises to those of another, the more likely is the spread of infection to healthy birds on an adjacent farm.

Some highly concentrated poultry areas have developed because of some favorable condition such as a close market, an available slaughter or processing plant, an accessible feed supply, low-cost land, or favorable climate or zoning. Usually, these areas deteriorate into problem zones of disease of one type or another and resemble huge "megafarms" with many managers, each vaccinating, treating, or exposing birds without regard to the programs of others. Since such areas are in competition for markets, several things may happen. Various advantages may offset disease losses, or the additional cost of production resulting from disease prices the product (meat, eggs) out of the market. In extreme cases, products cannot be marketed either because of the disease or the residues from drugs used to control disease. Producers who do not minimize losses go out of business; and many abandoned poultry farms are purchased or leased by other poultry producers. Some move their operations to a less concentrated area where they usually escape disease, unless they take their problems with them knowingly, or inadvertently through carelessness. Those who remain usually upgrade disease-prevention practices by redesigning houses and reprogramming the production cycle. Frequently, reprogramming proceeds to a system of a single age of fowl, permitting complete depopulation at the end of each rearing or laying cycle.

Another solution to area disease problems where farms are too close even for systematic depopulation to succeed is to develop a coordinated area depopulation and restocking program. All flocks in a reasonably defined geographic area may be marketed at the same time and the houses refilled at the same time. This is more adaptable to broiler production than egg production.

Most serious disease problems could be avoided if a philosophy of premise isolation prevailed from the beginning of an enterprise. No exact minimum distance from other poultry farms can be stated because this is influenced by prevailing winds, climate, type of houses, and other factors. The farther from other poultry farms, the less likelihood of contracting disease from them. Isolation can be effected by taking advantage of segregating space provided by natural or artificial barriers such as bodies of water, hills, cities or towns, or forests, or other interposing agriculture enterprises such as grain, vegetable, or fruit production.

One Age of Fowl per Farm. Removing carriers from a flock and premises is an effective way of preventing a recurrence of some diseases, but it is impossible or impractical for others. The best way to prevent infection from carrier birds is to remove the entire flock from the farm before any new replacements are added, and to rear young stock in complete isolation from older recovered birds on a separated farm segment or preferably on another farm and in an isolated area.

Where birds of different ages exist on a large farm, depopulation seems drastic; but considering mortality, poor performance, and endless drug expense, it could be the most economical solution. Farms and quarantinable farm divisions of up to 100,000 birds of one age prove that size is no deterrent to application of the sound principle of one age of bird per farm or quarantinable segment with programmed depopulation at the end of the production cycle.

Where only one age of bird is maintained, depopulation occurs each time pullets or poults are moved to the layer or breeder premises, each time the broilers or turkeys are moved to slaughter, and each time the old layers or breeders are sent to market. Should a disease occur, the flock can be quarantined, treated, and handled in the best way possible until its disposal. Depopulated premises are then cleaned out, washed, and disinfected, and left idle for as long as possible but at least for 2 wk before new healthy stock is introduced.

Depopulation is most effective in controlling disease agents that do not survive for long outside the bird. This applies to most respiratory infections (mycoplasma infections, infectious coryza, laryngotracheitis). It is least effective in controlling disease agents having a resistant state that survives for long periods in nature (intestinal parasites, clostridia).

Started-pullet and pullet-rearing premises are now an established specialized enterprise in the poultry industry. This system has made layer and breeder farm depopulation more practical and successful. As on multiple-age layer farms, serious disease problems may develop and persist on multiple-age rearing farms until they are reprogrammed for a single age or divided into quarantinable, isolated units.

In addition to sanitary practices, environmental factors (temperature, humidity) play an important role in the time interval necessary to prevent carryover of disease. Disease germs begin to die out slowly after elimination from the body. Some (coryza) die out very quickly; others (parasites, coccidia) survive for months or years, depending on whether they develop a resistant stage and on factors discussed under individual diseases. In general, the longer a premises remains vacant, the lower the number of surviving pathogens.

Functional Units. For certain economic reasons (breeding farm or small specialized market trade), it is not always possible to limit the entire farm to a single age of poultry. In such instances, it should be divided into separate quarantinable units or areas for different groups of birds (rearing area, pedigree unit, production groups, experimental birds) (Fig. 1.3). With a suitable arrangement, each area is periodically depopulated, cleaned, and sanitized, or can be if necessary. Much stricter security procedures for personnel, bird, and equipment movements are necessary for this type of operation. A very rigid monitoring system is also essential to detect any disease early enough to bring it under control while it is still confined to one quarantinable segment.

There is no reliable formula for minimum distances between houses or units. Windowless and temperature- and ventilation-controlled houses appear to prevent building-to-building and premise-to-premise spread better than open houses. Greater distance can compensate for some inadequacy in building design, human traffic control, and shared equipment. Since each premises and enterprise is different from all others, the poultry producer should seek advice from specialists whose business it is to study diseases and how to prevent and control them.

The most important factor in dividing the farm into segregated units is not so much to facilitate daily separation of farm personnel, equipment, and poultry, but to provide quarantinable units to prevent spread and facilitate elimination of disease, should it occur.

Building Construction

BIRDPROOFING. The first rule in poultry house construction is to exclude free-flying wild birds, since many carry mites and harbor them in their nests. In addition, many species have been found susceptible to some common viral and bacterial dis-

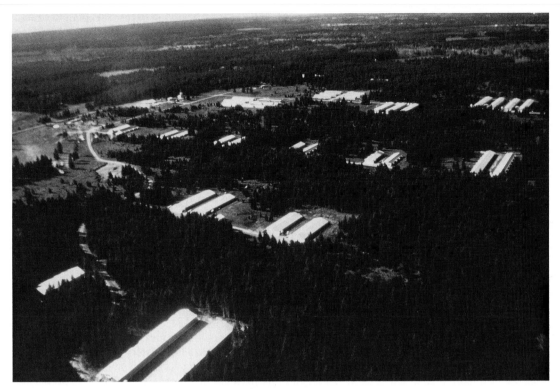

1.3. This isolated breeding farm benefits from several fundamental disease prevention and control principles. It is isolated from other poultry farms, is surrounded by forest land, and is divided into quarantinable sections separated by woods as well as distance.

eases of poultry and thus could act as carriers. Turkeys on range are especially vulnerable to infections carried by wild birds. For this reason and for generally improved sanitary practices, the trend is to house turkeys, especially breeder and young growing turkeys, in closed or partially closed birdproof houses. Ducks and other domestic waterfowl are also vulnerable to waterborne diseases and to diseases carried by wild birds, especially wild waterfowl and seabirds (gulls, terns, etc.).

Light- and temperature-controlled houses are usually birdproof by reason of their construction (Fig 1.4). Both ventilation and birdproofing are also achievable in open-type houses in hot climates. Birdproofing is also an important feature of other buildings on the farm, e.g., clean crate and wood shavings (bedding) storage.

ENTRANCES. An apron of concrete at the entrance to a poultry house helps prevent tracking of disease into the unit. Rain and sunshine help keep the apron cleaned and sterilized. A water faucet, boot brush, and covered pan of disinfectant available on the apron for disinfecting footwear are further aids in keeping litter and soil-borne diseases out of the house. Boots must be thoroughly cleaned

before the wearer steps into the pan of disinfectant. The disinfectant is useless, however, unless renewed frequently enough to ensure a potent solution at all times.

VENTILATION. Poultry buildings should be constructed to provide protection against the elements,

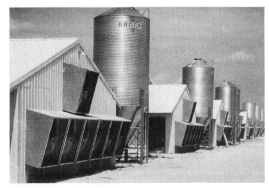

1.4. Light-, temperature-, and ventilation-controlled houses exclude wild birds and most flying insects. Concrete aprons and paved roadways help prevent tracking of soil-borne diseases into the premises.

yet not create stress conditions such as excess dust, insufficient ventilation with ammonia buildup, excessive draft, damp litter, and situations leading to injuries by mechanical equipment or sharp objects.

There are many advantages of windowless and temperature-controlled houses, but one serious drawback has been development in some instances of excessively dry and dusty litter. While Anderson et al. (4) could not demonstrate significant deleterious effects of short-term inhalation of dust by test chickens, it has been observed in practice that colibacillosis outbreaks are frequently associated with inhalation of excessive dust, which must be carried from the building with ventilating air. This may require increased air movement, and precautions must be taken to prevent a stream of incoming cold outside air from blowing directly onto chickens that are prevented, by pen (or cage) arrangement, from seeking shelter.

Coccidial oocysts require moisture to develop into the infective stage. Excessively dry litter inhibits their development and may so limit the number of infective oocysts that infection is too light for a good immune reaction. Conversely, improper ventilation can lead to excessively wet litter, which favors the survival and development of coccidia and other parasites.

Ammonia fumes develop in damp litter and droppings. If ventilation is poor and fumes accumulate, they may reach high enough concentration to inhibit growth and performance, cause keratoconjunctivitis, and exacerbate respiratory infections.

Litter will dry better if it can be stirred frequently, but in spite of all efforts, it may remain wet in winter or in humid climates. If wetness and excess ammonia concentration persist, litter should be replaced and ventilation improved.

Proper ventilation is an engineering science; a good policy is to seek professional advice before installing any system. The influence of such environmental conditions as temperature, humidity, radiation, and atmospheric pollutants on viral disease of poultry has been reviewed by Anderson and Hanson (3).

FLOORS AND CAGES. All surfaces inside the building should be of impervious material (such as concrete) to permit thorough washing and disinfection. It is impossible to sterilize a dirt floor!

Raised slatted floors have been used successfully for years for laying chickens, both for adults and for rearing birds. Such floors have alternating wooden pieces and spaces, each about ¾-in. wide (Fig. 1.5), to permit droppings to fall out of reach of birds and to prevent recycling infection of intestinal parasites and diseases. Since coccidial infection is thus avoided or greatly reduced, poor or no immunity to the parasite develops. This creates no problem for

pullets destined for cages or slat-floored laying houses, because immunity to coccidiosis during the laying period in such units would not be an important consideration. If such pullets were transferred to litter-floored laying houses, however, they would very likely become seriously infected with coccidiosis. Commercial meat birds are inclined to develop leg problems and breast blisters if raised on completely slatted or wire floors. A modification of this system, with part of the floor or yard raised slightly and covered with slats, has been used for broiler breeders. The value of this system is increased further by placing feed and water over the slatted area, which encourages collection of more droppings out of reach of birds.

Keeping laying hens in some type of cage has become an accepted practice in closed houses (Fig. 1.6) and open-type houses found in hot climates. Cages and wire floors are widely used also to rear pullets destined for cages as adults. The system is so successful in preventing intestinal diseases that birds have no opportunity to develop immunity to them. Coccidiosis is almost certain to occur if chickens or other poultry reared in cages are transferred to litter floors. Drugs can be used successfully to control coccidiosis in these birds, but legal restrictions on their use in meat and egg-producing fowl seriously curtail drug choices for this purpose in laying hens. There has been renewed interest in developing suitable cages for breeder turkeys and commercial broilers. Such a development would be a distinct aid in eliminating many disease problems of soil and litter origin.

FEEDERS AND WATERERS. Rats, mice, and other rodents should be kept out of feed because they may

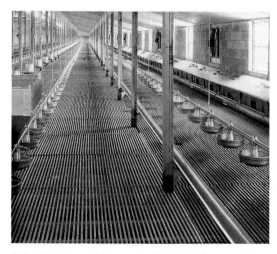

1.5. Slat floors aid in control of intestinal diseases and parasites. Droppings fall through open spaces and out of reach of the flock.

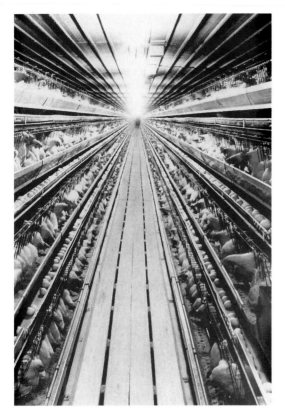

1.6. Poultry are kept in cages in well-built, ventilated, light- and temperature-controlled houses in many countries. Good housing reduces stresses associated with variations in weather, and cages reduce intestinal diseases and parasitism.

introduce and spread salmonellae or other disease agents that can be the source of an outbreak in the poultry flock.

Litter scratched into feed and water troughs and feed spilled in litter increase intake of litter and litter-borne disease agents; e.g., more coccidial oocysts and less coccidiostat are ingested, and a clinical infection may result. If poultry are permitted to consume litter, considerable mortality and depression can occur from impaction of the gizzard, and litter fragments may cause enteritis by mechanical irritation.

Feed troughs should have some type of guard to keep poultry out and should not be overfilled so that feed is spilled into litter. Feeders without guards permit defecation into feed, which encourages spread of diseases shed in feces. Wet feed in litter or yards attracts wild birds and rodents and provides a good medium for growth of molds, which can cause liver, kidney, immune system, and other damage to the well-being of poultry. Feeders used in turkey yards should be in a covered area designed to pro-

tect the feed from rainwater and sunlight to prevent mold growth and vitamin loss. Growing and laying cages for egg production flocks in light- and temperature-controlled houses eliminate most of the problems associated with litter. There are many good automated feeding and watering systems available commercially, but sometimes these are not installed or oriented as the manufacturer intended, and consequently health problems develop.

Roost areas over screened dropping pits are common in floor-laying and breeder hen houses to keep chickens away from their feces. Screened roost areas are also desirable in rearing houses for layers and breeders to prevent piling by the birds and excessive fouling of litter with feces, which in turn leads to packing and caking. Feeders and waterers over the pits keep the birds on the roost area much of the daytime as well as at night, so most droppings collect out of reach. Spilled water also falls under the roosts, so the litter area stays drier.

Waterers are frequently set or hung over the litter area. In this case, waterers should be managed so that spillage onto the litter is minimized. Waterers can be put into two basic categories: those that provide a constant reservoir of water, which is maintained automatically (troughs, cups, and hanging plastic bells) and nipple drinkers (Fig. 1.7), which supply water on demand when activated by a bird. Waterers that provide an open reservoir of water must be cleaned and disinfected regularly to prevent the buildup of potentially pathogenic organisms in the water supply. These waterers are also more prone to spillage and the associated problems of wet litter. Starting day-old birds is somewhat easier with waterers that have an open and visible water reservoir. The advantages of nipple drinkers are found in the significant improvement they offer in providing water free of organisms commonly found in the poultry house environment and in decreased water spillage. The drier litter conditions afforded by nipple drinkers result in decreased multiplication or maturation of coccidia, bacteria, and fungi in the litter. Broiler production managers report a decreased incidence of infectious disease with the conversion of poultry buildings to nipple drinkers. Nipple drinkers have been developed that are suitable for most types of poultry production.

FEED AND WATER MEDICATION. In spite of all precautions, poultry may become sick. This should be recognized from the start, and facilities for quick treatment by medication in water or feed should be provided long before it is needed. When birds are grouped by tens of thousands in one big pen, segregation and treatment of individuals is impractical; mass medication and vaccination are essential if any treatment is to be given.

Feed medication is not the best method of treat-

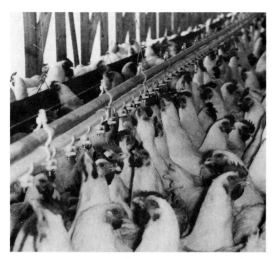

1.7. Nipple drinkers are effective in preventing microbiological contamination of clean water and help maintain dry litter conditions.

ment because of the inappetence of sick birds and their inability to compete for feed. Water medication is somewhat better because the sick will frequently drink when they will not eat, but the medicaments that can be administered in water are limited. Mass medication, while not completely successful in curing the sick, may hold the disease in check until the host can respond with a successful immune response. Provision should also be made for mass vaccination through drinking water, as this is an accepted and successful labor-saving practice. If drinking water is chlorinated or otherwise treated, the sanitizing agent may destroy the vaccine, so provision must be made to permit use of untreated or distilled water for mixing and administering water vaccines.

Several methods can be used to reduce, remove, or neutralize chlorine in chlorinated water supplies. The only practical method for dealing with this problem on poultry farms is to add protein to the water when mixing water vaccines. A common practice is to add 1 lb of nonfat dried milk to 50 gal water in tanks or canned liquid nonfat milk mixed with vaccine in a proportioner.

If a building is constructed with a bulk water tank for gravity-flow watering devices, the tank should be of plastic or lined with some nonreactive protective substance, and be readily accessible for cleaning and for mixing medicaments. If the watering devices are operated on high pressure, the pipe leading into the pen should have a bypass system with proper valve arrangement so that a medicament proportioner can be installed quickly when needed. A metering device to measure feed and water consumption is useful to keep track of the health of the flock. Float-regulated or continuous-flow wa-

ter troughs can spread disease within a house. Infectious coryza has been observed to spread down cage rows of chickens in the direction of water flow. Use of a watering system with nipple drinkers for individual cage units will aid in preventing spread of disease.

Bulk feed delivery, metal bulk storage tanks, and automatic feeders are common in modern poultry operations. These eliminate the possibility of rodent contamination, since feed is always in closed tanks rather than in bags or open bins; but the system leads to difficulties when short-term emergency medication in feed is desirable and the bulk tank is full. Two alternative systems are useful: an additional smaller bulk tank may be installed just for emergency medicated feed, or a small dispensing tank may be interposed between the bulk tank and feed troughs so emergency medicated feed can be put in the smaller tank by hand. Though rarely, if ever, used in commercial poultry operations any longer, disposable paper bags have been developed that eliminate the danger of used feed bags as a mechanical carrier of disease from farm to farm. Users of such prebagged rations should be certain that the feed has recently been milled and is not old, with the risk of lowered vitamin potency.

Personnel Control

COMPANY AND FARM PERSONNEL. Managers, supervisors, and owners are sometimes the worst offenders at breaking sanitation rules. These people frequently visit many different types of poultry enterprises, farms, and farm units, and disease agents do not respect authority or ownership. Such personnel, like veterinarians, should set a good example for the workers. One of the most important aspects of disease control is an awareness on the part of everyone—owner; workforce; feed and supply delivery people; egg, bird, and litter haulers; and all who visit or work on poultry farms—that each has an important role in the disease-prevention program. Assembling the workforce for occasional educational conferences on health goals and reasons for procedures will foster awareness. This is as important as the preventive measure established. It is also a good occasion to use the biosecurity action tapes mentioned previously in this chapter.

In designing buildings and farm layout and in programming production and management, it is important to make every disease-preventive practice as easy and efficient as possible. Any procedures that are difficult will probably be done incorrectly.

VISITORS AND CUSTOMERS. For some types of poultry enterprise, it is deemed necessary to show the birds, premises, or procedures to visitors. In such cases, an observation booth, platform, or fenced area should be provided. Such an area should be sealed off from the poultry pens or hatchery. For maximum security, the entry, access road, and observation area should be completely separated from the work area.

Visitors can be a minimum hazard if proper provisions are made to accommodate them and they cooperate fully with strict sanitary rules. When they must enter the poultry quarters, it is most important that they wear disinfected rubber overshoes and other footwear; in addition, they should wear protective clothing such as clean, laundered, or new disposable coveralls and hat. Disposable plastic boots may become punctured when used on gravel or other sharp surfaces; therefore, only heavy gauge (3 mil or greater) plastic disposable boots should be used. These sanitary precautions are most essential when entering floor brooding and rearing houses, but will help keep disease out of any house or pen.

SANITARY ENVIRONMENTS

Grounds Around Buildings

RODENT CONTROL. Piles of trash and unused equipment are good hiding and breeding places for rats, mice, and ground squirrels, which may serve as reservoirs of disease and contaminate troughs with their excrement. Rodents are reluctant to travel over open spaces that do not provide protective cover. A 20-m band of short-mowed grass or gravel tends to discourage the migration of rodents into a poultry building from surrounding areas. Feed spilled or left in stored troughs is an attractive food supply; when it is exhausted, rodents will find any available route into the building where they have intimate contact with poultry. Even if buildings are rodent-proof, excrement can be tracked in on footwear. It is more difficult to get rid of rodents once the premises are infested than to keep them out initially.

INSECT CONTROL. Many parasites and disease agents are harbored from one generation to another in resident insects (Marek's disease), require an insect for an intermediate stage of development (tapeworms), or are simply carried from bird to bird mechanically or by biting (fowl pox virus). Countermeasures against insects are part of the sanitary environment and cleanup.

Some methods used to keep insects away from buildings are an apron of treated soil to prevent growth of all vegetation, an apron of hard surface material, or a border of well-mowed green grass. Spraying the area around buildings with an insecticide also prevents insect buildup, but the other methods have the additional advantage of reducing fire hazards to the buildings.

A good practice during cleanup is to spray the grounds, litter, and buildings with an insecticide immediately after removing fowl, then allow a few days for effective insect kill before removing litter preparatory to cleaning and disinfection. This is especially important when there is a history of an insect-borne disease in the previous brood. After cleaning, the building should be sprayed again with an insecticide having a residual effect to prevent reinfestation. Professional, integrated rodent and insect control services are available in some locations. They may provide cost-effective convenience.

Dead-Bird Disposal

FOCI OF INFECTION. When birds die owing to disease agents, carcasses remain a source of infection for penmates and other poultry on the same or other farms. Also, hopelessly sick birds discharge infectious material into the environment and should be removed from the flock and killed in a manner that will not permit the discharge of blood or exudates (see Diagnostic Procedures). Whether the result of a serious clinical infection or just the usual expected mortality, all carcasses should be disposed of by one of the following methods to prevent dissemination of disease.

COOKING OR RENDERING. Freshly dead poultry, like livestock, can be rendered into fertilizer or other products. The rendering temperature should be sufficient for sterilization, and the truck bed used to transport the carcasses washed and disinfected. Cans used to haul the carcasses should be steam-cleaned and sterilized. Again, it should be remembered that commercial or contract haulers of dead carcasses may introduce another disease from some other outbreak unless strict precautionary measures are taken.

BURNING. Burning is the most dependable way of destroying infectious material. Many smokeless, odorless incinerators for disposal of animal carcasses are available commercially. These devices are expensive, but are handy and suitable for some purposes. Homemade incinerators of various types have also been used successfully, but they may create objectionable odors and are unlikely to meet government air pollution standards.

BURYING. For losses creating a serious disposal problem, where environmental regulations allow, a deep hole may be dug and the carcasses buried so animals cannot get at them. The best and easiest way is to use a backhoe and dig a deep narrow trench. Each day's collection of dead birds can be deposited and covered until the trench is filled.

PIT OR TANK DISPOSAL. For small losses and normal attrition, a decomposition pit can be used

(Fig. 1.8A). A bigger and less elaborate one than that shown can be built, but precautions should be taken to assure that it is not located where it will contaminate drinking water supplies, that the roof or walls will not cave in, that animals will not dig into it, that flies and other insects cannot get into it, and above all that children cannot fall into it. The pit cover should be sealed with tar paper or plastic and be strong enough to hold at least a foot of soil overlay. Where ground water levels are close to the surface (deltas, lowlands, shorelines), underground pits may be undesirable. An alternative is an above-ground dead-bird composting unit.

COMPOSTING. Aerobic, thermophilic batch composting of poultry carcasses is a method of disposal developed at the University of Maryland (31). Compost mixtures of straw, whole poultry carcasses, manure, and water in the proportions of 1:1:1.5:0.5, respectively (⅓ of water added to each layer), decompose rapidly and odorlessly. Composts heat rapidly, attain temperatures of between 145 and 165 F, and reduce soft tissues completely within 14 days. Compost structures and management procedures are simple (Fig. 1.8B). Pathogen survival studies suggest the process is biologically "clean." Attempts to isolate coliform and *Salmonella*-like bacteria, and IBD virus have yielded negative results. Composting may be an effective alternative to more traditional dead-bird disposal methods, especially where water tables are near the surface.

Buildings and Runs

CLEAN BUILDINGS. A clean sanitized environment is good insurance against disease outbreaks from any cause. Stringent sanitary practices are frequently ineffective because disease is tracked in after the buildings and equipment are cleaned and disinfected, or because some step in the total program was omitted and a focus of infection was preserved.

LITTER REMOVAL. When a house is depopulated, the litter or droppings should be removed preparatory to cleaning. With development of huge specialized poultry farms, proper and economical disposal of litter and poultry manure has become a serious problem. There is no clear-cut answer. A general recommendation is to remove it far enough from the buildings so that insects will not crawl or fly back into the houses, and to dry it, compost it, or spread it onto fields and work it into the soil. If cleaning is done while chickens are still present (cages), remember that contracted personnel, trucks, and equipment may recently have been on another farm where a disease outbreak occurred.

In some cases, the nature of a disease may dictate

that some extra precautions (wetting down or soaking with disinfectant, delaying removal, burying, burning) be taken with litter, even though expensive. Any treatment of manure or litter must consider residual effects of the applied compounds on plant life when treated manure is spread on the land. For most disease agents, composting of litter or

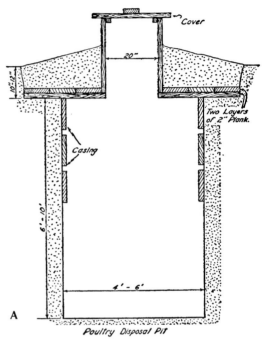

A

Poultry Disposal Pit

1.8. *A.* Poultry disposal pit. Such a pit can be made any size that is convenient. *B.* A simple above-ground poultry carcass composter of 200 ft³ (5.7 m³) capacity. Five such bins will process 1000 lb (455 kg) of carcasses per day. (Courtesy Poult Sci Dept, Univ Maryland)

SIMPLE   POULTRY   COMPOSTER
200 Cu Ft CAPACITY. FIVE BINS
WILL PROCESS ca. 1,000 LBS OF
MORTALITY PER DAY.

B

PRESSURE–TREATED
LUMBER
[DRAWING NOT TO SCALE]

COMPOST MIXTURE
RATIO OF 1: 1: 1.5: 0.5, STRAW:
POULTRY: MANURE: WATER
[By Volume]

droppings is sufficient. Whatever is done, one must be aware that wherever litter is spilled or piled, it remains as a disease reservoir for varying lengths of time.

OUTSIDE RUNS. In the case of outside runs such as turkey and game bird ranges, the topsoil should be scraped off and hauled some distance from the poultry. Sunlight and soil activity combine over a long period to destroy most pathogens. Anything that can be done to aid the destruction process is helpful. Removal of organic residues such as leaf beds and manure accumulations helps to reduce the danger for future broods. It is best to rotate the ranges or dirt yards so they stand idle for one complete flock cycle.

WASHING AND DISINFECTING. Once the litter or cage droppings have been removed, cleaning and transfer equipment, feeders, waterers, egg collecting equipment, walls, floors, roosts or cages, outside concrete or suspended runs, and entries to buildings should be washed thoroughly and disinfected. If the supply of water is limited and washing is not possible, dry cleaning may suffice if it is thorough and includes scraping and sweeping or vacuuming surfaces, corners, ledges, nests, and feeders. The amount of disinfectant used on dry-cleaned surfaces must be increased over that required for washed surfaces.

If possible to do so efficiently, it is preferable to clean the house without removing equipment. If not, all portable equipment should be removed, soaked with water, then thoroughly washed and dried. A high-pressure water hose is effective. Equipment that cannot be removed should be washed in place and then the entire inside building surface washed clean. If the building has been constructed to facilitate good cleaning, it can be done easily. If not, satisfactory cleaning may not be accomplished at all or only with great effort and expense. A large concrete apron equipped with racks and a high-pressure hose is a good place to clean and stack equipment.

After washing, disinfection is in order (see Disinfectants). There are many good disinfectants sold under trade names; follow the manufacturers' recommendations. The important thing is that the surfaces be clean before application. Disinfectants applied to dirt-encrusted surfaces are ineffective and wasted. Not only are they inactivated by organic material in the dirt, but they never reach the infectious agents beneath it. Thorough washing removes most infectious agents from the house and equipment and leaves a clean surface so the disinfectant can reach those that remain. Two to 4 wk of idleness or "down time" before a new flock is moved in is additional insurance against carryover of disease;

however, "down time" should be considered as an adjunct to, and not a substitute for, thorough cleaning, washing, and disinfection.

BUILT-UP LITTER AND UNCLEANED BUILDINGS. Commercial producers demand chicks and poults that are free of pathogenic microbial agents acquired through egg transmission or from unsanitary hatchery or delivery environments. To maintain this status, it is preferable to place these healthy new flocks in cleaned and disinfected buildings with fresh clean litter. Providing these ideal conditions is expensive because of labor and litter costs. Also, suitable litter materials are becoming less plentiful. In keeping with the constant necessity to reduce production costs and cope with shortages, rearing of several successive flocks on the same (built-up) litter has become an economically acceptable practice with broilers, where the life span is very short and single ages of birds per farm permit complete depopulation at the end of each brood. The litter in turkey grow-out buildings is also frequently used for several successive flocks. This trend has become commonplace with the use of litter-processing machinery, which can break up caked litter and produce a litter with acceptable production characteristics. The continual reuse of such built-up litter will result in an increase of microbial pathogens and parasites within the litter. Commercial producers recognize, however, that cleaning and disinfecting a house or group of houses may become necessary any time excessive economic losses are attributable to a disease that may carry over to the next brood.

The practice of reusing litter is much less attractive for rearing egg-production flocks, where the life span usually exceeds 18 mo; it is not acceptable for rearing breeding flocks that produce hatching eggs for new generations. In any case, those who reuse litter should be fully aware of the possible hazards involved and should follow other sound disease control practices to minimize the dangers.

When old litter must be reused, it is good insurance to remove any caked or excessively fouled litter, accumulated feathers, and decomposed carcasses. A layer of fresh clean litter should then be placed under the heating brooders and over the area to which the young will be confined or will spend most of their time the 1st wk or 2 of life. One disadvantage of multiple brooding on the same litter is the excessive dust that accumulates. Inhalation of the dust provides an avenue of entry to the respiratory tract for bacteria and fungal spores.

HATCHERY MANAGEMENT. The building and equipment in which the fertile egg is converted to a day-old chick, poult, or other fowl and the equipment used to process and deliver it to the farm must be clean and sanitary. An individual hatched from a pathogen-free egg will remain pathogen-free only if it hatches in a clean hatcher, is put in a clean box and held in a clean room where it can breathe clean air, and then is hauled to the farm in a clean delivery van.

Design and Location.
A hatchery should be located away from sources of poultry pathogens such as poultry farms, processing plants, necropsy laboratories, rendering plants, and feed mills. It is not good practice to retail poultry equipment and supplies from a hatchery building, since this draws producers and service workers who may introduce contaminating material.

A good hatchery design has a one-way traffic flow from the egg-entry room through egg-traying, incubation, hatching, and holding rooms to chick-loading area. The cleanup area and hatch-waste discharge should be off the hatching room, with a separate load-out area. Each hatchery room should be designed for thorough washing and disinfecting. The ventilation system is equally important and must be designed to prevent recirculation of contaminated and dust-laden air. Gentry et al. (19) found that hatcheries with poor floor designs and faulty traffic patterns were highly contaminated compared with those with one-way flow.

Importance of Good Sanitation.
Factors that aid in obtaining pathogen-free chicks and poults are hatchery cleanliness and sanitation, well-arranged traffic flow, and well-controlled ventilation.

Techniques have been devised for evaluating the sanitary status of commercial hatcheries by culturing fluff samples (52), detecting microbial populations in hatchery air samples (14, 19, 25), and culturing various surfaces in the hatchery (27). By relating results of these techniques to hatchery management, it has been observed by Magwood (26) that bacterial counts of eggshells dropped quickly in clean air and low counts persisted on all surfaces to completion of hatching. Chute and Barden (13) found fungal flora of hatcheries to be related to management and sanitation programs.

To minimize bacterial contamination of eggs and hatching chicks, hatchery premises must be kept free of reservoirs of contamination, which readily become airborne (26). Trays used for hatching should be thoroughly cleaned with water and then disinfected before eggs are placed in them. This can be done by dipping in a tank of suitable disinfectant (see Disinfectants), washing with hot water or steam followed with disinfectant spray, or fumigating with formaldehyde in the hatcher. Trays and eggs are frequently fumigated together immediately after eggs are transferred to the hatcher. Fumigation is sometimes done during the hatch (at about 10% hatch), but concentrations low enough to avoid harming the hatching chick probably serve only to give the down a pleasing yellow color. Formaldehyde fumigation in one case increased the severity of mold infection rather than overcoming it (53). Wright (50) emphasized the practical meaning of hatchery sanitation and how to attain it. He concluded that no fumigation program should be used to replace cleanliness, but rather to supplement it.

As chicks hatch, the exposed embryo fluids collect bacteria from contaminated shells, trays, and ventilating air. The combination of the nutritious fluids and warm temperature forms an excellent environment for bacteria and they multiply very rapidly (19). The cleaner the air and environment to begin with, the more the bacterial buildup is delayed and, as the hatch progresses, the less likely is the navel to become infected (omphalitis).

BREEDER CODES.   The breeder code is a designation used to denote the source of hatching eggs. It usually denotes breeders of the same age on the same or different farms, all breeders on a particular farm, or any other grouping. There is a tendency to keep breeders in larger flocks and to avoid as much as practicable the mixing of hatching eggs from flocks of many different microbial, nutritional, and genetic backgrounds. If breeders are kept free of disease and fed a good ration, hatching eggs are produced clean and properly disinfected, and chicks are hatched and handled in clean surroundings, keeping chicks of different breeder codes separated has little practical meaning other than providing that all have more nearly the same level of maternal antibodies against the same diseases. This may permit a more uniform response to vaccines applied to chicks the first 2–3 wk of life when maternal antibodies have a protective effect.

Occasionally, a disease is believed to be egg transmitted from a breeder flock to the offspring. When this occurs, the disease nearly always appears in several offspring flocks derived from the same breeder flock(s) and delivered to different farms. On the other hand, a hatch of chicks is frequently divided into deliveries to several farms and a disease occurs in only those delivered to one farm. This indicates that the disease is farm associated and not hatchery or breeder-flock associated.

CHICK SEXERS.   Unless the output of one hatchery is so great as to demand their full time, chick sexers may go from one hatchery to another, which introduces the possibility of carrying disease. Most sexers are aware of this hazard and are eager to follow proper procedures. If sexers must also service other hatcheries, facilities should be provided so that their equipment can remain at the hatchery. They should have a clean area in which to change clothes and wash themselves and their equipment and should have clean protective garments to wear.

Their habits should be at least as clean as those of the hatchery crew.

FLOCK MANAGEMENT

Handling the Young. Chicks and poults hatch with a reserve food supply in unabsorbed yolk sufficient to sustain them for about 72 hr. Some offspring actually hatch 1 or 2 days before they are taken from the hatcher; therefore, they should receive feed and water as soon as possible, preferably within 24 hr after removal.

BROODER TEMPERATURE. Chilling, overheating, starvation, and dehydration are serious stress producers and can precipitate active disease from latent infections that might otherwise be overcome by the young without detectable symptoms. In a randomly split hatch of chicks from the same group of dams, those delivered to one farm can suffer much greater mortality than those delivered to others. This is associated with differences in environmental stresses and exposure to disease. Young chicks and poults should be kept at a comfortable temperature at all times. The brooder temperature is usually started at 35 C and gradually reduced as the birds mature. While thermometers are helpful, strict adherence to thermometer temperatures without regard to obvious discomfort of chicks or poults is poor practice. An uncomfortable bird lets the caretaker know about it. Its peeping should be heeded and the cause of discomfort corrected, regardless of thermometer reading.

COCCIDIOSTATS. Floor-reared poultry receive coccidiostatic drugs in feed from the 1st day to prevent coccidiosis (broilers, turkeys, replacement pullets destined for cage adult housing) or to keep the disease under control until birds develop active immunity (breeder flocks, replacement pullets destined for floor adult housing).

Immunity, however, depends on a number of factors. The amount of feed and coccidiostat intake may vary among birds, and the number of viable sporulated oocysts will vary with differing humidity, temperature, and litter conditions, even in different areas of large buildings. Depending on the relationship of these variable factors, the coccidial infection may be too mild to elicit good immunity, or it may be so severe that a frank outbreak occurs. There is no special management formula to overcome this dilemma other than a keen awareness of the variable factors and an attempt to maintain the proper physical environment to favor the degree of infection desired (see Chapter 34).

FEED AND WATER CONSUMPTION AND MEDICATION. Scientific feed formulation is the business of highly trained nutrition experts, and quality feeds are the rule, not the exception. Poultry eat the feed, not the formula, however, and occasionally problems arise that are traceable to feed (accidental omission of an ingredient, low-potency vitamin supplement, moldy or toxic contamination of an ingredient).

More important in everyday disease control are variations in feed consumption associated with hot or cold weather; housing changes, breed, type, strain, and age of bird; body weight; rate of lay; energy and fiber content of feed, and particle size of feed ingredients. With a 10–20% lower feed consumption associated with one of these factors, there is also a lower intake of coccidiostat or other medicament in feed by the same amount. Conversely, an increase in total feed consumption as a result of one of these factors increases total intake of all feed ingredients, including drugs.

Increased water intake during hot weather can spell disaster through overconsumption of water medication, but a given concentration of a drug in water may fail to control a disease under circumstances in which consumption is very low, as in very cold weather. Also, if natural sources of water are available, particularly for range turkeys, the intake by some birds from the trough may be light. Many are the tragedies from overdosing due to carelessness; miscalculation; or failure to consider feed and water intake, weather, and other variables. When drugs are used in feed, great care should be exercised in adding the same or other drugs to water.

IMMUNIZATION. Some diseases are so ubiquitous and easily and rapidly spread that it is possible to avoid them only with extreme precautions, and little can be done to alter the course of an outbreak should it occur. Yet prevention through vaccination is relatively harmless and inexpensive. This is particularly true of Marek's disease, IBD, Newcastle disease, infectious bronchitis, and avian encephalomyelitis. For these diseases, vaccination at the appropriate time is good common sense and a means of preventing spread of virulent forms.

Encounters with virulent and devastating disease agents have become less frequent. Reliance on emergency drug treatments has declined as a result of increased knowledge of diseases, widespread saturation of the poultry population with mild and attenuated immunizing agents, elimination of egg-borne diseases, improved genetic resistance to disease, and improved health-protecting management practices. As a consequence, minor health improvements have become more significant.

SURGICAL PROCEDURES. Beak trimming is commonly practiced on growing flocks, particularly those destined for cages as adults. When this is done properly, there is no serious adverse effect;

however, proper beak trimming is more an art than a science, and many birds are permanently handicapped when it is not done properly.

If the operation is done correctly, after the beak tip is removed, the remaining growing tip is cauterized sufficiently with the hot cutter blade to prevent bleeding and regrowth, but not so much that the bird develops a sensitive or abnormal beak that interferes with eating and drinking. Proper beak trimming promotes maximum performance. Done improperly, it is probably the greatest single management cause of unsatisfactory performance of laying and breeding stock. Poor performance resulting from improper beak trimming must not be attributed to some mysterious disease. For more detail on cannibalism and beak trimming, see Chapter 35. Similarly, other surgical procedures such as removing wattles, combs, or toenails of certain toes must be done by one trained in the procedure if harm to the bird is to be avoided.

Adult Flocks. Modern laying strains are bred for high egg production, and broiler stocks for rapid growth and good feed conversion. The most important management factor is maintaining feed, water, and environmental conditions at the optimum condition for hen conform, which in turn results in maximum efficient production and growth. The same is required of meat birds, turkeys, and other types of breeder hens. The egg production or efficiency of feed use will be a good indicator of the success of the management and the welfare of the flock. Many conditions arise that hamper performance, and it is important not only to keep disease out, but to prevent conditions causing discomfort.

BREEDER FLOCK MANAGEMENT. The breeder flock should be managed so that egg-borne diseases are prevented by whatever techniques are available.

Diet, Health, Parental Immunity. A breeder ration must contain a higher level of many nutrients than does a laying ration. Laying rations sufficient to sustain egg production are not always adequate to sustain good hatchability and health of young offspring. Many times, production is satisfactory in breeder hens, but their embryos or chicks show symptoms and lesions of vitamin deficiency. The breeder ration must be adequate for development of the embryo and the chick as well as performance of the breeder hen.

Breeder hens in poor health for any reason frequently fail to supply the embryo with some vital nutritional factor or perhaps pass some toxic material to the egg; thus, the hatch is poor or chicks are of low quality and must be culled. While this occasionally happens with apparently healthy birds also, a healthy breeder flock is the best insurance of good quality offspring. Holding hatching eggs too long or under improper storage temperature, humidity, and environment can result in poor quality chicks.

Baby poultry are delivered into many types of environment. In some areas, husbandry methods are such that birds are exposed to disease from the 1st day of life. In some cases, exposure of very young poultry lacking any maternal antibodies to a disease can lead to significant mortality or economic loss (infectious bronchitis, avian encephalomyelitis, IBD, duck virus hepatitis). Where exposure is apt to occur at a very early age, maternal antibody can be a significant aid to prevention of disease. On the other hand, a high level of maternal antibodies can interfere with early immunization. How much maternal immunity is desirable and against how many diseases are debatable subjects and will vary according to the area where poultry are raised and the type of rearing facility (cage vs. floor).

Maternal immunity is dissipated gradually and usually does not last more than 2–4 wk after hatch. In modern, well-run layer and breeder replacement-rearing facilities chicks and poults are well protected, not only against the elements, but also against introduction of disease from outside sources for several weeks or beyond the time that a high initial maternal immunity would be protective. Maternal immunity in chicks is of less concern in such cases. This is not so likely to be true of inadequately sanitized and poorly managed pullet-rearing or broiler grow-out farms, where exposure can occur as early as the 1st day of life to a disease agent carried over from the previous brood in reused built-up litter. In these cases, protective maternal antibodies become a very important consideration in preventing disease or reducing losses, and vaccinating breeder dams with killed vaccines to give high maternal antibody protection for the offspring has become common practice. Lesions and residues from the carrier for killed vaccines injected into the breast muscle has been cause for carcass condemnation at slaughter.

Interior Egg-borne Diseases. Various techniques are used for preventing disease agents from being transmitted from dam to offspring via the egg. The ideal situation is to have breeders free of all pathogens. For most viral diseases, there is still no practical way of obtaining this utopian situation. For others (avian encephalomyelitis), the probability of the infection occurring during the egg-laying period, with resultant egg transmission, is too great to permit the clean but susceptible status (see Chapter 21).

IMMUNIZATION. In addition to immunization of breeders against several common diseases to prevent adverse effects of inopportune infections on egg production, they are immunized against avian encephalomyelitis during the growing period to ensure that they do not become naturally infected during the period they are producing hatching eggs. While this may not be an absolute guarantee against egg transmission of the virus, it has been a practical means of preventing its serious dissemination through infected offspring. Reluctance to use the vaccine in breeder flocks only encourages this type of dissemination.

TESTING AND REMOVAL OF CARRIERS. Carriers of some transovarially transmitted diseases can be detected by serologic means, and this procedure has been used to eliminate possible egg shedders from breeding flocks. This has proved most successful for pullorum disease and fowl typhoid. The method has been so effective that its application in infected breeder flocks, along with management techniques, has been largely responsible for eradication of these diseases from most commercial poultry enterprises in the United States and many other countries.

TESTING AND SLAUGHTER OF INFECTED FLOCKS. Where infected breeders are detected, the entire flock may be discarded. This method is indicated in circumstances whereby testing is not likely to detect all infected birds. It is a costly procedure and not warranted unless there is a definite advantage for the offspring and reasonable assurance that they will not become infected from other sources after delivery to the farm. It has been used successfully for eliminating mycoplasma-infected turkey and chicken breeder flocks.

DESTRUCTION OF AGENT INSIDE THE EGG. A pressure differential between the atmosphere and the inside of the egg has been used to force antibiotics through the shell of incubating eggs to prevent transmission of pathogenic *Mycoplasma* spp. from dam to offspring. This is done by dipping warm eggs into cold antibiotic solutions or using special vacuum machines (2). Antibiotics have also been injected directly into eggs for this purpose (29).

Elevating the egg temperature has also been used to destroy mycoplasmas inside the egg (54). In this procedure, incubator temperature (and internal egg temperature) is gradually raised over a 12- to 14-hr period to the maximum embryo survival temperature, approximately 46.9 C, and then cooled immediately and rapidly to normal incubation temperatures. The procedure usually lowers hatchability.

TREATMENT OF OFFSPRING. Offspring from infected dams may be treated with high levels of antibiotics by injection or feeding or both. This is unreliable, but can be a significant adjunct to other methods and can greatly assist in overcoming economic losses from egg-transmitted diseases that are drug sensitive.

Eggshell-borne Diseases. Several procedures are used to overcome shell contamination that arises from intestinal contents and other environmental sources. Control involves preventing shell contamination or destroying organisms before they penetrate the shell.

Egg penetration by bacteria occurs more readily if the shell becomes porous. This occurs in the late life of the breeder hen or when there is a deficiency or imbalance between calcium, phosphorus, and Vitamin D. Respiratory virus infections can also result in porous and poor shells.

VACCINATION AND SEROLOGIC MONITORING

The Avian Immune System. An understanding of the avian immune system is essential to vaccination and serologic monitoring programs. The avian immune system is complex and involves numerous types of cells and chemical mediators. The primary function of the immune system is to provide the bird with the ability to resist the invasion by, and injurious effects of, infectious disease agents. A crucial aspect of the immune system is that it has an immunologic memory. This allows a bird to respond to the second challenge of a particular disease agent with a more rapid and effective immune response.

The immune system is typically characterized as providing both humoral immunity and cell-mediated immunity. These types of immune response are also called bursal-derived and thymus-derived immunity, respectively. Humoral immunity is associated with the immunoglobulins (antibodies) produced when a bird has been exposed to a particular disease agent. These antibodies are capable of neutralizing, or assisting in the neutralization of, specific infectious disease agents. Antibodies are produced by B lymphocytes that originate from the bursa of Fabricius. Cell-mediated immunity is less easily characterized as it involves numerous different cell types and modes of actions. Examples of cell-mediated immunity are the phagocytosis and destruction of infectious organisms by macrophages, the regulation of the immune response by T helper cells, the killing of certain virus-infected cells by cytotoxic T cells, or the destruction of tumor cells by natural killer cells. The effective use of vaccines takes advantage of both humoral and cell-mediated immunity. The monitoring of immunity resulting from vaccination or disease challenge typically depends on the detection of antibodies in the blood, which are produced by the humoral immune response.

Types of Vaccines. Poultry vaccines are typically characterized as viable (live) or inactivated products. Viable vaccines are available for numerous viral, bacterial, and coccidial organisms. Viable products are most commonly administered by mass vaccination techniques, such as aerosolization or administration in the drinking water, which makes them practical for broiler or turkey production flocks. An exception is Marek's disease vaccine, which must be injected. The immunity provided by viable vaccines may be short- or long-lived. Repeated vaccinations, with increasingly virulent vaccines, may be necessary to provide long-term immunity with some agents. Care must be taken with viable vaccines to assure that both the appropriate vaccine and the correct vaccine dosage are used. Severe vaccine reactions can result in unacceptable morbidity and mortality if too virulent a vaccine strain is used in young poultry or if the dose administered is too high.

A second generation of viable vaccines is emerging with the development of genetically engineered, live-virus-vector vaccines. These recombinant vaccines use a live-virus vaccine, such as fowl poxvirus or turkey herpesvirus, as a vector to transport the gene coding for the protective antigen of a second infectious agent, for which immunity is desired. Examples of these vaccines include a recombinant fowl poxvirus vaccine expressing genes to protect against H5N2 avian influenza (7) and a recombinant fowl poxvirus expressing Newcastle disease virus antigen (11). Both of these recombinant vaccines are protective against pathogenic virus challenge under experimental conditions. The efficacy and cost effectiveness of recombinant vaccines under field conditions is yet to be determined. This type of vaccine may offer significant protection against disease with a minimal adverse vaccine reaction.

Inactivated vaccines, also called nonviable vaccines, killed virus vaccines, or bacterins (in the case of bacteria), often offer the advantage of providing long-term immunity. These vaccines must be administered by subcutaneous or intramuscular injection, and in some cases they are the final vaccination after one or more "priming" vaccinations with live vaccines. The labor and vaccine costs associated with these products make them most practical for use in layer and breeder flocks in which long-term protection against disease and/or decreased egg production are desired.

The primary goal of a vaccination program is to prevent disease and the decreased productivity associated with the infection by disease agents. In broiler and turkey flocks, a vaccine program is designed to protect against the disease agents that are a significant threat to the productivity of a flock in a specific geographic area. A universally effective vaccination program cannot be designed, owing to differences in disease challenge. Certain regions, with a long history of poultry production, may re-

quire a vaccination program with repeated vaccinations against numerous different pathogenic agents, due to the certainty of heavy disease challenge. New poultry farms, geographically isolated from other poultry operations, may have the opportunity to decrease the costs of production with a more limited vaccination program.

The goal of a vaccination program for layers is to prevent disease and provide long-term protection against decreased egg production and egg quality. The vaccination of breeder flocks must encompass the goals set for layer flocks, and also ensure that antibody levels against selected viruses are high enough to provide progeny with a uniform protective immunity during the 1st weeks of life in the form of maternally derived antibodies. Due to the high value and life span of layer and breeder flocks, the vaccination programs designed for these birds are typically more intensive and comprehensive than those used for broilers.

Vaccine Failure.   Numerous factors can cause a vaccine failure. One of the most common causes of vaccine failure is the inappropriate administration of the vaccine. Certain live vaccines, such as Marek's disease vaccine, are easily killed, and failure to follow the manufacturer's recommended handling practices will result in the inactivation of the virus prior to administration. Viable vaccines administered in the drinking water can, likewise, be destroyed before they reach the bird if they are mishandled or if water sanitizers have not been removed from the water prior to the addition of the vaccine. Vaccines that are administered by intramuscular or subcutaneous injection can also fail if vaccinators do not deliver the vaccine to the appropriate vaccination site.

While the most common cause of vaccine failure is an inadequacy or error in vaccine delivery, there are numerous instances of vaccines simply not providing adequate protection. In some cases, the field strain of an organism is of very high virulence and the vaccine strain is highly attenuated. In this situation, the flock may be effectively immunized, but the immunity is insufficient to protect against disease completely. Many infectious agents have several different serotypes and vaccine failure may be the result of the antigens in the vaccine serotype being different and not providing protection against the particular serotype of the agent causing the field challenge. It is not uncommon for a vaccine break to occur with infectious bronchitis virus when the field challenge is of a serotype different from that of the vaccine used (6).

Management conditions play an important role in the prevention of vaccine failures. If infectious disease agents are allowed to build up on a farm over successive flocks without clean-out and disinfection, it is possible that the challenge dose of a particular infectious agent will be so great, or so soon, that a normally effective vaccination program will be overwhelmed. The immune status of the breeder flock also can be involved in a vaccine failure. If the breeder flock provides progeny with high levels of maternal antibodies, vaccination during the first 2 wk of life may result in the vaccine being neutralized. The timing of the vaccination of young poultry with viable vaccines must always take the presence or absence of maternal antibodies into consideration.

Certain infectious disease agents and mycotoxins are immunosuppressive and may result in vaccine failure. Infectious bursal disease virus (Chapter 29), infectious anemia (Chapter 30), and Marek's disease virus (Chapter 17) are examples of agents that may cause severe immunosuppression in chickens. One mycotoxin, aflatoxin, has been shown experimentally to be immunosuppressive and has been implicated in decreased resistance to disease (see Chapter 36).

Evaluation of a Vaccination Program.
To assure that a vaccination program is effective, it must undergo regular evaluation. A logical criterion for the evaluation of any vaccination program is the prevention of morbidity and mortality. A more subtle, but equally important, criterion is the evaluation of production parameters; specifically, feed conversion, rate of gain, livability, condemnation, egg production, and egg quality of the flock must meet or exceed accepted production standards (6). Production can also be affected by numerous environmental and nutritional parameters, so if production is poor, all of these factors, including the vaccination program, must be considered.

SEROLOGIC MONITORING. A vaccination program is incomplete if it does not include regular serologic monitoring. In broiler and turkey production flocks, an effective monitoring program can be the regular sampling and testing of blood as they are slaughtered at the processing plant. This serologic monitoring will establish a baseline of antibody titers that are the result of both vaccination and field challenge. Changes in the usually observed antibody titers may indicate a decrease in the efficacy of vaccine administration or an increased field challenge by a particular pathogen. A regular serologic monitoring program is also helpful to determine whether a flock has been exposed to a new pathogen, not previously present in the region.

Serologic monitoring of layer flocks should be performed before the flock is placed in the layer building, with periodic serologic monitoring throughout the production cycle. This type of program will assess both the efficacy of vaccine ad-

ministration and the disease challenge the flock experiences in the field. Breeder flocks should be monitored in the same way as layer flocks and, in certain instances, breeders can be revaccinated during production to boost the maternal antibody titers of their progeny if they are found to be low.

INTERPRETATION OF SEROLOGIC DATA. It is usually impossible to differentiate between antibodies that are produced by vaccination versus those induced by field exposure to a given infectious agent. The only difference that may be observed is that the antibody titer following a field challenge may be higher than that observed following vaccination. A valid interpretation of serologic results requires a complete knowledge of the flock's vaccination history.

It usually takes poultry 1 to 3 wk to produce detectable levels of antibodies in their serum. It is possible, therefore, to collect blood during the middle of a disease outbreak and not be able to detect any antibodies to the causative disease agent. If this same flock is tested 2 wk later, however, serum-antibody levels will be high. A useful practice in establishing a disease diagnosis is to take acute and convalescent serum samples from the flock as it is undergoing an unknown disease challenge. Typically, the acute serum sample collected during the initial phase of the disease outbreak will be negative for antibodies to the suspected disease agent. The convalescent serum sample, taken shortly after the flock has recovered, if positive, will provide a definitive diagnosis when interpreted in conjunction with the clinical signs and lesions of the case. An important concept in the interpretation of serologic results is that a single positive serologic test only indicates that the flock was exposed to that disease agent during its life.

Different laboratories often conduct serologic tests using different reagents or techniques. Because of this, comparing antibody titers (a titer is a measure of the level or concentration of antibody in the serum) reported from different laboratories may be confusing. It is best to use one laboratory for a given test so that a familiar range for negative, low, or high titers is established. With experience and training, production managers can become skilled at the interpretation of serologic results. In the initial phases of establishing a serology monitoring program, it is important to consult with a poultry veterinarian to develop guidelines for the interpretation of test results.

MANAGEMENT OF HATCHING EGGS

Clean Hatching Eggs.
Very dirty eggs should not be used for hatching. If they must be used, they should be dry-cleaned when gathered.

The cleaner the shell surface, the less likelihood there will be for bacterial contamination and shell penetration.

The most important consideration in hatching egg sanitation is to manage the flock so that eggs are clean when gathered. Many factors enter into accomplishing this goal. Sloping wire-bottom roll-away nests, with or without automatic collecting devices, generally result in clean eggs and a minimum of bacterial contamination.

Clean eggs can also be produced in conventional box-type nests if nesting material is diligently kept clean by continually replacing soiled material. Egg breakage can be reduced by providing sufficient nests for the peak laying period.

The number of floor and yard eggs can be reduced by proper design and location of nests when maturing pullets need them; location and design will vary with the type of house. Nests should be darkened and ventilated, and hens must be prevented from roosting in them at night because they contaminate the area with fecal deposits.

Keeping the litter dry is an aid in preventing soiled nests and nest material. Proper design and construction of the breeder house to create conditions conducive to keeping litter dry aids disease control at the hatching-egg level. Table-egg breeding stock performs satisfactorily in litterless housing—either all slat or sloping wire-floor houses—and this largely eliminates dirty eggs resulting from tracking litter and feces into the nests. Heavy breeds and turkeys do not perform as well on these floors, so combinations of part slat and part litter are used to aid in litter management.

Measures should be taken to prevent *Salmonella* infections by using *Salmonella*-free feed ingredients particularly meat meal, eliminating these pathogens from mixed feed (pelleting), keeping feed clean by good feeding practices and storage facilities, and keeping natural carriers (rodents, wild birds, pets) out of pens and houses. Preventing salmonellosis and other types of enteric infections also helps prevent wet droppings, which contribute to wet litter.

Above all, eggs should be gathered frequently, especially in the early part of the day when most hens visit the nests. They should be gathered in clean, dry equipment and held in a dry, dust-free area.

Fumigation of Eggs.   The shell surface of hatching eggs should be disinfected immediately after gathering (on-farm fumigation). If fumigation cannot be done on the farm, it should be done as soon as possible thereafter, preferably before eggs enter the hatchery building or at the entrance to the egg-processing area. The more delayed the fumigation, the less effective it is because the bacteria will

have had longer to penetrate the shell. Unfumigated eggs raise the possibility of carrying some serious infection into the hatchery when susceptible newly hatched chicks are present (see Disinfectants, Formaldehyde).

Washing and Liquid Sterilization.   Washing eggs with warm detergent solution at a temperature (43–51.8 C) always higher than that of the eggs entering the washing machine—at least 16.6 C higher but not to exceed 54 C—followed by sanitizing the shells with a chlorine compound, quaternary ammonia product, or other sanitizing agent is routine for commercial eggs. The procedure has been employed successfully with hatching eggs, but some real disasters have occurred where thousands of eggs were contaminated rather than sanitized when dirty water was used, especially in recirculating washing machines. Even if eggs are washed properly, very dirty eggs should be cleaned first by sanding to prevent excessive pollution of the washing solution and equipment. If the iron content of the wash water exceeds 5 ppm, it favors multiplication of certain types of bacteria and creates a serious egg spoilage problem. A complete review of egg sanitizing agents is presented by Scott and Swetnam (43).

If egg washing is done, it should be only with a type of machine (brush conveyor type using flow-through wash water principle) that will ensure against contamination with dirty wash or rinse water. Very careful supervision is also necessary to see that all equipment is working properly at all times and is cleaned daily. In some types of machines, if the washing system fails, a few eggs can contaminate the water and thus contaminate thousands of others before the problem is detected and corrected. Contaminated eggs in the incubator set off a chain reaction of egg explosions that contaminate surrounding eggs, causing more "exploders" and more contamination. While washing and liquid sterilization of hatching eggs can be done satisfactorily, the procedure is subject to operational difficulties and should not be attempted on a routine basis without full knowledge of the hazards involved.

Whenever cold eggs are moved into a warm, humid atmosphere, moisture condenses on the cold shells (called "sweating"). This moisture provides a medium for growth of bacteria and fungi already present on dirty or unsanitized shells, or originates in contaminated warm air around the eggs. Cold eggs should, therefore, be warmed to room temperature in clean, low humidity air before placing in an incubator.

STORAGE FACILITIES.   After fumigation or other shell sterilization, hatching eggs are frequently stored in a cool room (about 10 C) at the hatchery until set. Cool rooms should be clean and free of mold and bacteria and periodically disinfected to prevent recontamination of shells. Clinical histories indicate that infection in young chicks may sometimes be traceable to fungus-contaminated hatching eggs; infections have been produced experimentally by contaminating shells with fungus spores (53). See Chapter 3 for additional discussion on egg-handling procedures to control salmonellae.

Because of possible adverse health considerations resulting from inhalation of formaldehyde fumes, hatchery personnel should be alert for any new and effective shell sterilization compounds and methods that may become available.

HANDLING DISEASE OUTBREAKS

Observe the Normal. Good poultry producers watch feed and water consumption and egg production at all times, but more important, they observe normal sounds and actions of the flock. They sense immediately when any of these conditions are abnormal and interpret them as signs of abnormal health. When this happens, it should be assumed that an infectious disease has gained entry and may be tracked elsewhere during the investigation period. In a modern factorylike poultry operation, any disease creates serious disruption in the economical operation of the farm and the plants processing products from it. Serious infectious diseases can create havoc. The following steps should be followed when disease is suspected.

Look for Noninfectious Conditions. Take precautions against tracking an infectious disease that may be present, but investigate management errors immediately. A high percentage of so-called disease problems referred to laboratories for diagnosis are noninfectious conditions related to management: beak trimming errors; consumption of litter and trash; feed and water deprivation; chilling of chicks; injury from rough handling, automatic equipment, or drug injection; electrical failures; cannibalism; smothering; overcrowding; poor arrangement of feeders, waterers, and ventilators; inexpensive low-quality feed ingredients; ingredients causing feed refusal; improper particle size of feed ingredients; and rodent and predator attacks (1, 9). Zander observed a severe drop in egg production in a pathogen-free flock after a 48-hr failure of a mechanical feeder (55). Bell (8) observed marked reduction in lay from water deprivation related to a beak trimming system that resulted in long lower beaks, making it difficult to obtain water when the level was low. These are conditions that do not require services of a diagnostic laboratory. External parasites (mites, lice, ticks) can be determined by producers if they examine affected birds.

Quarantine the Flock. In the event that no management factors can be found, the next step is to set up a quarantine of the pen, building, farm unit area, or entire farm, depending upon its design and programming. If this emergency was anticipated when the farm was laid out and programmed originally, the quarantine will be a minor problem. If the basic principle of "a single age in quarantinable units" was disregarded in original farm planning, a disease outbreak can be an economic disaster. Separate caretakers should be established for affected birds, or at least sick ones should be visited last.

SUBMIT SPECIMENS OR CALL A VETERINARIAN. The owner or caretaker should submit typical specimens to a diagnostic laboratory or call a veterinarian to visit the farm and establish the diagnosis. Owners should seek professional diagnosis, rather than trying to hide some disease because of possible public recrimination. Veterinarians and caretakers can and should help dispel this apprehension by maintaining high ethical standards and refraining from discussing one producer's problems with others. Yet, there comes a time when all producers must be apprised of a problem. Service workers are frequently requested to examine the flock, select specimens for the laboratory, and initiate first-aid procedures until the veterinarian can be called or visited. If so, they should wear protective footwear and clothing when they enter the house. No other farm should be visited en route to the laboratory.

DIAGNOSIS. It is important to get a diagnosis as soon as possible. The course of action will be determined by the nature of the disease. A producer should not procrastinate for any reason when a disease threatens, or it may get completely out of hand before a diagnosis is made. It is not always possible to treat a disease or check its deleterious effects; but to plan effectively for the future, it is important to identify any and all diseases that occur. A veterinarian should also be aware of the owner's economic plight at such times and render advice and assistance as quickly as information is available or a judgment can be made.

SPECIAL PRECAUTIONS. In addition to causing serious losses in poultry, some diseases (ornithosis, erysipelas, fungus infections) are especially hazardous for humans. When these conditions are suspected or diagnosed, extra precautions must be taken to ensure against human infection. The proper government health authorities should be notified of ornithosis outbreaks, and all handling and processing personnel should be apprised of the disease, hazards, and necessary precautions.

In some states, certain diseases (*Salmonella* infections, ornithosis, laryngotracheitis) must be reported immediately to the state animal disease control authorities so that proper investigation and action can be taken to protect the human population and the poultry industry. Common sense dictates that when a condition suggestive of an exotic disease such as velogenic viscerotropic Newcastle disease, fowl typhoid, or avian influenza is encountered, the proper regulatory authorities should be informed.

Nursing Care.   Whether the flock consists of a few hundred individuals or tens of thousands, nursing care plays an important role in the outcome of disease. Additional heat should be supplied to young chicks that begin huddling because of sickness. Clean and fresh (or medicated) water should be available at close range. Temporary, more accessibly located waterers are sometimes necessary during sickness. If water founts are normally located where chickens must jump onto some raised device or turkeys must cross through hot sunlight to reach them, the sick will not have the energy or initiative to seek water. They will soon become dehydrated, an early step on the road to death. Turkey yards should be well drained because birds tend to drink from the closest puddles, which may be thoroughly polluted.

The same principles are true for feed. Sick birds can be encouraged to eat if the caretaker will proceed through the house, stirring feed and rattling feed hoppers or adding small quantities of fresh feed. Sometimes a little molasses in feed or water (1 pt/gal) will encourage consumption. Some antibiotics appear to stimulate feed consumption when included in the diet; however, any additive that proves distasteful to the bird should be removed immediately.

Sometimes birds become so depressed and moribund that the caretaker must walk among them frequently to rouse them so that they will eat or drink.

Hopelessly sick and crippled birds should be killed in a manner to preclude or control the discharge of blood or exudates (see Diagnostic Procedures). Dead and destroyed birds should be disposed of immediately (see Dead-Bird Disposal).

DRUGS.   No drugs should be given until a diagnosis is obtained or a veterinarian consulted. If the wrong drug is given, it can be a waste of money, or it may be harmful or even disastrous. If an infectious disease is found and corrective drugs are indicated, they should be used very carefully according to directions.

Strict regulations govern use of drugs in mixed feeds for food-producing animals. For information, write to the U.S. Food and Drug Administration (FDA), 5600 Fishers Lane, Rockville, MD 20857. A handy reference is the annually updated *Feed Ad-*

ditive Compendium published by Miller Publishing Co., Minnetonka, MN. Feed manufacturers must have FDA clearance to include most drugs in mixed feeds. When treated flocks are to be marketed, a specified period (depending on the drug used) must follow cessation of treatment to allow dissipation of drug residues from tissues before slaughter. If the flock is producing table eggs when treated, the drug must be one permitted for use in laying flocks, or eggs must be discarded during, and for varying lengths of time after, treatment, a costly alternative.

If the flock is producing hatching eggs when it becomes infected and there is danger that egg transmission of the infectious agent from dams to offspring may occur (salmonellosis, mycoplasmosis, avian encephalomyelitis), eggs should not be used for hatching until the danger has passed. It should also be kept in mind that in fertile eggs, residues of drugs used to treat breeders may occasionally cause abnormalities in some embryos.

DISPOSITION OF THE FLOCK.   The flock should not be moved or handled until it has recovered, unless the move is to a more favorable environment as part of the therapy. After treatment, if any, has been completed and the flock appears to be completely healthy, it may be marketed or moved to permanent quarters if such a move is part of the management program. Some healthy carriers may remain. If the flock is moved to another depopulated farm, this will present no problem except that occasionally a disease may flare up from stress of handling and moving. If the recovered flock is moved to a multiple-age farm, carriers can introduce the disease into susceptible flocks already there. If the recovered flock is already in permanent quarters having multiple ages, newly introduced flocks may be exposed and contract the disease, a common occurrence especially with respiratory and litter-borne diseases.

DIAGNOSTIC PROCEDURES.   There are many satisfactory diagnostic and necropsy methods. The techniques and instruments used by one pathologist may vary considerably from those used by another. Some suggestions are offered here to guide the student and beginner. The goal of the necropsy is to determine the cause of impaired performance, signs, or mortality by examining tissues and organs, and to obtain the best specimens possible to carry out microbiologic, serologic, histopathologic, or animal inoculation tests. It is important that in the process, infectious materials do not endanger the health of humans, livestock, or other poultry. By proceeding in an orderly fashion, possible clues are less apt to be overlooked, and tissues will not be grossly contaminated prior to examination. Remember that a blood sample or tissue specimen determined later to be superfluous can always be discarded. It's better to save tissues, then discard if they are later determined to be unnecessary or unimportant to the diagnosis.

A key to good poultry diagnosis is the art of "seeing the forest as well as the trees." Try to identify the most significant flock problem(s), rather than becoming engrossed in individual bird disorders. Watch for telltale patterns of pathology as presented by the total diagnostic consignment.

The techniques and procedures necessary to make an accurate diagnosis and identify specific disease agents are found in the technical information contained in succeeding chapters of this book and in the following excellent reference manuals: *A Laboratory Manual for Isolation and Identification of Avian Pathogens* (38), *Avian Disease Manual* (49), *Avian Histopathology* (41), and *Color Atlas of Diseases of the Domestic Fowl and Turkey* (39). *Avian Hematology and Cytology* (12) should be consulted for detailed information on avian blood elements and methods for preparation and study. New information is continually being presented in the following journals, *Avian Diseases, Avian Pathology,* and *Poultry Science,* in the proceedings of several regional poultry disease conferences, and in other avian pathology and science journals.

Anamnesis.   The pathologist who has not seen the farm or the flock before attempting to diagnose the problem and recommend corrective measures is at a disadvantage. This can be partially overcome by getting a complete history of the disease and all pertinent events leading to the outbreak. The more information pathologists have about the history and environment, the more directly they can proceed to solution of problems. Unfortunately, the history includes only the situations, events, and signs that the caretaker, owner, service worker, or neighbor has observed and remembered. Knowledge of management factors such as ventilation; feeding and watering systems, accurate records of egg production, feed consumption, feed formulation, and body weight; lighting program; beak trimming practices; brooding and rearing procedures; routine medication and vaccination used; age; previous history of disease; farm location; and unusual weather or farm events may make the difference between diagnosis of the flock problem and the finding of a few miscellaneous conditions in a sample that may or may not be representative. Duration of the signs, the number sick and dead, and when and where they were found dead can be important clues.

Poultry producers have developed a high degree of knowledge about poultry diseases and usually recognize those resulting in dramatic or clear-cut signs and lesions. The veterinarian, therefore, is often confronted with obscure, undramatic, and complicated disease cases requiring extensive investiga-

tion. Even if all indications are that reduced performance is most likely due to a management factor, the veterinarian must check all reasonable disease possibilities. This requires a systematic approach to be sure nothing is overlooked.

External Examination.   Look for external parasites. Lice and northern fowl mites (*Ornithonyssus silviarum*) can be found on the affected chicken. If red mites (*Dermanyssus gallinae*) or blue bugs (*Argas persicus*) are suspected, examination of roosting areas and cracks and crevices in the houses and around the yards must be made, because these species do not stay on birds. See Chapter 32 for diagnosis and identification of external parasites.

The general attitude of live birds and all abnormal conditions should be carefully noted. It is very important to observe evidence of incoordination, tremors, paralytic conditions, abnormal gait and leg weakness, depression, blindness, and respiratory signs before the specimens are killed. It is very helpful to place birds in a cage where they can be observed after they have become accustomed to the surroundings and perform at their best. It is sometimes advisable to save some of the affected birds to observe possible recovery from a transitory condition (transient paralysis), respiratory infection, chemical toxicity, feed or water deprivation on the farm, or overheating during transport to the laboratory.

Examination should be made for tumors, abscesses, skin changes, beak condition, evidence of cannibalism, injuries, diarrhea, nasal and respiratory discharges, conjunctival exudates, feather and comb conditions, dehydration, and the body fleshing condition. These are all useful clues.

Blood Samples.   Blood specimens may be taken at this time (or immediately after the bird is killed). Frequently, it is desirable to have two (paired) blood samples several days apart to determine a rising or falling titer of antibodies to some disease (Newcastle disease) in the serum. In this case, a blood specimen may be taken from the main (brachial) wing vein or jugular vein or by heart puncture and the bird saved for a second sample.

Venipuncture of the brachial vein is usually the simplest and best method for obtaining blood from turkeys, chickens, and most fowl under field condition, especially when the bird is to be returned to the flock. Ducks are bled from the saphenous vein near the hock. Expose the vein to view by plucking a few feathers from the ventral surface of the humeral region of the wing. The vein will be seen lying in the depression between the biceps brachialis and triceps humeralis muscles. It is more easily seen if the skin is first dampened with 70%

alcohol or other colorless disinfectant. To facilitate venipuncture, extend both wings dorsally by gripping them firmly together in the area of the wing web with the left hand. Insert the needle into the vein of the right wing holding the syringe in the right hand (Fig. 1.9). The needle should be inserted opposite to the direction of blood flow.

Heart puncture can be made anteromedially between the sternum and metasternum (23), laterally through the rib cage, or anteroposteriorly through the thoracic inlet. Only through experience can one learn exactly where and at what angle to insert the needle. It is best to practice these techniques on freshly killed specimens before attempting to bleed live birds. A general rule for the lateral puncture is to form an imaginary vertical line at the anterior end of, and at a right angle with, the keel, then palpate along that line. The heartbeat can be felt and the needle inserted to the proper depth.

For heart puncture through the thoracic inlet, the bird should be held on its back with the keel up. The crop and contents are then pressed out of the way with a finger while the needle is guided along the ventral angle of the inlet. After penetrating the inlet, the needle is directed horizontally and posteriorly along the midline until reaching the heart.

The site for heart puncture between the sternum and metasternum is (in a mature chicken) about an inch above and posterior to the anterior point of the keel. The needle is directed at approximately a 45 degree angle in the anteromedial direction toward the opposite shoulder joint. The needle should pass through the angle formed by the sternum and metasternum and directly into the heart. For further details and illustrations, see Hofstad (23).

The size and length of the needle required for heart and venipuncture will depend on the size of the bird: for young chicks and poults, a ¾-in. 20-gauge needle, for mature chickens, a 2-in. 20-gauge needle. Mature turkeys may require larger needles. For quick and accurate bleeding, it is essential that the needle be sharp. Very slight vacuum should be developed intermittently to determine when vein or heart puncture has occurred. After vein puncture, steady slight vacuum should be continuous to withdraw blood. If vacuum is too great, the vessel wall may be drawn into the needle and plug the beveled opening. It is sometimes necessary to rotate the needle and syringe to be sure the beveled opening is free in the lumen of the vessel.

For most serologic studies, the serum from 2 mL blood is adequate. The blood should be removed aseptically and placed in a clean vial, which is then laid horizontally, or nearly so, until the blood clots. An occasional sample may require a long time to clot. This is especially true of turkey blood. Clotting can be hastened by adding a drop of tissue extract, made by killing and pooling a number of 10- to 12-day-old chicken embryos, grinding in a Waring blender, and freezing for future use. After the clot is firm, the vial may be returned to the vertical position to permit serum to collect in a pool at the bottom. Plastic vials are also available for blood collection. The clot does not adhere to the vial, and special positioning during clotting is unnecessary. Frequently, the serum from fat hens will appear milky due to lipids. Placing vials in an incubator will hasten syneresis. A fresh blood sample should never be refrigerated immediately after collection, as this will hinder the clotting process. Sera should not be frozen if agglutination tests are to be performed as this frequently causes false-positive reactions.

If an unclotted blood sample is required, it should be drawn into sodium citrate solution at the rate of 1.5 mL 2% solution/10 mL fresh blood, or deposited in a vial containing sodium citrate powder at the rate of 3 mg/1 mL whole blood, and the mixture quickly shaken. One way to prepare tubes for collecting sterile citrated blood is to add the proper amount of 2% sodium citrate solution to the col-

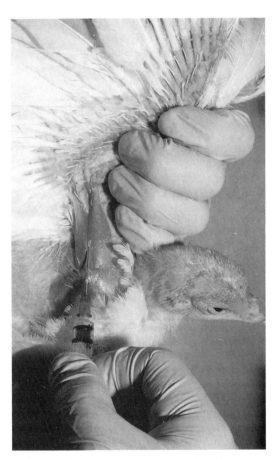

1.9.   Obtaining a blood sample from the wing vein.

lecting tubes ahead of time, then sterilize the solution and evaporate the moisture in an oven.

Blood-collecting vials containing the anticoagulant heparin can also be obtained commercially from laboratory supply companies. For certain types of serologic tests, fresh blood can be absorbed on the tips of filter paper strips, dried, and sent to the diagnostic laboratory, where antibodies can be recovered for testing by placing pieces of the treated paper into saline solution (Fig. 1.10).

If a blood parasite or blood dyscrasia is suspected, smears of whole blood should be made on clean glass slides previously warmed to promote rapid drying. For staining techniques, see Campbell (12).

A drop of blood for a wet mount or smear may be obtained from very small chicks by pricking the vein on the posteromedial side of the leg or by pricking or cutting the immature comb.

Killing Birds for Necropsy

CERVICAL DISLOCATION. Several methods can be used to kill fowl, and each has certain advantages. The objective is to kill the bird instantaneously so it will not suffer in the process. The quickest way to kill a small bird is illustrated in Fig. 1.11. Cervical dislocation, as described, is considered a humane method of poultry euthanasia by the American Veterinary Medical Association (AVMA) (5)

Bovine Burdizzo castration forceps can be used for killing large chickens and turkeys. It is difficult for one person to perform this operation and hold the bird at the same time, but it is quite easily done with the aid of an assistant. This technique also prevents agonal regurgitation and aspiration of crop contents into the respiratory passages if the forceps are left clamped until reflex muscle spasms cease. The neck of a young chick can also be broken easily by pressing it firmly against a sharp table edge,

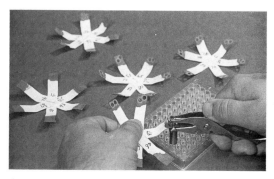

1.10. Blood absorbed on filter paper strips. For antibody testing, serum is recovered by punching out a piece of blood-soaked paper into saline solution. (Beard)

or by pinching between thumb and index finger, or by using the inside, noncutting angles of a surgical scissor such as a small Burdizzo.

ELECTROCUTION. Electrocution is a satisfactory method also. Clamps fixed to the end of electrical wires are fastened to the cloaca and mouth (this will assure moist contacts). The wires are then attached by means of a standard plug directly to 110-V alternating house current. A switch is thrown to feed the electric current through the wires. With this system, the bird rarely struggles and thus does not stir up dust or regurgitate crop contents. There is also less danger of agonal hemorrhages occurring or loss of blood when tissue specimens are desired. Obvious hazards to personnel and of short circuits on metal table tops should be recognized.

OTHER. Specimens selected for diagnosis may also be killed by intravenous injection of euthanasia solutions. Another method that would be satisfactory is asphyxiation by placing the specimen in a chamber filled with carbon dioxide (CO_2). Local availability of a CO_2 source may limit utilization of this technique.

Other methods of euthanasia can be found in a report of the AVMA (5). The method selected will depend upon the existing situation: species, size, and number of birds to be necropsied, or sacrificed; tissues, fluids, and cultures to be taken, etc.

Necropsy Precautions.

If there is reason to suspect that birds to be necropsied are infected with disease that may be contagious for humans (ornithosis, erysipelas, equine encephalitis), stringent health precautions are essential. The carcass and the necropsy table surface should be wet thoroughly with a disinfectant. Good rubber gloves should be worn, and care should be taken that neither the pathologist nor assistants puncture the skin of their hands or inhale dust or aerosols from tissues or feces. It is advisable to wear a fine-particle respiratory mask to prevent inhalation of contaminated dust. All laboratory personnel who may come in contact with carcasses, tissues, or cultures should be informed of their possible infectious nature and precautions to be taken.

With some notable exceptions (see specific diseases), most commonly encountered poultry disease agents are not considered pathogenic for humans. Nevertheless, it is wise to wear rubber gloves at all times while performing necropsies. For a review of poultry diseases in public health, see Galton and Arnstein (18). Examining specimens on metal trays that will fit into an autoclave facilitates quick sterilization of carcasses after necropsy.

Adequate instruments for routine work are necropsy shears to cut bones, enterotome scissors to

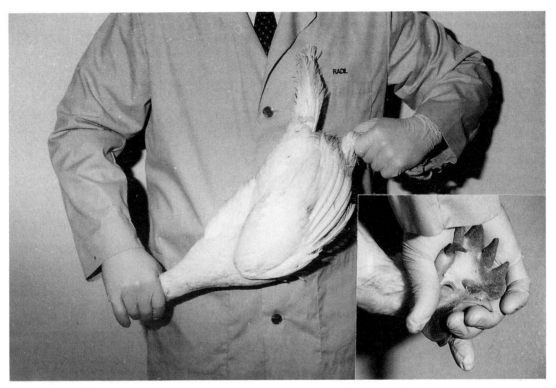

1.11. To euthanize a chicken or a small turkey, the bird is held as illustrated. The legs are held in a fixed position by one hand. The thumb and index finger of the other hand circle the base of the skull and the middle and ring fingers are held under the beak. Cervical dislocation is accomplished by the rapid extension of the arm holding the head with a simultaneous dorsal flexion of the head (*inset*).

incise the gut, a necropsy knife to cut skin and muscle, and a scalpel for fine examination of tissues. These should be supplemented with forceps, sterile syringes, needles, vials, and petri dishes for collecting blood samples and tissue specimens as the situation dictates.

Necropsy Technique

INTERNAL ORGANS. The specimen is laid on its back and each leg in turn drawn outward away from the body while the skin is incised between the leg and abdomen. Each leg is then grasped firmly in the area of the femur and bent forward, downward, and outward until the head of the femur is broken free of the acetabular attachment so that the leg will lie flat on the table (Fig. 1.12A).

The skin is cut between the two previous incisions at a point midway between keel and vent. The cut edge is then forcibly reflected forward, cutting as necessary, until the entire ventral aspect of the body, including the neck, is exposed (Fig. 1.12B). Hemorrhages of the musculature, if present, can be detected at this stage.

Either of two procedures is now used to expose the viscera. The poultry shears are used to cut through the abdominal wall transversely midway between keel and vent and then through breast muscles on each side (Fig. 1.12C). Bone shears are used to cut the rib cage and then the coracoid and clavicle on both sides (Fig. 1.12D). With some care, this can be done without severing the large blood vessels. The process may also be done equally well in reverse order, cutting through the clavicle and coracoid and then through the rib cage and abdominal wall on each side. The sternum and attached structures can now be removed from the body and laid aside. The organs are now in full view and may be removed as they are examined (Fig. 1.12E,F).

If a blood sample has not previously been taken and the bird was killed just prior to necropsy, a sample can be promptly taken by heart puncture before clotting occurs. Large veins leading into the leg may be incised, allowing blood to pool in the region for subsequent collection.

Laboratory Procedures

IMPRESSION SMEARS. If the foregoing procedures have all been done aseptically, the internal or-

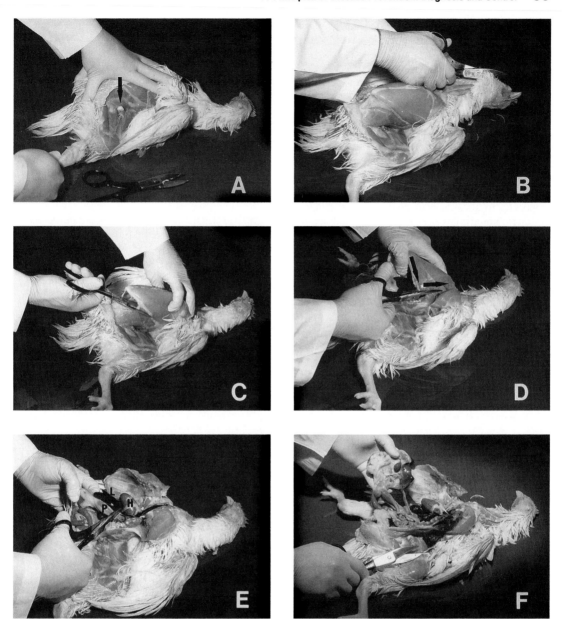

1.12. Each pathologist will develop his/her own systematic technique for conducting a
necropsy. A sturdy pair of poultry shears is usually sufficient to conduct a necropsy.
Other instruments such as scissors, forceps and scalpel may be helpful in collecting small
or delicate samples. A knife may be needed to cut through joints and bone. The illustrated
technique will aid the beginner. *A.* The skin and fascia between the leg and abdomen are
cut and the legs are pulled and twisted to disarticulate the head of the femur (*arrow*) from
the hip. *B.* The skin from the vent to the beak is incised and reflected. *C.* The body cavity
is entered at the ventral tip of the sternum. The incision is made at the margin of the pectoral muscle and continues through 2–3 ribs. A similar incision is made on the opposite
side of the breast. *D.* The shears are reoriented (*arrows*) and the incision is continued
through bone and muscle to the thoracic inlet. The breast is broken over to the opposite
side (or removed) exposing the viscera. At this point of the necropsy, microbiological
samples are collected. *E.* The intestinal viscera are freed by cutting through the esophagus and vessels of the liver just anterior to the proventriculus and liver. Heart (H), liver
(L), and proventriculus (P) are indicated. *F.* The intestines can be removed by gentle trac-
tion which tears mesenteric and air sac attachments. The lungs, heart, and kidneys remain
in the body cavity for later examination.

gans will not be contaminated; if exudates suggest the need, impression smears with sterile slides can now be taken.

BACTERIAL CULTURES. If gross lesions indicate bacterial cultures are needed, they can be made from unexposed surfaces of the viscera without searing the surface. If contamination has occurred, the surface of the organs should be seared with a hot spatula or other iron designed for that purpose before inserting a sterile culture loop. Care must be taken not to sear and heat the tissue excessively. It is often desirable to transfer large tissue samples aseptically to a sterile petri dish and take them to the microbiology laboratory for initial culture in cleaner surroundings.

BILE SAMPLES. If infection with a campylobacter species is suspected, a bile sample for wet mount examination or bacterial culture can be made at this point.

RESPIRATORY VIRUS ISOLATION. If a respiratory disease is suspected and virus culture or bird passage is desirable, an intact section of lower trachea, the bronchi, and upper portions of the lungs is removed aseptically with sterile scissors and forceps and transferred to a sterile mortar and pestle for grinding or to a sterile petri dish for temporary storage and later grinding. Other tissues (air sac tissue) can be added aseptically to the sample or transferred to other sterile containers for separate study. The trachea can now be incised; if exudate is present, it can be added to the above collection or saved in separate vials.

Grinding of such specimens is facilitated by adding a portion of sterile sand or, preferably, Alundum (mesh #60) to the mortar contents. Ground tissues are then transferred to sterile covered centrifuge tubes and spun at low speeds to prepare a supernatant fluid free of particulate matter for inoculation into embryos, nutrient media, cell cultures, or experimental birds.

Similar procedures can be followed for initial virus isolation from various parenchymatous organs.

SALMONELLA CULTURES. All other visceral organs should be examined for abnormalities (microabscesses, discoloration, swelling, friability). If abnormalities are observed, inoculum from the affected tissues should be transferred to suitable solid or liquid media for culture before the intestinal tract is opened. Once opened, gross contamination of other organs with gut contents is almost certain to occur. If *Salmonella* infection is suspected, selected sections of the gut are removed with sterile forceps and scissors and placed directly into a sterile mortar

and pestle or into a sterile petri dish for later culture. For routine examination, a single section comprising the lower ileum, proximal portions of the ceca and cecal "tonsils," and proximal portion of the large intestine may be used. All are minced and ground aseptically to produce an inoculum. Additional areas of the intestinal tract or tissues of other visceral organs may be added to the gut collection or cultured separately. Alternatively, sterile swabs may be used to obtain samples from the exposed gut lining for *Salmonella* cultures. See Chapter 3 and *Isolation and Identification of Avian Pathogens* (38) for detailed culture technique.

MISCELLANEOUS. After necessary cultures have been made, the intestine may be examined for inflammation, exudates, parasites, foreign bodies, malfunctions, tumors, and abscesses. The various nerves, bone structure, marrow condition, and joints can now be examined. The sciatic nerve can be examined by dissecting away the musculature on the medial side of the thigh. Inside the body cavity, the sciatic plexus is obscured by kidney tissue. These nerves can best be exposed by scraping away the tissue with the blunt end of a scalpel. Nerves of the brachial plexuses are easily found on either side near the thoracic inlet and should be examined for enlargement. Examination of vagus nerves in their entirety should be made, otherwise, short enlargements may be missed.

The ease or difficulty with which bones can be cut with the bone shears is indicative of their condition. The costochondral junctions should be palpated and examined for enlargement ("beading") and the long bones cut longitudinally through the epiphysis to examine for abnormal calcification. Rigidity of the tibiotarsus or metatarsus should be tested by bending and breaking to check for nutritional deficiency. A healthy bone will make an audible snap when it breaks. Bones from a chicken deficient in vitamin D or minerals may be so lacking in mineral elements that they can be bent at any angle without breaking.

Joint exudate, if present, can be removed after first plucking the feathers and searing the overlying skin with a hot iron. After searing, the skin may be incised with a sterile scalpel and exudate removed with a sterile inoculating loop or swab. Paranasal sinus exudates can be removed and examined in a similar manner.

EXPOSURE AND REMOVAL OF BRAIN. Removing the intact brain is not easy, since meningeal layers are attached firmly to bony structures in some places. The following technique can be performed quickly and is satisfactory for examination and removal of the brain in most instances.

Remove the head at the atlanto-occipital junction

and remove the lower mandible. Sear the cut surface and trim away excess loose tissue. Reflect the skin forward over the skull and upper mandible and hold it firmly in that position with one hand. Sterile instruments should be used for the succeeding steps if a portion of the brain is desired for animal inoculation, virus isolation, or fungal or bacterial culture.

With the sterilized tips of heavy-jawed bone shears or strong surgical scissors, nip just through the bone to the cranial cavity on both sides of the head, beginning at the occipital foramen and proceeding forward laterally to the midpoint at the anterior edge of the cranial cavity (Fig. 1.13A). Lift off the cut portion of bone and expose the entire brain (Fig. 1.13B).

If a portion is needed for culture or animal inoculation (e.g., avian encephalomyelitis virus suspect) and also one for histopathologic examination (e.g., vitamin E deficiency), cut the brain medially from anterior to posterior along the midline with a sharp, sterile scalpel blade. With sterile, sharp curved scissors, cut the nerves and attachments carefully from one of the brain halves while the head is tipped upside down, so that the loosened portion falls into a jar of formalin as it is freed (Fig. 1.13C). The second half can now be removed aseptically (but without concern for preservation of tissue structure) to a sterile petri dish or sterile mortar and pestle. Be careful not to contaminate brain tissue intended for virus isolation with instruments that have been in contact with formalin. The separate halves may also be removed in reverse order (Fig. 1.13D). If all of the brain is required for either purpose, proceed with proper precautions for the purpose intended. If the brain is destined only for sectioning, it may be fixed in situ and then removed. Large brain portions should be incised longitudinally to permit good penetration of fixative.

TISSUES FOR HISTOPATHOLOGIC EXAMINATION. Frequently, stained tissue sections are needed. The quality of the slide is no better than the quality of

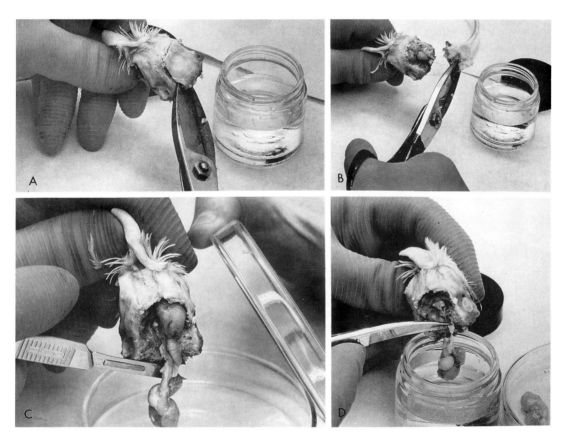

1.13. With a little practice, the brain can be removed with a minimum of trauma. *A.* Incise bone all the way around the periphery of the cranial cavity with heavy bone shears. *B.* Remove loosened portion of the bony skull. *C.* Incise brain longitudinally with sterile, sharp scalpel and remove one-half for sterile culture technique. *D.* Remove second half by dropping it into 10% formalin for histologic techniques.

the specimen and the care taken to preserve it. For good preservation, the tissue pieces from killed birds should be saved immediately after death, especially brain and kidney tissues, which deteriorate rapidly. Specimens should be small to allow quick penetration of fixative, gently incised with a sharp scalpel or razor blade to preserve tissue structure, and preserved in 10 times their own volume of 10% formalin or other fixative. Bone pieces should be sawed with a sharp bone saw unless thin or soft enough to cut with scissors or scalpel. After proper labeling and dating, they should be sent immediately to the processing laboratory.

Lung tissue usually floats on the surface of the fixing solution because of trapped air. Satisfactory fixation can be accomplished by placing absorbent cotton over the tissue, which serves to keep it immersed. Methods to exhaust air from air spaces in lung tissue by creating a vacuum over the fixative can be used, but are less satisfactory and may result in artifacts.

After fixing, bone tissue must be decalcified by immersion in a decalcification solution made by mixing equal parts of aqueous 8% hydrochloric acid and aqueous 8% formic acid (37). Decalcification typically takes 1–3 days, the length of time depending on the size and density of the bone sample.

If eye tissue is to be saved for sectioning, the whole eye should be removed and all ocular muscles trimmed off the globe to allow for rapid penetration by the fixative.

Any tissue held too long in formalin fixative becomes excessively hard. If processing is to be delayed, tissues should be transferred to 70% alcohol after 48 hr in fixative. Textbooks on histologic techniques (36, 37, 46) should be consulted for detailed procedures.

PROGRESSIVE EXAMINATION HINTS. The following procedures during the course of necropsy may be helpful to the beginner in checking for some commonly encountered diseases. They are not intended as definitive diagnostic methods. To arrive at a diagnosis, the student and beginning diagnostician must refer to the characteristic signs and lesions, diagnostic procedures, and characteristics of the infectious agent discussed under the specific diseases in succeeding chapters, and also to the manual, *Isolation and Identification of Avian Pathogens* (38).

Coccidia. Observe and note the subserosa before incising the intestine. Make wet mount smears of mucosal scrapings from various segments of the intestine and cecal contents and examine directly under the microscope for suspended oocysts and merozoites and stages undergoing development in epithelial cells (tissue stages).

Other Protozoa. Make wet mounts of affected areas, adding a little warm physiologic saline solution if necessary to provide fluid, and examine under a microscope for hexamita, histomonads, and trichomonads.

Capillarids and Ascarid Larvae. Collect mucous exudate and deep mucosal scrapings, and press into a thin layer between two thick pieces of plate glass. Examine before a strong light or under low-power magnification for the presence of parasites. Under magnification, look for double-poled, lemon-shaped eggs in the female capillarids.

Fungi. Make wet mount smears of scrapings of affected areas and add 20% sodium or potassium hydroxide. Digest with frequent warming for 15 min or more and examine under high-power magnification for mold hyphae.

Campylobacter. Examine fresh bile wet mounts under dark-field or phase illumination. Only positive findings may have significance.

Bacteremia and Blood Parasites. Make fresh mounts, preferably with citrated blood, and examine under light- and dark-field illumination for viable organisms. Make fresh blood smears and air dry for staining by Giemsa's, Gram's, Wright's, or other method.

Exudates. If infectious coryza is suspected, make thin smears of clear nasal or sinus exudate for staining by Giemsa's, Gram's, methylene blue, or other method. Inoculate appropriate media or susceptible chickens for isolation of the organism.

Abscesses. Select appropriate culture media suitable for growth of a variety of infectious organisms that may be suspected of causing the abscess. Sear and incise the surface of the abscess and inoculate culture media with the extracted material, using a sterile inoculating loop or swab. Make smears from the abscess on clean glass slides, diluting with a drop of water if the material is too thick. Air dry and flame slides, and make Gram's, acid-fast, or any other stain as desired.

Embryo Inoculation for Virus Isolation. For routine virus isolation, centrifuged and/or filtered fine-ground suspensions of suspect tissues (trachea, bronchi, lung, liver, spleen, kidney, brain, bone marrow) or body fluids and exudates may be inoculated into the chorioallantoic cavity and yolk sac and onto the chorioallantoic membrane (CAM) of embryos at various stages of incubation. See specific diseases for virus culture techniques. Also see *A Laboratory Manual for the Isolation and Identification of Avian Pathogens* (38) for selection of the proper age of embryo and route of inoculation for various disease agents as well as detailed inoculation procedures. Embryos from specific pathogen-free dams should be used for culture to be sure any agent recovered originated in the inoculum and not in the dams that produced the eggs. Equally important is assurance that negative cultures are due to absence of infectious agents in inoculum, rather than to interference of passive antibodies in eggs. Since the purpose of virus isolation is to determine which may be present, it is advisable to inoculate various ages of embryo by the various routes. Several blind passages may be necessary before the culture attempt can reasonably be considered negative. A simple technique that does not require dropping the CAM has been described (21).

The CAM may be drawn away from the shell (dropped) to facilitate inoculation. First, drill or punch a small hole in the shell over the air cell, then slowly drill or punch a second hole through the shell at a point on the side over the embryo. Applying mild suction through a rubber tube over the hole into the air cell causes the CAM to drop away from the inner shell membrane under the second drilled hole. A bright candling light should be used while suction is applied to determine when the CAM has dropped.

For yolk sac inoculation, the needle can be directed through the air cell and directly to the center of the egg. Some yolk may be withdrawn into the syringe to verify the location of the needle.

For chorioallantoic cavity inoculation, a hole is drilled over the edge of the air cell at a spot previously marked with the aid of a candling light. The cavity lies adjacent to the shell and can be easily penetrated from that point. All holes should be sealed with suitable sterile material before reincubating.

Cell culture procedures are becoming more common in diagnostic laboratories. Technicians with this capability may inoculate the cell cultures directly with tissue extracts or body fluids, or they may use embryos for primary screening and transfer embryo fluids or extracts to cell culture for further study and identification.

DISPOSING OF THE SPECIMEN. If a disease infectious for humans is suspected, the carcass should be autoclaved, incinerated, or otherwise rendered incapable of causing infection to laboratory or other personnel. Similar precautions should be followed during disposal of carcasses infected with a virulent poultry pathogen that presents a health hazard to the industry. The necropsy area, instruments, and gloves should then be cleaned, washed, and disinfected.

COMMUNICATION. Flock owners are not interested in technical data. They want to know what the problem is and what should be done to correct it and/or how to prevent reoccurrences. Sometimes technical data are necessary to clarify the diagnosis, but the report should be in language and terms that they will understand. A minimum of complicated scientific and medical technology words should be used. When medical terms are apt to be confusing, they should always be explained in lay terms.

The report should include the necropsy findings, results of laboratory studies, (histopathologic, serologic, cultural), diagnosis (temporary or final), and conclusions and recommendations. The owner is seeking professional advice. The veterinarian should give his/her best conclusions and recommendations based on the facts available. A verbal report or telephone call to the flock owner, manager, or service worker soon after completion of the necropsy and initial tests is highly advisable. A tentative diagnosis can be offered pending further confirmation.

FLOCK PROFILING. Today's disease problems often represent the sum of various subclinical disorders occurring at different times throughout the life of a flock. Acquisition of the fullest understanding of this sequential collection of serologic and other data concerning multiple pathogens requires disciplined and careful organization. The systematic, graphic presentation of this data is commonly called a "flock profile." The establishment of such profiles is facilitated by enzyme-linked immunosorbent assay (ELISA) technology, because a single basic test system is used to monitor for a broad array of diseases (44).

Snyder et al. (45) demonstrated the value of correlating ELISA profiling data with flock performance. The further evolution and diagnostic advantages of the graphic presentation of ELISA-based flock profiling data in combination with gross and microscopic pathology data was described by Mallinson et al. (28). The method has broad applicability to epizootiologic investigations, field research, and quality control. Baseline profiles can be established both as targets for vaccination goals and as a base from which deviations from the norm may be demonstrated when a field problem is subsequently encountered. Several flock-profiling kits and systems are now commercially available. Their value is enhanced when good data retrieval and graphic presentation of data (Fig. 1.14) is combined with the diagnostician's veterinary skills and experience in assimilating medical information and establishing a plausible diagnosis.

DISINFECTANTS. To disinfect is to free from pathogenic substances or organisms or to render them inert; a disinfectant is an agent or substance that disinfects chiefly by destroying infective agents (pathogenic microorganisms) or rendering them inactive; disinfection is the act or process of destroying pathogenic microorganisms. To sanitize is to reduce microbial populations and keep them from multiplying.

Properties. Among the properties of an ideal disinfectant are low cost per unit of disinfecting value, ready solubility in hard water, relative safety for humans and animals, ready availability, nondestructibility to utensils and fabrics, stability when exposed to air, absence of objectionable or lingering odor, no residual toxicity, effectiveness for a large variety of infectious agents, and no deleterious accumulation of any portion of the disinfectant in meat or eggs. For any disinfectant to be effective in economical quantities it must be applied to surfaces that have first been freed of debris and organic material by thorough scraping, scrubbing, brushing, and dusting and washing with soap or detergent solutions. Many disinfectants are highly efficient but only when these basic cleaning prerequisites have first been met.

Types. Many disinfectants of similar composition are sold under different trade names. Before buying a product with an unfamiliar name, compare types and values with a well-known product. Directions for dilutions given by the manufacturer should be closely followed. Complete discussions of various disinfectants and sterilization methods should be consulted (10, 40). Additional references on disinfectants and their use (20, 35) and textbooks on pharmacology and therapeutics should be consulted.

The virucidal activity of several commercial disinfectants against velogenic viscerotropic Newcastle disease have been determined (51). A list of 48 commercial disinfectants approved for use against avian influenza virus is available from USDA, APHIS, VS Emergency Programs, 4700 River Road, Riverdale, MD 20737-1231. The list provides product names, basic formulations, and dilutions along with the names, addresses, and telephone numbers of appropriate distributors or formulators.

PHENOL (CARBOLIC ACID). Phenol is a chemical substance obtained from coal tar. In its pure form, it occurs as colorless crystals having a characteristic and familiar odor (lysol soap). It is usually sold in water solutions and is too expensive for general poultry house use. It is, however, the chemical used as a basis for determining the phenol coefficients of various disinfectants (relative ability to kill specific test organisms when compared with that of phenol). O'Connor and Rubino (33) present a complete discussion of the phenolic compounds. Commercial disinfectants containing phenolic compounds have been developed and marketed at cost values, which permits wider use in poultry operations. Some have

residual activity persisting after they have dried, giving the advantage of continued suppression of bacterial and viral populations on sprayed surfaces.

CRESOLS. Cresol extracts of coal tar products are compounds closely related chemically to phenol and having similar bactericidal properties. They are thick yellow or brown liquids, miscible with water but only slightly soluble. They form the basis for a large number of commercial brands made by combining cresol with soap.

BISPHENOLS. Bisphenols are compounds composed of two phenol molecules modified and joined by various chemical linkages. Halogens, particularly chlorine, have been combined with bisphenols to increase their effectiveness; some of the chlorophenols have high antifungal activity. Bisphenols are frequently combined with other phenolic compounds in disinfectants. Additional information on these compounds is available (33).

PINE OIL. Pine oil has proved satisfactory as a disinfectant and has the advantage of being less injurious to the skin than cresol compounds. The odor is also less objectionable and in fact is rather pleasant, which enhances its desirability for use in offices and lavatory areas. Since it is insoluble in water, it is used in the emulsion form with soap or other emulsifying agent.

HYPOCHLORITES AND CHLORINATED LIME. Chlorine is the basis of disinfectants known as hypochlorites, which contain about 70% available chlorine. Hypochlorites (16), are available as powders containing calcium hypochlorite and sodium hypochlorite (NaOCl) combined with hydrated trisodium phosphate and as liquids containing NaOCl. Chlorinated lime (bleaching powder), prepared by saturating slaked lime with chlorine gas, was one of the earliest recognized disinfectants. It has been largely supplanted by the more readily available hypochlorites.

Products containing NaOCl are essentially liquids ranging in concentrations from 1 to 15%. The 15% solutions are used to prepare 5% solutions with water for bleaches and sanitizing agents. Germicidal potency of hypochlorites is dependent upon concentration of available chlorine and the pH (acidity) of the solution or upon the amount of hypochlorous acid formed, which, in turn, is dependent upon both factors. The influence of pH, especially in dilute solutions, is even greater than the percentage of available chlorine. Increasing the pH decreases the biocidal activity of chlorine, and decreasing the pH increases the activity. Germicidal activity is speeded up by raising the temperature.

If used according to directions, hypochlorites are highly efficient. Their principal use in the poultry industry is for egg washing and sanitizing and for disinfecting limited areas such as incubators, incubator and hatcher trays, and other areas around the hatchery, egg breaking areas, small brooders, and water and feed containers. They can also be used on cement surfaces. All surfaces to be disinfected with hypochlorite solutions must first be thoroughly cleaned to ensure the greatest efficiency. Stock supplies should be kept in dark, cool places, and containers should be tightly sealed when not in use. Fresh solutions must be prepared daily and periodically tested to assure that proper levels of available chlorine remain. A simple swimming pool test kit may prove helpful for such monitoring. Recently purchased or stored hypochlorites have been found to have wide ranges of concentration values.

All products containing chlorine must be handled with care because free chlorine is destructive to fabrics, leather, and metal.

ORGANIC IODINE COMBINATIONS. Iodine has long been recognized as an effective disinfectant. Many of the disadvantages of earlier products have been overcome by combining iodine in organic complexes, sometimes called tamed iodine. The term *iodophor* refers to a combination of iodine with a solubilizing agent that slowly liberates free iodine when diluted with water. The term most frequently refers to formulas consisting of iodine complexed with certain types of surfactants that have detergent properties. These complexes are said to enhance the bactericidal activity of iodine and render it nontoxic, nonirritating, and nonstaining when used as directed. The detergent also makes the products water soluble and stable under usual conditions of storage. There is no offensive odor, and the detergent properties impart cleansing activity. See Gottardi (22) for additional information on iodine compounds.

A group of commercial iodophors have been developed and marketed for a wide variety of disinfectant uses. Some of these products have a built-in indicator of germicidal activity; as the solution is used up, the normal amber color fades. When the solution is colorless, it is no longer effective. The products can be mixed in cold and hard water. Organic iodine products have a wide variety of uses in the industry. They can be applied without hazard to nearly all surfaces and are useful for disinfecting hatchery and incubator surfaces, incubator and hatcher trays, egg breaking areas, feeders and fountains, footwear, and poultry buildings. Like other disinfectants, these compounds are most effective on clean surfaces.

QUICKLIME (UNSLAKED LIME, CALCIUM OXIDE). The action of quicklime depends on liberation of heat and oxygen when the chemical comes in contact with water. On the poultry farm, its use is lim-ited to small yard areas that are damp and cannot be exposed to the sun, disinfection of drains and fecal matter, and whitewashes. As quicklime has a caustic action, birds should be kept away from it until it has become thoroughly dry.

FORMALDEHYDE. Formaldehyde (CH_2O) is a gas. It is sold commercially in a 40% solution (37% by weight) with water, under the name of formalin. It may also be purchased in the form of a powder known as paraformaldehyde (paraform, triformal, formaldegen). When heated, this powder liberates CH_2O. A suitable heating device is a thermostatically controlled electric pan with a timer that can be controlled from outside the fumigation chamber. Manufacturer's directions on amounts to use for each type of equipment and the means of liberating the gas must be carefully observed.

Formaldehyde is often generated by adding formalin to potassium permanganate ($KMnO_4$) in an earthenware crock or metal container. Because of the heat generated by the chemical reaction, glass containers should not be used. The container should be deep and have a volume several times that of the combined chemicals, because considerable bubbling and splattering takes place. The ratio in liquid measure of formalin is approximately twice the dry measure of $KMnO_4$ (1 g $KMnO_4$/2 mL formalin). If too much formalin is used, the excess will remain in the vessel. If too much $KMnO_4$ is used, the excess remains unchanged and is wasted. Potassium permanganate is poisonous. Both these compounds must be kept in accident-proof containers in a safe place away from work traffic.

A suitable fumigation cabinet must have a source of heat, a fan to circulate the warm humid air and fumigant, a source of humidifying moisture, and a method of generating formaldehyde gas. The box should be airtight, and have an exhausting device from the fumigation box to the outside of the building. It is much safer to locate fumigation chambers outside of any building and away from human traffic.

Though it is a powerful disinfectant, CH_2O has many disadvantages, especially its volatility, pungent odor, caustic action, and tendency to harden the skin—properties that make it disagreeable to apply. It is extremely irritating to the conjunctiva and mucous membranes, and some people are very sensitive to it. Because of this and other toxic properties, precautions must be taken to prevent its escape into areas where people work. Its chief advantages are that it can be used as a gas or vapor for fumigation of hatching eggs. It is a good disinfectant in the presence of some organic matter, and it does not injure equipment with which it comes in contact. The maximum atmospheric concentration permitted in work areas by some Occupational Safety and Health Administration (OSHA) regulations is 2 ppm. Suitable gas masks should be readily available near fumigation boxes. Formaldehyde can be neutralized with ammonium hydroxide by using a solution of approximately 30% and a quantity not to exceed one-half of the quantity of formalin used in the fumigation. Ammonia may be released by sprinkling or spraying in the intake air during evacuation of the fumigation box after the surfaces have dried completely.

Formaldehyde gas is widely used in poultry enterprises for fumigation of hatching eggs to destroy potential pathogenic shell contaminants. See Chapter 3 for detailed information on fumigation to control salmonellae. It is also used at the end of cleanup to fumigate the inside of incubators and hatchers and their contents.

Fumigation of incubators and eggs has been an established practice in the industry and has varied little over the years. Various recommendations have been made for quantities, humidity, temperature, and time for adequate sterilization of shells of hatching eggs. Frequent recommendations specify the following: 60 g $KMnO_4$:120 mL formalin/100 ft^3 (2.8 m^3) cabinet space, 21.1 C, 70% humidity, and 20 min fumigation time. The higher the humidity and temperature, the more effective the fumigation. When fumigation is completed, exhaust ducts are opened and the gas thoroughly exhausted before anyone opens the door to the cabinet.

In modern enterprises, hatching eggs are frequently handled only once and are placed directly into plastic holders (flats), which then travel in stacks through the fumigation, transportation, and storage route and eventually into the incubators. Entire racks, dollies, or pallets of closely stacked flats of eggs are thus fumigated in large boxes. In order to generate adequate concentration of CH_2O and have it penetrate and disinfect the egg shells in the centers of these stacks there should be increased quantity of chemicals (75 g. $KMnO_4$:150 mL formalin/100 ft^3), higher humidity (up to 90%), higher temperature (up to 32.2 C), longer time (up to 30 min), and vigorous agitation of the gas during fumigation so that it will penetrate the spaces and effectively sanitize surfaces of eggs in the centers of such large stacks. Pressed paper egg flats tend to trap CH_2O and continue to release the gas during storage and processing; therefore, CH_2O fumigation should be confined to eggs in plastic flats or wire containers.

CH_2O fumigation is sometimes used to disinfect the inside and contents (including eggs at 18 days of incubation) of hatching machines. Since these machines are inside of the building, this should not be done unless provision is made for adequate ventilation of the gas to the outside of the building when fumigation is completed.

Certain precautions are necessary after fumigation of hatching eggs. The incoming air for exhaustion must be clean, otherwise the humid surface of the egg can become recontaminated. During extremely cold weather, outside air must be warmed before entering the fumigation chamber to avoid overchilling eggs. While humidity is essential for disinfective activity of the CH_2O, the surface of eggs should not become visibly wet during fumigation and should be dry when the eggs leave the fumigator.

Fumigation should not be done in incubators because of the danger of injuring embryos (see Chapter 3). Also, it should not be done at such high concentration after the hatch begins because of the danger of injuring chicks or poults. Formaldehyde may be generated in hatchers by using approximately 20 mL formalin solution/100 ft^3. The formalin is soaked into enough cheesecloth so that it does not drip, and the cloth is hung in the circulating currents in the box. Effectiveness of this method is limited because of the low concentration.

ANTIFUNGAL IMIDAZOLES. The use of formaldehyde may pose some health and safety concerns for hatchery personnel. An effective substitute for formaldehyde used to control *Aspergillus* spp. in the hatchery is imazalil or enilconazole (nonproprietary names for phytopharmaceutical and veterinary uses, respectively) (48). The imidazoles are fungistatic at low concentrations by inhibiting ergosterol synthesis, and fungicidal at high concentrations by causing direct membrane damage (42). Imazalil is intended for use on clean hatchery surfaces or equipment and is delivered in an aqueous spray or by smoke propellant canisters. The antifungal properties of imazalil must be complemented with the use of antibacterial disinfectants for a complete hatchery sanitation program.

COPPER SULFATE (BLUESTONE). Although copper sulfate ($CuSO_4$) and other salts of copper have a marked toxic effect upon some of the lower forms of life, they are not considered good general disinfectants. Copper sulfate is toxic to algae and fungi and has been used in attempts to stop or prevent outbreaks of fungal diseases. It has been used in the feed at 0.5 lb/ton and sometimes 1 lb/ton for short periods without noticeable toxicity to chickens. Poultry will usually drink water containing $CuSO_4$ at no greater concentration than 1:2000, but a concentration greater than 1:500 may be toxic when given in the only source of water. Turkeys do not like water containing $CuSO_4$ and will seek other supplies if available. A 0.5% solution may be of value for disinfecting feed hoppers, water fountains, and surrounding areas associated with outbreaks of fungal disease.

QUATERNARY AMMONIUM SURFACTANT DISINFECTANTS. Quaternary ammonium products (quats) are considered to be good disinfectants when used according to directions. They are non-corrosive, water clear, odorless, cationic (+ charged ions), nonirritating to the skin, good deodorants, and have a marked detergent action. They contain no phenols, halogens, or heavy metals and are highly stable and relatively nontoxic. Most quats cannot be used in soapy solutions. All surfaces to be disinfected must be thoroughly rinsed with water to remove any residue of soap or anionic (− charged ions) detergent before using quats for sterilizing purposes. Some hard-water minerals may interfere with their action. See Merianos (30) for more information on these compounds.

Quats are used for washing eggs and disinfecting hatchery surfaces, incubator and hatcher trays, egg breaking equipment and areas, feeders and waterers, and footwear, among other uses.

SUNLIGHT AND ULTRAVIOLET RADIATION. Solar radiation has disinfecting properties; however, since the material to be treated must be in thin layers and exposed to direct rays, this method is limited to impervious surfaced yards, concrete and blacktop aprons, and equipment that can be thoroughly cleaned before being exposed. The construction of most poultry houses prevents efficient disinfection by the sun. A cement platform fully exposed to the sun makes a convenient place for treating movable equipment. If properly constructed with a drain, such a platform can be used as a washing and disinfection rack. A concrete apron before the poultry house entry will be washed by rains or can be washed by hose to take advantage of the disinfecting power of the sun's rays on the clean surface.

There are many types of germicidal (ultraviolet, or UV) lamps, but not enough scientific evidence is available to warrant a recommendation for their general use in hatcheries or on poultry farms. A complete review of the use of UV radiation in microbiologic laboratories is available (34).

HOT WATER. Hot water adds to the efficiency of most disinfectants, and if applied in the form of boiling water or live steam, is effective without addition of any chemical. Detergents added to systems for generating and disseminating hot water and steam will increase cleaning and decontaminating efficiency. Live steam must be applied directly and at close range to the part to be disinfected.

DRY HEAT. Dry heat in the form of a flame is effective if the flame comes in contact with the pathogen to be killed. All methods involving direct flame are fire hazards and not recommended except possibly on cement surfaces. In tightly controlled circumstances, flames might be used to eliminate hard-to-remove feathers and fluff accumulations.

Other commercial disinfectants, mostly organic compounds, are available under trade names. Many are combinations of several individual disinfectants with complementary properties. Some also have long residual activity. To choose disinfectants wisely, one must continually keep abreast of new product development through current scientific and lay publications.

Residues of disinfectants used to sanitize drinking fountains should be rinsed off with fresh water before water vaccines are given, since they can inactivate the vaccine virus.

DISINFESTANTS (PARASITICIDES, INSECTICIDES, PESTICIDES)

Properties. Disinfestants destroy animal parasites such as lice, mites, ticks, and fleas. They also destroy other undesirable insects (flies, beetles, ants, sow bugs). Some pesticides are highly toxic to humans and livestock. Their use (preferably by a licensed expert as part of a professional, integrated, insect and rodent control service) is recommended only as an adjunct to a properly conducted total sanitary control program. Many disinfectants are also destructive to lice, mites, and other similar parasites, but must come in contact with them. Many pesticides, however, are useless as disinfectants.

Suitable insecticides are those that can be used on or around poultry without causing toxic effects to humans or birds from contact or ingestion and that do not accumulate to harmful levels in edible tissues or eggs as a result of ingestion or absorption.

The list of available and permissible commercial insecticides has declined greatly and changes frequently. A regularly updated bulletin, *Livestock and Livestock Building Pest Management*, is available from the Ohio State University Extension. Many, widely used in the past, have been prohibited for use around food animals because of the deposition of insecticides in fatty tissues and eggs. Others have been abandoned because populations of insects become resistant to them. It is necessary, therefore, to keep informed on available effective insecticides through current government, university, and industry literature. In some situations, it may be cost effective to contract this complex changing activity through an agency providing professional insect and pest control services. Biosecurity measures for the agency employees and equipment must be considered when contemplating such contract services.

The limited number of available commercial parasiticides, their active chemical properties, limitations, tolerances, and various applications, are discussed in detail in Chapter 32. See also Chapter 36 for toxic effects of some insecticides.

Unlike flies, which travel to insecticide baits or over insecticide-treated surfaces, bird ectoparasites are best controlled by bringing the insecticide into

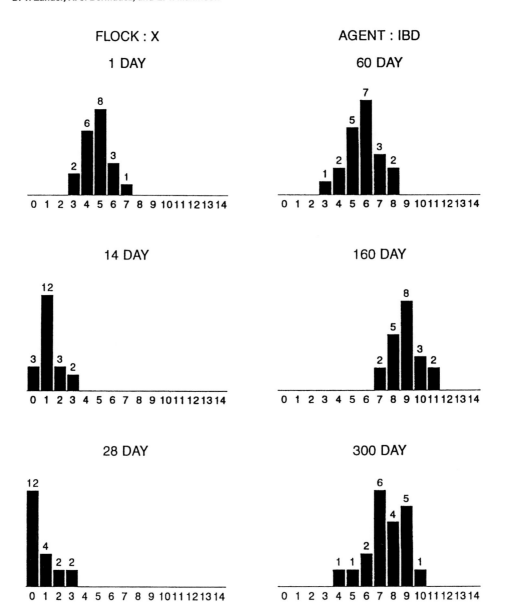

1.14. Temporal graphic distribution of infectious bursal disease (IBD) enzyme-linked immunosorbent assay (ELISA) group titer levels at 1, 14, 28, 60, 160, and 300 days of age for an IBD-vaccinated broiler breeder flock. Numbers on the X-axis represent group titer levels obtained by ELISA. Titers of 0 are group 0, 1–350 are group 1, 351–1500 are group 2, 1501–2500 are group 3, 2501–3550 are group 4, etc., with titers of > 12,500 comprising group 14. Numbers above each bar represent the number of samples reacting at each level on the indicated day of age.

contact with the parasite. A wide assortment of housing types and production systems are in use. One application method or system is seldom suitable for all types of housing. The type and form of parasiticide best suited for a particular type of housing and management system should be determined and then used according to directions on the label. Fogging and misting can be effective only if the insecticide can be confined in the building and/or applied (blown) into cracks and crevices and on feathers where parasites are congregated. Otherwise, the effort and expense are largely wasted. Pyrethrum preparations containing synergists can be used in light- and temperature-controlled houses, but the automatic ventilation system must be bypassed and hand controlled during treatment. In high-rise houses, one must be sure to compensate for the large volume of space under the floors by using additional insecticide in a space-calculated application.

A common error is to assume that one application of insecticide will accomplish the objective. Parasite eggs are seldom destroyed; they remain to generate a new population, which must be attacked with a second application 2–3 wk after the first. In addition, no system, application, or insecticide will result in a 100% parasite kill. Once the parasite gains a foothold, it must be attacked repeatedly. Frequently, alternating insecticides and methods is necessary to effect control. Do not be misled by statements that the birds learn to live with their parasites. Such thinking encourages continuous poor bird performance and a host of problems.

Handling Precautions. Possible hazards to humans and animals from many of the modern pesticides must always be remembered when considering their use. It is best to wear a suitable mask, rubber gloves, and protective clothing when applying insecticides. The most important precaution in handling chemical insecticides is to read the directions, hazards, and antidotes on labels of containers before any use.

A basic rule in handling insecticides is to keep them properly labeled and stored in a locked building reserved for that purpose. Disposal of empty containers and discarded leftover insecticides is becoming more of a hazard and responsibility. Large drums should be returned to the supplier or heated to red heat for 5–10 min. Paper and plastic containers should be burned. Small glass and metal containers should be broken or punctured so that no one will use them for any purpose. In addition to the human hazard, discarded insecticides must not pollute lakes or streams nor become a hazard for honeybees. A safe policy is to check with the local environmental protection agency (EPA) for recommendations.

Types

CRUDE OIL, DISTILLATES, SIMILAR COMPOUNDS. Petroleum oils applied to clean buildings and equipment prior to introducing a new flock have been widely used to control lice, mites, and ticks. Oily residues get on the parasites and cause suffocation. They have been effective in getting at parasites in cracks and crevices of the building, but they cannot be applied to parasites on birds. Carbolinium, a wood preservative, also repels mites and other insects for long periods after it is applied. These products are quite messy and smelly and not as effective as many newer products.

NICOTINE SULFATE. A 40% solution of nicotine sulfate has been widely used to control lice and mites. It is sprayed or painted on perches or floors of cages shortly before the flock settles for the night. In heavily infested birds, it is daubed on the fluff feathers. A 2% nicotine sulfate dust is also available for mite control. It can be dusted into the fluff feathers with a garden duster. The insect-killing properties depend on a substance that volatilizes at body temperature and penetrates the feathers to attack the parasites. In very cold weather, volatilization may not occur unless the treated surface is close enough to the bird to be warmed by the body heat. This product is not well adapted for control of turkey parasites where roosting areas are not enclosed.

Though it has been largely replaced by newer products, it remains a very effective parasiticide for lice and mites and is often used when others fail. Whenever nicotine products, particularly the concentrated ones, are applied, workers should be well protected with coveralls, hats, respirators, goggles, and rubber gloves. If the concentrate is spilled, any contaminated clothing should be removed immediately and thoroughly washed, and any contaminated skin area should be washed immediately with soap and water.

SPACE DIFFUSION INSECTICIDES. Pyrethrum products are released as a fog or mist, and the volatile compound permeates the room. Pyrethrum, an extract from plants, has low toxicity for higher forms of life but high toxicity for insects. It is relatively costly and may fail to penetrate adequately through feathers of birds and into insect hiding places. Synthetic forms of pyrethrum are now available commercially.

Vapona or DDVP, a preparation of dichlorvos, is sometimes impregnated into special materials from which it slowly vaporizes and diffuses through the air. This has greatest application in storage and other rooms that are closed and unventilated for long periods (overnight).

SYSTEMIC INHIBITORS. Sulfaquinoxaline, used so extensively in feed and water for control of coccidiosis and many bacterial infections, was found to rid birds of northern fowl mites (17). The product or its metabolites apparently creates body conditions objectionable to the parasites (possibly odors), which drive them off the birds. The drug has since been banned from feed for hens laying eggs for human consumption, but other products have been reported to exert similar effects, and some may exert an unsuspected mite-repelling action. Drugs providing this type of mite control seem most effective when incorporated in feed prior to infestation and least effective as a treatment after infestation has become established.

DUSTS AND SPRAYS. Nearly all insecticides adaptable to control of parasites on fowl can be obtained as ready-to-use dusts or in the form of wettable powders, emulsifiable concentrates, or liquid suspensions, all of which can be prepared as sprays. Each has advantages, and suggested uses are supplied with the insecticide.

Chickens dust themselves instinctively. In litter-floor houses, insecticide dusts can be added to litter to control mites, according to specifications of the manufacturer. Special dust boxes with added insecticide can be placed in large cages and wire- or slat-floored houses to accomplish the same objective. Dusts can also be applied to birds in cages by using a dust applicator. The dust must be blown into the feathers to get at the parasites. Although laborious, dusting individual birds can be effective.

The most common method of applying insecticides is by spray. The mixture must be agitated during application to maintain a constant concentration and prevent separation. Sprays are mostly applied to floors and walls, but some can be sprayed on the birds.

None of the insecticides is perfect, and resistance is already known to have developed against some of them. New products are constantly being developed and tested for effectiveness. Poultry producers should be alert for products, preparations, and local vendors of professional pest-control services most suitable for their type of management system.

The best parasite control is to prevent the initial infestation through wise management practices. Once again, parasite infestations, like bacterial and viral diseases, can be most successfully controlled and eradicated from single-age farms or quarantinable units as part of a total, integrated system of "disease-prevention management" (biosecurity).

REFERENCES

1. Adams, A.W. 1973. Consequences of depriving laying hens of water a short time. Poultr Sci 52:1221–1223.
2. Alls, A.A., W.J. Benton, W.C. Krauss, and M.S. Cover. 1963. The mechanics of treating hatching eggs for disease prevention. Avian Dis 7:89–97.
3 Anderson, D.P., and R.P. Hanson. 1965. Influence of environment on virus diseases of poultry. Avian Dis 9:171–182.
4. Anderson, D.P., C.W. Beard, and R.P. Hanson. 1966. Influence of poultry house dust, ammonia, and carbon dioxide on resistance of chickens to Newcastle disease virus. Avian Dis 10:117–188.
5. AVMA. 1993. Report of the American Veterinary Medical Association Panel on Euthanasia. J Am Vet Med Assoc 202:229–249.
6. Beard, C.W. 1979. Avian Immunoprophylaxis. Avian Dis 23:327–334.
7. Beard, C.W., W.M. Schnitzlein, and D.N. Tripathy.

1991. Protection of chickens against highly pathogenic avian influenza virus (H5N2) by recombinant fowlpox viruses. Avian Dis 35:356–359.
8. Bell, D. 1966. Water shortages can cut egg production. Poultr Trib 72:30.
9. Bierer, B.W., T.H. Eleazer, and D.E. Roebuck. 1965. Effect of feed and water deprivation on chickens, turkeys, and laboratory mammals. Poultr Sci 44:768–773.
10. Block, S.S. 1991. Disinfection, Sterilization, and Preservation. Lea and Febiger, Philadelphia, PA.
11. Boursnell, M.E.G., P.F. Green, A.C.R. Samson, J.I.A. Campbell, A. Deuter, R.W. Peters, N.S. Millar, P.T. Emmerson, and M.M. Binns. 1990. A recombinant fowlpox virus expressing the hemagglutinin-neuraminidase gene of Newcastle disease virus (NDV) protects chickens against challenge by NDV. Virology 178:297–300.
12. Campbell, T.W. 1995. Avian Hematology and Cytology, 2nd e d. Iowa State University Press, Ames, IA.
13. Chute, H.L., and E. Barden. 1964. The fungous flora of chick hatcheries. Avian Dis 8:13–19.
14. Chute, H.L., and M. Gershman. 1961. A new approach to hatchery sanitation. Poultr Sci 40:568–571.
15. Chute, H.L., D.R. Stauffer, and D.C. O'Meara. 1964. The production of specific pathogen-free (SPF) broilers in Maine. Maine Agric Exp Stn Bull 633.
16. Dychdala, G.R. 1991. Chlorine and chlorine compounds. In S.S. Block (ed.). Disinfection, Sterilization, and Preservation. Lea and Febiger, Philadelphia, PA, pp. 131–151.
17. Furman, D.P., and V.S. Stratton. 1963. Control of northern fowl mites, Ornithonyssus sylviarum, with sulphaquinoxaline. J Econ Entomol 56:904–905.
18. Galton, M.M., and P. Arnstein. 1960. Poultry diseases in public health. US Public Health Serv Publ 767.
19. Gentry, R.F., M. Mitrovic, and G.R. Bubash. 1962. Application of Andersen sampler in hatchery sanitation. Poultr Sci 41:794–804.
20. Glick, C.A., G.G. Gremillion, and G.A. Bodmer. 1961. Practical methods and problems of steam and chemical sterilization. Proc Anim Care Panel 11:37–44.
21. Gorham, J.R. 1957. A simple technique for the inoculation of the chorioallantoic membrane of chicken embryos. Am J Vet Res 18:691–692.
22. Gottardi, W. 1991. Iodine and iodine compounds. In S.S. Block (ed.). Disinfection, Sterilization, and Preservation. Lea and Febiger, Philadelphia, PA, pp. 152–166.
23. Hofstad, M.S. 1950. A method of bleeding chickens from the heart. J Am Vet Med Assoc 116:353–354.
24. Jensen, M.M. 1988. Update on usage and effectiveness of coryza, cholera, and staphylococcal vaccines. Proc 37th West Poultr Dis Conf, Veterinary Extension, University of California, Davis, pp. 54–56.
25. Magwood, S.E. 1964. Studies in hatchery sanitation. 1. Fluctuations in microbial counts of air in poultry hatcheries. Poultr Sci 43:441–449.
26. Magwood, S.E. 1964. Studies in hatchery sanitation. 3. The effect of air-borne bacterial populations on contamination of egg and embryo surfaces. Poultr Sci 43:1567–1572.
27. Magwood, S.E., and H. Marr. 1964. Studies in hatchery sanitation. 2. A simplified method for assessing bacterial populations on surfaces within hatcheries. Poultr Sci 43:1558–1566.
28. Mallinson, E.T., D.B. Snyder, W.W. Marquardt, and S.L. Gorham. 1988. In B.A. Morris, M.N. Clifford, and R. Jackman (eds.). Immunoassays for Veterinary and Food Analysis-1. Elsevier, London, and New York, pp. 109–117.
29. McCapes, R.H., R. Yamamoto, G. Ghazikhanian, W.M. Dungan, and H.B. Ortmayer. 1977. Antibiotic egg injection to eliminate disease. I. Effect of injection methods on turkey hatchability and Mycoplasma meleagridis infection. Avian Dis 21:57–68.
30. Merianos, J.J. 1991. Quaternary ammonium antimicrobial compounds. In S.S. Block (ed.). Disinfection, Steril-

ization, and Preservation. Lea and Febiger, Philadelphia, PA, pp. 225–255.

31. Murphy, D.W. 1988. Composting as a dead bird disposal method. Poultr Sci 67(Suppl 1):124.

32. North, M.O., and D.D. Bell. 1990. Commercial Chicken Production Manual, 4th ed. Chapman & Hall, New York, NY.

33. O'Connor, D.O., and J.R. Rubino. 1991. Phenolic compounds. In S.S. Block (ed.). Disinfection, Sterilization, and Preservation. Lea and Febiger, Philadelphia, PA, pp. 204–224.

34. Phillips, G.B., and E. Hanel. 1960. Use of ultraviolet radiation in microbiological laboratories [abst]. US Gov Res Rep 34:122.

35. Phillips, C.R., and B. Warshowsky. 1958. Chemical disinfectants. Annu Rev Microbiol 12:525.

36. Preece, A. 1965. A Manual for Histological Techniques, 2nd ed. Little, Brown & Co., Boston.

37. Prophet, E. B., B. Mills, J.B. Arrington, and L.H. Sobin. 1992. Laboratory Methods in Histotechnology. American Registry of Pathology, Washington, DC.

38. Purchase, H.G., L.H. Arp, C.H. Domermuth, J.E. Pearson. 1989. A Laboratory Manual for Isolation and Identification of Avian Pathogens, 3rd ed. American Association of Avian Pathologists, Kennett Square, PA.

39. Randall, C.J., 1991. Color Atlas of Diseases and Disorders of the Domestic Fowl and Turkey. Iowa State University Press, Ames, IA.

40. Reddish, G.F. 1957. Antiseptics, Disinfectants, Fungicides and Sterilization, 2nd ed. Lea and Febiger, Philadelphia, PA.

41. Riddell, C. 1987. Avian Histopathology. American Association of Avian Pathologists, Kennett Square, PA.

42. Russell, A.D. 1991. Principles of antimicrobial activity. In S.S. Block (ed.). Disinfection, Sterilization, and Preservation. Lea and Febiger, Philadelphia, PA, pp. 29–58.

43. Scott, T.A., and C. Swetnam. 1993. Screening sanitizing agents and methods of application for hatching eggs. II. Effectiveness against microorganisms on the egg shell. J Appl Poultr Res 2:7–11.

44. Snyder, D.B., 1986. Latest developments in the enzyme-linked immunosorbent assay (ELISA). Avian Dis 30:19–23.

45. Snyder, D.B., W.W. Marquardt, E.T. Mallinson, E. Russek-Cohen, P.K. Savage, and D.C. Allen. 1986. Rapid serological profiling by enzyme-linked immunosorbent assay. IV. Association of infectious bursal disease serology with broiler flock performance. Avian Dis 30:139–148.

46. Thompson, S.W. 1966. Selected Histochemical and Histopathological Methods. Charles C. Thomas, Springfield, IL.

47. Utterback, W.W., and J.H. Schwartz. 1973. Epizootiology of velogenic viserotropic Newcastle disease in Southern California, 1971–1973. J Am Vet Med Assoc 163:1080–1088.

48. Van Cutsem, J. 1983. Antifungal activity of enilconazole on experimental aspergillosis in chickens. Avian Dis 27:36–42.

49. Whiteman, C.E., and A.A. Bickford. 1996. Avian Disease Manual, 4th ed. American Association of Avian Pathologists, Kennett Square, PA (in press).

50. Wright, M.L. 1958. Hatchery sanitation. Can J Comp Med Vet Sci 22:62–66.

51. Wright, H.S. 1974. Virucidal activity of commercial disinfectants against velogenic viserotropic Newcastle disease virus. Avian Dis 18:526–530.

52. Wright, M.L., G.W. Anderson, and N.A. Epps. 1959. Hatchery sanitation. Can J Comp Med Vet Sci 23:288–290.

53. Wright, M.L., G.W. Anderson, and J.D. McConachie. 1961. Transmission of aspergillosis during incubation. Poultr Sci 40:727–731.

54. Yoder, H.W., Jr. 1970. Preincubation heat treatment of chicken hatching eggs to inactivate Mycoplasma. Avian Dis 14:75–86.

55. Zander, D.V. 1977. Unpublished observations.

2 Nutritional Diseases

NUTRITIONAL DISEASES

Richard E. Austic and Milton L. Scott

INTRODUCTION. More than 36 nutrients are absolutely essential and must be in the diet in appropriate concentrations and balance in order to maximize the ability of poultry to express their genetic potential to grow and reproduce. Often, it is the task of the veterinarian to determine whether an ailment is nutritional in its origin or whether nutrition is a contributing factor to a specific clinical problem. Whenever a serious deficiency of one of the essential nutrients occurs, signs develop that are often characteristic. These are frequently preceded or accompanied by nonspecific signs such as retarded and uneven growth, rough feather development, decreased egg production, and lowered hatchability. When a deficiency is partial, these may be the only signs observed. This makes it difficult to recognize a partial nutritional deficiency, since nonspecific signs may be brought about by a number of causes, including infectious diseases and toxicants.

The quantitative nutrient requirements of the young growing chick and turkey and for light breeds of laying hens are quite well established (5, 111); however, the requirements of growing chicks and poults after the first few weeks of age and the requirements of male and female broiler and turkey breeding fowls for many nutrients have not been determined experimentally.

Food substances of importance in nutrition of poultry are proteins and amino acids, carbohydrates, fats, vitamins, essential inorganic elements, and water.

PROTEINS AND AMINO ACIDS. The protein requirement represents the collective need for 10 absolutely essential amino acids (arginine, histidine, isoleucine, leucine, lysine, methionine, phenylalanine, threonine, tryptophan, and valine), two amino acids (cysteine and tyrosine) that can be synthesized from essential amino acids, two amino acids that are essential for the young chick (glycine or serine, proline), plus additional amino acids to satisfy the nitrogen requirement for synthesis of nonessential amino acids, purines, pyrimidines, and other nitrogenous compounds.

Practical ingredients are usually limiting in one or more amino acids. In rations composed of corn and soybean meals as sources of protein, methionine supplementation is usually necessary. Lysine may be slightly deficient in such diets for starting broilers or turkeys unless alternate lysine-rich protein sources or feed-grade lysine are included. Diets based on cereal grains and other protein concentrates such as cottonseed meal, safflower meal, or peanut meal may require both lysine and methionine supplementation. Other amino acids such as threonine, tryptophan, arginine, and isoleucine can become limiting when unusual protein sources are used or when the dietary protein level is reduced.

In contrast to the specific signs that may occur as a result of vitamin or mineral deficiencies, the effects of essential amino acid deficiencies are nonspecific: reduced growth, reduced feed consumption, decreased egg production and egg size, and loss of body weight in adults. Marginal amino acid deficiencies often result in increased food intake or maintenance of food intake, with concomitant reduction of body weight gain and lean tissue growth resulting in increased body fat. Severe deficiencies also result in altered body composition. Some amino acids have additional effects. Methionine deficiency may exacerbate choline or vitamin B_{12} deficiencies owing to its role in methyl group metabolism. Lysine deficiency causes impaired pigmentation of Bronze turkey poults, the biochemical basis of which is unknown (58), and can result in stunting and retarded development in chicks (Fig. 2.1). Arginine deficiency tends to cause the wing feathers to curl upward, giving the chick a distinct ruffled appearance. Several other amino acids have been reported to affect feather growth and structure (133).

When animals are provided with dietary protein in excess of their requirements, the surplus protein is catabolized and the nitrogen released is converted

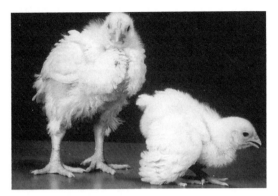

2.1. Lysine deficiency. Stunting and retarded development are apparent in this chick (*right*) fed a diet without sufficient lysine when compared with the normal control chick (*left*) fed adequate lysine. (Swayne)

to uric acid. A large excess of protein may cause hyperuricemia and articular gout, particularly in birds that are genetically susceptible (12, 126, 151).

CARBOHYDRATES. This food component is the primary source of metabolizable energy in practical poultry diets. Starch and sucrose are readily used by the chick. Intestinal lactase activity is low in chickens; this limits the amount of milk sugar (lactose) that can be tolerated. Milk by-products such as whey are excellent sources of B vitamins and although beneficial at low levels, excessive levels in the diet cause growth depression and severe diarrhea. The latter condition, characteristic of lactose intolerance in many species, is caused by influx of water into the lower digestive tract and by microbial fermentation of undigested lactose.

FATS. Fats are important in the diet of poultry as concentrated sources of energy and sources of the essential nutrients, linoleic acid and arachidonic acid. Linoleic acid cannot be synthesized but can be converted to arachidonic acid, by poultry or other monogastric animals. Both fatty acids are important constituents of cell organelles, membranes, and adipose tissue and have additional physiologic roles as precursors of prostaglandins. Lack of these fatty acids in the diet of young chicks results in suboptimal growth and enlarged fatty livers (74). Essential fatty acid deficiency in laying hens results in lowered egg production, egg size, and hatchability (107). Reduced concentrations of arachidonic acid and increased concentrations of eicosatrienoic acid in tissue and egg lipids are a characteristic sign of essential fatty deficiency.

Unsaturated fatty acids may undergo oxidative rancidity, with multiple effects: essential fatty acids are destroyed; aldehydes that are formed may react with free amino groups in proteins, reducing amino acid availability; and the active peroxides generated during rancidification may destroy activities of vitamins A, D, and E and water-soluble vitamins such as biotin. Producers of vitamin A supplements have enhanced the stability of this vitamin by mechanical means, wherein minute droplets of vitamin A are enveloped in a stable fat, gelatin, or wax, forming a small bead that prevents most of the vitamin from coming into contact with oxygen until it is digested in the intestinal tract. The addition of synthetic antioxidants to poultry feeds provides further protection of vitamin A and other essential nutrients.

VITAMINS. The term *vitamin* refers to a heterogeneous group of fat-soluble and water-soluble chemical compounds essential in nutrition that bear no structural or necessary functional relationship to each other. All recognized vitamins with the exception of vitamin C are dietary essentials for poultry. Although amounts of various vitamins needed in poultry diets range from parts per million to parts per billion, each is required for normal metabolism and health.

A marked deficiency of a single vitamin in the diet of a chick or poult results in breakdown of the metabolic process in which that particular vitamin is concerned. This causes a vitamin-deficiency disease, which in some instances exhibits characteristic macroscopic or microscopic changes. In several instances, a single disease may result from a deficiency of any one of several nutrients. Perosis, for example, occurs in young chicks or poults when the diet is deficient in manganese or any one of the following vitamins: choline, nicotinic acid, pyridoxine, biotin, or folic acid. Perosis is an anatomic deformity of leg bones of young chickens, turkeys, pheasants, and other birds, which is characterized by enlargement of the tibiometatarsal joint, twisting or bending of the distal end of the tibia and proximal end of the metatarsus, and, finally, slipping of the gastrocnemius tendon from its condyles. This last lesion causes complete crippling in the affected leg; if both legs are affected, death usually results since the chick or poult cannot secure food and water. Analysis of the diet may be the only way to determine whether a specific nutritional deficiency is responsible for the condition.

Vitamins A and D and riboflavin are most likely to be deficient if special attention is not given to provide them when feed is formulated. Because of continued extraction and purification of many common ingredients, however, and the tendency to omit animal proteins and high-fiber ingredients such as alfalfa meal and wheat mill by-products from diets, amounts of several other vitamins have decreased to sometimes deficient levels. These are vitamins E, B_{12}, and K; pantothenic acid, nicotinic acid, biotin, and choline. Poultry rations are usually formulated to contain more than adequate amounts of all vitamins, providing margins of safety to compensate for possible losses during feed processing, transportation, and storage, and variations in feed composition and environmental conditions.

Vitamin A.   Vitamin A is essential in poultry diets for growth, optimal vision, and integrity of mucous membranes. Since epithelial linings of alimentary, urinary, genital, and respiratory systems are composed of mucous membranes, these are the tissues in which lesions of vitamin A deficiency are most readily observed.

Vitamin A aldehyde, or retinal, is a component of visual pigments in sensory cells of the retina within which *cis–trans* isomerization of the isoprenoid side chain plays an essential role in the detection of light. Vitamin A functions in morphogenesis during embryonic development, the maintenance of epithelial tissues, mucus production, bone growth, immunity, and a variety of other essential processes. Vitamin A alcohol (retinol) and retinal are oxidized to retinoic acid which, in turn, mediates the effects of vitamin A by regulating gene expression.

Signs of Deficiency.

When adult chickens or turkeys are fed a diet severely deficient in vitamin A, signs and lesions usually develop within 2–5 mo, depending on the amount stored in liver and other tissues of the body. As deficiency progresses, chickens become emaciated and weak and their feathers are ruffled. Egg production decreases sharply, the length of time between clutches increases, and hatchability is decreased. A watery discharge from the nostrils and eyes is noted, and eyelids are often stuck together. As the deficiency continues, milky white, caseous material accumulates in the eyes. At this stage of the disease, eyes fill with this white exudate to such an extent that it is impossible for the chicken to see unless the mass is removed; in many cases, the eye is destroyed. Most signs in adult turkeys are similar to those in chickens (72).

The incidence and severity of blood spots in eggs of chickens is increased in vitamin A deficiency (20). The amount of vitamin A required to minimize blood spot incidence may be slightly higher than the requirement for good production and health of the laying hens (71, 128).

Vitamin A deficiency signs in chicks and poults are characterized by cessation of growth, drowsiness, weakness, incoordination, emaciation, and ruffled plumage. If deficiency is severe, they may show ataxia not unlike that of vitamin E deficiency (71), although the two conditions can be differentiated by histologic examination of the brain (3). Periorbital edema may occur (Fig. 2.2A). In acute vitamin A deficiency, lacrimation usually occurs, and a caseous material may be seen under the eyelids. Xerophthalmia is a lesion of vitamin A deficiency; not all chicks and poults exhibit this because in acute deficiency, they often die of other causes before eyes become affected. Increased testes weight, spermatogenesis, and comb development may occur in young cockerels marginally deficient in vitamin A (114). Vitamin A–deficient cocks have decreased sperm counts, reduced sperm motility, and a high incidence of abnormal sperm (121).

Pathology.

Vitamin A–deficiency lesions first appear in the pharynx and are largely confined to mucous glands and their ducts. The original epithelium is replaced by a keratinizing epithelium that blocks ducts of the mucous glands, causing them to become distended with secretions and necrotic materials. Squamous metaplasia can be found in nasal mucosa (Fig. 2.2B). Small white pustules are found in the nasal passages, mouth, esophagus, and pharynx and may extend into the crop. Pustules range in size from microscopic lesions to 2 mm in diameter (Fig. 2.2C). As the deficiency progresses, lesions enlarge, are raised above the surface of the mucous membrane, and have a depression in the center. Small ulcers surrounded by inflammatory products may appear at the site of these lesions. This condition resembles certain stages of fowl pox, and the two conditions can be differentiated only by microscopic examination. Bacterial and viral infections often occur because of breakdown of the mucous membrane.

Clinical signs and lesions of vitamin A deficiency of the respiratory tract are variable; it is difficult to differentiate this condition from infectious coryza, fowl pox, and infectious bronchitis. In vitamin A deficiency, thin membranes and nasal plugs are usually limited to the cleft palate and its adjacent epithelium. They may be removed easily without bleeding. Atrophy and degeneration of the respiratory mucous membrane and its glands occur. Later, the original epithelium is replaced by a stratified squamous keratinizing epithelium. In early stages of vitamin A deficiency in chickens, turbinates are filled with seromucoid water-clear masses that may be forced out of the nodules and cleft palate by application of slight pressure. The vestibule becomes plugged and overflows into paranasal sinuses. Exudate may also fill sinuses and other nasal cavities, causing swelling of one or both sides of the face. Mucous membranes, cleared of inflammatory products, appear thin, rough, and dry.

Similar lesions may frequently be found in trachea and bronchi. In early stages, these may be difficult to see. As the condition progresses, the mucous membrane is covered with a dry, dull fine film that is slightly uneven, whereas normal membrane is even and moist. In some cases, small nodulelike particles may be found in or beneath the mucous membrane in the upper part of the trachea.

Chronic vitamin A deficiency causes damage to the kidney tubules, which leads to azotemia and visceral gout in severe cases (151).

Histopathology. The first histologic lesion of vitamin A deficiency is atrophy and deciliation of columnar-ciliated epithelium of the respiratory tract (148). Nuclei often present marked karyorrhexis. A pseudomembrane formed by the atrophying and degenerating ciliated cells may hang as tufts on the basement membrane; later these are sloughed. During this process, new cylindric or polygonal cells may be formed singly or in pairs and appear as islands beneath the epithelium. These new cells proliferate and their nuclei enlarge, containing less chromatin as they develop. Cell boundaries are less clearly defined; finally, the columnar ciliated epithelial lining of nasal cavities and communicating sinuses, trachea, bronchi, and submucous glands are transformed into a stratified squamous keratinizing epithelium. Lesions in glands of tongue, palate, and esophagus (Fig. 2.2D) are similar to those of the respiratory tract (149).

Histopathologic examination of tissues from nasal passages of chicks serves as a sensitive indicator of borderline deficiencies of vitamin A (82). Chicks receiving suboptimal levels show lesions that resemble in basic character, but not in severity, those described by Seifried (148) for complete deficiency of vitamin A.

According to Wolbach and Hegsted (185, 186), vitamin A deficiency in young chicks and ducks causes marked retardation and suppression of endochondral bone growth. The proliferating zone is reduced. Hypertrophied cells accumulate, surrounded by uncalcified matrix. Vascular invasion of the epiphyseal cartilage is reduced and exhibits irregular patterns such as branching. The number of endosteal and periosteal osteoblasts is decreased, leading to impaired bone growth and thinning of bone cortex. Bone remodeling is inhibited. Disproportionate growth of brain and spinal cord relative to that of the axial skeleton appears to cause compression of brain tissue. Increased cerebrospinal fluid pressure is one of the earliest signs of vitamin A deficiency (189).

An increased frequency of atretic ovarian follicles containing hemorrhages either throughout the follicle or between the theca interna and granulosa cell layer has been observed in chickens exposed to vitamin A deficiency over a period of 5 to 8 months (22). Vitamin A deficiency has been reported to decrease hatchability of chicken and turkey eggs, and to increase mortality of chicks and poults that do hatch (9, 71). Thompson et al. (166) produced a severe vitamin A deficiency in developing embryos

by supplementing breeder diets with retinoic acid. This form of vitamin A permits egg production but does not support embryonic development. Embryos die—always in the same stage of development. The complete trunk and head are formed, and the head is rotated slightly to one side. No differentiation of major blood vessels occurs, and an expanded area of vasculosa is seen forming a "blood ring" at the sinus terminalis.

Hypervitaminosis A. Baker et al. (16) reported that the administration of 200 mg retinyl acetate per kg of body weight per day to growing chickens adversely affects skeletal development. Chicks have lighter and shortened tibiae exhibiting widened epiphyseal growth plates with irregular tunneling by blood vessels. Widening results from increased numbers of hyperplastic chondrocytes. Bones exhibit reduced osteoblastic activity and increased bone and blood alkaline phosphatase activity. Ventricular dilation and brain swelling are also observed.

Tang et al. (163) administered 330 or 660 IU vitamin A per kg body weight per day to commercial broilers. Chicks had an unsteady gait and were reluctant to walk within a few days of treatment with excess vitamin A. They became anorexic by 9 days and developed conjunctivitis, adhesions of the eye-

2.2. *A-D.* Vitamin A deficiency. *A.* Periorbital edema and lack of pigmentation. (Swayne) *B.* Squamous metaplasia of nasal mucosa. (Swayne, Barnes) *C.* Vitamin A deficiency. Distended, impacted mucosal glands resembling pustules in the esophagus. (Barnes) *D.* Squamous metaplasia has replaced all but a few focal areas of normal mucosa in the base of this esophageal gland. Distention has resulted from occlusion of opening and accumulation of keratin and cellular debris in the lumen. Inflammation resulting in formation of a pustule will occur if contents contact surrounding tissues. (Barnes) *E-G.* Rickets. *E.* Soft, thick ribs form a flattened thorax in this severely affected 8-day-old broiler chicken. Vertebra are also short and thick. In less affected birds, enlargement at junctions of ribs with vertebrae and sternum, folding of sternal portions of caudal ribs resulting in a flat, broad thorax, and occasionally pathologic rib fractures may be seen. (Munger) *F.* Beak of affected chicken is soft and easily bent. (Swayne) *G.* Field or infectious rickets in turkeys occurs secondarily to intestinal disease. In this affected poult, there is excess, hypertrophic cartilage that is poorly vascularized because of a compression-induced fold fracture involving trabeculae at the physeal–metaphyseal junction. (Barnes) *H.* Osteopenia ("Cage-Layer Fatigue"). Pathologic fracture of rib with imperfect callus formation. There is minimal mineral being deposited at the fracture site. (Barnes)

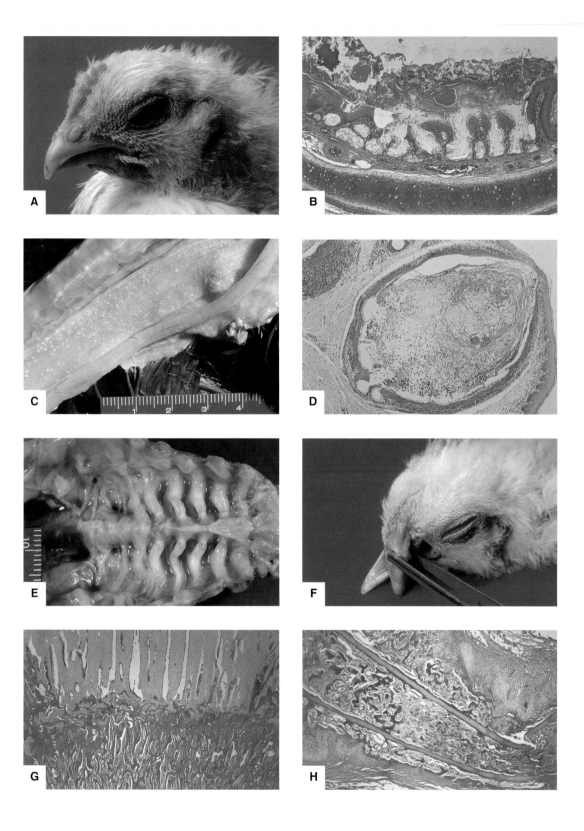

lids, and encrustations around the mouth. Tibiae had widened epiphyseal growth plates due primarily to accumulation of hypertrophic chondrocytes. These investigators reported other abnormalities of the tibia including hyperosteoidosis and metaphyseal sclerosis. Frontal bones of the skull were thinner and more porous and exhibited thickened osteoid seams.

Signs of hypervitaminosis A in leghorn chicks differed from those of broiler chicks administered similar levels of vitamin A (163). The epiphyseal growth plates in tibiae from leghorn chicks were normal in width but contained a narrower proliferative/maturation zone and a wider hypertrophic zone. Osteoid seams were normal. Leghorns had normal parathyroid morphology, whereas parathyroid hyperplasia was observed in broiler chicks.

It must be noted that the reported histopathology of hypervitaminosis A is not entirely consistent among laboratories. The nature of the cell population contributing to widening of the epiphyseal growth plate differed in the preceding studies (16, 163). Wolbach and Hegstead (187, 188), moreover, reported that vitamin A excess caused narrowing of the growth plate in their early studies involving young chicks and ducks.

Treatment of Deficiency. Poultry found to be severely deficient in vitamin A should be given a stabilized vitamin A preparation at a level of approximately 10,000 IU vitamin A/kg of ration. Absorption of vitamin A is rapid; therefore, chickens or turkeys not in advanced stages of deficiency should respond promptly, except for blindness, which may be permanent.

VITAMIN D. Vitamin D is required by poultry for proper metabolism of calcium and phosphorus in the formation of normal skeleton, hard beaks and claws, and strong eggshells. It functions in the regulation of calcium metabolism by stimulating the intestinal absorption of calcium, influencing osteoblast and osteoclast activity, and increasing renal tubular reabsorption of calcium in response to metabolic demands for calcium.

Vitamin D can be synthesized from 7-dehydrocholesterol in the skin under the influence of ultraviolet light. Although this synthesis can reduce the dietary requirement for vitamin D to some extent (52), it is not sufficient to satisfy the requirements of fowl under normal conditions of poultry and egg production.

The metabolically active form of vitamin D is formed by two enzymatic hydroxylations of cholecalciferol (vitamin D_3), the first yielding 25-hydroxycholecalciferol in liver, and the second yielding 1,25-dihydroxycholecalciferol in kidney (45). The latter appears to be a regulatory step, influenced by calcium status and activated by low blood phosphate or parathyroid hormone. Its product is much more potent in promoting calcium absorption and bone mobilization than its precursors, vitamin D_3 and 25-hydroxycholecalciferol. Many other hydroxylation products of 25-hydroxycholecalciferol have been identified. Their biologic roles are unknown (7).

Signs of Deficiency. In confined laying hens, signs of deficiency begin to occur as soon as 2 wk after they are deprived of vitamin D. The first sign is marked increase in number of thin-shelled and soft-shelled eggs, followed soon after by marked decrease in egg production. Biochemical indicators include a rapid decrease in the concentrations of 25-hydroxycholecalciferol and 1,25-dihydroxycholecalciferol in the blood, followed soon thereafter by a decrease in blood calcium concentration (169, 168). Egg production and eggshell strength may vary in a cyclic manner. Several cycles of decreased egg production and shell strength may each be followed by periods of relatively normal production and shell strength.

Individual hens may show temporary loss of use of the legs, with recovery after laying an egg that is usually shell-less. During periods of extreme leg weakness, hens show a characteristic posture that has been described as a "penguin-type squat." Later, beak, claws, and keel become very soft and pliable. The sternum usually is bent and ribs lose their normal rigidity and turn inward at the junction of the sternal and vertebral portions, producing a characteristic inward curve of the ribs along the sides of the thorax.

Vitamin D metabolism has been implicated in problems of eggshell quality. Soares et al. (153) recently reported that two strains of chickens that had been selected for divergence in eggshell strength and thickness differed in their blood concentrations of 1,25-dihydroxycholecalciferol: the strain having higher eggshell quality also had significantly higher concentrations of the vitamin D metabolite. When hens of a commercial strain of leghorns received 30 μg of vitamin D_3 or 5 μg of 1a-hydroxycholecalciferol (a putative synthetic precursor of 1,25-dihydroxycholecalciferol), the latter resulted in greater tibial calcium and phosphorus content, tibial breaking strength, and eggshell mineralization. Bar et al. (18) reported that the inclusion of 2 or 5 μg/kg of 1,25-dihydroxycholecalciferol in the diet of aging hens increased shell weight and density in the first egg of the clutch and decreased the rate of decline of both measures in subsequent eggs of the clutch. Other studies (167, 168, 169) confirm that 1,25-dihydroxycholecalciferol supports egg production and is effective in promoting eggshell mineralization and minimizing eggshell breakage when it is used at a concentration of 5 µg/kg in the diet of leghorn hens.

Hatchability is markedly reduced by vitamin D deficiency. Chicks and poults that do not hatch have a high incidence of chondrodystrophy in which the upper or lower mandible is shortened to the extent that occlusion of the mandibles is abnormal (155, 161). The synthetic vitamin D analogues 25-hydroxycholecalciferol, 1a-hydroxycholecalciferol, and 1,25-dihydroxycholecalciferol support adequate egg production and eggshell strength but only 25-hydroxycholecalciferol is effective in supporting hatchability (1, 7). Evidence strongly suggests that the other two analogues are poorly transported into the egg (8, 53, 152). Manley and coworkers (101) reported that the addition of 1100 ICU of 25-hydroxycholecalciferol to diets of turkey hens that already contained 2200 ICU of vitamin D_3 improved the hatchability of fertile eggs. This interesting observation appears at odds with other evidence that 900 IU of vitamin D_3 per kilogram of diet is adequate for hatchability of turkey eggs (155).

In addition to retarded growth, the first sign of vitamin D deficiency in chicks or poults is rickets, characterized by a severe bone weakness. Between 2 and 3 wk of age beaks and claws become soft and pliable and birds walk with obvious effort and take a few unsteady steps before squatting on their hocks, which they rest upon while swaying slightly from side to side. Feathering is poor. A marked increase in serum phosphatase is perhaps the first indicator of a borderline rachitic condition.

Pathology. In laying and breeding chicken and turkey hens receiving deficient vitamin D, characteristic changes observed on necropsy are confined to bones and parathyroid glands. The latter become enlarged from hypertrophy and hyperplasia. Bones are soft and break easily. Well-defined knobs are present on the inner surface of the ribs at the costochondral junction (rachitic rosary) (Fig. 2.2E). Many ribs show evidence of pathologic fracture in this region. In chronic vitamin D deficiency, marked skeletal distortions become apparent. The spinal column may bend downward in the sacral and coccygeal region; the sternum usually shows a lateral bend and an acute dent near the middle of the breast. These changes reduce the size of the thorax with consequent crowding of vital organs. The beak may be soft and pliable (Fig. 2.2F).

The most characteristic internal signs of vitamin D deficiency in chicks and poults are a beading of the ribs at their juncture with the spinal column and a bending of the ribs downward and posteriorly (Fig. 2.2E). Poor calcification can be observed at the epiphysis of the tibia or femur (Fig. 2.3). Bones of vitamin D–deficient chicks have a reduced calcium content with an increased proportion of osteoid, and a greater proportion of bone mineral is present as a low density amorphous form of calcium phosphate (47). The ratio of dihydroxylysinonorleucine to hydroxylysinonorleucine in bone collagen is increased (106).

Vitamin D deficiency results in widening of the epiphyseal plate, hypertrophy, and softening of bone. Enlargement of the epiphyseal plate is due initially to widening of the proliferating and hypertrophic zones; as the deficiency progresses, it may be primarily the former (76, 95). Long and coworkers (95) noted that the hypertrophic zone exhibits irregular contours—wider in some areas and narrower in others—among and within affected birds. The widening of the proliferating zone appears to be the result of delayed chondrocyte hypertrophy rather than increased chondrocyte replication (86). As the deficiency progresses, the columns of chondrocytes in the degenerating hypertrophic zone of the epiphyseal plate become shortened and thickened and exhibit an irregular pattern of invasion by metaphyseal blood vessels. Irregular patterns of cartilage and bone development occur in the primary and secondary spongiosa (76, 95). Porosity of cortical bone, sometimes leading to fractures (Fig. 2.2G), increases due to resorption of bone in haversion canals. Fractures also may occur elsewhere (Fig. 2.2H).

The histopathology of rickets differs significantly depending on the cause of the disease (86, 95, 96, 97). Refer to the section on calcium and phosphorus for further information on this topic.

Another skeletal disorder, tibial dyschondroplasia, is frequently observed in broiler chickens (refer to Chapter 35 for a description of the pathology). It has been produced experimentally by decreasing the ratio of calcium to phosphorus in the diet (49, 129) or by altering the ratio of these two nutrients and increasing the dietary concentration of chloride (50). This condition persists even when experimental diets contain generous levels of vitamin D_3. The incidence and severity of tibial dyschondroplasia was reduced or prevented when the diets were supplemented with 1,25-dihydroxycholecalciferol (50, 51, 129), suggesting that the metabolic conversion of vitamin D_3 to 1,25-dihydroxycholecalciferol is not sufficient under some conditions to meet the need for this metabolite for normal bone development (50).

Hypervitaminosis D. Very high levels of vitamin D_3—4 million IU or more/kg diet—cause renal damage from dystrophic calcification of kidney tubules. Calcification may be less often observed in the aorta and other arteries. A moderate excess of vitamin D has been reported to increase the incidence of eggshell pimpling (62). The latter appears

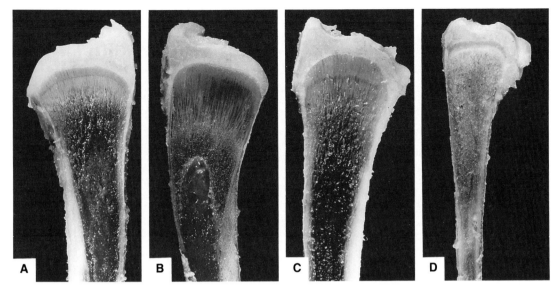

2.3. Effects of nutrient deficiencies on tibiotarsal bones of broiler chickens. (Swayne) *A.* Control fed an adequate diet. *B.* Phosphorus deficiency. Prominent wide zone of hypertrophy. *C.* Calcium/phosphorus deficiency. Widened zone of proliferation. *D.* Lysine deficiency. Hypoplasia.

to be due to excessive localized calcareous deposits on and within the eggshell that when scraped off the shell, often expose the underlying eggshell membranes.

Treatment of Deficiency. Hooper et al. (73) found that feeding a single massive dose of 15,000 IU vitamin D_3 cured rachitic chicks more promptly than when generous levels of the vitamin were added to feed. This single oral dose protected cockerels against rickets for 8 wk and pullet chicks for 5 wk. In giving massive doses to rachitic chicks, it should be remembered that excess vitamin D can be harmful. The dose should be scaled to the degree of deficiency, and excessive amounts of vitamin D should not be added to feed.

VITAMIN E. Vitamin E deficiency produces encephalomalacia, exudative diathesis, and nutritional myopathy (muscular dystrophy) in chicks; enlarged hocks and dystrophy of the gizzard musculature in turkeys; and nutritional myopathy in ducks. Vitamin E also is required for normal embryonic development in chickens, turkeys, and probably ducks.

In its alcoholic form, vitamin E is a very effective antioxidant. It is an important protector in feeds of the essential fatty acids and other highly unsaturated fatty acids as well as vitamins A and D_3, carotenes, and xanthophylls. Selenium (Se) at dietary concentrations of 0.04–0.1 ppm have been shown to prevent or cure exudative diathesis in vitamin E–deficient chicks (142, 143). Selenium at 0.1–0.2 ppm effectively prevents myopathies of gizzard and heart in young poults (147).

Vitamin E plays multiple roles in poultry nutrition. It is required not only for normal reproduction but also as nature's most effective antioxidant for prevention of encephalomalacia, in a specific role interrelated with action of selenium for prevention of exudative diathesis and turkey myopathies, and in another role interrelated with selenium and cystine for prevention of nutritional myopathy.

Signs and Pathology of Deficiency. No outward signs occur in mature chickens or turkeys receiving very low levels of vitamin E over prolonged periods. Hatchability of eggs from vitamin E–deficient chickens or turkeys, however, is reduced markedly (77). Embryos from hens fed rations low in vitamin E may die as early as the 4th day of incubation or considerably later, depending on severity of the deficiency. Turkey embryos may have bilateral cataracts that can cause blindness (55). Testicular degeneration occurs in males deprived of vitamin E for prolonged periods (4).

ENCEPHALOMALACIA IN CHICKS. Encephalomalacia is a nervous derangement characterized by ataxia or paresis (Fig. 2.4A), backward or downward retractions of the head (sometimes with lateral twisting), forced movements, increasing incoordination, rapid contraction and relaxation of the legs, and finally complete prostration and death. Even under these conditions, complete paralysis of wings or legs is not observed. The deficiency usually manifests itself between the 15th and 30th days of the chick's life, although it has been known to occur as early as the 7th and as late as the 56th day.

The cerebellum, striatal hemispheres, medulla oblongata, and mesencephalon are affected most commonly in the order named (120). In chicks killed soon after appearance of signs of encephalomalacia, the cerebellum is softened and swollen and the meninges are edematous (Fig. 2.4B). Minute hemorrhages are often visible on the surface of the cerebellum. The convolutions are flattened. As much as four-fifths of the cerebellum may be affected, or lesions may be so small they cannot be recognized grossly. A day or 2 after signs of encephalomalacia appear, necrotic areas present a green-yellow opaque appearance. One or 2 days later, the cerebellum may become pale and shrunken (Fig. 2.4C).

In the corpus striatum, necrotic tissue is frequently pale, swollen, and wet and in early stages becomes sharply delineated from remaining normal tissue. The greater portion of both hemispheres may be destroyed. In other cases lesions are apparent only on microscopic examination. Medullary lesions are not so readily noted in a macroscopic examination.

Histologically, lesions include circulatory disturbances (ischemic necrosis), demyelination, and neuronal degeneration (Fig. 2.4D,E). Meningeal, cerebellar, and cerebral vessels are markedly hyperemic, and a severe edema usually develops. Capillary thrombosis often results in necrosis of varying extent. In the normal chick cerebellum, myelinated tracts exhibit a strongly positive reaction with Luxol fast blue, whereas in affected chicks the staining reaction is markedly diminished, diffusely or locally accentuated. Degenerative neuronal changes occur everywhere but are most prominent in Purkinje cells and in large motor nuclei. Ischemic cell change is most frequently encountered. Cells are shrunken and intensely hyperchromatic, and the nucleus is typically triangular. Peripheral chromatolysis with the Nissl substance packed along the periphery of the cell nucleus is also common.

Signs of encephalomalacia in turkey poults are similar to those observed in chicks (78). Poults with paresis usually do not have brain lesions but have poliomyelomalacia (Fig. 2.4F).

EXUDATIVE DIATHESIS IN CHICKS. Exudative diathesis is an edema of subcutaneous tissues (Fig. 2.5) associated with abnormal permeability of capillary walls. In severe cases, chicks stand with their legs far apart as a result of accumulation of fluid under the ventral skin. This green-blue viscous fluid is easily seen through the skin, since it usually contains some blood components from slight hemor-

rhages that appear throughout the breast and leg musculature and in the intestinal walls. Distention of the pericardium and sudden deaths have been noted. Chicks suffering from exudative diathesis show a low ratio of albumin to globulins in blood (61).

Onset of exudative diathesis coincides with appearance of peroxides in tissues. Plasma activities of selenium-dependent glutathione peroxidase decrease sharply (115). Glutathione peroxidase catalyzes the neutralization of hydrogen peroxide and lipoperoxides that can cause oxidative damage to structural elements of the cell, particularly membrane lipids. Noguchi et al. (115) proposed that vitamin E in the capillary membranes and the selenium-containing enzyme glutathione peroxidase of plasma protect the capillary membrane against oxidative damage. This may explain the dual role of vitamin E and selenium in prevention of exudative diathesis and other vitamin E/selenium-responsive diseases (145, 158). Another selenium-dependent enzyme, phospholipid hydroperoxide glutathione peroxidase, probably also is involved in protection of membranes from oxidative damage (31).

2.4. *A-F.* Nutritional encephalomalacia (vitamin E deficiency). *A.* Paresis in one poult and another with pronounced neurologic signs. While either clinical manifestation can be seen in turkeys, the latter is seen in chickens ("Crazy Chick Disease"). (Barnes) *B.* Birds with neurologic signs have cerebellar swelling, edema, hemorrhage, and attenuation of folia. Coning of the swollen cerebellum into the foramen magnum is often seen. Lesions in the cerebrum also may occur but are not common. (Barnes) *C.* This bird with chronic nutritional encephalomalacia survived 3 days after onset of signs. Affected areas are now pale and shrunken. (Barnes) *D.* Severe malacia of cerebellum. Variable portions of affected outer folia are sharply separated from inner normal tissue. There is congestion and hemorrhage. At higher magnification characteristic fibrin thrombi in small vessels would be seen. Inflammatory cells are minimal to absent. (Barnes) *E.* Increased swollen astrocytes replace much of the normal cerebellar architecture in this bird with chronic encephalomalacia. Only isolated parts of the granular layer and individual Purkinje cells remain. (Barnes) *F.* Poults with paresis usually do not have brain lesions but have bilateral poliomyelomalacia as seen here. (Barnes) *G.* Nutritional myopathy. Degeneration of muscle fibers can result from inadequate vitamin E and/or selenium. These are seen as pale, often fusiform, linear streaks in skeletal muscle. Fibrosis, intramuscular fat deposition, and other myopathies can produce similar changes. (Barnes) *H.* Gizzard myopathy. Deficiency of vitamin E and/or selenium can produce myopathic changes in smooth muscle as well as cardiac and skeletal muscle. Lesions are seen as extensive, pale areas in gizzard musculature. Turkeys are more commonly affected. (Munger)

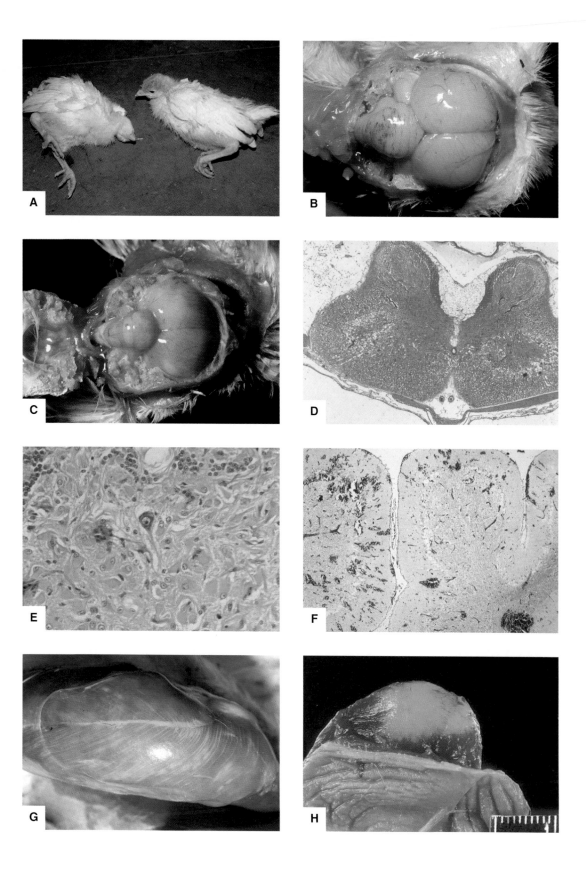

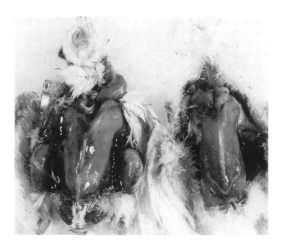

2.5. Exudative diathesis in chicks.

NUTRITIONAL MYOPATHY (MUSCULAR DYSTRO-PHY) IN CHICKENS, DUCKS, AND TURKEYS. When vitamin E deficiency is accompanied by a sulfur amino acid deficiency, chicks show signs of nutritional myopathy—particularly of the breast muscle—at about 4 wk of age. The condition is characterized by light-colored streaks of easily distinguished affected bundles of muscle fibers in the breast (Fig. 2.4G). A similar dystrophy occurs throughout all skeletal muscles of the body in vitamin E–deficient ducks.

The initial histologic change is hyaline degeneration. Mitochondria undergo swelling, coalesce, and form intracytoplasmic globules. Later, muscle fibers are disrupted transversely. Extravasation separates groups of muscle fibers and individual fibers. The transuded plasma usually contains erythrocytes and heterophilic leukocytes. In more chronic conditions, reparative processes dominate the picture. There is a pronounced proliferation of cell nuclei and also fibroplasia, leaving a scar in the degenerate muscle.

Vitamin E and selenium deficiency in chickens and especially in turkeys may result in an extreme myopathy of the gizzard (Fig. 2.4H) and heart muscles (147).

ENLARGED HOCK DISORDER IN TURKEYS. Turkeys receiving diets low in vitamin E and also containing readily oxidizable fats or oils may develop characteristic hock enlargements and bowed legs at approximately 2–3 wk of age (141). If poults are allowed to continue on these diets, hock enlargements usually disappear by the time the poults are 6 wk of age, only to reappear in more severe form when they reach 14–16 wk, especially in toms raised on wire or slat floors. Creatine excretion is increased and muscle creatine levels are reduced. The need for vitamin E may be related to a protec-

tion of biotin that otherwise might be destroyed in the presence of rancidifying fats or oils (144).

Treatment of Deficiency. If not too far advanced, exudative diathesis and nutritional myopathy in chicks are readily reversed by administration of proper levels of vitamin E and selenium by injection, by oral dosing, or in feed. Encephalomalacia may or may not respond to treatment with vitamin E, depending on the extent of damage to the cerebellum. Gizzard myopathy in turkeys is prevented by supplementing deficient diets with vitamin E or selenium. It is not affected by the dietary level of sulfur amino acids.

VITAMIN K. Vitamin K is required for synthesis of prothrombin. It is a cofactor in the posttranslational carboxylation of glutamic acid in prothrombin and a protein in bone, osteocalcin. The product, γ-carboxyglutamic acid, is anionic at physiologic pH and functions in the binding of Ca^{2+} to protein during blood-clotting. In the absence of vitamin K, an abnormal prothrombin lacking γ-carboxyglutamic acid is secreted into the blood by the liver (59). Since prothrombin is an important part of the blood-clotting mechanism, deficiency of vitamin K results in markedly prolonged blood-clotting time; an affected chick or poult may bleed to death from a slight bruise or other injury. Vitamin K deficiency reduces the γ-carboxyglutamic acid content of bone in laying hens and growing chicks (87).

Signs and Pathology of Deficiency. Signs of vitamin K deficiency occur most frequently 2–3 wk after chicks are placed on a vitamin K–deficient diet. Presence of sulfaquinoxaline in feed or drinking water may increase incidence and severity of the condition. Large hemorrhages appear on the breast, legs, and wings, and/or in the abdominal cavity. Chicks show an anemia that may result partly from loss of blood but also from development of a hypoplastic bone marrow. Although blood-clotting time is a fairly good measure of vitamin K deficiency, a more accurate one is obtained by determining prothrombin time. Inadequate vitamin K in breeder diets causes increased embryo mortality late in incubation. Dead embryos appear hemorrhagic.

Treatment of Deficiency. Within 4–6 hr after vitamin K is administered to deficient chicks, blood clots normally, but recovery from anemia or disappearance of hemorrhages cannot be expected to take place promptly.

THIAMIN (VITAMIN B₁). Thiamin is converted in the body to an active form, thiamin pyrophosphate, which is an important cofactor in oxidative decarboxylation reactions and aldehyde exchanges in carbohydrate metabolism. Deficiency of thiamin leads to extreme anorexia, polyneuritis, and death.

Signs and Pathology of Deficiency.

Polyneuritis is observed in mature chickens approximately 3 wk after they are placed on a thiamin-deficient diet. In young chicks, it may appear before 2 wk of age. Onset is sudden in young chicks but more gradual in mature birds. Anorexia is followed by loss of weight, ruffled feathers, leg weakness, and an unsteady gait. Adult chickens often show a blue comb. As the deficiency progresses, apparent paralysis of muscles occurs, beginning with the flexors of the toes and progressing upward, affecting the extensor muscles of legs, wings, and neck. The chicken characteristically sits on its flexed legs and draws back the head in a "stargazing" position (Fig. 2.6). Retraction of the head is due to paralysis of the anterior muscles of the neck. The chicken soon loses the ability to stand or sit upright, and it topples to the floor, where it may lie with the head still retracted.

The body temperature may drop to as low as 35.6 C. A progressive decrease in respiration rate occurs. Adrenal glands hypertrophy more markedly in females than males. The cortex is affected to a greater extent than the medulla. Apparently, the degree of hypertrophy determines the degree of edema, which occurs chiefly in the skin. The epinephrine content of the adrenal increases as the organ hypertrophies. Atrophy of genital organs is more pronounced in males than females. The heart shows a slight degree of atrophy; the right side may be dilated, the auricle being more frequently affected than the ventricle. Atrophy of the stomach and intestinal walls may be sufficiently severe to be easily noted.

Crypts of Lieberkühn in the duodenum of deficient chicks become dilated (Fig. 2.7) (63). Mitosis of epithelial cells in the crypts decreases markedly; in advanced stages of deficiency the mucosal lining

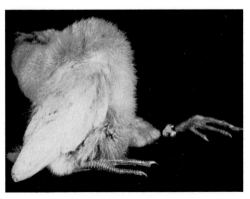

2.6. Typical stargazing pose displayed by chick suffering from thiamin deficiency.

disappears, leaving a connective tissue framework. Necrotic cells and cell debris accumulate in the enlarged crypts. Exocrine cells of the pancreas show cytoplasmic vacuolation with formation of hyaline bodies.

Treatment of Deficiency.

Chickens suffering from thiamin deficiency respond in a matter of a few hours to oral administration of the vitamin. Since thiamin deficiency causes extreme anorexia, supplementing feed with the vitamin is not a reliable treatment until after chickens have recovered from acute deficiency.

RIBOFLAVIN (VITAMIN B₂).

Riboflavin is a cofactor in many enzyme systems in the body. Examples of riboflavin-containing enzymes are: NAD- and NADP-cytochrome reductases, succinic dehydrogenase, acyl dehydrogenase, diaphorase, xanthine oxidase, L- and D-amino acid oxidases, L-hydroxy acid oxidases and histaminase, some of which are vitally associated with oxidation-reduction reactions involved in cell respiration.

Signs and Pathology of Deficiency.

When chicks are fed a diet deficient in riboflavin, they grow very slowly and become weak and emaciated; their appetite is fairly good; diarrhea develops between the 1st and 2nd wk. Chicks do not walk except when forced to, and then they frequently walk on their hocks with the aid of their wings. Leg paralysis may be more prevalent than curled toe paralysis (38). Toes are curled inward when both walking and resting (Fig. 2.8). Chicks are usually found in a resting position. The wings often droop as though it were impossible to hold them in the normal position. Leg muscles are atrophied and flabby, and the skin is dry and harsh. Young chicks in advanced stages of deficiency do not move around but lie with their legs sprawled out.

A deficiency of riboflavin in the diet of hens results in decreased egg production, increased embryonic mortality, and an increase in size and fat content of the liver. Hatchability of eggs decreases within 2 wk after hens are fed a riboflavin-deficient diet but improves to near normal levels within 7 days after adequate amounts of riboflavin are added to the diet. Embryos that fail to hatch from eggs of hens fed diets low in this vitamin are dwarfed and show a high incidence of edema, degeneration of Wolffian bodies, and defective down. The down is referred to as "clubbed" and results from failure of the down feathers to rupture the sheaths, causing feathers to coil in a characteristic way.

Riboflavin deficiency in young turkeys is characterized by poor growth, poor feathering, and leg paralysis (139) and by encrustations in the corners

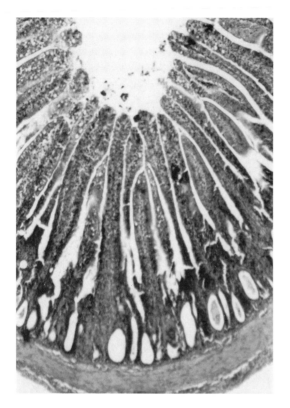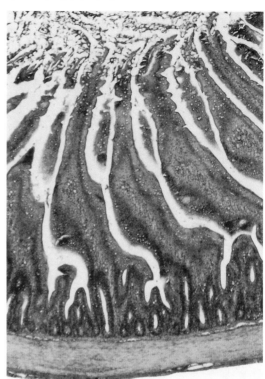

2.7. Duodenum from thiamin-deficient chick, with severe dilation of crypts of Lieberkühn (*left*). Control (*right*). ×30.

of the mouth and on the eyelids. Severe dermatitis of the feet and shanks—marked by edematous swelling, desquamation, and deep fissures—appears in some deficient poults (104).

In severe cases of riboflavin deficiency, chicks show marked swelling and softening of sciatic and brachial nerves. Sciatic nerves usually undergo the most pronounced changes, sometimes reaching a diameter four to five times normal size. Histologic

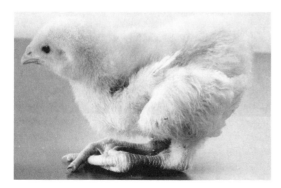

2.8. Curled-toe paralysis (riboflavin deficiency). Typical signs include poor growth, reluctance to stand or walk, sitting on hocks, and toes curled inward. (Swayne)

examination of affected nerves shows degenerative changes in myelin sheaths of the main peripheral nerve trunks (Fig. 2.9). This may be accompanied by axis cylinder swelling and fragmentation. Schwann cell proliferation, myelin changes, gliosis, and chromatolysis occur in the spinal cord. In cases of curled-toe paralysis, degeneration of the neuromuscular end plate and muscle tissues is often found. Riboflavin is probably also essential for myelin metabolism of the main peripheral nerve trunks. No gross dystrophy develops, although muscle fibers are in some cases completely degenerated. The sciatic nerve exhibits myelin degeneration in one or more branches. Similar changes are apparent in the brachial nerve trunks.

The nervous system of embryos that fail to hatch from eggs laid by hens fed riboflavin-deficient diets has degenerative changes very much like those described in riboflavin-deficient chicks (54).

Chicks fed riboflavin-deficient diets develop pancreatic and duodenal lesions as described for thiamin deficiency in addition to the more classic nervous signs (63).

Treatment of Deficiency. Two 100-μg doses of riboflavin should be sufficient for treatment of riboflavin-deficient chicks or poults, followed by in-

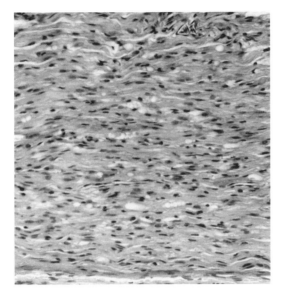

2.9. Curled-toe paralysis. Peripheral neuropathy characterized by axonal swelling and degeneration, Schwann cell activation and proliferation, and myelin degeneration. ×70. (Swayne, Barnes)

corporation of an adequate level in the ration. When the curled-toe deformity is of long standing, however, irreparable damage has occurred and administration of riboflavin no longer cures the condition.

PANTOTHENIC ACID.   Pantothenic acid is a component of coenzyme A, which is involved in the formation of citric acid in the Krebs cycle, synthesis and oxidation of fatty acids, oxidation of keto acids resulting from deamination of amino acids, acetylation of choline, and many other reactions.

Signs and Pathology of Deficiency.

Signs of pantothenic acid deficiency in chicks are difficult to differentiate from those of biotin deficiency; deficiencies of either result in dermatitis, broken feathers, perosis, poor growth, and mortality. Pantothenic acid–deficient chicks are characterized by retarded and rough feather growth. Chicks are emaciated, and definite crusty scablike lesions appear in corners of the mouth. Eyelid margins are granular, and small scabs develop on them. Eyelids frequently are stuck together by a viscous exudate; they are contracted and vision is restricted. There is slow sloughing of the keratinizing epithelium of the skin. Outer layers of skin between the toes and on bottoms of the feet sometimes peel off; small cracks and fissures appear at these points. These cracks and fissures enlarge and deepen, so chicks move about very little. In some cases, skin layers of the feet of deficient chicks cornify and wartlike protuberances develop on the balls of the feet.

Necropsy shows the presence of a puslike substance in the mouth and an opaque gray-white exudate in the proventriculus (131). The liver is hypertrophied and may vary in color from a faint to dirty yellow. The spleen is slightly atrophied. Kidneys are somewhat enlarged. Nerves and myelinated fibers of the spinal cord show myelin degeneration (127). These degenerating fibers occur in all segments of the cord down to the lumbar region.

Pantothenic acid is required in the diet of breeding hens for normal hatchability of eggs (60). Beer et al. (21) observed that the peak day of embryonic mortality depends on the degree of pantothenic acid deficiency and that borderline deficiencies produce extremely weak chicks that fail to survive unless injected immediately with pantothenic acid (200 μg intraperitoneally). Subcutaneous hemorrhage and severe edema are signs of pantothenic acid deficiency in the developing chicken embryo (21).

Pantothenic acid deficiency in chicks produces duodenal and pancreatic lesions as described under thiamin deficiency (but of lesser extent), dermatosis, and severe ataxia progressing to inability to stand. In addition, there is pronounced lymphocytic necrosis and lymphoid depletion in the bursa of Fabricius, thymus, and spleen (63).

Treatment of Deficiency.

Pantothenic acid deficiency appears to be completely reversible, if not too far advanced, by oral treatment or injection with the vitamin followed by restoration of an adequate level in the diet.

NICOTINIC ACID (NIACIN).   Nicotinic acid is the vitamin component in two important coenzymes, nicotinamide adenine dinucleotide (NAD) and nicotinamide adenine dinucleotide phosphate (NADP), that are extensively involved in carbohydrate, fat, and protein metabolism. They are especially important in metabolic reactions that furnish energy. One or both coenzymes take part in the anaerobic and aerobic oxidation of glucose, glycerol synthesis and catabolism, fatty acid synthesis and oxidation, and oxidation of acetyl coenzyme A via the Krebs cycle.

Niacin–Tryptophan–Pyridoxine Interrelationships.

Tryptophan pyrrolase catalyzes the initial reaction in the major metabolic pathway of tryptophan catabolism. Picolinic carboxylase regulates an important branchpoint in the pathway at which an intermediate either enters a sequence of reactions resulting in its degradation to carbon dioxide, water, and ammonia or enters a biosynthetic pathway leading to NAD synthesis. Picolinic carboxylase catalyzes the first reaction in the degradative pathway, whereas the first reaction in the NAD pathway occurs nonenzymatically. High picolinic carboxylase activity limits the synthesis of NAD from tryptophan.

Key enzymes in the metabolism of tryptophan require vitamin B_6 as a cofactor and limit the overall pathway in vitamin B_6 deficiency. Briggs et al. (28) first showed that niacin requirements of chicks and hens depend on the level of tryptophan in the diet. When tryptophan is marginally adequate, chickens are able to synthesize approximately 1 mg of niacin from 45 mg of dietary tryptophan (17, 35, 48). Ducks, in contrast, are much less efficient: approximately 1 mg niacin can be synthesized from 175 mg of dietary tryptophan (35). This difference in efficiency of conversion of tryptophan to niacin is reflected in a markedly higher niacin requirement for ducks than chicks. It has been attributed to relatively high picolinic carboxylase activity in ducks (35, 48).

Signs and Pathology of Deficiency. The main sign of nicotinic acid deficiency in young chicks, turkeys, and ducks is an enlargement of the hock joint and bowing of the legs similar to perosis (146). The main difference between this condition and the perosis of manganese or choline deficiency is that in nicotinic acid deficiency, the Achilles tendon rarely slips from its condyles. Scott (141) showed that both nicotinic acid and vitamin E are required for prevention of the disorder in turkeys. Briggs (27) described further signs of nicotinic acid deficiency as inflammation of the mouth, diarrhea, and poor feathering. Hock disorders and lesions of the mouth were prominent lesions in ducks and chicks, respectively, in recent studies by Chen (35). Niacin/tryptophan deficiency in chicks produces duodenal and pancreatic lesions comparable to those of thiamin deficiency (63).

Ringrose et al. (132) observed reduced feed consumption and body weight, decreased rate of egg production, and reduced hatchability of eggs when hens were fed a semipurified diet based on casein and gelatin as the sources of protein and lacking in supplemental niacin. No signs of pathology were observed. Although no evidence has been obtained of any need to supplement practical diets of mature chickens with nicotinic acid (2), niacin supplementation was reported to increase egg size with turkey breeders (68).

Treatment of Deficiency. Supplementing a deficient ration with required amounts of nicotinic acid has little or no effect on cases that have progressed to the extent that the tendon has slipped from its condyles (perosis) or on advanced cases of enlarged hock disorder in adult tom turkeys.

PYRIDOXINE (VITAMIN B_6). Pyridoxine is required in several enzymes, particularly those involved in transamination and decarboxylation of amino acids. The coenzymes are pyridoxal phosphate and pyridoxamine phosphate.

Signs and Pathology of Deficiency. Pyridoxine-deficient chicks show depressed appetite, poor growth, perosis, and characteristic nervous signs. Chicks show jerky, nervous movements of the legs when walking and often undergo extreme spasmodic convulsions that usually terminate in death. During these convulsions chicks may run aimlessly about, flapping their wings and falling to their sides or rolling completely over on their backs, where they perform rapid jerking motions with their feet and heads. These signs may be distinguished from those of encephalomalacia (vitamin E deficiency) by the relatively greater intensity of activity of the chicks during a seizure, which results in complete exhaustion and often death.

Gries and Scott (64) observed that chicks fed very low levels of pyridoxine (up to 2.2 mg B_6/kg diet) combined with a high protein level (31%) have classic nervous signs. Intermediate levels (2.5–2.8 mg B_6/kg diet) combined with 31% protein cause severe perosis but no nervous signs. The consequence is bone curvature. If the diet contains 22% protein, even the lowest levels of pyridoxine (1.9 mg/kg diet) fail to induce nervous signs, perosis, or even lowered growth rate. The function of pyridoxine in amino acid metabolism is reflected in an increased requirement when high levels of protein are fed.

Symptoms of pyridoxine deficiency in ducklings are reported to include poor growth and food consumption, hyperexcitability, weakness, microcytic hypochromic anemia, convulsions, and death (190).

In adult birds, pyridoxine deficiency causes marked reduction of egg production and hatchability, as well as decreased feed consumption, loss of weight, and death. The injection of pyridoxine into the fertile egg has increased the hatchability of eggs from turkey breeders that had received in their diets more than twice the concentration of pyridoxine estimated as the requirement by the National Research Council (135). This suggests that the requirement of breeders under some conditions may be higher than the dietary level of pyridoxine used under practical conditions.

BIOTIN. Biotin is a cofactor in carboxylation and decarboxylation reactions involving fixation of carbon dioxide. These reactions have important roles in anabolic processes and in nitrogen metabolism.

Signs and Pathology of Deficiency. In biotin deficiency, the dermatitis of the feet and skin around the beak and eyes is similar to that of pantothenic acid deficiency. Thus, in making a differential diagnosis, it is usually necessary to examine composition of the diet.

Perosis is a sign of biotin avitaminosis in growing chickens and turkeys. Biotin deficiency signs in chicks include various other abnormalities of the tibia. Bain et al. (15) reported that chicks fed a purified diet devoid of biotin had shortened tibiae, higher bone density and bone ash, and an abnormal pattern of bone modeling: the median side of the middiaphyseal cortex was thicker than the lateral side in chicks fed the biotin-free diet, whereas the opposite pattern existed for chicks fed the same diet supplemented with adequate biotin. This raises the possibility that biotin may have a role in varus deformities of the limb (15). Changes in tibial concentrations of fatty acids that are prostaglandin precursors correlate with bone abnormalities in biotin-deficient chicks, suggesting that altered prostaglandin synthesis may be a contributing factor in altered bone modeling patterns of the tibiotarsus in biotin deficiency (171).

Biotin is essential for embryonic development (39, 40). Embryos from hens fed biotin-deficient diets developed syndactylia, an extensive webbing between the third and fourth toes. Many embryos that fail to hatch are chondrodystrophic—characterized by reduced size, a parrot beak, severely crooked tibia, shortened or twisted tarsometatarsus, shortened bones of the wing and skull, and shortening and bending of the scapula. Two peaks of embryonic mortality may occur: one during the 1st wk and a second during the last 3 days of incubation.

Robel and Christensen (134) reported that the injection of 87 μg of D-biotin into eggs of large white turkey hens that had been held under commercial conditions resulted in approximately 4–5% higher hatchability of their eggs. The reason for the improvement is not known; however, the authors suggest that biotin levels or biotin availability in the egg may have been low.

Fatty liver and kidney syndrome (FLKS) is a biotin-responsive condition that has been observed in broiler chicks. Chicks exhibit depressed growth; fatty infiltrations of liver, kidney, and heart; decreased plasma glucose; increased plasma-free fatty acids; and increased ratio of C16:1 to C18:0 fatty acids in liver and adipose tissue (123, 175). High dietary protein or fat reduces or eliminates mortality, whereas high protein or fat increases the signs of biotin deficiency. Fasting exacerbates FLKS and its associated mortality (175). Fasting decreases blood glucose concentrations and increases plasma-free fatty acids. Pyruvic carboxylase, a biotin-containing enzyme, is decreased in activity in FLKS biotin deficiency (123). It has been suggested that biotin deficiency impairs gluconeogenesis as a result of low activity of this enzyme, leading to increased

conversion of pyruvate to fatty acids. Chicks having FLKS frequently do not have the characteristic signs of biotin deficiency. This may be a temporal phenomenon wherein the changes in tissue metabolism leading to FLKS occur rapidly in biotin-depleted chicks, but the classic signs of biotin deficiency require a longer period of time to develop (29).

Biotin has been suspected of having a role in "acute death syndrome" (or "sudden death syndrome") in broiler chickens. Biotin deficiency alters the unsaturated fatty acid profile in tissue lipids in such a manner as to suggest that it impairs the conversion of linoleic acid to arachidonic acid (170). The latter is a precursor of the prostaglandins, prostocyclin I_2 and thromboxane A_2, which have marked effects on the vascular system. The concentration of biotin in liver was reported to be depressed in chicks that exhibited acute death syndrome (85). The role of biotin in acute death syndrome, however, remains obscure.

Biotin bioavailability for chickens and turkeys varies greatly among practical feed ingredients (57, 108, 176). Biotin is no more than 10% available in some grains but almost completely available in others. This is an important consideration in formulating diets to satisfy the biotin requirements of poultry.

Treatment of Deficiency. Patrick et al. (122) and Jukes and Bird (79) reported that injection or oral administration of a few micrograms of biotin was sufficient to prevent biotin deficiency signs in chicks and turkey poults.

FOLIC ACID (FOLACIN). Folic acid is a part of the enzyme system involved in single-carbon metabolism. It is involved in synthesis of purines and the methyl groups of such important metabolites as choline, methionine, and thymine. Folic acid, therefore, is required for normal nucleic acid metabolism and formation of the nucleoproteins required for cell multiplication.

Signs and Pathology of Deficiency. Folic acid deficiency in chicks is characterized by poor growth, very poor feathering, anemia, and perosis. Folic acid is required for pigmentation in feathers of Rhode Island Red and black leghorn chicks. Thus, folic acid, lysine, copper, and iron appear to be required for prevention of achroma of feathers in colored poultry.

A deficiency in the breeding diet of chickens or turkeys causes a marked increase in embryonic mortality. Embryos die soon after pipping the air cell. According to Sunde et al. (159, 160), a deformed upper mandible and bending of the tibiotarsus are lesions of embryonic deficiency. Poults show a characteristic cervical paralysis and die within 2 days after the onset of these signs unless folic acid is administered immediately. Poults show only a slight anemia.

Folic acid deficiency in chicks causes megaloblastic arrest of erythrocyte formation in bone marrow, which results in a severe macrocytic anemia as one of the first signs in chicks. White cell formation also is reduced, causing a marked agranulocytosis.

Folic Acid–Choline Interrelationship.
Folic acid has a central role in methyl group metabolism. Young et al. (191) observed that when a diet for chicks is deficient in folic acid, an increase in the dietary level of choline reduces, but does not completely prevent, the incidence and severity of perosis. A growth depression has been observed in chicks fed a practical diet that was low in folic acid and marginally deficient in methionine and choline. Supplementation of the diet with folic acid or methionine and choline stimulated growth under these conditions (125).

Treatment of Deficiency.
A single intramuscular (IM) injection of 50–100 µg pure pteroylglutamic (folic) acid causes a peak reticulocyte response within 4 days in severely anemic folic acid-deficient chicks (136). Hemoglobin values and growth rates return to normal within 1 wk. Addition of 500 µg folic acid/100 g feed caused recovery comparable to that obtained with injection of the vitamin.

VITAMIN B_{12} (COBALAMIN).
Vitamin B_{12} is involved in nucleic acid and methyl synthesis and carbohydrate and fat metabolism. One of its main enzyme functions involves isomerization of methylmalonyl coenzyme A to form succinyl CoA.

Signs and Pathology of Deficiency.
Signs of vitamin B_{12} deficiency are slow growth, decreased efficiency of feed utilization, mortality, and reduced egg size and hatchability. Specific signs for vitamin B_{12} deficiency have not been demonstrated in growing or mature poultry. Vitamin B_{12} deficiency has been reported to cause myelin degeneration in chicks. Some investigators have detected increased total phospholipids and decreased levels of galactolipids from deficient chicks, suggesting impaired myelin-maturation (83). Perosis may occur in vitamin B_{12}-deficient chicks or poults when their diets lack choline, methionine, or betaine as sources of methyl groups. Addition of vitamin B_{12} may prevent perosis under these conditions because of its effect on the synthesis of methyl groups.

Vitamin B_{12}-deficient embryos have a peak in mortality at the 17th day of incubation, reduced size, myoatrophy of the legs, diffuse hemorrhages, perosis, edema, and fatty liver (113, 118).

Treatment of Deficiency.
Peeler et al. (124) showed that IM injection of 2 µg vitamin B_{12}/hen increased hatchability of eggs from vitamin B_{12}-deficient hens from approximately 15% to 80% within 1 wk. Addition of 4 mg vitamin B_{12}/ton breeding ration is sufficient to maintain maximum hatchability and to produce chicks having sufficient stores of the vitamin to prevent any deficiency during the first few weeks of life. Similar injections of young chicks followed by supplementation of the chick ration also will correct the deficiency.

CHOLINE.
Choline is present in acetylcholine in body phospholipids and acts as a methyl source in synthesis within the body of methyl-containing compounds such as methionine, creatine, carnitine, and N-methylnicotinamide. Choline per se does not act as a methyl donor but first must be oxidized to the compound betaine, which can then donate one of its three methyl groups to a methyl-acceptor such as homocysteine or glycocyamine for formation of methionine or creatine, respectively.

Signs and Pathology of Deficiency.
In addition to poor growth, the outstanding sign of choline deficiency in chicks and poults is perosis (Figs. 2.10 and 2.11). Young turkeys have a high requirement for choline and, therefore, will show a high incidence of severe perosis unless special care is taken to supplement the diet with choline. Perosis is first characterized by pinpoint hemorrhages and a slight puffiness about the hock joint, followed by an apparent flattening of the tibiometatarsal joint caused by rotation of the metatarsus. The metatarsus continues to twist and may become bent or bowed until it is out of alignment with the tibia. When this condition exists, the leg cannot adequately support the weight of the bird. The articular cartilage is deformed and the Achilles tendon slips from its condyles.

When laying pullets that have received high-choline rearing diets are fed severely deficient diets, percentage of fat in the liver increases. In livers of choline-deficient chickens, fat content is higher in females than males. Choline deficiency is, however, rare in adult chickens and turkeys fed practical rations. Nesheim et al. (112) showed that pullets fed high choline levels during the 8- to 20-wk growing period are more likely to show fatty livers when placed on purified low-choline laying diets than pullets fed minimum levels during the same growth period. These results indicate that maturing chick-

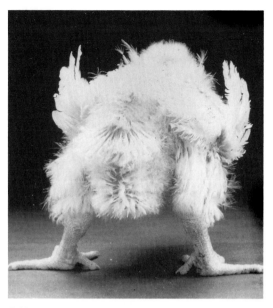

2.10. Choline deficiency. Stunting, poor feathering, and short, thick, bowed legs typical of chondrodystrophy are seen in a bird that had been fed a choline-deficient diet. (Swayne)

ens can synthesize choline but will not fully develop this ability if given diets containing ample amounts.

Treatment of Deficiency. If choline deficiency is noted in chicks or poults before severe signs of perosis have developed, the deficiency can be cured by supplementing the ration with sufficient choline to meet the requirements. Once the tendon has slipped in chicks or poults suffering from choline deficiency, the damage is irreparable.

ESSENTIAL INORGANIC ELEMENTS.
Essential mineral elements are as important as

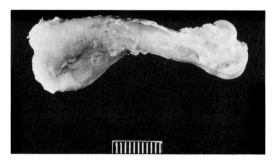

2.11. Choline deficiency. Perosis and deformity of tibiotarsus from broiler chicken given a diet lacking adequate choline. (Swayne)

amino acids and vitamins in maintenance of life, well-being, and production in poultry. They enter into composition of bones and give the skeleton the rigidity and strength needed to support the soft tissues. Minerals combine with protein, lipids, and other substances that make up the soft tissues. They take part in maintenance of osmotic pressure and acid-base balance and exert specific effects on the ability of muscles and nerves to respond to stimuli. Minerals also are necessary for activation of many enzymes of the body.

The inorganic elements essential for maintenance of well-being are calcium; phosphorus; magnesium; potassium; sodium; chlorine; and the trace elements manganese, iron, copper, zinc, iodine, molybdenum, and selenium. Fluorine in small amounts is a constant constituent of several tissues, particularly bones. Traces of this element may be essential or at least beneficial for some species, but no direct evidence has been obtained with poultry. Analyses of individual mineral constituents in the body of chickens show that major portions of calcium, phosphorus, magnesium, and zinc are present in bones. Other essential elements are distributed largely in muscles, other soft tissues, and body fluids.

CALCIUM AND PHOSPHORUS. Calcium (Ca) and phosphorus (P) are closely associated in metabolism, particularly in bone formation. The major portion of dietary calcium is used for bone formation in growing chicks or poults and for eggshell formation in mature hens. Calcium also is essential for clotting of blood, and it is required along with sodium and potassium for normal beating of the heart. Calcium is an important factor in the regulation of cellular metabolism and processes.

In addition to its role in bone formation, phosphorus is an essential component of purine nucleotides and other phosphorylated compounds involved in the transfer or conservation of free energy in biochemical reactions. It exercises important functions in metabolism of carbohydrates and fats, and it enters into composition of important constituents of all living cells. Salts formed from it play an important part in maintenance of the acid-base balance.

The utilization of calcium and phosphorus depends on presence of an adequate amount of vitamin D in the diet. In vitamin D deficiency, the deposition of these minerals in bones of growing chicks and poults is reduced, bones become depleted of mineral, and the quantity of calcium in eggshells is decreased.

According to Long and associates (95, 96, 97), deficiencies of calcium and phosphorus in the diet of growing broiler chicks cause rickets that differs in histopathology and that differs from the rickets of vitamin D deficiency. Tibiae from chicks that had been fed a diet containing 0.3% Ca from the time of hatching showed, by 2 wk, a widening of the proliferating prehypertrophic zone of epiphyseal cartilage and irregular contours in the boundary between the zones of proliferating and hypertrophic cartilage (96). Irregular cartilage columns and elongated epiphyseal vessels were present. By 4 wk, the epiphyseal growth plate had widened and, in some cases, extended as a cartilaginous plug into the metaphysis. Histologically, the proliferating and hypertrophic zones were irregular and often contained areas of nonviable cells. The hypertrophied zone was markedly widened in some chicks by 4 wk. Metaphyseal blood vessels invaded along the lateral, but not the apical, region of the cartilaginous plug; cartilage columns of the metaphysis were thickened and irregular. The investigators note that the pathology is similar to that of tibial dyschondroplasia.

According to Long et al. (97), phosphorous deficiency (0.2% available dietary P) and calcium excess (2.24% Ca and 0.45% available P) resulted in similar abnormalities of the tibia. Several histologic abnormalities were observed, but most conspicuous was a marked lengthening of the cartilage columns of the degenerating hypertrophied epiphyseal cartilage and metaphyseal primary spongiosa. Some chicks were unable to stand at 4 wk, displaying a spraddle-legged posture. Folding fractures and bowing or rotation of the tibiotarsus were frequently observed.

Julian (81) observed that phosphorus-deficient chicks had increased respiratory rates and were polycythemic. Blood CO_2 and O_2 were decreased, presumably due to poor rib strength and infolding, which interfered with respiratory movements of the rib cage. Birds died of right ventricular failure, often accompanied by ascites.

In laying hens, calcium deficiency results in reduced egg production and thin-shelled eggs as well as a tendency to deplete calcium content of the bones, first by complete removal of the medullary bone, followed by a gradual removal of the cortical bone. Finally, bones become so thin that spontaneous fractures may occur, especially in vertebrae, tibia, and femur. This condition may be associated with a syndrome commonly termed "cage layer fatigue" (130). While a marginal calcium deficiency has often been found to be a triggering agent in cage layer fatigue, the syndrome apparently is not due to a simple deficiency of calcium but also involves other etiologic factors not yet identified.

Excess Calcium. Shane et al. (150) fed leghorn pullets diets containing 3.0% Ca and 0.4% P from 8 to 20 wk of age. Nephrosis and visceral gout were observed in the high calcium treatment by 16 wk of age. Wideman et al. 1985 (177) provided replacement pullets diets containing excess (3.25%) or adequate (1.0%) levels of calcium in combinations with moderate (0.6%) or low (0.4%) available phosphorus from 7 wk until 18 wk of age. All birds received a commercial layer diet during the laying period. Pullets fed on the 3.25% Ca diets developed a high incidence of urolithiasis by 18 wk, which persisted or increased in the laying period through 51 wk of age. Low levels of dietary phosphorus during the rearing period exacerbated the effect of excess calcium.

MAGNESIUM. Magnesium (Mg) is essential for carbohydrate metabolism and for activation of many enzymes, especially those involved in phosphorylation reactions. It is essential for bone formation, about two-thirds being present in bone chiefly as a carbonate. Eggshells contain about 0.4% Mg.

Almquist (6) observed that chicks fed a magnesium-deficient diet grew slowly for approximately 1 wk and then ceased growing and became lethargic. When disturbed, these chicks frequently passed into a brief convulsion accompanied by gasping and finally into a comatose state sometimes ending in death. Magnesium deficiency signs of poults are similar to those of chicks (157). Hypomagnesemia and hypocalcemia are associated with severe magnesium deficiency in chicks. Tibiae have decreased magnesium and increased calcium content and exhibit abnormalities (172, 173) including thickening of trabeculae, increased retention of cartilage cores, and the occurrence of elongated and inactive osteocytes in the metaphysis. Deficient chicks have thickening of the cortex, the presence of elongated inactive osteocytes, and enlargement of Haversion canals within the diaphysis. The epiphyseal plate, however, appears normal. The parathyroid appears hyperactive, perhaps in response to the hypocalcemia that is characteristic of magnesium deficiency (173).

Excess Magnesium. Ordinary feeds supply enough magnesium in practical poultry diets to meet requirements. It is possible, however, that under certain conditions rations may contain excess magnesium, producing detrimental effects including reduced growth rate and bone ash in chicks and decreased egg size, eggshell thinning, and diarrhea in hens (36, 105, 156).

SODIUM AND CHLORINE (SALT). Sodium (Na) as chloride (Cl), carbonate, and phosphate is found chiefly in blood and body fluids. Sodium is connected intimately with maintenance of membrane potentials, cellular transport processes, and the regulation of the hydrogen ion concentration of blood. Chloride, the major mineral anion in extracellular fluid, plays a role in fluid and ionic balance.

Signs of Deficiency. Animals receiving diets deficient in sodium not only fail to grow but also develop softening of bones, corneal keratinization, gonadal inactivity, adrenal hypertrophy, changes in cellular function, impairment of food utilization, and decrease in both plasma and special fluid volumes. Cardiac output drops; mean arterial pressure falls; the hematocrit increases; elasticity of subcutaneous tissue decreases; adrenal function is impaired; and a state of shock results, which if uncorrected, terminates in death.

Chicks fed a diet containing no added salt show retarded growth with decreased efficiency of food utilization. Lack of salt in the diet of laying hens results in an abrupt decrease of egg production and reduced egg size, loss of weight, and cannibalism. Salt deprivation in turkeys impairs egg production and hatchability (67). Leach and Nesheim (91) observed that chicks fed a purified diet containing 0.24% Na and 0.4% potassium required 0.12% chlorine. They produced chloride deficiency by feeding young chicks a purified diet containing 190 mg Cl/kg diet. Chicks exhibited extremely poor growth rate, high mortality, hemoconcentration, dehydration, and reduced blood chloride. In addition, deficient chicks showed nervous signs characteristic of Cl deficiency. When startled, they fell forward with their legs outstretched behind them and lay paralyzed for several minutes, then appeared quite normal until frightened again (Fig. 2.12).

Excess Salt. Large amounts of salt in the ration are toxic to chickens. The lethal dose is approximately 4 g/kg body weight. Young chicks appear to be more susceptible to toxic effects of salt than are older chickens. Signs of salt intoxication include inability to stand, intense thirst, pronounced muscular weakness, and convulsive movements preceding death. There are lesions in many organs, particularly hemorrhages and severe congestion in the gastrointestinal tract, muscles, liver, and lungs. Excess sodium resulted in ascites, right ventricular hypertrophy, and right ventricular failure in broiler chickens (Fig. 2.13) (80). Matterson et al. (102) fed day-old poults graded quantities of salt for 23 days and observed 25% edema and 25% mortality at 4.0% salt but none at 2.0%. Swayne et al. (162), however, described a case of accidental salt poisoning in 5- to 11-day-old poults in which a diet contained 1.85% salt. Signs included respiratory distress, ascites, hydropericardium, hydrothorax, and sudden death.

POTASSIUM. Potassium is found primarily in the cellular compartment of the body; soft tissues of the chicken contain more than three times as much potassium as sodium. As a major cation in intracellular fluid, potassium has an essential role in the maintenance of membrane potential and cellular fluid balance. Potassium participates directly in numerous biochemical reactions and is necessary for normal heart activity, reducing contractility of the heart muscle and favoring relaxation.

Signs of Deficiency. The main effect of potassium deficiency is overall muscle weakness characterized by weak extremities, poor intestinal tone with distention, cardiac weakness, and weakness of the respiratory muscles and their ultimate failure. Severely affected individuals may exhibit tetanic seizures followed by death. Low levels of potassium in laying diets cause decreased egg production and eggshell thinning (89). A low potassium level in the vital organs of animals may occur during severe stress. Plasma potassium is elevated, causing the kidney (acting under influence of the adrenocortical hormone) to discharge potassium into the urine. During adaptation to stress, the muscle will begin to retrieve its lost potassium. As liver glycogen is restored, potassium returns to the liver.

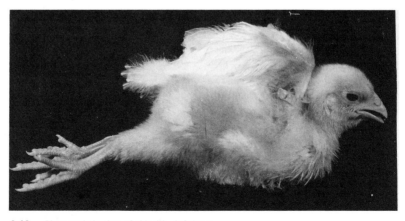

2.12.   Characteristic sign of chloride deficiency.

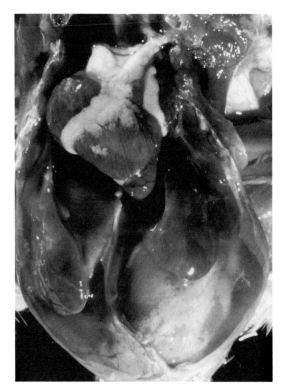

2.13. Sodium excess. Cardiomegaly, especially involving the right ventricle, ascites, and fibrin masses in the body cavity and on the liver capsule, occurred in this chicken given excess sodium. (Swayne)

This may result in temporary prolongation of the general potassium deficiency throughout the body. High temperature results in increased loss of potassium in the urine (44).

An all vegetable diet low in potassium produced low plasma potassium concentrations and a high incidence of sudden death syndrome at the onset of egg production in broiler breeder pullets that had undergone restricted feeding (75). The hypothesis that low dietary potassium leads to this syndrome, however, has not been subjected to testing.

DIETARY BALANCE OF MACROMINERALS. Studies in many laboratories during the past 2 decades have determined that the balance among dietary minerals has a profound effect on acid-base balance and certain developmental, metabolic, and physiologic functions in poultry (109). Balance has been expressed in several ways. One expression is dietary undetermined anion (dUA), sometimes referred to as mineral cation–anion balance (14). It is defined as follows: dUA = [Na+K+Ca+Mg] − [Cl+P+S], in which all values are expressed in milliequivalents per kg of diet and valences are assumed to be +1 for Na and K, +2 for Ca and Mg,

−1 for Cl, −1.75 for P and −2 for S. P and S are assumed to be inorganic. Trace minerals are excluded because of their insignificant contributions to the overall mineral balance. Another term, *dietary electrolyte balance*, emphasizes the balance among the strong electrolytes (Na+K−Cl).

A positive value of dUA represents the net dietary concentration of organic anions. If the value is negative, a very unusual condition, it is a measure of the net hydrogen ion content of the diet. Minerals differ in their chemical properties and metabolism. Therefore, while dUA provides an indication of the qualitative effect, it is not an accurate predictor of the quantitative effect of the diet on acid-base balance.

Diets rich in mineral anions, particularly Cl, tend to cause metabolic acidosis and result in disturbances of Ca metabolism, increased incidence and severity of tibial dyschondroplasia in immature fowls, and reduced eggshell calcification in laying hens. Effects on tibial development (49, 66, 92, 140) and eggshells (13) are exacerbated when calcium is limiting.

A dietary combination of excessive calcium and low phosphorus results in the excretion of an alkaline urine (177), as would be predicted from dUA. The urolithiasis observed in replacement pullets by Wideman et al. (177) under these conditions may be due in part to the increased pH of urine. Alkaline conditions favor the precipitation of divalent mineral salts. Increasing the dietary acid load has been used to reduce uroliths (178) in poultry and some mammals. The potentially adverse effects of low dUA on bone development and eggshell quality should be considered before such treatment is attempted.

MANGANESE. Manganese (Mn) is an activator of several enzymes and is required for normal growth and reproduction and prevention of perosis.

In addition to its perosis-preventing properties, manganese is necessary for formation of normal bones. Wilgus et al. (182, 183) observed that leg bones of chicks fed perosis-producing diets frequently were thickened and shortened. Manganese deficiency impairs endochondral bone growth. Cells of the epiphyseal growth plate are arranged irregularly and the extracellular matrix is greatly reduced (88). Manganese is essential for the activity of glycosyltransferases; a deficiency of manganese impairs the synthesis of the glycosaminoglycan molecules that are components of proteoglycans in the cartilage of the epiphyseal growth plate (90, 94). Bone of manganese-deficient ducks, consequently, contains a reduced concentration of hexosamine (90). Manganese also has been reported to be necessary for maximum eggshell quality.

Lyons and Insko (100) found that manganese deficiency resulted in very low hatchability of fertile eggs and chondrodystrophy in embryos. The peak of mortality for such embryos occurred on the 20th and 21st days of incubation. Chondrodystrophic embryos were characterized by very short, thickened legs, short wings, parrot beak, globular contour of head, protruding abdomen, and retarded down and body growth. Marked edema was noted in about 75% of these embryos. The manganese content of eggs producing chondrodystrophic embryos was less than that of normal eggs.

Chicks hatched from eggs produced by hens fed a diet deficient in manganese sometimes exhibit ataxia, particularly when excited (34). The head may be drawn forward and bent underneath the body or retracted over the back. Ataxic chicks grow normally and reach maturity but fail to recover completely. They also retain the short bones characteristic of embryos and newly hatched chicks from manganese-deficient dams (33).

IODINE.   Traces of iodine (I) are required for normal functioning of the thyroid gland in poultry as in other animals. Thyroxine contains approximately 65% I and acts as an important regulating agent in body metabolism. When the intake of iodine is suboptimal, the thyroid tissue enlarges and goiter results.

Wilgus et al. (184) reported that iodine deficiency results in an enlarged thyroid and, in some cases, lower body weight in growing chicks. They observed congenital goiter in baby chicks hatched from hens receiving 0.025 ppm I in the ration. Rogler et al. (137) observed mortality late in incubation. Hatching time was delayed. Embryo size was reduced and yolk sac resorption was retarded. Use of 0.25% iodized salt in chicken and turkey rations should prevent development of iodine deficiency. This would supply 0.175 ppm in addition to that contained in the diet. Christensen and Ort (37) recently reported that dietary supplements of iodine increased the permeability of eggshells and the hatchability of turkey eggs.

Iodine deficiency in poultry has been largely prevented by widespread use of iodine either in iodized salt or as part of the trace mineral premix.

COPPER.   Copper (Cu) is essential for formation of hemoglobin. In the absence of copper, dietary iron is absorbed and deposited in the liver and elsewhere but hemoglobin synthesis does not occur. Copper deficiency in chicks results in anemia, characterized by reduced numbers of circulating erythrocytes, and impaired feather pigmentation in colored breeds of fowl (42).

Copper is a component of several enzymes that participate in redox reactions. Lysyl oxidase is a copper-containing enzyme that catalyzes oxidation of lysine residues in formation of the cross-linking structure desmosine in elastin. Copper deficiency decreases the cross-linking. This weakens the structure of elastin, leading to aortic rupture in poultry. Thinning of the tertiary bronchial mantle in lungs may also result from decreased cross-linking of elastin (30); however, observations on birds fed high levels of cadmium appear inconsistent with this view (93). Copper deficiency has been reported to decrease cross-linking in bone collagen and to increase bone fragility (119, 138). Copper is a component of superoxide dismutase and cytochrome oxidase, both of which have decreased activities in copper-deficient chicks (23).

A deficiency of copper in laying hens causes reduced egg production, increased egg size, and abnormal eggshell calcification. Eggshell abnormalities include shell-less eggs, misshapen eggs, wrinkled eggshells, and reduced eggshell thickness. The palisade layer of the eggshell appears normal; however, the mammillary layer has enlarged mammillary knobs and increased spacing between knobs. This may be related to an abnormal structure of eggshell membranes caused by a decrease in lysine cross-linking (19).

Excess Copper.   Excessive dietary levels of copper have been reported to cause abnormalities of the gizzard. Fisher et al. (56) reported that dietary copper levels ranging from 205 ppm to 605 ppm resulted in a rough thickened gizzard lining in broiler chicks, the severity of the lesion increasing as the copper level of the diet increased. The highest copper level caused markedly thickened and folded linings having a warty appearance. Histologic examination revealed thickening of the koilin layer, sloughing of epithelial cells into the area under the koilin layer and the inclusion of clusters of sloughed cells within the koilin layer. Wight et al. (181) observed similar lesions in chicks receiving 2000 and 4000 ppm copper. They noted gizzard erosions and fissures in the gizzard lining, hemorrhages under the koilin layer, and a mucoid material adhering to the mucosa of the proventriculus.

IRON.   Iron (Fe) is an essential component of heme, the porphyrin nucleus of hemoglobin and the cytochromes, and is a component of several enzymes including catalase, peroxidase, phenylalanine hydroxylase, tyrosinase, and proline hydroxylase.

Iron deficiency results in a hypochromic, microcytic anemia and reduced concentration of nonheme iron in plasma and prevents normal feather pigmentation in breeds having colored plumage (42, 70). A deficiency in laying hens also causes anemia in the developing chick embryo and reduced hatchability (110). Chicks that survive incubation are weak and listless; however, they recover when given supplemental iron.

The hemoglobin level of hens falls with the beginning of egg production, but this apparently is not related to the iron or copper content of the diet. Since the hemoglobin level rises rapidly with onset of broodiness, it is more probable that low levels prevailing in egg production are caused by changes in hormone activity rather than iron or copper deficiencies. A deficiency of iron has been reported to decrease the synthesis of niacin from tryptophan in chicks (117).

ZINC. Traces of zinc (Zn) appear to be necessary for life in all animals. It is a constituent of the enzyme carbonic anhydrase and is necessary for activation of several other enzymes.

Deficiency signs include retarded growth; poor feathering; enlarged hocks (Fig. 2.14); short, thickened long bones; scaling of the skin and dermatitis, particularly on the feet; and an awkward arthritic gait (116, 192). Zinc-deficient chicks exhibit increased hematocrit, which is due to redistribution of body water rather than altered water intake (26).

Histologic lesions include hyperkeratinization of skin of the shank and feet and parakeratosis of the esophagus. Nucleoli of the crop epithelium are enlarged and contain increased amounts of RNA. Alkaline phosphatase and alcohol dehydrogenase, two zinc-containing enzymes, exhibit reduced activities in the crop and esophagus (180). Reduced alkaline phosphatase activity is also observed in epiphyseal cartilage. Starcher et al. (154) found that activity of

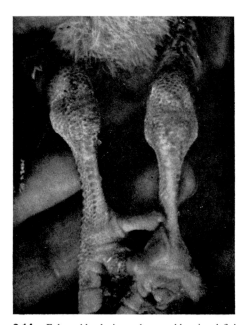

2.14. Enlarged hocks in poult caused by zinc deficiency.

the zinc-dependent enzyme collagenase is reduced in the tibia during zinc deficiency. They suggest that effects of zinc on bone may be the result of decreased bone collagen turnover. Bettger et al. (24, 25) reported evidence of an interrelationship between vitamin E and zinc. Leg abnormalities, arthritic gait, and epidermal lesions were reduced by vitamin E and exacerbated by polyunsaturated fatty acids.

Ducks exhibit poor growth and epidermal lesions of the feet, particularly interdigital webs (179). Pathology of the epidermis is evident in the interdigital web, mucous membrane of the tongue, and epithelium in other parts of the gastrointestinal tract. Hyperkeratosis and acanthosis characterize the tongue and interdigital web lesions. Intercellular spacing between prickle cells and basal cells is increased and number of desmosomes is diminished. Prickle cells have an abnormal structure, enlarged nuclei and nucleoli, and decreased content of free ribosomes, tonofilaments, and other structures.

The zinc requirement of poults is higher than for chicks. Thus, poults are more likely to show enlarged hocks and poor feathering of zinc deficiency unless special supplements are added to the diet. The most dramatic embryonic abnormalities resulting from nutritional deficiency appear when the breeding diet contains excess calcium and phosphorus, is high in phytic acid, and is deficient in zinc. Zinc-deficient embryos may have only a head and complete viscera but no spinal column beyond a few vertebrae, and no wings, body wall, or legs (84).

Chickens maintained on a zinc-deficient diet are unable to produce antibodies against T cell–dependent antigens even though lymphocytes are capable of immunoglobulin production (32).

Excess Zinc. Excessive dietary levels of zinc (e.g., 20,000 ppm as zinc oxide) induce molt in laying hens (41). Zinc results in abrupt decline in egg production and onset of molt followed by rapid resumption of egg laying after dietary zinc concentrations are returned to normal. Excess zinc results in inanition, which is presumably responsible for initiating the molt (103). High levels of zinc result in accumulation of zinc in tissues and pathologic changes in the gizzard and pancreas. Chicks exhibit a rough, pale gizzard lining, which may show evidence of fissures and, less frequently, ulceration (46, 181). Histologic examination reveals epithelial desquamation and infiltration of inflammatory cells. Pancreases exhibit dilated acinar lumina and degenerative changes in acinar cells. The latter include loss of zymogen granules, vacuolization of the cytoplasm, the presence of hyaline bodies and other electron-dense debris (181).

Large excesses of dietary zinc such as those used

to induce a molt result in reduced activity of the selenium-dependent enzyme, plasma glutathione peroxidase. Selenium administration restores glutathione peroxidase activity but fails to prevent pathologic changes in the gizzard and pancreas (181). Lesser excesses of zinc (i.e., up to 2000 ppm) did not affect plasma or hepatic glutathione peroxidase activity, but interfered with exocrine function of the pancreas and reduced the plasma and tissue concentrations of a-tocopherol in chicks fed a purified diet but not in chicks fed a practical diet (98, 99).

SELENIUM. Selenium has been shown to be an essential mineral element for both chicks and poults. It is a constituent of the enzymes, glutathione peroxidase and phospholipid hydroperoxide glutathione peroxidase, which serve to protect tissues against oxidative damage, and it is a component of iodothyronine 5'-deiodinase, an enzyme that is involved in the conversion of thyroxine to its active form (31). Selenium prevents development of exudative diathesis in young chickens and myopathy of gizzard and heart in young turkeys (142, 143, 147). Selenium-deficient ducklings have reduced plasma glutathione peroxidase activity and exhibit low body weight gain and increased mortality. Ducklings that succumb to selenium deficiency may exhibit necrosis of several tissues including the gizzard, heart, skeletal muscle and smooth muscle of the intestine, and show signs of hydropericardium and ascites (43). Vitamin E and selenium have a mutual sparing effect in prevention of these diseases (see Vitamin E).

Chicks severely deficient in selenium exhibit poor growth and feathering, impaired fat digestion, pancreatic atrophy and fibrosis (164, 165), and reduced activity of selenium-dependent glutathione peroxidase activity in the pancreas (174). Gries and Scott (65) performed a time-sequence study of pancreatic lesions, which began at 6 days of age with vacuolation and hyaline body formation in the exocrine pancreas. As the deficiency progressed, cytoplasm degenerated until acini were represented by rings of cells with a central lumen embedded in fibrous tissue (Fig. 2.15). Addition of 0.1 ppm Se as Na_2SeO_3 to the diet caused complete pancreatic acinar regeneration within 2 wk and a marked clinical recovery. High dietary levels of vitamin E (15 to 20 times the amount needed for prevention of other vitamin E–deficiency diseases) protect against the pancreatic degeneration caused by selenium deficiency (174).

High plasma tocopherol levels were maintained by feeding 100 IU vitamin E/kg and bile salts to enhance its absorption. This greatly reduced incidence of exudative diathesis, which did not appear until the pancreas in chicks had degenerated severely.

WATER. Water holds a unique position in nutrition mainly due to its physical properties. Because of its solvent and polar properties, it acts as a transport medium for other nutrients and products of metabolism and enhances cell reactions. Because of its high specific heat, it can absorb the heat of reactions produced in oxidation of carbohydrates and fats with little rise in temperature. Water evaporates readily, removing many calories from the body as

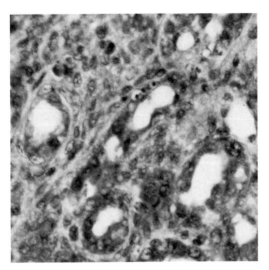 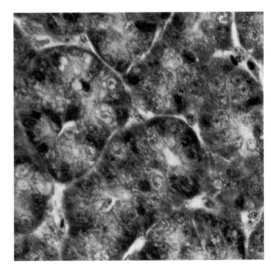

2.15. Pancreas from selenium-deficient chick. Acini consist of degenerating cells forming central lumen with extensive interstitial fibrosis (*left*). Control (*right*). ×250.

latent heat of vaporization. These and many other functions explain why the animal is able to exist much longer without food than without water.

Unlike larger farm animals, chickens and turkeys must have access to a continuous water supply, since they drink only small amounts at a time. An insufficient amount results in decreased growth and egg production.

The quantity of water drunk by chicks is correlated directly with salt content of the diet (69). Austic (11) reported that equimolar additions to the diet of sodium and potassium in the form of bicarbonate salts resulted in similar increases in water intake of broiler chicks. When added to the diet as calcium chloride in substitution for calcium carbonate, chloride increased water intake, but only about one-half as much as equivalent amounts of sodium and potassium. Excess dietary protein and deficiencies of amino acids result in increased water intake (10). The effect of protein is presumably due to increased excretion of nitrogen and minerals such as phosphorus and sulfur that are constituents of protein.

REFERENCES

1. Abdulrahim, S.M., M.B. Patel, and J. McGinnis. 1979. Effects of vitamin D_3 and D_3 metabolites in production parameters and hatchability of eggs. Poult Sci 58:858–863.
2. Adams, R.L., and C.W. Carrick. 1967. A study of the niacin requirement of the laying hen. Poult Sci 46:712–718.
3. Adamstone, F.B. 1947. Histologic comparisons of the brains of vitamin A-deficient and vitamin E-deficient chicks. Arch Pathol 43:301–312.
4. Adamstone, F.B., and L.E. Card. 1934. The effects of vitamin E deficiency on the testis of the male fowl (Gallus domesticus). J Morphol 56:339–359.
5. Agricultural Research Council. 1975. Nutrient requirement of farm livestock. No. 1. Poultry. Agricultural Research Council (London).
6. Almquist, H.J. 1942. Magnesium requirement of the chick. Proc Soc Exp Biol Med 49:544–545.
7. Ameenuddin, S., M.L. Sunde, and M.E. Cook. 1985. Essentiality of vitamin D_3 and its metabolites in poultry nutrition: a review. World Poult Sci J 41:52–63.
8. Ameenuddin, S., M.L. Sunde, and H.F. DeLuca. 1987. Lack of response of bone mineralization of chicks fed egg yolks from hens on dietary 1,25-dihydroxycholecalciferol. Poult Sci 66:1829–1834.
9. Asmundson, V.S., and F.H. Kratzer. 1952. Observations of vitamin A deficiency in turkey breeding stock. Poult Sci 31:71–73.
10. Austic, R.E. 1979. Nutritional influences on water intake in poultry. Proc Cornell Nutr Conf. Syracuse, NY, pp. 37–41.
11. Austic, R.E. 1981. Sodium, potassium and chlorine ratios in broiler nutrition. Proc Carolina Poult Nutr Conf. Charlotte, NC, pp. 1–5.
12. Austic, R.E., and R.K. Cole. 1972. Impaired renal clearance of uric acid in chickens having hyperuricemia and articular gout. Am J Physiol 223:525–530.
13. Austic, R.E., and K. Keshavarz. 1988. Interaction of dietary calcium and chloride and the influence of monovalent minerals on eggshell quality. Poult Sci 67:750–759.
14. Austic, R.E., and J.F. Patience. 1988. Undetermined anion in poultry diets: influence on acid-base balance, metabolism and physiological performance. CRC Crit Rev Poult Biol 1:315–345.

15. Bain, S.D., J.W. Newbrey, and B.A. Watkins. 1988. Biotin deficiency may alter tibiotarsal bone growth and modeling in broiler chicks. Poult Sci 67:590–595.
16. Baker, J.R., J. McC. Howell, and J.N. Thompson. 1967. Hypervitaminosis A in the chick. Br J Exp Pathol 48:507–512.
17. Baker, D.H., N.K. Allen, and A.J. Kleiss. 1973. Efficiency of tryptophan as a niacin precursor in the young chick. J Anim Sci 36:299–302.
18. Bar, A., S. Striem, J. Rosenberg, and S. Hurwitz. 1988. Egg shell quality and cholecalciferol metabolism in aged laying hens. J Nutr 118:1018–1023.
19. Baumgartner, S., D.J. Brown, E. Salevsky, Jr., and R.M. Leach, Jr. 1978. Copper deficiency in the laying hen. J Nutr 108:804–811.
20. Bearse, G.F., C.F. McClary, and H.C. Saxena. 1953. Blood spot incidence and the vitamin A level of the diet. Poult Sci 32:888.
21. Beer, A.E., M.L. Scott, and M.C. Nesheim. 1963. The effects of graded levels of pantothenic acid on the breeding performance of White Leghorn pullets. Br Poult Sci 4:243–253.
22. Bermudez, A.J., D.E. Swayne, M.W. Squires, and M.J. Radin. 1993. Effects of vitamin A deficiency on the reproductive system of mature White Leghorn hens. Avian Dis 37–183.
23. Bettger, W.J., J.E. Savage, and B.L. O'Dell. 1979. Effects of dietary copper and zinc on erythrocyte superoxide dismutase activity in the chick. Nutr Rep Int 19:893–900.
24. Bettger, W.J., P.G. Reeves, J.E. Savage, and B.L. O'Dell. 1980. Interaction of zinc and vitamin E in the chick. Proc Soc Exp Biol Med 163:432–436.
25. Bettger, W.J., P.G. Reeves, E.A. Moscatelli, J.E. Savage, and B.L. O'Dell. 1980. Interaction of zinc and polyunsaturated fatty acids in the chick. J Nutr 110:50–58.
26. Bettger, W.J., J.E. Savage, and B.L. O'Dell. 1981. Extracellular zinc concentration and water metabolism in chicks. J Nutr 111:1013–1019.
27. Briggs, G.M. 1946. Nicotinic acid deficiency in turkey poults and the occurrence of perosis. J Nutr 31:79–84.
28. Briggs, G.M., A.C. Groschke, and R.J. Lillie. 1946. Effect of proteins low in tryptophane on growth of chickens and on laying hens receiving nicotinic acid-low rations. J Nutr 32:659–675.
29. Bryden, W.L. 1991. Tissue depletion of biotin in chickens and the development of deficiency lesions and the fatty liver and kidney syndrome. Avian Pathol 20:259–269.
30. Buckingham, K., C.S. Heng-Khoo, M. Dubick, M. Lefevre, C. Cross, L. Julian, and R. Rucker. 1981. Copper deficiency and elastin metabolism in avian lung. Proc Soc Exp Biol Med 166:310–319.
31. Burk, R.F., and K.E. Hill. 1993. Regulation of selenoproteins. Annu Rev Nutr 13:65–81.
32. Burns, R.B. 1983. Antibody production suppressed in the domestic fowl (Gallus domesticus) by zinc deficiency. Avian Pathol 12:141–146.
33. Caskey, C.D., and L.C. Norris. 1940. Micromelia in adult fowl caused by manganese deficiency during embryonic development. Proc Soc Exp Biol Med 44:332–335.
34. Caskey, C.D., L.C. Norris, and G.F. Heuser. 1944. A chronic congenital ataxia in chicks due to manganese deficiency in the maternal diet. Poult Sci 23:516–520.
35. Chen, B.-J. 1989. Studies on the conversion of tryptophan to niacin in chickens and ducks. Ph.D. Thesis. Cornell University, Ithaca, NY.
36. Chicco, C.F., C.B. Ammerman, P.A. van Walleghem, P.W. Waldroup, and R.H. Harms. 1967. Effects of varying dietary ratios of magnesium, calcium, and phosphorus in growing chicks. Poult Sci 46:368–373.
37. Christensen, V.L., and J.F. Ort. 1988. Effect of dietary iodine on the permeability and hatchability of large white turkey eggs [abst]. Poult Sci 67(Suppl):67.

38. Chung, T.K., and D.H. Baker. 1990. Riboflavin requirement of chicks fed purified amino acid and conventional corn-soybean meal diets. Poult Sci 69:1357–1363.

39. Couch, J.R., W.W. Cravens, C.A. Elvehjem, and J.G. Halpin. 1948. Relation of biotin to congenital deformities in the chick. Anat Rec 100:29–48.

40. Cravens, W.W., W.H. McGibbon, and E.E. Sebesta. 1944. Effect of biotin deficiency on embryonic development in the domestic fowl. Anat Rec 90:55–64.

41. Creger, C.R., and J.T. Scott. 1980. Using zinc oxide to rest laying hens. Poult Dig 39:230–232.

42. Davis, P.N., L.C. Norris, and F.H. Kratzer. 1962. Iron deficiency studies in chicks using treated isolated soybean protein diets. J Nutr 78:445–453.

43. Dean, W.F., and G.F. Combs, Jr. 1981. Influence of dietary selenium on performance, tissue selenium content, and plasma concentrations of selenium-dependent glutathione peroxidase, vitamin E, and ascorbic acid in ducklings. Poult Sci 60:2655–2663.

44. Deetz, L.E., and R.C. Ringrose. 1976. Effect of heat stress on the potassium requirement of the hen. Poult Sci 55:1765–1770.

45. DeLuca, H.F. 1971. Vitamin D: a new look at an old vitamin. Nutr Rev 29:179–181.

46. Dewar, W.A., P.A.L. Wight, R.A. Pearson, and M.J. Gentle. 1983. Toxic effects of high concentrations of zinc oxide in the diet of the chick and laying hen. Br Poult Sci 24:397–404.

47. Dickson, I.R., and E. Kodicek. 1979. Effect of vitamin D deficiency on bone formation in the chick. Biochem J 182:429–435.

48. DiLorenzo, R.N. 1972. Studies of the genetic variation in tryptophan-nicotinic acid conversion in chicks. Ph.D. Thesis. Cornell University, Ithaca, NY.

49. Edwards, H.M., Jr. 1984. Studies on the etiology of tibial dyschondroplasia in chickens. J Nutr 114:1001–1013.

50. Edwards, H.M., Jr. 1990. Efficacy of several vitamin D compounds in the prevention of tibial dyschondroplasia in broiler chickens. J Nutr 120:1054–1061.

51. Edwards, H.M., Jr., M.A. Elliot, and S. Sooncharernying. 1992. Effect of dietary calcium on tibial dyschondroplasia. Interaction with light, cholecalciferol, 1,25-dihydroxycholecalciferol, protein, and synthetic zeolite. Poult Sci 71:2041–2055.

52. Edwards, H.M., Jr., M.A. Elliot, S. Sooncharernying, and W.M. Britton. 1994. Quantitative requirement for cholecalciferol in the absence of ultraviolet light. Poult Sci 73:288–294.

53. Elaroussi, M.A., H.F. DeLuca, L.R. Forte, and H.V. Biellier. 1993. Survival of vitamin D-deficient embryos: time and choice of cholecalciferol or its metabolites for treatment in ovo. Poult Sci 72:1118–1126.

54. Engel, R.W., P.H. Phillips, and J.G. Halpin. 1940. The effect of a riboflavin deficiency in the hen upon embryonic development of the chick. Poult Sci 19:135–142.

55. Ferguson, T.M., R.H. Rigdon, and J.R. Couch. 1956. Cataracts in vitamin E deficiency; An experimental study in the turkey embryo. Am Med Assoc Arch Ophthalmol (New York) 55:346–355.

56. Fisher, C., A.P. Laursen-Jones, K.J. Hill, and W.S. Hardy. 1973. The effect of copper sulphate on performance and the structure of the gizzard in broilers. Br Poult Sci 14:55–68.

57. Frigg, M. 1984. Available biotin content of various feed ingredients. Poult Sci 63:750–753.

58. Fritz, J.C., J.H. Hooper, J.L. Halpin, and H.P. Moore. 1946. Failure of feather pigmentation in bronze poults due to lysine deficiency. J Nutr 31:387–396.

59. Garvey, W.T., and R.E. Olson. 1978. In vitro vitamin K-dependent conversion of precursor to prothrombin in chick liver. J Nutr 108:1078–1086.

60. Gillis, M.B., G.F. Heuser, and L.C. Norris. 1948. Pantothenic acid in the nutrition of the hen. J Nutr 35:351–363.

61. Goldstein, J., and M.L. Scott. 1956. An electrophoretic study of exudative diathesis in chicks. J Nutr 60:349–359.

62. Goodson-Williams, R., D.A. Roland, Sr., and J.A. McGuire. 1986. Effects of feeding graded levels of vitamin D_3 on egg shell pimpling in aged hens. Poult Sci 65:1556–1560.

63. Gries, C.L., and M.L. Scott. 1972. The pathology of thiamin, riboflavin, pantothenic acid and niacin deficiencies in the chick. J Nutr 102:1269–1285.

64. Gries, C.L., and M.L. Scott. 1972. The pathology of pyridoxine deficiency in chicks. J Nutr 102:1259–1267.

65. Gries, C.L., and M.L. Scott. 1972. Pathology of selenium deficiency in the chick. J Nutr 102:1287–1296.

66. Halley, J.T., T.S. Nelson, L.K. Kirby, and Z.B. Johnson. 1987. Effect of altering dietary mineral balance on growth, leg abnormalities, and blood base excess in broiler chicks. Poult Sci 66:1684–1692.

67. Harms, R.H., R.E. Buresh, and H.R. Wilson. 1985. Sodium requirement of the turkey hen. Br Poult Sci 26:217–220.

68. Harms, R.H., N. Ruiz, R.E. Buresh, and H.R. Wilson. 1988. Effect of niacin supplementation of a corn-soybean meal diet on performance of turkey breeder hens. Poult Sci 67:336–338.

69. Heuser, G.F. 1952. Salt additions to chick rations. Poult Sci 31:85–88.

70. Hill, C.H., and G. Matrone. 1961. Studies on copper and iron deficiencies in growing chickens. J Nutr 73:425–431.

71. Hill, F.W., M.L. Scott, L.C. Norris, and G.F. Heuser. 1961. Reinvestigation of the vitamin A requirements of laying and breeding hens and their progeny. Poult Sci 40:1245–1254.

72. Hinshaw, W.R., and W.E. Lloyd. 1934. Vitamin-A deficiency in turkeys. Hilgardia 8:281–304.

73. Hooper, J.H., J.L. Halpin, and J.C. Fritz. 1942. The feeding of single massive doses of vitamin D to birds [abst]. Poult Sci 21:472.

74. Hopkins, D.T., and M.C. Nesheim. 1967. The linoleic acid requirement of chicks. Poult Sci 46:872–881.

75. Hopkinson, W.I. 1991. Reproduction of the sudden death syndrome of broiler breeders: A relative potassium imbalance. Avian Pathol 10:403–408.

76. Itakura, C., K. Yamasaki, and M. Goto. 1978. Pathology of experimental vitamin D deficiency rickets in growing chickens. 1. Bone. Avian Pathol 7:491–513.

77. Jensen, L.S., M.L. Scott, G.F. Heuser, L.C. Norris, and T.S. Nelson. 1956. Studies on the nutrition of breeding turkeys. I. Evidence indicating a need to supplement practical turkey rations with vitamin E. Poult Sci 35:810–816.

78. Jortner, B.S., J.B. Meldrum, C.H. Domermuth, and L.M. Potter. 1985. Encephalomalacia associated with hypovitaminosis E in turkey poults. Avian Dis 29:488–498.

79. Jukes, T.H., and F.H. Bird. 1942. Prevention of perosis by biotin. Proc Soc Exp Biol Med 49:231–232.

80. Julian, R.J. 1987. The effect of increased sodium in the drinking water on right ventricular hypertrophy, right ventricular failure and ascites in broiler chickens. Avian Pathol 16:61–71.

81. Julian, R.J., J. Summers, and J.B. Wilson. 1986. Right ventricular failure and ascites in broiler chicks caused by phosphorus-deficient diets. Avian Dis 30:453–459.

82. Jungherr, E. 1943. Nasal histopathology and liver storage in subtotal vitamin A deficiency of chickens. Conn Agric Exp Stn Bull No. 250, pp.1–36.

83. Kalemegham, R., and K. Krishnaswamy. 1975. Myelin lipids in vitamin B_{12} deficiency in chicks. Life Sci 16:1441–1445.

84. Kienholz, E.W., D.E. Turk, M.L. Sunde, and W.G. Hoekstra. 1961. Effects of zinc deficiency in the diets of hens. J Nutr 75:211–221.

85. Kratzer, F.H., J.L. Buenrostro, and B.A. Watkins, 1985. Biotin related abnormal fat metabolism in chickens and its consequences. Ann N Y Acad Sci 447:401–402.

86. Lacy, D.L., and W.E. Huffer. 1982. Studies on the pathogenesis of avian rickets. I. Changes in epiphyseal and metaphyseal vessels in hypocalcemic and hypophosphatemic rickets. Am J Pathol 109:288–301.

87. Lavelle, P.A., Q.P. Lloyd, C.V. Gay, and R.M. Leach, Jr. 1994. Vitamin K deficiency does not functionally impair skeletal metabolism of laying hens and their progeny. J Nutr 124:371–377.

88. Leach, R.M., Jr. 1968. Effect of manganese upon the epiphyseal growth plate in the young chick. Poult Sci 47:828–830.

89. Leach, R.M., Jr. 1974. Studies on the potassium requirement of the laying hen. J Nutr 104:684–686.

90. Leach, R.M., Jr. 1986. Chapter 6, Mn(II) and glycosyltransferases essential for skeletal development. In V.L. Schramm and F.C. Wedler (eds.). Manganese in Metabolism and Enzyme Function. Academic Press, Inc., pp. 81–91.

91. Leach, R.M., Jr., and M.C. Nesheim. 1963. Studies on chloride deficiency in chicks. J Nutr 81:193–199.

92. Leach, R.M., Jr., and M.C. Nesheim. 1972. Further studies on tibial dyschondroplasia (cartilage abnormality) in young chicks. J Nutr 102:1673–1680.

93. Lefevre, M., H. Heng, and R.B. Rucker. 1982. Dietary cadmium, zinc and copper: effects on chick lung morphology and elastin cross-linking. J Nutr 112:1344–1352.

94. Liu, A.C.-H., B.S. Heinrichs, and R.M. Leach, Jr. 1994. Influence of manganese deficiency on the characteristics of proteoglycans of avian epiphyseal growth plate cartilage. Poult Sci 73:663–669.

95. Long, P.H., S.R. Lee, G.N. Rowland, and W.M. Britton. 1984. Experimental rickets in broilers: gross, microscopic, and radiographic lesions. III. Vitamin D deficiency. Avian Dis 28:933–943.

96. Long, P.H., S.R. Lee, G.N. Rowland, and W.M. Britton. 1984. Experimental rickets in broilers: gross, microscopic, and radiographic lesions. II. Calcium deficiency. Avian Dis 28:921–932.

97. Long, P.H., S.R. Lee, G.N. Rowland, and W.M. Britton. 1984. Experimental rickets in broilers: gross, microscopic, and radiographic lesions. I. Phosphorus deficiency and calcium excess. Avian Dis 28:460–474.

98. Lü, J., and G.F. Combs, Jr. 1988. Effect of excess dietary zinc on pancreatic exocrine function in the chick. J Nutr 118:681–689.

99. Lü, J., and G.F. Combs, Jr. 1988. Excess dietary zinc decreases tissue a-tocopherol in chicks. J Nutr 118:1349–1359.

100. Lyons, M., and W.M. Insko, Jr. 1937. Chondrodystrophy in the chick embryo produced by manganese deficiency in the diet of the hen. Ky Agric Exp Stn Bull No. 371, pp. 61–75.

101. Manley, J.M., R.A. Voitle, and R.H. Harms. 1978. The influence of hatchability of turkey eggs from the addition of 25-hydroxycholecalciferol to the diet. Poult Sci 57:290–292.

102. Matterson, L.D., H.M. Scott, and E. Jungherr. 1946. Salt tolerance of turkeys. Poult Sci 25:539–541.

103. McCormick, C.C., and D.L. Cunningham. 1984. High dietary zinc and fasting as methods of forced resting: a performance comparison. Poult Sci 63:1201–1206.

104. McGinnis, J., and J.S. Carver. 1947. The effect of riboflavin and biotin in the prevention of dermatitis and perosis in turkey poults. Poult Sci 26:364–371.

105. McWard, G.W. 1967. Magnesium tolerance of the growing and laying chicken. Br Poult Sci 8:91–99.

106. Mechanic, G.L. 1977. The qualitative and quantitative crosslink chemistry of collagen matrices. Adv Exp Med Biol 86B:699–708.

107. Menge, H.C., C. Calvert and C.A. Denton. 1965. Further studies of the effect of linoleic acid on reproduction in the hen. J Nutr 86:115–119.

108. Misir, R., and R. Blair. 1988. Biotin bioavailability of protein supplements and cereal grains for starting turkey poults. Poult Sci 67:1274–1280.

109. Mongin, P. 1981. Recent advances in dietary anion-cation balance: applications in poultry. Proc Nutr Soc 40:285–294.

110. Morck, T.A., and R.E. Austic. 1981. Iron requirements of white leghorn hens. Poult Sci 60:1497–1503.

111. National Research Council. 1994. Nutrient requirements of poultry. National Academy of Sciences. Washington, DC.

112. Nesheim, M.C., R.M. Leach, Jr., and M.J. Norvell. 1967. The effect of rearing diet on choline deficiency in hens. Proc 1967 Cornell Nutr Conf. Buffalo, NY, pp. 57–60.

113. Noble, R.C., and J.H. Moore. 1966. Some aspects of the lipid metabolism of the chick embryo. In C. Horton-Smith and E.C. Amoroso (eds.). Physiology of the Domestic Fowl. Oliver and Boyd, London, pp. 87–102.

114. Nockels, C.F., and E.W. Kienholz. 1967. Influence of vitamin A deficiency on testes, bursa fabricius, adrenal and hematocrit in cockerels. J Nutr 92:384–388.

115. Noguchi, T., A.H. Cantor, and M.L. Scott. 1973. Mode of action of selenium and vitamin E in prevention of exudative diathesis in chicks. J Nutr 103:1502–1511.

116. O'Dell, B.L., P.M. Newberne, and J.E. Savage. 1958. Significance of dietary zinc for the growing chicken. J Nutr 65:503–518.

117. Oduho, G.W., Y. Han, and D.H. Baker. 1994. Iron deficiency reduces the efficacy of tryptophan as a niacin precursor. J Nutr 124:444–450.

118. Olcese, O., J.R. Couch, J.H. Quisenberry, and P.B. Pearson. 1950. Congenital anomalies in the chick due to vitamin B_{12} deficiency. J Nutr 41:423–431.

119. Opsahl, W., H. Zeronian, M. Ellison, D. Lewis, R.B. Rucker, and R.S. Riggins. 1982. Role of copper in collagen cross-linking and its influence on selected mechanical properties of chick bone and tendon. J Nutr 112:708–716.

120. Pappenheimer, A.M., M. Goettsch, and E. Jungherr. 1939. Nutritional encephalomalacia in chicks and certain related disorders of domestic birds. Conn Agric Exp Stn Bull 229.

121. Paredes, J.R., and T.P. Garcia. 1959. Vitamin A as a factor affecting fertility in cockerels. Poult Sci 38:3–7.

122. Patrick, H., R.V. Boucher, R.A. Dutcher, and H.C. Knandel. 1941. Biotin and prevention of dermatitis in turkey poults. Proc Soc Exp Biol Med 48:456–458.

123. Pearce, J., and D. Balnave. 1978. A review of biotin deficiency and the fatty liver and kidney syndrome in poultry. Br Vet J 134:598–609.

124. Peeler, H.T., R.F. Miller, C.W. Carlson, L.C. Norris, and G.F. Heuser. 1951. Studies of the effect of vitamin B_{12} on hatchability. Poult Sci 30:11–17.

125. Pesti, G.M., G.N. Rowland, and K.-S. Ryu. 1991. Folate deficiency in chicks fed diets containing practical ingredients. Poult Sci 70:600–604.

126. Peterson, D.W., W.H. Hamilton, and A.L. Lilyblade. 1971. Hereditary susceptibility to dietary induction of gout in selected lines of chickens. J Nutr 101:347–354.

127. Phillips, P.H., and R.W. Engel. 1939. Some histopathological observations on chicks deficient in the chick antidermatitis factor in pantothenic acid. J Nutr 18:227–232.

128. Reid, B.L., B.W. Heywang, A.A. Kurnick, M.G. Vavich, and B.J. Hulett. 1965. Effect of vitamin A and ambient temperature on reproductive performance of white leghorn pullets. Poult Sci 44:446–452.

129. Rennie, S., C.C. Whitehead, and B.H. Thorp. 1993. The effect of dietary 1,25-dihydroxycholecalciferol in preventing tibial dyschondroplasia in broilers fed on diets imbalanced in calcium and phosphorus. Br J Nutr 69:809–816.

130. Riddell, C., C.F. Helmboldt, E.P. Singsen, and L.D. Matterson. 1968. Bone pathology of birds affected with cage layer fatigue. Avian Dis 12:285–297.

131. Ringrose, A.T., L.C. Norris, and G.F. Heuser. 1931. The occurrence of a pellagra-like syndrome in chicks. Poult Sci 10:166–177.

132. Ringrose, R.C., A.G. Manoukas, R. Hinkson, and A.E. Teeri. 1965. The niacin requirement of the hen. Poult Sci 44:1053–1065.

133. Robel, E.J. 1977. A feather abnormality in chicks fed diets deficient in certain amino acids. Poult Sci 56:1968–1971.

134. Robel, E.J., and V.L. Christensen. 1987. Increasing hatchability of turkey eggs with biotin egg injections. Poult Sci 66:1429–1430.

135. Robel, E.J., and V.L. Christensen. 1991. Increasing hatchability of turkey eggs by injecting eggs with pyridoxine. Br Poult Sci 32:509–513.

136. Robertson, E.I., G.F. Fiala, M.L. Scott, L.C. Norris, and G.F. Heuser. 1947. Response of anemic chicks to pteroylglutamic acid. Proc Soc Exp Biol Med 64:441–443.

137. Rogler, J.C., H.E. Parker, F.N. Andrews, and C.W. Carrick. 1959. The effects of an iodine deficiency on embryo development and hatchability. Poult Sci 38:398–405.

138. Rucker, R.B., R.S. Riggins, R. Laughlin, M. M.Chan, M. Chen, and K. Tom. 1975. Effects of nutritional copper deficiency on the biomechanical properties of bone and arterial elastin metabolism in the chick. J Nutr 105:1062–1070.

139. Ruiz, N., and R.H. Harms. 1989. Riboflavin requirement of turkey poults fed a corn-soybean meal diet from 1 to 21 days of age. Poult Sci 68:715–718.

140. Sauveur, B., and P. Mongin. 1978. Tibial dyschondroplasia, a cartilage abnormality in poultry. Ann Biol Anim Biochem Biophys 18:87–98.

141. Scott, M.L. 1953. Prevention of the enlarged hock disorder in turkeys with niacin and vitamin E. Poult Sci 32:670–677.

142. Scott, M.L. 1962. Anti-oxidants, selenium and sulfur amino acids in the vitamin E nutrition of chicks. Nutr Abstr Rev 32:1–8.

143. Scott, M.L. 1962. Vitamin E in health and disease of poultry. Vitam Horm 20:621–632.

144. Scott, M.L. 1968. Rediscovery of biotin as a factor for prevention of leg weakness in turkeys. Feedstuffs 40:24–26.

145. Scott, M.L. 1980. Advances in our understanding of vitamin E. Fed Proc 39:2736–2739.

146. Scott, M.L., and G.F. Heuser. 1954. Studies on leg weakness in turkeys, ducks and geese. Proc 10th World Poult Congr. Edinburgh, Scotland, pp. 255–258.

147. Scott, M.L., G. Olson, L. Krook, and W.R. Brown. 1967. Selenium-responsive myopathies of myocardium and of smooth muscle in the young poult. J Nutr 91:573–583.

148. Seifried, O. 1930. Studies on A-avitaminosis in chickens. I. Lesions of the respiratory tract and their relation to some infectious diseases. J Exp Med 52:519–531.

149. Seifried, O. 1930. Studies on A-avitaminosis in chickens. II. Lesions of the upper alimentary tract and their relation to some infectious diseases. J Exp Med 52:533–538.

150. Shane, S.M., R.J. Young, and L. Krook. 1969. Renal and parathyroid changes produced by high calcium intake in growing pullets. Avian Dis 13:558–567.

151. Siller, W.G. 1981. Renal pathology of the fowl—A review. Avian Pathol 10:187–262.

152. Soares, J.H., Jr., M.R. Swerdel, and M.A. Ottinger. 1979. The effectiveness of vitamin D analog 1a-OH-D_3 in promoting fertility and hatchability in the laying hen. Poult Sci 58:1004–1006.

153. Soares, J.H., Jr., M.A. Ottinger, and E.G. Buss. 1988. Potential role of 1,25 dihydroxycholecalciferol in egg shell calcification. Poult Sci 67:1322–1328.

154. Starcher, B.C., C.H. Hill, and J.G. Madaras. 1980. Effect of zinc deficiency on bone collagenase and collagen turnover. J Nutr 110:2095–2102.

155. Stevens, V.I., R. Blair, R.E. Salmon, and J.P. Stevens. 1984. Effect of varying levels of dietary vitamin D_3 on turkey hen egg production, fertility and hatchability, embryo mortality and incidence of embryo beak malformations. Poult Sci 63:760–764.

156. Stillmak, S.J., and M.L. Sunde. 1971. The use of high magnesium limestone in the diet of the laying hen. I. Egg production. Poult Sci 50:553–564.

157. Sullivan, T.W., 1964. Studies on the dietary requirement and interaction of magnesium with antibiotics in turkeys to 4 weeks of age. Poult Sci 43:401–405.

158. Sunde, R.A., and W.G. Hoekstra. 1980. Structure, synthesis and function of glutathione peroxidase. Nutr Rev 38:265–273.

159. Sunde, M.L., W.W. Cravens, H.W. Bruins, C.A. Elvehjem, and J.G. Halpin. 1950. The pteroylglutamic acid requirement of laying and breeding hens. Poult Sci 29:220–226.

160. Sunde, M.L., W.W. Cravens, C.A. Elvehjem, and J.G. Halpin. 1950. The effect of folic acid on embryonic development of the domestic fowl. Poult Sci 29:696–702.

161. Sunde, M.L., C.M. Turk, and H.F. DeLuca. 1978. The essentiality of vitamin D metabolites for embryonic chick development. Science 200:1067–1069.

162. Swayne, D.E., A. Shlosberg, and R.B. Davis. 1986. Salt poisoning in turkey poults. Avian Dis 30:847–852.

163. Tang, K.-N., G.N. Rowland, and J.R. Veltmann, Jr. 1985. Vitamin A toxicity: comparative changes in bone of the broiler and leghorn chicks. Avian Dis 29:416–429.

164. Thompson, J.N., and M.L. Scott. 1969. Role of selenium in the nutrition of the chick. J Nutr 97:335–342.

165. Thompson, J.N., and M.L. Scott. 1970. Impaired lipid and vitamin E absorption related to atrophy of the pancreas in selenium-deficient chicks. J Nutr 100:797–809.

166. Thompson, J.N., J. McC. Howell, G.A.J. Pitt, and C.I. Houghton. 1965. Biological activity of retinoic acid ester in the domestic fowl: production of vitamin A deficiency in the early chick embryo. Nature (London) 205:1006–1007.

167. Tsang, C.P.W. 1992. Calcitriol reduces egg breakage. Poult Sci 71:215–217.

168. Tsang, C.P.W., and A.A. Grunder. 1993. Effect of dietary contents of cholecalciferol, 1a,25-dihydroxycholecalciferol and 24,25-dihydroxycholecalciferol on blood concentrations of 25-hydroxycholecalciferol, 1a,25-dihydroxycholecalciferol, total calcium and eggshell quality. Br Poult Sci 34:1021–1027.

169. Tsang, C.P.W., A.A. Grunder, and R. Narbaitz. 1990. Optimal dietary level of 1a,25-dihydroxycholecalciferol for eggshell quality in laying hens. Poult Sci 69:1702–1712.

170. Watkins, B.A., and F.H. Kratzer. 1987. Dietary biotin effects on polyunsaturated fatty acids in chick tissue lipids and prostaglandin E_2 levels in freeze-clamped hearts. Poult Sci 66:1818–1828.

171. Watkins, B.A., S.D. Bain, and J.W. Newhrey. 1989. Eicosanoic fatty acid reduction in the tibiotarsus of biotin-deficient chicks. Calcif Tissue Int 45:41–46.

172. Weaver, V.M., and J. Welsh. 1993. 1,25-dihydroxycholecalciferol supplementation prevents hypocalcemia in magnesium-deficient chicks. J Nutr 123:764–771.

173. Welsh, J., R. Schwartz, and L. Krook. 1981. Bone pathology and parathyroid gland activity in hypocalcemic magnesium-deficient chicks. J Nutr 111:514–524.

174. Whitacre, M.E., G.F. Combs, Jr., S.B. Combs, and R.S. Parker. 1987. Influence of dietary vitamin E on nutritional pancreatic atrophy in selenium-deficient chicks. J Nutr 117:460–467.

175. Whitehead, C.C., D.W. Bannister, A.J. Evans, W.G. Siller, and P.A.L. Wight. 1976. Biotin deficiency and fatty liver and kidney syndrome in chicks given purified diets containing different fat and protein levels. Br J Nutr 35:115–125.

176. Whitehead, C.C., J.A. Armstrong, and D. Waddington. 1982. The determination of the availability to chicks of biotin in feed ingredients by a bioassay based on the response of blood pyruvate carboxylase (EC 6.4.1.1) activity. Br J Nutr 48:81–88.

177. Wideman, R.F., Jr., J.A. Closser, W.B. Roush, and B.S. Cowen. 1985. Urolithiasis in pullets and laying hens: role of dietary calcium and phosphorus. Poult Sci 64:2300–2307.

178. Wideman, R.F., B.C. Ford, J.J. DiLner, W.W. Robey, and A.G. Yersin. 1994. Responses of laying hens to diets containing up to 2% DL-methionine or equimolar (2.25%) 2-hydroxy-4-(methylthio)butanoic acid. Poult Sci 73:259–267.

179. Wight, P.A.L., and W.A. Dewar. 1976. The histopathology of zinc deficiency in ducks. J Pathol 120:183–191.

180. Wight, P.A.L., and W.A. Dewar. 1979. Some histochemical observations on zinc deficiency in chickens. Avian Pathol 8:437–451.

181. Wight, P.A.L., W.A. Dewar, and C.L. Saunderson. 1986. Zinc toxicity in the fowl: ultrastructural pathology and relationship to selenium, lead and copper. Avian Pathol 15:23–38.

182. Wilgus, H.S., Jr., L.C. Norris, and G.F. Heuser. 1937. The role of manganese and certain other trace elements in the prevention of perosis. J Nutr 14:155–167.

183. Wilgus, H.S., Jr., L.C. Norris, and G.F. Heuser. 1937. The effect of various calcium and phosphorus salts on the severity of perosis. Poult Sci 16:232–237.

184. Wilgus, H.S., Jr., G.S. Harshfield, A.R. Patton, L.P. Ferris, and F.X. Gassner. 1941. The iodine requirements of growing chickens [abst]. Poult Sci 20:477.

185. Wolbach, S.B., and D.M. Hegsted. 1952. Vitamin A deficiency in the chick. Skeletal growth and the central nervous system. Arch Pathol 54:13–29.

186. Wolbach, S.B., and D.M. Hegsted. 1952. Vitamin A deficiency in the duck. Skeletal growth and the central nervous system. Arch Pathol 54:548–563.

187. Wolbach, S.B., and D.M. Hegsted. 1952. Hypervitaminosis A and the skeleton of growing chicks. Arch Pathol 54:30–38.

188. Wolbach, S.B., and D.M. Hegsted. 1953. Hypervitaminosis A in young ducks. The epiphyseal cartilages. Arch Pathol 55:47–54.

189. Woolam, D.H.M., and J.W. Millen. 1955. Effect of vitamin A deficiency on the cerebro-spinal fluid pressure of the chick. Nature (London) 175:41–42.

190. Yang, C.-P., and S.-L. Jenq. 1989. Pyridoxine deficiency and requirement in mule ducklings. J Chin Agric Chem Soc 27:450–459.

191. Young, R.J., L.C. Norris, and G.F. Heuser. 1955. The chicks requirement for folic acid in the utilization of choline and its precursors betaine and methylaminoethanol. J Nutr 55:353–362.

192. Young, R.J., H.M. Edwards, Jr., and M.B. Gillis. 1958. Studies on zinc in poultry nutrition. II. Zinc requirement and deficiency symptoms of chicks. Poult Sci 37:1100–1107.

INTERACTIONS BETWEEN NUTRITION AND INFECTIOUS DISEASE

Kirk C. Klasing

INTRODUCTION. There are extremely important interactions, synergisms, and antagonisms between nutrition and immunity that markedly affect productivity of poultry. Two types of interactions occur. First, nutrition can impact the immunocompetence of birds and, thus, their resistance to infectious disease. Second, immune responses due to infectious challenges impact growth, reproduction, metabolism, and nutrient requirements. Pathology from infectious organisms can impact the digestion and metabolism of nutrients. Further, these important interactions can lead to a malnutrition–infection cycle. Malnutrition results in increased incidence, duration, or lethality of infectious diseases, and infections cause anorexia and malnutrition. Regardless of whether the cycle begins by poor nutrition or by inadequate control of disease, the immune system and nutrient status can simultaneously deteriorate, resulting in opportunistic infections and poor production.

In poultry, there are over 35 required nutrients and dozens of economically important infectious diseases, resulting in many hundreds of specific nutrient–disease combinations. Although there is little specific information on many of these combinations, the interactions between nutrition and immunity can be reduced to the underlying mechanisms and principles. When considering the impact of infection on nutrient requirements, there are many changes that are mediated by the immune system and are common to most disease organisms. Similarly, when considering the impact of nutrition on immunity and disease resistance, there are several mechanisms and actions that can be generalized across most nutrients. For any nutrient–disease interaction of interest, these generalized changes and actions must be interpreted in light of the pathology specific to that pathogen and nutrient combination.

NUTRITION VERSUS IMMUNOCOMPETENCE. Severe, chronic deficiencies of most nutrients impair the immune response and increase susceptibility to infectious diseases. This is not surprising given the continued development and maturation of the immune system following hatching and the high rate of cell division and large number of enzyme cofactors that are needed to elicit an immune response. Severe nutrient deficiencies are particularly deleterious to the immune system when they occur early in life during the development of the primary lymphoid organs and the maturation of the immune system. In mammals, nutrient deficiencies that are especially damaging to the immune system and that presumably result in greater incidence of infection include those of linoleic acid, vitamins A and E, iron, selenium, and the B vitamins. The literature in poultry is incomplete, but a similar pattern may occur (7, 10, 34). For example, vitamin A deficiency reduces antibody responses, causes lymphocyte depletion of lymphoid organs and tissues resulting in lower thymic and bursal weights (9), and causes a deterioration of the mucosal epithelium that provides a barrier to invading microorganisms. In disease-challenge models, deficient vitamin A intake increases the incidence of Newcastle disease virus–induced mortality (49). White leghorn chicks with vitamin E or selenium deficiencies have decreased humoral immune responses at low, but not high, immunogen doses (36). In young chicks, both nutrients have to be supplemented in order to stimulate immunity above the level observed in chicks with a combined deficiency (36), and when supplemented together, vitamin E and selenium decrease the mortality and weight loss due to malabsorption (infectious stunting) syndrome (6). Chicks deficient in vitamin E and selenium have impaired development of the bursa, spleen, and thymus. Supplementation of vitamins and trace minerals is relatively inexpensive. Their levels in modern poultry diets are rarely deficient and more commonly contain many times the requirement set by the National Research Council (NRC). High levels of vitamin A, however, interfere with vitamin E absorption, and the potential for deleterious interactions in commercial diets exists. For example, Veltman et al. (56) found that supplementing broiler diets with vitamin A exacerbated the morbidity due to malabsorption syndrome presumably by an interaction with vitamin D or vitamin E, which precipitates a deficiency.

Fortunately, severe deficiencies of nutrients are rarely seen in modern animal production due to the scientific formulation of diets. From a practical point of view, several nutrients can markedly modulate immune responses and disease resistance when dietary levels are varied over ranges that are marginally below to well above those required to meet typical dietary recommendations. The mechanisms through which nutrients can impact the immune system are diverse.

Mechanisms of Nutritionally Induced Changes in Immunity

IMPACT OF NUTRITION ON SUBSTRATE SUPPLY. Nutrient recommendations are typically developed using indices of productivity such as growth or egg production as the criteria for adequacy. Immunocompetence is often not examined. Fortunately, for most nutrients, the levels that optimize growth or reproduction are also adequate for optimal immunocompetence. The binding affinities of transport proteins on the cell membranes of leukocytes suggest that the immune system has a high priority for circulating nutrients and is able to compete favorably with many other tissues when nutrient levels are low. In this regard, the leukocytes have a high position in the hierarchy of competition for nutrient use. During an immune response, leukocytes release cytokines such as interleukins 1 and 6. These cytokines act systemically to mobilize large quantities of nutrients from other tissues, especially skeletal muscle and bone (see below). Thus, the immune system can liberate nutrients in amounts proportional to the size of the immune response, buffering marginal dietary deficiencies due to faulty formulation.

During the immune response, the need for nutrients for the clonal proliferation of responding leukocytes and for the production of antibody and other effector molecules is small in comparison to the amount liberated from other tissues. During the acute phase of an immune response, the greatest nutritional need is for the synthesis and release of acute phase proteins by the liver (12). This process requires approximately 10 times more energy and amino acids than are needed by responding leukocytes. Synthesis of acute-phase proteins is comparatively more sensitive than specific immunity to deficiencies of several nutrients including amino acids and trace minerals (21, 31).

There are not many examples in which the dietary level of a nutrient required to supply adequate substrate to the immune system to optimize disease resistance is higher than the level set by the NRC as the requirement. Potential nutrients in which a margin of safety may be needed to improve immunocompetence include vitamin E (see next section) and possibly methionine and arginine. Levels of arginine well above that required to maximize body weight gain of New Hampshire chicks augment nitric oxide production and decrease the growth profile of Rous sarcoma virus–induced tumors (52). Methionine is the first limiting amino acid in most commercial feeds and the most likely nutrient to be marginally deficient. Tsiagbe et al. (53) observed that the requirement for methionine to support maximal humoral and cell-mediated immune responses is greater than that for growth, but other investigators have not observed this relationship (3). Methionine-deficient diets do not result in more severe lesion scores during coccidiosis infections than diets that meet the requirement (39), and either a methionine- or lysine-deficient diet markedly decreases the morbidity associated with an *Eimeria acervulina* infection as indicated by better weight gain (60).

The literature is replete with other examples whereby marginal deficiencies of nutrients actually increase indices of immunity and disease resistance. For example, modern broiler chicks fed diets typically used during the late 1950s that are low in energy and marginally deficient in sulfur amino acids and several trace minerals had improved indices of humoral immunity and macrophage function compared with chicks fed a modern diet meeting all NRC requirements (43). Hill and Garren (16) demonstrated that decreasing the protein level in the diet from 30% to 20% to 10% of the diet resulted in progressively decreasing rates of mortality of chicks from *Salmonella gallinarum* infection. Boyd and Edwards (4) observed decreased mortality with protein-deficient diets following challenges with either *S. gallinarum* or Newcastle disease virus. Protein-deficient diets also reduced the severity of disease and the mortality level from *E. tenella* infection due to the lack of trypsin activity in the intestinal tract and a decrease in excystation of the oocysts (5).

NUTRIENTS AS IMMUNOREGULATORY AGENTS. Dietary manipulations of some nutrients result in immunoregulatory consequences due to the participation of the nutrient or its products in communication within and between leukocytes. The best example of this is the role of essential and other dietary fatty acids in cellular communication, membrane fluidity, and second messenger elaboration. After consumption, these fatty acids are either incorporated directly into membranes or they are elongated and further desaturated prior to incorporation into membranes. A portion of dietary linoleic acid, the most prevalent n-6 fatty acid in feed, is metabolized to arachidonic acid prior to incorporation into membranes. Arachidonic acid is the precursor for eicosanoids, such as the prostaglandins, thromboxanes, and leukotrienes. The amount and potency of eicosanoid production is related to membrane concentration of arachidonic acid and, consequently, the dietary levels of linoleic acid. The dietary concentration of n-3 fatty acids, such as linolenic and eicosapentenoic acids modifies the rate at which arachidonic acid is converted to eicosanoids. Thus, the ratio of dietary n-3 to n-6 fatty acids determines the type and rate of eicosanoid production in leukocytes and accessory cells, and modulates the immune response. This interpretation is probably an oversimplification, since these two fatty acid classes also determine membrane fluidity and receptor-binding activities and participate in second messenger generation.

In growing white leghorn chicks, feeding dietary n-3 fatty acids from fish oil enhances the antibody response of chicks to sheep red blood cells but suppresses rates of lymphocyte proliferation after mitogen stimulation (11). Macrophage function and the regulatory roles of macrophages are also sensitive to dietary fat source. The release of interleukin-1 by *Staphylococcus aureus*–stimulated macrophages from broiler chicks fed high levels of n-6 fatty acids was markedly increased compared with that seen with chicks fed diets high in n-3 fatty acids (33). Indicators of the acute-phase response to *S. typhimurium* lipopolysaccharide were also elevated in diets with high ratios of n-6 to n-3 fatty acids. Practical feed ingredients high in n-6 fatty acids include corn, vegetable oils, restaurant grease, and poultry fat. Fish fat, fish meal, and linseed oil are the major dietary sources of n-3 fatty acids. Lard and tallow are not particularly rich sources of either of the immunoregulatory fatty acids.

Research with laboratory rodents demonstrated that other nutrients have immunoregulatory roles within the range of dietary levels commonly fed. These include arginine, vitamin C, vitamin D (in the 1,25 configuration), vitamin E, and vitamin A. Vitamin C and vitamin E appear to exert at least some of their positive effects by serving as antioxidants and maintaining the stability of leukocyte membranes in the face of high levels of reactive oxygen intermediates at inflammatory sites. Vitamin E and vitamin A, however, have immunoregulatory action on avian leukocytes that is independent of their antioxidant functions. Vitamin E decreases prostaglandin E_2 release and modulates cytokine release, and vitamin A increases antigen-specific responses in T cells via the retinoic acid receptor (13, 44). In both cases, the immunomodulatory effects are large and occur with vitamin levels well above the established requirement.

Translation of the regulatory shifts due to nutrients into disease resistance has not been well studied except in the case of vitamin E. The addition of vitamin E to the diet of broiler chicks and turkeys in excess of that required for normal growth and reproduction stimulates humoral immunity and reduces the severity of an *Escherichia coli* infection as indicated by mortality and weight gain (40). Likewise, supplementation of diets fed to commercial broiler flocks with 178 IU/kg vitamin E decreases the morbidity of subclinical infectious bursal disease compared with diets containing 48 IU/kg (37). The NRC requirement is 10 mg/kg.

INFLUENCE OF NUTRITION ON HORMONAL MILIEU. The immune system is not an autonomous system but is influenced by other physiologic systems (35). Leukocytes have receptors for many of the hormones involved in homeostasis. The nutritionally responsive hormones insulin, glucagon, corticosterone, growth hormone, insulin-like growth factor-1, thyroxin, and the catecholamines regulate the activity of immune cells. A diet-induced change in the relative concentration of these hormones can impact leukocytes during the critical early phase of the immune response when the cells that recognize antigen commit to cell cycling, cytokine production, and initiation of the immune response.

In broiler chicks, short periods (24 hr) of feed deprivation enhance both cellular and humoral immune responses. Conversely, overconsumption of feed impairs immunoglobulin production and delayed-type hypersensitivity. Overconsumption results in a high insulin to glucagon ratio, which presumably mediates this effect (25). Meal frequency and diet composition are often varied to accomplish various management goals in poultry production. For example, growing broiler breeder chicks are commonly placed on a skip-a-day feeding regimen to improve viability and productivity. Some of the improvement is due to increased humoral immunity and an inhibition of the age-related involution of the thymus and bursa. Feeding a restricted amount of feed daily also improves viability, productivity, and resistance to infections (24, 41). In growing Plymouth Rock chickens, feed restriction to 60% of ad libitum intake improves resistance to *E. tenella* (61) and marble spleen disease (62). Restricted feeding of a diet low in nutrient density increases the dose of *S. enteritidis* required to establish an infection. Prolonged periods of starvation, however, result in greatly elevated corticosterone levels and eventually impair both cellular and humoral immune responses. White leghorn hens fasted for 14 days to force a molt have depressed cell-mediated immunity and decreased peripheral blood CT4+ helper T lymphocytes and are more susceptible to *S. enteritidis* infections (19, 20).

IMPACT ON THE PATHOLOGY DUE TO AN IMMUNE RESPONSE. When the immune system responds against invading pathogens, it produces a wide variety of noxious agents including proteolytic and other hydrolytic enzymes, reactive oxygen intermediates, and reactive nitrogen derivatives, which destroy bacteria, parasites, or infected cells. These defensive agents can injure normal host cells and result in various types of pathology. Several nutrients can modulate the degree of pathology induced by an immune response. For example, antioxidants such as vitamins E and C and xanthophils protect host cells from the damaging effects of superoxides and limit the extent of pathology. The quantity of these antioxidants in tissues is directly affected by dietary levels. A deficiency in vitamin E or selenium results in peroxidation of membrane lipids

during an inflammatory response to *S. minnesota* lipopolysaccharide (51). Similarly, the antiinflammatory effects of n-3 fatty acids can reduce the level of intestinal pathology associated with *E. tenella* infection in broiler chicks (32).

NUTRITIONAL IMMUNITY. Pathogens often require a host source of nutrients for their replication and virulence. The host animal can sometimes decrease the rate of replication of bacteria and parasites by withholding nutrients. For example, in broiler chicks and white leghorn hens, iron is removed from the circulation and sequestered into compartments that are nutritionally unavailable to bacteria and parasites (14). Iron becomes the first limiting nutrient for the growth of the pathogen. In mammals, replenishing the iron lost in biologic fluids by injections or very high dietary supplementation increases the mortality and morbidity due to a variety of disease organisms. Tuft and Nockels (54) have shown that feeding ethylenediaminetetraacetic acid (EDTA) increases the deposition of iron in tissues of chicks and increases its plasma level. This predisposes chicks to increased mortality after a challenge with *E. coli*, presumably by making iron or zinc more available for the replication and virulence of the pathogen.

FEEDSTUFF-SPECIFIC EFFECTS. The use of some feedstuffs results in an increased incidence of infectious disease due to nonnutrient effects in the intestine. Components of the feedstuff that are not enzymatically digested in the upper gastrointestinal tract provide nutrients to microflora in the ileum, cecum, and large intestine, influencing the ecology within these organs. Changes in the types of gastrointestinal microflora due to dietary fiber have been well documented, although the association of these changes with incidence of infectious disease is not well characterized. Some nonstarch polysaccharides such as ß-glucans markedly affect the viscosity of the digesta in the lower gastrointestinal tract, and other components of fiber can physically cause erosion of the epithelia. Barley, which is high in nonstarch polysaccharides, has been associated with increased incidence of necrotic enteritis and elevated numbers of *Clostridium perfringens* in the ileum (18, 23).

The presence of unstabilized, rancid fat in the diet increases numbers of *E. coli* and lowers numbers of lactobacilli in the small intestine (Dibner 1995). Fat sources with high levels of free fatty acids, polyunsaturated fatty acids, and low levels of antioxidants are especially susceptible to oxidative rancidity. Lectins that are especially rich in legumes can stimulate intestinal epithelial cells, affecting motility and modulating the associated microflora.

A wide variety of mycotoxins found in feeds also have marked effects on intestinal microflora and on gastrointestinal morphology and physiology.

EFFECT OF INFECTIOUS DISEASE ON PRODUCTIVITY AND NUTRIENT NEEDS.

During many infectious agent challenges, monocytes and macrophages recognize foreign organisms and release interleukin-1, interleukin-6, and tumor necrosis factor. Each of these monokines has a specific role in the regulation of the immune response by acting in the local area of challenge. They also act systemically by binding to receptors on cells of all tissues. Lastly, they can have indirect systemic effects by altering levels of hormones such as insulin, glucagon, and corticosterone. Through their systemic actions, leukocytic cytokines orchestrate metabolic changes that underlie the classic acute-phase symptoms of anorexia, lethargy, fever, increased blood heterophil counts, muscle catabolism, and bone resorption (26, 28). The metabolic changes represent a homeorhetic response that alters the partitioning of dietary nutrients away from growth, skeletal muscle accretion, or reproduction in favor of metabolic process that support the immune response and disease resistance. Such changes form the basis of impaired growth, feed utilization, and altered nutritional requirements of sick birds. The decreased feed intake accounts for about 70% of the decreased growth, while the remainder is due to metabolic inefficiencies caused by the immune response (29).

The impact of an immune response to a pathogen challenge on productivity is proportional to the intensity and duration of the challenge. Each disease organism has its own pathologic effect on specific organs, which modifies the generic response. Many pathogens synthesize toxins that cause additional pathology. Consequently, the total impact of an infectious challenge on metabolism and nutrition is the sum of generalized effects of the immune system responding to the presence of the pathogen plus specific effects due to the destructive actions of the pathogen itself.

Nutrient recommendations such as those set by NRC are usually based on needs by healthy animals raised under excellent management. The established requirements often do not include a "margin of safety" for deviations from the ideal situation. The use of these recommended values requires adjustments for stresses experienced in practical production situations. Modification of nutrient requirements due to an infectious challenge should be considered during at least two separate situations. First, diet changes may be necessary during the challenge when growth is slowed and the immune system is responding vigorously, and second, dietary changes may be needed following elimination of the challenging organism when pathologic insults are repaired and compensatory growth typically occurs. Thus, in the normal animal we feed for normal growth, in the infected animal we feed for the immune response, and in the convalescing bird we feed for accelerated growth and tissue repair. There is a plethora of information on nutrition in the healthy bird and little information on the disease-stressed or the convalescing animal (25). In fact, there is a general reluctance to publish the results of experiments designed to determine nutrient requirements if a disease situation develops.

Because the most deleterious aspect of a disease challenge on growth and reproduction is due to decreased feed intake, manipulations of the nutrient density of the diet would appear prudent. Increasing the energy density of a ration with carbohydrates while keeping required nutrients at a constant percent of the energy improved energy intake and the rate of gain of broiler chicks challenged with *S. typhimurium* lipopolysaccharide (2). Conversely, the negative impact of an immune response on intake and rate of gain of broiler chicks is more evident at lower dietary energy. This interaction between dietary energy level and performance during an immunologic challenge was not seen in turkey poults (42).

The requirement for lysine and methionine is decreased during an immune challenge in young broiler chicks, probably as a result of slower growth rates and decreased skeletal muscle accretion (27). Following the disease process, compensatory growth induces an increase in amino acid requirements. In practice, if only one diet is to be fed, the amino acid fortification that supports maximal growth across the different physiologic states may be greater than that commonly recommended. Though additional amino acid fortification may be necessary to support intermittent periods of compensatory growth, this may not always be a least-cost level because there is a surfeit of amino acids during periods when birds are actually being challenged and when they are healthy. Thus, in the case of amino acids, a margin of safety may be needed to permit accelerated growth following disease challenges, but it is not needed during the course of the disease unless pathology specific to the pathogen adds to the requirement (30).

As discussed in previous sections, maximal disease resistance often occurs at dietary energy and protein levels well below those that maximize performance. In the case of especially pathogenic disease organisms, feeding diets that give maximal gain and feed efficiency during the course of an infectious challenge may be contraindicated.

Quantitative changes in the requirement of trace

minerals as the result of a disease challenge have not been subjected to detailed study in poultry but can be surmised from known changes in metabolism, absorption, and excretion. Low circulating levels of iron and zinc are an integral part of the immune response brought about by interleukins 1 and 6 and do not, in themselves, indicate higher requirements. The increased use of zinc, manganese, and copper for hepatic acute-phase protein synthesis indicates a severalfold increase in the requirement at the tissue level (14). In the short term, this increased tissue requirement is met largely by a redistribution within the body. In the case of copper, increased fortification of trace minerals over the requirement of nonstressed animals does not augment these redistributions (31). Preventing the decrease in circulating iron or zinc may impair resistance to some (54), but not all, pathogens (15). Increased excretion of zinc and copper and decreased absorption of iron indicate (17) a net loss of trace minerals during the immune response. Thus, good mineral stores prior to the disease challenge are important, and an increase in the requirement for trace minerals is indicated following an infectious challenge.

Changes in the need for vitamins during infectious disease are not well understood. In the case of fat-soluble vitamins (A, D, E, and K) and xanthophils, absorption is impaired due to poorer fat absorption. Newcastle disease virus infection compromises vitamin A status of white leghorn chicks by interfering with retinol-binding protein metabolism in liver and by increasing the rate of utilization and catabolism of retinol and retinol-binding protein in extrahepatic tissues (49). Infectious bronchitis also increases the utilization of vitamin A by tissues, and reovirus infection appears to impair vitamin A status through decreasing absorption and increasing endogenous losses (58). Needs for antioxidants at the tissue level are also increased because of the higher burden of reactive oxygen intermediates emanating from the immune system (12, 51). Together, these changes would indicate increased dietary needs during a disease challenge.

The nutritional modifications discussed above represent best guesses to maximize gain and feed efficiency during a generalized immune response. The specific pathology associated with a disease state may cause additional changes in nutrient requirements. This is especially true for diseases that affect the gastrointestinal tract and impair nutrient absorption or increase the endogenous loss of nutrients (47). Nutrient absorption during coccidiosis is related to the nutrient studied, the stage of infection, and the severity of infection (55). Each species of *Eimeria* tends to localize in a specific region of the intestinal tract resulting in disruptions of digestive, absorptive, and secretory functions specific for that region. Compensatory changes occurring in unin-

fected regions mitigate some of the negative impact (46). Changes in intestinal morphology, including shortening of villi, loss of microvilli, decrease in villous surface area, and reduction of mucosal thickness are probably related to impaired digestive and absorptive capacities. A decreased rate of passage of feed through the gastrointestinal tract and retention of food in the crop and gizzard probably also contribute to lower digestibility of feed (38). The leakage of plasma proteins into the intestinal tract is also a major factor affecting the apparent digestibility of protein (22). The net result of coccidial-induced intestinal pathology is impaired absorption of protein and energy, causing a reduction in the metabolizable energy value of the diet (48). Although the combination of impaired absorption and increased endogenous losses would point to higher amino acid requirements, this is not the case. Methionine requirements of young growing chicks are not increased during coccidial infection (39, 59), apparently because decreased digestibility is offset by lower needs due to slower growth rates. The intestine closely regulates the absorption of trace minerals to prevent toxicities when feed or water levels are high. In the case of copper absorption, this regulation is impaired due to a mixed coccidial infection, increasing the likelihood of copper toxicity in turkey poults (57). *E. acervulina* infection of broiler chicks does not increase the toxicity of high dietary levels of zinc or increase the zinc requirement (50).

Malabsorption syndrome results in pathology in most regions of the gastrointestinal tract and does not appear to permit compensatory adaptations during or after acute infections. Thus, the magnitude of digestive disturbances is greater than in coccidiosis. Experimentally induced malabsorption syndrome in turkey poults results in a 40% reduction in growth, impaired conversion of absorbed nutrients into weight gain, and loss of enteric digestive enzymes (1, 47). Some of these effects can be alleviated by feeding a complex diet devoid of soymeal instead of a typical corn–soymeal diet. Changes in nutrient requirements during malabsorption syndrome result from the balance between increased needs due to poor utilization of dietary nutrients and decreased needs resulting from poor growth rates; such changes need to be quantified by further investigation.

Subclinical Challenges versus Productivity. There is little doubt that most infectious diseases decrease the productivity of poultry. Decreased performance is also associated with subclinical challenges, even from organisms not usually considered to be pathogenic. Chicks housed in germ-free environments grow 15% faster than those raised in conventional environments where they are continuously exposed to microflora. Chicks housed in disinfected quarters grow faster and convert a higher percent of their feed into body mass than chicks housed in less sanitary conditions, even in the absence of infectious diseases and pathogenic agents. The differences become larger and more devastating as sanitary conditions worsen.

Broiler chicks raised in environments with poor sanitation have markedly higher levels of circulating interleukin-1 than chicks raised with excellent sanitation. Presumably, the high burden of microbes, dust, and dander chronically stimulates the immune system and induces the release of interleukin-1. As described above, high circulating levels of interleukin-1 result in slower growth. Feeding antibiotics to chicks in a dirty environment decreases the amount of circulating interleukin-1 to levels similar to those in chicks raised in a clean environment. Feeding antibiotics results in little or no improvement in growth rate or changes in circulating interleukin-1 levels in clean environments. Thus, it appears that antibiotics may act by limiting the number of times, and the vigor with which, the immune system must respond to dispose of frequent microbial challenges in the intestines (45). In turkeys, this is manifested as improved growth and decreased intestinal thickness, intestinal lymphoid mass, and numbers of lymphocytes (8).

REFERENCES

1. Angel, C.R., J.L. Sell, and D.W. Trampel. 1990. Stunting syndrome in turkeys. Development of an experimental model. Avian Dis 34:447–453.
2. Benson, B.N., C.C. Calvert, E. Roura and K.C. Klasing. 1993. Dietary energy source and density modulate the expression of immunologic stress in chicks. J Nutr 93:1714–1723.
3. Bhargava, K.K., R.P. Hanson, and M.L. Sunde. 1970. Effects of methionine and valine on growth and antibody production in chicks infected with live or killed Newcastle disease virus. J Nutr 95:184–190.
4. Boyd, F.M., and H.M. Edwards, Jr. 1963. The effect of dietary protein on the course of various infections in the chick. J Infect Dis 121:53–56.
5. Britton, W.M., C.H. Hill, and C.W. Barber. 1964. A mechanism of interaction between dietary protein levels and coccidiosis in chicks. J Nutr 82:306–310.
6. Colnago, G.L., T. Gore, L.S. Jensen, and P.L. Long. 1982. Amelioration of pale bird syndrome in chicks by vitamin E and selenium. Avian Dis 27:312–318.
7. Cook, M.E. 1991. Nutrition and the immune response of the domestic fowl. Crit Rev Poult Biol 3:167–190.
8. Cook, J., S.A. Naqi, N. Sahin, and G. Wagner. 1984. Distribution of immunoglobulin-bearing cells in the gut-associated lymphoid tissues of the turkey: Effect of antibiotics. Am J Vet Res 45:2189–2192.
9. Davis, C.Y., and J.L. Sell. 1983. Effect of all-trans retinol and retinoic acid nutriture on the immune system in chicks. J Nutr 113:1914–1919.
10. Dietert, R.R., K.A. Golemboski, and R.E. Austic. 1994. Environment-immune interactions. Poult Sci 73:1062–1076.
11. Fritsche, K.L., N.A. Cassity, and S. Huang. 1991. Effect of dietary fat source on antibody production and lymphocyte proliferation in chickens. Poult Sci 70:611–617.

12. Grimble, R.F. 1992. Dietary manipulation of the inflammatory response. Proc Nutr Soc 51:285–294.
13. Halevy, O., Y. Arazi, D. Melamed, A. Friedman, and D. Sklan. 1994. Retinoic acid receptor-alpha gene expression is modulated by dietary vitamin A and by retinoic acid in chicken T lymphocytes. J Nutr 124:2139–2146.
14. Hallquist, N.A., and K.C. Klasing. 1994. Serotransferrin, ovatransferrin and metallothionein levels during an immune response in chickens. Comp Biochem Physiol 108B:375–384.
15. Hill, C.H. 1979. Dietary influences on resistance to Salmonella infection in chicks. Fed Proc 38:2129–2133.
16. Hill, C.H., and H.W. Garren. 1961. Protein levels and survival time of chicks infected with Salmonella gallinarum. J Nutr 61:28–32.
17. Hill, C.H., I.M. Smith, H. Mohammadi, and S.T. Licence. 1977. Altered absorption and regulation of iron in chicks with acute Salmonella gallinarum infection. Res Vet Sci 22:371–375.
18. Hofshagen, M., and M. Kaldhusdal. 1992. Barley inclusion and avoparcin supplementation in broiler diets. 1. Effect on small intestinal bacterial flora and performance. Poult Sci 71:959–969.
19. Holt, P.S. 1992. Effect of induced molting on B cell and CT4 and CT8 T cell numbers in spleens and peripheral blood of white leghorn hens. Poult Sci 71:2027–2034.
20. Holt, P.S., R.J. Buhr, D.L. Cunningham, and R.E. Porter. 1994. Effect of two different molting procedures on a Salmonella enteritidis infection. Poult Sci 73:1267–1275.
21. Hunter, E.A.L., and R.F. Grimble. 1994. Cysteine and methionine supplementation modulate the effect of tumor necrosis factor alpha on protein synthesis, glutathione and zinc concentration of liver and lung in rats fed a low protein diet. J Nutr 124:2319–2328.
22. Joyner, L.P., D.S.P. Patterson, S. Berrett, C.D.H. Boarer, F.H. Cheong, and C.C. Norton. 1975. Amino-acid malabsorption and intestinal leakage of plasma-proteins in young chicks infected with Eimeria acervulina. Avian Pathol 4:17–33.
23. Kaldhusdal, M., and M. Hofshagen. 1992. Barley inclusion and avoparcin supplementation in broiler diets. 2. Clinical, pathological, and bacteriological findings in a mild form of necrotic enteritis. Poult Sci 71:1145–1153.
24. Katanbaf, M.N., E.A. Dunnington, and P.B. Siegel. 1989. Restricted feeding in early and late-feathering chickens. 1. Growth and physiological responses. Poult Sci 68:344–351.
25. Klasing, K.C. 1988. Influence of acute starvation or acute excess intake on immunocompetence of broiler chicks. Poult Sci 67:626–634.
26. Klasing, K.C. 1988. Nutritional aspects of leukocytic cytokines. J Nutr 118:1–11.
27. Klasing, K.C., and D.M. Barnes. 1988. Decreased amino acid requirements of growing chicks due to immunologic stress. J Nutr 118:1158–1164.
28. Klasing, K.C., and B.J. Johnstone. 1991. Monokines in growth and development. Poult Sci 70:1781–1789.
29. Klasing, K.C., D.E., Laurin, R.K. Peng, & D.M. Fry. 1987. Immunologically mediated growth depression in chicks: Influence of feed intake, corticosterone, and interleukin-1. J Nutr 117:1629–1637.
30. Klasing, K.C., B.J. Johnstone, and B.N. Benson. 1991. Implications of an immune response on growth and nutrient requirements of chicks. In W. Haresign and D.J.A. Cole (eds.). Recent Advances in Animal Nutrition. Butterworth, London, pp. 135–147.
31. Koh, T. S., R. K. Peng, and K. C. Klasing. 1996. Dietary Copper Level Affects Copper Metabolism during Lipopolysaccharide-Induced Immunological Stress in Chicks. Poult Sci 75:867-872.
32. Korver, D.R., and K.C. Klasing. 1995. Fish oil and fenleuton, a lipoxygenase inhibitor, improve growth of

broiler chicks challenged with coccidia. Poult Sci 74:60.

33. Korver, D.R., and K.C. Klasing. 1995. n-3 polyunsaturated fatty acids improve growth rate of broiler chickens and decrease interleukin-1 production. Poult Sci 74:43.

34. Latshaw, D.J. 1991. Nutrition — mechanisms of immunosuppression. Vet Immunol Immunopathol 30:111–120.

35. Marsh, J.A., and C.G. Scanes. 1994. Neuroendocrine-immune interactions. Poult Sci 73:1049–1061.

36. Marsh, J.A., R.R. Dietert, and G.F. Combs, Jr. 1981. Influence of dietary selenium and vitamin E on the humoral immune response of the chick. Proc Soc Exp Biol Med 166:228–236.

37. McIlroy, S.G., E.A. Goodall, D.A. Rice, M.S. McNulty, and D.G. Kennedy. 1993. Improved performance in commercial broiler flocks with subclinical infectious bursal disease when fed diets containing increased concentrations of vitamin E. Avian Pathol 22:81–94.

38. McKenzie, M.E., G.L. Colnago, and P.L. Long. 1987. Gut stasis in chickens infected with Eimeria. Poult Sci 66:264–269.

39. Murillo, M.G., L.S. Jensen, M.D. Ruff, and A.P. Rahn. 1976. Effect of dietery methionine status on response of chicks to coccidial infection. Poult Sci 55:642–649.

40. Nockels, C.F. 1988. The role of vitamins in modulating disease resistance. Vet Clin North Am Food Anim Pract 4:531–537.

41. O'Sullivan, N.P., E.A. Dunnington, and P.B. Siegel. 1991. Growth and carcass characteristics of early- and late-feathering broilers reared under different feeding regimens. Poult Sci 70:1323–1332.

42. Piquer, F.J., J.L. Sell, M.F. Soto-Salanova, L. Vilaseca, P.E. Palo, and K. Turner. 1995. Effects of early immune stress and changes in dietary metabolizable energy on the development of newly hatched turkeys. 1. Growth and nutrient utilization. Poult Sci 74:983–997.

43. Qureshi, M.A., and G.B. Havenstein. 1994. A comparison of the immune performance of a 1991 commercial broiler with a 1957 randombred strain when fed "typical" 1957 and 1991 broiler diets. Poult Sci 73:1805–1812.

44. Romach, E.H., S. Kidao, B.G. Sanders, and K. Kline. 1993. Effects of RRR-alpha-tocopheryl succinate on IL-1 and PGE2 production by macrophages. Nutr Cancer 20:205–214.

45. Roura, E., J. Homedis, and K.C. Klasing. 1992. Prevention of immunologic stress contributes to the growth-permitting ability of dietary antibiotics in chicks. J Nutr 122:2383–2390.

46. Ruff, M.D., and G.C. Wilkins. 1980. Total intestinal absorption of glucose and L-methionine in broilers infected with Eimeria acervulina, E. mitavi, E. maxima or E. brunetti. Parasitology 80:555–569.

47. Sell, J.L., and R.C. Angel. 1990. Nutritional aspects of selected enteric disorders with emphasis on young poultry. Crit Rev Poult Biol 2:277–292.

48. Sharma, V.D., and M.A. Fernando. 1975. Effect of Eimeria acervulina infection on nutrient retention with special reference to fat malabsorption in chickens. Can J Comp Med 39:146–151.

49. Sijtsma, S.R., C.E. West, J.H.W.M. Rombout, and A.J. van der Zipp. 1989. Effect of Newcastle disease virus infection on vitamin A metabolism in chickens. J Nutr 119:940–947.

50. Southern, L.L., and D.H. Baker. 1983. Zinc toxicity, zinc deficiency and zinc-copper interrelationship in Eimeria acervulina-infected chicks. J Nutr 113:688–696.

51. Sword, J.T., A.L. Pope, and W.G. Hoekstra. 1991. Endotoxin and lipid peroxidation in vivo in selenium- and vitamin E-deficient and -adequate rats. J Nutr 121:251–257.

52. Taylor, R.L., Jr., R.E. Austic, and R.R. Dietert. 1992. Dietary arginine influences rous sarcoma growth in a major histocompatibility B complex progressor genotype. Proc Soc Exp Biol Med 199:38–43.

53. Tsiagbe, V.K., M.E. Cook, A.E. Harper, and M.L. Sunde. 1987. Enhanced immune responses in broiler chicks fed methionine-supplemented diets. Poult Sci 66:1147–1154.

54. Tufft, L.S., Nockels, C.F. 1991. The effects of stress, Escherichia coli, dietary ethylenediaminetetraacetic acid, and their interaction on tissue trace elements in chicks. Poult Sci 70:2439–2449

55. Turk, D.E. 1974. Intestinal parasitism and nutrient absorption. Fed Proc 33:106–111.

56. Veltmann Jr., J.R., L.S. Jensen, and G.N. Rowland. 1984. Exacerbative effect of vitamin A on malabsorption syndrome in chicks. Avian Dis 29:446–452.

57. Ward, T.L., K.L. Watkins, and L.L. Southern. 1995. Interactive effects of dietary copper, water copper, and Eimeria spp. infection on growth, water intake, and plasma and liver copper concentrations of poults. Poult Sci 74:502–509.

58. West, C.E., S.R.Sijtsma, B. Kouwenhoven, J.H.W.M. Rombout, and A.J. van der Zijpp. 1992. Epithelia-damaging virus infections affect vitamin A status in chickens. J Nutr 122:333–339.

59. Willis, G.M., and D.H. Baker. 1981. Eimeria acervulina infection in the chicken: Sulfur amino acid requirement of the chick during acute coccidiosis. Poult Sci 60:1892–1897.

60. Willis, G.M., and D.H. Baker. 1981. Interaction between dietary protein/amino acid level and parasitic infection: Morbidity in amino acid deficient or adequate chicks inoculated with Eimeria acervulina. J Nutr 111:1157–1163.

61. Zulkifli, I., E.A. Dunnington, W.B. Gross, A.S. Larsen, A. Martin, and P.B. Siegel. 1993. Responses of dwarf and normal chickens to feed restriction, Eimeria tenella infection, and sheep red blood cell antigen. Poult Sci 72:1630–1640.

62. Zulkifli, I., E.A. Dunnington, W.B. Gross, and P.B. Siegel. 1994. Food restriction early or later in life and its effect on adaptability, disease resistance, and immunocompetence of heat-stressed dwarf and nondwarf chickens. Br Poult Sci 35:203–213.

3 *Salmonella* Infections

INTRODUCTION

Richard K. Gast

Infections with bacteria of the genus *Salmonella* are responsible for a variety of acute and chronic diseases in poultry. Infected poultry, moreover, comprise one of the most important reservoirs of salmonellae that can be transmitted through the food chain to humans. Isolations of *Salmonella* are reported more often from poultry and poultry products than from any other animal species. This likely reflects not only the high prevalence of *Salmonella* infections in poultry, but also the very large numbers of commercially raised chickens and turkeys, and the application of active nationwide programs for identifying infected flocks.

The genus *Salmonella* (of the family Enterobacteriaceae), named for the eminent United States Department of Agriculture (USDA) veterinarian and bacteriologist Daniel E. Salmon, consists of more than 2300 serologically distinguishable variants. These serotypes are usually named for the place of initial isolation. Although recent taxonomic refinements have indicated that all salmonellae can be grouped into only five subgenera (1), the distinctions between serotypes are often epidemiologically relevant. Accordingly, *Salmonella* isolates are still most often described primarily in terms of their traditional serotype nomenclature.

Infections of poultry with salmonellae can be grouped into three categories, each of which is the subject of a separate section of this chapter. The first section discusses infections with the two nonmotile serotypes, *S. pullorum* and *S. gallinarum,* which are generally host-specific for avian species. Pullorum disease, caused by *S. pullorum,* is an acute systemic disease of chicks and poults. Fowl typhoid, caused by *S. gallinarum,* is an acute or chronic septicemic disease that most often affects mature birds. Both of these diseases have been responsible for serious economic losses to poultry producers in the past, and have been addressed by the implementation of extensive testing and eradication programs.

The second section of this chapter discusses infections with a group of motile *Salmonella* serotypes referred to collectively as paratyphoid salmonellae. This diverse group of serotypes is principally of concern as a cause of food-borne disease in humans. Although paratyphoid infections of poultry are very common, they seldom cause acute systemic disease except in highly susceptible young birds subjected to stressful conditions. More often, paratyphoid *Salmonella* infections of chickens and turkeys are characterized by asymptomatic colonization of the intestinal tract, sometimes persisting until slaughter and leading ultimately to contamination of the finished carcass. Some serotypes, especially *S. enteritidis,* can be deposited in the contents of clean and intact eggs. Improper food handling before consumption can permit the multiplication of *Salmonella* to levels capable of causing severe gastrointestinal disease in human consumers. Heightened concerns about the microbial safety of foods have led to the initiation of numerous testing efforts to detect paratyphoid salmonellae in poultry flocks and poultry products.

The third section of this chapter discusses infections with the various motile serotypes of the subgenus *S. arizonae,* which was formerly designated *Arizona hinshawii.* This group of organisms, although biochemically distinct, causes a disease that is not clinically distinguishable from other *Salmonella* infections. Arizonosis is of particular economic significance in turkeys.

The dimensions of the poultry *Salmonella* problem have expanded considerably in recent years. In the past, the primary motivation for controlling *Salmonella* infections in poultry was to reduce disease losses. Today, public health concerns, political pressures, and consumer demands have increasingly made prevention of food-borne transmission of disease to humans an urgent priority for poultry producers. Pullorum disease and fowl typhoid have been attacked effectively in the United States by a strategy of testing and eradication. The paratyphoid salmonellae, however, are not host specific and are found nearly ubiquitously in domestic animals, wild animals, and humans. In addition, the interna-

The contributions of the authors of this chapter in previous editions, notably, K.V. Nagaraja, B.S. Pomeroy, G.H. Snoeyenbos, and J.E. Williams, are gratefully acknowledged.

tional scope of the modern poultry industry has created new and more complex opportunities for the spread of *Salmonella*. With so many potential sources of introduction of paratyphoid salmonellae into poultry flocks, the strategy for controlling these organisms may have to be correspondingly broader than has been applied to the avian-adapted serotypes. The combined application of an array of control measures, including testing programs, the production of *Salmonella*-free feed, the elimination of

biological vectors (pests), effective cleaning and disinfection of poultry houses, and prophylactic treatment of poultry to reduce their susceptibility to infection, may be necessary to achieve tangible progress in reducing the overall incidence of salmonellae in poultry and poultry products.

REFERENCES

1. Krieg, N.R. and J.G. Holt. 1984. Bergey's Manual of Systematic Bacteriology, vol 1. Williams and Wilkins, Baltimore, MD.

PULLORUM DISEASE AND FOWL TYPHOID

H. L. Shivaprasad

INTRODUCTION. Because of the many similarities between pullorum disease and fowl typhoid in terms of history, clinical signs, epizootiology, lesions, and control and eradication procedures, these two diseases are described here together. Differences between these two diseases and their causative organisms are pointed out where appropriate.

Pullorum disease (PD) is caused by the bacterium *Salmonella pullorum* and fowl typhoid (FT) is caused by *S. gallinarum*. They are septicemic diseases affecting primarily chickens and turkeys, but other birds such as quail, pheasants, ducks, peacocks, and guinea fowl are susceptible. Both diseases can be transmitted through the egg by transovarian infection. *S. pullorum* and *S. gallinarum* are highly host adapted and they seldom cause significant clinical signs, morbidity, or mortality in hosts other than chickens and turkeys. In some areas of the world, including parts of Europe, *S. pullorum* and *S. gallinarum* are considered to be the same species.

Bacillary white diarrhea was a term used to designate PD before 1929, but the term *pullorum disease* has since gained universal acceptance. There have been no reported outbreaks of FT in commercial poultry in the United States since 1980 (5, 75). PD was once enzootic in many areas of the world. The incidence of PD in the United States is so rare that it was once thought that the disease had been eradicated from the commercial poultry population. The impact of PD was felt recently, however, when a series of outbreaks occurred in a completely inte-

grated broiler operation involving five states (Delaware, Maryland, North Carolina, Alabama, and Florida) (59, 84). The outbreaks occurred in 1990 and 1991 and eventually involved 19 breeder flocks and more than 261 grow-out facilities in those five states.

The elimination of PD and FT from commercial flocks in the United States is largely due to the pullorum–typhoid control program, the National Poultry Improvement Plan (NPIP), instituted by a voluntary organization (7). Even though PD is rare in commercial chickens, the disease still occurs in backyard flocks (8, 36, 110, 88). The major economic loss from PD over the last 20 yr has been the cost involved in testing breeding flocks of chickens and turkeys to ensure that they are free of the infection.

Occasional infections of PD in humans have been produced by massive exposure following ingestion of contaminated foods or experimental challenge (68, 71). The clinical signs are characterized by rapid onset of acute enteritis, followed by prompt recovery without treatment. *S. gallinarum* is rarely isolated from humans and is of little public health significance (6, 78).

HISTORY. Only the salient features of these two diseases are provided here. Further information on the history of these two diseases can be found in previous editions of this book, as well as in a historical review by Bullis (27).

The etiologic agent of PD was described by Rettger in 1899 and the disease was called fatal septicemia of young chicks (79). Later, the disease was designated as bacillary white diarrhea to distinguish it from other diseases of chicks (80). It was known at that time that PD was widespread in the United

The author thanks Drs. K. V. Nagaraja, B.S. Pomeroy and G.H. Snoeyenbos for material from previous editions incorporated into this chapter.

States and in many other countries throughout the world. Mortality associated with this disease in chicks ranged up to 100% (81), seriously threatening the chicken industry. Between 1900 and 1910, it was proved that PD was an egg-borne infection. In 1913, the practical application of the macroscopic tube agglutination test for detection of carriers of the organism was described (60). Standard methods of diagnosis of pullorum disease in barnyard fowl were formulated by the Conference of Research Workers in Animal Diseases of North America and later adopted by the USA Livestock Association, now the United States Animal Health Association (USAHA), in 1932 (3, 4). A modified whole blood test method in which stained antigen is employed was developed in 1931 (86). It has been widely used because of its simplicity.

The NPIP is administered by state agencies cooperating with the USDA, and was established in 1935, designed in part to control PD in chickens. Pullorum disease was first recognized in turkeys in 1928, and by 1940, the disease was widespread in turkeys and responsible for severe economic losses (72). A National Turkey Improvement Plan, similar to NPIP, was organized in 1943. A series of modifications of these plans over a number of years has helped in the eradication of PD in commercial poultry.

Fowl typhoid, a disease very closely related to PD and caused by *S. gallinarum,* was first recognized in 1888, even before PD (62). Initially, the causative agent was named *Bacillus gallinarum* and later changed to *B. sanguinarium* (62). The name fowl typhoid was applied in 1902 and it was soon used in other parts of the world such as Germany and Holland. Control of FT was included in the NPIP in 1954. This resulted in the treatment of FT in the same category as PD and is one of the main reasons for the near eradication of FT in commercial poultry and its low incidence in all poultry, as reported from year to year.

INCIDENCE AND DISTRIBUTION.

PD and FT are worldwide in distribution. Pullorum disease is rare in commercial poultry in the United States and perhaps other parts of the world. It is still common in backyard chickens, however, and a recent outbreak of PD in commercial chickens in the United States has been documented (59, 84).

There is a low incidence of FT in countries such as Canada, United States, and several European countries. On the other hand, Mexico, Central and South America, and Africa have reported dramatic increases in the incidence of FT in poultry flocks (14, 23, 24, 66, 90). Recently, there have been a few outbreaks of FT in commercial poultry in Denmark and Germany (32).

ETIOLOGY

Classification. *S. pullorum* and *S. gallinarum* are both members of the family Enterobacteriaceae and are highly host adapted. They are among the few members of the genus that are nonmotile, and they belong to the serogroup D according to the Kauffman White scheme. *Bergey's Manual* once used the designation *Salmonella gallinarum* for both *S. pullorum* and *S. gallinarum,* resulting in confusion; however, they are now listed as *S. gallinarum–pullorum.*

It has been reported that the nonmotile salmonellae such as *S. pullorum* and *S. gallinarum* are monophyletic and that their most recent common ancestor was nonmotile (65). Since diverging from this ancestor, the pullorum lineage has evolved more rapidly than the gallinarum lineage. This was shown by multilocus enzyme electrophoresis and by estimation of the chromosomal genotypic diversity for *S. gallinarum* and *S. pullorum* (65). It has also been shown by multilocus enzyme electrophoresis that *S. enteritidis,* as a polyphyletic serotype, is closely related to *S. pullorum* and *S. gallinarum* (99).

Morphology and Staining. The organisms are gram-negative, nonsporogenic, nonmotile, and facultatively anaerobic. They are slender rods, 1.0–2.5 µm in length and 0.3–1.5 µm in width. The bacilli mostly occur singly, but occasionally two or more can be found united.

Growth Requirements. *S. pullorum* and *S. gallinarum* grow readily on beef agar or broth or other nutrient media. They are aerobic or facultatively anaerobic, and grow best at 37 C. The organisms will grow in selective enrichment media such as selenite-F and tetrathionate broths, and differential plating media such as MacConkey, bismuth sulfite, and brilliant green agars. It has been shown that *S. pullorum* occasionally fails to grow on certain selective media such as brilliant green or salmonella–shigella agar but grows satisfactorily on bismuth sulfite and MacConkey agars (29). *S. pullorum* appears to grow slower than *S. gallinarum* and this has been attributed to its inability to assimilate oxidatively a variety of amino acids (100).

Colony Morphology. There are very few differences in colonial morphology between *S. pullorum* and *S. gallinarum.* On meat extract or infusion agar (pH 7.0–7.2), colonies can appear small, discrete, smooth, blue-gray or grayish white, glistening, homogenous, and entire. *S. pullorum* growth is luxuriant and markedly translucent on liver infusion agar. Covered colonies remain small (1 mm or less), but isolated colonies may have a diameter of 3–4 mm or more. Surface markings may appear as the colonies increase in size and age, but as a rule, young colonies in a heavily seeded plate change little with age. Occasionally, morphologically abnormal strains are encountered. Inoculation of gelatin slants yields grayish-white surface growth with filiform growth in the stab and no liquefaction. Growth in broth is turbid with heavy flocculent sediment.

Resistance to Chemical and Physical Agents. In general, the resistance of these organisms is about the same as that of members of the paratyphoid groups (see 76, 97). They may survive for several years in a favorable environment, but they are less resistant than paratyphoid salmonellae to heat, chemicals, and adverse environmental factors. For example, S. gallinarum was killed within 10 min at 60 C, within a few min by direct exposure to sunlight, in 3 min by 1:1000 phenol, 1:20,000 dichloride of mercury, or 1% potassium permanganate, and in 1 min by 2% formalin (see 76). Agar cultures may rapidly lose their pathogenic character. Orr and Moore (73) found that S. gallinarum retained viability up to 43 days subject to daily freezing and thawing. Organisms in the liver survived more than 148 days at -20 C even though they were accidentally thawed twice. S. gallinarum can survive in the feces from infected chickens up to 10.9 days when kept in a range house and 2 days less in the open (93).

Biochemical Properties. There are more similarities than differences between S. pullorum and S. gallinarum in their biochemical properties (21, 107, 30). Both organisms can ferment arabinose, dextrose, galactose, mannitol, mannose, rhammose, and xylose to produce acid, with or without gas production. Substances not fermented include lactose, sucrose, and salicin. One important biochemical difference between these two organisms is that S. gallinarum ferments dulcitol, whereas S. pullorum does not. Also, S. pullorum only occasionally ferments maltose. The major difference between the two organisms is, however, that S. pullorum cultures produce rapid decarboxylation of ornithine, whereas cultures of S. gallinarum do not. In addition, S. gallinarum uses citrate, D(-) sorbitol, L(-) fucose, D(-) tartrate, and cysteine hydrochloride gelatin (30). Some of these differences are helpful in differentiating the two organisms; however, variation in the behavior in some strains can occasionally be observed, especially in regard to gas production.

Ribotyping by the use of the enzyme *EcoRI* has also been suggested as an important tool to differentiate between S. pullorum and S. gallinarum (31).

Antigenic Structure and Toxins. Both S. pullorum and S. gallinarum possess the O antigens 1, 9, 12. Variation involving antigen 12 occurs in S. pullorum, but there is no evidence for such in S. gallinarum. The first evidence of antigenic variation in S. pullorum was found when infected progeny were negative using a standard agglutination test. Sera from infected chicks agglutinated homologous-strain antigen, but not standard antigens. This antigenic variation, characteristic of S. pullorum, was studied extensively (34, 35, 117, 121). The antigenic composition of S. pullorum was shown to be $9,12_1,12_2,12_3$; the variation involved antigens 12_2 and 12_3. Standard strains contain a large amount of 12_3 and a very small amount of 12_2, but in variant strains the content of the two antigens is reversed. It was recognized that standard strains of S. pullorum contained a small percentage of cells with strong 12_2 antigen and this was considered to be a normal form of the organism. Later, it was shown that the initial field isolates were usually rather unstable unless they were in the variant form. Extensive examination of individual colonies, sometimes through successive transfers, was necessary to determine accurately the antigenic form of a culture. Most isolates tend to stabilize during passage on artificial media. Standard-form cultures usually contain a small percentage of 12_2-predominant colonies even after long artificial cultivation. Variant forms of cultures are often pure or nearly pure for 12_2 and 12_3 factors. Colonies of intermediate strains are usually mixtures of 12_2- and 12_3-predominant colonies, or rarely are uniform and contain appreciable amounts of both factors in individual colonies. Strains may also vary in content of the O-1 antigen.

Early reports indicated that as many as one-third of the S. pullorum isolates from some areas of the United States were of the variant type; by 1950, only 13% of total isolates were of that type (115), a reduction believed to be the result of extensive use of polyvalent testing antigens.

Tests to differentiate standard, intermediate, and variant types of S. pullorum have been described (113, 114). Phage typing of S. pullorum can be used for type identification, epidemiologic investigations, and genetic studies (108, 109, 30).

S. pullorum and S. gallinarum, being gram-negative bacteria, probably elaborate endotoxins. Unfortunately, this has not been studied extensively. S. pullorum contains a thermostable toxin to which rodents, but not chicks, are susceptible. Similarly, there are reports that S. gallinarum contains a toxin that was lethal to a rabbit (96). Endotoxins from S. gallinarum have been shown to cause clinical illness within a few hr after intravenous injection in chicks (95). Most of the clinical signs subsided within 24-48 hr. Storing S. gallinarum at -75 or -20 C did not have any effect on the pathogenicity (95).

Like most pathogenic microorganisms, S. gallinarum, and probably S. pullorum, may lose virulence rapidly in artificial media; hence, cultures should be passaged serially in their natural host, the chicken, before testing the pathogenicity of the organisms. Pathogenicity of such cultures is best maintained in the lyophilized or frozen state. This may explain why various investigators have found wide variation in virulence among cultures of *S. gallinarum*.

It has also been shown that particular genes are responsible for efficient adherence and entry of various salmonellae into cultured epithelial cells (1). When a mutated version of one of these genes was introduced into different *Salmonella* strains, some of these salmonellae (including *S. gallinarum*) were rendered deficient for adherence and invasion of cultured cells. There is also evidence that an 85-kb plasmid plays a role in virulence of *S. pullorum* and *S. gallinarum* in chickens (13, 12, 30).

PATHOGENESIS AND EPIZOOTIOLOGY

Natural Hosts.   Chickens are the natural hosts for both *S. pullorum* and *S. gallinarum*; however, naturally occurring outbreaks of PD and FT have been described in turkeys, guinea fowl, quail, pheasants, sparrows, and parrots (see 76, 97). In addition, naturally occurring outbreaks of PD have been described in canaries and bullfinches, and FT has been described in ring doves, ostriches, and peafowl. The susceptibility of ducks, geese, and pigeons to *S. gallinarum* has been variable, but they appear to be resistant to this pathogen.

Significant differences in susceptibility to PD among breeds of chickens have been described (87). The lighter breeds, particularly leghorns, appear to be more resistant than the heavy breeds. PD-resistant and PD-susceptible lines of Rhode Island Reds, New Hampshires, and crosses between the two were developed based on the selection for high and low body temperature during the first 6 days of life (58). Differences in resistance to *S. pullorum* and *S. gallinarum* have also been shown in inbred lines of chickens (28). It appears that a greater percentage of females than males stay as reactors, probably due to the sequestered nature of local infection of the ovarian follicles.

AGE OF HOSTS COMMONLY INFECTED.   Mortality from PD is usually confined to the first 2-3 wk of age. Acute infections in older chickens, particularly among brown egg–producing strains, have been occasionally reported. Similarly, mortality due to PD in semimature and mature turkeys has been observed. A certain percentage of chickens and turkeys that survive the initial infection become carriers with or without the presence of lesions.

Although FT is frequently referred to as a disease of adult birds, there are also many reports of high mortality in young chicks (16, 17, 64, 67). Fowl typhoid can cause mortality as high as 26% in chicks during the 1st month of life. As in PD, FT losses begin at hatching time; however, in FT they also continue to laying age. There are reports of certain strains of *S. gallinarum* producing lesions in chicks indistinguishable from those associated with PD (98).

Unusual Hosts.   Pullorum disease has been described as a naturally occurring or experimental infection in mammals including chimpanzees, rabbits, guinea pigs, chinchillas, pigs, kittens, foxes, dogs, swine, mink, cows, and wild rats. *S. gallinarum* was able to be cultured for up to 121 days from the feces of experimentally infected rats (9). Human salmonellosis caused by *S. pullorum* has occasionally been reported (6, 68, 71). According to a Centers for Disease Control and Prevention report (6), there were 18 *S. pullorum* isolates and 8 *S. gallinarum* isolates out of a total of 458,081 *Salmonella* isolates from humans between 1982 and 1992. Experimental reproduction of salmonellosis with four strains of *S. pullorum* in humans with large numbers (billions) of bacteria produced only transient illness with prompt recovery (71).

Transmission.   Like many other bacterial diseases, PD and FT can be transmitted in several ways. The infected bird (reactor and carrier) is by far the most important means of perpetuation and spread of the organism. The primary role of infected hatching eggs in the transmission of these two diseases was recognized in the early course of investigations. Birds may infect not only their own generation, but also succeeding ones through egg transmission. Egg transmission may result from contamination of the ovum following ovulation (16, 17), but localization of *S. pullorum* or *S. gallinarum* in the ovules before ovulation is also likely and probably constitutes the chief mode of transmission.

Transmission through shell penetration and feed contamination by *S. pullorum* has been reported but appears to be of minor importance (118). The number of eggs infected with *S. pullorum* or *S. gallinarum* can be as high as 33% of the total laid by an infected hen. Contact transmission of infected chicks or pullets can be an important route of dissemination of *S. pullorum* and *S. gallinarum*. This can happen in the hatcher and can only be partially prevented by formaldehyde fumigation (56). Mortality as high as 60.9% of the exposed flock due to *S. gallinarum* has been reported (44). Transmission may also occur within a flock as a result of cannibalism of infected birds, egg eating, and through wounds on the skin. Feces from infected birds are also a source of bacteria for infected birds. Contaminated feed, water, and litter can also be sources of both *S. pullorum* and *S. gallinarum*. Attendants, feed dealers, chicken buyers, and visitors who move from house to house and from farm to farm may carry infection unless precautions are taken to disinfect footwear, hands, and clothing. Similarly, trucks, crates, and feed sacks may also be contaminated. Wild birds, mammals, and flies may be important mechanical spreaders of the organisms.

Egg transmission can be influenced by levels of agglutinins in the yolk (112). Agglutinins against *S. pullorum* may be critical in the prevention of embryonic mortality in infected eggs, thus allowing successful egg transmission.

Clinical Signs.

PD is considered principally a disease of chicks and poults, whereas FT is encountered more frequently in growing and adult chickens and turkeys. The signs noted in young chicks and poults due to both diseases, however, are very similar as a result of the transovarian transmission of these diseases. Occasional cases of PD can be subclinical even though the disease may originate by egg transmission.

CHICKS AND POULTS. If birds are hatched from infected eggs, moribund and dead birds may be observed in the incubator or within a short time after hatching. The birds can manifest somnolescence, weakness, loss of appetite, poor growth, and adherence of chalky white material to the vent. Death may soon follow. In some cases, evidence of PD is not observed until 5 to 10 days after hatching, but the disease gains momentum during the following 7–10 days. The peak of mortality usually occurs during the 2nd or 3rd wk of life. In these situations, the birds exhibit lassitude and inclination to huddle together under heaters; droopy wings; and distorted body appearance.

Labored breathing or gasping may be observed as a result of extensive pathology of the lungs. Survivors may be greatly retarded in their growth and appear underdeveloped and poorly feathered. These birds may not mature into vigorous or well-developed laying or breeding birds. Flocks that have passed through a serious outbreak usually have a high percentage of carriers at maturity.

Blindness, as well as swelling of the tibiotarsal and the humeroradial and ulnar articulations, due to *S. pullorum* infection in chicks, has been described (18, 37, 38, 59, 84). In certain instances, a relatively high incidence of localization of infection in the joint, which can produce lameness and obvious swelling, has been reported in chicks. In the recent outbreaks of PD in the eastern part of the United States, synovitis, or swelling of the hock joint, due to *S. pullorum* was commonly seen (84). Similar lesions in turkey poults have also been reported. This suggests that some strains of *S. pullorum* may have a predilection for these sites.

GROWING AND MATURE FOWL. Infected birds may or may not exhibit any signs and cannot be detected by their physical appearance, especially in the case of PD. Acute outbreaks in chickens may begin by a sudden drop in feed consumption, with birds being droopy, with ruffled feathers and pale and shrunken combs. Other signs, such as a drop in egg production, decreased fertility, and diminished hatchability, can sometimes be observed in both PD and FT, depending upon the severity of infection. Death may occur within 4 days of exposure, but usually occurs after 5–10 days. There may be an increase in body temperature of 1–3 degrees within 2–3 days after exposure. Unusual cases of PD in semimature and mature flocks have been described (36). Anorexia, diarrhea, depression, and dehydration are the prominent signs.

Signs due to PD and FT in turkeys may consist of increased thirst, inappetence, listlessness, tendency to separate from healthy birds, and green to greenish-yellow diarrhea, but losses may occur with no apparent clinical signs. Body temperature increases several degrees initially. The initial outbreaks usually cause the greatest mortality followed by intermittent recurrence and less severe loss (55).

Morbidity and Mortality.

Both morbidity and mortality are highly variable in chickens and are influenced by age, strain susceptibility, nutrition, flock management, and characteristics of exposure. Mortality from PD may vary from 0 to 100%. The greatest losses usually occur during the 2nd wk after hatching, with a rapid decline between the 3rd and 4th wk of age in PD. Mortality ranging from 10 to 93% due to FT have been reported in chicks (52).

Morbidity is often much higher than mortality with some of the affected birds recovering spontaneously. Birds hatched from an infected flock and raised on the same premises exhibit less mortality than those subjected to the stress of shipping. In turkeys, losses may be as severe as in chickens.

Gross Lesions

CHICKS. In peracute cases, birds that die suddenly

3.1. Gross lesions associated with *Salmonella pullorum* (A–F) and *S. arizonae* (G) infections in chickens. A. Enlarged liver showing congestion and small necrotic foci (Glass). B. Heart from young chick with white nodules representing myocarditis. Such nodules can be confused for tumors such as Marek's disease (Chin). C. Nodular lesions in the heart; note the thickened yellowish pericardium (*reflected*). D. Swollen hock joint containing yellow viscous fluid (Peckham). E. Ovarian lesions and salpingitis. F. Lungs with pyrogranulomatous pneumonia due to pullorum disease in a chick (Peckham). G. Turkey poult with exudate in the anterior chamber of the eye due to arizonosis.

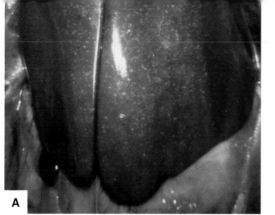

A

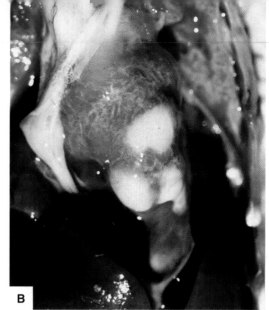

B

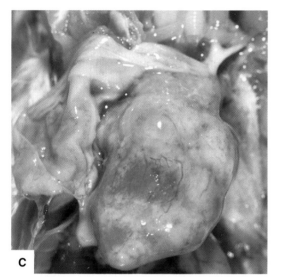

C

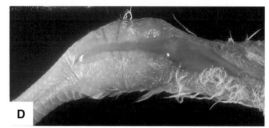

D

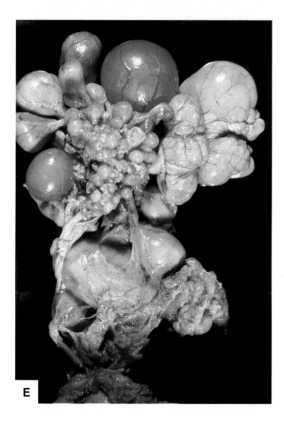

E

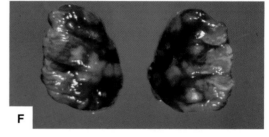

F

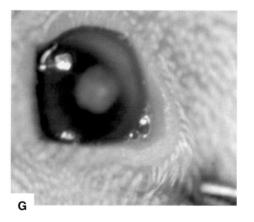

G

in the early stages of brooding may show no gross lesions. In acute cases, enlarged and congested liver, spleen, and kidneys can be seen. Livers sometimes have white foci (Fig. 3.1A). The yolk sac and its contents may or may not reveal any alterations, but in protracted cases, interference with yolk absorption may occur. In such cases, the yolk sac contents may be of creamy or caseous consistency. Occasionally, those birds with respiratory signs may have white nodules in the lung (Fig. 3.1F) and white nodules sometimes resembling Marek's disease tumors may be present in the cardiac muscle (Fig. 3.1B) or pancreas. Occasionally, nodules in the heart may get so large that they can cause distortion in the shape of the heart (Fig. 3.1C). This, in turn, may lead to chronic passive congestion of the liver and ascites. The pericardium may be thickened and may contain yellow or fibrinous exudate. Similar nodules may be present in the muscle of the gizzard and occasionally in the wall of the ceca and large intestine. The ceca may contain caseous cores. Some birds may exhibit swollen joints containing yellow viscous fluid (19) (Fig. 3.1D); this was one of the most commonly reported gross lesions in a recent outbreak of PD in commercial broilers (84). Among the joints, the hock joint is most commonly involved, but other joints such as the wing joint and the foot pad may also be swollen. Other changes that can be seen are exudate in the peritoneum, thickening of the wall of the intestine, and exudate in the anterior chamber of the eye.

Enlarged spleens, gray necrotic foci with petechial hemorrhages in lungs, and pale or discolored livers were observed in bobwhite quail inoculated with *S. pullorum* (26).

ADULT CHICKENS. Lesions may be minimal in some birds even though they may be active serologic reactors. Sometimes, only a minimal lesion, such as a small nodular or regressing ovarian follicle, can be found. Lesions found most frequently in chronic carrier hens, however, are a few misshapen, discolored cystic ova among a few normal-appearing ovules (Fig. 3.1E). The involved ova may contain oily and caseous material enclosed in a thickened capsule. These degenerative ovarian follicles may be closely attached to the ovary, but frequently they are pedunculated and may become detached from the ovarian mass. In such cases, they may become embedded in the inner lining of the abdominal cavity. Often, the oviduct contains caseous exudate in the lumen. Ovary and oviduct dysfunction may lead to abdominal ovulation or oviduct impaction, which in turn may bring about extensive peritonitis and adhesions of the abdominal viscera. Fibrinous peritonitis and perihepatitis with or without involvement of the reproductive tract can sometimes be seen. Ascites also may develop, especially

in turkeys. Sometimes it is difficult to culture *Salmonella* from such advanced lesions.

Frequently, pericarditis is observed in both females and males. Changes in the pericardium, epicardium, and pericardial fluid appear to depend on the duration of the disease. In some cases, the pericardium exhibits only a slight translucency, and the pericardial fluid may be increased and turbid. In the more advanced stages, the pericardial sac is thickened and opaque, and the pericardial fluid is greatly increased in amount, containing considerable exudative material. This may be followed by permanent thickening of the pericardium and epicardium and partial obliteration of the pericardial cavity by adhesions. Occasionally, small cysts containing amber, caseous material may be found embedded in the abdominal fat or attached to the gizzard and intestine. Pancreas may frequently be infected.

In the male, testes may have white foci or nodules (43). Occasionally, caseous granulomas can be found in the lungs and air sacs (36).

TURKEYS. Lesions in turkeys are similar to those observed in chickens (54). Enlarged mahogany or brown-streaked livers, enlarged spleens, areas of necrosis in the heart, and grayish lungs are characteristic lesions of FT in turkey poults. Ulceration extending from the duodenum to the ceca, although uncommon in chickens, is a common lesion in turkeys. In adult carriers, there is a predilection of infection for the reproductive organs similar to that seen in chickens.

DUCKS AND GUINEA FOWL. Lesions due to FT in ducklings and adult ducks are similar to those in chickens. In guinea fowl, FT lesions involve the respiratory tract and are characterized by congested lungs and increased mucus in the nasal cleft and trachea.

Histopathology. A very limited amount of information on microscopic lesions is available for PD or FT. Most of the PD lesions described are from field cases, which might have been complicated by other bacterial and/or viral agents (33, 104); however, the lesions can be summarized as follows. In peracute cases, only severe vascular congestion in various organs, especially liver, spleen, and kidney can be discerned. In acute to subacute cases, there is multifocal necrosis of hepatocytes (Fig. 3.2) with accumulation of fibrin and infiltration of heterophils in the liver. Periportal infiltration of heterophils mixed with a few lymphocytes and plasma cells can also be seen in the liver. In chronic cases, especially in cases in which there are large nodules in the heart, the liver will have chronic passive congestion with interstitial fibrosis. The spleen may have severe congestion or fibrin exudation of vascular sinuses in acute stages, and severe hyperplasia of the mononuclear phagocytic system cells in later stages. Ceca in young chicks may have extensive necrosis of the mucosa and submucosa, with accumulation of necrotic debris mixed with fibrin and heterophils in the lumen.

The most characteristic microscopic lesions, however, are in the heart and gizzard. In the heart, they initially consist of necrosis of myofibers with infiltration of heterophils mixed with lymphocytes and plasma cells. In later stages, these cells are replaced by massive numbers of fairly uniform-appearing cells of the histiocytic type (Fig. 3.3). These cells are fairly large, with irregular vesicular nuclei and faintly staining foamy eosinophilic cytoplasm. They may be arranged in solid sheets, forming nodules that often protrude from the epicardial surface. These nodules, both grossly and histologically, can be confused with lymphoid tumors caused by Marek's disease virus and possibly retroviruses. A similar process can be seen in the gizzard and pancreas. The lesions in the pancreas can be so severe that the entire normal architecture is destroyed.

Other changes, such as serositis of various organs such as the pericardium, pleuroperitoneum, synovium, and serosa of the intestinal tract and mesen-

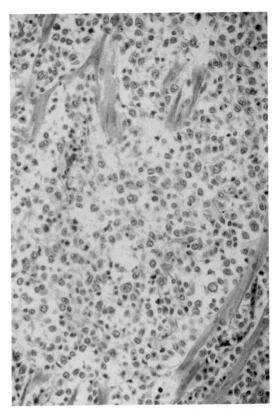

3.3. Myocardium from a *Salmonella pullorum*-infected chick showing infiltration with histiocytic-type cells, ×62.

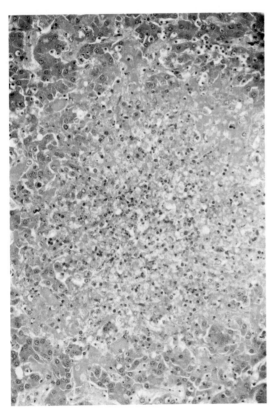

3.2. Liver revealing focal degeneration and necrosis, ×51.

tery can be seen in a high percentage of cases (104). In acute stages, these lesions can be associated with heterophils and fibrin, but in later stages, only lymphocytes, plasma cells, and histiocytic cells can be found.

Microscopic lesions in the ovary range from acute fibrinosuppurative inflammation to severe pyogranulomatous inflammation of the ovules (Fig. 3.4). The pyogranulomatous inflammation is characterized by infiltration of heterophils mixed with fibrin and bacterial colonies in the coagulated yolk material. This, in turn, is surrounded by successive layers of multinucleated giant cells and a mixed population of inflammatory cells including macrophages, plasma cells, heterophils, and lymphocytes. In males, degeneration and necrosis and inflammation of the epithelial cells lining the seminiferous tubules can be seen (63). Other, but less common, changes are catarrhal bronchitis, catarrhal enteritis, and interstitial inflammation of the lungs and kidneys. Minimal and nonspecific changes in endocrine glands such as the thyroid, adrenal, and pituitary glands due to FT have been described (41).

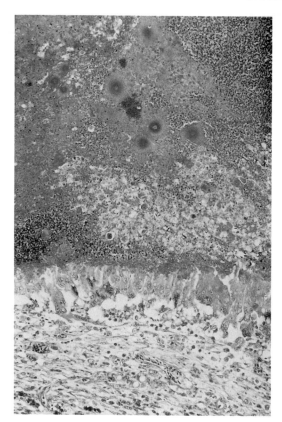

3.4. Ovule from an adult hen with pullorum disease showing fibrinosuppurative inflammation and bacterial colonies, ×20.

Immunity. Very little information regarding immunity to PD and FT is available, due in part to the great success in eradication of the infections by elimination of the carriers. Chicks orally infected at 4 days of age did not produce detectable agglutinating antibodies until 20–40 days of age, but mature birds produced agglutinating antibodies within 3–10 days following infection. In chicks, maximum antibody production was not reached until 100 days after infection. The possible role of agglutinating antibodies in modifying the course of infection in the host is little understood. Some of the earlier work done with *S. gallinarum* suggested that antigen–antibody reactions occur during acute infections. This could result in an anaphylactic type of hypersensitivity, which could in turn produce signs and death. This is less likely, however, in the context of our present understanding of the signs and pathogenesis of anaphylaxis. Even though anaphylactic reactions in birds have not been studied extensively, affected birds generally die within a few hours due to extensive pulmonary edema. Using a bactericidal assay for the presence of antibody, it

was demonstrated that 1-day-old chicks had little natural antibody against *S. gallinarum,* whereas adults had higher levels (57). It is probable that immunity to *S. pullorum* and *S. gallinarum* is not dependent on a humoral immune mechanism, but instead on a cell-mediated mechanism.

It has been suggested that the differences among various salmonellae, including *S. pullorum* and *S. gallinarum,* in their ability to survive and multiply in visceral organs (especially in spleen and liver) is attributed to an unknown control mechanism involving the reticuloendothelial system of the host (15).

DIAGNOSIS. A definitive diagnosis of PD or FT requires isolation and identification of *S. pullorum* or *S. gallinarum,* respectively. A tentative diagnosis, however, can be made based on flock history, clinical signs, mortality, and lesions. Positive serologic findings can also be of major value in detecting infection; however, positive results should not be considered adequate for a definite diagnosis because of the delay of 3 to 10 or more days in appearance of agglutinating antibodies following infection and also because of cross-reactions with other salmonellae such as *S. enteritidis* (42, 89, 111).

Isolation of *S. pullorum* and *S. gallinarum.* Acute PD and FT are characterized by systemic infections; causative organisms can be isolated from most body tissues. The liver, spleen, and ceca are usually involved and are the preferred organs to culture. Lesions may occur in lungs, heart, gizzard, pancreas, or yolk sac and these are also dependable sites for isolation. In mature birds, if lesions are present in the reproductive organs, ovarian follicles and testes can be cultured. Other sites for culturing are peritoneum, synovial fluid, and the interior of the eye. Beef extract or infusion, or tryptose agar, in tubes or petri dishes, are all satisfactory for primary isolation. Enrichment broths or selective media may also be used if tissues are decomposed.

Birds with chronic PD or FT detected by serologic tests may or may not have gross lesions. If such birds are submitted to the laboratory as carriers, detailed culturing of internal organs is necessary. A detailed outline for examination of such specimens is given in the NPIP (7). This procedure may be summarized briefly as follows.

Grossly normal or diseased internal organs should be cultured directly on veal infusion (VI) and brilliant green (BG) agar plates and incubated for 48 hr at 37 C. In addition, portions of the internal organs should be pooled, ground, or blended, in 10 times their volume of VI broth; 10 mL aliquots of the suspension are transferable to 100 mL of both VI and tetrathionate BG (TBG) broth and incubated for 24 hr at 37 C. The broths are then plated on VI and BG agar and incubated and examined after 24 and 48 hr. If contamination with proteus or pseudomonas is a problem, platings can be done on BG sulfapyridine (BGS) agar.

The digestive tract should be cultured using individual cotton swabs for the upper, middle, and lower intestinal tract, including both the ceca and the rectum–cloaca area. The swabs should be deposited in 10 mL TBG broth, incubated, and plated as previously described for the internal organs. In addition, portions of the gut should be pooled, ground, or blended, in 10 times their volume of TBG broth. Ten milliliters of the suspension from the digestive tract are transferred to 100 mL TBG broth and incubated at 42 or 37 C for 24 hr. The higher incubation temperatures for TBG broth reduce populations of competitive contaminants common in gut tissue.

Suspect colonies are transferred to triple sugar–iron (TSI) agar and lysine–iron (LI) agar and incubated at 37 C for 24 hr. Cultures revealing typical reactions of salmonellae or arizonae on TSI or LI agar slants should be identified by appropriate biochemical and other tests. All *Salmonella* cultures should be serologically typed.

Use of nonselective media demands careful aseptic techniques but has the advantage of more dependably securing isolation of *S. pullorum* and *S. gallinarum*. Also, other bacteria capable of producing cross-reactions with pullorum–typhoid antigen may be more dependably demonstrated.

Identification of Cultures.

The colonies of *S. pullorum* may appear small, smooth, and translucent on nutrient media after 24 hr of incubation. With *S. gallinarum,* colonies are smooth, blue-gray, moist, circular, and entire. Careful initial culture of tissues on nonselective media should usually result in pure cultures. If pure cultures are not secured, or

if an enriched medium has been used, it is often advantageous to transfer individual colonies to TSI agar slants for preliminary differentiation. *S. pullorum* and *S. gallinarum* produce a red slant with a yellow butt that shows delayed blackening from H_2S production. Reactions listed in Table 3.1, which can be determined within 24 hr, provide identification of a number of other common pathogens and allow differentiation between the two organisms.

Additional differentiation tests described under etiology may be necessary to identify isolates that produce nontypical reactions (chiefly fermentation of maltose or no gas production). Decarboxylation of ornithine by *S. pullorum* is the single most dependable test for differentiating maltose-fermenting *S. pullorum* strains from *S. gallinarum.*

Serology.

Serologic tests to detect PD and FT include the macroscopic tube agglutination (TA) test, rapid serum (RS) test, stained antigen whole blood (WB) test, and microagglutination (MA) test using tetrazolium-stained antigens (see 76, 97). Standard procedure in the United States for detection of breeding flocks chronically infected with *S. pullorum* and *S. gallinarum* is to use the standard strains of *S. pullorum* (1, 9, 12_3) for tube and serum plate antigens and both standard (1, 9, 12_3) and variant (1, 9, 12_2) strains of *S. pullorum* for the polyvalent rapid whole blood plate antigens. These antigens will detect flocks infected with either *S. pullorum* or *S. gallinarum.*

Techniques and procedures for official testing of chicken and turkey breeding flocks and interpretation of tests are described in detail in the latest version of the NPIP (7) (see also Prevention and Control, Serologic Tests).

Enzyme-linked immunosorbent assays (ELISA) for detecting *S. pullorum* and *S. gallinarum* antibodies have been developed by using lipopolysaccharides from these salmonellae as antigens (14, 69, 70). This technique can be used for screening

Table 3.1. Biochemical reactions useful in differentiating *Salmonella pullorum* and *S. gallinarum*

Reactant or characteristic	S. pullorum	S. gallinarum
Dextrose	Fermented with gas	Fermented with no gas
Lactose	Not fermented	Not fermented
Sucrose	Not fermented	Not fermented
Mannitol	Fermented with gas	Fermented with no gas
Maltose	Usually not fermented	Fermented with no gas
Dulcitol	Not fermented	Fermented with no gas
Ornithine	Fermented	Not fermented
Indole	Not produced	Not produced
Urea	Not hydrolyzed	Not hydrolyzed
Motility	Nonmotile	Nonmotile
Agglutination	Positive with group D	Positive with group D

large numbers of blood samples. As with other techniques, the ELISA technique may show positive reactions to other salmonellae, especially those belonging to group D (14, 69, 70).

Differential Diagnosis. Clinical signs and lesions produced by PD or FT are not pathognomonic. Other *Salmonella* infections may produce similar lesions in the liver, spleen, and intestine that cannot be distinguished grossly or microscopically from those produced by PD or FT. Aspergillus or other fungi may produce similar lesions in the lungs. *S. pullorum* and *S. gallinarum* can localize in major joints and tendon sheaths of chicks. Signs and lesions from these may resemble those produced by organisms such as *Mycoplasma synoviae, Staphylococcus aureus, Pasteurella multocida, or Erysipelothrix rhusiopathiae.* Sometimes the white nodules in the heart of young chicks may resemble Marek's disease tumors. Local infections with *S. pullorum* and *S. gallinarum* in adult carriers, particularly of the ovary, may appear identical to those produced by other bacterial infections such as coliforms, staphylococci, *P. multocida,* streptococci, and other salmonellae. Birds of any age may be infected with *S. pullorum* or *S. gallinarum* but fail to show grossly discernable lesions. A definitive diagnosis of PD and FT can only be made following isolation and identification of *S. pullorum* and *S. gallinarum,* respectively.

TREATMENT. Reasonably effective prophylactic and therapeutic drugs have been developed against PD and FT. In Canada and the United States, every effort is being made to eradicate these diseases. Various sulfonamides followed by nitrofurans and several other antibiotics have been found to be effective in reducing mortality from PD and FT; however, no drug or combination of drugs has been found capable of eliminating infection from a treated flock. Sulfonamides, in particular, frequently suppress growth and may interfere with feed and water intake and egg production.

Sulfonamides that have been used in treatment of PD and FT include sulfadiazine, sulfamerazine, sulfathiazole, sulfamethazine, and sulfaquinoxaline (2). Sulfadiazine, sulfamethazine, and sulfamerazine at a maximum drug level of 0.75% in starter mash, used for either 5 or 10 days starting at 1 day of age, was effective in preventing chick mortality. Mortality recurred, however, in all groups beginning 5 days after drug withdrawal (22). Sulfamerazine at 0.5% level in mash for the first 5 days reduced mortality of poults from infected breeders (72). Sulfaquinoxaline at 0.1% in the feed can be used for 2 to 3 days and 0.05% for 2 additional days, if necessary, to treat FT. The water-soluble form may be used at the level of 0.04% for 2–3 days

and repeated if necessary. The withdrawal period is a minimum of 10 days before slaughter for food (75). Most of the studies have indicated, however, that appreciable numbers of infected birds remain among medicated survivors (22, 77).

Numerous reports have indicated the effectiveness of nitrofurans in the treatment of PD and FT. Furazolidone at the concentration of 0.04% in feed for a 10- to 14-day period was highly effective in preventing mortality in carriers among chicks (45, 92, 119, 120). It has also been suggested that furazolidone may interfere with antibody production and that it is contraindicated for at least 6 wk before testing for PD (53). Other reports indicated using furazolidone either at 0.011% or 0.066% in feed may reduce the mortality due to PD, but some birds remain infected (39, 82). For FT, use of furazolidone at a 0.011% level in the feed for 2 wk, followed by use at a 0.0055% level continuously until the flock is marketed, is suggested (75). The withdrawal period is a minimum of 5 days before slaughtering for food. Furazolidone water medication has also been shown to be effective in reducing mortality in chicks infected with *S. pullorum* (20). The approval of furazolidone in the treatment of various poultry diseases in the United States has been withdrawn by the Food and Drug Administration since 1993.

Various antibiotics such as chloramphenicol at a concentration of 0.5% in feed for 10 days, chlortetracycline at a 200 mg/kg level in the feed, and the aminoglycoside apramycin for a 5-day treatment at either 150 or 225 mg/L in drinking water were effective in reducing morbidity and mortality (46, 92, 105). None of these antibiotics, however, was totally effective in eliminating *S. pullorum*. Spraying eggs with neomycin sulfate prior to incubation has also been helpful in controlling PD in chicks (101).

In addition to chlortetracycline, other antibiotics such as streptomycin and chloromycetin have been tried in treatment of FT; however, none have been approved for use in poultry raised for food in the United States (75).

Variable drug resistance to chlortetracycline and nitrofurazone have been reported among isolates of *S. pullorum* (61, 85). Similar drug resistance to furazolidone by certain strains of *S. gallinarum* has been reported (51, 94, 102, 103).

PREVENTION AND CONTROL. It has long been established that chicken and turkey flocks can be developed and maintained free of PD and FT by adhering to well-defined procedures. Both PD and FT are good examples of diseases that have decreased in incidence over the years by application of basic management procedures. In the simplest sense, it can be stated that the only requirement is to establish breeding flocks free of *S. pullorum* and *S.*

gallinarum and to hatch and rear their progeny under circumstances that preclude direct or indirect
contact with infected chickens or turkeys.

Management Procedures.   Methods of management broadly designed to prevent the introduction of infectious agents are also usually specifically applicable to preventing the introduction of *S.
pullorum* and *S. gallinarum.* That egg transmission
plays a dominant role in the spread of these two diseases makes it mandatory that only eggs from
flocks known to be free of PD and FT be introduced
into hatcheries. Under the NPIP, chicken and turkey
breeding flocks and their progeny may be recognized as free of PD and FT. Chickens and turkeys
are the primary hosts of *S. pullorum* and *S. gallinarum*; free-flying birds and other fowl are not major reservoirs of infection. Thus, eradication of
these diseases from chicken and turkey breeding
flocks will go a long way toward their total elimination from commercial poultry flocks.

Management practices should be broadly applied
to prevent introduction of PD or FT. Elimination of
carriers must be carried out regularly.

1. Chicks and poults should be obtained from
   sources free of PD and FT.
2. There should be no mixing of pullorum-free and
   typhoid-free stock with other poultry or confined
   birds not known to be free of the diseases.
3. Chicks and poults should be placed in an environment that can be cleaned and sanitized to
   eliminate any residential salmonellae from previous flocks (see Resistance to Chemical and
   Physical Agents).
4. Chicks and poults should receive pelletized,
   crumbled feed to minimize the introduction of *S.
   pullorum* and *S. gallinarum* and other salmonellae through contaminated feed ingredients. Use
   of feed ingredients free of salmonellae is highly
   desirable.
5. Introduction of salmonellae from outside
   sources must be minimized by the use of a sound
   biosecurity program.
   a. Free-flying birds are commonly found to be
      carriers of salmonellae, although *S. pullorum*
      or *S. gallinarum* are rarely encountered. Poul-
      try houses should be birdproof.
   b. Rats, mice, rabbits, cats, dogs, and pests may
      be carriers of salmonellae but are rarely
      found to be infected with *S. pullorum* or *S.
      gallinarum.* Nevertheless, poultry houses
      should be rodentproof.
   c. Insect control is important, particularly
      against flies, poultry mites, and the lesser
      mealworm. These pests may provide a means
      of survival of salmonellae and other avian
      pathogens in the environment.

d. Potable drinking water must be used, or chlorinated water should be provided. In some areas, a danger is posed by surface water collected in open ponds for use as drinking
   water for livestock and poultry.
e. Mechanical carriers of the organism include
   footwear and clothing of humans, as well as
   poultry equipment, processing trucks, and
   poultry crates. Every precaution should be
   made to prevent introduction of *S. pullorum*
   or *S. gallinarum* by fomites.
f. Proper disposal of dead birds is essential.

Elimination of Carriers.   The foundation of
the PD control program was established in 1913 by
use of TA for detecting infected chickens (60). The
test was promptly applied in state programs to eliminate the disease from flocks by detection and removal of reactors.

Early field testing results indicated that removal
of reactors following a single test usually was not
sufficient for complete elimination of infected birds
from a flock. Such results may be expected because
of three possible intercurrent characteristics: 1)
serum agglutinin titers of infected birds tend to fluc-
tuate and may for brief periods fail to produce significant agglutination at the usual dilution of 1:25 or
1:50; 2) there is a delay of at least several days between infection and the development of agglutinins;
and 3) following the removal of reactors, environmental contamination may serve as a source of infection for other birds at a later date.

SEROLOGIC TESTS.   As noted above, in addition
to the TA test, others such as RS, WB, and MA tests
were developed (83, 86, 116). All of these are effective in detecting carriers. The MA test is as dependable as the TA test and offers an important advantage in economy. The NPIP (7), which details
testing methods, accepts four tests for testing chickens: standard TA test, WB test, RS test, and MA
test. Of the four, only the WB test is not accepted
for turkeys, as it was found not satisfactory. Testing
for accreditation is allowed after chickens and
turkeys reach approximate immunologic maturity at
16 wk of age.

In contrast to requirements in the United States
for producing antigen from cells grown on the surface of appropriate agar, a different WB test antigen
was developed in Japan, where it is officially used
(106). This antigen is prepared from cultures grown
in a continuous-flow, broth-culture system, in
which it is necessary to blend sublots to secure desired agglutinability. An ELISA test is also available for screening of flocks for PD and FT (14, 69,
70).

Serologic evidence of infection should be confirmed by bacteriologic examination of one or more
reactors. If only suspicious reactions are observed

in a flock, the birds reacting most strongly should be submitted to a laboratory for retesting and a careful bacteriologic examination. In routine testing, flocks should not be interpreted as infected solely on the basis of doubtful or atypical reactions, because such reactions may result from infections other than *S. pullorum* or *S. gallinarum* (42, 89, 111).

NONPULLORUM–NONGALLINARUM REACTORS. Nonpullorum, and possibly nongallinarum, reactions occasionally cause problems of interpretation (40, 111). A variety of bacteria possessing antigens in common with, or closely related to, those of *S. pullorum* may infect birds and produce an agglutinin response. It was reported that nonpullorum reactions occur more frequently with variant than with standard-form antigen. Infections with coliforms, micrococci, and streptococci, particularly those belonging to the Lancefield Group D, were found to be responsible for a large percentage of nonpullorum reactions in chickens. Infections with other bacteria such as *Staphylococcus epidermidis*, *Micrococcus* spp., *Aerobacter aerogenus*, *Proteus* spp., *Escherichia coli*, and species of *arizonae*, *providentia*, and *citrobacter*, were responsible for many nonpullorum reactions. Other salmonellae, particularly those in Group D, such as *S. enteritidis*, may also produce cross-reactions. Nonpullorum reactors range from a few birds in a flock to as high as 30–40%. The character of the agglutination may be variable. Detailed bacteriologic examination of representative reactors is often the only dependable method of determining the infection status of a flock, and it is usually the only method of distinguishing between infections by *S. pullorum* and *S. gallinarum*.

NATIONAL CONTROL PROGRAM. The NPIP (7) details specific criteria for establishing and maintaining official United States pullorum–typhoid-clean flocks and hatcheries. These criteria are based on farm and hatchery management to prevent direct or indirect contact with infected stock and annual testing of all, or a representative portion, of the birds in the flocks.

If an attempt is made to free a flock of infection, retesting of the infected flock should be done at 2- to 4-wk intervals until two consecutive negative tests of the entire flock are secured at not less than a 21-day interval. In the majority of cases, infection can be eliminated from the flock through short-interval testing. Two or three retests are often sufficient to detect all infected birds; occasionally, however, infection continues to spread within a flock and the disease cannot be eliminated by repeated testing.

AREA ERADICATION. The essentials of an eradi-cation program for an area are the following:

1. PD and FT must be mandatory reportable diseases.
2. Outbreaks must be placed under quarantine, and infected flocks marketed under supervision.
3. All reports of PD and FT must be investigated by an authorized state or federal official.
4. Importation regulations must require shipments of poultry and hatching eggs to be from sources considered free of PD and FT.
5. Regulations must require poultry going to public exhibition to be from flocks free from PD and FT.
6. Total participation of poultry breeding flocks and hatcheries must be required in a pullorum–typhoid control program such as NPIP programs or the equivalent.

Forty-two states in the United States had qualified under the above program as pullorum–typhoid-clean states by 1995; however, a reservoir of PD still exists in small flocks. This reservoir of infection may be larger than indicated, since not all states have a program to test noncommercial and exhibition poultry. Experience indicates that the usual separation of commercial and noncommercial poultry is quite effective in preventing transmission of *S. pullorum* and *S. gallinarum* between these populations. Nevertheless, infected backyard flocks pose some danger to commercial flocks. It is necessary to continue to test commercial breeding flocks to enable earlier identification of accidental infections from noncommercial poultry.

Immunization. Since PD has been mostly eradicated from commercial flocks over the years and the eradication program is in place, there is very little incentive for the production of vaccines to control PD. Fowl typhoid, however, continues to be a problem in some parts of the world. There is no federally licensed *S. gallinarum* killed bacterin produced in the United States, and live modified vaccines used in other countries are not permitted in the United States. Various investigators have evaluated killed and modified live vaccines. With the upsurge of FT in many countries, studies on the use of the 9R strain as live oral or injectable vaccine, with or without oil adjuvants, have been reported with variable results (48, 49, 50, 91, 74). Similarly, outer membrane proteins from *S. gallinarum* have been reported to offer better protection than the 9R live vaccine in terms of clearance of the pathogenic strain from internal organs (23, 25). More recently, immunization against FT by the use of mutant strains of *S. gallinarum* and a virulence-plasmid–cured derivative of *S. gallinarum* appear to be promising in protecting birds challenged with *S. gallinarum* (10, 11, 47).

REFERENCES

1. Altmeyer, R.M., J.K. McNern, J.C. Bossio, I. Rosenshine, B.B. Finlay, and J.E. Galan. 1993. Cloning and molecular characterization of a gene involved in salmonella adherence and invasion of cultured epithelial cells. Mol Microbiol 7:89–98.

2. Anderson, G.W., J.B. Cooper, J.C. Jones, and C.L. Morgan. 1948. Sulfonamides in the control of pullorum disease. Poult Sci 27:172–175.

3. Anonymous. 1930. Eastern states conference on laboratory workers in pullorum disease control. J Am Vet Med Assoc 77:259–263.

4. Anonymous. 1933. Report of the conference of official research workers in animal diseases of North America on standard methods of pullorum disease in barnyard fowl. J Am Vet Med Assoc 82:487–491.

5. Anonymous. 1987. 1986 Summary of commercial poultry disease reports. Avian Dis 31:926–978.

6. Anonymous. 1992. Salmonella Surveillance, Annual Summary. Centers for Disease Control and Prevention, Atlanta, GA.

7. Anonymous. 1994. The National Poultry Improvement Plan and Auxiliary Provisions. United States Department of Agriculture, Animal and Plant Health Inspection Service, Hyattsville, MD.

8. Anonymous. 1994. Salmonella Serotyping Results. National Veterinary Services Laboratory, Ames, IA.

9. Badi, M.A., N. Iliadis, and K. Sarris. 1992. Natural and experimental infection of rodents (Rattus norvegicus) with Salmonella gallinarum. Berl Munch Tierarztl Wochenschr 105:264–267.

10. Barrow, P.A. 1990. Immunity to experimental fowl typhoid in chickens induced by a virulence plasmid-cured derivative of Salmonella gallinarum. Infect Immun 58:2283–2288.

11. Barrow, P.A. 1992. In-vitro and in-vivo characteristics of TnphoA mutant strains of Salmonella serotype gallinarum not invasive for tissue culture cells. J Med Microbiol 36:389–397.

12. Barrow, P.A., and M.A. Lovell. 1988. The association between a large molecular mass plasmid and virulence in a strain of Salmonella pullorum. J Gen Microbiol 134:2307–2316.

13. Barrow, P.A., J.M. Simpson, M.A. Lovell, and M.M. Binns. 1987. Contribution of Salmonella gallinarum large plasmid toward virulence in fowl typhoid. Infect Immun 55:388–392.

14. Barrow, P.A., A. Berchieri, Jr., and O. Al-Haddad. 1992. Serological response of chickens to infection with Salmonella gallinarum-S. pullorum detected by enzyme-linked immunosorbent assay. Avian Dis 36:227–236.

15. Barrow, P.A., M.B. Huggins, and M.A. Lovell. 1994. Host specificity of Salmonella infection in chickens and mice is expressed in vivo primarily at the level of the reticuloendothelial system. Infect Immun 62:4602–4610.

16. Beach, J.R., and D.E. Davis. 1927. Acute infection in chicks and chronic infection of the ovaries of hens caused by the fowl typhoid organisms. Hilgardia 2:411–424.

17. Beaudette, F.R. 1925. The possible transmission of fowl typhoid through the egg. J Am Vet Med Assoc 67:741–745.

18. Beaudette, F.R. 1930. Fowl typhoid and bacillary white diarrhea. Proc 11th Int Vet Congr 3:705–723.

19. Beaudette, F.R. 1936. Arthritis in a chick caused by Salmonella pullorum. J Am Vet Med Assoc 89:89–91.

20. Bierer, B.W. 1961. Furaltadone water medication against naturally induced Salmonella pullorum infection in stressed floor broilers. Avian Dis 5:333–336.

21. Blaxland, J.D., W.J. Sojka, and A.M. Smither. 1956. A study of Salmonella pullorum and Salmonella gallinarum strains isolated from field outbreaks of disease. J Comp Pathol Ther 66:270–277.

22. Bottorff, C.A., and J.S. Kiser. 1947. The use of sulfonamides in the control of pullorum disease. Poult Sci 26:335–339.

23. Bouzoubaa, K. 1988. Membrane proteins from Salmonella gallinarum for protection against fowl typhoid. PhD Thesis. Institute of Agronomy and Veterinary Medicine, Hassan II, Rabat, Morocco.

24. Bouzoubaa, K., and K.V. Nagaraja. 1984. Epidemiological studies on the incidence of salmonellosis in chicken breeder/hatchery operations in Morocco. In G.H. Snoeyenbos (ed.). Proc Int Symp Salmonella, New Orleans. American Association of Avian Pathologists, Kennett Square, PA, p. 337.

25. Bouzoubaa, K., K.V. Nagaraja, J.A. Newman, and B.S. Pomeroy. 1987. Use of membrane proteins from Salmonella gallinarum for prevention of fowl typhoid infection in chickens. Avian Dis 31:699–704.

26. Buchholz, P.S., and A. Fairbrother. 1992. Pathogenicity of Salmonella pullorum in northern bobwhite quail and mallard ducks. Avian Dis 36:304–312.

27. Bullis, K. 1977. The history of avian medicine in the U.S. II. Pullorum disease and fowl typhoid. Avian Dis 21:422–435.

28. Bumstead, N., and P. Barrow. 1993. Resistance to Salmonella gallinarum, S. pullorum, and S. enteritidis in inbred lines of chickens. Avian Dis 37:189–193.

29. Carlson, V.L., and G.H. Snoeyenbos. 1974. Comparative efficacies of selenite and tetrathionate broths for the isolation of salmonella serotypes. Am J Vet Res 35:711–718.

30. Christensen, J.P., J.E. Olsen, H.C. Hansen, and M. Bisgaard. 1992. Characterization of Salmonella enterica serovar gallinarum biovars gallinarum and pullorum by plasmid profiling and biochemical analysis. Avian Pathol 21:461–470.

31. Christensen, J.P., J.E. Olsen, and M. Bisgaard. 1993. Ribotypes of Salmonella enterica serovar gallinarum biovars gallinarum and pullorum. Avian Pathol 22:725–738.

32. Christensen, J.P., M.N. Skov, K.H. Hinz, and M. Bisgaard. 1994. Salmonella enterica serovar gallinarum biovar gallinarum in layers: Epidemiological investigations of a recent outbreak in Denmark. Avian Pathol 23:489–501.

33. Doyle, L.P., and F.P. Mathews. 1928. The pathology of bacillary white diarrhea in chicks. Purdue Univ Agric Exp Stn Res Bull 323.

34. Edwards, P.R., and D.W. Bruner. 1946. Form variation in Salmonella pullorum and its relation to X strains. Cornell Vet 36:318–324.

35. Edwards, P.R., D.W. Bruner, E.R. Doll, and G.S. Hermann. 1948. Further notes on variation in Salmonella pullorum. Cornell Vet 38:257–262.

36. Erbeck, D.H., B.G. McLaughlin, and S.N. Singh. 1993. Pullorum disease with unusual signs in two backyard chicken flocks. Avian Dis 37:895–897.

37. Evans, W.M., D.W. Bruner, and M.C. Peckham. 1955. Blindness in chicks associated with salmonellosis. Cornell Vet 45:239–247.

38. Ferguson, A.E., M.C. Connell, and B. Truscott. 1961. Isolation of Salmonella pullorum from the joints of broiler chicks. Can Vet J 2:143–145.

39. Francis, D.W. 1960. Treatment of natural infection of Salmonella pullorum in day-old chicks with furazolidone. Avian Dis 4:63–73.

40. Garrard, E.H., W.H. Burton, and J.A. Carpenter. 1948. Non-pullorum agglutination reactions. Proc 8th World's Poult Congr, pp. 626–631.

41. Garren, H.W., and C.W. Barber. 1955. Endocrine and lymphatic gland changes occurring in young chickens with fowl typhoid. Poult Sci 34:1250–1258.

42. Gast, R.K., and C.W. Beard. 1990. Serological detection of experimental Salmonella enteritidis infections in laying hens. Avian Dis 34:721–728.

43. Gauger, H.C. 1934. A chronic carrier of fowl typhoid

with testicular focalization. J Am Vet Med Assoc 84:248–251.

44. Gordeuk, S., Jr., P.J. Glantz, E.W. Callenbach, and W.T.S. Thorp. 1949. Transmission of fowl typhoid. Poult Sci 28:385–391.

45. Gordon, R.F., and J. Tucker. 1955. The treatment of chronic carriers of Salmonella pullorum with furazolidone. Vet Rec 67:116–118.

46. Grausgruber, W., and R. Kissling. 1964. Influence of antibiotic food supplements on bacteriological and serological diagnosis of pullorum disease. Wien Tieraerztl Monatsschr 51:814–822.

47. Griffin, H.G., and P.A. Barrow. 1993. Construction of an aroA mutant of Salmonella serotype gallinarum: Its effectiveness in immunization against experimental fowl typhoid. Vaccine 11:457–462.

48. Gupta, B.R., and B.B. Mallick. 1976. Immunization against fowl typhoid. 1. Live oral vaccine. Indian J Anim Sci 46:502–505.

49. Gupta, B.R., and B.B. Mallick. 1976. Immunization against fowl typhoid. 2. Live adjuvant vaccine. Indian J Anim Sci 46:546–551.

50. Gupta, B.R., and B.B. Mallick. 1977. Use of 9R strain of S. gallinarum as vaccine against S. pullorum infection in chicks. India Vet J 54:331–333.

51. Hall, C.F., and H.T. Cartrite. 1961. Observations on strains of Salmonella gallinarum apparently resistant to furazolidone. Avian Dis 5:382–392.

52. Hall, W.J., D.H. Legenhausen, and A.D. McDonald. 1949. Studies on fowl typhoid. 1. Nature and dissemination. Poult Sci 28:344–362.

53. Henderson, W., G.L. Morehouse, and R.F. Cross. 1960. The effect of furazolidone on Salmonella pullorum and agglutination titers in chickens. Avian Dis 4:223–230.

54. Hewitt, E.A. 1928. Bacillary white diarrhea in baby turkeys. Cornell Vet 18:272–276.

55. Hinshaw, W.R. 1930. Fowl typhoid of turkeys. Vet Med 25:514–517.

56. Hinshaw, W.R., C.W. Upp, and J.M. Moore. 1926. Studies on transmission of bacillary white diarrhea in incubators. J Am Vet Assoc 68:631–641.

57. Horsfall, D.J., Rowley, and C.R. Jenkins. 1970. The titre of bactericidal antibody against Salmonella gallinarum in chicks. Immunology 18:595–598.

58. Hutt, F.B., and R.D. Crawford. 1960. On breeding chicks resistant to pullorum disease without exposure thereto. Can J Genet Cytol 2:357–370.

59. Johnson, D.C., M. David, and S. Goldsmith. 1992. Epizootiological investigation of an outbreak of pullorum disease in an integrated broiler operation. Avian Dis 36:770–775.

60. Jones, F.S. 1913. The value of the macroscopic agglutination test in detecting fowls that are harboring Bacterium pullorum. J Med Res 27:481–495.

61. Karyagin, V.V. 1964. Development of resistance of Salmonella pullorum. I. To biomycin. II. To Furazolidone. Nauchn Tr, pp. 31–49.

62. Klein, E. 1889. Über eine epidemische Krankheit der Hühner, verursacht durch einer Bacillus–Bacillus gallinarum. Zentralbl Bakteriol Parasitenkd Abt I Orig 5:689–693.

63. Kokosharov, T., I. Petkov, and I. Dzhurova. 1984. Cocks with experimentally induced acute typhoid. Vet Med Nauki 21:18–26.

64. Komarov, A. 1932. Fowl typhoid in baby chicks. Vet Rec 12:1455–1457.

65. Li, J., N.H. Smith, K. Nelson, P.B. Crichton, D.C. Old, T.S. Whittam, and R.K. Selander. 1993. Evolutionary origin and radiation of the avian-adapted non-motile salmonellae. J Med Microbiol 38:129–39.

66. Lucio, B., M. Padron, and A. Mosqueda. 1984. Fowl typhoid in Mexico. In G.H. Snoeyenbos (ed.). Proc Int Symp Salmonella, New Orleans. American Association of Avian Pathologists, Kennett Square, PA, pp. 382–383.

67. Martinaglia, G. 1929. A note on Salmonella gallinarum infection of ten-day-old chicks and adult turkeys. J S Afr Vet Med Assoc 1:35–36.

68. McCullough, N.B., and C.W. Eisele. 1951. Experimental human salmonellosis. IV. Pathogenicity of strains of Salmonella pullorum obtained from spray-dried whole egg. J Infect Dis 89:259–265.

69. Minga, U.M., and C. Wray. 1992. A disc ELISA for the detection of Salmonella group D antibodies in poulty. Res Vet Sci 52:384–386.

70. Minga, U.M., C. Wray, and P.S. Gwakisa. 1992. Serum, disc and egg ELISA for the serodiagnosis of Salmonella gallinarum and S. enteritidis infections in chickens. Scand J Immunol 11:157–159.

71. Mitchell, R.B., F.C. Garlock, and R.H. Broh-Kahn. 1946. An outbreak of gastro-enteritis presumably caused by Salmonella pullorum. J Infect Dis 79:57–62.

72. Mullen, F.E. 1946. Sulfamerazine as a prophylactic in pullorum disease in poults. J Am Vet Med Assoc 108:163–164.

73. Orr, B.B, and E.N. Moore. 1953. Longevity of Salmonella gallinarum. Poult Sci 32:800–805.

74. Padmanaban, V.D., K.R. Mittal, and B.R. Gupta. 1981. Cross protection against fowl typhoid: Immunization trials and humoral immune response. Dev Comp Immunol 5:301–312.

75. Pomeroy, B.S. 1984. Fowl Typhoid. In M.S. Hofstad, H.J. Barnes, B.W. Calnek, W.M. Reid, and H.W. Yoder, Jr. (eds.). Diaeases of Poultry, 8th ed. Iowa State University Press, Ames, IA, pp 79–91.

76. Pomeroy, B.S., and K.V. Nagaraja. 1991. Fowl typhoid. In B.W. Calnek, H.J. Barnes, C.W. Beard, W.M. Reed, and H.W. Yoder, Jr. (eds.). Diseases of Poultry, 9th Ed. Iowa State University Press, Ames, IA, pp. 87–99.

77. Pomeroy, B.S., R. Fenstermacher, and M.H. Roepke. 1948. Sulfonamides in the control of salmonellosis of chicks and poults. J Am Vet Med Assoc 112:296–303.

78. Popp, L. 1947. Fowl typhoid organisms as the cause of gastroenteritis in man [abst]. J Am Vet Med Assoc 111:314.

79. Rettger, L.F. 1900. Septicemia among young chickens. NY Med J 71:803–805.

80. Rettger, L.F. 1909. Further studies on fatal septicemia in young chickens or "white diarrhea." J Med Res 21:115–123.

81. Rettger, L.F., and W.N. Plastridge. 1932. Pullorum disease of domestic fowl. Monogr Storrs Agric Exp Stn Bull 178.

82. Richey, D.J., and C.L. Morgan. 1960. The effects of furazolidone on chicken Salmonella pullorum carriers. Avian Dis 4:48–63.

83. Runnels, R.A., C.J. Coon, H. Farley, and F. Thorp. 1927. An application of the rapid-method agglutination test to the diagnosis of bacillary white diarrhea infection. J Am Vet Med Assoc 70:660–662.

84. Salem, M., E.M. Odor, and C. Pope. 1992. Pullorum disease in Delaware roasters. Avian Dis 36:1076–1080.

85. Sarkisov, A.Kh., and E.T. Trishkina. 1966. Antibiotic sensitivity of Salmonella pullorum isolated from chicks on farms where antibiotics have been used over a long period. Tr Vses Inst Eksp Vet 32:224–230.

86. Schaffer, J.M., A.D. MacDonald, W.J. Hall, and H. Bunyea. 1931. A stained antigen for the rapid whole blood test for pullorum disease. J Am Vet Med Assoc 79:236–240.

87. Severens, J.M., E. Roberts, and L.E. Card. 1944. A study of the defense mechanism involved in hereditary resistance to pullorum disease of the domestic fowl. J Infect Dis 75:33–46.

88. Shivaprasad, H.L. 1995. Unpublished data.

89. Shivaprasad, H.L., J.F. Timoney, S. Morales, B. Lucio, and R.C. Baker. 1990. Pathogenesis of Salmonella enteritidis infection in laying chickens. I. Studies on egg transmission, clinical signs, fecal shedding, and serologic responses. Avian Dis 34:548–557.

90. Silva, E.N. 1984. The Salmonella gallinarum problem in Central and South America. In G.H. Snoeyenbos (ed.). Proc Int Symp Salmonella, New Orleans. American Association of Avian Pathologists, Kennett Square, PA, pp. 150–156.

91. Silva, E.N., G.H. Snoeyenbos, O.M. Weinack, and C.F. Smyser. 1981. Studies on the use of 9R strain of Salmonella gallinarum as a vaccine in chickens. Avian Dis 25:38–52.

92. Smith, H.W. 1954. The treatment of Salmonella pullorum infection in chicks with furazolidone, sulphamerazine, and chloramphenicol. Vet Rec 493–496.

93. Smith, H.W. 1955. The longevity of Salmonellarum in the faeces of infected chickens. J Comp Pathol Ther 65:267–270.

94. Smith, H.W., J.F. Tucker, and M. Lovell. 1981. Furazolidone resistance in Salmonella gallinarum: The relationship between in vitro and in vivo determinations of resistance. J Hyg (Camb) 87:71–81.

95. Smith, I.M., S.T. Licence, and R. Hill. 1978. Haematological, serological and pathological effects in chicks of one or more intravenous infections of Salmonella gallinarum endotoxin. Res Vet Sci 24:154–160.

96. Smith, T.H., and C. Ten Broeck. 1915. Agglutination affinities of a pathogenic bacillus from fowls (fowl typhoid) (Bacterium Sanguinarium Moore) with the typhoid bacillus of man. J Med Res 31:503–521.

97. Snoeyenbos, G.H. 1991. Pullorum disease. In B.W. Calnek, H.J. Barnes, C.W. Beard, W.M. Reed, and H.W. Yoder, Jr. (eds.). Diseases of Poultry, 9th Ed. Iowa State University Press, Ames, IA, pp. 73–86.

98. St. John-Brooks, R., and M. Rhodes. 1923. The organisms of the fowl typhoid group. J Pathol Bacteriol 26:433–439.

99. Stanley, J., and N. Baquar. 1994. Phylogenetics of Salmonella enteritidis. Int J Food Microbiol 21:79–87.

100. Stokes, J.L., and H.G. Bayne. 1961. Oxidative assimilation of amino acids by salmonellae in relation to growth rates. J Bacteriol 81:118–125.

101. Stuart, E.E., and R.D. Keenum. 1970. Preincubation treatment of chicken hatching eggs infected with Salmonella pullorum. Avian Dis 14:87–95.

102. Stuart, E.E., R.D. Keenum, and H.W. Bruins. 1962. Experimental studies on an isolate of Salmonella gallinarum apparently resistant to furazolidone. Avian Dis 7:294–303.

103. Stuart, E.E., R.D. Keenum, and H.W. Bruins. 1967. The emergence of a furazolidone-resistant strain of Salmonella gallinarum. Avian Dis 11:139–45.

104. Suganuma, Y. 1960. Histopathological studies of serositis of pullorum disease. Jpn J Vet Sci 22:175–182.

105. Tacconi, G., G. Astrybal, and G. Bertorotta. 1987. Evaluation of the efficacy of apromycin against Salmonella pullorum infection in chickens. Avian Pathol 16:319–326.

106. Tanaka, S. 1975. Production of pullorum antigen by continuous submerged culture. Jpn Agric Res Q 9:60–65.

107. Trabulsi, L.R., and P.R. Edwards. 1962. The differentiation of Salmonella pullorum and Salmonella gallinarum by biochemical methods. Cornell Vet 52:563–569.

108. Tsubokura, M. 1965. Studies of Salmonella pullorum phage. I. Isolation of phages and their properties. Jpn J Vet Sci 27:179–188.

109. Tsubokura, M. 1966. Studies on Salmonella pullorum phage. V. Conversion of subtypes of S. pullorum by phage. Jpn J Vet Sci 28:35–40.

110. Van Buskirk, M.A. 1987. A pullorum disease outbreak in a pullorum-free state. Proc 59th Northeast Conf Avian Dis, Atlantic City, NJ, pp. 40–42.

111. Waltman, W.D., and A.M. Horne. 1993. Isolation of salmonella from chickens reacting in the pullorum-typhoid agglutination test. Avian Dis 37:805–810.

112. Watanabe, S., T. Nagai, K. Hashimoto, T. Kume, and R. Sakazaki. 1960. Studies on salmonella infection in hens' eggs during incubation. VII. Transmission to eggs of agglutinins and immunity from hens infected with S. pullorum. Bull Natl Inst Anim Health (Tokyo) 39:37–41.

113. Williams, J.E. 1953. Antigenic studies using ammonium sulfate. I. The relative sedimentation effect of ammonium sulfate on the various antigenic types of Salmonella pullorum. Am J Vet Res 14:458–462.

114. Williams, J.E. 1953. Antigenic studies using ammonium sulfate. II. The macroscopic ammonium sulfate sedimentation test for distinguishing the antigenic forms of Salmonella pullorum. Am J Vet Res 14:465–470.

115. Williams, J.E., and A.D. MacDonald. 1955. The past, present, future of salmonella antigens for poultry. Proc Annu Meet Am Vet Med Assoc, pp. 333–339.

116. Williams, J.E. and A.D. Whittemore. 1971. Serological diagnosis of pullorum disease with the microagglutination system. Appl Microbiol 21:394–399.

117. Williams, J.E., B.S. Pomeroy, R. Fenstermacher, and A. Holland. 1949. The incidence of variant pullorum in Minnesota. Cornell Vet 39:129–135.

118. Williams, J.E., L.H. Dillard, and G.O. Hall. 1968. The penetration patterns of Salmonella typhimurium through the outer structures of chicken eggs. Avian Dis 12:445–466.

119. Wilson, J.E. 1955. The use of furazolidone in the treatment of infections of day-old chicks with S. pullorum, S. gallinarum, S. typhimurium, and S. thompson. Vet Rec 67:849–853.

120. Wilson, J.E. 1956. The treatment of carriers of Salmonella pullorum and Salmonella gallinarum with furazolidone. Vet Rec 68:748–751.

121. Younie, A.R. 1941. Fowl infection like pullorum disease. Can J Comp Med Vet Sci. 5:164–167.

PARATYPHOID INFECTIONS

Richard K. Gast

INTRODUCTION. Motile *Salmonella* serotypes other than those in the *S. arizonae* subgenus are often referred to as paratyphoid (PT) salmonellae. These organisms can infect a very wide variety of hosts (including humans), in some instances resulting in relatively asymptomatic intestinal carriage and in other instances producing clinical disease. First reported in avian species a century ago in an outbreak of infectious enteritis in pigeons (221), PT infections continue to cause significant disease losses in young poultry. More recently, PT salmonellae have been the subject of intensified interest as agents of food-borne disease transmission to humans. Commercial poultry constitute one of the largest and most important reservoirs of salmonellae that can be introduced into the human food supply. Contaminated poultry meat and eggs have consistently been among the most frequently implicated sources of human *Salmonella* outbreaks. Controlling PT infections has thus become an important objective for the poultry industry from both the public health and economic perspectives.

Public Health Significance.

Although many other pathogens have recently received considerable attention, salmonellae remain among the leading sources of food-borne illness throughout much of the world. For example, nearly 84% of food-borne human illnesses in Scotland between 1980 and 1989 for which a causative agent was established were attributed to salmonellae (239). Between 1973 and 1987, 51% of human food-borne bacterial disease cases in the United States were caused by salmonellae. (23). According to the Centers for Disease Control and Prevention, salmonellosis may affect as many as 1–5 million people each year in the United States; about 20,000 hospitalizations and 500 deaths associated with *Salmonella* are reported annually (255). *Salmonella* outbreaks can have particularly severe consequences in highly vulnerable populations. Of 52 food-borne disease outbreaks in nursing homes in the United States between 1975 and 1987 that had known causes, 52% of the outbreaks and 81% of the deaths were associated with *Salmonella* (195).

Poultry products are consistently identified as important sources of salmonellae that cause illness in humans. More than one-third of food-borne salmonellosis outbreaks in humans in the United States between 1983 and 1987 were associated with poultry meat or eggs (297). The percentage of *Salmonella* outbreaks in England and Wales that were associated with poultry meat rose from less than 13% in 1959–62 to more than 32% in 1984–85 (158). Between 1985 and 1991, 82% of *S. enteritidis* outbreaks in the United States that could be attributed to a specific food vehicle were associated with eggs (218).

Economic Significance.

Infections of domestic poultry with salmonellae are expensive both for the poultry industry and for society as a whole. The costs associated with PT infections in poultry fall into two broad categories. The first concerns the expenses associated with human illnesses caused by the consumption of contaminated poultry products. The total combined costs associated with medical care and lost productivity resulting from food-borne *Salmonella* infections of humans in the United States have been estimated at up to $3.5 billion for 1993 (318).

The second category of costs associated with salmonellae in poultry involves various direct expenses producers face as a consequence of *Salmonella* infections in their flocks. During the first few days after hatching, *Salmonella* infections acquired vertically from parents or horizontally in the hatchery can cause significant growth depression or even mortality in young chicks or poults. Although birds quickly become far less susceptible to salmonellae during the 1st wk of life, other diseases or stressful conditions can predispose poultry to severe *Salmonella* infections. Likewise, infection with *Salmonella* can increase the susceptibility of birds to other pathogens. Infections of mature poultry with salmonellae can also be costly to producers in terms of the efforts required to prevent the transmission of infection to progeny or to humans. Control measures such as biosecurity practices, cleaning and disinfecting of facilities, rodent control programs, vaccination, and testing all can significantly increase production costs. Moreover, negative publicity generated by media reports regarding *Salmonella* contamination of particular foods can significantly affect consumer demand for those items and, thereby, ultimately affect the profitability of producers.

INCIDENCE AND DISTRIBUTION. Found in virtually every part of the world, salmonellae infect or are carried by an extremely wide variety of hosts, including wild animals, domestic animals, and humans. Information about the incidence and serotype distribution of salmonellae in domestic animal populations is essential for understanding the relationships within and between the reservoirs of salmonellae in animals and humans that are ultimately responsible for zoonotic disease transmission.

Incidence of Salmonellae in Poultry and Poultry Products.

Advances in poultry production practices, changes in consumer lifestyles and preferences, and heightened nutritional awareness have all combined to make poultry products a leading source of protein for much of the world. The incidence of *Salmonella* infection in poultry flocks and the associated incidence of *Salmonella* contamination of poultry products are thus of considerable public health significance. Although salmonellae have been found in poultry flocks of various species, including both meat-type and egg-type breeds, estimates of the incidence of salmonellae in birds or their environments have varied considerably.

Surveys of meat-type poultry have reported the isolation of salmonellae from the feces of 94% of broiler flocks sampled in the Netherlands (319) and from the environments of 87% of turkey flocks sampled in Canada (167). The actual prevalence of infection within *Salmonella*-positive flocks, however, has often been observed to be relatively low (171, 286). Surveys of egg-type poultry have reported the recovery of salmonellae from the feces of 47% of flocks sampled in the Netherlands (319) and from either feces or eggbelt samples from nearly 53% of flocks sampled in Canada (251). In studies of pooled cecal samples from spent egg-laying flocks in the United States, salmonellae were detected in all of 81 flocks from nine southern states (327) and in 86% of 406 houses from several regions (88).

In surveys of poultry products, salmonellae have been isolated from 57% of chicken carcasses in Portugal (201), 43% of ready-to-cook broiler carcasses obtained from retail stores in Ohio (33), and 29% of frozen broiler carcasses obtained from retail stores in Arkansas (169). Contamination of eggs with salmonellae has also become an important issue in recent years. In a study of more than 1000 unpasteurized liquid egg samples collected at 20 egg-breaking plants throughout the United States, Ebel et al. (89) found salmonellae in 52% of the samples.

Distribution of *Salmonella* Serotypes.

Although more than 2300 serotypes of *Salmonella* have been identified, only about 10% of these have been isolated from poultry. Moreover, an even smaller subset of serotypes accounts for the vast majority of poultry *Salmonella* isolates. The distribution of *Salmonella* serotypes from poultry sources varies geographically and changes over time. The degree of relatedness between the poultry

and human reservoirs of salmonellae is partly illustrated by similarities in the distribution of serotypes.

Although the frequency of isolation of various *Salmonella* serotypes from poultry changes from year to year, several serotypes are consistently found at a high incidence. Based on data from clinical and environmental isolates submitted to the U.S. Department of Agriculture (USDA) National Veterinary Service Laboratory between July 1990 and June 1993, the most commonly identified serotypes in chickens in the United States were (in descending order of incidence) *S. heidelberg*, *S. enteritidis*, *S. hadar*, *S. montevideo*, *S. kentucky*, and *S. typhimurium* (97, 98, 99). These reports also indicated that the most commonly isolated PT salmonellae in turkeys in the United States during the same period were *S. reading*, *S. heidelberg*, *S. hadar*, *S. agona*, *S. senftenberg*, and *S. saintpaul*. The significance of the poultry *Salmonella* reservoir for public health can be illustrated by considering the serotypes commonly isolated from humans. In 1991, the serotypes most often reported to the Centers for Disease Control and Prevention from human sources in the United States were *S. typhimurium*, *S. enteritidis*, *S. heidelberg*, *S. hadar*, *S. newport*, and *S. agona* (24).

Because of the unique epidemiologic association of *S. enteritidis* with disease transmission via contaminated eggs, the specific prevalence of this one serotype has been a topic of considerable interest in recent years. A Canadian report indicated that environmental samples from 2.7% of 295 layer flocks and 3% of 294 broiler flocks were positive for *S. enteritidis* (250). In two nationwide surveys in the United States, *S. enteritidis* was found in pooled cecal samples from 27% of 406 laying houses tested (88) and from 13% of 1002 pooled samples of unpasteurized liquid egg (89). The increasing public health significance of *S. enteritidis* was shown in a survey of the frequency of reporting of human infections with various *Salmonella* serotypes in 21 nations (261). Only 10% of these nations reported *S. enteritidis* as their most common serotype in 1979, but by 1987 this figure had increased to 43%.

ETIOLOGY

Classification and Nomenclature.

The genus *Salmonella* is a member of the bacterial family Enterobacteriaceae and is divided into five biochemically distinct subgenera (184). The various motile and non–host-adapted serotypes of subgenus I are often referred to as PT salmonellae. The degree of genetic relatedness among the salmonellae is so great that some researchers have suggested that the genus actually consists of only a single species (93), but the names of individual serotypes remain in common usage to facilitate diagnostic classification and epidemiologic analysis.

Morphology and Staining.
Salmonellae are straight, non–spore-forming rods, measuring about 0.7–1.5 x 2.0–5.0 μm. Salmonellae are gram-negative, but cells can readily be stained with common dyes such as methylene blue or carbolfuchsin. Paratyphoid salmonellae are usually peritrichously flagellated and motile, although naturally occurring nonmotile mutants are occasionally encountered. Typical *Salmonella* colonies on agar media are about 2 to 4 mm in diameter, round with smooth edges, slightly raised, and glistening.

Growth Requirements.
Salmonellae are facultatively anaerobic and can grow well under both aerobic and anaerobic conditions. The optimum temperature to support the growth of salmonellae is 37 C, but some growth is generally observed over a range of about 5 to 45 C. Salmonellae can grow within a pH range of about 4.0 to 9.0, with an optimum pH of about 7.0. The nutritional requirements of salmonellae are relatively simple, and most culture media that supply sources of carbon and nitrogen can support their growth. The viability of *Salmonella* cultures can be maintained for many years in simple media, such as peptone agar (184) or nutrient agar, which have been stab-inoculated, sealed, and held at room temperature.

Biochemical Properties.
The biochemical properties characteristic of most PT (subgenus I) *Salmonella* strains are described by Krieg and Holt (184) and Ewing (93). Typical PT salmonellae ferment glucose (to produce both acid and gas), dulcitol, mannitol, maltose, and mucate, but do not ferment lactose, sucrose, malonate, or salicin. They can produce hydrogen sulfide on many types of media, decarboxylate ornithine and lysine, utilize citrate as a sole source of carbon, and reduce nitrates to nitrites. Paratyphoid salmonellae do not hydrolyze urea or gelatin and do not produce indole.

Paratyphoid salmonellae can be distinguished from *S. arizonae* (*Salmonella* subgenus III), *S. pullorum,* and *S. gallinarum* on the basis of several biochemical differences. For example, *S. arizonae* strains cannot ferment dulcitol but usually can ferment malonate, *S. pullorum* strains cannot ferment mucate or dulcitol, and *S. gallinarum* strains cannot decarboxylate ornithine or produce gas from glucose fermentation. In addition, PT salmonellae are usually motile, but *S. pullorum* and *S. gallinarum* are nonmotile.

Antigenic Structure.
The traditional Kauffmann-White schema for antigenic classification of salmonellae is based on both somatic and flagellar antigens (93). The somatic "O" antigens are determined by polysaccharides associated with the body of the cell and are identified by arabic numerals. Serogroups (designated with upper-case letters) of salmonellae are defined by particular somatic antigens that are unique to members of the group. Most *Salmonella* isolates found in poultry belong to Serogroups B, C, or D. The "H" antigens are determined by flagellar proteins and are usually identified by lower-case letters. Flagellar antigens sometimes occur in two different phases. The serotype of a particular *Salmonella* isolate is determined by the combination of O and H antigens that it expresses. Serotyping of isolates is generally accomplished using agglutination tests with batteries of specific antisera. Slide agglutination tests are first used to establish the somatic antigen content and the flagellar antigen content is then determined using tube agglutination tests.

Resistance to Physical and Chemical Agents

HEAT, IRRADIATION, AND OTHER PHYSICAL AGENTS. With the exception of a few distinctively thermoresistant strains (such as *S. senftenberg* 775W), salmonellae are generally quite susceptible to destruction by heat. For example, cooking to an internal temperature of 79 C in conventional or convection ovens always eliminated inoculated *S. typhimurium* from roasting chickens (269). Exposure of ground chicken meat to a temperature of 60 C eliminated *S. typhimurium* contamination (at a level of 10^8 cells/g) within 5 minutes (22). The heat resistance of *S. enteritidis* can be increased by prior exposure to alkaline conditions (163), and decreased by prior refrigeration (156, 263). Salmonellae strains of several serotypes have been able to survive cooking methods for eggs that allow some of the yolk to remain liquid (12, 161). Liquid whole egg is pasteurized in the United States according to USDA specifications that require a minimum treatment time of 3.5 minutes at 60 C (11). Steam pelleting treatment of poultry feed under precisely defined conditions has been reported to eliminate both inoculated and naturally occurring salmonellae (213, 270).

Irradiation has received considerable attention as a potential method for eliminating salmonellae from foods and feedstuffs. Most salmonellae strains appear to be highly susceptible to the lethal effects of irradiation (302). Gamma radiation has been successfully applied to reducing the levels of *Salmonella* contamination in poultry meat (301, 304), egg products (211, 265), and poultry feeds (193). Combined heat and radiation treatments have been shown to be more effective in eliminating salmonellae than either treatment alone (265, 303). Several other physical agents, including electrical stimulation (196, 275), ultraviolet radiation (325), and ultrasonic wave treatment (346) have also been reported to be lethal for salmonellae.

CHEMICAL DISINFECTANTS. A wide variety of chemical disinfectants have been assessed for their efficacy against salmonellae. The application of hydrogen peroxide (226), acetic acid (84), lactic acid (168), potassium sorbate (223), chlorine (223), or trisodium phosphate (175) have all been reported to reduce the incidence or level of *Salmonella* contamination on broiler carcasses. Fumigating with formaldehyde (335) or hydrogen peroxide (272), or spraying with polyhexamethylene biguanide hydrochloride (73), has been shown to be effective in controlling salmonellae on hatching eggs. Both ozone and formaldehyde fumigation have similarly been reported to be effective poultry hatchery disinfectants (332).

Studies of the efficacy of chemical treatment of poultry feeds to inhibit salmonellae have produced variable results. Inclusion of an organic acid mixture in feed was reported to reduce significantly the eventual level of salmonellae in feed contaminated with mouse droppings containing *S. typhimurium* (189). Smyser and Snoeyenbos (277), however, studied 12 compounds as potential antagonists of salmonellae in poultry feed (including organic acids) and found that only formalin was consistently effective.

The application of chemical disinfectants to poultry houses is also of uncertain effectiveness. Phenols and quaternary ammonium compounds are often used for this purpose, but cleaning and disinfection has not always been successful in eliminating salmonellae from contaminated houses (209, 282). Formaldehyde fumigation has been found to be highly effective for this purpose (337), but safety considerations have limited its availability and use.

ENVIRONMENTAL FACTORS. The environmental persistence of PT salmonellae is a significant factor in the epidemiology of these organisms in poultry by creating opportunities for horizontal transmission of infection within and between flocks. Smyser et al. (278) reported the isolation of *S. heidelberg* from contaminated litter after 7 mo of holding at room temperature. Williams and Benson (338) observed the survival of *S. typhimurium* for 16 mo in feed and 18 mo in litter stored at 25 C. Water activity has been identified as an important supporting factor in allowing the persistence of salmonellae in poultry houses (242). Although salmonellae can sometimes persist for long periods in poultry litter, used litter has also occasionally been reported to exert an inhibitory effect on *Salmonella* growth or survival (312). Turnbull and Snoeyenbos (313) suggested that this effect might result from a pH increase over time due to dissolved ammonia. The survival of salmonellae on eggs during and after washing has been shown to be dependent on the pH, temperature, and presence of egg solids in the washwater (190) and on the rate of cooling after washing (42).

Pathogenicity

TOXINS. Three general categories of toxins have been reported to play roles in the pathogenicity of PT salmonellae. Endotoxin is associated with the lipid A portion of *Salmonella* cell wall lipopolysaccharide (LPS). If released into the bloodstream of an infected animal when bacterial cells are lysed, endotoxin can produce fever. Intravenously administered *S. enteritidis* endotoxin was found by Turnbull and Snoeyenbos (314) to cause liver and spleen lesions in 2-wk-old chickens. Lipopolysaccharide also contributes to the resistance of the bacterial cell wall to attack and digestion by host phagocytes. Loss of the ability to synthesize complete LPS has been associated with a loss of virulence for *S. enteritidis* in mice (45) and an impaired ability of *S. typhimurium* to colonize the ceca and invade to the spleen in broiler chicks (74).

Two proteinaceous toxins have also been identified in salmonellae. Enterotoxin activity by salmonellae induces a secretory response by epithelial cells that results in fluid accumulation in the intestinal lumen (183). A heat-labile enterotoxin was detected in 44% of 123 *S. typhimurium* strains from animal sources (214). The heat-stable cytotoxin of salmonellae causes structural damage to intestinal epithelial cells, perhaps by inhibiting protein synthesis (181).

Adherence, Invasiveness, and Intracellular Survival.

The adherence of PT salmonellae to intestinal epithelial cells is the pivotal first step in the sequence of events that produces disease. Adherence has been associated with type 1 fimbriae (5, 198) and with a mannose-resistant hemagglutinin (101). Although adherence evidently does not require metabolically active salmonellae, the subsequent bacterial invasion of host cells requires protein synthesis by live salmonellae (186, 200). The overall virulence of salmonellae depends heavily on the initial degree of mucosal invasiveness (4). Putative mechanisms for *Salmonella* invasion of intestinal cells have included type 1 fimbriae (92) and various bacterial proteins induced by contact with epithelial cell surfaces (102).

Adherence and invasiveness of salmonellae can be influenced by culture growth conditions. Logarithmically growing *Salmonella* cells are more invasive in tissue culture than are cells in the stationary phase of growth, and salmonellae grown anaerobically have been shown to be both more adherent and more invasive than salmonellae grown aerobically (92, 191). Rapidly growing *S. typhimurium* cells have been reported to kill mice faster after intravenous injection than do cells in a slower phase of growth (27).

The replication of salmonellae within host cells has also been found to be necessary for the full expression of pathogenicity (194). Mutants of *S. typhimurium* that were unable to survive within host macrophages (100) or to resist the antimicrobial effects of host peptides (127) were reported to exhibit reduced virulence in mice. The production of iron-chelating siderophores may also contribute to the in vivo survival of salmonellae (349).

PLASMIDS. Plasmids are extrachromosomal DNA elements that have often been associated with bacterial pathogenicity. Serotype-specific plasmids of characteristic molecular weights have been directly linked with virulence for a number of salmonellae. Considerable homology has been demonstrated between virulence-associated plasmids of different serotypes (36, 344, 345). Strains of *S. typhimurium* and *S. enteritidis* cured of their virulence-associated plasmids have been found to be significantly less lethal for mice (46, 49, 137, 228). Plasmid-mediated virulence among *S. typhimurium* and *S. enteritidis* isolates has been variously associated with invasion of mesenteric lymph nodes, the liver, and the spleen in mice (128, 293), in vivo growth within cells of infected mice (129, 154, 260), immunosuppression (144), and serum resistance (292). Analysis and characterization of the plasmid content of *S. enteritidis* isolates from diverse poultry sources has proven to be of significant value in establishing epidemiologic relationships (85, 274).

The pathogenicity of salmonellae, however, does not always require the presence of the serotype-specific plasmids. Some strains of *S. typhimurium*, for example, have been shown to retain their invasiveness in cell culture assays (37, 153) and their lethality for infected mice (244) in the absence of virulence-associated plasmids. Moreover, although a serotype-specific plasmid was found to be essential for the full expression of virulence by *S. enteritidis* in mice, curing this plasmid did not affect *S. enteritidis* colonization and invasion of the tissues of orally inoculated chickens (130).

Pathogenicity Differences of Strains, Serotypes, and Phage Types. Paratyphoid salmonellae strains are often found to differ in their ability to cause disease or death in young poultry. Several investigators (58, 138, 276) have reported significant differences in mortality between groups of chicks orally inoculated with isolates representing diverse *Salmonella* serotypes. However, tremendous variation in lethality for chicks has also been observed within single *Salmonella* serotypes, sometimes even among strains of the same phage type (16, 276). Pathogenicity differences have also been noted between the various phage types of *S. enteritidis,* with phage type 4 often associated with a particularly high level of invasiveness (13, 143) and lethality (13, 114, 253) for newly hatched chicks. Differences in virulence within the phage types of *S. enteritidis* (including phage type 4), however, have also been demonstrated (112, 114, 253). Variation between strains of *S. enteritidis,* crossing phage-type boundaries, has also been reported in the frequency of deposition in the contents of eggs laid by experimentally infected hens (112, 273).

The bacterial characteristics responsible for the observed pathogenicity differences between *Salmonella* strains are still incompletely understood. Nolan et al. (237) compared *Salmonella* isolates of identical serotypes obtained from healthy and ill chickens and found differences in the utilization of carbon sources, mannose-sensitive hemagglutination of erythrocytes, and invasiveness in cell culture. However, Barrow et al. (17) concluded that flagellar and somatic antigens, mannose-sensitive hemagglutinins, and the serotype-specific plasmid of *S. typhimurium* were all unessential for intestinal colonization. Petter (246) associated invasive properties of *S. enteritidis* variants with quantitative and qualitative differences in LPS expression.

PATHOGENESIS AND EPIZOOTIOLOGY.
Paratyphoid salmonellae can be isolated from an extremely wide variety of host species, including humans and other mammals, birds, reptiles, and insects. The many interconnections between these reservoirs often impair efforts to reduce the incidence of *Salmonella* infections in humans and domestic animals. Poultry have often been identified as one of the most important reservoirs of salmonellae that ultimately cause human infections. Although chickens and turkeys are susceptible to a broad range of *Salmonella* serotypes, the resulting infection process is determined less by the serotype involved than by factors such as the age of the affected birds, the infecting dose, and predisposing conditions. Paratyphoid salmonellae can be introduced into poultry flocks by several different sources and can likewise be spread within and between flocks by a number of mechanisms.

Paratyphoid Infections in Young Poultry.
Paratyphoid infections often have very different consequences for newly hatched poultry than for more mature birds. In very susceptible young chicks and poults, PT infection can sometimes lead

to illness and death at high frequencies. Older birds are far less susceptible to the lethal effects of PT salmonellae and may experience intestinal colonization and even systemic dissemination without significant morbidity or mortality. The development of resistance to salmonellae in young birds has often been attributed to the acquisition of protective microflora that either compete with salmonellae for intestinal receptor sites or produce antagonistic factors that inhibit *Salmonella* growth (285, 290). Gast and Beard (107) accordingly observed that significantly more orally administered *S. typhimurium* cells adhered in the ceca of 2-day-old chicks than in those of 3- to- 7-day-old chicks.

The usual outcomes of PT infections in chicks and poults fall into three general categories (271). Intestinal colonization is normally the first step in the infection process for orally introduced PT salmonellae, frequently leading to the persistent shedding of salmonellae in the feces. In many infected birds, invasion beyond the gastrointestinal tract results in *Salmonella* multiplication in reticuloendothelial tissue of the liver and spleen (16) and eventual dissemination to colonize a variety of internal tissue sites. Finally, extensive bacteremia sometimes occurs, occasionally causing a high incidence of mortality. The incidence of both mortality (95) and intestinal colonization (262) in chicks correlate strongly with the dose of orally administered salmonellae.

Mortality associated with naturally occurring PT infections in poultry is often observed to reach peak levels at about 3 to 7 days of age (222). Studies of experimental PT infections in young poultry have consistently shown that newly hatched birds are highly susceptible to salmonellae, but this susceptibility decreases over time. Fagerberg et al. (95) found that oral doses of 10^9 *S. typhimurium* cells were lethal for 50% of 1-day-old broiler chicks, 20% of 3-day-old chicks, and no 7-day-old chicks. Smith and Tucker (276) saw mortality associated with *S. typhimurium* inoculation of chicks drop precipitously from 79% at 1 day of age to only 3% at 2 days. A steep reduction in susceptibility to PT-associated mortality has also been reported in turkey poults (31).

The frequency of both intestinal colonization (262) and invasion to internal organs (314) are higher in newly hatched chicks than in older birds. The persistence of salmonellae in various colonization sites is also influenced by the age of the birds when infected. Horizontal contact exposure of chicks within 24 hr of hatching has been reported to result in fecal shedding of *S. enteritidis* for at least 28 wk (230). Gast and Beard (107) determined that cecal colonization with *S. typhimurium* persisted for 7 wk after oral inoculation significantly more often when chicks were infected at 1 day of age than at 7

days. Gorham et al. (125) likewise observed an age-related decrease in the persistence of *S. enteritidis* in the internal organs of inoculated chicks.

Paratyphoid Infections in Mature Poultry.
Morbidity or mortality are not consistently associated with PT infections in mature poultry. Experimental infections of adult chickens with large oral doses of PT salmonellae have often been reported to cause no evident signs of clinical illness (35, 159). Timoney et al. (309) noted that although oral inoculation of laying hens with *S. enteritidis* often resulted in bacteremia and extensive systemic dissemination to internal organ sites, the birds remained clinically normal except for some brief mild diarrhea. Humphrey et al. (162) observed, however, that six of ten 1-year-old hens died after oral inoculation with a phage type 4 *S. enteritidis* isolate.

The two most consistently observed features of PT infections in mature poultry are intestinal colonization and systemic dissemination to internal organs. During approximately the first 2 wk following experimental oral infection of chickens or turkeys, PT salmonellae can generally be isolated from the intestinal tracts and voided feces of a high percentage of inoculated birds (35, 110, 348). Although the incidence of intestinal colonization and fecal shedding steadily declines thereafter, some *S. enteritidis* strains have been shown to persist in the intestinal tract of laying chickens for several months after oral inoculation (108, 110, 273).

Gut colonization by PT salmonellae is usually followed by invasion of the intestinal epithelium and dissemination to internal tissues. Various PT serotypes, including *S. infantis, S. typhimurium,* and *S. heidelberg,* have been found in internal sites such as the liver, spleen, lung, ovary, oviduct, and peritoneum of naturally and experimentally infected chickens and turkeys (35, 281, 348). Invasiveness and systemic dissemination have been documented very extensively for *S. enteritidis.* After experimental oral inoculation of laying hens, *S. enteritidis* has been isolated from numerous internal tissues, including the liver, spleen, ovary, oviduct, heart blood, and peritoneum (110, 309). Dissemination of *S. enteritidis* to diverse internal organs, including the ovary and oviduct, has also been recorded following conjunctival inoculation (165) or exposure to contaminated aerosols (21). The isolation of *S. enteritidis* from a wide range of internal organs has similarly been reported in naturally infected poultry (152, 151, 252).

Another aspect of infections of mature chickens with some PT salmonellae that is of particular concern from a public health perspective is the production of *Salmonella*-contaminated eggs. In the late 1980s, considerable epidemiologic evidence began to accumulate indicating that the contaminated contents of clean and intact eggs were responsible for the transmission of *S. enteritidis* infection to humans (217, 287). Investigations of laying flocks implicated as the sources of eggs that caused human outbreaks have detected *S. enteritidis* isolates of the same phage types found in affected humans, often with identical plasmid profiles or fingerprints, in environmental samples, tissue samples, and eggs (86, 140, 306).

S. enteritidis has been found in the contents of eggs laid by commercial layers (152) and broiler breeders (199), but the incidence of *S. enteritidis* contamination of eggs has generally been found to be extremely low. In studies of 17 naturally infected laying flocks in the United Kingdom, Humphrey et al. (160, 164) found *S. enteritidis* in the contents of less than 1% of the eggs sampled. In two Canadian layer flocks that yielded *S. enteritidis* isolates from both environmental and tissue samples, less than 0.06% of the eggs sampled were contaminated with *S. enteritidis* (252). Naturally contaminated eggs have generally been found to contain very small numbers of *S. enteritidis* (160, 164), but the *S. enteritidis* population in eggs can expand to more dangerous levels if eggs are held at growth-supporting temperatures (113, 164). Contamination of egg contents by *S. enteritidis* has also been demonstrated in experimentally infected laying hens (273, 309). Gast and Beard (108) isolated *S. enteritidis* from the albumen of 19% and yolks of 16% of eggs laid within 4 wk after the administration of a large oral dose to hens.

Predisposing Factors.

A number of factors have been demonstrated to increase the likelihood or severity of PT infection in poultry. Several other infectious agents have been reported to influence the course of infection with salmonellae. Prior infection with several species of coccidia, including *Eimeria tenella*, *E. maxima*, and *E. acervulina*, can increase the ability of salmonella serotypes such as *S. typhimurium*, *S. enteritidis*, *S. agona*, and *S. infantis* to colonize the intestinal tracts of chickens (8, 256, 294). The mechanisms for this effect may be related to decreased levels of *Salmonella*-inhibiting volatile fatty acids and increased oxidation-reduction potential in the intestine related to coccidial infection (7). Infection with *E. tenella*, however, was observed by Tellez et al. (299) to decrease the frequency by invasion of subsequently administered *S. enteritidis* to the internal organs of chicks, perhaps by increasing the thickness of the intestinal lamina propria. Infections of poultry with immunosuppressive viruses or bacteria can also affect the outcome of *Salmonella* infections. Exposure to reticuloendotheliosis virus at 1 day of age increased mortality among chicks inoculated intraperitoneally with *S. typhimurium* at 1, 7, or 14 days of age (224). Exposure of 1-day-old chicks to infectious bursal disease virus led to increased mortality following *S. typhimurium* infection 3 wk later, although viral infection of 3-wk-old chicks did not affect their susceptibility to subsequent infection with *S. typhimurium* (347). Suppression of cell-mediated immunity by *Corynebacterium parvum* led to increased morbidity in chicks subsequently infected with *S. typhimurium* (60).

Environmental and management factors can also influence the susceptibility of poultry to PT salmonellae. Exposure to stressful conditions has often been shown to facilitate or exacerbate *Salmonella* infections. For example, lowering the brooding temperature of chicks by 5 to 8 C was found to increase significantly mortality among newly hatched chicks inoculated with *S. worthington* (300). Water deprivation before inoculation of 7-wk-old chickens increased the duration of fecal shedding of orally administered *S. typhimurium* (34). Forced molting of laying hens by feed deprivation has been reported to increase the incidence and level of fecal shedding (149), the incidence and severity of intestinal lesions (147, 254), and the frequency of horizontal transmission (146) following oral inoculation with *S. enteritidis*. Molting also reduced the infectious dose of *S. enteritidis* necessary to establish intestinal colonization in hens (145) and increased the likelihood of recurrence of previous *S. enteritidis* infections (148).

Sources, Vectors, and Transmission.

Paratyphoid salmonellae can be introduced into poultry flocks from many different sources. The extremely wide host range of PT salmonellae creates an equally large number of reservoirs of infectious organisms that can be transmitted to chickens or turkeys. Among the most frequently implicated sources of infection are contaminated feed and various animal and insect vectors. Paratyphoid salmonellae can be transmitted vertically to the progeny of infected breeder flocks and horizontally within and between flocks.

Contaminated feeds, particularly those containing animal proteins, have often been identified as likely sources of introduction of PT salmonellae to poultry flocks. Zecha et al. (350) reported that four of eight *Salmonella* serotypes isolated from a turkey breeding facility over a 5-yr period had also been isolated from samples of pelleted feed. MacKenzie and Bains (202) noted that *Salmonella* serotypes not previously detected in the flocks of a broiler company in Australia were detected first in raw feed ingredients, and then later appeared in live birds and processed carcasses. Cox et al. (70) collected poultry feed from commercial mills in the United States and found salmonellae in 92% of meat and bone meal samples and in 58% of finished feed (mash) samples, but in no samples of pelleted feed. Experimental inoculation studies have demonstrated that chicks can readily become infected with PT salmonellae from their feed, even when contamination levels are very low (142, 266).

Biologic vectors can both disseminate and amplify salmonellae in poultry flocks. Insects, including cockroaches (182) and lesser mealworms (212), can carry *Salmonella* organisms internally and externally and spread them throughout poultry houses. Mice have been identified as particularly important vectors for *S. enteritidis* in laying flocks. Henzler and Opitz (139) cultured mice and environmental samples from laying farms to isolate *S. enteritidis*. They detected *S. enteritidis* in 24% of the mice from environmentally contaminated laying farms, but in none of the mice from farms with environments free of *S. enteritidis*. They noted that a single mouse fecal pellet could contain 10^5 *S. enteritidis* cells.

Vertical transmission of PT salmonellae to the progeny of infected breeder flocks can result from the production of eggs contaminated by salmonellae in the contents or on the surface. Experimentally infected hens were observed by Gordon and Tucker (123) to transmit *S. menston* to their offspring. The same *Salmonella* serotypes responsible for mortality in naturally infected chicks and poults have often also been isolated from their parent flocks (185, 222). In a survey of 10 farms in France, Lahellec et al. (188) concluded that the greatest contribution to the eventual distribution of *Salmonella* serotypes in broiler houses came from the chicks themselves and not from their environment.

Egg shells are often contaminated with PT salmonellae by fecal contamination during oviposition. The penetration of salmonellae into or through the shell and shell membranes can result in direct transmission of infection to the developing embryo or can lead to exposure of the chick to infectious *Salmonella* organisms when the shell structure is disrupted during hatching. Some PT serotypes, particularly *S. enteritidis*, can be deposited in the contents of eggs before oviposition. The resulting transovarian transmission of infection to progeny is an important aspect of the epidemiology of *S. enteritidis* in chickens.

Regardless of the mechanism or site of egg contamination, any PT salmonellae carried in or on eggs can be spread extensively in the hatchery. As chicks or poults pip through egg shells, salmonellae are released into the air and circulated around hatching cabinets on contaminated fluff and other hatching debris. Bailey et al. (10) reported that 17% of egg shell samples and 21% of chick rinse samples obtained from commercial broiler hatcheries in the United States were positive for PT salmonellae.

Cox et al. (71) likewise isolated salmonellae (of 12 different serotypes) from more than 75% of samples of egg fragments, belting material, and paper pads from three broiler hatcheries. Newly hatched birds, lacking protective intestinal microflora, are highly susceptible to intestinal colonization by salmonellae. Cason et al. (41) observed that nearly 44% of chicks from uncontaminated eggs, hatched along with eggs dipped before incubation in a solution containing *S. typhimurium*, were found to carry *S. typhimurium* in their intestinal tracts upon removal from the hatcher. Bhatia and McNabb (30) found the same *Salmonella* serotypes in hatchery fluff and meconium as were later detected in broiler house litter and finished broiler carcasses.

After introduction into poultry, PT salmonellae can spread horizontally within and between flocks. Snoeyenbos et al. (280) noted that 10 *Salmonella* serotypes spread rapidly from infected day-old chicks to penmates reared on litter. Gast and Beard (108, 110) reported that *S. enteritidis* could be found in the feces and internal organs of uninoculated laying hens housed in cages adjacent to those of orally inoculated birds. Contaminated poultry house environments are often implicated as among the principal sources of PT salmonellae (185). Lahellec and Colin (187) concluded that *Salmonella* serotypes present in broiler houses or introduced into houses by vectors during the rearing period were more likely to appear on processed carcasses than were serotypes originating in the hatchery. In a Dutch study, cumulative infection curves for laying flocks showed an increasing incidence of *S. enteritidis* over time during the laying cycle, suggesting that infection was more likely acquired from farm environments than from breeding stock (321). Horizontal transmission can be mediated by direct bird-to-bird contact, ingestion of contaminated feces or litter, contaminated water (123, 231), personnel and equipment (350), and a variety of other mechanisms.

Clinical Signs.   Paratyphoid infection of poultry is usually associated with disease only in very young birds. The contamination of eggs with salmonellae may lead to a high level of embryo mortality and the rapid death of newly hatched birds before clinical signs are observed. Signs of disease are rarely observed after the first 2 wk of life, although morbidity and mortality can be high during that period and significant growth retardation can occur. The course of illness is normally relatively brief in individual birds. Signs of severe PT infection in young poultry are generally similar to those observed in connection with other avian *Salmonella* infections (pullorum disease, fowl typhoid, and avian arizonosis) and with other bacteria that can cause acute septicemia. Although clinical disease is not normally associated with PT infections in mature poultry, some *S. enteritidis* strains have been found to cause anorexia, diarrhea, and reduced egg production in experimentally infected laying hens (108, 112, 229, 273).

Typical signs of PT infection in chicks and poults include progressive somnolence with closed eyes, drooping wings, and ruffled feathers (336). Anorexia and emaciation are common (16). Affected birds are often seen to shiver and huddle near heat sources. Profuse watery diarrhea is frequently observed, often resulting in dehydration and pasting of the vent area (219, 336). Blindness (245) and lameness (245, 336) have occasionally been associated with PT infections.

Gross Lesions and Histopathology.
In severe outbreaks of PT infection in newly hatched poultry, rapidly developing septicemia can cause a high incidence of mortality with few or no apparent lesions. When the course of disease is longer, severe enteritis is often accompanied by focal necrotic lesions in the mucosa of the small intestine. Cheesy cecal cores (16, 126, 336) are often observed. Spleens and livers are commonly swollen and congested, with evident hemorrhagic streaks or necrotic foci (245, 336). Kidneys may also sometimes be enlarged and congested (219). Fibrinopurulent perihepatitis and pericarditis have been reported on numerous occasions (13, 126, 245, 336). Unabsorbed, coagulated yolk material may be present in the yolk sac (13, 126, 245). Other lesions occasionally observed include hypopyon, panophthalmitis, purulent arthritis (245), airsacculitis, (126), and omphalitis (28).

The invasion of intestinal epithelial cells by salmonellae leads to a series of pathologic changes that affects intestinal fluid and electrolyte regulation. This process can ultimately cause cell death and thereby produce and exacerbate diarrhea. Oral inoculation of laying hens with *S. enteritidis* can produce inflammation of the epithelium and lamina propria of the colon and ceca related to heterophilic infiltration (147, 254). Epithelial cells can be invaded throughout the intestinal tract, but the ceca and the ileocecal junction are often sites of particular affinity for salmonellae (314). In addition, epithelial invasion may also allow the removal of salmonellae through the basement membrane into the lamina propria by macrophages (249). Humphrey et al. (166) recovered *S. enteritidis* from several internal organ sites of a few laying hens within as little as 1 hr after oral inoculation. The ability of salmonellae to survive and multiply in internal organs, particularly the liver and spleen, has been correlated with the comparative virulence of salmonellae in different host species (20). Intracellular replication in the spleens of mice has been shown to offer a

protected site where bacterial multiplication can continue without exposure to host defense mechanisms (87). Slight inflammatory processes with heterophil infiltration ranging from focal to diffuse in distribution have been observed in the ovaries and oviducts of flocks naturally infected with *S. enteritidis* (151).

Immunity.
The immune response of poultry to PT salmonellae acts to minimize the duration and severity of infection and helps protect against reinfection. This response also permits the serologic detection of infected flocks and serves as the basis for efforts to protect birds against infection by vaccination. The development of immunity was illustrated in a study conducted by Hassan et al. (135), in which oral reinfection of chickens with *S. typhimurium* (10 wk after the initial inoculation) resulted in reduced fecal shedding and more rapid clearance from tissues than was observed in previously uninfected birds. Administering immunosuppressive agents to chicks has been reported to increase mortality associated with PT infection (91, 351), but such treatments apparently have very little effect on intestinal colonization by salmonellae (61). Hassan and Curtiss (132) have recently provided evidence that *S. typhimurium* infection of chickens can cause lymphocyte depletion, atrophy of lymphoid organs, and immunosuppression that may facilitate the establishment of a persistent carrier state.

Paratyphoid salmonellae can elicit strong antibody responses from infected poultry. For example, experimental infection of chicks with *S. typhimurium* induced strong IgG, IgA, and IgM responses in serum, intestinal contents, and bile which could be detected by antigens composed of whole bacterial cells, LPS, flagella, and outer-membrane proteins (135). When laying hens were orally infected with *S. enteritidis,* serum antibodies were produced by most birds by 1 wk postinoculation and reached peak values at 1 wk postinoculation (109). High serum IgG titers have been detected in laying hens for at least 27 wk after experimental oral inoculation with *S. enteritidis* (15). In a naturally infected broiler breeder flock, 70% of the birds were found to be positive for serum antibodies to *S. enteritidis* LPS at 35 wk of age (59). Antibodies to *S. enteritidis* have also been found in the yolks of eggs laid by infected hens. Specific antibodies were found as early as 9 days postinoculation and reached peak levels at 3–5 wk postinoculation in eggs from hens experimentally infected with *S. enteritidis* (111). Antibodies to *S. enteritidis* have also been detected in eggs from naturally infected flocks (59).

Although less completely characterized than the antibody response, cell-mediated immunity to PT salmonellae has also been observed in poultry. Hassan et al. (135) detected a strong delayed hypersensitivity reaction, using either whole bacterial cells or outer membrane proteins, between 2 and 5 wk after experimental infection of chicks with *S. typhimurium*. Heterophils of chickens and turkeys are strongly phagocytic and bactericidal for salmonellae (288) and apparently play a vital role in restricting organ invasion during the early phases of *S. enteritidis* infection (179). Cytokines produced by sensitized T lymphocytes may play a particularly important role in conferring immunity on poultry, perhaps by expanding the pool of circulating phagocytic heterophils (178) and recruiting them to the site of infection (180). Prophylactic administration of these immune lymphokines to chicks has been shown to provide protection against organ invasion by *S. enteritidis* (298).

The relative contributions of the antibody response and the cell-mediated response in providing poultry with protective immunity against *Salmonella* infection are somewhat uncertain. Lee et al. (192) indicated that the development of high antibody levels in chickens experimentally infected with *S. typhimurium* did not seem to result in any significant reductions in the *Salmonella* levels in various tissue sites, but effective clearance of salmonellae from tissues was observed after the emergence of a strong cell-mediated response. On the other hand, Humphrey et al. (162) noted that a group of hens infected with *S. enteritidis* at 20 wk of age produced high levels of IgM antibodies and showed no adverse signs, whereas a group of hens infected at 1 year of age produced much lower levels of antibodies and accordingly experienced significant mortality. Research in mice has indicated that the opsonic activity of specific antibodies and the phagocytic and lytic activity of cellular effectors may both be necessary for the full expression of immunity (210).

Although the responsible mechanism has not been clearly defined, genetically based differences in the innate resistance of lines of chickens to *Salmonella* infection have been reported on several occasions. Chicks from different lines have been found to vary in their susceptibility to the lethal effects of *S. typhimurium* and *S. enteritidis* infection (25, 38). Differences in the incidences of fecal shedding, organ invasion, and egg contamination have been reported between lines of mature chickens infected with *S. enteritidis* (25, 197). Bumstead and Barrow (39) found that the patterns of susceptibility of six inbred lines of chickens to various host-adapted and PT *Salmonella* serotypes were all very similar, suggesting a common mechanism of resistance.

DIAGNOSIS. Although clinical observations may suggest the likelihood of a PT infection, final diagnosis depends on the isolation and identification of causative organisms. Using conventional culture methods, this requires 48 to 96 hr (and even longer for some culturing protocols). A concise summary of traditional methods for isolating salmonellae from poultry was provided by Mallinson and Snoeyenbos (205). A wide array of faster alternative strategies for detecting and identifying salmonellae have also been proposed in recent years. Serologic detection of specific antibodies is often employed effectively as a rapid preliminary screening device to identify flocks that have been exposed to salmonellae.

Isolation and Identification of Causative Agent

SAMPLE SELECTION. To identify PT infection in poultry flocks, samples are obtained and cultured from a variety of sources, principally including tissues, eggs, and the poultry house environment. The number of samples that must be processed to achieve a predetermined level of confidence of detection of PT infection in a flock is directly related to the size of the flock and inversely related to the actual prevalence of infection (1). In very large flocks estimated to have very low prevalences of *Salmonella* infection, samples from more than one bird are often pooled together before culturing to allow an adequate sample size to be attained within the limitations of existing laboratory resources.

As many PT *Salmonella* serotypes are highly invasive and can be systemically disseminated to numerous internal tissues, a diversity of different sites (including the liver, spleen, ovary, oviduct, testes, yolk sac, heart, heart blood, kidney, gall bladder, pancreas, synovia, and eye) can provide samples for diagnostic culturing. As lesions cannot be relied upon to indicate infected tissues, several different organs should be cultured from each bird (separately or together). Some highly invasive PT serotypes, particularly *S. enteritidis,* can be deposited in the contents of eggs before oviposition (108). Culturing eggs for *S. enteritidis,* therefore, has been applied as a test for assessing the potential threat to public health posed by infected laying flocks. Gast (103) reported that culturing pools of egg contents for *S. enteritidis* detected experimentally infected hens at a frequency similar to culturing fecal samples or testing for specific serum antibodies during the first 2 wk after inoculation.

Because infections of poultry with PT salmonellae almost invariably involve colonization of the intestinal tract, samples of intestinal tissues and contents are frequently the focus of *Salmonella*-culturing efforts. In a survey of birds submitted to a diagnostic laboratory (94), salmonellae were found exclusively in intestinal samples in 78% of the chickens and 70% of the turkeys. In experimentally inoculated laying hens, *S. enteritidis* was recovered more often from the intestinal tract than from any other tissue sampled (110). Most recommendations for culturing intestinal samples indicate that the caudal ileum, ceca, cecal tonsils, and cecal contents are the sites most likely to offer the maximum probability of recovering salmonellae (34, 96, 314). Cloacal swabs (108) or samples of voided feces (103) have been used to provide evidence of persistent intestinal colonization by salmonellae in individual birds. The often intermittent pattern of shedding of salmonellae in the feces of infected birds tends to diminish the overall reliability of cloacal swabs for diagnosing infection (203, 341).

Fecal shedding of salmonellae into the poultry house environment by infected birds makes culturing environmental samples a useful diagnostic tool. Moreover, environmental samples also provide an opportunity to monitor for the introduction of salmonellae into poultry houses by vectors, personnel, equipment, and other sources. Although sampling fresh feces themselves likely provides the most sensitive test for the shedding of salmonellae (141), sampling litter can sometimes provide a comparable level of detection (264). Olesiuk et al. (240) reported that experimental *S. typhimurium* infection in laying flocks was detected more consistently over a period of 1 yr by culturing floor litter than by any other testing approach. In a naturally infected laying flock, Snoeyenbos et al. (279) found that salmonellae were most often recovered from nest litter samples. Drag-swab samples, obtained by dragging moistened gauze pads across the floor of poultry houses, have been reported to detect salmonellae with greater sensitivity than litter sampling (176). The use of multiple-swab assemblies can further improve the sensitivity of this method (40).

Numerous other environmental sampling approaches, including the culturing of cage surfaces, water sources, eggbelts, trapped rodents, and dust have also been suggested. Dust can remain contaminated with salmonellae even after cleaning and disinfection of poultry houses (141). Hatcher fluff is frequently contaminated with salmonellae, offering an opportunity for early detection of infection in flocks (220, 264). Culturing poultry feed for salmonellae is often important in establishing the source of infection of a flock with a particular serotype (279).

STANDARD CULTURE METHODS FOR *SALMONELLA* DETECTION. Although a very diverse assortment of culture conditions have been proposed for the isolation and identification of PT salmonellae, most standard methods follow a general scheme that involves four principal stages. First, nonselective preenrichment is used to encourage the growth of very small numbers of salmonellae or to allow the recovery of injured *Salmonella* cells. Preenrich-

ment is not advisable when testing samples (such as intestinal contents or feces) with large numbers of competing organisms that might overgrow salmonellae in the nonselective broth. Second, selective enrichment is used to allow additional expansion of the *Salmonella* population while suppressing the growth of other organisms. Third, plating on selective agar media is used to obtain isolated colonies, each derived from a single cell. Nonselective agar plating media are also sometimes used with swabs from internal organs. Fourth, colonies with appearances characteristic of salmonellae are subjected to biochemical and serologic tests to confirm their genus and serotype identity. Virtually all proposed methods require the last two of these steps, but enrichment requirements vary according to the nature of the sample.

Tissue samples (except for samples of intestinal tissues or contents) from infected birds generally contain relatively few competing organisms. Swab or loop samples taken from internal organs are often transferred directly to plates of both selective and nonselective agar media, without broth enrichment. Excised tissue samples, and any samples derived from the intestinal tract, are generally transferred initially into selective enrichment broth.

Because fecal contamination may result in the presence of diverse flora, eggshells are generally sampled without preenrichment. The surface of eggshells can be sampled by immersion in selective broth media or the entire shell (including interior structures and shell membranes) can be sampled by aseptic breaking to release the contents followed by manual crushing and addition of selective enrichment broth (108, 104). Before culturing egg contents for contamination by salmonellae, the shell exterior must be disinfected to prevent fecal contaminants of the shell from being transferred to the contents during breaking.

Because of the very low prevalence of salmonellae (primarily *S. enteritidis*) in egg contents, and because *Salmonella* contaminants tend to be present in eggs in very small numbers, the entire liquid contents of 10–20 eggs are often pooled together for sampling to minimize demands on laboratory resources. Egg contents pools are generally incubated before further culturing to allow the *Salmonella* population to expand to a consistently detectable level (106, 115). Iron supplementation of whole egg pools can increase the multiplication of some *S. enteritidis* strains during incubation (76, 115, 116). Preenrichment of egg contents has been shown to lead to a greater sensitivity of *S. enteritidis* detection than direct selective enrichment (105, 291), probably by allowing very small initial levels of salmonellae to expand to levels that will survive the harsher conditions of selective enrichment (50). Direct plating of incubated egg pools onto selective agar media can markedly reduce the time, media, and labor demands of culturing, but does so at a significant loss in detection sensitivity (105, 115).

Environmental samples are generally collected in sterile plastic bags and cultured by transfer into selective enrichment broth. Litter or fluff samples can be collected from several sites in each house. Various environmental surfaces can be sampled using moistened gauze pads. Similarly moistened drag swabs can be drawn across floor litter or dropping pits. Feed should be tested by collecting several representative samples from each lot and transferring into selective enrichment broth. Preenrichment of poultry feed samples has been reported to be unnecessary or even counterproductive (68, 69, 78).

Culture media are generally incubated for 24 hr at 37 C. Longer (48-hr) incubation in nonselective media has been reported to be useful for recovering small numbers of *S. enteritidis* from egg contents (108, 157). Shorter (6-hr) selective enrichment has been used successfully to recover salmonellae from animal feeds (78), but such abbreviated selective enrichment is likely inadequate to suppress competing microflora in more heavily contaminated samples (79). Incubation of selective enrichment cultures at elevated temperatures (42–43 C) has been recommended to suppress the growth of competing microflora, especially in intestinal samples or samples containing fecal material (80, 82, 205). Delayed secondary enrichment, in which selective enrichment broth cultures are held for an additional 5 days at room temperature to allow salmonellae an extended opportunity to grow to detectable levels, has been found to improve the recovery of PT salmonellae from poultry diagnostic and environmental samples (326, 328).

CULTURE MEDIA. A diverse array of media has been developed and recommended for isolating and identifying salmonellae. Although some evidence has suggested that proper media selection is somewhat contingent upon the type of sample being tested, several media have been consistently effective in a variety of applications. Formulations and preparations for most standard *Salmonella* media are provided in Atlas and Parks (6), and most preparations are commercially available in dehydrated form from several manufacturers.

Suggested broth media for the preenrichment of samples for salmonellae include buffered peptone water and trypticase soy broth. Stephenson et al. (291) reported that, of five preenrichment media tested, trypticase soy broth provided the greatest sensitivity of detection of *S. enteritidis* in artificially contaminated egg yolks.

Selective broth media most often used for isolating PT salmonellae in recent years include tetrathionate (TT) broth, selenite-cystine (SC) broth, and Rappaport-Vassiliadis (RV) broth.

Tetrathionate broth preparations have been found to yield a higher frequency of *Salmonella* detection than RV broth or SC broth from a variety of types of samples, including cloacal swabs, intestinal tissues, pooled egg contents, poultry feeds, and various foods (68, 79, 83, 105, 311). Rappaport-Vassiliadis broth has been effectively used to isolate salmonellae from raw chicken and egg contents pools (2, 157, 324).

A large number of agar media are available for the isolation of PT salmonellae. Among the most commonly used plating media are brilliant green (BG) agar, XLD agar, XLT4 agar, bismuth sulfite agar, and Hektoen enteric agar. Brilliant green agar remains the most widely used medium for *Salmonella* isolation from poultry sources and has been shown to be effective in application to diverse tissue, environmental, egg, and feed samples (68, 105, 326, 327). XLT4 agar has been successfully applied to detect salmonellae efficiently from poultry house environmental drag swabs (216). The addition of novobiocin to agar plating media has been demonstrated to improve *Salmonella* recovery by suppressing the growth of some competing organisms (notably *Proteus*) that might otherwise overgrow the salmonellae (295, 296). Samples should always be streaked onto two different media, preferably with dissimilar indicator systems for differentiating salmonellae from other organisms.

CONFIRMATION OF GENUS AND SEROTYPE. Colonies on selective agar plates that have the characteristic appearance of PT salmonellae must be tested further to confirm their genus identity and to determine their serotype. The combined use of triple sugar–iron agar and lysine–iron agar provides an effective presumptive test for identifying PT salmonellae. Additional differentiation of PT salmonellae from other organisms can be accomplished by determining the fermentation pattern of each isolate for a set of six particular carbohydrates, as described by Cox and Williams (67). The serogroup of each isolate can be determined by slide agglutination tests with polyvalent antisera to groups of somatic O antigens, and the serotype can then be determined by slide agglutination tests with monovalent antisera to specific O antigens and tube agglutination tests with antisera to flagellar H antigens.

RAPID DETECTION TECHNOLOGIES. Obtaining negative results from conventional culturing methods for salmonellae requires several days for most types of samples, and confirming positive results adds even more time. Many comparatively more rapid techniques have been proposed and investigated in recent years, but none have yet achieved particularly wide acceptance. Most of the rapid methods reduce the time requirements of testing by 1 or more days, and many are amenable to some degree of automation. Concerns about rapid methods include their typically high cost, their usual dependence on enrichment to achieve sufficient cell densities to allow detection, and their frequent inability to demonstrate a specificity of detection comparable to that of conventional culturing. Although properties as diverse as the ability to exhibit motility (257) or to cause specific changes in the electrical impedance of media (247) have been successfully used to enrich for or identify salmonellae, most efforts to develop rapid *Salmonella*-detection methods have centered around the use of specific antibodies or DNA probes.

Specific antibodies to *Salmonella* antigens have been used to develop a variety of enzyme-linked immunosorbent assay (ELISA) methods. These tests, using polyclonal antibodies to *Salmonella* LPS or flagella, have been reported to detect salmonellae in eggs, tissues, cloacal swabs, environmental drag swabs, litter, and feed (136, 206, 258). Monoclonal antibodies to outer membrane proteins or flagella have been used as the basis for ELISA tests to specifically detect *S. enteritidis* in eggs, tissues, and environmental samples (172, 173). Although not apparently quite as sensitive as conventional culture methods (296), ELISA tests are usually reported to detect salmonellae at a frequency comparable to standard methods, and to do so at least 1 day sooner. One or more initial enrichment culturing steps, however, are generally necessary to allow the expansion of the *Salmonella* population into the range detectable by ELISA, which is often estimated at between 10^5 and 10^7 salmonellae per mL (29, 136, 172). Like conventional culturing methods, ELISA tests are also somewhat prone to false-positive results from competing flora able to grow in enrichment media (26).

Another application of antibodies for detecting salmonellae involves coating small magnetic beads with specific antibodies. When mixed with the sample to be tested, the antibody-coated beads will bind to any *Salmonella* target antigens present and a magnetic field can then be applied to recover the bead–antibody–antigen complex. In essence, immunomagnetic separation thus serves as an alternative to broth enrichment for concentrating salmonellae, but with the advantages of requiring less time and having no adverse effect on sublethally injured cells. A method using immunomagnetic separation to concentrate salmonellae before plating on selective agar detected a higher frequency of *Salmonella* contamination in samples of poultry meat, tissues, eggshells, and cloacal or fecal swabs than did either traditional selective enrichment or motility-based enrichment (75). Immunomagnetic separation has also been used to detect small levels of *S.*

enteritidis contamination in pools of egg contents by both culturing and ELISA (76, 150).

Another approach to rapid testing for salmonellae in poultry, which has received considerable attention in recent years, involves using probes for particular DNA sequences unique to salmonellae. Hybridization of the probe with DNA extracted from the sample indicates a positive result. DNA probes, in both radiolabeled and colorimetric assays, have been applied to the detection of salmonellae in drag-swab environmental samples from poultry houses with a high degree of specificity (131). The sensitivity of detection of salmonellae by DNA hybridization is similar to that of ELISA, and thus generally also requires one or more enrichment culturing steps. Moreover, DNA hybridization assays are often procedurally complex and are rather expensive in comparison to other available methods. The development of polymerase chain reaction (PCR) technology, however, has allowed the specific amplification of particular target segments of DNA, thereby enabling hybridization reactions with probes to detect salmonellae in feces and environmental drag-swab samples with a very high level of sensitivity (51, 52). Carefully chosen DNA probes can be used along with PCR to detect salmonellae with specific characteristics, such as those carrying particular virulence genes (204).

Serologic Diagnosis of Infection. Specific antibodies to PT salmonellae have been detected in the sera of infected poultry with a high degree of sensitivity using several different agglutination and ELISA methods. Detectable serum antibody titers are often still present long after all salmonellae have evidently been cleared from tissues and fecal shedding has ceased (134, 329, 340). Various tests for serum antibodies to salmonellae have been applied effectively for detecting both naturally (47, 151, 252, 323) and experimentally (14, 109) infected poultry. Because antibody tests only demonstrate prior exposure to salmonellae, and do not provide unequivocal evidence of a currently ongoing infection in a flock, positive serologic results must generally be followed by bacteriologic culturing for confirmation. Other problems with serologic testing include the possibility that subclinical infections will lead to fecal shedding without sufficient invasion and dissemination to elicit a detectable antibody response (240), the general immunologic unresponsiveness of very young birds to *Salmonella* infection (329), and cross-reactions between antibodies to similar PT serotypes (235).

The various agglutination tests have been applied successfully for detecting chickens naturally or experimentally infected with *S. enteritidis* or *S. typhimurium* on many occasions (48, 109, 151, 252, 341). The principal agglutination test formats include rapid whole-blood plate, serum plate, tube agglutination, microagglutination, and microantiglobulin tests. All of these tests rely on the ability of specific antibodies to cause visible agglutination when mixed with antigen preparations of killed whole *Salmonella* cells. Except for the tube test, all agglutination assays use stained antigens to improve the ease of visualization of the agglutination reaction. The rapid whole-blood plate test is the most widely used method for detecting antibodies to *S. pullorum* or *S. gallinarum* (317). Tube agglutination tests are used extensively for confirming rapid whole-blood plate test results for *S. pullorum* and *S. gallinarum* (317), but have not been widely applied to detecting PT salmonellae.

Microagglutination tests for PT salmonellae are conducted in 96-well disposable plastic plates (317). Microantiglobulin tests enhance the sensitivity of microagglutination tests by using an additional incubation period with a secondary antibody directed against chicken immunoglobulins to increase the overall agglutination of the target antigen (339). The microantiglobulin test has frequently been reported to provide greater sensitivity for detecting PT infections than other agglutination test methods (53, 235, 342, 341).

Paratyphoid salmonellae infections in poultry have also been effectively detected using various ELISA approaches. For example, ELISA tests with LPS, flagella, or outer membrane proteins as antigens have been successfully used to identify chickens infected naturally or experimentally with *S. typhimurium* or *S. enteritidis* (14, 174, 233, 235, 310). By using very precisely defined antigens, ELISA tests often achieve a high degree of specificity and are thus frequently associated with fewer false-positive results due to cross-reactions between serotypes than are agglutination reactions (134, 174, 322). Screening for serum antibodies using a flagella-based ELISA test has been used satisfactorily for detecting *S. enteritidis* in Dutch breeder flocks (323).

Antibodies deposited in egg yolks can also be used to detect poultry infected with PT salmonellae. Both microantiglobulin (111) and ELISA (14, 77, 234) tests have been applied to find antibodies to *S. enteritidis* and *S. typhimurium* in eggs from naturally and experimentally infected chickens. Gast and Beard (111) reported that the presence of specific antibodies in eggs from commercial laying flocks in the United States was directly correlated with the presence of *S. enteritidis* in tissue samples from those flocks. Van de Giessen et al. (320) found a direct relationship between specific egg-yolk antibody titers and the incidence of shedding of *S. enteritidis* in the feces of laying flocks in the Netherlands.

PREVENTION AND CONTROL. Efforts to establish critical control points for preventing PT infections in poultry are handicapped by the diversity of sources from which salmonellae can be introduced into flocks or houses. Effective prevention and control programs, therefore, must involve coordinated and simultaneous attacks on the problem from several directions. Eggs and chicks or poults should be secured only from demonstrably *Salmonella*-free breeding flocks. Hatching eggs should be properly disinfected and hatched according to stringent sanitation standards. Poultry houses should be thoroughly cleaned and disinfected by recommended procedures between flocks. Rodent and insect control measures should be incorporated into house design and management and verified by periodic testing. Rigidly enforced biosecurity practices should be implemented to restrict entry onto poultry housing premises to only authorized personnel and equipment, and to prevent horizontal transmission of salmonellae between houses. Only pelleted feed or feed containing no animal protein should be used, to minimize the likelihood of using contaminated rations. Treatments such as medication, competitive exclusion cultures, or vaccination can be applied to reduce the susceptibility of birds to *Salmonella* infection. Finally, the *Salmonella* status of poultry and their environment should be monitored by frequent testing. Such multifaceted prevention and control programs have reportedly been successful in addressing *Salmonella* problems in both chickens (90, 215) and turkeys (248).

Increased international interest in controlling PT infections, especially *S. enteritidis,* has led to the development and implementation of many testing and monitoring programs in recent years (3). In the United States, the National Poultry Improvement Plan (NPIP) defines stringent sanitation and testing standards for breeder flocks to prevent the transmission of *S. enteritidis* infection to egg-laying stock (317). Participation in this plan requires compliance with standards for feed selection and handling, disinfection of hatching eggs, and hatchery sanitation. The NPIP testing for *S. enteritidis* involves bacteriologic monitoring of the environment and serologic monitoring of birds, with culturing of tissues from selected birds used for confirmation. A similar protocol, involving screening for infection with drag-swab samples of the manure pit and confirmation of infection by sampling tissues from selected hens, has been used by the USDA to test epidemiologically implicated laying flocks for *S. enteritidis* (315). More recent programs to assure the microbiologic safety of eggs have continued the use of environmental sampling as a screening device, but instituted egg culturing as the confirming step in place of culturing tissues (316).

Medication. Although medication is often used to prevent or treat PT infections, the efficacy and wisdom of using this approach are still topics of considerable debate. Antibiotics were used effectively both as therapeutic and prophylactic agents as part of control efforts for *S. enteritidis* in broiler and broiler breeder flocks in Northern Ireland (215). Combined administration of polymyxin B sulfate and trimethoprim to chicks both prevented and cleared experimental infections with *S. enteritidis* (122). Various antimicrobial agents, including tetracyclines, neomycin, bacitracin, and sulfa drugs (except in laying chickens) are approved and regularly used in poultry (225). Injectable gentamicin and spectinomycin are approved for use in controlling yolk sac infections acquired at the hatchery (225), especially in turkey poults.

Williams and Whittemore (343) reported that adding any of five different antimicrobial agents to the drinking water of chicks reduced the frequency of isolation of subsequently administered *S. typhimurium* from cloacal swabs. However, as birds removed from antimicrobial treatment were found to be active carriers of salmonellae, the investigators concluded that drug excretion was often interfering with recovery of the infecting organism from fecal material, and thereby resulting in a misleading impression that treatment was efficacious. Olesiuk et al. (241) similarly found that five antimicrobial agents had only very limited value for preventing or eliminating experimental *S. typhimurium* infection. The administration of some antibiotics has been reported to increase the susceptibility of poultry to *Salmonella* infection, perhaps by suppressing the growth of other microflora capable of exerting inhibitory activity against salmonellae (207, 208). Antibiotics are also sometimes added to poultry feeds at subtherapeutic levels to promote growth. Both therapeutic and subtherapeutic antibiotic administration has been shown to select for drug-resistant strains of salmonellae, thereby potentially compromising the effectiveness of those drugs in both animals and humans (117, 118, 177). Multiple resistant salmonellae, insensitive to the effects of several antimicrobial agents, have become increasingly prevalent among poultry isolates in both the United Kingdom and North America (81, 305).

Competitive Exclusion. Newly hatched chicks and poults are highly susceptible to infection by PT salmonellae, but quickly become more resistant. This age-associated decrease in susceptibility to salmonellae is largely attributable to the acquisition of protective intestinal microflora from the environment. The evident ability of other intestinal bacteria to exert inhibitory effects against salmonellae has served as the basis for the development of a diverse group of treatments often referred to collectively as competitive exclusion (CE). Competitive exclusion treatments involve administering defined or undefined bacterial cultures to poultry in order to diminish intestinal colonization by salmonellae.

The efficacy of CE treatment has been illustrated repeatedly in both chickens and turkeys, using intestinal or fecal material from mature birds or undefined anaerobic cultures derived from such material. Administration of CE cultures has been shown to diminish both intestinal colonization by various PT salmonellae and subsequent invasion to internal tissues (238, 259, 268, 283, 284). Used litter can also be used as a source of CE cultures (62, 63). In field trials in commercial broiler chicken flocks in several nations, treatment with CE cultures led to significant reductions in the incidence of salmonellae in live birds and on carcasses (32, 124, 333, 334). After antibiotic therapy to treat *Salmonella* infections in replacement pullet flocks, administration of a CE preparation was used effectively for providing a complete intestinal microflora to prevent reinfection with salmonellae (170). In some instances, treatment with CE cultures has been observed to enhance the clearance of preexisting *Salmonella* infections (330, 352).

Competitive exclusion cultures have been shown to be effective against salmonellae following administration to poultry in a variety of forms, including crop gavage, application to the vent lip, whole-body spraying or droplet application, addition to drinking water, encapsulation in lyophilized alginate beads added to the feed, and in ovo inoculation into the air cell (64, 65, 72, 267). Considerable research has sought to identify the microflora constituents responsible for protection against salmonellae. A defined mixture of microorganisms would likely produce a given level of protection with greater consistency than undefined cultures and would also provide a greater assurance of safety than is available with mixtures of unknown organisms. The protective efficacy of mixtures of small numbers of intestinal bacteria is usually very limited (289), but more diverse defined mixtures can provide significant protection (66, 121, 236, 289).

Several factors have been identified that affect the overall usefulness of CE cultures for controlling PT salmonellae infections in poultry. Although CE treatment generally reduces the incidence of intestinal colonization by salmonellae, it does not prevent it altogether. Moreover, the protective efficacy of CE cultures can sometimes be overcome by severe challenge with salmonellae (283). Administration of CE cultures can thus contribute significantly to an overall *Salmonella* control effort, but proper cleaning and disinfection, biosecurity, rodent reduction, and other similar measures are still necessary to minimize the chances of exposure to salmonellae (243). Factors that disrupt the normal intestinal microflora, such as antibiotic administration and feed or water deprivation, can also interfere with the protective capabilities of CE cultures (9, 155, 331).

Vaccination. Vaccination to reduce the susceptibility of poultry to PT infection has been examined using both killed and live preparations. Live *Salmonella* vaccines have often been associated with a stronger or longer-lasting protective response in poultry, perhaps because relevant antigens may be adversely affected during the preparation of killed vaccines, or because live vaccines present relevant antigens to the host immune system more persistently (18). Killed vaccines may also fail to elicit fully the cell-mediated portion of the protective response (227). Nevertheless, both killed and live vaccines have been associated with significant protection against salmonellae, although neither type of vaccine has consistently been shown to provide an impenetrable barrier against infection. Moreover, feed or water deprivation and environmental stresses such as heat may compromise the effectiveness of vaccines (232). Like competitive exclusion, therefore, vaccination is most effectively used in conjunction with management practices that reduce opportunities for flocks to be exposed to PT salmonellae.

Interest in the use of killed vaccines (bacterins) in poultry has been renewed in recent years by escalating concerns about *S. enteritidis*. Subcutaneous administration of adjuvanted oil-emulsion bacterins to laying hens has been reported to reduce significantly the incidence of fecal shedding and the numbers of *S. enteritidis* shed in the feces, the frequency of isolation of *S. enteritidis* from various internal tissues, and the incidence of production of eggs with contaminated contents following subsequent oral challenge (119, 120, 232). Chickens vaccinated with bacterins have been reported to exhibit reductions in mortality, lesions, clinical signs, and organ invasion for up to 12 wk postvaccination when challenged with *S. enteritidis* by intravenous or intramuscular routes (307, 308). Subunit vaccines, composed of *Salmonella* outer-membrane proteins incorporated into lipid-conjugated immunostimulating complexes, have been efficacious against *S. enteritidis* and *S. heidelberg* in turkeys (43, 44).

Live attenuated vaccines need to persist in tissues long enough to induce a protective immune response, but should be avirulent and eventually cleared from vaccinated birds. Paratyphoid *Salmonella* vaccine strains attenuated by several different approaches have been tested for their protective efficacy in poultry. Oral or intramuscular administration of various *aroA*-mutants of *S. enteritidis* (auxotrophs that do not grow well in vivo because of

their inability to synthesize particular aromatic compounds) has been reported to reduce fecal shedding, horizontal transmission, and egg contamination after oral challenge and organ colonization or invasion after intravenous challenge (19, 54, 55, 56). This protection has been found to persist for up to 23 wk after administration of the vaccine strain (57). Oral immunization with *aroA S. enteritidis* strains did not cross-protect very effectively against *S. typhimurium* challenge (56, 57). An orally administered Δ*cya* Δ*crp S. typhimurium* strain (a double mutant with deletions of both adenylate cyclase and the cyclic AMP receptor protein) provided very strong protection against intestinal colonization and organ invasion by *S. typhimurium* and also some degree of protection against salmonellae from other serogroups (133).

REFERENCES
1. Aho, M. 1992. Problems of Salmonella sampling. Int J Food Microbiol 15:225–235.
2. Allen, G., V.R. Bruce, P. Stephenson, F.B. Satchell, and W.H. Andrews. 1991. Recovery of Salmonella from high-moisture foods by abbreviated selective enrichment. J Food Prot 54:492–495.
3. Altekruse, S., J. Koehler, F. Hickman-Brenner, R.V. Tauxe, and K. Ferris. 1993. A comparison of Salmonella enteritidis phage types from egg-associated outbreaks and implicated laying flocks. Epidemiol Infect 110:17–22.
4. Amin, I.I., G.R. Douce, M.P. Osborne, and J. Stephen. 1994. Quantitative studies of invasion of rabbit ileal mucosa by Salmonella typhimurium strains which differ in virulence in a model of gastroenteritis. Infect Immun 62:569–578.
5. Aslanzadeh, J., and L.J. Paulissen. 1990. Adherence and pathogenesis of Salmonella enteritidis in mice. Microbiol Immunol 34:885–893.
6. Atlas, R.M., and L.C. Parks. 1993. Handbook of microbiological media. CRC Press, Boca Raton, FL.
7. Baba, E., T. Fukata, and A. Arakawa. 1985. Factors influencing enhanced Salmonella typhimurium infection in Eimeria tenella-infected chickens. Am J Vet Res 46:1593–1596.
8. Baba, E., M. Yaono, T. Fukata, and A. Arakawa. 1985. Infection by Salmonella typhimurium, S. agona, S. enteritidis, or S. infantis of chicks with cecal coccidiosis. Br Poult Sci 26:505–511.
9. Bailey, J.S., L.C. Blankenship, N.J. Stern, N.A. Cox, and F. McHan. 1988. Effect of anticoccidial and antimicrobial feed additives on prevention of Salmonella colonization of chicks treated with anaerobic cultures of chicken feces. Avian Dis 32:324–329.
10. Bailey, J.S., N.A. Cox, and M.E. Berrang. 1994. Hatchery-acquired Salmonellae in broiler chicks. Poult Sci 73:1153–1157.
11. Baker, R.C. 1990. Survival of Salmonella enteritidis on and in shelled eggs, liquid eggs, and cooked egg products. Dairy Food Environ Sanit 10:273–275.
12. Baker, R.C., S. Hogarty, W. Poon, and D.V. Vadehra. 1983. Survival of Salmonella typhimurium and Staphylococcus aureus in eggs cooked by different methods. Poult Sci 62:1211–1216.
13. Barrow, P.A. 1991. Experimental infection of chickens with Salmonella enteritidis. Avian Pathol 20:145–153.
14. Barrow, P.A. 1992. Further observations on the serological response to experimental Salmonella typhimurium in chickens measured by ELISA. Epidemiol Infect 108:231–241.

15. Barrow, P.A. and M.A. Lovell. 1991. Experimental infection of egg-laying hens with Salmonella enteritidis phage type 4. Avian Pathol 20:335–348.

16. Barrow, P.A., M.B. Huggins, M.A. Lovell, and J.M. Simpson. 1987. Observations on the pathogenesis of experimental Salmonella typhimurium infection in chickens. Res Vet Sci 42:194–199.

17. Barrow, P.A., J.M. Simpson, and M.A. Lovell. 1988. Intestinal colonisation in the chicken by food-poisoning Salmonella serotypes: Microbial characteristics associated with faecal excretion. Avian Pathol 17:571–588.

18. Barrow, P.A., J. Hassan, and A. Berchieri, Jr. 1990. Reduction in faecal excretion of Salmonella typhimurium strain F98 in chickens vaccinated with live and killed S. typhimurium organisms. Epidemiol Infect 104:413–426.

19. Barrow, P.A., M.A. Lovell, and A. Berchieri. 1991. The use of two live attenuated vaccines to immunize egg-laying hens against Salmonella enteritidis phage type 4. Avian Pathol 20:681–692.

20. Barrow, P.A., M.B. Huggins, and M.A. Lovell. 1994. Host specificity of Salmonella infection in chickens and mice is expressed in vivo primarily at the level of the reticuloendothelial system. Infect Immun 62:4602–4610.

21. Baskerville, A., T.J. Humphrey, R.B. Fitzgeorge, R.W. Cook, H. Chart, B. Rowe, and A. Whitehead. 1992. Airborne infection of laying hens with Salmonella enteritidis phage type 4. Vet Rec 130:395–398.

22. Bayne, H.G., J.A. Garibaldi, and H. Lineweaver. 1965. Heat resistance of Salmonella typhimurium and Salmonella senftenberg 775 W in chicken meat. Poult Sci 44:1281–1284.

23. Bean, N.H. and P.M. Griffin. 1990. Foodborne disease outbreaks in the United States, 1973–1987: Pathogens, vehicles, and trends. J Food Prot 53:804–817.

24. Bean, N.H. and M.E. Potter. 1992. Salmonella serotypes from human sources, January 1991 through December 1991. Proc 96th Annu Meet U.S. Anim Health Assoc. U.S. Animal Health Association, Richmond, VA, pp. 488–491.

25. Beaumont, C., J. Trotais, P. Colin, J.F. Guillot, F. Ballatif, C. Mouline, F. Lantier, I. Lantier, O. Girard, and P. Pardon. 1994. Comparison of resistance of different poultry lines to intramuscular or oral inoculation by Salmonella enteritidis. Vet Res 25:412.

26. Beckers, H.J., P.D. Tips, P.S.S. Soentoro, E.H.M. Delfgou-Van Asch, and R. Peters. 1988. The efficacy of enzyme immunoassays for the detection of salmonellas. Food Microbiol 5:147–156.

27. Benjamin, W.H., Jr., B.S. Posey, and D.E. Briles. 1986. Effects of the in vitro growth phase on the pathogenesis of Salmonella typhimurium in mice. J Gen Microbiol 132:1283–1295.

28. Berchieri, A., Jr. A.M. De Carvalho, S.A. Fernandes, and A.M. Iba. 1993. Detection of Salmonella typhimurium in a broiler chicken flock. Rev Microbiol São Paulo 24:212–213.

29. Beumer, R.R., E. Brinkman, and F.M. Rombouts. 1991. Enzyme-linked immunoassays for the detection of Salmonella spp.: A comparison with other methods. Int J Food Microbiol 12:363–374.

30. Bhatia, T.R.S. and G.D. McNabb. 1980. Dissemination of Salmonella in broiler chicken operations. Avian Dis 24:616–624.

31. Bierer, B.W. 1960. Effect of age factor on mortality in Salmonella typhimurium infection in turkey poults. J Am Vet Med Assoc 137:657–658.

32. Blankenship, L.C., J.S. Bailey, N.A. Cox, N.J. Stern, R. Brewer, and O. Williams. 1993. Two-step mucosal competitive exclusion flora treatment to diminish Salmonellae in commercial broiler chickens. Poult Sci 72:1667–1672.

33. Bokanyi, R.P., Jr., J.F. Stephens, and D.N. Foster. 1990. Isolation and characterization of Salmonella from broiler carcasses or parts. Poult Sci 69:592–598.

34. Brownell, J.R., W.W. Sadler, and M.J. Fanelli. 1969. Factors influencing the intestinal infection of chickens with Salmonella typhimurium. Avian Dis 13:804–816.

35. Brown, D.D., J.G. Ross, and A.F.G. Smith. 1976. Experimental infection of poultry with Salmonella infantis. Res Vet Sci 20:237–243.

36. Buisán, M., J.M. Rodríguez-Peña, and R. Rotger. 1994. Restriction map of the Salmonella enteritidis virulence plasmid and its homology with the plasmid of Salmonella typhimurium. Microb Pathog 16:165–169.

37. Bukholm, G., and K.J. Figenschau. 1988. Invasiveness of enterobacteria related to the presence of high molecular weight plasmids. Acta Pathol Microbiol Immunol Scand 96:30–36.

38. Bumstead, N., and P.A. Barrow. 1988. Genetics of resistance to Salmonella typhimurium in newly hatched chicks. Br Poult Sci 29:521–529.

39. Bumstead, N., and P. Barrow. 1993. Resistance to Salmonella gallinarum, S. pullorum, and S. enteritidis in inbred lines of chickens. Avian Dis 37:189–193.

40. Caldwell, D.J., B.M. Hargis, D.E. Corrier, J.D. Williams, L. Vidal, and J.R. DeLoach. 1994. Predictive value of multiple drag-swab sampling for the detection of Salmonella from occupied or vacant poultry houses. Avian Dis 38:461–466.

41. Cason, J.A., J.S. Bailey, and N.A. Cox. 1994. Transmission of Salmonella typhimurium during hatching of broiler chicks. Avian Dis 38:583–588.

42. Catalano, C.R., and S.J. Knabel. 1994. Destruction of Salmonella enteritidis by high pH and rapid chilling during simulated commercial egg processing. J Food Prot 57:592–595.

43. Charles, S.D., K.V. Nagaraja, and V. Sivanandan. 1993. A lipid-conjugated immunostimulating complex subunit vaccine against Salmonella infection in turkeys. Avian Dis 37:477–484.

44. Charles, S.D., I. Hussain, C.-U. Choi, K.V. Nagaraja, and V. Sivanandan. 1994. Adjuvanted subunit vaccines for the control of Salmonella enteritidis infection in turkeys. Am J Vet Res 55:636–642.

45. Chart, H., B. Row, E.J. Threlfall, and L.R. Ward. 1989. Conversion of Salmonella enteritidis phage type 4 to phage type 7 involves loss of lipopolysaccharide with concomitant loss of virulence. FEMS Microbiol Lett 60:37–40.

46. Chart, H., E.J. Threlfall, and B. Rowe. 1989. Virulence of Salmonella enteritidis phage type 4 is related to the possession of a 38 MDa plasmid. FEMS Microbiol Lett 58:299–304.

47. Chart, H., B. Rowe, A. Baskerville, and T.J. Humphrey. 1990. Serological response of chickens to Salmonella enteritidis infection. Epidemiol Infect 104:63–71.

48. Chart, H., B. Rowe, A. Baskerville, and T.J. Humphrey. 1990. Serological analysis of chicken flocks for antibodies to Salmonella enteritidis. Vet Rec 127:501–502.

49. Chart, H., E.J. Threlfall, and B. Rowe. 1991. Virulence studies of Salmonella enteritidis phage types. Lett Appl Microbiol 12:188–191.

50. Chen, H., A.D.E. Fraser, and H. Yamazaki. 1993. Evaluation of the toxicity of Salmonella selective media for shortening the enrichment period. Int J Food Microbiol 18:151–159.

51. Cohen, N.D., E.D. McGruder, H.L. Neibergs, R.W. Behle, D.E. Wallis, and B.M. Hargis. 1994. Detection of Salmonella enteritidis in feces from poultry using booster polymerase chain reaction and oligonucleotide primers specific for all members of the genus Salmonella. Poult Sci 73:354–357.

52. Cohen, N.D., D.E. Wallis, H.L. Neibergs, A.P. McElroy, E.D. McGruder, J.R. DeLoach, D.E. Corrier, and B.M. Hargis. 1994. Comparison of the polymerase chain reaction using genus-specific oligonucleotide primers and microbio-

logic culture for the detection of Salmonella in drag-swabs from poultry houses. Poult Sci 73:1276–1281.

53. Cooper, G.L., R.A. Nicholas, and C.D. Bracewell. 1989. Serological and bacteriological investigations of chickens from flocks naturally infected with Salmonella enteritidis. Vet Rec 125:567–572.

54. Cooper, G.L., R.A.J. Nicholas, G.A. Cullen, and C.E. Hormaeche. 1990. Vaccination of chickens with a Salmonella enteritidis aro A live oral salmonella vaccine. Microb Pathog 9:255–265.

55. Cooper, G.L., L.M. Venables, R.A.J. Nicholas, G.A. Cullen, and C.E. Hormaeche. 1992. Vaccination of chickens with chicken-derived Salmonella enteritidis phage type 4 aro A live oral salmonella vaccines. Vaccine 10:247–254.

56. Cooper, G.L., L.M. Venables, R.A. J. Nicholas, G.A. Cullen, and C.E. Hormaeche. 1993. Further studies of the application of live Salmonella enteritidis aroA vaccines in chickens. Vet Rec 133:31–36.

57. Cooper, G.L., L.M. Venables, M.J. Woodward, and C.E. Hormaeche. 1994. Vaccination of chickens with strain CVL30, a genetically defined Salmonella enteritidis aroA live oral vaccine candidate. Infect Immun 62:4747–4754.

58. Cooper, G.L., L.M. Venables, M.J. Woodward, and C.E. Hormaeche. 1994. Invasiveness and persistence of Salmonella enteritidis, Salmonella typhimurium, and a genetically defined S. enteritidis aroA strain in young chickens. Infect Immun 62:4739–4746.

59. Corkish, J.D., R.H. Davies, C. Wray, and R.A.J. Nicholas. 1994. Observations on a broiler breeder flock naturally infected with Salmonella enteritidis phage type 4. Vet Rec 134:591–594.

60. Corrier, D.E., and R.L. Ziprin. 1989. Suppression of resistance to Salmonella typhimurium in young chickens inoculated with Corynebacterium parvum. Avian Dis 33:787–791.

61. Corrier, D.E., M.H. Elissalde, R.L. Ziprin, and J.R. DeLoach. 1991. Effect of immunosuppression with cyclophosphamide, cyclosporin, or dexamethasone on Salmonella colonization of broiler chicks. Avian Dis 35:40–45.

62. Corrier, D.E., A. Hinton, Jr., B. Hargis, and J.R. DeLoach. 1992. Effect of used litter from floor pens of adult broilers on Salmonella colonization of broiler chicks. Avian Dis 36:897–902.

63. Corrier, D.E., B.M. Hargis, A. Hinton, Jr., and J.R. DeLoach. 1993. Protective effect of used poultry litter and lactose in the feed ration on Salmonella enteritidis colonization of Leghorn chicks and hens. Avian Dis 37:47–52.

64. Corrier, D.E., A.G. Hollister, D.J. Nisbet, C.M. Scanlan, R.C. Beier, and J.R. DeLoach. 1994. Competitive exclusion of Salmonella in Leghorn chicks: Comparison of treatment by crop gavage, drinking water, spray, or lyophilized alginate beads. Avian Dis 38:297–303.

65. Corrier, D.E., D.J. Nisbet, A.G. Hollister, R.C. Beier, C.M. Scanlan, B.M. Hargis, and J.R. DeLoach. 1994. Resistance against Salmonella enteritidis cecal colonization in Leghorn chicks by vent lip application of cecal bacteria culture. Poult Sci 73:648–652.

66. Corrier, D.E., D.J. Nisbet, C.M. Scanlan, G. Tellez, B.M. Hargis, and J.R. DeLoach. 1994. Inhibition of Salmonella enteritidis cecal and organ colonization in Leghorn chicks by a defined culture of cecal bacteria and dietary lactose. J Food Prot 56:377–381.

67. Cox, N.A. and J.E. Williams. 1976. A simplified biochemical system to screen salmonella isolates from poultry for serotyping. Poult Sci 55:1968–1971.

68. Cox, N.A., J.S. Bailey, and J.E. Thomson. 1982. Effect of various media and incubation conditions on recovery of inoculated Salmonellae from poultry feed. Poult Sci 61:1314–1321.

69. Cox, N.A., J.S. Bailey, and J.E. Thomson. 1983. Comparison of preenrichment to direct enrichment and the effect of pyruvate in media for recovery of Salmonellae in feed. Poult Sci 62:947–951.

70. Cox, N.A., J.S. Bailey, J.E. Thomson, and B.J. Juven. 1983. Salmonella and other Enterobacteriaceae found in commercial poultry feed. Poult Sci 62:2169–2175.

71. Cox, N.A., J.S. Bailey, J.M. Mauldin, and L.C. Blankenship. 1990. Presence and impact of Salmonella contamination in commercial broiler hatcheries. Poult Sci 69:1606–1609.

72. Cox, N.A., J.S. Bailey, L.C. Blankenship, and R.P. Gildersleeve. 1992. In ovo administration of a competitive exclusion culture treatment to broiler embryos. Poult Sci 71:1781–1784.

73. Cox, N.A., J.S. Bailey, M.E. Berrang, R.J. Buhr, and J.M. Mauldin. 1994. Chemical treatment of Salmonella-contaminated fertile hatching eggs using an automated egg spray sanitizing machine. J Appl Poult Res 3:26–30.

74. Craven, S.E. 1994. Altered colonizing ability for the ceca of broiler chicks by lipopolysaccharide-deficient mutants of Salmonella typhimurium. Avian Dis 38:401–408.

75. Cudjoe, K.S., R. Krona, and E. Olsen. 1994. IMS: A new selective enrichment technique for detection of Salmonella in foods. Int J Food Microbiol 23:159–165.

76. Cudjoe, K.S., R. Krona, B. Grøn, and E. Olsen. 1994. Use of ferrous sulphate and immunomagnetic separation to recover Salmonella enteritidis from raw eggs. Int J Food Microbiol 23:149–158.

77. Dadrast, H., R. Hesketh, and D.J. Taylor. 1990. Egg yolk antibody detection in identification of Salmonella infected poultry. Vet Rec 126:219.

78. D'Aoust, J.-Y., A. Sewell, and A. Boville. 1983. Rapid cultural methods for detection of Salmonella in feeds and feed ingredients. J Food Prot 46:851–855.

79. D'Aoust, J.-Y., A. Sewell, and A. Jean. 1990. Limited sensitivity of short (6 h) selective enrichment for detection of foodborne Salmonella. J Food Prot 53:562–565.

80. D'Aoust, J.-Y., A.M. Sewell, and E. Daley. 1992. Inadequacy of small transfer volume and short (6 h) selective enrichment for the detection of foodborne Salmonella. J Food Prot 55:326–328.

81. D'Aoust, J.-Y., A.M. Sewell, E. Daley, and P. Greco. 1992. Antibiotic resistance of agricultural and foodborne Salmonella in Canada:1986–1989. J Food Prot 55:428–434.

82. D'Aoust, J.-Y., A. Sewell, and A. Jean. 1992. Efficacy of prolonged (48h) selective enrichment for the detection of foodborne Salmonella. Int J Food Microbiol 15:121–130.

83. D'Aoust, J.-Y., A. M. Sewell, and D.W. Warburton. 1992. A comparison of standard cultural methods for the detection of foodborne Salmonella. Int J Food Microbiol 16:41–50.

84. Dickens, J.A. and A.D. Whittemore. 1994. The effect of acetic acid and air injection on appearance, moisture pickup, microbiological quality, and Salmonella incidence on processed poultry carcasses. Poult Sci 73:582–586.

85. Dorn, C.R., R. Silapanuntakul, E.J. Angrick, and L.D. Shipman. 1992. Plasmid analysis and epidemiology of Salmonella enteritidis infection in three commercial layer flocks. Avian Dis 36:844–851.

86. Dorn, C.R., R. Silapanuntakul, E.J. Angrick, and L.D. Shipman. 1993. Plasmid analysis of Salmonella enteritidis isolated from human gastroenteritis cases and from epidemiologically associated poultry flocks. Epidemiol Infect 111:239–243.

87. Dunlap, N.E, W.H. Benjamin, Jr., A.K. Berry, J.H. Eldridge, and D.E. Briles. 1992. A `safe-site' for Salmonella typhimurium is within splenic polymorphonuclear cells. Microb Pathogen 13:181–190.

88. Ebel, E.D., M.J. David, and J. Mason. 1992. Occurrence of Salmonella enteritidis in the U. S. commercial egg industry: Report on a national spent hen survey. Avian Dis 36:646–654.

89. Ebel, E.D., J. Mason, L.A. Thomas, K.E. Ferris, M.G. Beckman, D.R. Cummins, L. Scroeder-Tucker, W.D. Sutherlin, R.L. Glasshoff, and N.M. Smithhisler. 1993. Occurrence of Salmonella enteritidis in unpasteurized liquid egg in the United States. Avian Dis 37:135–142.

90. Edel, W. 1994. Salmonella enteritidis eradication programme in poultry breeder flocks in The Netherlands. Int J Food Microbiol 21:171–178.

91. Elissalde, M.H., R.L. Ziprin, W.E. Huff, L. F. Kubena, and R. B. Harvey. 1994. Effect of Ochratoxin A on Salmonella-challenged broiler chicks. Poult Sci 73:1241–1248.

92. Ernst, R.K., D.M. Dombroski, and J.M. Merrick. 1990. Anaerobiosis, type 1 fimbriae, and growth phase are factors that affect invasion of HEp-2 cells by Salmonella typhimurium. Infect Immun 58:2014–2016.

93. Ewing, W.H. 1986. Edwards and Ewing's Identification of Enterobacteriaceae, 4th ed. Elsevier, New York, NY.

94. Faddoul, G.P. and G.W. Fellows. 1966. A five-year survey of the incidence of Salmonellae in avian species. Avian Dis 10:296–304.

95. Fagerberg, D.J, C.L. Quarles, J.A. Ranson, R.D. Williams, L.P. Williams, Jr., C.B. Hancock, and S.L. Seaman. 1976. Experimental procedure for testing the effects of low level antibiotic feeding and therapeutic treatment on Salmonella typhimurium var. copenhagen infection in broiler chicks. Poult Sci 55:1848–1857.

96. Fanelli, M.J, W.W. Sadler, C.E. Franti, and J.R. Brownell. 1971. Localization of Salmonellae within the intestinal tract of chickens. Avian Dis 15:366–375.

97. Ferris, K.E., and D.A. Miller. 1991. Salmonella serotypes from animals and related sources reported during July 1990–June 1991. Proc 95th Annu Meet U.S. Anim Health Assoc. U.S. Animal Health Association, Richmond, VA, pp. 440–454.

98. Ferris, K.E., and D.A. Miller. 1992. Salmonella serotypes from animals and related sources reported during July 1991–June 1992. Proc 96th Annu Meet U.S. Anim Health Assoc. U.S. Animal Health Association, Richmond, VA, pp. 492–504.

99. Ferris, K.E., and L.A. Thomas. 1993. Salmonella serotypes from animals and related sources reported during July 1992–June 1993. Proc 97th Annu Meet U.S. Anim Health Assoc. U.S. Animal Health Association, Richmond, VA, pp. 524–539.

100. Fields, P.I., R.V. Swanson, C.G. Haidaris, and F. Heffron. 1986. Mutants of Salmonella typhimurium that cannot survive within the macrophage are avirulent. Proc Natl Acad Sci USA 83:5189–5193.

101. Finlay, B.B., and S. Falkow. 1988. Virulence factors associated with Salmonella species. Microbiol Sci 5:324–328.

102. Finlay, B.B., F. Heffron, and S. Falkow. 1989. Epithelial cell surfaces induce Salmonella proteins required for bacterial adherence and invasion. Science 243:940–943.

103. Gast, R.K. 1993. Detection of Salmonella enteritidis in experimentally infected laying hens by culturing pools of egg contents. Poult Sci 72:267–274.

104. Gast, R.K. 1993. Immersion in boiling water to disinfect egg shells before culturing egg contents for Salmonella enteritidis. J Food Prot 56:533–535.

105. Gast, R.K. 1993. Evaluation of direct plating for detecting Salmonella enteritidis in pools of egg contents. Poult Sci 72:1611–1614.

106. Gast, R.K. 1993. Recovery of Salmonella enteritidis from inoculated pools of egg contents. J Food Prot 56:21–24.

107. Gast, R.K., and C.W. Beard. 1989. Age-related changes in the persistence and pathogenicity of Salmonella typhimurium in chicks. Poult Sci 68:1454–1460.

108. Gast, R.K., and C.W. Beard. 1990. Production of Salmonella enteritidis-contaminated eggs by experimentally infected hens. Avian Dis 34:438–446.

109. Gast, R.K., and C.W. Beard. 1990. Serological detection of experimental Salmonella enteritidis infections in laying hens. Avian Dis 34:721–728.

110. Gast, R.K., and C.W. Beard. 1990. Isolation of Salmonella enteritidis from internal organs of experimentally infected hens. Avian Dis 34:991–993.

111. Gast, R.K., and C.W. Beard. 1991. Detection of Salmonella serogroup D-specific antibodies in the yolks of eggs laid by hens infected with Salmonella enteritidis. Poult Sci 70:1273–1276.

112. Gast, R.K., and C.W. Beard. 1992. Evaluation of a chick mortality model for predicting the consequences of Salmonella enteritidis infections in laying hens. Poult Sci 71:281–287.

113. Gast, R.K., and C.W. Beard. 1992. Detection and enumeration of Salmonella enteritidis in fresh and stored eggs laid by experimentally infected hens. J Food Prot 55:152–156.

114. Gast, R.K., and S.T. Benson. 1995. The comparative virulence for chicks of Salmonella enteritidis phage type 4 isolates and isolates of phage types commonly found in poultry in the United States. Avian Dis 39:567–574.

115. Gast, R.K., and P.S. Holt. 1995. Iron supplementation to enhance the recovery of Salmonella enteritidis from pools of egg contents. J Food Prot 58:268–272.

116. Gast, R.K., and P.S. Holt. 1995. Differences in the multiplication of Salmonella enteritidis strains in liquid whole egg: Implications for detecting contaminated eggs from commercial laying flocks. Poultry Sci 74:893–897.

117. Gast, R.K., and J.F. Stephens. 1988. Effects of kanamycin administration to poultry on the proliferation of drug-resistant Salmonella. Poult Sci 67:689–698.

118. Gast, R.K., J.F. Stephens, and D.N. Foster. 1988. Effects of kanamycin administration to poultry on the interspecies transmission of drug-resistant Salmonella. Poult Sci 67:699–706.

119. Gast, R.K., H.D. Stone, P.S. Holt, and C.W. Beard. 1992. Evaluation of the efficacy of an oil-emulsion bacterin for protecting chickens against Salmonella enteritidis. Avian Dis 36:992–999.

120. Gast, R.K., H.D. Stone, and P.S. Holt. 1993. Evaluation of the efficacy of oil-emulsion bacterins for reducing fecal shedding of Salmonella enteritidis by laying hens. Avian Dis 37:1085–1091.

121. Gleeson, T.M., S. Stavric, and B. Blanchfield. 1989. Protection of chicks against Salmonella infection with a mixture of pure cultures of intestinal bacteria. Avian Dis 33:636–642.

122. Goodnough, M.C., and E.A. Johnson. 1991. Control of Salmonella enteritidis infections in poultry by polymyxin B and trimethoprim. Appl Environ Microbiol 57:785–788.

123. Gordon, R.F., and J.F. Tucker. 1965. The epizootiology of Salmonella menston infection of fowls and the effect of feeding poultry food artificially infected with Salmonella. Br Poult Sci 6:251–264.

124. Goren, E., W.A. deJong, P. Dorrnebal, N.M. Bolder, R.W.A.W. Mulder, and A. Jansen. 1988. Reduction of salmonella infection of broilers by spray application of intestinal microflora: A longitudinal study. Vet Q 10:249–255.

125. Gorham, S.L., K. Kadavil, H. Lambert, E. Vaughan, B. Pert, and J. Abel. 1991. Persistence of Salmonella enteritidis in young chickens. Avian Pathol 20:433–437.

126. Gorham, S.L., K. Kadavil, E. Vaughan, H. Lambert, J. Abel, and B. Pert. 1994. Gross and microscopic lesions in young chickens experimentally infected with Salmonella enteritidis. Avian Dis 38:816–821.

127. Groisman, E.A., C. Parra-Lopez, M. Salcedo, C.J. Lipps, and F. Heffron. 1992. Resistance to host antimicrobial peptides is necessary for Salmonella virulence. Proc Natl Acad Sci USA 89:11,939–11,943.

128. Gulig, P.A., and R. Curtiss III. 1987. Plasmid-associ-

ated virulence of Salmonella typhimurium. Infect Immun 55:2891–2901.

129. Gulig, P.A., and T.J. Doyle. 1993. The Salmonella typhimurium virulence plasmid increases the growth rate of Salmonellae in mice. Infect Immun 61:504–511.

130. Halavatkar, H., and P.A. Barrow. 1993. The role of a 54-kb plasmid in the virulence of strains of Salmonella Enteritidis of phage type 4 for chickens and mice. J Med Microbiol 38:171–176.

131. Hasan, J.A.K., I.T. Knight, C.R. Tate, E.T. Mallinson, R.G. Miller, R.R. Colwell, and S.W. Joseph. 1991. Evaluation of radiolabeled and colorimetric DNA probes in comparison with an antigen screening assay for the detection of Salmonella from poultry samples. Avian Dis 35:397–402.

132. Hassan, J.O., and R. Curtiss III. 1994. Virulent Salmonella typhimurium-induced lymphocyte depletion and immunosuppression in chickens. Infect Immun 62:2027–2036.

133. Hassan, J.O., and R. Curtiss III. 1994. Development and evaluation of an experimental vaccination program using a live avirulent Salmonella typhimurium strain to protect immunized chickens against challenge with homologous and heterologous Salmonella serotypes. Infect Immun 62:5519–5527.

134. Hassan, J.O., P.A. Barrow, A.P.A. Mockett, and S. McLeod. 1990. Antibody response to experimental Salmonella typhimurium infection in chickens measured by ELISA. Vet Rec 126:519–522.

135. Hassan, J.O., A.P.A. Mockett, D. Catty, and P.A. Barrow. 1991. Infection and reinfection of chickens with Salmonella typhimurium: Bacteriology and immune responses. Avian Dis 35:809–819.

136. Hassan, J.O., A.P.A. Mockett, S. McLeod, and P.A. Barrow. 1991. Indirect antigen-trap ELISAs using polyclonal antisera for detection of group B and D Salmonellas in chickens. Avian Pathol 20:271–282.

137. Helmuth, R., R. Stephan, C. Bunge, B. Hoog, A. Steinbeck, and E. Bulling. 1985. Epidemiology of virulence-associated plasmids and outer membrane protein patterns within seven common Salmonella serotypes. Infect Immun 48:175–182.

138. Henderson, W., J. Ostendorf, Jr., and G.L. Morehouse. 1960. The relative pathogenicity of some Salmonella serotypes for chicks. Avian Dis 4:103–109.

139. Henzler, D.J., and H. M. Opitz. 1992. The role of mice in the epizootiology of Salmonella enteritidis infection on chicken layer farms. Avian Dis 36:625–631.

140. Henzler, D.J., E. Ebel, J. Sanders, D. Kradel, and J. Mason. 1994. Salmonella enteritidis in eggs from commercial chicken layer flocks implicated in human outbreaks. Avian Dis 38:37–43.

141. Higgins, R., R. Malo, E. René-Roberge, and R. Gauthier. 1982. Studies on the dissemination of Salmonella in nine broiler-chicken flocks. Avian Dis 26:26–33.

142. Hinton, M. 1988. Salmonella infection in chicks following the consumption of artificially contaminated feed. Epidemiol Infect 100:247–256.

143. Hinton, M., E.J. Threlfall, and B. Rowe. 1990. The invasive potential of Salmonella enteritidis phage types for young chickens. Lett Appl Microbiol 10:237–239.

144. Hoertt, B.E., J. Ou, D.J. Kopecko, L.S. Baron, and R.L. Warren. 1989. Novel virulence properties of the Salmonella typhimurium virulence-associated plasmid: Immune suppression and stimulation of splenomegaly. Plasmid 21:48–58.

145. Holt, P.S. 1993. Effect of induced molting on the susceptibility of white leghorn hens to a Salmonella enteritidis infection. Avian Dis 37:412–417.

146. Holt, P.S., and R.E. Porter, Jr. 1992. Effect of induced molting on the course of infection and transmission of Salmonella enteritidis in white leghorn hens of different ages. Poult Sci 71:1842–1848.

147. Holt, P.S., and R.E. Porter, Jr. 1992. Microbiological and histopathological effects of an induced-molt fasting procedure on a Salmonella enteritidis infection in chickens. Avian Dis 36:610–618.

148. Holt, P.S., and R.E. Porter, Jr. 1993. Effect of induced molting on the recurrence of a previous Salmonella enteritidis infection. Poult Sci 72:2069–2078.

149. Holt, P.S., R.J. Buhr, D.L. Cunningham, and R.E. Porter, Jr. 1994. Effect of two different molting procedures on a Salmonella enteritidis infection. Poult Sci 73:1267–1275.

150. Holt, P.S., R.K. Gast, and C.R. Greene, 1995. Rapid detection of Salmonella enteritidis in pooled liquid egg samples using a magnetic bead-ELISA system. J Food Prot 58:967–972.

151. Hoop, R.K., and A. Pospischil. 1993. Bacteriological, serological, histological and immunohistochemical findings in laying hens with naturally acquired Salmonella enteritidis phage type 4 infection. Vet Rec 133:391–393.

152. Hopper, S.A., and S. Mawer. 1988. Salmonella enteritidis in a commercial layer flock. Vet Rec 123:351.

153. Horiuchi, S., N. Goto, Y. Inagaki, and R. Nakaya. 1991. The 106-kilobase plasmid of Salmonella braenderup and the 100-kilobase plasmid of Salmonella typhimurium are not necessary for the pathogenicity in experimental models. Microbiol Immunol 35:187–198.

154. Hovi, M., S. Sukupolvi, M.F. Edwards, and M. Rhen. 1988. Plasmid-associated virulence of Salmonella enteritidis. Microb Pathog 4:385–391.

155. Humbert, F., G. Salvat, F. Lalande, P. Colin, and C. Lahellec. 1990. Rapid detection of Salmonella from poultry meat products using the 1.2. Test. Lett Appl Microbiol 10:245–249.

156. Humphrey, T.J. 1990. Heat resistance in Salmonella enteritidis phage type 4: The influence of storage temperatures before heating. J Appl Bacteriol 69:493–497.

157. Humphrey, T.J., and A. Whitehead. 1992. Techniques for the isolation of salmonellas from eggs. Br Poult Sci 33:761–768.

158. Humphrey, T.J., G.C. Mead, and B. Rowe. 1988. Poultry meat as a source of human salmonellosis in England and Wales. Epidemiol Infect 100:175–184.

159. Humphrey, T.J., A. Baskerville, H. Chart, and B. Rowe. 1989. Infection of egg-laying hens with Salmonella enteritidis PT4 by oral inoculation. Vet Rec 125:531–532.

160. Humphrey, T.J., A. Baskerville, S. Mawer, B. Rowe, and S. Hopper. 1989. Salmonella enteritidis phage type 4 from the contents of intact eggs: A study involving naturally infected hens. Epidemiol Infect 103:415–423.

161. Humphrey, T.J., M. Greenwood, R.J. Gilbert, B. Rowe, and P.A. Chapman. 1989. The survival of salmonellas in shell eggs cooked under simulated domestic conditions. Epidemiol Infect 103:35–45.

162. Humphrey, T.J., H. Chart, A. Baskerville, and B. Rowe. 1991. The influence of age on the response of SPF hens to infection with Salmonella enteritidis PT4. Epidemiol Infect 106:33–43.

163. Humphrey, T.J., N.P. Richardson, A.H.L. Gawler, and M.J. Allen. 1991. Heat resistance of Salmonella enteritidis PT4: The influence of prior exposure to alkaline conditions. Lett Appl Microbiol 12:258–260.

164. Humphrey, T.J., A. Whitehead, A.H.L. Gawler, A. Henley, and B. Rowe. 1991. Numbers of Salmonella enteritidis in the contents of naturally contaminated hens' eggs. Epidemiol Infect 106:489–496.

165. Humphrey, T.J., A. Baskerville, H. Chart, B. Rowe, and A. Whitehead. 1992. Infection of laying hens with Salmonella enteritidis PT4 by conjunctival challenge. Vet Rec 131:386–388.

166. Humphrey, T.J., A. Baskerville, A. Whitehead, B. Rowe, and A. Henley. 1993. Influence of feeding patterns on the artificial infection of laying hens with Salmonella enteri-

tidis phage type 4. Vet Rec 132:407–409.

167. Irwin, R.J., C. Poppe, S. Messier, G.G. Finley, and J. Oggel. 1994. A national survey to estimate the prevalence of Salmonella species among Canadian registered commercial turkey flocks. Can J Vet Res 58:263–267.

168. Izat, A.L., M. Colberg, R.A. Thomas, M.H. Adams, and C.D. Driggers. 1990. Effects of lactic acid in processing waters on the incidence of Salmonellae on broilers. J Food Qual 13:295–306.

169. Izat, A.L., J.M. Kopek, and J.D. McGinnis. 1991. Incidence, numbers, and serotypes of *Salmonella* on frozen broiler chickens at retail. Poult Sci 70:1438–1440.

170. Johnson, C.T. 1992. The use of an antimicrobial and competitive exclusion combination in Salmonella-infected pullet flocks. Int J Food Microbiol 15:293–298.

171. Jones, F.T., R.C. Axtell, D.V. Rives, S.E. Scheideler, F.R. Tarver, Jr., R.L. Walker, and M.J. Wineland. 1991. A survey of Salmonella contamination in modern broiler production. J Food Prot 54:502–507,513.

172. Keller, L.H., C.E. Benson, V. Garcia, E. Nocks, P. Battenfelder, and R.J. Eckroade. 1993. Monoclonal antibody-based detection system for Salmonella enteritidis. Avian Dis 37:501–507.

173. Kerr, S., H.J. Ball, D.P. Mackie, D.A. Pollock, and D.A. Finlay. 1992. Diagnostic application of monoclonal antibodies to outer membrane proteins for rapid detection of salmonella. J Appl Bacteriol 72:302–308.

174. Kim, C.J., K.V. Nagaraja, and B.S. Pomeroy. 1991. Enzyme-linked immunosorbent assay for the detection of Salmonella enteritidis infection in chickens. Am J Vet Res 52:1069–1074.

175. Kim, J.-W., M.F. Slavik, M.D. Pharr, D.P. Raben, C.M. Lobsinger, and S. Tsai. 1994. Reduction of Salmonella on post-chill chicken carcasses by trisodium phosphate (Na₃PO₄) treatment. J Food Safety 14:9–17.

176. Kingston, D.J. 1981. A comparison of culturing drag swabs and litter for identification of infections with Salmonella spp. in commercial chicken flocks. Avian Dis 25:513–516.

177. Kobland, J.D., G.O. Gale, R.H. Gustafson, and K.L. Simkins. 1987. Comparison of therapeutic versus subtherapeutic levels of chlortetracycline in the diet for selection of resistant Salmonella in experimentally challenged chickens. Poult Sci 66:1129–1137.

178. Kogut, M.H., E.D. McGruder, B.M. Hargis, D.E. Corrier, and J.R. DeLoach. 1994. Dynamics of avian inflammatory response to Salmonella-immune lymphokines: Changes in avian blood leukocyte populations. Inflammation 18:373–388.

179. Kogut, M.H., G.I. Tellez, E.D. McGruder, B.M. Hargis, J.D. Williams, D.E. Corrier, and J.R. DeLoach. 1994. Heterophils are decisive components in the early responses of chickens to Salmonella enteritidis infections. Microb Pathog 16:141–151.

180. Kogut, M.H., E.D. McGruder, B.M. Hargis, D.E. Corrier, and J.R. DeLoach. 1995. Characterization of the pattern of inflammatory cell influx in chicks following the intraperitoneal administration of live Salmonella enteritidis and Salmonella enteritidis-immune lymphokines. Poult Sci 74:8–18.

181. Koo, F.C. J.W. Peterson, C.W. Houston, and N.C. Molina. 1984. Pathogenesis of experimental salmonellosis: Inhibition of protein synthesis by cytotoxin. Infect Immun 43:93–100.

182. Kopanic, R.J., Jr., B.W. Sheldon, and C.G. Wright. 1994. Cockroaches as vectors of Salmonella: Laboratory and field trials. J Food Prot 57:125–132.

183. Koupal, L.P., and R.H. Deibel. 1975. Assay, characterization, and localization of an enterotoxin produced by Salmonella. Infect Immun 11:14–22.

184. Krieg, N.R., and J.G. Holt. 1984. Bergey's Manual of Systematic Bacteriology, vol 1. Williams and Wilkins, Baltimore, MD.

185. Kumar, M.C., M.D. York, J.R. McDowell, and B.S. Pomeroy. 1971. Dynamics of Salmonella infection in fryer roaster turkeys. Avian Dis 15:221–232.

186. Kusters, J.G., G.A.W.M. Mulders-Kremers, C.E.M. van Doornik, and B.A.M. van der Zeijst. 1993. Effects of multiplicity of infection, bacterial protein synthesis, and growth phase on adhesion to and invasion of human cell lines by Salmonella typhimurium. Infect Immun 61:5013–5020.

187. Lahellec, C., and P. Colin. 1985. Relationship between serotypes of salmonellae from hatcheries and rearing farms and those from processed poultry carcasses. Br Poult Sci 26:179–186.

188. Lahellec, C., P. Colin, G. Bennejean, J. Pacquin, A. Guillerm, and J.C. Debois. 1986. Influence of resident Salmonella on contamination of broiler flocks. Poult Sci 65:2034–2039.

189. Larsen, G.J., A.M. Rolow, and C.E. Nelson. 1993. The effect of organic acids on Salmonella contamination originating from mouse fecal pellets. Poult Sci 72:1797–1799.

190. Leclair, K., H. Heggart, M. Oggel, F.M. Bartlett, and R.C. McKellar. 1994. Modelling the inactivation of Listeria monocytogenes and Salmonella typhimurium in simulated egg wash water. Food Microbiol 11:345–353.

191. Lee, C.A., and S. Falkow. 1990. The ability of Salmonella to enter mammalian cells is affected by bacterial growth state. Proc Natl Acad Sci USA 87:4304–4308.

192. Lee, G.M., G.D.F. Jackson, and G.N. Cooper. 1981. The role of serum and biliary antibodies and cell-mediated immunity in the clearance of S. typhimurium from chickens. Vet Immunol Immunopathol 2:233–252.

193. Leeson, S., and M. Marcotte. 1993. Irradiation of poultry feed I. Microbial status and bird response. World's Poult Sci 49:19–33.

194. Leung, K.Y., and B.B. Finlay. 1991. Intracellular replication is essential for the virulence of Salmonella typhimurium. Proc Natl Acad Sci USA 88:11,470–11,474.

195. Levine, W.C., J.F. Smart, D.L. Archer, N.H. Bean, and R.V. Tauxe. 1991. Foodborne disease outbreaks in nursing homes, 1975 through 1987. J Am Med Assoc 266:2105–2109.

196. Li, Y.M.F. Slavik, C.L. Griffis, J.T. Walker, J.W. Kim, and R.E. Wolfe. 1994. Destruction of Salmonella in poultry chiller water using electrical stimulation. Trans Am Soc Agric Eng 37:211–215.

197. Lindell, K.A., A.M. Saeed, and G.P. McCabe. 1994. Evaluation of resistance of four strains of commercial laying hens to experimental infection with Salmonella enteritidis phage type eight. Poult Sci 73:757–762.

198. Lindquist, B.L., E. Lebenthal, P.-C. Lee, M.W. Stinson, and J.M. Merrick. 1987. Adherence of Salmonella typhimurium to small-intestinal enterocytes of the rat. Infect Immun 55:3044–3050.

199. Lister, S.A. 1988. Salmonella enteritidis infection in broilers and broiler breeders. Vet Rec 123:350.

200. MacBeth, K.J., and C.A. Lee. 1993. Prolonged inhibition of bacterial protein synthesis abolishes Salmonella invasion. Infect Immun 61:1544–1546.

201. Machado, J., and F. Bernardo. 1990. Prevalence of Salmonella in chicken carcasses in Portugal. J Appl Bacteriol 69:477–480.

202. MacKenzie, M.A., and B.S. Bains. 1976. Dissemination of Salmonella serotypes from raw feed ingredients to chicken carcasses. Poult Sci 55:957–960.

203. Magwood, S.E., and C.H. Bigland. 1962. Salmonellosis in turkeys: Evaluation of bacteriological and serological evidence in infection. Can J Comp Med Vet Sci 26:151–159.

204. Mahon, J., and A.J. Lax. 1993. A quantitative polymerase chain reaction method for the detection in avian fae-

ces of salmonellas carrying the spvR gene. Epidemiol Infect 111:455–464.

205. Mallinson, E.T. and G.H. Snoeyenbos. 1989. Salmonellosis. In H.G. Purchase, L.H. Arp, C.H. Domermuth, and J.E. Pearson (eds). A Laboratory Manual for the Isolation and Identification of Avian Pathogens, 3rd ed. Kendall/Hunt Publishing, Dubuque, IA, pp. 3–11.

206. Mallinson, E.T., C.R. Tate, R.G. Miller, B. Bennett, and E. Russek-Cohen. 1989. Monitoring poultry farms for Salmonella by drag-swab sampling and antigen-capture immunoassay. Avian Dis 33:684–690.

207. Manning, J.G., B.M. Hargis, A. Hinton, Jr., D.E. Corrier, J.R. DeLoach, and C.R. Creger. 1992. Effect of nitrofurazone or novobiocin on Salmonella enteritidis cecal colonization and organ invasion in leghorn hens. Avian Dis 36:334–340.

208. Manning, J.G., B.M. Hargis, A. Hinton, Jr., D.E. Corrier, J.R. DeLoach, and C.R. Creger. 1994. Effect of selected antibiotics and anticoccidials on Salmonella enteritidis cecal colonization and organ invasion in Leghorn chicks. Avian Dis 38:256–261.

209. Mason, J. 1994. Salmonella enteritidis control programs in the United States. Int J Food Microbiol 21:155–169.

210. Mastroeni, P., B. Villarreal-Ramos, and C.E. Hormaeche. 1993. Adoptive transfer of immunity to oral challenge with virulent Salmonellae in innately susceptible BALB/c mice requires both immune serum and T cells. Infect Immun 61:3981–3984.

211. Matic, S., V. Mihokovic, B. Katusin-Razem, and D. Razem. 1990. The eradication of Salmonella in egg powder by gamma irradiation. J Food Prot 53:111–114.

212. McAllister, J.C., C.D. Steelman, and J.K. Skeeles. 1994. Reservoir competence of the lesser mealworm (Coleoptera: Tenebrionidae) for Salmonella typhimurium (Eubacteriales: Enterobacteriaceae). J Med Entomol 31:369–372.

213. McCapes, R.H., H.E. Ekperigin, W.J. Cameron, W.L. Ritchie, J. Slagter, V. Stangeland, and K.V. Nagaraja. 1989. Effect of a new pelleting process on the level of contamination of poultry mash by Escherichia coli and Salmonella. Avian Dis 33:103–111.

214. McDonough, P.L., R.H. Jacobson, and J.F. Timoney. 1989. Virulence determinants of Salmonella typhimurium from animal sources. Am J Vet Res 50:662–670.

215. McIlroy, S.G., R.M. McCracken, S.D. Neilland, and J.J. O'brien. 1989. Control, prevention and eradication of Salmonella enteritidis infection in broiler and broiler breeder flocks. Vet Rec 125:545–548.

216. Miller, R.G., C.R. Tate, E.T. Mallinson, and J.A. Scherrer. 1991. Xylose-lysine-tergitol 4: An improved selective agar medium for the isolation of Salmonella. Poult Sci 70:2429–2432.

217. Mishu, B., P.M. Griffin, R.V. Tauxe, D.N. Cameron, R.H. Hutcheson, and W. Schaffner. 1991. Salmonella enteritidis gastroenteritis transmitted by intact chicken eggs. Annals Intern Med 115:190–194.

218. Mishu, B., J. Koehler, L.A. Lee, D. Rodrigue, F.H. Brenner, P. Blake and R.V. Tauxe. 1994. Outbreaks of Salmonella enteritidis infections in the United States, 1985–1991. J Infect Dis 169:547–552.

219. Mitrovic, M. 1956. First report of paratyphoid infection in turkey poults due to Salmonella reading. Poult Sci 35:171–174.

220. Miura, S., G. Sato, and T. Miyamae. 1964. Occurrence and survival of Salmonella organisms in hatcher chick fluff from commercial hatcheries. Avian Dis 8:546–554.

221. Moore, V.A. 1895. On a pathogenic bacillus of the hog-cholera group associated with a fatal disease in pigeons. USDA BAI Bull 8:71–76.

222. Morris, G.K., B.L. McMurray, M.M. Galton, and J.G. Wells. 1969. A study of the dissemination of salmonel-

losis in a commercial broiler chicken operation. Am J Vet Res 30:1413–1421.

223. Morrison, G.J., and G.H. Fleet. 1985. Reduction of Salmonella on chicken carcasses by immersion treatments. J Food Prot. 48:939–943.

224. Motha, M.X.J., and J.R. Egerton. 1983. Effect of reticuloendotheliosis virus on the response of chickens to Salmonella typhimurium infection. Res Vet Sci 34:188–192.

225. Muirhead, S. 1994. Feed Additive Compendium. Miller Publishing, Minnetonka, MN.

226. Mulder, R.W.A.W., M.C. van der Hulst, and N.M. Bolder. 1987. Salmonella decontamination of broiler carcasses with lactic acid, L-cysteine, and hydrogen peroxide. Poult Sci 66:1555–1557.

227. Muotiala, A., M. Hovi, and P.H. Makela. 1989. Protective immunity in mouse salmonellosis: Comparison of smooth and rough live and killed vaccines. Microb Pathog 6:51–60.

228. Nakamura, M., S. Sato, T. Ohya, S. Suzuki, and S. Ikeda. 1985. Possible relationship of a 36-megadalton plasmid to virulence in mice. Infect Immun 47:831–833.

229. Nakamura, M., N. Nagamine, S. Suzuki, M. Norimatsu, K. Oishi, M. Kijima, Y. Tamura, and S. Sato. 1993. Long-term shedding of Salmonella Enteritidis in chickens which received a contact exposure within 24 hrs of hatching. Jpn Vet Med Sci 55:649–653.

230. Nakamura, M., N. Nagamine, M. Norimatsu, S. Suzuki, K. Ohishi, M. Kijima, Y. Tamura, and S. Sato. 1993. The ability of Salmonella enteritidis isolated from chicks imported from England to cause transovarian infection. J Vet Med Sci 55:135–136.

231. Nakamura, M., N. Nagamine, T. Takahashi, S. Suzuki, M. Kijima, Y. Tamura, and S. Sato. 1994. Horizontal transmission of Salmonella enteritidis and effect of stress on shedding in laying hens. Avian Dis 38:282–288.

232. Nakamura, M., N. Nagamine, T. Takahashi, S. Suzuki, and S. Sato. 1994. Evaluation of the efficacy of a bacterin against Salmonella enteritidis infection and the effect of stress after vaccination. Avian Dis 38:717–724.

233. Nicholas, R.A.J. 1992. Serological response of chickens naturally infected with Salmonella typhimurium detected by ELISA. Br Vet J 148:241–248.

234. Nicholas, R.A.J., and S.J. Andrews. 1991. Detection of antibody to Salmonella enteritidis and S. typhimurium in the yolk of hens' eggs. Vet Rec 128:98–100.

235. Nicholas, R.A.J., and G.A. Cullen. 1991. Development and application of an ELISA for detecting antibodies to Salmonella enteritidis in chicken flocks. Vet Rec 128:74–76.

236. Nisbet, D.J, D.E. Corrier, C.M. Scanlan, A.G. Hollister, R.C. Beier, and J.R. DeLoach. 1993. Effect of a defined continuous-flow derived bacterial culture and dietary lactose on Salmonella typhimurium colonization in broiler chickens. Avian Dis 37:1017–1025.

237. Nolan, L.K., R.E. Wooley, J. Brown, and J.P. Payeur. 1991. Comparison of phenotypic characteristics of Salmonella spp isolated from healthy and ill (infected) chickens. Am J Vet Res 52:1512–1517.

238. Nuotio, L., C. Schneitz, U. Halonen, and E. Nurmi. 1992. Use of competitive exclusion to protect newly-hatched chicks against intestinal colonisation and invasion by Salmonella enteritidis PT4. Br Poult Sci 33:775–779.

239. Oboegbulem, S.I., P.W. Collier, J.C.M. Sharp, and W.J. Reilly. 1993. Epidemiological aspects of outbreaks of food-borne salmonellosis in Scotland between 1980 and 1989. Rev Sci Tech 12:957–967.

240. Olesiuk, O.M., V.L. Carlson, G.H. Snoeyenbos, and C.F. Smyser. 1969. Experimental Salmonella typhimurium infection in two chicken flocks. Avian Dis 13:500–508.

241. Olesiuk, O.M., G.H. Snoeyenbos, and C.F. Smyser. 1973. Chemotherapy studies of Salmonella typhimurium in chickens. Avian Dis 17:379–389.

242. Opara, O.O., L.E. Carr, E. Russek-Cohen, C.R. Tate, E.T. Mallinson, R.G. Miller, L.E. Stewart, R.W. Johnston, and S.W. Joseph. 1992. Correlation of water activity and other environmental conditions with repeated detection of Salmonella contamination on poultry farms. Avian Dis 36:664–671.

243. Opitz, H.M., M. El-Begearmi, P. Flegg, and D. Beane. 1993. Effectiveness of five feed additives in chicks infected with Salmonella enteritidis phage type 13a. J Appl Poult Res 2:147–153.

244. Ou, J.T. and L.S. Baron. 1991. Strain Differences in expression of virulence by the 90 kilobase pair virulence plasmid of Salmonella serovar typhimurium. Microb Pathog 10:247–251.

245. Padron, M.N. 1990. Salmonella typhimurium outbreak in broiler chicken flocks in Mexico. Avian Dis 34:221–223.

246. Petter, J.G. 1993. Detection of two smooth colony phenotypes in a Salmonella enteritidis isolate which vary in their ability to contaminate eggs. Appl Environ Microbiol 59:2884–2890.

247. Pless, P., K. Futschik, and E. Schopf. 1994. Rapid detection of Salmonellae by means of a new impedance-splitting method. J Food Prot 57:369–376.

248. Pomeroy, B.S., K.V. Nagaraja, L.T. Ausherman, I.L. Peterson, and K.A. Friendshuh. 1989. Studies on feasibility of producing Salmonella-free turkeys. Avian Dis 33:1–7.

249. Popiel, I. and P.C.B. Turnbull. 1985. Passage of Salmonella enteritidis and Salmonella thompson through chick ileocecal mucosa. Infect Immun 47:786–792.

250. Poppe, C. 1994. Salmonella enteritidis in Canada. Int J Food Microbiol 21:1–5.

251. Poppe, C., R.J. Irwin, C.M. Forsberg, R.C. Clarke, and J. Oggel. 1991. The prevalence of Salmonella enteritidis and other Salmonella spp. among Canadian registered commercial layer flocks. Epidemiol Infect 106:259–270.

252. Poppe, C., R.P. Johnson, C.M. Forsberg, and R.J. Irwin. 1992. Salmonella enteritidis and other Salmonella in laying hens and eggs from flocks with Salmonella in their environment. Can J Vet Res 56:226–232.

253. Poppe, C., W. Demczuk, K. McFadden, and R.P. Johnson. 1993. Virulence of Salmonella enteritidis phagetypes 4, 8, and 13 and other Salmonella spp. for day-old chicks, hens and mice. Can J Vet Res 57:281–287.

254. Porter, R.E., Jr. and P.S. Holt. 1993. Effect of induced molting on the severity of intestinal lesions caused by Salmonella enteritidis infection in chickens. Avian Dis 37:1009–1016.

255. Potter, M.E. 1992. The changing face of foodborne disease. J Am Vet Med Assoc 201:250–253.

256. Qin, A.R., T. Fukata, E. Baba, and A. Arakawa. 1995. Effect of Eimeria tenella infection on Salmonella enteritidis infection in chickens. Poult Sci 74:1–7.

257. Read, S.C., R.J. Irwin, C. Poppe, and J. Harris. 1994. A comparison of two methods for isolation of Salmonella from poultry litter samples. Poult Sci 73:1617–1621.

258. Rigby, C.E. 1984. Enzyme-linked immunosorbent assay for detection of Salmonella lipopolysaccharide in poultry specimens. Appl Environ Microbiol 47:1327–1330.

259. Rigby, C.E., and J.R. Pettit. 1980. Observations on competitive exclusion for preventing Salmonella typhimurium infection of broiler chickens. Avian Dis 24:604–615.

260. Riikonen, P., P.H. Mäkelä, H. Saarilahti, S. Sukupolvi, S. Taira, and M. Rhen. 1992. The virulence plasmid does not contribute to growth of Salmonella in cultured murine macrophages. Microb Pathog 13:281–291.

261. Rodrigue, D.C., R.V. Tauxe, and B. Rowe. 1990. International increase in Salmonella enteritidis: A new pandemic? Epidemiol Infect 105:21–27.

262. Sadler, W.W., J.R. Brownell, and M.J. Fanelli. 1969.

263. Saeed, A.M., and C.W. Koons. 1993. Growth and heat resistance of Salmonella enteritidis in refrigerated and abused eggs. J Food Prot 56:927–931.

264. Sato, G., S. Matsubara, S. Etoh, and H. Kodama. 1971. Cultivation of samples of hatcher chick fluff, floor litter and feces for the detection of Salmonella infection in chicken flocks. Jpn J Vet Res 19:73–80.

265. Schaffner, D.F., M.K. Handy, R.T. Toledo, and M.L. Tift. 1989. Salmonella inactivation in liquid whole egg by thermoradiation. J Food Sci 54:902–905.

266. Schleifer, J., B.J. Juven, C.W. Beard, and N.A. Cox. 1984. The susceptibility of chicks to Salmonella montevideo in artificially contaminated poultry feed. Avian Dis 28:497–503.

267. Schneitz, C. 1992. Automated droplet application of a competitive exclusion preparation. Poult Sci 71:2125–2128.

268. Schneitz, C., and L. Nuotio. 1992. Efficacy of different microbial preparations for controlling Salmonella colonisation in chicks and turkey poults by competitive exclusion. Br Poult Sci 33:207–211.

269. Schnepf, M., and W.E. Barbeau. 1989. Survival of Salmonella typhimurium in roasting chickens cooked in a microwave, convection microwave, and a conventional electric oven. J Food Safety 9:245–252.

270. Shackelford, A.D., L.C. Blankenship, O.W. Charles, and J.A. Dickens. 1987. Experimental two-stage pellet mill conditioner with paddle shaft steam injection. Poultry Sci 66:1737–1743.

271. Shaffer, M F., K.C. Milner, D.I. Clemmer, and J.F. Bridges. 1957. Bacteriologic studies of experimental Salmonella infections in chicks. II. J Infect Dis 100:17–31.

272. Sheldon, B.W., and J. Brake. 1991. Hydrogen peroxide as an alternative hatching egg disinfectant. Poult Sci 70:1092–1098.

273. Shivaprasad, H.L., J.F. Timoney, S. Morales, B. Lucio, and R.C. Baker. 1990. Pathogenesis of Salmonella enteritidis infection in laying chickens. I. Studies on egg transmission, clinical signs, fecal shedding, and serologic responses. Avian Dis 34:548–557.

274. Singer, J.T., H.M. Opitz, M. Gershman, M.M. Hall, I.G. Muniz, and S.V. Rao. 1992. Molecular characterization of Salmonella enteritidis isolates from Maine poultry and poultry farm environments. Avian Dis 36:324–333.

275. Slavik, M.F., C. Griffis, Y. Li, and P. Engler. 1991. Effect of electrical stimulation on bacterial contamination of chicken legs. J Food Prot 54:508–513.

276. Smith, H.W., and J.F. Tucker. 1980. The virulence of salmonella strains for chickens: Their excretion by infected chickens. J Hyg, Camb 84:479–488.

277. Smyser, C.F., and G.H. Snoeyenbos. 1979. Evaluation of organic acids and other compounds as Salmonella antagonists in meat and bone meal. Poult Sci 58:50–54.

278. Smyser, C.F., N. Adinarayanan, H. van Roekel, and G.H. Snoeyenbos. 1966. Field and laboratory observations on Salmonella heidelberg infections in three chicken breeding flocks. Avian Dis 10:314–329.

279. Snoeyenbos, G.H., V.L. Carlson, B.A. McKie, and C.F. Smyser. 1967. An epidemiological study of salmonellosis of chickens. Avian Dis 11:653–667.

280. Snoeyenbos, G.H., V.L. Carlson, C.F. Smyser, and O.M. Olesiuk. 1969. Dynamics of Salmonella infection in chicks reared on litter. Avian Dis 13:72–83.

281. Snoeyenbos, G.H., C.F. Smyser, and H. van Roekel. 1969. Salmonella infections of the ovary and peritoneum of chickens. Avian Dis 13:668–670.

282. Snoeyenbos, G.H., B.A. McKie, C.F. Smyser, and C.R. Weston. 1970. Progress in identifying and maintaining Salmonella-free commercial chicken breeding flocks. 1. 1967–1969. Avian Dis 14:683–696.

Influence of age and inoculum level on shed pattern of Salmonella typhimurium in chickens. Avian Dis 13:793–803.

283. Snoeyenbos, G.H., O.M. Weinack, and C.F. Smyser. 1978. Protecting chicks and poults from Salmonellae by oral administration of "normal" gut microflora. Avian Dis 22:273–287.

284. Snoeyenbos, G.H., O.M. Weinack, A.S. Soerjadi-Liem, B.M. Miller, D.E. Miller, D.E. Woodward, and C.R. Weston. 1985. Large-scale trials to study competitive exclusion of Salmonella in chickens. Avian Dis 29:1004–1011.

285. Soerjadi-Liem, A.S., and R.B. Cumming. 1984. Studies on the incidence of Salmonella carriers in broiler flocks entering a poultry processing plant in Australia. Poult Sci 63:892–895.

286. Soerjadi, A.S., S.M. Stehman, G.H. Snoeyenbos, O.M. Weinack, and C.F. Smyser. 1981. Some measurements of protection against paratyphoid Salmonella and Escherichia coli by competitive exclusion in chickens. Avian Dis 25:706–712.

287. St. Louis, M.E., D.L. Morse, M.E. Potter, T.M. DeMelfi, J.J. Guzewich, R.V. Tauxe, and P.A. Blake. 1988. The emergence of Grade A eggs as a major source of Salmonella enteritidis infections: New implications for the control of salmonellosis. J Am Med Assoc 259:2103–2107.

288. Stabler, J.G., T.W. McCormick, K.C. Powell, and M.H. Kogut. 1994. Avian heterophils and monocytes: Phagocytic and bactericidal activities against Salmonella enteritidis. Vet Microbiol 38:293–305.

289. Stavric, S., T.M. Gleeson, B. Blanchfield, and H. Pivnick. 1985. Competitive exclusion of Salmonella from newly hatched chicks by mixtures of pure bacterial cultures isolated from fecal and cecal contents of adult birds. J Food Prot 48:778–782.

290. Stavric, S., T.M. Gleeson, B. Blanchfield, and H. Pivnick. 1987. Role of adhering microflora in competitive exclusion of Salmonella from young chicks. J Food Prot 50:928–932.

291. Stephenson, P., F.B. Satchell, G. Allen, and W.H. Andrews. 1991. Recovery of Salmonella from eggs. J AOAC Int 74:821–826.

292. Sukupolvi, S., P. Riikonen, S. Taira, H. Saarilahti, and M. Rhen. 1992. Plasmid-mediated serum resistance in Salmonella enterica. Microb Pathog 12:219–225.

293. Suzuki, S., K. Ohishi, T. Takahashi, Y. Tamura, M Muramatsu, M. Nakamura, and S. Sato. 1992. The role of 36 megadalton plasmid of Salmonella Enteritidis for the pathogenesis in mice. J Vet Med Sci 54:845–850.

294. Takimoto, H., E. Baba, T. Fukata, and A. Arakawa. 1984. Effects of infection of Eimeria tenella, E. acervulina, and E. maxima upon Salmonella typhimurium infection in chickens. Poult Sci 63:478–484.

295. Tate, C.R., R.G. Miller, E.T. Mallinson, L.W. Douglass, and R.W. Johnston. 1990. The isolation of Salmonellae from poultry environmental samples by several enrichment procedures using plating media with and without novobiocin. Poult Sci 69:721–726.

296. Tate, C.R., R.G. Miller, and E.T. Mallinson. 1992. Evaluation of two isolation and two nonisolation methods for detecting naturally occurring Salmonellae from broiler flock environmental drag-swab samples. J Food Prot 55:964–967.

297. Tauxe, R.V. 1991. Salmonella: A postmodern pathogen. J Food Prot 54:563–568.

298. Tellez, G.I., M.H. Kogut, and B.M. Hargis. 1993. Immunoprophylaxis of Salmonella enteritidis infection by lymphokines in Leghorn chicks. Avian Dis 37:1062–1070.

299. Tellez, G.I., M.H. Kogut, and B.M. Hargis. 1994. Eimeria tenella or Eimeria adenoeides: Induction of morphological changes and increased resistance to Salmonella enteritidis infection in leghorn chicks. Poult Sci 73:396–401.

300. Thaxton, P., R.D. Wyatt, and P.B. Hamilton. 1975. The effect of environmental temperature on paratyphoid infection in the neonatal chicken. Poult Sci 53:88–94.

301. Thayer, D.W. and G. Boyd. 1991. Effect of ionizing radiation dose, temperature, and atmosphere on the survival of Salmonella typhimurium in sterile, mechanically deboned chicken meat. Poult Sci 70:381–388.

302. Thayer, D.W., G. Boyd, W.S. Muller, C.A. Lipson, W.C. Hayne, and S.H. Baer. 1990. Radiation resistance of Salmonella. J Ind Microbiol 5:383–390.

303. Thayer, D.W., S. Songprasertchai, and G. Boyd. 1991. Effects of heat and ionizing radiation on Salmonella typhimurium in mechanically deboned chicken meat. J Food Prot 54:718–724.

304. Thayer, D.W., C.Y. Dickerson, D.R. Rao, G. Boyd, and C.B. Chawan. 1992. Destruction of Salmonella typhimurium on chicken wings by gamma radiation. J Food Sci 57:586–589.

305. Threlfall, E.J., B. Rowe, and L.R. Ward. 1993. A comparison of multiple drug resistance in salmonellas from humans and food animals in England and Wales, 1981 and 1990. Epidemiol Infect 111:189–197.

306. Threlfall, E.J, M.D. Hampton, H. Chart, and B. Rowe. 1994. Use of plasmid profile typing for surveillance of Salmonella enteritidis phage type 4 from humans, poultry and eggs. Epidemiol Infect 112:25–31.

307. Timms, L.M., R.N. Marshall, and M.F. Breslin. 1990. Laboratory assessment of protection given by an experimental Salmonella enteritidis PT4 inactivated, adjuvant vaccine. Vet Rec 127:611–614.

308. Timms, L.M., R.N. Marshall, and M.F. Breslin. 1994. Laboratory and field trial assessment of protection given by a Salmonella enteritidis PT4 inactivated, adjuvant vaccine. Br Vet J 150:93–102.

309. Timoney, J.F., H.L. Shivaprasad, R.C. Baker, and B. Rowe. 1989. Egg transmission after infection of hens with Salmonella enteritidis phage type 4. Vet Rec 125:600–601.

310. Timoney, J.F., N. Sikora, H.L. Shivaprasad, and M. Opitz. 1990. Detection of antibody to Salmonella enteritidis by a gm flagellin-based ELISA. Vet Rec 127:168–169.

311. Truscott, R.B. 1983. A comparison of two enrichment and two plating media for the isolation of Salmonella sp. from broilers. Can J Comp Med 47:373–374.

312. Tucker, J.F. 1967. Survival of Salmonellae in built-up litter for housing of rearing and laying fowls. Br Vet J 123:92–103.

313. Turnbull, P.C.B. and G.H. Snoeyenbos. 1973. The roles of ammonia, water activity, and pH in the salmonellacidal effect of long-used poultry litter. Avian Dis 17:72–86.

314. Turnbull, P.C.B. and G.H. Snoeyenbos. 1974. Experimental salmonellosis in the chicken. 1. Fate and host response in alimentary canal, liver, and spleen. Avian Dis 18:153–177.

315. U.S. Department of Agriculture. 1991. Chickens affected by Salmonella enteritidis. Fed Reg 56:3730–3743.

316. U.S. Department of Agriculture. 1993. Chicken disease caused by Salmonella enteritidis. Fed Reg 58:41,048–41,061.

317. U.S. Department of Agriculture. 1994. National Poultry Improvement Plan and Auxiliary Provisions. United States Department of Agriculture, Animal and Plant Health Inspection Service, Hyattsville, MD.

318. U.S. Department of Agriculture. 1995. Pathogen reduction; hazard analysis and critical control point (HACCP) systems. Fed Reg 60:6774–6889.

319. Van de Giessen, A.W., R. Peters, P.A.T.A. Berkers, W.H. Jansen, and S.H.W. Notermans. 1991. Salmonella contamination of poultry flocks in the Netherlands. Vet Q 13:41–46.

320. van de Giessen, A.W., J.B. Dufrenne, W.S. Ritmeester, P.A.T.A. Berkers, W.J. van Leeuwen, and S.H.W. Notermans. 1992. The identification of Salmonella enteritidis-infected poultry flocks associated with an outbreak of human salmonellosis. Epidemiol Infect 109:405–411.

321. van de Giessen, A.W., A.J.H.A. Ament, and S.H.W.

Notermans. 1994. Intervention strategies for Salmonella enteritidis in poultry flocks: A basic approach. Int J Food Microbiol 21:145–154.

322. van Zijderveld, F.G., A.M. van Zijderveld-van Bemmel, and J. Anakotta. 1992. Comparison of four different enzyme-linked immunosorbent assays for serological diagnosis of Salmonella enteritidis infections in experimentally infected chickens. J Clin Microbiol 30:2560–2566.

323. van Zijderveld, F.G., A.M. van Zijderveld-van Bemmel, R.A.M. Brouwers, T.S. de Vries, W.J.M. Landman, and W.A. de Jong. 1993. Serological detection of chicken flocks naturally infected with Salmonella enteritidis, using an enzyme-linked immunosorbent assay based on monoclonal antibodies against the flagellar antigen. Vet Q 15:135–137.

324. Vassiliadis, P., V. Kalapothaki, D. Trichopoulos, C. Mavrommatti, and C. Serie. 1981. Improved isolation of Salmonellae from naturally contaminated meat products by using Rappaport-Vassiliadis enrichment broth. Appl Environ Microbiol 42:615–618.

325. Wallner-Pendleton, E.A., S.S. Sumner, G.W. Froning, and L.E. Stetson. 1994. The use of ultraviolet radiation to reduce Salmonella and psychrotrophic bacterial contamination on poultry carcasses. Poult Sci 73:1327–1333.

326. Waltman, W.D., A.M. Horne, C. Pirkle, and T. Dickson. 1991. Use of delayed secondary enrichment for the isolation of Salmonella in poultry and poultry environments. Avian Dis 35:88–92.

327. Waltman, W.D., A.M. Horne, C. Pirkle, and D.C. Johnson. 1992. Prevalence of Salmonella enteritidis in spent hens. Avian Dis 36:251–255.

328. Waltman, W.D., A.M. Horne, and C. Pirkle. 1993. Influence of enrichment incubation time on the isolation of Salmonella. Avian Dis 37:884–887.

329. Weinack, O.M., C.F. Smyser, and G.H. Snoeyenbos. 1979. Evaluation of several methods of detecting Salmonellae in groups of chickens. Avian Dis 23:179–193.

330. Weinack, O.M., G.H. Snoeyenbos, A.S. Soerjadi-Liem, and C.F. Smyser. 1985. Influence of temperature, social, and dietary stress on development and stability of protective microflora in chickens against S. typhimurium. Avian Dis 29:1177–1183.

331. Weinack, O.M., G.H. Snoeyenbos, A.S. Soerjadi-Liem, and C.F. Smyser. 1985. Therapeutic trials with native intestinal microflora for Salmonella typhimurium infections in chickens. Avian Dis 29:1230–1234.

332. Whistler, P.E., and B.W. Sheldon. 1989. Comparison of ozone and formaldehyde as poultry hatchery disinfectants. Poult Sci 68:1345–1350.

333. Wierup, M., M. Wold-Troell, E. Nurmi, and M. Hakkinen. 1988. Epidemiological evaluation of the Salmonella-controlling effect of a nationwide use of a competitive exclusion culture in poultry. Poult Sci 67:1026–1033.

334. Wierup, M., H. Wahlström, and B. Engström. 1992. Experience of a 10-year use of competitive exclusion treatment as part of the Salmonella control programme in Sweden. Int J Food Microbiol 15:287–291.

335. Williams, J.E. 1970. Effect of high-level formaldehyde fumigation on bacterial populations on the surface of chicken hatching eggs. Avian Dis 14:386–392.

336. Williams, J.E. Observations on Salmonella thompson as a poultry pathogen. 1972. Avian Pathol 1:69–73.

337. Williams, J.E. 1980. Formalin destruction of Salmonellae in poultry litter. Poult Sci 59:2717–2724.

338. Williams, J.E., and S.T. Benson. 1978. Survival of Salmonella typhimurium in poultry feed and litter of three temperatures. Avian Dis 22:742–747.

339. Williams, J.E., and A.D. Whittemore. 1972. Microantiglobulin test for detecting Salmonella typhimurium agglutinins. Appl Microbiol 23:931–937.

340. Williams, J.E., and A.D. Whittemore. 1975. Influence of age on the serological response of chickens to Salmonella typhimurium infection. Avian Dis 19:745–760.

341. Williams, J.E., and A.D. Whittemore. 1976. Comparison of six methods of detecting Salmonella typhimurium infection of chickens. Avian Dis 20:728–734.

342. Williams, J.E., and A.D. Whittemore. 1976. Field applications of MA and MAG tests for detection of avian salmonellosis. Proc 80th Annu Meet U.S. Anim Health Assoc. U.S. Animal Health Association, pp. 297–303.

343. Williams, J.E., and A.D. Whittemore. 1980. Bacteriostatic effect of five antimicrobial agents on Salmonellae in the intestinal tract of chickens. Poult Sci 59:44–53.

344. Williamson, C.M., G.D. Baird, and E.J Manning. 1988. A common virulence region on plasmids from eleven serotypes of Salmonella. J Gen Microbiol 134:975–982.

345. Woodward, M.J, I. McLaren, and C. Wray. 1989. Distribution of virulence plasmids within Salmonellae. J Gen Microbiol 135:503–511.

346. Wrigley, D.M., and N.G. Llorca. 1992. Decrease of Salmonella typhimurium in skim milk and egg by heat and ultrasonic wave treatment. J Food Prot 55:678–680.

347. Wyeth, P.J. 1975. Effect of infectious bursal disease on the response of chickens to S. typhimurium and E. coli infections. Vet Rec 96:238–243.

348. Yamamoto, R., H.E. Adler, W.W. Sadler, and G.F. Stewart. 1961. A study of Salmonella typhimurium infection in market-age turkeys. Am J Vet Res 22:382–387.

349. Yancey, R.J., S.A.L. Breeding, and C.E. Lankford. 1979. Enterochelin (enterobactin): Virulence factor for Salmonella typhimurium. Infect Immun 24:174–180.

350. Zecha, B.C., R.H. McCapes, W.M. Dungan, R.J. Holte, W.W. Worcester, and J.E. Williams. 1977. The Dillon Beach Project—a five year epidemiological study of naturally occurring Salmonella infection in turkeys and their environment. Avian Dis 21:141–159.

351. Ziprin, R.L., D.E. Corrier, and M.H. Elissalde. 1989. Maturation of resistance to Salmonellosis in newly hatched chicks: Inhibition by cyclosporine. Poultry Sci 68:1637–1642.

352. Ziprin, R.L., D.E. Corrier, and J.R. DeLoach. 1993. Control of established Salmonella typhimurium intestinal colonization with in vivo-passaged anaerobes. Avian Dis 37:183–188.

ARIZONOSIS

H. L. Shivaprasad, K. V. Nagaraja, B. S. Pomeroy, and J. E. Williams

INTRODUCTION. Arizonosis is an acute septicemic disease, primarily of young turkey poults, caused by the bacterium *Salmonella arizonae*. *S. arizonae* is one of the most frequently identified *Salmonella* serotypes in turkeys in the United States (28) and is related to significant morbidity and mortality. The disease is clinically indistinguishable from salmonellosis, and is referred to as arizona infection or avian arizonosis (AA). Avian arizonosis is of considerable economic significance to the turkey industry of North America and certain parts of the world through reduced egg production and hatchability (16, 17, 35, 47, 57, 83, 87).

S. arizonae represents an antigenically diverse group of bacteria (over 300 serotypes have been identified), which can be distinguished biochemically from other species in the genus *Salmonella*. Historically, the organisms now classified as *S. arizonae* were included in the genus *Arizona,* and have commonly been referred to as the arizona group, arizonas, and paracolons. In 1982, the International Subcommittee on Taxonomy of Enterobacteriaceae decided that the arizona group should be classed as two subspecies of the genus *Salmonella* based on the relatedness of their DNA with that of *Salmonella* spp. Earlier reviews on the arizona group and arizonosis have been published (3, 4, 42).

HISTORY. Caldwall and Ryerson were the first to isolate the *Salmonella*-like organisms from diseased reptiles from the semiarid regions surrounding Tucson, Arizona (8). It is probable, however, that the bacteria were isolated earlier from poultry. Lewis and Hitchner (62) had previously reported recovery of slow lactose-fermenting bacteria from a disease of chicks resembling salmonellosis. This infection was probably due to a member of the arizona group, and may represent the first report of AA. In Great Britain, the first report of avian arizonosis in poultry was in 1968 (53).

INCIDENCE AND DISTRIBUTION. Avian arizonosis occurs worldwide wherever poultry is raised. At one time, *S. arizonae* 18:Z4,Z32 was endemic in turkey flocks of North America. Very high rates of isolation were reported in California in 1968 and 1969, but decreased considerably by 1972 (65). It has been eliminated from the turkey industry in Great Britain (5, 53, 88).

ETIOLOGY

Classification. Since 1939, many attempts have been made to find a generally acceptable taxonomic position for this group of bacteria; several classification systems have been used and a wide variety of names and designations has been applied to the organisms.

Edwards and associates (cited in 64), established the biochemical and antigenic similarity of the arizonae and salmonellae. Enough differences were found between the groups, however, to justify classification of the arizonae in a separate genus. Kauffmann and Edwards (55) first employed the name *Arizona arizonae,* which was also used by Ewing (21) for members of the genus *Arizona* (genus II of the tribe Salmonellae). A new type species name *Arizona hinshawii* had been proposed by Ewing (23) to pay honor to the pioneering work of W.R. Hinshaw on AA in turkeys, reptiles, and other animals. Kauffmann (54) subsequently included the arizonae in his subgenus III of the genus *Salmonella,* designating them *S. arizonae* and listing their antigenic formulas only in the simplified Kauffmann-White scheme. The arizonae have been classified in the *Salmonella* genus in the 8th edition of *Bergey's Manual* (7) and all organisms in the group are designated *Salmonella arizonae.*

Ewing and his colleagues (22, 25, 26, 27, 64) have further clarified the definition by which the biochemical and antigenic characteristics of members of the genus *Arizona* may be readily differentiated from other Enterobacteriaceae. The terminology used by Centers for Disease Control and Prevention will be followed in this subchapter, e.g., *S. arizonae,* 18:Z4,Z32 (see Antigenic Structure).

Morphology and Staining. The *S. arizonae* resemble other enteric organisms. They are gram-negative nonsporogenic bacilli that are motile by peritrichous flagella.

Growth Requirements. Members can be readily cultivated on ordinary liquid and solid laboratory media, revealing an abundant growth similar to that of the salmonellae. Most cultures grow very well on *Salmonella–Shigella* and brilliant green (BG) agars, as well as other solid media recommended for isolation of salmonellae. On initial isolation, colonies usually resemble those of salmonellae but may develop an indicator change typical of lactose fermenters after incubation for several days or weeks. Rapid lactose-fermenting strains, rare in poultry, cannot be distinguished from normal coliforms, which are usually inhibited by these media. Routine use of bismuth sulfite plating medium was recommended (19, 42, 64) to aid in preliminary recognition of lactose-fermenting arizona strains before they are possibly discarded as coliforms.

Biochemical Properties. Cultures possessing the following biochemical characteristics are almost invariably classifiable serologically as members of *S. arizonae* (24, 26, 12).

Dextrose	Fermented with gas
Lactose	Fermented, as a rule, slowly or promptly
Sucrose	Not fermented, as a rule
Mannitol	Fermented with gas
Maltose	Fermented with gas
Dulcitol	Not fermented
Inositol	Not fermented
Indole	Not produced, as a rule
Methyl red	Positive
Voges-Proskauer	Negative
Jordan's tartrate	No reaction
Hydrogen sulfide	Positive
Urea	Not hydrolyzed
Gelatin	Liquified slowly
Potassium cyanide	Negative, as a rule
Nitrates	Reduced
Motility	Positive
Betagalactosidase	Positive
Decarboxylases	
Lysine	Positive
Arginine	Positive, usually delayed
Ornithine	Positive
Malonate	Positive
Phenylalanine deaminase	Negative

Most isolates from poultry, unlike salmonellae, ferment lactose usually within 7–10 days' incubation. Failure of cultures to ferment dulcitol and inositol or to use D-tartrate, their slow liquefaction of gelatin, and their positive reactions in sodium malonate and betagalactosidase are most useful in distinguishing them from other members of the *Salmonella* group.

CITROBACTER. For purposes of classification and identification, the *S. arizonae* must be differentiated not only from other salmonellae, but also from the antigenically related genus *Citrobacter* of the tribe Salmonellae. Members of this genus are not known to be pathogenic for poultry, but from a diagnostic standpoint they may be confused with *Salmonella* cultures on initial isolation from fecal specimens. The former Bethesda-Ballerup "paracolons" (*P. intermedium*) are included in the genus *Citrobacter* along with cultures previously classified as *Escherichia freundii*.

Resistance to Chemical and Physical Agents. Arizonae are readily destroyed by heat and common disinfectants, but have survived in contaminated water for 5 mo, in contaminated feed for 17 mo, in soil on turkey ranges for 6–7 mo, and for 5 to 25 or more wk on materials and utensils in poultry houses (2, 31, 56, 57, 76, 80). Resistance properties are very similar to those of salmonellae.

Antigenic Structure. *S. arizonae* strains are related serologically to the salmonellae and other Enterobacteriaceae, and procedures for study and identification of their antigenic structure are identical to those for paratyphoid organisms. Thirty-four somatic (O) and 43 flagellar (H) antigens have been demonstrated.

The serotype nomenclature system used in designating members of the genus *Salmonella* has been applied to *S. arizonae*. In writing antigenic formulas, commas are used to separate O antigen factors, a colon to distinguish the O and H antigens, commas to separate H antigenic factors within a single phase, and a hyphen or dash to separate the first phase from the second and the second from the third, etc. Thus the monophasic type species would be designated *S. arizonae* 18:Z4,Z32.

Evolution of the nomenclature for salmonellae has resulted in some confusion over the identification of strains. Two serotypes that were previously designated as 7:1,7,8 and 7:1,2,6 are now recognized as 18:Z4,Z32 and 18:Z4,Z23, respectively. Confusion also exists because, even though there are only 34 O and 43 H antigens, sometimes an isolate is designated as 65:Z52,Z53. The latter is the designation that conforms to the system recognized by The Centers for Disease Control and Prevention, and the World Health Organization.

Pathogenicity. *S. arizonae* can invade the bloodstream, especially of young fowl; high mortality has been reported (16). Lewis and Hitchner (62) recorded mortality of 32–50% from the infection in chicks. Others have observed mortality generally between 10 and 50%, with chicks or poults especially susceptible within the 1st few days after hatching, and with mortality continuing for up to 3–4 wk (1, 15, 44, 57, 75, 87). Geissler and Youssef

(30) inoculated or dipped chicken eggs with *S. arizonae*; 100% and 40–79% of embryos in the respective groups died during the incubation period. Hatchability for the latter group varied from 0 to 21–70%, with evidence that the organisms penetrated to the inner structures of the eggs.

Worcester (98) noted that *S. arizonae* can penetrate the wall of the intestinal tract and stay there indefinitely.

PATHOGENESIS AND EPIZOOTIOLOGY

Natural and Experimental Hosts. *S. arizonae* recognize no host barriers and are widely distributed in nature in a variety of avian, mammalian, and reptilian species (9, 15, 16, 17, 64, 78, 84, 96, 97).

Among poultry, AA is most frequently encountered in turkeys. Greenfield (39) noted that AA in chickens does not appear to be economically important, although chickens are affected by AA both naturally and experimentally (15, 62, 86).

Dougherty (10) isolated *S. arizonae* from duck livers, revealing lesions very similar to those produced by paratyphoid infections.

For a review of AA as a human disease causing gastroenteritis and frequently more serious enteric fever and focal infections, see Guckian et al. (45), Martin et al. (64), Williams and Hobbs (94), Johnson et al. (52), and Weiss et al. (90).

Transmission, Carriers, and Vectors. The transmission cycle of AA in poultry is identical with that established for motile salmonellae (see Paratyphoid Infections). Infected adult birds are frequently intestinal carriers and spreaders of *S. arizonae* for long periods (14). Wild birds (67), rats and mice (35), and reptiles (46, 48) have been cited as common sources of the organisms for poultry flocks.

Intestinal infections have been reported (47, 82), and Adler and Rosenwald (1) reported that AA in adult turkeys is confined primarily to the intestinal tract.

Transmission of AA through eggs has been reported by many workers (6, 14, 15, 16, 17, 37, 47), and recovery of *S. arizonae* from ovaries of adult turkeys (29, 47, 83) suggests that transovarian transmission can occur. Direct contamination of the ovary by systemic infection can follow ingestion of the organisms (58, 83, 85). Perek et al. (74) isolated *S. arizonae* from semen of cockerels.

S. arizonae from fecal contamination have a penetration pattern through the shell and shell membranes of chicken eggs very similar to that of *S. typhimurium* when incubated at 37.2 C, resulting in frequent presence of the organisms in chicken and turkey eggs (14, 37, 83, 93). Fecal contamination

may spread the infection from other animal species to poultry. Goetz (35) found an AA infection rate of 90% in rats and 50% in mice on the premises of a turkey farm where the infection was a problem in poults. Various types of wild birds, reptiles, and many common animal species can also infect poultry flocks.

AA is transmitted in the incubator and brooder by direct contact and through contaminated feed and water (20, 57).

Signs. Although signs of AA in poultry are not specific, infected poults and chicks may appear listless and develop diarrhea, leg paralysis, twisted necks, and pasting of the down around the vent. There may be blindness caused by caseous material covering the retina (57, 86). Infected birds tend to sit on their hocks and huddle together. Nervous signs, including convulsions, may follow brain infection in poults (51, 73). Sato and Adler (83) noted that clinical signs of AA are rarely seen in adult turkeys and they seldom die from this infection.

Gross Lesions and Histopathology. Gross and microscopic lesions due to AA in poults have been well described (36, 79, 86, 91). Lesions in poults, either naturally or experimentally infected with *S. arizonae*, are comparable to lesions induced by paratyphoid organisms. Livers are enlarged and mottled with white foci. Also, there are retained yolks, caseous exudate in the abdominal cavity, discolored hearts, and exudate on the meninges of the brain. One of the most frequently noted pathologic changes is the presence of exudate in the vitreous of one or both eyeballs in poults (Fig. 3.1G, in Pullorum Disease and Fowl Typhoid subchapter). Microscopically, this exudate is composed of a large number of degranulating heterophils mixed with fibrin and numerous bacteria. In the brain, there is severe meningitis with infiltration of heterophils mixed with some fibrin and bacterial colonies (Fig. 3.5). Similar exudate can also be seen in the ventricles, and there is malacia, inflammation and vascular thrombosis in the cerebral cortex. Interestingly, changes in other organs are minimal, such as necrosis of hepatocytes, increased numbers of reticuloendothelial cells in the spleen, and vascular congestion in various organs.

Lesions typical of generalized septicemia, including peritonitis, retained yolk sacs, enlarged, yellowish mottled livers and discolored hearts, were also described in experimentally infected chicks by Lewis and Hitchner (62). Goetz and Quortrup (36) described caseous cores in the ceca similar to those seen in pullorum disease. Hinshaw and McNeil (47) observed that *S. arizonae*-infected adult turkeys had a small amount of caseous exudate in the abdominal cavity and cystic ovules.

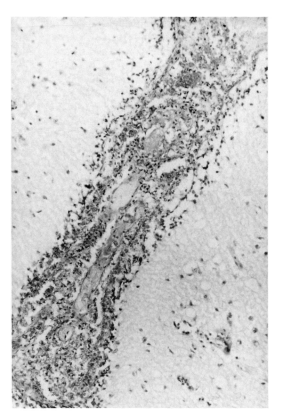

3.5. Brain with meningitis and encephalitis associated with *Salmonella arizonae* infection, ×300.

DIAGNOSIS. High mortality, neurologic signs, and blindness in turkey poults can be used for a presumptive diagnosis of AA. These clinical signs, as well as lesions, however, can be seen in other *Salmonella* infections, including those of paratyphoid organisms. Neurologic signs can also be caused by Newcastle disease, aspergillosis, and vitamin E deficiency (encephalomalacia). Blindness in turkey poults can be due to aspergillosis. Therefore, AA must be confirmed by isolation and identification of the causative bacteria. The organisms can usually be recovered from liver, spleen, heart blood, unabsorbed yolk sac, intestine, lung, kidney, brain, and eye.

Isolation and Identification of Causative Agent. Cultural procedures identical to those outlined and discussed under Paratyphoid Infections are employed for isolation and identification of arizonae. Standard methods for isolation and biochemical or serologic identification of *S. arizonae* from poultry tissues, eggs and embryos, and environmental samples have been described (19, 24, 88, 95). Bismuth sulfite medium can be used for plating

enrichment broths in addition to BG sulfa if desired. The two serotypes of *S. arizonae* common in turkeys are slow lactose fermenters and, therefore, identical to paratyphoids on initial isolation on BG agar.

Selenite cystine broth may be used in enrichment of fecal and organic tissue cultures (57, 82, 83). Selenite broth incubated at 43 C yielded fewer isolations of arizonae than did tetrathionate or selenite F broth at 35 C (40).

Forty-nine strains of *S. arizonae* isolated from turkeys all had similar cultural and biochemical characteristics, varying only in use of citrate and melibiose (89). Most *S. arizonae* strains were sensitive only to chloramphenicol and nalidixic acid among the antibiotics tested. Kumar et al. (59) found that selenite BG with sulfapyridine (SBGS) and tetrathionate BG broths gave comparable results with *S. arizonae,* but at 48 hr there was considerable reduction in recovery of arizonae from SBGS in tubes initially inoculated with high numbers of organisms. Littell (63) described a differential plating medium for isolation of *S. arizonae* that produces a uniform reaction of both lactose-negative and lactose-positive *S. arizonae,* and differentiates them from other salmonellae.

Snoeyenbos and Smyser (87) believed that litter culturing may aid epidemiologic studies and identify infected turkey flocks as part of a control program. Greenfield and Bigland (41) noted that culture of turkey litter might be a useful means of detecting insidious AA.

Culture of turkey shell membranes and shells is recommended over yolk material for rapid detection of arizonae-contaminated eggs (11, 43, 77).

Serology. Serologic analysis of cultures is essential in epizootiologic studies of AA of fowl; cultures can be submitted to the Salmonella Serotyping Laboratory, National Veterinary Services Laboratories P.O. Box 844, Ames, IA 50010, for biochemical characterization and antigenic typing.

Edwards and Galton (13) noted that it is essential to use a polyvalent *S. arizonae* antiserum in preliminary examination of cultures, since arizona types may not be agglutinated by *Salmonella* polyvalent antiserum. Kowalski and Stephens (57) employed formalinized broth cultures and *S. arizonae* poly-monophasic antiserum in serologic identification of arizonae cultures. Snoeyenbos and Smyser (87) used *S. arizonae* flagellar polyvalent, *Salmonella* flagellar Z32, and *Salmonella* somatic 18 antisera in screening cultures suspected to be *S. arizonae.*

TREATMENT. Chemotherapy may reduce losses in acute outbreaks of AA and may be recommended to prevent spread of the disease in market flocks. Williams (92) reviewed various treatments for AA. In the United States, the only drugs approved by the Food and Drug Administration for treatment of AA are furazolidone and antibiotic injectables, gentamicin and spectinomycin. These injectables, given at the hatchery, have dramatically controlled the acute losses and morbidity that may occur during the first 3 wk of age. Isolates of *S. arizonae* resistant to gentamicin have been reported (18, 49).

Ghazikhanian et al. (34) reviewed the program of a primary breeder to reduce and eliminate *S. arizonae* from a basic breeding operation. A combination antibiotic hatching-egg treatment (dipped and injected) was successful in producing *S. arizonae*-free pedigree stock (33, 66). In addition to the egg treatment program, an autogenous oil-emulsion *S. arizonae* bacterin was used on infected flocks to reduce transmission. Because of contamination of ranges, a new capital building program was initiated (total confinement, paved floors, birdproof). A cleaning and disinfecting program was initiated after each depopulation and the facilities were monitored to determine the effectiveness of the program. Finally, special emphasis was placed on frequent egg-collection practices. Only pelleted feed containing no animal or poultry by-products was used. The program has been highly successful.

PREVENTION AND CONTROL. Because *S. arizonae* is egg transmitted, primary breeding stock must be developed free of *S. arizonae*. The control program at the multiplier breeder level is dependent on having available *S. arizonae*-free stock. Management procedures outlined under Paratyphoid Infections are applicable for the control and reduction of AA. The program outlined by Ghazikhanian et al. (34) for the primary breeder level is applicable to the multiplier level except for the treatment of hatching eggs with antibiotics. Total confinement, birdproof and rodentproof buildings that can be cleaned and disinfected, quality feed and feed ingredients, and microbiologic monitoring at the hatchery and breeder farm levels are essential.

Serologic Testing. Serologic tests have not been entirely effective in detecting or controlling AA in turkeys (1, 76, 98).

Methods for preparing and using *S. arizonae* antigens for serologic testing of chickens and turkeys have been outlined (4).

Timms (88) found that the most reliable and satisfactory methods for detecting *S. arizonae* at various stages of infection in adult turkeys were the rapid serum plate (SP) test and the somatic tube agglutination (TA) test. The rapid whole-blood (WB) test was found to be a useful tool in testing large numbers of birds in the field, but it required confirmation by the TA test. Uses of the agar gel diffu-

sion, indirect hemagglutination, immunofluorescent, and H agglutination tests in providing supporting evidence of infection were discussed. Lamont and Timms (61) reported use of O and H TA tests, rapid WB test, and agar gel precipitin tests for detection of AA in turkeys. They also found the rapid WB test particularly useful for flock screening.

Sato and Adler (82, 83) used a formalin-treated broth culture of actively motile arizona strains in preparing H antigen, and ethanol-treated cell suspension from beef heart infusion agar for O antigen. They found that naturally infected turkeys had positive O agglutination reactions at some time during the period they were observed; however, some of the same birds were negative when tested with H antigen. The H agglutinins disappeared earlier than O agglutinins. Not all infected birds revealed positive O agglutinin tests at time of necropsy. There was little correlation between serologic results and persistence of infection.

Kumar et al. (60) developed a tetrazolium-stained microagglutination (MA) test antigen for detection of *S. arizonae* infections in turkeys. The MA test was demonstrated to be far more sensitive and superior to the TA and SP tests in detecting turkeys infected with *S. arizonae*. Attempts to detect infection with the microantiglobulin test were unsuccessful.

Adult carriers may lack detectable antibodies 12–14 wk after exposure, and infected turkey hens go through an antibody-negative phase at 16–20 wk of age when most breeder flocks are tested (60, 88). When the ovary becomes activated following a lighting regime at 28–32 wk of age, antibodies may be detectable. At that stage in the breeding cycle, it is too late to eliminate the flocks. Greenfield (38) noted that antibody titers do not persist for lengthy periods and may not be detectable in birds with subclinical infections.

An enzyme-linked immunosorbent assay (ELISA) using outer membrane proteins extracted from *S. arizonae* as antigens was found by Nagaraja et al. to be sensitive and specific for the detection of *S. arizonae* infection in breeder flocks of turkeys (69, 71). It was considered to be a valuable tool to determine which breeder flock is infected, allowing the hatchery program to be adjusted to reduce *S. arizonae* dissemination at the time of hatching.

Immunization. Several types of bacterins have been applied to turkey breeding stock. Holte (50) found that vaccinated breeders exposed to *S. arizonae* 18:Z4,Z32 had reduced shedding and were protected from systemic infection, thus preventing egg transmission of arizonae. Parental immunity was found to be transmitted to poults of vaccinated hens.

Sato and Adler (81) found varying degrees of protection afforded by arizona bacterins in both mice and turkeys. A formalin-treated whole culture in aluminum hydroxide gel provided the best protection, based on the number of organisms that migrated to the spleen following intramuscular challenge. In turkeys, a chrome-alum–treated arizona bacterin provided protection against both oral and intraperitoneal challenge (68). Fecal shedding for the first 3 wk after challenge may be reduced by immunization with bacterins (1).

Gerlach et al. (32) found serum from nonimmunized turkey hens had both bacteriostatic and bactericidal effects on cultures of *S. arizonae* 18:Z4,Z32, but there was no inhibitory activity in the serum of birds vaccinated with arizona bacterin or in serum from naturally infected breeders. Inhibition of growth was not associated with presence of agglutinating antibodies; in fact, the opposite appeared to be true. In contrast, a bactericidal substance in the albumen of eggs from vaccinated turkeys was reported (1).

Ghazikhanian et al. (34) reported encouraging results using oil-emulsion bacterins; egg transmission following challenge was reduced from 12% in nonvaccinated controls to 2% in vaccinated turkeys. Vaccination against *S. arizonae* infection with a mineral oil-adjuvanted vaccine was evaluated in turkey breeder flocks under laboratory and field situations by Nagaraja et al. (70, 72). The results were encouraging; it was possible to obtain *S. arizonae*-free progeny from vaccinated breeder flocks held in infected environments.

REFERENCES

1. Adler, H.E., and A.S. Rosenwald. 1968. Paracolon control—What we know and need to know. Turkey World 43:18.
2. Anonymous. 1967. Salmonella and Arizona group of infections of Avian origin. 1966 Annual Report of the Food Protein Toxicology Center. University of Calif, Davis, pp. 24–29.
3. Anonymous. 1976. Proc Salmonella Symp. American Association of the Avian Pathologists, Kennett Square, PA.
4. Anonymous. 1984. In G.H. Snoyenbos (ed.). Proc Int Symp Salmonella, New Orleans. American Association of Avian Pathologists, Kennett Square, PA.
5. Anonymous. 1986. Animal salmonellosis. Annual summaries, survey of drug resistance in Salmonellae. Ministry of Agriculture Fisheries and Food. Welsh Office Agriculture Department. Department of Agriculture and Fisheries for Scotland.
6. Bruner, D.W., and M.C. Peckham. 1952. An outbreak of paracolon infection in turkey poults. Cornell Vet 42:22–24.
7. Buchanan, R.E., and N.E. Gibbons. 1974. Bergey's Manual of Determinative Bacteriology, 8th ed. Williams & Wilkins, Baltimore, MD, pp. 290–340.
8. Caldwell, M.E., and D.L. Ryerson. 1939. Salmonellosis in certain reptiles. J Infect Dis 65:242–245.
9. Cambre, R.C., D.E. Green, E.E. Smith, R.J. Montali, and M. Bush. 1980. Salmonellosis and arizonosis in the reptile collection at the National Zoological Park. J Am Vet Med Assoc 177:800–803.
10. Dougherty, E. 1953. Disease problems confronting the duck industry. Proc 90th Annu Meet Am Vet Med Assoc, pp. 359–365.
11. Dovadola, E., and F. Carlotto. 1969. Bacteriological survey for arizona infection in turkey eggs. Results and discussion. Vet Ital 20:304–311.
12. Edwards, P.R., and W.H. Ewing. 1972. Identification of Enterobacteriaceae. Burgess Publishing, Minneapolis, MN.
13. Edwards, P.R., and M.M. Galton. 1967. Salmonellosis. Adv Vet Sci 11:1–63.
14. Edwards, P.R., W.B. Cherry, and D.W. Bruner. 1943. Further studies on coliform bacteria serologically related to the genus Salmonella. J Infect Dis 73:229–238.
15. Edwards, P.R., M.G. West, and D.W. Bruner. 1947. Arizona group of paracolon bacteria. Ky Agric Exp Stn Bull 499.
16. Edwards P.R., A.C. McWhorter, and M.A. Fife. 1956. The Arizona group of enterobacteriaceae in animals and man. Bull WHO 14:511–528
17. Edwards, P.R., M.A. Fife, and C.H. Ramsey. 1959. Studies on the arizona group of enterobacteriaceae. Bacteriol Rev 23:155–174.
18. Ekperigin, H.E., S. Jang, and R.H. McCapes. 1983. Effective control of a gentamicin-resistant Salmonella arizonae infection in turkey poults. Avian Dis 27:822–829.
19. Ellis, E.M., J.E. Williams, E.T. Mallinson, G.H. Snoeyenbos, and W.J. Martin. 1976. Culture Methods for the Detection of Animal Salmonellosis and Arizonosis. Iowa State University Press, Ames, IA, pp. 9–87.
20. Erwin, L.E. 1955. Examination of prepared poultry feeds for the presence of salmonella and other enteric organisms. Poult Sci 34:215–216.
21. Ewing, W.H. 1963. An outline of nomenclature for the family Enterobacteriaceae. Int Bull Bacteriol Nomencl Taxon 13:95–110.
22. Ewing, W.H. 1967. Revised Definitions for the Family Enterobacteriaceae, Its Tribes and Genera. U.S. Department of Health Education and Welfare, NCDC, Atlanta, GA.
23. Ewing, W.H. 1969. Arizona hinshawii. Int J Syst Bacteriol 19:1.
24. Ewing, W.H. 1986. Edwards and Ewing's Identification of Enterobacteriaceae. Elsevier Science, New York.
25. Ewing, W.H., and M.M. Ball. 1966. The Biochemical Reactions of Members of the Genus Salmonella. U.S. Department of Health Education and Welfare, NCDC, Atlanta, GA.
26. Ewing, W.H., and M.A. Fife. 1966. A summary of the biochemical reactions of Arizona arizonae. Int J Syst Bacteriol 16:427–433.
27. Ewing, W.H., M.A. Fife, and B.R. Davis. 1965. The Biochemical Reactions of Arizona arizonae. U.S. Department of Health Education and Welfare, NCDC, Atlanta, GA.
28. Ferris, K., and W.M. Frerichs. 1987. Salmonella serotypes from animals and related sources reported during the fiscal year 1987. Proc 92nd Annu Meet US Anim Health Assoc. U.S. Animal Health Association, Richmond, VA, pp. 349–362.
29. Gauger, H.C. 1946. Isolation of a type 10 paracolon bacillus from an adult turkey. Poult Sci 25:299–300.
30. Geissler, H., and Y.I. Youssef. 1979. The effect of infection with Arizona hinshawii on chicken embryos. Avian Pathol 8:157–161.
31. Geissler, H., and Y.I. Youssef. 1981. Persistence of Arizona hinshawii in or on materials used in poultry houses. Avian Pathol 10:359–363.
32. Gerlach, H., H.E. Adler, and A.S. Rosenwald. 1968. Research Note: Observations on immune factors associated with arizona group infection in turkeys. Avian Dis 12:681–686.
33. Ghazikhanian, G.Y., R. Yamamoto, R.H. McCapes, W.M. Dungan, and H.B. Ortmayer. 1980. Combination dip

and injection of turkey eggs with antibiotics to eliminate Mycoplasma meleagridis infection from a primary breeding stock. Avian Dis 24:57–70.

34. Ghazikhanian, G.Y., B.J. Kelly, and W.M Dungan. 1984. Salmonella arizonae control program. In G.H. Snoeyenbos (ed.). Proc Int Symp on Salmonella. American Association of Avian Pathologists, Kennett Square, PA, pp. 142–149.

35. Goetz, M.E. 1962. The control of paracolon and paratyphoid infections in turkey poults. Avian Dis 6:93–99.

36. Goetz, M.E., and E.R. Quortrup. 1953. Some observations of the problem of Arizona paracolon infections in poults. Vet Med 48:58–60.

37. Goetz, M.E., E.R. Quortrup, and J.E. Dunsing. 1954. Investigations of arizona paracolon infections in poults. J Am Vet Med Assoc 124:120–121.

38. Greenfield, J. 1972. Studies on Arizona in turkeys: Isolation and antibiotic control. Diss Abstr Int B, pp. 489–490.

39. Greenfield, J. 1976. Proc Salmonella Symposium. American Association of Avian Pathologists, Kennett Square, PA, pp. 70–78.

40. Greenfield, J., and J.C. Bankier. 1969. Isolation of salmonella and arizona using enrichment media incubated at 35 and 43 C. Avian Dis 13:864–871.

41. Greenfield, J., and C.H. Bigland. 1971b. Isolation of arizona from specimens grossly contaminated with competitive bacteria. Avian Dis 15:604–608.

42. Greenfield, J., C.H. Bigland, and T.W. Dukes. 1971a. The genus Arizona with special reference to Arizona disease in turkeys. Vet Bull 41:605–612.

43. Greenfield, J., C.H. Bigland, and H.D. McCausland. 1971b. Culture of shell and shell membranes for efficient isolation of arizona from turkey hatching eggs. Avian Dis 15:82–88.

44. Greenfield, J., C.H. Bigland, H.D. McCausland, and C.W. Wood. 1972. Control of arizona disease in turkeys by poult injection. Poult Sci 51:523–526.

45. Guckian, J.E., E.H. Byers, and J.E. Perry. 1967. Arizona infection of man. Arch Int Med 119:170–175.

46. Hinshaw, W.R., and E. McNeil. 1944. Gopher snakes as carriers of salmonellosis and paracolon infections. Cornell Vet 34:248–254.

47. Hinshaw, W.R., and E. McNeil. 1946a. The occurrence of type 10 paracolon in turkeys. J Bacteriol 51:281–286.

48. Hinshaw, W.R., and E. McNeil. 1947. Lizards as carriers of salmonella and paracolon bacteria. J Bacteriol 53:715–718.

49. Hirsh, D.C., J.S. Ikeda, L.D. Martin, B.J. Kelly, and G.Y. Ghazikhanian. 1983. R Plasmid-mediated gentamicin resistance in salmonella isolated from turkeys and their environment. Avian Dis 27:766–772.

50. Holte, R.J.A. 1965. Paracolon arizona immunization trials in turkeys. Proc 69th Annu Meet US Livest Sanit Assoc, pp. 539–542.

51. Jamison, S.L. 1956. Paracolon infections. Pac Poult 62:40–42.

52. Johnson, R.H., L.I. Lutwick, G.A. Huntley, and K.L. Vosti. 1976. Arizona hinshaawii infections. New cases, antimicrobial sensitivities and literature review. Ann Intern Med 85:587–592.

53. Jordan, F.T.W., P.H. Lamont, L. Timms, and D.A.P. Grattan, 1976. The eradication of Arizona 7:1,7,8 from a turkey breeding flock. Vet Rec 99:413–415.

54. Kauffmann, F. 1966. The Bacteriology of Enterobacteriaceae. Williams & Wilkins, Baltimore, MD.

55. Kauffmann, F., and P.R. Edwards. 1952. Classification and Nomenclature of Enterobacteriaceae. Int Bull Bacteriol Nomencl Taxon 2:2–8.

56. Kowalski, L.M., and J.F. Stephens. 1967. Persistence of Arizona paracolon 7:1,7,8 in feed and water. Poult Sci 46:1586–1587.

57. Kowalski, L.M., and J.F. Stephens. 1968. Arizona 7:1,7,8 infection in young turkeys. Avian Dis 12:317–326.

58. Kumar, M.C., S.C. Nivas, A.K. Bahl, M.D. York, and B.S. Pomeroy. 1974. Studies on natural infection and egg transmission of Arizona hinshawii 7:1,7,8 in turkeys. Avian Dis 18:416–426.

59. Kumar, M.C., M.D. York, and B.S. Pomeroy. 1976. Comparison of tetrathionate and selenite enrichment broth for isolations of Arizona hinshawii 7:1,7,8 and various serotypes of salmonella. Proc 19th Annu Meet Am Assoc Vet Lab Diagn, pp. 179–188.

60. Kumar, M.C., M.D. York, and B.S. Pomeroy. 1977. Development of microagglutination test for detecting Arizona hinshawii 7:1,7,8 infection in turkeys. Am J Vet Res 38:255–257.

61. Lamont, P.H., and L. Timms. 1972. Experimental infection of turkey poults with Arizona serotype 7:1,7,8. Br Vet J 128:129–137.

62. Lewis, K.H., and E.R. Hitchner. 1936. Slow lactose fermenting bacteria pathogenic for baby chicks. J Infect Dis 59:225–235.

63. Littell, A.M. 1977. Plating medium for differentiation of Salmonella arizonae from other salmonellae. Appl Environ Microbiol 33:485–487.

64. Martin, W.J., M.A. Fife, and W.H. Ewing. 1967. The Occurrence and Distribution of the Serotypes of Arizona. U.S. Department of Health Education and Welfare, NCDC, Atlanta, GA.

65. Mayeda, B., R.H. McCapes, and W.F. Scott. 1978. Protection of day-old poults against Arizona hinshawii challenge by preincubation streptomycin egg treatment. Avian Dis 22:61–70.

66. McCapes, R.H., R. Yamamoto, H.B. Ortmayer and W.F. Scott. 1975. Injecting antibiotics into turkey hatching eggs to eliminate Mycoplasma meleagridis infection. Avian Dis 19:506–514.

67. McClure, H.E., W.C. Eveland and A. Kase. 1957. The occurrence of certain Enterobacteriaceae in birds. Am J Vet Res 18:207–209.

68. Miyamae, T., and H.E. Adler. 1967. Comparative studies on immunogenicity of Arizona (7:1,7,8) adjuvant bacterins in mice and turkeys. Avian Dis 11:380–392.

69. Nagaraja, K.V., D.A. Emery, L.F. Sherlock, J.A. Newman and B.S. Pomeroy. 1984. Detection of Salmonella arizonae in turkey flocks by ELISA. Proc Am Assoc Vet Lab, pp. 185–203.

70. Nagaraja, K.V., M.C. Kumar, J.A. Newman and B.S. Pomeroy. 1985. Control of Salmonella arizonae infection in turkey breeder flocks by immunization. J Am Vet Med Assoc 187:309.

71. Nagaraja, K.V., L.T. Ausherman, D.A. Emery, and B.S. Pomeroy. 1986. Update on Enzyme-Linked Immunosorbent Assay for its field application in the detection of Salmonella arizonae infection in breeder flocks of turkeys. Proc Am Assoc Vet Diag, pp. 347–356.

72. Nagaraja, K.V., C.J. Kim and B.S. Pomeroy. 1988. Prophylactic vaccines for the control and reduction of salmonella in turkeys. Proc 92nd Annu Meet US Anim Health Assoc, U.S. Animal Health Association, Richmond, VA, pp. 347–348.

73. Perek, M. 1957. Isolation of a paracolobactrum organism pathogenic to chickens. J Infect Dis 101:8–10.

74. Perek, M., M. Elian, and E.D. Heller. 1969. Bacterial flora of semen and contamination of the reproductive organs of the hen following artificial insemination. Res Vet Sci 10:127–132.

75. Renault, L., J. Vaissaire, C. Maire, and P. Motte. 1972. Identification of Arizona arizonae from turkeys in France. Bull Acad Vet Fr 45:53–55.

76. Rosenwald, A.S. 1965. New facts on paracolon control. Poult Meat 2:25.

77. Saif, Y.M., L.C. Ferguson, and K.E. Nestor. 1971. Treatment of turkey hatching eggs for control of Arizona infection. Avian Dis 15:448–461.

78. Sambyal, D.S., and V.K. Sharma. 1972. Screening of free-living animals and birds for Listeria, Brucella and Salmonella infections. Br Vet J 128:50–55.

79. Sari, I., M. Lakatos, S. Toth, Z. Nemes, and G. Szeifert. 1979. Arizona salmonellosis of turkeys in Hungary. II. Aetiology and histopathology. Magy Allatorv Lapja 34:610–615.

80. Sato, G. 1967. Detection of salmonella and arizona organisms from soil of empty turkey yards. Jpn J Vet Res 15:53–55.

81. Sato, G., and H.E. Adler. 1966a. A study on the efficacy of arizona bacterin in turkeys. Avian Dis 10:239–246.

82. Sato, G., and H.E. Adler. 1966b. Bacteriological and serological observations on turkeys naturally infected with Arizona 7:1,7.8. Avian Dis 10:291–295.

83. Sato, G., and H.E. Adler. 1966c. Experimental infection of adult turkeys with arizona group organisms. Avian Dis 10:329–336.

84. Sharma, V.K., Y.K. Kaura, and I.P. Singh. 1970. Arizona infection in snakes, rats and man. Indian J Med Res 58:409–412.

85. Silva, E.N., and O. Hipólito. 1978. Salmonella strains isolated from the digestive tract of breeding chickens and apparently normal turkeys and in chick embryos. Proc 16th World's Poult Congr, pp. 701–706.

86. Silva, E.N., O. Hipolito, and R. Grecchi. 1980. Natural and experimental Salmonella arizonae 18:z4,z32 (Ar. 7:1,7,8) infection in broilers. Bacteriological and histological survey of eye and brain lesions. Avian Dis 24:631–636.

87. Snoeyenbos, G.H., and C.F. Smyser. 1969. Research Note—Isolation of Arizona 7:1,7,8 from litter of pens housing infected turkey. Avian Dis 13:223–224.

88. Timms, L. 1971. Arizona infection in turkeys in Great Britain. J Med Lab Technol [Br] 28:150–156.

89. Valeri, A., C. Marenzi, F. Enice, and T. Rampin. 1976. Study of biochemical characteristics of Salmonella arizonae isolates from turkeys. Clin Vet 99:422–429.

90. Weiss, S.H., M.J. Blaser, F.P. Paleologo, R.E. Black, A.C. McWhorter, M.A. Asbury, G.P. Carter, R.A. Feldman and D.J. Brenner. 1986. Occurrence and distribution of serotypes of the Arizona subgroup of Salmonella strains in the United States from 1967 to 1976. J Clin Microbiol 23:1056–1064.

91. West, J.L., and G.C. Mohanty. 1973. Arizona hinshawii infection in turkey poults: Pathologic changes. Avian Dis 17:314–324.

92. Williams, J.E. 1984. Avian Arizonosis. In M.S. Hofstad, H.J. Barnes, B.W. Calnek, W.M. Reid, and H.W. Yoder, Jr. (eds.). Diseases of Poultry, 8th ed. Iowa State University Press, Ames, IA, pp. 130–140.

93. Williams, J.E., and L.H. Dillard. 1968. Penetration of chicken egg shells by members of the Arizona group. Avian Dis 12:645–649.

94. Williams, L.P., and B.C. Hobbs. 1975. Enterobacteriaceae Infections. In W.T. Hubbert, W.F. McCulloch, and P.R. Schnurrenberger (eds.). Diseases Transmitted from Animals to Man. Charles C. Thomas, Springfield, IL, pp. 33–109.

95. Williams, J.E., E.T. Mallinson, and G.H. Snoeyenbos. 1980. Salmonellosis and arizonosis. In S.B. Hitchner, C.H. Domermuth, H.G. Purchase, and J.E. Williams (eds.). Isolation and Identification of Avian Pathogens. American Association of Avian Pathologists, Kennett Square, PA, pp. 1–8.

96. Windingstad, R.W., D.O. Trainer, and R. Duncan. 1977. Salmonella enteritidis and Arizona hinshawii isolated from wild sandhill cranes. Avian Dis 21:704–707.

97. Winsor, D.K., A.P. Bloebaum, and J.J. Mathewson. 1981. Gram-negative aerobic, enteric pathogens among intestinal microflora of wild turkey vultures (Cathartes aura) in west central Texas. Appl Environ Microbiol 42:1123–1124.

98. Worcester, W.W. 1965. Californian report results of test on paracolon control. Feedstuffs 37:6.

4 Colibacillosis

H. John Barnes and W. B. Gross

INTRODUCTION. Colibacillosis refers to any localized or systemic infection caused entirely or partly by *Escherichia coli,* including colisepticemia, coligranuloma (Hjarre's disease), air sac disease (chronic respiratory disease, CRD), avian cellulitis (inflammatory process), swollen-head syndrome, peritonitis, salpingitis, osteomyelitis/synovitis, panophthalmitis, and omphalitis/yolk sac infection. Colibacillosis in mammals is most often a primary enteric disease, whereas colibacillosis in poultry is typically a secondary localized or systemic disease occurring when host defenses have been impaired or overwhelmed. Other opportunistic bacteria, which can be identified by culture, may play a similar role to that of *E. coli* in secondary infections. Collectively, infections caused by *E. coli* are responsible for significant economic losses to the poultry industry. For example, 43% of broiler carcasses condemned for disease at processing had lesions consistent with colisepticemia (98).

Most *E. coli* serotypes isolated from poultry are pathogenic only for birds and are not recognized as important causes of infections in other animals including humans. Chickens, however, are susceptible to colonization with *E. coli* O157:H7, an important enterohemorrhagic pathogen of humans. Natural contamination of chicken meat with this organism has been found, and a food-borne outbreak of diarrheal disease was associated with contaminated turkey (8, 22, 32, 80). Characteristics of virulent *E. coli* in birds and other animals are often shared (e.g., K1 antigen), and avian strains can potentially be a source of genes and plasmids that encode for antimicrobial resistance and virulence factors (14, 51). Serotypes associated with diarrheal disease in humans (14) and strains that produce both heat-labile and heat-stable enterotoxins have been isolated from chickens in southeast Asia (1).

For recent reviews on colibacillosis in poultry see (6, 7, 38).

INCIDENCE AND DISTRIBUTION. The various serotypes of *E. coli* are intestinal inhabitants of animals including humans and probably infect most mammals and birds; therefore, they have a cosmopolitan distribution. Clinical disease is reported most often in chickens, turkeys, and ducks.

E. coli is a common inhabitant in the intestinal tracts of poultry at concentrations up to 10^6/g.

Higher numbers are found in younger birds, birds without an established normal flora, and in the lower intestinal tract (21, 54, 95). Its presence in drinking water is considered indicative of fecal contamination. Among normal chickens, 10–15% of intestinal coliforms belong to potentially pathogenic serotypes (45). Intestinal strains are not necessarily the same serotype as those from the pericardial sac of the same bird. Egg transmission of pathogenic *E. coli* is common and can be responsible for high chick mortality. Pathogenic coliforms are more frequent in the gut of newly hatched chicks than in eggs from which they hatched (46), suggesting rapid spread after hatching. The most important source of egg infection seems to be fecal contamination of the surface with subsequent penetration of the shell and membranes. Coliform bacteria can be found in litter and fecal matter. Dust in poultry houses may contain 10^5–10^6 *E. coli*/g. These bacteria persist for long periods, particularly when dry (44). There was a reduction of 84–97% in 7 days following wetting of dust with water. Feed is often contaminated with pathogenic coliforms, but these can be destroyed by hot pelleting processes. Rodent droppings often contain pathogenic coliforms. Pathogenic serotypes can also be introduced into poultry flocks through contaminated well water (62).

ETIOLOGY. *E. coli* is a gram-negative, non–acid-fast, uniform staining, non–spore-forming bacillus, usually $2–3 \times 0.6$ µm. The organism may be variable in size and shape. Many strains are motile and have peritrichous flagella. In one study (76), 57% of 607 isolates were motile.

Growth Requirements. *E. coli* grows on ordinary nutrient media at temperatures of 18–44 C or lower. On agar plates incubated for 24 hr at 37 C, colonies are low, convex, smooth, and colorless. They are usually 1–3 mm in diameter with granular structure and an entire margin. *E. coli* grows well in broth, producing turbid growth.

Biochemical Properties. Acid and gas are produced in glucose, maltose, mannitol, xylose, glycerol, rhamnose, sorbitol, and arabinose, but not in dextrin, starch, or inositol. A few strains ferment lactose slowly or not at all; fermentation of adonitol, sucrose, salicin, raffinose, and dulcitol is variable. *E. coli* produces positive methyl red and negative Voges-Proskauer reactions; hydrogen sulfide is not produced on Kligler's iron medium. It does not grow in the presence of potassium cyanide, hydrolyze urea, liquefy gelatin, or grow in citrate medium (28). *E. coli* isolates from poultry have biochemical properties similar to those from other sources (4).

Antigenic Structures.

Various serotypes of *E. coli* are classified according to the Ewing scheme (27). Knowledge about the antigenic structure of *E. coli* and its antigenic relationship to other species has been reviewed (78). Currently, 173 O, 74 K, 53 H, and 17 F antigens are recognized (56, 96). Rough strains autoagglutinate and cannot be serotyped (96).

O (SOMATIC) ANTIGEN. The O antigen is the endotoxin liberated following lysis of smooth cells. It is composed of a polysaccharide–phospholipid complex with a protein fraction resistant to boiling. Methods for preparation and use of O antisera, which agglutinate antigen at high titers (usually over 1:2560) when the antigen-antibody mixture is incubated at 50 C for 24 hr, have been described (27, 78, 96).

K (CAPSULAR) ANTIGEN. K antigens are polymeric acids containing 2% reducing sugars. They are associated with virulence, are on the surface of the cell, interfere with O agglutination, and can be removed by heating for 1 hr at 100 C; however, some strains require heating for 2.5 hr at 121 C. On the basis of heat stability, K antigens are subdivided into L, A, and B forms. Antisera are prepared in rabbits by inoculating live organisms intravenously. Tube agglutination titers are determined by incubating antigen-antibody mixtures at 37 C for 2 hr and overnight at 4 C. Titers are low (1:100–1:400). Most of these antigens can be identified by the slide agglutination test using appropriately diluted serum (96).

H (FLAGELLAR) ANTIGEN. H antigens are not often used in antigenic identification of *E. coli* isolates and are not correlated with pathogenicity. They are proteins that are destroyed by heating to 100 C. Tube agglutination tests are read after incubation at 37 C for 2 hr.

F (PILUS) ANTIGEN. F antigens are involved in attachment to cells. Pili are classified as being mannose sensitive or mannose resistant depending on whether or not agglutination is inhibited or unaffected respectively when mannose is present. While often associated with *E. coli* virulence in mammals,

the significance of pili in poultry disease is not as clear.

SEROTYPES. Surveys have been made in many parts of the world to determine serotypes most frequently associated with poultry disease. Over many years, the most common serotypes have been O1, O2, O35, and O78 (47, 78). Many other serotypes have been found less frequently while some pathogenic isolates do not belong to known serotypes or are untypeable.

OTHER CHARACTERISTICS. In addition to serotyping, isolates of *E. coli* can be further characterized by antibiotic resistance, toxigenicity, presence of adhesins including piliation, cell attachment, hemagglutination, lysogeny (phage typing), and occurrence of plasmids. DNA probes and polymerase chain reactions have been developed to detect specific genes important in virulence (56, 96). Multilocus enzyme electrophoresis identified specific genotypes, which demonstrated that relatively few clonal types are responsible for different forms of colibacillosis in chickens and turkeys in widespread geographic areas (56, 89). Virulence varied little among isolates within a clonal group but varied considerably between clonal groups.

PATHOGENESIS AND EPIZOOTIOLOGY.

Seventy-four (48%) of 154 *E. coli* serotypes caused pericarditis and mortality in 3-wk-old chicks following inoculation of air sacs and/or death of 13-day-old embryos following allantoic inoculation (76). Other serotypes might have been found pathogenic if other routes of inoculation had been used.

Bacterial Virulence Factors.

A number of potential virulence factors have been identified in strains of *E. coli* isolated from diseased birds (Table 4.1). Other than the ability to cause mortality in embryos or chicks, no single virulence factor has been identified that will distinguish all pathogenic strains from nonpathogenic isolates. Resistance to complement (serum resistance), which may often be mediated by presence of K1 capsular antigen, appears to correlate with virulence in most strains (65, 66, 91, 93). Virulent strains are capable of persisting in the intestinal tract longer and in greater numbers than avirulent ones; this may be related to colicin production by normal intestinal *E. coli* (54, 95).

Pathogenic and nonpathogenic isolates of *E. coli* are similar in biochemical characteristics and drug sensitivities (15, 74). Hemolysins, heat-stable toxins, metabolic activity, motility, R-plasmids, and phage resistance generally do not correlate with virulence (47, 48, 85, 92).

Host Susceptibility Factors.

Compared

Table 4.1. Factors that may correlate with virulence of *Escherichia coli* for poultry

Factor[a]	References
Genetically related clonal groups	(89)
Certain O serotypes	
(O1, O2, O35, O78)	(15, 47,78)
K1 and K80 capsular antigens	(12, 90)
Adonitol fermentation	(74)
Antibiotic resistance	(14, 91)
Congo red dye uptake	(9, 81)
Presence of large plasmids	(85, 90, 91)
Colicin production (esp. ColV)	(85, 95)
Presence of siderophores (aerobactin)	(12, 52, 85, 90, 91)
Presence of pili	(19, 23, 41, 91, 97)
Motility	(91)
Outer membrane proteins (*tra*T, *iss*)	(67)
Smooth lipopolysaccharide (endotoxin)	(93)
Cell adherence (esp. avian cells)	(12, 97)
Complement resistance	(65, 66, 85, 91, 93)
Resistance to phagocytosis or killing	(5)
Cytotoxins	(1, 26)
Ability to invade cells and tissues	(85)
Ability to persist in	
circulation or tissues	(5, 20)

[a]No single factor identifies all virulent strains, and conflicting correlations between most factors and virulence have often been found.

with bacterial virulence factors, host susceptibility factors are probably a greater determinant of colibacillosis occurrence (Table 4.2). Normal, healthy birds with intact defenses are remarkably resistant to naturally occurring *E. coli* exposure including virulent strains. Infection occurs when skin or mucosal barriers are compromised (e.g., unhealed navel; wounds, mucosal damage from viral, bacterial, or parasitic infections; and lack of normal flora), the mononuclear–phagocytic system is impaired (e.g., viral infections, toxins, and nutritional deficiencies), there is immunosuppression (e.g., viral infections, toxins), exposure is overwhelming (e.g., environmental contamination, poor ventilation, contaminated water), or birds are exposed to abnormal stress (too little or too much). Infection with infectious bronchitis virus in chickens, infection with hemorrhagic enteritis virus in turkeys, and exposure of avian species to ammonia are the most common factors that predispose to colibacillosis. Interactions between infectious bronchitis virus and *E. coli* have been studied extensively and used to determine virulence of both organisms and efficacy of vaccination programs (16, 63).

Moderate stress was reported to increase resistance, possibly as a result of the development of immunity following contact of organisms with the immune system (54), or as a result of developing and exercising defense mechanisms and maintaining them in a state of readiness (37). Similarly, provoking mild, nonspecific inflammation of the respiratory system was reported to increase resistance to *E. coli* infection (83). Individual survival likely derives from utilization of feed-derived resources for antibacterial defense rather than growth (39). Because the vast majority of colibacillosis cases occur secondarily to one or more other factors, predisposing causes must be identified and corrected before the disease can be effectively controlled.

Table 4.2. Factors that alter host susceptibility to *Escherichia coli* infections in poultry

Increased Susceptibility	Decreased Susceptibility
Viruses	Immunity
Adenovirus	Passive
Chicken infectious	Active
anemia virus	Immunostimulants (?)
Hemorrhagic enteritis virus	Phagocyte priming
Infectious bronchitis virus	
Infectious bursal	Physiologic
disease virus	Genetics
Infectious laryngotracheitis	Age—older
virus	Sex—Female
Influenza virus	Moderate stress
Newcastle disease virus	Socialization
Reovirus	Deoxycorticosterone
Turkey rhinotracheitis virus	Normal intestinal flora
Bacteria	Nutrition
Bordetella avium	High protein
Chlamydia psittaci (?)	Vitamin A
Clostridium perfringens (?)	ß-carotene
Mycoplasma gallisepticum	Vitamin C
M. meleagridis	Vitamin E
M. synoviae	High iron—oral
Parasites	
Ascaridia dissimilis (larvae)	
Eimeria brunetti	
Eimeria tenella	
Cryptosporidium baileyi	
Histomonas meleagridis	
Toxins	
Ammonia	
Cyclophosphamide	
Iron—parenteral	
Mycotoxins (?)	
Physiologic	
Age—young	
Low protein feed	
Stress—minimal or severe	
Sex—male	
Environmental	
Contaminated water	
Dry, dusty conditions	
Feed/water restriction	
Inadequate ventilation	
Overcrowding	
Poor litter conditions	
Temperature extremes	

Sources: (7, 11, 64, 68, 84)

Embryo and Early Chick Mortality. Between 0.5 and 6% of eggs from normal hens contain *E. coli.* Experimentally inoculated hens may shed *E. coli* in up to 26% of their eggs. Pathogenic strains accounted for 43 of 245 isolates from dead embryos (44). Normal contents of yolk sacs change from viscid, yellow–green to watery, yellow–brown or caseous material when contaminated with *E. coli* (Fig. 4.1A). The bacterium can occasionally be isolated from normal-appearing yolk. *Escherichia coli* was present in yolk sacs of about 70% of chicks with "mushy chick disease," which was characterized by edema and infected yolk (43). Other commonly isolated bacteria included *Proteus* spp., *Bacillus* spp., and enterococci.

Fecal contamination of eggs is considered to be the most important source of infection. Other sources may be ovarian infection or salpingitis. The incidence of infection increases shortly after hatching and is reduced after about 6 days.

Yolk sac of embryos is the focus of infection. Many embryos die before hatching, particularly late in incubation. Some die at or shortly after hatching, with losses continuing up to 3 wk. As few as 10 organisms of serotype O1a:K1:H7 caused 100% mortality in day-old chicks when injected into the yolk sac (76). Chicks with yolk sac infection also often have inflammation of the navel (omphalitis) (Fig. 4.1B). Chicks or poults living more than 4 days may have pericarditis as well as infected yolks, indicating systemic spread of the organism from the yolk sac. There may be no embryo or chick mortality, the only manifestation of infected yolk sacs being retained infected yolk and reduced weight gain (34).

The microscopic reaction in the wall of infected yolk sacs appears to be mild. The wall is edematous. There is an outer connective tissue zone followed by a layer of inflammatory cells containing heterophils and macrophages, a layer of giant cells, a zone of necrotic heterophils and masses of bacteria, and then the inner infected yolk contents. A few plasma cells may be found in some yolk sacs.

Omphalitis and yolk sac infection have been experimentally reproduced in ducks by exposing eggs to *E. coli* broth cultures (75). Dipping eggs at 18 days of incubation resulted in a higher incidence of infection than dipping at 1 day. Low brooding temperature or fasting increases the incidence of infection and mortality.

Respiratory Tract Infection. *E. coli* often infects respiratory tracts of birds concurrently infected with various combinations of infectious bronchitis viruses (IBV) and Newcastle disease viruses (NDV), including vaccine strains, and mycoplasmas.

Apparently, the damaged respiratory tract becomes extremely susceptible to invasion by *E. coli*

(33). The resulting disease is commonly called air sac disease or chronic respiratory disease (CRD). In addition to airsacculitis, which may spread to adjacent tissues, pneumonia, pleuropneumonia, pericarditis, and perihepatitis are also frequently present (Figs. 4.1C-F). Less commonly, salpingitis, panophthalmitis, and infections in bones and synovial structures may occur following sepsis. Air sac disease occurs chiefly in 4- to 9-wk-old broiler chickens. Considerable economic losses result from morbidity, mortality, and condemnation of birds at processing.

Lesions of uncomplicated coliform infection can easily be reproduced by inoculating pathogenic *E. coli* into the air sac (18). Airsacculitis occurs within 1.5 hr. Bacteremia and pericarditis may develop in 6 hr. In birds that survive, lesions are well developed 48 hr postinoculation. Most mortality occurs during the first 5 days. Recovery is usually rapid if birds survive initial infection, although a few with persistent anorexia become emaciated and die.

Mycoplasmal infection increases susceptibility to *E. coli* about 12–16 days postinoculation, and susceptibility persists for at least 30 days. Infection

4.1. Colibacillosis. *A.* Yolk sac infection in a 4-day-old leghorn chick. Yolk sac is distended, hyperemic (note prominent vessels), and filled with abnormal brown, watery contents. (Munger). *B.* Omphalitis and yolk sac infection in a group of 3-day-old leghorn chicks. Navels are inflamed and yolk sacs are distended with abnormal contents. (Munger). *C.* Advanced air sac disease in a 20-day-broiler chicken. Polyserositis (pericarditis, perihepatitis, peritonitis, airsacculitis) have occurred as a result of systemic spread of *Escherichia coli.* (Munger). *D.* Pleuropneumonia and airsacculitis in a broiler chicken caused by *E. coli* infection. *E.* Experimental colibacillosis in a turkey. Extension of inflammation between superficial and deep pectoral muscles from airsacculitis involving the interclavicular air sac. Detecting this type of lesion is important during inspection at processing. *F.* Microscopic appearance of pneumonia caused by *E. coli* in a broiler chicken. Exudate fills the lumen of several affected parabronchi (compare with unaffected parabronchi at the *top* of the figure). Exudate has expanded some atria. Some atria have ruptured permitting extension of the inflammatory process through the capillary bed into the interstitium. The process has involved almost all of one lobule with extension to the adjacent pleural surface. ×10. *G.* Pericarditis and green discoloration of the liver in a turkey that survived the acute septic phase of colibacillosis. Pericardium is thickened and exudate in the pericardial sac is beginning to undergo fibrosis. Green discoloration of the liver can indicate inflammation elsewhere in the bird, especially in turkeys. *H.* Salpingitis in a young bird caused by *E. coli.* This lesion occurs infrequently but is often associated with airsacculitis involving the left abdominal air sac.

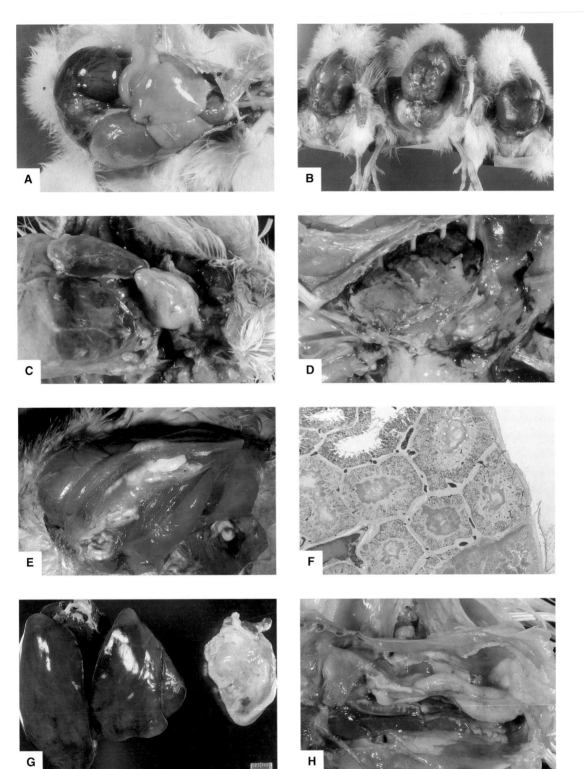

with IBV or NDV in addition to mycoplasma further decreases resistance to *E. coli* and the period of increased susceptibility begins earlier and persists longer.

Susceptibility is increased when only IBV or NDV infection occurs. Five days after administration of a vaccine strain of NDV, clearance of aerosol-administered *E. coli* is reduced. Microscopically, the pseudostratified, columnar epithelium of the trachea is replaced by 3–8 layers of immature, nonciliated cells (29). Mixed IBV–*E. coli* infections are more severe than those caused by single agent infections (64, 77).

Inhaled coliform-contaminated dust has been considered one of the most important sources for infecting susceptible air sacs. Exposure to chicken-house dust and ammonia results in deciliation of the upper respiratory tract of birds (61, 69) permitting inhaled *E. coli* to colonize and cause respiratory infection.

Pathology.   Infected air sacs are thickened and often have caseous exudate on the respiratory surface. Microscopically, the earliest changes consist of edema and heterophil infiltration. Mononuclear phagocytes are frequently seen 12 hr after inoculation. Later, mononuclear phagocytes become common, with giant cells along margins of necrotic areas. There is fibroblast proliferation and accumulation of vast numbers of necrotic heterophils in caseous exudate. Lesions of predisposing respiratory disease are usually present and consist of lymphoid follicles, epithelial hyperplasia, and epithelium-lined air passages that may contain heterophils.

PERICARDITIS.   Most *E. coli* serotypes cause pericarditis following septicemia. Pericarditis is usually associated with myocarditis and results in marked changes in the electrocardiogram (35), often before macroscopic lesions appear. The pericardial sac becomes cloudy and epicardium becomes edematous and covered with a light-colored exudate. The pericardial sac often fills with a light-yellow, fibrinous exudate (Fig. 4.1C). Microscopically, at first there are many heterophils in the epicardium. In less than 24 hr, macrophages become more numerous. Within the myocardium, particularly close to the epicardium, there are accumulations of lymphoid cells, and by 7–10 days there are many plasma cells. Subsequently, exudate in the pericardial sac undergoes organization (Fig. 4.1G), which can eventually result in constrictive pericarditis and liver fibrosis due to chronic passive congestion in survivors. Pericarditis–myocarditis results in reduction of carotid artery blood pressure from a norm of about 150 mmHg down to about 40 mmHg just before death.

SALPINGITIS.   When the left abdominal air sac is infected by *E. coli,* females may develop chronic salpingitis characterized by a large caseous mass in a dilated, thin-walled oviduct (Fig. 4.1H). The caseous mass contains necrotic heterophils and bacteria that persist for months. Size of the caseous mass may increase with time. Affected birds frequently die during the first 6 mo postinfection; those surviving rarely lay eggs. Salpingitis may also occur following entry of coliform bacteria from the cloaca in laying hens and ducks and geese (Fig. 4.2A) (10).

Tissue reaction in the oviduct is surprisingly mild consisting largely of heterophil accumulation just under the epithelium. High estrogenic activity seems to be associated with coliform growth in the oviduct. Infection can be reproduced by injecting large (10^9) doses of bacteria into the uterus or oviduct. Stilbestrol implants increase susceptibility and result in increased numbers of coliforms in the oviduct.

PERITONITIS.   Coliform infection of the peritoneal cavity occurs in laying hens and is characterized by acute mortality, fibrin, and free yolk (Fig. 4.2B). Infection occurs when bacteria ascending through the oviduct grow rapidly in yolk material that has been deposited in the peritoneal cavity (40).

ACUTE SEPTICEMIA.   An acute infectious disease resembling fowl typhoid and fowl cholera from which *E. coli* can be isolated is sometimes seen in mature and growing chickens and turkeys. Affected birds are in good physical condition and have full crops, which indicates the acute nature of the infection. The most characteristic lesions are green liver, marked splenomegaly, and congested muscles (Fig. 4.2C). In some cases, multiple, pale, foci in the liver have been described. Microscopically, these are areas of acute necrosis initially but with time evolve into granulomatous hepatitis in survivors (Fig. 4.2D). As in coliform septicemia associated with respiratory disease, there is a tendency toward pericarditis and peritonitis. Acute septicemia occurs most often in turkeys following infection with hemorrhagic enteritis virus.

SYNOVITIS/OSTEOMYELITIS.   Isolates of *E. coli* have been recovered from joint infections of chickens (Fig. 4.2E). Lesions can be reproduced following intravenous inoculation of a broth culture of certain isolates. Synovitis is frequently a sequel to septicemia and may occur in birds with insufficient immunity. Many birds recover in about 1 wk, while others remain chronically infected and may become emaciated. Lesions may develop in joint spaces of articulating thoracolumbar vertebrae causing spondylitis and progressive paresis and paralysis

(Fig. 4.3). Hematogenous spread of *E. coli* following hemorrhagic enteritis virus infection of turkeys resulted in synovitis, osteomyelitis, and green liver discoloration in turkeys (25).

PANOPHTHALMITIS. Panophthalmitis is an uncommon sequela of *E. coli* septicemia. There is hypopyon, usually of one eye, which is blind (Fig. 4.2F). Most birds die shortly after onset of lesions, although some recover. Microscopically, there are infiltrations of heterophils and mononuclear phagocytes throughout the eye, and giant cells form around necrotic areas. The choroid becomes hyperemic, and there is complete destruction of the retina.

COLIGRANULOMA (HJARRE'S DISEASE). Coligranuloma of chickens and turkeys is characterized by granulomas in liver, ceca, duodenum, and mesentery, but not spleen (Fig. 4.4). It is a relatively uncommon coliform disease; however, individual flocks may have mortality as high as 75%. Serosal lesions resembling leucosis tumors are sometimes caused by *E. coli*. There is confluent coagulation necrosis involving as much as half the liver. Only scattered heterophils are seen, and at the edge of the necrotic areas there are a few giant cells. This lesion is possibly the precursor to Hjarre's disease. Pyogranulomatous typhlitis and hepatitis characterized by cecal cores and ruptured ceca have recently been described in turkeys, which may be related to coligranuloma (58).

SWOLLEN-HEAD SYNDROME. Swollen-head syndrome (SHS) is an acute to subacute cellulitis involving the periorbital and adjacent subcutaneous tissues of the head (Fig. 4.2G). It was first described in broilers in South Africa associated with *E. coli* and an unidentified coronavirus infection (59). Swollen-head syndrome has subsequently been described in most intense poultry-producing areas of the world. In common with other forms of colibacillosis, different predisposing agents have been identified. Although *E. coli* is most frequently associated with the disease, other bacteria have occasionally been recovered from affected birds. Where it occurs, avian pneumovirus (turkey rhinotracheitis virus) and, in other areas, infectious bronchitis virus, often in conjunction with poor ventilation and high ammonia levels, are the most frequent predisposing factors (24).

Although the pathogenesis of SHS has not been established, conjunctival-associated lymphoid tissue inflamed from virus infection and/or ammonia irritation may serve as the site through which bacteria gain access to subcutaneous tissues. Periorbital inflammation is typically seen early in the disease and similarly affected bronchial-associated lymph-oid tissue has been shown to be an area where *E. coli* penetrates the mucosa (36). Lesions have been reproduced by scarifying the conjunctival mucosa and instilling a pure culture of *E. coli* (59). Possible infection via the eustachian tube has also been suggested (24). A similar condition in turkeys in which an adenovirus is suspected to be the predisposing cause has recently been identified in the north-central United States. *E. coli* can also complicate avian pneumovirus infections in turkeys (see Chapter 20).

AVIAN CELLULITIS. Avian cellulitis, also known as inflammatory process, infectious process, or IP, is a chronic skin disease affecting the abdomen of broiler chickens, characterized by sheets of caseated, heterophilic exudate in subcutaneous tissues. Lesions are located in the skin between the thigh and midline (Fig. 4.2H). They are usually discovered at processing and have become an increasingly important cause of carcass condemnation since the disease was first described in 1984 (73). *E. coli* is most often isolated from the lesions, although a variety of other bacteria occasionally have been recovered. Most *E. coli* isolates are serotypes O2, O78, or are untypeable, and produce aerobactin and colicin. They are similar to isolates from other types of colibacillosis. Avian cellulitis has been as-

4.2. Colibacillosis. A. Large caseated masses distending the oviduct of this mature laying hen are characteristic of salpingitis caused by *Escherichia coli*. Salpingitis in the adult female most likely results from an ascending infection from the cloaca. B. Goose breeder with acute peritonitis. Yolk was demonstrated in the peritoneum and *E. coli* was isolated. C. Acute *E. coli* septicemia in a turkey. Spleen is markedly enlarged and severely congested. Note it is approximately the same size as the proventriculus. Liver is also enlarged and congested, and there is evidence of early pericarditis and peritonitis. D. Experimental colibacillosis in a turkey. Liver from a bird that survived the acute septicemic phase has multiple pale foci, which were determined microscopically to be focal areas of early heterophilic, granulomatous hepatitis. E. Advanced tenosynovitis/arthritis involving the hock joint and flexor tendons of a lame commercial broiler. *E. coli* and *Staphylococcus* spp. were isolated from the lesion. F. Panophthalmitis affecting the eye of a turkey that survived an earlier episode of colisepticemia. This lesion is uncommon and affects only one eye. The organism can be isolated from the eye for an extended period after it is no longer present in other tissues. G. Swollen-head syndrome in a broiler chicken. There is conjunctival inflammation and periorbital swelling due to cellulitis. Evidence of exposure to high ammonia levels and infection with infectious bronchitis virus and *E. coli* were found in this flock. (Munger) H. Avian cellulitis (inflammatory process). Subcutaneous yellow, caseous exudate is present over the abdomen of this affected bird.

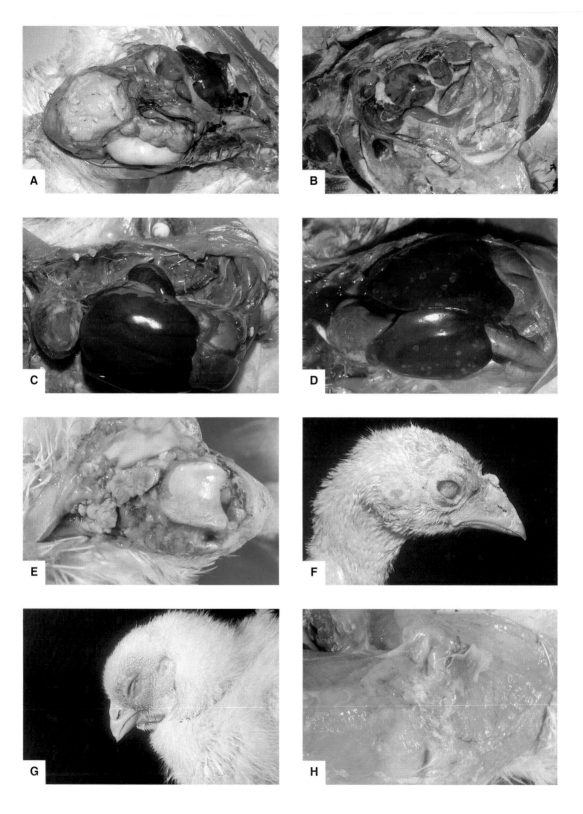

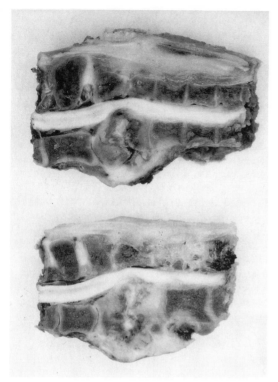

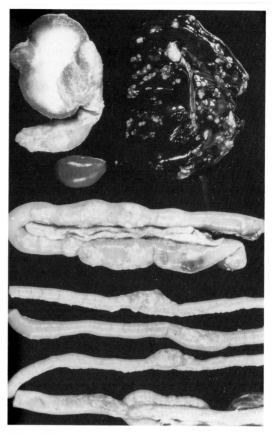

4.3. Spondylitis involving articulating thoracolumbar vertebrae of two lame turkeys (fixed tissues). Pressure from the lesion on the spinal cord has caused demyelination of the ventral tracts. *Escherichia coli* is a common cause of this lesion, but other bacteria that can localize in bones and synovial tissues may also be a cause.

4.4. Coligranuloma in a market-age turkey. Numerous, nodular lesions are located in gastrointestinal tissues including liver, but they do not involve the spleen. A mucoid *Escherichia coli* was isolated.

sociated with earlier outbreaks of colibacillosis in some flocks (70).

Avian cellulitis has been experimentally reproduced by applying cultures to skin scratches. Lesions occurred most frequently in birds exposed to isolates epidemiologically related to naturally occurring infections compared with birds exposed to isolates from airsacculitis or feces (71). Overcrowding, poor litter quality, and chick quality have also been identified as possible factors contributing to avian cellulitis. A mild, localized, cellulitis surrounding the navel can occur as a result of omphalitis.

ENTERITIS. Primary enteritis in poultry caused by *E. coli* has been considered rare, if it occurred at all. Recently, however, enterotoxigenic *E. coli* (ETEC) that elaborate toxins capable of causing fluid accumulation in ligated intestinal loops of chickens have been recovered from chickens with diarrhea (1). As well, naturally occurring and experimental infections of chickens and a pigeon with attaching, ef-

facing *E. coli* (AEEC) have been identified (31, 86). Infections with infectious bursal disease virus in chickens and adenovirus infection in the pigeon were considered possible predisposing factors to AEEC infection.

COLIFORM SEPTICEMIA OF DUCKS. Coliform septicemia of ducks is characterized by moist, granular to curdlike exudate of variable thickness causing pericarditis, perihepatitis, and airsacculitis. A characteristic odor is often noted at necropsy. Liver is frequently swollen, dark, and bile stained, and spleen is swollen and dark. *E. coli* (usually O78) can usually be recovered from any internal organs (53). *Riemerella anatipestifer* can cause similar lesions, which can be identified by appropriate cultural procedures (see Chapter 6).

Coliform septicemia occurs throughout the growing season but becomes more frequent in late fall and winter. All ages of ducklings are susceptible. Distribution of losses suggests individual farms, rather than hatcheries, are the source of infection (53).

DIAGNOSIS

Isolation and Identification of Causative Agent.
Material should be streaked on eosin-methylene blue (EMB), MacConkey, or tergitol-7 agar, as well as noninhibitory media. Care must be taken to avoid fecal contamination of samples. A presumptive diagnosis of *E. coli* infection can be made if most of the colonies are characteristically dark with a metallic sheen on EMB agar, bright pink with precipitate in medium on MacConkey agar, and yellow on tergitol-7 agar. Rarely, strains of *E. coli* can be slow lactose fermenters and appear as nonlactose-fermenting colonies. A definite diagnosis of *E. coli* can be made based on the organism's characteristics (see Etiology).

Antigenic identification and determination of virulence factors of the isolate might be helpful, particularly when done as part of an epidemiologic investigation. The correlation between virulence and complement resistance suggests this may be a good method for screening isolates for possible disease association. A relatively simple rapid turbidimetric assay has been described (72).

Survival after challenge correlated better with antibody titers detected by an enzyme-linked immunosorbent assay (ELISA) than by the standard indirect hemagglutination procedure (55).

Differential Diagnosis.
Lesions similar to those resulting from *E. coli* infection can be caused by many other organisms. Synovitis and arthritis can also be caused by viruses, mycoplasmas, staphylococci, salmonellae, *Streptobacillus moniliformis,* and other organisms. A great variety of organisms such as *Aerobacter* spp., *Klebsiella* spp., *Proteus* spp., salmonellae, *Bacillus* spp., staphylococci, enterococci, or clostridia are frequently isolated (often as mixed cultures) from yolk sacs of embryos and chicks (43). Pericarditis can also be caused by chlamydia. Peritonitis is sometimes caused by pasteurellae or streptococci. Airsacculitis can be caused by other bacteria, mycoplasmas, and chlamydia. Acute septicemic diseases may result from pasteurellae, salmonellae, streptococci, and other organisms. Liver granulomas have many causes, including anaerobic bacteria belonging to the genera *Eubacterium* and *Bacteroides.*

TREATMENT.
E. coli may be sensitive to many drugs such as ampicillin, chloramphenicol, chlortetracycline, neomycin, nitrofurans, gentamicin, ormethiprim-sulfadimethoxine, nalidixic acid, oxytetracycline, polymyxin B, spectinomycin, streptomycin, and sulfa drugs. Recently, fluoroquinolones (enrofloxacin, sarafloxacin) have be-

come available in the United States for treatment of colibacillosis in poultry, which have generally proved to be highly efficacious. Anticoccidials can also have antimicrobial activity—monensin reduced colonization of chickens with *E. coli* O157:H7 to undetectable levels 14 days postexposure compared with unmedicated controls and chickens receiving other coccidiostats (79).

Isolates of *E. coli* from poultry are frequently resistant to one or more drugs, especially if they have been widely used in the poultry industry over a long period (e.g., tetracyclines). It is imperative to determine drug sensitivity of *E. coli* strains involved in a disease outbreak so that ineffective drugs can be avoided. Even a highly effective drug may not result in improvement of the flock if too little is used or it is incapable of reaching the site of infection. Underdosing stimulates development of resistance. When chicks were given feeds with increasing low concentrations of ampicillin (1.7 and 5 g/ton), development of resistance was directly correlated to amount of antibiotic in the feed (2).

PREVENTION AND CONTROL.
Effective inactivated vaccines against serotypes O2:K1 and O78:K80 have been produced (3, 13, 17). Both homologous and heterologous protection were provided by a vaccine prepared by ultrasonic inactivation of the organism followed by irradiation (57). An inactivated O78 vaccine protected ducks (75). Multivalent vaccines made from pili containing low levels (180 µg) of protein per dose reduced the severity of challenge infection (42). Absorbed sera indicate pili of serotypes O1, O2, and O78 are antigenically different (82). Passive immunization results in increased resistance to aerosol challenge and clearance of bacteria from blood (60). Use of an inactivated vaccine in breeders provided passive protection against homologous challenge in progeny, which was complete for 2 wk and partial for several additional weeks posthatch (49).

A live vaccine prepared from a naturally occurring, nonpathogenic, piliated strain (BT-7) was efficacious when used in chickens older than 14 days of age. Protection against both homologous and heterologous strains was demonstrated (30). A *carAB* mutation of a virulent O2 serotype caused defective utilization of arginine and pyrimidines, increasing their requirement by the mutant. As low levels of these substances are generally available in vivo, the organism was unable to sustain itself, which resulted in a self-limiting infection. The mutant strain was found to be stable, immunogenic, and attenuated. Turkeys orally vaccinated with the mutant were protected against colibacillosis in a hemorrhagic enteritis virus-parent wild-type strain challenge model (50).

E. coli infection of the respiratory tract of birds can be reduced by raising mycoplasma-free birds and reducing exposure of birds to viruses causing respiratory diseases. Proper ventilation will reduce respiratory tract damage and exposure.

There are no known methods for reducing the level of pathogenic *E. coli* in the intestinal tract and feces, although consideration that 1) pelleted feed has fewer *E. coli* than mash, 2) rodent droppings are a source of pathogenic *E. coli,* and 3) contaminated water can contain high numbers of the organism should not be overlooked. Chlorination of drinking water and use of closed (nipple) watering systems have decreased the occurrence of colibacillosis and condemnations for airsacculitis. Pathogenic strains of *E. coli* can be competitively excluded from intestines of chicks by seeding them with native microflora from resistant chickens (87). Infection with *Mycoplasma gallisepticum* and/or infectious bronchitis virus induces protected chickens to shed *E. coli* (88).

The most important source for transmission of pathogenic *E. coli* between flocks is fecal contamination of hatching eggs. Transmission can be reduced by collecting eggs frequently, keeping nest material clean, not using floor eggs, discarding cracked eggs or those with obvious fecal contamination, and fumigating or disinfecting eggs within 2 hr after they are laid. If infected eggs are broken during incubation or hatching, the contents are a serious source of infection to others, especially when personnel and egg-handling equipment are contaminated. Eggs are particularly susceptible just before hatching. Methods for preventing incubator and hatcher dissemination are unknown. However, venting incubators and hatchers to the outside and having as few breeder flocks as possible represented in each unit will help reduce losses. Contaminated chicks survive better if kept warm and not starved. High protein diets and increased vitamin E levels apparently favor survival.

REFERENCES

1. Akashi, N., S. Hitotsubashi, H. Yamanaka, Y. Fujii, T. Tsuji, A. Miyama, J.E. Joya, and K. Okamoto. 1993. Production of heat-stable enterotoxin II by chicken clinical isolates of Escherichia coli. FEMS Microbiol Lett 109:311–316.
2. Al-Sam, S., A.H. Linton, P.M. Bennett, and M. Hinton. 1993. Effects of low concentrations of ampicillin in feed on the intestinal Escherichia coli of chicks. J Appl Bacteriol 75:108–112.
3. Arp, L.H. 1982. Effect of passive immunization on phagocytosis of blood-borne Escherichia coli in spleen and liver of turkeys. Am J Vet Res 43:1034–1040.
4. Arp, L.H. 1989. Colibacillosis. In H.G. Purchase, L.H. Arp, C.H. Domermuth, and J.E. Pearson (eds.). A Laboratory Manual for the Isolation and Identification of Avian Pathogens, 3rd ed. American Association of Avian Pathologists, Kennett Square, PA, pp. 12–13.
5. Arp, L.H., and N.F. Cheville. 1981. Interaction of blood-borne Escherichia coli with phagocytes of spleen and liver in turkeys. Am J Vet Res 42:650–657.
6. Barnes, H.J. 1994. Pathogenesis of respiratory Escherichia coli and Pasteurella multocida infections in poultry. Symposium on Respiratory Diseases of Chickens and Turkeys, Annu Meet Am Assoc Avian Pathol and Am Vet Med Assoc, July 10, 1994, San Francisco, CA, pp. 26–39.
7. Barnes, H.J., and F. Lozano. 1994. Colibacillosis in poultry. In Pfizer Veterinary Practicum, Pfizer Animal Health. Lee's Summit, MO, 45 pp.
8. Beery, J.T., M.P. Doyle, and J.L Schoeni. 1985. Colonization of chicken cecae by Escherichia coli associated with hemorrhagic colitis. Appl Environ Microbiol 49:310–315.
9. Berkhoff, H.A., and A.C. Vinal. 1986. Congo red medium to distinguish between invasive and non-invasive Escherichia coli pathogenic for poultry. Avian Dis 30:117–121.
10. Bisgaard, M. 1995. Salpingitis in web-footed birds: Prevalence, aetiology and significance. Avian Pathol 24:443–452.
11. Boyd, F.M., and H.M. Edwards, Jr. 1963. The effect of dietary protein on the course of various infections in the chick. J Infect Dis 112:53–56.
12. Brée, A., M. Dho, and J.P. Lafont. 1989. Comparative infectivity for axenic and specific-pathogen-free chickens of O2 Escherichia coli strains with or without virulence factors. Avian Dis 33:134–139.
13. Cessi, D. 1979. Prophylaxis of Escherichia coli infection in fowls with emulsified vaccines. Clin Vet 102:270–278.
14. Chulasiri, M., and O. Suthienkul. 1989. Antimicrobial resistance of Escherichia coli isolated from chickens. Vet Microbiol 21:189–194.
15. Cloud, S.S., J.K. Rosenberger, P.A. Fries, R.A. Wilson, and E.M. Odor. 1985. In vitro and in vivo characterization of avian Escherichia coli. I. Serotypes, metabolic activity, and antibiotic sensitivity. Avian Dis 29:1084–1093.
16. Cook, J.K.A., M.B. Huggins, and M.M. Ellis. 1991. Use of an infectious bronchitis virus and Escherichia coli model infection to assess the ability to vaccinate successfully against infectious bronchitis virus in the presence of maternally-derived immunity. Avian Pathol 20:619–626.
17. Deb, J.R., and E.G. Harry. 1978. Laboratory trials with inactivated vaccines against Escherichia coli 02:K1 infection in fowls. Res Vet Sci 24:308–313.
18. DeRosa, M., M.D. Ficken, and H.J. Barnes. 1992. Acute airsacculitis in untreated and cyclophosphamide-pretreated broiler chickens inoculated with Escherichia coli or Escherichia coli cell-free culture filtrate. Vet Pathol 29:68–78.
19. Dho, M., and J.P. Lafont. 1982. Escherichia coli colonization of the trachea in poultry: Comparison of virulent and avirulent strains in gnotoxenic chickens. Avian Dis 26:787–797.
20. Dho, M., and J.P. Lafont. 1984. Adhesive properties and iron uptake ability in Escherichia coli lethal and nonlethal for chicks. Avian Dis 28:1016–1025.
21. Dominick, M.A., and A.E. Jensen. 1984. Colonization and persistence of Escherichia coli in axenic and monoaxenic turkeys. Am J Vet Res 45:2331–2335.
22. Doyle, M.O., and J.L Schoeni. 1987. Isolation of Escherichia coli O157:H7 from retail fresh meats and poultry. Appl Environ Microbiol 53:2394–2396.
23. Dozois, C.M., N. Chanteloup, M. Dho-Moulin, A. Brée, C. Desautels, and J.M. Fairbrother. 1994. Bacterial colonization and in vivo expression of F1 (type 1) fimbrial antigens in chickens experimentally infected with pathogenic Escherichia coli. Avian Dis 38:231–239.
24. Droual, R., and P.R. Woolcock. 1994. Swollen head syndrome associated with E. coli and infectious bronchitis virus in the Central Valley of California. Avian Pathol 23:733–742.
25. Droual, R., R.P. Chin, and M. Rezvani. 1996. Synovitis, osteomyelitis, and green liver in turkeys associated with Escherichia coli. Avian Dis 40:417–424.
26. Emery, D.A., K.V. Nagaraja, D.P. Shaw, J.A. Newman, and D.G. White. 1992. Virulence factors of Escherichia coli associated with colisepticemia in chickens and turkeys. Avian Dis 36:504–511.
27. Ewing, W.H., H.W. Tatum, B.R. Davis, and R.W. Reavis. 1956. Studies on the serology of the Escherichia coli

group. U.S. Department of Health Education & Welfare, Public Health Service, Atlanta, GA, p. 42.

28. Farmer, J.J., III, and M.T. Kelly. 1991. Enterobacteriaceae. In A. Balow, W.J. Hausler, Jr., K.L. Herrmann, H.D. Isenberg, and H.J. Shadomy (eds.). Manual of Clinical Microbiology, 5th ed. American Society of Microbiologists, Washington, DC, pp. 360–383.

29. Ficken, M.D., J.F. Edwards, J.C. Lay, and D.E. Tveter. 1987. Tracheal mucus transport rate and bacterial clearance in turkeys exposed by aerosol to La Sota strain of Newcastle disease virus. Avian Dis 31:241–248.

30. Frommer, A., P.J. Freidlin, R.R. Bock, G. Leitner, M. Chaffer, and E.D. Heller. 1994. Experimental vaccination of young chickens with a live, non-pathogenic strain of Escherichia coli. Avian Pathol 23:425–433.

31. Fukui, H., M. Sueyoshi, M. Haritani, M. Nakazawa, S. Naitoh, H. Tani, and Y. Uda. 1995. Natural infection with attaching and effacing Escherichia coli (O 103:H⁻) in chicks. Avian Dis 39:912–918.

32. Griffin, P.M., and R.V. Tauxe. 1991. The epidemiology of infections caused by Escherichia coli O157:H7, other enterohemorrhagic E. coli and the associated hemolytic uremic syndrome. Epidemiol Rev 13:60–98.

33. Gross, W.B. 1961. The development of "air sac disease." Avian Dis 5:431–439.

34. Gross, W.B. 1964. Retained caseous yolk sacs caused by Escherichia coli. Avian Dis 8:438–441.

35. Gross, W.B. 1966. Electrocardiographic changes of Escherichia coli-infected birds. Am J Vet Res 27:1427–1436.

36. Gross, W.B. 1990. Factors affecting the development of respiratory disease complex in chickens. Avian Dis 34:607–610.

37. Gross, W.B. 1992. Effect of short-term exposure of chickens to corticosterone on resistance to challenge exposure with Escherichia coli and antibody response to sheep erythrocytes. Am J Vet Res 53:291–293.

38. Gross, W.B. 1994. Diseases due to Escherichia coli in poultry. In C.L. Gyles (ed.). Escherichia coli in Domestic Animals and Humans. CAB Int'l, Wallingford, United Kingdom, pp. 237–260.

39. Gross, W.B. 1995. Relationship between body-weight gain after movement of chickens to an unfamiliar cage and response to Escherichia coli challenge infection. Avian Dis 39:636–637.

40. Gross, W.B., and P.B. Siegel. 1959. Coliform peritonitis of chickens. Avian Dis 3:370–373.

41. Gyimah, J.E., and B. Panigrahy. 1988. Adhesin-receptor interactions mediating the attachment of pathogenic Escherichia coli to chicken tracheal epithelium. Avian Dis 32:74–78.

42. Gyimah, J.E., B. Panigrahy, and J.D. Williams. 1986. Immunogenicity of an Escherichia coli multivalent pilus vaccine in chickens. Avian Dis 30:687–689.

43. Harry, E.G. 1957. The effect on embryonic and chick mortality of yolk contamination with bacteria from the hen. Vet Rec 69:1433–1440.

44. Harry, E.G. 1964. The survival of E. coli in the dust of poultry houses. Vet Rec 76:466–470.

45. Harry, E.G., and L.A. Hemsley. 1965. The association between the presence of septicaemia strains of Escherichia coli in the respiratory and intestinal tracts of chickens and the occurrence of coli septicaemia. Vet Rec 77:35–40.

46. Harry, E.G., and L.A. Hemsley. 1965. The relationship between environmental contamination with septicaemia strains of Escherichia coli and their incidence in chickens. Vet Rec 77:241–245.

47. Heller, E.D., and N. Drabkin. 1977. Some characteristics of pathogenic Escherichia coli strains. Br Vet J 133:572–578.

48. Heller, E.D., and M. Perek. 1968. Pathogenic Escherichia coli strains prevalent in poultry flocks in Israel. Br Vet J 124:509–513.

49. Heller, E.D., G. Leitner, N. Drabkin, and D. Melamed. 1990. Passive immunisation of chicks against Escherichia coli. Avian Pathol 19:345–354.

50. Kwaga, J.K.P., B.J. Allan, J.V. van den Hurk, H. Seida, and A.A. Potter. 1994. A carAB mutant of avian pathogenic Escherichia coli serogroup O2 is attenuated and effective as a live oral vaccine against colibacillosis in turkeys. Infect Immun 62:3766–3772.

51. Lafont, J.-P., A. Brée, and M. Plat. 1984. Bacterial conjugation in the digestive tracts of gnotoxenic chickens. Appl Environ Microbiol 47:639–642.

52. Lafont, J.-P., M. Dho, M. d'Hauteville, A. Brée, and P.J. Sansonetti. 1987. Presence and expression of aerobactin genes in virulent avian strains of Escherichia coli. Infect Immun 55:193–197.

53. Leibovitz, L. 1972. A survey of the so-called "anatipestifer syndrome." Avian Dis 16:836–851.

54. Leitner, G., and E.D. Heller. 1992. Colonization of Escherichia coli in young turkeys and chickens. Avian Dis 36:211–220.

55. Leitner, G., D. Melamed, N. Drabkin, and E.D. Heller. 1990. An enzyme-linked immunosorbent assay for detection of antibodies against Escherichia coli: Association between indirect hemagglutination test and survival. Avian Dis 34:58–62.

56. Lior, H. 1994. Classification of Escherichia coli. In C.L. Gyles (ed.). Escherichia coli in Domestic Animals and Humans. CAB Int'l, Wallingford, United Kingdom, pp. 31–72.

57. Melamed, D., G. Leitner, and E.D. Heller. 1991. A vaccine against avian colibacillosis based on ultrasonic inactivation of Escherichia coli. Avian Dis 35:17–22.

58. Morishita, T.Y., and A.A. Bickford. 1992. Pyogranulomatous typhlitis and hepatitis of market turkeys. Avian Dis 36:1070–1075.

59. Morley, A.J., and D.K. Thomson. 1984. Swollen-head syndrome in broiler chickens. Avian Dis 28:238–243.

60. Myers, R.K., and L.H. Arp. 1987. Pulmonary clearance and lesions of lung and air sac in passively immunized and unimmunized turkeys following exposure to aerosolized Escherichia coli. Avian Dis 31:622–628.

61. Nagaraja, K.V., D.A. Emery, K.A. Jordan, V. Sivanandan, J.A. Newman, and B.S. Pomeroy. 1984. Effect of ammonia on the quantitative clearance of Escherichia coli from lungs, air sacs, and livers of turkeys aerosol vaccinated against Escherichia coli. Am J Vet Res 45:392–395.

62. Nagi, M.S., and L.G. Raggi. 1972. Importance to "airsac" disease of water supplies contaminated with pathogenic Escherichia coli. Avian Dis 16:718–723.

63. Nakamura, K., J.K.A. Cook, J.A. Frazier, and M. Narita. 1992. Escherichia coli multiplication and lesions in the respiratory tract of chickens inoculated with infectious bronchitis virus and/or E. coli. Avian Dis 36:881–890.

64. Nakamura, K., K. Imai, and N. Tanimura. 1996. Comparison of the effects of infectious bronchitis and infectious laryngotracheitis on the chicken respiratory tract. J Comp Pathol 114:11–21.

65. Nolan, L.K., R.E. Wooley, J. Brown, K.R. Spears, H.W. Dickerson, and M. Dekich. 1992. Comparison of a complement resistance test, a chicken embryo lethality test, and the chicken lethality test for determining virulence of avian Escherichia coli. Avian Dis 36:395–397.

66. Nolan, L.K., R.E. Wooley, and R.K. Cooper. 1992. Transposon mutagenesis used to study the role of complement resistance in the virulence of an avian Escherichia coli isolate. Avian Dis 36:398–402.

67. Nolan, L.K., R.E. Wooley, C.W. Giddings, and J. Brown. 1994. Characterization of an avirulent mutant of a virulent avian Escherichia coli isolate. Avian Dis 38:146–150.

68. Norton, R.A., B.A. Hopkins, J.K. Skeeles, J.N. Beasley, and J.M. Kreeger. 1992. High mortality of domestic

turkeys associated with Ascaridia dissimilis. Avian Dis 36:469–473.

69. Oyetunde, O.O.F., R.G. Thomson, and H.C. Carlson. 1978. Aerosol exposure of ammonia, dust and Escherichia coli in broiler chickens. Can Vet J 19:187–193.

70. Peighambari, S.M., J.-P. Vaillancourt, R.A. Wilson, and C.L. Gyles. 1995. Characteristics of Escherichia coli isolates from avian cellulitis. Avian Dis 39:116–124.

71. Peighambari, S.M., R.J. Julian, J.-P. Vaillancourt, and C.L. Gyles. 1995. Escherichia coli cellulitis: Experimental infections in broiler chickens. Avian Dis 39:125–134.

72. Pelkonen, S., and J. Finne. 1987. A rapid turbidimetric assay for the study of serum sensitivity of Escherichia coli. FEMS Microbiol Lett 42:53–57.

73. Randall, C.J., P.A. Meakins, M.P. Harris, and D.J. Watt. 1984. A new skin disease in broilers? Vet Rec 114:246.

74. Rosenberger, J.K., P.A. Fries, S.S. Cloud, and R.A. Wilson. 1985. In vitro and in vivo characterization of avian Escherichia coli. II. Factors associated with pathogenicity. Avian Dis 29:1094–1107.

75. Sandhu, T.S., and H.W. Layton. 1985. Laboratory and field trials with formalin-inactivated Escherichia coli (078)-Pasteurella anatipestifer bacterin in white Pekin ducks. Avian Dis 29:128–135.

76. Siccardi, F.J. 1966. Identification and disease producing ability of Escherichia coli associated with E. coli infection of chickens and turkeys. MS thesis, University of Minnesota, St. Paul, MN.

77. Smith, H.W., J.K.A. Cook, and Z.E. Parsell. 1985. The experimental infection of chickens with mixtures of infectious bronchitis virus and Escherichia coli. J Gen Virol 66:777–786.

78. Sojka, W.J. 1965. Escherichia coli in domestic animals and poultry. Commonwealth Agricultural Bureau, Farnham Royal, England.

79. Stanley, V.G., S. Woldesenbet, and C. Gray. 1996. Sensitivity of Escherichia coli O157:H7 strain 932 to selected anticoccidial drugs in broiler chickens. Poult Sci 75:42–46.

80. Stavric, S., B. Buchanan, and T.M. Gleeson. 1993. Intestinal colonization of young chicks with Escherichia coli O157:H7 and other verotoxin-producing serotypes. J Appl Bacteriol 74:557–563.

81. Stebbins, M.E., H.A. Berkhoff, and W.T. Corbett. 1992. Epidemiological studies of Congo red Escherichia coli in broiler chickens. Canadian J Vet Res 56:220–225.

82. Suwanichkul, A., B. Panigrahy, and R.M. Wagner. 1987. Antigenic relatedness and partial amino acid sequences of pili of Escherichia coli serotypes O1, O2, and O78 pathogenic for poultry. Avian Dis 31:809–813.

83. Toth, T.E., H. Veit, W.B. Gross, and P.B. Siegel. 1988. Cellular defense of the avian respiratory system: Protection against Escherichia coli airsacculitis by Pasteurella multocida-activated respiratory phagocytes. Avian Dis 32:681–687.

84. Van den Hurk, J.V., B.J. Allan, C. Riddell, T. Watts, and A.A. Potter. 1994. Effect of infection with hemorrhagic enteritis virus on susceptibility of turkeys to Escherichia coli. Avian Dis 38:708–716.

85. Vidotto, M.C., E.E. Müller, J.C. de Freitas, A.A. Alfieri, I.G. Guimarães, and D.S. Santos. 1990. Virulence factors of avian Escherichia coli. Avian Dis 34:531–538.

86. Wada, Y., H. Kondo, M. Nakazawa, and M. Kubo. 1995. Natural infection with attaching and effacing Escherichia coli and adenovirus in the intestine of a pigeon with diarrhea. J Vet Med Sci 57:531–533.

87. Weinack, O.M., G.H. Snoeyenbos, C.F. Smyser, and A.S. Soerjadi. 1981. Competitive exclusion of intestinal colonization of Escherichia coli in chicks. Avian Dis 25:696–705.

88. Weinack, O.M., G.H. Snoeyenbos, C.F. Smyser, and A.S. Soerjadi-Liem. 1984. Influence of Mycoplasma gallisepticum, infectious bronchitis, and cyclophosphamide on chickens protected by native intestinal microflora against Salmonella typhimurium or Escherichia coli. Avian Dis 28:416–425.

89. White, D.G., M. Dho-Moulin, R.A. Wilson, and T.S. Whittam. 1993. Clonal relationships and variation in virulence among Escherichia coli strains of avian origin. Microb Pathog 14:399–409.

90. Wittig, W., R. Prager, E. Tietze, G. Seltmann, and H. Tschäpe. 1988. Aerobactin-positive Escherichia coli as causative agents of extra-intestinal infections among animals. Arch Exp Veterinaermed 42:221–229.

91. Wooley, R.E., K.R. Spears, J. Brown, L.K. Nolan, and O.J. Fletcher. 1992. Relationship of complement resistance and selected virulence factors in pathogenic avian Escherichia coli. Avian Dis 36:679–684.

92. Wooley, R.E., K.R. Spears, J. Brown, L.K. Nolan, and M.A. Dekich. 1992. Characteristics of conjugative R-plasmids from pathogenic avian Escherichia coli. Avian Dis 36:348–352.

93. Wooley, R.E., L.K. Nolan, J. Brown, P.S. Gibbs, C.W. Giddings, and K.S. Turner. 1993. Association of K-1 capsule, smooth lipopolysaccharides, traT gene, and colicin V production with complement resistance and virulence of avian Escherichia coli. Avian Dis 37:1092–1096.

94. Wooley, R.E., L.K. Nolan, J. Brown, P.S. Gibbs, and D.I. Bounous. 1994. Phenotypic expression of recombinant plasmids pKT107 and pHK11 in an avirulent avian Escherichia coli. Avian Dis 38:127–134.

95. Wooley, R.E., J. Brown, P.S. Gibbs, L.K. Nolan, and K.R. Turner. 1994. Effect of normal intestinal flora of chickens on colonization by virulent colicin V-producing, avirulent, and mutant colicin V-producing avian Escherichia coli. Avian Dis 38:141–145.

96. Wray, C., and M.J. Woodward. 1994. Laboratory diagnosis of Escherichia coli infections. In C.L. Gyles (ed.). Escherichia coli in Domestic Animals and Humans. CAB Int'l, Wallingford, United Kingdom, pp. 595–628.

97. Yerushalmi, Z., N.I. Smorodinsky, M.W. Naveh, and E.Z. Ron. 1990. Adherence pili of avian strains of Escherichia coli O78. Infect Immun 58:1129–1131.

98. Yogaratnam, V. 1995. Analysis of the causes of high rates of carcass rejection at a poultry processing plant. Vet Rec 137:215–217.

5 Fowl Cholera

Richard B. Rimler and J. R. Glisson

INTRODUCTION. Fowl cholera (FC) (avian cholera, avian pasteurellosis, avian hemorrhagic septicemia) is a contagious disease affecting domesticated and wild birds. It usually appears as a septicemic disease associated with high morbidity and mortality, but chronic or benign conditions often occur. This disease is of historical importance because of its role in early development of bacteriology and because it was one of four diseases the Veterinary Division of the United States Department of Agriculture (USDA) was created to investigate.

HISTORY. Several epornitics among fowl occurred in Europe during the latter half of the 18th century. The disease was studied in France by Chabert in 1782, and in 1836 by Mailet, who first used the term *fowl cholera.* Huppe in 1886 referred to "hemorrhagic septicemia," and Lignieres in 1900 used the term *avian pasteurellosis.* Benjamin in 1851 gave a good description of the disease and demonstrated that it could be spread by cohabitation. With this knowledge of the disease he formulated procedures for its prevention. At about the same time, Renault, Reynal, and Delafond demonstrated its transmissibility to various species by inoculation. In 1877 and 1878, Perroncito of Italy and Semmer of Russia observed in tissues of affected birds a bacterium that had a rounded form and occurred singly or in pairs. In 1879, Toussaint isolated the bacterium and proved it was the sole cause of the disease (43).

Pasteur (105) isolated the organism and grew pure cultures in chicken broth. In further studies, Pasteur (106, 107) used the FC organism to perform his classic experiments in attenuation of bacteria for use in producing immunity. Salmon (133) appears to have been the first to study the disease in the United States. A good description of disease signs was reported, however, as early as 1867 in Iowa, where losses of chickens, turkeys, and geese had occurred (7).

INCIDENCE AND DISTRIBUTION. Fowl cholera occurs sporadically or enzootically in most countries. At some times it causes high mortality; at others, losses are nominal. Alberts and Graham (2) reported a loss of 68% within 6 days in a flock of 5½-mo-old turkeys. Vaught et al. (141) reported that over 1000 wild geese died of FC in one night. In studying the chronic respiratory form in chickens, Hall et al. (46) observed that mortality was low, but infection persisted for at least 4 yr.

Fowl cholera is more prevalent in late summer, fall, and winter. This seasonal occurrence is one of circumstance rather than lowered resistance, except that chickens become more susceptible as they reach maturity.

ETIOLOGY

Classification. *Pasteurella multocida* is the causative agent of FC. When pronouncing *multocida*, the accent should be on the *ci* (15) rather than on the *to* as given in the 7th and 8th editions of *Bergey's Manual.* In the past, the bacterium has been given many names, including *Micrococcus gallicidus,* 1883; *M. cholerae gallinarum,* 1885; *Octopsis cholerae gallinarum,* 1885; *Bacterium cholerae gallinarum,* 1886; *Bacillus cholerae gallinarum,* 1886; *P. cholerae-gallinarum,* 1887; *Coccobacillus avicidus,* 1888; *P. avicida,* 1889; *Bacterium multicidum,* 1899; *P. avium,* 1903; *Bacillus avisepticus,* 1903; *Bacterium avisepticum,* 1903; *Bacterium avisepticus,* 1912; and *P. aviseptica,* 1920 (15, 18).

For a while, each isolate of *P. multocida* was named according to the animal from which it was isolated, such as *P. avicida* or *P. aviseptica, P. muricida* or *P. muriseptica.* In 1929, it was suggested that all isolates be referred to as *P. septica* (146). This name was used mainly in the United Kingdom, and can be found in recent literature. *Pasteurella multocida,* proposed by Rosenbusch and Merchant (131), is now accepted as the official name in *Bergey's Manual* and is used exclusively throughout the world.

Morphology and Staining. *P. multocida* is a gram-negative, nonmotile, non–spore-forming rod occurring singly, in pairs, and occasionally as chains or filaments. It measures 0.2–0.4 x 0.6–2.5 μm, but tends to become pleomorphic after repeated subculture. A capsule can be demonstrated in recently isolated cultures, using indirect methods of staining (Fig. 5.1). In tissues, blood, and recently isolated cultures the organism stains bipolar (Fig. 5.2). Pili have been reported (41, 115).

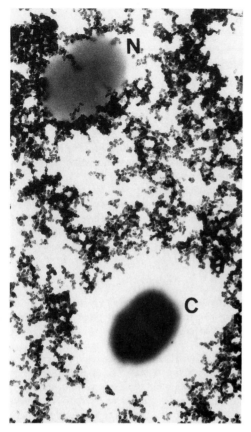

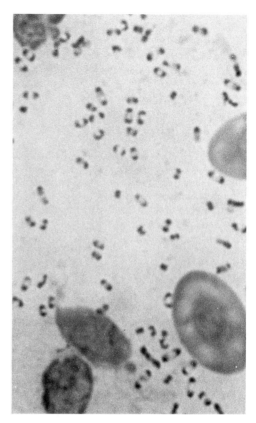

5.1. Electron photomicrograph of *Pasteurella multocida*–encapsulated cell (*C*) and nonencapsulated cell (*N*) suspended in India ink. ×19,000.

5.2. *Pasteurella multocida* in liver imprint from chicken with acute FC (note bipolarity). Wright's stain, ×2500.

Growth Requirements. *P. multocida* grows aerobically or anaerobically. The optimal growth temperature is 37 C. The optimal pH range is 7.2–7.8, but growth can occur in the range 6.2–9.0, depending upon composition of the medium. In liquid media, maximum growth is obtained in 16–24 hr. The broth becomes cloudy, and in a few days a sticky sediment collects. With some isolates a flocculent precipitate occurs.

The bacterium will grow on meat infusion media; growth is enhanced when the medium is enriched with peptone, casein hydrolysate, or avian serum. Blood or serum from some animals inhibits growth of *P. multocida*. Inhibition is greatest from blood of horses, cattle, sheep, and goats; blood of chickens, ducks, swine, and water buffalo has little or no inhibitory action (132). Several selective media for isolation have been described (22, 23, 38, 82, 94, 138). Chemically defined media have been described by Jordan (76), Watko (143), Wessman and Wessman (145) and Flossmann et al. (36). Berkman (11) found that pantothenic acid and nicotinamide are essential for growth. Dextrose starch agar with

5% avian serum is an excellent medium for isolating and growing *P. multocida*.

Colonial Morphology and Related Properties. Colonial morphology observed with obliquely transmitted light is one of the most useful characteristics in the study of *P. multocida*. On primary isolation from birds with FC, colonies may be iridescent, sectored with various intensities of iridescence, or blue with little or no iridescence (Fig. 5.3). Iridescence is related to the presence of a capsule. The term *fluorescent* used to describe colonies in older literature should be considered synonymous with the term *iridescent*; the latter is the appropriate term.

The composition of the medium determines to a certain extent the degree and type of iridescence. Occasionally an isolate produces blue colonies; when serum is added to the medium, sectored or iridescent colonies are sometimes produced. Examination of 18- to 24-hr colonies with a stereomicroscope using obliquely transmitted light (Fig. 5.4) is helpful when observing colonial morphology (64). Iridescent colonies on primary isolation from acute

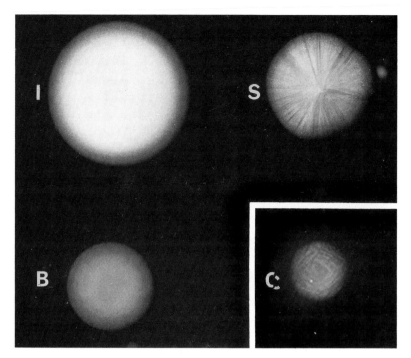

5.3. *Pasteurella multocida* 20-hr colonies on dextrose starch agar viewed with obliquely transmitted lighting (see Fig. 5.4); (*I*) iridescent, (*S*) sectored, (*B*) blue, and (*C*) rough. ×20.

cases of FC are circular (2–3 mm), smooth, convex, translucent, glistening, and butyrous, and show a tendency to coalesce. As the colony ages, it usually loses these distinguishing properties, becomes larger and viscous, and may adhere to the medium when picked with an inoculating needle. Blue colonies often isolated from birds with the chronic type of cholera or derived by dissociation of iridescent colonies are circular (1–2 mm), smooth, slightly convex or flat, translucent, butyrous, and discrete. The watery mucoid colonies produced by encapsulated strains from the respiratory tract of cattle, swine, sheep, rabbits, and humans are not iridescent but gray (58).

Anderson et al. (5) observed that a highly virulent isolate, which produced smooth colonies, later dissociated on subculture and produced rough colonies. Organisms from the smooth colonies were approximately 3–4 million times more virulent for pigeons than those from rough colonies. Hughes (66) studied the colonial morphology of 210 cultures from cases of FC and distinguished three types. The iridescent type was associated with outbreaks of acute FC and was highly virulent. The blue type was of low virulence and occurred in flocks in which cholera was enzootic. The third type was intermediate in its properties of iridescence and virulence.

Heddleston et al. (59) reported that a virulent isolate of *P. multocida* of avian origin produced iridescent colonies that dissociated in vitro and produced blue colonies. Organisms from blue colonies also mutated and produced gray colonies, which have not been reported in primary cultures from birds. Cells from iridescent colonies occurred singly or in pairs, did not agglutinate in immune serum, were encapsulated, and were virulent for chickens, turkeys, rabbits, and mice when administered on mucous membranes of the upper air passages. Cells

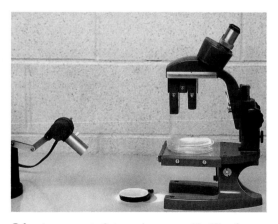

5.4. Arrangement of stereomicroscope with obliquely transmitted light for evaluation of colonial morphology.

from blue colonies occurred singly or in pairs, were agglutinated by immune serum, were unencapsulated, and were avirulent when applied to mucous membranes of chickens and mice, but were virulent for rabbits and slightly virulent for turkeys. Cells from gray colonies occurred only as chains and were unencapsulated and avirulent. Killed organisms from all three colonial forms induced immunity in chickens. Antigens extracted with hot saline from highly virulent encapsulated cells of iridescent colonies by Yaw and Kakavas (147) actively immunized chickens and mice, whereas less virulent unencapsulated cells from blue colonies immunized chickens more effectively than mice.

Physiologic Properties. The physiologic properties of *P. multocida* are used for identification. *P. multocida* does not produce gas but produces oxidase, catalase, peroxidase, and a characteristic odor. Unlike most gram-negative bacteria, it is sensitive to penicillin. The results of 29 other physiologic tests with 948 cultures of avian origin are shown in Table 5.1.

Significant differential characteristics are listed in Table 5.2.

Resistance to Chemical and Physical Agents. *P. multocida* is easily destroyed by or-

Table 5.1. Physiologic properties of 948 *Pasteurella multocida* cultures of avian origin

Test	% Positive
Arabinose	7.4
Dextrin	0.6
Dulcitol	2.6
Fructose	100.0
Galactose	99.8
Gelatin	0.0
Glucose	100.0
Glycerol	93.3
Hemolysis	0.0
Hydrogen sulfide	97.5
Indol	99.6
Inositol	0.0
Inulin	0.0
Lactose	1.6
Litmus milk	0.7
MacConkey agar	0.1
Maltose	0.0
Mannitol	99.5
Mannose	99.6
Motility	0.0
Nitrate reduction	100.0
Raffinose	2.7
Rhamnose	0.0
Salicin	0.0
Sorbitol	97.6
Sucrose	100.0
Trehalose	4.1
Urease	0.0
Xylose	77.4

Source: From (55).

Table 5.2. Differential tests for *Pasteurella multocida*, *P. haemolytica*, and *P. gallinarum*

Test	*P. multocida*	*P. haemolytica*	*P. gallinarum*
Hemolysis	−	+	−
MacConkey agar	−	+U	−
Indol	+	−	−
Motility	−	−	−
Gelatin	−	−	−
Catalase	+	+U	−
Oxidase	+	+	+
Urease	−	−	−
Glucose	+	+	+
Lactose	−U	+U	−
Sucrose	+	+	+
Maltose	−U	−U	+

Note: U = usually.

dinary disinfectants, sunlight, drying, or heat, being killed within 15 min at 56 C and 10 min at 60 C. A 1% solution of formaldehyde, phenol, sodium hydroxide, betapropiolactone, or glutaraldehyde and a 0.1% solution of benzalkonium chloride killed within 5 min 4.4×10^8 organisms of *P. multocida*/ml suspended in 0.85% saline solution at 24 C.

Das (22) observed that cotton swabs saturated with blood from infected mice contained viable organisms after 118 hr but not after 166 hr (at which time the swabs were completely dry); films of blood on glass contained viable organisms after 24 but not 30 hr. Das also reported that infected blood sealed in glass tubes and held in a cold room contained viable organisms after 221 days. Skidmore (137) observed that the organism survived in dried turkey blood on glass for 8 but not 30 days at room temperature. In studies of the influence of environment on the incidence of FC, Van Es and Olney (140) found the infection hazard had apparently disappeared from a poultry yard 2 wk after occurrence of the last death and removal of birds.

Influence of temperature on viability and virulence of *P. multocida* was studied by Nobrega and Bueno (100), who observed that broth cultures stored in sealed tubes at an average room temperature of 17.6 C were still virulent after 2 yr; at 2–4 C they were nonviable after 1 yr. With controlled experiments Dimov (28) observed that *P. multocida* died rapidly in soils with moisture content of less than 40%. At a moisture content of 50% and temperature of 20 C, it survived for 5–6 days at pH 5.0, 15–100 days at pH 7.0, and 24–85 days at pH 8.0. A culture survived without loss of virulence for 113 days in soil with 50% moisture at 3 C and pH 7.15.

Cultures may be maintained without dissociation or loss of virulence in the lyophilized state or sealed in glass tubes and stored at 4 C or colder (144). Lyophilized cultures tested after 26 yr were still virulent for chickens, and a culture sealed in a rubber-stoppered bottle containing beef infusion broth with

50% horse serum and held at room temperature was virulent after 26 yr (51).

Serotyping and Other Methods of Grouping Strains.

Serologic typing is based on methods that detect specific capsule and somatic antigens. Specific capsule serogroup antigens are recognized using passive hemagglutination tests (19). Five serogroups (A, B, D, E, and F) are currently recognized (127). Carter (19) studied numerous isolates from various animals and found serogroups A and D were isolated from fowl and other animals. In a study of isolates representing a variety of avian hosts, Rhoades and Rimler (118) found organisms belonging to serogroups A, B, D, and F. Presumptive identification of serogroups A, D, and F can be determined by capsule depolymerization with specific mucopolysaccharidases (125).

Somatic serotyping has been done by tube agglutination test (96) and gel diffusion precipitin test methods (61). Comparison studies by Brogden and Packer (16) indicated that a serotype determined by one method did not correlate with a serotype determined by the other method. Often, cultures that represented a single somatic serotype in a particular test represented more than one serotype in the other test. Because of its simplicity, the gel diffusion precipitin test is used routinely in the United States, and its popularity is increasing throughout the world. The test uses antisera prepared in chickens and heat-stable antigens extracted from formalinized saline suspensions of the bacteria. The heat-stable antigens form lines of identity with lipopolysaccharide–protein complexes from culture supernatants (61). Somatic serotype specificity seems to be determined by the lipopolysaccharide component of a complex (123). Heddleston et al. (61) found there was good, though not absolute, correlation between the gel diffusion precipitin test and the immune response in chickens and turkeys. Rimler and Phillips (126) found that lipopolysaccharide combined with carrier protein protected chickens against FC. To date, 16 somatic serotypes have been described (17). All of these somatic serotypes have been isolated from avian hosts. Rosenbusch and Merchant (131) placed isolates of *P. multocida* into three groups on the basis of fermentation of xylose, arabinose, and dulcitol. Group I fermented arabinose and dulcitol but not xylose; group II fermented xylose but not arabinose or dulcitol; group III was variable but more nearly like group I. Dorsey (31) studied fermentation reactions of 409 isolates of fowl origin and found that 81.42% were of group I, 16.87% of group II, and 1.71% of group III; 23 isolates could not be grouped on the basis of these reactions. Donahue and Olson (29) studied 214 isolates from turkeys: 0.47% were in group I; 83.64% in group II; 1.4% in group III; and 14% did not correlate with any of the groups.

Phage sensitivity as a basis for grouping *P. multocida* has been investigated. Rifkind and Pickett (122) found that 84 of 118 isolates from various hosts were sensitive to one or more of 16 bacteriophages. Kirchner and Eisenstark (80) examined 25 cultures of avian origin and found that 11 were lysogenic. They divided the 11 bacteriophages into five groups based on their host range, and into three groups based on plaque morphology. Karaivanov and Mraz (79) identified 87% of 77 cultures of *P. multocida* using one strain of bacteriophage. Saxena and Hoerlein (134) demonstrated lysogeny in 63 of 112 cultures from various hosts. One phage caused lysis of 8 different cultures; many were lysogenic for only 1 or 2 cultures. Gadberry and Miller (37) showed that 32 of 61 isolates were sensitive to 1 or more of 3 phages. Isolates of *P. haemolytica, P. gallinarum, P. ureae, P. pneumotropica,* and 3 species of the genus *Yersinia* were resistant to lysis. Results of these investigations demonstrated the possibility of a phage grouping system for *P. multocida.*

Pathogenicity.

Pathogenicity or virulence of *P. multocida* in relation to FC is complex and variable, depending on the strain, host species, and variations within the strain or host and conditions of contact between the two. The ability of *P. multocida* to invade and reproduce in the host is enhanced by the presence of a capsule (see Fig. 5.1) that surrounds the organism (86). Loss of ability of a virulent strain to produce the capsule results in loss of virulence (59). Many isolates from cases of fowl cholera have large capsules but are of low virulence. Therefore, virulence is apparently related to some chemical substance associated with the capsule, rather than with its physical presence.

P. multocida usually enters tissues of birds through mucous membranes of the pharnyx or upper air passages, but it may also enter through the conjunctiva or cutaneous wounds. Hughes and Pritchett (67) were unable to infect chickens by placing a culture in a gelatin capsule and inserting it into the esophagus, but chickens were infected when culture was dropped on the roof of the nasal cleft. Arsov (8) infected birds by mouth, using ^{35}P-labeled culture, and observed that the portal of infection was the mucous membrane of the mouth and pharnyx but not the esophagus, crop, or proventriculus. The eustachian tube was suggested by Olson and McCune (102) as the most likely route of infection, since it localizes in air spaces of the cranial bone, middle ear, and meninges.

Turkeys are much more susceptible than chickens to infection with *P. multocida,* and mature chickens are more susceptible than young ones (50). Hungerford (68) observed heavy losses in mature chickens, but no losses in birds up to 16 wk of age in a case involving 90,000 birds. When testing infectivity of an isolate or susceptibility of a host, cohabitation is the most natural method of exposure. Unless the host is highly susceptible and the isolate highly invasive, however, results may be slow. Therefore, it is often advantageous to swab the nasal cleft with cotton saturated with the culture; if a more severe exposure is required, culture can be injected parenterally.

Toxicity.   A dried culture filtrate of *P. multocida* was first demonstrated to produce signs of toxicity in chickens by Pasteur (105). Salmon (133) repeated this work and described signs resulting from toxicity similar to those observed in cases of acute FC. Kyaw (83), using the developing chick embryo in the study of pathogenesis, suggested that a toxin was produced in vivo by *P. multocida.* Rhoades (117) observed severe general passive hyperemia in chickens that died from acute FC. This lesion was considered to be indicative of shock and was attributed to action of endotoxin.

Endotoxins.   Endotoxins are produced by all *P. multocida,* both virulent and nonvirulent. They may contribute to virulence; however invasion and multiplication of a strain are necessary for production of sufficient quantities of endotoxin in vivo to contribute to pathologic processes.

Pirosky (111) obtained an endotoxin from *P. multocida* of avian origin by the trichloroacetic acid extraction procedure of Boivin. Heddleston and Rebers (55) demonstrated that a loosely bound endotoxin could be washed from *P. multocida* with cold formalinized saline solution. This endotoxin was a nitrogen-containing phosphorylated lipopolysaccharide, readily inactivated under mild acid conditions. Signs of acute FC were induced in chickens by injection of fractional amounts of endotoxin. The LD_{50} for chicken embryos was 5.2 µg via the chorioallantoic membrane; the LD_{50} for mice was 194 µg via the peritoneal cavity. One dose of 1.9 mg injected intravenously killed five of six 19-day-old turkeys; the median death time was only 3 hr. The endotoxin was present in the vascular system of turkeys with FC and could be detected with the Limulus lysate test and antiserum in the gel diffusion precipitin test. The serologic specificity of the endotoxin was associated with the lipopolysaccharide. Free endotoxin induced active immunity.

Purified lipopolysaccharides of each of the Heddleston serotypes were prepared by Rimler et al. (128). The lipopolysaccharides were similar to those of other gram-negative bacteria. Wk-old poults were relatively resistant to the lethal effects of purified lipopolysaccharides from two highly pathogenic FC strains of *P. multocida* (119). In poults, the lipopolysaccharides did not provoke a dermal Shwartzman reaction and lethality was not enhanced by a liver-damaging substance, a histamine-releasing substance, or surgical bursectomy.

Protein Toxins.   Heat-labile protein toxins have been found in serogroup A and D strains isolated from different animal species. Nielsen et al. (99) found 6 of 10 turkey strains produced heat-labile protein toxins; the strains were not serotyped. Four serogroup D strains isolated from turkeys were found to contain a heat-labile toxin (120). Sonicated suspensions of these strains produced necrotic lesions in turkey skin and were lethal to poults. Antiserum prepared against the heat-labile toxin from a swine strain neutralized the ability of the avian strain sonicated material to produce skin necrosis (121). Baba and Bito (9) chemically purified a protein toxin from an avian strain.

PATHOGENESIS AND EPIZOOTIOLOGY

Natural and Experimental Hosts.   Most reported outbreaks of FC affected chickens, turkeys, ducks, or geese. However, this disease also affects other types of poultry, game birds raised in captivity, companion birds, birds in zoos, and wild birds. The wide range of avian hosts in which FC has been reported suggests that all types of birds are susceptible.

Among types of poultry, turkeys are most affected. Most or all in an infected flock may die within a few days. The disease usually occurs in young mature turkeys, but all ages are highly susceptible. Under experimental conditions 90–100% of mature turkeys may die within 48 hr when exposed to a highly virulent strain of *P. multocida* by swabbing the palatine cleft or by contact with infected birds.

The disease in turkeys was first reported in detail by DeVolt and Davis (27), who described an outbreak in a flock of 175 turkeys in Maryland, where the mortality was 17%. Alberts and Graham (2) described outbreaks in four flocks of turkeys in which mortality was 17–68%. They emphasized that environmental stressors such as changes in climate, nutrition, injury, and excitement may have influenced the incidence and course of the disease.

Death losses from FC in chickens usually occur in laying flocks, because this age bird is more susceptible than younger chickens. Chickens less than 16 wk of age are generally quite resistant. Fowl cholera in young chickens usually is caused by serotype 1 and often occurs in conjunction with some other malady. Recent outbreaks of FC in six flocks of 20- to 46-day-old broilers, however, resulted from infections with serotypes 3; 1,3; and 3,4. Experimental challenge of 5-wk-old broilers with two representative strains (serotypes 3 and 1,3) resulted in mortality and lameness. In naturally infected chickens, mortality usually ranges from 0 to 20%, but greater losses have been reported. Reduced egg production and persistent localized infection often occur. Chickens are more susceptible to FC after withdrawal of feed and water or after abrupt change of diet (14). Heat or rough treatment on a shaking machine increased the incidence in chickens exposed experimentally (77, 78).

Under experimental conditions, 90–100% of mature chickens exposed by swabbing the palatine cleft may die within 24–48 hr, depending on the strain of *P. multocida* used, but only 10–20% usually die within a 2-wk period when exposed by contact with infected birds. Pritchett et al. (113) observed mortality of 35–45% in three houses of pullets. In one house, 45% of the birds died within 4 wk. In a flock of 45 birds that had survived an acute outbreak the previous year, no losses were observed, but the number of birds with localized lesions increased during winter. In South Carolina and adjoining areas, FC exists mainly as a persistent, subacute chronic disease that clinically resembles avian monocytosis (12).

Domestic geese and ducks are also highly susceptible to FC. Curtice (21) reported the disease in geese in Rhode Island, where about 3200 of a flock of 4000 died in a short period. Van Es and Olney (140) recognized the marked susceptibility of geese to FC, in using them to test for persistence of viable organisms in lots after removal of infected chickens. Fowl cholera in ducks is a serious problem on Long Island, where it was diagnosed on 32 of 68 commercial duck farms. Losses usually occur in ducks over 4 wk of age, and mortality may reach 50% (33).

Birds of prey, waterfowl, and other birds kept in zoologic gardens occasionally succumb to infection; *P. multocida* has been isolated from over 50 species of feral birds. During a 2½-yr survey, Faddoul et al. (34) isolated *P. multocida* from 13 (seven species) of 248 feral birds submitted to the diagnostic laboratory. Jaksic et al. (74) described an acute epornitic among pheasants, in which 1700 died. An outbreak in the San Francisco Bay area was reported to have been responsible for an estimated loss of 40,000 waterfowl (130). Gershman et al. (39) observed a serious outbreak among eider ducks (*Somateria mollissima*) in their nesting area 6 mi off the coast of Maine, where over 200 birds died and more than 100 nests were lost. Over 60,000 waterfowl died of FC during the winter of 1956–57 at the Muleshoe National Wildlife Refuge in Texas (75). Rosen (129) reported that there are two areas in the United States where fowl cholera is enzootic in waterfowl: the Muleshoe National Wildlife Refuge and the north central area of California. Both locations have had periodic outbreaks since 1944.

P. multocida from birds with FC will usually kill rabbits and mice, but other mammals are resistant to infection. According to Heddleston and Watko (57), rabbits, mice, pigeons, and sparrows died of acute septicemia when exposed intranasally to an isolate of *P. multocida* from an acute case of FC; rats, ferrets, guinea pigs, a sheep, a pig, and a calf did not show any clinical response to the same organism. One of 5 rats, 1 of 2 mink, and 11 of 19 mice fed viscera of infected chickens developed nasal infection, pneumonia, and fatal septicemia, respectively. A calf died of acute septicemia less than 18 hr after intramuscular (IM) exposure. Guinea pigs exposed by IM inoculation developed necrosis at the inoculation site; those exposed intraperitoneally usually died.

Horses, cattle, sheep, pigs, dogs, and cats are refractory to oral inoculation, and subcutaneous (SC) inoculation results in localized abscesses. All of these animals, however, may succumb to intravenous inoculation.

Transmission, Carriers, and Vectors. How FC is introduced into a flock is often impossible to determine. Chronically infected birds are considered to be a major source of infection. The only limit to the duration of the chronic carrier state is the life span of the infected bird. Free-flying birds having contact with poultry may be a source of FC organisms. Transmission of the organism through the egg seldom, if ever, occurs. A study of more than 2000 fresh and embryonated eggs from chickens infected with chronic FC yielded no evidence that *P. multocida* was transmitted through the egg (136).

Pritchett et al. (113, 114) and Pritchett and Hughes (112) examined three infected commercial flocks of white leghorns for *P. multocida*, and found that many birds harbored the organism in nasal clefts. Presence of the bacterium was related to severity of upper respiratory infection in the flocks. They concluded that the enzootic focus of infection was healthy nasal carriers. These studies, as well as those of Van Es and Olney (140) and Hall et al. (46), proved that survivors of an epornitic of FC may be reservoirs of infection. Dorsey and Harshfield (32) reported a higher incidence of FC during late summer and fall in South Dakota. Carrier birds among the older flock, held over for a 2nd yr, provided a reservoir of infection for young susceptible pullets housed with them.

Most species of farm animals may be carriers of *P. multocida*. Generally, these organisms, except for those from swine and possibly those from cats, are avirulent for fowl. Iliev et al. (70) isolated *P. multocida* from tonsils of 34 of 75 slaughtered cattle, 14 of 27 sheep, and 102 of 162 pigs. Isolates from cattle and sheep were not pathogenic for fowl, but all 18 isolates from pigs in areas where FC was common were highly pathogenic for fowl. Only 2 of 47 isolates from pigs in areas having low incidence of FC were pathogenic. Iliev et al. (71) also reported that healthy pigs that were carriers of *P. multocida* transmitted infection to fowl in the same enclosure.

Two isolates, serotypes 1:A and 5:A, from lungs of pigs with pneumonia, were studied by Murata et al. (95). Serotype 5:A was highly virulent for chickens, and serotype 1:A was avirulent. They found no cross-immunity in chickens between the 2 serotypes.

Gregg et al. (44) isolated two cultures from raccoons that were pathogenic for turkeys. They suggested that raccoons are a reservoir of *P. multocida* and the organisms may be transmitted to turkeys via the raccoon bite.

Contaminated crates, feed bags, or any equipment used previously for poultry may serve in introducing FC into a flock. Organisms are disseminated throughout the carcasses of birds that die of acute FC, and may serve as an infection source, especially since fowl tend to consume such carcasses. Hendrickson and Hilbert (63) were able to isolate *P. multocida* from the blood of a naturally infected chicken for 49 days preceding death. They noticed rapid increase in the number of organisms immediately preceding and following death, and that the organisms remained viable 2 mo at 5–10 C. Serdyuk and Tsimokh (135) demonstrated experimentally that sparrows, pigeons, and rats could become infected with *P. multocida* when exposed to chickens with FC and that they in turn could infect susceptible chickens. Sparrows and pigeons carried organisms without showing clinical signs, but 10% of infected rats developed acute pasteurellosis.

The possibility that insects may serve as vectors of FC has been investigated. Skidmore (137) experimentally transmitted FC to turkeys by feeding them flies that had previously fed on infected blood. He pointed out that under natural conditions, ingestion of flies might be a means of introducing the disease into a flock. Transmission by flies, however, is probably not common, as indicated by studies of Van Es and Olney (140). Although FC was maintained in two lots of chickens during the height of the fly season, there was no spread of the disease to adjoining lots separated only by poultry netting. Iovcev (73) observed that larvae, nymphs, and adult ticks (*Argas persicus*) contained *P. multocida* after feeding on infected hens. Petrov (109) demonstrated that the red mite (*Dermanyssus gallinae*) became infected with *P. multocida* after feeding on infected birds, but the mite did not transmit the organism.

Heddleston and Wessman (58) showed that 27 cultures of *P. multocida* from the upper respiratory tract of humans were not pathogenic for turkeys. Humans can become infected, however, and may infect poultry via excretion from the nose or mouth.

Dissemination of *P. multocida* within a flock is primarily by excretions from the mouth (Fig. 5.5), nose, and conjunctiva of diseased birds that contaminate their environment, particularly feed and water. Feces very seldom contain viable *P. multocida*;

however, Reis (116) found the organism in feces from 1 of 9 birds just before death. In the remaining 8 birds, the organisms were isolated only in feces collected from the cloacae of dead birds. Iliev et al. (72) demonstrated that *P. multocida* labeled with ^{32}P was inactivated in the proventriculus, and feces contained no viable *P. multocida*. Turkeys drinking from the same water trough with those experimentally infected with *P. multocida* developed FC (103).

Signs of Infection

ACUTE. Signs of infection in acute FC are often present for only a few hr before death. Unless infected birds are observed during this period, death may be the first indication of disease. Signs that often occur are fever, anorexia, ruffled feathers, mucous discharge from the mouth, diarrhea, and increased respiratory rate. Cyanosis often occurs immediately prior to death and is most evident in unfeathered areas of the head, such as comb and wattles. Fecal material associated with the diarrhea is initially watery and whitish in color, but later becomes greenish and contains mucus. Birds that survive the initial acute septicemic stage may later succumb to debilitating effects of emaciation and dehydration, may become chronically infected, or may recover.

CHRONIC. Chronic FC may follow an acute stage of the disease or result from infection with organ-

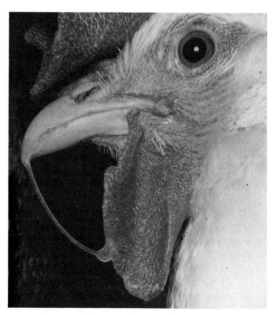

5.5. Acute FC; mucous excretion from the mouth contains large numbers of *Pasteurella multocida* that can contaminate feed and water.

isms of low virulence. Signs are generally related to localized infections. Wattles (Fig. 5.6), sinuses, leg or wing joints, foot pads, and sternal bursae often become swollen. Exudative conjunctival (Fig. 5.7) and pharyngeal lesions may be observed, and torticollis (Fig. 5.8) sometimes occurs. Tracheal rales and dyspnea may result from respiratory tract infections. In the past the term *roup* was used to indicate a condition in which signs were associated with chronic infections of cephalic mucous membranes. The term was not limited to FC, but included other diseases as well. Chronically infected birds may succumb, remain infected for long periods, or recover.

Gross and Microscopic Lesions.
Lesions of FC are not constant but vary in type and severity. The greatest variation is related to the course of the disease, whether acute or chronic. Although it is convenient for descriptive purposes to refer to either acute or chronic FC, it is sometimes difficult to categorize the disease in this manner. Signs of infection and lesions that occur may be intermediate to those described for acute and chronic forms.

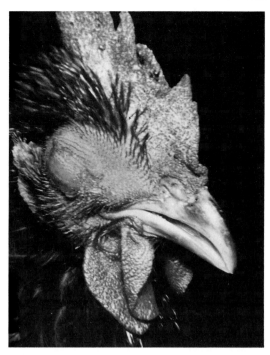

5.7. Chronic FC; serous inflammation of conjunctiva.

ACUTE. When the course of the disease is acute, most of the postmortem lesions are associated with vascular disturbances. General hyperemia usually occurs, is most evident in veins of the abdominal viscera, and may be quite pronounced in small vessels of the duodenal mucosa (Fig. 5.9). Large numbers of bacteria can usually be observed microscopically in the hyperemic vessels. Petechial and ecchymotic hemorrhages are frequently found and may be widely distributed. Subepicardial (Fig. 5.10A) and subserosal hemorrhages are common, as are hemorrhages in the lung, abdominal fat, and intestinal mucosa. Increased amounts of pericardial and peritoneal fluid frequently occur. Disseminated

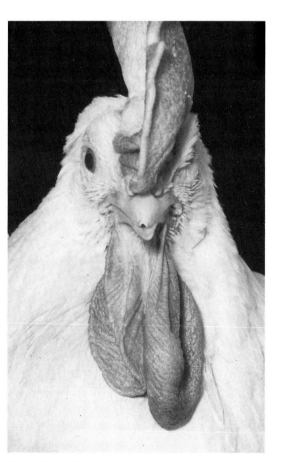

5.6. Chronic FC; swollen wattle resulting from localized infection.

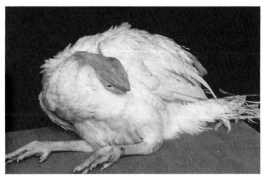

5.8. Chronic FC; torticollis resulting from meningeal infection.

intravascular clotting or fibrinous thrombosis has been observed in chickens and ducks that died from acute experimentally induced FC (69, 104).

Livers of acutely affected birds may be swollen, and usually contain multiple small focal areas of coagulative necrosis (Fig. 5.10B) and heterophilic infiltration (Fig. 5.11). Some of the less virulent *P. multocida* do not produce necrotic foci in the liver. Heterophilic infiltration also occurs in lungs and certain other parenchymatous organs (117). Lungs of turkeys are affected more severely than those of chickens, with pneumonia being a common sequela. Large amounts of viscid mucus may be observed in the digestive tract, particularly in the pharynx, crop, and intestine.

Ovaries of laying hens are commonly affected. Mature follicles often appear flaccid; thecal blood vessels, which are normally easily observed, are less evident (Fig. 5.10E). Yolk material from ruptured follicles may be found in the peritoneal cavity. Immature follicles and ovarian stroma are often hyperemic.

CHRONIC. Chronic FC is usually characterized by localized infections, in contrast to the septicemic nature of the acute disease. These generally become suppurative and may be widely distributed anatomically. They often occur in the respiratory tract and may involve any part, including sinuses and pneumatic bones (Fig. 5.12). Pneumonia (Fig. 5.10C,D) is an especially common lesion in turkeys. Infections of the conjunctiva and adjacent tissues occur (see Fig. 5.7), and facial edema may be observed.

5.10. *A.* Acute FC; subepicardial hemorrhages in a turkey. *B.* Acute FC; multiple necrotic foci in turkey liver. *C.* Acute FC; turkey lung with extensive hemorrhage and patchy areas of necrosis (*arrow*) and emphysema. *D.* Submassive necrosis with fibrous exudate on pleural surface. *E.* Acute FC; flaccid ovarian follicle (*arrow*) with thecal blood vessels less evident than normal. *F.* Chronic FC; caseous exudate in sternal bursa (*A*) and hock joint (*B*) of a turkey.

Localized infections may also involve the hock joints (Fig. 5.10F), foot pads, peritoneal cavity, and oviduct.

Chronic localized infections can involve the middle ear and cranial bones and have been reported to result in torticollis. In turkeys, torticollis and eventual death can be associated with infections of the cranial bones, middle ear, and meninges. In a study of naturally infected turkeys exhibiting torticollis, Olson (101) described lesions at these sites. The outstanding gross lesion was yellowish caseous exudate in air spaces of the calvarial bones. Heterophilic infiltration and fibrin were consistently observed in the air spaces, middle ear, and

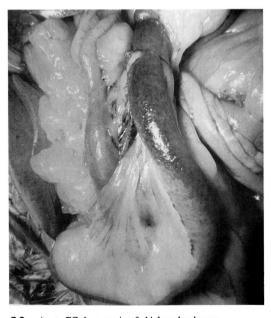

5.9. Acute FC; hyperemia of chicken duodenum.

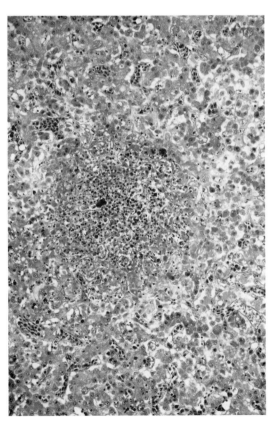

5.11. Acute FC; coagulative necrosis and heterophilic infiltration in turkey liver. H & E, ×600.

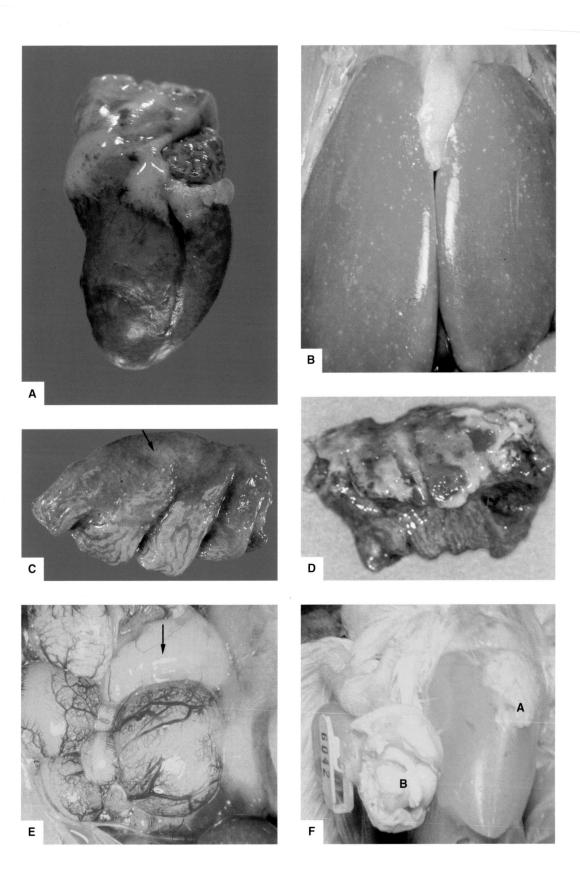

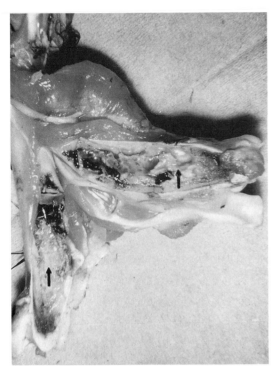

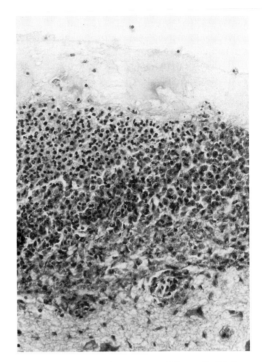

5.12. Chronic FC; caseous exudate (*arrows*) in turkey humerus.

5.13. Chronic FC; fibrinoheterophilic meningitis in turkey. H & E, ×400.

meninges. Multinuclear giant cells were often associated with necrotic masses of heterophils in air spaces. Similar lesions were found in experimentally exposed turkeys (102). Localized meningeal infections (Fig. 5.13) without involvement of cranial bones or the middle ear have been observed in turkeys exhibiting torticollis, as have cerebellar infections (35).

Immunity. Pasteur (107) used an avirulent culture attenuated by prolonged growth on artificial medium and produced immunity that protected fowl against subsequent exposure. In field use, his method did not prove practical because uniform attenuation could not be obtained and heavy losses sometimes occurred in vaccinated flocks.

Since Pasteur's classic work there have been numerous attempts to produce efficient vaccines against FC, but results have not been consistent. There can be little doubt, however, that a substantial, but not absolute, immunity can be induced in fowl by using killed *P. multocida* vaccines under controlled conditions (10, 52). Killed *P. multocida* vaccines are usually prepared by growing selected immunogenic strains on a suitable medium and suspending in formalinized saline solution. The killed organisms are usually incorporated with an adjuvant and injected subcutaneously.

Under field conditions, losses from FC sometimes occur in vaccinated flocks. This failure may be due to improperly prepared or administered vaccine or immune impaired birds. Heddleston and Reisinger (56) demonstrated that stress caused by changing the social or peck order of vaccinated males, as well as fowl pox infection in chickens at time of vaccination and exposure, significantly reduced the efficacy of vaccination. In experimental studies (110), the manifestation of acquired resistance was impaired in turkeys vaccinated against *P. multocida* while receiving aflatoxin in their feed. It was also observed that an isolate of *P. multocida* recovered from an FC outbreak in previously vaccinated turkeys differed serologically from the culture used in preparing vaccine (60).

In experimental studies, Heddleston and Rebers (54) showed that bacterins prepared with tissues from infected turkeys or live *P. multocida* administered in drinking water will induce immunity in turkeys against a different immunogenic type. A bacterin prepared with bacteria grown on conventional agar media did not induce cross-immunity. These studies indicate that *P. multocida* produces a wider spectrum of immunogens in vivo than in vitro. Rimler (124) showed that turkeys vaccinated with in vivo–grown *P. multocida* and challenged with the homologous strain produced serum that passively immunized poults against five different serotypes. Bierer and others at Clemson University stimulated renewed interest in live FC vaccine administered in drinking water. Bierer and Derieux (13) demonstrated good immunity in 14-wk-old turkeys that were given a live culture of *P. multocida* (CU strain, previously CS-148) in drinking water 2 wk before challenge exposure. The vaccine, however, killed 4.2% of 120 turkeys. Best results were obtained by inoculating 8-wk-old turkeys with a killed bacterin and then administering the live vaccine 2 wk later; the live vaccine killed only 2.5% of 120 turkeys. Derieux and Bierer (26) stated that good immunity may be obtained in 6-wk-old turkeys by administering 2 doses of vaccine in drinking water on the same day and repeating the vaccination 4 wk later. No data were given, however, as to duration of immunity or number of turkeys killed by vaccination. The CU strain administered in drinking water was immunologically less effective in chickens than in turkeys. It was more effective in chickens by wing-web or SC inoculation than in drinking water (25). Live vaccines are commercially available for oral administration to turkeys and parenteral administration to chickens.

Maheswaran et al. (85) also induced immunity in turkeys with live vaccines via drinking water; they suggested that the vaccine induced localized, but not systemic, protection. In other studies, Heddleston et al. (62) showed that serum from birds vaccinated via drinking water would induce passive immunity in chicks and turkeys.

Passive immunity for prevention of FC was studied in 1892 by Kitt, who used immune horse serum. This method was employed frequently, but because of the short duration of passive immunity it is presently used little if at all. Bolin and Eveleth (14) reported that *P. multocida* antiserum prepared in chickens gave maximum protection 16–24 hr after injection; protection began to decline after 48 hr and had disappeared after 192 hr.

DIAGNOSIS.   A presumptive diagnosis of FC may be made from clinical observations, necropsy findings, or isolation of *P. multocida*; a conclusive diagnosis should be based on all three. Signs and lesions of the disease were described previously.

Isolation and Identification.   *P. multocida* can be isolated readily from viscera of birds that die of acute FC, and usually from lesions of chronic cases; it is less likely to be isolated from dehydrated, emaciated survivors of an acute outbreak. A tentative diagnosis of acute FC can be made by demonstrating bipolar organisms in liver imprints (see Fig. 5.2) using Wright's stain. Immunofluorescent microscopy can be used to identify *P. multocida* in tissue or exudate (87).

Bone marrow, heart blood, liver, meninges, or lo-calized lesions are preferred for culturing. To isolate *P. multocida,* sear the tissue or exudate with a spatula and obtain a specimen by inserting a sterile cotton swab or wire loop through the seared surface. If birds are living, squeeze mucus from the nostril or insert a cotton swab into the nasal cleft. Transfer the specimen to peptone broth and streak on dextrose starch agar containing 5% chicken serum or other suitable media. Specimens may also be streaked on MacConkey and blood agar media to aid in identification.

Colonies characteristic of *P. multocida* (described under Etiology) are transferred to dextrose starch agar slants incubated 18–24 hr. Tubes of phenol red broth base containing 1% glucose, lactose, sucrose, mannitol, and maltose respectively are then inoculated with growth from the slant. Fermentation of glucose, sucrose, and mannitol without gas is characteristic of *P. multocida.* Lactose is usually not fermented, but some avian isolates will ferment it. Inoculate 2% tryptose in 0.85% saline solution, incubate 24 hrs at 37 C and test for indole (Kovac's test). Indole is almost always produced by *P. multocida.* There should be no hemolysis of blood and no growth on MacConkey agar (Table 5.2).

Inoculation of animals may be used as an aid in isolating *P. multocida* from contaminated materials. Rabbits, hamsters, or mice are inoculated subcutaneously or intraperitoneally with 0.2 mL exudate or minced tissue. If *P. multocida* is present, the animal usually dies within 24–48 hr, and the organism can be isolated in pure culture from heart, blood, or liver.

Serologic diagnosis of FC by rapid whole-blood agglutination, serum plate agglutination, or agar diffusion tests has limited value in chronic cholera, and no value with the acute form of the disease.

Differential Diagnosis.   *P. gallinarum* and *P. haemolytica* are two closely related bacteria that may be isolated from diseased poultry and incorrectly identified as *P. multocida* (53). *P. gallinarum* was first described by Hall et al. (46), who isolated it along with *P. multocida* from chickens with other maladies characterized by inflammation of the upper respiratory tract. The gel diffusion precipitin test shows a common antigen between *P. gallinarum* and *P. multocida.* Clark and Godfrey (20) found *P. gallinarum* associated with a respiratory disease complex of chickens in southern California. Gilchrist (40), in a survey of avian respiratory diseases in New South Wales, reported finding *P. gallinarum, P. haemolytica,* and *P. multocida.* Harbourne (48) isolated *P. haemolytica* on four occasions from livers of young chickens and turkeys. *P. haemolytica* was isolated from young chickens with salpingitis, which was often accompanied by nasal catarrh, helminth infection, or leukosis; the organism was also isolated from lungs of fowl with chronic respiratory disease and infectious bronchitis (98). Matthes et al. (88) isolated *P. haemolytica* from chickens with a septicemia. Chloramphenicol was effective in treatment. Hacking and Pettit (45) reported on 8 cases of *P. haemolytica* in pullets and laying hens: 5 cases involved egg production, with some birds showing peritonitis or salpingitis; 3 cases involved mortality; some birds had enteritis, enteritis and hepatitis, or respiratory infection. In most cases, *P. haemolytica* was thought to be a secondary pathogen.

Differential characteristics of various species of *Pasteurella* that may be isolated from poultry are listed in Table 5.2.

TREATMENT. Antibacterial chemotherapy has been used extensively in treatment of FC with varying success, depending to a large extent on the promptness of treatment and drug used. Sensitivity testing is often advantageous, since strains of *P. multocida* vary in susceptibility to chemotherapeutic agents (30, 142) and resistance to treatment may develop, especially during prolonged use of these agents.

Sulfonamides. Several of the sulfonamides have been employed both experimentally and in naturally occurring outbreaks. The main disadvantages of the sulfonamides are their bacteriostatic instead of bactericidal action, inability to cure localized abscesses, and toxic effect on birds. Kiser et al. (81) reported 63–85% reduction in mortality from experimentally produced FC compared with untreated controls when using sulfamethazine and sodium sulfamethazine. In naturally occurring outbreaks, mortality was reduced 45–75%. Favorable results were obtained with 0.5–1% of the drug in food, or 0.1% in drinking water.

Alberts and Graham (3) employed 0.5% sulfamerazine in mash feed for 5 days in a field outbreak of FC in turkeys. Mortality was 1.9% in the treated group compared with 50% in untreated birds. Fowl cholera recurred four times after cessation of treatment, and each time losses were arrested after turkeys were again given the sulfamerazine-mash mixture. In experimental infection in turkeys, sodium sulfamerazine at oral dosage rates of 143 and 107.25 mg/kg body weight effectively reduced mortality. In chickens, 0.2% sodium sulfamerazine in drinking water or 0.4% sulfamerazine in mash checked mortality in an established outbreak 2 days after treatment was started (1). Sulfaquinoxaline in amounts of 0.01–0.05% in drinking water was completely prophylactic in experimental FC when treatment was started 24 hr before birds were inoculated. Peterson (108) treated two naturally occurring outbreaks in turkey flocks successfully with 1:2000–1:4000 dilution of the drug in drinking water. He found sulfamethazine and sodium sulfamerazine also were markedly effective in reducing experimental FC; sulfadiazine, sulfathiazole, and sulfanilamide were much less so. Sulfaquinoxaline was used by Delaplane (24) at the rate of 0.1% or 0.05% in mash in prophylaxis of FC in chickens. Nelson (97) reported favorable results in controlling mortality in turkeys with a concentration of 0.025% sulfaquinoxaline in drinking water for 5–7 days; he stated also that its administration 1 day out of 4 usually controls later mortality and permits the grower to finish birds for market. Dorsey and Harshfield (32) confirmed the usefulness of several sulfonamide drugs in checking losses from FC if treatment is carried out in early stages of an outbreak. They also noted frequent recurrence of mortality after treatment was discontinued, and unsatisfactory results of treatment after the disease had become chronic.

Sulfaethoxypyridazine was reported by Stuart et al. (139) to be effective in controlling FC in chickens and turkeys. Effectiveness of the drug was dependent in part on size of dose, and duration and promptness of treatment. Sulfadimethoxine, used alone or potentiated with ormetoprim, was found to be safe, palatable, and effective against experimentally induced FC in chickens and turkeys (90, 91, 92, 93, 139). Anderson et al. (6) reported that sulfachloropyrazine administered in drinking water was effective in preventing mortality in experimentally exposed chickens.

Antibiotics. Streptomycin given IM in a dose of 150,000 µg prevented deaths in adult turkeys when administered before or at the time of inoculation of *P. multocida*. When treatment was delayed for 6–24 hr or dosage was reduced, chronic infection resulted (89). Penicillin, streptomycin, penicillin and streptomycin, and oxytetracycline (administered IM at the time of experimental exposure of chickens) all possessed activity as therapeutic agents (12). Chlortetracycline reduced losses in chicks about 80% when given at the rate of 40 mg/kg body weight IM 30 min after parenteral inoculation of the organism (84). Chicks that received mash containing 1 mg/g had 50% fewer losses than untreated controls. In an outbreak of FC in pheasants, however, Alberts and Graham (4) did not observe any beneficial results when 1 mg/g mash was fed. When chlortetracycline was given IM, a slight reduction in mortality was recorded. Novobiocin administered in feed or water reduced death losses in experimentally exposed turkeys (47). Chloramphenicol (20 mg/kg body weight) in a single IM injection was effective in treating FC, but in flocks where FC and fowl typhoid or fowl pox were concurrently present, chloramphenicol treatment was not successful (65). A chloramphenicol–dexamethasone–pyribenzamine combination was used successfully with vaccination in treatment of FC in breeding turkeys. Respiratory problems, which occurred 1 wk after the initial outbreak, responded readily to IM administration of this drug combination (42). Water-soluble erythromycin at the rate of 1 lb/50 gal drinking water halted mortality in two flocks of Muscovy ducklings infected with *P. multocida* (49).

Antibiotics used in rations at very low levels for promotion of growth, according to the experiments of Dorsey and Harshfield (32), did not significantly influence the course of FC infection in inoculated birds. At therapeutic levels, birds that received penicillin and streptomycin in feed died at about the same rate as controls. No deaths occurred in groups that received sulfaquinoxaline or sulfamerazine. These workers found oxytetracycline and chlortetracycline effective also in preventing mortality in experimental FC in a small flock of laying birds; mortality was 80% in an untreated group compared with 12% in a group receiving mash containing oxytetracycline at the level of 500 g/ton. In six naturally occurring outbreaks, oxytetracycline at this level in feed checked mortality, but losses returned in three flocks after withdrawal of the antibiotic.

PREVENTION AND CONTROL

Management Procedures. Prevention of FC can be effected by eliminating reservoirs of *P. multocida* or by preventing their access to poultry flocks. Good management practices, with emphasis on sanitation as prescribed by Zander, Bermudez, and Mallinson (see Chapter 1), are the best means of preventing FC. Unlike many bacterial diseases, FC is not a disease of the hatchery. Infection therefore occurs after birds are in the hands of the producer, and consideration must be given to the many ways that infection might be introduced into a flock.

The primary source of infection is usually sick birds or those that have recovered and still carry the causative organism. Only young birds should be introduced as new stock; they should be raised in a clean environment completely isolated from other birds. Isolation should be extended to housing. Unless separate houses can be provided for 1st- and 2nd-yr layer flocks, the older flock should be marketed in its entirety. Different species of birds should not be raised on the same premises. The danger of mixing birds from different flocks cannot be overemphasized. Farm animals (particularly pigs, dogs, and cats) should not have access to the poultry area. Water fountains should be self-cleaning and feeders covered to prevent contamination as much as possible.

That *P. multocida* has been recovered from many species of free-flying birds warrants consideration of this source of infection to poultry, with measures taken to prevent their association with the flock. Raising turkeys in areas where FC is a serious prob-

lem may warrant their confinement in houses from which free-flying birds, rodents, and other animals can be excluded. If an outbreak of FC occurs, the flock should be quarantined and disposed of as soon as economically feasible. All housing and equipment should be cleaned and disinfected before repopulation.

Immunization. Vaccination should be considered in areas where FC is prevalent, but it should not be substituted for good sanitary practice. Commercially produced bacterins and live vaccines are available. Bacterins usually contain whole cells of serotypes 1, 3, and 4 emulsified in an oil adjuvant. Autogenous local strains are also commonly used. Three live vaccines available for use in the United States are CU, a strain of low virulence; M-9, a mutant of CU with very low virulence; and PM-1, a mutant of CU intermediate in virulence between CU and M-9. Bacterins are inoculated SC in both chickens and turkeys. Live vaccines are administered in the drinking water to turkeys and by wing-web stab in chickens.

Bacterins, live vaccines, or both are used with broiler breeders. Usually two doses of bacterin are given, the first at 8–10 wk of age and the second at 18–20 wk of age. Protection occurs only against serotypes contained in the bacterin and does not give solid immunity for an entire laying cycle. Live vaccine, when given to broiler breeders, is usually given in a schedule similar to that of bacterin. Live vaccination results in a long-term, broad-spectrum protection, but the vaccines often cause chronic FC. A third program involves administration of bacterin at 8–10 wk of age, followed by live vaccine at 18–20 wk of age. This program usually gives broad protection and minimizes live vaccine–induced disease.

Meat turkeys are almost exclusively vaccinated with live vaccines. The first vaccination is at 6–8 wk, followed every 4–6 wk with another vaccination until market age. Bacterins are used in breeder turkeys, and they are vaccinated 2–5 times before the onset of egg production, with the first vaccination beginning at 6–8 wk.

REFERENCES

1. Alberts, J.O. 1950. The prophylactic and therapeutic properties of sulfamerazine in fowl cholera. Am J Vet Res 11:414–420.
2. Alberts, J.O., and R. Graham. 1948. Fowl cholera in turkeys. North Am Vet 29:24–26.
3. Alberts, J.O., and R. Graham. 1948. Sulfamerazine in the treatment of fowl cholera in turkeys. Am J Vet Res 9:310–313.
4. Alberts, J.O., and R. Graham. 1951. An observation on aureomycin therapy of fowl cholera in pheasants. Vet Med 46:505–506.
5. Anderson, L.A.P., M.G. Coombes, and S.M.K. Mallick 1929. On the dissociation of Bacillus avisepticus. Indian J Med Res 29:611–622.

6. Anderson, N.G., W.C. Alpaugh, and C.O. Baughn. 1974. Effect of sulfachloropyrazine in the drinking water of chickens infected experimentally with fowl cholera. Avian Dis 18:410–415.

7. Anonymous. 1867. Poultry Diseases, USDA Monthly Rep, pp. 216–217.

8. Arsov, R. 1965. The portal of infection in fowl cholera. Nauchni Tr Vissh Vet Med Inst 14:13–17.

9. Baba, T., and Y. Bito. 1966. Studies on the toxin of Pasteurella multocida. Jpn J Bacteriol 21:711–714.

10. Bairey, M.H. 1975. Immune response to fowl cholera antigens. Ann J Vet Res 36:575–578.

11. Berkman, S. 1942. Accessory growth factor requirements of the members of the genus Pasteurella. J Infect Dis 71:201–211.

12. Bierer, B.W. 1962. Treatment of avian pasteurellosis with injectable antibiotics. J Am Vet Med Assoc 141:1344–1346.

13. Bierer, B.W., and W.T. Derieux. 1972. Immunologic response of turkeys to an avirulent Pasteurella multocida vaccine in the drinking water. Poult Sci 51:408–416.

14. Bolin, F.M., and D.F. Eveleth. 1951. The use of biological products in experimental fowl cholera. Proc 88th Annu Meet Am Vet Med Assoc, pp. 110–112.

15. Breed, R.S., E.G.D. Murray, and N.R. Smith. 1957. Bergey's Manual of Determinative Bacteriology, 7th ed. Williams & Wilkins, Baltimore, MD.

16. Brogden, K.A., and R.A. Packer. 1979. Comparison of Pasteurella multocida serotyping systems. Am J Vet Res 40:1332–1335.

17. Brogden, K.A., K.R. Rhoades, and K.L. Heddleston. 1978. A new serotype of Pasteurella multocida associated with fowl cholera. Avian Dis 22:185–190.

18. Buchanan, R.E., J.G. Holt, and E.F. Lessel. 1966. Index Bergeyana. Williams & Wilkins, Baltimore, MD.

19. Carter, G.R. 1955. Studies on Pasteurella multocida. I. A hemagglutination test for the identification of serological types. Am J Vet Res 16:481–484.

20. Clark, D.S. and J.F. Godfrey. 1960. Atypical Pasteurella infections in chickens. Avian Dis 4:280–290.

21. Curtice, C. 1902. Goose septicemia. Univ RI Agric Exp Stn Bull 86:191–203.

22. Das, M.S. 1958. Studies on Pasteurella septica (Pasteurella multocida). Observations on some biophysical characteristics. J Comp Pathol Ther 68:288–294.

23. de Jong, M.F., and G.H.A. Borst. 1985. Selective media for the isolation of P. multocida and B. bronchiseptica. Vet Rec 116:167.

24. Delaplane, J.P. 1945. Sulfaquinoxaline in preventing upper respiratory infection of chickens inoculated with infective field material containing Pasteurella avicida. Am J Vet Res 6:207–208.

25. Derieux, W.T. 1978. Responses of young chickens and turkeys to virulent and avirulent Pasteurella multocida administered by various routes. Avian Dis 22:131–139.

26. Derieux, W.T., and B.W. Bierer. 1975. The CU strain of Pasteurella multocida. Proc 24th West Poult Dis Conf, pp. 64–66.

27. DeVolt, H.M., and C.R. Davis. 1932. A cholera-like disease in turkeys. Cornell Vet 22:78–80.

28. Dimov, I. 1964. Survival of avian Pasteurella multocida in soils at different acidity, humidity and temperature. Nauchni Tr Vissh Vet Med Inst Sofia 12:339–345.

29. Donahue, J.M., and L.O. Olson. 1972. Biochemic study of Pasteurella multocida from turkeys. Avian Dis 16:501–505.

30. Donahue, J.M., and L.O. Olson. 1972. The in vitro sensitivity of Pasteurella multocida of turkey origin to various chemotherapeutic agents. Avian Dis 16:506–511.

31. Dorsey, T.A. 1963. Studies on fowl cholera. I. A biochemic study of avian Pasteurella multocida strains. Avian Dis 7:386–392.

32. Dorsey, T.A., and G.S. Harshfield. 1959. Studies on control of fowl cholera. South Dakota State Univ Agric Exp Stn Bull 23:1–18.

33. Dougherty, E. 1953. Disease problems confronting the duck industry. Proc 90th Annu Meet Am Vet Med Assoc, pp 359–365.

34. Faddoul, G.P., G.W. Fellows, and J. Baird. 1967. Pasteurellosis in wild birds in Massachusetts. Avian Dis 11:413–418.

35. Fenstermacher, R., and B.S. Pomeroy. 1941. Encephalitis-like symptoms in turkeys associated with a Pasteurella sp. Cornell Vet 31:295–301.

36. Flossmann, K.D., Feist, H., Hofer, M., and W. Erler. 1974. Untersuchungen uber chemisch definierte nahrmedien fur Pasteurella multocida und P. haemolytica. Z Allg Mikrobiol 14:29–38.

37. Gadberry, J.L., and N.G. Miller. 1977. Use of bacteriophages as an adjunct in the identification of Pasteurella multocida. Am J Vet Res 38:129–130.

38. Garlinghouse, L.E., DiGiacomo, R.F., Van Hoosier, G.L. and J. Condon. 1971. Selective media for Pasteurella multocida and Bordetella bronchiseptica. J Lab Anim Sci 31:39–42.

39. Gershman, M., J.F. Witter, H.E. Spencer, and A. Kalvaitis. 1964. Epizootic of fowl cholera in the common eider duck. J Wildl Manage 28:587–589.

40. Gilchrist, P. 1963. A survey of avian respiratory disease. Aust Vet J 39:140–144.

41. Glorioso, J.C., G.W. Jones, H.G. Rush, L.J. Pentler, C.A. Darif and J.E. Coward. 1982. Adhesion of type A Pasteurella multocida to rabbit pharyngeal cells and its possible role in rabbit respiratory tract infection. Infect Immun 35:1103–1109.

42. Grant, G., A.M. Russell, and D.McK. Fraser. 1968. Treatment of fowl cholera. Vet Rec 83:419.

43. Gray, H. 1913. Some diseases of birds. In E.W. Hoare (ed.). A System of Veterinary Medicine, vol. 1. Alexander Eger, Chicago, pp. 420–432.

44. Gregg, D.A., L.O. Olson, and E.L. McCune. 1974. Experimental transmission of Pasteurella multocida from raccoons to turkeys via bite wounds. Avian Dis 18:559–564.

45. Hacking, W.C., and J.R. Pettit. 1974. Pasteurella hemolytica in pullets and laying hens. Avian Dis 18:483–486.

46. Hall, W.J., K.L. Heddleston, D.H. Legenhausen, and R.W. Hughes. 1955. Studies on pasteurellosis: I. A new species of Pasteurella encountered in chronic fowl cholera. Am J Vet Res 16:598–604.

47. Hamdy, A.H., and C.J. Blanchard. 1970. Effect of novobiocin on fowl cholera in turkeys. Avian Dis 14:770–778.

48. Harbourne, J.F. 1962. A hemolytic coccobacillus recovered from poultry. Vet Rec 74:566–567.

49. Hart, L. 1963. Treatment of duck cholera with erythromycin. Aust Vet J 39:92–93.

50. Heddleston, K.L. 1962. Studies on pasteurellosis. V. Two immunogenic types of Pasteurella multocida associated with fowl cholera. Avian Dis 6:315–321.

51. Heddleston, K.L. 1970. Personal communication.

52. Heddleston, K.L. 1972. Avian Pasteurellosis. In M.S. Hofstad, B.W. Calnek, C.F. Helmboldt, W.M. Reid, and H.W. Yoder, Jr. (eds.). Diseases of Poultry, 6th ed. Iowa State University Press, Ames, IA, pp. 219–241.

53. Heddleston, K.L. 1975. Pasteurellosis. In S.B. Hitchner, C.H. Domermuth, H.G. Purchase, and J.E. Williams (eds.). Isolation and Identification of Avian Pathogens. American Association of Avian Pathologists, Kennett Square, PA, pp. 38–51.

54. Heddleston, K.L., and P.A. Rebers. 1972. Fowl cholera: cross-immunity induced in turkeys with formalin-killed in-vivo-propagated Pasteurella multocida. Avian Dis 16:578–586.

55. Heddleston, K.L., and P.A. Rebers. 1975. Properties of

free endotoxin from Pasteurella multocida. Am J Vet Res 36:573–574.

56. Heddleston, K.L., and R.C. Reisinger. 1960. Studies on pasteurellosis. IV. Killed fowl cholera vaccine adsorbed on aluminum hydroxide. Avian Dis 4:429–435.

57. Heddleston, K.L., and L.P. Watko. 1963. Fowl cholera: susceptibility of various animals and their potential as disseminators of disease. Proc 67th Annu Meet US Livest Sanit Assoc, pp. 247–251.

58. Heddleston, K.L., and G. Wessman. 1975. Characteristics of Pasteurella multocida of human origin. J Clin Microbiol 1:377–383.

59. Heddleston, K.L., L.P. Watko, and P.A. Rebers. 1964. Dissociation of a fowl cholera strain of Pasteurella multocida. Avian Dis 8:649–657.

60. Heddleston, K.L., J.E. Gallagher, and P.A. Rebers. 1970. Fowl cholera: immune responses in turkeys. Avian Dis 14:626–635.

61. Heddleston, K.L., J.E. Gallagher, and P.A. Rebers. 1972. Fowl cholera: gel diffusion precipitin test for serotyping Pasteurella multocida from avian species. Avian Dis 16:925–936.

62. Heddleston, K.L., P.A. Rebers, and G. Wessman. 1975. Fowl cholera: immunologic and serological response in turkeys to live Pasteurella multocida vaccine administered in the drinking water. Poult Sci 54:217–221.

63. Hendrickson, J.M., and K.F. Hilbert. 1932. The persistence of P. avium in the blood and organs of fowls with spontaneous fowl cholera. J Infect Dis 50:89–97.

64. Henry, B.S. 1933. Dissociation in the genus Brucella. J Infect Dis 52:374–402.

65. Horvath, Z., M. Padanyi, and Z. Palatka. 1962. Chloramphenicol in the treatment of fowl cholera. Magy Allatory Lapja 17:332–336.

66. Hughes, T.P. 1930. The epidemiology of fowl cholera. II. Biological properties of P. avicida. J Exp Med 51:225–238.

67. Hughes, T.P., and I.W. Pritchett. 1930. The epidemiology of fowl cholera. III. Portal of entry of P. avicida; reaction of the host. J Exp Med 51:239–248.

68. Hungerford, T.G. 1968. A clinical note on avian cholera. The effect of age on the susceptibility of fowls. Aust Vet J 44:31–32.

69. Hunter, B. and G. Wobeser. 1980. Pathology of experimental avian cholera in mallard ducks. Avian Dis 24:403–414.

70. Iliev, T., R. Arsov, I. Dimov, G. Girginov, and E. Iovcev. 1963. Swine, cattle, and sheep as carriers and latent sources of pasteurella infection for fowl. Nauchni Tr Vissh Vet Med Inst Sofia 11:281–288.

71. Iliev, T., R. Arsov, E. Iovcev, and G. Girginov. 1963. Role of swine in the epidemiology of fowl cholera. Nauchni Tr Vissh Vet Med Inst Sofia 11:289–293.

72. Iliev, T., R. Arsov, and V. Lazarov. 1965. Can fowls, carriers of Pasteurella, excrete the organism in faeces? Nauchni Tr Vissh Vet Med Inst 14:7–12.

73. Iovcev, E. 1967. The role of Argas persicus in the epidemiology of fowl cholera. Angew Parasitol 8:114–117.

74. Jaksic, B.L., M. Dordevic, and B. Markovic. 1964. Fowl cholera in wild birds. Vet Glas 18:725–730.

75. Jensen, W.I., and C.S. Williams. 1964. Botulism and fowl cholera. In J. P. Linduska (ed.). Waterfowl Tomorrow. US Government Printing Office, Washington, D.C., pp. 333–341

76. Jordan, R.M.M. 1952. The nutrition of Pasteurella septica. II. The formation of hydrogen peroxide in a chemically-defined medium. Br J Exp Pathol 33:36–45.

77. Juszkiewicz, T. 1966. Hyperthermia and prednisolone acetate as provocative factors of Pasteurella multocida infection in chickens. Pol Arch Weter 10:141–151.

78. Juszkiewicz, T. 1966. Effects of shaking and premedication with methylprednisolone on some biochemical indices associated with Pasteurella multocida infection of cockerels. Pol Arch Weter 10:129–140.

79. Karaivanov, L., and O. Mraz. 1973. Use of phagodiagnostics in Pasteurella multocida. Acta Vet (Brno) 42:195–200.

80. Kirchner, C., and A. Eisenstark. 1956. Lysogeny in Pasteurella multocida. Am J Vet Res 17:547–548.

81. Kiser, J.S., J. Prier, C.A. Bottorff, and L.M. Greene. 1948. Treatment of experimental and naturally occurring fowl cholera with sulfamethazine. Poult Sci 27:257–262.

82. Knight, D.P., Paine, J.E., and D.C.E. Speller. 1983. A selective medium for Pasteurella multocida and its use with animal and human species. J Clin Pathol 36:591–594.

83. Kyaw, M.H. 1944. Pathogenesis of Pasteurella septica infection in developing chick embryo. J Comp Pathol 54:200–206.

84. Little, P.A. 1948. Use of Aureomycin in some experimental infections in animals. Ann NY Acad Sci 51:246–253.

85. Maheswaran, S.K., J.R. McDowell, and B.S. Pomeroy. 1973. Studies on Pasteurella multocida. I. Efficacy of an avirulent mutant as a live vaccine in turkeys. Avian Dis 17:396–405.

86. Manninger, R. 1919. Concerning a mutation of the fowl cholera bacillus. Zentralbl Bakteriol Abt I Orig 83:520–528.

87. Marshall, J.D. 1963. The use of immunofluorescence for the identification of members of the genus Pasteurella in chemically fixed tissues. PhD Diss., Univ Maryland.

88. Matthes, S., H. Loliger, and H.J. Schubert. 1969. Enzootisches Auftreten der Pasteurella hemolytica beim Huhn. Dtsch Tierarztl Wochenschr 76:94–95.

89. McNeil, E., and W.R. Hinshaw. 1948. The effect of streptomycin on Pasteurella multocida in vitro, and on fowl cholera in turkeys. Cornell Vet 38:239–246.

90. Mitrovic, M. 1967. Chemotherapeutic efficacy of sulfadimethoxine against fowl cholera and infectious coryza. Poult Sci 46:1153–1158.

91. Mitrovic, M., and J.C. Bauernfeind. 1971. Efficacy of sulfadimethoxine in turkey diseases. Avian Dis 15:884–893.

92. Mitrovic, M., G. Fusiek, and E.G. Schildknecht. 1969. Antibacterial activity of sulfadimethoxine potentiated mixture (Ro 5-0013) in chickens. Poult Sci 48:1151–1155.

93. Mitrovic, M., G. Fusiek, and E.G. Schildknecht. 1971. Antibacterial activity of sulfadimethoxine potentiated mixture (Rolfenaid) in turkeys. Poult Sci 50:525–529.

94. Morris, E.J. 1958. Selective media for some Pasteurella species. J Gen Microbiol 19:305–311.

95. Murata, M., T. Horiuchi, and S. Namioka. 1964. Studies on the pathogenicity of Pasteurella multocida for mice and chickens on the basis of O-groups. Cornell Vet 54:293–307.

96. Namioka, S., and M. Murata. 1961. Serological studies on Pasteurella multocida. II. Characteristics of somatic (O) antigen of the organism. Cornell Vet 51:507–521.

97. Nelson, C.L. 1955. The veterinarian in poultry practice. Proc 92nd Annu Meet Am Vet Med Assoc, pp. 306–310.

98. Nicolet, J., and H. Fey. 1965. Role of Pasteurella haemolytica in salpingitis of fowls. Schweiz Arch Tierheilkd 107:329–334.

99. Nielsen, J.P., Bisgaard, M., and K.B. Pedersen. 1986. Production of toxin in strains previously classified as Pasteurella multocida. Acta Pathol Microbiol Immunol Scand Sect B 94:203–204.

100. Nobrega, R., and R.C. Bueno. 1950. The influence of the temperature on the viability and virulence of Pasteurella avicida. Boll Soc Paulista Med Vet 8:189–194.

101. Olson, L.D. 1966. Gross and histopathological description of the cranial form of chronic fowl cholera in turkeys. Avian Dis 10:518–529.

102. Olson, L.D., and E.L. McCune. 1968. Experimental production of the cranial form of fowl cholera in turkeys. Am J Vet Res 29:1665–1673.

103. Pabs-Garnon, L.F., and M.A. Soltys. 1971. Methods

of transmission of fowl cholera in turkeys. Am J Vet Res 32:1119–1120.

104. Park, P.Y. 1982. Disseminated intravascular coagulation in experimental fowl cholera of chickens. Korean J Vet Res 22:211–219.

105. Pasteur, L. 1880a. Sur les maladies virulents et en particulier sur la maladie appelee vulgairement cholera des poules. CR Acad Sci 90:239–248, 1030–1033.

106. Pasteur, L. 1880b. De l'attenuation du virus du cholera des poules. CR Acad Sci 91:673–680.

107. Pasteur, L. 1881. Sur les virus-vaccins du cholera des poules et du charbon. CR Travaux Congr Int Dir Stn Agron Sess Versailles, pp. 151–162.

108. Peterson, E.H. 1948. Sulfonamides in the prophylaxis of experimental fowl cholera. J Am Vet Med Assoc 113:263–266.

109. Petrov, D. 1975. Studies on the gamasid red mite of poultry, Dermanyssus gallinae, as a carrier of Pasteurella multocida. Vet Med Nauk (Bulg) 12:32–36.

110. Pier, A.C., K.L. Heddleston, S.J. Cysewski, and J.M. Patterson. 1972. Effect of aflatoxin on immunity in turkeys. II. Reversal of impaired resistance to bacterial infection by passive transfer of plasma. Avian Dis 16:381–387.

111. Pirosky, I. 1938. Sur l'antigen glucidolipidique des Pasteurella. CR Soc Biol 127:98–100.

112. Pritchett, I.W., and T.P. Hughes. 1932. The epidemiology of fowl cholera. VI. The spread of epidemic and endemic strains of Pasteurella avicida in laboratory populations of normal fowl. J Exp Med 55:71–78.

113. Pritchett, I.W., F.R. Beaudette, and T.P. Hughes. 1930. The epidemiology of fowl cholera. IV. Field observations of the "spontaneous" disease. J Exp Med 51:249–258.

114. Pritchett, I.W., F.R. Beaudette, and T.P. Hughes. 1930. The epidemiology of fowl cholera. V. Further field observations of the spontaneous disease. J Exp Med 51:259–274.

115. Rebers, P.A., A.E. Jensen, and G.A. Laird. 1988. Expression of pili and capsule by the avian strain P-1059 of Pasteurella multocida. Avian Dis 32:313–318.

116. Reis, J. 1941. On the presence of Pasteurella avicida in feces of infected birds. Arq Inst Biol (San Paulo) 12:307–309.

117. Rhoades, K.R. 1964. The microscopic lesions of acute fowl cholera in mature chickens. Avian Dis 8:658–665.

118. Rhoades, K.R., and R.B. Rimler. 1987. Capsular groups of Pasteurella multocida isolated from avian hosts. Avian Dis 31:895–898.

119. Rhoades, K.R., and R.B. Rimler. 1987. Effects of Pasteurella multocida endotoxins on turkey poults. Avian Dis 31:523–526.

120. Rhoades, K.R., and R.B. Rimler. 1988. Toxicity and virulence of capsular serogroup D Pasteurella multocida strains isolated from turkeys. J Am Med Assoc 192:1790.

121. Rhoades, K.R. and R.B. Rimler. 1988. Unpublished data.

122. Rifkind, D., and M.J. Pickett. 1954. Bacteriophage studies on the hemorrhagic septicemia Pasteurellae. J Bacteriol 67:243–246.

123. Rimler, R.B. 1984. Comparisons of serologic responses of white leghorn and New Hampshire red chickens to purified lipopolysaccharides of Pasteurella multocida. Avian Dis 28:984–989.

124. Rimler, R.B. 1987. Cross-protection factor(s) of Pasteurella multocida: Passive immunication of turkeys against fowl cholera caused by different serotypes. Avian Dis 31:884–887.

125. Rimler, R.B. 1994. Presumptive identification of Pasteurellla multocida serogroups A, D, and F by capsule depolymerisation with mucopolysaccharidases. Vet Rec 134:191–192.

126. Rimler, R.B., and M. Phillips. 1986. Fowl cholera: protection against Pasteurella multocida by ribosome-lipopolysaccharide vaccine. Avian Dis 30:409–415.

127. Rimler, R.B., and K.R. Rhoades. 1987. Serogroup F, a new capsule serogroup of Pasteurella multocida. J Clin Microbiol 25:615–618.

128. Rimler, R.B., Rebers, P.A., and Phillips, M. 1984. Lipopolysaccharides of the Heddleston serotypes of Pasteurella multocida. Am J Vet Res 45:759–763.

129. Rosen, M. 1971. Avian Cholera. In J.W. Davis, L.H. Karstad, D.O. Trainer, and R.C. Anderson (eds.). Infectious and Parasitic Diseases of Wild Birds. Iowa State Univ Press, Ames, IA, pp. 59–74.

130. Rosen, M.N., and A.I. Bischoff. 1949. The 1948–49 outbreak of fowl cholera in birds in the San Francisco Bay area and surrounding counties. Calif Fish Game 35:185–192.

131. Rosenbusch, C., and I.A. Merchant. 1939. A study of the hemorrhagic septicemia Pasteurellae. J Bacteriol 37:69–89.

132. Ryu, E. 1961. Studies on Pasteurella multocida. VI. The relationship between inhibitory action of blood and susceptibility of animals to Past. multocida. Jpn J Vet Sci 23:357–361.

133. Salmon, D.E. 1880. Investigations of fowl cholera. Rep US Comm Agric, pp. 401–445.

134. Saxena, S.P., and A.B. Hoerlein. 1959. Lysogeny in Pasteurella. I. Isolation of bacteriophages from Pasteurella strains isolated from shipping fever and those from other infectious processes. J Vet Anim Husb 3:53–66.

135. Serdyuk, H.G., and P.F. Tsimokh. 1970. Role of free-living birds and rodents in the distribution of pasteurellosis. Veterinariia 6:53–54.

136. Simms, B.T. 1951. Rep Chief Bureau Anim Indust, USDA, pp. 44–45.

137. Skidmore, L.V. 1932. The transmission of fowl cholera to turkeys by the common house fly (Musca domestics Linn) with brief notes on the viability of fowl cholera microorganisms. Cornell Vet 22:281–285.

138. Smith, I.M., and A.J. Baskerville. 1983. A selective medium for isolation of P. multocida in nasal specimens from pigs. Br Vet J 139:476–486.

139. Stuart, E.E., R.D. Keenum, and H.W. Bruins. 1966. Efficacy of sulfaethoxypyridazine against fowl cholera in artificially infected chickens and turkeys, and its safety in laying chickens and broilers. Avian Dis 10:135–145.

140. Van Es, L., and J.F. Olney. 1940. An inquiry into the influence of environment on the incidence of poultry diseases. Univ Neb Agric Exp Stn Res Bull 118:17–21.

141. Vaught, R.W., H.C. McDougle, and H.H. Burgess. 1967. Fowl cholera in waterfowl at Squaw Creek National Wildlife Refuge, Missouri. J Wildl Manage 31:248–253.

142. Walser, M.M., and R.B. Davis. 1975. In vitro characterization of field isolates of Pasteurella multocida from Georgia turkeys. Avian Dis 19:525–532.

143. Watko, L.P. 1966. A chemically defined medium for growth of Pasteurella multocida. Can J Microbiol 12:933–937.

144. Watko, L.P., and K.L. Heddleston. 1966. Survival of shell-frozen, freeze-dried, and agar slant cultures of Pasteurella multocida. Cryobiology 3:53–55.

145. Wessman, G.E., and G. Wessman. 1970. Chemically defined media for Pasteurella multocida and Pasteurella ureae, and a comparison of their thiamine requirements with those of Pasteurella haemolytica. Can J Microbiol 16:751–757.

146. Wilson, G.S., and A.A. Miles. 1964. Topley and Wilson's Principles of Bacteriology and Immunity. Williams & Wilkins, Baltimore, MD.

147. Yaw, K.E., and J.C. Kakavas. 1957. A comparison of the protection-inducing factors in chickens and mice of a type 1 strain of Pasteurella multocida. Am J Vet Res 18:661–664.

6 Riemerella anatipestifer Infection

T. S. Sandhu and Richard B. Rimler

INTRODUCTION. *Riemerella* (*Pasteurella*) *anatipestifer* (RA) infection is a contagious disease of domestic ducks, turkeys, and various other birds. It is also known as new duck disease, duck septicemia, anatipestifer syndrome, anatipestifer septicemia, and infectious serositis. In geese, RA infection has been called goose influenza or septicemia anserum exsudativa (32). It occurs as an acute or chronic septicemia characterized by fibrinous pericarditis, perihepatitis, airsacculitis, caseous salpingitis, and meningitis. The respiratory tract may also be infected without showing clinical signs. *R. anatipestifer* infection accounts for major economic losses to the duck industry due to high mortality, weight loss, and condemnations.

HISTORY AND DISTRIBUTION. *R. anatipestifer* infection was first described in 1932 in White Pekin ducks from three farms on Long Island, New York (26). The report referred to a new disease, which became known in the area as "new duck disease." The disease started in 7- to 10-wk-old ducks with about 10% mortality, and later spread to younger ducklings of about 3 wk of age. Six years later, the disease was observed in ducks from a commercial farm in Illinois and was reported as "duck septicemia" (18). The designation "infectious serositis" was given by Dougherty et al. (14) after a comprehensive pathologic study. The term *R. anatipestifer infection* was recommended by Leibovitz (31) to identify the disease specifically caused by *R. anatipestifer* and to differentiate it from other infections with similar pathology. A similar disease, septicemia anserum exsudativa, was described in geese by Riemer (43). The causative agent, *Pasteurella septicaemiae*, is identical to RA on the basis of reported characteristics (27, 53).

The disease occurs worldwide and has been recognized in countries that have intensive duck production (46).

ETIOLOGY

Classification. The causative bacterium was isolated and characterized by Hendrickson and Hilbert (26), who called it *Pfeifferella anatipestifer.* Bruner and Fabricant (10) studied and compared its characteristics with those of *Brucella, Pasteurella, Moraxella, Actinobacillus,* and *Haemophilus.* They concluded that the organism had more in common with *Moraxella* spp. and suggested the name *Moraxella anatipestifer.* It was listed in the seventh edition of *Bergey's Manual of Determinative Bacteriology* as *Pasteurella anatipestifer* (8). Because of its uncertain taxonomic status, it was placed as species *incertae sedis* in the eighth (53) and ninth (34) editions of *Bergey's Manual of Systematic Bacteriology.* Comparison of DNA base composition, DNA–DNA homology, and cellular fatty-acid profile has indicated its exclusion from the genus *Moraxella* as well as *Pasteurella* (5, 34). Piechulla et al. (41) have suggested the transfer of RA to the *Flavobacterium/Cytophaga* group on the basis of low but significant DNA binding and production of menaquinones and branched-chain fatty acids. Segers et al. (52) reported significant differences between RA and its close genotypic relatives *Flavobacterium* and *Weeksella.* They suggested placing this organism in a separate genus *Riemerella,* in honor of Riemer (43) who first described the disease "septicemia anserum exsudativa" in geese in 1904, and named it *Riemerella anatipestifer* on the basis of DNA-ribosomal RNA hybridization analysis, protein and fatty-acid profiles, and phenotypic characteristics such as lack of pigment production and presence of respiratory quinone "menaquinone 7."

Morphology and Staining. *R. anatipestifer* is a gram-negative, nonmotile, non–spore-forming rod occurring singly, in pairs, and occasionally in chains. The cells vary from 0.2 to 0.4 µm in width and 1 to 5 µm in length. Many cells stain bipolar with Wright's stain, and a capsule can be demonstrated in preparations with India ink.

Growth Requirements and Colonial Morphology. The organism grows well on chocolate agar, blood agar, or trypticase soy agar. Growth on trypticase soy agar can be enhanced by the addition of 0.05% yeast extract and 5% newborn calf serum. Growth is more abundant with increased carbon dioxide (18). Hendrickson and Hilbert (26) described the organism as a strict aerobe on the ba-

161

sis of results obtained with the pyrogallic acid and sodium hydroxide procedure for removing oxygen. However, since carbon dioxide would also be depleted by reacting with the sodium hydroxide, neither oxygen nor carbon dioxide was available to the organism. Although some strains of RA grew at an incubation temperature of 45 C, no growth was observed at 4 C or 55 C (4); maximum growth usually occurs in 48–72 hr when incubated at 37 C in a candle jar.

Colonies on blood agar, when grown 24 hr at 37 C in a candle jar, are 1–2 mm in diameter, convex, entire, transparent, glistening, and butyrous. Some strains produce slimy growth. Colonies on clear media are iridescent when observed with obliquely transmitted light. Incubation in the candle jar is recommended for good growth as it increases carbon dioxide and moisture, both of which are favorable for growth.

Biochemical Characteristics. Carbohydrates are not fermented, although some researchers have reported acid production in glucose, maltose, inositol, and fructose by some strains (2, 4). Gelatin is usually liquified, and litmus milk may slowly turn alkaline. Indole and hydrogen sulfide are not produced. Nitrate is not reduced to nitrite, and starch is not hydrolyzed. There is no growth on MacConkey agar and no hemolysis of blood agar. *R. anatipestifer* is oxidase- and catalase-positive; phosphatase is produced (20). Some strains produce urease and arginine dihydrolase.

R. anatipestifer is positive for acid and alkaline phosphatase, ester lipase C8 (APIZYME system), leucine-, valine- and cystine-arylamidases, phosphoamidase, α-glucosidase and estrase C4; while negative for the following enzyme activities: α- and ß-galactosidases, ß-glucronidase, ß-glucosidase, α-mannosidase, ß-glucosaminidase, lipase C14, fucosidase, and ornithine and lysine decarboxylases (41, 52).

Resistance to Chemical and Physical Agents.   Most RA strains do not survive on solid media for more than 3–4 days at 37 C or room temperature; cultures in broth may be viable for 2–3 wk when stored at 4 C. Incubation at 55 C for 12–16 hr resulted in nonviability of the organism (4). *R. anatipestifer* has been reported to survive in tap water and turkey litter for 13 and 27 days, respectively (6). It is sensitive to penicillin, novobiocin, chloramphenicol, lincomycin, streptomycin, erythromycin, ampicillin, bacitracin, neomycin, and tetracycline, but resistant to kanamycin and polymyxin B (4). *R. anatipestifer* is relatively resistant to gentamicin.

Serotype Classification. *R. anatipestifer* isolates have been serotyped using agglutination and agar-gel precipitin (AGP) reactions. Both these tests involve surface antigens that are presumed to be polysaccharides (9). Plate agglutination is rapid and convenient; tube agglutination is favored over AGP as it is quantitative in terms of antibody titers.

To date, 19 serotypes have been reported. Based on agglutination reactions, Harry identified 16 serotypes (A through P), 4 of which (E, F, J, and K) were lost during storage, while serotypes G and N were found to be identical to serotypes I and O, respectively (7, 19). Seven serotypes (1 through 7) were differentiated using AGP reaction (9). Subsequently, Bisgaard (7) reported serotypes 1, 2, 3, 4, 5, and 6 to be serologically identical to Harry's types A, I/G, L, H, M, and B, respectively. He also suggested numerical designation of serotypes to avoid confusion and to standardize serotype nomenclature for recognition of new serotypes. He identified 2 new serotypes (12 and 13). Serotype 7 was reported to be identical to serotype O/N, and a new serotype (8) was isolated (50). Sandhu and Leister (51) revised the typing scheme proposed by Bisgaard. They redesignated Harry's serotypes C and D as types 9 and 10, excluded serotype 4, which was not RA, and reported 5 new serotypes (11, 14, 15, 16, 17). Loh et al. (33) reported serotypes 13 and 17 to be identical. They redesignated Harry's type P as serotype 4, and added 3 new serotypes (17, 18, and 19), which were isolated from ducks in Singapore. All serotypes reacted specifically with homologous-type antisera with the exception of serotype 5, which gave minor cross-reactions with serotypes 2 and 9 (33, 50).

PATHOGENESIS AND EPIZOOTIOLOGY

Natural and Experimental Hosts.   *R. anatipestifer* infection is primarily a disease of domestic ducks. Ducklings of 1–8 wk of age are highly susceptible. Ducklings under 5 wk of age usually die 1–2 days after signs appear; older birds may survive longer. The disease is rare in breeder ducks. Naturally occurring outbreaks of RA have been reported in turkeys (25, 57). Serious outbreaks in turkeys in the United States and other countries showed that RA is a potential pathogen of domestic turkeys (17, 38, 39, 54). *R. anatipestifer* has also been isolated from pheasants (11), chickens (44), guinea fowl and quail (39), partridge (56) and other waterfowl (15, 29, 37, 42, 55).

Adverse environmental conditions or concomitant disease often predispose the birds to outbreaks of RA infection. Mortality may vary from 5 to 75%.

The disease can be produced in healthy ducks by exposure to RA. There is wide variation, however, in severity of the disease depending on the strain of the organism and the route of exposure. Mortality can be produced most consistently by injection of the organism intravenously, subcutaneously, into the foot pad, or into the infraorbital sinus. The disease can also be reproduced by intraperitoneal, intramuscular, or intratracheal routes of exposure. Attempts to produce the disease by oral inoculation have been unsuccessful (3, 22).

Chickens, geese, pigeons, rabbits, and mice were reported to be refractory to infection with RA; guinea pigs succumbed to inoculation of large doses intraperitoneally (18, 26). Heddleston (24) observed, however, that 8×10^6 organisms inoculated into the foot pad killed 5 of 7 day-old chicks; 4×10^6 organisms produced the same signs and lesions in 2-wk-old White Chinese goslings as were produced in White Pekin ducklings. Infection takes place via the respiratory tract (31) or through wounds of the skin, particularly of the feet (3). Cooper (12) suggested that the disease in turkeys may be transmitted by arthropod vectors based on its seasonal occurrence and the apparent affinity of RA for host erythrocytes.

Signs. Signs most often observed are listlessness, ocular and nasal discharge, mild coughing and sneezing, greenish diarrhea, ataxia, tremor of head and neck, and coma. Affected ducklings show inability to move with the brood. Surviving ducks may be stunted (40).

Lesions. The most obvious gross lesion in ducks is fibrinous exudate, which involves serosal surfaces in general, but is most evident in the pericardial cavity and over the surface of the liver (Figs. 6.1, 6.2, 6.3); similar lesions have been reported in turkeys and other birds. In addition to fibrin, the exudate contains a few inflammatory cells, primarily mononuclear cells and heterophils.

Fibrinous airsacculitis is common. Both abdominal and thoracic air sacs may be involved. Mononuclear cells are the predominant cell type in the exudate. Multinuclear giant cells and fibroblasts may be observed in chronic cases (14). Lungs of infected ducks may be unaffected; there may be interstitial cellular infiltration and proliferation of lymphoid nodules adjacent to parabronchi (40); or there may be an acute fibrinopurulent pneumonia (18).

Liver lesions observed in the acute stage of the disease are mild periportal mononuclear leukocytic infiltration, cloudy swelling and hydropic degeneration of parenchymal cells. In less acute cases, moderate periportal lymphocytic infiltration may be observed (40).

Infections of the central nervous system can produce a fibrinous meningitis. Spleens may be enlarged and mottled. Mucopurulent exudate in nasal sinuses and caseous exudate in oviducts have been observed in RA infection (14). Jortner et al. (28) studied lesions in the central nervous system of naturally infected ducklings and described diffuse fibrinous meningitis with leukocytic infiltration in and

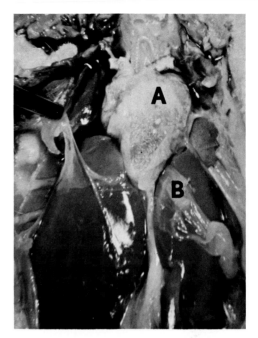

6.1. *Riemerella anatipestifer* infection. Fibrinous epicarditis (*A*), pericarditis, and perihepatitis (*B*). Forceps hold exudate from surface of liver.

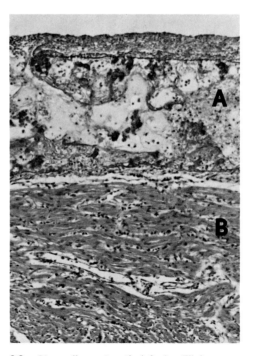

6.2. *Riemerella anatipestifer* infection. Fibrinous exudate (*A*) over surface of heart (*B*). H & E,

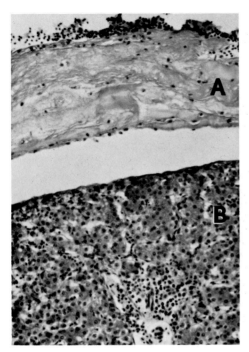

6.3. *Riemerella anatipestifer* infection. Fibrinous exudate (*A*) over surface of liver (*B*). H & E, ×300.

around the walls of meningeal blood vessels. Extensive exudate was observed in the ventricular system. Slight to moderate leukocytic and microglial infiltrates were observed in subpial and periventricular brain tissue.

Chronic localized infections usually occur in skin and occasionally in joints. Skin lesions are in the form of necrotic dermatitis on the lower back or around the vent. Yellowish exudate is observed between skin and fat layers.

IMMUNITY. Ducklings that recover from the disease are resistant to subsequent infection (2, 18, 26). Inactivated bacterins have been used in ducks to prevent RA infection. Ducks vaccinated with formalin-inactivated bacterins and subsequently challenged with strains representing serotypes 1, 2, and 5 developed homologous, but not heterologous, protection. A trivalent bacterin containing these strains provided protection against challenge with each, but the protection lasted only a short time (45). Harry and Deb (21) evaluated effectiveness of several types of bacterins and conducted a field trial with a formalin-inactivated bacterin. A single dose of oil-emulsion bacterin provided longer lasting immunity in ducklings (16, 45). One-day-old ducklings exposed to live avirulent strains by aerosol or through the drinking water were resistant when challenged at 3–4 wk of age with virulent homolo-

gous strains (47). Passive protection of progeny may be obtained by immunization of the female breeder ducks; this protection may last for about 2 wk. Maternally immune ducklings responded successfully to active immunization with a live or inactivated vaccine (48).

DIAGNOSIS. Although a presumptive diagnosis may be made from clinical signs and necropsy findings, a definite diagnosis should be based on isolation and identification of RA.

Isolation and Identification. The bacterium can be isolated most readily when birds are in the acute stage of the disease. Suitable tissues for culturing the organism are heart blood, brain, air sacs, bone marrow, lung, liver, and exudates from the lesions. Specimens should be taken aseptically, streaked over blood agar or trypticase soy agar containing 0.05% yeast extract, and incubated in a candle jar at 37 C for 24–72 hr. Addition of newborn calf serum (5%) and gentamicin (5 mg/1000 mL) to plate medium is helpful for isolation of RA from contaminated specimens. Isolated colonies should be selected for inoculation of the differential media and identified on the basis of characteristics described under Etiology. Serotype identification can be established by the rapid slide or tube agglutination test with specific antisera.

Immunofluorescent procedures can be used to identify RA in tissue or exudate from infected birds (35). Hatfield et al. (23) described an enzyme-linked immunosorbent assay (ELISA) that was more sensitive than the agglutination test to detect serum antibodies in ducks.

Differential Diagnosis. *R. anatipestifer* infection should be differentiated from other septicemic diseases caused by *Pasteurella multocida*, *Escherichia coli*, *Streptococcus faecium*, and salmonellae. Since these diseases produce gross lesions indistinguishable from those caused by RA, diagnosis must include isolation and identification of the causal organism. Differential diagnosis of RA should also include chlamydiosis, especially in turkeys and in areas where the latter is a serious problem.

TREATMENT. Antibiotics and sulfa drugs have been tried for treatment of RA with varying degrees of success. Sulfamethazine, 0.2 to 0.25%, in drinking water or feed, was reported to prevent the onset of clinical signs in ducks exposed experimentally to RA (2). Sulfaquinoxaline at levels of 0.025 or 0.05% in feed was effective in reducing mortality in field and experimental infections (13, 49). Medicated feeds containing novobiocin (0.0303–0.0368%) or lincomycin (0.011–0.022%) were reported to be highly effective in reducing mortality when started 3 days prior to experimental infection. A combination of sulfadimethoxine and ormetoprim, when administered at 0.02–0.12% levels in feed, prevented or reduced mortality and gross lesions in experimentally exposed ducks (36, 49). Tetracyclines were of little value for treatment of RA infection (1, 49). Subcutaneous injection of lincomycin–spectinomycin, penicillin, or a combination of penicillin and dihydrostreptomycin were reported to be effective in reducing mortality in artificially infected ducklings (49).

PREVENTION AND CONTROL

Management Procedures. The most important aspects of prevention are good management and sanitation practices. This includes proper ventilation, especially in houses where ducks are raised in total confinement. Predisposing factors such as stress due to overcrowding or exposure to hot or cold weather should be avoided. Strict measures should be taken to prevent spread of infection from diseased to healthy flocks. If ducks are raised on wire, the floors should be periodically washed and sanitized to avoid accumulation of manure and to reduce the exposure to infection.

Immunization. Inactivated bacterins have been reported to prevent or reduce mortality due to RA (21, 30, 45). Since immunity induced by bacterins is serotype specific, an ideal bacterin should contain cells of predominant serotypes to provide an effective protection. A bacterin containing serotypes 1, 2, and 5 has been used in the United States. Ducklings are vaccinated at 2 and 3 wk of age to provide adequate protection up to market age (30). A single inoculation of oil-emulsified bacterin has been reported to produce better and longer lasting protection, but it may cause unfavorable lesions at the site of inoculation (16, 45).

A live RA vaccine, developed against serotypes 1, 2, and 5, has been reported to provide significant protection against experimental or field infections with virulent organisms when administered to 1-day-old ducklings by aerosol or in drinking water (47). A single vaccination provided protection for at least 42 days. The vaccine strains grew in the upper respiratory tract, and produced a humoral antibody response. The vaccine was reported to be avirulent to 1-day-old ducklings when administered by aerosol or injection into the infraorbital sinus, and was safe in ducks up to 10 back-passages using the contact-exposure method.

REFERENCES

1. Ash, W.J. 1967. Antibiotics and infectious serositis in White Pekin ducklings. Avian Dis 11:38–41.
2. Asplin, F.D. 1955. A septicaemic disease of ducklings. Vet Rec 67:854–858.
3. Asplin, F.D. 1956. Experiments on the transmission of a septicaemic disease of ducklings. Vet Rec 68:588–590.
4. Bangun, A., D.N. Tripathy, and L.E. Hanson. 1981. Studies of Pasteurella anatipestifer: An approach to its classification. Avian Dis 25:326–337.
5. Bangun, A., J.L. Johnson, and D.N. Tripathy. 1987. Taxonomy of Pasteurella anatipestifer. 1. DNA base composition and DNA-DNA hybridization analysis. Avian Dis 31:43–45.
6. Bendheim, U., and A. Even-Shoshan. 1975. Survival of Pasteurella multocida and Pasteurella anatipestifer in various natural media. Refu Vet 32:40–46.
7. Bisgaard, M. 1982. Antigenic studies on Pasteurella anatipestifer, species incertae sedis, using slide and tube agglutination. Avian Pathol 11:341–350.
8. Breed, R.S., E.F. Lessel, Jr., and E. Heist Clise. 1957. Genus I. Pasteurella Trevisan, 1887. In R.S. Breed, E.G.D. Murray, and N.R. Smith (eds.). Bergey's Manual of Determinative Bacteriology, 7th ed. Williams & Wilkins, Baltimore, MD, pp.395–402.
9. Brogden, K.A., K.R. Rhoades, and R.B. Rimler. 1982. Serologic types and physiologic characteristics of 46 avian Pasteurella anatipestifer cultures. Avian Dis 26:891–896.
10. Bruner, D.W., and J. Fabricant. 1954. A strain of Moraxella anatipestifer (Pfeifferella anatipestifer) isolated from ducks. Cornell Vet 44:461–464.
11. Bruner, D.W., C.I. Angstrom, and J.I. Price. 1970. Pasteurella anatipestifer infection in pheasants. A case report. Cornell Vet 60:491–494.
12. Cooper, G.L. 1989. Pasteurella anatipestifer infections in California turkey flocks: Circumstantial evidence of a mosquito vector. Avian Dis 33:809–815.
13. Dean, W.F., J.I. Price, and L. Leibovitz. 1973. Effect of feed medicaments on bacterial infections in ducklings. Poult Sci 52:549–558.
14. Dougherty, E., L.Z. Saunders, and E.H. Parsons. 1955. The pathology of infectious serositis of ducks. Am J Pathol 31:475–487.
15. Eleazer, T.H., H.G. Blalock, J.S. Harrell, and W.T. Derieux. 1973. Pasteurella anatipestifer as a cause of mortality in semiwild pen-raised mallard ducks in South Carolina. Avian Dis 17:855–857.
16. Floren, U., P.K. Storm, and E.F. Kaleta. 1988. Pasteurella anatipestifer sp.i.c. bei Pekingenten: Pathogenitätsprüfungen und immunisierung mit einer inaktivierten, homologen, monovalenten (serotyp 6/B) ölemulsionsvakzine. Dtsch Tierarztl Wochenschr 95:210–214.
17. Frommer, A., R. Bock, A. Inbar, and S. Zemer. 1990. Muscovy ducks as a source of Pasteurella anatipestifer infection in turkey flocks. Avian Pathol 19:161–163.
18. Graham, R., C.A. Brandly, and G.L. Dunlap. 1938. Studies on duck septicemia. Cornell Vet 28:1–8.
19. Harry, E.G. 1969. Pasteurella (Pfeifferella) anatipestifer serotypes isolated from cases of antipestifer septicaemia in ducks. Vet Rec 84:673.
20. Harry, E.G. 1981. Personal communication.
21. Harry, E.G., and J.R. Deb. 1979. Laboratory and field trials on a formalin inactivated vaccine for the control of Pasteurella anatipestifer septicaemia in ducks. Res Vet Sci 27:329–333.
22. Hatfield, R.M., and B.A. Morris. 1988. Influence of the route of infection of Pasteurella anatipestifer on the clinical and immune responses of White Pekin ducks. Res Vet Sci 44:208–214.
23. Hatfield, R.M., B.A. Morris, and R.R. Henry. 1987. Development of an enzyme-linked immunosorbent assay for the detection of humoral antibody to Pasteurella anatipestifer. Avian Pathol 16:123–140.
24. Heddleston, K.L. 1972. Infectious serositis. In M.S. Hofstad, B.W. Calnek, C.F. Helmboldt, W.M. Reid, H.W. Yoder, Jr. (eds.). Diseases of Poultry, 6th ed. Iowa State University Press, Ames, IA, pp. 246–251.

25. Helfer, D.H., and C.F. Helmboldt. 1977. Pasteurella anatipestifer infection in turkeys. Avian Dis 21:712–715.

26. Hendrickson, J.M., and K.F. Hilbert. 1932. A new and serious septicemic disease of young ducks with a description of the causative organism, Pfeifferella anatipestifer, N.S. Cornell Vet 22:239–252.

27. Hinz, K.-H., H. Grebe, and M. Knapp. 1976. Morzxella septicaemiae-Infektion bei Gänsen. Zentralbl Veterinaermed Med [B] 23:341–345.

28. Jortner, B.S., R. Porro, and L. Leibovitz. 1969. Central-nervous-system lesions of spontaneous Pasteurella anatipestifer infection in ducklings. Avian Dis 13:27–35.

29. Karstad, L., P. Lusis, and J.R. Long. 1970. Pasteurella anatipestifer as a cause of mortality in captive wild waterfowl. J Wildl Dis 6:408–413.

30. Layton, H.W., and T.S. Sandhu. 1984. Protection of ducklings with a broth-grown Pasteurella anatipestifer bacterin. Avian Dis 28:718–726.

31. Leibovitz, L. 1972. A survey of the so-called "anatipestifer syndrome." Avian Dis 16:836–851.

32. Levine, N.D. 1965. Goose influenza (septisemia anseru exsudative). In H.E. Biester, and L.H. Schwarte (eds.). Diseases of Poultry, 5th ed. Iowa State University Press, Ames, IA, pp. 469–471.

33. Loh, H., T.P. Teo, and H. Tan. 1992. Serotypes of Pasteurella anatipestifer isolates from ducks in Singapore: A proposal of new serotypes. Avian Pathol 21:453–459.

34. Mannheim, W. 1984. Family III. Pasteurellaceae Pohl 1981a, 382. In N.R. Krieg and J.G. Holt (eds. Bergey's Manual of Systematic Bacteriology, 9th ed., vol. 1. Williams & Wilkins, Baltimore. MD, pp. 550–557.

35. Marshall, J.D., Jr., P.A. Hansen, and W.C. Eveland. 1961. Histobacteriology of the genus Pasteurella. 1. Pasteurella anatipestifer. Cornell Vet 51:24–34.

36. Mitrovic, M., E.G. Schildknecht, G. Maestrone, and H.G. Luther. 1980. Rofenaid in the control of Pasteurella anatipestifer and Escherichia coli infections in ducklings. Avian Dis 24:302–308.

37. Munday, B.L., A. Corbould, K.L. Heddleston, and E.G. Harry. 1970. Isolation of Pasteurella anatipestifer from black swan (Cygnus atratus). Aust Vet J 46:322–325.

38. Nagaraja, K.V. 1988. Personal communication.

39. Pascucci, S., L. Giovannetti, and P. Massi. 1989. Pasteurella anatipestifer infection in guinea fowl and Japanese quail (Coturnix coturnix japonica). Proc 9th Int Congr World Vet Poultry Assoc. Brighton, England, p. 47.

40. Pickrell, J.A. 1966. Pathologic changes associated with experimental Pasteurella anatipestifer infection in ducklings. Avian Dis 10:281–288.

41. Piechulla, K., S. Pohl, and W. Mannheim. 1986. Phenotypic and genetic relationships of so-called Moraxella (Pasteurella) anatipestifer to the Flavobacterium/Cytophaga group. Vet Microbiol 11:261–270.

42. Pierce, R.L., and M.W. Vorhies. 1973. Pasteurella anatipestifer infection in geese. Avian Dis 17:868–870.

43. Riemer. 1904. Kurze Mitteilung über eine bei Gänsen beobachtete exsudative septikämie und deren Erreger. Zentralbl Bakteriol I Abt I Orig 37:641–648.

44. Rosenfeld, L.E. 1973. Pasteurella anatipestifer infection in fowls in Australia. Aust Vet J 49:55–56.

45. Sandhu, T. 1979. Immunization of White Pekin ducklings against Pasteurella anatipestifer infection. Avian Dis 23:662–669.

46. Sandhu, T.S. 1986. Important diseases of ducks. In D.J. Farrell and P. Stapleton (eds.). Duck Production Science and World Practice. University of New England, Australia, pp. 111–134.

47. Sandhu, T.S. 1991. Immunogenicity and safety of a live Pasteurella anatipestifer vaccine in White Pekin ducklings: Laboratory and field trials. Avian Pathol 20:423–432.

48. Sandhu, T.S. 1992. Unpublished data.

49. Sandhu, T.S., and W.F. Dean. 1980. Effect of chemotherapeutic agents on Pasteurella anatipestifer infection in White Pekin ducklings. Poult Sci 59:1027–1030.

50. Sandhu, T., and E.G. Harry. 1981. Serotypes of Pasteurella anatipestifer isolated from commercial White Pekin ducks in the United States. Avian Dis 25:497–502.

51. Sandhu, T.S., and M. Leister. 1991. Serotypes of Pasteurella anatipestifer isolates from poultry in different countries. Avian Pathol 20:233–239.

52. Segers, P., W. Mannheim, M. Vancanneyt, K. DeBrandt, K.-H. Hinz, K. Kersters, and P. Vandamme. 1993. Riemerella anatipestifer gen. nov., comb. nov., the causative agent of septicemia anserum exsudativa, and its phylogenetic affiliation within the Flavobacterium-Cytophaga rRNA homology group. Int J Syst Bacteriol 43:768–776.

53. Smith, J.E. 1974. Genus Pasteurella Trevisan 1987. In R.E. Buchanan and N.E. Gibbons (eds.). Bergey's Manual of Determinative Bacteriology, 8th ed. Williams and Wilkins, Baltimore, MD, pp. 370–373.

54. Smith, J.M., D.D. Frame, G. Cooper, A.A. Bickford, G.Y. Ghazikhanian, and B.J. Kelly. 1987. Pasteurella anatipestifer infection in commercial meat-type turkeys in California. Avian Dis 31:913–917.

55. Wobeser, G., and G.E. Ward. 1974. Pasteurella anatipestifer infection in migrating whistling swans. J Wildl Dis 10:466–470.

56. Wyffels, R., and N.E. Hommez. 1990. Pasteurella anatipestifer geisoleerd uit ademhalingsletsels bij grijze patrijzen (Perdix perdix). Vlaam Diergeneeskd Tijdschr 59:105–106.

57. Zehr, W.J., and J. Ostendorf, Jr. 1970. Pasteurella anatipestifer in turkeys. Avian Dis 14:557–560.

7 Tuberculosis

Charles O. Thoen

INTRODUCTION. Tuberculosis of poultry is a contagious disease caused by *Mycobacterium avium*. It is characterized by its chronicity; persistence in a flock when once established; and tendency to induce unthriftiness, decreased egg production, and finally death. Although the incidence of tuberculosis in chickens has been reduced to a low level, tuberculosis remains an important problem in captive exotic birds. The importance of tuberculosis in birds in zoo aviaries is compounded by lack of efficacious vaccines or suitable drug-treatment regimens.

The literature contains a number of instances in which it was claimed that *M. avium* was responsible for a tuberculous infection in humans. In the United States, the first case of avian tuberculosis (AT) in humans (with adequate proof) was published in 1947 (16).

With decline in the incidence of tuberculosis in humans, increasing interest is directed toward mycobacteria other than *M. tuberculosis,* so that more isolations of *M. avium* are being recognized (14, 64, 76). Moreover, available information indicates that *M. avium* infection is common in patients with acquired immune deficiency syndrome (AIDS) (12, 15, 34, 74). *M. avium* serovar 1, the organism most commonly isolated from wild birds, has been isolated from patients with AIDS (21, 26). *M. avium* serovar 2, the organism most commonly isolated from chickens, is not often isolated from humans.

HISTORY. Avian tuberculosis in chickens was first recognized as a related but separate entity by Cornil and Megnin (10). Koch (36) maintained for many years that tubercle bacilli were always the same regardless of the species in which they might occur. Rivolta and later Maffucci (40), however, showed that the microorganism of AT in chickens is dissimilar to that of bovine tuberculosis. Koch (37) finally abandoned his previous position and declared that tuberculosis of poultry is unlike tuberculosis of humans, and that the disease in humans is dissimilar to that of cattle.

Although AT in chickens has long been recognized as a contagious disease, it has continued to spread throughout most of the world. With the available information on the nature of AT, its eradication is entirely feasible. The more important reasons for its elimination are 1) affected birds are unthrifty, 2) tuberculous chickens are undesirable for human food, 3) diseased birds produce fewer eggs, 4) tuberculous chickens are the source of tuberculosis of sheep and especially of swine, 5) avian tubercle bacilli are capable of sensitizing cattle to mammalian tuberculin, and 6) avian tubercle bacilli have been isolated from lesions in humans.

The occurrence of AT in birds in zoo aviaries has become of additional importance because the disease causes increased economic losses. Certain species of exotic birds have increased in value as they near extinction, thereby increasing the significance of mortalities from AT. Management problems concerning control of the disease are magnified, since exotic species are often maintained for years. A major obstacle to the elimination of AT from zoologic gardens is related to the ability of the organism to survive in the soil and to the lack of adequate procedures for cleaning and disinfecting contaminated premises.

INCIDENCE AND DISTRIBUTION. Avian tuberculosis in chickens is worldwide in distribution, but occurs most frequently in the North Temperate Zone. The highest incidence of infection in the United States is in flocks of the north central states–North Dakota, South Dakota, Kansas, Nebraska, Minnesota, Iowa, Missouri, Wisconsin, Illinois, Michigan, Indiana, and Ohio. Incidence of the disease in western and southern states is low. The explanation for this is not entirely obvious, although there are several possible contributing factors such as climate, flock management, and duration of infection. The necessity of keeping birds closely confined during winter provides favorable conditions for spread of the disease.

The difficulty of tuberculin-testing all chickens in the United States, or even a majority of the flocks, makes it impossible to obtain exact data on incidence of *M. avium* infection of chickens. In 1992, AT was the cause for condemning 0.02% of the mature chickens slaughtered under federal inspection (41). This figure may be misleading, however, because the chickens may not be representative of the average farm flock. Furthermore, visual inspection may not disclose all infected birds. There has been significant reduction in the prevalence of AT, owing in considerable part to the changing concept of poultry husbandry. Increasing emphasis has

167

been placed on the desirability of maintaining all-pullet flocks, rather than older hens.

In Canada, the incidence of AT in chickens varies greatly in different areas—from 1 to 26%. It occurs in some Latin American countries, but the incidence is variable—low in Brazil, common in Uruguay, widespread in Venezuela as of 1946, and reported in Argentina.

Considerable information exists on occurrence of AT in certain European countries. It is said to be rare in Finland (73), but not uncommon in Norway (18) and Denmark (2); AT occurs in Germany (44, 52) and Great Britain (39). In Australia, AT is unknown in Queensland and West Australia, but occurs in other states. In South Africa, the incidence in poultry is low (35). Infections probably occur in domestic and wild fowl in other countries, but the incidence and distribution cannot be determined because bacteriologic studies are not universally done. In Kenya, AT has been reported in lesser flamingoes (9). Disease in swine from *M. avium* has been reported in countries other than the foregoing (59) and in humans (38). Further discussion on the prevalence of tuberculosis in animals may be found in Thoen et al. (68).

Age in Relation to Incidence.

Avian tuberculosis appears to be less prevalent in young fowl not because the younger birds are more resistant to infection, but because in older birds the disease has had a greater opportunity to become established through a longer period of exposure. Although tuberculosis lesions are usually less severe in young chickens than adult birds, extensive or generalized AT in young chickens has been observed. Such birds are an important source of dissemination of virulent tubercle bacilli and must be considered a menace to other fowl and susceptible mammals.

Schack-Steffenhagen and Seeger (48) found *M. avium* in livers of 3.38% of mature chickens imported into Germany from Holland and the United States, but could not demonstrate the microorganisms in broilers. They concluded that tuberculosis is more common in older birds.

Tuberculosis causes important death losses in captive wild birds of zoo aviaries (45). The significance of these findings is emphasized by reports of disease in valuable endangered species. Numerous reports are also available on tuberculosis in pet birds.

ETIOLOGY.

The most common cause of AT in chickens in the United States is *M. avium* serovars 1 and 2 (60). In Europe, *M. avium* serovar 3 has been isolated from birds; however, this organism has not been isolated from domestic birds in the United States (50). Serovar 3 was cultured from a tree duck being held for importation into the United States (66). Some other serovars of *M. avium* (such as 4 and 8) isolated from humans and swine have not been found to cause progressive disease in chickens or captive wild birds (68).

The most characteristic feature of *M. avium* is its acid-fastness. The organisms are bacillary in character; clublike, curved, and crooked forms are also seen in some preparations. Cords are not formed. Branching infrequently occurs. Most of the bacteria have rounded ends and vary in length from 1 to 3 μm. Spores are not produced, and the organism is nonmotile. Spherical or conical granules occur in the cytoplasm anywhere along the length of the bacterium.

Cultural Distinctions.

The avian tubercle bacillus is not as exacting in its temperature requirements as *M. tuberculosis* and *M. bovis* (56). *M. avium* will grow at temperatures ranging from 25 to 45 C, although the most favorable temperature range is 39–45 C. *M. avium* is aerobic. On original isolation, growth is enhanced by an atmosphere of 5–10% carbon dioxide (30).

For original isolation from naturally infected material, one of the special media designed for culturing tubercle bacilli is desirable. Both glycerinated and nonglycerinated media are satisfactory, but colonies are larger if the medium contains glycerin. Some strains of *M. avium* require mycobactin as a growth factor for initial and subsequent growth (42). On media containing whole egg or egg yolk and incubated at 37.5–40 C, the bacteria usually become evident in 10 days to 3 wk as small, slightly raised, discrete, grayish white colonies. If the inoculum is rich in bacteria, colonies will be numerous and may tend to coalesce. Colonies are hemispheric and do not penetrate the medium. They gradually change from grayish white to light ocher and become darker as age of the culture increases. Karlson et al. (32) described a culture of *M. avium* that was bright yellow but typical in all other respects.

Subcultures on solid media show evidence of growth usually within 6–8 days and reach maximal development in 3–4 wk. Such cultures usually appear moist and unctuous, the surface eventually becoming roughened. The growth is creamy or sticky and is readily removable from the underlying medium. In liquid media, growth occurs at the bottom as well as at the surface. Growth usually may be dispersed readily by shaking to form a turbid suspension, which is in contrast to the flocculent growth of mammalian tubercle bacilli.

A definite relationship appears to exist between type of colony and virulence (4). Studies comparing cultures isolated from tuberculous chickens and certain similar nonchromogenic mycobacteria from humans showed that pure cultures with smooth transparent colonies were virulent for chickens; in contrast, variants with smooth-domed or rough colonies were avirulent for chickens regardless of source. The loss of virulence in *M. avium* has been associated with change from transparent to domed colonies on culture media (58).

Biochemical Properties.

Cultures of *M. avium* and certain nonchromogenic strains from humans and swine have been studied with an attempt to delineate differences. There appear to be no significant biochemical distinctions between *M. avium* serovars 1, 2, and 3 (avian tubercle bacilli), known to be virulent for chickens, and serovars 4–20, previously called *M. intracellulare,* having little virulence for chickens (44, 68). *M. avium,* however, has features that separate it from other species or groups of mycobacteria (13).

M. avium does not produce niacin, does not hydrolyze Tween-80, is peroxidase-negative, produces catalase, does not have urease or arylsulfatase, and does not reduce nitrate; there are variations in these features, particularly in results of tests for arylsulfatase. Mycobacteria possess amidases that appear to be specific for certain species or closely related groups; e.g., avian tubercle bacilli are singularly lacking in certain amidases except for pyrazinamidase and nicotinamidase. Detailed discussions of the biochemical features of *M. avium* and related microorganisms may be found in Karlson and Thoen (30).

Sensitivity to Antituberculosis Drugs.

Generally, *M. avium* is more resistant to the commonly used antituberculosis drugs as compared to *M. tuberculosis* and *M. bovis.* On approximately 50 strains of *M. avium* from chickens and swine and 11 from humans, the authors found that in egg yolk agar, most strains will grow in the presence of 10 mg, but not in 50 mg, of streptomycin/mL, in more than 10 mg of *p*-aminosalicylic acid/mL, and in more than 40 mg isoniazid/mL medium. On the same kind of medium, a relative resistance was shown to ethambutol, thionamide, viomycin, and pyrazinamide. The inhibitory concentration is variable, depending on the medium and procedure. Other reports are in agreement that *M. avium* has a high degree of resistance to antituberculosis agents (13). However, synergistic effects of antimycobacterial drug combinations (i.e., ethambutol and rifampicin) on *M. avium* complex have been reported (25).

Serovars.

The notable contributions of Schaefer (49) have demonstrated a number of serovars of *M. avium* that appear to be stable even during years of artificial culture. These studies indicate that strains of *M. avium* can be identified by serologic procedures, including those that have lost their virulence for fowl. A numbering scheme has been developed for reporting *M. avium* serotypes (78) that are more recently referred to as serovars. Serovars 1 and 2 occur mainly in animals, whereas 4–20 are commonly found in humans (61). Some serovars of *M. avium* found in swine (serovars 4 and 8) have also been isolated from humans (77). Ability to identify stable serovars of *M. avium* provides a means for studying origin and distribution of specific strains.

A micromethod has been developed for identifying serovars of *M. avium,* enabling savings in time and materials compared with the tube agglutination test (65). The method is simple and can be conducted in microtiter plates.

PATHOGENESIS AND EPIZOOTIOLOGY

Natural and Experimental Hosts

FOWL. All species of birds can be infected with *M. avium.* Generally speaking, domesticated fowl or captive wild birds are affected more frequently than those living in wild state. Avian tuberculosis may occur in ducks, geese, swans, peacocks, pigeons, turkeys, and captive and wild birds. Parrots and canaries may also be infected. Reports of AT in domestic fowl other than chickens have been made by Scrivner and Elder (53), Feldman (16), and Francis (19).

Although uncommon among wildfowl, the disease may be expected to develop in wild birds that frequent farm premises where AT is prevalent in chickens. Pheasants seem to be unusually susceptible to infection by the avian tubercle bacillus (55). The disease has also been observed in sparrows, crows, barn owls, cowbirds, blackbirds, eastern sparrow hawks, starlings, wood pigeons, and whooping cranes.

RATITES. Avian tuberculosis has been reported in ostriches, emus, and rheas housed in zoologic parks. Recently, AT was diagnosed in a 3-yr-old female emu in a commercial flock (54). Lesions 1–2.5 cm in diameter appearing as tan to yellow colored nodules were observed in the spleen, liver and kidney. Similar lesions were observed in the mesentery, pleura, and intestinal serosa, and in the marrow cavity of a tibiotarsal bone. On histologic examination, multifocal granulomas were observed in tissues and were characterized by central areas of caseous necrosis surrounded by a wide band of macrophages and multinucleated giant cells. Lymphocytes and fibroblasts were observed on the periphery. Few acid-fast bacilli were found in appropriately stained sections. Delayed-type hypersensitivity (DTH) responses to *M. avium* purified protein derivative tuberculin were reported in 25% of the adult emus.

TURKEYS. Turkeys are not commonly affected with AT. The disease in most instances is contracted from infected chickens and is chronic in character. Information regarding AT in turkeys has been contributed by Hinshaw et al. (24), who examined a total of 88 birds at necropsy; AT was found in 45 (51.15%). The disease was found in only 1 of 11 birds less than 1 yr of age, whereas 28 (65.12%) of 43 over 2 yr of age were tuberculous. Additional information on the disease in turkeys may be found in Feldman (16) and Francis (19).

WILD BIRDS. Accounts of AT in wild birds, and reviews of the literature may be found in Feldman (16), McDiarmid (43), Francis (19), Hoybraten (27), Bickford et al. (6), Schaefer et al. (50) and Karlson (29).

Avian tuberculosis is common among birds in many zoologic gardens. In the unnatural environment of captivity, the incidence frequently equals or even exceeds that for domestic fowl (45). The infectious agent in nearly all instances is *M. avium* serovar 1 or serovar 2 (63). Tuberculosis in parrots may also be due to *M. tuberculosis* (1).

MAMMALS. The avian tubercle bacillus has a definite pathogenicity for some important species of domesticated mammals, and at least a slight pathogenicity for others (18, 19, 22, 39, 61). This should be recognized if the problem of eliminating tuberculosis is to be attacked and eventually solved.

Under conditions of natural exposure, it is very exceptional for extensive tuberculosis caused *M. avium* to develop in mammals other than rabbits and swine (61). Infection may occur, but the disease in most mammals remains localized; however, microorganisms may multiply in tissues for a considerable period and induce sensitivity to tuberculin. Although spontaneous infection of mammals may not be of comparable severity to that that develops in fowl, it is possible to produce extensive changes in many species of mammals by introducing the infective agent artificially. The relative pathogenicity of *M. avium* for many of the domesticated mammals is summarized in Table 7.1.

In the United States and Europe, *M. avium* serovar 2 is the most common cause of tuberculous lesions in swine (28, 59, 75). Tuberculosis will remain an unnecessary economic burden on the swine industry until it is eliminated from chickens and other barnyard fowl. There has been a gradual but definite decrease of tuberculosis in swine in the United States (69, 70, 71). One reason for the decrease may be the lower incidence of AT in poultry as a result of the increasing practice of maintaining one-age flocks.

Table 7.1. Comparative pathogenicity of *Mycobacterium avium* for certain mammals

Animal	Susceptibility
Cat	Highly resistant
Cattle	Infection occurs; usually localized
Deer	Infection reported
Dog	Highly resistant
Goat	Assumed to be relatively resistant
Guinea pig	Relatively resistant
Hamster	Susceptible (intratesticularly)
Horse	Infection reported
Llamas	Susceptible
Marsupial	Infection reported
Mink	Readily infected
Monkey	Susceptible
Mouse	Relatively resistant
Rabbit	Readily infected
Rat	Relatively resistant
Sheep	Moderately susceptible
Swine	Readily infected

Transmission. The tremendous number of tubercle bacilli exuded from ulcerated tuberculous lesions of the intestine in poultry creates a constant source of virulent bacteria. Although other sources of infection exist, none equals infective fecal material in dissemination of AT. Fecal discharges may contain tubercle bacilli from lesions of the liver and mucosa of the gallbladder expelled through the common duct. The respiratory tract is also a potential source of infection, especially if lesions occur in tracheal mucosa.

The contaminated environment containing bacilli-laden soil and litter is the factor of greatest importance in transmission of the disease to uninfected animals. The longer the premises have been occupied by infected birds and the more concentrated the poultry population, the more prevalent the infection is likely to be.

Avian tubercle bacilli may persist in soil for a long time. Schalk et al. (51) found a contaminated barnyard to have viable and virulent *M. avium* in litter and soil 4 yr after the removal of an infected flock. These workers also demonstrated that bacteria remained viable in carcasses buried 3-ft deep for 27 mo. Virulent strains of *M. avium* have been found to survive in sawdust for 168 days at 20 C and 244 days at 37 C (52). This ability to survive outside the host presents a serious hazard to swine and to domestic and wild fowl.

ROLE OF EGGS. The possibility that AT might be transmitted through eggs from tuberculous hens has long been pertinent. It has been demonstrated many times that some artificially inoculated eggs will hatch, and that chicks hatched from such eggs will be infected with tubercle bacilli. Such observations are of doubtful importance to the fundamental question: Are eggs from naturally infected chickens likely to produce tuberculous chicks? The most convincing evidence to the contrary is furnished by Fitch and Lubbenhusen (17) and Schalk et al. (51), who raised many hundreds of chicks hatched from eggs of naturally infected hens without AT being observed in a single instance. Similar conclusions were reached by others (16, 19). *M. avium*, however, has been isolated by culture of eggs from naturally infected chickens. In Germany, Fritzsche and Allam (20) found that avian tubercle bacilli were demonstrable in 3.55% of 899 eggs from 58 flocks in which AT existed. In contrast, of 650 eggs from seven commercial poultry farms, only 0.31% had *M. avium;* these came from a single large farm where a few tuberculin-positive chickens were found. Also, these workers found that avian tubercle bacilli would not survive in eggs after 6 min of boiling; in preparation of scrambled eggs, 2 min of frying was sufficient to kill the bacteria. Studies in Poland by Bojarski (7) revealed that *M. avium* could be cultured from 8% of 175 eggs from naturally infected hens. Avian tubercle bacilli were recovered by culture, however, from 8 of 24 (33.3%) eggs from artificially infected hens.

OTHER SOURCES. Other sources of dissemination of avian tubercle bacilli are carcasses of tuberculous fowl that die of the disease and offal from chickens dressed for food. It is also conceivable that cannibalism might play a part in transmission.

Avian tubercle bacilli may be carried by persons whose shoes have become soiled with fecal matter. Equipment used in care and maintenance of infected poultry (crates and feed sacks) also might be responsible for transfer of infective bacteria from diseased to healthy flocks.

Wild birds and pigeons may be infected with *M. avium* and are, therefore, capable of spreading *M. avium* to poultry flocks. Swine may have ulcerative intestinal lesions from avian tubercle bacilli and thus constitute a source of infection for other animals and birds. Birds such as sparrows, starlings, and pigeons that feed in farmyards are also potential sources.

Signs. Few signs of the disease in chickens are pathognomonic; however, if the disease is prevalent in a flock, several or most of the signs may be evident in different birds.

Ordinarily, if the infection has progressed sufficiently to affect physical condition, the bird will be less lively than its penmates. The affected fowl fatigues easily and appears depressed. Although appetite usually remains good, progressive and striking loss of weight commonly occurs, especially noticeable in the breast muscles. The pectoral muscles are often atrophied, and the breastbone becomes very prominent and may be deformed. In extreme instances, most of the body fat eventually disappears, and the face of the affected bird appears smaller than normal.

Feathers assume a dull and ruffled appearance. Comb, wattle, and earlobes often become anemic and thinner than normal, and the uncovered epidermis has a peculiar dryness. Occasionally, however, the comb and wattles have a bluish discoloration. Icterus, indicative of hepatic changes, may be noted.

Even though the disease is severe, the temperature of the affected bird remains within the normal range. In many instances, the bird reveals a unilateral lameness and walks with a peculiar jerky hopping gait, probably the result of tuberculous involvement of the humeral scapulocoracoid articulation, which may rupture and discharge fluid of caseous material. Paralysis from tuberculous arthritis sometimes occurs.

If the affected chicken is greatly emaciated, one may detect nodular masses along the intestine by palpation of the abdomen. The great hypertrophy of the liver of many tuberculous birds, however, may make this procedure difficult or impossible. Most tuberculous chickens have lesions along the intestinal tract; if these are ulcerative, severe diarrhea results. The enteric disturbance induces extreme weakness, and the affected bird assumes a sitting position as a result of exhaustion.

Affected birds may die within a few months or live for many, depending on severity or extent of the disease. A bird may die suddenly as a consequence of hemorrhage from rupture of the affected liver or spleen.

Gross Lesions. Lesions are seen most frequently in liver, spleen, intestines, and bone marrow. The bacillemia, which probably occurs intermittently and perhaps early in most instances, provides for a generalized distribution of lesions. None of the tissues, with the possible exception of the central nervous system, appears to be immune from infection. Some of the organs, such as heart, ovaries, testes, and skin, are affected infrequently and cannot be considered organs of predilection. Francis (19) reviewed the available literature and found that for turkeys, ducks, and pigeons, lesions predominate in liver and spleen but occur also in many other organs.

Avian tuberculosis in fowl is characterized by occurrence of irregular grayish yellow or grayish white nodules of varying sizes in organs of predilection such as spleen, liver, and intestine (Fig. 7.1A, B, D). Involvement of liver and spleen results in hypertrophy, which is often significant; fatal hemorrhage from rupture may result. The tuberculous nodule varies in size from a barely discernible structure to a huge mass that may measure several centimeters in diameter. Large nodules frequently have an irregular knobby contour, with smaller granulations or nodules often present over the surface. Lesions near the surface in such organs as liver and spleen are enucleated easily from adjacent tissues. Nodules are firm but can be incised easily, since mineral salts are not present. On cross section, a fibrous nodule containing a variable number of small yellowish foci or a single soft yellowish central region, which is frequently caseous, may be observed. The latter is surrounded by a fibrous capsule, the continuity of which often is interrupted by small circumscribed necrotic foci. The fibrous capsule varies in thickness and consistency, depending on size and duration of lesion. It is barely discernible or apparently absent in small lesions and measures 0.1–0.2 cm in thickness in larger nodules.

The number of lesions is also variable, ranging from a few to innumerable. It is rather common to observe a few nodular lesions in organs such as liver and spleen associated with an enormous number of lesions of minute to moderate size. Variation in size is a consequence of successive episodes of reinfection from previously established lesions, usually of the same organ. Involvement of lungs is usually less severe than that of liver or spleen.

The marked tendency of the disease to disseminate to several organs indicates that tuberculous bacillemia is common. This tendency of the bacilli to circulate within the bloodstream provides the explanation for frequent involvement of bone marrow (Figs. 7.1C, 7.2). Infection of bone marrow probably occurs very early in the course of the disease.

In chickens, the tubercle may be observed experimentally 14–21 days postinfection as a closely packed collection of pale-staining cells with vesiculated nuclei. These epithelioid cells are derived from fixed tissue elements known as histiocytes. The latter cells phagocytose tubercle bacilli early in the reactive process.

The cellular mass or primary tubercle gradually expands as histiocytes proliferate at the periphery; within 3–4 wk, signs of retrogression can be detected in epithelioid cells in the central zone. This retrogression is due partly to the avascularity of the structure and partly to the toxic substances of the tubercle bacilli. As the cellular mass becomes larger, epithelioid cells have tendency to fuse and form syncytia. Outlines of the individual cells become less distinct or disappear. This is followed within a week or so by a necrobiotic change resembling coagulation necrosis. Nuclei or epithelioid cells become pyknotic and may disappear; the cellular mass, except the peripheral portion, becomes fused and stains deeply with eosin. The tubercle bacilli have multiplied and appear singly or in clumps throughout the necrotic tissue.

While the epithelioid cells in the central zone undergo necrobiotic changes, there persists an outer zone of epithelioid syncytia appearing as a mantle around the entire periphery. From these, giant cells are developed, the nuclei of which are situated distally to the central zone of necrosis; the cells are arranged rather frequently in palisade formation. Immediately peripheral to the zone of giant cells there is a more or less diffuse collection of epithelioid cells and their progenitors, histiocytes (Fig. 7.3). Fibrocytes and minute blood vascular channels also occur near the outer portion of the peripheral area. Although bacilli are more numerous in the central or necrotic zone of the tubercle, they are also found in large numbers in the epithelioid zone adjacent and distal to giant cells.

The final phase in formation of a tubercle is development of a zone of encapsulation consisting of fibrous connective tissue, histiocytes, some lymphocytes, and an occasional eosinophilic granulocyte. New tubercles develop in the epithelioid zone immediately peripheral to giant cells. Consequently, a tubercle, as recognized grossly, consists of the original or parent tubercle and several smaller or adjacent ones.

The nature of the degenerative process in the central zone of the tubercle is somewhat unusual in that the integrity of the cells is maintained for a considerable period before disintegration. Caseous necrosis eventually occurs and may affect all or part of the central zone.

Calcification of the tubercle rarely occurs in fowl. Amyloidlike degeneration of portions of the surrounding parenchymal element sometimes is observed in liver, spleen, and kidney.

Acid-fast bacilli occur in great numbers in smears of lesions and appropriately stained sections (Fig. 7.4).

Microscopically, lesions of AT in turkeys vary considerably. In some, tubercles like those seen in AT of chickens are present. In other instances, lesions are diffuse, with extensive destruction of surrounding parenchyma. Cytoplasmic masses or large giant cells may be numerous, and large numbers of eosinophilic granulocytes are commonly present. Some lesions become circumscribed by a broad, dense zone of fibrous connective tissue.

Detailed descriptions of gross and microscopic lesions of AT in the different organs of birds can be found in Feldman (16), Francis (19), and Thoen et al. (68).

Pathogenesis. The capacity of *M. avium* to produce progressive disease may be related to cell wall constituents and certain complex lipids present in the cell wall, such as cord factor, sulfur-containing glycolipids (sulfatides), or strongly acidic lipids (47, 62). It appears, however, that the effect of these components alone or together on phagosome–lysosome fusion cannot account for virulence. Delayed-type hypersensitivity develops following exposure to mycobacteria; once captivated, macrophages demonstrate an increased capacity to kill intracellu-

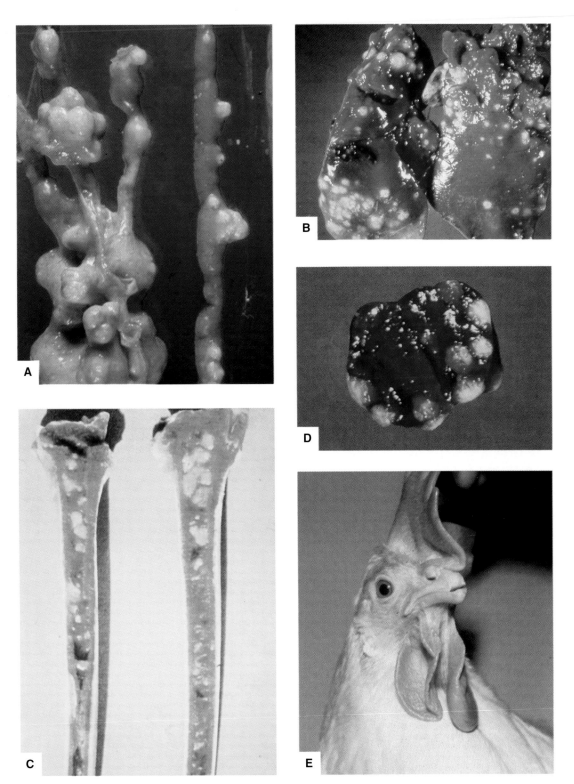

7.1. *A-D.* Tuberculous lesions in intestine (*A*), liver (*B*), bone marrow (*C*) (Peckham); and spleen (*D*) of naturally infected chickens. Note the variation in size of lesions in the liver and spleen. *E.* Positive reaction in the left wattle of tuberculous chicken 48 hr after intradermal injection of avian tuberculin. (Peckham)

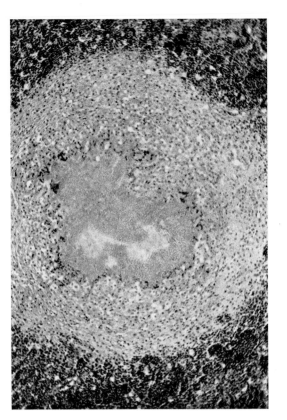

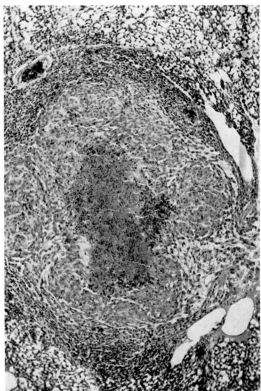

7.2. Small tuberculous nodule in bone marrow of a naturally infected chicken. Central necrotic region is surrounded by zone of dense connective tissue. ×100.

7.3. Developing tubercle in lung of chicken. ×100.

lar *M. avium.* The DTH responses are mediated by lymphocytes, which release lymphokines that act to attract, immobilize, and activate blood-borne mononuclear cells at the site where virulent bacilli or their products exist. Tumor necrosis factor, alone or in combination with interleukin-2, but not γ interferon, is associated with macrophage killing of *M. avium* serovar 1 (5). The DTH that develops contributes to accelerated tubercle formation and is, in part, responsible for cell-mediated immunity in tuberculosis. Activated macrophages that lack sufficient subcellular microbicidal components to kill virulent tubercle bacilli are destroyed by the intracellular growth of the organism, and a lesion develops. Available information indicates a combination of toxic lipids and factors released by virulent *M. avium* may 1) cause disruption of the phagosome, 2) inhibit phagolysosome formation, 3) interfere with release of hydrolytic enzymes from the attached lysosomes, and/or 4) inactivate lysosomal enzymes released into the cytoplasmic vacuole. Available information suggests that toxic oxygen metabolites are not responsible for killing activated macrophages. However, the significance of hydrogen peroxide, activated oxygen radical(s) and nitric

oxide in resistant macrophages of birds exposed to virulent *M. avium* remains to be elucidated (62).

DIAGNOSIS.   A presumptive diagnosis of AT in fowl can usually be made on the basis of gross lesions (8). Finding acid-fast organisms, however, in smears of infected liver, spleen, or other organs stained with a stain such as Ziehl-Neelsen is very helpful in diagnosis. Inoculation of suitable media to isolate and identify the causative agent is necessary for definite diagnosis of AT (30).

Tuberculin Test.   When administered properly, the tuberculin test provides a satisfactory procedure for determining presence of AT in a flock.

TECHNIQUE.   Equipment consists of a sterile tuberculin syringe (1-mL capacity) and a supply of sterile 25–26 gauge hypodermic needles 0.5 in. (1.3 cm) in length. Absorbent cotton and 70% alcohol should also be available. Tuberculin should be that prepared for intradermic use from avian tubercle bacilli. That prepared from mammalian strains of tubercle bacilli may elicit positive reactions in tuberculous chickens, but results are generally unsat-

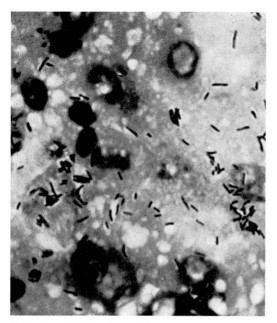

7.4. Numerous tubercle bacilli in smear preparation from small lesion of lung of naturally infected chicken. Ziehl-Neelsen stain, ×1600.

isfactory. The reactions to avian tuberculin are usually more pronounced.

The bird should be restrained so that the head is entirely immobile. The surface of the wattle should be cleaned with alcohol; other attempts to clean or disinfect the skin are unnecessary. The needle is inserted carefully into the lateral aspect of the dermis, and 0.03–0.05 mL tuberculin is injected into the tissue. The purified protein derivative tuberculin presently supplied by the U.S. Department of Agriculture (USDA) is prepared from synthetic liquid culture medium on which *M. avium* strain D-4 has grown for 8 wk (3). The tuberculoproteins are precipitated using ammonium sulfate. The protein concentration is adjusted to 1 mg phosphorus/mL with phosphate-buffered saline. A small bleb or diffuse blanched area will appear where tuberculin was deposited. Although fairly satisfactory results may follow if tuberculin is injected into subcutaneous tissue, it is a better practice to inject it intradermally.

REACTION.   After 48 hr the chickens are examined. The opposite uninfected wattle is used for comparison. A positive reaction is indicated by soft swelling in tissues of the injected wattle (Fig. 7.1E). Some reactions are small; others result in pronounced swelling that increases the thickness of the wattle one to five times. The swelling is due largely to edema that occurs in the zone of connective tissue lying between layers of the dermis. To a lesser

extent, swelling is due to increased width of the corium, which is filled with closely packed mononuclear histiocytic cells, a few eosinophilic granulocytes, and a variable number of lymphoid cells and lymphocytes. After 48 hr, the swelling gradually subsides and usually disappears within 5 days.

Sometimes a negative reaction will appear in a bird that is definitely tuberculous; conversely, a positive result is sometimes obtained in chickens in which signs of AT cannot be demonstrated. In the latter instance, failure to find lesions does not imply that tubercle bacilli are not present in tissues of the chicken. In the early stage of the disease, lesions are likely to be too small to be noted grossly or too few to be found by ordinary methods of examination. A definitely positive tuberculin test indicates that the bird has been exposed to avian tubercle bacilli.

Tuberculin is a bacteria-free concentrated filtrate prepared from a liquid culture of tubercle bacilli and, as used for diagnosis of AT in chickens, may be considered harmless to normal birds (23). If retests are done after an interval of 1 mo, false-positive reactions will not occur. In chickens, the usual diagnostic dose of tuberculin does not sensitize the nontuberculous bird to subsequent injections of the same product.

The tuberculin test has been used to a limited extent in diagnosing AT of turkeys. For the most part, however, results have been less satisfactory than for chickens. Certain difficulties are encountered also in tuberculin testing of pigeons and ducks. For pigeons, Svrcek et al. (57) applied the test in the submandibular area. For Japanese quail, tuberculin may be injected intradermally in the area around the vent (33). The test is of limited value in diagnosing AT in these birds.

Usefulness of the tuberculin test in diagnosis of AT in turkeys has not been adequately established. Hinshaw et al. (24), using avian tuberculin, injected the snood, mucosa of the cloaca, wattle, skin of the edge of the wing web, and skin at the center of the wing web. Test results indicated that reactions in the wattle agreed with the findings at necropsy in only 11.1% of the birds, and that there was agreement between the tuberculin reaction in the wing web and findings at necropsy in 75.68% of the birds. From the meager information available, one must conclude that the intradermic tuberculin test has been less reliable for detecting AT in turkeys than in chickens. It would seem desirable to investigate reliability of the rapid agglutination test as a means of detecting AT in live turkeys.

Serology

ENZYME-LINKED IMMUNOSORBENT ASSAY.   Enzyme-linked immunosorbent assay (ELISA) has been described for use in detecting mycobacterial antibodies in sera of chickens experimentally inoculated with *M. avium* serovar 2 (67). Positive ELISA reactions were observed in uninfected controls. Tuberculin skin tests did not induce positive reactions in uninfected chickens. As well, ELISA has been used for detecting antibodies in sera of tuberculous birds maintained in captivity. Since only a small amount of serum is required, the ELISA method may be of practical value for diagnosis of AT in small species as well as exotic birds without wattles. Its reagents can be readily standardized. Moreover, the test is a rapid, simple procedure that can be readily automated to allow for screening large numbers of birds.

Serologic procedures offer certain practical advantages. Birds need to be handled only once, and samples of blood submitted for agglutination tests for pullorum disease may be examined for presence of specific mycobacterial antibodies. A recent report reveals that an ELISA was sensitive and specific for detecting AT in barnacle geese (11).

RAPID AGGLUTINATION TEST. A whole-blood agglutination test of possible diagnostic value for AT in fowl was described by Karlson et al. (31). The antigen is a 10% suspension of avian tubercle bacilli in 0.85% sodium chloride solution containing 0.5% phenol. Blood is obtained by pricking the comb with a sharp instrument such as an 18-gauge needle. A drop of fresh blood is mixed with a drop of antigen on a warm plate. Appearance of agglutination in 1 min is considered a positive test.

In chickens, the whole-blood agglutination test may have a reliability comparable to that of the tuberculin test. Hiller et al. (23) compared the agglutination test and the tuberculin test in flocks where, on the same farm, so-called nonspecific tuberculin reactions were found in cattle. In 290 flocks, 38.3% of the birds reacted to the serologic test compared with 18.4% to the tuberculin test; 77.2% had postmortem or bacteriologic evidence of AT. It was concluded that the agglutination test was more useful than the tuberculin test for detecting infected birds in a diseased flock; however, occurrence of false-positive agglutination reactions in healthy birds is a drawback.

Differential Diagnosis. The most expedient way to diagnose the disease is by necropsy. Lesions are rather characteristic, but other conditions must be differentiated. These include neoplasia, enterohepatitis, and possibly fowl cholera and fowl typhoid. Presence of numerous acid-fast bacilli in lesions is especially significant because they do not occur in any other known disease of chickens. Proof of diagnosis depends on laboratory studies to establish the microorganism as *M. avium*.

TREATMENT. Antituberculosis drugs are not often used to treat domestic fowl. Combinations of these drugs, however, have been utilized in treatment of certain exotic birds maintained in captivity (72). Clinical remission was observed in three birds that received a combination of isoniazid (30 mg/kg), ethambutol (30 mg/kg), and rifampicin (45 mg/kg). The recommended duration of therapy was 18 mo, provided there were no adverse side effects. Additional investigations are needed to develop suitable regimens for treatment of tuberculosis in various exotic birds.

PREVENTION AND CONTROL. Importance of the poultry and swine industries makes it imperative that measures be developed for control and eradication. The disease is not diagnosed in commercial poultry in the United States, but it is found occasionally in backyard flocks.

The tuberculin test is of considerable practical value. Removal of chickens that react eliminates many foci of infection. The test enables detection of many infected fowl before the disease reaches a severe or chronic state; if repeated tests are made and reactors removed, dissemination of the bacteria to the environment may be reduced. The whole-blood agglutination test also may serve to detect infected birds. Hiller et al. (23) concluded that this rapid serologic test was more useful than the tuberculin test for detecting tuberculous chickens in a diseased flock.

If the residual flock is permitted to occupy the same contaminated premises, a continuing source of infection remains. This provides opportunity for new infections to occur indefinitely, since avian tubercle bacilli may remain viable and virulent in the soil for years. Neither the tuberculin nor the agglutination test can be depended upon for detection of every tuberculous fowl. As long as one infected bird remains in a flock, dissemination of the disease to healthy fowl is possible. Consequently, means other than the tuberculin test must be used if a more satisfactory control of AT is to be expected.

It has been stated frequently that AT can be controlled if all birds in the flock are disposed of after the first laying season. The practice is commendable, especially because it is economically sound from the point of view of egg production. Older birds usually produce fewer eggs; furthermore, mortality from nonbacterial disease such as neoplasia is greater among older hens than pullets. Another factor in favor of disposal of old stock is that AT is usually more severe in older birds, which as a consequence are more likely to become depots of dissemination.

Use of vaccines containing inactivated and/or live mycobacteria for protecting chickens against tuberculosis has been evaluated (46). The best results were obtained in chickens vaccinated with live *M. intracellulare* serovar 6 (*M. avium* serovar 6) given orally. These fowl showed 70% protection after intramuscular (IM) challenge with *M. avium.* Encouraging results were also reported in chickens after combined IM vaccination with inactivated plus live *M. intracellulare* serovar 7 and serovar Darden (*M. avium* serovars 7 and 19). Additional investigations are needed to confirm the efficacy of various vaccines in exotic birds.

Procedures for establishing and maintaining AT-free flocks should include the following: 1) Abandon old equipment and establish other facilities on new soil. Ordinarily, it is impractical to render an infected environment satisfactorily safe by disinfection. 2) Provide proper fencing or other measures to prevent unrestricted movement of chickens, thus preventing exposure from previously infected premises. 3) Eliminate the old flock, burning carcasses of birds that show lesions of tuberculosis. 4) Establish a new flock in the new environment from AT-free stock. 5) Eliminate from swine herds all reactors to avian and mammalian tuberculin. If chickens in a clean flock are prevented from access to an infected environment, and are protected against accidental exposure to an infected environment and accidental exposure to tubercle bacilli, it is reasonable to believe they will remain free from AT.

The measures just described are not complicated. Additional profits that will accrue from an AT-free flock maintained in a hygienic environment will compensate for the initial expense and work. The general health of birds will be better, and disease other than AT will be controlled more satisfactorily. Benefits will also be reflected in a decrease in tuberculosis in swine. The importance of AT in infection of swine is such that if chickens were maintained entirely separate and apart, the incidence of tuberculosis of swine from *M. avium* would be reduced.

Recommendations for control of AT in exotic birds include the following: 1) Prevent contact with tuberculous birds; premises and housing previously used by them are to be avoided. 2) Quarantine additions to the aviary for 60 days and retest with avian tuberculin. Studies should be made to confirm the validity of vaccination trials made in chickens for protection of various exotic species against the disease.

REFERENCES

1. Ackerman, L.J., S.C. Benbrook, and B.C. Walton. 1974. Mycobacterium tuberculosis infection in a parrot (Amazona farinosa). Annu Rev Respir Dis 109:388–390.

2. Andersen, S. 1965. The distribution of avian tuberculosis in Denmark. Medlemsbl Dan Dyrlaegeforen 2:54–59.

3. Angus, R.D. 1978. Production of reference PPD tuberculins for veterinary use in the United States. J Biol Stand 6:221–228.

4. Belisle, J.T. and P.J. Brennan. 1994. Molecular basis of colony morphology in Mycobacterium avium. Res Microbiol 145:237–242.

5. Bermudez, L., and L. Young. 1988. Tumor necrosis factor, alone or in combination with IL-2, but not IFN-gamma, is associated with macrophage killing of Mycobacterium avium complex. J Immunol 140:3006–3013.

6. Bickford, A.A., G.H. Ellis, and H.E. Moses. 1966. Epizootiology of tuberculosis in starlings. J Am Vet Med Assoc 149:312–318.

7. Bojarski, J. 1968. Occurrence of Mycobacterium in eggs of tuberculin-positive hens. Med Weter 24:21–23.

8. Bush, M.A., R.J. Montali, C.O. Thoen, E.E. Smith, W. Peritino, and D.W. Johnson. 1978. Avian tuberculosis: Status of antemortem diagnostic procedures. Proc 1st Int Birds Captivity Symp, pp. 185–195.

9. Cooper, J.E., L Karstad, and E. Boughton. 1975. Tuberculosis in lesser flamingos in Kenya. J Wild Dis 11:32–36.

10. Cornil, V., and P. Megnin. 1884. Tuberculose et diphtherie des gallinaces. CR Soc Biol 36:617-621.

11. Cromie, R.L., M.J. Brown, N.A. Forbes, J. Morgan, and J.L. Stanford. 1993. A comparison and evaluation of techniques for diagnosis of avian tuberculosis in wildfowl. Avian Pathol 22:617–630.

12. Denis, M. 1994. Immunomodulatory events in Mycobacterium avium infections. Res Microbiol 145:225–229.

13. Engbaek, H.C., E.H. Runyon, and A.G. Karlson. 1971. Mycobacterium avium Chester: Designation of neotype strain. Int J Syst Bacteriol 21:192–196.

14. Falk, G.A., S.J. Hadley, F.E. Sharkey, M. Liss, and C. Muschenheim. 1973. Mycobacterium avium infections in man. Am J Med 54:801–810.

15. Falkingham III, J.O., 1994. Epidemiology of Mycobacterium avium infections in the pre- and post- HIV era. Res Microbiol 145:169–172.

16. Feldman, W.H. 1938. Avian Tuberculosis Infections. Williams & Williams, Baltimore, MD.

17. Fitch, C.P., and R.E. Lubbenhusen. 1928. Completed experiments to determine whether avian tuberculosis can be transmitted through eggs of tuberculous fowls. J Am Vet Med Assoc 72:636–649.

18. Fodstad, F.H. 1967. A survey of mycobacterial infections detected in animals in Norway in 1966. Medlemsbl Nor Veterinaerforen 19:314–327.

19. Francis, J. 1958. Tuberculosis in Animals and Man: A Study in Comparative Pathology. Cassell, London.

20. Fritzsche, K., and M.S.A.M. Allam. 1965. The contamination of hen eggs with mycobacteria. Arch Lebensmittelhyg 16:248–250.

21. Good, R.C. 1985. Opportunistic pathogens in the genus Mycobacterium. Annu Rev Microbiol 39:347–369.

22. Gunnes, G., K. Nord, S. Vatn, and F. Saxegaard. 1995. A case of generalized avian tuberculosis in a horse. Vet Rec 136:565–566.

23. Hiller, K., T. Schliesser, G Fink, and P. Dorn. 1967. Zur serologischen Diagnose der Huhnertuberkulose. Berl Munch Tierarztl Wochenschr 80:212–216.

24. Hinshaw, W.R., K.W. Niemann, and W.H. Busic. 1932. Studies of tuberculosis of turkeys. J Am Vet Med Assoc 80:765–777.

25. Hoffner, S.E., S.B. Svenson, and G. Kallenius. 1987. Synergistic effects of antimycobacterial drug combinations on Mycobacterium avium complex determined radiometrically in liquid medium. Eur J Clin Microbiol 6:530–535.

26. Horsburgh, C.R., Jr., U.G. Mason, D.C. Farhi, and M.D. Iseman. 1985. Disseminated infection with Mycobacterium avium-intracellulare. Medicine 64:36–48.

27. Hoybraten, P. 1959. Tuberkulose tiefeller nos fuglen. Nord Vet Med 11:780–786.

28. Jorgensen, J.B. 1978. Serological investigation of strains of Mycobacterium avium and Mycobacterium intracellulare isolated from animals and nonanimal sources. Nord Vet Med 30:155–162.

29. Karlson, A.G. 1978. Avian Tuberculosis. In R.J. Montali (ed.). Mycobacterial Infections of Zoo Animals. Smithsonian Institution Press, Washington, DC, pp. 21–24.

30. Karlson, A.G. and C.O Thoen. 1991. Tuberculosis. In H.G. Purchase, C.H. Domermuth, L.A. Arp, and J.E. Pearson (eds.). A Laboratory Manual for the Isolation and Identification of Avian Pathogens, 3rd ed. Kendall/Hunt Publishing Co. Dubuque, IA, pp. 52–56.

31. Karlson, A.G., M.R. Zinober, and W.H. Feldman. 1950. A whole blood rapid agglutination test for avian tuberculosis. Am J Vet Res 11:137–141.

32. Karlson, A.G., C.L. Davis, and M.L. Cohn. 1962. Skotochromogenic Mycobacterium avium from a trumpeter swan. Am J Vet Res 23:575–579.

33. Karlson, A.G., C.O. Thoen, and R. Harrington. 1970. Japanese quail: Susceptibility to avian tuberculosis. Avian Dis 14:39–44.

34. Kiehn, T., F. Edwards, P. Brannon, A. Tsang, M. Maio, J. Gold, E. Whimbey, B. Wong, K. McClatchy, and D. Armstrong. 1985. Infections caused by Mycobacterium avium complex in immunocompromised patients: Diagnosis by blood culture and fecal examination, antimicrobial susceptibility tests, and morphological and seroagglutination characteristics. J Clin Microbiol 21:168–173.

35. Kleeberg, H.H. 1975. Tuberculosis and other Mycobacterioses. In W.T. Hubbert, W.F. McCulloch, and P.R. Schnurrenberger (eds.). Diseases Transmitted from Animals to Man, 6th ed. Charles C. Thomas, Springfield, IL, pp. 303–360.

36. Koch, R. 1890. Ueber bakteriologische Forschung. Wien Med Bl 13:531–535.

37. Koch, R. 1902. Address before the second general meeting. Trans Br Congr Tuberc 1:23–35.

38. Kubin, M., and E. Matuskova. 1968. Serological typing of mycobacteria for tracing possible sources of avian mycobacterial infections in man. Bull WHO 39:657–662.

39. Lesslie, I.W., and K.J. Birn. 1967. Tuberculosis in cattle caused by the avian type tubercle bacillus. Vet Rec 80:559–564.

40. Maffucci, A. 1890. Beitrag zur Aetiologie der Tuberkulose (Huhnertuberculose). Zentralbl Allg Pathol Pathol Anat 1:409–416.

41. Masters, B. 1996. Personal communication.

42. Matthews, P.R.J., J.A. McDiarmid, P. Collins, and A. Brown. 1977. The dependence of some strains of Mycobacterium avium of mycobactin for initial and subsequent growth. J Med Microbiol 2:53–57.

43. McDiarmid, A. 1948. The occurrence of tuberculosis in the wild wood-pigeon. J Comp Pathol Ther 58:128–133.

44. Meissner, G., K.H. Schroder, G.E. Amadio, W. Anz, S. Chaparas, H.W.B. Engel, P.A. Jenkins, W. Kappler, H.H. Kleeberg, E. Kubala, M. Kubin, D. Lauterbach, A. Lind, M. Magnusson, Z.D. Mikova, S.R. Pattyn, W.B. Schaefer, J.L. Stanford, M. Tsukamura, L.G. Wayne, I. Willers and E. Wolinsky. 1974. A cooperative numerical analysis of nonscoto- and nonphoto-chromogenic slowly growing mycobacteria. J Gen Microbiol 83:207–235.

45. Montali, R.J., M. Bush, C.O. Thoen, and E. Smith. 1976. Tuberculosis in captive exotic birds. J Am Vet Med Assoc 169:920–927.

46. Rossi, L. 1974. Immunizing potency of inactivated and living Mycobacterium avium and Mycobacterium intracellulare vaccines against tuberculosis of domestic fowls. Acta Vet Brno 43:133–138.

47. Rostagi, N., and W.W. Barrow. 1994. Cell envelope constituents and the multifaceted nature of Mycobacterium avium pathogenicity and drug resistance. Res Microbiol 145:243–252.

48. Schack-Steffenhagen, G., and J. Seeger. 1967. Untersuchungen uber das Vorkommen von Geflugeltuberkelbakterien beiauslandischen Schlachthuhnern. Zentralbl Bakteriol Parasitenkd Abt I Orig 202:204–211.

49. Schaefer, W.B. 1965. Serologic identification and classification of the atypical mycobacteria by their agglutination. Am Rev Respir Dis 92:85–93.

50. Schaefer, W.B., J.V. Beer, N.A. Wood, E. Boughton, P.A. Jenkins, and J. Marks. 1973. A bacteriological study of endemic tuberculosis in birds. J Hyg (Camb) 71:549–557.

51. Schalk, A.F., L.M. Roderick, H.L. Fousr, and G.S. Harshfield. 1935. Avian tuberculosis: collected studies. North Dakota Agric Exp Stn Tech Bull 279.

52. Schliesser, T., and A. Weber. 1973. Untersuchungen uber die Tenazitat von Mykobakterien der Gruppe III nach runyon in Sagemehleinstreu. Zentralbl Veterinaermed [B] 20:710–714.

53. Scrivner, L.H., and C. Elder. 1931. Cutaneous and subcutaneous tuberculosis in turkeys. J Am Vet Med Assoc 79:244–247.

54. Shane, S.M., Camus, A., Strain, M.G., Thoen, C.O., and Tully, T.N. 1993. Tuberculosis in Commercial Emus (Dromaius novaehollandiae). Avian Dis 37:1172–1176.

55. Singbeil, B.A., Bickford, A.A., and Stolz, J.H. 1993. Isolation of Mycobacterium avium from ringneck pheasants (Phasianus colchicus). Avian Dis 37:612–615.

56. Stenburg, H., and A. Turunen. 1968. Differentiation of Mycobacteria isolated from domestic animals. Zentralbl Veterinaermed [B] 15:494–503.

57. Svrcek, S., O.J. Vrtiak, B. Kapitancik, T. Pauer, and Z. Koppel. 1966. Wild birds and domestic pigeons as sources of avian tuberculosis. Rozhl Tuberk 26:659–67.

58. Thoen, C.O. 1979. Factors associated with pathogenicity of mycobacteria. In R. Schlessinger (ed.). Microbiology-979. American Society of Microbiologists, Washington, DC, pp. 162–167.

59. Thoen, C.O., 1992. Tuberculosis. In A.D. Leman, B. Straw, W.L. Mengeling, S. D'Allaire and D.J. Taylor (eds.). Diseases of Swine, 7th ed. Iowa State University Press, Ames, IA, pp. 617–626.

60. Thoen, C.O., 1994. Mycobacterium avium infections in animals. Res Microbiol 145:173–177.

61. Thoen, C.O., 1994. Tuberculosis in Wild and Domestic Mammals. In B.R. Bloom (ed). Tuberculosis: Pathogenesis, Prevention and Control. American Society of Microbiologists, Washington DC, pp. 157–162.

62. Thoen, C.O., and R. Chiodini. 1993. Mycobacterium. In C.L. Gyles and C.O. Thoen (eds.). Pathogenesis of Bacterial Infections in Animals. Iowa State University Press, Ames, IA, pp. 44–56.

63. Thoen, C.O., and E.M. Himes. 1981. Tuberculosis. In J.W. Davis, L.H. Karstad, and D.O. Trainer (eds.). Infectious Diseases of Wild Mammals, 2nd ed. Iowa State University Press, Ames, IA, pp 263–274.

64. Thoen, C.O., and D.E. Williams. 1994. Tuberculosis, Tuberculoidosis and Other Mycobacterial Infections. In G.W. Beran (ed.). Handbook of Zoonoses, Section A, 2nd ed. CRC Press, Boca Raton, FL, pp. 41–60.

65. Thoen, C.O., J.L. Jarnagin, and M.L. Champion. 1975. Micromethod for serotyping strains of Mycobacterium avium. J Clin Microbiol 1:469–471.

66. Thoen, C.O., E.M. Himes, and J.H. Campbell. 1976. Isolation of Mycobacterium avium serotype 3 from a white-headed tree duck. Avian Dis 20:587–592.

67. Thoen, C.O., W.G. Eacret, and E.M. Himes. 1978. An enzyme-labeled antibody test for detecting antibodies in chickens infected with Mycobacterium avium serotype 2. Avian Dis 22:162–168.

68. Thoen, C.O., E.M. Himes, and A.G. Karlson. 1984. Mycobacterium avium complex. In G.P. Kubica and L.G. Wayne (eds.). The Mycobacteria: A Sourcebook. Marcel Dekker, New York, pp. 1251–1275.

69. USDA. 1973. Statistical Summary. Federal Meat and Poultry Inspection for Calendar Year 1972. MPI-I.

70. USDA. 1979. Statistical Summary. Federal Meat and Poultry Inspection for Calendar Year 1978. MPI-I.

71. USDA. 1985. Statistical Summary. Federal Meat and Poultry Inspection for Calendar Year 1984. MPI-I.

72. Vanderheyden, N. 1986. Avian tuberculosis: Diagnosis and attempted treatment. Proc 1986 Annu Meet Assoc Avian Vet, pp. 203–211.

73. Vasenius, H. 1965. Tuberculosislike lesions in slaughter swine in Finland. Nord Vet Med 17:17–21.

74. Wallace, J.M., and J.B. Hannah. 1988. Mycobacterium avium complex infections in patients with the acquired immunodeficiency syndrome. Chest 93:926–932.

75. Weber. A., T. Schliesser, J.M. Schultze, and U. Bertelsmann. 1976. Serologische Typendifferenzierung aviarer Mykobacterienstamme isoliert von Schlachtrindern. Zentralbl Bakterial [orig A] 235:202–206.

76. Wiesenthal, A.M., K.E. Powell, J. Kopp, and J.W. Spindler. 1982. Increase in Mycobacterium avium complex isolation among patients admitted to a general hospital. Public Health Rep 97:61–65.

77. Wolinsky, E. 1979. Nontuberculous mycobacteria and associated diseases. Am Rev Respir Dis 119:107–159.

78. Wolinsky, E., and W.B. Schaefer. 1973. Proposed numbering scheme for mycobacterial serotypes by agglutination. Int J Syst Bacteriol 23:182–183.

8 Infectious Coryza

Pat J. Blackall, Masakazu Matsumoto, and Richard Yamamoto

INTRODUCTION. Infectious coryza (IC) is an acute respiratory disease of chickens caused by *Haemophilus paragallinarum*. The clinical syndrome has been described in the early literature as roup, contagious or infectious catarrh, cold, and uncomplicated coryza (138). The disease was named infectious coryza because it was infectious and affected primarily the nasal passages (3). The greatest economic losses result from poor growth performance in growing birds and marked reduction (10–40%) in egg production in layers. The disease is limited primarily to chickens and has no public health significance.

HISTORY. As early as 1920, Beach (2) believed that IC was a distinct clinical entity. The etiologic agent eluded identification for a number of years, since the disease was often masked in mixed infections and with fowl pox in particular. In 1932, De Blieck (37) isolated the causative agent and named it *Bacillus hemoglobinophilus coryzae gallinarum*.

INCIDENCE AND DISTRIBUTION. Infectious coryza is a disease of economic significance in many parts of the world. In the United States, the disease is most prevalent in California and the southeastern states.

ETIOLOGY

Classification. Based on studies conducted during the 1930s, the causative agent of IC was classified as *H. gallinarum* because of its requirement for both X-(hemin) and V-(nicotinamide adenine dinucleotide) factors for growth (43, 120). Since 1962, however, Page (91) and others (13, 50, 87, 99) found that all isolates recovered from cases of IC required only the V-factor for growth. This led to the proposal and general acceptance of a new species, *H. paragallinarum* (146), for organisms requiring only the V-factor. *H. gallinarum* and *H. paragallinarum* are identical in all other growth characteristics and disease-producing potential (99). These observations, in addition to the apparent abrupt change in the X-factor requirement of all isolates recovered worldwide since 1962, have led some workers to question the validity of tests used by earlier workers in classifying their isolates as *H.*

gallinarum (99). Indeed, it has been suggested that the early descriptions of the causative agent of IC as an X- and V-factor–dependent organism were incorrect (15).

More recently, V-factor independent isolates of *H. paragallinarum* have been recovered from chickens with coryza in South Africa (29, 53, 84). Thus, it is apparent that classification of hemophili based strictly on in vitro growth factor requirements may be misleading, as suggested by Kilian and Biberstein (69).

Morphology and Staining. *H. paragallinarum* is a gram-negative nonmotile bacterium. In 24-hr cultures, it appears as short rods or coccobacilli 1–3 mm in length and 0.4–0.8 mm in width, with a tendency for filament formation. A capsule may be demonstrated in virulent strains (46, 113). The organism undergoes degeneration within 48–60 hr, showing fragments and ill-defined forms. Subcultures to fresh medium at this stage will again yield the typical rod-shaped morphology. Bacilli may occur singly, in pairs, or as short chains (120).

Growth Requirements. The reduced form of NAD (NADH) (1.56–25 µg/mL medium) (91, 103) or its oxidized form (20–100 µg/mL) (109) is necessary for the in vitro growth of most isolates of *H. paragallinarum*. The exceptions are the isolates described in South Africa that are NAD independent (29, 53, 84). Sodium chloride (NaCl) (1.0–1.5%) (103) is essential for growth. Chicken serum (1%) is required by some strains (46), whereas others merely show improved growth with this supplement (13). Brain heart infusion, tryptose agar, and chicken-meat infusion are some basal media to which supplements are added (46, 74, 109). More complex media are used to obtain dense growth of organisms for characterization studies (4, 98, 99). The pH of various media varies from 6.9 to 7.6. A number of bacterial species excrete V-factor that will support growth of *H. paragallinarum* (91).

The determination of the growth factor requirements of the avian haemophili is not an easy process. Commercial growth factor disks used for this purpose may yield a high percentage of cultures that falsely appear to be both X- and V-factor dependent (12). The brand of disks and the medium to be used should be carefully checked for their suitability. For well-equipped laboratories, the porphyrin test (68) is recommended for X-factor testing; the use of purified hemin and NAD as supplements to otherwise complete media may also be considered.

The organism is commonly grown in an atmosphere of 5% carbon dioxide; however, carbon dioxide is not an essential requirement, since the organism is able to grow under reduced oxygen tension or anaerobically (43, 91).

The minimal and maximal temperatures of growth are 25 and 45 C, respectively, the optimal range being 34–42 C. The organism is commonly grown at 37–38 C.

Colony Morphology. Tiny dewdrop colonies up to 0.3 mm in diameter develop on suitable media. In obliquely transmitted light, mucoid (smooth) iridescent and rough noniridescent and other intermediate colony forms have been observed (48, 99, 112, 110).

Biochemical Properties. The ability to reduce nitrate to nitrite, and ferment glucose without the formation of gas is common to all the avian haemophili. Oxidase activity, the presence of the enzyme alkaline phosphatase, and a failure to produce indole or hydrolyse urea or gelatin are also uniform characteristics (8). Considerable confusion surrounds the carbohydrate fermentation patterns of the avian haemophili. Much of the variability recorded in the literature may be due to the use of different basal media. False-negative results are mainly associated with poor growth and can also be a significant problem (4). In general, recent studies have used a medium consisting of a phenol red broth containing 1% (w/v) NaCl, 25 µg/mL NADH, 1% (v/v) chicken serum and 1% (w/v) carbohydrate. For routine identification, the use of the phenol red broth just described and a dense inoculum is a most suitable approach for determining carbohydrate fermentation patterns. For large studies, a replica plating technique (4) may be more suitable.

A range of organisms that superficially resemble *H. paragallinarum* can be found in chickens. In particular, organisms once known as *Haemophilus avium* are common in chickens and are regarded as nonpathogenic (51). Based on DNA hybridization studies, isolates of *H. avium* were found to be comprised of at least three DNA homology groups (85). They have been named *Pasteurella avium, P. volantium,* and *Pasteurella* species A. Not all isolates of *H. avium*, however, can be assigned to these three new taxa solely on the basis of phenotypic properties (7). Table 8.1 presents those properties that allow a full identification of the avian haemophili.

The failure of *H. paragallinarum* to ferment either galactose or trehalose and its lack of catalase clearly separate this organism from the other avian haemophili. The properties shown in the table for *H. paragallinarum* have been found to be typical of isolates from Argentina, Australia, Brazil, China, Germany, Japan, and the United States (27, 13, 32, 51, 71, 87, 99, 130). The main characteristics that differentiate the NAD-independent from the NAD-dependent *H. paragallinarum* are that the former does not have ß-galactosidase activity and does not ferment maltose (84).

Resistance to Chemical and Physical Agents. *H. paragallinarum* is a delicate organism that is inactivated rather rapidly outside the host. Infectious exudate suspended in tap water is inactivated in 4 hr at ambient temperature; when suspended in saline, the exudate is infectious for at least 24 hr at 22 C. Exudate or tissue remains infectious when held at 37 C for 24 hr and, on occasion, up to 48 hr; at 4 C, exudate remains infectious for several days. At temperatures of 45–55 C, hemophili are killed within 2–10 min. Infectious embryonic fluids treated with 0.25% formalin are inactivated within 24 hr at 6 C, but the organism survives for several days under similar conditions when treated with thimerosal, 1:10,000 (139).

The organism may be maintained on blood agar plates by weekly passages. Young cultures maintained in a "candle jar" will remain viable for 2 wk at 4 C. Chicken embryos 6–7 days old may be inoculated with single colonies or broth cultures via the yolk sac; yolk from embryos dead in 24–48 hr will contain a large number of organisms which may be frozen at -20 to -70 C or lyophilized (138).

Antigenic Structure. Page (91, 92) classified his organisms of *H. paragallinarum* with the plate agglutination test into serovars A, B, and C. While Page's serovar A strain 0083 and B strain 0222 are available today, all the serovar C strains were lost during the mid-1960s. Matsumoto and Yamamoto (81) isolated strain Modesto which was later classified as a strain of serovar C by Rimler et al. (102).

Based on Page's typing scheme and using an agglutination test, isolates from Germany were classified as serovars A and B (47), from Spain as A, B and C (93), from Australia, South Africa and Indonesia as A and C (11, 126), and from Malaysia as serovar A (145).

It is also possible to use a hemagglutination inhibition (HI) test to serotype isolates by the Page scheme (18). Using this HI approach, isolates from China were classified as serovar A (32), and from Argentina and Brazil as serovars A, B, and C (27, 130).

Table 8.1. Differential tests for the avian haemophili

Property	Hemophilus paragallinarum	H. avium	Pasteurella avium	P. volantium	Pasteurella species A
Pigment	–	Yellow V	–	Yellow U	–
Catalase	–	+	+	+	+
Growth in air	–	+	+	+	+
ONPG	+	V	–	+	V
Acid from					
Arabinose	–	V	–	–	+
Galactose	–	+	+	+	+
Maltose	+	V	–	+	V
Mannitol	+	V	–	+	V
Sorbitol	V	V	–	V	–
Sucrose	V	+	+	+	+
Trehalose	–	+	+	+	+

U = usually; V = variable; + = positive; – = negative.

A third method of assigning isolates of *H. paragallinarum* to a Page serovar is based on the use of a panel of monoclonal antibodies developed by workers in Japan (23). Drawbacks with the monoclonal antibody approach are that a serovar B–specific monoclonal antibody is not available, some Page serovar A strains from South America fail to react with the serovar A monoclonal antibody (27, 130), and there is no commercial source for the antibodies.

There have been suggestions that Page serovar B is not a true serovar, but rather consists of variants of serovar A or C that have lost their type-specific antigen (74, 113). Recent studies, however, have conclusively shown that Page serovar B is a true serovar (135).

In independent studies from Japan, Kato and Tsubahara (66) described three serovars, I, II, and III; but later studies have suggested that serovars II and III were variants of serovar I (60, 111). Sawata et al. (111) extended Kato and Tsubahara's study and identified two serovars, 1 and 2. Serovar 1 was represented by strain 221 from Kato and Tsubahara (66), and the new serovar, serovar 2, was represented by strain H-18. Later, serovars 1 and 2 were shown to correspond to Page's serovars A and C (74, 113).

The importance of the Page scheme is that several studies have shown a correlation between Page serovars and immunotype specificity (14, 73, 102). Chickens vaccinated with a bacterin prepared from one serovar were protected only against homologous challenge. A recent study has shown that cross-protection within Page serovar B is only partial (136).

Kume et al. (75) proposed an alternative serologic classification based on an HI test using potassium thiocyanate-treated and -sonicated cells, rabbit hyperimmune serums, and glutaraldehyde-fixed chicken erythrocytes. In essence, Page's serovars A, C, and B were elevated to serogroups I, II, and III, and seven serovars (HA-1 to HA-7) were recognized among the three serogroups: three each for I and II and one for III. Of interest was the finding that the serovars seemed to be unique to the geographic origin of the strains. Many isolates that were nontypable in the Page scheme by agglutination tests were easily typed using the Kume scheme (42). An eighth and a ninth serovar have been recognized in Australia (19, 42). The terminology of the Kume scheme has recently been altered to allow for the addition of further serovars (19). Under this altered nomenclature, the three serogroups, I, II, and III, are renamed A, C, and B, thus emphasizing that Kume serogroups A, B, and C match Page serovars A, B, and C. Within each of the serogroups, the serovars are numbered sequentially, allowing new serovars to be added in numerical order. Thus, the nine currently recognized Kume serovars are A-1, A-2, A-3, A-4, B-1, C-1, C-2, C-3, and C-4 (19). The Kume scheme has not been widely applied, as it is technically demanding to perform.

As the Kume serogroups match the Page serovars, it is reasonable to assume that there is no cross-protection across Kume serogroups. There have not been extensive studies examining the cross-protection within the Kume serogroups. By reexamining past publications in the light of the Kume scheme, plus some recent experiments, it has been determined that Kume serovars C-1 and C-2 are cross-protective, and that Kume serovars C-2 and C-4 are cross-protective (9, 14, 74).

Another serotyping scheme, based on heat-stable determinants detected in an agar-gel precipitin (AGP) test, has been described (49). The six serovars recognized by this scheme do not correlate with immunotypes, and the scheme is not widely used.

A serum bactericidal test capable of classifying

isolates to Kume serogroups A and C (corresponding to Page serovars A and C) has also been described (117).

Strain Classification. Typing of *H. paragallinarum* isolates below species level has traditionally been done by serotyping (see Antigenic Structure). Typing by carbohydrate fermentation patterns and antimicrobial resistance patterns can be done, but yields few subtypes (17). Both soluble whole-cell proteins and outer-membrane proteins have been shown to exist in only two major banding patterns (16, 21), and these techniques have not been used for typing purposes. DNA fingerprinting by restriction endonuclease analysis has been shown to be a suitable typing technique with patterns being stable in vitro and in vivo (20, 22). Restriction endonuclease analysis has proven useful in epidemiologic studies (20), as well as confirming that the recent NAD-independent *H. paragallinarum* isolates from South Africa are clonal in nature (83). The technique of multilocus enzyme electrophoresis has been used to examine the genetic diversity of *H. paragallinarum* isolates (28). A panel of monoclonal antibodies has been used to differentiate field isolates from the serovar A and B vaccine strains of *H. paragallinarum* (131). This same panel of antibodies was used to type the non-NAD–requiring isolates of *H. paragallinarum* into serovar A (30).

Pathogenicity. A range of factors has been associated with the pathogenicity of *H. paragallinarum*. Considerable attention has been paid to HA antigens. In both Page serovar A and C, mutants lacking HA activity have been used to demonstrate that the HA antigen plays a key role in colonization (110, 137).

The capsule has also been associated with colonization, and has been suggested to be the key factor in the lesions associated with IC (110, 119). The capsule of *H. paragallinarum* has been shown to protect the organism against the bactericidal activity of normal chicken serum (118). It has been suggested that a toxin released from capsular organisms during in vivo multiplication was responsible for the clinical disease (76).

H. paragallinarum is capable of acquiring iron from chicken and turkey transferrin, suggesting that iron sequestration may not be an adequate host defense mechanism (89). In contrast, two strains of *H. avium* were unable to acquire iron from these transferrins despite apparently having the same receptor proteins (89).

Crude polysaccharide extracted from *H. paragallinarum* is toxic to chickens and may be responsible for the toxic signs that may follow administration of bacterin (59). The role, if any, of this component in the natural occurrence of the disease is unknown.

PATHOGENESIS AND EPIZOOTIOLOGY

Natural and Experimental Hosts. The chicken is the natural host for *H. paragallinarum*. All ages are susceptible (140), but the disease is usually less severe in juvenile birds. The incubation period is shortened, and the course of the disease tends to be longer in mature birds.

While there have been reports of IC due to *H. paragallinarum* in a number of bird species other than chickens, reviewed by Yamamoto (140), these reports need to be interpreted carefully. As a range of hemophilic organisms, none of which are *H. paragallinarum*, have been described in birds other than chickens (39, 45, 94), only those studies that involve detailed bacteriology can be regarded as definitive proof of the presence of *H. paragallinarum* in birds other than chickens. The following species are refractory to experimental infection: turkey, pigeon, sparrow, duck, crow, rabbit, guinea pig, and mouse (138, 139).

Transmission, Carriers, and Vectors. Chronic or healthy carrier birds have long been recognized as the main reservoir of infection. The recent application of molecular fingerprinting techniques has confirmed the role of carrier birds in the spread of IC (20). Infectious coryza seems to occur most frequently in fall and winter, although such seasonal patterns may be coincidental to management practices (e.g., introduction of susceptible replacement pullets onto farms where IC is present). On farms where multiple-age groups are brooded and raised, spread of the disease to successive age groups usually occurs within 1–6 wk after such birds are moved from the brooder house to growing cages near older groups of infected birds (34). Infectious coryza is not an egg-transmitted disease.

Whereas the sparrow could not be implicated as a vector, epidemiologic studies suggested that the organism may be introduced onto isolated ranches by the airborne route (141).

Incubation Period. The characteristic feature is a coryza of short incubation that develops within 24–48 hr after inoculation of chickens with either culture or exudate. The latter will more consistently induce disease (99). Susceptible birds exposed by contact to infected cases may show signs of the disease within 24–72 hr.

The duration of the disease varies with the inoculum and virulence of the organism (110). Early studies showed that the organism rapidly lost virulence following serial passages on artificial media (88); consequently, the culture-induced coryza was of much shorter duration (6–14 days) than that produced by infectious sinus exudate (50 days or more) (88, 120). The virulence of attenuated laboratory cultures also could be increased to simulate the exudate-induced disease by rapid serial passages through chickens (120). Since these studies were performed before the existence of *Mycoplasma gallisepticum* was recognized, however, the prolonged course of the exudate-induced disease could have resulted from a concurrent infection with this and possibly other agents. A coryza in specific-pathogen-free chickens of short incubation (2 days) and long duration (36 days or more) has since been demonstrated in mixed infections of *H. paragallinarum* and *M. gallisepticum* (1). In the absence of a concurrent infection, IC usually runs its course within 2–3 wk.

Signs. The most prominent features are involvement of nasal passage and sinuses with a serous to mucoid nasal discharge, facial edema, and conjunctivitis. Figure 8.1 illustrates the typical facial edema. Swollen wattles may be evident, particularly in males. Rales may be heard in birds with infection of the lower respiratory tract.

A swollen head–like syndrome associated with *H. paragallinarum* has been reported in broilers in the absence of pneumovirus, but in the presence or absence of other bacterial pathogens such as *M. synoviae* and *M. gallisepticum* (40, 107). Arthritis and septicemia have been reported in broiler and layer flocks, respectively, in which the presence of other pathogens has contributed to the disease complex (107).

Birds may have diarrhea, and feed and water consumption usually is decreased; in growing birds this means an increased number of culls, and in laying flocks a reduction in egg production (10 to 40%). A foul odor may be detected in flocks in which the disease has become chronic and complicated with other bacteria.

Morbidity and Mortality. The virulence of the organism may alter the course of the disease. While highly toxigenic strains such as described by Delaplane et al. (38) may cause high mortality, IC is usually characterized by low mortality and high morbidity. Variations in age and breed may also influence the clinical picture (5). Complicating factors such as poor housing, parasitism, and inadequate nutrition may add to severity and duration of the disease. When complicated with other diseases such as fowl pox, infectious bronchitis, laryngotracheitis, chronic respiratory disease, and pasteurellosis, IC is usually more severe and prolonged, with resulting increased mortality (107, 138).

Gross Lesions. *H. paragallinarum* produces an acute catarrhal inflammation of mucous membranes of nasal passages and sinuses. There is frequently a catarrhal conjunctivitis and subcutaneous edema of face and wattles. Typically, pneumonia and airsacculitis are rarely present; however, reports of recent outbreaks in broilers have indicated significant levels of condemnations (up to 69.8%) due to airsacculitis, even in the absence of any other recognized viral or bacterial pathogens (40, 52).

Histopathology. Fujiwara and Konno (44) studied the histopathologic response of chickens from 12 hr to 3 mo after intranasal inoculation. Es-

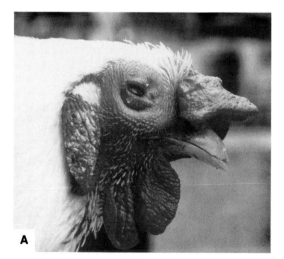 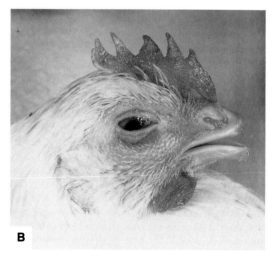

A **B**

8.1. Chickens artificially infected with *Haemophilus paragallinarum*. *A.* Mature male with coryza and facial edema. *B.* Mature female showing conjunctivitis, nasal discharge and open-mouth breathing.

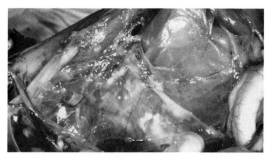

8.2. Field infection with IC showing caseopurulent air sac lesions.

sential changes in the nasal cavity, infraorbital sinuses, and trachea consisted of sloughing, disintegration, and hyperplasia of mucosal and glandular epithelia, and edema and hyperemia with heterophil infiltration in the tunica propria of the mucous membranes. Pathologic changes first observed at 20 hr reached maximum severity by 7–10 days, with subsequent repair occurring within 14–21 days. In birds with involvement of the lower respiratory tract, acute catarrhal bronchopneumonia was observed, with heterophils and cell debris filling the lumen of secondary and tertiary bronchi; epithelial cells of air capillaries were swollen and showed hyperplasia. Catarrhal inflammation of air sacs was characterized by swelling and hyperplasia of the cells, with abundant heterophil infiltration. In addition, a pronounced infiltration of mast cells was observed in the lamina propria of the mucous membrane of the nasal cavity (119). The products of mast cells, heterophils, and macrophages may be responsible for the severe vascular changes and cell damage leading to coryza. A dissecting fibrinopurulent cellulitis similar to that seen in chronic fowl cholera has been reported in broiler and layer chickens (40).

Immunity.   Chickens that have recovered from active infection possess varying degrees of immunity to reexposure. Pullets that have experienced IC during their growing period are generally protected against a later drop in egg production. Resistance to reexposure among individual birds may develop as early as 2 wk after initial exposure by the intrasinus route (108).

It has been shown that experimentally infected chickens develop a cross-serovar (Page scheme) immunity (100). In contrast, as discussed earlier, bacterins provide only serovar-specific immunity (14, 73, 102). This suggests that cross-protective antigens are expressed in vivo that are either not expressed or expressed at very low levels in vitro.

The protective antigens of *H. paragallinarum*

have not been definitively identified. It has been suggested that the capsule of *H. paragallinarum* contains protective antigens (116). Using both Page serovar A and C strains, a crude polysaccharide extract was shown to provide serovar-specific protection (59).

Considerable attention has been paid to the role of HA antigens as protective antigens. It has been long noted that for Page serovar A organisms, there is a close correlation between HI titer and both protection (73, 90) and nasal clearance of the challenge organism (76) in vaccinated chickens. Purified HA antigen from a Page serovar A organism has been shown to be protective (58). Takagi and colleagues have shown that a monoclonal antibody specific for the HA of Page serovar A provides passive protection, and that the HA antigen purified by use of this antibody is also protective (124, 127).

Based on studies conducted to date, there is considerable evidence that the protective antigens of *H. paragallinarum* are surface located. The antigens implicated have been the antigens detected during Page serotyping, HA antigens, and some component or components of the polysaccharide content of the cell. It seems probable that a number of different antigens (outer-membrane proteins, polysaccharides, lipopolysaccharides) are all likely to be involved.

DIAGNOSIS

Isolation and Identification of Causative Agent.   Many different media have been developed to support growth of *H. paragallinarum*. (74, 90, 99). While *H. paragallinarum* is considered to be a fastidious organism, it is not difficult to isolate, requiring simple media and procedures. Specimens should be taken from two or three chickens in the acute stage of the disease (1–7 days' incubation). The skin under the eyes is seared with a hot iron spatula and an incision made into the sinus cavity with sterile scissors. A sterile cotton swab is inserted deep into the sinus cavity where the organism is most often found in pure form. Tracheal and air sac exudates also may be taken on sterile swabs. The swab is streaked on a blood agar plate, which is then cross-streaked with a *Staphylococcus* culture and incubated at 37 C in a large screw-cap jar in which a candle is allowed to burn out. *Staphylococcus epidermidis* (91) or *S. hyicus* (13), which are commonly used as "feeders," should be pretested because not all strains actively produce the V-factor.

At the simplest level, IC may be diagnosed on the basis of a history of a rapidly spreading disease in which coryza is the main manifestation, combined with the isolation of a catalase-negative bacterium showing satellitic growth. Better equipped laboratories should attempt a more complete biochemical identification as described earlier. Additional studies of this nature are essential when isolates of NAD-independent *H. paragallinarum* are suspected. A DNA probe, specific for *H. paragallinarum,* has been described and could be used in laboratories with appropriate technical support (33). Serotyping of *H. paragallinarum* isolates is important for epidemiologic investigations and to assist in management programs based on vaccination (see Antigenic Structure).

Another efficient diagnostic procedure is to inoculate the sinus exudate or culture into two or three normal chickens by the intrasinus route. The production of a coryza in 24–48 hr is diagnostic; however, the incubation period may be delayed up to 1 wk if only a few organisms are present in the inoculum, such as in long-standing cases.

Serology. Commonly used serologic tests include plate or tube agglutination (56, 74, 142) AGP (56, 108) and HI (56, 73).

Since common antigens are shared by the three serovars, an agglutination antigen prepared from one serovar may be used to detect antibodies to all three serovars. Agglutinins are detected 7–14 days postinfection and may persist up to 1 yr or longer. The test may be used to check flocks for evidence of past infection and to follow the antibody response in bacterin efficacy studies.

Autoagglutination and nonagglutination observed with some antigen preparations may be rendered satisfactory in some cases by treating the cells with trypsin (57) and hyaluronidase (102), respectively. Others have found that trypsin destroys functional determinant groups (110).

A serovar-specific agglutination test was devel-

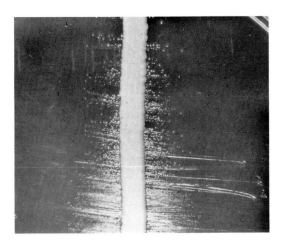

8.3. Satellite phenomenon. Tiny dewdrop colonies of *Haemophilus paragallinarum* growing adjacent to *Staphylococcus* culture (broad streak) on a blood agar plate.

oped by adsorbing polysaccharide antigens onto latex particles (133); this test seems to be effective in detecting recent infections (3 wk).

The AGP test will detect antibodies 2 wk postinfection or postvaccination and for at least 11 wk (56,108).

A test to detect HI antibodies to serovar A strains uses whole bacterial cells and fresh chicken erythrocytes. Kato's strain 221 is commonly used as the antigen, although other strains of serovar A will hemagglutinate chicken erythrocytes (74, 99). Many factors such as type of basal media and chicken serum concentration used, and length of incubation of cultures will influence the yield and quality of the HA antigen (55, 121). The chicken erythrocyte phenotype can influence reactivity of the HA antigen (60). Treatment of the erythrocytes with trypsin or formalin will increase the sensitivity of the test (61). Glutaraldehyde-fixed erythrocytes also have been used (116). Trypsin and hyaluronidase treatment of cells of strain 221 will enhance its HA activity (54, 55, 110, 115); hyaluronidase treatment, which removes the hyaluronic acid capsule, will also render some nonhemagglutinating strains to hemagglutinate (99). The HI test does not detect antibody as early as agglutination or AGP in infected or immunized birds (56, 65). The test detects antibodies to the serovar-specific antigen that is closely correlated with protective immunity (65, 70, 76, 90, 114).

The finding that serovar C strains can be made to hemagglutinate by the use of potassium thiocyanate-treated and -sonicated cells and glutaraldehyde-fixed chicken erythrocytes has yielded a test that detects antibodies to the serovar-specific HA antigen. While somewhat controversial (123), this test has been used to evaluate protective potency of serovar C bacterins (114, 134). For both of the HI tests, it may be necessary to pretreat the sera with erythrocytes to eliminate nonspecific hemagglutinins. Early developmental work on an enzyme-linked immunosorbent assay (ELISA) has been reported (96).

Differential Diagnosis. Infectious coryza must be differentiated from other diseases such as chronic respiratory disease, chronic fowl cholera, fowl pox, swollen head syndrome, and A-avitaminosis, which produce similar clinical signs. Since *H. paragallinarum* infections often occur in mixed infections, one should consider the possibility of other bacteria or viruses as complicating IC, particularly if mortality is high and the disease takes a prolonged course (see Pathogenicity; Morbidity and Mortality).

TREATMENT. Various sulfonamides and antibiotics are useful in alleviating the severity and course of IC. It should be noted drug resistance does develop (6, 97). Relapse often occurs after treatment is discontinued and the carrier state is not eliminated (139). Erythromycin and oxytetracycline are two commonly used antibiotics.

Drugs in combination found effective in treatment of IC include sulfachloropyrazine–sulfadimidine (31), chlortetracycline–sulfadimethoxine (67), sulfachloropyridazine–trimethoprim (77, 95, 122), sulfadimethoxine–trimethoprim (106), and sulfamonomethoxine–ormetoprim (79, 129). Dihydrostreptomycin and some sulfa drugs act synergistically (31, 64). A range of new generation antibiotics have been shown to have promise in the treatment of IC (78, 105, 128, 143). Strains of *H. paragallinarum* resistant to various antibiotics did not carry plasmids (6).

PREVENTION AND CONTROL

Management Procedures.   Since recovered carrier birds are the main source of infection, practices such as buying breeding males or started chicks from unknown sources should be discouraged.

Only day-old chicks should be secured for replacement purposes unless the source is known to be free of IC. Isolation rearing and housing away from old stock are desirable practices. To eliminate the agent from a farm, it is necessary to depopulate the infected or recovered flock(s) because birds in such flocks remain reservoirs of infection. After cleaning and disinfection of the equipment and houses, the premises should be allowed to remain vacant for 2–3 wk before restocking with clean birds.

Immunization.   Commercial IC bacterins are widely available. As the literature of the various factors influencing the efficacy of bacterins has recently been reviewed (10), only key points are considered here. While bacterins have been prepared from chicken embryos (34), broth (35), and cell culture (132), most commercial products are currently based on broth-grown cultures. They must contain at least 10^8 colony-forming units/mL to be effective (81). The following section reviews only the literature on broth-based bacterins.

There is disagreement in the literature as to the effect of different inactivating agents on the efficacy of bacterins. Thimerosal has been shown to be effective (14, 36, 81), as has formalin (35, 101). In three studies directly comparing formalin and thimerosal, formalin reduced the efficacy of the vaccines, although there was evidence that the effect was adjuvant specific. The use of formalin, compared with thimerosal, resulted in a reduction of the efficacy of aluminum hydroxide–based vaccines in two studies (14, 36), but had no such effect

in a third (80). Similarly, formalin, compared with thimerosal, impaired the efficacy of a vaccine containing chrome alum as an adjuvant (81), and another based on mineral oil (36). These studies suggest that while vaccines containing formalin as the inactivating agent can be protective, it is possible that a similar vaccine containing thimerosal would be even more efficient.

A number of adjuvants have been shown to be effective for IC bacterins, in particular, aluminium hydroxide gel and mineral oil (63, 24, 35, 36, 73, 80, 81, 98). The report of mineral oil being less effective than aluminium hydroxide gel (98) may result from a formulation problem rather than any inherent deficiency in the ability of mineral oil to act as an effective adjuvant. As with any bacterin that contains adjuvants, particularly mineral oil, the potential adverse reaction at the site of injection (41) should be considered when using such products.

Bacterins are generally injected in birds between 10 and 20 wk of age and yield optimal results when given 3–4 wk prior to an expected natural outbreak. Two injections given approximately 4 wk apart before 20 wk of age seem to result in better performance of layers than a single injection. When administered to growing birds, the bacterin reduces losses from complicated respiratory disease. Both subcutaneous and intramuscular routes have been effective (14, 36, 81). Injection of the bacterin into the leg muscle gave better protection than when injected into the breast muscle (62). The intranasal route was not effective (14). Oral delivery of an IC bacterin was effective, but this route required 100 times as many cells as with the parenteral route (86). Significant immunity has been demonstrated for about 9 mo following vaccination (14, 72, 81).

As inactivated IC bacterins provide protection only against the Page serovars included in the vaccine, it is vital that bacterins contain the serovars present in the target population. The confirmed existence of Page serovar B as a true serovar with full pathogenicity, as well as its widespread occurrence (see Antigenic Structure), means that this serovar must be included in inactivated bacterins in areas where serovar B is present. However, since different strains of serovar B provide only partial cross-protection among themselves (136), it may be necessary to prepare an autogenous bacterin for use in areas where the B serovar is endemic.

Since dissociation of *H. paragallinarum* is a common phenomenon (112), care should be taken in selecting the proper seed culture, media, and incubation period to obtain the most immunogenic product.

Mixed bacterins containing inactivated infectious bronchitis virus, Newcastle disease virus, and *H. paragallinarum* have been described (90, 144). A combined *H. paragallinarum–M. gallisepticum* bacterin was reported to provide protection against transient and chronic coryza (104). However, antibody response to *H. paragallinarum* was suppressed in chickens inoculated with a similar product (82).

Another approach to control IC in endemic areas has been the practice of controlled exposure. The usual procedure is to vaccinate birds between 15 and 18 wk of age with bacterin, and then expose them to the live virulent organism at 20 wk. Autogenous organisms or isolates of known characteristics should be used. Vaccination with live viruses should be avoided during controlled exposure. Individual birds showing severe signs may be treated with antibiotics. Controlled exposure should be performed under careful veterinary supervision.

Attenuated strains of *H. paragallinarum,* if available, could form the basis of a live vaccine, a preferred alternative to controlled exposure. Preliminary work on the production of attenuated, immunogenic *H. paragallinarum* strains has been reported (25, 26). A study with a serovar A recombinant vaccine that expresses HA activity and induces protective immunity in chickens also appears promising (125).

REFERENCES

1. Adler, H.E., and R. Yamamoto. 1956. Studies on chronic coryza (Nelson) in the domestic fowl. Cornell Vet 46:337–343.
2. Beach, J.R. 1920. The diagnosis, therapeutic, and prophylaxis of chicken-pox (contagious epithelioma) of fowls. J Am Vet Med Assoc 58:301–312.
3. Beach, J.R., and O.W. Schalm. 1936. Studies of the clinical manifestations and transmissibility of infectious coryza of chickens. Poult Sci 15:466–472.
4. Blackall, P.J. 1983. An evaluation of methods for the detection of carbohydrate fermentation patterns in avian Haemophilus species. J Microbiol Methods 1:275–281.
5. Blackall, P.J. 1983. Development of a vaccine against infectious coryza. In Disease Prevention and Control in Poultry Production. Proc #66. Postgraduate Committee on Veterinary Science, University of Sydney, pp. 99–104.
6. Blackall, P.J. 1988. Antimicrobial drug resistance and the occurrence of plasmids in Haemophilus paragallinarum. Avian Dis 32:742–747.
7. Blackall, P.J. 1988. Biochemical properties of catalase-positive avian haemophili. J Gen Microbiol 134:2801–2805.
8. Blackall, P. J. 1989. The avian haemophili. Clin Microbiol Rev 2:270–277.
9. Blackall, P.J. 1991. An evaluation of the cross protection afforded by inactivated infectious coryza vaccines. Aust Vet J 68:266–267.
10. Blackall, P.J. 1995. Vaccines against infectious coryza. World's Poult Sci J 51:17–26.
11. Blackall, P.J., and L.E. Eaves. 1988. Serological classification of Australian and South African isolates of Haemophilus paragallinarum. Aust Vet J 65:362–363.
12. Blackall, P.J., and J.G. Farrah. 1985. An evaluation of commercial discs for the determination of the growth factor requirements of the avian haemophili. Vet Microbiol 10:125–131.
13. Blackall, P.J., and G.G. Reid. 1982. Further characterization of Haemophilus paragallinarum and Haemophilus avium. Vet Microbiol 7:359–367.
14. Blackall, P.J., and G.G. Reid. 1987. Further efficacy studies on inactivated, aluminum-hydroxide-adsorbed vaccines against infectious coryza. Avian Dis 31:527–532.
15. Blackall, P.J., and R. Yamamoto. 1989. "Haemophilus gallinarum"—a re-examination. J Gen Microbiol 135:469–474.
16. Blackall, P.J., and R. Yamamoto. 1989. Whole-cell protein profiles of Haemophilus paragallinarum as detected by polyacrylamide gel electrophoresis. Avian Dis 33:168–173.
17. Blackall, P.J., L.E. Eaves, and D.G. Rogers. 1989. Biotyping of Haemophilus paragallinarum by hemagglutination serotyping, carbohydrate fermentation, and antimicrobial drug resistance patterns. Avian Dis 33:491–496.
18. Blackall, P.J., L.E. Eaves, and G. Aus. 1990. Serotyping of Haemophilus paragallinarum by the Page scheme: Comparison of the use of agglutination and hemagglutination-inhibition tests. Avian Dis 34:643–645.
19. Blackall, P.J., L.E. Eaves, and D.G. Rogers. 1990. Proposal of a new serovar and altered nomenclature for Haemophilus paragallinarum in the Kume hemagglutinin scheme. J Clin Microbiol 28:1185–1187.
20. Blackall, P.J., C.J. Morrow, A. McInnes, L.E. Eaves, and D.G. Rogers. 1990. Epidemiologic studies on infectious coryza outbreaks in northern New South Wales, Australia, using serotyping, biotyping, and chromosomal DNA restriction endonuclease analysis. Avian Dis 34:267–276.
21. Blackall, P.J., D.G. Rogers, and R. Yamamoto. 1990. Outer-membrane proteins of Haemophilus paragallinarum. Avian Dis 34:871–877.
22. Blackall, P.J., L.E. Eaves, and C.J. Morrow. 1991. Comparison of Haemophilus paragallinarum isolates by restriction endonuclease analysis of chromosomal DNA. Vet Microbiol 27:39–47.
23. Blackall, P.J., Y.-Z. Zheng, T. Yamaguchi, Y. Iritani, and D.G. Rogers. 1991. Evaluation of a panel of monoclonal antibodies in the subtyping of Haemophilus paragallinarum. Avian Dis 35:955–959.
24. Blackall, P.J., L.E. Eaves, D.G. Rogers, and G. Firth. 1992. An evaluation of inactivated infectious coryza vaccines containing a double-emulsion adjuvant system. Avian Dis 36:632–636.
25. Blackall, P.J., M. Rafiee, R.J. Graydon, and D. Tinworth. 1993. Towards a live infectious coryza vaccine. Proc 10th World Vet Poult Assoc Congr, p. 99.
26. Blackall, P.J., M. Rafiee, R.J. Graydon, and D. Tinworth. 1994. Progress towards a live infectious coryza vaccine. Proc 43rd West Poult Dis Conf, pp. 65–66.
27. Blackall, P.J., E.N. Silva, Y. Yamaguchi, and Y. Iritani. 1994. Characterization of isolates of avian haemophili from Brazil. Avian Dis 38:269–274.
28. Bowles, R., P.J Blackall, H.R. Terzolo, and V.E. Sandoval. 1993. An assessment of the genetic diversity of Australian and overseas isolates of Haemophilus paragallinarum by multilocus enzyme electrophoresis. Proc 10th World Vet Poult Assoc Congr, p. 148.
29. Bragg, R.R., L. Coetzee, and J.A. Verschoor. 1993. Plasmid encoded NAD-independence in some South African isolates of Haemophilus paragallinarum. Onderstepoort J Vet Res 60:147–152.
30. Bragg, R.R., L. Coetzee, and J.A. Verschoor. 1993. Monoclonal antibody characterization of South African field isolates of Haemophilus paragallinarum. Onderstepoort J Vet Res 60:181–187.
31. Buys, S.B. 1972. Haemophilus coryza: Therapy with selected drugs. J S Afr Vet Assoc 43:383–389.
32. Chen, X., P. Zhang, P.J. Blackall, and W. Feng. 1993. Characterization of Haemophilus paragallinarum isolates from China. Avian Dis 37:574–576.
33. Chen, X., J. Miflin, P. Zhang, and P. Blackall. 1995. DNA based tests for the identification of Haemophilus paragallinarum. Proc 44th West Poult Dis Conf, pp. 110–111.
34. Clark, D.S., and J.F. Godfrey. 1961. Studies of an inactivated Hemophilus gallinarum vaccine for immunization of chickens against infectious coryza. Avian Dis 5:37–47.

35. Coetzee, L., E. J. Rogers, and L. Velthuysen. 1983. The production and evaluation of a Haemophilus paragallinarum (infectious coryza) oil emulsion vaccine in laying birds. In Disease Prevention and Control in Poultry Production. Proc #66. Postgraduate Committee on Veterinary Science, University of Sydney, pp. 277–283.

36. Davis, R.B., R.B. Rimler, and E.B. Shotts, Jr. 1976. Efficacy studies on Haemophilus gallinarum bacterin preparations. Am J Vet Res 37:219–222.

37. De Blieck, L. 1932. A haemoglobinophilic bacterium as the cause of contagious catarrh of the fowl (coryza infectiosa gallinarum). Vet J 88:9–13.

38. Delaplane, J.P., L.E. Erwin, and H.O. Stuart. 1934. A hemophilic bacillus as the cause of an infectious rhinitis (coryza) of fowls. R I Agric Exp Stn Bull 244.

39. Devriese, L.A., N. Viaene, E. Uyttebroek, R. Froyman, and J. Hommez. 1988. Three cases of infection by Haemophilus-like bacteria in psittacines. Avian Pathol 17:741–744.

40. Droual, R., A.A. Bickford, B.R. Charlton, G.L. Cooper, and S.E. Channing. 1990. Infectious coryza in meat chickens in the San Joaquin Valley of California. Avian Dis 34:1009–1016.

41. Droual, R., A.A. Bickford, B.R. Charlton, and D.R. Kuney. 1990. Investigation of problems associated with intramuscular breast injection of oil-adjuvanted killed vaccines in chickens. Avian Dis 34:473–478.

42. Eaves, L.E., D.G. Rogers, and P.J. Blackall. 1989. Comparison of hemagglutinin and agglutinin schemes for the serological classification of Haemophilus paragallinarum and proposal of a new hemagglutinin serovar. J Clin Microbiol 27:1510–1513.

43. Eliot, C.P., and M.R. Lewis. 1934. A hemophilic bacterium as a cause of infectious coryza in the fowl. J Am Vet Med Assoc 84(N.S.37):878–888.

44. Fujiwara, H., and S. Konno. 1965. Histopathological studies on infectious coryza of chickens. I. Findings in naturally infected cases. Natl Inst Anim Health Q (Tokyo) 5:36–43.

45. Grebe, H.H., and K.-H. Hinz. 1975. Vorkommen von Bakterien der Gattung Haemophilus bei verschiedenen Vogelarten. Zentralbl Veterinaermed [B] 22:749–757.

46. Hinz, K.-H. 1973. Beitrag zur Differenzierung von Haemophilus-Stämmen aus Hühnern. I. Mitteilung: Kulturelle und Biochemische Untersuchungen. Avian Pathol 2:211–229.

47. Hinz, K.-H. 1973. Beitrag zur Differenzierung von Haemophilus-Stämmen aus Hühnern. II. Mitteilung: Serologische Untersuchungen im Objektträger-Agglutinations-Test. Avian Pathol 2:269–278.

48. Hinz, K.-H. 1976. Beitrag zur Differenzierung von Haemophilus-Stämmen aus Hühnern. IV. Mitteilung: Untersuchungen Über die Dissoziation von Haemophilus paragallinarum. Avian Pathol 5:51–66.

49. Hinz, K.-H. 1980. Heat-stable antigenic determinants of Haemophilus paragallinarum. Zentralbl Veterinaermed [B] 27:668–676.

50. Hinz, K.-H. 1980. Differentiation of Haemophilus paragallinarum and Haemophilus avium by phenotypical characteristics. Proc 2nd Int Symp Vet Lab Diag 3:347–350.

51. Hinz, K.-H., and C. Kunjara. 1977. Haemophilus avium, a new species from chickens. Int J Syst Bacteriol 27:324–329.

52. Hoerr, F.J., M. Putnam, S. Rowe-Rossmanith, W. Cowart, and J. Martin. 1994. Case report: Infectious coryza in broiler chickens in Alabama. Proc 43rd West Poult Dis Conf, p 42.

53. Horner, R.F., G.C. Bishop, and C. Haw. 1992. An upper respiratory disease of commercial chickens resembling infectious coryza, but caused by a V-factor independent bacterium. Avian Pathol 21:421–427.

54. Iritani, Y., and S. Hidaka. 1976. Enhancement of

hemagglutinating activity of Haemophilus gallinarum by trypsin. Avian Dis 20:614–616.

55. Iritani, Y., S. Hidaka, and K. Katagiri. 1977. Production and properties of hemagglutinin of Haemophilus gallinarum. Avian Dis 21:39–49.

56. Iritani, Y., G. Sugimori, and K. Katagiri. 1977. Serologic response to Haemophilus gallinarum in artificially infected and vaccinated chickens. Avian Dis 21:1–8.

57. Iritani, Y., K. Katagiri, and K. Tsuji. 1978. Slide-agglutination test of Haemophilus gallinarum antigen treated by trypsin to inhibit spontaneous agglutination. Avian Dis 22:793–797.

58. Iritani, Y., K. Katagiri, and H. Arita. 1980. Purification and properties of Haemophilus paragallinarum hemagglutinin. Am J Vet Res 41:2114–2118.

59. Iritani, Y., S. Iwaki, and T. Yamaguchi. 1981. Biological activities of crude polysaccharide extracted from two different immunotype strains of Hemophilus gallinarum in chickens. Avian Dis 25:29–37.

60. Iritani, Y., S. Iwaki, T. Yamaguchi, and T. Sueishi. 1981. Determination of types 1 and 2 hemagglutinins in serotypes of Haemophilus paragallinarum. Avian Dis 25:479–483.

61. Iritani, Y., T. Yamaguchi, K. Katagiri, and H. Arita. 1981. Hemagglutination inhibition of Haemophilus paragallinarum type 1 hemagglutinin by lipopolysaccharide. Am J Vet Res 42:689–690.

62. Iritani, Y., K. Kunihiro, T. Yamaguchi, T. Tomii, and Y. Hayashi. 1984. Difference of immune efficacy of infectious coryza vaccine by different site of injection in chickens. J Jpn Soc Poult Dis 20:182–185.

63. Jacobs, A.A.C., W. Cuenen, and P.K. Storm. 1992. Efficacy of a trivalent Haemophilus paragallinarum vaccine compared to bivalent vaccines. Vet Microbiol 32:43–49.

64. Kato, K. 1968. Infectious coryza in chickens. VII. Effectiveness of sulfamonomethoxine in the treatment of experimental Haemophilus infections. J Jpn Vet Med Assoc 21:349–358.

65. Kato, K. 1970. Nature of hemagglutination inhibition antibody response and its relationship to protection in infectious coryza. Jpn J Vet Sci (Suppl) 32:263.

66. Kato, K., and H. Tsubahara. 1962. Infectious coryza of chickens. II. Identification of isolates. Bull Natl Inst Anim Health 45:21–26. [Engl summ Natl Inst Anim Health Q (Tokyo) 2:239].

67. Kato, K., H. Tsubahara, and O. Taniguchi. 1967. Infectious coryza of chickens. VI. Therapeutic effect of chlortetracycline-sulfadimethoxine tablets (CTC-SD) on chickens experimentally infected with Haemophilus gallinarum and on chickens involved in mixed infection with H. gallinarum and Mycoplasma gallisepticum. Bull Natl Inst Anim Health 55:35–39. [Engl summ Natl Inst Anim Health Q (Tokyo) 7:233].

68. Kilian, M. 1974. A rapid method for the differentiation of Haemophilus strains. Acta Pathol Microbiol Immunol Scand Sect B 82:835–842.

69. Kilian, M., and E.L. Biberstein. 1984. Haemophilus. In N.R. Kreig, and J.G. Holt (eds.). Bergey's Manual of Systematic Bacteriology, 1st ed. Williams & Wilkins, Baltimore, MD, pp. 558–569.

70. Kume, K., and A. Sawata. 1984. Immunologic properties of variants dissociated from serotype 1 Haemophilus paragallinarum strains. Jpn J Vet Sci 46:49–56.

71. Kume, K., A. Sawata, and Y. Nakase. 1978. Haemophilus infections in chickens. 1. Characterization of Haemophilus paragallinarum isolated from chickens affected with coryza. Jpn J Vet Sci 40:65–73.

72. Kume, K., A. Sawata, and Y. Nakase. 1980. Haemophilus infections in chickens. 3. Immunogenicity of serotypes 1 and 2 strains of Haemophilus paragallinarum. Jpn J Vet Sci 42:673–680.

73. Kume, K., A. Sawata, and Y. Nakase. 1980. Relation-

ship between protective activity and antigen structure of Haemophilus paragallinarum serotypes 1 and 2. Am J Vet Res 41:97–100.

74. Kume, K., A. Sawata, and Y. Nakase. 1980. Immunologic relationship between Page's and Sawata's serotype strains of Haemophilus paragallinarum. Am J Vet Res 41:757–760.

75. Kume, K., A. Sawata, T. Nakai, and M. Matsumoto. 1983. Serological classification of Haemophilus paragallinarum with a hemagglutinin system. J Clin Microbiol 17:958–964.

76. Kume, K., A. Sawata, and T. Nakai. 1984. Clearance of the challenge organisms from the upper respiratory tract of chickens injected with an inactivated Haemophilus paragallinarum vaccine. Jpn J Vet Sci 46:843–850.

77. Linster, N., and K.-H. Hinz. 1983. In-vivo efficacy of sulfachlorpyridazine and the combination sulfachlorpyridazine-trimethoprim against Haemophilus paragallinarum. Dtsch Tieraertl Wochenschr 90:170–173.

78. Lublin, A., S. Mechani, M. Malkinson, and Y. Weisman. 1993. Efficacy of norfloxacin nicotinate treatment of broiler breeders against Haemophilus paragallinarum. Avian Dis 37:673–679.

79. Lu, Y.S., D.F. Lin, H.J. Tsai, K.S. Tsai, Y.L. Lee, and T. Lee. 1983. Drug sensitivity test of Haemophilus paragallinarum isolated in Taiwan. Taiwan J Vet Med Anim Husb 41:73–76.

80. Matsumoto, M., and R. Yamamoto. 1971. A broth bacterin against infectious coryza: Immunogenicity of various preparations. Avian Dis 15:109–117.

81. Matsumoto, M., and R. Yamamoto. 1975. Protective quality of an aluminum hydroxide absorbed broth bacterin against infectious coryza. Am J Vet Res 36:579–582.

82. Matsuo, K., C. Kuniyasu, S. Yamada, S. Susumi, and S. Yamamoto. 1978. Suppression of immunoresponses to Haemophilus gallinarum with nonviable Mycoplasma gallisepticum in chickens. Avian Dis 22:552–561.

83. Miflin, JK., R.F. Horner, P.J. Blackall, X. Chen, G.C. Bishop, C.J Morrow, T. Yamaguchi, and Y. Iritani. 1995. Phenotypic and molecular characterization of V-factor (NAD)-independent Haemophilus paragallinarum. Avian Dis 39:304–308.

84. Mouahid, M., M. Bisgaard, A.J. Morley, R. Mutters, and W. Mannheim. 1992. Occurrence of V-factor (NAD) independent strains of Haemophilus paragallinarum. Vet Microbiol 31:363–368.

85. Mutters, R., K. Piechulla, K.-H. Hinz, and W. Mannheim. 1985. Pasteurella avium (Hinz and Kunjara 1977) comb. nov. and Pasteurella volantium sp. nov. Int J Syst Bacteriol 35:5–9.

86. Nakamura, T., S. Hoshi, Y. Nagasawa, and S. Ueda. 1994. Protective effect of oral administration of killed Haemophilus paragallinarum serotype A on chickens. Avian Dis 38:289–292.

87. Narita, N., O. Hipolito, and J.A. Bottino. 1978. Studies on infectious coryza of chickens. I. The biochemical and serological characteristics of 17 Haemophilus strains isolated in Brazil. Proc 16th World's Poult Congr, pp. 685–692.

88. Nelson, J.B. 1933. Studies on an uncomplicated coryza of the domestic fowl. I. The isolation of a bacillus which produces a nasal discharge. J Exp Med 58:289–295.

89. Ogunnariwo, J.A., and A.B. Schryvers. 1992. Correlation between the ability of Haemophilus paragallinarum to acquire ovotransferrin-bound iron and the expression of ovotransferrin-specific receptors. Avian Dis 36:655–663.

90. Otsuki, K., and Y. Iritani. 1974. Preparation and immunological response to a new mixed vaccine composed of inactivated Newcastle disease virus, inactivated infectious bronchitis virus, and inactivated Haemophilus gallinarum. Avian Dis 18:297–304.

91. Page, L.A. 1962. Haemophilus infectious in chickens. I. Characteristics of 12 Haemophilus isolates recovered from diseased chickens. Am J Vet Res 23:85–95.

92. Page, L.A., A.S. Rosenwald, and F.C. Price. 1963. Haemophilus infections in chickens. IV. Results of laboratory and field trials of formalinized bacterins for the prevention of disease caused by Haemophilus gallinarum. Avian Dis 7:239–256.

93. Pages Mante, A., and L. Costa Quintana. 1986. Efficacy of polyvalent inactivated oil vaccine against avian coryza. Med Vet 3:27–36.

94. Piechulla, K., K.-H. Hinz, and W. Mannheim. 1985. Genetic and phenotypic comparison of three new avian Haemophilus-like taxa and of Haemophilus paragallinarum Biberstein and White 1969 with other members of the family Pasteurellaceae Pohl 1981. Avian Dis 29:601–612.

95. Poernomo, P., and P. Ronohardjo. 1987. Efficacy of cosumix plus in broilers with coryza (Haemophilus paragallinarum infection). Penyakit Hewan 19:6–10.

96. Raie, N., M. Manzer, D.H.Read, J.T. Barton, and S.K. Heitala. 1993. Preliminary evaluation of antigens for use in a newly developed ELISA for detection of antibodies to Hemophilus paragallinarum in chickens. Proc 42nd West Poult Dis Conf, p. 59.

97. Reece, R.L., and P.J. Coloe. 1985. The resistance to anti-microbial agents of bacteria isolated from pathological conditions of birds in Victoria, 1978 to 1983. Aust Vet J 62:379–381.

98. Reid, G.G., and P.J. Blackall. 1987. Comparison of adjuvants for an inactivated infectious coryza vaccine. Avian Dis 31:59–63.

99. Rimler, R. B. 1979. Studies of the pathogenic avian haemophili. Avian Dis 23:1006–1018.

100. Rimler, R.B., and R.B. Davis. 1977. Infectious coryza: In vivo growth of Haemophilus gallinarum as a determinant for cross protection. Am J Vet Res 38:1591–1593.

101. Rimler, R.B., E.B. Shotts Jr, and R.B. Davis. 1975. A growth medium for the production of a bacterin for immunization against infectious coryza. Avian Dis 19:318–322.

102. Rimler, R.B., R.B. Davis, and P.K. Page. 1977. Infectious coryza: Cross-protection studies, using seven strains of Haemophilus gallinarum. Am J Vet Res 38:1587–1589.

103. Rimler, R.B., E.B. Shotts, Jr., J. Brown, and R.B. Davis. 1977. The effect of sodium chloride and NADH on the growth of six strains of Haemophilus species pathogenic to chickens. J Gen Microbiol 98:349–354.

104. Rimler, R.B., R.B. Davis, R.K. Page, and S.H. Kleven. 1978. Infectious coryza: Preventing complicated coryza with Haemophilus gallinarum and Mycoplasma gallisepticum bacterins. Avian Dis 22:140–150.

105. Sakaguchi, Y., K. Kouno, T. Kojima, H. Yoshida, M. Nakai, S. Matsumoto, H. Katae, and S. Nakamura. 1988. Esafloxacin, a new quinolone derivative: Its in vitro antibacterial activity against chicken pathogens. Proc 18th World's Poult Congr, pp. 1265–1266.

106. Sakai, T., and S. Nagao. 1987. Experimental infection of chickens with Haemophilus paragallinarum and therapeutic efficacy of TA-068W. Bull Coll Agric Vet Med Nihon Univ 44:228–235.

107. Sandoval, V.E., H.R. Terzolo, and P.J. Blackall. 1994. Complicated infectious coryza cases in Argentina. Avian Dis 38:672–678.

108. Sato, S., and M. Shifrine. 1964. Serologic response of chickens to experimental infection with Hemophilus gallinarum, and their immunity to challenge. Poult Sci 43:1199–1204.

109. Sato, S., and M. Shifrine. 1965. Application of the agar gel precipitation test to serologic studies of chickens inoculated with Haemophilus gallinarum. Avian Dis 9:591–598.

110. Sawata, A., and K. Kume. 1983. Relationships between virulence and morphological or serological properties of variants dissociated from serotype 1 Haemophilus paragallinarum strains. J Clin Microbiol 18:49–55.

111. Sawata, A., K. Kume, and Y. Nakase. 1978. Haemophilus infections in chickens. 2. Types of Haemophilus paragallinarum isolates from chickens with infectious coryza, in relation to Haemophilus gallinarum strain No.221. Jpn J Vet Sci 40:645–652.

112. Sawata, A., K. Kume, and Y. Nakase. 1979. Antigenic structure and relationship between serotypes 1 and 2 of Haemophilus paragallinarum. Am J Vet Res 40:1450–1453.

113. Sawata, A., K. Kume, and Y. Nakase. 1980. Biologic and serologic relationships between Page's and Sawata's serotypes of Haemophilus paragallinarum. Am J Vet Res 41:1901–1904.

114. Sawata, A., K. Kume, and Y. Nakase. 1982. Hemagglutinin of Haemophilus paragallinarum serotype 2 organisms: Occurrence and immunologic properties of hemagglutinin. Am J Vet Res 43:1311–1314.

115. Sawata, A., K. Kume, and T. Nakai. 1984. Hemagglutinin of Haemophilus paragallinarum serotype 1 organisms. Jpn J Vet Sci 46:21–29.

116. Sawata, A., K. Kume, and T. Nakai. 1984. Relationship between anticapsular antibody and protective activity of a capsular antigen of Haemophilus paragallinarum. Jpn J Vet Sci 46:475–486.

117. Sawata, A., K. Kume, and T. Nakai. 1984. Serologic typing of Haemophilus paragallinarum based on serum bactericidal reactions. Jpn J Vet Sci 46:909–912.

118. Sawata, A., K. Kume, and T. Nakai. 1984. Susceptibility of Haemophilus paragallinarum to bactericidal activity of normal and immune chicken sera. Jpn J Vet Sci 46:805–813.

119. Sawata, A., T. Nakai, K. Kume, H. Yoshikawa, and T. Yoshikawa. 1985. Intranasal inoculation of chickens with encapsulated or nonencapsulated variants of Haemophilus paragallinarum: Electron microscopic evaluation of the nasal mucosa. Am J Vet Res 46:2346–2353.

120. Schalm, O.W., and J.R. Beach. 1936. Studies of infectious coryza of chickens with special reference to its etiology. Poult Sci 15:473–482.

121. Sueishi, T., Y. Hayashi, and Y. Iritani. 1982. Use of gonococcal agar medium for preparation of antigen of Haemophilus paragallinarum hemagglutinin. Avian Dis 26:186–190.

122. Sumano Lopez, H., and L. Ocampo Camberos. 1987. Comparative pharmacokinetics of three sulfonamide-trimethoprim combinations in healthy White Leghorn pullets and pullets with infectious coryza (Haemophilus gallinarum). Vet Mexico 18:21–26.

123. Takagi, M., S. Ohta, and K. Kato. 1986. Haemagglutination inhibition antibody response in chickens to inactivated infectious coryza serotype C vaccine. Bull Natl Inst Anim Health 89:11–17.

124. Takagi, M., N. Hirayama, H. Makie, and S. Ohta. 1991. Production, characterization and protective effect of monoclonal antibodies to Haemophilus paragallinarum serotype A. Vet Microbiol 27:327–338.

125. Takagi, M., K. Ohmae, N. Hirayama, and S. Ohta. 1991. Expression of hemagglutinin of Haemophilus paragallinarum serotype A in Escherichia coli. J Vet Med Sci 53:917–920.

126. Takagi, M., T. Takahashi, N. Hirayama, Istiananingsi, S. Mariana, K. Zarkasie, Sumadi, M. Ogata, and S. Ohta. 1991. Survey of infectious coryza of chickens in Indonesia. J Vet Med Sci 53:637–642.

127. Takagi, M., N. Hirayama, T. Simazaki, K. Taguchi, R. Yamaoka, and S. Ohta. 1993. Purification of hemagglutinin from Haemophilus paragallinarum using monoclonal antibody. Vet Microbiol 34:191–197.

128. Takahashi, I., T. Yoshida, Y. Honma, and E. Saito. 1990. Comparison of the susceptibility of Haemophilus paragallinarum to ofloxacin and other existing antimicrobial agents. J Jpn Vet Med Assoc 43:187–191.

129. Takahata, T., M. Takei, and M. Kato. 1988. Efficacy of the combination of sulfamonomethoxine and ormetoprim against experimentally induced infectious coryza in chickens. Proc 18th World's Poult Congr, pp. 1282–1283.

130. Terzolo, H.R., F.A. Paolicchi, V.E. Sandoval, P.J. Blackall, T. Yamaguchi, and Y. Iritani. 1993. Characterization of isolates of Haemophilus paragallinarum from Argentina. Avian Dis 37:310–314.

131. Verschoor, J.A., L.Coetzee, and L. Visser. 1989. Monoclonal antibody characterization of two field strains of Haemophilus paragallinarum isolated from vaccinated layer hens. Avian Dis 33:219–225.

132. Wichmann, R.W., and A.C. Wichmann. 1983. The cultivation of Haemophilus gallinarum (Haemophilus paragallinarum) in tissue culture and the use of these cultures in the preparation of a bacterin for the prevention of infectious coryza. Proc 32rd West Poult Dis Conf, pp. 7–10.

133. Yamaguchi, T., S. Iwaki, and Y. Iritani. 1981. Latex agglutination test for measurement of type-specific antibody to Haemophilus paragallinarum in chickens. Avian Dis 25:988–995.

134. Yamaguchi, T., Y. Iritani, and Y. Hayashi. 1988. Serological response of chickens either vaccinated or artificially infected with Haemophilus paragallinarum. Avian Dis 32:308–312.

135. Yamaguchi, T., P.J. Blackall, S. Takigami, Y. Iritani, and Y. Hayashi. 1990. Pathogenicity and serovar-specific hemagglutinating antigens of Haemophilus paragallinarum serovar B strains. Avian Dis 34:964–968.

136. Yamaguchi, T., P.J. Blackall, S. Takigami, Y. Iritani, and Y. Hayashi. 1991. Immunogenicity of Haemophilus paragallinarum serovar B strains. Avian Dis 35:965–968.

137. Yamaguchi, T., M. Kobayashi, S. Masaki, and Y. Iritani. 1993. Isolation and characterisation of a Haemophilus paragallinarum mutant that lacks a hemagglutinating antigen. Avian Dis 37:970–976.

138. Yamamoto, R. 1972. Infectious coryza. In M.S. Hofstad, B.W. Calnek, C.F. Helmboldt, W.M. Reid, and H.W. Yoder, Jr. (eds.). Diseases of Poultry, 6th ed. Iowa State University Press, Ames, IA, pp. 272–281.

139. Yamamoto, R. 1978. Infectious coryza. In M.S. Hofstad, B. W. Calnek, C.F. Helmbolt, W.M. Reid, and H.W. Yoder, Jr. (eds.). Diseases of Poultry, 7th ed. Iowa State University Press, Ames, IA, pp. 225–232.

140. Yamamoto, R. 1991. Infectious coryza. In B.W. Calnek, H.J. Barnes, C.W. Beard, W.M. Reid, and H.W. Yoder, Jr. (eds.). Diseases of Poultry, 9th ed. Iowa State University Press, Ames, IA, pp. 186–195.

141. Yamamoto, R., and G. T. Clark. 1966. Intra- and interflock transmission of Haemophilus gallinarum. Am J Vet Res 27:1419–1425.

142. Yamamoto, R., and D. T. Somersett. 1964. Antibody response in chickens to infection with Haemophilus gallinarum. Avian Dis 8:441–453.

143. Yamamoto, K., S. Tateyama, T. Sakai, N. Watanabe, N. Watanabe, Y. Hattori, M. Suzuki, and M. Kozasa. 1988. Myplabin® (miporamicin), a new macrolide antibiotic. II. Clinical effects of Myplabin® premix against respiratory mycoplasmosis and infectious coryza in chickens. Proc 18th World's Poult Congr, pp. 1256–1258.

144. Yoshimura, M., S. Tsubaki, T. Yamagami, R. Sugimoto, S. Ide, Y. Nakase, and S. Masu. 1972. The effectiveness of immunization to Newcastle disease, avian infectious bronchitis, and avian infectious coryza with inactivated combined vaccines. Kitasato Arch Exp Med 45:165–179.

145. Zaini, M.Z., and Y. Iritani. 1992. Serotyping of Haemophilus paragallinarum in Malaysia. J Vet Med Sci 54:363–365.

146. Zinneman, K., and E.L. Biberstein. 1974. Haemophilus. In R.E. Buchanan, and N.E. Gibbons (eds.). Bergey's Manual of Determinative Bacteriology, 8th ed. Williams & Wilkins, Baltimore, MD, pp. 364–370.

9 Mycoplasmosis

INTRODUCTION
S. H. KLEVEN

Mycoplasmas are very small prokaryotes totally devoid of cell walls, bounded by a plasma membrane only (33). This accounts for the "fried egg" type of colonial morphology, resistance to antibiotics that affects cell wall synthesis, and complex nutritional requirements. Mycoplasmas tend to be quite host specific; some infect only a single species of animal, while others may have the ability to infect several different animal species. They are found in humans, many animal species, plants, and insects. In general, mycoplasmas colonize mucosal surfaces and most species are noninvasive.

HISTORY. The first successful cultivation of a mycoplasma, the agent of bovine pleuropneumonia, was reported by Nocard and Roux in 1898 (28). *Mycoplasma* spp. were probably first encountered in chickens during the 1930s by Nelson (26, 27), and the condition designated "chronic respiratory disease" was described in 1943 by Delaplane and Stuart (9). The infection in turkeys was described by Dodd (12) in 1905 and was named "infectious sinusitis" in 1938 by Dickinson and Hinshaw (10). Markham and Wong (24) and Van Roekel and Olesiuk (39) reported in the early 1950s on the successful cultivation of the organisms from chickens and turkeys and noted their similarity.

It became apparent during early studies by Adler et al. (1) that mycoplasma isolates represented different serotypes, which are now designated as different species. Yamamoto and Adler (40, 41) characterized 5 serotypes; Kleckner (21) described 8 serotypes, which he designated serotypes A–H. Twelve serotypes (A–L) were characterized by Yoder and Hofstad (43), and 19 (A-S) by Dierks et al. (11). Numerous characteristics were described, but the final serotyping procedure was based primarily on agglutination titrations and growth inhibition by specific hyperimmune sera. Several of those 19 serotype designations were either deleted or combined as further research employing additional serologic procedures was evaluated.

CHARACTERIZATION. Mycoplasma species from avian sources generally require a protein-rich medium containing 10–15% added animal serum. Further supplementation with some yeast-derived component is often beneficial. Growth of *M. synoviae* requires the addition of nicotinamide adenine dinucleotide (NAD) (see *M. synoviae* section). A medium described by Frey (17) or a medium described by Bradbury (2) is commonly used for the cultivation of avian mycoplasmas.

Mycoplasma organisms tend to grow rather slowly, usually prefer 37–38 C, and are rather resistant to thallium acetate and penicillin, which are frequently employed in media to retard growth of contaminant bacteria and fungi. Colonies form on agar media after 3–10 days at 37 C; however, non-pathogenic species such as *M. gallinarum* and *M. gallinaceum* may develop colonies within 1 day (*M. gallinarum* and *M. gallinaceum* are frequently isolated as contaminants during attempts to isolate pathogenic avian mycoplasmas). Typical colonies are small (0.1–1.0 mm), smooth, circular, and somewhat flat with a more dense central elevation (see Fig. 9.1). Variations in colony morphology have been described, but cannot be relied upon to differentiate the various species. Individual cells vary from 0.2 to 0.5 μm and are basically coccoid to coccobacilliform, but slender rods, filaments, and ring forms have been described.

Fermentation of carbohydrates is variable, but all species may be divided into those that ferment glucose with acid production and those that do not. Glucose is frequently added to broth media to enhance growth of the carbohydrate-fermenting species and to provide an indication of growth when glucose fermentation produces acid in media containing added phenol red. Phosphatase activity is often present, as is arginine decarboxylase. Most species that do not ferment glucose use the amino acid arginine as their major source of energy. *M. iowae* and some other species, however, ferment glucose and hydrolyze arginine.

One useful characteristic of *M. gallisepticum, M. meleagridis,* and *M. synoviae* is hemagglutination of erythrocytes from chickens or turkeys. Hemag-

The contributions of Dr. H. W. Yoder, Jr. to the previous edition of this chapter are gratefully acknowledged.

glutinating antigens are used for hemagglutination-inhibition serologic tests for these three pathogenic species.

Direct staining of mycoplasma colonies on agar surfaces or colony imprints with specific fluorescent antibody (8, 37) is most commonly used to determine the species of avian mycoplasma isolates. Other suitable methods include growth inhibition (7), immunodiffusion (29), and others. More recently, molecular methods such as sequencing of the rRNA gene (18), DNA probes (19), polymerase chain reaction (23, 25, 44), and a polymerase chain reaction that amplifies the rRNA gene followed by restriction fragment length polymorphism analysis (14) have been used.

CLASSIFICATION. Mycoplasmas are members of the class Mollicutes, Order I, Mycoplasmatales. Genus I, *Mycoplasma,* has 85 or more species, a DNA G+C content of 23–40%, a genome size of 600–1350 kb, requires cholesterol for growth, occurs in humans and animals, and has a usual optimum growth temperature of 37 C. Genus II, *Ureaplasma,* is differentiated on the basis of hydrolysis of urea. Acholeplasmas are classified in Order III, Acholeplasmatales, family I, Acholeplasmataceae, genus I, *Acholeplasma.* They are characterized by lack of a growth requirement for cholesterol (38).

Earlier serotype designations (see History) have now been replaced by species names, beginning with *M. gallinarum* (16), *M. gallisepticum* and *M.*

iners (13), *M. meleagridis* (42), *M. synoviae* (30), and *M. anatis* (34). *M. gallopavonis, M. iowae, M. pullorum, M. gallinaceum,* and *M. columbinasale* were named in 1982 (20). *M. columbinum* was named for an isolate from the trachea of pigeons and *M. columborale* from the oropharynx of pigeons (35). *M. lipofaciens* was named for an isolate from the sinus of a chicken (4). *M. glycophilum* was named for an isolate obtained from the oviduct of a chicken (15), *M. cloacale* was described as an isolate from the cloaca of turkeys (3), and *M. anseris* was reported from geese (5). *Ureaplasma gallorale* was named for an isolate from the oropharynx of a chicken (22), but there are no reported isolations of this species from the United States.

Recently, *M. imitans,* a new mycoplasma species related to *M. gallisepticum,* was isolated from ducks, geese, and partridges in France and England (6). There are also recent descriptions of *M. corogypsi,* isolated from a black vulture (31), *M. falconis* from Saker falcons, *M. gypis* from Griffon vultures, and *M. buteonis* from buteos (32).

In addition, there are numerous mycoplasma isolates from various species of birds, including strain 1220, a pathogen of domestic geese (36), isolates from various ratites, as well as unidentified isolates from domestic poultry.

Most of the species of mycoplasma isolated from avian sources are included in the ninth edition of *Bergey's Manual* (33). A summary of the characteristics of mycoplasma species isolated from avian sources is presented in Table 9.1.

Table 9.1. Characteristics of avian mycoplasmas

Species	Usual host	Glucose fermentation	Arginine hydrolysis	Phosphatase activity
A. laidlawii[a]	Various	+	−	+ or −
M. anatis	Duck	+	−	+
M. anseris	Hawk	−	+	−
M. buteonis	Goose	+	−	−
M. cloacale	Buteo hawk	−	+	−
M. columbinasale	Turkey	−	+	+
M. columbinum	Pigeon	−	+	−
M. columborale	Pigeon	+	−	−
M. corogypsi	Black vulture	+	−	−
M. falconis	Saker falcon	−	+	−
M. gallinaceum	Chicken	+	−	−
M. gallinarum	Chicken	−	+	−
M. gallisepticum	Chicken, turkey	+	−	−
M. gallopavonia	Turkey	+	−	−
M. glycophilum	Chicken	+	−	+ or −
M. gypis	Griffon vulture	−	+	+
M. imitans	Duck, goose, partridge	+	−	−
M. iners	Chicken	−	+	−
M. iowae	Turkey	+	+	−
M. lipofaciens	Chicken	+	+	−
M. meleagridis	Turkey	−	+	+
M. pullorum	Chicken	+	−	−
M. synoviae	Chicken, turkey	+	−	−
U. gallorale[b]	Chicken	−	−	?

[a]*Acholeplasma* species do not require sterols for growth.

[b]*Ureaplasma* species are characterized by splitting of urea.

REFERENCES

1. Adler, H.E., R. Yamamoto, and J. Berg. 1957. Strain differences of pleuropneumonia-like organisms of avian origin. Avian Dis 1:19–27.

2. Bradbury, J.M. 1977. Rapid biochemical tests for characterization of the Mycoplasmatales. J Clin Microbiol 5:531–534.

3. Bradbury, J., and M. Forrest. 1984. Mycoplasma cloacale, a new species isolated from a turkey. Int J Syst Bacteriol 34:389–392.

4. Bradbury, J., M. Forrest, and A. Williams. 1983. Mycoplasma lipofaciens, a new species of avian origin. Int J Syst Bacteriol 33:329–335.

5. Bradbury, J.M., F.T.W. Jordan, T. Shimizu, L. Stipkovits, and Z. Varga. 1988. Mycoplasma anseris sp. nov. found in geese. Int J Syst Bacteriol 38:74–76.

6. Bradbury, J.M., O.M.S. Abdulwahab, C.A. Yavari, J.P. Dupiellet, and J.M. Bové. 1993. Mycoplasma imitans sp-nov is related to Mycoplasma gallisepticum and found in birds. Int J Syst Bacteriol 43:721–728.

7. Clyde, W.A., Jr. 1964. Mycoplasma species identification based upon growth inhibition by specific antisera. J Immunol 92:958–965.

8. Corstvet, R.E., and W.W. Sadler. 1964. The diagnosis of certain avian diseases with the fluorescent antibody technique. Poult Sci 43:1280–1288.

9. Delaplane, J.R, and H.O. Stuart. 1943. The propagation of a virus in embryonated chicken eggs causing a chronic respiratory disease of chickens. Am J Vet Res 4:325–332.

10. Dickinson, E.M., and W.R. Hinshaw. 1938. Treatment of infectious sinusitis of turkeys with argyrol and silver nitrate. J Am Vet Med Assoc 93:151–156.

11. Dierks, R.E., J.A. Newman, and B.S. Pomeroy. 1967. Characterization of avian Mycoplasma. Ann NY Acad Sci 143:170–189.

12. Dodd, S. 1905. Epizootic pneumo-enteritis of the turkey. J Comp Pathol Ther 18:239–245.

13. Edward, D.G., and A.D. Kanarek. 1960. Organisms of the pleuropneumonia group of avian origin: their classification into specie. Ann NY Acad Sci 79:696–702.

14. Fan, H., S.H. Kleven, and M.W. Jackwood. 1994. Application of polymerase chain reaction with arbitrarily primers to strain identification of Mycoplasma gallisepticum. IOM Lett 3:443.

15. Forrest, M., and J. Bradbury. 1984. Mycoplasma glycophilum, a new species of avian origin. J Gen Microbiol 130:597–603.

16. Freundt, E.A. 1955. The classification of the pleuropneumonia group of organisms (Borrelomycetales). Int Bull Bacteriol Nomencl Taxon 5:67–68.

17. Frey, M.L., R.P. Hanson, and D.P. Anderson. 1968. A medium for the isolation of avian mycoplasmas. Am J Vet Res 29:2163–2171.

18. Grau, O., F. Laigret, P. Carle, J.G. Tully, D.L. Rose, and J.M. Bové. 1991. Identification of a plant-derived mollicute as a strain of an avian pathogen Mycoplasma iowae, and its implications for mollicute taxonomy. Int J Syst Bacteriol 41:473–478.

19. Hyman, H.C., S. Levisohn, D. Yogev, and S. Razin. 1989. DNA probes for Mycoplasma gallisepticum and Mycoplasma synoviae: Application in experimentally infected chickens. Vet Microbiol 20:323–338.

20. Jordan, F.T.W., H. Erno, G.S. Cottew, K.H. Hinz, and L. Stipkovits. 1982. Characterization and taxonomic description of five Mycoplasma serovars (serotypes) of avian origin and their elevation to species rank and further evaluation of the taxonomic status of Mycoplasma synoviae. Int J Syst Bacteriol 32:108–115.

21. Kleckner, A.L. 1960. Serotypes of avian pleuropneumonia-like organisms. Am J Vet Res 21:274–280.

22. Koshimizu, K., R. Harasawa, I.J. Pan, H. Kotani, M. Ogata, E.B. Stephens, and M.F. Barile. 1987. Ureaplasma gallorale sp. nov. from the oropharynx of chickens. Int J Syst Bacteriol 37:333–338.

23. Lauerman, L.H., F.J. Hoerr, A.R. Sharpton, S.M. Shah, and V.L. van Santen. 1993. Development and application of a polymerase chain reaction assay for Mycoplasma synoviae. Avian Dis 37:829–834.

24. Markham, F.S., and S.C. Wong. 1952. Pleuropneumonia-like organisms in the etiology of turkey sinusitis and chronic respiratory disease of chickens. Poult Sci 31:902–904.

25. Nascimento, E.R., R. Yamamoto, K.R. Herrick, and R.C. Tait. 1991. Polymerase chain reaction for detection of Mycoplasma gallisepticum. Avian Dis 35:62–69.

26. Nelson, J.B. 1933. Studies on an uncomplicated coryza of the domestic fowl. II. The relation of the 'Bacillary' coryza to that produced by exudate. J Exp Med 58:297–304.

27. Nelson, J.B. 1939. Growth of the fowl coryza bodies in tissue culture and in blood agar. J Exp Med 69:199–209.

28. Nocard, E., and E.R. Roux. 1898. Le microbe de la peripneumonia. Ann Inst Pasteur Paris 12:240–262.

29. Nonomura, I., and H.W. Yoder, Jr. 1977. Identification of avian Mycoplasma isolates by the agar gel precipitin test. Avian Dis 21:370–381.

30. Olson, N.O., K.M. Kerr, and A. Campbell. 1964. Control of infectious synovitis. 13. The antigen study of three strains. Avian Dis 8:209–214.

31. Panangala, V.S., J.S. Stringfellow, K. Dybvig, A. Woodard, F. Sun, D.L. Rose, and M.M. Gresham. 1993. Mycoplasma corogypsi sp. nov, a new species from the footpad abscess of a black vulture, Coragyps atratus. Int J Syst Bacteriol 43:585–590.

32. Poveda, J.B., J. Giebel, J. Flossdorf, J. Meier, and H. Kirchhoff. 1994. Mycoplasma buteonis sp. nov., Mycoplasma falconis sp. nov., and Mycoplasma gypis sp. nov., 3 species from birds of prey. Int J Syst Bacteriol 44:94–98.

33. Razin, S., and E.A. Freundt. 1984. The Mycoplasmas. In Krieg, N.R. and J.G. Holt (ed.). Bergey's Manual of Systematic Bacteriology, 9th ed., vol. 1. Williams & Wilkins, Baltimore, pp. 740–793.

34. Roberts, D.H. 1964. The isolation of an influenza A virus and a mycoplasma associated with duck sinusitis. Vet Rec 76:470–473.

35. Shimizu, T., H. Erno, and H. Nagatomo. 1978. Isolation and characterization of Mycoplasma columbinum and Mycoplasma columborale, two new species from pigeons. Int J Syst Bacteriol 28:538–546.

36. Stipkovits, L., R. Glavits, E. Ivanics, and E. Szabo. 1993. Additional data on Mycoplasma disease of goslings. Avian Pathol 22:171–176.

37. Talkington, F.D., and S.H. Kleven. 1983. A classification of laboratory strains of avian Mycoplasma serotypes by direct immunofluorescence. Avian Dis 27:422–429.

38. Tully, J.G., J.M. Bové, F. Laigret, and R.F. Whitcomb. 1993. Revised taxonomy of the class mollicutes—proposed elevation of a monophyletic cluster of arthropod-associated mollicutes to ordinal rank (entomoplasmatales ord nov), with provision for familial rank to separate species with nonhelical morphology (Entomoplasmataceae fam Nov) from helical species (Spiroplasmataceae), and emended descriptions of the order Mycoplasmatales, family Mycoplasmataceae. Int J Syst Bacteriol 43:378–385.

39. Van Roekel, H., and O.M. Olesiuk. 1953. The etiology of chronic respiratory disease. Proc 90th Annu Meet Am Vet Med Assoc, pp. 289–303.

40. Yamamoto, R., and H.E. Adler. 1958. Characterization of pleuropneumonia-like organisms of avian origin. 1. Antigenic analysis of seven strains and their comparative pathogenicity for birds. J Infect Dis 102:143–152.

41. Yamamoto, R., and H.E. Adler. 1958. Characteristics of pleuropneumonia-like organisms of avian origin. II. Cultural, biochemical, morphological and further serological studies. J Infect Dis 102:243–250.

42. Yamamoto, R., C.H. Bigland, and H.B. Ortmayer. 1965. Characteristics of Mycoplasma meleagridis, sp. n., isolated from turkeys. J Bacteriol 90:47–49.

43. Yoder, H.W., Jr., and M.S. Hofstad. 1964. Characterization of avian Mycoplasma. Avian Dis 8:481–512.

44. Zhao, S., and R. Yamamoto. 1993. Detection of Mycoplasma meleagridis by polymerase chain reaction. Vet Microbiol 36:91–97.

MYCOPLASMA GALLISEPTICUM INFECTION

David H. Ley and Harry W. Yoder, Jr.

INTRODUCTION.   *Mycoplasma gallisepticum* (MG) infection is commonly designated as chronic respiratory disease (CRD) of chickens and infectious sinusitis of turkeys. It is characterized by respiratory rales, coughing, and nasal discharge, and, frequently in turkeys, sinusitis. Clinical manifestations are usually slow to develop and the disease has a long course. Air sac disease designates a severe airsacculitis that is the result of *M. gallisepticum* infection complicated by some respiratory virus infection and usually *Escherichia coli* (see also section on *M. synoviae*).

Economic and Public Health Significance.
Airsacculitis in chickens, and airsacculitis and sinusitis in turkeys can cause significant condemnations at slaughter. Most of this loss is related directly or indirectly to *M. gallisepticum* infection, with or without complicating factors. Economic losses from downgrading of carcasses, reduced feed and egg production efficiency, and increased medication costs are additional factors that make this one of the costliest disease problems confronting the industry. Prevention and control programs, which may include vaccination, account for additional costs. The disease is of no public health significance.

HISTORY.   The first accurate description of the disease in turkeys was probably made in 1905 by Dodd (49) in England under the name "epizootic pneumoenteritis." Dickinson and Hinshaw (46) named the disease "infectious sinusitis" of turkeys in 1938.

Nelson (122) described coccobacilliform bodies associated with an infectious coryza in chickens in 1935. Later, he associated them with the coryza of slow onset and long duration and eventually was able to grow the coccobacilliform bodies in embryonating eggs, tissue culture, and cell-free medium.

In 1943, Delaplane and Stuart (45) cultivated an agent in embryos isolated from chickens with CRD, and later from turkeys with sinusitis. In the early 1950s, Markham and Wong (110) and Van Roekel and Olesiuk (158) reported the successful cultivation of the organisms from chickens and turkeys, noting their similarity, and suggested they were members of the pleuropneumonia group (*Mycoplasma* spp.).

INCIDENCE AND DISTRIBUTION.   The disease has become an important flock problem in

chickens and turkeys in all areas of the United States. It appears to be worldwide in distribution.

The incidence has decreased considerably during the past 25 yr of extensive control programs within the poultry industry. However, the continuation of MG infection in many large multiple-age commercial egg production units is a major problem, and is discussed further under Prevention and Control. There is some evidence that MG is also present in small backyard poultry flocks (113).

ETIOLOGY

Classification.   *M. gallisepticum* is a pathogenic species within the genus *Mycoplasma* of the family Mycoplasmataceae (95).

Morphology and Staining.   The organism stains well with Giemsa stain, but is weakly gramnegative. It is generally coccoid, approximately 0.25–0.5 µm. *M. gallisepticum* shows a filamentous or flask-shaped polarity of the cell body. This polarity appears prior to division (118) and is due to the presence of well-organized terminal organelles or blebs (109). It has been theorized that such structures govern motility or host–pathogen interactions and, ultimately, pathogenicity (31, 97). Cell division by binary fission is synchronous with DNA replication (129). Tajima et al. (146) described capsular material associated with MG cells in contact with chicken tracheal epithelium based on electron microscopy (EM) studies. Further reports on the interaction of MG cells with tracheal epithelium are discussed under Histopathology.

Growth Requirements.   *M. gallisepticum* requires a rather complex medium usually enriched with 10–15% heat-inactivated swine, avian, or horse serum. Several types of liquid or agar media will support growth of mycoplasmas of avian origin, with certain purposes altering the final choice. Media and techniques for MG culture and antigen production have been described (67, 91, 160). Growth generally is optimal in medium at approximately pH 7.8 incubated at 37–38 C. Colonies form on agar medium containing the usual mycoplasma ingredients, but require prolonged incubation (2–5 days) in a very moist atmosphere.

Frey et al. (62) developed a medium (see *M. synoviae* section) that incorporated all essential ingredients including yeast autolysate and dextrose. When prepared with 10–15% swine serum, it is a convenient and very efficient medium for cultivation of most mycoplasmas. Inclusion of phenol red and dextrose makes it possible to detect growth in tubes employed in mass culturings, as does addition of 0.0025% 2,3,5-triphenyl tetrazolium chloride as an indicator (173).

M. gallisepticum may also be propagated in embryonated chicken eggs (see Pathogenicity; Isolation and Identification of Causative Agent).

Colony Morphology. *M. gallisepticum* can be grown on serum-enriched agar medium inoculated directly or following passage from broth or agar cultures. It often is very difficult to obtain colony growth directly from clinical specimens. Inoculated agar plates must be incubated at 37 C in a very moist atmosphere for 3–5 days. Evidence of colony growth is best studied with the aid of a dissecting microscope with indirect lighting. Characteristic colonies appear as tiny, smooth, circular, translucent masses with a dense, raised central area (Fig. 9.1). They rarely are more than 0.2–0.3 mm in diameter and frequently occur in ridges along the streak line, since closely adjacent colonies readily coalesce. Variations in colonies of isolates representing numerous species of avian mycoplasma have been noted (47, 173), but the species designa-

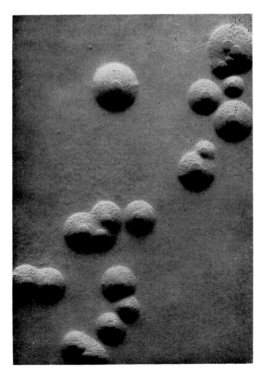

9.1. Colonies of *Mycoplasma gallisepticum* on 20% chicken serum agar plates. ×40. (Hofstad)

tion of an organism cannot be determined by its colony characteristics.

Biochemical Properties. Biochemical and related biologic properties of MG have been reported by numerous workers. It ferments glucose and maltose, with production of acid but not gas. It does not ferment lactose, dulcitol, or salicin. Sucrose is rarely fermented; results with galactose, fructose, trehalose, and mannitol are variable. It does not hydrolyze arginine, and is phosphatase-negative. It reduces 2,3,5-triphenyl tetrazolium (becomes red) and neotetrazolium (becomes blue). *M. gallisepticum* causes complete hemolysis of horse erythrocytes incorporated into agar medium, and agglutinates turkey and chicken erythrocytes. See further discussion of the hemagglutination-inhibition (HI) test under Serology.

Resistance to Chemical and Physical Agents. It is assumed that most of the commonly employed chemical disinfectants are effective against MG. Inactivation has been produced by phenol, formalin, ß-propiolactone, and merthiolate. Its resistance to penicillin and low concentration (1:4000) of thallous acetate make these valuable additives to mycoplasma culture media as inhibitors of bacterial and fungal contamination.

The organism remained viable in chicken feces 1–3 days at 20 C, on muslin cloth 3 days at 20 C or 1 day at 37 C, and in egg yolk 18 wk at 37 C or 6 wk at 20 C (36). Broth suspensions of infective chorioallantoic membrane (CAM) lost their infectivity after 1 hr of exposure at 46 C, after 20 min at 50 C, or by the 3rd wk at 5 C (74). However, other workers (125) found allantoic fluid remained infective 4 days in the incubator, 6 days at room temperature, and 32–60 days in the refrigerator. *M. gallisepticum* was inactivated in infected chicken hatching eggs that just reached 45.6 C during a 12- to 14-hr heating procedure (167). Broth cultures remained viable 2–4 yr when stored at -30 C, and viable *M. gallisepticum* were recovered from lyophilized broth culture stored at 4 C at least 7 yr and from lyophilized infective chicken turbinates stored at 4 C for 13–14 yr (173). Yoder (171) found that numerous broth cultures of MG and various other serotypes that had been frozen at -60 C since 1965 were viable upon subculturing more than 20 yr later. Lyophilized broth cultures including MG, *M. synoviae* (MS), and *M. meleagridis* (MM) were routinely found to be viable when subcultured at 10 to 15 yr. Kleven (90) studied the stability of F strain MG in powdered skim milk, phosphate-buffered saline (PBS), tryptose phosphate broth, and distilled water stored at 4, 22, and 37 C. It was stable in all diluents for 24 hr when stored at 4 or 22 C. When stored at 37 C, it was stable in PBS for up to 24 hr.

Strain Classification. Various strains within MG should not be confused with the numerous serotypes that have been characterized from avian sources within the entire genus *Mycoplasma*. Certain isolates of *M. gallisepticum* have come to be known more commonly by their isolate designations that sometimes are called strains. The S6 strain of Zander (3, 57, 178) was an early pathogenic isolate from the brain of a turkey with infectious sinusitis. The A5969 strain was given that designation by Jungherr et al. (80) for a pathogenic culture supplied by Van Roekel. The A5969 strain has become a standard strain for various antigen productions. The F strain of MG, which is so commonly used in current live culture vaccination programs (35, 64, 133), is a relatively mild strain that apparently originated from studies by van der Heide (157) employing the Connecticut F strain. The original F isolate, however, was described by Yamamoto and Adler (166) as a typical pathogenic strain. That strain was used by Luginbuhl et al. (103) in Connecticut for live culture vaccination of young broiler breeder replacement flocks to reduce possible egg transmission of MG in the subsequent breeder flocks. The R strain of MG was isolated by Dale Richey at the University of Georgia Poultry Disease Research Center in 1963 from a chicken with airsacculitis. The R strain has been widely used for bacterin production and as a pathogenic strain for MG challenge studies (64, 131, 168, 175).

M. gallisepticum isolates from both chickens and turkeys have been described as variant, or atypical, because they are often difficult to isolate, and are less pathogenic, transmissible, and immunogenic than expected of field isolates (15, 48, 107, 170).

A mycoplasma strain designated 4229T, isolated in 1984 from the turbinate of a duck in France, and similar isolates from geese in France and from a partridge in England, were originally identified as MG by immunofluorescence and growth-inhibition tests (26). Subsequent serologic and molecular studies, however, indicated only a partial relationship to MG, and DNA–DNA hybridization studies revealed only approximately 40 to 46% genetic homology (26). A new species name, *Mycoplasma imitans*, was proposed for this organism that cross-reacts serologically with MG (26).

M. gallisepticum strains designated 6/85 (56) and ts-11 (162, 163) have recently been used in commercially produced live culture vaccines.

Pathogenicity

INOCULUM. Isolates of MG vary widely in their relative pathogenicity, depending on the nature of the isolate, its method of propagation, the number of passages through which it has been maintained, the challenge route, and the dosage. Infective yolk from inoculated embryonated chicken eggs was often considered to be more infective than broth-passaged mycoplasma.

CHICKENS AND TURKEYS. Turkeys are more susceptible to MG than chickens; inoculated turkeys develop more severe sinusitis, airsacculitis, and tendovaginitis. The live F strain of MG was relatively more pathogenic for turkeys than usually noted in chickens (99, 100). Inoculation by the eye drop, intranasal, or intratracheal routes often results in fewer and milder lesions than intrasinus on intra–air sac inoculation. Turkeys sometimes do not develop sinusitis unless cultures are injected directly into the sinus (48). *M. gallisepticum* infection is frequently associated with a complexity of environmental and disease agents involved, as discussed further under Morbidity and Mortality.

EMBRYONATED CHICKEN EGGS. Inoculation of broth cultures or exudates containing MG into 7-day-old embryonated chicken eggs via the yolk sac route usually results in embryo deaths within 5–7 days. One or more yolk passages may be necessary before typical deaths and lesions are produced. Dwarfing, generalized edema, liver necrosis, and enlarged spleens are most typical. The organism reaches its highest concentration in the yolk sac, yolk, and CAM just prior to embryo death. Studies showed that MG strains varied in their in ovo pathogenicity, and that there was no correlation between in ovo pathogenicity and other in vivo or in vitro methods for pathogenicity evaluation (98). Embryo mortality due to virulent MG was prevented in eggs containing maternal MG antibodies, although MG could be reisolated from the yolk sac membrane of live embryonated eggs after 17 days of incubation.

Inoculation of embryonated chicken eggs is rarely employed for the isolation of avian mycoplasma now that adequate media are available.

PATHOGENESIS AND EPIZOOTIOLOGY

Natural and Experimental Hosts. *M. gallisepticum* infection occurs naturally in chickens and turkeys; however, MG has also been isolated from naturally occurring infections in pheasants (*Phasianus colchicus*), chukar partridge (*Alectoris graeca*), peafowl (*Pavo cristatus*), bobwhite quail (*Colinus virginianus*) and Japanese quail (*Coturnix coturnix japonica*). *M. gallisepticum* was isolated from a golden pheasant (*Chrysolophus pictus*) in Australia by Reece et al. (130), and was also isolated from a yellow-naped Amazon parrot (*Amazona ochrocephala auropalliata*) by Bozeman et al. (24). The isolation of MG from ducks has been reported from England (78) and from Yugoslavia (21). Reports on the isolation of MG from geese have come from France (34) and from Yugoslavia (22). A report by Davidson et al. (44) concerning MG isolated from wild turkeys (*Meleagris gallopavo*) notes that involved turkeys were in confinement, not free-living in their natural habitat. A follow-up survey of the same population 8 yr later found no conclusive evidence that MG was present, indicating that MG did not persist or spread in this wild turkey population (104). Other surveys of wild turkeys have found MG sero-negative (75, 105) and sero-positive (38, 63) populations. However, MG has rarely been isolated from wild turkeys, perhaps due in part to the common occurrence of other *Mycoplasma* spp., especially *M. gallopavonis* (38, 63).

There are reports of mycoplasma isolations from various other free-flying birds, but the significance of occasionally reported MG has not been clearly established. Similarly, attempts to determine the pathogenicity of MG for various free-flying birds have not been very conclusive. Budgerigars (*Melopsittacus undulatus*), experimentally infected with MG for use as a model to assess the efficacy of inhalant therapy, developed clinical signs and lesions of the trachea and air sac with no mortality (32).

Transmission. Direct contact of susceptible birds with infected carrier chickens or turkeys causes outbreaks of the disease; spread may also occur by contaminated airborne dust, droplets, or feathers. Spread by contact with contaminated equipment is commonly assumed, but has not been well documented. Lateral spread of MG in small flocks of chickens has been described in four phases: phase 1, a latent phase (12–21 days) before antibody was first detected in inoculated birds; phase 2, a period (1–21 days) in which infection gradually appeared in 5–10% of the population; phase 3, a period (7–32 days) in which 90–95% of the remaining population developed antibody; phase 4, a terminal phase (3–19 days) in which the remainder of the population became positive (114). Increasing the population density increased the rate at which lateral spread occurred. Infection is often transmitted through the egg in chickens and turkeys. *M. gallisepticum* was isolated from the oviduct of infected chickens and semen of infected roosters (173). Egg transmission has been successfully produced following experimental infection of susceptible chickens (23, 59, 64, 174, 175). Culturing the vitelline membrane of fresh eggs provided more isolations of MG than did culture of 18-day-old embryos (138).

Incubation Period. Early investigators found the incubation period to vary from 6 to 21 days in experimental transmission. Sinusitis often develops

in experimentally inoculated turkeys within 6–10 days. Under natural conditions, it is very difficult to determine the exact date of exposure; so many variable factors seem to influence the onset and extent of clinical infection that meaningful incubation periods cannot be stated. Numerous chicken and turkey flocks develop clinical infection near the onset of egg production, suggesting a low level of inherent infection (probably due to egg transmission) that precipitates from a series of stressing events. This apparent long extension of the incubation period is especially common in offspring of infected chickens or turkeys hatched from eggs dipped in antibiotic solutions for control of MG infection. The possible role of contamination from other sources of infection is not always clear and can rarely be proved beyond reasonable doubt. Many isolates of MG seem to represent this type of infection with delayed onset in which serologic evidence first appears between the 26th and 38th wk of age, usually without clinical signs (107, 156, 170).

Signs

CHICKENS. The most characteristic signs of the naturally occurring disease in adult flocks are tracheal rales, nasal discharge, and coughing. Feed consumption is reduced and birds lose weight. In laying flocks, egg production declines but is usually maintained at a lowered level (117). However, flocks may have serologic evidence of infection with no obvious clinical signs, especially if they encountered the infection at a younger age and have partially recovered. Male birds frequently have the most pronounced signs, and the disease is often more severe during winter. In broiler flocks, most outbreaks occur between 4 and 8 wk of age. Signs are frequently more marked than those observed in mature flocks. Severe outbreaks observed in broilers are frequently due to complications (see Morbidity and Mortality).

Cases of keratoconjunctivitis apparently caused by MG were reported in commercial layer chickens in Japan, first appearing around 30 days of age (124). Chickens showed swelling of the facial skin and the eyelids, increased lacrimation, congestion of conjunctival vessels, and respiratory rales. Conjunctivitis developed in chickens following conjunctival inoculation of Australian field strains of MG combined with infectious bronchitis virus (142).

TURKEYS. Nasal discharge with foaming of eye secretions frequently precedes the more typical swelling of the paranasal sinuses from sinusitis. Sometimes partial to complete closing of the eyes results from severe sinus swelling (Fig. 9.2). Appetite remains near normal as long as the bird can

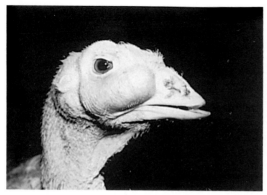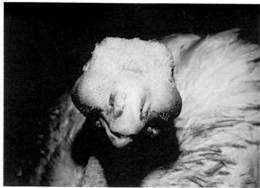

9.2.   Turkey with advanced case of infectious sinusitis showing marked swelling of infraorbital sinuses and nasal exudate.

see to eat. As the disease progresses, the affected birds become thin. Tracheal rales, coughing, and labored breathing may become evident if tracheitis or airsacculitis is present. An encephalitic form of MG has been reported in 12- to 16-wk-old commercial meat turkeys displaying torticollis and opisthotonos (37). In breeding flocks, there may be a drop in egg production or at least a lowered production efficiency.

Morbidity and Mortality

CHICKENS. The infection usually affects nearly all chickens in a flock, but is variable in severity and duration. It tends to be more severe and of longer duration in the cold months and affects younger birds more severely than mature birds, although there may be a considerable loss from lowered egg production.

While MG is considered the primary cause of chronic respiratory disease, other organisms frequently cause complications. Severe air sac infection, frequently designated as complicated CRD, or air sac disease, is undoubtedly the condition more commonly encountered in the field. Newcastle disease (ND) or infectious bronchitis (IB) may precipitate outbreaks of MG infection. *Escherichia coli* has been found to be a frequent complicating organism. The effect of MG, *E. coli,* and IB virus (IBV) infections alone or together in chickens was studied by Gross (66) and Fabricant and Levine (58). They reproduced a severe air sac infection when all three agents were combined. They further noted that *E. coli* could not readily infect the air sacs unless they were previously invaded by MG alone or in combination with either IBV or ND virus (NDV). Investigators have noted increased severity and duration of the disease when both MG and IBV were present (142).

Mortality may be negligible in adult flocks, but there can be a reduction in the number of birds in production (28). In broilers the mortality may range from low in uncomplicated disease to as much as 30% in complicated outbreaks and especially during the colder months. Retarded growth, downgrading of carcasses, and condemnations constitute further losses.

TURKEYS. The disease affects most turkeys in a flock, although some may not exhibit sinusitis, and the lower respiratory form of the infection may be most prominent. The infection will last for weeks and months in untreated flocks. Clinical signs, morbidity, and mortality associated with MG infection in turkeys may be highly variable. Typically, meat turkeys experience outbreaks between 8 and 15 wk of age. Initially, mild respiratory signs may progress in 2–7 days to a severe cough in 80–90% of the flock. Swollen sinuses with nasal discharge may affect 1–70% of birds in affected flocks. Condemnations primarily result from airsacculitis and related systemic effects, rather than from sinusitis.

Gross Lesions.   Gross lesions consist primarily of catarrhal exudate in nasal and paranasal passages, trachea, bronchi, and air sacs. Sinusitis is usually most prominent in turkeys, but is also observed in chickens and other affected avian hosts. Air sacs frequently contain caseous exudate, although they may only present a "beaded" or lymphofollicular appearance. Some degree of pneumonia may be observed. In severe cases of typical air sac disease in chickens, there is fibrinous or fibrinopurulent perihepatitis and pericarditis along with massive airsacculitis. *M. gallisepticum*-induced salpingitis of chickens and turkeys was reported by Domermuth et al. (51). Commercial layer chickens with MG-associated keratoconjunctivitis had marked edema in the facial subcutis and eyelids, with occasional corneal opacity (124).

Histopathology. The microscopic pathology in chickens and turkeys was studied by Van Roekel et al. (159) and in turkeys by Hitchner (72). They found marked thickening of the mucous membrane of the affected tissues from infiltration with mononuclear cells and hyperplasia of the mucous glands (Fig. 9.3). Focal areas of lymphoid hyperplasia were commonly found in the submucosa (Fig. 9.4). In the lungs, in addition to pneumonic areas and lymphofollicular changes, granulomatous lesions were also found. Detailed examination of MG-infected chicken air sacs via light microscopy, scanning EM, and histomorphic evaluation was reported by Trampel and Fletcher (155). Ultrastructural details of the interaction of MG with the tracheal epithelium of chickens was studied by Tajima et al. (145). Similar studies with infected tracheal ring explants were reported by Abu-Zahr and Butler (2) and Takagi and Arakawa (147). Dykstra et al. (52) employed EM, including scanning studies, to show the cytopathologic changes induced in chicken tracheal epithelium and in tracheal ring cultures inoculated with pathogenic MG. They described release of mucous granules followed by exfoliation of ciliated and nonciliated epithelial cells, and infrequent loss of cilia from individual cells. Repair of the epithelial surface was effected by basilar epithelial cells differentiating and filling in the spaces formed by exfoliated cells. During infection, there was increasing epithelial thickness due to cellular infiltration and edema (52).

Histologic examination of brains in cases of encephalitic MG revealed moderate to severe encephalitis with lymphocytic cuffing of vessels, fibrinoid vasculitis, focal parenchymal necrosis, and meningitis (37).

Conjunctivitis associated with MG was characterized by epithelial hyperplasia, severe cell infiltration, and edema of the subepithelial and central fibrovascular connective tissue stroma, which resulted in marked thickening of the eyelids (124). In the subepithelial lamina propria, proliferation of plasma cells and lymphocytes accompanying germinal centers was marked and resulted in irregular elevations of the overlying hyperplastic epithelial layer (124).

Immunity. Birds that have recovered from clinical signs of the disease have some degree of immunity. Such flocks, however, carry the organism and can transmit the disease to susceptible stock by contact or by egg transmission to their progeny. A review of the early literature concerning the immune response to MG is included in the report by Luginbuhl et al. (103). Adler et al. (4) determined the importance of the bursa of Fabricius in development of resistance and serologic response to the organism. Increasing antibody titers to MG have been found in tracheal washings of infected chickens with a concomitant decrease in organisms and tracheal lesion scores (164). Antibodies persisted in recovered chickens, and upon reexposure, they had a faster rate of MG elimination and less severe tracheal lesions than observed after the first exposure.

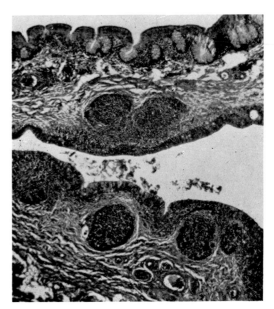

9.4. Section of sinus in chicken. Subepithelial infiltration of mononuclear cells and lymphofollicular reaction.

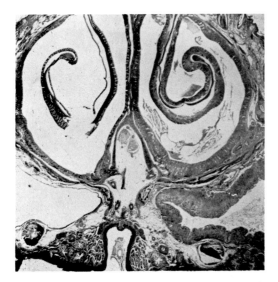

9.3. Section through nasal passages and sinuses of experimentally infected chicken. Unilateral mucosal thickening of sinus and nasal passage. ×6. (Van Roekel)

These results and others suggest that antibodies in respiratory secretions play a role in resistance to MG (54, 164, 165). Respiratory tract antibodies produced in response to MG infection inhibited attachment of the organism to tracheal epithelial cells (12), which may be one important mechanism of immune-mediated protection.

There has been considerable effort to identify MG antigens, especially those with adhesin or hemagglutinin properties, which may play key roles in the pathogenesis of, and immune response to, infection. *M. gallisepticum* proteins or lipoproteins with molecular weights ranging from 60 to 75 kD have been described as immunodominant adhesins or hemagglutinins (11, 14, 15, 18, 27, 43, 61, 111). A hemagglutinin of 67 kD from the S6 strain of MG was found to be encoded by a family of genes, whose hypothetical function is immune evasion (112). Further discussion is presented under Immunization.

DIAGNOSIS

Isolation and Identification of Causative Agent.
Suspensions of tracheal or air sac exudates, turbinates, lungs, or fluid sinus exudate may be inoculated directly to mycoplasma broth or agar medium (91). Swabs can also be taken from the trachea or choanal cleft (palatine fissure) for MG culture (29). In Frey's medium (62) supplemented with 10–15% horse or swine serum, extraneous bacterial contamination is usually controlled by inclusion of thallous acetate (1:4000) and penicillin (up to 2000 IU/mL). *M. gallisepticum* has been isolated from rooster semen (173) and from oviducts (51, 173). Although *M. meleagridis* is frequently isolated from turkey cloacal swabs, MG has been similarly isolated from the cloacal areas of turkeys (161) and chickens (7, 106).

Direct plating of exudates or tissue swabs onto agar plates may result in colonies after 4–5 days of incubation, but initial isolation in broth is generally a more sensitive method. Cultures should be incubated at least 5–7 days at 37 C. Growth may not be evident, but 2 or 3 serial passages at 3- to 7-day intervals may increase the number of isolations. Inclusion of triphenyl tetrazolium or phenol red with sufficient dextrose provides a growth indicator system. *M. gallisepticum* reduces 2,3,5-triphenyl tetrazolium to produce a red color in the medium, or it ferments dextrose to change phenol red to a yellow color as the medium becomes acid.

Enriched agar medium may be inoculated from broth cultures to study colonial morphology and to perform immunofluorescence tests. Inoculated plates must be incubated at 37 C in a very moist atmosphere 3–7 days before typical mycoplasma colonies are sufficiently large to be observed with a dissecting microscope. Sinuses, air sacs, or tendon sheaths of young chickens or turkeys may be inoculated to determine pathogenicity of the culture. Sections prepared for histopathology may also be of aid in making a diagnosis.

The inoculation of 7-day-old embryonated chicken eggs via the yolk sac with original exudates may be employed as a further means of isolating MG, but the inoculum must be free from fungal and bacterial contamination. Death of embryos should occur within 5–8 days, but one serial passage or more of harvested yolk material might be required before embryo deaths and typical lesions are noted.

Proof that mycoplasma isolates are MG has commonly been determined by antibody-based procedures. Antigens can be prepared and then tested with known MG antiserum, although such testing of recently isolated cultures is rarely very satisfactory. Another method is to test the serum from experimentally inoculated chickens or turkeys with known MG antigen. Direct immunofluorescence employing colonies on the surface of agar plates, or colony imprints, has been very effective for culture identification (119, 148, 149). These techniques and their modifications are especially useful for identification of MG in cultures containing other mycoplasma species (20, 119).

The agar gel precipitin test has also been used to identify cultures (16, 123). The direct immunoperoxidase test system was reported to be effective for the identification of MG and MS cultures (77), but that procedure is more commonly employed in an enzyme-linked immunosorbent assay (ELISA) procedure for detecting antibodies in serum.

M. gallisepticum strains can be differentiated from one another by direct comparison of protein banding patterns resulting from sodium dodecyl sulfate–polyacrylamide gel electrophoresis (SDS-PAGE), or restriction fragment length polymorphism (RFLP) of DNA, which has greater sensitivity (88, 92, 93, 137). These methods are especially useful for identification of vaccine strains of MG (85, 153) and for epidemiologic investigations of MG outbreaks. DNA and ribosomal RNA gene probes have also been used to speciate MG and identify vaccine strains (50, 60, 76, 87, 84, 120, 136, 177). Polymerase chain reaction (PCR) technology has increased the sensitivity of organism detection based on specific sequences of nucleotides (121, 141) and been used in commercial test kits.

Serology.
Serologic procedures are useful for flock monitoring in MG control programs and to aid in diagnosis when infection is suspected. A positive serologic test, together with history and signs typical of the disease, would allow a presumptive diagnosis pending isolation and identification of the organisms.

The tube agglutination test was a common procedure, especially within the MG control program in turkeys during the 1960s and 1970s, but is rarely used anymore. Serum plate agglutination (SPA) antigen, for the detection of antibodies to MG, is commercially available. Because the SPA test is quick, relatively inexpensive, and sensitive it has been widely used as an initial screening test for flock monitoring and serodiagnosis. However, nonspecific reactors occur in some flocks infected with *M. synoviae*, or those recently vaccinated with oil-emulsion vaccines and/or vaccines of tissue-culture origin against various agents (25, 39, 65, 132, 172). Certain nonspecific SPA reactions may be reduced by diluting the test serum (134) or producing SPA antigen in medium containing liposomes instead of swine serum (5).

The HI test has been commonly used to confirm reactors detected by SPA or, more recently, ELISA. The HI test, however, is time consuming, the reagents are not commercially available, and the test is not very sensitive (48, 73, 92, 135).

The ELISA has been used by several researchers to devise a test that would be more sensitive and more specific for MG antibodies than either the SPA or HI test (13, 42, 70, 108, 151). Commercial ELISA test kits are being used increasingly as an initial screening test for flock monitoring and serodiagnosis. Efforts continue to improve MG ELISA sensitivity and specificity by identifying and purifying specific immunodominant MG proteins for use as ELISA antigen (14, 126). As well, ELISAs have been used to detect MG antibodies in respiratory tract washings (11, 164) and egg yolk samples (116). Studies comparing egg yolk and serum for the detection of MG antibodies by ELISA or HI found comparable results, indicating that egg yolk samples could be used instead of serum samples for flock screening (33, 116, 175). Dot immunobinding assays for the detection of MG antibodies have also been described (10, 41, 139).

During the 1970s, atypical MG serologic test results were encountered in some chicken breeding flocks with histories of being free of MG. The usually normal-appearing flocks started to have a small percentage of MG SPA test reactors at 28–36 wk of age. Hemagglutination-inhibition titers rarely exceeded 1:80, and the percent of SPA reactors often did not exceed 20–40% of the flock during several months of study (107, 170). Low-virulence "variant" MG strains that were difficult to isolate and apparently egg transmitted were considered responsible (156, 170). Turkeys have also been infected with MG isolates of low virulence, low transmissibility, and poor immunogenicity (48). Antigenic variation of MG isolates, demonstrated by immunoblots (14, 15, 140) and agglutination (128) or HI assays (48, 92, 111), is at least partly responsible for atypical reactors.

Differential Diagnosis

CHICKENS. Care must be taken to differentiate *M. gallisepticum* infection from other common respiratory diseases of chickens. Newcastle disease and IB or their antibodies may be present as separate entities or as part of the complicated CRD problem. Infectious coryza and fowl cholera (FC) usually can be identified by bacterial culture. *M. synoviae* infection may be present alone or in addition to MG. Application of both serologic and cultural test procedures may be necessary in some cases.

TURKEYS. Presence of a respiratory disease including sinusitis in a turkey flock may at times be due to FC, chlamydiosis, cryptosporidiosis, MS infection, or vitamin A deficiency as well as the more usual MG. Specific cultural and serologic procedures are needed to differentiate them. Avian influenza A infection might also be considered.

TREATMENT. *M. gallisepticum* is susceptible to several antibiotics including streptomycin, oxytetracycline, chlortetracycline, erythromycin, magnamycin, spiramycin, tylosin, lincomycin, and spectinomycin (40, 154). Some MG isolates, however, have been reported to be rather resistant to streptomycin, erythromycin, spiramycin, and tylosin.

Attempts to treat CRD with various antibiotics and chemicals during the 1960s produced variable results. In many cases, it is doubtful if small increases in weight gain or egg production, and moderate reduction of carcass condemnations, were sufficient to cover medication costs. However, some more commonly employed treatments that tend to provide favorable results include use of oxytetracycline or chlortetracycline at 200 g/ton feed for at least several days. Tylosin has been injected subcutaneously at 3–5 mg/lb body weight or administered at 2–3 g/gal drinking water for 3–5 days. Administration of very low levels of tylosin in feed to MG-exposed layers in multiple-age complexes was found to lessen egg production losses (127). Tiamulin, and tiamulin plus salinomycin, were reported to be effective treatments in chickens or turkeys (9, 19, 143).

A combination of lincomycin and spectinomycin was effective in controlling experimental complicated airsacculitis in young chickens (69). Danofloxacin, a quinolone antimicrobial, has shown efficacy in chickens experimentally infected with MG (79, 83, 152).

Attempts to eliminate egg transmission of MG by medication of breeder flocks or their progeny with streptomycin, dihydrostreptomycin, oxytetracycline, chlortetracycline, erythromycin, or tylosin have generally been able to produce considerable reduction in rate of MG infection but generally were not adequate to obtain entirely infection-free flocks.

Egg dipping with a temperature or pressure differential has been used as a means of getting antibiotics into hatching eggs to eliminate egg-transmitted MG (6, 58, 68, 144). In general, these methods greatly reduced, but sometimes did not completely eliminate, the possibility of egg transmission. The influence on hatchability was not consistently favorable, and bacterial contamination was troublesome at times. However, egg dipping in antibiotic solutions has made it possible to obtain sufficient *M. gallisepticum*-free flocks to provide the poultry industry with a nucleus for producing clean progeny for large flocks, resulting in *M. gallisepticum*-free chicken and turkey breeder flocks in the United States. Serologic testing and selection of negative flocks for breeders are practical only when clean breeder flocks are established and reproduced.

An alternative approach for breaking the egg transmission cycle was reported by Yoder (167). Room temperature (25.6 C) eggs were heated in a forced-air incubator during a 12- to 14-hr period to reach an internal temperature of 46.1 C. Hatchability was sometimes reduced 8–12%, but MG and MS appeared to be inactivated. Similar success was reported by Meroz et al. (115) in Israel. Field studies have been extensive, with adequate success apparent in many cases and only 2–3% reduction of hatchability (169).

PREVENTION AND CONTROL. Because MG can be egg transmitted, maintaining chicken and turkey flocks free of MG infection is only possible by obtaining replacement flocks that are known to be free of the infection, and rearing them in strict isolation to avoid introduction of the disease. Establishing the MG-clean status of breeder flocks and maintaining that status can be accomplished by participation in control programs. Turkey and chicken breeders have generally adopted the various state-supported MG control programs within the National Poultry Improvement Plan (8).

Immunization

INACTIVATED *M. GALLISEPTICUM* BACTERINS. Interest in MG vaccines originated in the late 1970s as it became apparent that MG infection was enzootic in some multiple-age, egg-laying complexes. *M. gallisepticum* bacterins with oil-emulsion adjuvant were reported to protect young chickens from intrasinus challenge with virulent MG, and commercial egg layers from MG-induced drops in egg production (71). Some investigators found that such bacterins could protect broilers from airsacculitis (82, 176) or layers from reductions in egg produc-

tion (175), while others did not detect much efficacy in commercial egg layers with enzootic MG infection (86). Vaccination with bacterins has been shown to reduce, but usually not eliminate, colonization by MG following challenge (150, 165, 175, 176). To enhance the performance of inactivated MG vaccines, various adjuvants and antigen delivery systems, including liposomes and iota carrageenan, have been investigated (17, 53, 55). Inactivated MG vaccines have been produced commercially.

LIVE *M. GALLISEPTICUM* VACCINES. Studies using live MG cultures (Connecticut F strain) in young replacement pullets prior to housing in multiple-age egg-laying complexes were first reported by van der Heide (157) and Carpenter (35). There are numerous reports on the use of live F strain MG vaccine (28, 30, 64), which has been produced commercially and used extensively in multiple-age laying complexes. In broilers, vaccination with F strain provided some protection from airsacculitis following aerosol challenge with virulent R strain (97, 100, 133). The biologic mechanism underlying protection by F strain was found not to involve competition for adherence sites or blockage by prior colonization, and F strain vaccination did not prevent colonization by the challenge strain of MG (97). F strain can be transmitted through the egg (100) and from bird to bird. Kleven (89), however, reported that pullets given live F strain by the eye-drop route did not readily transmit the infection to broilers in pens in the same house when separated by an isle or empty pen. Studies (35, 117) have shown that F strain vaccinated laying hens produce more eggs than do unvaccinated hens in flocks with enzootic MG, but not as many as do MG-clean flocks. Field-strain MG was displaced from a multiple-age layer complex following 2 yr of continuous use of F strain vaccine in replacement pullets (94). The vaccinal F strain of MG was found to be pathogenic in turkeys following experimental infection (100), and it has been associated with MG outbreaks in meat and breeder turkeys under field conditions (99). Recently, live MG vaccines using strains 6/85 and ts-11 have been reported to possess little or no virulence for chickens and turkeys (1, 56, 162). These have been produced commercially.

LIVE CULTURE VACCINATION. Early studies on the use of live cultures of MG in young replacement pullets prior to being housed in large multiple-age egg-laying complexes was reported in 1977 by van der Heide (157). He employed the rather mild Connecticut F strain of MG, as did Carpenter et al. (35) in Pennsylvania. Numerous other studies concerning live F strain MG vaccination have been published.

Glisson and Kleven (64) studied the relative efficacy of live F strain and MG bacterin in protecting MG-challenged hens against production losses or egg transmission of MG. All vaccinated groups had better egg production and less egg transmission than controls. Hens vaccinated with two doses of MG bacterin had the longest lag before egg transmission. In a large-scale field study, Branton and Deaton (28) evaluated the use of live F strain MG in three strains of commercial egg layers in an endemic MG complex. Egg weight and eggshell strength were similar for all three strains of chickens with no differences from the unvaccinated controls. Less mortality in F strain–vaccinated hens of some strains gives the appearance of better egg production, based on production per hen housed. Further studies (30) showed that vaccination with live F strain at 45 wk of age (post–production peak) had no effect on oviduct function as judged by eggshell strength and thickness, and egg quality. Egg transmission of live F strain MG did not occur in hens vaccinated by ocular exposure, but did occur in hens given F strain by aerosol. However, egg transmission was considerably greater when live R strain was administered by either route (101). Other reports (102, 133) showed protection against airsacculitis in broilers aerosol-challenged with virulent R strain following ocular vaccination with live F strain. Levisohn and Dykstra (97) also found that F strain could protect against airsacculitis induced by MG challenge, but F strain colonization on the tracheal epithelium did not block infection by the pathogenic MG strain. Kleven (89) reported that pullets given live F strain by ocular inoculation did not readily transmit the infection to broilers in pens in the same house when separated by an isle or empty pen.

Carpenter et al. (35) reported on the relative performance of MG-clean and F strain–vaccinated laying hens on farms in Pennsylvania with endemic MG infection. They concluded that on the average, layers maintained free of MG infection laid 15.7 more eggs, and F strain–vaccinated layers 7.0 more eggs, per hen housed, than did the MG-infected layers. Similarly, Mohammed et al. (117) determined the economic impact of MG and MS infection in commercial layers in California. They concluded that MG-infected flocks produced 5–12 fewer eggs per hen and F strain–vaccinated flocks 6 eggs less per hen, compared with uninfected flocks. They estimated that the total loss due to MG infection in commercial layers in California for 1984 was approximately $7 million.

Young chicks immunized with selected temperature-sensitive mutants of the S6 strain of MG by intranasal inoculation and then challenged via the air sac with virulent S6 were noted to have less airsacculitis than controls (81, 96).

REFERENCES

1. Abd-el-Motelib, T.Y., and S.H. Kleven. 1993. A comparative study of Mycoplasma gallisepticum vaccines in young chickens. Avian Dis 37:981–987.

2. Abu-Zahr, M.N., and M. Butler. 1978. Ultrastructural features of Mycoplasma gallisepticum in tracheal explants under transmission and stereoscan electron microscopy. Res Vet Sci 24:248–253.

3. Adler, H.E., R. Yamamoto, and J. Berg. 1957. Strain differences of pleuropneumonia-like organisms of avian origin. Avian Dis 1:19–27.

4. Adler, H.E., B.J. Bryant, D.R. Cordy, M. Shifrine, and A.J. DaMassa. 1973. Immunity and mortality in chickens infected with Mycoplasma gallisepticum: Influence of the Bursa of Fabricius. J Infect Dis (Suppl) 127:61–68.

5. Ahmad, I., S.H. Kleven, A.P. Avakian, and J.R. Glisson. 1988. Sensitivity and specificity of Mycoplasma gallisepticum agglutination antigens prepared from medium with artificial liposomes substituting for serum. Avian Dis 32:519–526.

6. Alls, A.A., W.J. Benton, W.C. Krauss, and M.S. Cover. 1963. The mechanics of treating hatching eggs for disease prevention. Avian Dis 7:89–97.

7. Amin, M.M., and F.T.W. Jordan. 1979. Infection of the chicken with a virulent or avirulent strain of Mycoplasma gallisepticum alone and together with Newcastle disease virus or E. coli or both. Vet Microbiol 4:35–45.

8. Anonymous. 1994. The National Poultry Improvement Plan and Auxiliary Provisions. United States Department of Agriculture, Animal and Plant Health Inspection Service, Hyattsville, MD.

9. Arzey, G.G., and K.E. Arzey. 1992. Successful treatment of mycoplasmosis in layer chickens with single dose therapy. Aust Vet J 69:126–128.

10. Avakian, A.P., and S.H. Kleven. 1990. Evaluation of sodium dodecyl sulfate-polyacrylamide gel electrophoresis purified proteins of Mycoplasma gallisepticum and M. synoviae as antigens in a dot-enzyme-linked immunosorbent assay. Avian Dis 34:575–584.

11. Avakian, A.P., and D.H. Ley. 1993. Protective immune response to Mycoplasma gallisepticum demonstrated in respiratory-tract washings from M. gallisepticum-infected chickens. Avian Dis 37:697–705.

12. Avakian, A.P., and D.H. Ley. 1993. Inhibition of Mycoplasma gallisepticum growth and attachment to chick tracheal rings by antibodies to a 64-kilodalton membrane protein of M. gallisepticum. Avian Dis 37:706–714.

13. Avakian, A.P., S.H. Kleven, and J.R. Glisson. 1988. Evaluation of the specificity and sensitivity of two commercial enzyme-linked immunosorbent assay kits, the SP agglutination test, and the hemagglutination-inhibition test for antibodies formed in response to Mycoplasma gallisepticum. Avian Dis 32:262–272.

14. Avakian, A.P., S.H. Kleven, and D.H. Ley. 1991. Comparison of Mycoplasma gallisepticum strains and identification of immunogenic integral membrane proteins with Triton X-114 by immunoblotting. Vet Microbiol 29:319–328.

15. Avakian, A.P., D.H. Ley, and M.A. McBride. 1992. Humoral immune response of turkeys to strain S6 and a variant Mycoplasma gallisepticum studied by immunoblotting. Avian Dis 36:69–77.

16. Aycardi, E.R., D.P. Anderson, and R.P. Hanson. 1971. Classification of avian Mycoplasmas by gel diffusion and growth inhibition tests. Avian Dis 15:434–447.

17. Barbour, E.K., J.A. Newman, V. Sivanandan, D.A. Halvorson, and J. Sasipreeyajan. 1987. Protection and immunity in commercial chicken layers administered Mycoplasma gallisepticum liposomal bacterins. Avian Dis 31:723–729.

18. Barbour, E.K., J.A, Newman, J. Sasipreeyajan, A.C. Caputa, and M.A. Muneer. 1989. Identification of the antigenic components of the virulent Mycoplasma gallisepticum

(R) in chickens: Their role in differentiation from the vaccine strain (F). Vet Immunol Immunopathol 21:197–206.

19. Baughn, C.O., W.C. Alpaugh, W.H. Linkenheimer, and D.C. Maplesden. 1978. Effect of Tiamulin in chickens and turkeys infected experimentally with avian Mycoplasma. Avian Dis 22:620–626.

20. Bencina, D., and J.M. Bradbury. 1992. Combination of immunofluorescence and immunoperoxidase techniques for serotyping mixtures of Mycoplasma species. J Clin Microbiol 30:407–410.

21. Bencina, D., T. Tadina, and D. Dorrer. 1988. Natural infection of ducks with Mycoplasma synoviae and Mycoplasma gallisepticum and mycoplasma egg transmission. Avian Pathol 17:441–449.

22. Bencina, D., T. Tadina, and D. Dorrer. 1988. Natural infection of geese with Mycoplasma gallisepticum and Mycoplasma synoviae and egg transmission of the mycoplasmas. Avian Pathol 17:925–928.

23. Benton, W.J., M.S. Cover, and F.W. Melchior. 1967. Mycoplasma gallisepticum in a commercial laryngotracheitis vaccine. Avian Dis 11:426–429.

24. Bozeman, L.H., S.H. Kleven, and R.B. Davis. 1984. Mycoplasma challenge studies in budgerigars (Melopsittacus undulatus) and chickens. Avian Dis 28:426–434.

25. Bradbury, J.M., and F.T.W. Jordan. 1972. Studies on the absorption of certain medium proteins to Mycoplasma gallisepticum and their influence on agglutination and haemagglutination reactions. J Hyg, Camb 70:267–278.

26. Bradbury, J.M., O.M. Abdul-Wahab, C.A. Yavari, J.P. Dupiellet, and J.M. Bove. 1993. Mycoplasma imitans sp. nov. is related to Mycoplasma gallisepticum and found in birds. Int J Syst Bacteriol 43:721–728.

27. Bradley, L.D., D.B. Snyder, and R.A. Van Deusen. 1988. Identification of species-specific and interspecies-specific polypeptides of Mycoplasma gallisepticum and Mycoplasma synoviae. Am J Vet Res 49:511–515.

28. Branton, S.L., and J.W. Deaton. 1985. Egg production, egg weight, eggshell strength, and mortality in three strains of commercial layers vaccinated with F strain Mycoplasma gallisepticum. Avian Dis 29:832–837.

29. Branton, S.L., H. Gerlach, and S.H. Kleven. 1984. Mycoplasma gallisepticum isolation in layers. Poult Sci 63:1917–1919.

30. Branton, S.L., B.D. Lott, J.W. Deaton, J.M. Hardin, and W.R. Maslin. 1988. F strain Mycoplasma gallisepticum vaccination of post-production-peak commercial leghorns and its effect on egg and eggshell quality. Avian Dis 32:304–307.

31. Bredt, W. 1973. Motility of mycoplasmas. Ann NY Acad Sci 225:246–250.

32. Brown, M.B., and G.D. Butcher. 1991. Mycoplasma gallisepticum as a model to assess efficacy of inhalant therapy in budgerigars (Melopsittacus undulatus). Avian Dis 35:834–839.

33. Brown, M.B., M.L. Stoll, A.E. Scasserra, and G.D. Butcher. 1991. Detection of antibodies to Mycoplasma gallisepticum in egg yolk versus serum samples. J Clin Microbiol 29:2901–2903.

34. Buntz, B., J.M. Bradbury, A. Vuillaume, and D. Rousselot-Paillet. 1986. Isolation of Mycoplasma gallisepticum from geese. Avian Pathol 15:615–617.

35. Carpenter, T.E., E.T. Mallinson, K.F. Miller, R.F. Gentry, and L.D. Schwartz. 1981. Vaccination with F-strain Mycoplasma gallisepticum to reduce production losses in layer chickens. Avian Dis 25:404–409.

36. Chandiramani, N.K., H. Van Roekel, and O.M. Olesiuk. 1966. Viability studies with Mycoplasma gallisepticum under different environmental conditions. Poult Sci 45:1029–1044.

37. Chin, R.P., B.M. Daft, C.U. Meteyer, and R. Yamamoto. 1991. Meningoencephalitis in commercial meat turkeys associated with Mycoplasma gallisepticum. Avian Dis 35:986–993.

38. Cobb, D.T., D.H. Ley, and P.D. Doerr. 1992. Isolation of Mycoplasma gallopavonis from free-ranging wild turkeys in coastal North Carolina seropositive and culture-negative for Mycoplasma gallisepticum. J Wildl Dis 28:105–109.

39. Cullen, G.A., and L.M. Timms. 1972. Diagnosis of Mycoplasma infection in poultry previously vaccinated with killed adjuvant vaccines. Br Vet J 128:94–100.

40. Cummings, T.S., S.H. Kleven, and J. Brown. 1986. Effect of medicated feed on tracheal infection and population of Mycoplasma gallisepticum in chickens. Avian Dis 30:580–584.

41. Cummins, D.R., D.L. Reynolds, and K.R. Rhoades. 1990. An avidin-biotin enhanced dot-immunobinding assay for the detection of Mycoplasma gallisepticum and M. synoviae serum antibodies in chickens. Avian Dis 34:36–43.

42. Czifra, G., B. Sundquist, T. Tuboly, and L. Stipkovits. 1993. Evaluation of a monoclonal blocking enzyme-linked immunosorbent assay for the detection of Mycoplasma gallisepticum-specific antibodies. Avian Dis 37:680–688.

43. Czifra, G., T. Tuboly, B.G. Sundquist, and L. Stipkovits. 1993. Monoclonal antibodies to Mycoplasma gallisepticum membrane proteins. Avian Dis 37:689–696.

44. Davidson, W.R., V.F. Nettles, C.E. Couvillion, and H.W. Yoder. 1982. Infectious sinusitis in wild turkeys. Avian Dis 26:402–405.

45. Delaplane, J.P., and H.O. Stuart. 1943. The propagation of a virus in embryonated chicken eggs causing a chronic respiratory disease of chickens. Am J Vet Res 4:325–332.

46. Dickinson, E.M., and W.R. Hinshaw. 1938. Treatment of infectious sinusitis of turkeys with argyrol and silver nitrate. J Am Vet Med Assoc 93:151–156.

47. Dierks, R.E., J.A. Newman, and B.S. Pomeroy. 1967. Characterization of avian Mycoplasma. Ann NY Acad Sci 143:170–189.

48. Dingfelder, R.S., D.H. Ley, J.M. McLaren, and C. Brownie. 1991. Experimental infection of turkeys with Mycoplasma gallisepticum of low virulence, transmissibility, and immunogenicity. Avian Dis 35:910–919.

49. Dodd, S. 1905. Epizootic pneumo-enteritis of the turkey. J Comp Pathol Ther 18:239–245.

50. Dohms, J.E., L.L. Hnatow, P. Whetzel, R. Morgan, and C.L. Keeler, Jr. 1993. Identification of the putative cytadhesin gene of Mycoplasma gallisepticum and its use as a DNA probe. Avian Dis 37:380–388.

51. Domermuth, C.H., W.B. Gross, and R.T. Dubose. 1967. Mycoplasmal salpingitis of chickens and turkeys. Avian Dis 11:393–398.

52. Dykstra, M.J., S. Levisohn, O.J. Fletcher, and S.H. Kleven. 1985. Evaluation of cytopathologic changes induced in chicken tracheal epithelium by Mycoplasma gallisepticum in vivo and in vitro. Am J Vet Res 46:116–122.

53. Elfaki, M.G., S.H. Kleven, L.H. Jin, and W.L. Ragland. 1992. Sequential intracoelomic and intrabursal immunization of chickens with inactivated Mycoplasma gallisepticum bacterin and iota carrageenan adjuvant. Vaccine 10:655–662.

54. Elfaki, M.G., G.O. Ware, S.H. Kleven, and W.L. Ragland. 1992. An enzyme-linked immunosorbent assay for the detection of specific IgG antibody to Mycoplasma gallisepticum in sera and tracheobronchial washes. J Immunoassay 13:97–126.

55. Elfaki, M.G., S.H. Kleven, L.H. Jin, and W.L. Ragland. 1993. Protection against airsacculitis with sequential systemic and local immunization of chickens using killed Mycoplasma gallisepticum bacterin with iota carrageenan adjuvant. Vaccine 11:311–317.

56. Evans, R.D., and Y.S. Hafez. 1992. Evaluation of a Mycoplasma gallisepticum strain exhibiting reduced virulence for prevention and control of poultry mycoplasmosis. Avian Dis 36:197–201.

57. Fabricant, J. 1958. A re-evaluation of the use of media

for the isolation of pleuropneumonia-like organisms of avian origin. Avian Dis 2:409–417.

58. Fabricant, J., and P.P. Levine. 1962. Experimental production of complicated chronic respiratory disease infection ("air sac" disease). Avian Dis 6:13–23.

59. Fabricant, J., and P.P. Levine. 1963. Infection in young chickens for the prevention of egg transmission of Mycoplasma gallisepticum in breeders. Proc 17th World Vet Congr, pp. 1469–1474.

60. Fernandez, C., J.G. Mattsson, G. Bolske, S. Levisohn, and K.E. Johansson. 1993. Species-specific oligonucleotide probes complementary to 16S rRNA of Mycoplasma gallisepticum and Mycoplasma synoviae. Res Vet Sci 55:130–136.

61. Forsyth, M.H., M.E. Tourtellotte, and S.J. Geary. 1992. Localization of an immunodominant 64 kDa lipoprotein (LP 64) in the membrane of Mycoplasma gallisepticum and its role in cytadherence. Mol Microbiol 6:2099–2106.

62. Frey, M.L., R.P. Hanson, and D.P. Anderson. 1968. A medium for the isolation of avian Mycoplasmas. Am J Vet Res 29:2163–2171.

63. Fritz, B.A., C.B. Thomas, and T.M. Yuill. 1992. Serological and microbial survey of Mycoplasma gallisepticum in wild turkeys (Meleagris gallopavo) from six western states. J Wildl Dis 28:10–20.

64. Glisson, J.R., and S.H. Kleven. 1984. Mycoplasma gallisepticum vaccination: Effects on egg transmission and egg production. Avian Dis 28:406–415.

65. Glisson, J.R., J.F. Dawe, and S.H. Kleven. 1984. The effect of oil-emulsion vaccines on the occurrence of nonspecific plate agglutination reactions for Mycoplasma gallisepticum and M. synoviae. Avian Dis 28:397–405.

66. Gross, W.B. 1961. The development of "air sac disease." Avian Dis 5:431–439.

67. Hall, C.F. 1962. Mycoplasma gallisepticum antigen production. Avian Dis 6:359–362.

68. Hall, C.F., A.I. Flowers, and L.C. Grumbles. 1963. Dipping of hatching eggs for control of Mycoplasma gallisepticum. Avian Dis 7:178–183.

69. Hamdy, A.H. 1970. Therapeutic effect of Lincospectin on airsacculitis in chickens. Avian Dis 14:706–714.

70. Higgins, P.A., and K.G. Whithear. 1986. Detection and differentiation of Mycoplasma gallisepticum and M. synoviae antibodies in chicken serum using enzyme-linked immunosorbent assay. Avian Dis 30:160–168.

71. Hildebrand, D.G., D.E. Page, and J.R. Berg. 1983. Mycoplasma gallisepticum—Laboratory and field studies evaluating the safety and efficacy of an inactivated MG Bacterin. Avian Dis 27:792–802.

72. Hitchner, S.B. 1949. The pathology of infectious sinusitis of turkeys. Poult Sci 28:106–118.

73. Hitchner, S.B., C.H. Domermuth, G. Purchase, and J.E. Williams (eds.). 1980. Isolation and Identification of Avian Pathogens, 2nd ed. American Association of Avian Pathologists, Kennett Square, PA.

74. Hofstad, M.S. 1959. Chronic respiratory disease. In H.E. Biester, and L.H. Schwarte (eds.). Diseases of Poultry, 4th ed. Iowa State University Press, Ames, IA, pp. 320–330.

75. Hopkins, B.A., J.K. Skeeles, G.E. Houghten, D. Slagle, and K. Gardner. 1990. A survey of infectious diseases in wild turkeys (Meleagridis gallopavo silvestris) from Arkansas. J Wildl Dis 26:468–472.

76. Hyman, H.C., S. Levisohn, D. Yogev, and S. Razin. 1989. DNA probes for Mycoplasma gallisepticum and Mycoplasma synoviae: Application in experimentally infected chickens. Vet Microbiol 20:323–337.

77. Imada, Y., I. Nonomura, S. Hayashi, and S. Tsurubuchi. 1979. Immunoperoxidase technique for identification of Mycoplasma gallisepticum and M. synoviae. Nat Inst Anim Health Q (Tokyo) 19:40–46.

78. Jordan, F.T.W., and M.M. Amin. 1980. A survey of mycoplasma infections in poultry. Res Vet Sci 28:96–100.

79. Jordan, F.T., B.K. Horrocks, S.K. Jones, A.C. Cooper, and C.J. Giles. 1993. A comparison of the efficacy of danofloxacin and tylosin in the control of Mycoplasma gallisepticum infection in broiler chicks. J Vet Pharmacol Therapeut 16:79–86.

80. Jungherr, E.L., R.E. Luginbuhl, M. Tourtellotte, and W.E. Burr. 1955. Significance of serological testing for chronic respiratory disease. Proc 92nd Annu Meet Am Vet Med Assoc, pp. 315–321.

81. Karaca, K., and K.M. Lam. 1986. Effect of temperature-sensitive Mycoplasma gallisepticum vaccine preparations and routes of inoculation on resistance of white leghorns to challenge. Avian Dis 30:772–775.

82. Karaca, K., and K.M. Lam. 1987. Efficacy of commercial Mycoplasma gallisepticum bacterin (MG-Bac) in preventing air-sac lesions in chickens. Avian Dis 31:202–203.

83. Kempf, I., F. Gesbert, M. Guittet, G. Bennejean, and A.C. Cooper. 1992. Efficacy of danofloxacin in the therapy of experimental mycoplasmosis in chicks. Res Vet Sci 53:257–259.

84. Khan, M.I., and S.H. Kleven. 1993. Detection of Mycoplasma gallisepticum infection in field samples using a species-specific DNA probe. Avian Dis 37:880–883.

85. Khan, M.I., and R. Yamamoto. 1989. Differentiation of the vaccine F-strain from other strains of Mycoplasma gallisepticum by restriction endonuclease analysis. Vet Microbiol 19:167–174.

86. Khan, M.I., D.A. McMartin, Y. Yamamoto, and H.B. Ortmayer. 1986. Observations on commercial layers vaccinated with Mycoplasma gallisepticum (MG) bacterin on a multiple-age site endemically infected with MG. Avian Dis 30:309–312.

87. Khan, M.I., B.C. Kirkpatrick, and R. Yamamoto. 1987. A Mycoplasma gallisepticum strain-specific DNA probe. Avian Dis 31:907–909.

88. Khan, M.I., K.M. Lam, and R. Yamamoto. 1987. Mycoplasma gallisepticum strain variations detected by sodium dodecyl sulfate-polyacrylamide gel electrophoresis. Avian Dis 31:315–320.

89. Kleven, S.H. 1981. Transmissibility of the F strain of Mycoplasma gallisepticum in leghorn chickens. Avian Dis 25:1005–1018.

90. Kleven, S.H. 1985. Stability of the F strain of Mycoplasma gallisepticum in various diluents at 4, 22, and 37 C. Avian Dis 29:1266–1268.

91. Kleven, S.H., and H.W. Yoder, Jr. 1989. Mycoplasmosis. In H.G. Purchase, L.H. Arp, C.H. Domermuth, and J.E. Pearson (eds.). A Laboratory Manual for the Isolation and Identification of Avian Pathogens, 3rd ed. American Association of Avian Pathologists, Kennett Square, PA, pp. 57–62.

92. Kleven, S.H., C.J. Morrow, and K.G. Whithear. 1988. Comparison of Mycoplasma gallisepticum strains by hemagglutination-inhibition and restriction endonuclease analysis. Avian Dis 32:731–741.

93. Kleven, S.H., G.F. Browning, D.M. Bulach, E. Ghiocas, C.J. Morrow, and K.G. Whithear. 1988. Examination of Mycoplasma gallisepticum strains using restriction endonuclease DNA analysis and DNA-DNA hybridisation. Avian Pathol 17:559–570.

94. Kleven, S.H., M.I. Khan, and R. Yamamoto. 1990. Fingerprinting of Mycoplasma gallisepticum strains isolated from multiple-age layers vaccinated with live F strain. Avian Dis 34:984–990.

95. Kreig, N.R., and J.G. Holt. 1984. Bergey's Manual of Systematic Bacteriology, 9th ed, vol. 1. Williams and Wilkins, Baltimore, MD, pp. 740–793.

96. Lam, K.M., K. Karaca, and A.A. Bickford. 1986. Response of chickens to inoculation with a temperature-sensitive mutant of Mycoplasma gallisepticum. Avian Dis 30:382–388.

97. Levisohn, S., and M.J. Dykstra. 1987. A quantitative study of single and mixed infection of the chicken trachea by

Mycoplasma gallisepticum. Avian Dis 31:1–12.

98. Levisohn, S., J.R. Glisson, and S.H. Kleven. 1985. In Ovo pathogenicity of Mycoplasma gallisepticum strains in the presence and absence of maternal antibody. Avian Dis 29:188–197.

99. Ley, D.H., A.P. Avakian, and J.E. Berkhoff. 1993. Clinical Mycoplasma gallisepticum infection in multiplier breeder and meat turkeys caused by F strain: Identification by sodium dodecyl sulfate-polyacrylamide gel electrophoresis, restriction endonuclease analysis, and the polymerase chain reaction. Avian Dis 37:854–862.

100. Lin, M.Y., and S.H. Kleven. 1982. Pathogenicity of two strains of Mycoplasma gallisepticum in turkeys. Avian Dis 26:360–364.

101. Lin, M.Y., and S.H. Kleven. 1982. Egg transmission of two strains of Mycoplasma gallisepticum in chickens. Avian Dis 26:487–495.

102. Lin, M.Y., and S.H. Kleven. 1982. Cross-immunity and antigenic relationships among five strains of Mycoplasma gallisepticum in young leghorn chickens. Avian Dis 26:496–507.

103. Luginbuhl, R.E., M.E. Tourtellotte, and M.N. Frazier. 1967. Mycoplasma gallisepticum-control by immunization. Ann NY Acad Sci 143:234–238.

104. Luttrell, M.P., S.H. Kleven, and W.R. Davidson. 1991. An investigation of the persistence of Mycoplasma gallisepticum in an Eastern population of wild turkeys. J Wildl Dis 27:74–80.

105. Luttrell, M.P., T.H. Eleazer, and S.H. Kleven. 1992. Mycoplasma gallopavonis in eastern wild turkeys. J Wildl Dis 28:288–291.

106. MacOwan, K.J., C.J. Randall, and T.F. Brand. 1983. Cloacal infection with Mycoplasma gallisepticum and the effect of inoculation with H120 Infectious Bronchitis vaccine virus. Avian Pathol 12:497–503.

107. Mallinson, E.T., and M. Rosenstein. 1976. Clinical, cultural, and serologic observations of avian mycoplasmosis in two chicken breeder flocks. Avian Dis 20:211–215.

108. Mallinson, E.T., D.B. Snyder, W.W. Marquardt, E. Russek-Cohen, P.K. Savage, D.C. Allen, and F.S. Yancey. 1985. Presumptive diagnosis of subclinical infections utilizing computer-assisted analysis of sequential enzyme-linked immunosorbent assays against multiple antigens. Poult Sci 64:1661–1669.

109. Maniloff, J., and D.C. Quinlan. 1973. Biosynthesis and subcellular organization of nucleic acids in Mycoplasma gallisepticum strain A5969. Ann NY Acad Sci 225:181–189.

110. Markham, F.S, and S.C. Wong. 1952. Pleuropneumonia-like organisms in the etiology of turkey sinusitis and chronic respiratory disease of chickens. Poult Sci 31:902–904.

111. Markham, P.F., M.D. Glew, M.R. Brandon, I.D. Walker, and K.G. Whithear. 1992. Characterization of a major hemagglutinin protein from Mycoplasma gallisepticum. Infect Immun 60:3885–3891.

112. Markham, P.F., M.D. Glew, K.G. Whithear, and I.D. Walker. 1993. Molecular cloning of a member of the gene family that encodes pMGA, a hemagglutinin of Mycoplasma gallisepticum. Infect Immun 61:903–909.

113. McBride, M.D., D.W. Hird, T.E. Carpenter, K.P. Snipes, C. Danaye-Elmi, and W.W. Utterback. 1991. Health survey of backyard poultry and other avian species located within one mile of commercial California meat-turkey flocks. Avian Dis 35:403–407.

114. McMartin, D.A., M.I. Khan, T.B. Farver, and G. Christie. 1987. Delineation of the lateral spread of Mycoplasma gallisepticum infection in chickens. Avian Dis 31:814–819.

115. Meroz, M., D. Hadash, and Y. Samberg. 1973. Elimination of avian Mycoplasma organisms by heat treatment of eggs prior to incubation—some technical aspects. Refu Vet 30:101–109.

116. Mohammed, H.O., R. Yamamoto, T.E. Carpenter, and H.B. Ortmayer. 1986. Comparison of egg yolk and serum for the detection of Mycoplasma gallisepticum and M. synoviae antibodies by enzyme-linked immunosorbent assay. Avian Dis 30:398–408.

117. Mohammed, H.O., T.E. Carpenter, and R. Yamamoto. 1987. Economic impact of Mycoplasma gallisepticum and M. synoviae in commercial layer flocks. Avian Dis 31:477–482.

118. Morowitz, H.J., and J. Maniloff. 1966. Analysis of the life cycle of Mycoplasma gallisepticum. J Bacteriol 91:1638–1644.

119. Morse, J.W., J.T. Boothby, and R. Yamamoto. 1986. Detection of Mycoplasma gallisepticum by direct immunofluorescence using a species-specific monoclonal antibody. Avian Dis 30:204–206.

120. Nascimento, E.R., R. Yamamoto, K.R. Herrick, and R.C. Tait. 1991. Polymerase chain reaction for detection of Mycoplasma gallisepticum. Avian Dis 35:62–69.

121. Nascimento, E.R., R. Yamamoto, and M.I. Khan. 1993. Mycoplasma gallisepticum F-vaccine strain-specific polymerase chain reaction. Avian Dis 37:203–211.

122. Nelson, J.B. 1935. Cocco-bacilliform bodies associated with an infectious fowl coryza. Science 82:43–44.

123. Nonomura, I., and H.W. Yoder, Jr. 1977. Identification of avian Mycoplasma isolates by the agar gel precipitin test. Avian Dis 21:370–381.

124. Nunoya, T., T. Yagihashi, M. Tajima, and Y. Nagasawa. 1995. Occurrence of keratoconjunctivitis apparently caused by Mycoplasma gallisepticum in layer chickens. Vet Pathol 32:11–18.

125. Olesiuk, O.M., and H. Van Roekel. 1952. Cultural attributes of the chronic respiratory disease agent [abst]. Proc 24th Annu Conf Northeast Lab Workers in Pullorum Disease Control.

126. Opitz, H.M., and M.J. Cyr. 1986. Triton X-100-solubilized Mycoplasma gallisepticum and M. synoviae ELISA antigens. Avian Dis 30:213–215.

127. Ose, E.E., R.H. Wellenreiter, and L.V. Tonkinson. 1979. Effects of feeding tylosin to layers exposed to Mycoplasma gallisepticum. Poult Sci 58:42–49.

128. Panangala, V.S., M.A. Morsy, M.M. Gresham, and M. Toivio-Kinnucan. 1992. Antigenic variation of Mycoplasma gallisepticum, as detected by use of monoclonal antibodies. Am J Vet Res 53:1139–1144.

129. Quinlan, D.C., and J. Maniloff. 1973. Deoxyribonucleic acid synthesis in synchronously growing Mycoplasma gallisepticum. J Bacteriol 155:117–120.

130. Reece, R.L., L. Ireland, and D.A. Barr. 1986. Infectious sinusitis associated with Mycoplasma gallisepticum in game-birds. Aust Vet J 63:167–168.

131. Rimler, R.B., R.B. Davis, R.K. Page, and S.H. Kleven. 1978. Infectious coryza: Preventing complicated coryza with Haemophilus gallinarum and M. gallisepticum bacterins. Avian Dis 22:140–150.

132. Roberts, D.H. 1970. Nonspecific agglutination reactions with Mycoplasma gallisepticum antigens. Vet Rec 87:125–126.

133. Rodriguez, R., and S.H. Kleven. 1980. Evaluation of a vaccine against Mycoplasma gallisepticum in commercial broilers. Avian Dis 24:879–889.

134. Ross, T., M. Slavik, G. Bayyari, and J. Skeeles. 1990. Elimination of mycoplasmal plate agglutination cross-reactions in sera from chickens inoculated with infectious bursal disease viruses. Avian Dis 34:663–667.

135. Ryan, T.B. 1973. The use of microtiter hemagglutination-inhibition in Mycoplasma gallisepticum testing program. Proc US Anim Health Assoc 77:593–595.

136. Santha, M., K. Burg, I, Rasko, and L. Stipkovits. 1987. A species-specific DNA probe for the detection of Mycoplasma gallisepticum. Infect Immun 55:2857–2859.

137. Santha, M., K. Lukacs, K. Burg, S. Bernath, I. Rasko,

and L. Stipkovits. 1988. Intraspecies genotypic heterogeneity among Mycoplasma gallisepticum strains. Appl Environ Microbiol 54:607–609.

138. Sasipreeyajan, J., D.A. Halvorson, and J.A. Newman. 1987. Comparison of culturing Mycoplasma gallisepticum from fresh eggs and 18-day-old embryos. Avian Dis 31:556–559.

139. Shimizu, T., T. Takahata, and M. Kato. 1990. Detection of serum antibodies against Mycoplasma gallisepticum and Mycoplasma synoviae by a dot-immunobinding technique. Jap J Vet Sci 52:191–197.

140. Silveira, R.M., E.K. Marques, N.B. Nardi, and L. Fiorentin. 1993. Monoclonal antibodies species-specific to Mycoplasma gallisepticum and M. synoviae. Avian Dis 37:888–890.

141. Slavik, M.F., R.F. Wang, and W.W. Cao. 1993. Development and evaluation of the polymerase chain reaction method for diagnosis of Mycoplasma gallisepticum infection in chickens. Mol Cell Probes 7:459–463.

142. Soeripto, K.G. Whithear, G.S. Cottew, and K.E. Harrigan. 1989. Virulence and transmissibility of Mycoplasma gallisepticum. Aust Vet J 66:65–72.

143. Stipkovits, L., E. Csiba, G. Laber, and D.G. Burch. 1992. Simultaneous treatment of chickens with salinomycin and tiamulin in feed. Avian Dis 36:11–16.

144. Stuart, E.E., and H.W. Bruins. 1963. Preincubation immersion of eggs in erythromycin to control chronic respiratory disease. Avian Dis 7:287–293.

145. Tajima, M., T. Nunoya, and T. Yagihashi. 1979. An ultrastructural study on the interaction of Mycoplasma gallisepticum with the chicken tracheal epithelium. Am J Vet Res 40:1009–1014.

146. Tajima, M., T. Yagihashi, and T. Nunoya. 1985. Ultrastructure of mycoplasmal capsules as revealed by stabilization with antiserum and staining with ruthenium red. Jpn J Vet Sci 47:217–223.

147. Takagi, H., and A. Arakawa. 1980. The growth and cilia stopping effect of Mycoplasma gallisepticum 1RF in chicken tracheal organ cultures. Res Vet Sci 28:80–86.

148. Talkington, F.D., and S.H. Kleven. 1983. A classification of laboratory strains of avian Mycoplasma serotypes by direct immunofluorescence. Avian Dis 27:422–429.

149. Talkington, F.D., and S.H. Kleven. 1984. Research note: Additional information on the classification of avian Mycoplasma serotypes. Avian Dis 28:278–280.

150. Talkington, F.D., and S.H. Kleven. 1985. Evaluation of protection against colonization of the trachea following administration of Mycoplasma gallisepticum bacterin. Avian Dis 29:998–1003.

151. Talkington, F.D., and S.H. Kleven, and J. Brown. 1985. An enzyme-linked immunosorbent assay for the detection of antibodies to Mycoplasma gallisepticum in experimentally infected chickens. Avian Dis 29:53–70.

152. Tanner, A.C., A.P. Avakian, H.J. Barnes, D.H. Ley, T.T. Migaki, and R.A. Magonigle. 1993. A comparison of danofloxacin and tylosin in the control of induced Mycoplasma gallisepticum infection in broiler chicks. Avian Dis 37:515–522.

153. Thomas, C.B., P. Sharp, B.A. Fritz, and T.M. Yuill. 1991. Identification of F strain Mycoplasma gallisepticum isolates by detection of an immunoreactive protein. Avian Dis 35:601–605.

154. Timms, L.M., R.N. Marshall, and M.F. Breslin. 1989. Evaluation of the efficacy of chlortetracycline for the control of chronic respiratory disease caused by Escherichia coli and Mycoplasma gallisepticum. Res Vet Sci 47:377–382.

155. Trampel, D.W., and O.J. Fletcher. 1981. Light microscopic, scanning electron microscopic, and histomorphometric evaluation of Mycoplasma gallisepticum induced airsacculitis in chickens. Am J Vet Res 42:1281–1289.

156. Truscott, R.B., A.E. Ferguson, H.L. Ruhnke, J.R. Pettit, A. Robertson, and G. Speckmann. 1974. An infection in chickens with a strain of Mycoplasma gallisepticum of low virulence. Can J Comp Med 38:341–343.

157. van der Heide, L. 1977. Vaccination can control costly chronic respiratory disease in poultry. Res Report, Conn Storrs Agric Exp Stn 47:26.

158. Van Roekel, H., and O.M. Olesiuk. 1953. The etiology of chronic respiratory disease. Proc 90th Annu Meet Am Vet Med Assoc, pp. 289–303.

159. Van Roekel, H., J.E. Gray, N.L. Shipkowitz, M.K. Clarke, and R.M. Luchini. 1957. Etiology and pathology of the chronic respiratory disease complex in chickens. Univ Mass Agric Exp Stn Bull 486.

160. Vardaman, T.H. 1967. A culture medium for the production of Mycoplasma gallisepticum antigen. Avian Dis 11:123–129.

161. Varley, J., and F.T.W. Jordan. 1978. The response of turkey poults to experimental infection with strains of M. gallisepticum of different virulence and with M. gallinarum. Avian Pathol 7:383–395.

162. Whithear, K.G., Soeripto, K.E. Harrigan, and E. Ghiocas. 1990. Safety of temperature sensitive mutant Mycoplasma gallisepticum vaccine. Aust Vet J 67:159–165.

163. Whithear, K.G., Soeripto, K.E. Harrigan, and E. Ghiocas. 1990. Immunogenicity of a temperature sensitive mutant Mycoplasma gallisepticum vaccine. Aust Vet J 67:168–174.

164. Yagihashi, T., and M. Tajima. 1986. Antibody responses in sera and respiratory secretions from chickens infected with Mycoplasma gallisepticum. Avian Dis 30:543–550.

165. Yagihashi, T., T. Nunoya, S. Sannai, and M. Tajima. 1992. Comparison of immunity induced with a Mycoplasma gallisepticum bacterin between high- and low-responder lines of chickens. Avian Dis 36:125–133.

166. Yamamoto, R., and H.E. Adler. 1956. The effect of certain antibiotics and chemical agents on pleuropneumonia-like agents of avian origin. Am J Vet Res 17:538–542.

167. Yoder, H.W., Jr. 1970. Preincubation heat treatment of chicken hatching eggs to inactivate Mycoplasma. Avian Dis 14:75–86.

168. Yoder, H.W., Jr. 1979. Serologic response of chickens vaccinated with inactivated preparations of Mycoplasma gallisepticum. Avian Dis 23:493–506.

169. Yoder, H.W., Jr. 1985. Unpublished data.

170. Yoder, H.W., Jr. 1986. A historical account of the diagnosis and characterization of strains of Mycoplasma gallisepticum of low virulence. Avian Dis 30:510–518.

171. Yoder, H.W., Jr. 1988. Unpublished data.

172. Yoder, H.W., Jr. 1989. Nonspecific reactions to Mycoplasma serum plate antigens induced by inactivated poultry disease vaccines. Avian Dis 33:60–68.

173. Yoder, H.W., Jr., and M.S. Hofstad. 1964. Characterization of avian Mycoplasma. Avian Dis 8:481–512.

174. Yoder, H.W., Jr., and M.S. Hofstad. 1965. Evaluation of tylosin in preventing egg transmission of Mycoplasma gallisepticum in chickens. Avian Dis 9:291–301.

175. Yoder, H.W., Jr., and S.R. Hopkins. 1985. Efficacy of experimental inactivated Mycoplasma gallisepticum oil-emulsion bacterin in egg layer chickens. Avian Dis 29:322–334.

176. Yoder, H.W., Jr., S.R. Hopkins, and B.W. Mitchell. 1984. Evaluation of inactivated Mycoplasma gallisepticum oil-emulsion bacterins for protection against airsacculitis in broilers. Avian Dis 28:224–234.

177. Yogev, D., S. Levisohn, S.H. Kleven, D. Halachmi, and S. Razin. 1988. Ribosomal RNA gene probes to detect intraspecies heterogeneity in Mycoplasma gallisepticum and M. synoviae. Avian Dis 32:220–231.

178. Zander, D.V. 1961. Origin of S6 strain Mycoplasma. Avian Dis 5:154–156.

MYCOPLASMA MELEAGRIDIS INFECTION

Richard Yamamoto and G. Yan Ghazikhanian

INTRODUCTION. *Mycoplasma meleagridis* (MM) (N strain PPLO, H serotype) is a specific pathogen of turkeys. It is the cause of an egg-transmitted disease in which the primary lesion is an airsacculitis in the progeny. Other manifestations include decreased hatchability, skeletal abnormalities, and poor growth performance.

Economic and Public Health Significance. Economic losses caused by MM in turkeys have been associated primarily with egg-borne infections. During the early 1980s when the prevalence of MM was very high, the monetary cost to the U.S. turkey industry resulting from MM-related hatchability losses and cost of egg treatment to control egg-borne infections was estimated at $9.4 million per year (24). Currently, the economic losses due to MM infection in turkeys have been reduced significantly with the availability of MM-free eggs and poults supplied by major turkey breeders. *M. meleagridis* infections in turkeys have no public health significance.

HISTORY. In 1958, Adler et al. (3) were the first investigators to show that airsacculitis in poults hatched from infected eggs could be associated with a mycoplasma other than *M. gallisepticum*. The mycoplasma, later named *M. meleagridis,* was isolated from the air sac lesions of poults originating from eight breeding flocks from four states. The clinical syndrome of airsacculitis and/or associated skeletal abnormalities has been called day-old type airsacculitis (72), airsacculitis deficiency syndrome (98), and turkey syndrome-65 (TS-65) (131).

INCIDENCE AND DISTRIBUTION. Early studies showed that MM was a common pathogen of turkeys with a worldwide distribution (3, 9, 56, 78, 102, 113, 121, 127, 131). These prevalence studies, together with the knowledge that MM was transmitted through the egg, led major primary breeders in the mid-1970s to initiate programs to eradicate the agent from their stocks (54). With the success of these programs, the prevalence of MM has been reduced significantly within the past 15 yr in the major turkey-producing areas in the world (see Eradication).

ETIOLOGY

Classification. *M. meleagridis* (146) was designated as the N strain by Adler et al. (3) and placed

in the H serotype by Kleckner (66), Yoder and Hofstad (155), and Dierks et al. (34).

Morphology and Staining. Giemsa-stained smears of broth cultures of MM show coccoid bodies approximately 0.4 µm in diameter, similar to those of *M. gallisepticum* (146, 155). They appear singly, in pairs, or in small clusters. Ultrastructure studies (126) showed that MM did not possess bleb structures typical of *M. gallisepticum*, but had thicker fibrils in the central nuclear area. In both species, ribosomes were distributed in uniform rinds around the cell peripheries. Similar studies by others (55) revealed that the predominant morphotype of MM was a spherical form ranging from 200 to 700 nm in diameter. Other forms (chains of *Streptococcus*-like cells) suggested replication by binary fission. Similar forms, including short filaments, have been observed by scanning electron microscopy (61). An acidic mucopolysaccharide capsule was demonstrated. The DNA of type strain 17529 has a guanine and cytosine (GC) base composition of 27.0 to 28.1% and a genome size of 4.2 ± 0.5 x 10^8 daltons, both figures being at the lower range exhibited by mycoplasma (4).

Growth Requirements. *M. meleagridis* is a facultative anaerobe. Growth is optimal at 37–38 C and slight at 40–42 C. Most isolates do not adapt readily to broth media (41, 134). Serum or serum fraction (Difco) is an essential ingredient for growth. Swine and horse sera are satisfactory, but chicken and turkey sera are not (134).

A number of media have been described for cultivation of MM (134). A satisfactory broth consists of PPLO broth powder (Difco) (2.1%), yeast autolysate (Sigma) (1%), and heat-inactivated (56 C for 30 min) horse serum (15%) (83, 104, 146). For solid medium, Bacto agar (1.2%) is added to the formulation. The pH of the final medium is 7.5–7.8. Fresh yeast extract (44) may be substituted for the dehydrated product. Another commonly used medium is Frey's FM (45) described under *Mycoplasma synoviae* Infection. A broth medium, designated SP-4, containing cell culture medium components also supports excellent growth of MM (41).

The fastidious nature of this organism is exemplified in the observation that from time to time, certain batches of media do not support growth of the organism. In such cases, the source of the problem often can be traced to any one of the ingredients including the water used in the medium.

Colonial Morphology.   Colonies on agar medium after 2–3 days incubation appear small and flat (0.04–0.2 mm in diameter), with rough-appearing centers of ill-defined nipples. Nippling of the colonies is more prominent in laboratory-adapted strains than in fresh isolates (146).

Biochemical Properties.   The organism does not ferment dextrose or other carbohydrates or reduce tetrazolium salts (146, 155) but uses arginine (60) and has phosphatase activity (63). Horse erythrocytes incorporated into turkey meat infusion agar is hemolyzed by MM (155).

Resistance to Chemical and Physical Agents.   Very little is known about resistance of MM to chemical and physical agents. It is assumed, however, that most chemical disinfectants would be effective against it (21).

In broth at pH 8.4–8.7, MM may survive up to 25–30 days at high titers, 10^7 colony-forming units (CFU)/mL (33). Freshly seeded cultures on agar will survive for at least 6 days at room temperature (146, 65). The organism survives for at least 6 hr in the air (8). In vitro inactivation of four strains of MM at 45 C varied from 6 to 24 hr, while at 47 C inactivation of two strains occurred between 40 and 120 min (76).

Isolates of MM may be maintained for at least 2 mo by mincing colonies on agar in 3% sucrose and freezing at -20 to -70 C. Yoder and Hofstad (155) found broth-overlaid agar slant cultures to be viable after at least 2 yr storage at -30 C. Lyophilized cultures remain viable indefinitely (135). The organism does not decline in substantial numbers in turkey semen during cryopreservation and subsequent thawing (42).

Antigenic Structure.   *M. meleagridis* is antigenically unrelated to all other avian mycoplasmas. The agglutination (3, 155), fluorescent antibody (FA) (30), antiglobulin (2), growth and metabolic inhibition (34, 41, 77, 93), and complement fixation (46, 91) tests have been used to identify MM.

A few isolates possess hemagglutination activity (103, 125, 146). When hemagglutinating and non-hemagglutinating strains of MM were compared by polyacrylamide gel electrophoresis and simple and two-dimensional immunoelectrophoresis, minor antigenic differences were observed in the latter test only (41). Rhoades (109) showed that the determinant group(s) responsible for hemagglutination differed from that of agglutination.

The organism possesses a heat-stable lipid or polysaccharide toxin that causes an increase in ceruloplasmin activity when injected intravenously into chickens (32). The relationship of this toxin to the capsular material described by Green and Hanson (55) and to hemagglutinating activity is not known. However, hemagglutinating activity is not an essential component for virulence, since strains lacking this activity may be highly pathogenic (146, 152).

Pathogenicity.   Pathogenic and nonpathogenic strains of MM were described by Ghazikhanian and Yamamoto (51, 52). Of three strains studied, one failed to multiply in vivo, another multiplied but failed to produce lesions, while the third multiplied and produced airsacculitis. Zhao et al. (158) showed by sodium dodecyl sulfate–polyacrylamide gel electrophoresis (SDS–PAGE) that these strains differed in their cell protein profiles. Strain variations may account for the variability in clinical manifestations attributed to this organism (39).

PATHOGENESIS AND EPIZOOTIOLOGY

Natural and Experimental Hosts.   *M. meleagridis* is a specific pathogen of turkeys. When injected into turkey embryos by the yolk sac route, the organism produces a high incidence of airsacculitis but causes minimal mortality (138). The high infectivity and low mortality caused by MM in turkey embryos under experimental and natural conditions indicate that it has attained an ideal host–parasite relationship.

When inoculated into the yolk sac of chicken embryos, MM multiplies to high titers without causing high mortality (140, 155). Turkeys of all ages are susceptible to air sac infection with MM when inoculated via the air sac or trachea (71, 84, 137). Chickens are refractory to infection with MM (1, 136). Reports concerning the presence of MM in Japanese quail, peacocks, and pigeons (134) have not been confirmed.

Transmission

VERTICAL TRANSMISSION.   *M. meleagridis* is perpetuated primarily through egg transmission. Infection of the female reproductive tract occurs as an endogenous infection during embryonic development (80), as an ascending infection from foci in the cloaca or bursa of Fabricius after the occluding plate is perforated at sexual maturity (79), or by insemination of hens with MM-containing semen (71, 83, 85, 133, 148). Infection rates of 19–57% have been found in flocks in which cultures were taken from the vagina of virgin females. While such hens contribute to the overall egg-transmission rate, particularly when the incidence is high, insemination with mycoplasma-contaminated semen plays a major role in sustaining the egg-transmission rate during the laying season (68, 71, 144). The egg-transmission rate among individual hens may vary from

10 to 60% (148). There is apparently, however, no regular pattern as to sequence of infected eggs laid (83). Transmission starts out at a low rate during the first 2–3 wk of lay, reaches a maximum at midseason, and gradually declines toward the end of the laying season (16, 71). There seems to be some intracyclic fluctuation in the transmission pattern during the laying season (71, 148), but it has not been possible to relate such changes to the insemination schedule.

Egg transmission does not occur in hens in which the organism is found only in the upper respiratory tract (sinus) (71, 83, 133) and is minimal in hens infected via air sac and subsequently inseminated with clean semen (71).

A comparative study of persistence of MM, *M. synoviae,* and *M. gallisepticum* in the genitalia of adult turkeys indicated that MM favored this environment more than the others (143).

Although the exact site in the reproductive system where the organism infects the developing egg is not known, it appears not to be in the ovary; several studies have generally failed to yield the organism from the ova of hens known to be transmitting the organism through their eggs (83, 133, 148). Furthermore, egg transmission occurs at a high rate in the absence of active abdominal airsacculitis.

The organism has been recovered from various sites of the oviduct, with the greatest frequency from the vagina and uterus (85, 148). In hens repeatedly inseminated with MM-contaminated semen, high levels of infection in the uterovaginal region were not sustained, although such hens did transmit the organism through their eggs (135). In hens inseminated with contaminated semen, the organism was found as high as the magnum (71). The organism has been isolated from the shell membrane and vitelline membrane-yolk of preincubated eggs from naturally infected turkeys, but at higher rates from the latter (10–12%) than former (2–4%) sites (54). Mycoplasma counts of 10^3 to 10^5 CFU/vitelline membrane have been obtained (135). Thus, while the organism has the potential to infect the developing egg at various sites in the oviduct, the critical site appears to be in the area of the fimbria or magnum.

As is the case with the female, cloacal infection detected in the male at the time of hatch can persist through sexual maturity; semen taken from such males will contain the organism (133, 150). The organism remains localized in the cloaca and phallus and does not ascend the vas deferens or testes (104, 133). Isolation rates of MM from the phallus or semen of naturally infected male flocks have ranged from 13 to 32%. Histologic study of the phallus and accessory organs suggests that a possible site of lo-

calization is the region of the submucosal gland (47).

HORIZONTAL TRANSMISSION.   Direct and indirect transmission of MM may occur at any stage of the bird's life. Direct transmission by the airborne route may occur within a hatchery (71) or flock (142) or on occasion between flocks separated by ¼ mile (54). Airborne transmission in mature turkeys usually results in a high infection rate (up to 100%), which remains localized in the sinus and trachea (71, 83). In young birds during the brooding and growing periods, however, the organism may localize in the genitalia of approximately 5% of the birds infected by the respiratory route (142).

Indirect transmission results from management practices including sexing, vaginal palpation, artificial insemination, and vaccination whereby mycoplasmas are manually carried from infected to noninfected turkeys via contaminated hands, clothing, and equipment (54, 83).

Airborne transmission apparently is of little significance once a bird has reached sexual maturity. Thus, egg transmission does not occur in noninfected females that have been placed in cages adjacent to infected females. Similarly, clean males held in the same room with phallus-infected males produce MM-free semen throughout the production period (133, 135). The transmission cycle of MM is graphically shown in Figure 9.5.

Signs.   Despite a high rate of airsacculitis in poults originating from infected dams, respiratory signs are rarely observed. Lateral transmission that may occur by direct or indirect means in adult birds may lead to a high infection rate, but rarely to clinical disease. Thus, *M. meleagridis* commonly occurs as a silent infection in adult birds.

While not a consistent feature of the disease, the syndrome called TS-65 (also called airsacculitis deficiency syndrome) may be associated with MM egg-borne infection (101). The syndrome, which includes signs of bowing, twisting, and shortening of the tarsometatarsal bone and hock joint swelling, has been reproduced experimentally in MM-free poults (13, 90, 129, 132, 151). Deformation of cervical vertebrae (22, 86), stunting, and abnormal feathering (13) are additional features of the disease.

M. meleagridis acts synergistically in producing severe airsacculitis with *M. iowae* (112) and sinusitis with *M. synoviae* (108). In a flock naturally infected with MM and *M. synoviae,* sinusitis was estimated to be 2.1% in males and 0.13% in females (108). While it is generally believed that neither agent alone is capable of producing sinusitis, field

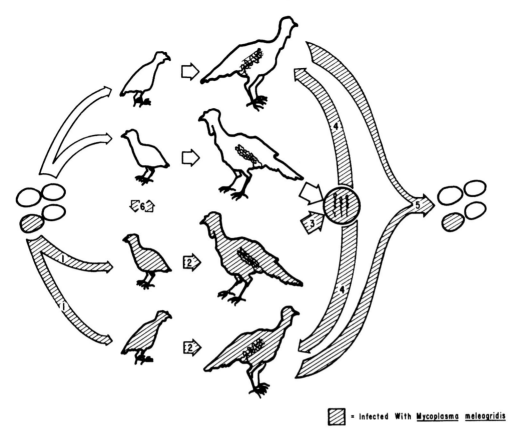

= Infected With <u>Mycoplasma meleagridis</u>

9.5.   Transmission cycle of *Mycoplasma meleagridis*. (*1*) Infected eggs yield poults in which the organism is widely distributed in the body. (*2*) Genital infection may persist in both males and females through sexual maturity. (*3*) Semen from infected males contaminates clean semen when pooled. (*4*) Biweekly insemination of hens ensures a high rate of oviduct infection. (*5*) The egg-transmission rate is approximately 25% during the season's lay. (*6*) Lateral transmission may also contribute to genital infection.

cases have been encountered in which only MM has been isolated from sinus exudate (29).

Morbidity and Mortality

REPRODUCTIVE PERFORMANCE. *M. meleagridis* does not adversely affect egg production or fertility and does not cause early incubation mortality (28, 141). It causes late incubation (25–28 days) mortality in artificially (24, 141) and naturally (35) infected turkey embryos. It has been estimated that MM causes a loss in hatchability of 5–6% of fertile eggs set under commercial conditions (37). Edson (35), using risk analysis, determined the mortality rates of embryos naturally infected with MM and/or an unidentified mycoplasma. The analysis showed that embryos infected with MM, unidentified mycoplasma, and both agents were 5, 7, and 25 times more likely to die than the mycoplasma-free embryos. The unidentified mycoplasma was later identified as *M. iowae* (135), a common mycoplasma of turkeys known to reduce hatchability (111).

AIR SAC LESIONS AND CONDEMNATIONS. During the mid-1960s, MM-associated airsacculitis was reported to be one of the major causes of condemnation of fryer-roaster turkeys in the United States (5, 73). Air sac lesion rates of 10–25% in first-run poults from MM-infected flocks over a season's production were reported under experimental and commercial conditions (43, 71, 83, 148).

Since air sac lesions caused by uncomplicated MM infection regress within 15–16 wk (9, 150), it appears that other agents or factors may be involved in the overall picture. Anderson et al. (5) observed a twofold or greater increase in incidence of air sac lesions caused by MM in turkeys raised to 12 wk of age in a high-dust environment.

Brown and Nestor (20) suggested that turkeys selected for low plasma ACTH following cold stress were more resistant to MM infection than those selected for high ACTH levels. Saif et al. (116) reproduced complicated airsacculitis with MM and *Escherichia coli* in poults. Mixed infections of MM and *M. iowae* also accentuate the severity of air sac lesions (112). Therefore, a number of interacting factors may aggravate MM-induced air sac lesions in young turkeys.

SKELETAL ABNORMALITIES AND GROWTH PERFORMANCE. In affected flocks, MM-associated skeletal abnormalities (i.e., TS-65 syndrome) may be observed in poults between 1–6 wk of age (131). Five to 10% of the poults may show clinical signs, but on occasion the percentage may reach higher levels. Not all cases progress to an irreversible state (131). Incidence of the disease seems to increase with progression of the laying season. Mortality is due primarily to cannibalism of affected birds. The problem is not associated with a particular strain of bird, but the male seems to be more susceptible.

Peterson (97) found a positive association of skeletal lesions, airsacculitis, and high agglutination titers to MM in poults with the TS-65 syndrome, which supports the view that the syndrome is initiated by a generalized egg-borne infection (132). It was further hypothesized, based on in vitro and in vivo studies, that the organism may deprive the embryo of biotin, resulting in abnormal bone development (13, 15). Others have postulated that the organism may compete for arginine, an essential amino acid for proper bone development (151). In vitro studies indicated, however, that MM strains of varying virulence did not differ in their arginine requirement; also, significant differences in plasma arginine concentration between noninfected and infected poults with leg abnormalities were not observed (60).

Nelson et al. (90) distributed MM-free and -infected eggs in large numbers to 11 cooperators in eight states to study the leg weakness syndrome under commercial conditions. The results indicated that the total daily mortality, number of cull poults, and skeletal deformity were much lower in poults hatched from MM-free eggs. A significant advantage in weight gain was also observed with MM-free vs. infected poults (12, 92, 131).

Conversely, others (23, 26, 27) were unable to demonstrate any economic advantage of MM-free over MM-infected turkeys. Possible reasons for the divergent results are not clear, but factors such as differences in the genetic makeup of the bird, virulence of MM strains, environmental stresses, and secondary infections may influence the picture.

Gross Lesions.   While gross lesions, if any, in poults at time of hatch from infected dams are limited to the air sacs, the organism may be widely distributed in various tissues including feathers, skin, sinus, trachea, lungs, air sacs, bursa of Fabricius, intestine, cloaca, (11, 99, 106) and hock joints (135). The air sac lesions are characterized by thickening of the air sac walls with adherence of a yellow exudate to the tissue and, occasionally, presence of variously sized flecks of caseous material free in the lumen (3). Extension of such lesions to the abdominal air sacs is a common occurrence by 3–4 wk of age. It is also possible for the organism to be present in air sacs of day-old poults exhibiting no lesions; in such cases, air sac lesions may develop in 3–5 wk (9). Lesions produced by MM when not mixed with *M. iowae* are not as extensive or fulminating as those described for *M. gallisepticum* (34, 72). Figure 9.6 shows a poult, hatched from an MM-infected egg, with caseopurulent airsacculitis.

Skeletal lesions, when present, are usually associated with severe airsacculitis (97). Sternal bursitis (137), synovitis (116), and ascites (129) are additional lesions observed in experimental infections. The sinusitis produced by MM and *M. synoviae* in mixed infections contains clear mucus to caseous exudate (108). Leg abnormalities in poults hatched from MM-infected eggs are shown in Figure 9.7.

Histopathology.   In embryonic infection with MM, exudative airsacculitis and pneumonia were the only inflammatory lesions seen. Lesions that developed at 25–28 days of age were related to maturation of inflammatory cells. Air sac lesions consisted predominantly of heterophils with some mononuclear cells, including lymphocytes and varying amounts of fibrin and cellular debris. Epithelial necrosis was seen in severely affected air

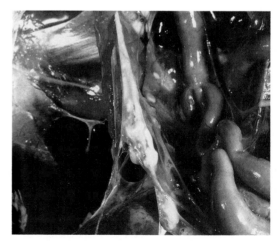

9.6.   Airsacculitis in a 4-wk-old poult caused by eggborne *Mycoplasma meleagridis* infection.

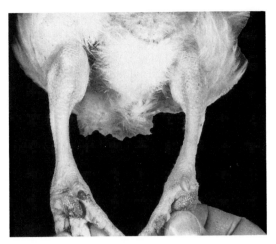

9.7. Bowing of tarsometatarsal bones of a 3-wk-old poult hatched from a *Mycoplasma meleagridis*-infected egg.

sacs. Mononuclear cells and fibrin were the prominent features of lung lesions (52, 106). Significant or marked microscopic changes in other organs in embryos or poults were not observed despite invasion of the organism into many of these sites (52).

In 7-wk-old poults infected with MM by the air sac route, lymphocytic perivascular infiltration and fibrinocellular exudate were observed in 2 days. Some areas of the air sac epithelium became hyperplastic and others underwent necrosis at about 4–8 days. Lymphoid follicles were observed in 16 days. When examined by electron microscopy, the follicles were found to be surrounded by encapsulated collagen bundles and composed of hemocytoblasts of bursal origin presumed to be involved in antibody formation (107). Essentially similar sequential changes were observed by others in poults infected as embryos or at 1–3 days of age (6, 52, 87).

Wise et al. (131) indicated that gross and microscopic long-bone lesions of TS-65 were similar to those observed in perosis of dietetic origin. The main lesions were seen in proximal ends of the long bones. Cartilage farthest from blood vessels descending into the proliferative zone from the cartilaginous epiphysis lacked cell density and contained abnormal-appearing chondrocytes. In long-standing cases of 6–8 wk or longer, growth plates often were normal, suggestive of repair even though the bones were grossly deformed. These cellular changes in the proliferative zone of the growth plates were seen in all long bones examined, suggestive of a generalized response. It was postulated that MM causes a secondary block of nutrients to the growth plates.

A secondary lesion in the medial side of the proximal end of the tarsometatarsal bone of chronic cases with varus deformity was described as a dyschondroplasia or chondrodystrophy resulting from partial failure of the metaphyseal blood supply at the growth plates (131).

Mild mononuclear cell infiltration was observed in the periarticular region of the hock joint in 2-wk-old poults inoculated with MM intravenously (100).

The most prominent lesion in hens infected by the vaginal route was focal encapsulated accumulation of lymphocytes present most frequently in the fimbria, uterus, and vagina. Plasma cells and heterophils were also present in significant numbers in the lamina propria of the reproductive tract. The encapsulated follicles were believed to be active in antibody formation (105). Similar lesions in the reproductive tract of turkeys infected with MM were described by Ball et al. (7).

Gerlach et al. (47) examined histologically the phallus and accessory structures of males experimentally infected with MM. The only significant change was an extensive lymphofollicular formation in the region of the mucous-type glands in the submucosa of the lymphfold.

Immunity

ACTIVE. Turkeys inoculated intravenously or by the respiratory route with MM were resistant to reinfection when challenged by the same routes 21 wk later. There was no correlation, however, between antibody titer and resistance (84). Repeated injections of 20-wk-old hens with live organisms failed to induce protective immunity or reduce egg transmission (128).

When hens that had been vaginally infected artificially with MM culture or with contaminated semen were subsequently inseminated with clean semen, the organism was eliminated from the vagina within 4–14 wk, while hens continuously inseminated with contaminated semen maintained a high incidence of infection (68, 71). On the other hand, insemination with clean semen of virgin hens known to be vaginal carriers of MM resulted in a high egg-transmission rate and persistence of oviduct infection (35, 144). In the first-mentioned studies, it appears that an active immune mechanism was functioning to eliminate the organism after removal of the source of infection, i.e., contaminated semen. Persistence of infection in the latter study may be an expression of immune tolerance in hens infected by egg transmission.

Yamamoto et al. (149) found that hens infected with MM via the oviduct during one breeding season were free of MM at the start of the second laying season; among five adult males infected via the phallus, the organism persisted for 55–344 days. These findings are consistent with the observation that the decline in the egg-transmission rate during the latter part of the laying season may be related to an active immune response. A study by Ortiz et al. (94) suggested that MM infection of the bursa of Fabricius during embryonic development causes an impairment of the secondary antibody response to innate or inactivated antigens.

PASSIVE. Maternal antibodies (agglutinins) may be detected in a high percentage of poults from infected dams and persist for approximately 2 wk posthatching. Such antibodies are not protective against development of air sac lesions in infected embryos (84, 148). Conversely, purified IgM and IgG antibodies when injected into the yolk sac of infected embryos significantly reduced embryo mortality and the incidence of leg deformities in hatched poults, but they did not reduce air sac lesions or isolation rates when compared with the controls (17).

DIAGNOSIS

Isolation and Identification of Causative Agent.
M. meleagridis may be readily isolated on several commercially available and laboratory-prepared media (see Growth Requirements). Thallium acetate (1:4000) and penicillin (1000 units/mL) are inhibitors added to agar plates, slants, and broth. Polymyxin B (100 units/mL) may be added to the broth portion of the overlay to facilitate isolation of MM from highly contaminated sources such as the cloaca and phallus. Mycostatin (50 units/mL) may be added to the agar and broth to inhibit fungi (85). M. meleagridis may be selectively isolated from specimens containing mixed cultures by adding to the medium immune serum against the undesired mycoplasma (18). The organism may be isolated from vitelline membrane, air sacs, intestine, and many other sites of infected embryos (see Gross Lesions). It may also be isolated from the kidneys of poults infected by the air sac route (129).

For large sampling studies in the field (e.g., cultures from the trachea, palatine cleft, vagina, or phallus), placing swab specimens in overlay broth (3) facilitates transport to the laboratory; the broth also serves as an initial enrichment (95). At necropsy, the organism may be isolated from various sites of the respiratory (including sinus) and reproductive systems.

Once growth is apparent in original isolation medium, usually after 4–6 days of incubation, agar plates are streaked and placed in a sealed container with added moisture. Plates are incubated at 37 C for 5–7 days before being examined for colonies under the dissecting microscope, and are incubated at least 10 days before being discarded as negative.

M. meleagridis may be differentiated from other chicken and turkey mycoplasmas by its inability to utilize glucose and its ability to metabolize arginine and phosphate (60, 63, 121, 155). Definitive identification, however, must be based on serologic methods. The direct (30) and indirect (18) FA, growth inhibition (34), and immunoperoxidase (62, 120) tests are commonly used for this purpose.

DNA-based tests have recently been developed for the direct detection of the organism in clinical specimens (156, 157).

Serology.
The rapid plate (RP) and tube agglutination (TA) tests are effective in detecting MM infections. Antibodies are detected in poults hatched from infected eggs in 3 wk and in turkeys infected by contact in 4–5 wk. Birds with active air sac lesions may have high agglutinin titers, while those with localized infections in the sinus or phallus may be negative or show low titers (1, 84, 150). The RP test may be quantified by performing it on serially diluted serums. A reaction at a dilution of 1:5 is significant (150, 152), but for flock diagnosis, some samples should react at 1:10 or higher. Each lot of antigen should be pretested with a standard positive serum for its reactive quality at higher serum dilutions.

The hemagglutination-inhibition (HI) test (103, 125) is another useful test for detecting antibodies to MM infections. While nonhemagglutinating laboratory strains of MM do not elicit high HI antibody responses in turkeys, the HI test is very effective in detecting such antibodies in naturally infected birds (109). Apparently, field infections with MM occur with strains possessing hemagglutinating activity, but this characteristic is quickly lost for most strains when they are cultivated on laboratory media (109). Furthermore, since the antigenic determinant(s) responsible for hemagglutination differs from that of agglutination (109), it is possible to find individual turkeys in an infected flock whose serum will be positive in the HI and negative in the TA tests; the reverse situation may also occur (152).

Yamamoto et al. (152) adapted the HI test to the microtest system. Using four units of antigen, titers of 1:40 were considered suspects and 1:80 or greater as reactors. When used as a confirmatory test to the RP test, a positive HI signifies infection, while a negative HI requires a more conservative interpretation and may involve use of other confirmatory tests or follow-up testing for final diagnosis (153). The micro-HI test has been used to identify false-positive RP reactions (135) in flocks recently vaccinated with Erysipelothrix vaccine (14).

Kleven and Pomeroy (67) found that the RP test detected IgM, the TA test detected both IgM and IgG, and the HI test detected IgG most efficiently. However, the early HI antibody response of turkeys to high doses of MM given intravenously was of the IgM class (110).

Other tests developed for mass screening are the microagglutination (139), enzyme-linked immunosorbent assay (ELISA) (96), and avidin-biotin enhanced dot-immunobinding assay (31).

Differential Diagnosis.
Air sac lesions caused by MM must be differentiated from those caused by *M. gallisepticum*, other *Mycoplasma* serotypes, and possibly other agents. The possibility of a mixed infection of MM with *M. synoviae* or *M. iowae* should be considered if embryo mortality, sinusitis, or airsacculitis is observed. *M. meleagridis*-associated skeletal abnormalities must be differentiated from similar lesions caused by *M. iowae* or of dietetic origin.

TREATMENT.
Antibiotics having in vitro activity against MM include gentamicin (118), tylosin, chloramphenicol, tetracycline (147), spectinomycin–lincomycin (57), tiamulin, spectinomycin and spiramycin (75), doxycycline and the fluoroquinolones (124), and josamycin (122). In trials conducted with turkey embryos, tylosin was the most active; tetracycline, chlortetracycline, and streptomycin were variable; and erythromycin showed no activity against two isolates of MM (147).

A combination of lincomycin and spectinomycin administered at 2 g/gal of water for 5 days (58) or tiamulin at a concentration of 0.025% in the drinking water for 3 days (123) had therapeutic activity against MM infections. Enrofloxacin was effective in reducing mortality of poults having complicated MM infections (19). Parenteral injections or water medication with tylosin of turkeys in production did not reduce egg transmission (16, 73). Dipping of hatching eggs in antibiotic solution, however, significantly reduced the incidence of air sac infection (10, 73, 97, 117) concomitant with improved hatchability (73, 117), improved performance (10, 89), reduced incidence of skeletal deformities (89, 97), and reduced condemnation at processing (73, 89).

During the late 1960s to early 1980s, before MM-free eggs and poult were available, it was a common practice for multiplier breeders to dip their eggs in antibiotic solution. Tylosin (3000 ppm) or gentamicin (500 ppm) along with a disinfectant such as quaternary ammonium compound (250 ppm) were used in dip solutions. Currently, most major U.S. multiplier breeder companies dip their eggs only when faced with a potential MM break (49).

The procedures for dipping of hatching eggs in antibiotic solution are described under *Mycoplasma gallisepticum* Infection.

PREVENTION AND CONTROL

Management Procedures.
While early studies placed much emphasis on the control of MM infections in turkeys by use of various antibiotic treatment regimens (see Treatment), the goal of primary breeder organizations was to eradicate the agent from their stocks. Since virtually all breeding stocks were infected, a program of test and slaughter—which had been so effective in the control of *M. gallisepticum*—was not a practical approach for eradicating MM (145). Experimental studies demonstrated that administration of antibiotics into eggs either by dipping or by inoculation into the air cell (59) or the small end (40, 81, 82) were useful methods to reduce the egg-transmission rate. Heat treatment of eggs (154) was not effective in eliminating MM from turkey eggs (56, 64, 131). Tylosin (69) or gentamicin (115) was not effective, but spectinomycin (0.6 mg/mL of diluent) (114) was effective in eliminating MM from turkey semen. These studies laid the foundation for effective eradication programs that followed.

Immunization.
Vaccines are not available for prevention of MM infection in turkeys.

Eradication.
The basic principles and procedures for producing MM-free breeders include: 1) Reduction of genital infection to minimal levels by serology and culture. The egg-transmission rate can be reduced significantly by using males that are not genital carriers. Males that yield three consecutive negative cultures from the phallus or semen are usually free of infection. The infection rate can be reduced even further by eliminating vaginal carriers. Even a single sampling will identify most carriers. Cultures from males are taken a few weeks before their use as breeders, while those from females are taken from the cloaca before or from the vagina during egg production. Special care must be taken to prevent cross-contamination when specimens are taken for culture or during insemination (36). 2) Treatment of eggs with an effective antibiotic(s) by dipping and/or injection. Since these procedures may reduce hatchability by 10% or more, pretrials should be conducted before embarking on a large program. The possibility of developing antibiotic resistant strains of MM should be kept in mind, particularly at the primary breeder level where treated birds must be recycled in the operation (50, 81, 132). 3) Hatching of eggs in MM-free hatchers and isolation rearing of the turkeys. Since MM can be introduced onto a farm in a number of ways (see Transmission) and usually occurs as an inapparent infection, it is essential that a high level of biosecurity be maintained. 4) Serologic and cul-

tural monitoring of the treated flock at 16 wk of age and periodic intervals thereafter, and elimination of infected groups.

Using the principles just outlined, MM-free turkeys have been produced experimentally (133) and commercially (53, 54, 74, 92, 130). A treatment regimen that was used to eradicate MM from a primary breeder organization consisted of dipping eggs in a solution of gentamicin sulfate (750–900 ppm) followed by injection with a solution containing 0.6 mg gentamicin and 2.4 mg tylosin/dose into the small end of the egg (54).

Edson et al. (38) developed an equation based on the Poisson distribution to predict the chance of success of eradicating MM: $p(0) = e^{-na\beta h}$, where the probability of success $p(0)$ was described by n, the number of eggs treated; a, the pretreatment infection rate of the eggs; β, the treatment failure rate; and h, the hatchability of treated eggs. Decreasing the size of any or all of the four parameters increases likelihood of eradication. This predictive equation is a useful quantitative tool for management decision-making. Currently, three primary breeder organizations that are the major genetic source for commercial turkeys worldwide are free of MM (49).

An economic decision analysis was described by Carpenter et al. (25) to assist commercial multiplier breeders to determine the economic advantage of eradicating MM.

A program for certifying freedom from MM infection of turkey breeding stocks under the National Poultry Improvement Plan (NPIP) was initiated on January 1, 1983 (119). According to the 1994 NPIP testing summary, 97.3% of 594 multiplier breeder flocks representing 4.7 million breeders (with a potential production of 331 million meat turkeys) qualified as "U.S. MM Clean" (88). These data and a recent industry-based survey conducted by Ghazikhanian (49) suggest that significant progress has been made in reducing the prevalence of MM in the turkey industry since MM-free stock first became available in the early 1980s (48, 54, 70).

REFERENCES

1. Adler, H. 1958. A PPLO slide agglutination test for the detection of infectious sinusitis of turkeys. Poult Sci 37:1116–1123.

2. Adler, H.E., and A.J. DaMassa. 1964. Enhancement of Mycoplasma agglutination titers by use of anti-globulin. Proc Soc Exp Biol Med 116:608–610.

3. Adler, H.E., J. Fabricant, R. Yamamoto, and J. Berg. 1958. Symposium on chronic respiratory diseases of poultry. I. Isolation and identification of pleuropneumonia-like organisms of avian origin. Am J Vet Res 19:440–447.

4. Allen, T.C. 1971. Base composition and genome size of Mycoplasma meleagridis deoxyribonucleic acid. J Gen Microbiol 69:285–286.

5. Anderson, D.P., R.R. Wolfe, F.L. Cherms, and W.E. Roper. 1968. Influence of dust and ammonia on the development of air sac lesions in turkeys. Am J Vet Res 29:1049–1058.

6. Arya, P.L., J.H. Sautter, and B.S. Pomeroy. 1971. Patho-

genesis and histopathology of airsacculitis in turkeys produced by experimental inoculation of day-old poults with Mycoplasma meleagridis. Avian Dis 15:163–176.

7. Ball, R.A., V.B. Singh, and B.S. Pomeroy. 1969. The morphologic response of the turkey oviduct to certain pathogenic agents. Avian Dis 13:119–133.

8. Beard, C.W., and D.P. Anderson. 1967. Aerosol studies with avian Mycoplasma. I. Survival in the air. Avian Dis 11:54–59.

9. Bigland, C.H. 1969. Natural resolution of air sac lesions caused by Mycoplasma meleagridis in turkeys. Can J Comp Med 33:169–172.

10. Bigland, C.H. 1970. Experimental control of Mycoplasma meleagridis in turkeys by the dipping of eggs in tylosin and spiramycin. Can J Comp Med 34:26–30.

11. Bigland, C.H. 1972. The tissue localization of Mycoplasma meleagridis in turkey embryos. Can J Comp Med 36:99–102.

12. Bigland, C.H., and M.L. Benson. 1968. Mycoplasma meleagridis ("N"-strain mycoplasma-PPLO): Relationship of airsac lesions and isolations in day-old turkeys (Meleagridis gallopavo). Can Vet J 9:138–141.

13. Bigland, C.H., and F.T.W. Jordan. 1974. Experimental relationship of biotin and Mycoplasma meleagridis in the etiology of turkey syndrome 1965. Proc 23rd West Poult Dis Conf and 8th Poult Health Symp, Davis, CA, pp. 55–61.

14. Bigland, C.H., and J.J. Matsumoto. 1975. Nonspecific reaction to Mycoplasma antigens caused in turkey sera by Erysipelothrix insidiosa bacterins. Avian Dis 19:617–621.

15. Bigland, C.H., and M.W. Warenycia. 1978. Effects of biotin, folic acid and pantothenic acid on the growth of Mycoplasma meleagridis, a turkey pathogen. Poult Sci 57:611–618.

16. Bigland, C.H., W. Dungan, R. Yamamoto, and J.C. Voris. 1964. Airsacculitis in poults from different strains of turkeys. Avian Dis 8:85–92.

17. Bigland, C.H., M.W. Warenycia, and M. Denson. 1979. Specific immune gammaglobulin in the control of Mycoplasma meleagridis. Poult Sci 58:319–328.

18. Bradbury, J. M., and M. McClenaghan. 1982. Detection of mixed Mycoplasma species. J Clin Microbiol 16:314–318.

19. Braunius, W.W. 1987. Effect of Baytril (Bay Vp 2674) on young turkeys with respiratory infection. Tijdschr Diergeneeskd 112:531–533.

20. Brown, K.I., and K.E. Nestor. 1974. Interrelationships of cellular physiology and endocrinology with genetics. 2. Implications of selection for high and low adrenal response to stress. Poult Sci 53:1297–1306.

21. Brunner, H., and G. Laber. 1985. Chemotherapy of Mycoplasma infections. In S. Razin and M.F. Barile (eds.). The Mycoplasma IV Mycoplasma Pathogenicity. Academic Press, Orlando, FL, pp. 403–450.

22. Cardona, C.J., and A.A. Bickford. 1993. Wry necks associated with Mycoplasma meleagridis infection in a backyard flock of turkeys. Avian Dis 37:240–242.

23. Carpenter, T.E. 1983. A microeconomic evaluation of the impact of Mycoplasma meleagridis infection in turkey production. Prev Vet Med 1:289–301.

24. Carpenter, T.E., R.K. Edson, and R. Yamamoto. 1981a. Decreased hatchability of turkey eggs caused by experimental infection with Mycoplasma meleagridis. Avian Dis 25:151–156.

25. Carpenter, T.E., R. Howitt, R. McCapes, R. Yamamoto, and H.P. Riemann. 1981b. Formulating a control program against Mycoplasma meleagridis using economic decision analysis. Avian Dis 25:260–271.

26. Carpenter, T.E., H.P. Riemann, and C.E. Franti. 1982a. The effect of Mycoplasma meleagridis infection and egg dipping on the weight-gain performance of turkey poults. Avian Dis 26:272–278.

27. Carpenter, T.E., H.P. Riemann, and R.H. McCapes. 1982b. The effect of experimental turkey embryo infection

with Mycoplasma meleagridis on weight, weight gain, feed consumption, and conversion. Avian Dis 26:689–695.

28. Cherms, F.L., and M.L. Frey. 1967. Mycoplasma meleagridis and fertility in turkey breeder hens. Avian Dis 11:268–274.

29. Chin, R.P. 1988. Personal communication.

30. Corstvet, R.E., and W.W. Sadler. 1964. The diagnosis of certain avian diseases with the fluorescent antibody technique. Poult Sci 43:1280–1288.

31. Cummins, D.R., and D.L. Reynolds. 1990. Use of an avidin-biotin enhanced dot-immunobinding assay to detect antibodies for avian mycoplasma in sera from Iowa market turkeys. Avian Dis 34:321–328.

32. Curtis, M.J., and G.A. Thornton. 1973. The effect of heat killed Mycoplasma gallisepticum and M. meleagridis on plasma caeruloplasmin activity in the fowl. Res Vet Sci 15:399–401.

33. DaMassa, A.J., and H.E. Adler. 1969. Effect of pH on growth and survival of three avian and one saprophytic Mycoplasma species. Appl Microbiol 17:310–316.

34. Dierks, R.E., J.A. Newman, and B.S. Pomeroy. 1967. Characterization of Avian Mycoplasma. Ann NY Acad Sci 143:170–189.

35. Edson, R.K. 1980. Mycoplasma meleagridis infection of turkeys: Motivation, methods, and predictive tools for eradication. PhD dissertation, University of California, Davis, CA.

36. Edson, R.K., D. Massey, R. Yamamoto, and H.B. Ortmayer. 1978. Factors affecting the spread of Mycoplasma meleagridis during artificial insemination. Proc 18th Annu Turkey Meet, University of California, Fresno, CA.

37. Edson, R.K., R. Yamamoto, H.B. Ortmayer, and D.E. Massey. 1979. The effect of Mycoplasma meleagridis on hatchability of turkey eggs. Proc 28th West Poult Dis Conf and 13th Poult Health Symp, Davis, CA, pp. 24–29.

38. Edson, R.K., R. Yamamoto, and T.B. Farver. 1987. Mycoplasma meleagridis of turkeys: Probability of eliminating egg-borne infection. Avian Dis 31:264–271.

39. El-Ebeedy, A.A., M.E.S. Easa, M.Z. Sabey, M.A. Hafez, A.M. Ammar, and A. Rashwan. 1982. Pathological changes in air sacs and lungs of turkey poults after experimental inoculation with different isolates of Mycoplasma meleagridis. J Egypt Vet Med Assoc 42:91–100.

40. Elmahi, M.M., and M.S. Hofstad. 1979. Prevention of egg transmission of Mycoplasma meleagridis by antibiotic treatment of naturally and experimentally infected turkey eggs. Avian Dis 23:88–94.

41. Elmahi, M.M., R.F. Ross, and M.S. Hofstad. 1982. Comparison of seven isolates of Mycoplasma meleagridis. Vet Microbiol 7:61–76.

42. Ferrier, W.T., H.B. Ortmayer, F.X. Ogasawara, and R. Yamamoto. 1982. The survivability of Mycoplasma meleagridis in frozen-thawed turkey semen. Poult Sci 61:379–381.

43. Fox, M.L., and C.H. Bigland. 1970. Differences between cull and normal turkeys in natural infection with Mycoplasma meleagridis at one day of age. Can J Comp Med 34:285–288.

44. Freundt, E.A. 1983. Culture media for classic mycoplasmas. In S. Razin and J.G. Tully (eds.). Methods in Mycoplasmology, vol I. Mycoplasma Characterization. Academic Press, New York, NY, pp. 127–135.

45. Frey, M.L., R.P. Hanson, and D.P. Anderson. 1968. A medium for the isolation of avian Mycoplasmas. Am J Vet Res 29:2163–2171.

46. Frey, M.L., S.T. Hawk, and P.A. Hale. 1972. A division by micro-complement fixation tests of previously reported avian mycoplasma serotypes into identification groups. Avian Dis 16:780–792.

47. Gerlach, H., R. Yamamoto, and H.B. Ortmayer. 1968. Zur Pathologie der Phallus-Infektion der Puten mit Mycoplasma meleagridis. Arch Gefluegelkd 32:396–399.

48. Ghazikhanian, G.Y. 1983. Progress in maintaining Mycoplasma meleagridis-negative turkey breeding flocks.

Avian Dis 27:326–329.

49. Ghazikhanian, G.Y. 1994. Personal communication.

50. Ghazikhanian, G., and R. Yamamoto. 1969. Tylosin resistant strains of Mycoplasma meleagridis. Proc 18th West Poult Dis Conf, Davis, CA, pp. 36–37.

51. Ghazikhanian, G., and R. Yamamoto. 1974a. Characterization of pathogenic and nonpathogenic strains of Mycoplasma meleagridis: In ovo and in vitro studies. Am J Vet Res 35:425–430.

52. Ghazikhanian, G., and R. Yamamoto. 1974b. Characterization of pathogenic and nonpathogenic strains of Mycoplasma meleagridis: Manifestations of disease in turkey embryos and poults. Am J Vet Res 35:417–424.

53. Ghazikhanian, G., R. Yamamoto, R.H. McCapes, W.M. Dungan, C.T. Larsen, and H.B. Ortmayer. 1980a. Antibiotic egg injection to eliminate disease. II. Elimination of Mycoplasma meleagridis from a strain of turkeys. Avian Dis 48–56.

54. Ghazikhanian, G., R. Yamamoto, R.H. McCapes, W.M. Dungan, and H.B. Ortmayer. 1980b. Combination dip and injection of turkey eggs with antibiotics to eliminate Mycoplasma meleagridis infection from a primary breeding stock. Avian Dis 24:57–70.

55. Green, F. III, and R.P. Hanson. 1973. Ultrastructure and capsule of Mycoplasma meleagridis. J Bacteriol 116:1011–1018.

56. Grimes, T.M. 1972. Means of obtaining Mycoplasma-free turkeys in Australia. Aust Vet J 48:124.

57. Hamdy, A.H., C.J. Farho, C.J. Blanchard, and M.W. Glenn. 1969. Effect of lincomycin and spectinomycin on airsacculitis of turkey poults. Avian Dis 13:721–728.

58. Hamdy, A.H., Y.M. Saif, and C.W. Kasson. 1982. Efficacy of lincomycin-spectinomycin water medication on Mycoplasma meleagridis airsacculitis in commercially reared turkey poults. Avian Dis 26:227–233.

59. Hofstad, M.S. 1974. The injection of turkey hatching eggs with tylosin to eliminate Mycoplasma meleagridis infection. Avian Dis 18:134–138.

60. Ibrahim, A.A., and R. Yamamoto. 1977a. Arginine catabolism by Mycoplasma meleagridis and its role in pathogenesis. Infect Immun 18:226–229.

61. Ibrahim, A.A., and R. Yamamoto. 1977b. Morphology and growth cycle of Mycoplasma meleagridis viewed by scanning-electron microscopy. Avian Dis 21:415–421.

62. Imada, Y., I. Uchida, and K. Hashimoto. 1987. Rapid identification of mycoplasma by indirect immunoperoxidase test using small square filter paper. J Clin Microbiol 25:17–21.

63. Jordan, F.T.W. 1983. Recovery and identification of avian mycoplasmas. In J.G. Tully, and S. Razin (eds.). Methods in Mycoplasmology, vol 2. Diagnostic Mycoplasmology. Academic Press, New York, pp. 69–79.

64. Jordan, F.T.W., and M.M. Amin. 1978. The influence of preincubation heating of turkey eggs on Mycoplasma infection. Avian Pathol 7:349–355.

65. Jordan, F.T.W., B.L. Nutor, and S. Bozkur. 1982. The survival and recognition of Mycoplasma meleagridis grown at 37°C and then maintained at room temperature. Avian Pathol 11:123–129.

66. Kleckner, A.L. 1960. Serotypes of avian pleuropneumonia-like organisms. Am J Vet Res 21:274–280.

67. Kleven, S.H., and B.S. Pomeroy. 1971a. Characterization of the antibody response of turkeys to Mycoplasma meleagridis. Avian Dis 15:291–298.

68. Kleven, S.H., and B.S. Pomeroy. 1971b. Role of the female in egg transmission of Mycoplasma meleagridis in turkeys. Avian Dis 15:299–304.

69. Kleven, S.H., B.S. Pomeroy, and R.C. Nelson. 1971. Ineffectiveness of antibiotic treatment of semen in the prevention of egg transmission of Mycoplasma meleagridis in turkeys. Poult Sci 50:1522–1526.

70. Kolb, G.E. 1983. Mycoplasma meleagridis eradication status in commercial turkeys. Avian Dis 27:329.

71. Kumar, M.C., and B.S. Pomeroy. 1969. Transmission of Mycoplasma meleagridis in turkeys. Am J Vet Res 30:1423–1436.

72. Kumar, S., R.E. Dierks, J.A. Newman, C.I. Pfow, and B.S. Pomeroy. 1963. Airsacculitis in turkeys. I. A study of airsacculitis in day-old poults. Avian Dis 7:376–385.

73. Kumar, M.C., S. Kumar, R.E. Dierks, J.A. Newman, and B.S. Pomeroy. 1966. Airsacculitis in turkeys. II. Use of tylosin in the control of the egg transmission of Mycoplasma spp. other than Mycoplasma gallisepticum in turkeys. Avian Dis 10:194–198.

74. Kumar, M.C., B.S. Pomeroy, W.M. Dungan, and C.T. Larsen. 1974. Development of Mycoplasma gallisepticum, M. synoviae, and M. meleagridis-free primary turkey breeding flocks. Proc 15th World's Poult Congr, New Orleans, LA, pp. 353–355.

75. Levisohn, S. 1981. Antibiotic sensitivity patterns in field isolates of Mycoplasma gallisepticum as a guide to chemotherapy. Isr J Med Sci 17:661–666.

76. Matsumoto, M., and R. Yamamoto. 1971. Inactivation of Mycoplasma meleagridis by immune serum or heat treatment. Proc 20th West Poult Dis Conf and 5th Poult Health Symp, Davis, CA, pp. 70–74.

77. Matsumoto, M., and R. Yamamoto. 1973. Demonstration of complement-dependent and independent systems in immune inactivation of Mycoplasma meleagridis. J Inf Dis 127:S43–S51.

78. Matzer, N. 1972. Mycoplasma melagridis in Guatemalan turkeys. Avian Dis 16:945–948.

79. Matzer, N., and R. Yamamoto. 1970. Genital pathogenesis of Mycoplasma meleagridis in virgin turkey hens. Avian Dis 14:321–329.

80. Matzer, N., and R. Yamamoto. 1974. Further studies on the genital pathogenesis of Mycoplasma meleagridis. J Comp Pathol 84:271–278.

81. McCapes, R.H., R. Yamamoto, H.B. Ortmayer, and W.F. Scott. 1975. Injecting antibiotics into turkey hatching eggs to eliminate Mycoplasma meleagridis infection. Avian Dis 19:506–514.

82. McCapes, R.H., R. Yamamoto, G. Ghazikhanian, W.M. Dungan, and H.B. Ortmayer. 1977. Antibiotic egg injection to eliminate disease. I. Effect of injection methods on turkey hatchability and Mycoplasma meleagridis infection. Avian Dis 21:57–68.

83. Mohamed, Y.S., and E.H. Bohl. 1967. Studies on the transmission of Mycoplasma meleagridis. Avian Dis 11:634–641.

84. Mohamed, Y.S., and E.H. Bohl. 1968. Serologic studies on Mycoplasma meleagridis in turkeys. Avian Dis 12:554–566.

85. Mohamed, Y.S., S. Chema, and E.H. Bohl. 1966. Studies on Mycoplasma of the "H" serotype (Mycoplasma meleagridis) in the reproductive and respiratory tracts of turkeys. Avian Dis 10:347–352.

86. Moorhead, P.D., and Y.S. Mohamed. 1968. Case Report: Pathologic and Microbiologic studies of crooked-neck in a turkey flock. Avian Dis 12:476–482.

87. Moorhead, P.D., and Y.M. Saif. 1970. Mycoplasma meleagridis and Escherichia coli infections in germ-free and specific pathogen free turkey poults: Pathologic manifestations. Am J Vet Res 31:1645–1653.

88. National Poultry Improvement Plan. 1995. Tables on Hatchery and Flock Participation. United States Department of Agriculture, Animal Plant Inspection Service, Veterinary Service, Conyers, GA, p. 4.

89. Nelson, R.C. 1971. Evaluation of egg dipping (1967–70). Proc Symp on Leg Weakness in Turkeys. Iowa State University Press, Ames, IA, pp. 13–21

90. Nelson, R.C., W.M. Dungan, and C.T. Larsen. 1974. Comparison of the performance of Mycoplasma meleagridis-free and infected poults. Proc 23rd West Poult Dis Conf and 8th Poult Health Symp, Davis, CA, pp. 66–69.

91. Newman, J.A. 1967. The detection and control of My-

coplasma meleagridis. PhD Dissertation, University of Minnesota, St. Paul, MN.

92. O'Brien, J.D.P. 1979. Effect of Mycoplasma meleagridis on hatchability. Proc 28th West Poult Dis Conf and 13th Poult Health Symp, University of California, Davis, CA, pp. 29–31.

93. Ogra, M.S., and E.H. Bohl. 1970. Growth-inhibition test for identifying Mycoplasma meleagridis and its antibody. Avian Dis 14:364–373.

94. Ortiz, A.M., R. Yamamoto, A.A. Benedict, and A.P. Mateos. 1981. The immunosuppressive effect of Mycoplasma meleagridis on nonreplicating antigens. Avian Dis 25:954–963.

95. Ortmayer, H.B. 1970. A cultural field screening procedure for detection of Mycoplasma meleagridis in the reproductive tract of turkeys. MS Thesis, University of California, Davis, CA.

96. Ortmayer, H.B., and R. Yamamoto. 1981. Mycoplasma meleagridis antibody detection by enzyme-linked immunosorbent assay (ELISA). Proc 30th West Poult Dis Conf and 15th Poult Health Symp, Davis, CA, pp. 63–66.

97. Peterson, I.L. 1968. Field significance of Mycoplasma meleagridis infection. Poult Sci 47:1708–1709.

98. Pohl, R. 1969. Airsacculitis and pantothenic acid-biotin deficiency in turkeys in New Zealand. NZ Vet J 7:183.

99. Reis, R., and R. Yamamoto. 1971. Pathogenesis of single and mixed infections caused by Mycoplasma meleagridis and Mycoplasma gallisepticum in turkey embryos. Am J Vet Res 32:63–74.

100. Reis, R., J.M L. DaSilva, and R. Yamamoto. 1970. Pathologic changes in the joint and other organs of turkey poults after intravenous inoculation of Mycoplasma meleagridis. Avian Dis 14:117–125.

101. Report of Working Party. (R.F. Gordon, chairman). 1965. A new syndrome in turkey poults. Vet Rec 77:1292.

102. Resende, M., R. Reis, and P.P. Ornellas-Santos. 1969. Mycoplasma of poultry origin. III. Identification of Mycoplasma meleagridis. Arq Esc Vet 21:157–161.

103. Rhoades, K.R. 1969a. A hemagglutination-inhibition test for Mycoplasma meleagridis antibodies. Avian Dis 13:22–26.

104. Rhoades, K.R. 1969b. Experimentally induced Mycoplasma meleagridis infection of turkey reproductive tracts. Avian Dis 13:508–519.

105. Rhoades, K.R. 1971a. Mycoplasma meleagridis infection: Reproductive tract lesions in mature turkeys. Avian Dis 15:722–729.

106. Rhoades, K.R. 1971b. Mycoplasma meleagridis infection: Development of lesions and distribution of infection in turkey embryos. Avian Dis 15:762–774.

107. Rhoades, K.R. 1971c. Mycoplasma meleagridis infection: Development of air sac lesions in turkey poults. Avian Dis 15:910–922.

108. Rhoades, K. 1977. Turkey sinusitis: Synergism between Mycoplasma synoviae and Mycoplasma meleagridis. Avian Dis 21:670–674.

109. Rhoades, K.R. 1978a. Comparison of Mycoplasma meleagridis antibodies demonstrated by tube agglutination and hemagglutination-inhibition test. Avian Dis 22:633–638.

110. Rhoades, K.R. 1978b. Inhibition of avian mycoplasmal hemagglutination by IgM type antibody. Poult Sci 57:608–610.

111. Rhoades, K.R. 1981a. Pathogencity of strains of the I J K N Q R group of avian mycoplasmas for turkey embryos and poults. Avian Dis 25:104–111.

112. Rhoades, K.R. 1981b. Turkey airsacculitis: Effect of mixed mycoplasmal infections. Avian Dis 25:131–135.

113. Rosenfeld, L.E., and T.M. Grimes. 1972. Natural and experimental cases of airsacculitis associated with Mycoplasma meleagridis infections in turkeys. Aust Vet J 48:240–243.

114. Rott, M., H. Pfutzner, H. Gigas, and B. Mach. 1989. Die nachweishaufigkeit von Mycoplasma meleagridis bei re-

produktionsputen in abhangigkeit vom legealter. Arch Exper Vet Med Leipzig 43:737–741.

115. Saif, Y.M., and K.I. Brown. 1972. Treatment of turkey semen to eliminate Mycoplasma meleagridis. Turkey Res, Ohio Agric Res Cent, Wooster, OH, pp. 49–50.

116. Saif, Y.M., P.D. Moorhead, and E.H. Bohl. 1970a. Mycoplasma meleagridis and Escherichia coli infections in germfree and specific pathogen free turkey poults: Production of complicated airsacculitis. Am J Vet Res 31:1637–1643.

117. Saif, Y M., K.E. Nestor, and K.E. McCracken. 1970b. Tylosin tartrate absorption of turkey and chicken eggs dipped using pressure and temperature differentials. Poult Sci 49:1641–1649.

118. Saif, Y.M., L.C. Ferguson, and K.E. Nestor. 1971. Treatment of turkey hatching eggs for control of Arizona infection. Avian Dis 15:448–461.

119. Schar, R.D., and I.L. Peterson. 1982. The national poultry improvement plan—an update (with reference to the control of salmonellosis and mycoplasmosis). Proc US Anim Health Assoc 86:445–453.

120. Sharp, P., P. VanEss, B. Ji, and C.B. Thomas. 1991. Immunobinding assay for the speciation of avian mycoplasmas adapted for use with a 96-well filtration manifold. Avian Dis 35:332–336.

121. Shimizu, T., and T. Yagihashi. 1980. Isolation of Mycoplasma meleagridis from turkeys in Japan. Jpn J Vet Sci 42:41–47.

122. Sokkar, I.M., A.M. Soliman, S. Mousa, and M.Z. El-Demerdash. 1986. In-vitro sensitivity of mycoplasma and associated bacteria isolated from chickens and turkeys and ducks at the area of Upper Egypt. Assiut Vet Med J 15:243–250.

123. Stipkovits, L., G. Laber, and E. Schultze. 1977. Prophylactical and therapeutical efficacy of tiamuline in mycoplasmosis of chickens and turkeys. Poult Sci 56:1209–1215.

124. Takahata, T., R. Yamamoto, and H.B. Ortmayer. 1994. Unpublished data.

125. Thornton, G.A., D.R. Wise, and M.K. Fuller. 1975. A Mycoplasma meleagridis haemagglutination-inhibition test. Vet Rec 96:113–114.

126. Uppal, P.K., D.R. Wise, and M.K. Boldero. 1972. Ultrastructural characteristics of Mycoplasma gallisepticum, M. gallinarum and M. meleagridis. Res Vet Sci 13:200–201.

127. Vlaovic, M.S., and C.H. Bigland. 1971a. A review of mycoplasma infections relative to Mycoplasma meleagridis. Can Vet J 12:103–109.

128. Vlaovic, M.S., and C.H. Bigland. 1971b. The attempted immunization of turkey hens with viable Mycoplasma meleagridis. Can J Comp Med 35:338–341.

129. Wise, D.R., and M.K. Fuller. 1975a. Experimental reproduction of turkey syndrome '65 with Mycoplasma meleagridis and Mycoplasma gallisepticum and associated changes in serum protein characteristics. Res Vet Sci 19:201–203.

130. Wise, D.R., and M.K. Fuller. 1975b. Eradication of Mycoplasma meleagridis from a primary turkey breeder enterprise. Vet Rec 96:133–134.

131. Wise, D.R., M.K. Boldero, and G.A. Thornton. 1973. The pathology and aetiology of turkey syndrome '65 (T.S.65). Res Vet Sci 14:194–200.

132. Wise, D.R., M.K. Fuller, and G.A. Thornton. 1974. Experimental reproduction of turkey syndrome '65 with Mycoplasma meleagridis. Res Vet Sci 17:236–241.

133. Yamamoto, R. 1967. Localization and egg transmission of Mycoplasma meleagridis in turkeys exposed by various routes. Ann NY Acad Sci 143:229–233.

134. Yamamoto, R. 1978. Mycoplasma meleagridis infection. In M.S. Hofstad, B.W. Calnek, C.F. Helmboldt, W.M. Reid, and H.W. Yoder, Jr. (eds.). Diseases of Poultry, 7th ed. Iowa State University Press, Ames, IA, pp. 250–260.

135. Yamamoto, R. 1991. Mycoplasma meleagridis infection In B.W. Calnek, H.J. Barnes, C.W. Beard, W.M. Reid, and H.W. Yoder, Jr. (eds.). Diseases of Poultry, 9th ed. Iowa

State University Press, Ames, IA, pp. 212–223.

136. Yamamoto, R., and C.H. Bigland. 1964. Pathogenicity to chicks of Mycoplasma associated with turkey airsacculitis. Avian Dis 8:523–531.

137. Yamamoto, R., and C.H. Bigland. 1965. Experimental production of airsacculitis in turkey poults by inoculation with "N"-type Mycoplasma. Avian Dis 9:108–118.

138. Yamamoto, R., and C.H. Bigland. 1966. Infectivity of Mycoplasma meleagridis for turkey embryos. Am J Vet Res 27:326–330.

139. Yamamoto, R., and A. Ortiz. 1974. Microtiter agglutination test for Mycoplasma meleagridis. Proc 15th World's Poult Congr, New Orleans, LA, pp. 171–172.

140. Yamamoto, R., and H.B. Ortmayer. 1966. Pathogenicity of Mycoplasma meleagridis for turkey and chicken embryos. Avian Dis 10:268–272.

141. Yamamoto, R., and H.B. Ortmayer. 1967a. Effect of Mycoplasma meleagridis on reproductive performance. Poult Sci 46:1340.

142. Yamamoto, R., and H.B. Ortmayer. 1967b. Hatcher and intraflock transmission of Mycoplasma meleagridis. Avian Dis 11:288–295.

143. Yamamoto, R., and H.B. Ortmayer. 1967c. Localization and persistence of avian mycoplasma in the genital system of the mature turkey. J Am Vet Med Assoc 150:1371.

144. Yamamoto, R., and H.B. Ortmayer. 1969. Egg transmission of Mycoplasma meleagridis in naturally infected turkeys under different mating systems. Poult Sci 48:1893.

145. Yamamoto, R., and H.B. Ortmayer. 1971. Control of Mycoplasma meleagridis (N-strain). Proc 19th World Vet Congr 2:498–501.

146. Yamamoto, R., C.H. Bigland, and H.B. Ortmayer. 1965. Characteristics of Mycoplasma meleagridis sp.n., isolated from turkeys. J Bacteriol 90:47–49.

147. Yamamoto, R., C.H. Bigland, and H.B. Ortmayer. 1966a. Sensitivity of Mycoplasma meleagridis to various antibiotics. Poult Sci 45:1139.

148. Yamamoto, R., C.H. Bigland, and I.L. Peterson. 1966b. Egg transmission of Mycoplasma meleagridis. Poult Sci 45:1245–1257.

149. Yamamoto, R., H.B. Ortmayer, and C.S. Joshi. 1968. Persistence of Mycoplasma meleagridis in the genitalia of experimentally infected turkeys. Poult Sci 47:1734.

150. Yamamoto, R., H.B. Ortmayer, and M. Matsumoto. 1970. Standardization and application of Mycoplasma meleagridis agglutination test. Proc 14th World's Poult Congr Sci Comm 3:139–148.

151. Yamamoto, R., F.H. Kratzer, and H.B. Ortmayer. 1974. Recent research on Mycoplasma meleagridis. Proc 23rd West Poult Dis Conf and 8th Poult Health Symp, Davis, CA, pp. 53–54.

152. Yamamoto, R., H.B. Ortmayer, and R.K. Edson. 1978. Micro-hemagglutination-inhibition test for Mycoplasma meleagridis. Proc 16th World's Poult Congr 9:1417–1427.

153. Yamamoto, R., H.B. Ortmayer, and R.K. Edson. 1979. Serology of Mycoplasma meleagridis. Proc 28th West Poult Dis Conf and 13th Poult Health Symp, Davis, CA, p. 23.

154. Yoder, H.W., Jr. 1970. Preincubation heat treatment of chicken hatching eggs to inactivate mycoplasma. Avian Dis 14:75–86.

155. Yoder, H.W., Jr., and M.S. Hofstad. 1964. Characterization of avian mycoplasma. Avian Dis 8:481–512.

156. Zhao, S., and R. Yamamoto. 1993a. Species-specific recombinant DNA probes for Mycoplasma meleagridis. Vet Microbiol 35:179–185.

157. Zhao, S., and R. Yamamoto. 1993b. Detection of Mycoplasma meleagridis by polymerase chain reaction. Vet Microbiol 36:91–97.

158. Zhao, S., R. Yamamoto, G.Y. Ghazikhanian, and M.I. Khan. 1988. Antigenic analysis of three strains of Mycoplasma meleagridis of varying pathogenicity. Vet Microbiol 18:373–377.

MYCOPLASMA SYNOVIAE INFECTION

S. H. Kleven

INTRODUCTION. *Mycoplasma synoviae* (MS) infection most frequently occurs as a subclinical upper respiratory infection. It may cause air sac infection when combined with Newcastle disease (ND), infectious bronchitis (IB), or both. At other times, MS becomes systemic and results in infectious synovitis, an acute to chronic infectious disease of chickens and turkeys, involving primarily the synovial membranes of joints and tendon sheaths producing an exudative synovitis, tenovaginitis, or bursitis.

HISTORY. Infectious synovitis was first described and associated with a mycoplasma by Olson et al. (67, 68). A respiratory form of *M. synoviae* infection occurs (70) and air sac infection results with some isolates of MS when combined with ND and IB vaccination (50). See Jordan (39, 40) and Timms (90) for reviews of the MS literature.

INCIDENCE AND DISTRIBUTION. Infectious synovitis was observed primarily in growing birds 4–12 wk of age in broiler-growing regions of the United States during the 1950s and 1960s. From the 1970s to the 1990s, the synovitis form was rarely observed in chickens in the United States, but the respiratory form was seen more frequently. Infection without apparent clinical signs is not unusual. *M. synoviae* infection occurs frequently in multiage commercial layers (58, 73). Infectious synovitis usually appears in turkeys when they are 10–20 wk old. Breeding stock from all major commercial breeds of chickens and turkeys is largely free of infection. *M. synoviae* is worldwide in distribution.

ETIOLOGY

Classification. Mycoplasma colonies were observed as satellites adjacent to *Micrococcus* colonies by Chalquest and Fabricant (18), who identified the requirement for nicotinamide adenine dinucleotide (NAD). It was designated as serotype S by Dierks et al. (23). Olson et al. (71) studied several isolates and proposed the name *M. synoviae,* which was subsequently confirmed as a separate species (41).

Identification is based on typical colony and cell morphology, biochemical characteristics, special requirements for growth, and serologic reactions. Immunofluorescence of mycoplasma colonies is the most rapid and reliable method for identification of field isolates.

Morphology and Staining. In Giemsa-stained preparations, *M. synoviae* cells appear as pleomorphic coccoid bodies approximately 0.2 μm in diameter. Ultrastructural studies of avian synovium reveal MS in endocytotic vesicles. The mycoplasma cells are round or pear shaped with granular ribosomes. They are 300–500 nm in diameter, lack a cell wall, and are bounded by a triple-layered unit membrane (97). An extracellular surface layer has been demonstrated by electron microscopy by ruthenium red and negative staining (1).

Growth Requirements. Nicotinamide adenine dinucleotide is required for growth (18); however, it may be possible to substitute nicotinamide for the more expensive NAD for production of antigens (22). Serum is essential for growth, and swine serum is preferred (17). Growth on agar is accomplished by incubation of plates in a closed container to prevent dehydration of the agar. The optimum temperature is 37 C.

On primary isolation, tissue antigens, toxins, and antibodies may be present; therefore, a small inoculum, transfer within 24 hr, or making dilutions of the inoculum in broth is recommended. Transfers are made with a pipette using a 10% inoculum. Inoculation of broth medium with a cotton swab from the trachea, choanal cleft, or synovial or air sac lesion is satisfactory. Direct plating onto agar plates may result in colonies at 3–5 days of incubation, but isolation in broth is more sensitive. Broth cultures should be incubated until a color change of the phenol red indicator from red to orange or yellow is noted (usually after 3–7 days); the culture should then be transferred to an agar plate and subcultured into another broth culture. *M. synoviae* is sensitive to low pH; therefore, cultures incubated for more than a few hr after the phenol red indicator has changed to yellow (pH <6.8) may no longer be viable. Plates are observed for the presence of mycoplasma colonies after 3–5 days using a microscope with indirect or low-intensity lighting at a magnification of approximately x30.

Excellent growth is obtained using a modification of Frey's medium (27) (Table 9.2). For agar plates, use 1% of a purified agar such as ionagar #2, Noble agar, or Difco purified agar. All components except cysteine, NAD, serum, and penicillin are sterilized by autoclaving at 121 C for 15 min. Cool to 50 C and aseptically add the above components, which have been sterilized by filtration and warmed to 50 C. Pour plates to a depth of approximately 5 mm. Phenol red may be eliminated from agar plates.

Table 9.2.   Modified Frey's medium

Mycoplasma broth base (BBL)	22.5 g
Glucose	3 g
Swine serum	120 mL
Nicotinamide adenine dinucleotide (NAD)	0.1 g
Cysteine hydrochloride	0.1 g
Phenol red (1%)	2.5 mL
Thallium acetate (1%)[a]	5 mL
Potassium penicillin G[a]	1,000,000 units
Distilled H$_2$O	1000 mL
Adjust pH to 7.8 with 20% NaOH and filter sterilize.	

[a]For potentially contaminated specimens, an extra 20 mL of 1% thallium acetate and 2,000,000 units of penicillin per liter may be added. Ampicillin (200 mg/L to 1 g/L) may be substituted for penicillin.

Colony Morphology.   Colonies on solid media are best observed with a dissecting microscope at x30 using indirect lighting; they appear as raised, round, slightly latticed colonies with or without centers. Colonies range from less than 1 to 3 mm in diameter, depending on number of colonies present, suitability of medium, and age of culture. Growth is seen on solid medium in 3–5 days.

Biochemical Properties.   Biochemical characteristics of *M. synoviae* have been described (18, 23). *M. synoviae* ferments glucose and maltose with production of acid but not gas in suitably enriched media. It does not ferment lactose, dulcitol, salicin, or trehalose. *M. synoviae* is phosphatase negative and produces film and spots (41). Some isolates are capable of hemagglutinating chicken and turkey erythrocytes. Its ability to reduce tetrazolium salts is very limited.

Resistance to Chemical and Physical Agents.   Resistance to disinfectants has not been determined but is probably similar to other mycoplasmas. Day-old chicks placed in contaminated chicken houses which had been cleaned and disinfected and maintained empty for 1 wk did not become infected (28). *M. synoviae* is not stable at pH 6.8 or lower. It is sensitive to temperatures above 39 C. It will withstand freezing; however, the titer is reduced. End points have not been reached, but in yolk material *M. synoviae* is viable at least 7 yr at −63 C and after 2 yr at −20 C. Broth cultures maintained frozen at −70 C or lyophilized cultures maintained at 4 C are viable for several years. Survival occurred up to 3 days at room temperature on feathers and up to 12 hr in the nasal cavity of a volunteer, while survival was less than 1 day on most other materials (20).

Antigenic Structure.   Serum plate agglutination (SPA) (69), tube agglutination (TA) (95), hemagglutination (94), agar gel precipitin (AGP) (85), and enzyme-linked immunosorbent assay (ELISA) (35, 74, 77) antigens have been studied. Studies utilizing Western blots have characterized the major immunogenic membrane antigens of MS (3, 4, 5). A major immunogenic protein, p41, showed promise as an antigen in a dot ELISA, while p53 and p22 did not perform well (3). The molecular size of the major membrane proteins varied among MS strains (5).

Available information indicates a single serotype of *M. synoviae* (23, 71), and DNA–DNA hybridization techniques show little heterogeneity among MS strains (104, 105). *M. synoviae* strains can be differentiated using restriction endonuclease analysis of DNA (55, 60). A simpler more rapid procedure for differentiation of MS strains is the polymerase chain reaction (PCR) utilizing arbitrary primers (24).

Serum from chickens infected with MS occasionally agglutinates *M. gallisepticum* plate antigen (71, 72). The reverse occurs less frequently. Roberts and Olesuik (84) suggested that the cross-reactions were related to presence of the rheumatoid factor and could be stimulated by tissue reactions. Cross-reactions are minimal when the hemagglutination inhibition (HI) or TA test is used. There are also epitopes shared by *M. gallisepticum* and MS (2, 105). Species-specific monoclonal antibodies against MS have been produced (37). A 55,000-mW antigen associated with hemagglutination, which shows homology with the P1 protein of *M. pneumoniae,* has been identified (61), and the protein has been cloned and partially sequenced (62). Immunoglobulin G Fc receptors have been identified (53).

Pathogenicity.   There is considerable variation among isolates in their ability to produce disease; many isolates cause little or no clinical disease. Passage in embryos, tissue culture, or broth reduces its ability to produce typical infection. Embryo passage appears to have less effect on pathogenicity than broth passage. *M. synoviae* isolated from air sac lesions are more apt to cause airsacculitis, while those isolated from synovia are more apt to produce synovitis (51). Airsacculitis is exacerbated by ND–IB vaccination (50, 88) or any respiratory infection. The severity of the airsacculitis depends on the virulence of the infectious bronchitis virus used in conjunction with MS (36). Air sac lesions are greatly enhanced by cold environmental temperatures (103). Infectious bursal disease causes immunosuppression in chickens, and dual infection with MS results in more severe air sac lesions (31). Nervous signs with lesions of meningeal vasculitis have been seen in MS-infected turkeys displaying severe synovitis (19).

PATHOGENESIS AND EPIZOOTIOLOGY

Natural and Experimental Hosts. Chickens, turkeys, and guinea fowl (76) are the natural hosts of *M. synoviae*. Ducks (9, 91), geese (10), pigeons (8, 79), Japanese quail (8), and red-legged partridge (78) have been found to be naturally infected. Pheasants and geese (87), ducks (100), and budgerigars (13) are susceptible by artificial inoculation. *M. synoviae* was isolated from house sparrows (*Passer domesticus*) in Spain (78); Kleven and Fletcher (49) found that sparrows could be artificially infected, but were quite resistant. Rabbits, rats, guinea pigs, mice, pigs, and lambs are not susceptible to experimental inoculation (68).

Natural infection in chickens has been observed as early as 1 wk, but acute infection is generally seen when chickens are 4–16 wk old and turkeys are 10–24 wk old. Acute infection occasionally occurs in adult chickens. Chronic infection follows the acute phase and may persist for the life of the flock. The chronic stage may be seen at any age and in some flocks may not be preceded by an acute infection.

Airsacculitis occurs in day-old and older turkeys in MS-infected flocks. Air sac inoculation of mycoplasma-free turkeys results in airsacculitis (30, 82). Inoculation of 18-day-old chicken embryos via the yolk-sac resulted in synovitis and airsacculitis in the chicks (14). *M. synoviae* may be isolated from lesions during the acute phase of the disease, but infection of the upper respiratory tract is permanent (50).

Transmission. Lateral transmission occurs readily by direct contact. *M. synoviae* has been demonstrated in the respiratory tract of contact control chickens 1–4 wk following infection of the principals (70). Spread between batteries in the same room occurs. In many respects, the spread appears to be similar to that of *M. gallisepticum* (65) except that it is more rapid. However, slow-spreading infections have been reported (98). Transmission occurs via the respiratory tract, and usually 100% of the birds become infected, although none or only a few develop joint lesions.

Vertical transmission occurs in naturally and artificially infected chickens (16); however, many flocks hatched from infected dams remain free of infection. Vertical transmission plays a major role in spread of MS in chickens and turkeys. Thus, all eggs used for live virus vaccine production should be obtained from MS-free flocks. Experimental infection of broiler breeders resulted in MS in the trachea of day-old progeny, infertile eggs, and dead-in-shell embryos 6–31 days postinoculation (93). When commercial breeder flocks become infected during egg production, egg-transmission rate appears to be highest during the first 4–6 wk after infection; transmission thereafter may cease, but infected flocks may shed at any time.

Incubation Period. Infectious synovitis has been seen in 6-day-old chicks, suggesting that the incubation period can be relatively short in birds infected by egg transmission. The incubation period following contact exposure is generally 11–21 days. Antibodies may be detected before clinical disease becomes evident. In birds experimentally infected by inoculation at 3–6 wk of age with joint exudate from infected birds or yolk from infected embryos, the order of susceptibility and incubation period is as follows: foot pad, 2–10 days; intravenous, 7–10 days; intracranial, 7–10 days; intraperitoneal, 7–14 days; intrasinus, 14–20 days; and conjunctival instillation, 20 days. Birds are also susceptible to intramuscular inoculation. Intratracheal inoculation results in infection of the trachea and sinus as early as 4 days and readily spreads to contact birds. Air sac lesions are at a maximum 17–21 days after aerosol challenge (50). The incubation period varies with titer and pathogenicity of the inoculum.

Signs

CHICKENS. The first observable signs in a flock affected with infectious synovitis are pale comb, lameness, and retarded growth. As the disease progresses, feathers become ruffled and the comb shrinks. In some cases, the comb is bluish red. Swellings usually occur around joints, and breast blisters are common. Hock joints and foot pads are principally involved, but in some birds most joints are affected; however, birds are occasionally found with a generalized infection but not with apparent swelling of the joints. Birds become listless, dehydrated, and emaciated. Although birds are severely affected, many continue to eat and drink if placed near feed and water. A greenish discoloration of droppings, which contain large amounts of uric acid or urates, is frequently seen. Acute signs described above are followed by slow recovery; however, synovitis may persist for the life of the flock. In other instances, the acute phase is absent or not noticed and only a few chronically infected birds are seen in a flock. Chickens infected via the respiratory tract may show slight rales in 4–6 days or may be asymptomatic.

Air sac infection may occur at any age, but is most often observed as a cause of condemnation in broilers (47). Under field conditions, most air sac lesions resulting from *M. synoviae* infection occur in winter. Progeny of MS-infected breeders may have increased air sac condemnations, reduced weight gains, and reduced feed efficiency.

Experimental aerosol inoculation of hens with MS resulted in a detectable drop in egg production in 1 wk postchallenge, by 2 wk production dropped

18%, and by 4 wk production returned to normal (56). With naturally occurring infection of adults, however, there is ordinarily little or no effect on egg production or egg quality (59, 73), although instances of egg production losses in commercial layers have been observed.

TURKEYS. *M. synoviae* generally causes the same type of signs in turkeys as in chickens. Lameness is the most prominent sign. Warm fluctuating swellings of one or more joints of lame birds are usually found. Occasionally, there is enlargement of the sternal bursa. Severely affected birds lose weight, but many less severely affected make satisfactory weight gains when separated from the flock. In experimentally infected turkeys (68), the first noticeable sign is failure to grow.

Respiratory signs are not usually observed in turkeys, but MS has been isolated from sinus exudates obtained from turkey flocks exhibiting a very low incidence of sinusitis. Rhoades (81) described a synergistic effect of MS and *M. meleagridis* in producing sinusitis in turkeys. Foot pad inoculation of turkeys may result in total cessation of egg production.

Morbidity and Mortality

CHICKENS. Morbidity in flocks with clinical synovitis varies from 2 to 75%, with 5–15% being most usual. Respiratory involvement is generally asymptomatic, but 90–100% of the birds may be infected. Mortality is usually less than 1%, ranging up to 10%. In experimentally infected chickens, mortality may vary from 0 to 100%, depending on route of inoculation and dose of inoculum.

TURKEYS. Morbidity in infected flocks is usually low (1–20%), but mortality from trampling and cannibalism may be significant.

Gross Lesions

CHICKENS. In early stages of the infectious synovitis form of the disease, chickens frequently have a viscous creamy to gray exudate involving synovial membranes of the tendon sheaths, joints, and keel bursa, and hepatosplenomegaly (Fig. 9.8). Kidneys are usually swollen, mottled, and pale. As the disease progresses caseous exudate may be found involving tendon sheaths, joints, and extending into muscle and air sacs. Articular surfaces, particularly of the hock and shoulder joints, become variably thinned to pitted over time (Fig. 9.9). Generally no gross lesions are seen in the upper respiratory tract. In the respiratory form of the disease, airsacculitis may be present.

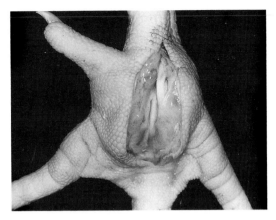

9.8. Incised swollen foot pad of 8-wk-old turkey with granulation tissue and purulent exudate surrounding digital flexors. Similar lesions can be seen in chickens.

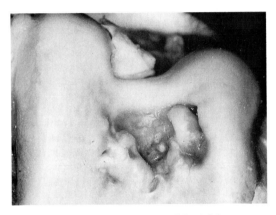

9.9. Ulceration of articular surface of distal tibiotarsus from a chicken with infectious synovitis.

TURKEYS. Swellings of the joints may not be as prominent as in chickens, but fibrinopurulent exudate is frequently present when the joints are opened. Lesions in the respiratory tract are variable.

Histopathology. The histopathology of infectious synovitis (43, 46, 87) in chickens and respiratory disease caused by *M. synoviae* in chickens (26) and turkeys (30, 83) has been described.

The joints, particularly of the foot and hock, have an infiltrate of heterophils and fibrin into joint spaces and along tendon sheaths. The synovial membranes are hyperplastic with villous formation and a diffuse to nodular subsynovial infiltrate of lymphocytes and macrophages (Fig. 9.10). Cartilage surfaces, over time, become discolored, thinned, or pitted. Air sacs may have a mild lesion consisting of edema, capillary proliferation, and the

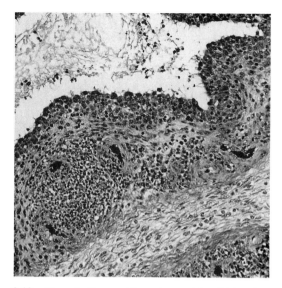

9.10. Hyperplastic synovial membrane with multiple sub-synovial lympoid aggregates from a 7-wk-old turkey with infectious synovitis.

accumulation of heterophils and necrotic debris on the surface, to more severe lesions with hyperplasia of epithelial cells, a diffuse infiltrate of mononuclear cells and caseous necrosis. Other lesions reported to be associated with infectious synovitis are hyperplasia of the macrophage–monocyte system associated with the sheathed arteries of the spleen; lymphoid infiltrates in the heart, liver, and gizzard; and thymic and bursal atrophy. Cardiac pathology has been described in detail (45).

Immunity. Chickens exposed intranasally to *M. synoviae* were resistant to subsequent foot pad challenge (70). Chickens immunized intranasally with a temperature-sensitive mutant of MS were protected against airsacculitis for at least 21 wk (64). Prior exposure to MS-H, a temperature-sensitive mutant strain, protected against subsequent challenge with a virulent synovitis-producing field strain (86). Parenteral inoculation of MS frequently overwhelms the bird before adequate resistance can develop. Resistance to lesions induced by MS is bursa dependent (52, 96), while thymus-dependent lymphocytes may be needed for the development of macroscopic synovial lesions (52).

DIAGNOSIS

Isolation and Identification. Positive diagnosis may be made by isolation and identification of *M. synoviae*. Isolation from lesions in acutely infected birds is not difficult, but in the chronic stages of infection viable organisms may be no longer pre-sent in lesions. Isolation from the upper respiratory tract is more reliable in chronically infected birds. (For medium and isolation methods, see Growth Requirements.) The fluorescent antibody technique using colony imprints (21) or intact colonies (89) may be used for the identification.

Direct detection of MS DNA in tissues or culture medium utilizing DNA probes has been described (25, 38, 44, 106). It is a simple, rapid method of detection, but sensitivity may not be adequate. Polymerase chain reaction is a simple, rapid, and highly sensitive method of detection of MS DNA in tissues or culture medium (29, 54, 107), and PCR kits (92) are commercially available. The PCR procedures are comparable in sensitivity to isolation and identification.

Serology. Antigen is available commercially for the serum plate agglutination test. Adequate directions for use are given with each package. Generally 0.02 mL serum is mixed with an equal amount of antigen on a glass plate, which is gently rotated and observed for agglutination. Antigen should be tested with known positive and negative serums each day. Approximately 2–4 wk are required for antibodies to develop in infected birds (69).

Nonspecific reactors occur in some flocks when using the SPA test (32, 102), especially in flocks that have been vaccinated with oil emulsion vaccines against various agents. *M. gallisepticum* antigen may be agglutinated on occasion, but reaction is somewhat delayed and usually lower in titer (72). To confirm specificity of the reaction, the HI test is used (94).

An indirect immunoperoxidase test utilizing intact Mycoplasma colonies as substrate has been utilized to detect antibodies in serum, respiratory secretions, synovial fluids, bile, harderian gland, oviduct, and yolk (7, 11, 12).

Enzyme-linked immunosorbent assay (35, 74, 77) is commonly used as a diagnostic test and for routine testing of flocks, and may replace serum plate agglutination as the primary serologic test. ELISA kits are available commercially.

Further confirmation of serologic results may be made by isolation and identification of *M. synoviae* from the upper respiratory tract (85) or by PCR.

Turkeys produce a low level of antibody following respiratory infection; therefore, agglutination may not be effective in determining the *M. synoviae* status of a flock. Significant antibodies develop following foot pad inoculation only (30, 80). Various commercial agglutination antigens vary in their ability to detect agglutinins in turkeys. Individual infected turkeys may not develop detectable antibodies(75). Culture and HI testing may be required in some cases to detect infection.

Differential Diagnosis. A presumptive diagnosis may be made on the basis of pale comb, droopiness, emaciation, leg weakness, breast blisters, enlarged foot pads or hock joints, splenomegaly, and enlarged liver or kidneys. Bacteria as causes of synovitis or arthritis must be eliminated by bacteriologic procedures. *Staphylococcus aureus, Escherichia coli,* pasteurellae, and salmonellae may also be present as primary causes of synovitis. *M. gallisepticum* may also be a cause of breast blisters and joint lesions (68, 71).

Fibrosis of metatarsal extensor or digital flexor tendons and lymphocytic infiltration of the myocardium associated with the viral arthritis agent help to differentiate it from *M. synoviae* (57). Serum from viral tenosynovitis-infected chickens does not agglutinate MS antigen, but one must bear in mind that MS agglutinins may be present without obvious joint involvement.

In cases with respiratory involvement, *M. gallisepticum* and other causes of respiratory disease should be eliminated.

TREATMENT. *M. synoviae* is susceptible in vitro to several antibiotics, including chlortetracycline, danofloxacin, enrofloxacin, lincomycin, oxytetracycline, spectinomycin, spiromycin, tetracycline, tiamulin, and tylosin (15, 42, 48, 99). In contrast to *M. gallisepticum,* MS isolates appear to be resistant to erythromycin (99). Acquired antibiotic resistance has not been reported for MS, although earlier isolates seem to respond more poorly to chlortetracycline than later isolates (66). Generally, suitable medication is of value in preventing airsacculitis or synovitis, but treatment of existing lesions is less effective. Antibiotic medication will not eliminate MS infection from the flock.

A summary of data obtained from field and experimental studies indicates that chlortetracycline (50–100 g/ton of feed) given continuously will provide satisfactory control of infectious synovitis in chickens. Higher concentrations (approximately 200 g/ton) are required to control synovitis after infection has occurred. In turkeys, prophylactic levels of 200 g/ton are required. Effectiveness of chlortetracycline may be related to the MS isolate involved (66).

Soluble lincomycin–spectinomycin (2 g/gal of drinking water) is of value in preventing airsacculitis in broilers (33) and turkey poults (34). Tiamulin in the drinking water (0.006–0.025%) has been shown to be effective in preventing airsacculitis and synovitis in chickens (6). Other products have been used, but their value in treatment of MS has not been adequately studied.

PREVENTION AND CONTROL. *M. synoviae* is egg transmitted, and the only effective method of control is to select chickens or turkeys from MS-free flocks. Most primary breeding stocks are free of infection, and MS-free sources of replacement breeding stocks should be available. Effective biosecurity measures should be used to prevent introduction of the infection.

Outbreaks of MS infection in broilers can often be traced to a specific breeder flock. Often, by the time the infected breeder flock is found, egg transmission is low or no longer of clinical significance. The decision to slaughter infected parent breeder flocks is usually made on an economic basis. If such flocks are kept for egg production, progeny should be hatched separately and isolated from MS-free flocks.

Antibiotic treatment of breeders is not effective in eliminating MS, although the level of egg transmission may be reduced.

Treatment of eggs with antibiotics such as tylosin by egg dipping, or egg inoculation with tylosin and gentamycin (63), or heat treatment (101) of hatching eggs has been used in breeding flocks to prevent egg transmission of MS. Exposure of breeders before the onset of egg production with virulent MS will reduce egg transmission. This should only be used in flocks in which infection will almost certainly occur. An inactivated, oil emulsion bacterin is commercially available, but its role in the control of MS has not been adequately studied. A live temperature-sensitive MS vaccine strain, MS-H, has been evaluated extensively in field trials in Australia, but it is not yet commercially available (86).

REFERENCES

1. Ajufo, J.C., and K.G. Whithear. 1980. The surface layer of Mycoplasma synoviae as demonstrated by the negative staining technique. Res Vet Sci 29:268–270.

2. Avakian, A.P., and S.H. Kleven. 1990. The humoral immune response of chickens to Mycoplasma gallisepticum and potential causes of false positive reactions in avian Mycoplasma serology. 1989. Zentralbl Bakteriol Mikrobiol Hyg (Suppl 20):500–512.

3. Avakian, A.P., and S.H. Kleven. 1990. Evaluation of SDS-polyacrylamide gel electrophoresis purified proteins of Mycoplasma gallisepticum and Mycoplasma synoviae as antigens in a dot ELISA. Avian Dis 34:575–584.

4. Avakian, A.P., and S.H. Kleven. 1990. The humoral immune response of chickens to Mycoplasma gallisepticum and Mycoplasma synoviae studied by immunoblotting. Vet Microbiol 24:155–170.

5. Avakian, A.P., D.H. Ley, and S.H. Kleven. 1992. Comparison of Mycoplasma synoviae isolates by immunoblotting. Avian Pathol 21:633–642.

6. Baughn, C.O., W.C. Alpaugh, W.H. Linkenheimer, and D.C. Maplesden. 1978. Effect of Tiamulin in chickens and turkeys infected experimentally with avian mycoplasma. Avian Dis 22:620–626.

7. Bencina, D., and J.M. Bradbury. 1991. Indirect immunoperoxidase assay for the detection of antibody in chicken Mycoplasma infections. Avian Pathol 20:113–124.

8. Bencina, D., T. Tadina, and D. Dorrer. 1987. Mycoplasma species isolated from six avian species. Avian Pathol 16:653–664.

9. Bencina, D., T. Tadina, and D. Dorrer. 1988. Natural

infection of ducks with Mycoplasma synoviae and Mycoplasma gallisepticum and Mycoplasma egg transmission. Avian Pathol 17:441–449.

10. Bencina, D., T. Tadina, and D. Dorrer. 1988. Natural infection of geese with Mycoplasma gallisepticum and Mycoplasma synoviae and egg transmission of the Mycoplasmas. Avian Pathol 17:925–928.

11. Bencina, D., I. Mrzel, A. Svetlin, D. Dorrer, and T. Tadina-Jaksic. 1991. Reactions of chicken biliary immunoglobulin A with avian mycoplasmas. Avian Pathol 20:303–313.

12. Bencina, D., A. Svetlin, D. Dorrer, and T. Tadina-Jaksic. 1991. Humoral and local antibodies in chickens with mixed infection with three Mycoplasma species. Avian Pathol 20:325–334.

13. Bozeman, L.H., S.H. Kleven, and R.B. Davis. 1984. Mycoplasma challenge studies in budgerigars (Melopsittacus undulatus) and chickens. Avian Dis 28:426–434.

14. Bradbury, J.M., and L.J. Howell. 1975. The response of chickens to experimental infection `in ovo' with Mycoplasma synoviae. Avian Pathol 4:277–286.

15. Bradbury, J.M., C.A. Yavari, and C.J. Giles. 1994. In vitro evaluation of various antimicrobials against Mycoplasma gallisepticum and Mycoplasma synoviae by the micro-broth method, and comparison with a commercially-prepared test system. Avian Pathol 23:105–115.

16. Carnaghan, R.B.A. 1961. Egg transmission of infectious synovitis. J Comp Pathol 71:279–285.

17. Chalquest, R.R. 1962. Cultivation of the infectious-synovitis-type pleuropneumonia-like organisms. Avian Dis 6:36–43.

18. Chalquest, R.R., and J. Fabricant. 1960. Pleuropneumonia-like organisms associated with synovitis in fowls. Avian Dis 4:515–539.

19. Chin, R.P., C.U. Meteyer, R. Yamamoto, H.L. Shivaprasad, and P.N. Klein. 1991. Isolation of Mycoplasma synoviae from the brains of commercial meat turkeys with meningeal vasculitis. Avian Dis 35:631–637.

20. Christensen, N.H., C.A. Yavari, A.J. McBain, and J.M. Bradbury. 1994. Investigations into the survival of Mycoplasma gallisepticum, Mycoplasma synoviae and Mycoplasma iowae on materials found in the poultry house environment. Avian Pathol 23:127–143.

21. Corstvet, R.E., and W.W. Sadler. 1964. The diagnosis of certain avian diseases with the fluorescent antibody technique. Poult Sci 43:1280–1288.

22. DaMassa, A.J., and H.E. Adler. 1975. Growth of Mycoplasma synoviae in a medium supplemented with nicotinamide instead of B-nicotinamide adenine dinucleotide. Avian Dis 19:544–555.

23. Dierks, R.E., J.A. Newman, and B.S. Pomeroy. 1967. Characterization of avian mycoplasma. Ann NY Acad Sci 143:170–189.

24. Fan, H., S.H. Kleven, and M.W. Jackwood. 1994. Application of polymerase chain reaction with arbitrarily primers to strain identification of Mycoplasma gallisepticum. IOM Lett 3:443.

25. Fernández, C., J.G. Mattsson, G. Bölske, and K.-E. Johansson. 1993. Species-specific oligonucleotide probes complementary to 16S rRNA of Mycoplasma gallisepticum and Mycoplasma synoviae. Res Vet Sci 55:130–136.

26. Fletcher, O.J., D.P. Anderson, and S.H. Kleven. 1976. Histology of air sac lesions induced in chickens by contact exposure to Mycoplasma synoviae. Vet Pathol 13:303–314.

27. Frey, M.L., R.P. Hanson, and D.P. Anderson. 1968. A medium for the isolation of avian mycoplasmas. Am J Vet Res 29:2163–2171.

28. Furuta, K., Y. Makino, K. Komi, Y. Nakamura, and S. Oda. 1985. Sanitization of a chicken house contaminated with Mycoplasmas. Jpn Poult Sci 22:126–133.

29. Garcia, M., M.W. Jackwood, S.H. Kleven, S. Levisohn, and K.-E. Johansson. 1994. Detection of Mycoplasma gallisepticum, M. synoviae, and M. iowae by polymerase chain reaction and species-specific oligonucleotide probes. IOM Lett 3:480.

30. Ghazikhanian, G., R. Yamamoto, and D.R. Cordy, 1973. Response of turkeys to experimental infection with Mycoplasma synoviae. Avian Dis 17:122–136.

31. Giambrone, J.J., C.S. Eidson, and S.H. Kleven. 1977. Effect of infectious bursal disease on the response of chickens to Mycoplasma synoviae, Newcastle disease virus, and infectious bronchitis virus. Am J Vet Res 38:251–253.

32. Glisson, J.R., J.F. Dawe, and S.H. Kleven. 1984. The effect of oil-emulsion vaccines on the occurrence of nonspecific plate agglutination reactions for Mycoplasma gallisepticum and M. synoviae. Avian Dis 28:397–405.

33. Hamdy, A.H., S.H. Kleven, E.L. McCune, B.S. Pomeroy, and A.C. Peterson. 1976. Efficacy of Linco-spectin water medication on Mycoplasma synoviae airsacculitis in broilers. Avian Dis 20:118–125.

34. Hamdy, A.H., Y.M. Saif, and C.W. Kasson. 1982. Efficacy of lincomycin-spectinomycin water medication on Mycoplasma meleagridis airsacculitis in commercially reared turkey poults. Avian Dis 26:227–233.

35. Higgins, P.A., and K.G. Whithear. 1986. Detection and differentiation of Mycoplasma gallisepticum and Mycoplasma synoviae antibodies in chicken serum using enzyme-linked immunosorbent assay. Avian Dis 30:160–168.

36. Hopkins, S.R., and H.W. Yoder, Jr. 1982. Influence of infectious bronchitis strains and vaccines on the incidence of Mycoplasma synoviae airsacculitis. Avian Dis 26:741–752.

37. Hwang, Y.S., V.S. Panangala, C.R. Rossi, J.J. Giambrone, and L.H. Lauerman. 1989. Monoclonal antibodies that recognize specific antigens of Mycoplasma gallisepticum and M. synoviae. Avian Dis 33:42–52.

38. Hyman, H.C., S. Levisohn, D. Yogev, and S. Razin. 1989. DNA probes for Mycoplasma gallisepticum and Mycoplasma synoviae: Application in experimentally infected chickens. Vet Microbiol 20:323–338.

39. Jordan, F.T.W. 1975. Avian mycoplasma and pathogenicity—A review. Avian Pathol 4:165–174.

40. Jordan, F.T.W. 1981. Mycoplasma-induced arthritis in poultry. Israel J Med Sci 17:622–625.

41. Jordan, F.T.W., H. Erno, G.S. Cottew, K.H. Hinz, and L. Stipkovits. 1982. Characterization and taxonomic description of five Mycoplasma serovars (Serotypes) of avian origin and their elevation to species rank and further evaluation of the taxonomic status of Mycoplasma synoviae. Int J Syst Bacteriol 32:108–115.

42. Jordan, F.T.W., S. Gilbert, D.L. Knight, and C.A. Yavari. 1989. Effects of Baytril, Tylosin, and Tiamulin on avian mycoplasmas. Avian Pathol 18:659–673.

43. Kawakubo, Y., K. Kume, and M. Yoshioka. 1980. Histo- and immuno-pathological studies on experimental Mycoplasma synoviae infection of the chicken. J Comp Pathol 457–467.

44. Kempf, I., F. Gesbert, M. Guittet, J.P. Le Pennec, and G. Bennejean. 1991. Sondes nucléiques spécifiques de Mycoplasma gallisepticum et Mycoplasma synoviae: Préparation et intérêt. Revue de Médecine Vétérinaire 142:887–892.

45. Kerr, K.M., and N.O. Olson. 1967. Cardiac pathology associated with viral and mycoplasmal arthritis in chickens. Ann NY Acad Sci 143:204–217.

46. Kerr, K.M., and N.O. Olson. 1970. Pathology of chickens inoculated experimentally or contact-infected with Mycoplasma synoviae. Avian Dis 14:291–320.

47. King, D.D., S.H. Kleven, D.M. Wenger, and D.P. Anderson. 1973. Field studies with Mycoplasma synoviae. Avian Dis 17:722–726.

48. Kleven, S.H., and D.P. Anderson. 1971. In vitro activity of various antibiotics against Mycoplasma synoviae. Avian Dis 15:551–557.

49. Kleven, S.H., and W.O. Fletcher. 1983. Laboratory infection of house sparrows (Passer domesticus) with Mycoplasma gallisepticum and Mycoplasma synoviae. Avian Dis 27:308–311.

50. Kleven, S.H., D.D. King, and D.P. Anderson. 1972. Airsacculitis in broilers from Mycoplasma synoviae: Effect on air sac lesions of vaccinating with infectious bronchitis and Newcastle virus. Avian Dis 16:915–924.

51. Kleven, S.H., O.J. Fletcher, and R.B. Davis. 1975. Influence of strain of Mycoplasma synoviae and route of infection on development of synovitis or airsacculitis in broilers. Avian Dis 19:126–135.

52. Kume, K., Y. Kawakubo, C. Morita, E. Hayatsu, and M. Yoshioka. 1977. Experimentally induced synovitis of chickens with Mycoplasma synoviae: Effects of bursectomy and thymectomy on course of the infection for the first four weeks. Am J Vet Res 38:1595–1600.

53. Lauerman, L.H., and R.A. Reynolds-Vaughn. 1991. Immunoglobulin G Fc receptors of Mycoplasma synoviae. Avian Dis 35:135–138.

54. Lauerman, L.H., F.J. Hoerr, A.R. Sharpton, S.M. Shah, and V.L. van Santen. 1993. Development and application of a polymerase chain reaction assay for Mycoplasma synoviae. Avian Dis 37:829–834.

55. Ley, D.H., and A.P. Avakian. 1992. An outbreak of Mycoplasma synoviae infection in North Carolina turkeys: Comparison of isolates by sodium dodecyl sulfate-polyacrylamide gel electrophoresis and restriction endonuclease analysis. Avian Dis 36:672–678.

56. Lott, B.D., J.H. Drott, T.H. Vardaman, and F.N. Reece. 1978. Effect of Mycoplasma synoviae on egg quality and egg production of broiler breeders. Poult Sci 57:309–311.

57. MacDonald, J.W., C.J. Randall, M.D. Dagless, and D.A. McMartin. 1978. Observations on viral tenosynovitis (viral arthritis) in Scotland. Avian Pathol 7:471–482.

58. Mohammed, H.O., T.E. Carpenter, R. Yamamoto, and D.A. McMartin. 1986. Prevalence of Mycoplasma gallisepticum and M. synoviae in commercial layers in southern and central California. Avian Dis 30:519–526.

59. Mohammed, H.O., T.E. Carpenter, and R. Yamamoto. 1987. Economic impact of Mycoplasma gallisepticum and M. synoviae in commercial layer flocks. Avian Dis 31:477–482.

60. Morrow, C.J., K.G. Whithear, and S.H. Kleven. 1990. Restriction endonuclease analysis of Mycoplasma synoviae strains. Avian Dis 34:611–616.

61. Morsy, M.A., V.S. Panangala, and P.C. Hu. 1993. Identification and characterization of a Mycoplasma synoviae 55,000-molecular-weight antigen associated with hemagglutinin. Avian Dis 37:1097–1104.

62. Morsy, M.A., V.S. Panangala, V.L. van Santen, and R.C. Bird. 1993. Cloning and partial sequence analysis of a Mycoplasma synoviae DNA fragment encoding epitopes shared with the major adhesin P1 protein of Mycoplasma pneumoniae. Avian Dis 37:1105–1112.

63. Nascimento, E.R., and M.G.F. Nascimento. 1994. Eradication of Mycoplasma gallisepticum and M. synoviae from a chicken flock in Brazil. Proc West Poult Dis Conf 43:58–59.

64. Nonomura, I., and Y. Imada. 1982. Temperature-sensitive mutant of Mycoplasma synoviae. I. Production and selection of a nonpathogenic but immunogenic clone. Avian Dis 26:763–775.

65. Olson, N.O., and K.M. Kerr. 1967. The duration and distribution of synovitis-producing agents in chickens. Avian Dis 11:578–585.

66. Olson, N.O., and S.P. Sahu. 1976. Efficacy of chlortetracycline against Mycoplasma synoviae isolated in two periods. Avian Dis 20:221–229.

67. Olson, N.O., J.K. Bletner, D.C. Shelton, D.A. Munro, and G.C. Anderson. 1954. Enlarged joint condition in poultry caused by an infectious agent [abst]. Poult Sci 33:1075.

68. Olson, N.O., D.C. Shelton, J.K. Bletner, D.A. Munro, and G.C. Anderson. 1956. Studies of infectious synovitis in chickens. Am J Vet Res 17:747–754.

69. Olson, N.O., K.M. Kerr, and A. Campbell. 1963. Control of infectious synovitis. 12. Preparation of an agglutination test antigen. Avian Dis 7:310–317.

70. Olson, N.O., H.E. Adler, A.J. DaMassa, and R.E. Corstvet. 1964. The effect of intranasal exposure to Mycoplasma synoviae and infectious bronchitis on development of lesions and agglutinins. Avian Dis 8:623–631.

71. Olson, N.O., K.M. Kerr, and A. Campbell. 1964. Control of infectious synovitis. 13. The antigen study of three strains. Avian Dis 8:209–214.

72. Olson, N.O., R. Yamamoto, and H. Ortmayer. 1965. Antigenic relationship between mycoplasma synoviae and Mycoplasma gallisepticum. Am J Vet Res 26:195–198.

73. Opitz, H.M. 1983. Mycoplasma synoviae infection in Maine's egg farms. Avian Dis 27:324–326.

74. Opitz, H.M., J.B. Duplessis, and M.J. Cyr. 1983. Indirect micro enzyme linked immunosorbent assay ELISA for the detection of antibodies to Mycoplasma synoviae and Mycoplasma gallisepticum. Avian Dis 27:773–786.

75. Ortiz, A., and S.H. Kleven. 1992. Serological detection of Mycoplasma synoviae infection in turkeys. Avian Dis 36:749–752.

76. Pascucci, S., N. Maestrini, S. Govoni, and A. Prati. 1976. Mycoplasma synoviae in the guinea-fowl. Avian Pathol 5:291–297.

77. Patten, B.E., P.A. Higgins, and K.G. Whithear. 1984. A urease-ELISA for the detection of mycoplasma infections in poultry. Aust Vet J 61:151–155.

78. Poveda, J.B., J. Carranza, A. Miranda, A. Garrido, M. Hermoso, A. Fernandez, and J. Domenech. 1990. An epizootiological study of avian Mycoplasmas in Southern Spain. Avian Pathol 19:627–633.

79. Reece, R.L., L. Ireland, and P.C. Scott. 1986. Mycoplasmosis in racing pigeons. Aust Vet J 63:166–167.

80. Rhoades, K.R. 1975. Antibody responses of turkeys experimentally exposed to Mycoplasma synoviae. Avian Dis 19:437–442.

81. Rhoades, K.R. 1977. Turkey sinusitis: Synergism between Mycoplasma synoviae and Mycoplasma meleagridis. Avian Dis 21:670–674.

82. Rhoades, K.R. 1981. Turkey airsacculitis: Effect of mixed mycoplasmal infections. Avian Dis 25:131–135.

83. Rhoades, K.R. 1987. Airsacculitis in turkeys exposed to Mycoplasma synoviae membranes. Avian Dis 31:855–860.

84. Roberts, D.H., and O.M. Olesuik. 1967. Serological studies with Mycoplasma synoviae. Avian Dis 11:104–119.

85. Sahu, S.P., and N.O. Olson. 1976. Evaluation of broiler breeder flocks for nonspecific Mycoplasma synoviae reaction. Avian Dis 20:49–64.

86. Scott, P.C., J. Jones, C.J. Morrow, D.H. Ley, and K.G. Whithear. 1994. Experiences with a live attenuated Mycoplasma synoviae vaccine. Proc West Poult Dis Conf 43:97–98.

87. Sevoian, M., G.H. Snoeyenbos, H.I. Basch, and I.M. Reynolds. 1958. Infectious synovitis. I. Clinical and pathological manifestations. Avian Dis 2:499–513.

88. Springer, W.T., C. Luskus, and S.S. Pourciau. 1974. Infectious Bronchitis and mixed infections of Mycoplasma synoviae and Escherichia coli in gnotobiotic chickens. I. Synergistic role in the airsacculitis syndrome. Infect Immun 10:578–589.

89. Talkington, F.D., and S.H. Kleven. 1983. A classification of laboratory strains of avian Mycoplasma serotypes by direct immunofluorescence. Avian Dis 27:422–429.

90. Timms, L.M. 1978. Mycoplasma synoviae: A review. Vet Bull 48:187–198.

91. Tiong, S.K. 1990. Mycoplasmas and acholeplasmas isolated from ducks and their possible association with pasteurellas. Vet Rec 127:64–66.

92. Tyrrell, P., and P. Anderson. 1994. Efficacy of sample pooling for the detection of Mycoplasma gallisepticum and Mycoplasma synoviae utilizing PCR. Proc West Poult Dis Conf 43:62.

93. Vardaman, T.H. 1976. The resistance and carrier status of meat-type hens exposed to Mycoplasma synoviae. Poult Sci 55:268–273.

94. Vardaman, T.H., and H.W. Yoder, Jr. 1969. Preparation of Mycoplasma synoviae hemagglutinating antigen and its use in the hemagglutination-inhibition test. Avian Dis 13:654–661.

95. Vardaman, T.H., and H.W. Yoder, Jr. 1971. Preparation of Mycoplasma synoviae antigen for the tube agglutination test. Avian Dis 15:462–466.

96. Vardaman, T.H., K. Landaeth, S. Whatley, L.J. Dreesen, and B. Glick. 1973. Resistance to Mycoplasma synoviae is bursal dependent. Infect Immun 8:674–676.

97. Walker, E.R., M.H. Friedman, N.O. Olson, S.P. Sahu, and H.F. Mengoli. 1978. An ultrastructural study of avian synovium infected with an arthrotropic Mycoplasma, Mycoplasma synoviae. Vet Pathol 15:407–416.

98. Weinack, O.M., G.H. Snoeyenbos, and S.H. Kleven. 1983. Strain of Mycoplasma synoviae of low transmissibility. Avian Dis 27:1151–1156.

99. Whithear, K.G., D.D. Bowtell, E. Ghiocas, and K.L. Hughes. 1983. Evaluation and use of a micro-broth dilution procedure for testing sensitivity of fermentative avian mycoplasmas to antibiotics. Avian Dis 27:937–949.

100. Yamada, S., and K. Matsuo. 1983. Experimental infection of ducks with Mycoplasma synoviae. Avian Dis 27:762–765.

101. Yoder, H.W., Jr. 1970. Preincubation heat treatment of hatching eggs to inactivate mycoplasma. Avian Dis 14:75–86.

102. Yoder, H. W., Jr. 1989. Nonspecific reactions to mycoplasma serum plate antigens induced by inactivated poultry disease vaccines. Avian Dis 33:60–68.

103. Yoder, H.W., Jr., L.N. Drury, and S.R. Hopkins. 1977. Influence of environment on airsacculitis: Effects of relative humidity and air temperature on broilers infected with Mycoplasma synoviae and infectious bronchitis. Avian Dis 21:195–208.

104. Yogev, D., S. Levisohn, S.H. Kleven, D. Halachmi, and S. Razin. 1988. Ribosomal RNA gene probes to detect intraspecies heterogeneity in Mycoplasma gallisepticum and M. synoviae. Avian Dis 32:220–231.

105. Yogev, D., S. Levisohn, and S. Razin. 1989. Genetic and antigenic relatedness between Mycoplasma gallisepticum and Mycoplasma synoviae. Vet Microbiol 19:75–84.

106. Zhao, S., and R. Yamamoto. 1990. Recombinant DNA probes for Mycoplasma synoviae. Avian Dis 34:709–716.

107. Zhao, S., and R. Yamamoto. 1993. Detection of Mycoplasma synoviae by polymerase chain reaction. Avian Pathol 22:533–542.

MYCOPLASMA IOWAE INFECTION

S. H. Kleven and C. Baxter-Jones

INTRODUCTION. *Mycoplasma iowae* is generally associated with reduced hatchability and embryo mortality in turkeys. It has been shown experimentally to induce mortality in turkey and chicken embryos and mild to moderate airsacculitis and leg abnormalities in chickens and turkeys.

HISTORY. The Iowa 695 strain of avian mycoplasma was isolated and characterized by Yoder and Hofstad (41) and was subsequently designated avian serotype I (42). Avian mycoplasma serotypes I, J, K, N, Q, and R were classified into separate groups by Dierks et al.(17), and they were later characterized as a single, related group (2, 3, 19). The organism was later named *Mycoplasma iowae* (23).

INCIDENCE AND DISTRIBUTION. In addition to North America, *M. iowae* has been reported in western Europe (22), eastern Europe (5), and India (33). It is presumed to be worldwide in distribution.

ETIOLOGY

Classification. *M. iowae* identification is based on colony and cell morphology typical of mycoplasmas, special requirements for growth, and

serologic reactions. Immunofluorescence of mycoplasma colonies (39) is the most rapid and reliable method for identification of field isolates.

Morphology and Staining. As with other mycoplasmas, with Giemsa staining or dark-field examination, *M. iowae* organisms appear coccobacillary in form and show some pleomorphism. By electron microscopy, pleomorphism is evident and cells are bounded by a triple-layered cell membrane and lack a cell wall (23).

Growth Requirements. Like other mycoplasmas, *M. iowae* has complex growth requirements. Cholesterol is required for growth. Incubation is at 37 C, and growth occurs either aerobically or with added CO_2 (23). Recovery of *M. iowae* from tissues appears to be more successful by direct plating on agar than by inoculation of broth (1). Although several formulations of mycoplasma medium have been used successfully, the formulation described by Bradbury (7) works well. Field isolates of *M. iowae* may be intolerant of certain media components, and it is advisable to perform quality control checks of yeast extract and serum batches before use, with cultures of the organism that have not been serially passaged in artificial media.

Colony Morphology. Colonies are characteristic of mycoplasmas and show typical fried egg morphology on solid media and are 0.1–0.3 mm in diameter (41).

Biochemical Properties. *M. iowae* ferments glucose aerobically and anaerobically, utilizes arginine, does not utilize urea, is phosphatase negative, does not produce film and spots, and does not reduce tetrazolium chloride (23). It has the ability to grow in the presence of 0.5 to 1.0% bile salts (36).

Resistance to Chemical and Physical Agents. Resistance of *M. iowae* to disinfectants has not been determined, but it is probably similar to that of other mycoplasmas. *M. iowae* appears to be hardier than *M. gallisepticum* or *M. synoviae* (16), surviving for up to 5 days on feathers and 6 days on human hair and several other materials. This may have implications for terminal site disinfection, especially with the existence of an oral/fecal mode of transmission. Practically, however, the organisms appear to be inactivated by proper cleaning and disinfection.

Antigenic Structure. The antigenic structure of *M. iowae* has not been well studied. Agglutination (41) and enzyme-linked immunosorbent assay (ELISA) (24) have been studied, but the antibody response is not strong (14, 15), and nonspecific reactions have been a problem with ELISA (24). Antigenic structure has been studied utilizing monoclonal antibodies (32). There appears to be significant antigenic diversity among strains of *M. iowae* (8, 21, 32, 43).

Pathogenicity. There is variability in the pathogenicity and virulence of *M. iowae* strains (34, 41). Experimental infection with *M. iowae* causes dose-related mortality in chicken and turkey embryos (13, 20, 30, 34, 41). Under field conditions, it is responsible for embryo mortality and reduced hatchability in turkeys. The hatchability loss is widely variable and dependent on the extent of vertical transmission. Discernible hatchability losses are not always encountered in eggs from infected turkey breeder flocks. On other occasions, however, the losses can be quite severe and prolonged. The reasons for these observed differences are not known but could include the variance in pathogenicity of *M. iowae* strains, incubation conditions, and the susceptibility of breeds of turkeys.

Artificial challenge with *M. iowae* induces mild to moderate airsacculitis in turkeys (17, 34, 41), as well as leg lesions in both chickens and turkeys (10, 15, 12, 41). Artificial inoculation of 1-day-old broiler breeder chickens resulted in stunting and poor feathering in addition to leg lesions (11). Production of a challenge model that induces persistent infection for the purpose of evaluating antimicrobials has been difficult; a procedure involving inoculation of the lung of day-old poults has been recommended for such purposes (26). There are few clinical reports, however, describing airsacculitis or leg problems in chickens or turkeys, or embryo mortality in chickens under field circumstances. An outbreak associated with *M. iowae* in commercial turkey poults exhibiting leg weakness and dehydration has been described (40).

PATHOGENESIS AND EPIZOOTIOLOGY

Natural and Experimental Hosts. The natural host is the turkey, but isolation of *M. iowae* from chickens is not uncommon (5, 41). *M. iowae* has also been isolated from yellow-naped Amazon parrots (6).

Transmission, Carriers, and Vectors. Only avian species are known to be infected with *M. iowae*. Unlike other avian mycoplasmas, *M. iowae* exhibits a predilection for the digestive tract (31). Egg transmission occurs in turkeys (41, 30). Infection may be spread venereally, and under modern methods of insemination, infected semen may play a role in dissemination (35).

Horizontal transmission may occur, but the organism does not spread rapidly in young flocks. Before achieving reproductive maturity, very few birds may be identified as culture-positive within a flock.

After laying begins following artificial insemination and for a few weeks thereafter, a high percentage of birds may become culture-positive. The organism can be recovered from both cloacal and vaginal sites. Infection may be spread by the venereal route (28), particularly following hand contact with the vagina at artificial insemination. Infected semen may also play a role in facilitating spread of the organism. The patterns of vertical transmission have been well characterized (20). Within any infected flock, it is possible to identify individuals that do not lay any infected eggs. Other birds lay only one or a few infected eggs, while the remainder lay many infected eggs. It is the latter group that is important in determining the extent of vertical transmission.

Signs. No clinical signs are observed in live turkeys, although there is one report of an association of *M. iowae* with leg weakness in young poults (40). Eggs from infected turkey breeders may have reduced hatchability (usually 2–5%). Affected embryos usually die during the last 10 days of incubation, typically from days 18–24, although death may occur later.

Gross Lesions. Lesions in affected embryos consist primarily of stunting and congestion, with various degrees of hepatitis, edema, and splenomegaly (41, 30). Sometimes affected embryos exhibit a down abnormality, "swollen down plumule," particularly in severe cases. These lesions cannot be considered pathognomonic and may be very similar to those observed when embryos are overheated in the incubator (18). Airsacculitis in inoculated chickens and turkeys is ordinarily mild to moderate and similar to lesions caused by other mycoplasmas (17, 34, 41). Inoculation of day-old poults results in stunting, poor feathering, tenosynovitis, and leg abnormalities including chondrodystrophy, rotated tibia, toe deviations, and sometimes erosion of the articular cartilage of the hock joint and rupture of the digital flexor tendon (15, 41). Similar leg lesions may be observed in experimental chicks, including rupture of the digital flexor tendon, but lesions ordinarily are less severe than in turkeys (14). Inoculation of turkey poults with *M. iowae* may result in bursal atrophy (9). Lesions have not been reported under field conditions, perhaps because infected embryos do not hatch.

Histopathology. After inoculation of day-old poults, lesions of the spleen consist of reticular cells with macrophages, plasma cells, and heterophils in the parenchyma. The bursa of Fabricius has localized congestion with infiltration of plasma cells, heterophils, and reticular cells. Macrophages, lymphocytes, heterophils, and plasma cells are seen in the lamina propria of the duodenum, ileum, and cecal tonsils. There is little obvious change observed in cartilage and tendon except for edema in the tendon sheaths (15). After air sac inoculation of turkey poults, lesions consist of thickened air sacs that contain large numbers of inflammatory cells, primarily lymphocytes. In some areas, lymphoid follicles are observed. Exudate on the mucosal surface contains fibrin and inflammatory cells (34).

Immunity. Very little information is available on immunity to *M. iowae,* although antibody responses have been observed (41, 24). Equally, there is very little information on the age susceptibility of turkeys. It is difficult or impossible to infect some individuals within a flock of adult breeder turkeys (4). Breeders that become infected and vertically transmit the organism to their eggs usually resolve the infection. This may occur in a few weeks or sometimes can take 2–3 months. Embryo mortality usually subsides immediately before resolution of the infection. That an immune response is involved is suggested by the finding of growth-inhibiting and metabolism-inhibiting antibodies in the serum of these hens (4).

DIAGNOSIS

Isolation and Identification. *M. iowae* is present in high numbers in dead embryos (13, 30). After inoculation of turkey poults, *M. iowae* can be isolated from a variety of tissues, especially from the gastrointestinal tract or from cloacal swabs, but isolations become less frequent with age, and organisms could not be recovered after 12 wk (15, 37). Isolation of *M. iowae* from oviduct, semen, and phallus of adult chickens and turkeys has been reported (33, 35, 41). Cotton swabs from the appropriate tissue are streaked on agar plates and incubated 4–5 days or longer at 37 C. Typical mycoplasma colonies can be readily identified by immunofluorescence (39).

Polymerase chain reaction has been used for direct detection of *M. iowae* DNA (29, 44), but this is not yet a routine procedure for field situations.

Serology. Although agglutination, metabolism inhibition, indirect hemagglutination, and ELISA tests have been used for experimental infections (28, 24, 38, 41), the serologic response is weak, and there is no reliable serologic test available for widespread clinical use.

Differential Diagnosis. *M. iowae* infection should be considered in cases of low hatchability in turkeys, especially when there is evidence of late embryo mortality. Although it is not recognized as a significant cause of clinical tenosynovitis, *M. iowae* should be considered as a possibility in cases where there is no apparent explanation for leg problems including tenosynovitis, especially in young turkeys.

TREATMENT. Treatment of clinical disease in turkeys associated with *M. iowae* is not an issue because it is not typically associated with clinical disease. Jordan (25) did show the effectiveness of different antibiotics in reducing levels of infection.

Attempts have been made, however, to reduce vertical transmission in commercial flocks to alleviate hatchability losses. *M. iowae* appears to be unusually resistant to the commonly used antimicrobials. The quinoline class of antibiotics, particularly enrofloxacin (Bayer), have sometimes been effective when administered to laying hens in the drinking water, early during production. Eggs from medicated turkeys have been shown to be resistant to in ovo challenge with *M. iowae* (27). Egg treatment with enrofloxacin has, however, been more commonly employed. Hatching eggs from affected flocks are vacuum dipped in a solution of the antibiotic. This product is not generally available for food animal use in some countries.

PREVENTION AND CONTROL. There is no reliable serologic testing procedure for *M. iowae* to screen commercial flocks. Culture and isolation may also be impractical before birds begin production because of the difficulties involved in isolating the organism and the poor horizontal spread. It is often possible, however, to detect infection in toms and hens before the onset of reproduction.

Clean flocks can be maintained free of *M. iowae* infection by preventing fomite transmission. Special attention should be given when birds reach reproductive age, especially during artificial insemination. It should be noted, however, that *M. iowae* does not always appear to be associated with hatchability losses.

Residual site infection is not known to be a problem where effective terminal cleaning and disinfection procedures are employed. The possibility of contaminated fomites should be borne in mind, however, if adequate cleaning is not achieved between successive flocks.

REFERENCES

1. Amin, M.M., and F.T.W. Jordan. 1978. A comparative study of some cultural methods in the isolation of avian mycoplasma from field material. Avian Pathol 7:455–470.

2. Aycardi, E.R., D.P. Anderson, and R.P. Hanson. 1971. Classification of avian Mycoplasmas by gel diffusion and growth inhibition tests. Avian Dis 15:434–447.

3. Barber, T.L., and J. Fabricant. 1971. A suggested reclassification of avian mycoplasma serotypes. Avian Dis 15:125–138.

4. Baxter-Jones, C. 1995. Unpublished data.

5. Bencina, D., I. Mrzel, T. Tadina, and D. Dorrer. 1987. Mycoplasma spp in chicken flocks with different management systems. Avian Pathol 16:599–608.

6. Bozeman, L.H., S.H. Kleven, and R.B. Davis. 1984. Mycoplasma challenge studies in budgerigars (Melopsittacus undulatus) and chickens. Avian Dis 28:426–434.

7. Bradbury, J.M. 1977. Rapid biochemical tests for characterization of the Mycoplasmatales. J Clin Microbiol 5:531–534.

8. Bradbury, J.M. 1983. Mycoplasma iowae—an avian Mycoplasma with unusual properties. Yale J Biol Med 56:912.

9. Bradbury, J.M. 1984. Effect of Mycoplasma iowae infection on the immune system of the young turkey. Isr J Med Sci 20:985–988.

10. Bradbury, J.M., and A. Ideris. 1982. Abnormalities in turkey poults following infection with Mycoplasma iowae. Vet Rec 110:559–560.

11. Bradbury, J.M., and D.F. Kelly. 1991. Mycoplasma iowae infection in broiler breeders. Avian Pathol 20:67–78.

12. Bradbury, J.M., and J.D. McCarthy. 1981. Rupture of the digital flexor tendons of chickens after infection with Mycoplasma iowae. Vet Rec 109:428–429.

13. Bradbury, J.M., and J.D. McCarthy. 1983. Pathogenicity of Mycoplasma iowae for chick embryos. Avian Pathol 12:483–496.

14. Bradbury, J.M., and J.D. McCarthy. 1984. Mycoplasma iowae infection in chicks. Avian Pathol 13:529–543.

15. Bradbury, J.M., A. Ideris, and T.T. Oo. 1988. Mycoplasma iowae infection in young turkeys. Avian Pathol 17:149–171.

16. Christensen, N.H., C.A. Yavari, A.J. McBain, and J.M.

Bradbury. 1994. Investigations into the survival of Mycoplasma gallisepticum, Mycoplasma synoviae and Mycoplasma iowae on materials found in the poultry house environment. Avian Pathol 23:127–143.

17. Dierks, R.E., J.A. Newman, and B.S. Pomeroy. 1967. Characterization of avian mycoplasma. Ann NY Acad Sci 143:170–189.

18. French, N.A. 1994. Effect of incubation-temperature on the gross pathology of turkey embryos. Br Poult Sci 35:363–371.

19. Frey, M.L., S.T. Hawk, and P.A. Hale. 1972. A division by microcomplement fixation tests of previously reported avian Mycoplasma serotypes into identification groups. Avian Dis 16:780–792.

20. Grant, M. 1987. Significance, epidemiology and control methods of Mycoplasma iowae in turkeys. Ph.D. thesis. Council for National Academic Awards.

21. Grau, O., F. Laigret, P. Carle, J.G. Tully, D.L. Rose, and J.M. Bové. 1991. Identification of a plant-derived mollicute as a strain of an avian pathogen Mycoplasma iowae, and its implications for mollicute taxonomy. Int J Syst Bacteriol 41:473–478.

22. Jordan, F.T.W., and M.M. Amin. 1980. A survey of mycoplasma infections in domestic poultry. Res Vet Sci 28:96–100.

23. Jordan, F.T.W., H. Erno, G.S. Cottew, K.H. Hinz, and L. Stipkovits. 1982. Characterization and taxonomic description of 5 mycoplasma serovars (serotypes) of avian origin and their elevation to species rank and further evaluation of the taxonomic status of Mycoplasma synoviae. Int J Syst Bacteriol 32:108–115.

24. Jordan, F.T.W., B.K. Horrocks, and R. Froyman. 1993. A model for testing the efficacy of enrofloxacin (Baytril) administered to turkey hens in the control of Mycoplasma iowae infection in eggs and embryos. Avian Dis 37:1057–1061.

25. Jordan, F.T.W., B.K. Horrocks, and S.K. Jones. 1991. A comparison of Baytril, Tylosin, and Tiamulin in the Control of Mycoplasma iowae infection of turkey poults. Avian Pathol 20:283–289.

26. Jordan, F.T.W., B.K. Horrocks, S.K. Jones, and C.M. Clee. 1992. The production of Mycoplasma iowae infection of turkey poults suitable for monitoring antimicrobials. Avian Pathol 21:307–313.

27. Jordan, F.T.W., C. Yavari, and D.L. Knight. 1987. Some observations on the indirect ELISA for antibodies to Mycoplasma iowae serovar I in sera from turkeys considered to be free from Mycoplasma infections. Avian Pathol 16:307–318.

28. Kempf, I., A. Blanchard, F. Gesbert, M. Guittet, and G. Bennejean. 1994. Comparison of antigenic and pathogenic properties of Mycoplasma iowae strains and development of a PCR-based detection assay. Res Vet Sci 56:179–185.

29. Kempf, I., M. Guittet, F.X. Le Gros, D. Toquin, and G. Bennejean. 1989. Mycoplasma iowae: Field and laboratory studies to evaluate egg transmission in turkeys. Avian Pathol 18:299–305.

30. McClenaghan, M., J.M. Bradbury, and J.N. Howse. 1981. Embryo mortality associated with avian Mycoplasma serotype I. Vet Rec 108:459–460.

31. Mirsalimi, S.M., S. Rosendal, and R.J. Julian. 1989. Colonization of the intestine of turkey embryos exposed to Mycoplasma iowae. Avian Dis 33:310–315.

32. Panangala, V.S., M.M. Gresham, and M.A. Morsy. 1992. Antigenic heterogeneity in Mycoplasma iowae demonstrated with monoclonal antibodies. Avian Dis 36:108–113.

33. Rathore, B.S., G.C. Mohanty, and B.S. Rajya. 1979. Isolation of mycoplasma from oviducts of chickens and their pathogenicity. Indian J Microbiol 19:192–197.

34. Rhoades, K.R. 1981. Turkey airsacculitis: Effect of mixed mycoplasmal infections. Avian Dis 25:131–135.

35. Shah-Majid, M., and S. Rosendal. 1986. Mycoplasma iowae from turkey phallus and semen. Vet Rec 118:435.

36. Shah-Majid, M., and S. Rosendal. 1987. Evaluation of growth of avian mycoplasmas on bile salt agar and in bile broth. Res Vet Sci 43:188–190.

37. Shah-Majid, M., and S. Rosendal. 1987. Oral challenge of turkey poults with Mycoplasma iowae. Avian Dis 31:365–369.

38. Shah-Majid, M., and S. Rosendal. 1992. Serological response of turkeys to the intravaginal inoculation of Mycoplasma iowae. Vet Rec 131:420.

39. Talkington, F.D., and S.H. Kleven. 1983. A classification of laboratory strains of avian Mycoplasma serotypes by direct immunofluorescence. Avian Dis 27:422–429.

40. Trampel, D.W., and F. Goll,Jr. 1994. Outbreak of Mycoplasma iowae infection in commercial turkey poults. Avian Dis 38:905–909.

41. Yoder, H.W.,Jr., and M.S. Hofstad. 1962. A previously unreported serotype of avian mycoplasma. Avian Dis 6:147–160.

42. Yoder, H.W.,Jr., and M.S. Hofstad. 1964. Characterization of avian mycoplasma. Avian Dis 8:481–512.

43. Zhao, S., and R. Yamamoto. 1989. Heterogeneity of Mycoplasma iowae determined by restriction enzyme analysis. J Vet Diagn Invest 1:165–169.

44. Zhao, S., and R. Yamamoto. 1993. Amplification of Mycoplasma iowae using polymerase chain reaction. Avian Dis 37:212–217.

OTHER MYCOPLASMAL INFECTIONS

S. H. Kleven

MYCOPLASMA IMITANS. *Mycoplasma imitans* is of interest because of its close relationship to *M. gallisepticum*. It has been isolated from ducks and geese in France and from a partridge in England. *M. imitans* strains share many phenotypic properties with *M. gallisepticum,* including biochemical reactions, hemadsorption, hemagglutination, and presence of an attachment organelle. The original isolates were initially identified as *M. gallisepticum* on the basis of immunofluorescence and growth-inhibition tests. Further serologic studies indicated that it had only a partial relationship to *M. gallisepticum,* and DNA hybridization studies with the type strains of *M. gallisepticum* showed a DNA homology of 40–46%. Preliminary studies have indicated that it may be pathogenic (4).

A polymerase chain reaction (PCR) procedure developed by Garcia et al. (11) and a PCR which amplifies the 16s rRNA gene followed by restriction fragment-length polymorphism (RFLP) analysis, which are used to identify the species of avian *Mycoplasma* isolates (10), do not differentiate between *M. gallisepticum* and *M. imitans*. A commercially available PCR kit for *M. gallisepticum* (IDEXX, Westbrook, Maine), however, does differentiate between the two species.

Although *M. imitans* has not yet been reported in the United States, and it has not been found in commercial poultry flocks, there is concern about possible misidentification of isolates as *M. gallisepticum* and possible serologic cross-reactions in testing of field flocks.

MYCOPLASMA GALLINARUM INFECTION. *M. gallinarum* has not been considered to be one of the pathogenic avian mycoplasma species, but there is one report of consistent isolation from air sacs and tracheas from a series of broiler flocks that were having higher than normal condemnations due to airsacculitis. One of those isolates had the ability to induce airsacculitis when given in conjunction with Newcastle disease–infectious bronchitis vaccine (17). *M. gallinarum* and *M. gallinaceum* are often isolated as contaminants during attempts to isolate pathogenic avian mycoplasmas.

It was originally classified as avian serotype B (6, 34) and was named *Mycoplasma gallinarum* (8). It grows well on all commonly used avian mycoplasma media, and has characteristics common to all mycoplasmas, including cell and colony morphology, absence of a cell wall, and a requirement for cholesterol. It does not ferment glucose, but reduces tetrazolium, is positive for arginine decarboxylase, and exhibits the film and spots (1). There is genetic heterogeneity among various strains (7) as measured by RFLP analysis of genomic DNA.

M. gallinarum is ordinarily isolated primarily from chickens, but it has also been found in turkeys (2, 13). It has been isolated from jungle fowl (22), ducks (9), and pigeons (21). It is considered to be worldwide in distribution. *M. gallinarum* is commonly isolated as a contaminant during attempts to isolate *M. gallisepticum* or *M. synoviae*, especially from adult chickens. Isolation of *M. gallinarum* from chicken embryos (2) and demonstration of the organism in oviducts (5, 33) suggest the possibility of egg transmission. It is readily identified by immunofluorescence of colonies on agar (31). No serologic test is available.

AVIAN UREAPLASMAS.

Ureaplasmas differ from mycoplasmas primarily in their ability to hydrolyze urea (19). There are several reports of isolation of avian ureaplasmas (12, 18). These organisms subsequently received the name *Ureaplasma gallorale* (19). There are no reports of avian ureaplasma isolation in North America.

Very little is known about the pathogenicity. Artificial challenge of chickens produced no clinical signs or macroscopic lesions (18). Turkeys and chickens challenged with a turkey ureaplasma isolated in Hungary developed fibrinous airsacculitis and serologic responses (24). Ureaplasmas were also isolated in Eastern Europe from turkeys that were experiencing problems with reduced fertility (25).

MYCOPLASMA INFECTIONS OF GEESE.

Three serologically and biochemically distinct mycoplasma species were isolated from geese in Europe (27). One of these has been further characterized and named *Mycoplasma anseris* (3), another was subsequently identified as *Mycoplasma cloacale* (28), and the third was designated strain 1220. Two other isolates, strains 1223 and 1225, also represent two additional species isolated from geese (32).

Clinically, strain 1220 has been associated with reductions in egg production, egg transmission, infertility, inflammation of the cloaca and phallus, and lack of weight gain in hatched goslings (26, 28, 29), but proof of etiology is unclear because mixed mycoplasma species were isolated. Strain 1220, on experimental inoculation of goose embryos and day-old goslings, resulted in embryo mortality and reduced growth of young goslings (29). Strain 1220 has also been implicated in a field syndrome of goslings with respiratory and nervous signs (30). More work needs to be done to clarify the role of these mycoplasmas in the field syndromes described.

MYCOPLASMA INFECTIONS OF PIGEONS.

There are three species of *Mycoplasma* primarily associated with pigeons: *M. columbinasale* (15), *M. columborale,* and *M. columbinum* (23). One or more of these *Mycoplasma* species have been isolated from normal birds (2, 14), as well as birds showing signs of respiratory disease (16, 20, 21). An isolate of *M. columborale* reproduced airsacculitis in chickens (20). Medication of pigeons infected with *M. columborale* with tylosin elicited a favorable response (20, 21). Even though there has been isolation of these organisms from birds showing respiratory signs, and there have been favorable responses to medication, there is no conclusive proof that pigeon mycoplasmas are etio-logically involved in naturally occurring respiratory disease of pigeons.

REFERENCES

1. Barber, T., and J. Fabricant. 1971. A suggested reclassification of avian mycoplasma serotypes. Avian Dis 15:125–138.
2. Bencina, D., D. Dorrer, and T. Tadina. 1987. Mycoplasma species isolated from six avian species. Avian Pathol 16:653–664.
3. Bradbury, J.M., F.T.W. Jordan, T. Shimizu, L. Stipkovits, and Z. Varga. 1988. Mycoplasma anseris sp. nov. found in geese. Int J Syst Bacteriol 38:74–76.
4. Bradbury, J.M., O.M.S. Abdulwahab, C.A. Yavari, J.P. Dupiellet, and J.M. Bové. 1993. Mycoplasma imitans sp-nov is related to Mycoplasma gallisepticum and found in birds. Int J Syst Bacteriol 43:721–728.
5. De Las Mulas, J.M., A. Fernandez, M.A. Sierra, J.B. Poveda, and J. Carranza. 1990. Immunohistochemical demonstration of Mycoplasma gallinarum and Mycoplasma gallinaceum in naturally infected hen oviducts. Res Vet Sci 49:339–345.
6. Dierks, R.E., J.A. Newman, and B.S. Pomeroy. 1967. Characterization of avian mycoplasma. Ann NY Acad Sci 143:170–189.
7. Dovc, P., D. Bencina, and I. Zajc. 1991. Genotypic heterogeneity among strains of Mycoplasma gallinarum. Avian Pathol 20:705–711.
8. Edward, D.G., and E.A. Freundt. 1956. The classification and nomenclature of organisms of the pleuropneumonia group. J Gen Microbiol 14:197–207.
9. El-Ebeedy, A.A., I. Sokkar, A. Soliman, A. Rashwan. and A. Ammar. 1987. Mycoplasma infection of ducks. I. Incidence of mycoplasmas, acholeplasmas and associated E. coli and fungi at Upper Egypt. Isr J Med Sci 23:529.
10. Fan, H., S.H. Kleven, and M.W. Jackwood. 1994. Application of polymerase chain reaction with arbitrarily primers to strain identification of Mycoplasma gallisepticum. IOM Lett 3:443.
11. Garcia, M., M.W. Jackwood, S.H. Kleven, S. Levisohn, and K.-E. Johansson. 1994. Detection of Mycoplasma gallisepticum, M. synoviae, and M. iowae by polymerase chain reaction and species-specific oligonucleotide probes. IOM Lett 3:480.
12. Harasawa, R., K. Koshimizu, I.-J. Pan, and M.F. Barile. 1985. Genomic and phenotypic analyses of avian ureaplasma strains. Jpn J Vet Sci 47:901–909.
13. Jordan, F.T.W., and M.M. Amin. 1980. A survey of mycoplasma infections in domestic poultry. Res Vet Sci 28:96–100.
14. Jordan, F.T.W., J.N. Howse, M.P. Adams, and O.O. Fatunmbi. 1981. The isolation of Mycoplasma columbinum and M. columborale from feral pigeons. Vet Rec 109:450.
15. Jordan, F.T.W., H. Erno, G.S. Cottew, K.H. Hinz, and L. Stipkovits. 1982. Characterization and taxonomic description of five Mycoplasma serovars (serotypes) of avian origin and their elevation to species rank and further evaluation of the taxonomic status of Mycoplasma synoviae. Int J Syst Bacteriol 32:108–115.
16. Keymer, I.F., R.H. Leach, R.A. Clarke, M.E. Bardsley, and R.R. McIntyre. 1984. Isolation of Mycoplasma spp. from racing pigeons (Columba livia). Avian Pathol 13:65–74.
17. Kleven, S.H., C.S. Eidson, and O.J. Fletcher. 1978. Airsacculitis induced in broilers with a combination of Mycoplasma gallinarum and respiratory viruses. Avian Dis 22:707–716.
18. Koshimizu, K., H. Kotani, T. Magaribuchi, T. Yagihashi, K. Shibata, and M. Ogata. 1982. Isolation of ureaplasmas from poultry and experimental infection in chickens. Vet Rec 110:426–429.

19. Koshimizu, K., R. Harasawa, I.-J. Pan, H. Kotani, M. Ogata, E.B. Stephens, and M.F. Barile. 1987. Ureaplasma gallorale sp. nov. from the oropharynx of chickens. Int J Syst Bacteriol 37:333–338.

20. MacOwan, K.J., H.G.R. Jones, C.J. Randall, and F.T.W. Jordan. 1981. Mycoplasma columborale in a respiratory condition of pigeons and experimental airsacculitis of chickens. Vet Rec 109:562.

21. Reece, R.L., L. Ireland, and P.C. Scott. 1986. Mycoplasmosis in racing pigeons. Aust Vet J 63:166–167.

22. Shah-Majid, M. 1987. A case-control study of Mycoplasma gallinarum in the male and female reproductive tract of indigenous fowl. Isr J Med Sci 23:530.

23. Shimizu, T., H. Erno, and H. Nagatomo. 1978. Isolation and characterization of Mycoplasma columbinum and Mycoplasma columborale, two new species from pigeons. Int J Syst Bacteriol 28:538–546.

24. Stipkovits, L., A. Rashwan, and M.Z. Sabry. 1978. Studies on pathogenicity of turkey ureaplasma. Avian Pathol 7:577–582.

25. Stipkovits, L., P.A. Brown, R. Glavits, and R.J. Julian. 1983. The possible role of ureaplasma in a continuous infertility problem in turkeys. Avian Dis 27:513–523.

26. Stipkovits, L., J.M. Bové, M. Rousselot, P. Larrue, M. Labat, and A. Vuillaume. 1984. Studies on mycoplasma infection of laying geese. Avian Pathol 14:57–68.

27. Stipkovits, L., Z. Varga, M. Dobos-Kovacs, and M. Santha. 1984. Biochemical and serological examination of some Mycoplasma strains of goose origin. Acta Vet Hung 32:117–125.

28. Stipkovits, L., Z. Varga, G. Czifra, and M. Dobos-Kovacs. 1986. Occurrence of Mycoplasmas in geese affected with inflammation of the cloaca and phallus. Avian Pathol 15:289–299.

29. Stipkovits, L., Z. Varga, R. Glavits, F. Ratz, and E. Molnar. 1987. Pathological and immunological studies on goose embryos and one-day-old goslings experimentally infected with a Mycoplasma strain of goose origin. Avian Pathol 16:453–468.

30. Stipkovits, L., R. Glavits, E. Ivanics, and E. Szabo. 1993. Additional data on Mycoplasma disease of goslings. Avian Pathol 22:171–176.

31. Talkington, F.D., and S.H. Kleven. 1983. A classification of laboratory strains of avian Mycoplasma serotypes by direct immunofluorescence. Avian Dis 27:422–429.

32. Varga, Z., L. Stipkovits, M. Dobos-Kovacs, and G. Czifra. 1989. Biochemical and serological study of two Mycoplasma strains isolated from geese. Arch Exper Vet Med Leipzig 43:733–736.

33. Wang, Y., K.G. Whithear, and E. Ghiocas. 1990. Isolation of Mycoplasma gallinarum and Mycoplasma gallinaceum from the reproductive tract of hens. Aust Vet J 67:31–32.

34. Yoder, H.W., Jr., and M.S. Hofstad. 1964. Characterization of avian mycoplasma. Avian Dis 8:481–512.

10 Campylobacteriosis

Simon M. Shane

INTRODUCTION. Campylobacteriosis has emerged as a significant zoonotic condition associated with a wide range of food and companion animals (111), in addition to infecting exotic and free-living avian and mammalian species (12). The occurrence of a disease, termed avian vibrionic hepatitis (AVH), was extensively documented during the 10-yr period commencing in 1965 (43). This condition was retrospectively attributed to *Campylobacter jejuni* infection (94), although contemporary epidemiologic evidence fails to support any association between *C. jejuni* and the classic syndrome characterized by hepatopathy (124).

Since various species of domestic poultry serve as reservoir hosts of *C. jejuni* (63, 88), infection is significant primarily in relation to food-borne enterocolitis (37) in consumers of broilers (49), turkeys (2), and potentially eggs (114).

AVIAN VIBRIONIC HEPATITIS

This syndrome was originally described in New Jersey as a chronic hepatodegeneration characterized by low morbidity and variable mortality in mature egg-production flocks by Tudor (134). Subsequent studies in Texas by Delaplane et al. (26) yielded an agent from field cases that could be propagated in 7-day chicken embryos inoculated via the yolk sac. An apparently similar syndrome, avian infectious hepatitis (AIH), was first reported from five flocks in Massachusetts with 35% depression in egg production, morbidity of 10%, and cumulative flock mortality of 15% by Winterfield and Sevoian (143). Gross lesions comprised focal to diffuse hepatic necrosis and subcapsular hemorrhage. Histologic examination revealed lymphocytic and granulocytic foci and bile duct proliferation. It was possible to reproduce hepatopathy in young chicks and mature hens using yolk fluid from embryonated eggs inoculated with liver homogenate from field cases (109). Subsequent work showed the agent to be between 0.3 and 0.5-μ long and sensitive to oxytetracycline and furazolidone (144). Studies on the isolation of the AIH agent confirmed the suitability of the embryonic yolk sac for propagation (108). Investigations performed on isolates derived from field cases of AIH in Iowa by Hofstad et al. (52) yielded a curved, vibriolike microorganism (VLO) that was lethal to embryos. This agent was also sensitive to tetracyclines and furazolidone.

During 1955–1958, similar VLOs were isolated by Peckham (93) from 29 field cases of hepatitis syndrome, which was diagnosed on the basis of flock history, clinical signs, and gross lesions. These VLOs were isolated either by inoculating embryonated eggs with a suspension of liver from affected birds, or by culturing bile on blood agar medium. It is considered significant that liver necrosis could be induced in susceptible chicks after four passages of the agent on blood agar incubated at 37 C under microaerobic conditions. Based on the characterization of the microorganism and its resemblance to isolates obtained from field cases by other workers, the syndrome was termed avian vibrionic hepatitis.

The isolation of a group of thermophilic VLOs from cases of human enterocolitis (64) stimulated comparisons between these organisms and avian isolates derived from cases of AIH/AVH (32). Both groups of microaerophilic curved rods produced catalase and were less tolerant to sodium chloride than VLOs of human origin.

A relationship between the VLOs and the hepatitis syndrome was indicated by the results of studies conducted in New York State (48). Vibriolike organisms were recovered from 47% of bile samples obtained from 30 field cases classified as presumptive AIH/AVH on the basis of history, clinical observations, and gross lesions. In contrast, VLOs were cultured from only 2% of 173 submissions not corresponding to the profile for AIH/AVH. Both brilliant green agar and blood agar were suitable to culture VLOs from bile, and yielded a 32% recovery rate, compared with 35% using embryos.

Studies on field isolates derived from laying flocks in Ontario showed that VLOs isolated from either bile or cecal contents of specific birds showed identical biochemical and serologic criteria. It was also noted that VLOs derived from various submissions showed differences in pathogenicity and ability to colonize the cecum (133). In a recent study on the prevalence of *C. jejuni* in broilers from 44 farms sampled at the time of processing, 21% of 223 livers showing gross necrotic lesions yielded three biotypes of *C. jejuni.* In comparison, an isolation rate of 12% was obtained from 50 unaffected livers, with biotype 2 predominating. These observations would not, however, support the authors' contention that *C. jejuni* was responsible for hepatic lesions (16).

In assessing the literature relating to the AIH/AVH complex, it is evident that a field syndrome in commercial laying hens occurred prior to and during the mid-1960s. The syndrome was characterized by low morbidity and mortality with degeneration of the liver as the principal diagnostic feature. The current enigma facing pathologists and epidemiologists is the complete disappearance of the condition as a clinical entity from the United States and western Europe.

Studies conducted during the past few years have failed to reproduce hepatopathy using strains of *C.*

jejuni derived either from humans or avian species (103, 104). It is noted that only enteritis, characterized by diarrhea, can be induced by infecting newly hatched chicks (141) or poults (69), as well as mammalian food animals (30), exotics (74), and companion species (31).

Necrotic hemorrhagic hepatitis-splenomegaly of commercial laying hens has been described in Canada and regions of the United States. As yet, no etiology has been defined, but *C. jejuni* has been isolated from livers of affected birds (99).

There are two speculative explanations for the disappearance of the AIH/AVH complex. The original condition may have been caused by a pathogen other than the VLO that was isolated; however, the experimental reproduction of the condition with an agent cultured on artificial media tends to disprove this hypothesis (93). It is more probable that the VLO interacted synergistically as an opportunist with some other pathogen (142), analogous to the association between *C. jejuni* and parvovirus in dogs (34) or with immunosuppressive or debilitating agents in humans (77). The primary pathogen or cofactor may have subsequently been eliminated by comprehensive immunization programs introduced during the mid-1960s. There is no conclusive experimental evidence to indicate the VLOs isolated from cases of AIH/AVH complex were in fact campylobacters. Attempts in 1985 to propagate and characterize the agent recovered from frozen lyophilized yolk material stored since 1960 were unsuccessful (21).

CAMPYLOBACTERIOSIS

ETIOLOGY. Campylobacteriosis is attributed to infection by thermophilic members of the genus *Campylobacter* (107). The three species of clinical significance, *C. jejuni, C. coli,* and *C. laridis,* are microaerophilic, gram-negative, spiral, uniflagellate organisms, which demonstrate characteristic darting motility when examined under dark-field illumination (118).

Classification. The nomenclature of the genus *Campylobacter* has been subject to frequent changes in response to emerging biochemical and taxonomic criteria. Various classification schemes for the genus have been described (40, 60) that clearly designate *C. jejuni,* the predominant organism isolated from avian hosts, as a separate and valid species (121), and not a subspecies of *C. fetus*

as in early literature. The phylogeny of the campylobacters has been evaluated on the basis of 16S ribosomal ribonucleic acid sequencing, with *C. jejuni, C. coli,* and *C. laridis* included in Homology Group I (132). *Campylobacter jejuni* is the most frequently occurring member of the thermophilic triad, but *C. coli* may occasionally be isolated from the intestinal tract of poultry and derived meat products (84, 102). *Campylobacter laridis,* previously referred to as an NARTC (nalidixic acid-resistant thermophilic campylobacter) (7), is the remaining species in the related thermophilic group and is isolated mainly from free-living marine birds such as gulls (*Larus* spp.) (58).

Morphology and Staining. Campylobacters are spirally curved rods which appear S-shaped or in "gull-wing" forms, and range in size from 0.2 to 0.8 μ in diameter and 0.5 to 6.0 μ in length. All species are motile and possess a single polar flagellum, although bipolar cells are occasionally observed (120). Campylobacters are gram-negative, but require a fuchsin-based counterstain because of their relative inability to take up saffranin (106).

Growth Requirements. The campylobacters of clinical significance show optimal growth on artificial media at 43 C (118), although minimal growth occurs at 37 C.

Campylobacters are microaerophilic, and satisfactory propagation requires an atmosphere comprising 5% oxygen, 10% carbon dioxide, and 85% nitrogen (98). Purchase of a commercial gas mixture is recommended for laboratories conducting routine isolation of campylobacters. An analysis of alternative methods to achieve a microaerobic environment, including commercial gas packs, torbal and candle jars, or application of Fortner's principle, has demonstrated various disadvantages relating to decreased growth, extended incubation periods, or high cost (44).

Appropriate methods of transport and storage of campylobacters are necessary because these organisms are sensitive to desiccation. An enriched semisolid brucella medium incorporating 10% ovine blood can be used to maintain viability of cultures for transport at 25 C for up to 3 wk (139). Six alternative transport media were compared in a structured study of C. jejuni survival. Cary-Blair medium with decreased agar content was superior to Stuart's medium for storage periods exceeding 7 days at 25 C (76). Both Stuart's fluid medium and Cary-Blair semisolid transport medium are commercially available in plastic tubes with accompanying rayon-tipped swabs to facilitate sampling of biologic material for subsequent submission to a diagnostic laboratory.

During the late 1970s, selective media containing antimicrobial compounds were introduced, simplifying the isolation and propagation of campylobacters (91). Commercial media contain brucella agar, blood agar base, ovine, bovine or equine blood, and various antibiotic additives, including bacitracin, novobiocin, trimethoprim, actidone, cycloheximide, cephalothin, and colistin. Differences in source of blood and antibiotic content of media have been evaluated under field and laboratory conditions. Medium BU-40 was shown to be superior to both Skirrow's and Butzler's media in terms of efficiency of isolation of C. jejuni (82). Preston medium, a selective agar incorporating lysed horse blood and antibiotics yielded higher isolation rates of C. jejuni than Skirrow's, Butzler's, Blaser's, or Campy-BAP media. Recovery can be enhanced by preincubation in Preston enrichment broth (15). A semisolid medium has been developed for transport and enrichment of fecal specimens, which enhances the rate of recovery of C. jejuni from patients receiving antibiotic therapy and from their contacts (19). A blood-free selective medium containing charcoal has been shown to be as effective in isolating C. jejuni as conventional Skirrow's medium (62). Campy-Choc Agar, a charcoal- and blood-free medium, compared favorably with three conventional media which yielded a 0.3% C. jejuni isolation rate in a survey of 2890 human fecal specimens (137).

The current status of isolating enteric pathogens, including campylobacters, has been extensively reviewed with specific reference to selection and preparation of samples, preenrichment, and selective plating. Despite the introduction of immunoassays and gene probes, conventional media provide acceptable selectivity and inhibition for diagnostic and survey purposes (38).

Colonial Morphology. The incubation period for detecting colonial growth generally exceeds 24 hr. With a low concentration of organisms in the inoculum, or when an inhibitory medium is used, incubation for up to 72 hr may be required to observe colony formation (82). On primary isolation, colonies may be either flat, translucent, and gray with a tendency to coalesce, or be raised, opaque, and brown-gray with discrete margins (120). The presence of swarming colonies is attributed to higher moisture content of freshly prepared media in contrast to the discrete colonies formed on media that has aged for a few days prior to inoculation (17). Colonies are nonhemolytic on blood agar (121).

Biochemical Properties. As campylobacters are unable to ferment carbohydrates, energy is derived from the degradation of amino acids. The three thermophilic species of clinical significance all reduce selenite, are oxidase and catalase positive, and indole negative (118). Differentiation between C. jejuni, C. coli, and C. laridis is based on nalidixic acid sensitivity and hippurate hydrolysis (Table 10.1). The additional properties of DNA hydrolysis and rapid production of hydrogen sulfide were incorporated into an extended biotyping scheme for the three species (Table 10.2).

An evaluation of various biochemical characteristics of 264 cultures permitted differentiation between eight species or subspecies of Campylobacter (51, 71).

Other sources have defined up to eight biotypes of C. jejuni based on hydrolysis of DNA and hippurate, and growth on charcoal-yeast extract agar (51). Details concerning biochemical reactions of the thermophilic campylobacters have been com-

Table 10.1. Differentiation among catalase-positive *Campylobacter* species according to biochemical characteristics

Species	Growth at 25 C	Growth at 42 C	Nalidixic acid sensitivity[a]	Hippurate hydrolysis
C. fetus	+	–	R	–
C. coli	+	+	S	–
C. jejuni	–	+	S	+
C. laridis	–	+	R	–

Source: (119).
[a]R = resistant; S = sensitive.

Table 10.2. Biotyping scheme for *Campylobacter jejuni*, *C. coli*, and *C. laridis*

Test	*C. jejuni*				*C. coli*		*C. laridis*	
	I[a]	II	III	IV	I	II	I	II
Hippurate hydrolysis	+	+	+	+	–	–	–	–
Rapid H$_2$S test	–	–	+	+	–	–	+	+
DNA hydrolysis	–	+	–	+	–	+	–	+

Source: (71).
[a]Biotype.

prehensively reviewed with specific reference to differential characteristics to distinguish between field isolates (40, 118, 121).

Resistance to Physical and Chemical Agents and Antibiotics

PHYSICAL AGENTS. Campylobacters are extremely sensitive to desiccation. A suspension of *C. jejuni* impregnated onto a filter paper strip will not survive beyond 2 hr at 20 C (76). Infectivity is retained for up to 4 wk in water at 4 C (9), but *C. jejuni* can remain viable in milk for 3 wk at 4 C and for 24 hr at 25 C (100).

A comprehensive study on the survival of *C. jejuni* in biologic systems showed the organism could multiply in bile stored for 2 months at 37 C, but was rapidly destroyed in human urine at the same temperature. At 4 C, *C. jejuni* retained viability for 3 wk in feces and 5 wk in urine (10). *C. jejuni* persisted for a 10-day period on chicken portions stored at either –9 C or –12 C, and contamination could be detected after 182 days storage at –20 C (145).

Lyophilized cultures of *C. jejuni* in Brucella broth containing 0.16% agar and blood retain viability for many years. When cryoprotective agents such as dimethyl sulfoxide or glycerol are added to heavy suspensions of the organism in brucella broth, survival exceeds 3 yr at –80 C (121).

Irradiation pasteurization at a dose of 1.0 kGy from a cobalt-60 source effectively eliminated *C. jejuni* surface contamination at a level of 10^3 colony-forming units (CFU)/cm^2 (146).

CHEMICAL RESISTANCE. The in vitro sensitivity of *C. jejuni* to various disinfectants was assessed using three strains of the organism isolated from diarrheic human patients. A 1:200,000 solution of 5% sodium hypochlorite and a 2.5% solution of 10% formaldehyde both destroyed *C. jejuni* within 15 min. Contact with 0.15% organic phenol, a 1:50,000 quaternary-ammonium compound, or 0.125% glutaraldehyde killed a 10^7 CFU suspension of *C. jejuni* within 1 min (140). Resistance to chemical agents is increased by the protective action of biological material. In a comparative study of the efficacy of chemical disinfectants used in the food industry, it was shown that 3% succinic acid, 0.5% glutaraldehyde, and 25 ppm poly-(hexamethylenebiguanide hydrochloride) were all able to reduce significantly the level of *C. jejuni* contamination on the surface of chicken drumsticks. Chlorine levels below 120 ppm were ineffective under conditions simulating immersion in poultry processing plant tanks (146).

ANTIBIOTIC SENSITIVITY. The antibiotic sensitivity of the three thermophilic campylobacters has been extensively documented (61, 121). A study conducted in Sweden showed close similarity in antibiotic sensitivity between approximately 75 isolates derived from diarrheic human patients and from processed broilers. The majority of isolates were sensitive to erythromycin and doxycycline, although a high proportion of strains were resistant to the tetracyclines, and an acceptable response to gentamicin, chloramphenicol, and carbenicillin was obtained (129). Similar results were achieved in an investigation involving 276 food animal isolates, including 107 derived from chickens and 403 human fecal isolates from patients admitted to a hospital in Brussels. Furazolidone was shown to be the most effective compound, with most human and animal isolates also sensitive to erythromycin and gentamicin. Approximately 26% of the chicken strains were resistant to tetracycline (136). In evaluating the efficacy of 16 antimicrobial compounds against 103 clinical isolates of *C. jejuni*, kanamycin and gentamicin were shown to be completely effective, in contrast to tetracycline, penicillin G, and erythromycin. Approximately 38%, 36%, and 13% of the isolates were resistant to these three compounds, respectively (79). The biochemical mechanisms and genetic aspects of antibiotic resistance in campylobacters have been comprehensively reviewed in relation to quinolones, tetracyclines, aminoglycosides, and macrolides (131).

Serotyping. A significant advance in serotyping *C. jejuni* was achieved with the introduction of the Penner scheme based on soluble, heat-stable "O" antigens derived from surface lipopolysaccharides (95). Antisera produced in rabbits can be applied to a passive hemagglutination technique to identify 60 serotypes of *C. jejuni.* Subsequent studies showed that *C. jejuni* and *C. coli* have individual antigens, with minimal commonality between species (96). The alternative Lior serotyping scheme is based on heat-labile "H" antigens (72). This system is read using slide agglutination and requires multiple absorption of heterogenous antisera. In a comparison between the two schemes, the Penner technique was found to be marginally more specific than the Lior system and, although requiring more equipment, was faster under practical conditions in a diagnostic laboratory (92).

Bacterial restriction endonuclease DNA analysis (BRENDA) has been used to differentiate campylobacters. An epidemiologic study has demonstrated that 50% of a sample of 316 isolates of *C. jejuni,* representing 11 of 60 BRENDA types, were common to both humans and poultry (57).

PATHOGENESIS AND EPIZOOTIOLOGY

Natural Hosts.   Poultry serve as primary reservoir hosts of thermophilic campylobacters (41). Up to 90% of broilers may be infected (8), while 100% of turkeys (70, 74, 76) and 88% of domestic ducks (97) may harbor the organisms.

Various species of *Campylobacter* have been isolated from free-ranging pigeons in the United States (75) and Japan (65). Infection has been recorded among game birds, including partridges, pheasants (138), and quail (80). Campylobacters have been isolated from marine birds such as puffins (59) and gulls (58), from waders (39), and migratory Anseriformes (89). Approximately 8% of samples taken from eight species (Columbiformes and Passeriformes) in a Japanese investigation yielded *C. jejuni.* It was noted that numerically higher recovery rates were obtained from scavengers and omnivores than from granivores (54). The prevalence of *C. jejuni* in avian species is a function of the intensity of surveillance, since diligent collection and culturing will generally reveal intestinal infection in many orders of exotic and domestic birds within a specific area (3, 147).

Experimental Hosts.   The wide range of laboratory animal species susceptible to *C. jejuni* includes rabbits, mice, rats, hamsters, and primates (33). Animal models for campylobacter enterocolitis in humans include mice (13), hamsters (35), and ferrets (36).

Campylobacters can be propagated in vitro in tissue culture systems, including Chinese hamster ovary cells (45), HeLa cells (28), and human epithelial cell lines (18). Fertile chicken eggs serve as a convenient system for isolation and propagation of campylobacters. Both *C. jejuni* and *C. coli* infection of embryos can be achieved by either the chorioallantoic route or by direct intravenous injection on the 11th day of incubation (29). The embryo system can be used as a model to differentiate between the relative virulence of various strains of *C. jejuni* and *C. coli* derived from cases of human and animal enterocolitis. Fecal isolates of *C. jejuni* obtained from chickens and turkeys are lethal when introduced via the yolk sac route into embryonated eggs of the corresponding species (69).

Transmission.   Despite the fact that C. jejuni is prevalent as an intestinal commensal in floor-housed turkeys, broiler breeders, and layer-type breeder chickens, there is no evidence to show that campylobacters can be transmitted vertically by either transovarian infection or by penetration of the egg shell after oviposition. An extensive survey failed to demonstrate *C. jejuni* in fertile turkey eggs and poults derived from a flock known to carry the organism (1). Another study showed that *C. jejuni* did not penetrate the shells of eggs produced by cage-housed hens, despite recovery of the organism from the intestinal tract and feces (27). Infrequent isolation of *C. jejuni* from the inner and outer membranes of refrigerated eggs is attributable to shell damage. Failure to demonstrate *C. jejuni* within or on the surface of table eggs was confirmed in field studies conducted on three farms in Louisiana (114) and on 23 units in New York (6). It is possible to induce egg-penetration by immersion in a suspension of *C. jejuni* (86) or by using either temperature or pressure differential techniques (22). It is concluded that under practical commercial conditions, desiccation will destroy organisms on the surface of clean eggs within a short period following oviposition. Artificial contamination of eggs with a fecal suspension of *C. jejuni* showed that viability did not exceed 16 hr, and that 50% of the artificially contaminated egg shells were free of viable campylobacters within 10 hr (114). Rejection of grossly soiled eggs, physical removal of small quantities of fecal material adherent to the shell surface, and fumigation or chemical disinfection within 2 hr of collection will all reduce the possibility of egg-borne transmission of campylobacters (115).

Experiments have conclusively demonstrated that contamination of feed and water by chronic intestinal carriers transmits *C. jejuni* to susceptible contacts (81). This study also showed that intestinal infection persisted for at least 63 days in broilers housed on wire-mesh floors, which prevented coprophagy.

Houseflies (*Musca domestica*) can acquire *C. jejuni* from contaminated litter and are capable of transmitting infection to susceptible chicks under controlled experimental conditions (113). A field investigation that revealed 50% of houseflies in the vicinity of a poultry farm were infected with *C. jejuni* (101) and the recovery of the organism from cockroaches (135) imply that insects may play a role in transmission of campylobacteriosis.

The presence of *C. jejuni* in the feces of domestic sparrows captured in a turkey house suggests the role of free-living birds in introducing infection into commercial poultry flocks (1, 122).

Surveys on broilers (85) and turkey flocks (1) showed that chicks and poults remain uninfected for up to 3 wk when placed into thoroughly disinfected houses containing new litter. Both *C. jejuni* and *C. coli* can be introduced into houses by nonconfined companion animals, vermin, and footwear contaminated with feces and litter (4). Campylobacters are spread rapidly within flocks by horizontal, fecal-oral infection. Consumption of fecally contaminated feed and litter and nonchlorinated water dispensed from trough-type drinkers contribute to dissemination of the organism (41). Poultry strains of *C. jejuni* have a marked capacity to spread horizontally among chicks in hatchers during the last 24 hr of incubation, and with subsequent posthatch processing. Artificial infection of one chick in a hatcher resulted in recovery of *C. jejuni* from 70% of the intestines of contact chicks after 24 hr (23).

Incubation Period. *Campylobacter jejuni* colonized the intestinal tracts of 62% of a batch of susceptible day-old broiler chicks within 24 hr of administration of either 10^2 CFU by the intracloacal route, or 10^4 CFU instilled into the crop. The proportion of chicks yielding *C. jejuni* on cloacal swabs increased to 88 and 97%, respectively, on the 3rd and 4th days postinfection (116). In Japanese quail, *C. jejuni* could be recovered from feces (4 CFU/g) 1 day after receiving an oral dose of 10^8 CFU (78).

Clinical Signs. The severity of clinically detectable changes, usually confined to depression and diarrhea, is dependent on infective dose, strain of *C. jejuni* or *C. coli,* and age of the host. Concurrent environmental stress factors or intercurrent disease and immunosuppression may exacerbate the pathogenicity of *C. jejuni.*

A pathogenic, invasive strain of *C. jejuni* isolated from diarrheic human patients in Mexico produced diarrhea in 88% of a batch of day-old chicks which received 10^8 organisms orally. Within 24 to 72 hr, affected chicks showed depression, fecal saturation of the vent plumage, and watery droppings, which persisted for 8 days. Mortality of 32% was recorded in infected chicks from which *C. jejuni* could be isolated from the heart blood and intestinal tract (103). Infection of holoxenic (conventionally-reared) chicks with *C. jejuni* in a trial designed to investigate competitive exclusion, resulted in transient diarrhea (123). Similar observations were made in broiler chicks that were inoculated with 10^3 to 10^6 CFU of *C. jejuni* derived from diarrheic patients in Bangladesh (104).

In contrast, experimental infections have not produced any clinical abnormalities in broiler chicks aged either 2-3 days or 3 wk, although intestinal colonization was achieved by inoculation via both the oral and cloacal routes (116). In a comparison of age susceptibility, diarrhea was induced in chicks within 12 hr of hatch compared with birds 3 days of age which were unaffected by an oral dose of 10^9 CFU. Signs of *C. jejuni* infection included diarrhea, characterized by the presence of mucus and blood, commencing 6 hr after inoculation and extending for 10 days. Recurrence of diarrhea was noted in the subjects housed on raised wire-mesh floors, which inhibited coprophagy (141).

C. jejuni isolated from feces of turkeys produced transient foamy diarrhea and depressed 21-day body weight in poults infected at either 2 or 4 days of age with 5×10^6 CFU by the oral route. In contrast, chicken-origin *C. jejuni* was apathogenic when introduced into 2- and 3-day-old chicks (69). Intestinal colonization of non–clinically affected broilers may be influenced by genetic factors presumably associated with the major histocompatibility complex controlled by immune-response genes designated "Gregion" (128).

Gross Lesions. The principal change associated with *C. jejuni* infection in chicks comprises distention of the intestinal tract extending from the distal duodenal loop to the bifurcation of the ceca. Accumulation of mucus and watery fluid occurs (104), and depending on the cytotoxic properties of the *Campylobacter* involved, hemorrhages may be present (141), consistent with observations in human campylobacteriosis (66).

The presence of red or yellow mottling of the liver parenchyma was noted in newly hatched chicks subjected to contact infection by toxigenic and invasive strains of *C. jejuni* during the last 24 hr of incubation (23). This observation may relate to an experiment in which focal hepatic necrosis was induced in 60% of a batch of experimentally infected chicks which received the immunosuppressive agent cyclophosphamide. Untreated control chicks infected with *C. jejuni* failed to show liver lesions (124). It is likely that an intact and functional immune system is required to prevent dissemination of the organism from the intestinal tract (14).

Histologic Lesions. Histologic changes attributed to *C. jejuni* infection include congestion and mononuclear cell infiltration of the lamina propria and destruction of mucosal cells in the entire intestinal tract. Edema of the mucosa was noted in the ileum and ceca, with accumulation of mucus, erythrocytes, mononuclear cells, and a few polymorphonuclear cells in the lumen. Within 48 hr of infection, hyperplasia and villous atrophy were evident in the distal jejunum. Electron microscopy revealed the presence of campylobacters within and between cells of the epithelium and lamina propria (141).

In mild cases characterized by distention of the jejunum, microscopic changes were confined to submucosal edema with gram-negative curved rods adherent to the brush border and within enterocytes (104).

DIAGNOSIS. Thermophilic campylobacters can be isolated from feces, and cecal and jejunal contents. With systemic infection, the organism can also be recovered from liver tissue, bile, and blood. Because of the sensitivity of campylobacters to desiccation, special precautions are required when submitting fecal or other biologic material to a diagnostic laboratory. It is advisable to sample using a commercially available transport system comprising a rayon-tipped swab, which is inserted into a tube containing Cary-Blair medium. Bile samples can be obtained by direct aspiration from the gallbladder using a sterile tuberculin syringe.

Isolation of thermophilic campylobacters requires incubation of cultures for 48–72 hr at 43 C in a microaerobic atmosphere. Selective media are required to suppress the growth of contaminants in fecal and other biologic samples (91). Differentiation between *C. jejuni, C. coli,* and *C. laridis,* and their biotypes, can be achieved applying the criteria of incubation temperature, nalidixic acid sensitivity, hippurate hydrolysis, and hydrogen sulfide production (71, 119). A serotyping scheme, such as the Penner system, can be used to identify specific organisms for epidemiologic investigations (96).

A 45-kD outer-membrane protein of *C. jejuni* can be detected in cultures of the organism by applying on oligonucleotide probe in a dot-hybridization assay (67).

PUBLIC HEALTH SIGNIFICANCE. Human campylobacteriosis is a food-borne condition of emerging significance (11, 24, 110, 112). During 1984, the *Campylobacter* isolation rate in the United States attained 4.9/100,000 population, with *C. jejuni* representing 99% of the species cultured (130). This estimate grossly understates the actual prevalence of campylobacteriosis, which may be responsible for 2.1 million cases annually in the United States (83). Projections of cost associated with diagnosis and treatment of human campylobacteriosis, including lost productivity and deaths, range from 700 million to 1400 million dollars per annum.

Early studies on the epidemiology of intestinal campylobacteriosis in human populations demonstrated that consumption of chicken meat was a significant risk factor (12, 87, 117). The high carriage rate of campylobacters in the intestinal tract of broilers (47) and turkeys (73) contributes to contamination during processing (42). This is reflected in high levels of *C. jejuni* on poultry meat (90). Recovery of campylobacters from chicken carcasses is approximately six times higher than from pork or beef, and ranges from 30% to 100% of specimens surveyed (125).

The association of campylobacters with poultry meat represents a significant potential for human food-borne infection under conditions of defective handling, inadequate refrigeration, and improper preparation (25, 53). The correlation between specific *C. jejuni* and *C. coli* serotypes in poultry and in diarrheic humans has been documented, with Penner groups 2, 5, 7, 9, and 22 predominating (5). The staff of poultry processing plants are exposed to campylobacteriosis by handling contaminated material, and the condition may be regarded as an occupational disease (46, 56). An outbreak of *Campylobacter* enteritis in Sweden involved 71% of a group of 24 temporary workers who became ill within 2 wk of commencing employment in a poultry plant. In contrast, only 30% of the long-term employees were infected (20). The dynamics of *Campylobacter* contamination of poultry meat and its relationship to human intestinal infection have been extensively documented following completion of a comprehensive epidemiologic study conducted in King County, Washington (49, 50).

Based on field surveys showing a low prevalence of egg shell contamination with *C. jejuni,* and the sensitivity of the organism to desiccation and approved industrial egg-washing compounds, it is unlikely that campylobacteriosis is attributable to consumption of commercially produced table eggs (55).

PREVENTION AND CONTROL. It is impractical to apply preventive action to reduce *Campylobacter* infection in broiler flocks reared on litter. Although extreme biosecurity measures may limit the introduction of campylobacters into breeding farms, current practices in the U.S. broiler industry contribute to infection before depletion. Under commercial conditions, unrestricted movement of personnel, recycling of litter, and the use of earth-floor convection-ventilated housing subject to ingress by flies, vermin, and possibly wild birds, all contribute to colonization of the intestinal tract with *C. jejuni* and *C. coli* (112). Since coprophagy ensures rapid horizontal spread within a flock (81), the expedient of multitier mesh-floor growing would be required to reduce or obviate transmission. Thorough decontamination, including removal of litter and disinfection of equipment and buildings, followed by a rest period of at least 7 days, will effectively eliminate residual campylobacters in poultry housing (37).

Despite early studies showing the inhibition of *Campylobacter* colonization of the intestinal tract by competitive exclusion flora (124), recent trials have shown variable results in reducing infection rates (116). Defined cultures comprising *Citrobacter diversus, Klebsiella pneumonia,* and *Escherichia coli* in combination with 2.5% dietary mannose significantly reduced intestinal colonization rates, but did not eliminate infection (105). These findings are attributed to the association of *C. jejuni* with the intraluminal mucin layer and failure of the organism to adhere to enterocytes (127).

Although it is unrealistic to achieve complete elimination of *Campylobacter* infection during the growing period, it is possible to ameliorate processing plant contamination by disinfecting transport coops and by withholding feed for at least 8 hr prior to flock depletion. Postprocessing decontamination of carcasses and portions with chemical solutions will reduce the level of *C. jejuni*. A 0.5% acetic or lactic acid rinse effectively limits levels of viable organisms under controlled laboratory conditions (126). Subsequent studies have shown that 120 ppm chlorine, warm succinic acid, and 0.5% glutaraldehyde all reduced *C. jejuni* contamination of drumsticks (146). Gamma radiation of poultry meat at subradicidation (pasteurization) levels of 1–5 kGy using a cobalt-60 source will eliminate campylobacters without inducing any undesirable organoleptic or biochemical changes in product (68).

REFERENCES

1. Acuff, G.R., C. Vanderzant, F.A. Gardner, and F.A. Golan. 1982. Examination of turkey eggs, poults and brooder house facilities for Campylobacter jejuni. J Food Prot 45:1279–1281.

2. Acuff, G.R., C. Vanderzant, M.O. Hanna, J.G. Ehlers, F.A. Golan, and F.A. Gardner. 1986. Prevalence of Campylobacter jejuni in turkey carcass processing and further processing of turkey products. J Food Prot 49:712–717.

3. Adekeye, J.O., P.A. Abdu, and E.K. Bawa. 1989. Campylobacter fetus subsp. jejuni in poultry reared under different management systems in Nigeria. Avian Dis 33:801–803.

4. Annan-Prah, A., and M. Janc. 1988. The mode of spread of Campylobacter jejuni/coli to broiler flocks. Zentralbl Veterinarmed [B] 35:11–18.

5. Annan-Prah, A., and M. Janc. 1988. Chicken-to-human infection with Campylobacter jejuni and Campylobacter coli: Biotype and serotype correlation. J Food Prot 51:562–564.

6. Baker, R.C., M.D.C. Paredes, and R.A. Qureshi. 1987. Prevalence of Campylobacter jejuni in eggs and poultry meat in New York State. Poult Sci 66:1766–1770.

7. Benjamin, J., S. Leaper, R.J. Owen, amd M.B. Skirrow. 1983. Description of Campylobacter laridis, a new

species comprising the nalidixic acid-resistant thermophilic Campylobacter (NARTC) group. Curr Microbiol 8:231–238.

8. Blaser, M.J. 1982. Campylobacter jejuni and food. Food Technol 36:89–92.

9. Blaser, M.J., F.M. LaForce, N.A. Wilson, and W.L.L. Wang. 1980. Reservoirs for human campylobacteriosis. J Infect Dis 141:665–669.

10. Blaser, M.J., H.L. Hardesty, B. Powers, and W-L.L. Wang. 1980. Survival of Campylobacter fetus subsp jejuni in biological milieus. J Clin Microbiol 11:309–313.

11. Blaser, M.J., P. Checko, C. Bopp, A. Bruce, and J.M. Hughes. 1982. Campylobacter enteritis associated with foodborne transmission. Am J Epidemiol 116:886–894.

12. Blaser, M.J., D.N. Taylor, and R.A. Feldman. 1983. Epidemiology of Campylobacter jejuni infections. Epidemiol Rev 5:157–176.

13. Blaser, M.J., D.J. Duncan, G.H. Warren, and W-L.L. Wang. 1983. Experimental Campylobacter jejuni infection of adult mice. Infect Immun 39:908–916.

14. Blaser, M.J., P.F. Smith, J.E. Repine, and K.A. Joiner. 1988. Pathogenesis of Campylobacter fetus infections. J Clin Invest 81:1434–1444.

15. Bolton, F.J., D. Coates, P.M. Hinchliffe, and L. Robertson. 1983. Comparison of selective media for isolation of Campylobacter jejuni/coli. J Clin Pathol 36:78–83.

16. Boukraa, L., S. Messier, and Y. Robinson. 1991. Isolation of campylobacter from livers of broiler chickens with and without hepatic lesions. Avian Dis 35:714–717.

17. Buck, G.E., and M.T. Kelly. 1981. Effect of moisture content of the medium on colony morphology of Campylobacter fetus subsp jejuni. J Clin Microbiol 14:585–586.

18. Bukholm, G., and G. Kapperud. 1987. Expression of Campylobacter jejuni invasiveness in cell cultures coinfected with other bacteria. Infect Immun 55:2816–2821.

19. Chan, F.T.H., and A.M.R. Mackenzie. 1986. Evaluation of primary selective media and enrichment methods for Campylobacter species isolation. Eur J Clin Microbiol 5:162–164.

20. Christenson, B., Å. Ringer, C. Blücher, H. Billaudelle, K.N. Gundtoft, G. Eriksson, and M. Böttiger. 1983. An outbreak of Campylobacter enteritis among the staff of a poultry abbatoir in Sweden. Scand J Infect Dis 15:167–172.

21. Clark, A.G. 1986. The effect of toxigenic and invasive human strains of Campylobacter jejuni on broiler hatchability and health. Proc 35th West Poult Dis Conf, pp. 25–27.

22. Clark, A.G., and D.H. Bueschkens. 1985. Laboratory infection of chicken eggs with Campylobacter jejuni by using temperature or pressure differentials. Appl Environ Microbiol 49:1467–1471.

23. Clark, A.G., and D.H. Bueschkens. 1988. Horizontal spread of human and poultry-derived strains of Campylobacter jejuni among broiler chicks held in incubators and shipping boxes. J Food Prot 51:438–441.

24. Cruickshank, J.G. 1986. Salmonella and Campylobacter infections: an update. J Small Anim Pract 27:673–681.

25. de Boer, E., and M. Hahne. 1990. Cross-contamination with Campylobacter jejuni and Salmonella spp. from raw chicken products during food preparation. J Food Prot 53:1067–1068.

26. Delaplane, J.P., H.A. Smith, and R.W. Moore. 1955. An unidentified agent causing a hepatitis in chickens. Southwest Vet 8:356–361.

27. Doyle, M.P. 1984. Association of Campylobacter jejuni with laying hens and eggs. Appl Environ Microbiol 47:533–536.

28. Fauchere, J.L., A. Rosenau, M. Veron, E.N. Moyen, S. Richard, and A. Pfister. 1986. Association with HeLa cells of Campylobacter jejuni and Campylobacter coli isolated from human feces. Infect Immun 54:283–287.

29. Field, L.H., V.L. Headley, J.L. Underwood, S.M. Payne, and L.J. Berry. 1986. The chicken embryo as a model

for Campylobacter invasion: Comparative virulence of human isolates of Campylobacter jejuni and Campylobacter coli. Infect Immun 54:118–125.

30. Firehammer, B.D., and L.L. Myers. 1981. Campylobacter fetus subsp jejuni: its possible significance in enteric disease of calves and lambs. Am J Vet Res 42:918–922.

31. Fleming, M.P. 1983. Association of Campylobacter jejuni with enteritis in dogs and cats. Vet Rec 113:372–374.

32. Fletcher, R.D., and W.N. Plastridge. 1964. Difference in physiology of Vibrio spp. from chickens and man. Avian Dis 8:72–75.

33. Fox, J.G. 1982. Campylobacteriosis—a "new" disease in laboratory animals. Lab Anim Sci 32:625–637.

34. Fox, J.G., R. Moore, and J.I. Ackerman. 1983. Campylobacter jejuni-associated diarrhea in dogs. J Am Vet Med Assoc 183:1430–1433.

35. Fox, J.G., S. Zanotti, H.V. Jordan, and J.C. Murphy. 1986. Colonization of Syrian hamsters with streptomycin resistant Campylobacter jejuni. Lab Anim Sci 36:28–31.

36. Fox, J.G., J.I. Ackerman, N. Taylor, M. Claps, and J.C. Murphy. 1987. Campylobacter jejuni infection in the ferret: An animal model of human campylobacteriosis. Am J Vet Res 48:85–90.

37. Franco, D.A. 1988. Campylobacter species: Considerations for controlling a foodborne pathogen. J Food Prot 51:145–153.

38. Fricker, C.R. 1987. The isolation of salmonellas and campylobacters. J Appl Bacteriol 63:99–116.

39. Fricker, C.R., and N. Metcalfe. 1984. Campylobacters in wading birds (Charadrii): Incidence, biotypes and isolation techniques. Zentralbl Bakteriol Mikrobiol Hyg [B] 179:469–475.

40. Garcia, M.M., M.D. Eaglesome, and C. Rigby. 1983. Campylobacters important in veterinary medicine. Vet Bull 53:793–818.

41. Genigeorgis, C. 1986. Significance of campylobacter in poultry. Proc 35th West Poult Dis Conf, pp. 54–59.

42. Genigeorgis, C., M. Hassuneh, and P. Collins. 1986. Campylobacter jejuni infection on poultry farms and its effect on poultry meat contamination during slaughtering. J Food Prot 49:895–903.

43. Gerlach, H., and I. Gylstorff. 1967. Untersuchungen über biochemische Eigenschaften, Pathogenität und Resistenzspektrum gegen Antibiotika bei Vibrio metschnikovi. Berl Munch Tierarztl Wochenschr 80:153–155, 161–164.

44. Goossens, H., M. De Boeck, H. Van Landuyt, and J.P. Butzler. 1984. Isolation of Campylobacter jejuni from human feces. In J.P. Butzler (ed.). Campylobacter Infection in Man and Animals. CRC Press, Inc, FL, pp. 39–50.

45. Goossens, H., E. Rummens, S. Cadranel, J-P. Butzler, and Y. Takeda. 1985. Cytotoxic activity on Chinese hamster ovary cells in culture filtrates of Campylobacter jejuni/coli. Lancet ii:511.

46. Grados, O., N. Bravo, J.P. Butzler, and G. Ventura. 1983. Campylobacter infection: an occupational disease risk in chicken handlers. Campylobacter II, Proc Int Workshop on Campylobacter Infect, Public Health Laoratory Service, London, p. 162.

47. Grant, I.H., N.J. Richardson, and V.D. Bokkenheuser. 1980. Broiler chickens as potential source of Campylobacter infections in humans. J Clin Microbiol 11:508–510.

48. Hagan, J.R. 1964. Diagnostic techniques in avian vibrionic hepatitis. Avian Dis 8:428–437.

49. Harris, N.V., D. Thompson, D.C. Martin, and C.M. Nolan. 1986. A survey of Campylobacter and other bacterial contaminants of pre-market chicken and retail poultry and meats, King County, Washington. Am J Public Health 76:401–406.

50. Harris, N.V., N.S. Weiss, and C.M. Nolan. 1986. The role of poultry and meats in the etiology of Campylobacter jejuni/coli enteritis. Am J Public Health 76:407–411.

51. Hébert, G.A., D.G. Hollis, R.E. Weaver, M.A. Lambert, M.J. Blaser, and C.W. Moss. 1982. 30 years of campylobacters: Biochemical characteristics and a biotyping proposal for Campylobacter jejuni. J Clin Microbiol 15:1065–1073.

52. Hofstad, M.S., E.H. McGehee, and P.C. Bennett. 1958. Avian infectious hepatitis. Avian Dis 2:358–364.

53. Istre, G.R., M.J. Blaser, P. Shillam, and R.S. Hopkins. 1984. Campylobacter enteritis associated with undercooked barbecued chicken. Am J Public Health 74:1265–1267.

54. Ito, K., Y. Kubokura, K. Kaneko, Y. Totake, and M. Ogawa. 1988. Occurrence of Campylobacter jejuni in free-living wild birds from Japan. J Wildl Dis 24:467–470.

55. Izat, A.L., and F.A. Gardner. 1988. Incidence of Campylobacter jejuni in processed egg products. Poult Sci 67:1431–1435.

56. Jones, D.M., and D.A. Robinson. 1981. Occupational exposure to Campylobacter jejuni infection. Lancet i:440–441.

57. Kakoyiannis, C.K., P.J. Winter, and R.B. Marshall. 1988. The relationship between intestinal Campylobacter species isolated from animals and humans as determined by BRENDA. Epidemiol Infect 100:379–387.

58. Kaneuchi, C., T. Imaizumi, Y. Sugiyama, Y. Kosako, M. Seki, T. Itoh, and M. Ogata. 1987. Thermophilic campylobacters in seagulls and DNA-DNA hybridization test of isolates. Jpn J Vet Sci 49:787–794.

59. Kapperud, G., O. Rosef, O.W. Rostad, and G. Lid. 1983. Isolation of Campylobacter fetus subsp jejuni from the common puffin (Fratercula arctica) in Norway. J Wildl Dis 19:64–65.

60. Karmali, M.A., and M.B. Skirrow. 1984. Taxonomy of the genus Campylobacter. In J.P. Butzler (ed.). Campylobacter Infection in Man and Animals. CRC Press, Boca Raton, FL, pp. 1–20.

61. Karmali, M.A., S. De Grandis, and P.C. Fleming. 1981. Antimicrobial susceptibility of Campylobacter jejuni with special reference to resistance patterns of Canadian isolates. Antimicrob Agents Chemother 19:593–597.

62. Karmali, M.A., A.E. Simor, M. Roscoe, P.C. Fleming, S.S. Smith, and J. Lane. 1986. Evaluation of a blood-free, charcoal-based, selective medium for the isolation of Campylobacter organisms from feces. J Clin Microbiol 23:456–459.

63. Kasrazadeh, M., and C. Genigeorgis. 1987. Origin and prevalence of Campylobacter jejuni in ducks and duck meat at the farm and processing plant level. J Food Prot 50:321–326.

64. King, E.O. 1957. Human infections with Vibrio fetus and a closely related vibrio. J Infect Dis 101:119–128.

65. Kinjo, T., M. Morishige, N. Minamoto, and H. Fukushi. 1983. Prevalence of Campylobacter jejuni in feral pigeons. Jpn J Vet Sci 45:833–835.

66. Klipstein, F.A., R.F. Engert, H. Short, and E.A. Schenk. 1985. Pathogenic properties of Campylobacter jejuni: Assay and correlation with clinical manifestations. Infect Immun 50:43–49.

67. Lam, K.M. 1992. Use of a 45 kDa protein in the detection of Campylobacter jejuni. Avian Pathol 21:643–650.

68. Lam, K.M., A.J. DaMassa, T.Y. Morashita, H.L. Shivaprasad, and A.A. Bickford. 1992. Pathogenicity of Campylobacter jejuni for turkeys and chickens. Avian Dis 36:359–363.

69. Lambert, J.D., and R.B. Maxcy. 1984. Effect of gamma radiation of Campylobacter jejuni. J Food Sci 49:665–667.

70. Lammerding, A.M., M.M. Garcia, E.D. Mann, Y. Robinson, W.J. Dorward, R.B. Truscott, and F. Tittiger. 1988. Prevalence of Salmonella and thermophilic Campylobacter in fresh pork, beef, veal and poultry in Canada. J Food Prot 51:47–52.

71. Lior, H. 1984. New, extended biotyping scheme for

Campylobacter jejuni, Campylobacter coli, and "Campylobacter laridis." J Clin Microbiol 20:636–640.

72. Lior, H., D.L. Woodward, J.A. Edgar, L.J. Laroche, and P. Gill. 1982. Serotyping of Campylobacter jejuni by slide agglutination based on heat-labile antigenic factors. J Clin Microbiol 15:761–768.

73. Luechtefeld, N.W., and W-L.L. Wang. 1981. Campylobacter fetus subsp jejuni in a turkey processing plant. J Clin Microbiol 13:266–268.

74. Luechtefeld, N.W., and W-L.L. Wang. 1982. Animal reservoirs of Campylobacter jejuni. In D.G. Newell (ed.). Campylobacter. Epidemiology, Pathogenesis and Biochemistry. MTP Press, Lancaster, UK, pp. 249–252.

75. Luechtefeld, N.W., R.C. Cambre, and W-L.L. Wang. 1981. Isolation of Campylobacter jejuni from zoo animals. J Am Vet Med Assoc 179:1119–1122.

76. Luechtefeld, N.W., W-L.L. Wang, M.J. Blaser, and L.B. Reller. 1981. Evaluation of transport and storage techniques for isolation of Campylobacter fetus subsp jejuni from turkey cecal specimens. J Clin Microbiol 13:438–443.

77. Mandal, B.K., P. De Mol, and J.P. Butzler. 1984. Clinical aspects of Campylobacter infections in humans. In J.P. Butzler (ed.). Campylobacter Infection in Man and Animals. CRC Press, Boca Raton, FL, pp. 21–31.

78. Maruyama, S., and Y. Katsube. 1988. Intestinal colonization of Campylobacter jejuni in young Japanese quails (Coturnix coturnix japonica). Jpn J Vet Sci 50:569–572.

79. Michel, J., M. Rogol, and D. Dickman. 1983. Susceptibility of clinical isolates of Campylobacter jejuni to sixteen antimicrobial agents. Antimicrob Agents Chemother 23:796–797.

80. Minakshi, S.C.D., and A. Ayyagari. 1988. Isolation of Campylobacter jejuni from quails: an initial report. Br Vet J 144:411–412.

81. Montrose, M.S., S.M. Shane, and K.S. Harrington. 1985. Role of litter in the transmission of Campylobacter jejuni. Avian Dis 29:392–399.

82. Morris, G.K., C.A. Bopp, C.M. Patton, and J.G. Wells. 1982. Media for isolating Campylobacter. Arch Lebensmittelhyg 33:151–153.

83. Morrison, R.M., and T. Roberts. 1985. Potential public health benefits of irradiating fresh chicken, pork and beef. In: Food Irradiation: New Perspectives on a Controversial Technology. U.S. Government Printing Office, Washington, DC, Serial 99–14, pp. 1038–1064.

84. Munroe, D.L., J.F. Prescott, and J.L. Penner. 1983. Campylobacter jejuni and Campylobacter coli serotypes isolated from chickens, cattle, and pigs. J Clin Microbiol 18:877–881.

85. Neill, S.D., J.N. Campbell, and J.A. Greene. 1984. Campylobacter species in broiler chickens. Avian Pathol 13:777–785.

86. Neill, S.D., J.N. Campbell, and J.J. O'Brien. 1985. Egg penetration by Campylobacter jejuni. Avian Pathol 14:313–320.

87. Norkrans, G., and Å. Svedhem. 1982. Epidemiological aspects of Campylobacter jejuni enteritis. J Hyg 89:163–170.

88. Oosterom, J., S. Notermans, H. Karman, and G.B. Engels. 1983. Origin and prevalence of Campylobacter jejuni in poultry processing. J Food Prot 46:339–344.

89. Pacha, R.E., G.W. Clark, E.A. Williams, and A.M. Carter. 1988. Migratory birds of central Washington as reservoirs of Campylobacter jejuni. Can J Microbiol 34:80–82.

90. Park, C.E., Z.K. Stankiewicz, J. Lovett, and J. Hunt. 1981. Incidence of Campylobacter jejuni in fresh eviscerated whole market chickens. Can J Microbiol 27:841–842.

91. Patton, C.M., S.W. Mitchell, M.E. Potter, and A.F. Kaufmann. 1981. Comparison of selective media for primary isolation of Campylobacter fetus subsp jejuni. J Clin Microbiol 13:326–330.

92. Patton, C.M., T.J. Barrett, and G.K. Morris. 1985. Comparison of the Penner and Lior methods for serotyping Campylobacter spp. J Clin Microbiol 22:558–565.

93. Peckham, M.C. 1958. Avian vibrionic hepatitis. Avian Dis 2:348–358.

94. Peckham, M.C. 1984. Avian vibrio infections. In M.S. Hofstad, H.J. Barnes, B.W. Calnek, W.M. Reid, and H.W. Yoder, Jr. (eds.). Diseases of Poultry, 8th ed. Iowa State University Press, Ames, IA, pp 221–231.

95. Penner, J.L., and J.N. Hennessy. 1980. Passive hemagglutination technique for serotyping Campylobacter fetus subsp jejuni on the basis of soluble heat-stable antigens. J Clin Microbiol 12:732–737.

96. Penner, J.L., J.N. Hennessy, and R.V. Congi. 1983. Serotyping of Campylobacter jejuni and Campylobacter coli on the basis of thermostable antigens. Eur J Clin Microbiol 2:378–383.

97. Prescott, J.F., and C.W. Bruin-Mosch. 1981. Carriage of Campylobacter jejuni in healthy and diarrheic animals. Am J Vet Res 42:164–165.

98. Prescott, J.F., and D.L. Munroe. 1982. Campylobacter jejuni enteritis in man and domestic animals. J Am Vet Med Assoc 181:1524–1530.

99. Read, D.H., B.M. Daft, J.T. Barton, P.R. Woolcock, G. Cutler, and F. Galey. 1994. Necrotic hemorrhagic hepatitis-splenomegaly syndrome: An unsolved sudden death syndrome in layer leghorn chickens. Proc 43rd Western Poult Dis Conf, pp. 8–9.

100. Robinson, D.A., and D.M. Jones. 1981. Milk-borne campylobacter infection. Br Med J 282:1374–1376.

101. Rosef, O., and G. Kapperud. 1983. House flies (Musca domestica) as possible vectors of Campylobacter fetus subsp jejuni. Appl Environ Microbiol 45:381–383.

102. Rosef, O., B. Gondrosen, and G. Kapperud. 1984. Campylobacter jejuni and Campylobacter coli as surface contaminants of fresh and frozen poultry carcasses. Int J Food Microbiol 1:205–215.

103. Ruiz-Palacios, G.M., E. Escamilla, and N. Torres. 1981. Experimental Campylobacter diarrhea in chickens. Infect Immun 34:250–255.

104. Sanyal, S.C., K.M.N. Islam, P.K.B. Neogy, M. Islam, P. Speelman, and M.I. Huq. 1984. Campylobacter jejuni diarrhea model in infant chickens. Infect Immun 43:931–936.

105. Schoeni, J.L., and A.C. Wong. 1994. Inhibition of Campylobacter jejuni colonization in chicks by defined competitive exclusion bacteria. Appl Environ Microbiol 60:1191–1197.

106. Schwartz, R.H., C. Bryan, W.J. Rodriguez, C. Park, and P. McCoy. 1983. Experience with the microbiologic diagnosis of Campylobacter enteritis in an office laboratory. Pediatr Infect Dis 2:298–301.

107. Sebald, M., and M. Véron. 1963. Teneur en bases de l'ADN et classification des vibrions. Ann Inst Pasteur (Paris) 105:897–910.

108. Sevoian, M., and B.W. Calnek. 1959. Avian infectious hepatitis. III. Treatment of chickens in egg production. Avian Dis 3:302–311.

109. Sevoian, M., R.W. Winterfield, and C.L. Goldman. 1958. Avian infectious hepatitis. I. Clinical and pathological manifestations. Avian Dis 2:3–18.

110. Shane, S.M. 1992. The significance of Campylobacter jejuni infection in poultry: A review. Avian Pathol 21:189–213.

111. Shane, S.M. 1994. Campylobacteriosis. In G.W. Beran, and J.H. Steele (eds.). Handbook of Zoonoses, 2nd ed. CRC Press, Boca Raton, FL, pp. 311–320.

112. Shane, S.M., and M.S. Montrose. 1985. The occurrence and significance of Campylobacter jejuni in man and animals. Vet Res Commun 9:167–198.

113. Shane, S.M., M.S. Montrose, and K.S. Harrington. 1985. Transmission of Campylobacter jejuni by the housefly (Musca domestica). Avian Dis 29:384–391.

114. Shane, S.M., D.H. Gifford, and K. Yogasundram. 1986. Campylobacter jejuni contamination of eggs. Vet Res Commun 10:487–492.

115. Shanker, S., A. Lee, and T.C. Sorrell. 1986. Campy-

lobacter jejuni in broilers: the role of vertical transmission. J Hyg 96:153–159.

116. Shanker, S., A. Lee, and T.C. Sorrell. 1988. Experimental colonization of broiler chicks with Campylobacter jejuni. Epidemiol Infect 100:27–34.

117. Skirrow, M.B. 1982. Campylobacter enteritis the first five years. J Hyg 89:175–184.

118. Skirrow, M.B., and J. Benjamin. 1980. '1001' Campylobacters: cultural characteristics of intestinal campylobacters from man and animals. J Hyg 85:427–442.

119. Skirrow, M.B., and J. Benjamin. 1980. Differentiation of enteropathogenic campylobacter. J Clin Pathol 33:1122.

120. Smibert, R.M. 1978. The genus Campylobacter. Ann Rev Microbiol 32:673–709.

121. Smibert, R.M. 1984. Genus Campylobacter Sebald and Veron 1963, 907^AL. In N.R. Krieg and J.G. Holt (eds.). Bergey's Manual of Systematic Bacteriology, vol 1. Williams & Wilkins, Baltimore, pp 111–118.

122. Smitherman, R.E., C.A. Genigeorgis, and T.B. Farver. 1984. Preliminary observations on the occurrence of Campylobacter jejuni at four California chicken ranches. J Food Prot 47:293–298.

123. Soerjadi, A.S., G.H. Snoeyenbos, and O.M. Weinack. 1982. Intestinal colonization and competitive exclusion of Campylobacter fetus subsp jejuni in young chicks. Avian Dis 26:520–524.

124. Soerjadi-Liem, A.S., G.H. Snoeyenbos, and O.M. Weinack. 1984. Comparative studies on competitive exclusion of three isolates of Campylobacter fetus subsp. jejuni in chickens by native gut microflora. Avian Dis 28:139–146.

125. Stern, N.J., M.P. Hernandez, L. Blankenship, K.E. Deibel, S. Doores, M.P. Doyle, H. Ng, M.D. Pierson, J.N. Sofos, W.H. Sveum, and D.C. Westhoff. 1985. Prevalence and distribution of Campylobacter jejuni and Campylobacter coli in retail meats. J Food Prot 48:595–599.

126. Stern, N.J., P.J. Rothenberg, and J.M. Stone. 1985. Enumeration and reduction of Campylobacter jejuni in poultry and red meats. J Food Prot 48:606–610.

127. Stern, N.S., J.S. Bailey, L.C. Blankenship, N.A. Cox, and F McHan. 1988. Colonization characteristics of Campylobacter jejuni in chick ceca. Avian Dis 32:330–334.

128. Stern, N.J., R.J. Meinersmann, N.A. Cox, J.S. Bailey, and L.C. Blakenship. 1990. Influence of host lineage on cecal colonization by Campylobacter jejuni in chickens. Avian Dis 34:602–606.

129. Svedhem, Å., B. Kaijser, and E. Sjögren. 1981. Antimicrobial susceptibility of Campylobacter jejuni isolated from humans with diarrhoea and from healthy chickens. J Antimicrob Chemother 7:301–305.

130. Tauxe, R.V., D.A. Pegues, and N. Hargrett-Bean. 1987. Campylobacter infections: The emerging national pattern. Am J Public Health 77:1219–1221.

131. Taylor, D.E., and P. Courvalin. 1988. Mechanisms of antibiotic resistance in Campylobacter species. Antimicrob Agents Chemother 32:1107–1112.

132. Thompson, L.M. III, R.M. Smibert, J.L. Johnson, and N.R. Krieg. 1988. Phylogenetic study of the genus Campylobacter. Int J Syst Bacteriol 38:190–200.

133. Truscott, R.B., and P.H.G. Stockdale. 1966. Correlation of the identity of bile and cecal vibrios from the same field cases of avian vibrionic hepatitis. Avian Dis 10:67–73.

134. Tudor, D.C. 1954. A liver degeneration of unknown origin in chickens. J Am Vet Med Assoc 125:219–220.

135. Umunnabuike, A.C., and E.A. Irokanulo. 1986. Isolation of Campylobacter subsp jejuni from Oriental and American cockroaches caught in kitchens and poultry houses in Vom, Nigeria. Int J Zoon 13:180–186.

136. Vanhoof, R., H. Goossens, H. Coignau, G. Stas, and J.P. Butzler. 1982. Susceptibility patterns of Campylobacter jejuni from human and animal origins to different antimicrobial agents. Antimicrob Agents Chemother 21:990–992.

137. Van Landuyt, H.W., J-M. Fossépré, and B. Gordts. 1987. A blood-free medium for isolation of thermophilic Campylobacter species. Eur J Clin Microbiol 6:201–203.

138. Volkheimer, A., and H-H. Wuthe. 1986. Campylobacter jejuni/coli bei Rebhühnern (Perdix perdix L.) und Fasanen (Phasianus colchicus L.). Berl Munch Tierarztl Woschenschr 99:374.

139. Wang, W-L.L., N.W. Luechtefeld, L.B. Reller, and M.J. Blaser. 1980. Enriched brucella medium for storage and transport of cultures of Campylobacter fetus subsp jejuni. J Clin Microbiol 12:479–480.

140. Wang, W-L.L., B.W. Powers, N.W. Luechtefeld, and M.J. Blaser. 1983. Effects of disinfectants on Campylobacter jejuni. Appl Environ Microbiol 45:1202–1205.

141. Welkos, S.L. 1984. Experimental gastroenteritis in newly-hatched chicks infected with Campylobacter jejuni. J Med Microbiol 18:233–248.

142. Winkenwerder, W., and T. Maciak. 1964. Vibrionenfunde bei Hühnern aus erkrankten Beständen und bei Schlachthühnern. Dtsch Tierarztl Wochenschr 71:625–627.

143. Winterfield, R.W., and M. Sevoian. 1957. Isolation of a causal agent of an avian hepatitis. Vet Med 53:273–274.

144. Winterfield, R.W., M. Sevoian, and C.L. Goldman. 1958. Avian infectious hepatitis. II. Some characteristics of the etiologic agent. Effect of various drugs on the course of the disease. Avian Dis 2:19–39.

145. Yogasundram, K., and S.M. Shane. 1986. The viability of Campylobacter jejuni on refrigerated chicken drumsticks. Vet Res Commun 10:479–486.

146. Yogasundram, K., S.M. Shane, R.M. Grodner, E.N. Lambremont, and R.E. Smith. 1987. Decontamination of Campylobacter jejuni on chicken drumsticks using chemicals and radiation. Vet Res Commun 11:31–40.

147. Yogasundram, K., S.M. Shane, and K.S. Harrington. 1989. Prevalence of Campylobacter jejuni in selected domestic and wild birds in Louisiana. Avian Dis 33:664–667.

11 Staphylococcosis

J. Kirk Skeeles

INTRODUCTION. *Staphylococcus aureus* infections are common in poultry; the most frequent sites being bones, tendon sheaths, and joints of the leg (Table 11.1). Staphylococcal infections occur less frequently in other locations including skin (39), sternal bursa (83), yolk sac (89), heart (6), vertebrae (9), eyelid (11), and as granulomas in the liver and lungs (3, 58). Staphylococcal septicemia, causing acute deaths in laying birds (7), seems to be prevalent in hot weather and resembles fowl cholera.

Economic and Public Health Significance. In addition to being a major disease-producing organism for poultry, approximately 50% of typical and atypical *S. aureus* strains produce enterotoxins capable of causing food poisoning in humans (25, 29, 37, 69). Staphylococcal food poisoning has been associated with poultry (78). Enterotoxin-producing *S. aureus* strains, which contaminate poultry carcasses at processing, have their origin from either contaminated equipment or people in the processing plant (1, 66, 80). In the processing of turkeys, an association has been made between green-discolored livers and internal staphylococcal or other bacterial infections (5, 12). While the correlation between bacterial infections and green-discolored livers is high, the reverse relationship is less certain, apparently because there are causes of liver discoloration in turkeys other than staphylococcosis.

HISTORY. Staphylococcosis in poultry and other avian species has been recognized for over 100 yr; most early reports describe arthritis and synovitis (35, 40, 42, 51).

INCIDENCE AND DISTRIBUTION. *Staphy-lococcus* spp. are ubiquitous, normal inhabitants of skin and mucous membranes, and are common organisms in environments where poultry are hatched, reared, or processed. Most staphylococcal species are considered to be normal flora, which help suppress other possible pathogens by their presence through interference or competitive exclusion. Some have the potential to be pathogenic and produce disease if allowed entry through the skin or mucous membranes.

Staphylococcus spp. and staphylococcosis have been associated with poultry throughout the world including Argentina (79), Australia (44), Belgium (17, 18), Bulgaria (4), Canada (59), China (10), Costa Rica (57), France (87), Germany (47, 48), Hungary (31), India (68), Italy (34), Japan (75), the Netherlands (66), Pakistan (82), Poland (91), Romania (55), Taiwan (84), the United Kingdom (81), and the United States (41).

ETIOLOGY

Classification. The genus *Staphylococcus* contains approximately 20 species. It is the most important genus in the family Micrococcaceae. The term *staphylococcus* refers to the morphology of the microorganisms in stained smears, which resemble grapelike clusters. Other genera in the family are considered to be nonpathogenic and include *Micrococcus, Planococcus* (see also Chapter 14), and *Stomatococcus* (45, 67).

Staphylococci isolated frequently from poultry include *S. aureus* and *S. epidermidis*. Another species, *S. gallinarum*, has been isolated from processed poultry (22). *S. hyicus* has been associated with fibrinoheterophilic blepharitis in chickens and turkeys (11) and was isolated from five of nine tibiotarsal growth plates of turkeys with stifle joint

Table 11.1. Staphylococcal-related infections in poultry

Location	Age	Lesion	Usual Outcome
Bone	Any, usually older	Osteomyelitis	Lameness
Joint	Any, usually older	Arthritis/Synovitis	Lameness
Yolk sac	Chicks, poults	Omphalitis	Death
Blood (septicemia)	Any	Generalized necrosis	Death
Skin	Young	Gangrenous dermatitis	Death
Feet	Mature	"Bumblefoot"	Lameness

osteoarthritis (77). *S. hyicus* is similar biochemically to *S. aureus*, but gives a delayed positive coagulase reaction. Other staphylococci, often encountered in humans and domestic animals and considered pathogenic for those species, are not believed to be important in poultry.

Morphology and Staining. *S. aureus* is the only staphylococcal species found in poultry considered to be pathogenic. Typical pathogenic *S. aureus* strains are gram-positive, coccoid in shape, and found in clusters when grown on solid media. In liquid media, they may occur in short chains. Older cultures (>24 hr) may stain gram-negative.

Growth Requirements. Staphylococci are readily isolated on 5% blood agar with growth evident in 18–24 hr.

Colony Morphology. Aerobic growth of *S. aureus* results, within 24 hr, in circular, smooth colonies, 1–3 mm in diameter, that are often pigmented white to orange (88).

Biochemical Properties. *S. aureus* is aerobic, facultatively anaerobic, ß-hemolytic, catalase-positive, fermentative for glucose and mannitol, and gelatinase-positive. Only coagulase-positive strains isolated from clinical material are considered pathogenic (88).

Resistance to Chemical and Physical Agents. Staphylococci are extremely hardy and remain viable for long periods of time on solid media or in exudate. Some strains are heat and disinfectant resistant (52). A resistance feature used to isolate *S. aureus* from heavily contaminated clinical material is its tolerance to high (7.5%) concentrations of NaCl (45, 67).

Antigenic Structure and Toxins. The antigenic nature of *S. aureus* is often complex. Strains may have a capsule consisting of glucosaminouronic acid, manosaminouronic acid, lysine, glutamic acid, glycine, alanine, or glucosamine; polysaccharide A consisting of linear ribitol teichoic acid, *N*-acetylglucosamine, and D-alanine; and protein-A, a cell-wall component that interacts nonspecifically with the Fc portion of immunoglobulin and may be a virulence factor. A variety of enzymes and toxins including hyaluronidase (spreading factor), deoxyribonuclease, fibrinolysin, lipase, protease, hemolysins, leukocidin, dermonecrotic toxin, hemolysins, exfoliative toxin, and enterotoxins can also contribute to a strain's pathogenicity and virulence (2, 56, 88).

Strain Classification. Chicken *S. aureus* strains have been typed using phages, as have *S. aureus* strains from humans (30, 72, 73, 74, 75). The ability to type with the International Series of *S. aureus* phages depends on where the organism was isolated. Strains isolated from diseased poultry are often untypable, while strains isolated from processed poultry are more likely to be typable with the International Series. *S. aureus* strains from processed poultry are thought to be human strains endemic to the processing plant, or from the hands of workers in the plant (48). Phage sets isolated from poultry strains of *S. aureus* can be used to type strains of poultry origin (30, 72). These have been used in studies involving *S. aureus* of poultry origin from various locations around the world with varying results (44, 75, 81). Phages tend to be specific for *S. aureus* of poultry origin and cannot be used to type strains from other species (74).

Several biotyping schemes have been devised that divide *S. aureus* strains into species-specific ecovars. Poultry strains have been biotyped using these classification schemes (19, 36). Strains have also been classified using antibiotic susceptibility patterns, plasmid profiles (45), and serotyping based on capsular polysaccharides (16).

Pathogenicity. Coagulase-positive isolates of *S. aureus* are considered to be pathogenic for poultry, while coagulase-negative strains are thought to be nonpathogenic.

PATHOGENESIS AND EPIZOOTIOLOGY

Natural and Experimental Hosts. All avian species are susceptible to staphylococcal infections.

Transmission, Carriers, and Vectors. For infection to occur, a breakdown in the natural defense mechanisms of the host must occur (2). In most cases, this would involve damage to an environmental barrier, such as a skin wound or inflamed mucous membrane. *S. aureus* enters through the breached barrier and travels to internal locations where a locus of infection (e.g., osteomyelitis) is established, usually in the metaphyseal area of a nearby joint (15, 61). In newly hatched chicks, the open navel provides a portal of entry leading to omphalitis and other types of infections. Minor surgical procedures (e.g., trimming of toes, beak, or comb; removal of the snood) and parenteral vaccinations may offer additional means of entry for staphylococci.

Another type of host defense impairment occurs following infectious bursal disease (71), chicken infectious anemia, or possibly Marek's disease virus infection, where the bursa of Fabricius or thymus is damaged and the immune system is compromised. Under these conditions, septicemic staphylococcal infections can occur and cause acute death. Gangrenous dermatitis (Chapter 12) caused by *S. aureus,* along with *Clostridium septicum,* can be seen following early infectious bursal disease virus infection (27, 70).

Recently *Escherichia coli* was discovered to be the predominant bacterial organism in livers of turkeys immediately following challenge with virulent hemorrhagic enteritis virus (HEV). However, when livers of survivors were cultured 2 wk postexposure, *Staphylococcus* spp. were the predominant bacteria (62). This suggests HEV, and possibly other similar viral, intestinal infections, may create portals of entry and provide the underlying basis for subsequent staphylococcal problems associated with older, commercial turkeys.

Susceptibility to staphylococcal infections also may be influenced genetically. Two related lines of New Hampshire chickens had significant differences in mortality following experimental infection (14).

Incubation Period.   The incubation period is short. In experimental chickens, clinical signs were evident 48–72 hr following intravenous inoculation. Experimentally, chickens can be readily infected by the intravenous route, but not by intratracheal or aerosol routes. The number of bacteria affects the ability to produce experimental disease consistently; at least 10^5 organisms/kg body weight are necessary (59, 60).

Signs.   Early clinical signs include ruffled feathers, limping on one leg, drooping of one or both wings, reluctance to walk, and fever (59). This can be followed by severe depression and death. Birds surviving the acute disease have swollen joints, sit on their hocks and keel bone, and are reluctant or unable to stand (24, 59). Clinical signs of septicemic staphylococcal infection and gangrenous dermatitis occur in birds in good condition, and may only be evident because of increased mortality in the flock (7, 27, 70).

Morbidity and Mortality.   Morbidity and mortality due to staphylococcosis is usually low, unless there has been massive contamination of chicks because of exposure to unusually high numbers of bacteria in the hatchery through environmental contamination, vaccination, or servicing procedures. Leg disorders are one of the most prevalent problems observed in broilers and turkeys. With the advent of further processing and need for birds with more breast meat, leg problems have become more prevalent. Several reports from diagnostic laboratories have indicated *S. aureus* is the most common bacterial agent isolated from affected legs and joints (46, 43).

Morbidity and mortality from septicemic staphylococcal infection are usually low. The number of chickens that develop gangrenous dermatitis is low, but usually all that develop lesions succumb to the infection (8, 27, 46).

Gross Lesions.   Gross lesions of osteomyelitis in bone consist of focal yellow areas of caseous exudate or lytic areas (Fig. 11.1A), which cause affected bones to be fragile. Bones and sites most frequently involved are the proximal tibiotarsus and proximal femur. Less commonly, the proximal tarsometatarsus, distal femur, distal tibiotarsus, proximal humerus, ribs, or spine may be involved. In affected birds, the femoral head often separates from the shaft by a fracture through the neck when the coxofemoral joint is disarticulated (femoral head necrosis) (Fig. 11.1C) (59, 61).

Arthritis, periarthritis, and synovitis are common. Affected joints are swollen and filled with inflammatory exudate as the infection (osteomyelitis) extends from nearby metaphyseal areas (Fig. 11.1D) (54, 61). Spondylitis involving articulating thoracolumbar vertebrae may cause lameness indirectly because of impingement on the spinal cord (9, 61).

Gross lesions of septicemic staphylococcal infection consist of necrosis and vascular congestion in many internal organs including liver (Fig. 11.1E), spleen, kidneys, and lungs (7). Dark, moist areas under the skin with crepitation are seen in gangrenous dermatitis (7, 27). Following mild trauma, gangrenous dermatitis lesions develop on the wing tips of birds infected with chicken infectious anemia virus (Chapter 30). This condition has been referred to as "blue-wing disease."

Staphylococcal-related hatchery infections are common and can cause increased mortality within the first few days after hatching. Chicks have wet navel areas and deteriorate rapidly. Internally, yolk sacs are enlarged with the contents having an abnormal color and consistency.

Plantar abscess is a common infection seen in mature chickens ("bumblefoot"); an infection that leads to massive swelling of the foot and lameness.

Partially, or less commonly, entirely green-discolored livers (Fig. 11.1F) have been associated with osteomyelitis and/or associated soft tissue lesions (e.g., arthritis, periarthritis, tenosynovitis) in commercial turkeys at processing. Carcasses with lesions from which staphylococci or other bacteria are isolated also have liver discoloration, but frequently turkeys with liver discoloration do not have demonstrable osteomyelitis or associated lesions, or, if present, bacteria cannot be isolated from the lesions (5, 12). Green liver discoloration has not been reproduced experimentally and the cause of this disorder is still unknown.

Liver spots are another common cause of condemnation in commercial turkeys. Most affected livers yielded no aerobic or facultatively anaerobic bacteria when two flocks with histories of high liver condemnation were examined, although *S. cohnii* and other staphylococci were isolated most frequently from the few culture-positive livers. Ascarid larval migration appeared to be the most likely cause of the liver lesions (65).

Histopathology. Histologically, staphylococcal lesions consist of necrosis; bacterial colonies composed of large numbers of gram-positive, coccoid bacteria, and heterophils (Fig. 11.1B) (23, 32, 59). Long-standing lesions are primarily granulomatous.

Immunity. Neither active nor passive immunity is important in preventing *S. aureus* infections in poultry. It has even been implied that specific antibody to *S. aureus* may promote development of *S. aureus*-related infections in chickens (26, 33). Whole-cell bacterins and toxoids have not proven to be effective in other species either (2, 56).

DIAGNOSIS

Isolation and Identification. *S. aureus* is diagnosed by culturing suspected clinical material including exudate from joints, yolk material, and stab swabs of internal organs. The basic medium for growing staphylococci is blood agar (preferably sheep or bovine). Organisms grow well with colonies 1–3 mm in diameter within 18–24 hr. Most *S. aureus* strains are ß-hemolytic, while other staphylococci are usually nonhemolytic. Heavily contaminated material should be streaked onto a selective medium inhibitory for gram-negative bacteria such as mannitol-salt or phenylethyl-alcohol agar (45, 67, 88).

Most *S. aureus* colonies will be pigmented. Colonies should be picked and gram stained. Staphylococci are gram-positive cocci. To differentiate pathogenic *S. aureus* from nonpathogenic *S. epidermidis,* coagulase and mannitol fermentation tests should be done. *S. aureus* is positive on both tests, while *S. epidermidis* is negative (Table 11.2). Several systems for identifying staphylococcal species are available commercially, but these are not used routinely for poultry isolates (45, 67).

Serology. Serology is not generally used for diagnosis of staphylococcosis, but a microagglutination test has been described (26).

Differential Diagnosis. Staphylococcosis can resemble infection with *E. coli, Pasteurella multocida, Salmonella gallinarum, Mycoplasma synoviae,* reoviruses, or any other infection of bones or joints that is hatchery related or causes septicemia.

11.1. Lesions of staphylococcosis. *A.* Osteomyelitis of proximal tibiotarsus in a 13-wk-old turkey. (Barnes) *B.* Focal osteomyelitis subjacent of physis of proximal tibiotarsus (×5). (Barnes) *C.* Bilateral osteomyelitis of femoral head due to *Staphylococcus aureus* infection in a 2-wk-old turkey. Note extension through joint into body cavity. *D.* Three-wk-old turkey. Swollen hock joint with extension of inflammatory exudate along tendon sheaths. (Munger) *E.* Leghorn, 20-wk-old. Multiple foci of necrosis in liver following septicemic staph infection. (Munger) *F.* Green liver discoloration seen in turkeys with osteomyelitis. (Barnes)

TREATMENT. *S. aureus* infection can be successfully treated, but sensitivity tests should always be performed, because antibiotic resistance is common (18, 21, 76, 90). Drugs used successfully for treatment include penicillin, streptomycin, tetracyclines, erythromycin, novobiocin, sulfonamides, lincomycin, and spectinomycin. Staphylococcal dermatitis has also been associated with use of a sulfa drug in broiler breeder pullets (28).

PREVENTION AND CONTROL

Management Procedures. Any management procedure reducing damage to host defense mechanisms will help prevent staphylococcosis. Because wounds are a portal of entry for *S. aureus* into the body, anything reducing the chance of injury will help prevent infection. Sharp objects such as splinters, jagged rocks, or metal edges that cut or puncture feet should be eliminated from areas where poultry are reared. Maintenance of good litter quality will reduce foot pad ulceration. Particular attention should be given to hatchery management and sanitation. *S. aureus* is found everywhere, and conditions in incubators and hatchers are ideal for bacterial growth. Recently hatched and hatching chicks with open navels and immature immune systems can easily be infected, leading to mortality and chronic infections shortly after hatching. Prevention of early infections with infectious bursal disease virus and chicken infectious anemia virus will also help prevent staphylococcosis (71).

Table 11.2. Differentiation of *Staphylococcus aureus* and *S. epidermidis* in poultry

Characteristic	S. aureus	S. epidermidis
Colony pigment	+	−
Hemolysis	+	−
Coagulase	+	−
D. mannitol fermentation	+	−

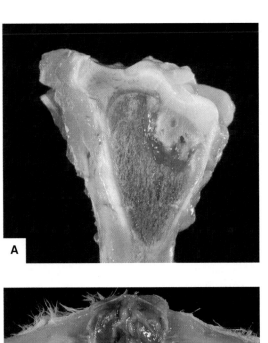

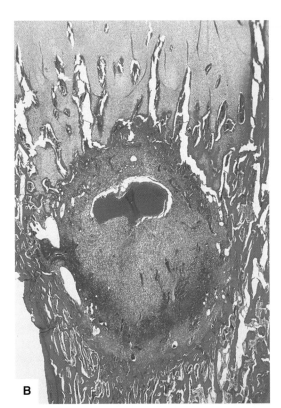

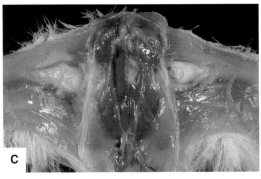

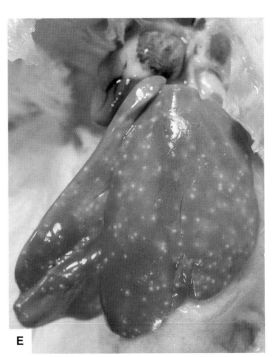

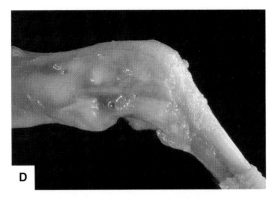

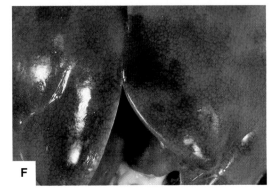

Poultry under mild stress are more resistant to experimental staphylococcosis than those not stressed (13, 38, 49, 59). Resistance is attributed to an increase in heterophil numbers, which occurs in birds under stress. The heterophil is thought to be the most important cell in controlling bacterial infections, particularly *S. aureus* (60).

Staphylococcal bacterins have been ineffective in preventing infections (2), but use of live, avirulent vaccines based on the principle of bacterial interference has shown promise. Avirulent *S. aureus* strain 502A has been utilized in humans to manage recurrent furunculosis and abort nursery outbreaks (56). One strain of staphylococcus was shown to interfere with colonization of other strains of *S. aureus* in chickens (20). Using the principle of bacterial interference, a live, avirulent vaccine for prevention of staphylococcosis in turkeys has been developed. A naturally occurring, coagulase-negative *S. epidermidis* isolate, designated strain 115, which colonizes cells and tissues in the respiratory tract and prevents adherence of virulent strains of *S. aureus* is used. In addition to interfering with colonization of virulent *S. aureus, S. epidermidis* 115 also secretes a stable, antibioticlike bacteriocin capable of inhibiting and killing virulent *S. aureus.* The vaccine is administered by aerosol at 1–10 days and again at 4–6 wk of age. Use of strain 115 in commercial flocks has reduced the number of turkeys with staphylococcosis and improved overall livability. Similar results were found when strain 115 was used in chickens (41, 50, 53, 63, 64, 86).

Competitive gut exclusion using *Lactobacillus acidophilus* was attempted to exclude *S. aureus* from experimentally infected, germ-free chickens. The treatment was effective in reducing *S. aureus* counts in crop contents, but counts in the ceca and rectum were unaffected (85).

REFERENCES

1. Adams, B.W., and G.C. Mead. 1983. Incidence and properties of Staphylococcus aureus associated with turkeys during processing and further-processing operations. J Hyg 91:479–490.
2. Anderson, J.C. 1986. Staphylococcus. In C.L. Gyles and C.O. Thoen (eds.). Pathogenesis of Bacterial Infections in Animals, 1st ed. Iowa State University Press, Ames, IA, pp. 14–20.
3. Arp, L.H., I.M. Robinson, and A.E. Jensen. 1983. Pathology of liver granulomas in turkeys. Vet Pathol 20:80–89.
4. Bajljosov, D., Z. Sachariev, and L. Georgiev. 1974. Characteristics of staphylococci isolated from slaughter fowl. Monatsh Veterinaeremed 29:692–694.
5. Bayyari, G.R., W.E. Huff, R.A. Norton, J.K. Skeeles, J.N. Beasley, N.C. Rath, and J.M. Balog. 1994. A longitudinal study of green-liver osteomyelitis complex in commercial turkeys. Avian Dis 38:744–754.
6. Bergmann, V., B. Köhler, and K. Vogel. 1980. Staphylococcus aureus infection of fowls on industrialized poultry units. I. Types of infection. Arch Exp Vet 34:891–903.
7. Bickford, A.A., and A.S. Rosenwald. 1975. Staphylococcal infections in chickens. Poult Dig July:285–287.
8. Bitay, Z., L. Quarini, R. Glavits, and R. Fischer. 1984. Staphylococcus infection in fowls. Magy Allatorv Lapja 39:86–91.
9. Carnaghan, R.B.A. 1966. Spinal cord compression in fowls due to spondylitis caused by Staphylococcus pyogenes. J Comp Pathol 76:9–14.
10. Chen, D.W., M.H. Gan, and R.P. Liu. 1984. Studies on staphylococcosis in chickens. III. Properties and pathogenicity of Staphylococcus aureus. Chinese J Vet Med 10:6–8.
11. Cheville, N.F., J. Tappe, M. Ackermann, and A. Jensen. 1988. Acute fibrinopurulent blepharitis and conjunctivitis associated with Staphylococcus hyicus, Escherichia coli, and Streptococcus sp. in chickens and turkeys. Vet Pathol 25:369–375.
12. Clark, R.S., H.J. Barnes, A.A. Bickford, R.P. Chin, and R. Droual. 1991. Relationship of osteomyelitis and associated soft-tissue lesions with green liver discoloration in turkeys. Avian Dis 35:139–146.
13. Coates, S.R., D.K. Buckner, and M.M. Jensen. 1977. The inhibitory effect of Corynebacterium parvum and Pasteurella multocida pretreatment on staphylococcal synovitis in turkeys. Avian Dis 21:319–322.
14. Cotter, P.F., and R.L. Taylor, Jr. 1991. Differential resistance to Staphylococcus aureus challenge in two related lines of chickens. Poult Sci 70:1357–1361.
15. Daum, R.S., H. Davis, S. Shane, D. Mulvihill, R. Campeau, and B. Farris. 1990. Bacteremia and osteomyelitis in an avian model of Staphylococcus aureus infection. J Orthop Res 8:804–813.
16. Daum, R.S., A. Fattom, S. Freese, and W. Karakawa. 1994. Capsular polysaccharide serotypes of coagulase-positive staphylococci associated with tenosynovitis, osteomyelitis, and other invasive infections in chickens and turkeys: Evidence for new capsular types. Avian Dis 38:762–771.
17. Devriese, L.A. 1980. Pathogenic staphylococci in poultry. World Poult Sci 36:227–236.
18. Devriese, L.A. 1980. Sensitivity of staphylococci from farm animals to antibacterial agents used for growth promotion and therapy: A ten year study. Ann Rech Vet 11:399–408.
19. Devriese, L.A. 1984. A simplified system for biotyping Staphylococcus aureus strains isolated from different animal species. J Appl Bacteriol 56:215–220.
20. Devriese, L.A., A.H. Devos, and J. Beumer. 1972. Staphylococcus aureus colonization on poultry after experimental spray inoculations. Avian Dis 16:656–665.
21. Devriese, L.A., A.H. Devos, J. Beumer, and R. Moes. 1972. Characterization of staphylococci isolated from poultry. Poult Sci 51:389–397.
22. Devriese, L.A., B. Poutrel, R. Kilpper-Balz, and K.H. Schleifer. 1983. Staphylococcus gallinarum and Staphylococcus caprae, two new species from animals. Int J Syst Bacteriol 33:480–486.
23. Emslie, K.R., and S. Nade. 1985. Acute hematogenous staphylococcal osteomyelitis. Comp Pathol Bull 17:2–3.
24. Emslie, K.R., N.R. Ozanne, and S.M.L. Nade. 1983. Acute haemotogenous osteomyelitis: An experimental model. Pathology 141:157–167.
25. Evans, J.B., G.A. Ananaba, C.A. Pate, and M.S. Bergdoll. 1983. Enterotoxin production by atypical Staphylococcus aureus from poultry. J Appl Bacteriol 54:257–261.
26. Forget, A., L. Meunier, and A.G. Borduas. 1974. Enhancement activity of homologous anti-staphylococcal sera in experimental staphylococcal synovitis of chicks: A possible role of immune adherence antibodies. Infect Immun 9:641–644.
27. Frazier, M.N., W.J. Parizek, and E. Garner. 1964. Gangrenous dermatitis of chickens. Avian Dis 8:269–273.
28. Froyman, R., L. Deruyttere, and L.A. Devriese. 1982. The effect of antimicrobial agents on an outbreak of staphy-

lococcal dermatitis in adult broiler breeders. Avian Pathol 11:521–525.

29. Gibbs, P.A., J.T. Patterson, and J. Harvey. 1978. Biochemical characteristics and enterotoxigenicity of Staphylococcus aureus strains isolated from poultry. J Appl Bacteriol 44:57–74.

30. Gibbs, P.A., J.T. Patterson, and J.K. Thompson. 1978. Characterization of poultry isolates of Staphylococcus aureus by a new set of poultry phages. J Appl Bacteriol 44:387–400.

31. Glavits, R., F. Ratz, T. Fehervari, and J. Povazsan. 1984. Pathological studies in chicken embryos and day-old chicks experimentally infected with Salmonella typhimurium and Staphylococcus aureus. Acta Vet Hung 32:39–49.

32. Griffiths, G.L., W.I. Hopkinson, and J. Lloyd. 1984. Staphylococcal necrosis of the head of the femur in broiler chickens. Aust Vet J 61:293.

33. Gross, W.G., P.B. Siegel, R.W. Hall, C.H. Domermuth, and R.T. Duboise. 1980. Production and persistence of antibodies in chickens to sheep erythrocytes. 2. Resistance to infectious diseases. Poult Sci 59:205–210.

34. Guarda, F., G. Cortellezzi, C. Cucco, and O. Massimino. 1979. Blindness due to Staphylococcus aureus in pullets. Clin Vet 102:315–324.

35. Gwatkin, R. 1940. An outbreak of staphylococcal infection in barred Plymouth rock males. Can J Comp Med 4:294–296.

36. Hajek, V., and E. Marsalek. 1971. The differentiation of pathogenic staphylococci and a suggestion for their taxonomic classification. Zentralbl Bakteriol [A] 217:176–182.

37. Harvey, J., J.T. Patterson, and P.A. Gibbs. 1982. Enterotoxigenicity of Staphylococcus aureus strains isolated from poultry: Raw poultry carcasses as a potential food-poisoning hazard. J Appl Bacteriol 52:251–258.

38. Heller, E.D., D.B. Nathan, and M. Perek. 1979. Short heat stress as an immunostimulant in chicks. Avian Pathol 8:195–203.

39. Hoffman, H.A. 1939. Vesicular dermatitis in chickens. J Am Vet Med Assoc 48:329–332.

40. Hole, N., and H.S. Purchase. 1931. Arthritis and periostitis in pheasants caused by Staphylococcus pyogenes aureus. J Comp Pathol Ther 44:252–257.

41. Jensen, M.M., W.C. Downs, J.D. Morrey, T.R. Nicoll, S.D. LeFevre, and C.M. Meyers. 1987. Staphylococcosis of turkeys. 1. Portal of entry and tissue colonization. Avian Dis 31:64–69.

42. Jungherr, E. 1933. Staphylococcal arthritis in turkeys. J Am Vet Med Assoc 35:243–249.

43. Kibenge, F.S.B., M.D. Robertson, G.E. Wilcox, and D.A. Pass. 1982. Bacterial and viral agents associated with tenosynovitis in broiler breeders in Western Australia. Avian Pathol 11:351–359.

44. Kibenge, F.S.B., G.E. Wilcox, and D. Perret. 1982. Staphylococcus aureus isolated from poultry in Australia. I. Phage typing and cultural characteristics. Vet Microbiol 7:471–483.

45. Kloos, W.E., and J.H. Jorgensen. 1985. Staphylococci. In E.H. Lenette, A. Balows, W.J. Hausler, Jr., and H.J. Shadomy (eds.). Manual of Clinical Microbiology, 4th ed. American Society of Microbiologists, Washington, DC, pp. 143–153.

46. Köhler, B., V. Bergmann, W. Witte, R. Heiss, and K. Vogel. 1978. Dermatitis bei broilen durch Staphylococcus aureus. Monatsch Veterinaermed 33:22–28.

47. Köhler, B., H. Nattermann, W. Witte, F. Friedrichs, and E. Kunter. 1980. Staphylococcus aureus infection of fowls on industrialized poultry units. II. Microbiological tests for S. aureus and other pathogens. Arch Exp Veterinaermed 34:905–923.

48. Kusch, D. 1977. Biochemical characteristics and phage-typing of staphylococci isolated from poultry. Zentralbl Bakteriol Parasit Infekt Hyg [IB] 164:360–367.

49. Larson, C.T., W.B. Gross, and J.W. Davis. 1985. Social stress and resistance of chicken and swine to Staphylococcus aureus challenge infections. Can J Comp Med 49:208–210.

50. LeFevre, S.D., and M.M. Jensen. 1987. Staphylococcosis of turkeys. 2. Assay of protein A levels of staphylococci isolated from turkeys. Avian Dis 31:70–73.

51. Lucet, A. 1892. De l'ostèo-arthrite aigue infectieuse des jeunes oies. Ann Inst Pasteur (Paris) 6:841–850.

52. Mead, G.C., and B.W. Adams. 1986. Chlorine resistance of Staphylococcus aureus isolated from turkeys and turkey products. Appl Microbiol 3:131–133.

53. Meyers, C.M., and M.M. Jensen. 1987. Staphylococcosis of turkeys. 3. Bacterial interference as a possible means of control. Avian Dis 31:74–79.

54. Miner, M.L., R.A. Smart, and A.E. Olson. 1968. Pathogenesis of staphylococcal synovitis in turkeys: Pathologic changes. Avian Dis 12:46–60.

55. Minzat, R.M., V. Volintir, S. Panaitescu, I. Javanescu, B. Kelciov, and E. Cretu. 1977. A peculiar form of staphylococcal infection in chickens. Lucr Stiint Inst Agron Timisoara, Ser Med Vet 14:141–144.

56. Morse, S.I. 1980. Staphylococci. In B.D. Davis, R. Dulbecco, H.N. Eisen, and H.S. Ginsberg (eds.). Microbiology, 3rd ed. Harper and Row Publishers, Philadelphia, PA, pp. 623–633.

57. Moya, S.F. 1986. Staphylococcus aureus as a potential contaminant of animal feeds. Ciencias Vet, Costa Rica 8:77–80.

58. Munger, L.L., and B.L. Kelly. 1973. Staphylococcal granulomas in a leghorn hen. Avian Dis 17:858–860.

59. Mutalib, A., C. Riddell, and A.D. Osborne. 1983. Studies on the pathogenesis of staphylococcal osteomyelitis in chickens. I. Effect of stress on experimentally induced osteomyelitis. Avian Dis 27:141–156.

60. Mutalib, A., C. Riddell, and A.D. Osborne. 1983. Studies on the pathogenesis of staphylococcal osteomyelitis in chickens. II. Role of the respiratory tract as a route of infection. Avian Dis 27:157–160.

61. Nairn, M.E. 1973. Bacterial osteomyelitis and synovitis of the turkey. Avian Dis 17:504–517.

62. Newberry, L.A., D.G. Lindsey, J.N. Beasley, R.W. McNew, and J.K. Skeeles. 1994. A summary of data collected from turkeys following acute hemorrhagic enteritis virus infection at different ages. Proc 45th NC Avian Dis Conf, Oct 9–11, Des Moines, IA, p. 63.

63. Nicoll, T.R., and M.M. Jensen. 1987. Preliminary studies on bacterial interference of staphylococcosis of chickens. Avian Dis 31:140–144.

64. Nicoll, T.R., and M.M. Jensen. 1987. Staphylococcosis of turkeys. 5. Large-scale control programs using bacterial interference. Avian Dis 31:85–88.

65. Norton, R.A., G.R. Bayyari, J.K. Skeeles, W.E. Huff, and J.N. Beasley. 1994. A survey of two commercial turkey farms experiencing high levels of liver foci. Avian Dis 38:887–894.

66. Notermans, S., J. Dufrenne, and W.J. van Leeuwen. 1982. Contamination of broiler chickens by Staphylococcus aureus during processing; incidence and origin. J Appl Bacteriol 52:275–280.

67. Pezzlo, Marie. 1992. Identification of commonly isolated aerobic gram-positive bacteria. In H.D. Isenberg, chief ed. Clinical Microbiology Procedures Handbook, vol 1. American Society for Microbiology, Washington, DC, pp. 1.20.1–1.20.12.

68. Rao, M.V.S., S.B. Kulshrestha, and S. Kumar. 1977. Biological properties and drug sensitivity reactions of intestinal staphylococci of poultry. Indian J Anim Sci 46:648–651.

69. Raska, K., V. Matejovska, D. Matejovska, M.S. Bergdoll, and P. Petrus. 1981. To the origin of contamination of foodstuffs by enterotoxigenic staphylococci. In J. Jel-

jaszewicz (ed.). Staphylococci and Staphylococcal Infections. Gustav Fischer Verlag, Stuttgart, pp. 381–385.

70. Rosenberger, J.K., S. Klopp, R.J. Eckroade, and W.C. Krauss. 1975. The role of the infectious bursal agent and several avian adenoviruses in the hemorrhagic-aplastic-anemia syndrome and gangrenous dermatitis. Avian Dis 19:717–729.

71. Santivatr, D., S.K. Maheswaran, J.A. Newman, and B.S. Pomeroy. 1981. Effect of infectious bursal disease virus infection on the phagocytosis of Staphylococcus aureus by mononuclear phagocytic cells of susceptible and resistant strains of chickens. Avian Dis 25:303–311.

72. Shimizu, A. 1977. Establishment of a new bacteriophage set for typing avian staphylococci. Am J Vet Res 38:1601–1605.

73. Shimizu, A. 1977. Isolation and characteristics of bacteriophages from staphylococci of chicken origin. Am J Vet Res 38:1389–1392.

74. Shimizu, A. 1977. Bacteriophage typing of chicken staphylococci by adapted phages. Jpn J Vet Sci 39:7–13.

75. Shimizu, A. 1979. Phage-typing results of Staphylococcus aureus isolated from poultry in Japan and Europe. Avian Dis 23:39–46.

76. Takahashi, I., T. Yokoyama, T. Uehara, and T. Yoshida. 1986. Susceptibility of S. aureus and Streptococcus isolates from diseased animals to commonly used antibacterial agents and nosiheptide. I. Susceptibility of S. aureus. Bull Nippon Vet Zootech No. 35:43–49.

77. Tate, C.R., W.C. Mitchell, and R.G. Miller. 1993. Staphylococcus hyicus associated with turkey stifle joint osteomyelitis. Avian Dis 37:905–907.

78. Terayama, T., H. Ushioda, M. Shingaki, M. Inaba, A. Kai, and S. Sakai. 1977. Coagulase types of Staphylococcus aureus from food poisoning outbreaks and types of incriminated foods. Ann Rpt Tokyo Metrop Res Lab Public Health 28:1–4.

79. Terzolo, H.R., J.A. Villar, A.S. Zamora, and A. Zoratti De Verona. 1978. Staphylococcus infection of fowls. Gaceta Vet 40:388–402.

80. Thompson, J.K., and J.T. Patterson. 1983. Staphylococcus aureus from a site of contamination in a broiler processing plant. Rec Agr Res 31:45–53.

81. Thompson, J.K., J.T. Patterson, and P.A. Gibbs. 1980. The use of a new phage set for typing poultry strains of Staphylococcus aureus obtained from seven countries. Br Poult Sci 21:95–102.

82. Vaid, M.Y., M.A. Muneer, M. Naeem, and H.A. Hashmi. 1979. A study on the incidence of Staphylococcus infections in poultry. Pak J Sci 31:155–158.

83. Van Ness, G. 1946. Staphylococcus citreus in the fowl. Poult Sci 25:647–648.

84. Wang, C.T., Y.C. Lee, and T.H. Fuh. 1977. Artificial infection of chicks with Staphylococcus aureus. J Chin Soc Vet Sci 3:1–6.

85. Watkins, B.A. and B.F. Miller. 1983. Competitive gut exclusion of avian pathogens by Lactobacillus acidophilus in gnotobiotic chicks. Poult Sci 62:1772–1779.

86. Wilkinson, D.M., and M.M. Jensen. 1987. Staphylococcosis of turkeys. 4. Characterization of a bacteriocin produced by an interfering staphylococcus. Avian Dis 31:80–84.

87. Willemart, J.P. 1980. Staphylococcal synovitis in poultry and its treatment with tiamulin. Bull Acad Vet Fr 53:209–213.

88. Willett, H.P. 1992. Staphylococcus. In W.K. Joklik, H.P. Willett, D.B. Amos and C.M. Wilfert (eds.). Zinsser Microbiology, 20th ed. Appleton & Lange, Norwalk, CT, pp. 401–416.

89. Williams, R.B., and L.L. Daines. 1942. The relationship of infectious omphalitis of poults and impetigo staphylogenes in man. J Am Vet Med Assoc 101:26–28.

90. Witte, W., and H. Kühn. 1978. Macrolide (antibiotic) resistance of Staphylococcus aureus strains from outbreaks of synovitis and dermatitis among chickens in large production units. Arch Exp Veterinaermed 32:105–114.

91. Wos, Z., and H. Jagodzinska. 1978. Characteristics of staphylococci found in chicken carcasses. Przem Spozyw 32:186–187.

12 Clostridial Diseases

INTRODUCTION

H. John Barnes

Clostridial infections associated with four disease conditions in poultry or game birds are described in this chapter. *Clostridium colinum* is the cause of ulcerative enteritis; *C. perfringens* and *C. septicum* have been isolated from cases of necrotic enteritis or gangrenous dermatitis; and *C. botulinum* is the etiology of botulism. Other clostridial species may be involved in sporadic or possibly emerging diseases including *C. fallax* (1), *C. novyi* (4), and *C. sporogenes* (5). Recently, *C. chauvoei* was identified in lesions of the comb and livers of chickens in two flocks with complex disease conditions (6), and from intestines and livers of ostriches in a zoologic collection with an unusual neuroparalytic disease (3). *C. difficile* caused severe enteritis and enterotoxemia, resulting in the death of 153 of 160 young ostrich chicks in one flock, and was suspected when a second flock experienced a similar disease with high mortality (2). The organism was isolated in culture and *C. difficile* enterotoxin was confirmed by enzyme-linked immunosorbent assay (ELISA). Toxins produced by clostridial organisms are responsible for the pathology of some of these condi-

tions; in other cases, the organisms are relatively innocuous unless there are cofactors such as dietary ingredients or changes, severe stress, coccidiosis, or immunosuppressive infections such as infectious bursal disease or chicken infectious anemia.

REFERENCES

1. Ellwood, D.C., and R.W. Halliwell. 1973. Clostridium fallax infection in poultry. Trop Anim Health Prod 5:202–204.
2. Frazier, K.S., A.J. Herron, M.E. Hines, II, J.M. Gaskin, and N.H. Altman. 1993. Diagnosis of enteritis and enterotoxemia due to Clostridium difficile in captive ostriches (Struthio camelus). J Vet Diagn Invest 5:623–625.
3. Lublin, A., S. Mechani, H.I. Horowitz, and Y. Weisman. 1993. A paralytic-like disease of the ostrich (Struthio camelus masaicus) associated with Clostridium chauvoei infection. Vet Rec 132:273–275.
4. Peterson, E.H. 1964. Clostridium novyi isolated from chickens. Poult Sci 43:1062–1063.
5. Peterson, E.H. 1967. The isolation of Clostridium sporogenes from the viscera of day old chicks. Poult Sci 46:527–529.
6. Prukner-Radovcic, E., L. Milakovic-Novak, S. Ivesa-Petricevic, and N. Grgic. 1995. Clostridium chauvoei in hens. Avian Pathol 24:201–206.

ULCERATIVE ENTERITIS (QUAIL DISEASE)

Herman A. Berkhoff

INTRODUCTION. Ulcerative enteritis (UE) is an acute bacterial infection in young chickens, turkeys, and upland game birds characterized by sudden onset and rapidly increasing mortality. The disease was first seen in enzootic proportions in quail and was therefore named quail disease. It has since been established that many avian species

other than quail are susceptible, and the earlier name has been superseded by ulcerative enteritis.

Infection of humans has not been reported.

HISTORY. Quail disease was first reported in the United States in 1907 (32). Several scattered outbreaks in quail and grouse (1, 18, 27, 28, 36)

The author wishes to acknowledge Dr. M.C. Peckham for his previous contribution to this chapter.

were reported during the next 2 decades. Subsequently, infection in wild and domestic turkeys (10, 39) was discovered. Other avian species found to be susceptible included pigeons (19), chickens (39), pheasants, blue grouse, and California quail (11).

Chronologic events leading to isolation and precise identification of the etiologic bacterium are detailed by Bass (2, 3), Peckham (33, 34), and Berkhoff et al. (7).

INCIDENCE AND DISTRIBUTION. Distribution of UE is worldwide; a number of reports have originated from England (20), Germany (38), and India (22, 40, 41).

Ulcerative enteritis is an important disease problem in some concentrated poultry-raising areas (9) and is a threat to gamebirds either in confinement or in the wild.

ETIOLOGY. Initially, a gram-positive, pleomorphic, aerobic, nonmotile bacterium isolated from the liver of a diseased quail was used to reproduce UE in quail. The organism was identified as *Corynebacterium perdicum*. It did not grow on solid media and grew poorly in fluid media. On subculture, the organism quickly lost virulence (30). Subsequently, a gram-negative, anaerobic bacillus was isolated from the intestine and liver of infected quail. Feeding quail thioglycolate broth cultures reproduced the clinical syndrome (3).

Peckham (33, 34) reported isolation of a gram-positive, anaerobic, spore-forming rod following yolk sac inoculation of chick embryos. This organism produced UE lesions in inoculated quail. It was reisolated from inoculated quail, fulfilling Koch's postulates. Similar anaerobes were isolated from chickens and turkeys affected with UE, and it was established that UE in chickens, turkeys, and quail was caused by the same organism (34). Berkhoff et al. (8) cultured the etiologic anaerobe on solid media, which allowed study of its biochemical characteristics.

Classification. The organism is a new species of *Clostridium* named *Clostridium colinum* (5, 8). On the basis of 16S rRNA sequence analysis, *C. colinum* has been placed into subcluster XIV-b with six other *Clostridium* spp. It is most closely related to *C. piliforme*, the noncultured causative agent of Tyzzer's disease (13).

Morphology and Staining. *C. colinum* is a 1 x 3–4 μm bacillus that occurs singly as a straight or slightly curved rod with rounded ends. Sporulation is rarely seen in artificial media, but if spores are present, they are oval and subterminal. Sporogenic cells are much longer and thicker than nonsporing cells (Fig. 12.1).

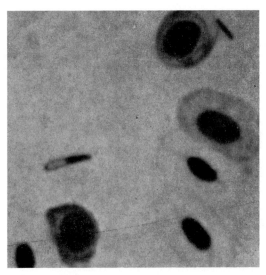

12.1.   Blood smear from quail with UE. Note two bacteria, one of which has a subterminal spore. (Peckham)

Growth Requirements. The organism is fastidious in its growth requirements, needing an enriched medium and anaerobic conditions. The best medium for isolating *C. colinum* is tryptose-phosphate agar (Difco) to which 0.2% glucose and 0.5% yeast extract are added. The pH is adjusted to 7.2 and the medium is then sterilized by autoclaving. After cooling to 56 C, 8% horse plasma is added, and the medium is poured into Petri dishes. Prereduced plates are inoculated with material from liver lesions and incubated anaerobically for 1–2 days at 35–42 C (17); colonies are white, circular, convex, and semitranslucent. Growth in broth media, prepared as above but without agar, can be detected as early as 12–16 hr postinoculation (PI). Actively growing cultures produce gas. Gas production continues for no more than 6–8 hr, after which growth settles to the bottom of the tube (5). Subcultures should be made from actively growing broth cultures still producing gas; later transfers may be unsuccessful.

Biochemical Characteristics. The following carbohydrates are fermented: glucose, mannose, raffinose, sucrose, and trehalose. Fructose and maltose are weakly fermented. Mannitol is fermented only by some strains, one of which is type strain (ATCC 27770). Carbohydrates not fermented are: arabinose, cellobiose, erythritol, glycogen, inositol, lactose, melezitose, melibiose, rhamnose, sorbitol, and xylose. Fermentation products of this organism are acetic and formic acids (5, 8).

Esculin is hydrolyzed. Starch hydrolysis is usually negative; only two strains have been found to cause starch hydrolysis. The type strain does not hydrolyze starch. Nitrite and indole are not produced. Milk is unchanged and casein is not digested. Good growth occurs in Chopped Meat Carbohydrate (CMC) broth. Pyruvate and lactate are not utilized. Gelatin is not liquefied. Catalase, urease, lipase, and lecithinase are not produced.

C. colinum resembles *C. difficile* most closely. These two organisms can be differentiated on cultural characteristics. *C. difficile* hydrolyzes gelatin and is unable to ferment raffinose, whereas *C. colinum* is inactive on gelatin and readily ferments raffinose (17).

Resistance to Chemical and Physical Agents.
The anaerobe, by virtue of its spore-forming characteristic, is extremely resistant to chemical agents and physical changes. Spores of *C. colinum* are resistant to octanol and chloroform (8). Yolk cultures have remained viable after 16 yr at −20 C and survive heating at 70 C for 3 hr, 80 C for 1 hr, and 100 C for 3 min (34).

Pathogenicity.
Pure cultures of *C. colinum* grown anaerobically were highly pathogenic for quail following oral inoculation. The experimental disease appeared either in an acute form with birds dying around 3 days PI, or in a more chronic form with deaths occurring after 1–2 wk (7).

PATHOGENESIS AND EPIZOOTIOLOGY

Natural and Experimental Hosts.
Ulcerative enteritis is found in a wide range of avian hosts, but quail are undoubtedly among the most susceptible species. Natural infections have been found in the following: bobwhite quail (*Colinus virginianus*), California quail (*Lophortyx california*), Gambel quail (*L. gambelii*), mountain quail (*Oreortyx picta*), scaled quail (*Callipepla squamata*), and sharp-tailed grouse (*Pedioecetes phasianellus*) (32); ruffed grouse (*Bonasa umbellus*) (28); domestic turkeys (*Meleagris gallopavo*) and chickens (*Gallus gallus*) (16, 39); European partridge (*Perdix perdix*) and wild turkeys (*M. gallopavo*) (16); chukar partridge (*Alectoris graeca*) (29); pigeons (*Columba livia*) (19); pheasants (*Phasianus colchicus*) and blue grouse (*Dendragapus obscurus*) (11); and crested quail (*L.c. californicus*) (20). An outbreak of UE in robins (*Turdus migratorius*), confirmed by isolation of *C. colinum* from the liver, was the first evidence that UE could affect passerine birds (42).

Although chickens are frequently infected naturally, experimental infections only can be readily produced in quail. Ulcerative enteritis is more frequently seen in young birds. It occurs in chickens 4–12 wk (34), turkeys 3–8 wk (10), and quail 4–12 wk of age. An outbreak has been reported in adult quail (23).

Outbreaks in chickens often accompany or follow coccidiosis, chicken infectious anemia, infectious bursal disease, or stress conditions. The importance of coccidiosis in outbreaks of UE in chickens was confirmed by producing UE in 5-wk-old chickens previously infected with *Eimeria brunetti* and *E. necatrix*, but not with either one alone (14).

Transmission.
Under natural conditions, UE is transmitted through droppings; birds become infected by ingesting contaminated feed, water, or litter. The organism produces spores, resulting in permanent contamination of premises after an outbreak has occurred. Oral administration of at least 10^7 viable cells of *C. colinum* is required to experimentally reproduce UE in quail (8).

The carrier status of recovered birds or survivors in a flock has not been critically studied. Chronic carriers, however, have been considered to be one of the most important factors in perpetuation of UE and a complement-fixation (CF) test to detect them has been used (31).

Incubation Period.
Following experimental infection in quail, the acute form of UE results in death within 1–3 days. The course of the disease in a flock generally lasts about 3 wk, with peak mortality occurring 5–14 days PI.

Signs.
Birds dying from acute disease may exhibit no premonitory signs. They are usually well muscled and fat and have feed in the crop. Quail often exhibit watery, white droppings. As UE progresses, infected birds become listless and humped up, with eyes partly closed, and feathers dull and ruffled. Extreme emaciation with atrophy of pectoral muscles is seen in birds affected 1 wk or longer.

Morbidity and Mortality.
Mortality in young quail may be as high as 100% in a matter of a few days. Chicken losses typically range from 2–10%.

Gross Lesions.
Acute lesions in quail are characterized by marked hemorrhagic enteritis in the duodenum. Small punctate hemorrhages may be visible through the serosa in the intestinal wall.

In birds that have survived infection for several days, inflammatory changes are followed by necrosis and ulceration, which may occur in any portion of the intestine and ceca. Early lesions are characterized by small yellow foci with hemorrhagic borders, which may be seen on serosal and mucosal surfaces. As ulcers increase in size, the hemorrhagic border tends to disappear. Ulcers may be lenticular or roughly circular in outline, sometimes coalescing to form large necrotic, diphtheritic patches. The lenticular shape is more common in the upper portion of the intestine. Ulcers may be deep in the mucosa; in older lesions they may be superficial and have raised edges. Ulcers in ceca may have a central depression filled with dark-staining material that cannot be rinsed off. Perforation of ulcers frequently occurs, resulting in peritonitis and intestinal adhesions. Gross lesions in the intestine are shown in Fig. 12.2A,B.

Liver lesions vary from light yellow mottling to large, irregular yellow areas along the edges. Other liver lesions are disseminated gray foci or small, yellow circumscribed foci, sometimes surrounded by a pale yellow halo (Fig. 12.2F). Spleen may be congested, enlarged, and hemorrhagic. Gross lesions are absent in other organs. Peckham (34) described an unusual lesion of UE in turkeys characterized by a necrotic, diphtheritic membrane occupying the middle third of the intestine. This combination of necrosis and sloughing of intestinal mucosa appeared similar to lesions produced by *E. brunetti* infection in chickens.

Histopathology. For a description of the histopathology of UE in quail, see (16). Intestinal sections from acute cases reveal desquamation of mucosal epithelium, edema of intestinal wall, vascular engorgement, and lymphocytic infiltration. The lumen of the intestine contains desquamated epithelium, blood cells, and fragments of mucosa. Early ulcers consist of small hemorrhagic, necrotic areas involving villi and extending into the submucosa. Cells adjacent to these areas exhibit coagulation necrosis with karyolysis and karyorrhexis. Lymphocytic and granulocytic infiltration occurs adjacent to necrosis. Small clumps of gram-positive bacteria are often present in necrotic tissue. Older ulcers appear as thick masses of granular, acidophilic, coagulated serum proteins mixed with cellular detritus and bacteria. Infiltrations of granulocytes and lymphocytes surround the ulcer. Microscopic pathology of the intestine is illustrated in Figure 12.2C, D, and E. Small blood vessels near ulcers and in liver are occasionally occluded by thrombi and bacteria. Liver lesions consist of poorly demarcated foci of coagulative necrosis, with minimal inflammatory reaction and occasional intralesional, gram-positive bacterial colonies, scattered throughout the parenchyma (20) (Fig. 12.2F,G,H).

Immunity. Active immunity seems to develop in birds that recover from naturally occurring infections. When survivors of a UE outbreak were subsequently challenged, there was no noticeable effect (24), whereas 85% of similarly challenged suscep-

tible controls died. It has been observed, however, that survivors in groups treated with antibiotics may remain highly susceptible to infection (26, 35).

DIAGNOSIS. Diagnosis of UE can be made on the basis of gross postmortem lesions. The presence of typical intestinal ulcerations accompanied by necrosis of the liver and an enlarged, hemorrhagic spleen suffices for clinical diagnosis. As an aid in diagnosis, necrotic liver tissue can be crushed between two slides, fixed by heat, and stained by Gram's method. Large, gram-positive rods, subterminal spores, and free spores can be seen. If necessary, *C. colinum* can be isolated from liver or spleen (see Isolation and Identification of Causative Agent).

A fluorescent antibody (FA) has been developed and found to be highly specific for diagnosis of UE; correlation between a presumptive diagnosis based on gross lesions and the FA test was 100% (6).

An agar gel immunodiffusion test has also been used for diagnosis of UE (4). Soluble bacterial antigens that reacted with antisera prepared against *C. colinum* were found in high concentrations in intestinal contents. These antigens were identical to bacterial antigens present in culture filtrates of *C. colinum*. Antigens were not, however, species-specific, as some strains of *C. perfringens* types A and C have cross-reacting antigens. Cross-reactivity among clostridial species makes this test unreliable for diagnostic purposes.

Isolation and Identification of Causative Agent. A clinical diagnosis of UE can be confirmed by isolation and identification of *C. colinum*. Because the organism is often present in the liver in pure culture, isolation from liver rather than from ulcerative, intestinal lesions is recommended. *C. perfringens* may be present as a secondary invader, but is easy to recognize (7, 17) (see Growth Requirements).

Differential Diagnosis. Among similar diseases that must be differentiated from UE are coccidiosis, necrotic enteritis, and histomoniasis. Frequently, coccidiosis in chickens, turkeys, and pheasants precedes or occurs concurrently with UE (Fig. 12.3). Both diseases may be present in the same or different specimens submitted for diagnosis (10, 11, 33). It is imperative that a differential diagnosis between coccidiosis and UE be made because medication for each disease is distinct. Furthermore, both diseases may occur simultaneously, necessitating use of two different medications.

A condition initially described as necrotic enteritis frequently occurs in broilers in densely populated areas. Although there was much controversy

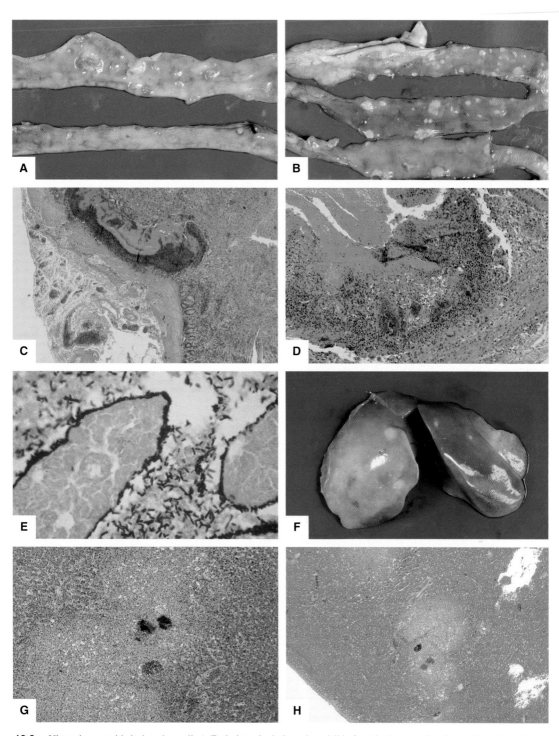

12.2. Ulcerative enteritis lesions in quail. *A.* Early intestinal ulceration visible from both mucosal and serosal surfaces. Note hyperemia around some lesions and occasional ulcers with marginal hemorrhage. *B.* More advanced ulcers filled with diptheretic, necrotic membranes. *C.* Transmural ulcer containing necrotic tissue and inflammatory exudate with adjacent focal peritonitis. *D.* Higher magnification of *C.* Note sharp demarcation between viable and necrotic tissue by a zone of inflammation, inflammatory exudate, and bacterial colonies. *E.* Gram-stained high-magnification of inflammatory zone showing numerous large gram-positive bacilli typical of *Clostridium colinum*. *F.* Areas of necrosis in chicken liver. *G.* Microscopic appearance of liver lesion. Note spreading areas of necrosis without distinct separation for normal tissue, minimal inflammatory response, and bacterial colonies. *H.* Gram stain of liver lesion. Note gram-positive staining colonies in necrotic foci.

that UE and necrotic enteritis are the same disease, it has been conclusively demonstrated (15) that they are distinct. Gross and histopathologic differentiation of necrotic enteritis and UE has been described (21) (see section on Necrotic Enteritis in this chapter).

Histomoniasis produces caseous cores in ceca and necrotic areas of varying size in the liver. This combination of cecal and liver lesions seen in chickens, turkeys, and other gallinaceous birds makes it imperative that cecal ulcerations and liver necrosis of UE be distinguished from histomoniasis. An enlarged hemorrhagic spleen and intestinal ulcerations are characteristic of UE. Histologic examination of the liver or ceca will reveal histomonads (see Chapter 34).

TREATMENT. Early attempts to use sulfonamides for treatment of UE were unsuccessful (12, 37). Streptomycin administered by injection or in feed or water has prophylactic and therapeutic value against UE in quail. Streptomycin at a level of 60 g/ton of feed or 1 g/gal of water gives complete protection when administered prophylactically (23, 24, 25, 26, 35). Addition of 100 g bacitracin/ton feed provides protection (35). Other chemotherapeutics reported to have efficacy for controlling UE in quail include furazolidone and chlortetracycline (CTC) (35).

The most effective drugs are bacitracin or streptomycin. Bacitracin is used in the feed at a concentration of 0.005–0.01%, streptomycin at 0.006%.

Either drug can be given in the drinking water prophylactically or therapeutically.

PREVENTION AND CONTROL

Management Procedures. Since the infectious organism is in the droppings and remains viable indefinitely in litter, it is recommended on problem farms to remove contaminated litter and use clean litter for each brood. In chickens, avoid stresses caused by overcrowding, keep coccidiosis under control, and use preventive measures against viral diseases, which may act as stressors and/or cause immunosuppression.

Game farm managers should exercise caution with regard to overgrazing ranges or overcrowding birds. Placing birds on 0.5-in. wire mesh is recommended on farms where the disease is a problem. Survivors of an outbreak may be carriers and should not be mixed with unexposed birds.

REFERENCES

1. Barger, E.H., S.E. Park, and R. Graham. 1934. A note on so-called quail disease. J Am Vet Med Assoc 84:776–783.
2. Bass, C.C. 1939. Observations on the specific cause and the nature of "quail disease" or ulcerative enteritis in quail. Proc Soc Exp Biol Med 42:375–380.
3. Bass, C.C. 1941. Specific cause and nature of ulcerative enteritis of quail. Proc Soc Exp Biol Med 46:250–52.
4. Berkhoff, G.A. 1975. Ulcerative enteritis—clostridial antigens. Am J Vet Res 36:583–585.
5. Berkhoff, H.A. 1985. Clostridium colinum sp. nov., nom. rev., the causative agent of ulcerative enteritis (quail disease) in quail, chickens, and pheasants. Int J Syst Bacteriol 35:155–159.

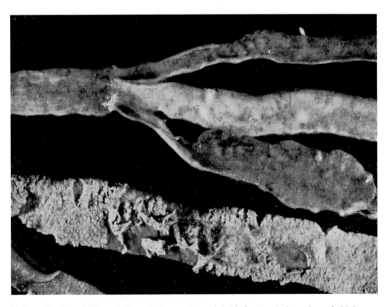

12.3. Combined UE and *Eimeria brunetti* coccidial infection in intestine of chicken. Note small ulcers in ceca and rectum. Diphtheritic membrane is due to coccidial infection. (Peckham)

6. Berkhoff, G.A., and C.L. Kanitz. 1976. Fluorescent antibody test in diagnosis of ulcerative enteritis. Avian Dis 20:525–533.

7. Berkhoff, G.A., S.G. Campbell, and H.B. Naylor. 1974. Etiology and pathogenesis of ulcerative enteritis ("quail disease"). Isolation of the causative anaerobe. Avian Dis 18:186–194.

8. Berkhoff, G.A., S.G. Campbell, H.B. Naylor, and L.DS. Smith. 1974. Etiology and pathogenesis of ulcerative enteritis ("quail disease"): Characterization of the causative anaerobe. Avian Dis 18:195–204.

9. Bryant, E.S., W. Gerencer, E.T. Mallinson, and G. Stein. 1973. Report of the committee on nomenclature and reporting of disease, Northeastern Conference on Avian Disease. Avian Dis 17:904–911.

10. Bullis, K.L., and H. Van Roekel. 1944. Uncommon pathological conditions in chickens and turkeys. Cornell Vet 34:312–319.

11. Buss, I.O., R.D. Conrad, and J.R. Reilly. 1958. Ulcerative enteritis in the pheasant, blue grouse and California quail. J Wildl Manage 22:446–449.

12. Churchill, H.M., and D.R. Coburn. 1945. Sulfonamide drugs in the treatment of ulcerative enteritis of quail. Vet Med 40:309–311.

13. Collins, M.D., P.A. Lawson, A. Willems, J.J. Cordoba, J. Fernandez-Garayzabal, P. Garcia, J. Cai, H. Hippe, and J.A. Farrow. 1994. The phylogeny of the genus Clostridium: Proposal of five new genera and eleven new species combinations. Int J Syst Bacteriol 44:812–826.

14. Davis, R.B. 1973. Ulcerative enteritis in chickens: Coccidiosis and stress as predisposing factors. Poult Sci 52:1283–1287.

15. Davis, R.B., J. Brown, and D.L. Dawe. 1971. Quail—biological indicators in the differentiation of ulcerative and necrotic enteritis of chickens. Poult Sci 50:737–740.

16. Durant, A.J., and E.R. Doll. 1941. Ulcerative enteritis in quail. Missouri Agr Exp Stn Res Bull 325:3–27.

17. Ficken, M.D., and H.A. Berkhoff. 1989. Clostridial infections. In H.G. Purchase, L.H. Arp, C.H. Domermuth, and J.E. Pearson (eds.). Isolation and Identification of Avian Pathogens. American Association of Avian Pathologists, Kennett Square, PA, pp. 47–51.

18. Gallagher, B.A. 1924. Ulcerative enteritis in quail. Am Game Prot Assoc Bull (Apr):14–15.

19. Glover, J.S. 1951. Ulcerative enteritis in pigeons. Can J Comp Med Vet Sci 15:295–297.

20. Harris, A.H. 1961. An outbreak of ulcerative enteritis amongst bobwhite quail (Colinus virginianus). Vet Rec 73:11–13.

21. Helmboldt, C.F., and E.S. Bryant. 1971. The pathology of necrotic enteritis in domestic fowl. Avian Dis 15:775–780.

22. Katiyar, A.K., A.G.R. Pillai, R.P. Awadhiya, and J.L. Vegad. 1986. An outbreak of ulcerative enteritis in chickens. Indian J Anim Sci 56:859–862.

23. Kirkpatrick, C.M., and H.E. Moses. 1953. The effects of streptomycin against spontaneous quail disease in bobwhites. J Wildl Manage 17:24–28.

24. Kirkpatrick, C.M., H.E. Moses, and J.T. Baldini. 1950. Streptomycin studies in ulcerative enteritis in bobwhite quail. I. Results of oral administration of the drug to manually exposed birds in the fall. Poult Sci 29:561–569.

25. Kirkpatrick, C.M., H.E. Moses, and J.T. Baldini. 1952. The effects of several antibiotic products in feed on experimental ulcerative enteritis in quail. Am J Vet Res 13:99–100.

26. Kirkpatrick, C.M., H.E. Moses, and J.T. Baldini. 1952. Streptomycin studies in ulcerative enteritis in bobwhite quail. II. Concentrations of streptomycin in drinking water suppressing the experimental disease. Am J Vet Res 13:102–104.

27. LeDune, E.K. 1935. Ulcerative enteritis in ruffed grouse. Vet Med 30:394–395.

28. Levine, P.P. 1932. A report on an epidemic disease in ruffed grouse. Trans 19th Am Game Conf, pp. 437–41.

29. Levine, P.P., and F.C. Goble. 1947. Diseases of grouse, pp. 401–442. In G. Bump et al. (eds.). The Ruffed Grouse. New York State Conservation Department, Albany, NY.

30. Morley, L.C., and P.W. Wetmore. 1936. Discovery of the organism of ulcerative enteritis. Proc N Am Wildl Conf, 74th Congr, 2nd sess. Senate Comm Print, Washington, DC, pp. 471–473.

31. Morris, J.A. 1948. The use of the complement fixation test in the detection of ulcerative enteritis in quail. Am J Vet Res 9:102–103.

32. Morse, G.B. 1907. Quail disease in the United States. United States Department of Agriculture, BAI Circ 109.

33. Peckham, M.C. 1959. An anaerobe, the cause of ulcerative enteritis ("quail disease"). Avian Dis 3:471–478.

34. Peckham, M.C. 1960. Further studies on the causative organism of ulcerative enteritis. Avian Dis 4:449–456.

35. Peckham, M.C., and R. Reynolds. 1962. The efficacy of chemotherapeutic drugs in the control of experimental ulcerative enteritis in quail. Avian Dis 6:111–118.

36. Pickens, E.N., H.M. DeVolt, and J.E. Shillinger. 1932. An outbreak of quail disease in bobwhite quail. Maryland Conservationist 9:18–19.

37. Rosen, M.N., and A.I. Bischoff. 1949. Field trials of sulfamethazine and sulfaquinoxaline in the treatment of quail ulcerative enteritis. Cornell Vet 39:195–197.

38. Schneider, J., and K. Haass. 1968. Beobachtungen zur ulceroesen enteritis (quail disease) bei huehnerkueken. Berl Munch Tieraerztl Wochenschr 81:466–468.

39. Shillinger, J.E., and L.C. Morley. 1934. Studies on ulcerative enteritis in quail. J Am Vet Med Assoc 84:25–35.

40. Shukla, P.K., and B.S. Rajya. 1968. Affections of the lower alimentary tract of domestic fowl. 1. On the occurrence and morphology of ulcerated enteritis simulating "quail disease." Indian Vet J 45:10–13.

41. Sing, N., M.S. Kwatra, and M.S. Oberoi. 1984. An outbreak of ulcerative enteritis ("quail's disease") in broilers in Punjab. Indian J Poult Sci 19:277–279.

42. Winterfield, R.W., and G.A. Berkhoff. 1977. Ulcerative enteritis in robins. Avian Dis 21:328–330.

NECROTIC ENTERITIS

Martin D. Ficken and Dennis P. Wages

HISTORY, INCIDENCE, AND DISTRIBUTION. Necrotic enteritis (NE) in domestic chickens was first described by Parish in 1961 (54, 55, 56), who reproduced the disease with a strain of *Clostridium welchii* (*C. perfringens*). It subsequently has been reported from most areas of the world where poultry is produced (7, 13, 19, 20, 38, 42, 44, 48, 51, 71). *Clostridium difficile* was isolated from a case of necrotic enteritis in a young ostrich (50).

ETIOLOGY. The cause of NE is *C. perfringens* types A (3, 9, 14, 41, 45, 52, 60, 70, 73) or C (22, 41, 51, 56, 60, 62). Some isolates of *C. perfringens* from cases of NE do not yield enough toxin in vitro to permit typing (41, 45). Alpha toxin produced by *C. perfringens* types A and C, and beta toxin produced by *C. perfringens* type C, are those believed responsible for intestinal mucosal necrosis, the characteristic lesion of NE. Both have been detected in feces of chickens with NE (41). Alpha toxin, obtained from broth culture supernatant fluids of type-A *C. perfringens*,(5, 52) is capable of producing characteristic intestinal lesions in conventional (5) or germ-free chickens (29).

C. perfringens can be readily isolated on blood agar plates incubated anaerobically at 37 C overnight. *C. perfringens* colonies on blood agar (with rabbit, human, or sheep blood) are surrounded by an inner zone of complete hemolysis and an outer zone of discoloration and incomplete hemolysis and are composed of short to intermediate, gram-positive rods without spores. Positive identification of the organism is made by inoculation of differential media (1). Most strains ferment glucose, maltose, lactose, and sucrose, do not ferment mannitol, and variably ferment salicin. Principal products of fermentation are acetic and butyric acids. Gelatin is hydrolyzed, milk is digested, and there is no indole production. Growth on egg yolk agar demonstrates presence of lecithinase and absence of lipase production. Subculturing on egg yolk agar plates, one-half of which have been spread with *C. perfringens* antitoxin, and incubating anaerobically overnight, will produce a zone of precipitation around colonies on control sides of the plate and little or no precipitation on sides spread with antitoxin (1).

PATHOGENESIS AND EPIZOOTIOLOGY. Naturally occurring outbreaks of NE have been reported in chickens from 2 wk to 6 mo of age. A majority of reports of NE have been in 2- to 5-wk-old broiler chickens raised on litter (7, 13, 31, 36, 38, 44, 48, 51, 71). However, outbreaks in 3- to 6-mo-old commercial layers raised in floor pens have also been reported (19, 42), and outbreaks of NE and coccidiosis have been reported in 12- to 16-wk-old cage-reared layer replacement pullets (18, 28). Subclinical NE in broiler chickens was significantly correlated with decreased growth rate and feed utilization, and occurred more frequently in flocks receiving high-barley diets (39).

Necrotic enteritis has been reported in turkey poults (25), 7-to 12-wk-old turkeys (32), and turkeys with concurrent ascarid infection (53) or coccidiosis (24).

C. perfringens can be found in feces, soil, dust, contaminated feed and litter, or intestinal contents (41, 43). In various outbreaks of NE, contaminated feed (20, 28, 73) and contaminated litter (72) have been incriminated as sources of infection.

Reports vary on the numbers of *C. perfringens* that can be consistently isolated from intestinal tracts of normal chickens. Some studies have found *C. perfringens* to be the principal obligate anaerobic bacterium in the intestinal tract of chickens (37, 63), whereas others have reported it only sporadically and in low numbers from small intestine of normal chickens ranging in age from recently hatched to 5 mo of age (11, 12, 61, 64, 69). Manipulating the diet can affect the population of *C. perfringens* in the intestinal tract (65), suggesting that *C. perfringens* numbers within the intestinal tract, and onset of intestinal clostridial disease in chickens, may be precipitated by the nature of the ration (51, 59). High levels of fishmeal (38, 70) or high levels of wheat (17) or barley (39) in the diet can predispose to and/or exacerbate outbreaks of NE.

Damage to the intestinal mucosa is another predisposing factor for NE (5, 70). Factors such as high-fiber litter (70) or various strains of coccidia (2, 6, 8, 9, 10, 36, 62) combined with higher than normal numbers of *C. perfringens* can result in NE. Necrotic enteritis has been experimentally reproduced in chickens (9, 21, 33, 34, 35, 57, 58), turkeys (26), and Japanese quail (22). In conventional chickens, the incidence can be from 1.3–37.3% and as high as 62.0% in specific-pathogen–free chicks (9). Necrotic enteritis can be reproduced by rearing chickens on litter in facilities where the disease has previously occurred (34, 35, 47, 72); feeding feed contaminated with *C. perfringens* (45, 70); administering vegetative cultures of *C. perfringens* intravenously (16), orally (16), or into the crop (9); administering intraduodenally broth cultures of *C. perfringens* (3), bacteria-free crude toxins of *C. perfringens* (4), or a combination of *C. perfringens* and its toxins (5, 10); or by dosing chickens with sporulated oocysts of *Eimeria* spp. and feeding vegetative cultures of *C. perfringens* or *C. perfringens*-contaminated feed (2, 8, 9, 10).

SIGNS AND LESIONS. Clinical signs in naturally occurring outbreaks include marked to severe depression, decreased appetite, reluctance to move, diarrhea, and ruffled feathers (7, 15, 36, 44, 51, 54, 71). Clinical illness is very short; often birds are just found acutely dead.

Gross lesions in naturally occurring outbreaks are usually confined to the small intestine, primarily jejunum and ileum (Fig. 12.4A,C) (7, 15, 36, 51, 71); however, cecal lesions have been described (46). Intestines are often friable and distended with gas. The mucosa is lined by a loosely to tightly adherent yellow or green pseudomembrane. Flecks of blood have been reported, but hemorrhage is not a prominent feature. Experimentally, gross lesions characterized by a gray, thickened mucosa in the duodenum and jejunum may be observed as early as 3 hr following inoculation of *C. perfringens* (3). By 5 hr, there is necrosis of the intestinal mucosa, which progresses over time to a severe fibrinonecrotic enteritis with formation of a diphtheritic membrane (9, 62). Swollen livers with necrotic foci may accompany *C. perfringens* infections (25).

Microscopic changes in natural outbreaks are characterized primarily by severe necrosis of the intestinal mucosa with an abundance of fibrin admixed with cellular debris adherent to the necrotic mucosa (Figs. 12.4B,D) (15, 36, 46, 51, 71). Initial lesions develop at the apices of villi, and are characterized by sloughing of epithelium and colonization of the exposed lamina propria with bacilli, accompanied by coagulation necrosis. Areas of necrosis are surrounded by heterophils. Progression of lesions usually occurs from villi apices to crypts. Necrosis may extend into the submucosa and muscular layers of the intestine. Numerous large bacilli are often observed attached to cellular debris. In birds that survive, regenerative changes consist of crypt epithelial cell proliferation with a corresponding increase in mitotic figures. Epithelial cells are primarily cuboidal, with a relative decrease in goblet and columnar epithelial cells. Villi are relatively short and flat. In many outbreaks, various sexual and asexual stages of coccidia are also found in the intestine (36, 46, 51).

Microscopic changes after experimental inoculation of *C. perfringens* (3) occur as early as 1 hr following challenge, and consist of slight edema and dilation of vessels in the lamina propria, sloughed epithelial cells in the intestinal lumen, and occasional heterophils and mononuclear cells in the lamina propria. By 3 hr, marked edema, resulting in detachment of the epithelial cell layer from the lamina propria, mostly at the apex of villi, has occurred. Mononuclear cell infiltration of the lamina propria is more marked than earlier. At 5 hr, there is marked coagulation necrosis of the epithelial cell layer and lamina propria at villous tips, resulting in villus shortening. Colonization of organisms may be prominent on necrotic tissues and apices of exposed lamina propria. Blood vessels are very congested; occasionally occluded by hyaline thrombi. By 8–12 hr, there is massive necrosis of villi, in some instances reaching to the crypts, characterized by areas of amorphous eosinophilic-staining material and cell nuclei. Fibrin and cellular debris are present in the lumen.

DIAGNOSIS. Diagnosis of NE can be made based on typical gross and microscopic lesions and isolation of the causative agent. In field cases of NE, *C. perfringens* can be readily isolated from intestinal contents, scrapings of intestinal wall, or hemorrhagic lymphoid nodules by anaerobic incubation overnight at 37 C on blood agar plates (27). Identification of *C. perfringens* can be done as described under Etiology.

Diseases that must be differentiated from NE are ulcerative enteritis (UE) and *Eimeria brunetti* infection. Ulcerative enteritis is caused by *C. colinum*

12.4. Necrotic enteritis (*A–D*). Gangrenous dermatitis (*E–H*). A. Necrotic enteritis in a 7-wk-old broiler breeder chicken with concurrent coccidiosis. Note the hyperemia and diffuse necrosis of the mucosa with multifocal ulceration. (Munger) B. Intestine of a turkey showing uniform diffuse coagulation necrosis of mucosa. Deeper viable mucosal tissue is demarcated from necrotic luminal mucosal tissue by a zone of intense hyperemia, hemorrhage, and inflammation, ×20. (Barnes) C. Necrotic enteritis in a 6-wk-old ostrich. *C. difficile* isolated. (Munger) D. Histologic lesions of the case in (*C*). Severe diffuse coagulation necrosis with separation from underlying viable tissue by an intense zone of inflammation. Note numerous large gram-positive bacilli primarily located at the interface of the necrotic and viable tissue. ×30 (Munger, Barnes) E. Gangrenous dermatitis affecting wing of a 12-day-old broiler. Spontaneous separation of epidermis revealing edematous, hyperemic, acutely inflamed dermis. (Munger) F. Broiler, 6-wk-old, with gangrenous dermatitis. Extensive discolored patches of necrotic skin are present on the abdomen. (Barnes) G. Same bird as in (*F*). Skin reflected to show discolored muscle and serosanguinous fluid expanding underlying dermis. (Barnes) H. Skin from a turkey with gangrenous dermatitis. Dermis beneath a normal epidermis is markedly expanded by fluid and gas. Cutaneous muscle is undergoing rhabdomyolysis. Cellular changes are minimal to absent, ×13. (Barnes)

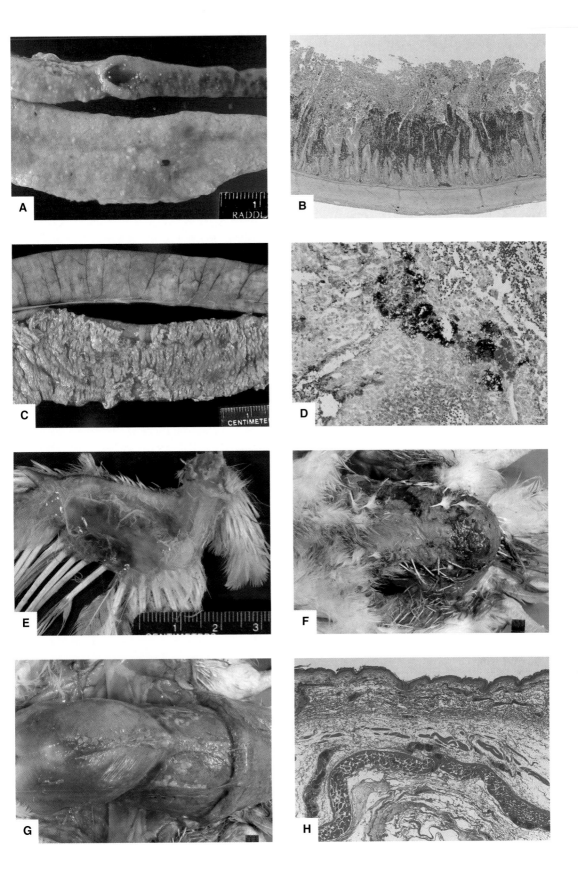

(see section on Ulcerative Enteritis in this chapter); characteristic gross lesions are multiple areas of necrosis and ulceration in the distal small intestine and ceca and areas of necrosis in the liver. As described previously, lesions of NE are usually confined to jejunum and ileum with little or no involvement of ceca or liver. These distinguishing characteristics should allow differentiation of NE and UE. Isolation and identification of the causative agent will confirm the diagnosis. *E. brunetti* infection (see Coccidiosis, Chapter 34) causes gross lesions similar to those produced by *C. perfringens*; however, microscopic examination of fecal smears, impressions, or intestinal sections should demonstrate the presence or absence of coccidia. Finally, NE and coccidiosis often occur simultaneously in a flock, and demonstration of one or both agents is warranted.

TREATMENT AND PREVENTION.
Experimentally, in vivo, a number of antibiotics placed in the feed reduce the numbers of *C. perfringens* shed in feces (66, 67, 68). These include virginiamycin, nitrovin, tylosin, penicillin, ampicillin, bacitracin, furazolidone, and efrotomycin.

Outbreaks of NE can be effectively treated by administration of lincomycin (34, 35), bacitracin (58), oxytetracycline (7), penicillin (42, 45), or tylosin tartrate (42) in the water. Bacitracin (57, 72), lincomycin (47), virginiamycin (23, 33), penicillin (51), avoparcin (39, 49, 57), and nitrovin (49) have been shown to be effective in preventing and controlling NE when placed in the feed.

Removal of fishmeal from the ration can help prevent clostridial infections in poultry (20). Probiotics such as *Lactobacillus acidophilus* and *Streptococcus faecium* reduce the severity of NE (30). Addition of *S. faecium* to cultures of *C. perfringens* results in a wide zone of inhibition (40).

REFERENCES
1. Allen, S. D. 1985. Clostridium. In E.H. Lennette, A. Balows, W.J. Hausler, Jr., and H.J. Shadomy (eds.). Manual of Clinical Microbiology, 4th ed. Am Soc Microbiol, Washington, DC, pp. 434–444.
2. Al-Sheikhly, F., and A. Al-Saieg. 1980. Role of coccidia in the occurrence of necrotic enteritis of chickens. Avian Dis 24:324–333.
3. Al-Sheikhly, F., and R.B. Truscott. 1977. The pathology of necrotic enteritis of chickens following infusion of broth cultures of Clostridium perfringens into the duodenum. Avian Dis 21:230–240.
4. Al-Sheikhly, F., and R.B. Truscott. 1977. The pathology of necrotic enteritis of chickens following infusion of crude toxins of Clostridium perfringens into the duodenum. Avian Dis 21:241–255.
5. Al-Sheikhly, F., and R.B. Truscott. 1977. The interaction of Clostridium perfringens and its toxins in the production of necrotic enteritis of chickens. Avian Dis 21:256–263.
6. Baba, E., A.L. Fuller, J.M. Gilbert, S.G. Thayer, and L.R. McDougald. 1992. Effects of E. brunetti infection and dietary zinc on experimental induction of necrotic enteritis in broiler chickens. Avian Dis 36:59–62.
7. Bains, B.S. 1968. Necrotic enteritis of chickens. Aust Vet J 44:40.
8. Balauca, N. 1976. Experimentelle reproduktion der nekrotischen enteritis beim huhn. I. Mitteilung. Mono- und polyinfektionen mit Clostridium perfringens und kokzidien unter berucksichtigung der kafighaltung. Arch Exp Veterinarmed 30:903–912.
9. Balauca, N. 1978. Experimentelle untersuchungen uber die Clostridien infektion und intoxikation bei geflugeln, unter besonderer berucksichtigung der kokzidiose. Arch Vet 13:127–141.
10. Balauca, N., B. Kohler, F. Horsch, R. Jungmann, and E. Prusas. 1976. Experimentelle reproduktion der nekrotischen enteritis des huhnes. II. Mitteilung. Weitere mono- und polyinfektionen mit Cl. perfringens und kokzidien unter besonderer berucksichtigung der bodenhaltung. Arch Exp Veterinarmed 30:913–923.
11. Barnes, E.M., G.C. Mead, D.A. Barnum, and E.G. Harry. 1972. The intestinal flora of the chicken in the period 2 to 6 weeks of age, with particular reference to the anaerobic bacteria. Br Poult Sci 13:311–326.
12. Barnes, E.M., C.S. Impey, and D.M. Cooper. 1980. Manipulation of the crop and intestinal flora of the newly hatched chick. Am J Clin Nutr 33:2426–2433.
13. Bernier, G., and R. Filion. 1971. Necrotic enteritis in broiler chickens. J Am Vet Med Assoc 158:1896–1897.
14. Bernier, G., R. Filion, R. Malo, and J.B. Phaneuf. 1974. Enterite necrotique chez le poulet de gril. II. Caracteres des souches de Clostridium perfringens isolees. Can J Comp Med 38:286–291.
15. Bernier, G., J.B. Phaneuf, and R. Filion. 1974. Enterite necrotique chez le poulet de gril. I. Aspect clinicopathologique. Can J Comp Med 38:280–285.
16. Bernier, G., J.B. Phaneuf, and R. Filion. 1977. Enterite necrotique chez le poulet de gril. III. Etude des facteurs favorisant la multiplication de Clostridium perfringens et la transmission experimentale de la maladie. Can J Comp Med 41:112–116.
17. Branton, S.L., F.N. Reece, and W.M. Hagler, Jr. 1987. Influence of a wheat diet on mortality of broiler chickens associated with necrotic enteritis. Poult Sci 66:1326–1330.
18. Broussard, C.T., C.L. Hofacre, R.K. Page, and O.J. Fletcher. 1986. Necrotic enteritis in cage-reared commercial layer pullets. Avian Dis 30:617–619.
19. Chakraborty, G.C., D. Chakraborty, D. Bhattacharyya, S. Bhattacharyya, U.N. Goswami, and H.M. Bhattacharyya. 1984. Necrotic enteritis in poultry in West Bengal. Indian J Comp Microbiol Immunol Infect Dis 5:54–57.
20. Char, N.L., D.I. Khan, M.R.K. Rao, V. Gopal, and G. Narayana. 1986. A rare occurrence of clostridial infections in poultry. Poult Advis 19:59–62.
21. Cowen, B.S., L.D. Schwartz, R.A. Wilson, and S.I. Ambrus. 1987. Experimentally induced necrotic enteritis in chickens. Avian Dis 31:904–906.
22. Cygan, Z., and J. Nowak. 1974. Nekrotyczne zapalenie jelit u kurczat. II. Wlasciwosci toksynogenne szczepow Cl. perfringens C i proby zakazenia przepiorek japonskich. Med Weter 30:262–265.
23. Davis, R., R.G. Oakley, M. Free, C. Miller, and R. Rivera. 1980. Profilaxis de la enteritis necrotica con la virginiamicina. Proc 29th West Poult Dis Conf, pp. 117–119.
24. Droual, R., H.L. Shivaprasad, and R.P. Chin. 1994. Coccidiosis and necrotic enteritis in turkeys. Avian Dis 38:177–183.
25. Eleazer, T.H., and J.S. Harrell. 1976. Clostridium perfringens in turkey poults. Avian Dis 20:774–776.
26. Fagerberg, D.J., B.A. George, W.R. Lance, and C.R. Miller. 1984. Clostridial enteritis in turkeys. Proc 33rd West Poult Dis Conf, pp. 20–21.
27. Ficken, M.D., and H.A. Berkhoff. 1989. Clostridial infections. In H.G. Purchase, L.H. Arp, C.H. Domermuth, and J.E. Pearson (eds.). Isolation and Identification of Avian

Pathogens. American Association of Avian Pathologists, Kennett Square, PA, pp. 47–51.

28. Frame, D.D., and A.A. Bickford. 1986. An outbreak of coccidiosis and necrotic enteritis in 16-week-old cage-reared layer replacement pullets. Avian Dis 30:601–602.

29. Fukata, T., Y. Hadate, E. Baba, T. Uemura, and A. Arakawa. 1988. Influence of Clostridium perfringens and its toxin in germ-free chickens. Res Vet Sci 44:68–70.

30. Fukata, T., Y. Hadate, E. Baba, and A. Arakawa. 1991. Influence of bacteria on Clostridium perfringens infection in young chickens. Avian Dis 35:224–247.

31. Gardiner, M.R. 1967. Clostridial infections in poultry in western Australia. Aust Vet J 43:359–360.

32. Gazdzinski, P., and R.J. Julian. 1992. Necrotic enteritis in turkeys. Avian Dis 36:792–798.

33. George, B.A., C.L. Quarles, and D.J. Fagerberg. 1982. Virginiamycin effects on controlling necrotic enteritis infection in chickens. Poult Sci 61:447–450.

34. Hamdy, A.H., R.W. Thomas, D.D. Kratzer, and R.B. Davis. 1983. Lincomycin dose response for treatment of necrotic enteritis in broilers. Poult Sci 62:585–588.

35. Hamdy, A.H., R.W. Thomas, R.J. Yancey, and R.B. Davis. 1983. Therapeutic effect of optimal lincomycin concentration in drinking water on necrotic enteritis in broilers. Poult Sci 62:589–591.

36. Helmboldt, C.F., and E.S. Bryant. 1971. The pathology of necrotic enteritis in domestic fowl. Avian Dis 15:775–780.

37. Johansson, K.R., and W.B. Sarles. 1948. Bacterial population changes in the ceca of young chickens infected with Eimeria tenella. J Bacteriol 56:635–647.

38. Johnson, D.C., and C. Pinedo. 1971. Gizzard erosion and ulceration in Peru broilers. Avian Dis 15:835–837.

39. Kaldhusdal, M., and M. Hofshagen. 1992. Barley inclusion and avoparcin supplementation in broiler diets. 2. Clinical, pathological and bacteriological findings in a mild form of necrotic enteritis. Poult Sci 71:1145–1153.

40. Kmet, V., J. Balascak, T. Dravecky, I. Koniarova, and R. Nemcova. 1992. Possibility of using probiotics in preventing necrotic enteritis in chickens. Veterinartvi 42:307–308.

41. Kohler, B., S. Kolbach, and J. Meine. 1974. Untersuchungen zur nekrotischen enteritis der huhner 2. Mitt.: Microbiologische aspekte. Monatsh Veterinaermed 29:385–391.

42. Kohler, B., G. Marx, S. Kolbach, and E. Bottcher. 1974. Untersuchungen zur nekrotischen enteritis der huhner 1. Mitt.: Diagnostik und bekampfung. Monatsh Veterinaermed 29:380–384.

43. Komnenov, V., M. Velhner, and M. Katrinka. 1981. Importance of feed in the occurrence of clostridial infections in poultry. Vet Glas 35:245–249.

44. Long, J.R. 1973. Necrotic enteritis in broiler chickens. I. A review of the literature and the prevalence of the disease in Ontario. Can J Comp Med 37:302–308.

45. Long, J.R., and R.B. Truscott. 1976. Necrotic enteritis in broiler chickens. III. Reproduction of the disease. Can J Comp Med 40:53–59.

46. Long, J.R., J.R. Pettit, and D.A. Barnum. 1974. Necrotic enteritis in broiler chickens. II. Pathology and proposed pathogenesis. Can J Comp Med 38:467–474.

47. Maxey, B.W., and R.K. Page. 1977. Efficacy of lincomycin feed medication for the control of necrotic enteritis in broiler-type chickens. Poult Sci 56:1909–1913.

48. Morch, J. 1974. Necrotic enteritis in broilers in Denmark. Proc XV World's Poult Congr Expos, pp. 290–292.

49. Morch, J. 1982. Undersgelser med vaekstfremmende foderadditiver specielt med henblik pa forebyggelse af nekrotiserende enteritis hos kyllinger. Nord Vet Med 34:377–387.

50. Munger, L.L. 1995. Personal communication.

51. Nairn, M.E., and V.W. Bamford. 1967. Necrotic enteritis of broiler chickens in western Australia. Aust Vet J 43:49–54.

52. Niilo, L. 1978. Enterotoxigenic Clostridium perfringens type A isolated from intestinal contents of cattle, sheep and chickens. Can J Comp Med 42:357–363.

53. Norton, R.A., B.A. Hopkins, J.K. Skeeles, J.N. Beasley, and J.M. Kreager. 1992. High mortality of domestic turkeys associated with Ascaridia dissimilis. Avian Dis 36:469–473.

54. Parish, W.E. 1961. Necrotic enteritis in the fowl (Gallus gallus domesticus). I. Histopathology of the disease and isolation of a strain of Clostridium welchii. J Comp Pathol 71:377–393.

55. Parish, W.E. 1961. Necrotic enteritis in the fowl. II. Examination of the causal Clostridium welchii. J Comp Pathol 71:394–404.

56. Parish, W.E. 1961. Necrotic enteritis in the fowl. III. The experimental disease. J Comp Pathol 71:405–413.

57. Prescott, J.F. 1979. The prevention of experimentally induced necrotic enteritis in chickens by avoparcin. Avian Dis 23:1072–1074.

58. Prescott, J.F., R. Sivendra, and D.A. Barnum. 1978. The use of bacitracin in the prevention and treatment of experimentally-induced necrotic enteritis in the chicken. Can Vet J 19:181–183.

59. Riddell, C., and X.M. Kong. 1992. The influence of diet on necrotic enteritis in broiler chickens. Avian Dis 36:469–503.

60. Seedy, E.L. 1990. Studies on necrotic enteritis in chickens. Vet Med J Giza 38:407–417.

61. Shane, S.M., D.G. Koetting, and K.S. Harrington. 1984. The occurrence of Clostridium perfringens in the intestine of chicks. Avian Dis 28:1120–1124.

62. Shane, S.M., J.E. Gyimah, K.S. Harrington, and T.G. Snider,III. 1985. Etiology and pathogenesis of necrotic enteritis. Vet Res Commun 9:269–287.

63. Shapiro, S.K., and W.B. Sarles. 1949. Microorganisms in the intestinal tract of normal chickens. J Bacteriol 58:531–544.

64. Smith, H.W. 1959. The effect of the continuous administration of diets containing tetracyclines and penicillin on the number of drug-resistant and drug-sensitive Clostridium welchii in the faeces of pigs and chickens. J Pathol Bacteriol 77:79–93.

65. Smith, H.W. 1965. The development of the flora of the alimentary tract in young animals. J Pathol Bacteriol 90:495–513.

66. Smith, H.W. 1972. The antibacterial activity of nitrovin in vitro: The effect of this and other agents against Clostridium welchii in the alimentary tract of chickens. Vet Rec 90:310–312.

67. Stutz, M.W., S.L. Johnson, and F.R. Judith. 1983. Effects of diet and bacitracin on growth, feed efficiency, and populations of Clostridium perfringens in the intestine of broiler chicks. Poult Sci 62:1619–1625.

68. Stutz, M.W., S.L. Johnson, F.R. Judith, and B.M. Miller. 1983. In vitro and in vivo evaluations of the antibiotic efrotomycin. Poult Sci 62:1612–1618.

69. Timms, L. 1968. Observations on the bacterial flora of the alimentary tract in three age groups of normal chickens. Br Vet J 124:470–477.

70. Truscott, R.B., and F. Al-Sheikhly. 1977. Reproduction and treatment of necrotic enteritis in broilers. Am J Vet Res 38:857–861.

71. Tsai, S.S., and M.C. Tung. 1981. An outbreak of necrotic enteritis in broiler chickens. J Chin Soc Vet Sci 7:13–17.

72. Wicker, D.L., W.N. Isgrigg, J.H. Trammell, and R.B. Davis. 1977. The control and prevention of necrotic enteritis in broilers with zinc bacitracin. Poult Sci 56:1229–1231.

73. Wijewanta, E.A., and P. Seneviratna. 1971. Bacteriological studies of fatal Clostridium perfringens type-A infection in chickens. Avian Dis 15:654–661.

GANGRENOUS DERMATITIS

Martin D. Ficken and Dennis P. Wages

HISTORY, INCIDENCE, AND DISTRIBUTION. In 1930, severe necrosis of muscle and subcutaneous tissue following intramuscular inoculation of *Clostridium welchii* (*C. perfringens*) isolated from heart blood and liver of two chickens was described (36). The next year (5), isolation of *C. perfringens, C. septicum,* and *C. novyi* from chickens dying of wound infections following collection of blood samples for pullorum testing was reported. The death of turkey breeder hens from wound infections occurring during mating caused by *C. perfringens, C. septicum,* and *C. sordellii* was reported in 1939 (14). Subcutaneous emphysema in chickens, from which *C. perfringens* and cocci were isolated, was described in Israel in 1950 (41). Since 1963, there have been reports of gangrenous dermatitis (GD) from various parts of the world including Argentina (4), Belgium (18), Egypt (2), Germany (24, 29), India (9), New Zealand (27), the United Kingdom (16), and the United States (17, 43). Gangrenous dermatitis also has been given a variety of names including necrotic dermatitis, gangrenous cellulitis, gangrenous dermatomyositis, avian malignant edema, gas edema disease, wing rot, and, in some instances, as a component of blue wing disease (39, 48, 7) (see Chapter 30, Chicken Infectious Anemia).

ETIOLOGY.   Causes of GD are *C. septicum* (16, 17, 23, 24, 44), *C. perfringens* type A (4, 9, 29, 49), and *Staphylococcus aureus* (6, 8, 18, 29), either singly or in combination (17, 25, 29, 43), with combined infections generally more severe.

S. aureus (see Staphylococcosis) and *C. perfringens* can be isolated and identified as described elsewhere (see the section on Necrotic Enteritis in this chapter). Culture for *C. septicum* should be carried out anaerobically on blood agar plates containing 2.5% agar, which will reduce swarming of *C. septicum* over the plate surface (15). Incubation is for 1–2 days at 37 C. Positive identification of the organism is made by inoculation of differential media (1). *C. septicum* ferments glucose, maltose, lactose, and salicin, but not sucrose or mannitol. Principal products of fermentation are acetic and butyric acids. Gelatin is hydrolyzed. Milk is not digested and indole is not produced. Growth on egg yolk agar demonstrates an absence of lecithinase and lipase production. Spores are oval and subterminal in location.

PATHOGENESIS AND EPIZOOTIOLOGY.
While natural outbreaks of GD have been reported

in chickens from 17 days to 20 wk of age, most have been in 4- to 8-wk-old broiler chickens (4, 6, 8, 16, 17, 23, 24, 25, 29, 43). The disease also has occurred in 6- to 20-wk-old commercial layers (17, 43), 20-wk-old broiler breeders (18), and chickens following caponization (49). In turkeys, fatalities in breeder hens due to clostridia and gram-positive cocci have been reported (14). Suspected cases of clostridial dermatitis have also been observed in turkeys on range and in breeder toms following semen collection (known locally as "bubbly tail"); however, the causative agent was not positively identified.

Clostridia are distributed in soil, feces, dust, contaminated litter or feed, and intestinal contents (1, 28). Staphylococci are ubiquitous and common inhabitants of skin and mucous membranes of poultry and areas where poultry are hatched, reared, and processed (see Chapter 11, Staphylococcosis).

In many instances, GD is believed to occur as a sequel to disease produced by other infectious agents such as infectious bursal disease (IBD) virus, chicken infectious anemia (parvovirus-like) virus (20, 39, 48, 7), reticuloendotheliosis virus (27), and avian adenovirus infections, including inclusion body hepatitis (IBH) virus (8, 16, 25, 31, 35, 42). Both GD and IBH occur as sequelae to IBD (13, 42, 45). In addition, some outbreaks of GD have been breeder flock–associated, i.e., progeny from a specific breeder flock consistently develop GD (19). Lack of antibody to IBD virus in broiler breeders correlates with increased susceptibility of their progeny to dermatitis (42).

Another condition predisposing chickens to GD is blue wing disease (BWD), which has been reported from Sweden (12)—where it was first described—Belgium, Denmark, Germany, Great Britain, Poland, and the United States. Characteristic lesions of BWD are intracutaneous, subcutaneous, and intramuscular hemorrhages and edema (11) with atrophy of thymus, spleen, and bursa of Fabricius (12). Numerous avian reoviruses and chicken infectious anemia virus (CIAV) have been isolated from chickens affected with BWD (12, 7), and the disease has been reproduced by dual infection with CIAV and a reovirus (12). GD often occurs secondarily to the skin hemorrhages. Apparently, a compromised immune system is the underlying predisposing factor allowing GD to occur.

Gangrenous dermatitis has been experimentally reproduced in chickens (17, 23, 24, 29, 43) and turkeys (43). In chickens, fatal disease, with lesions similar to those in naturally occurring outbreaks, followed intramuscular or subcutaneous inoculations of *C. septicum, C. perfringens* type A, or *S. aureus,* either singly or in combination, with combined infections being more severe. Intramuscular inoculations with *C. septicum* isolated from chickens caused death of turkeys within 24 hr with circumscribed lesions at the inoculation site.

Signs and Lesions. Clinical signs in naturally occurring outbreaks of GD include varying degrees of depression, incoordination, inappetence, leg weakness, and ataxia (16, 17, 23, 24, 43). Because the period of illness is short, usually less than 24 hr, birds are often just found acutely dead. Mortality ranges from 1 to 60% (16). Gross lesions consist of dark, moist areas of skin, usually devoid of feathers, overlying wings, breast, abdomen, or legs (see Fig. 12.4E,F [*Note:* Figure 12.4 can be found in the section entitled Necrotic Enteritis in this chapter]) (9, 16, 17, 23, 24, 43). Extensive blood-tinged edema, with or without gas (emphysema), is present beneath affected skin (Fig. 12.4G). Underlying musculature is discolored gray or tan, and may contain edema and gas between muscle bundles. In some cases, emphysema and serosanguineous fluid are present in subcutaneous tissue, but there is no loss of integrity in the overlying skin (25). Most cases report no internal lesions; however, discrete white foci (necrosis) in the liver (8, 43) and small flaccid bursae of Fabricius (8, 25), the latter presumably due to IBD virus infection, have been reported.

Microscopic changes are characterized by edema and emphysema (Fig. 12.4H) with numerous large, basophilic bacilli and/or small cocci within subcutaneous tissues (8, 43). Severe congestion, hemorrhage, and necrosis of underlying skeletal muscle is often present. Livers, if affected, contain small, randomly scattered, discrete areas of coagulation necrosis with intralesional bacteria. Cloacal bursal changes, in cases suspected to have concurrent IBD, are characterized by extensive follicular necrosis and atrophy (8, 25).

DIAGNOSIS. Diagnosis of GD can be made by the typical gross and microscopic lesions and isolation of the causative agent(s). In field cases of GD, staphylococci and clostridia can be isolated from exudates of skin and subcutaneous tissue or underlying muscle (8, 9, 17, 24, 43). Identification of the causative agent(s) can be done as described under Etiology.

Since occurrence of GD seems to be preceded by other infectious agents affecting immunologic defensive systems of the bird, diagnosis of the underlying etiology is necessary. Infections with IBD virus, avian adenoviruses, and CIAV and reoviruses

must be determined, as these can predispose GD.

A variety of skin conditions must be differentiated from GD. Dermatitis caused by mycotic agents, *Rhodotorula mucilaginosa* (3), *R. glutins* (37), *Candida albicans* (30), and *Aspergillus fumigatus* (50) can be differentiated from GD by demonstration of fungal elements in impression smears or tissue sections, and by isolation and identification of the agent. Contact, or ulcerative dermatitis ("breast burn") of broiler chickens (21, 33), and plantar pododermatitis of turkeys (32) are conditions characterized by erosions and ulcers accompanied by acute inflammatory changes over the breast, hock, and plantar surface of the feet. A strong correlation between wet or poor litter and these conditions is present (32, 34). Scabby hip dermatitis is a syndrome of broilers that, like contact dermatitis, is a nonspecific dermatitis with ulceration and secondary bacterial infection (22). Lesions originate as a scratch around the lumbar and sacral regions, and are strongly correlated with high stocking densities, resulting in feather breakage and entrance of bacteria into the dermis (22, 40). To differentiate GD from these conditions, demonstration of poor environmental conditions and/or overcrowding and lack of a primary infectious etiology is warranted. Vesicular lesions involving the wattles, comb, shanks, and feet have been described in chickens (26, 38, 46), and have been suspected or proven to be due to ingestion of the fungus *Cladosporium herbarum,* producing an ergotlike disease, or of *Ammi visnaga* seeds, which lead to photosensitization. These invariably occur only on unfeathered areas of the skin and should be easily differentiated. Squamous cell carcinoma of the skin of chickens, the cause of which is undetermined, leads to ulceration of the epidermis, which usually is infected with bacteria, and grossly may be difficult to differentiate from GD (47). Demonstration of cords and nests of neoplastic epithelial cells within the dermis by microscopy is necessary to diagnose this entity. Finally, a number of nutritional deficiencies and genetically slow-feathering male chickens may serve as underlying causes of dermatitis (10).

TREATMENT AND PREVENTION. Outbreaks of GD have been effectively treated by administration of chlortetracycline (23), oxytetracycline (43), erythromycin (43), penicillin (8, 9, 25), or copper sulfate (2) in the water, and chlortetracycline (24, 43) or furoxone (24) in the feed. However, in many instances, antibiotics used for control have had little success (16, 18, 19, 29). Failure of treatment is usually attributed to the underlying etiology, usually viral, which is not controlled. Administration of a mixed clostridial bacterin at 1 day of age has been shown to reduce losses in flocks due to GD (19); however, its use at present is not widespread. Management procedures to improve litter condition, reduce moisture and bacterial levels in the environment, and minimize trauma are useful adjuncts to treatment.

REFERENCES

1. Allen, S.D. 1985. Clostridium. In E.H. Lennette, A. Balows, W.J. Hausler, Jr., and H.J. Shadomy (eds.). Manual of Clinical Microbiology, 4th ed. American Society of Microbiologists, Washington, DC, pp. 434–444.
2. Awaad, M.H.H. 1986. A research note on the treatment of naturally induced gangrenous dermatitis in chickens by copper sulfate. Vet Med J Giza Egypt 34:121–124.
3. Beemer, A.M., S. Schneerson-Porat, and E.S. Kuttin. 1970. Rhodotorula mucilaginosa dermatitis on feathered parts of chickens: An epizootic on a poultry farm. Avian Dis 14:234–239.
4. Bianco, O., J. Quinones, J. Bergesio, M. Demo, and C. Pajaro. 1985. Dermatitis gangrenosa en pollos parrilleros: Dos brotes en Rio Cuarto. Vet Arg 19:879–883.
5. Bliek, L. de, and J. Jansen. 1931. Gasoedeem bij kippen na bloedtappen. Tijdschr Diergeneeskd 58:513–518.
6. Bootes, B.W., and G. Slennet. 1964. Staphylococcosis in chickens. Aust Vet J 40:238–239.
7. Bülow, V. von. 1991. Avian infectious anemia and related syndromes caused by chicken anemia virus. Crit Rev Poult Biol 3:1–17.
8. Cervantes, H.M., L.L. Munger, D.H. Ley, and M.D. Ficken. 1988. Staphylococcus-induced gangrenous dermatitis in broilers. Avian Dis 32:140–142.
9. Char, N.L., D.I. Khan, M.R.K. Rao, V. Gopal, and G. Narayana. 1986. A rare occurrence of clostridial infection in poultry. Poult Advis 19:59–62.
10. Clarke, W.E. 1974. Dermatitis in broiler chickens. Pract Nutr 8:5–7.
11. Engström, B.E., and M. Luthman. 1984. Blue wing disease of chickens: Signs, pathology and natural transmission. Avian Pathol 13:1–12.
12. Engström, B.E., O. Fossum, and M. Luthman. 1988. Blue wing disease of chickens: Experimental infection with a Swedish isolate of chicken anaemia agent and an avian reovirus. Avian Pathol 17:33–50.
13. Fadly, A.M., R.W. Winterfield, and H.J. Olander. 1976. Role of the bursa of Fabricius in the pathogenicity of inclusion body hepatitis and infectious bursal disease viruses. Avian Dis 20:467–477.
14. Fenstermacher, R., and B.S. Pomeroy. 1939. Clostridium infection in turkeys. Cornell Vet 29:25–28.
15. Ficken, M.D., and H.A. Berkhoff. 1989. Clostridial infections. In H.G. Purchase, L.H. Arp, C.H. Domermuth, and J.E. Pearson (eds.). Isolation and Identification of Avian Pathogens. American Association of Avian Pathologists, Kennett Square, PA, pp. 47–51.
16. Fowler, N.G., and S.N. Hussaini. 1975. Clostridium septicum infection and antibiotic treatment in broiler chickens. Vet Rec 96:14–15.
17. Frazier, M.N., W.J. Parizek, and E. Garner. 1964. Gangrenous dermatitis of chickens. Avian Dis 8:269–273.
18. Froyman, R., L. Deruyttere, and L.A. Devriese. 1982. The effect of antimicrobial agents on an outbreak of staphylococcal dermatitis in adult broiler breeders. Avian Pathol 11:521–525.
19. Gerdon, D. 1973. Effects of a mixed clostridial bacterin on incidence of gangrenous dermatitis. Avian Dis 17:205–206.
20. Goodwin, M.A., J. Brown, S.I. Miller, M.A. Smeltzer, and W.D. Waltman. 1989. Infectious anemia caused by a parvovirus-like virus in Georgia broilers. Avian Dis 33:438–445.
21. Greene, J.A., R.M. McCracken, and R.T. Evans.

1985. A contact dermatitis of broilers—clinical and pathological findings. Avian Pathol 14:23–38.
22. Harris, G.C., Jr., M. Musbah, J.N. Beasley, and G.S. Nelson. 1978. The development of dermatitis (scabby-hip) on the hip and thigh of broiler chickens. Avian Dis 22:122–130.
23. Helfer, D.H., E.M. Dickinson, and D.H. Smith. 1969. Clostridium septicum infection in a broiler flock. Avian Dis 13:231–233.
24. Hinz, K.H., M. Knapp, U. Lohren, and J. Batke. 1975. Gasodemerkrankung bei broilern. Dtsch Tierarztl Wochenschr 82:307–310.
25. Hofacre, C.L., J.D. French, R.K. Page, and O.J. Fletcher. 1986. Subcutaneous clostridial infection in broilers. Avian Dis 30:620–622.
26. Hoffman, H.A. 1939. Vesicular dermatitis in chickens. J Am Vet Med Assoc 95:329–332.
27. Howell, L.J., R. Hunter, and T.J. Bagust. 1982. Necrotic dermatitis in chickens. NZ Vet J 30:87–88.
28. Kohler, B., S. Kolbach, and J. Meine. 1974. Untersuchungen zur nekrotischen enteritis der huhner 2. Mitt.: Microbiologische aspekte. Monatsh Veterinaermed 29:385–391.
29. Kohler, B., V. Bergmann, W. Witte, R. Heiss, and K. Vogel. 1978. Dermatitis bei broilern durch Staphylococcus aureus. Monatsh Veterinaermed 33:22–28.
30. Kuttin, E.S., A.M. Beemer, and M. Meroz. 1976. Chicken dermatitis and loss of feathers from Candida albicans. Avian Dis 20:216–218.
31. Long, R.V. 1973. Necrotic dermatitis. Poult Dig 32:20–22.
32. Martland, M.F. 1984. Wet litter as a cause of plantar pododermatitis, leading to foot ulceration and lameness in fattening turkeys. Avian Pathol 13:241–252.
33. Martland, M.F. 1985. Ulcerative dermatitis in broiler chickens: The effects of wet litter. Avian Pathol 14:353–364.
34. McIlroy, S.G., E.A. Goodall, and C.H. McMurray. 1987. A contact dermatitis of broilers—epidemiological findings. Avian Pathol 16:93–105.
35. Monreal, G. 1984. Nachweis von neutralisierenden antikorpern gegen 11 serotypen der aviaren adenoviren. Arch Gefluegelkd 48:245–250.
36. Niemann, K. W. 1930. Clostridium welchii infection in the domesticated fowl. J Am Vet Med Assoc 77:604–606.
37. Page, R.K., O.J. Fletcher, C.S. Eidson, and G.E. Michaels. 1976. Dermatitis produced by Rhodotorula glutins in broiler-age chickens. Avian Dis 20:416–421.
38. Perek, M. 1958. Ergot and ergot-like fungi as the cause of vesicular dermatitis (sod disease) in chickens. J Am Vet Med Assoc 132:529–533.
39. Pope, C.R. 1991. Chicken anemia agent. Vet Immun Immunopathol 30:51–65.
40. Proudfoot, F.G., and H.W. Hulan. 1985. Effects of stocking density on the incidence of scabby hip syndrome among broiler chickens. Poult Sci 64:2001–2003.
41. Radan, M., and N. Rautenstein-Arasi. 1950. Anaerobic subcutaneous emphysema of poultry. Nature 166:442.
42. Rosenberger, J.K., S. Klopp, R.J. Eckroade, and W.C. Krauss. 1975. The role of the infectious bursal agent and several avian adenoviruses in the hemorrhagic-aplastic-anemia syndrome and gangrenous dermatitis. Avian Dis 19:717–729.
43. Saunders, J.R., and A.A. Bickford. 1965. Clostridial infections of growing chickens. Avian Dis 9:317–326.
44. Shirasaka, S., and Y. Benno. 1982. Isolation of Clostridium septicum from diseased chickens in broiler farms. Jpn J Vet Sci 44:807–809.
45. Shukla, R.P., B.P. Joshi, D.J. Ghadasara, and K.S. Prajapati. 1992. Pathological studies on outbreaks of gangrenous dermatitis in chickens. Indian Vet J 69:690–692.
46. Trenchi, H. 1960. Ingestion of Ammi visnaga seeds and photosensitization—the cause of vesicular dermatitis in fowls. Avian Dis 4:275–280.
47. Turnquest, R.U. 1979. Dermal squamous cell carci-

noma in young chickens. Am J Vet Res 40:1628–1633.
    48. Vielitz, E., and H. Landgraf. 1988. Anaemia-dermatitis of broilers: Field observations on its occurrence, transmission and prevention. Avian Pathol 17:113–120.
    49. Weymouth, D.K., M. Gershman, and H.L. Chute.

1963. Report of Clostridium in capons. Avian Dis 7:342–343.
    50. Yamada, S., S. Kamikawa, Y. Uchinuno, Y. Tominaga, K. Matsuo, H. Fujikawa, and K. Takeuchi. 1977. Avian dermatitis caused by Aspergillus fumigatus. J Jpn Vet Med Assoc 30:200–202.

BOTULISM

John E. Dohms

INTRODUCTION.   Botulism is an intoxication caused by exotoxin of *Clostridium botulinum.* Synonyms are "limberneck" and "Western duck sickness." Free-ranging and confinement-reared poultry, and feral birds can be affected. Most avian cases are caused by *C. botulinum* type C, although outbreaks due to other toxin types have been described (11, 34).

The public health significance of avian type C botulism outbreaks is considered minimal (4, 26). Four human type C botulism intoxications have been reported, but are not well documented (22, 26). No human cases of type C botulism have been associated with concurrent outbreaks of avian botulism (26, 51). Nonhuman primates, however, have succumbed to type C botulism after toxin inoculation (53), and captive monkeys died after eating chicken contaminated with type C toxin (48).

HISTORY.   Botulism was first reported in chickens in 1917 (9). Both chickens and humans developed the disease after ingestion of home-canned vegetables. Western duck sickness, first recognized in the United States in the early 1900s, was later found to be caused by *C. botulinum* type C toxin (17, 27). Botulism in chickens following ingestion of Lucilia fly larvae was reported in 1923. The first *C. botulinum* type C strains also were isolated from these invertebrates (3). For additional historical information, see (7, 11, 32, 43).

INCIDENCE AND DISTRIBUTION.   The disease has affected poultry and waterfowl worldwide (26). Although many early cases occurred in free-ranging poultry, and modern methods of poultry husbandry were thought to have reduced the incidence of botulism by preventing access to toxin-contaminated food, severe cases have been reported recently in confined broiler flocks (11, 39, 49). All types of wild birds and both avian and mammalian predators and scavengers have been affected during type C botulism outbreaks in wild birds (26). In these outbreaks, ducks have been most often affected (43). Botulism has been reported in pheas-

ants reared on game farms (43). Botulism in ducks, broiler chickens, and pheasants occurs more frequently and with greater severity during warmer months. However, outbreaks in broiler chickens also have been reported in winter (13, 40).

ETIOLOGY.   *C. botulinum* is a gram-positive, spore-forming bacterium capable of elaborating potent exotoxins under appropriate environmental conditions (34). The species consists of a diverse group of anaerobic bacteria including 4 cultural (I-IV) and 8 antigenically different toxigenic groupings (A, B, C alpha, C beta, D, E, F, and G). Human disease has been associated mainly with types A, B, E, and F, while A, C, and E have caused disease in birds (50). Cases of botulism in chickens, ducks, pheasants, and turkeys in natural or commercial settings have been caused primarily by the type C toxigenic group (11, 43, 49).

Morphology and Staining.   The gram-positive cells of *C. botulinum* type C measure 4–6 x 1.0 μm, often occurring singly or in short chains. The vegetative cell is motile. Subterminal or occasional terminal endospores are present in aging cultures (34). A cell-wall lysin is responsible for rapid autolysis of the organism and causes gram-variable staining in older cultures. Toxin is released during autolysis (5). Type C spores are more easily heat inactivated than type A and B spores (34), but are more resistant to heat than type E spores (46). The time required to cause a 10-fold reduction in spore viability at 101 C (D value) was 2.44 min for a terrestrial type C strain (46).

Culture group III contains nonproteolytic or weakly proteolytic type C and D toxigenic types (23, 51). *C. botulinum* requires an available water content (a_w) of 0.92 for growth and toxin production (41). The type C toxigenic group is further subdivided into C alpha and C beta subtypes based on their toxigenic properties (34).

Toxins.   Botulism toxins are among the most potent toxins known (31). Type C toxin is produced under anaerobic conditions at temperatures between 10 and 47 C with optimum toxin production between 35 and 37 C (34).

Type C alpha cultures produce three toxins; C1, C2, and small amounts of type D toxin (16). C1 and D toxin production is mediated by bacteriophage. Type C strains, cured of their prophage, can be converted to type D organisms by infection with phage purified from type D strains. The reciprocal is also true (16). Type C beta strains, lacking bacteriophage coding for C1 and D toxins, produce only C2 toxin; genes coding for C2 toxin are not phage associated (16). Because of the interconvertibility of C alpha and C beta strains, the relevance of C alpha and C beta toxigenic grouping has been questioned (16).

C1 and D, together with A, B, E, and F, toxins are synthesized as single nontoxic polypeptides that are cleaved by proteases to produce 140- to 167-kD dichain neurotoxins (47). A 98-kD heavy chain and a 53-kD light chain, held together by an interchain disulfide bond, are not toxic when dissociated (52).

Neurotoxin action occurs at the peripheral cholinergic nerve terminus. Free toxin binds to the cell membrane, translocates, and reacts intracellularly to block release of acetylcholine. When the cholinergic nerve ending is a motor endplate, muscle is paralyzed (47). Binary C2 toxin, though not neurotoxic, requires trypsin activation and causes increased membrane permeability in a variety of cultured tissues (37, 47). Ducks and geese inoculated intravenously with C2 toxin showed cardiopulmonary symptoms (25, 37). In mice, C2 toxin has enterotoxic properties (37). The role of C2 toxin in natural botulism outbreaks is presently unclear.

Chickens, turkeys, pheasants, and peafowl are susceptible to types A, B, C, and E, but not D or F, toxin (18). Chickens are most sensitive to types A and E given intravenously but relatively resistant to type C1 intoxication (12, 18, 35, 41, 42). In contrast, ducks and pheasants are more susceptible to C1 toxin (18, 20). Compared with other toxins, C1 and C2 are more readily absorbed by chickens when given orally (18). As broiler chickens age, they become less susceptible to C1 toxin. At hatching, the chicken lethal dose—50% (LD_{50})—$10^{3.0}$ mouse-LD_{50} per kg body weight compared with $10^{6.3}$ mouse-LD_{50} per kg body weight at 8 wk of age (12).

PATHOGENESIS AND EPIZOOTIOLOGY

Natural and Experimental Hosts.
Type C botulism has occurred in many species of birds including chickens, turkeys, ducks, pheasants, and ostriches (1). In wildlife outbreaks, 117 avian species in 22 families are believed to have been affected (26). Outbreaks in aviaries have occurred (49, 51). Mammalian species affected by type C toxin include mink, ferrets, cattle, pigs, dogs, horses, and a variety of zoo mammals (34). Fish succumbed to type C botulism during outbreaks on fish farms (51). Type C botulism in ruminants fed poultry manure has caused serious economic loss (15). Laboratory rodents are fully susceptible to type C toxin; mice are useful in the bioassay for toxin detection and typing.

In a study of 27 outbreaks in broiler chickens, ages ranged from 2 to 8 wk with a mean of 6.2 ± 1.7 wk (13). Outbreaks in older broiler chickens have been reported (4). Paradoxically, at these ages, broiler chickens are relatively resistant to C1 toxin (12).

Incubation Period.
Experimental subcutaneous, intravenous, or oral inoculation of type C toxin in chickens and ducks produced clinical signs identical to those observed in field outbreaks. Morbidity and mortality were dose related. With high levels of toxin, disease appears within hours. With low toxin doses, onset of paralysis occurs within 1–2 days (12, 18, 20, 24).

Transmission.
C. botulinum type C is distributed worldwide wherever large populations of wild and domestic birds are found. Type C organisms readily grow in the gastrointestinal tract of birds and are considered obligate parasites (51). Type C spores are commonly found in and around poultry and pheasant farms (13, 30, 49, 50). Presence of organisms in the gastrointestinal tract of wild and domestic birds, and resistance of spores to inactivation, favor spread of this organism (13, 26).

Signs.
Clinical signs of botulism in chickens, turkeys, pheasants, and ducks are similar (7, 11, 24, 43). In chickens, flaccid paralysis of legs, wings, neck, and eyelids are predominant features of the disease. Paralytic signs progress cranially from the legs to include wings, neck, and eyelids. Initially, affected birds are found sitting and are reluctant to move. If coaxed to walk, they appear lame. Wings droop when paralyzed. Limberneck, the original and common name for botulism, precisely describes the paralysis of the neck (Fig. 12.5). Because of eyelid paralysis, birds appear comatose and may seem dead. Gasping has been reported when birds are handled. Death results from cardiac and respiratory failure (51).

Affected chickens have ruffled feathers, which may fall out with handling. Quivering of certain feather tracts has been observed. Broiler chickens showing signs of botulism may have diarrhea with excess urates in the loose droppings.

Morbidity and Mortality.
Morbidity and mortality are related to the amount of acquired toxin. Low levels of intoxication produce little mortality

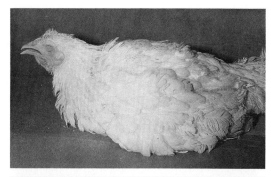

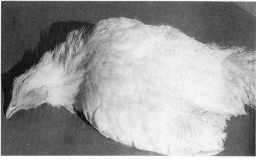

12.5. Botulism in chickens showing partial paralysis of wing and lower eyelid, difficult breathing caused by partial paralysis of respiratory muscles, and ruffled hackle feathers.

and morbidity, which can confuse diagnosis. In severe cases, up to 40% mortality has been observed in broiler flocks (11, 40).

Western duck sickness is one of the most devastating diseases of waterfowl. Mortality, although difficult to estimate in wild birds, was reportedly greater than 100,000 birds on separate occasions (7, 26). Such losses have a major impact on wildlife populations (26). In other cases, outbreaks in small lakes have been limited to the relatively few waterfowl in these habitats (2, 49). Mortality of pheasants reared on game farms has been as high as 40,000 birds (43).

Pathology. Birds with type C botulism lack gross or microscopic lesions. Occasionally, maggots or feathers can be found in the crop of affected birds.

Pathogenesis. Type C botulism can be caused by ingestion of preformed toxin. Because the organism is widely distributed in the gut, dead birds provide conditions for *C. botulinum* growth and toxin production. Greater than 2000 minimum lethal doses (MLD) of type C toxin per gram of carcass tissue have been found (4). Birds scavenging such carcasses can readily obtain enough toxin to become affected. Fly-blown carcasses may have

maggots containing varying levels of botulinal toxin. Maggots have been found to contain from 10^4–10^5 MLD of toxin (49). Maggots are readily devoured by chickens, pheasants, or ducks, which can lead to explosive botulism outbreaks. In aquatic environments, small crustaceans and insect larvae may contain *C. botulinum* in their gut. If large numbers die due to oxygen depletion, toxin can be produced within these invertebrates. Ingestion of toxin laden invertebrates has been proposed as the cause of type C botulism in ducks (43, 55). Lakes with shallow sloping banks that experience dramatic fluctuations in water level are most commonly associated with botulism outbreaks (26, 55).

Botulism caused by types A and E occurs rarely and generally has been associated with consumption of spoiled human food products fed to backyard chicken flocks (32). Botulism in sea gulls, loons, and grebes was caused by eating dead or dying fish contaminated with type E toxin (34). A type A botulism case in broiler chickens was due to a contaminated feed source (8).

The pathogenesis of botulism was once exclusively thought to be due to ingestion of preformed toxin. There is growing evidence that *C. botulinum* type C elaborates toxin in vivo to cause disease (49). The term *toxico-infection,* originally used by Russian researchers, was adapted to describe this form of the disease in broiler chickens (40, 51). In two cases of type C botulism in broiler chickens, carcasses were implicated as the toxin source (4, 21). In the majority of broiler chicken outbreaks, however, despite comprehensive searches, no toxin sources have been identified (13, 19, 39, 45, 49). The disease pattern in many of these outbreaks was inconsistent with food or water as toxin sources. Dead carcasses could not account for intoxications.

Type C botulism was reproduced in leghorn chickens and pheasants fed botulinal spores. Chickens and pheasants with their ceca ligated had a lower incidence of disease following spore challenge (30, 35) suggesting the cecum as the site of toxin production. In pheasants, the crop supported toxin production (10). Attempts to reproduce the toxicoinfectious form of botulism in broiler chickens have been unsuccessful (11, 30). Toxin is, however, produced in the cecum of broiler chickens, but not at levels sufficient to kill the host (30). An environmental, bacterial, phage, and/or host interaction may be required for toxicoinfectious botulism to occur in broilers.

Immunity. Because the toxigenic dose is lower than the immunogenic dose, chickens and ducks recovering from botulism do not develop immunity (6, 18). However, carrion-eating crows and turkey vultures possessed antibodies to botulinal toxin (38). This may partly explain why vultures were resistant to experimental inoculations of toxin (28).

DIAGNOSIS. The differential diagnosis of botulism is based on clinical signs and lack of gross or microscopic lesions. Definitive diagnosis requires detection of toxin in serum, crop, or gastrointestinal washings from morbid birds (11, 51).

Serum is the preferred diagnostic sample. Because *C. botulinum* is found in the gut of normal chickens, toxin can be produced in decaying body tissues. Therefore, finding toxin in tissues of dead birds does not confirm botulism.

The mouse bioassay is a sensitive and reliable method for confirming heat-labile toxin in serum (11). Groups of mice are inoculated with suspect serum samples. Other mice receive samples treated with type-specific antiserum. If toxin is present in the sample, signs and death of mice given untreated samples usually occur within 48 hr. Mice inoculated with specific antitoxin will be protected. Other in vitro methods of detecting toxin have been reviewed (36).

In waterfowl and some poultry outbreaks, toxin levels in blood may be too low to produce disease in mice. Concentration of serum, or repeated inoculations of mice with suspect serum, may be required to demonstrate toxin in these cases (20).

In advanced stages of the disease, clinical signs are obvious; during mild intoxications, only leg paralysis may be observed. The mild form of the disease must be differentiated from Marek's disease, drug and chemical toxicities, or appendicular skeletal problems. In these cases, the mouse bioassay is particularly helpful in diagnosis. Botulism in waterfowl must be differentiated from fowl cholera and chemical toxicity. Lead poisoning of water birds is commonly confused with botulism (43, 51).

Isolation of *C. botulinum* requires anaerobic culturing (23) and is of little help in diagnosis. The organism is widely distributed in gut, liver, and spleen of clinically normal chickens (12). Detection of the organism, however, in feed or environmental samples may prove useful in epidemiologic studies. The organism can be demonstrated in samples inoculated into cooked-meat medium and incubated anaerobically at 30 C (11). After 3–5 days' incubation, toxin can be detected using the mouse bioassay with specific typing antitoxins. Other modifications of this procedure are available (23, 51). The organism can be detected using the fluorescent antibody technique (33).

TREATMENT. Many sick birds, if isolated and provided with water and feed, will recover. Treatment of large numbers of morbid birds, however, is difficult, and various protocols have been used but are not verified experimentally. The success of these treatments is hard to establish because of the difficulty in experimentally reproducing toxicoinfectious botulism. The patterns of disease in untreated broiler houses can rise and fall during a given outbreak (13). Therefore, it is difficult to know whether a particular treatment is effective, or, if by chance, treatment precedes a drop in mortality that would have occurred anyway. However, several treatments have been reported to be of benefit. Treatment of affected broiler flocks with sodium selenite and vitamins A, D3, and E reduced mortality (45). Antibiotics including bacitracin (100 g/ton in feed), streptomycin (1 g/L in water), or periodic chlortetracycline treatments also reduced mortality (44). Penicillin was ineffective in controlling one outbreak (39), but has been found efficacious in other affected flocks (40). In vitro susceptibility of *C. botulinum* to 13 antibiotics was reviewed (44).

Inoculation with specific antitoxin neutralizes only free and extracellularly bound toxin and might be considered for treating valuable birds in zoologic collections. Ostriches showing clinical signs of botulism responded favorably within 24 hr after treatment with type C antitoxin (1). This is impractical in commercial poultry, duck, or pheasant outbreaks.

PREVENTION AND CONTROL. Management practices should emphasize removal of potential sources of the organism and its toxin from the environment. Prompt disposal of dead birds and culling of sick birds is very important in prevention and control. In problem areas, removal of contaminated litter and thorough disinfection using calcium hypochlorite, iodophor, or formalin disinfectants may help reduce spore numbers in the environment (44). In houses with dirt floors, complete destruction of these sporeformers is difficult. Disinfection of areas around poultry houses has been recommended (44). Spores may be located in soil outside of the poultry facility and can be transported back into houses. Fly control may be another means of reducing the risk of toxic maggots in the environment. During outbreaks, it has been suggested that feeding lower energy diets reduces mortality caused by toxicoinfectious botulism (45). Excess iron in feed or water has also been associated with some outbreaks (54).

Immunization. Active immunization with inactivated bacterin-toxoids has been successfully used in pheasant operations (29). Similarly formulated toxoids protect chickens and ducks from experimental botulism (6, 14). Vaccination of large numbers of broiler chickens, however, is costly, and vaccination of wildfowl is not practical.

REFERENCES

1. Allwright, D.M., M. Wilson, and W.J.J. van Rensburg. 1994. Botulism in ostriches (Struthio camelus). Avian Pathol 23:183–186.
2. Azuma, R., and T. Itoh. 1987. Botulism in waterfowl and distribution of C. botulinum type C in Japan. In M.W. Eklund and V.R. Dowell, Jr. (eds.). Avian Botulism: An International Perspective. Charles C. Thomas, Springfield, IL, pp. 167–187.

3. Bengtson, I.A. 1922. Preliminary note on a toxin-producing anaerobe isolated from the larvae of Lucilia caesar. Public Health Rep 37:164–170.

4. Blandford, T.B., and T.A. Roberts. 1970. An outbreak of botulism in broiler chickens. Vet Rec 87:258–261.

5. Bonventre, P.F., and L.L. Kempe. 1960. Physiology of toxin production by Clostridium botulinum types A and B. I. Growth, autolysis, and toxin production. J Bacteriol 79:18–23.

6. Boroff, D.A., and J.R. Reilly. 1959. Studies of the toxin of Clostridium botulinum. V. Prophylactic immunization of pheasants and ducks against avian botulism. J Bacteriol 77:142–146.

7. Clark, W.E. 1987. Avian botulism. In M.W. Eklund and V.R. Dowell, Jr. (eds.). Avian Botulism: An International Perspective. Charles C. Thomas, Springfield, IL, pp. 89–105.

8. De Fagonde, A.P., and H.F. Sardi. 1967. Botulismo aviar, primer caso comprobado en la Republica Argentina. Bull Off Int Epiz 67:1479–1491.

9. Dickson, E.C. 1917. Botulism, a case of limberneck in chickens. J Am Vet Med Assoc 50:612–613.

10. Dinter, Z., and K.E. Kull. 1954. Uber einen ausbruch des botulismus bei frasanenkuken. Nord Veterinaermed 6:866–872.

11. Dohms, J.E. 1987. Laboratory investigation of botulism in poultry. In M.W. Eklund and V.R. Dowell, Jr. (eds.). Avian Botulism: An International Perspective. Charles C. Thomas, Springfield, IL, pp. 295–314.

12. Dohms, J.E., and S.S. Cloud. 1982. Susceptibility of broiler chickens to Clostridium botulinum type C toxin. Avian Dis 26:89–96.

13. Dohms, J.E., P.H. Allen, and J.K. Rosenberger. 1982. Cases of type C botulism in broiler chickens. Avian Dis 26:204–210.

14. Dohms, J.E., P.H. Allen, and S.S. Cloud. 1982. The immunization of broiler chickens against type C botulism. Avian Dis 26:340–345.

15. Egyed, M.N. 1987. Outbreaks of botulism in ruminants associated with ingestion of feed containing poultry waste. In M.W. Eklund and V.R. Dowell, Jr. (eds.). Avian Botulism: An International Perspective. Charles C. Thomas, Springfield, IL, pp. 371–380.

16. Eklund, M.E., F. Poysky, K. Oguma, H. Iida, and K. Inoue. 1987. Relationship of bacteriophages to toxin and hemagglutinin production by Clostridium botulinum types C and D and its significance in avian botulism outbreaks. In M.W. Eklund and V.R. Dowell, Jr. (eds.). Avian Botulism: An International Perspective. Charles C. Thomas, Springfield, IL, pp. 191–222.

17. Giltner, L.T., and J.F. Couch. 1930. Western duck sickness and botulism. Science 72:660.

18. Gross, W.B., and L.DS. Smith. 1971. Experimental botulism in gallinaceous birds. Avian Dis 15:716–722.

19. Haagsma, J. 1974. An outbreak of botulism in broiler chickens. Tijdschr Diergeneesk 99:1069–1070.

20. Haagsma, J. 1987. Laboratory investigation of botulism in wild birds. In M.E. Eklund and V.R. Dowell, Jr. (eds.). Avian Botulism: An International Perspective. Charles C. Thomas, Springfield, IL, pp. 283–293.

21. Harrigan, K.E. 1980. Botulism in broiler chickens. Aust Vet J 56:603–605.

22. Holdeman, L.V. 1970. The ecology and natural history of Clostridium botulinum. J Wildl Dis 6:205–210.

23. Jansen, B.C. 1987. Clostridium botulinum type C, its isolation, identification, and taxonomic position. In M.W. Eklund and V.R. Dowell, Jr. (eds.). Avian Botulism: An International Perspective. Charles C. Thomas, Springfield, IL, pp. 123–132.

24. Jeffery, J.S., F.D. Galey, C.V. Meteyer, H. Kinde, and M. Rezvani. 1994. Type C botulism in turkeys: Determination of the median toxic dose. J Vet Diagn Invest 6:93–95.

25. Jensen, W.I., and R.M. Duncan. 1980. The susceptibility of the mallard duck (Anas platyrhynchos) to Clostridium botulinum C2 toxin. Jpn J Med Sci Biol 33:81–86.

26. Jensen, W.I. 1987. The global importance of type C botulism in wild birds. In M.W. Eklund and V.R. Dowell, Jr. (eds.). Avian Botulism: An International Perspective. Charles C Thomas, Springfield, IL, pp. 33–54.

27. Kalmbach, E.R. 1930. Western duck sickness produced experimentally. Science 72:658–660.

28. Kalmbach, E.R. 1939. American vultures and the toxin of Clostridium botulinum. J Am Vet Med Assoc 94:187–191.

29. Kurazono, H., K. Shimozawa, G. Sakaguchi, M. Takahashi, T. Shimizu, and H. Kondo. 1985. Botulism among penned pheasants and protection by vaccination with C1 toxoid. Res Vet Sci 38:104–108.

30. Kurazono, H., K. Shimozawa, and G. Sakaguchi. 1987. Experimental botulism in pheasants. In M.W. Eklund and V.R. Dowell, Jr. (eds.). Avian Botulism: An International Perspective. Charles C. Thomas, Springfield, IL, pp. 267–281.

31. Lamanna, C. 1959. The most poisonous poison. Science 130:763–772.

32. Levine, N.D. 1965. Botulism. In H.E. Biester and L.H. Schwarte (eds.). Diseases of Poultry, 5th ed. Iowa State University Press, Ames, IA, pp. 456–461.

33. Midura, T.F. 1987. Use of fluorescent antibody techniques in identification of Clostridium botulinum. In M.W. Eklund and V.R. Dowell, Jr. (eds.). Avian Botulism: An International Perspective. Charles C. Thomas, Springfield, IL, pp. 315–322.

34. Mitchell, W.R., and S. Rosendal. 1987. Type C botulism: The agent, host susceptibility, and predisposing factors. In M.W. Eklund and V.R. Dowell, Jr. (eds.). Avian Botulism: An International Perspective. Charles C. Thomas, Springfield, IL, pp. 55–71.

35. Miyazaki, S., and G. Sakaguchi. 1978. Experimental botulism in chickens: The cecum as the site of production and absorption of botulinal toxin. Jpn J Med Sci Biol 31:1–15.

36. Notermans, S., and S. Kozaki. 1987. In vitro techniques for detecting botulinal toxins. In M.W. Eklund and V.R. Dowell, Jr. (eds.). Avian Botulism: An International Perspective. Charles C. Thomas, Springfield, IL, pp. 323–336.

37. Ohishi, I., and B.R. Dasgupta. 1987. Molecular structure and biological activities of Clostridium botulinum C2 toxin. In M.W. Eklund and V.R. Dowell, Jr. (eds.). Avian Botulism: An International Perspective. Charles C. Thomas, Springfield, IL, pp. 223–247.

38. Ohishi, I., G. Sakaguchi, H. Riemann, D. Behymer, and B. Hurvell. 1979. Antibodies to Clostridium botulinum toxins in free-living birds and mammals. J Wildl Dis 15:3–9.

39. Page, R.K., and O.J. Fletcher. 1975. An outbreak of type C botulism in three-week-old broilers. Avian Dis 19:192–195.

40. Roberts, T.A., and I.D. Aitken. 1974. Botulism in birds and mammals in Great Britain and an assessment of the toxicity of Clostridium botulinum type C toxin in domestic fowl. In A.N. Barker, G.W. Gould, and J. Wolf (eds.). Spore Research 1973. Academic Press, London, pp. 1–9.

41. Roberts, T.A., and D.F. Collings. 1973. An outbreak of type-C botulism in broiler chickens. Avian Dis 17:650–658.

42. Roberts, T.A., A.I. Thomas, and R.J. Gilbert. 1973. A third outbreak of type C botulism in broiler chickens. Vet Rec 92:107–109.

43. Rosen, M.N. 1971. Botulism. In J.W. Davis, R.C. Anderson, L. Karstad, and D.O. Trainer (eds.). Infectious and Parasitic Diseases of Wild Birds. Iowa State University Press, Ames, IA, pp. 100–117.

44. Sato, S. 1987. Control of botulism in poultry flocks. In M.W. Eklund and V.R. Dowell, Jr. (eds.). Avian Botulism: An International Perspective. Charles C. Thomas, Springfield, IL, pp. 349–356.

45. Schettler, C.H. 1979. Clostridium botulinum type C toxin infection in broiler farms in North West Germany. Berl Munch Tierarztl Wochenschr 92:50–57.

46. Segner, W.P., and C.F. Schmidt. 1971. Heat resistance of spores of marine and terrestrial strains of Clostridium botulinum type C. Appl Microbiol 22:1030–1033.

47. Simpson, L.L. 1987. The pathophysiological actions of the binary toxin produced by Clostridium botulinum. In M.W. Eklund and V.R. Dowell, Jr. (eds.). Avian Botulism: An International Perspective. Charles C. Thomas, Springfield, IL, pp. 249–264.

48. Smart, J.L., T.A. Roberts, K.G. McCullagh, V.M. Lucke, and H. Pearson. 1980. An outbreak of type C botulism in captive monkeys. Vet Rec 107:445–446.

49. Smart, J.L., T.A. Roberts, and L. Underwood. 1987. Avian botulism in the British Isles. In M.W. Eklund and V.R. Dowell, Jr. (eds.). Avian Botulism: An International Perspective. Charles C Thomas, Springfield, IL, pp. 111–122.

50. Smith, L.DS. 1975. The Pathogenic Anaerobic Bacteria, 2nd ed. Charles C. Thomas, Springfield, IL, pp. 203–229.

51. Smith, G.R. 1987. Botulism in water birds and its relation to comparative medicine. In M.E. Eklund and V.R. Dowell, Jr. (eds.). Avian Botulism: An International Perspective. Charles C. Thomas, Springfield, IL, pp. 73–86.

52. Syuto, B., and S. Kubo. 1981. Separation and characterization of heavy and light chains from Clostridium botulinum type C toxin and their reconstitution. J Biol Chem 256:3712–3717.

53. Wagenaar, R.O., G.M. Dack, and D.P. Mayer. 1953. Studies on mink food experimentally inoculated with toxin-free spores of Clostridium botulinum types A, B, C, and E. Am J Vet Res 14:479–483.

54. Wages, D.P. 1995. Personal communication

55. Wobeser, G.A. 1987. Control of botulism in wild birds. In M.W. Eklund and V.R. Dowell, Jr. (eds.). Avian Botulism: An International Perspective. Charles C. Thomas, Springfield, IL, pp. 339–348.

13 Bordetellosis (Turkey Coryza)

J. Kirk Skeeles and Lawrence H. Arp

INTRODUCTION. Bordetellosis in poultry is a highly contagious upper respiratory tract disease caused by *Bordetella avium*. Colonization of ciliated epithelium by *B. avium* results in protracted inflammation and distortion of the respiratory mucosa. In young turkeys, the disease is characterized by an abrupt onset of sneezing accompanied by clear, oculonasal discharge, mouth breathing, submandibular edema, altered voice, tracheal collapse, stunted growth, and predisposition to other infectious diseases. A careful analysis of the economic impact of bordetellosis has not been made; however, impaired growth, and mortality resulting from secondary colisepticemia, probably cause several million dollars in losses annually to the turkey industry in the United States.

The disease is still commonly referred to as turkey coryza. Other synonyms that have been largely abandoned are alcaligenes rhinotracheitis (ART), adenovirus-associated respiratory disease, acute respiratory disease syndrome, *Bordetella avium* rhinotracheitis (BART), and turkey rhinotracheitis. The numerous names used for this disease reflect the confusion that has surrounded its etiology.

Members of the *Bordetella* genus are well known for their capacity to colonize ciliated epithelium and produce respiratory disease in vertebrates. Despite similarities between whooping cough of humans (caused by *B. pertussis*) and bordetellosis of turkeys, there is no evidence that *B. avium* can either colonize or produce disease in humans (39).

HISTORY. Turkey rhinotracheitis (coryza) attributable to a bacterium of the genus *Bordetella* was first reported by Filion et al. (38) from Canada in 1967. Nearly a decade later, a similar syndrome was recognized in Germany and in the United States, where the causative agent was identified as *Bordetella bronchiseptica*-like (52) and *Alcaligenes faecalis* (103), respectively. The name *Bordetella avium* was eventually proposed and generally accepted (71).

Initial investigations into the cause of turkey rhinotracheitis in the United States focused on viruses. Adenoviruses were frequently associated with the disease (21), but attempts to reproduce it experimentally often failed (30, 99). The postmortem finding of bursal atrophy led to speculation that infectious bursal disease virus (IBDV) may have a role in turkey rhinotracheitis (89, 100). Turkeys inoculated experimentally with IBDV failed, however, to develop clinical disease or lesions, and concurrent inoculation with IBDV and *B. avium* failed to exacerbate experimental bordetellosis (64). Other infectious agents, including mycoplasmas, paramyxoviruses, Yucaipa virus, and chlamydia (2), have been considered in the etiology of turkey rhinotracheitis (75). In 1985, an acute, highly contagious upper respiratory disease of turkeys was recognized in England and Wales (3). The cause of that disease, which also has been called turkey rhinotracheitis, has been shown to be a pneumovirus (27) (see Avian Pneumovirus Infections, Chapter 20).

INCIDENCE AND DISTRIBUTION. Bordetellosis is an important disease in major turkey-producing regions of the United States, Canada (23), Australia (18), and Germany (52). The etiology of turkey rhinotracheitis in Great Britain, France, Israel, and South Africa, however, may frequently include viruses and other bacteria in addition to *B. avium* (47, 75). Hopkins et al. (58) detected *B. avium* antibodies by enzyme-linked immunosorbent assay (ELISA) in 42 of 44 wild turkeys being translocated in Arkansas. Thus, *B. avium* may possibly be a significant problem in wild turkeys or it may be that wild turkeys act as a reservoir for the infection. McBride et al. (79) surveyed three backyard turkey flocks located within 1 mile of commercial turkey farms in California and found all turkeys sampled at each location to be seropositive to *B. avium* when tested by microagglutination.

ETIOLOGY. Bordetellosis of turkeys is caused by *Bordetella avium* alone or in combination with environmental stresses and other respiratory pathogens. Experimental transmission (98) of the disease to susceptible poults by Simmons et al. (101) in the United States clearly established the etiologic agent as a small gram-negative bacillus. The bacterium, tentatively identified as *Alcaligenes faecalis*, closely resembled *Bordetella bronchisep-*

275

tica except for its failure to split urea. A systematic study by Kersters et al. (71) compared 28 pathogenic turkey isolates from diverse sources with 50 culture-collection strains of closely related bacteria. Based on morphologic, physiologic, nutritional, serologic, electrophoretic, and DNA–RNA hybridization, they concluded that the bacterial cause of turkey rhinotracheitis represented a new species of *Bordetella*; the name *Bordetella avium* sp. nov. was proposed. Further molecular characterization of *B. avium* has confirmed its unique taxonomic position among species of the *Bordetella* and *Alcaligenes* genera (14, 54, 66, 86, 120).

Morphology and Growth.   *Bordetella avium* is a gram-negative, nonfermentative, motile, strictly aerobic bacillus (65, 71) (Table 13.1). It grows readily on MacConkey, Bordet-Gengou, veal infusion, trypticase soy blood agar, brain heart infusion (BHI), and many other solid media (4), but not on minimal essential medium (65). Trypticase soy and BHI broth support optimal growth when aeration is provided by agitation (9). Filamentous forms have been observed following growth of *B. avium* in broth media high in nutrients (31). Leyh et al. (73) have developed a defined minimal medium for growth of *B. avium* and detection of auxotrophic mutants. Biochemical properties of the organism are listed in Table 13.2.

Colony Morphology.   Most strains of *B. avium* produce small, compact, translucent, pearl-like colonies (type I) with entire edges and glistening surfaces (71). Type I colonies are typically 0.2 to 1 mm in diameter after 24 hr of incubation and 1 to 2 mm in diameter after 48 hr of incubation. Many

Table 13.1.   Physical properties of *Bordetella avium*

Characteristic	References
Gram-negative rod (0.4-0.5 μm x 1-2 μm)	71, 103
Strict aerobe	71, 103
Motile	71, 103
Capsulated	71, 103
Fimbriated (2 nm diameter)	63
Colonies, 0.2-1 mm at 24 hr; round, glistening, convex (some strains dissociate to larger colonies)	54, 71
Hemagglutination of guinea pig erythrocytes	39, 65
Erythrocytes of other species	54, 95
Growth temperature, optimal at 35 C, killed at 45 C	9
Generation time, 35 to 40 minutes at 35 C	9
Strict tropism for ciliated epithelium	7, 45
Toxins	
Dermonecrotic (heat labile) toxin	39, 92, 93
Heat stable toxin	106
Osteotoxin	42
Tracheal cytotoxin	42
Guanine + cytosine composition of DNA, 61.6-62.6 mol%	71

Table 13.2.   Biochemical properties of *Bordetella avium*

Biochemical Test	Results	References
Oxidase (Kovac's reagent)	Positive	71, 103, 120
Catalase	Positive	54, 103, 120
Urease	Negative	51, 71, 103
Nitrate reduced to nitrite	Negative	54, 71, 103
Growth on MacConkey agar (lactose not fermented)	Positive	71, 103
Triple sugar iron agar	Alkaline slant, no change in butt	14, 65, 103
Alkalinize amides and organic salts (Greenwood's low peptone)	Several positive	14, 18, 19, 54

isolates develop a slightly raised brown-tinged center when grown 48 hr on MacConkey agar (Fig. 13.1). A small percentage of strains dissociate into a larger colony type (type II). A third colony type, characterized by a serrated irregular edge, smooth surface, and larger size than type II colonies, has been reported (54).

Resistance to Chemical and Physical Agents.   Most commonly used disinfectants appear to kill *B. avium* when used according to manufacturers' recommendations. Survival of *B. avium* is prolonged by low temperatures, low humidities, and neutral pH (26). On simulated carrier materials such as dust and feces from turkey houses, the organism survived 25–33 days at 10 C and relative humidity 32–58%, whereas at 40 C with similar humidity the organism survived less than 2 days (26). Survival of the organism for at least 6 mo in undisturbed damp litter has been reported (13). In BHI broth culture, bacteria are killed within 24 hr at 45 C (9). Survival may be greatly prolonged at 10 C on smooth surfaces such as glass or aluminum (26). Fumigation of an uncleaned room with methyl bromide effectively stopped transmission of the disease to day-old susceptible poults (98).

Resistance to streptomycin, sulfonamides, and tetracycline by some strains of *B. avium* is encoded on up to five plasmids ranging in size from 16 to 51.5 kb (29, 76), however, most strains are sensitive

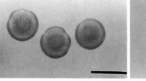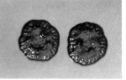

13.1.   Colonies of *Bordetella avium* strain 838 (*left*) and *B. avium*-like strain 007 (*right*) grown on MacConkey agar, 48 hr at 35 C. Note raised center in colonies of this *B. avium* strain. *Bar* = 1 mm.

in vitro to a large number of antibacterials. Treatment of *B. avium*-infected turkeys with oxytetracycline administered parenterally or by aerosol results in either no effect or a transient reduction in bacterial numbers even though the strain of *B. avium* was sensitive to oxytetracycline in vitro (36, 108, 119).

Antigenic Structure and Cell Surface Receptors. The antigenic structure of *B. avium* and related bacteria has been studied by agar gel precipitation, cross-agglutination, and Western immunoblotting (9, 48, 63, 65, 71). All evidence to date suggests that *B. avium* isolates from various sources are closely related antigenically (71). Using antisera produced in rabbits, Kersters et al. (71) identified six different surface antigens, three of which were cross-reactive among three strains of *B. avium.* In addition they found two or three precipitation lines in common with *B. bronchiseptica.* Further antigenic relatedness was demonstrated with *Alcaligenes denitrificans* and *Achromobacter xylosoxidans* (71). Jackwood et al. (65) have demonstrated antigenic cross-reactivity between *B. avium* and *B. avium*-like (see later discussion) bacteria. Using convalescent serum and tracheal washings in immunoblotting procedures, Hellwig and Arp (48) have shown that infected turkeys recognize at least 8 outer-membrane proteins of *B. avium.* These proteins range in size from about 14 to about 116 kd. Leyh and Griffith (72) examined the outer-membrane protein profiles of 50 virulent *B. avium* isolates and found 2 major sarkosyl-insoluble proteins of 21 and 37 kD, and at least 13 other lesser proteins, using sodium dodecyl sulfate–polyacryamide gel electrophoresis (SDS–PAGE). *B. avium* was found to have an electrophoresis profile distinctly different from those of both *B. avium*-like and *B. bronchiseptica* bacteria. Varley and Carter (121) examined seven *Bordetella* isolates from turkeys in the United Kingdom from the early 1980s using SDS–PAGE and compared those with known strains of *B. avium, B. bronchiseptica* and *Alcaligenes faecalis.* All electrophoretic profiles were similar to both known *B. avium* and *A. faecalis* strains, indicating the usefulness of the procedure in distinguishing between *Bordetella* sp. but not for *A. faecalis.* Gentry-Weeks et al. (41) identified five outer-membrane proteins with molecular masses of 21, 38, 40, 43, and 48 kD being produced in *Escherichia coli* into which genes from *B. avium* had been cloned. Moore and Jackwood (85) produced monoclonal antibodies to a whole-cell *B. avium* preparation that recognized a 41-kD protein. These monoclonal antibodies were used to inhibit *B. avium* guinea pig red blood cell hemagglutination and could also be utilized to demonstrate the binding of the 41-kD protein to guinea pig erythrocytes. Hemagglutination was also inhibited following treatment of *B. avium* with proteinase K and periodic acid, both of which cleave carbohydrates from protein. This strongly suggests that the *B. avium* hemagglutinin is a carbohydrate strongly associated with the 41-kD surface protein. In a related study, Arp et al. (11) demonstrated complete inhibition of guinea pig red blood cell hemagglutination by *B. avium* using the gangliosides GD_{1a} and GT_{1b} and partial inhibition of hemagglutination using *N*-acetylneuraminic acid. When these same compounds, along with bovine submaxillary mucin and horseshoe crab lectin, were used to treat *B. avium,* adherence to the tracheal mucosa in turkeys was inhibited in vivo. The authors speculated that these compounds may be chemically related to the receptors for *B. avium* on the tracheal mucosa.

Potential Virulence Factors. Major virulence factors of *B. avium* can be divided into those involved in adhesion, local mucosal injury, or systemic effects. Adhesion to cilia of respiratory epithelium is a consistent trait of *B. avium* and other species of *Bordetella.* The surface structures or molecules of *B. avium* responsible for adhesion have possibly been identified (11, 85), and the fimbriae (pili) and hemagglutinin may have roles (10, 62). Although fimbriae have been suggested as possible adhesive factors of *B. avium* (62), morphologically similar fimbriae are also common on adhesion-defective mutants and *B. avium*-like bacteria (49, 62). Hemagglutination (HA) of guinea pig erythrocytes correlates closely with virulence (39, 65), but appears to be unrelated to fimbriae (62). Two transposon-induced mutants selected for loss of HA activity had reduced adherence in vivo (10). Reversion of one mutant to HA-positive status resulted in reconstitution of adherence. As with other *Bordetella* species, it seems likely that more than one surface molecule is responsible for adhesion to cilia.

Several local effects have been attributed to toxins of *B. avium.* An acute cytotoxic and ciliostatic effect of *B. avium* on turkey tracheal organ cultures was reported by Gray et al. (44, 46) and others (77). Rimler (92) described a heat-labile toxin capable of killing mice and young turkeys. The toxin was later shown to produce necrotic and hemorrhagic lesions in the skin of turkeys and guinea pigs after intradermal injection and similar lesions in the liver and pancreas of turkeys following intraperitoneal injection (91, 93). Recent work has shown that *B. avium* produces a dermonecrotic toxin with physical, antigenic, and biologic properties comparable to those reported for the heat-labile toxin (39). The dermonecrotic toxin is a cell-associated, 155-kD protein with biologic activity comparable to dermonecrotic toxins of *B. pertussis* and *B. bronchiseptica* (39). A role for the dermonecrotic toxin has not been established in the pathogenesis of bordetellosis in turkeys; the toxin appears not to be responsible for ciliostasis (93) or local epithelial damage (115). Gentry-Weeks et al. (40) produced spontaneous-phase variants of *B. avium* that lacked dermonecrotic toxin and four outer-membrane proteins when grown in media containing nicotinic acid and $MgSO_4$. These variants had a different colony morphology but retained the ability to agglutinate guinea pig red blood cells. Passage in susceptible turkeys caused these variants to revert to the wild type.

Another toxin of *B. avium* implicated in local mucosal injury is the tracheal cytotoxin (TCT) isolated by Gentry-Weeks et al. (39). The TCT of *B. pertussis*, which is chemically identical to that produced by *B. avium*, has been shown to specifically damage ciliated epithelial cells leading to loss of epithelium and poor clearance of mucus (43). The TCT of *B. avium* is an anhydropeptidoglycan monomer with a mass of 921 d. Whether TCT is the mediator of cytotoxic activity reported earlier by Gray et al. (44, 46) is unclear.

Simmons et al. (106) have identified a *B. avium* heat-stable toxin capable of causing diarrhea and death in mice inoculated intraperitoneally; however, there is no evidence that the toxin produces adverse effects in poultry. None of 18 *B. avium* strains from Australia had the mouse-lethal toxin that was found in several reference strains from other turkey-producing areas in the world (20). An osteotoxin was recently found to be associated with *B. avium*. It has been identified as beta cystathionase and is lethal to MC3T3-E1 osteogenic cells, fetal bovine trabecular cells, UMR106-01 (BSP) rat osteosarcoma cells and embryonic bovine tracheal cells (42). This toxin might be responsible for the cartilage lesions that lead to tracheal softening and collapse. Examination of several *B. avium* strains for the production of extracytoplasmic adenylate cyclase (39, 93) or pertussis toxin (39) failed to detect either one by immunologic and functional assays. In a study to detect virulence genes of *B. pertussis* by Southern hybridization, it was determined that the bvgS gene was present but the bvgA was not (40). Earlier studies by Simmons et al. (105) suggested that *B. avium* produces a histamine-sensitizing factor similar to that produced by other *Bordetella* species.

A number of systemic pathophysiologic effects have been attributed to *B. avium* infection. These include elevation of serum corticosterone (83), enhanced leukocyte migration (80), altered electrocardiograms (123), reduced body temperature (32), reduced levels of monoamines in brain and lymphoid tissues (33, 34), reduced levels of liver tryptophan 2,3-dioxygenase (122), and reduced thyroid hormones in conjunction with fasting (35). Beginning with the original recognition of turkey rhinotracheitis in North Carolina, reports from flock service

people have suggested defective immune function in affected poults (102). Vaccination of these poults with live vaccines resulted in unexpected deaths. This background, along with the observation of reduced bursa size in some poults with rhinotracheitis (100), led to a series of experiments to determine effects of *B. avium* infection on immune function. Initial studies in poults infected with *B. avium* (102) found a decreased lymphocyte blastogenesis response to concanavalin A and depletion of thymic lymphocytes. Subsequent studies of cell-mediated immunity in *B. avium*-infected poults showed the reverse effect with enhanced graft-vs-host and delayed hypersensitivity responses (81, 82), both measures of cell-mediated immunity.

Pathogenicity and Strain Differences. Differences in pathogenicity have been reported among *B. avium* strains (95, 96). Differences in pathogenicity, associated with colony morphology and hemagglutination, led to categorization of isolates into various groups or types (14, 65, 95). Continuing study of the molecular characteristics of *B. avium* and related bacteria has identified several differentiating features of *B. avium* (Table 13.3). Strains previously referred to as "group 1" (95) and "type 1" (65) should now be called *B. avium*. The term "*B. avium*-like," as proposed by Jackwood et al. (66), will be reserved for nonpathogenic, avian isolates closely related to *B. avium*.

Studies of *B. avium* from various sources have revealed great similarity in electrophoretic patterns of outer-membrane proteins (49, 71, 121). Furthermore, antigenic profiles examined by cross-agglutination, agar gel precipitation, and Western immunoblotting showed little variation among *B. avium* strains (48, 71). *Bordetella avium* shares several cross-reactive antigens with *B. avium*-like and other *Bordetella* species (48, 65). Despite the apparent genetic and molecular similarity among *B. avium* strains, differences have been noted in toxin production (20, 92, 106), adherence to tracheal mucosa (10), plasmid profiles (67, 107), antibiotic sensitivity (67), pathogenicity (50, 96), and colony morphology (68, 71).

PATHOGENESIS AND EPIZOOTIOLOGY

Natural and Experimental Hosts. The natural host of *B. avium* is the turkey, although isolations of *B. avium* have also been made from chickens and other avian species (54, 104). Strains of *B. avium* isolated from avian species other than turkeys are pathogenic for day-old turkeys (54). A study of the prevalence of *B. avium* in North Carolina broiler flocks during the winter months revealed a 62% infection rate (16). Furthermore, there was a higher isolation rate from flocks with respira-

Table 13.3. Differentiation of *Bordetella avium* and *B. avium*-like bacteria

Characteristic	*B. avium*	*B. avium*-like
Pathogenicity	Positive	Negative
In vivo adhesion[a]	Positive	Negative
Hemagglutination[b]	Positive	Negative
Growth on minimal essential medium agar (65)	Negative	Positive
Growth in 6.5% NaCl broth (65)	Few positive	Most positive

Other distinguishing features:
  Outer membrane profiles on SDS-PAGE[c] (49, 65)
  Cellular fatty acid analyses (66, 86)
  Alkalinization of amides and organic acids (14, 17)

[a]Adhesion to turkey tracheal mucosa (5, 10).
[b]Hemagglutination of guinea pig erythrocytes (65) may be weak or inconsistent with some strains or organisms grown in liquid medium.
[c]SDS-PAGE, sodium dodecyl sulfate-polyacrylamide gel electrophoresis.

tory disease. Attempts to reproduce rhinotracheitis experimentally in chickens revealed that only 2 of 8 *B. avium* strains colonized the trachea and produced disease (15); however, a later study (14) suggested the isolations from chickens may have included both *B. avium* and *B. avium*-like bacteria. It appears turkey and chicken strains of *B. avium* are similar (71), and cross-infection can occur between the species (104). Bordetellosis in chickens tends to be less severe than in turkeys (84, 104). A strain of *B. avium*, pathogenic for turkeys and Japanese quail, failed to produce clinical disease in guinea pigs, hamsters, and mice (78). Naturally occurring infection with *B. avium* is typically recognized in turkeys 2- to 6-wk-old (23, 52, 90), although older turkeys and breeder flocks may also develop clinical disease (69, 70). Experimental inoculation of poults more than 1- to 2-wk-old frequently results in colonization, but with only mild disease.

Transmission and Carriers. Bordetellosis is highly contagious. The disease is readily transmitted to susceptible poults through close contact with infected poults or through exposure to litter or water contaminated by infected poults (98). Infection is not transmitted between adjacent cages, thus providing evidence against aerosol transmission (98). Litter contaminated by a flock infected with *B. avium* is likely to remain infective for 1 to 6 mo (13, 26). Although a carrier state has not been demonstrated in turkeys recovered from bordetellosis, the possibility seems likely.

Incubation Period. The incubation period is 7–10 days when susceptible poults are exposed to infected poults by close direct contact (98). In-

tranasal or intraocular inoculation of day-old poults with 10^5 to 10^7 colony-forming units of *B. avium* results in clinical signs (nasal exudate) of bordetellosis in 4 to 6 days (6, 45, 96).

Signs. An abrupt onset of sneezing (snick) in a high percentage of 2- to 6-wk-old turkeys over the course of a week is suggestive of bordetellosis. Older turkeys may also develop a dry cough (70). A clear nasal discharge can be expressed by placing gentle pressure over the bridge of the beak between the nostrils. During the first 2 wk of disease, the nares and feathers of the head and wings become crusted with wet, tenacious, brownish exudate (Fig. 13.2) and some birds develop submaxillary edema. Mouth breathing, dyspnea, and altered vocalization in the second week of clinical signs result when the nasal cavity and upper trachea become partially occluded with mucoid exudate. Tracheal softening can be palpated through the skin of the neck in some birds beginning in the 2nd week of disease. Behavioral changes include reduced activity, huddling, and decreased consumption of feed and water. Concurrent infections and poor weight gains contribute to poor flock performance and numerous birds with stunted growth (9). Signs of disease begin to subside after a course of 2–4 wk (45, 90, 96, 118).

Morbidity and Mortality. Bordetellosis in turkeys is typically characterized by high morbidity and low mortality. In turkeys 2–6 wk of age, morbidity reaches 80 to 100% (96), whereas the mortality rate is less than 10%. Infection of a breeder flock with *B. avium* resulted in only 20% morbidity with no mortality (70). High mortality rates (>40%)

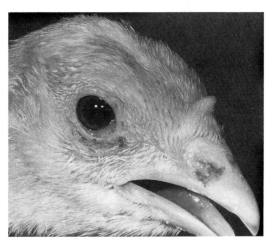

13.2. Clinical appearance of a poult with bordetellosis. Open-mouth breathing, dark stains around eye and nostril, and foamy exudate at the medial canthus of the eye.

in young turkeys are frequently associated with concurrent isolation of *Escherichia coli* (23, 96). Experimental studies of concurrent *B. avium* and *E. coli* infections in 2- to 4-wk-old turkeys revealed defective clearance of *E. coli* from tracheas (37, 116) and increased severity of airsacculitis attributable to *E. coli* (117). Adverse environmental temperatures (9), high humidity (109), poor air quality, and concurrent respiratory pathogens may increase mortality rates (96). Cook et al. (28) studied the interaction of turkey rhinotracheitis virus (TRTV), a pneumovirus, with *B. avium* and a *Pasteurella*-like organism in turkeys. When the TRTV was administered alone the virus could only be isolated from the trachea, but when given in combination with the bacteria it was capable of invasion and could be isolated from the heart, liver, spleen, kidney, and cecal tonsils. Hinz et al. (55) described an outbreak of *B. avium* in combination with *Chlamydia psittaci* in six different turkey flocks on a large multiple-age grow-out operation. Mortality in the affected flocks ranged from 7 to 20% and the high mortality was attributed to secondary infections from *Klebsiella pneumoniae, E. coli,* and *Pseudomonas fluoreszenz.*

Gross Lesions. Gross lesions are confined to the upper respiratory tract and vary with the duration of infection. Nasal and tracheal exudates change in character from serous initially to tenacious and mucoid during the course of disease. Tracheal lesions consisting of generalized softening and distortion of the cartilaginous rings, dorsal-ventral compression, and fibrinomucoid luminal exudate are highly suggestive of bordetellosis (6, 118). In isolated cases, there is severe infolding of the dorsal tracheal wall into the lumen immediately below the larynx (Fig. 13.3) (6, 119). In cross-section, tracheal rings appear to have thick walls and a diminished lumen. Distortion of tracheal cartilages persists at least 53 days postinfection (6). Accumulation of mucoid exudate in an area of tracheal infolding frequently leads to death by suffocation (6). Hyperemia of the nasal and tracheal mucosae and edema of interstitial tissues of the head and neck are apparent during the first 2 wk of infection.

Histopathology. Cilia-associated bacterial colonies, progressive loss of ciliated epithelium, and depletion of mucus from goblet cells are distinctive characteristics of bordetellosis (6). Colonization of ciliated epithelium begins on the nasal mucosa, progresses down the trachea, and moves into primary bronchi within 7 to 10 days. Bacteria adhere specifically to cilia and are never found attached to other cell types (7). As seen by scanning electron microscopy, surfaces of adherent bacteria are covered with numerous knoblike surface projections (Fig. 13.4). Colonized cells having in-

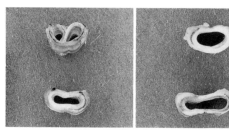

13.3. Cross sections of a collapsed trachea from a poult with bordetellosis. Section on the *top left*, taken immediately below the larynx, has extreme dorsal-ventral infolding. Other sections were taken at 5 cm intervals along the trachea. (Am J Vet Res)

creased eosinophilia of the apical cytoplasm may protrude slightly from the mucosa (119). Bacterial colonies (Fig. 13.5) are most apparent on the tracheal mucosa 1–2 wk after onset of clinical signs, before loss of ciliated cells is extensive (6, 7).

During the first 2 wk of signs, ciliated tracheal epithelium is gradually lost and replaced by nonciliated cuboidal epithelium (Fig. 13.6). These immature hyperplastic cells have basophilic cytoplasm with variable numbers of small mucous granules (6, 119). Late in the disease, squamous metaplasia of tracheal epithelium may occur (Fig. 13.7). Linear, eosinophilic inclusions occur in the cytoplasm of tracheal epithelium during the first 3 wk of disease (6, 7). Ultrastructurally, these inclusions are proteinaceous crystals composed of parallel filaments surrounded by membrane (7). During the 3rd and 4th wk of disease, the tracheal mucosa becomes distorted by numerous folds and mounds of dysplastic epithelium. Depending on the severity of the disease, the tracheal epithelium returns to normal 4–6 wk after the onset of signs (6, 45), when *B. avium* can no longer be isolated.

Discharge of copious mucoid exudates from the upper respiratory tract is accompanied by depletion of mucus from isolated goblet cells and mucous glands along the mucosa (6, 119). Alveolar glands become cystic and lined by immature epithelium with small mucous granules (Fig. 13.5). Goblet cells remain largely depleted of mucous granules from the 1st through the 3rd wk of clinical disease.

Cellular exudates in the tracheal lamina propria begin with multifocal infiltrates of heterophils and change to predominantly lymphocytes and plasma cells as clinical signs subside (6, 45). In the 3rd through 5th wk of disease, a diffuse increase in mucosal plasma cells is accompanied by multifocal lymphoid nodules in the submucosa. Mucosal surface exudates change from mucopurulent to fibrinopurulent after the 1st wk of disease (7).

Pulmonary lesions are restricted to primary bronchi and bronchus-associated lymphoid tissue

(117, 118). In contrast to the tracheal mucosa, the bronchial mucosa maintains a near normal appearance including ciliated columnar epithelium and goblet cells (118). Mild colonization of isolated ciliated cells by *B. avium* is accompanied by a mild infiltrate of heterophils. Bronchus-associated lymphoid tissue, normally found at the junction of primary and secondary bronchi, becomes apparent grossly and lymphoid nodules protrude into the bronchial lumen (118). Other changes of lymphoid tissues include depletion of cortical lymphocytes from the thymus during the early disease (102).

In summary, distinctive microscopic lesions of diagnostic value include cilia-associated bacterial colonies, cytoplasmic inclusions, cystic mucosal glands, and generalized loss of ciliated epithelium.

Immunity. Most turkeys develop a humoral immune response to infection with *B. avium* (6, 60, 113). Serum antibodies, detected by microtiter agglutination, appear within 2 wk after experimental exposure to *B. avium* and reach peak levels by 3–4 wk postexposure (6, 60). The period of peak antibody titer is followed within 1 wk by resolution of clinical disease and a decline in bacterial numbers in the trachea (6). This, combined with evidence for maternal immunity, suggests an important role for humoral immunity in prevention and recovery from infection (13, 53). Neighbor et al. (88) evaluated maternal antibody in poults from immunized and unimmunized hens. Resistance to clinical disease and gross lesions was greatest in poults with maternal antibody, as measured by ELISA. Convalescent serum and tracheal secretions from turkeys infected with *B. avium* inhibit adherence of the bacteria to

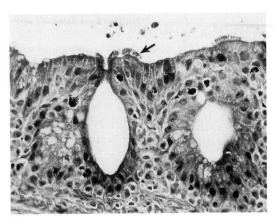

13.5. Trachea from a poult infected 3 wk previously with *Bordetella avium*. Characteristic lesions of bordetellosis include cilia-associated bacterial colonies (*arrow*), loss of ciliated epithelium, dilated mucous glands depleted of mucus, and interstitial infiltration of plasma cells and lymphocytes.

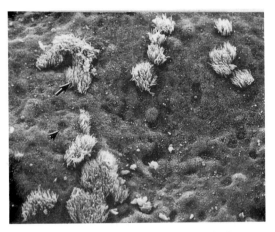

13.6. Loss of ciliated epithelium from the tracheal mucosal surface. Isolated clumps of ciliated cells (*arrow*) and dark pits left where ciliated cells have sloughed (*arrowhead*).

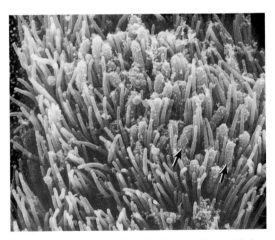

13.4. Numerous *Bordetella avium* bacteria (*arrows*) intimately associated with cilia of tracheal epithelial cells. The bacterial surfaces are covered with irregularly shaped, knoblike projections, which may contribute to adhesion.

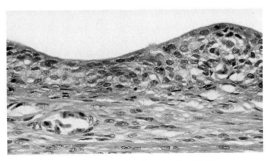

13.7. Squamous metaplasia of tracheal epithelium occurs in some poults late in the course of bordetellosis.

the tracheal mucosa in turkeys (8). Moreover, adherence of *B. avium* is inhibited whether convalescent serum is administered locally or parenterally. The passive administration of convalescent serum is believed to mimic many aspects of maternal immunity. Suresh et al. (113) evaluated antibody levels in serum, tracheal washings, and lacrimal secretions from turkeys experimentally infected with *B. avium*. Turkeys were sacrificed at weekly intervals through 8 wk postinoculation. Maternal antibody was undetectable by 3 wk of age and the appearance of serum and mucosal antibody was associated with clearance of *B. avium* from the trachea. Using serum and tracheal secretions collected from turkeys during a 4-wk course of infection, at least eight *B. avium* surface proteins were identified using Western immunoblots (48).

An active immune response is generated in most turkeys inoculated with live *B. avium* or various bacterins. The serum antibody response to a temperature-sensitive mutant of *B. avium* is variable depending on vaccination dosage, turkey age, and environmental factors affecting colonization (9, 25, 50, 56, 59, 61, 69). Recent studies have suggested that poults less than 3 wk of age respond poorly to *B. avium* vaccines (56, 61).

Infection with *B. avium* has been recognized as potentially immunosuppressive since Simmons et al. (102) reported thymic lesions and suppression of lymphocyte blastogenesis. Although subsequent tests have revealed no evidence for defects in cellular immunity (80, 81, 82), infection with *B. avium* apparently interferes with immunity to live *Pasteurella multocida* and hemorrhagic enteritis vaccines (94, 102). Reduced monoamine concentrations in brain and lymphoid tissues and elevated serum corticosterone have been recorded in turkeys infected with *B. avium* (33, 34, 83). Although such hormonal changes are probably not unique to bordetellosis, they may help explain the immunosuppression seen in the field.

Pathogenesis. Initial adhesion of bacteria to ciliated cells of the oronasal mucosa leads to progressive colonization from the upper trachea to the primary bronchi over the next week. Expansion of the bacterial population along the respiratory mucosa stimulates acute inflammation and release of mucus from goblet cells leading to sneezing, coughing, and nasal obstruction. Spread of infection against the flow of mucociliary clearance occurs as motile "swarmer" bacteria break free from microcolonies and move within the layer of mucin to other ciliated cells. Apparently, tracheal mucus does not contain receptor analogs to impede spread of the bacteria. During the next week, many of the cells colonized by *B. avium* slough into the tracheal lumen, leaving large surfaces devoid of cilia.

How *B. avium* damages the tracheal mucosa and cartilage remains unknown, but the tracheal cytotoxin may be involved. The formation of cytoplasmic protein crystals and delayed restitution of normal mucosa are suggestive of a toxin that alters cell growth and differentiation. The molecular basis for softening and collapse of tracheal rings may result from abnormal connective tissue metabolism leading to qualitative and quantitative changes in collagen and elastin (122).

As ciliated cells are progressively lost, the flow of mucus and exudates becomes sluggish, particularly in the upper trachea and nasal cavity. Obstruction of nasolacrimal ducts causes foamy ocular exudate to accumulate at the medial canthus of the eye. Signs of bordetellosis result from local and systemic products of the inflammatory response, soluble bacterial toxins, and physical obstruction of large air passages.

Within a week of the onset of clinical signs, local and systemic immune responses develop to *B. avium* antigens. Antibody transported from serum and antibody produced by submucosal plasma cells accumulates in respiratory secretions. Local antibody interacts with free "swarmer" *B. avium* cells to inhibit their motility and prevent adhesion to other ciliated cells. Colonies of bacteria among the cilia are largely protected from host defenses; however, numerous bacteria are shed along with colonized epithelial cells. The bacterial population diminishes over the next several weeks as colonized cells are lost and newly formed ciliated cells are protected from colonization by antibody.

Some convalescent birds are probably slow to clear all *B. avium* from their respiratory tissues, and serve as a source of infection for susceptible flocks. As mucosal immunity wanes over the next 4–8 wk, any residual population of *B. avium* in the nasal cavity or sinuses can again expand to produce clinical infection or be transmitted to susceptible birds.

DIAGNOSIS. The diagnosis of bordetellosis is currently based on clinical signs and lesions, isolation of *B. avium* from the respiratory tract, a positive serologic test, or some combination of these. Additional diagnostic techniques that have been developed include a monoclonal antibody–based latex bead agglutination test (112), an indirect fluorescent antibody staining technique using a monoclonal antibody (111), a capillary gas chromatography assay for cellular carbohydrates using per-acetylated aldonitriles and *O*-methyloximes (87), and a polymerase chain reaction technique (97).

Isolation and Identification of Causative Agent. Bacterial isolation is accomplished on MacConkey agar inoculated with a swab sample from the tracheal mucosa. Samples collected from the choanal opening and nostril, or by passing a swab into the trachea through the larynx, commonly yield large numbers of nonpathogenic bacteria (101, 110). When turkeys are available for necropsy examination, swab samples should be collected aseptically through an opening in the midcervical trachea. After 24 hr of incubation on MacConkey agar, colonies of *B. avium* are clear and pin-point in size. Although most contaminating bacteria form large mucoid colonies (often lactose fermenters) which mask *B. avium* in the more concentrated streak pattern, the minute colonies of *B. avium* may be recognized in the more diluted streak pattern. By incubating culture plates up to 48 hr, *B. avium* colonies are more easily recognized and may develop a brownish raised center (Fig. 13.1). Early in the course of infection, pure cultures can be obtained from the trachea, but in later stages, *E. coli* and other opportunistic bacteria may be isolated (96). Physical and biochemical characteristics that serve to distinguish *B. avium* from closely related bacteria are presented in Tables 13.2 and 13.3.

Serology. Serologic testing has proven to be useful experimentally and in the natural disease for detection of serum antibodies to *B. avium*. Jackwood and Saif (60) developed a microagglutination test (MAT) using a killed, neotetrazolium-chloride-stained *B. avium* antigen in a microtiter system. The MAT has been shown to correlate well with bacterial isolation. It seems likely that serologic tests remain positive for a period after *B. avium* can no longer be cultured. In a field study by Slavik et al. (110), flocks with a history of respiratory disease were more commonly positive serologically for *B. avium* even though bacteria were not isolated. In experimentally infected poults, antibody is detectable by the MAT from 2 wk post inoculation (PI) until at least 5–7 wk PI (6, 9, 60). Peak titers occur at about 3–4 wk PI. For each of the above tests, agglutination occurs at serum dilutions of from 1:320 to 1:512 (6, 60). Use of heterologous *B. avium* antigen has little effect on agglutination titers (9).

Hopkins et al. (57) developed an ELISA for detection of serum antibodies to *B. avium* using a whole-bacteria antigen, a 1:200 serum dilution, and a 1:3200 dilution of commercially available anti-turkey IgG conjugate. Serologic results obtained with ELISA correlate well with those from the MAT, but ELISA is more sensitive for detection of maternal antibody in day-old poults (57). Although *B. avium* has antigens in common with closely related *B. avium*-like bacteria, there is no evidence that these related bacteria cause a positive serologic reaction to *B. avium* in nature.

Several different variations of ELISA procedures have been developed for *B. avium* (12, 22, 88, 113, 114). The variations include a dot-immunobinding assay (114) and a particle concentration fluorescence immunoassay (22). All of these detect maternal antibody and are reproducible and sensitive. Recently a commercially available ELISA kit has become available and it has proven to be very useful (74).

Differential Diagnosis. Bordetellosis must be differentiated from other primary and secondary causes of rhinotracheitis. Mycoplasmosis, chlamydiosis, and respiratory cryptosporidiosis may mimic or contribute to many of the clinical signs of bordetellosis (2, 55, 70, 75). Of the viral agents, Newcastle disease virus, Yucaipa virus, adenovirus, influenza virus, and pneumovirus should be considered (27, 75). Although *B. avium* alone can produce all of the clinical signs and lesions of bordetellosis, in the natural disease, *B. avium* is more frequently accompanied by Newcastle disease, *Mycoplasma* spp., and opportunistic bacteria such as *E. coli*.

Currently, the greatest diagnostic challenge is to differentiate *B. avium* from *B. avium*-like bacteria in primary cultures. Distinguishing characteristics of these closely related bacteria are presented in Table 13.3, however pathogenicity testing in day-old poults is definitive. Intranasal inoculation of day-old poults with a 24-hr broth culture of *B. avium* is expected to produce clinical disease and nasal discharge in susceptible poults within 3 to 5 days.

TREATMENT. Treatment of bordetellosis with antibiotics administered in the water, by injection, or by aerosol has produced minimal clinical improvement in most cases. Treatment of an infected breeder flock with 1.8 g tetracycline-HCl and 2 x 10^6 IU potassium penicillin-G per gallon of drinking water for 3 days produced clinical improvement within 24 hr (70). Treatment of bordetellosis in young turkeys with an aerosol of oxytetracycline-HCl reduced mortality associated with subsequent Newcastle disease vaccination compared with untreated flocks (36). Although these clinical testimonials suggest a favorable response to treatment, it remains unclear whether clinical improvement results from antibacterial effects against *B. avium* or to secondary pathogens such as *E. coli*.

In a group of experimentally infected poults, parenteral administration of long-acting oxytetracycline had no apparent effect on *B. avium* infection (108). Treatment of experimental bordetellosis with oxytetracycline-HCl administered by aerosol caused a transient reduction of bacterial numbers in the trachea and a delay in clinical signs and lesion development (119). However, by 4 days after treatment, bacterial numbers and disease severity were similar between treated and nontreated groups (119).

Yersin et al. (124) was able to demonstrate up to a 40% reduction in the loss of cilia following treatment of *B. avium*-infected turkeys with niacin added to the drinking water at 70 mg/L. Niacin treatment also reduced clinical signs, increased body weight, and reduced adherence of bacteria to the tracheal epithelium when treated turkeys were compared with untreated infected turkeys. The authors speculate that the mechanism for this therapeutic effect may be the result of the inhibition of glucocorticoid-induced DNA strand breakage and subsequent ADP-ribosylation of nuclear DNA. This action would allow for continued protein synthesis necessary to maintain ATP-mediated functions in the cilia of the trachea.

PREVENTION AND CONTROL

Management Procedures. *Bordetella avium* is highly contagious by direct contact and through contamination of water, feed, and litter. Strict biosecurity measures are required to prevent infection of clean flocks, and rigorous cleanup procedures are required to eliminate the organism from contaminated premises. A minimal cleanup procedure for contaminated premises should include complete removal of litter, thorough washing of all surfaces, disinfection of watering systems and feeders, and application of a disinfectant followed by either formaldehyde fumigation or by application of a dilute formaldehyde solution to all surfaces. *Bordetella avium* is easily tracked from one facility to another, so the use of disinfectant foot baths, clean outer clothing, and even a required shower between visits to different houses and locations, is essential. Since the severity of bordetellosis is exacerbated by adverse environmental and infectious factors, attempts should be made to optimize temperature, humidity, and air quality while avoiding or delaying the use of live attenuated vaccines.

Immunization. Vaccines currently available commercially for prevention of bordetellosis in turkeys include a live temperature-sensitive (ts) mutant of *B. avium* (Art-Vax,™ American Scientific Laboratories, Madison, WI) and a whole cell bacterin (ADJUVAC-ART, Sanofi Animal Health, Inc., Overland Park, KS). The live ts-mutant vaccine was induced by nitrosoguanidine mutation of a virulent *B. avium* isolate obtained from North Carolina (24). Original studies indicated the ts mutant colonized the nasal mucosa and induced moderate levels of serum antibodies (24). Although subsequent use of the vaccine in Utah indicated substantial protection (25, 69), other controlled experiments indicated only moderate reduction in lesion severity or delayed onset of clinical disease (50, 56, 59, 61). The

ts mutant has the capacity to adhere to respiratory epithelium, but its slow growth rate may critically limit its ability to colonize and induce protective immunity (10, 9). Use of the ts-mutant vaccine according to label directions in day-old poults failed to prevent infection and disease; however, use of the vaccine in poults 3 wk of age and older prevented disease but not infection (56, 61). Concern exists that turkeys less than 3 wk of age may be unable to respond adequately to *B. avium* antigens or are unable to mount an adequate local immune response.

Houghten et al. (59) compared a spray method of vaccination with the method recommended by the manufacturer for the ts-mutant vaccine. Turkeys were immunized at 2 days of age, using a spray cabinet, followed 14 days later with another coarse spray exposure to the ts-mutant vaccine. Another group of turkeys was similarly immunized by eye-drop exposure followed 14 days later by oral exposure. The spray and eyedrop/oral methods of immunization were equally effective in reducing severity of tracheal lesions, but neither method prevented infection of the trachea by virulent challenge strains.

Several studies have indicated that breeder hen vaccination may be useful for prevention of bordetellosis in progeny poults (13, 53, 88). Vaccination of breeder hens with either heat-killed (53) or formalin-killed (13) adjuvanted bacterins delayed the onset and severity of clinical disease in challenge-exposed poults. Passive immunization of 3-wk-old poults with convalescent serum reduces adherence of *B. avium* to the tracheal mucosa in a dose- and time-dependent manner (8). Taken in total, these studies suggest that maternal antibody of the IgG class may confer temporary immunity to newly hatched poults. Additionally, vaccination of poults with purified pilus preparations and adjuvanted bacterins results in significant protection against *B. avium* colonization and clinical disease (1).

Since *B. avium* and *B. avium*-like bacteria are antigenically related, Jackwood and Saif (63) designed experiments to determine whether poults infected with nonpathogenic *B. avium*-like bacteria would develop immunity to *B. avium*. The *B. avium*-like bacteria failed to persist for a significant period in the respiratory tract and failed to induce either a serologic response or protection to *B. avium* challenge. Development of improved vaccines for bordetellosis requires better characterization of protective antigens of *B. avium* and an understanding of the turkey's immune response to them.

REFERENCES

1. Akeila, M.A., and Y.M. Saif. 1988. Protection of turkey poults from Bordetella avium infection and disease by pili and bacterins. Avian Dis 32:641–649.
2. Andral, B., C. Louzis, D. Trap, J.A. Newman, G. Bennejean, and R. Gaumont. 1985. Respiratory disease (rhinotracheitis) in turkeys in Brittany, France, 1981–1982. I. Field

observations and serology. Avian Dis 29:26–34.

3. Anon. 1985. Turkey rhinotracheitis of unknown aetiology in England and Wales: A preliminary report from the British Veterinary Poultry Association. Vet Rec 117:653–654.

4. Arp, L.H. 1986. Adherence of Bordetella avium to turkey tracheal mucosa: Effects of culture conditions. Am J Vet Res 47:2618–2620.

5. Arp, L.H., and E.E. Brooks. 1986. An in vivo model for the study of Bordetella avium adherence to tracheal mucosa in turkeys. Am J Vet Res 47:2614–2617.

6. Arp, L.H., and N.F. Cheville. 1984. Tracheal lesions in young turkeys infected with Bordetella avium. Am J Vet Res 45:2196–2200.

7. Arp, L.H., and J.A. Fagerland. 1987. Ultrastructural pathology of Bordetella avium infection in turkeys. Vet Pathol 24:411–418.

8. Arp, L.H., and D.H. Hellwig. 1988. Passive immunization versus adhesion of Bordetella avium to the tracheal mucosa of turkeys. Avian Dis 32:494–500.

9. Arp, L.H., and S.M. McDonald. 1985. Influence of temperature on the growth of Bordetella avium in turkeys and in vitro. Avian Dis 29:1066–1077.

10. Arp, L.H., R.D. Leyh, and R.W. Griffith. 1988. Adherence of Bordetella avium to tracheal mucosa of turkeys: Correlation with hemagglutination. Am J Vet Res 49:693–696.

11. Arp, L.H., E.L. Huffman, and D.H. Hellwig. 1993. Glycoconjugates as components of receptors for Bordetella avium on the tracheal mucosa of turkeys. Am J Vet Res 54:2027–2030.

12. Barbour, E.K., M.K. Brinton, S.D. Torkelson, J.B. Johnson, and P.E. Poss. 1991. An enzyme-linked immunosorbent assay for detection of Bordetella avium infection in turkey flocks: Sensitivity, specificity, and reproducibility. Avian Dis 35:308–314.

13. Barnes, H.J., and M.S. Hofstad. 1983. Susceptibility of turkey poults from vaccinated and unvaccinated hens to Alcaligenes rhinotracheitis (turkey coryza). Avian Dis 27:378–392.

14. Berkhoff, H.A., and G.D. Riddle. 1984. Differentiation of Alcaligenes-like bacteria of avian origin and comparison with Alcaligenes spp. reference strains. J Clin Microbiol 19:477–481.

15. Berkhoff, H.A., F.M. McCorkle, Jr., and T.T. Brown. 1983. Pathogenicity of various isolates of Alcaligenes faecalis for broilers. Avian Dis 27:707–713.

16. Berkhoff, H.A., H.J. Barnes, S.I. Ambrus, M.D. Kopp, G.D. Riddle, and D.C. Kradel. 1984. Prevalence of Alcaligenes faecalis in North Carolina broiler flocks and its relationship to respiratory disease. Avian Dis 28:912–920.

17. Blackall, P.J., and C.M. Doheny. 1987. Isolation and characterisation of Bordetella avium and related species and an evaluation of their role in respiratory disease in poultry. Aust Vet J 64:235–239.

18. Blackall, P.J., and J.G. Farrah. 1985. Isolation of Bordetella avium from poultry. Aust Vet J 62:370–372.

19. Blackall, P.J., and J.G. Farrah. 1986. An evaluation of two methods of substrate alkalinization for the identification of Bordetella avium and other similar organisms. Vet Microbiol 11:301–306.

20. Blackall, P.J., and D.G. Rogers. 1991. Absence of mouse-lethal toxins in Australian isolates of Bordetella avium. Vet Microbiol 27:393–396.

21. Blalock, H.G., D.G. Simmons, K.E. Muse, J.G. Gray, and W.T. Derieux. 1975. Adenovirus respiratory infection in turkey poults. Avian Dis 19:707–716.

22. Blore, P.J., M.F. Slavik, and N.K. Neighbor. 1991. Detection of antibody to Bordetella avium using a particle concentration fluorescence immunoassay (PCFIA). Avian Dis 35:756–760.

23. Boycott, B.R., H.R. Wyman, and F.C. Wong. 1984. Alcaligenes faecalis rhinotracheitis in Manitoba turkeys. Avian Dis 28:1110–1114.

24. Burke, D.S., and M.M. Jensen. 1980. Immunization against turkey coryza by colonization with mutants of Alcaligenes faecalis. Avian Dis 24:726–733.

25. Burke, D.S., and M.M. Jensen. 1981. Field vaccination trials against turkey coryza using a temperature-sensitive mutant of Alcaligenes faecalis. Avian Dis 25:96–103.

26. Cimiotti, W., G. Glunder, and K.-H. Hinz. 1982. Survival of the bacterial turkey coryza agent. Vet Rec 110:304–306.

27. Collins, M.S., and R.E. Gough. 1988. Characterization of a virus associated with turkey rhinotracheitis. J Gen Virol 69:909–916.

28. Cook, J.K.A., M.M. Ellis, and M.B. Higgins. 1991. The pathogenesis of turkey rhinotracheitis virus in turkey poults inoculated with the virus alone or together with two strains of bacteria. Avian Pathol 20:155–166.

29. Cutter, D.L., and G.H. Luginbuhl. 1991. Characterization of sulfonamide resistance determinants and relatedness of Bordetella avium R plasmids. Plasmid 26:136–140.

30. Dillman, R.C., and D.G. Simmons. 1977. Histopathology of a rhinotracheitis of turkey poults associated with adenoviruses. Avian Dis 21:481–491.

31. Domingo, D.T., M.W. Jackwood, and T.P. Brown. 1992. Filamentous forms of Bordetella avium: Culture conditions and pathogenicity. Avian Dis 36:707–713.

32. Edens, F.W., F.M. McCorkle, and D.G. Simmons. 1984. Body temperature response of turkey poults infected with Alcaligenes faecalis. Avian Pathol 13:787–795.

33. Edens, F.W., F.M. McCorkle, D.G. Simmons, and A.G. Yersin. 1987. Brain monoamine concentrations in turkey poults infected with Bordetella avium. Avian Dis 31:504–508.

34. Edens, F.W., F.M. McCorkle, D.G. Simmons, and A.G. Yersin. 1987. Effects of Bordetella avium on lymphoid tissue monoamine concentrations in turkey poults. Avian Dis 31:746–751.

35. Edens, F.W., J.D. May, A.G. Yersin, and H.M. Brown-Borg. 1991. Effect of fasting on plasma thyroid and adrenal hormone levels in turkey poults infected with Bordetella avium. Avian Dis 35:344–347.

36. Ficken, M.D. 1983. Antibiotic aerosolization for treatment of alcaligenes rhinotracheitis. Avian Dis 27:545–548.

37. Ficken, M.D., J.F. Edwards, and J.C. Lay. 1986. Clearance of bacteria in turkeys with Bordetella avium-induced tracheitis. Avian Dis 30:352–357.

38. Filion, P.R., S. Cloutier, E.R. Vrancken, and G. Bernier. 1967. Infection respiratoire du dindonneau causee par un microbe apparente au Bordetella bronchiseptica. Can J Comp Med Vet Sci 31:129–134.

39. Gentry-Weeks, C.R., B.T. Cookson, W.E. Goldman, R.B. Rimler, S.B. Porter, and R. Curtiss III. 1988. Dermonecrotic toxin and tracheal cytotoxin, putative virulence factors of Bordetella avium. Infect Immun 56:1698–1707.

40. Gentry-Weeks, C.R., D.L. Provence, J.M. Keith, and R. Curtiss, III. 1991. Isolation and characterization of Bordetella avium phase variants. Infect Immun 59:4026–4033.

41. Gentry-Weeks, C.R., A.L. Hultsch, S.M. Kelly, J.M. Keith, and R. Curtiss, III. 1992. Cloning and sequencing of a gene encoding a 21-kilodalton outer membrane protein from Bordetella avium and expression of the gene in Salmonella typhimurium. J Bacteriol 174:7729–7742.

42. Gentry-Weeks, C.R., J.M. Keith, and J. Thompson. 1993. Toxicity of Bordetella avium beta-cystathionase toward MC3T3-E1 osteogenic cells. J Biol Chem 268:7298–7314.

43. Goldman, W.E. 1986. Bordetella pertussis tracheal cytotoxin: Damage to the respiratory epithelium. In L. Leive and P.F. Bonventre (eds.). Microbiology—1986. Washington, DC, American Society for Microbiology, pp. 65–69.

44. Gray, J.G., J.F. Roberts, R.C. Dillman, and D.G. Simmons. 1981. Cytotoxic activity of pathogenic Alcaligenes faecalis in turkey tracheal organ cultures. Am J Vet Res 42:2184–2186.

45. Gray, J.G., J.F. Roberts, R.C. Dillman, and D.G. Simmons. 1983. Pathogenesis of change in the upper respiratory

tracts of turkeys experimentally infected with an Alcaligenes faecalis isolate. Infect Immun 42:350–355.

46. Gray, J.G., J.F. Roberts, and D.G. Simmons. 1983. In vitro cytotoxicity of an Alcaligenes faecalis and its relationship in in vivo tracheal pathologic changes in turkeys. Avian Dis 27:1142–1150.

47. Heller, E.D., Y. Weisman, and A. Aharonovovitch. 1984. Experimental studies on turkey coryza. Avian Pathol 13:137–143.

48. Hellwig, D.H., and L.H. Arp. 1990. Identification of Bordetella avium antigens recognized after experimental inoculation in turkeys. Am J Vet Res 51:1188–1191.

49. Hellwig, D.H., L.H. Arp, and J.A. Fagerland. 1988. A comparison of outer membrane proteins and surface characteristics of adhesive and non-adhesive phenotypes of Bordetella avium. Avian Dis 32:787–792.

50. Herzog, M., M.F. Slavik, J.K. Skeeles, and J.N. Beasley. 1986. The efficacy of a temperature-sensitive mutant vaccine against Northwest Arkansas isolates of Alcaligenes faecalis. Avian Dis 30:112–116.

51. Hinz, K.-H., and G. Glunder. 1986. Identification of Bordetella avium sp. nov. by the API 20 NE system. Avian Pathol 15:611–614.

52. Hinz, K.-H., G. Glunder, and H. Lunders. 1978. Acute respiratory disease in turkey poults caused by Bordetella bronchiseptica-like bacteria. Vet Rec 103:262–263.

53. Hinz, K.-H., G. Korthas, H. Luders, B. Stiburek, G. Glunder, H.E. Brozeit, and T. Redmann. 1981. Passive immunisation of turkey poults against turkey coryza (Bordetellosis) by vaccination of parent breeders. Avian Pathol 10:441–447.

54. Hinz, K.-H., G. Glunder, and K.J. Romer. 1983. A comparative study of avian Bordetella-like strains, Bordetella bronchiseptica, Alcaligenes faecalis and other related nonfermentable bacteria. Avian Pathol 12:263–276.

55. Hinz, K.-H., M. Rull, U. Heffels-Redmann, and M. Poeppel. 1992. Multicausal infectious respiratory disease of turkey poults. Dtsch Tierarztl Wochenschr 99:75–78.

56. Hofstad, M.S., and E.L. Jeska. 1985. Immune response of poults following intranasal inoculation with Art-vax™ vaccine and a formalin-inactivated Bordetella avium bacterin. Avian Dis 29:746–754.

57. Hopkins, B.A., J.K. Skeeles, G.E. Houghten, and J.D. Story. 1988. Development of an enzyme-linked immunosorbent assay for Bordetella avium. Avian Dis 32:353–361.

58. Hopkins, B.A., J.K. Skeeles, G.E. Houghten, D. Slagle, and K. Gardner. 1990. A survey of infectious diseases in wild turkeys (Meleagris gallopavo silvestris) from Arkansas (USA). J Wildl Dis 26:468–472.

59. Houghten, G.E., J.K. Skeeles, M. Rosenstein, J.N. Beasley, and M.F. Slavik. 1987. Efficacy in turkeys of spray vaccination with a temperature-sensitive mutant of Bordetella avium (Art Vax™). Avian Dis 31:309–314.

60. Jackwood, D.J., and Y.M. Saif. 1980. Development and use of a microagglutination test to detect antibodies to Alcaligenes faecalis in turkeys. Avian Dis 24:685–701.

61. Jackwood, M.W., and Y.M. Saif. 1985. Efficacy of a commercial turkey coryza vaccine (Art-Vax™) in turkey poults. Avian Dis 29:1130–1139.

62. Jackwood, M.W., and Y.M. Saif. 1987. Lack of protection against Bordetella avium in turkey poults exposed to B. avium-like bacteria. Avian Dis 31:597–600.

63. Jackwood, M.W., and Y.M. Saif. 1987. Pili of Bordetella avium: Expression, characterization, and role in in vitro adherence. Avian Dis 31:277–286.

64. Jackwood, D.J., Y.M. Saif, P.D. Moorhead, and R.N. Dearth. 1982. Infectious bursal disease virus and Alcaligenes faecalis infections in turkeys. Avian Dis 26:365–374.

65. Jackwood, M.W., Y.M. Saif, P.D. Moorhead, and R.N. Dearth. 1985. Further characterization of the agent causing coryza in turkeys. Avian Dis 29:690–705.

66. Jackwood, M.W., M. Sasser, and Y.M. Saif. 1986.

Contribution to the taxonomy of the turkey coryza agent: Cellular fatty acid analysis of the bacterium. Avian Dis 30:172–178.

67. Jackwood, M.W., Y.M. Saif, and D.L. Coplin. 1987. Isolation and characterization of Bordetella avium plasmids. Avian Dis 31:782–786.

68. Jackwood, M.W., D.A. Hilt, and P.A. Dunn. 1991. Observations on colonial phenotypic variation in Bordetella avium. Avian Dis 35:496–504.

69. Jensen, M.M., and M.S. Marshall. 1981. Control of turkey Alcaligenes rhinotracheitis in Utah with a live vaccine. Avian Dis 25:1053–1057.

70. Kelly, B.J., G.Y. Ghazikhanian, and B. Mayeda. 1986. Clinical outbreak of Bordetella avium infection in two turkey breeder flocks. Avian Dis 30:234–237.

71. Kersters, K., K.-H. Hinz, A. Hertle, P. Segers, A. Lievens, O. Siegmann, and J. De Ley. 1984. Bordetella avium sp. nov. isolated from the respiratory tracts of turkeys and other birds. Int J Syst Bacteriol 34:56–70.

72. Leyh, R., and R.W. Griffith. 1992. Characterization of the outer membrane proteins of Bordetella avium. Infect Immun 60:958–964.

73. Leyh, R.D., R.W. Griffith, and L.H. Arp. 1988. Transposon mutagenesis in Bordetella avium. Am J Vet Res 49:687–692.

74. Lindsey, D.G., P.D. Andrews, G.S. Yarborough, J.K. Skeeles, B. Glidewell-Erickson, G. Campbell, and M.B. Blankford. 1994. Evaluation of a commercial ELISA kit for detection and quantitation of antibody against Bordetella avium [abst 31]. Proc 75th Ann Meet Conf Res Workers Anim Dis. Chicago, IL.

75. Lister, S.A., and D.J. Alexander. 1986. Turkey rhinotracheitis: A review. Vet Bull 56:637–663.

76. Luginbuhl, G.H., D. Cutter, G. Campodonico, J. Peace, and D.G. Simmons. 1986. Plasmid DNA of virulent Alcaligenes faecalis. Am J Vet Res 47:619–621.

77. Marshall, D.R., D.G. Simmons, and J.G. Gray. 1984. Evidence for adherence-dependent cytotoxicity of Alcaligenes faecalis in turkey tracheal organ cultures. Avian Dis 28:1007–1015.

78. Marshall, D.R., D.G. Simmons, and J.G. Gray. 1985. An Alcaligenes faecalis isolate from turkeys: Pathogenicity in selected avian and mammalian species. Am J Vet Res 46:1181–1184.

79. McBride, M.D., D.W. Hird, T.E. Carpenter, K.P. Snipes, C. Danaye-Elmi, and W.W. Utterback. 1991. Health survey of backyard poultry and other avian species located within one mile of commercial California meat-turkey flocks. Avian Dis 35:403–407.

80. McCorkle, F.M., and D.G. Simmons. 1984. In vitro cellular migration of leukocytes from turkey poults infected with Alcaligenes faecalis. Avian Dis 28:853–857.

81. McCorkle, F.M., D.G. Simmons, and G.H. Luginbuhl. 1982. Delayed hypersensitivity response in Alcaligenes faecalis- infected turkey poults. Avian Dis 26:782–786.

82. McCorkle, F.M., D.G. Simmons, and G.H. Luginbuhl. 1983. Graft-vs-host response in Alcaligenes faecalis-infected turkey poults. Am J Vet Res 44:1141–1142.

83. McCorkle, F.M., F.W. Edens, and D.G. Simmons. 1985. Alcaligenes faecalis infection in turkeys: Effects on serum corticosterone and serum chemistry. Avian Dis 29:80–89.

84. Montgomery, R.D., S.H. Kleven, and P. Villegas. 1983. Observations on the pathogenicity of Alcaligenes faecalis in chickens. Avian Dis 27:751–761.

85. Moore, K.M., and M.W. Jackwood. 1994. Production of monoclonal antibodies to the Bordetella avium 41-kilodalton surface protein and characterization of the hemagglutinin. Avian Dis 38:218–224.

86. Moore, C.J., H. Mawhinney, and P.J. Blackall. 1987. Differentiation of Bordetella avium and related species by cellular fatty acid analysis. J Clin Microbiol 25:1059–1062.

87. Movalind, M., R. Mutters, and W. Mannheim. 1991. Rapid identification of Bordetella avium and related organisms on the basis of their cellular carbohydrate patterns. Avian Pathol 20:627–636.

88. Neighbor, N.K., J.K. Skeeles, J.N. Beasley, and D.L. Kreider. 1991. Use of an enzyme-linked immunosorbent assay to measure antibody levels in turkey breeder hens, eggs, and progeny following natural infection or immunization with a commercial Bordetella avium bacterin. Avian Dis 35:315–320.

89. Page, R.K., O.J. Fletcher, P.D. Lukert, and R. Rimler. 1978. Rhinotracheitis in turkey poults. Avian Dis 22:529–534.

90. Panigrahy, B., L.C. Grumbles, R.J. Terry, D.L. Millar, and C.F. Hall. 1981. Bacterial coryza in turkeys in Texas. Poult Sci 60:107–113.

91. Rhoades, K.R., and R.B. Rimler. 1987. The effects of heat-labile Bordetella avium toxin on turkey poults. Avian Dis 31:345–350.

92. Rimler, R.B. 1985. Turkey coryza: Toxin production by Bordetella avium. Avian Dis 29:1043–1047.

93. Rimler, R.B., and K.R. Rhoades. 1986. Turkey coryza: Selected tests for detection and neutralization of Bordetella avium heat-labile toxin. Avian Dis 30:808–812.

94. Rimler, R.B., and K.R. Rhoades. 1986. Fowl cholera: Influence of Bordetella avium on vaccinal immunity of turkeys to Pasteurella multocida. Avian Dis 30:838–839.

95. Rimler, R.B., and D.G. Simmons. 1983. Differentiation among bacteria isolated from turkeys with coryza (rhinotracheitis). Avian Dis 27:491–500.

96. Saif, Y.M., P.D. Moorhead, R.N. Dearth, and D.J. Jackwood. 1980. Observations on Alcaligenes faecalis infection in turkeys. Avian Dis 24:665–684.

97. Savelkoul, P.H.M., L.E.G.M. DeGroat, C. Boersma, I. Livey, C.J. Duggleby, B.A.M. Van der Zeijst, and W. Gaastra. 1993. Identification of Bordetella avium using the polymerase chain reaction. Microb Pathogen 15:207–215.

98. Simmons, D.G., and J.G. Gray. 1979. Transmission of acute respiratory disease (rhinotracheitis) of turkeys. Avian Dis 23:132–138.

99. Simmons, D.G., S.E. Miller, J.G. Gray, H.G. Blalock, and W.M. Colwell. 1976. Isolation and identification of a turkey respiratory adenovirus. Avian Dis 20:65–74.

100. Simmons, D.G., R.K. Page, P.V. Lukert, O.J. Fletcher, S.E. Miller, and R. C. Dillman. 1977. Bursal changes in turkey poults with acute respiratory disease. J Am Vet Med Assoc 171:1104–1105.

101. Simmons, D.G., J.G. Gray, L.P. Rose, R.C. Dillman, and S.E. Miller. 1979. Isolation of an etiologic agent of acute respiratory disease (rhinotracheitis) of turkey poults. Avian Dis 23:194–203.

102. Simmons, D.G., A.R. Gore, and E.C. Hodgin. 1980. Altered immune function in turkey poults infected with Alcaligenes faecalis, the etiologic agent of turkey rhinotracheitis (coryza). Avian Dis 24:702–714.

103. Simmons, D.G., L.P. Rose, and J.G. Gray. 1980. Some physical, biochemic, and pathologic properties of Alcaligenes faecalis, the bacterium causing rhinotracheitis (coryza) in turkey poults. Avian Dis 24:82–90.

104. Simmons, D.G., D.E. Davis, L.P. Rose, J.G. Gray, and G.H. Luginbuhl. 1981. Alcaligenes faecalis-associated respiratory disease of chickens. Avian Dis 25:610–613.

105. Simmons, D.G., L.P. Rose, F.M. McCorkle, and G.H. Luginbuhl. 1983. Histamine-sensitizing factor of Alcaligenes faecalis. Avian Dis 27:171–177.

106. Simmons, D.G., C. Dees, and L.P. Rose. 1986. A heat-stable toxin isolated from the turkey coryza agent, Bordetella avium. Avian Dis 30:761–765.

107. Simmons, D.G., L.P. Rose, F.J. Fuller, L.C. Maurer, and G.H. Luginbuhl. 1986. Turkey coryza: Lack of correlation between plasmids and pathogenicity of Bordetella avium. Avian Dis 30:593–597.

108. Skeeles, J.K., W.S. Swafford, D.P. Wages, H.M. Hellwig, M.F. Slavik, J.N. Beasley, G.E. Houghten, P.J. Blore, and D. Crawford. 1983. Studies on the use of a long-acting oxytetracycline in turkeys: Efficacy against experimental infections with Alcaligenes faecalis and Pasteurella multocida. Avian Dis 27:1126–1130.

109. Slavik, M.F., J.K. Skeeles, J.N. Beasley, G.C. Harris, P. Roblee, and D. Hellwig. 1981. Effect of humidity on infection of turkeys with Alcaligenes faecalis. Avian Dis 25:936–942.

110. Slavik, M.F., J.K. Skeeles, C.F. Meinecke, and L. Holloway. 1981. The involvement of Alcaligenes faecalis in turkeys submitted for diagnosis as detected by bacterial isolation and microagglutination test. Avian Dis 25:761–763.

111. Suresh, P. 1993. Detecting Bordetella avium in tracheal sections of turkeys by monoclonal antibody-based indirect fluorescence microscopy. Avian Pathol 22:791–795.

112. Suresh, P., and L.H. Arp. 1993. A monoclonal antibody-based latex bead agglutination test for the detection of Bordetella avium. Avian Dis 37:767–772.

113. Suresh, P., L.H. Arp, and E.L. Huffman. 1994. Mucosal and systemic humoral immune response to Bordetella avium in experimentally infected turkeys. Avian Dis 38:225–230.

114. Tsai, H.J., and Y.M. Saif. 1991. Detection of antibodies against Bordetella avium in turkeys by avidin-biotin enhancement of the enzyme-linked immunosorbent assay and the dot-immunobinding assay. Avian Dis 35:801–808.

115. Van Alstine, W.G., and L.H. Arp. 1987. Effects of Bordetella avium toxin on turkey tracheal organ cultures as measured with a tetrazolium-reduction assay. Avian Dis 31:136–139.

116. Van Alstine, W.G., and L.H. Arp. 1987. Influence of Bordetella avium infection on association of Escherichia coli with turkey trachea. Am J Vet Res 48:1574–1576.

117. Van Alstine, W.G., and L.H. Arp. 1987. Effects of Bordetella avium infection on the pulmonary clearance of Escherichia coli in turkeys. Am J Vet Res 48:922–926.

118. Van Alstine, W.G., and L.H. Arp. 1988. Histologic evaluation of lung and bronchus-associated lymphoid tissue in young turkeys infected with Bordetella avium. Am J Vet Res 49:835–839.

119. Van Alstine, W.G., and M.S. Hofstad. 1985. Antibiotic aerosolization: The effect on experimentally induced alcaligenes rhinotracheitis in turkeys. Avian Dis 29:159–176.

120. Varley, J. 1986. The characterisation of Bordetella/Alcaligenes-like organisms and their effects on turkey poults and chicks. Avian Pathol 15:1–22.

121. Varley, J., and S.D. Carter. 1992. Characterization of the proteins of Bordetella isolated from turkeys in the UK by polyacrylamide gel electrophoresis. Avian Pathol 21:137–140.

122. Yersin, A.G., F.W. Edens, and D.G. Simmons. 1990. Tryptophan 2,3-dioxygenase activity in turkey poults infected with Bordetella avium. Comp Biochem Physiol 97B:755–760.

123. Yersin, A.G., F.W. Edens, and D.G. Simmons. 1991. Effect of Bordetella avium infection on electrocardiograms in turkey poults. Avian Dis 35:668–673.

124. Yersin, A.G., F.W. Edens, and D.G. Simmons. 1991. Tracheal cilia response to exogenous niacin in drinking water of turkey poults infected with Bordetella avium. Avian Dis 35:674–680.

14 Other Bacterial Diseases

INTRODUCTION
H. John Barnes

Bacterial diseases cause significant economic losses in the poultry industry. Those that are common, widespread, or of major public health significance are covered in subchapters or chapters elsewhere in this text. Since the previous edition, *Ornithobacterium rhinotracheale* has been identified as a potential emerging bacterial pathogen causing respiratory disease (see Chapter 37), information on avian intestinal spirochetosis as a cause of production loss and diarrheal disease has increased to the point that it is covered in a separate section of this chapter, and *Helicobacter pullorum* (see below) is a newly recognized bacterium of poultry capable of causing food-borne illness in people. Bacterial diseases of sporadic occurrence, limited distribution, uncertain significance or potential public health significance, and those bacterial diseases of historical interest, are briefly discussed by etiology, disease, or pathologic lesion in this introduction.

ACINETOBACTER. *Acinetobacter lwoffi* and *A. calcoaceticus* were isolated from outbreaks of septicemia in hens. Mortality was approximately 15%, and multifocal necrosis of the liver was a prominent necropsy finding (32, 52). *Acinetobacter* has also been recovered from ducks with arthritis (15), septicemia, or airsacculitis (94).

ACTINOBACILLUS. *Actinobacillus* spp., distinct from *A. lignieresii* and *A. equuli,* have been isolated from a duck with septicemia and a goose with airsacculitis (33). Atypical *A. lignieresii,* currently identified as taxon 2 and taxon 3, were recovered frequently from lesions of salpingitis in egg-laying ducks and geese. Isolation of these organisms from the cloaca and penis of normal geese suggests that salpingitis probably results from an ascending infection (16).

ACTINOMYCES (CORYNEBACTERIUM). A chronic, disseminated granulomatous disease of turkeys in Canada suspected to be actinomycosis has been observed sporadically since 1955 (86). Serious outbreaks of osteomyelitis involving the proximal tibia, thoracic vertebra, and/or proximal tibiotarsi caused by *Actinomyces (Corynebacterium) pyogenes* in commercial male turkey flocks resulted in considerable economic loss. Lame birds in affected flocks averaged 20% (range, 5–50%), age averaged 16 wk (range, 12–20 wk), and weekly mortality averaged 2.8% (range, 0.5–10.5%). Hen flocks were not affected. Osteomyelitis was reproduced in 15-wk-old male turkeys inoculated intravenously with a representative isolate. Biochemical and serologic evaluation of isolates from nine flocks indicated they were either identical or very closely related. An agar-gel precipitin test was highly effective at detecting antibodies (9). Treatment of an affected flock with penicillin in the feed (100 g/ton) resulted in a gradual improvement in the flock after 8–10 days on medication (20).

Septicemia, visceral lesions in many organs, cutaneous abscesses, mortality of nearly 14%, and a decrease in egg production of over 27% occurred in caged layers infected with *A. pyogenes*. Portal of entry was through skin lesions caused by poor caging (27).

AEROBACTER. *Aerobacter* has been recovered occasionally from dead embryos (51).

AEROMONAS. *Aeromonas hydrophila,* either alone or in combination with other organisms, can cause localized and systemic infections in avian species including poultry (35, 89). *A. hydrophila* was occasionally recovered from ducks with salpingitis (16), septicemia, or airsacculitis (94), and *A. formicans* has been isolated infrequently from arthritic lesions in ducks at processing (15). *Aeromonas* has potential public health significance (47).

ANTHRAX. Anthrax occurs rarely in birds where the disease is endemic. Chickens are highly resistant. Ostriches are moderately susceptible, often with high mortality (44), while ducks have occasionally developed the disease (90). Ostriches in endemic areas should be vaccinated (44).

BACTEROIDES. *Bacteroides fragilis* has been occasionally isolated from salpingitis in laying hens (17).

BRUCELLA. Poultry can be experimentally and naturally infected with *Brucella* spp., and positive serologic tests have been found when free-ranging birds in contact with livestock have been tested (54, 90). There are no recent confirmed reports of *Brucella* infection in poultry; it is unlikely the organism has any importance in modern confinement poultry production.

CITROBACTER. *Citrobacter freundii* was rarely isolated from young ducks with salpingitis (16).

COWDRIA. Antibodies to *Cowdria ruminatum* were not detected in a survey of 216 ostriches on nine farms in Zimbabwe (53).

COXIELLA. There is serologic and cultural evidence of *Coxiella burnetii* infection in poultry, and chickens are susceptible to the organism following intraperitoneal inoculation (87). Antibodies to *C. burnetii* were not detected in a survey of 216 ostriches on nine farms in Zimbabwe (53).

EUBACTERIUM. See liver granulomas and related granulomatous diseases below.

FLAVOBACTERIUM. This organism has been recovered from ducks with arthritis (15) and from an adult goose with salpingitis (16). Heavy, pure cultures of *Flavobacterium meningosepticum* were obtained from a 5-wk-old ostrich chick that failed to grow and thrive and had airsacculitis, pneumonia, and thymic atrophy/hypoplasia (56).

FRANCISELLA. Birds are susceptible to tularemia. The disease has occurred in at least 25 avian species, primarily galliformes, including poultry, waterfowl, scavengers, and predatory wild birds. Major die-offs of blue grouse in the northwestern United States have resulted from tularemia, and *F. tularensis* has been isolated from them and infesting ticks (46). While a sporadic disease of significance in wild and free-ranging birds, which may play an important role in maintaining and disseminating the organism, tularemia is not known to occur or be important in commercial poultry.

HELICOBACTER. Bacteria previously identified as *Campylobacter*-like organisms form a distinct group based on DNA homology within the genus *Helicobacter*. A new species, *H. pullorum*, in the urease-negative, enteric group of helicobacters, which can be differentiated biochemically from other species, has been proposed. *H. pullorum* has been isolated from ceca of normal broilers, livers and intestines of layers with lesions characteristic of "vibrionic hepatitis," and people with gastroenteritis. It can be cultured using procedures for isolating campylobacters; however, it is inhibited by polymyxin B, which was used in some older media formulations. A polymerase chain reaction to detect the organism has been developed (21, 91). Another avian species (*H. pamatensis*) has been described from a tern (30) and other unnamed, distinct strains have been isolated from avian species (88).

KLEBSIELLA. *Klebsiella* is an environmental contaminant that occasionally causes embryo mortality and excess losses in young chickens and turkeys (74, 76, 83). Hygienic handling of hatching eggs and hatchery sanitation are necessary for prevention of these losses. Concurrent infection of young turkeys with *K. pneumoniae* increases the severity of respiratory disease resulting from *Bordetella avium* and *Chlamydia psittaci* infections (42). An outbreak of ocular disease caused by *Klebsiella* affected a flock of 4-wk-old chickens (59).

LISTERIA. Outbreaks of listeriosis caused by *L. monocytogenes* occur sporadically in many avian species including poultry (37). Human infection can result from contact with affected birds (38) or by consumption of contaminated poultry or products (63). In birds, the disease can occur as a septicemia with splenomegaly, necrotic areas in the liver and heart, and pericarditis (37), or as an encephalitic form without grossly visible lesions (25, 26). Emaciation and diarrhea are seen in birds with septicemia; depression, incoordination, ataxia, torticollis, opisthotonos, and other nervous signs are seen in the encephalitic form (25, 26). Microscopically, gliosis and satellitosis in the cerebellum and microabscesses containing gram-positive bacteria are present in the midbrain and medulla of birds with encephalitic listeriosis (26).

Listeria monocytogenes is commonly found in feces and soil in temperate areas of the world. Infection can follow inhalation, ingestion, or wound contamination. Cold, wet conditions causing excessively moist litter were associated with an outbreak of encephalitic listeriosis. The organism was isolated from litter, water, and soil samples (26).

Isolation of the organism may be difficult and require special procedures (11), although direct culture of brain stem was positive in four of five attempts in an outbreak of encephalitic listeriosis (25). Chicken embryos are readily infected and can be used for isolation.

Chickens (11) and turkeys (19) are relatively resistant but can be experimentally infected. Young birds and exposure to high numbers of organisms are more likely to result in colonization following oral challenge (7). The disease is more severe in young birds. *Listeria monocytogenes* has been used to study macrophage function in retrovirus infection (28) and cell-mediated responses in susceptible and resistant chickens exposed to Marek's disease virus (22).

Prevention of listeriosis depends on identifying and eliminating sources of infection. The organism is often resistant to most commonly used antibiotics; high levels of tetracyclines are usually recommended for treatment. Widespread use of antibiotics in feed may have had prophylactic value in listeriosis prevention in poultry (38).

LONG-SEGMENTED FILAMENTOUS ORGANISMS.

Long-segmented filamentous organisms (LSFOs) are gram-positive, unbranched bacteria commonly found in the jejunum and ileum of poultry and of a number of other animals, where they firmly attach to the brush border of enterocytes, displacing microvilli. In turkeys, LSFOs are 0.6 to 1.1 μm wide and up to 13.5 μm long (5). Chickens are refractory to infection with LSFOs from mice even following corticosteroid treatment, suggesting that there are different types or species of LSFOs and that rodents are not a likely source of infection for poultry (3). Often, LSFOs are markedly increased in young chickens, turkeys, and quail with gastrointestinal diseases, especially during winter (36). While most frequent in ill birds, LSFOs may not be pathogens, overgrowing when conditions are altered because of disease. High numbers of LSFOs were identified in jejuna of poults with experimental stunting syndrome (5), but subsequent studies using filtered inocula showed they were not the cause of the disease (85). Depressed growth (11–14%) occurred, however, when poults were inoculated with two isolates (67), and their presence has been associated with decreased carotenoid levels and skin pigmentation (4). Virginiamycin was partially effective in controlling the organisms and improving serum carotenoids (4).

MEGABACTERIA.

Megabacteria cause a progressively debilitating, gastrointestinal disease typical of malnutrition, which results in high mortality in juvenile ostriches. The characteristic large, gram-positive, PAS+ organisms can be found in fecal smears and in large numbers in the proventriculi of affected birds. Megabacteria need to be differentiated from *Candida,* which is similar in size and morphology. Variable inflammation of the proventriculus and ventriculus is seen microscopically. Antibiotic treatment does not alter the course of the disease (44, 45).

MORAXELLA.

Moraxella osloensis caused a choleralike disease in commercial turkeys. Affected birds had at least one consolidated, pneumonic lung, multiple hemorrhages and inflammation of serous membranes, and abnormal spleens and livers. The organism could be distinguished from *Pasteurella multocida* by its growth on eosin-methylene blue and MacConkey media. The disease was reproduced in experimentally inoculated turkeys (31). *Moraxella* sp. has also been recovered from salpingitis in layers (17).

NEISSERIA.

Diplococci consistent with *Neisseria* can cause pneumonia in young ostriches (44). *Neisseria* are also commonly identified in goose venereal disease (see below).

NOCARDIA.

Nocardia are branching, gram-positive filamentous bacteria that typically cause granulomatous lesions, especially in the respiratory system. The organism has rarely been isolated from avian species even though chickens are susceptible to experimental infection following oral or intraperitoneal inoculation (72).

PLANOCOCCUS.

Pure cultures of *Planococcus halophilus* were obtained from livers of 43-wk-old layers with multifocal, hepatic necrosis. Mortality of nearly 6% occurred in the flock during the month after onset of the disease. The isolate was resistant to most antimicrobials. Streptomycin was an exception; it was added to feed at 5 g/kg and successfully treated the flock. Feed, specifically fishmeal and marine byproducts, was considered to be the source of the organism, as it is normally found in a variety of marine animals. High ambient temperatures (up to 46 C) during the outbreak was thought to be a contributing factor (1).

PROTEUS.

Proteus was isolated from dead-in-shell chicken embryos (51, 74) and sick ducklings (81). Experimental inoculation of the organism from ducklings failed to cause disease. Penetration of eggs and survival within the egg are affected by temperature (2). Septicemia has occurred in quail (82) and broilers suspected of having immunologic deficiency (77). *Proteus vulgaris* can occasionally produce arthritis in ducks (15); *P. mirabilis* has been recovered from a low percent of salpingitis lesions in layers (17); swarming *Proteus* was isolated occasionally from young ducks with salpingitis (16); and *P. morganii* has been associated with respiratory disease in chickens. The latter isolate caused 50% mortality in experimentally inoculated 4-wk-old chickens (58).

PSEUDOMONAS.

Pseudomonas can cause localized or systemic diseases in young and growing poultry, invade fertile eggs causing death of embryos and newly hatched birds, and reduce shelf life of contaminated meat. The organisms are ubiquitous; often associated with soil, water, and humid environments. *Pseudomonas aeruginosa* is the most common pseudomonad causing infections. It can be highly virulent causing 100% mortality in experimentally inoculated chickens (58). *P. fluorescens*, however, can cause turkey embryo mortality following dipping of eggs in contaminated antibiotic solution (10), and it has been associated with multicausal respiratory disease of chickens (58) and turkeys (42). *P. stutzeri* has been isolated from chickens with respiratory disease but produced only low mortality in experimentally inoculated chickens (58). Pseudomonads are capable of digesting eggshell cuticle if the humidity is high (18). For a review of pseudomonas infections in domestic animals, see (60).

P. aeruginosa is a motile, gram-negative, non–spore-forming rod measuring 1.5–3 × 0.5–0.8 µm, occurring singly or in short chains. The organism is a strict aerobe that grows readily on common bacteriologic media, usually producing a water-soluble green pigment composed of fluorescein and pyocyanin. A characteristic fruity odor can often be recognized. Organisms are often resistant to many antimicrobials (58). For a detailed account of characteristics and differentiation of pseudomonads, see (34).

Pseudomonas is an opportunist that produces respiratory infections, including sinusitis in turkeys; conjunctivitis in chicks (79); or septicemia and its sequelae when introduced into tissues of susceptible birds. Chickens (8, 29, 64, 79), turkeys (39, 48), ducks (15, 81, 94), pheasants (43), and ostriches (44) have been affected. Although birds of any age can be infected, young birds are most susceptible, as are severely stressed or immunodeficient birds. Concurrent infections with viruses and other bacteria occur and may also affect susceptibility to *Pseudomonas* (77). Morbidity and mortality are usually 2–10% but can be much higher, approaching 100%.

Clinical signs include lassitude; lameness; incoordination; ataxia; swelling of head, wattles, and sinuses, hock joints or foot pads; diarrhea; and conjunctivitis (29, 39, 68, 79). Death usually occurs rapidly; often within 24–48 hr. Torticollis, indistinguishable from fowl cholera, occurs following *Pseudomonas* inoculation of turkeys via the eustachian tube (73).

Lesions are consistent with clinical findings and include subcutaneous edema and fibrin, occasionally with hemorrhage; exudate in affected joints; inflammation of serous membranes mimicking lesions of colisepticemia (airsacculitis, pericarditis, perihepatitis); pneumonia; swelling and necrotic foci in liver, spleen, kidney, and brain; conjunctivitis; sinusitis; and occasionally keratitis (29, 39, 58, 68). Heterophilic exudate in the pharynx and pulmonary foci are present in respiratory infections of pheasants (43). Large numbers of bacteria, often in and around affected blood vessels within most tissues, including brain, are typically seen microscopically.

Pseudomonas is among a variety of bacteria often recovered from dead embryos and sick newly hatched birds (51, 74, 81). With the exception of a respiratory outbreak in pheasants attributed to exploding contaminated eggs in the incubator, presence of *P. aeruginosa* in embryos is not considered a source of infection for older birds. Severe outbreaks have followed injection of large numbers of birds with contaminated vaccines (Fig. 14.1) (64, 93) and antibiotic solutions (23, 95). In these cases, contamination resulted from poor hygiene during mixing and handling, not from the products themselves. Contact with infected birds (68) and intense, continuous broiler production with different ages being raised at the same facility (29) can result in spread of *Pseudomonas* infection. In some outbreaks, the source of the organism and how it spread could not be determined.

Diagnosis requires isolation and identification of the organism. Various methods including serologic, phage, and aeruginocine typing methods are available (80) and may be useful in epidemiologic studies.

Prevention and control are based on identifying and eliminating the source of the organism. Good hygiene, especially in hatcheries and when birds are injected, is fundamental to *Pseudomonas* control. Cleaning and disinfection of equipment and use of sterile techniques in preparing vaccines and injectables will control *Pseudomonas* infections resulting from inoculation (23). Reduction of stress and prevention of other viral and bacterial infections will aid in reducing susceptibility to *Pseudomonas*. Antibiotics can be useful in reducing losses if initiated early in the disease. Because of the organism's resistance to many antibiotics (75, 79, 80), sensitivity testing of available drugs is essential. Isolates are generally susceptible to gentamicin. Supplemental vitamin A and potassium permanganate in the water were helpful adjuncts to antibiotic therapy in controlling conjunctivitis (79).

ROTHIA. *Rothia* spp. are aerobic actinomycetes that have been associated with chronic infections, most notably tooth decay, in humans and animals. They are closely related to *Actinomyces*. *Rothia* was the only bacterium isolated from osteomyelitis and joint lesions in four lame or recumbent tom turkeys in an affected flock. Intravenous inoculation of unaffected turkeys reproduced the clinical signs and lesions from which the organism was reisolated (10).

SHIGELLA. *Shigella boydii* has been isolated infrequently from poultry feces. Contamination of carcasses with *Shigella* by infected food handlers can occur, but the likelihood of poultry serving as a

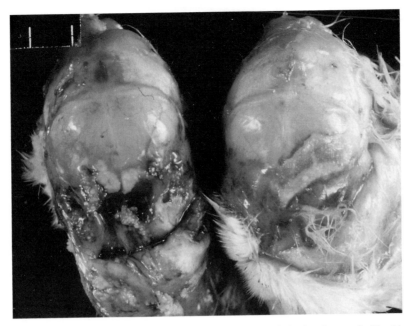

14.1. Subcutaneous lesions in the upper neck area of chicks following the use of a Marek's disease vaccine contaminated by *Pseudomonas*. (L. Munger)

source of shigellosis in humans is considered negligible (70).

STREPTOBACILLUS. *Streptobacillus moniliformis,* a gram-negative, often beaded, nonbranching, filamentous bacterium, can infect turkeys, usually following rat bites or exposure to infected rats. Polyarthritis and synovitis occur in infected birds; other tissues are usually normal. The disease can be reproduced in turkeys following experimental inoculation of the organism by intravenous, subcutaneous, and foot-pad routes, but not by oral administration. Diagnosis requires isolation and identification of the organism. Infection can be prevented through rodent control (65).

VIBRIO (CAMPYLOBACTER). Non-O1 *Vibrio cholerae* has been isolated from the liver of a goose that died following weight loss and lassitude of 2–3 days' duration, from nasal cavities of apparently healthy ducks, and from tissues of ducks with airsacculitis or septicemia (84, 94). Individuals working with ill birds having contact with coastal waters and shellfish need to be aware the birds could be a source of human *V. cholerae* infection (84).

Historically, a choleralike disease has been reported in poultry and zoo birds caused by *V. metschnikovii (metchnikovi)*, and campylobacters have been implicated as the cause of hepatitis in chickens (see Chapter 10). Neither of these diseases have apparently been reported recently, but *V.*

metschnikovii is still occasionally isolated from fowl (57).

DISEASES CAUSED BY OR ASSOCIATED WITH BACTERIA

Beak Necrosis. A gram-positive bacterium with affinity for keratin was associated with beak necrosis in a flock of broiler breeder hens. Nearly half of the flock was affected, and mortality was 10% (24).

Goose Venereal Disease. A venereal disease of unknown etiology affecting goose breeders in Europe, Russia, and the Middle East has been described. Initially, the base of the phallus becomes swollen and inflamed, with the process extending to the cloaca. Later, there is necrosis, ulceration, and eventually considerable scarring of the mucosa, often making reproduction impossible. Similar lesions may develop in the cloaca of the hens following breeding. Morbidity ranges from 20 to 100%, and newly introduced birds readily contract the disease. Increased infertility and gander mortality of approximately 5% are flock problems resulting from the disease (92).

A variety of bacteria, especially *Neisseria* and *Mycoplasma* spp. and *Candida albicans*, affecting the phallus of ganders and cloaca of hens have been associated with the disease (13, 62). The normal phallus microflora of unaffected ganders has been established (61). Microflora of the phallus of immature ganders was similar, with the exception of *Mycoplasma* and *C. albicans,* to that of affected ganders (14). Exposure of SPF Muscovy ducks to isolates from ganders alone and in various combinations failed to reproduce the disease consistently (62). Trauma is considered to play a part in development of the disease.

It is recommended that ganders be examined at each breeding season and affected birds removed from the flock (14).

Intracellular Infection in Ducks. Mortality in Muscovy ducks (*Cairina moschata*) caused by an intracellular organism primarily affecting endothelial cells in the lungs was initially attributed to *Haemoproteus* infection (49). Subsequent examination of additional cases, however, revealed that the organism was not a protozoan but probably a bacterium capable of forming spores or an unidentified microorganism. Muscovy ducks appear most susceptible and can contract the infection from asymptomatic infected Pekin ducks. Experimental transmission is possible using blood from an infected bird.

Lungs of affected ducks are dark red-purple, slightly edematous, and firm. Microscopically, air capillaries are obliterated because of marked swelling of endothelial cells, which are often packed with intracellular organisms, and interlobular septa are widened and contain inflammatory cells and edema. In tissue sections, organisms stain poorly with hematoxylin and eosin but are readily demonstrated with periodic-acid-Schiff or silver stains (50, 78).

Liver Granulomas and Related Granulomatous Disorders. Granulomas are occasionally seen in livers of turkeys at processing, requiring condemnation of the organ. The incidence may reach 50%. Lesions are grossly visible as firm, lobulated, roughly spherical, pale yellow to white masses ranging in size from a few millimeters to several centimeters. Advanced lesions have a rough appearance and may be "gritty" when cut. Bile stasis of adjacent normal hepatic tissue is often marked. A variety of bacteria have been isolated from the lesions including *Actinomyces* (86), *Catenabacterium, Corynebacterium, Eubacterium, Propionibacterium,* and *Staphylococcus* (55). Granulomatous lesions in liver and spleen can be reproduced experimentally following inoculation with *Eubacterium tortuosum* (6, 40). Coinoculation with other bacteria increases the likelihood of liver lesions. Often, mucosal ulcers in the lower intestinal tract can also be found in affected birds suggesting liver lesions develop from bacteria carried to the organ from the intestine via the bloodstream (6, 40, 55). *Eubacterium tortuosum* is considered to be part of the normal cecal flora (40).

In 7- to 8-wk-old turkeys, pyogranulomatous typhlitis and hepatitis characterized by cecal cores and rupture was associated with *Escherichia coli* and concurrent coccidia and hemorrhagic enteritis virus infections. Excess condemnations for granulomatous lesions did not occur at processing (66).

No causative organism was identified in granulomatous lesions affecting ceca and livers of older chickens from small flocks in Canada (69). Grampositive, filamentous bacteria morphologically distinct from *Eubacterium,* long-segmented filamentous organisms, *Actinomyces,* and *Nocardia* were present in sporadic cases of visceral granulomas in broiler chickens at processing in the United States (41).

Only a low percentage of hepatic foci ("white-spotted livers") cultured from turkey livers at processing yielded bacteria; *Escherichia coli* and *Salmonella* spp. were the organisms most commonly recovered (71). Foci were associated with *Ascaridia,* indicating they are different from liver granulomas caused by *Eubacterium* or other similar bacteria.

Turkey Osteomyelitis Complex. Turkeys with inflammatory lesions in the bones and/or joints have green discolored livers. Liver discoloration is used at processing to identify carcasses likely to be affected so that any abnormal tissue can be removed from the food chain. Culturing bones and livers of affected and unaffected birds from two flocks resulted in recovery of pleomorphic, gram-variable bacteria consistent with L-forms (cell-wall-deficient forms). Positive cultures were obtained more frequently from affected birds and bones than from unaffected birds or livers. The significance of these organisms in the disease is unknown, but the high number of isolates suggests these bacterial forms may be much more common in turkeys than is generally realized (12).

REFERENCES

1. Abdel Gabbar, K.M.A., P. Dewani, and B.M. Junejo. 1995. Possible involvement of Planococcus halophilus in an outbreak of necrotic hepatitis in chickens. Vet Rec 136:74.

2. Al Aboudi, A.R., I.M.S. Shnawa, A.A. Hassen, and R.B. Al-Sanjary. 1988. Penetration rate of Proteus organism through egg shell membranes at different temperatures. Iraqi J Vet Sci 1:1–8.

3. Allen, P.C. 1992. Comparative study of long, segmented, filamentous organisms in chickens and mice. Lab Anim Sci 42:542–547.

4. Allen, P.C. 1992. Effect of virginiamycin on serum carotenoid levels and long, segmented, filamentous organisms in broiler chicks. Avian Dis 36:852–857.

5. Angel, C.R., J.L. Sell, J.A. Fagerland, D.L. Reynolds, and D.W. Trampel. 1990. Long-segmented filamentous organisms observed in poults experimentally infected with stunting syndrome agent. Avian Dis 34:994–1001.

6. Arp, L.H., I.M. Robinson, and A.E. Jensen. 1983. Pathology of liver granulomas in turkeys. Vet Pathol 20:80–89.

7. Bailey, J.S., D.L. Fletcher, and N.A. Cox. 1990. Liste-

ria monocytogenes colonization of broiler chickens. Poult Sci 69:457–461.

8. Bapat, J.A., V.B. Kulkarni, and D.V. Nimje. 1985. Mortality in chicks due to Pseudomonas aeruginosa. Indian J Anim Sci 55:538–539.

9. Barbour, E.K., M.K. Brinton, A. Caputa, J.B. Johnson, and P.E. Poss. 1991. Characteristics of Actinomyces pyogenes involved in lameness of male turkeys in North-Central United States. Avian Dis 35:192–196.

10. Barnes, H.J. 1996. Unpublished data.

11. Basher, H.A., D.R. Fowler, F.G. Rodgers, A. Seaman, and M. Woodbine. 1984. Pathogenicity of natural and experimental listeriosis in newly hatched chicks. Res Vet Sci 36:76–80.

12. Bayyari, G.R., W.E. Huff, R.A. Norton, J.K. Skeeles, J.N. Beasley, N.C. Rath, and J.M. Balog. 1994. A longitudinal study of green-liver osteomyelitis complex in commercial turkeys. Avian Dis 38:744–754.

13. Behr, K.P., and K.-H. Hinz. 1989. Zur penisentzundung der ganter. Dtsch Tieraerztl Wochenschr 96:140–143.

14. Behr, K.P., K.-H. Hinz, and S. Rottmann. 1990. Phallus-inflammation of ganders: clinical observations and comparative bacteriological examinations of healthy and altered organs. Zentralbl Veterinaermed [B] 37:774–776.

15. Bisgaard, M. 1981. Arthritis in ducks. I. Aetiology and public health aspects. Avian Pathol 10:11–21.

16. Bisgaard, M. 1995. Salpingitis in web-footed birds: prevalence, aetiology and significance. Avian Pathol 24:443–452.

17. Bisgaard, M., and A. Dam. 1981. Salpingitis in poultry. II. Prevalence, bacteriology, and possible pathogenesis in egg-laying chickens. Nord Vet 33:81–89.

18. Board, R.G., S. Loseby, and V.R. Miles. 1979. A note on microbial growth on hen egg-shells. Br Poult Sci 20:413–420.

19. Bolin, F.M., and D.F. Eveleth. 1961. Experimental listeriosis of turkeys. Avian Dis 5:229–231.

20. Brinton, M.K., L.C. Schellberg, J.B. Johnson, R.K. Frank, D.A. Halvorson, and J.A. Newman. 1993. Description of osteomyelitis lesions associated with Actinomyces pyogenes infection in the proximal tibia of adult male turkeys. Avian Dis 37:259–262.

21. Burnens, A.P., J. Stanley, R. Morgenstern, and J. Nicolet. 1994. Gastroenteritis associated with Helicobacter pullorum. Lancet 344:1569–1560.

22. Carpenter, S.L., and M. Sevoian. 1983. Cellular immune response to Marek's disease: listeriosis as a model of study. Avian Dis 27:344–356.

23. Castro, A.G.M. de, A.M. de Carvalho, M. Hipólito, and A. Paludetti, Jr. 1989. Mortalidade em pinos de corte, provocada por Pseudomonas aeruginosa. Arq Inst Biol (São Paulo) 56:62.

24. Cheng, K.J., E.E. Gardiner, and J.W. Costerton. 1976. Bacteria associated with beak necrosis in broiler breeder hens. Vet Rec 99:503–504.

25. Cooper, G.L. 1989. An encephalitic form of listeriosis in broiler chickens. Avian Dis 33:182–185.

26. Cooper, G., B. Charlton, A.Bickford, C. Cardona, J. Barton, S. Channing-Santiago, and R. Walker. 1992. Listeriosis in California broiler chickens. J Vet Diagn Invest 4:343–345.

27. Corrales, W., L.M. Vivo, and E. Gutierriz. 1988. Abscesos en piel en una granja de ponedoras en jaula. Reporte de un caso. Rev Avic 32:15–27.

28. Cummins, T.J., I.M. Orme, and R.E. Smith. 1988. Reduced in vivo nonspecific resistance to Listeria monocytogenes infection during avian retrovirus-induced immunosuppression. Avian Dis 32:663–667.

29. Devriese, L.A., N.J. Viaene, and G. De Medts. 1975. Pseudomonas aeruginosa infection on a broiler farm. Avian Pathol 4:233–237.

30. Dewhirst, F.E., C. Seymour, G.J. Fraser, B.J. Paster, and J.G. Fox. 1994. Phylogeny of Helicobacter isolates from

bird and swine feces and description of Helicobacter pametensis sp. nov. Int J Syst Bacteriol 44:553–560.

31. Emerson, F.G., G.E. Kolb, and F.A. VanNatta. 1983. Chronic cholera-like lesions caused by Moraxella osloensis. Avian Dis 27:836–838.

32. Erganis,O., M. Corlu, O. Kaya, and M. Ates. 1988. Isolation of Acinetobacter calcoaceticus from septicaemic hens. Vet Rec 123:374.

33. Ganiere, J.P., P. Perreau, J. Brocas, and J. Chantal. 1982. Étude de deux souches "Actinobacillus species" d'origine aviaire. Rev Méd Vét 133:125–128.

34. Gilardi, G.L. 1991. Pseudomonas and related genera. In A. Balows, W.J. Hausler, Jr., K.L. Herrman, H.D. Isenberg, and H.J. Shadomy (eds.). Manual of Clinical Microbiology, 5th ed. American Society of Microbiologists, Washington, DC, pp. 429–441.

35. Glünder, G., and O. Siegmann. 1989. Occurrence of Aeromonas hydrophila in wild birds. Avian Pathol 18:685–695.

36. Goodwin, M.A., G.L. Cooper, J. Brown, A.A. Bickford, W.D. Waltman, and T.G. Dickson. 1991. Clinical, pathological, and epizootiological features of long-segmented filamentous organisms (bacteria, LSFOs) in the small intestines of chickens, turkeys, and quails. Avian Dis 35:872–876.

37. Gray, M.L. 1958. Listeriosis in fowls—A review. Avian Dis 2:296–314.

38. Gray, M.L., and A.H. Killinger. 1966. Listeria monocytogenes and listeric infections. Bacteriol Rev 30:309–382.

39. Hafez, H.M., H. Woernle, and G. Heil. 1987. Pseudomonas-aeruginosa-infektionen bei putenkuken und behandlungsversuche mit apramycin. Berl Munch Tierärztl Woshenschr 100:48–51.

40. Hafner, S., B.G. Harmon, S.G. Thayer, and S.M. Hall. 1994. Splenic granulomas in broiler chickens produced experimentally with inoculation with Eubacterium tortuosum. Avian Dis 38:605–609.

41. Hill, J.E., L.C. Kelley, and K.A. Langheinrich. 1992. Visceral granulomas in chickens infected with a filamentous bacteria. Avian Dis 36:172–176.

42. Hinz, K.-H., M. Ryll, U. Heffels-Redmann, and M. Pöppel. 1992. Multikausal bedingte infektiöse atemwegserkrankung junger mastputen. Dtsch Tieraerztl Wochenschr 99:75–78.

43. Honich, M. 1972. Facancsibek jarvanyszeru Pseudomonas aeruginosa fertozottsege. Magyar Allatorvosok Lapja 27:329–335.

44. Huchzermeyer, F.W. 1994. Ostrich Diseases. Bayer (South Africa) Animal Hlth.

45. Huchzermeyer, F.W., M.M. Henton, and R.H. Keffen. 1993. High mortality associated with megabacteriosis of proventriculus and gizzard in ostrich chicks. Vet Rec 133:143–144.

46. Jellison, W.L. 1974. Tularemia in North America, 1930–1974. Monograph, University of Montana, Missoula.

47. Jindal, N., S.R. Garg, and A. Kumar. 1993. Comparison of Aeromonas spp. isolated from human, livestock and poultry faeces. Isr J Vet Med 48:80–83.

48. Jones, J.C., and G.W. Anderson. 1948. Sulfamerazine in the treatment of a Pseudomonas infection of turkey poults. J Am Vet Med Assoc 113:458–459.

49. Julian, R.J., and D.E. Galt. 1980. Mortality in Muscovy ducks (Cairina moschata) caused by Haemoproteus infection. J Wildl Dis 16:39–44.

50. Julian, R.J., T.J. Beveridge, and D.E. Galt. 1985. Muscovy duck mortality not caused by Haemoproteus. J Wildl Dis 21:335–337.

51. Karim, M.R., and M.R. Ali. 1976. Survey of bacterial flora from chicken embryo and their effect on low hatchability. Bangladesh Vet J 10:15–18.

52. Kaya, O., M. Ates, O. Erganis, M. Corlu, and S. Sanlioglu. 1989. Isolation of Acinetobacter lwoffi from hens with septicemia. J Vet Med [B] 36:157–158.

53. Kelly, P.J., N. Masanvi, H.F. Cadman, S.M. Mahan, L.

Beati, and D. Raoult. 1996. Serosurvey for Cowdria ruminatum, Coxiella burnetii, and spotted fever group rickettsiae in ostriches (Struthio camelus) from Zimbabwe. Avian Dis 40:448–452.

54. Kulshreshtha, R.C., J. Singh, R. Verma, and N.K. Chandiramani. 1982. Seroprevalence of brucella infection in poultry. Indian J Poult Sci 17:299.

55. Langheinrich, K.A., and B. Schwab. 1972. Isolation of bacteria and histomorphology of turkey liver granulomas. Avian Dis 16:806–816.

56. Leard, T., and W. Maslin. 1993. Flavobacterium meningosepticum septicemia associated with thymic atrophy/hypoplasia in an ostrich chick. Vet Pathol 30:454.

57. Lee, J.V., T.J. Donovan, and A.L. Furniss. 1978. Characterization, taxonomy, and emended description of Vibrio metschnikovii. Int J Syst Bacteriol 28:99–111.

58. Lin, M.Y., M.C. Cheng, K.J. Huang, and W.C. Tsai. 1993. Classification, pathogenicity, and drug susceptibility of hemolytic gram-negative bacteria isolated from sick or dead chickens. Avian Dis 37:6–9.

59. Liu, S.G., M.H. Gan, and Z.M. Zhao. 1988. Studies on Klebsiella infection in chickens. I. Diagnosis and control of ophthalmia caused by Klebsiella. Chinese J Vet Med 14:7–9.

60. Lusis, P.I., and M.A. Soltys. 1971. Pseudomonas aeruginosa. Vet Bull 41:169–177.

61. Marius-Jestin, V., M. Le Menec, E. Thibault, J.C. Moisan, and R. L'Hospitalier. 1987. Normal phallus flora of the gander. J Vet Med [B] 34:67–78.

62. Marius-Jestin, V., E. Thibault, M. Le Menec, M. Lagadic, and G. Bennejean. 1987. Etiologie de la maladie vénérienne du jars—données complémentaires. Rec Méd Vét 163:645–653.

63. Marsden, J.L. 1994. Industry perspectives on Listeria monocytogenes in foods: raw meat and poultry. Dairy Food Environ Sanit 14:83–86.

64. Mireles, V., and C. Alvarez. 1979. Pseudomonas aeruginosa infection due to contaminated vaccination equipment. Proc 28th West Poult Dis Conf, pp. 55–57.

65. Mohamed, Y.S., P.D. Moorhead, and E.H. Bohl. 1969. Natural Streptobacillus moniliformis infection of turkeys, and attempts to infect turkeys, sheep, and pigs. Avian Dis 13:379–385.

66. Morishita, T.Y., and A.A. Bickford. 1992. Pyogranulomatous typhlitis and hepatitis of market turkeys. Avian Dis 36:1070–1075.

67. Morishita, T.Y., K.M. Lam, and R.H. McCapes. 1992. Isolation of two filamentous bacteria associated with enteritis in turkey poults. Poult Sci 71:203–207.

68. Mosqueda, T., G. Moedano, and J. Moreno. 1976. Pseudomonas aeruginosa as a source of nervous signs and lesions in young chicks. Proc 25th West Poult Dis Conf, pp. 68–69.

69. Mutalib, A.A., and C. Riddell. 1982. Cecal and hepatic granulomas of unknown etiology in chickens. Avian Dis 26:732–740.

70. National Research Council. 1987. Poultry inspection. In The Basis for a Risk-Assessment Approach. National Academy Press, Washington, DC, p. 72.

71. Norton, R.A., S.C. Ricke, J.N. Beasley, J.K. Skeeles, and F.D. Clark. 1996. A survey of sixty turkey flocks exhibiting hepatic foci taken at time of processing. Avian Dis 40:466–472.

72. Okoye, J.O.A., H.C. Gugnani, and C.N. Okeke. 1991. Experimental infection of chickens with Nocardia asteroides and Nocardia transvalensis. Avian Pathol 20:17–24.

73. Olson, L.D. 1970. A comparison of the growth of various microorganisms in air spaces of the turkey head. Avian Dis 14:676–682.

74. Orajaka, L.J.E., and K. Mohan. 1985. Aerobic bacterial flora from dead-in-shell chicken embryos from Nigeria. Avian Dis 29:583–589.

75. Panjnoo, J.L., S.P. Choudhary, and K.G. Narayan. 1994. Antimicrobial sensitivity of Pseudomonas aeruginosa. Indian Vet J 71:932–934.

76. Plesser, O., A. Even-Shoshan, and U. Bendheim. 1975. The isolation of Klebsiella pneumoniae from poultry and hatcheries. Refu Vet 32:99–105.

77. Randall, C.J., W.G. Siller, A.S. Wallis, and K.S. Kirkpatrick. 1984. Multiple infections in young broilers. Vet Rec 114:270–271.

78. Randall, C.J., S. Lees, G.A. Pepin, and H.M. Ross. 1987. An unusual intracellular infection in ducks. Avian Pathol 16:479–491.

79. Reddy, Y.K., and B. Mohan. 1993. An outbreak of purulent conjunctivitis in chicks. J Assam Vet Counc 3:62.

80. Sadasivan, P.R., V.A. Srinivasan, A.T. Venugopalan, and R.A. Balaprakasam. 1977. Aeruginocine typing and antibiotic sensitivity of Pseudomonas aeruginosa of poultry origin. Avian Dis 21:136–138.

81. Safwat, E.E.A., M.H. Awaad, A.M. Ammer, and A.A. El-Kinawy. 1984. Studies on Pseudomonas aeruginosa, Proteus vulgaris and S. typhi-murium infection in ducklings. Egypt J Anim Prod 24:287–294.

82. Sah, R.L., M.P. Mall, and G.C. Mohanty. 1983. Septicemic Proteus infection in Japanese quail chicks (Coturnix coturnix japonica). Avian Dis 27:296–300.

83. Sarakbi, T. 1989. Klebsiella—a killer in the hatchery. Int Hatchery Pract 3:19–21.

84. Schlater, L.K., B.O. Blackburn, R. Harrington, Jr., D.J. Draper, J. Van Wagner, and B.R. Davis. 1981. A non-O1 Vibrio cholerae isolated from a goose. Avian Dis 25:199–201.

85. Sell, J.L., D.L. Reynolds, and M. Jeffrey. 1992. Evidence that bacteria are not causative agents of stunting syndrome in poults. Poult Sci 71:1480–1485.

86. Senior, V.E., R. Lake, and C. Pratt. 1962. Suspected actinomycosis of turkeys. Can Vet J 3:120–125.

87. Sethi, M.S., B. Singh, and M.P. Yadev. 1978. Experimental infection of Coxiella burnetii in chicken: Clinical symptoms, serologic response, and transmission through egg. Avian Dis 22:391–395.

88. Seymour, C., R.J. Lewis, M. Kim, D.F. Gagnon, J.G. Fox, F.E. Dewhirst, and B.J. Paster. 1994. Isolation of Helicobacter strains from wild bird and swine feces. Appl Environ Microbiol 60:1025–1028.

89. Shane, S.M., and D.H. Gifford. 1985. Prevalence and pathogenicity of Aeromonas hydrophila. Avian Dis 29:681–689.

90. Snoeyenbos, G.H. 1965. Brucellosis, anthrax, pseudotuberculosis, tetanus, vibrio infection, avian vibrionic hepatitis, and spirochetosis. In H.E. Beister and L.H. Schwarte, eds. Diseases of Poultry, 5th ed. Iowa State University Press, Ames, pp. 427–450.

91. Stanley, J., D. Linton, A.P. Burnens, F.E. Dewhirst, S.L.W. On, A. Porter, R.J. Owen, and M. Costas. 1994. Helicobacter pullorum sp. nov.—genotype and phenotype of a new species isolated from poultry and from human patients with gastroenteritis. Microbiology 140:3441–3449.

92. Stipkovits, L., Z. Varga, G. Czifra, and M. Dobos-Kovacs. 1986. Occurrence of mycoplasmas in geese affected with inflammation of the cloaca and phallus. Avian Pathol 15:289–299.

93. Trenchi, H., M.T. Bellizzi, and C.G. de Sousa. 1981. Contaminacion en la vacunacion de Marek con Pseudomonas spp. (variedad acromogena). Gac Vet 43:982–989.

94. Watts, J.L., S.A. Salmon, R.J. Yancey, Jr., B. Nersessian, and Z.V. Kounev. 1993. Minimum inhibitory concentrations of bacteria isolated from septicemia and airsacculitis in ducks. J Vet Diagn Invest 5:625–628.

95. Williams, B.J., and H.L. Newkirk. 1966. Pseudomonas infection of one-day-old chicks resulting from contaminated antibiotic solutions. Avian Dis 10:353–356.

STREPTOCOCCOSIS

Dennis P. Wages

INTRODUCTION. Streptococcosis in avian species is worldwide in distribution, occurring as both acute septicemic and chronic infections with mortality ranging from 0.5% to 50%. Infection is considered secondary, since streptococci form part of the normal intestinal flora of most avian species, including wild birds (5). Streptococci are ubiquitous in nature and commonly found in various poultry environments. A low percentage (16.67%) of poultry meat contamination with *Streptococcus faecalis* has been found in ready-to-cook products; however, no incrimination of food poisoning in humans has been found (20).

HISTORY. Acute streptococcal infections of poultry were first described in chickens in 1902 (32) and 1908 (29) as apoplectiform septicemia. Chronic streptococcosis caused 50% mortality in a flock over a 4-mo period (23) and was the cause of mortality due to salpingitis and peritonitis in chickens (15). Streptococcosis in turkeys was reported as early as 1932 (40). Bacterial or vegetative endocarditis associated with streptococci was first reported in 1927 (28), and again in 1947 (34) and 1971 (26). For a historical review, see (33).

ETIOLOGY. The genus *Streptococcus* is composed of gram-positive, spherical bacteria occurring singly, in pairs or short chains, which are non-motile, non–spore-forming, facultative anaerobes. They are catalase-negative and ferment sugars, usually to lactic acid. Common avian isolates can be differentiated by their ability to ferment mannitol, sorbitol, and L-arabinose and by their growth on MacConkey agar (Table 14.1). The relationship of these characteristics to pathogenicity is unknown. *Streptococcus* spp. isolated from avian species and associated with disease include *S. zooepidemicus*

(occasionally referred to as *S. gallinarum*) from Lancefield antigenic serogroup type C, and *S. faecalis*, *S. faecium*, *S. durans*, and *S. avium* from Lancefield serogroup D (17). Lancefield serogroup D streptococci are commonly referred to as "fecal streps." It has been proposed that these streptococci should more appropriately be placed in the genus *Enterococcus* (8), but this has not been universally accepted. In this chapter, *S. faecalis* subsp. *faecalis*, *S. faecalis* subsp. *liquefaciens*, and *S. faecalis* subsp. *zymogenes* will all be considered as *S. faecalis*. A new species, *S. pleomorphus*, an obligate anaerobe in normal cecal contents of chickens, turkeys, and ducks has been described. Its possible role in disease for these species is undetermined (3). *S. mutans*, a common bacterium in the human oral cavity, has been associated with septicemia and mortality in geese; contaminated drinking water and poor quality litter were possible predisposing factors (24).

Both experimental and naturally occurring infections of *S. bovis* causing acute septicemia and joint infections have been found in racing pigeons (9, 11).

S. dysgalactiae has been cultured from broilers with cellulitis, a condition observed on the skin and subcutaneous tissue at processing (39).

Streptococcus spp. have been isolated from lesions of osteomyelitis in turkeys, along with *E. coli* and *Staphylococcus* spp. (7).

Bacterial endocarditis, commonly associated with streptococci, is caused by numerous bacteria in naturally occurring and experimental poultry infections. These include *S. faecalis* (12, 19, 26), *S. faecium* (36, 12), *S. durans* (12), *S. zooepidemicus* (33), *Staphylococcus aureus* and *Pasteurella multocida* (19). Of streptococci isolated from naturally occurring infections, *S. faecalis* has been the most

Table 14.1. Lancefield antigenic serogroups C and D in poultry: Differential characteristics

Species	Lancefield Antigenic Serogroup	Fermentation of:			Growth on MacConkey agar
		Mannitol	Sorbitol	L-arabinose	
Streptococcus avium	D	+	+	+	+
S. durans	D	–	–	–	+
S. faecalis	D	+	+	–	+
S. faecium	D	+	–	+	+
S. zooepidemicus[a]	C		+		–

Source: (13, 16, 17)

[a]Fermentation of mannitol and L-arabinose are not considered useful in the differentiation of this species.

common isolate, and the one most consistent in producing bacterial endocarditis in experimental infections via the intravenous route.

PATHOGENESIS AND EPIZOOTIOLOGY.

S. zooepidemicus occurs almost exclusively in mature chickens but has been documented as a cause of mortality in wild birds (25). Experimentally, rabbits, mice, turkeys, pigeons, ducks, and geese are susceptible. *S. faecalis* affects species of all ages; it is the most serious disease occurring in embryos and young chicks from fecal contaminated eggs (1, 2). *S. faecium* (36) and *S. mutans* (24) have been identified as causes of mortality in ducklings and goslings, respectively.

Transmission of streptococci occurs most commonly via oral and aerosol routes (5). Transmission can occur, however, through skin injuries, especially in caged layers. Most antigenic serogroup D streptococci are pathogenic when administered intravenously. Aerosol transmission of *S. zooepidemicus* and *S. faecalis* results in acute septicemia in chickens (1). High mortality from acute septicemia and liver granulomas occur after experimental oral inoculation with *S. faecalis* (21). *S. faecalis* has been incriminated as the cause of loss of intestinal epithelium integrity allowing bacteria, e.g., *Bacteroides* spp., *Catenabacterium* spp., *Eubacterium* spp., and *Streptococcus* spp., to produce liver granulomas in turkeys (31). These bacteria and *Proprionibacterium* spp., *Corynebacterium* spp., *Staphylococcus* spp., and *Lactobacillus* spp. can often be isolated from turkey liver granulomas (31). Concurrent enteric infections or any condition compromising the intestinal villous epithelium, allowing penetration of resident serogroup D streptococci, can result in septicemia and/or bacterial endocarditis. Incubation periods range from 1 day to several weeks, with 5–21 days being most common.

Experimental bacterial endocarditis (vegetative or valvular) results from intravenous exposure. *S. faecalis* isolates from intestines of apparently normal birds are capable of producing endocarditis (19). Endocarditis occurs when septicemic streptococcal infection progresses to a subacute or chronic stage (26).

Clinical Signs.

Streptococcal serogroup D infections in poultry can result in two distinct clinical forms of disease—acute and subacute/chronic. In the acute form, clinical signs are related to septicemia and include depression, lethargy, lassitude, pale comb and wattles, ruffled feathers, diarrhea, fine head tremors, and decrease or cessation of egg production. Often, only dead birds are found.

In the subacute/chronic form, depression, loss of body weight, lameness, and head tremors may be observed. Streptococci enhance the severity of fibrinopurulent blepharitis and conjunctivitis in chickens (6). Chickens experimentally inoculated intravenously with *S. faecalis* develop leukocytosis 2–3 days postinoculation; highest values occur in birds that develop endocarditis (19). Heterophils predominate, along with a slight monocytosis. Body temperatures are elevated and range from 108 to 110 F in birds with persistent bacteremia. Numbers of bacteria present in peripheral blood vary considerably. Clinically affected birds eventually die if not treated.

With *S. zooepidemicus* infections, clinical signs include lassitude, blood-stained tissue and feathers around the head, yellow droppings, emaciation, and pale combs and wattles.

Egg transmission or fecal contamination of hatching eggs results in late embryo mortality and an increased number of chicks or poults unable to "pip" or penetrate through the shell at hatch.

Lesions.

Gross lesions of *S. zooepidemicus* and serogroup D streptococci in acute disease are similar, characterized by splenomegaly, hepatomegaly (with or without miliary to 1 cm red, tan, or white foci), enlarged kidneys, and congestion of subcutaneous tissue (with or without sanguineous pericardial or subcutaneous fluid), and peritonitis. Omphalitis is observed in chicks or poults infected at hatching (2, 38).

Microscopically, the liver has dilated sinusoids congested with red blood cells and increased heterophils. If foci are present grossly, there are multiple areas of necrosis and/or infarction with heterophil accumulation and thrombosis. Splenomegaly is characterized by congestion and reticuloendothelial hyperplasia (21).

Lesions of chronic streptococcal infections include fibrinous arthritis and/or tenosynovitis, osteomyelitis, salpingitis, fibrinous pericarditis and perihepatitis, necrotic myocarditis, and valvular endocarditis (Fig. 14.2). Vegetative valvular lesions are usually yellow, white, or tan small, raised rough areas on the valvular surface (Fig. 14.3). Valve lesions are most consistently found on the mitral valve, and less frequently on the aortic or right atrioventricular valves. Additional gross lesions associated with valvular endocarditis include enlarged, pale, flaccid heart; pale to hemorrhagic areas in the myocardium, especially at the base of the valves, below the affected valve, or apex of the heart; infarcts in the liver, spleen, or heart and, less commonly, infarcts in the lung, kidney, and brain. Infarcts can be light colored or hemorrhagic with sharp margins. In the liver, infarcts are usually located near the ventral and posterior margins and are well demarcated, extending beneath the capsule into the parenchyma (19) (Fig. 14.4). Lesions of longer duration tend to have a sharp, narrow, lighter colored band just inside the infarct margin (26).

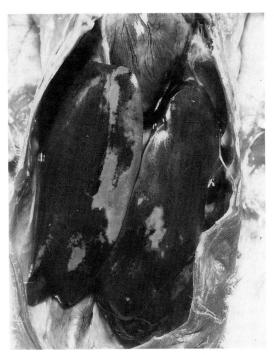

14.4. Bacterial endocarditis, showing infarcts of liver and myocardium.

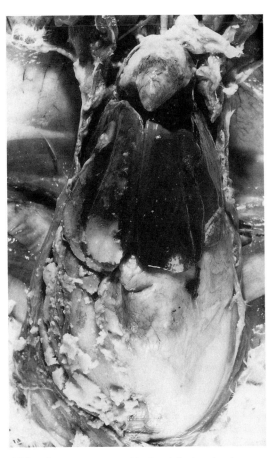

14.2. *Streptococcus zooepidemicus* infection showing perihepatitis and peritonitis. (Peckham, Avian Dis)

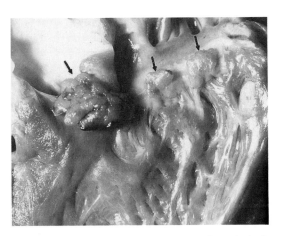

14.3. Bacterial endocarditis showing vegetations of mitral valve (*arrows*).

Microscopically, valvular lesions consist primarily of fibrin with bacteria, heterophils, macrophages, and fibroblasts. There is interstitial edema and infiltrative valvular distortion, with focal deposition of platelets and fibrin and subsequent microbial growth (19, 26). Cardiac histiocytes (Anichkov's myocytes) are numerous in the fibrous portion of the valve. Events leading to the vegetative valve lesion are 1) edema that loosens the valve surface epithelium, 2) fibrin deposition, and 3) bacterial attachment to the fibrin and colony formation. Other microscopic lesions related to endocarditis include cerebral vasculitis and infarcts, leptomeningitis, glomerulonephritis, and thrombosed pulmonary vessels (26). Cerebral lesions are usually confined to the corpus striatum. Focal granulomas can be found in virtually any tissue as a result of septic emboli. Liver infarcts are characterized by portal venous thrombosis followed by necrosis. Aggregates of bacteria are present throughout necrotic areas with a zone of heterophils just within the necrotic border, a characteristic feature of the lesion (Fig. 14.5). Gram-positive bacterial colonies are readily observed in thrombosed vessels and within necrotic foci with tissue gram stains.

DIAGNOSIS. Demonstration of bacteria typical of streptococci in blood films (Fig. 14.6) or impression smears of affected heart valves or lesions from

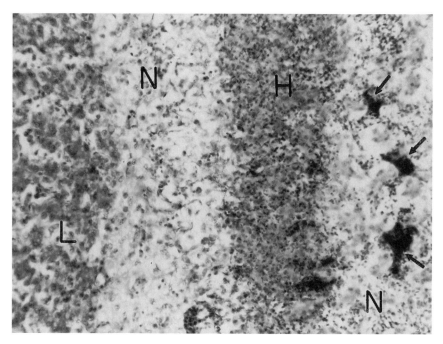

14.5. Margin of liver infarct associated with bacterial endocarditis, showing clumps of bacteria (*arrows*), necrotic area (N), zone of hecrotic heterophils (H), and relatively normal liver tissue (L). H & E, ×400.

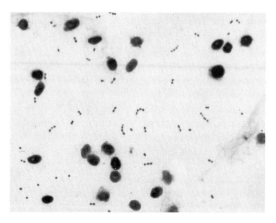

14.6. *Streptococcus zooepidemicus* in blood of naturally infected chicken. Gram, ×800. (Peckham, Avian Dis)

birds with typical signs and lesions will provide a presumptive diagnosis of streptococcosis.

Isolation of *S. zooepidemicus*, or any Lancefield serogroup D streptococci (without fecal contamination), from typical lesions in poultry with appropriate clinical signs will confirm streptococcosis. Streptococci are easily isolated on blood agar or more specific differential media (12), which should help differentiate species. Fermentation of manni-

tol, sorbitol, arabinose, and growth on MacConkey agar can also aid in differentiation of streptococci in Lancefield serogroup D and that of *S. zooepidemicus*. Preferred tissues for culture include liver, spleen, blood, yolk, embryo fluids, or any suspected lesion area. Diagnosis of bacterial endocarditis can be made based on valvular vegetations with secondary infarcts of myocardium, liver, and/or spleen. In suspected cases, it is important to culture lesions to establish a definitive diagnosis and rule out other bacteria.

Differential diagnosis includes other bacterial septicemic diseases, e.g., staphylococcosis, colibacillosis, pasteurellosis, and erysipelas.

TREATMENT. Treatment includes use of antibiotics such as penicillin, erythromycin, novobiocin, oxytetracycline, chlortetracycline, tetracycline, or nitrofurans in acute and subacute infections. Enrofloxacin has also shown in vitro sensitivity to *Streptococcus* spp. (30). Clinically affected birds respond well early in the course of the disease. As the disease progresses within a flock, treatment efficacy decreases. Novobiocin has been found to be efficacious in ducks with *S. faecium* infection (36). Dietary bacitracin decreases the incidence of some strains of serogroup D streptococci in young chickens (4). Certain streptococcal strains can develop resistance after exposure to antibiotics such as tylosin, but treatment with such antibiotics may not shift the overall number of resistant organisms (22). Antibacterial sensitivity should be performed on bacterial isolates in any clinical cases of streptococcosis. Serogroup D streptococci vary in their resistance and susceptibility to growth-promoting agents (14). Environmental forces, feeding schedules, stress, and interactions between different genotypes and housing influence the response of chickens to streptococcal infections (27, 37). There is no treatment for poultry with bacterial endocarditis.

In vitro sensitivity to *S. bovis* in pigeons has been demonstrated with penicillins, macrolides, lincomycin, tetracyclines, chloramphenicol, and nitrofurans (10). Ampicillin, in combination with corticosterone, is efficacious in treating *S. faecalis* infection in chickens (18).

Prevention and control requires reducing stress and preventing immunodepressive diseases and conditions. Proper cleaning and disinfection can reduce environmental streptococcal resident flora to minimize external exposure. The use of formaldehyde reduces the total count of *Streptococcus* spp. in the hatchers by as much as 85.7%. Reduction of seven log-10 bacterial counts has also been demonstrated compared with ozone use, which had bacterial-count reduction of four log-10 (35, 41).

REFERENCES

1. Agrimi, P. 1956. Studio sperimentale su alcuni focolai di streptococcosi nel pollo. Zooprofilassi 11:491–501.

2. Alaboudi, A.R., D.A. Hammed, H.A. Basher, and M.G. Hassen. 1992. Potential pathogenic bacteria from dead-in-shell chicken embryos. Iraqi J Vet Sci 5:109–114.

3. Barnes, E.M., C.S. Impey, B.J.H. Stevens, and J.L. Peel. 1977. Streptococcus pleomorphus sp.nov.: An anaerobic streptococcus isolated mainly from the caeca of birds. J Gen Microbiol 102:45–53.

4. Barnes, E.M., G.C. Mead, C.S. Impey, and B.W. Adams. 1978. The effect of dietary bacitracin on the incidence of Streptococcus faecalis subspecies liquefaciens and related streptococci in the intestines of young chicks. Poult Sci 19:713–723.

5. Brittingham, M.C., S.A. Temple, and R.M. Duncan. 1988. A survey of the prevalence of selected bacteria in wild birds. J Wildl Dis 24:299–307.

6. Cheville, N.F., J. Tappe, M. Ackermann, and A. Jensen. 1988. Acute fibrinopurulent blepharitis and conjunctivitis associated with Staphylococcus hyicus, Escherichia coli, and Streptococcus sp. in chickens and turkeys. Vet Pathol 25:369–375.

7. Clark, S.R., H.J. Barnes, A.A. Bickford, R.P. Chin, and R. Droual. 1991. Relationship of osteomyelitis and associated soft-tissue lesions with green liver discoloration in tom turkeys. Avian Dis 35:139–146.

8. Collins, M.D., D. Jones, J.A.E. Farrow, R. Kilpper-Balz, and K.H. Schleifer. 1984. Enterococcus avium nom. rev., comb. nov.; E. casseliflavus nom. rev., comb. nov.; E. durans nom. rev., comb. nov.; E. gallinarum comb. nov.; and E. malodoratus sp. nov. Int J System Bacteriol 34:220–223.

9. De Herdt, P., M. Desmidt, F. Haesebrouck, R. Ducatelle, and L.A. Devriese. 1992. Experimental Streptococcus bovis infections in pigeons. Avian Dis 36:916–925.

10. De Herdt, P., L.A. Devriese, B. De Groote, R. Ducatelle, and F. Haesebrouck. 1993. Antibiotic treatment of Streptococcus bovis infections in pigeons. Avian Pathol 22:605–615.

11. De Herdt, P., R. Ducatelle, F. Haesebrouck, L.A. Devriese, B. De Groote, and S. Roels. 1994. An unusual outbreak of Streptococcus bovis septicemia in racing pigeons (Columba livia). Vet Rec 134:42–43.

12. Domermuth, C.H., and W.B. Gross. 1969. A medium for isolation and tentative identification of fecal streptococci, and their role as avian pathogens. Avian Dis 13:394–399

13. Domermuth, C.H., and W.B. Gross. 1980. Streptococcosis, In S.B. Hitchner, C. H. Domermuth, H.G. Purchase, and J.E. Williams (eds.). Isolation and Identification of Avian Pathogens, 2nd ed. American Association of Avian Pathologists, Kennett Square, PA, pp. 31–32.

14. Dutta, G.N. and L.A. Devriese. 1982. Susceptibility of fecal streptococci of poultry origin to nine growth-promoting agents. Appl Environ Microbiol 44:832–837.

15. Edwards, P.R., and F.E. Hull. 1937. Hemolytic streptococci in chronic peritonitis and salpingitis of hens. J Am Vet Med Assoc 91:656–660.

16. Facklam, R.F., and R.B. Carey. 1985. Streptococci and aerococci. In E.H. Lennette, A. Balows, W.J. Hausler, Jr., and H.J. Shadomy (eds.). Manual of Clinical Microbiology, 4th ed. American Society of Microbiologists, Washington, DC, pp. 154–175.

17. Farrow, J.A.E., D. Jones, B.A. Phillips, and M.D. Collins. 1983. Taxonomic studies on some group D streptococci. J Gen Microbiol 129:1423–1432.

18. Glass, S.E. 1993. Personal communication.

19. Gross, W.B. 1991. Use of corticosterone and ampicillin for treatment of Streptococcus faecalis infection in chickens. Am J Vet Res 52:1288–1291.

20. Gross, W.B., and C.H. Domermuth. 1962. Bacterial endocarditis of poultry. Am J Vet Res 23:320–329.

21. Hefnawy, Y., and M. Sabah. 1990. Quality evaluation of ready to eat poultry in Assiut City. Assiut Vet Med J 23:119–125.

22. Hernandez D.J., E.D. Roberts, L.G. Adams, and T. Vera. 1972. Pathogenesis of hepatic granulomas in turkeys infected with Streptococcus faecalis var. liquefaciens. Avian Dis 15:201–216.

23. Hinton, M., A. Kaukas, S. K. Lim, and A. H. Linton. 1986. Preliminary observations on the influence of antibiotics on the ecology of Escherichia coli and the enterococci in the faecal flora of healthy young chickens. J Antimicrob Chemother 18:165–173.

24. Hudson, C.B. 1933. A specific infectious disease of chickens due to a hemolytic streptococcus. J Am Vet Med Assoc 82:218–231.

25. Ivanics, E., Z. Bitay, and R. Glavits. 1984. Streptococcus mutans infection in geese. Magy Allatorv Lapja 39:92–95.

26. Jensen. W.I. 1979. An outbreak of streptococcosis in eared grebes (Podiceps nigricollis). Avian Dis 23:543–546.

27. Jortner, B.S., and C.F. Helmboldt. 1971. Streptococcal bacterial endocarditis in chickens. Vet Pathol 8:54–62.

28. Katanbaf, M.N., P.B. Siegel, and W.B. Gross. 1987. Prior experience and response of chickens to a streptococcal infection. Poult Sci 66:2053–2055.

29. Kernkamp, H.C.H. 1927. Idiopathic streptococcic peritonitis in poultry. J Am Vet Med Assoc 23:585–596.

30. Mack, W.B. 1908. Apoplectiform septicemia in chickens. Am Vet Rev 33:330–332.

31. Mazurkiewicz, M., A. Latala, A. Wieliczko, A. Zalesinski, and M. Tomaszewski. 1990. Efficacy of Baytril in the control of bacterial diseases of poultry. Med Eterynaryjnego 46:286–289.

32. Moore, W.E.C., and W.B. Gross. 1968. Liver granulomas of turkeys—causative agents and mechanism of infection. Avian Dis 12:417–422.

33. Nogaard, V.A., and J.R. Mohler. 1902. Apoplectiform

septicemia in chickens. US Dep Agric BAI Bull 36.

34. Peckham M.C. 1966. An outbreak of streptococcosis (apoplectiform septicemia) in white rock chickens. Avian Dis 10:413–421.

35. Povar, M.L., and B. Brownstein. 1947. Valvular endocarditis in the fowl. Cornell Vet 37:49–54.

36. Rudy, A. 1991. The effects of microbial contamination of incubators on the health of broiler chicks in the first days of life. Zesz Nauk Akad Rolniczej we Wroclawin Weter 49:19–26.

37. Sandhu T.S. 1988. Fecal streptococcal infection of commercial white pekin ducklings. Avian Dis 32:570–573.

38. Siegel, P.B., M.N. Katanbaf, N.B. Anthony, D.E. Jones, A. Martin, W.B. Gross, and E.A. Dunnington. 1987.

Responses of chickens to Streptococcus faecalis: Genotype-housing interactions. Avian Dis 31:804–808.

39. Utoma, B.N., S. Poernoma, and Iskander. 1990. Bacteria isolated from chicken yolk sac infection at the Research Institute for Veterinary Science. Penyakit-Hewan 22:102–105.

40. Vaillancourt, J.P., A. Elfadil, and J.R. Bisaillon. 1992. Cellulitis in the broiler fowl. Med Vet Quebec 22:168–172.

41. Volkmar, F. 1932. Apoplectiform septicemia in turkeys. Poult Sci 11:297–300.

42. Whistler, P.E., and B.W. Sheldon. 1989. Biocidal activity of ozone versus formaldehyde against poultry pathogens inoculated in a prototype setter. J Poult Sci 68:1068–1073.

ERYSIPELAS

J. M. Bricker and Y. M. Saif

INTRODUCTION. Erysipelas in birds is generally an acute, fulminating infection of individuals within a flock. The infection and disease have been reported from many different vertebrate species, either as a contaminant (fish) or an infection. In birds, its primary economic importance is as a disease of turkeys. It is caused by *Erysipelothrix rhusiopathiae,* which also causes swine erysipelas in pigs and erysipeloid in humans. A second genomic species, *E. tonsillarum,* was described based on DNA homology studies with type strains of *E. rhusiopathiae* (75). Takahashi et al. (77) reported that none of 14 *E. tonsillarum* strains tested induced any signs of disease or lesions when inoculated intramuscularly (IM) into white leghorn chickens. These investigators suggested that *E. tonsillarum* should not be considered to be a potential pathogen for chickens. Although initially reported to be nonpathogenic for swine, some strains of *E. tonsillarum* have induced disease in this species (25). Recent evidence indicates there may be an additional distinct genomic species other than *E. rhusiopathiae* and *E. tonsillarum* (76). This chapter focuses on *E. rhusiopathiae* except where it is necessary to differentiate it from *E. tonsillarum.*

Outbreaks of economic significance are infrequent in avian species other than turkeys. Occasional losses of individual birds within a flock have been reported, and a few economically significant outbreaks in chickens and ducklings have occurred (49). *E. rhusiopathiae* has caused outbreaks of erysipelas in pheasants, ducks, geese, guinea fowl, chukars, grebes, and emus (13, 22, 32, 34, 38, 39, 42, 61, 83).

Erysipelas not only causes death but frequently affects the fertility of the male. Further marketing losses may result from lack of finish, condemnation, or downgrading resulting from postmortem evidence of septicemia. Affected chicken flocks have been reported to suffer depression of egg production.

Erysipeloid in humans may be a local or septicemic, and occasionally fatal, infection. It is particularly a disease of fish handlers, butchers, kitchen workers, veterinarians, and turkey growers. Silberstein (71) reported endocarditis and encephalitis in humans treated with penicillin. Presumptive diagnoses of the infection have been made in turkey flocks as a result of infection of a turkey handler or an insemination crew member. In most cases, the disease is preceded by an injury such as a cut. A thorough review of *E. rhusiopathiae* as an occupational pathogen has been compiled by Reboli and Farrar (62).

HISTORY. Sporadic cases of infection were reported in various avian species prior to 1936. Beaudette and Hudson (4) were the first to call attention to the economic significance of the disease in North American turkeys; other outbreaks were reported shortly thereafter. The disease is of economic concern to turkey growers in some parts of the United States. The infection has been reported from time to time in one or small groups of other species of birds; with the advent of widespread artificial insemination of turkeys, prevention of erysipelas became a problem facing producers of

The authors gratefully acknowledge the groundwork laid by the previous authors, Drs. A. S. Rosenwald and R. E. Corstvet.

turkey hatching eggs. With more confinement growing of turkeys, it has become a less important problem except in endemic areas.

Following the introduction of bacterins in the early 1950s and availability of penicillin as a treatment, various programs of preventive vaccination and/or treatment have been followed. Despite this, cases of postinsemination erysipelas occur in turkey hens.

INCIDENCE AND DISTRIBUTION. E. rhusiopathiae is worldwide in distribution. The adaptiveness of the organism is indicated by its ability to infect a wide variety of vertebrate species. It has been isolated from the tissues of birds, mammals, reptiles and amphibians, as well as the surface slime of fish.

Outbreaks of erysipelas in poultry occur sporadically, though locations exist in the world where the disease is endemic. Although the disease in turkeys has been reported more frequently among males than females, there is no evidence of differing susceptibility between sexes. Field observations suggest that the portal of entry (skin) is breached more frequently in the male, but incidence in hens has increased due to artificial insemination and frequent handling of females.

ETIOLOGY

Classification. E. rhusiopathiae (formerly E. insidiosa) belongs to the family Lactobacillaceae (12). The organism is a gram-positive bacillus, which tends to decolorize and form long filaments. It does not form spores, is not acid-fast, and is nonmotile. Barber (3) and Nelson and Shelton (56) reported that it resembles Listeria sp.; however, they demonstrated marked cultural differences between them. It resembles mycobacteria in that it has a high lipid content in its cell wall (almost 30%). Similar to some gram-negative bacteria, it has a rather low hexosamine content but differs from them in having a limited complement of amino acids (43).

Morphology and Staining. The cellular morphology of E. rhusiopathiae is variable. Cells taken from smooth colonies or isolated from the tissues of acutely infected birds are slender, straight or slightly curved rods measuring 0.2–0.4 by 0.8–2.5 μm, and may occur singly or in short chains. Organisms from older cultures or rough colonies are filamentous rods and may form masses that resemble mycelia. These filamentous rods usually appear somewhat thickened and may appear beaded following staining. The filamentous form begins to appear after several passages on artificial media. Both short rods and short filaments may be observed from a single colony (intermediate colony type). E.

rhusiopathiae stains gram-positive but tends to decolorize, a trait particularly noticeable in older cultures. E. tonsillarum is morphologically indistinguishable from E. rhusiopathiae.

Growth Requirements. E. rhusiopathiae is facultatively anaerobic and grows readily, though sparsely, on ordinary culture media and moderately well in thioglycollate broth and various other broths containing serum and serum components. It grows especially well in deep stabs of semisolid medium prepared by adding 0.5% agar to tryptose phosphate broth. Reduced oxygen or increased carbon dioxide (5–10%) enhances growth, but neither is necessary to support growth. Smith (72) described the appearance of growth in a meat infusion broth culture at 24 hr as "a faint opalescence..., which on shaking was resolved for the moment into delicate rolling clouds." The addition of serum to broth media supports heavier growth with a powdery sediment forming after 24 hr. Protein hydrolysates, glucose, and certain detergents such as Tween 80 also enhance growth. E. rhusiopathiae grows in a temperature range from 4 C (slow growth) to 42 C, with an optimal range of 35–37 C. The optimal pH for growth is mildly alkaline, pH 7.4–7.8. Oleic acid and riboflavin have been reported as essential for growth. The organism does not form a pellicle.

Colony Morphology. Three different colony types have been described for E. rhusiopathiae. Smooth colonies are dewy, colorless to bluish gray, and of pinpoint size (0.5–0.8 mm) with smooth edges. Most strains of E. rhusiopathiae and organisms isolated directly from infected tissues form this colony type. Some strains, however, form rough colonies that consist of long thickened filamentous rods. Rough colonies are opaque, flat, dry, and of pinhead size (1–2 mm) with irregular or lobed edges. The dissociation from smooth to rough colony type is described as intermediate colony type in which both short rods and short filaments may be identified. Most strains produce a narrow zone of alpha hemolysis in a medium containing 5–10% horse or bovine blood after 2–3 days' incubation at 37 C in an atmosphere of 5–10% carbon dioxide. A test-tube brush type of growth (lateral radiating projections) occurs 48 hr postinoculation in gelatin stab culture incubated at 21 C.

Biochemical Properties. E. rhusiopathiae ferments galactose, dextrose, fructose, maltose, lactose, and levulose without gas production. E. tonsillarum differs in its ability to ferment sucrose (76). Lead acetate agar or triple-sugar iron (TSI) agar is usually blackened, indicating hydrogen sulfide (H_2S) production, and xylose is occasionally fermented. Strains that do not produce H_2S have been isolated (6). Litmus milk is occasionally acidified slightly without coagulation. The organism is catalase negative, does not produce indole, does not reduce nitrites, is Voges-Proskauer and methyl red negative, does not hydrolyze esculin, and does not reduce 0.1% methylene blue. White and Shuman (88) found that the fermentation pattern varied with the medium, indicator, and method of measuring acid production; they stated that the most dependable medium was Andrade's base plus serum. Of three methods used to measure acid production (chemical indicator, change in pH, and production of titratable acidity) they found that the chemical indicator gave the most valid reproducible results.

Resistance to Chemical and Physical Agents.   *E. rhusiopathiae* is fairly resistant to various environmental and chemical factors. It is very resistant to desiccation and may survive the smoking and pickling processes used for processing meat and may remain viable in frozen or chilled meat, dried blood, decaying carcasses or fish meal. Apart from tissues, it is killed at 70 C in 5–10 minutes. Vallee (84) suggested that the organism remained viable in soil and multiplied in alkaline soils during warm weather. Wood (91), however, reported that under experimental conditions, *E. rhusiopathiae* was inactivated at different rates in soil when parameters of temperature, pH, and organic matter content were tested. Temperature exerted the greatest effect on viability. Populations of the pathogen survived 35 days at 3 C and 2 days at 30 C. Organisms did not survive longer than 11–18 days under various conditions of organic matter content and pH. *E. rhusiopathiae* is destroyed in a short time by a 1:1000 concentration of bichloride of mercury, 0.5% sodium hydroxide solution, 3.5% liquid cresol, or a 5% solution of phenol. The organism is resistant to 0.001% crystal violet, 0.5% potassium tellurite and can grow in the presence of 0.1% sodium azide.

Antigenic Structure and Toxins.   Sawada and Takahashi (68) vaccinated mice and swine with culture filtrate and found that they were protected against most serotypes of pathogenic *E. rhusiopathiae*. These studies and others indicate that essentially all strains of *E. rhusiopathiae* possess at least one or more common antigens (28, 73, 92). These antigens are heat labile and consist of protein or a complex of protein, carbohydrate, and lipid (89). Lachmann and Deicher (48) inferred the presence of a capsule following their discovery of a 14,000- to 22,000-MW surface polysaccharide. Shimoji et al. (69) demonstrated a capsule using transmission electron microscopy, which showed polar thickening on some *E. rhusiopathiae* strains.

A heat-stable antigen (cell wall peptidoglycan) is used to differentiate *E. rhusiopathiae* into serotypes. These antigens are easily extracted from the organism using acid or by autoclaving a washed whole cell inactivated culture for 1 hr at 121 C. Determination of serotype is accomplished with a double-diffusion gel system using specific hyperimmune rabbit sera. The preferred system for serotyping *E. rhusiopathiae* isolates is a numerical system described by Kuscera (47). Using the numerical system, strains previously designated as types A or B now become types 1 and 2, respectively. Although 26 serotypes of *E. rhusiopathiae* have been described (25), the recent identification of *E. tonsillarum* as a distinct species has led to a division of the serotyping scheme. Takahashi (76) reported that strains of serotypes 3, 7, 10, 14, 20, 22, and 25 are *E. tonsillarum* and that strains of *E. rhusiopathiae* belong to serotypes 1, 2, 4, 5, 6, 8, 9, 11, 12, 15, 16, 17, 19, 21 or type N. Strains not possessing a type-specific antigen are designated type N. Strains belonging to serotypes 13 and 18 exhibited low levels of DNA homology with *E. rhusiopathiae* and *E. tonsillarum* and possibly constitute a distinct genomic species. Subtypes of some serotypes were described, e.g., serotypes 1 and 2, and are designated by a number followed by a lower case letter. The majority of *E. rhusiopathiae* strains isolated from poultry fall into three major serotypes: types 1 (both subtypes 1a and 1b) and 2 and 5 (21, 24, 83, 95). Partridge et al. (60) cloned and characterized a bacterial-stress protein designated DnaK, which was highly expressed in *E. rhusiopathiae*. No flagella have been demonstrated on *E. rhusiopathiae,* and the organism produces no known toxins. Protective antigens are discussed under the section entitled Prevention and Control.

Strain Classification.   Strain classification is for the most part based on serologic, not biologic or biochemical, activity. White and Shuman (88) noted that the fermentation pattern of a particular strain did not vary to any great extent. There is no reported correlation between serologic grouping and biochemical pattern of strains of *E. rhusiopathiae* isolated from birds and production of the septicemic, urticarial, or endocardial form of erysipelas or of the carrier state (7, 87). Chooromoney et al. (14) analyzed strains of *Erysipelothrix* spp. by multilocus enzyme electrophoresis and indicated that serotyping was unreliable for epidemiologic studies, although serotype analysis was useful when one electrophoretic type contained multiple serotypes or subtypes or for strains isolated from different species and of varying virulence.

Pathogenicity.   *E. rhusiopathiae* is pathogenic for turkeys at any age or sex, following exposure by a variety of parenteral routes. Infection and disease are also produced in turkeys inoculated orally with chicken embryo yolk–propagated organisms (16) or when allowed to feed on viscera of turkeys that died from erysipelas. Several workers, however, have reported difficulty in reproducing consistent mortality with *E. rhusiopathiae* isolates of avian origin experimentally (2, 23). Reducing the number of passages on artificial media to an absolute minimum appears essential to maintaining virulence of the organism. Boyer and Brown (9) maintained virulence of an *E. rhusiopathiae* strain by storing infected liver at 4 C, which served as a source of the organism for further bird passage.

In addition to turkeys, other avian species are susceptible to infection with *E. rhusiopathiae,* both experimentally and under field conditions, and serious losses have been reported in chickens, ducks, and geese following naturally occurring outbreaks of the disease. Experimentally, Malik (52) demonstrated that virulent cultures of *E. rhusiopathiae* administered parenterally produced a septicemia in chickens less than 14 days old. In older chickens, however, septicemia could be produced only by intrapalpebral or subconjunctival installation of the pathogen along with injury to that tissue. Administration of hydrocortisone not only increased susceptibility to *E. rhusiopathiae* but shortened the course of infection and increased mortality, thus appearing to increase pathogenicity.

Parenteral injection of most avian strains of the organism regularly kills mice (*Mus musculus*), pigeons, and turkeys, but guinea pigs and chickens usually survive. Iliadis (40) reported that pigeons were more susceptible to intravenous than to oral inoculation.

The mechanism(s) by which the organism causes disease is still not very well understood. Takahashi et al. (74) reported a correlation between pathogenicity for mice and swine and the ability of *E. rhusiopathiae* to adhere to porcine kidney cells. The bacteria attached directly to the microvilli of the cells and adherence could be markedly reduced by heat or trypsin treatment of the bacteria. Other investigators have demonstrated that *E. rhusiopathiae* isolated from swine with endocarditis showed a higher degree of adherence to porcine heart valve tissue (10, 45). The enzyme hyaluronidase was initially thought to be involved in the virulence of *E. rhusiopathiae,* but later studies revealed no association with hyaluronidase production and pathogenicity of a particular strain (57). The enzyme neuraminidase, however, appears to correlate better with the virulence of *E. rhusiopathiae* isolates. This enzyme is produced during logarithmic growth, and the amount of enzyme activity was reported by Muller (54) to be lower in strains of lower virulence or avirulent strains compared with highly virulent isolates. No apparent relationship exists, however,

between the amount of neuraminidase activity and serotype. In a review of erysipelas, Wood (93) noted that a specific antibody to this enzyme from *E. rhusiopathiae* was identified in a commercial erysipelas antiserum produced in horses and from serum of rabbits hyperimmunized with *E. rhusiopathiae* neuraminidase. This rabbit preparation was shown to induce some protection in mice following challenge with the organism. *E. rhusiopathiae* neuraminidase has not been shown to have toxic activity and must be produced in large amounts to be active in pathogenesis, a condition that probably exists in the septicemic form of the disease.

Although earlier attempts failed to establish relationships between virulence and chemical structure, antigenic structure or morphology, Shimoji et al. (69) demonstrated, at least in part, that the virulence of *E. rhusiopathiae* for mice was associated with the presence of a capsule. Partridge et al. (60) suggested that expression of high levels of the DnaK protein may allow the organism to resist oxidation and survive the low pH environment of the phagolysosome following phagocytosis. Timoney (79) noted earlier that virulent *E. rhusiopathiae* were inefficiently inactivated in vitro by buffy-coat leukocytes obtained from swine. This investigator also examined the ability of macrophages to inactivate virulent *E. rhusiopathiae*; those from immune *E. rhusiopathiae*–infected mice inactivated more bacteria and did so at a faster rate than those from nonimmune mice (78). These studies suggest a cellular component in the immune response to *E. rhusiopathiae*. Though not completely clear, the pathogenicity of different isolates of *E. rhusiopathiae* may be related to their ability to produce various virulence factors to help them to resist or survive phagocytosis. These factors include specific attachment factors (capsule or adhesins), enzymes such as neuraminidase, and stress proteins.

PATHOGENESIS AND EPIZOOTIOLOGY.

Van Es and McGrath (85) cited Nocard and Leclainche as noting in 1903 that "at the present state of our knowledge it is impossible to explain the mysterious behavior of the contagion." Basically this is still true. Corstvet (16) found the organism shed in feces of a few birds up to 41 days postinoculation. In other experiments, the organism was found to persist in blood for several weeks postinoculation (20). It has been reported that the organism can survive in soil (8, 94) and that soil may serve as a source of the organism. Though soil is known to harbor the organism for long periods under certain conditions, and swine and sheep as well as various species of wildlife can harbor the organism, no clear-cut relationship has been established even between the presence of the infection in prior years among the same species (e.g., turkeys) and subsequent outbreaks among flocks (64). Wood (93) reported that survival time of the organism did not exceed 35 days in test soils maintained under different conditions of temperature, pH, moisture content, and organic matter content.

Natural and Experimental Hosts. The organism has been isolated in nature from turkeys, chickens, ducks, geese, emus, mud hens, eared grebes, parrots, sparrows, canaries, finches, thrushes, blackbirds, doves, quail, wild mallards, white storks, herring gulls, golden eagles, pheasant, starlings, peacocks, parakeets, swine, sheep, cattle, marine and freshwater fish, various captive wild birds and mammals, chipmunks, meadow and house mice, dolphins, and crocodiles (6, 8, 26, 31, 34, 41, 42, 44, 49, 94). From the reports, it appears that the susceptibilities of various avian populations differ. Genetic resistance may play a role in susceptibility to disease based on a report of an outbreak in turkeys with different genetic backgrounds (67). Experimental hosts are the pigeon, turkey, chicken, budgerigar, mouse, and rat (8, 29, 30).

Transmission, Carriers, and Vectors. The actual portal of entry and pathogenesis of *E. rhusiopathiae* infection in birds (and in animals other than humans) has not been definitely established. Contaminated material as the source of infection and entry through breaks in the mucous membranes or skin have been suggested.

Cannibalism and fighting among birds apparently result in increased losses. Permitting carcasses of infected dead birds to remain on the premises to be picked at or eaten by penmates also increases the spread and increases losses at unpredictable rates.

Experimentally, Corstvet (16) obtained up to 50% mortality in turkeys by oral inoculation of freshly isolated virulent organisms grown in chicken embryo yolk sac. Broth culture instilled orally, intranasally, or into the conjunctival sac (without damaging the membrane) was not infectious (33). Corstvet (16) and Bricker and Saif (11) found that subcutaneous (SC) inoculation of virulent cultures resulted in local multiplication followed by septicemia, with 80–100% mortality in susceptible turkeys.

Sadler and Corstvet (66) and Corstvet (20) showed that a few turkeys infected SC remained carriers for variable periods. Asymptomatic carriers of *E. rhusiopathiae* could not be detected before or after necropsy. The number of organisms used to challenge turkeys, route of inoculation (oral or parenteral), administration of antibiotics, time after vaccination and challenge, and age of the turkey apparently did not influence this carrier state, which is produced in very few birds. Isolations of *E. rhu-*

siopathiae from carriers are most frequent from cecal tonsils, liver, large intestine, heart, and blood (18, 20, 66). Xu et al. (95) reported a total of 95 isolates obtained from the pharynx of healthy chickens, ducks, and geese.

The role of vectors in transmission is not known. Wellmann (86) found that this pathogen could be transmitted mechanically from sick mice to pigeons by the stable fly, horsefly, mosquito, and other biting flies.

An outbreak of erysipelas in chickens in England was reported by Hall (36). Some pullets escaped from their pen, gained access to an area contaminated 8 yr previously with feces from pigs with erysipelas, and were returned to the same pens. Only chickens in these pens were affected; confined pullets not so exposed remained healthy.

Madsen (50) suggested that rain washing contaminated feces from a sheep corral initiated an outbreak in turkeys on range. Polner et al. (61) reported an outbreak in geese that had access to several hundred acres of pasture that was the initial site of a demolished pig farm, and which prior to the outbreak had been used for 5 yr for fattening sheep. Fishmeal and fish in general have been cited as probable sources of infection for avian species (8, 33, 55).

Incubation Period. In naturally occurring outbreaks, the incubation period cannot be readily ascertained. Experimental SC inoculation of turkeys with 104–106 organisms usually kills most of them in 44–70 hr; a few may die after 96–120 hr. With oral exposure, signs of disease generally occur 2–3 days later than with SC inoculation, and with a lower death rate. Occasionally, a turkey dies 2–3 wk after oral exposure. A SC inoculum of 102 instead of 104 or 106 organisms delays clinical signs by about 24 hr. The incubation period does not seem to vary among turkeys 7, 12, 16, and 20 wk of age or between sexes.

Signs

TURKEYS. Outbreaks usually start suddenly, with losses of one to several birds; owners may suspect that deaths are from poisoning, stampede injuries, or predators. A few droopy birds (especially toms) may be noticed, but these individuals are usually easily aroused. Just prior to death some birds may be very droopy, with unsteady gait. Some may have cutaneous lesions; affected males may have swollen purplish, turgid snoods (fleshy tubular appendage on dorsal surface of head). Some turkeys are now "desnooded" shortly after hatching; as a result, such lesions are infrequently seen. Gradual emaciation, weakness, and signs of anemia occur in some cases where endocarditis is the cause of death; other turkeys with vegetations (especially vaccinated birds) may die suddenly without signs, probably as a result of emboli. Sudden losses of hens 4–5 days after artificial insemination with peritonitis, perineal congestion, and skin discoloration have been reported.

OTHER BIRDS. Main clinical signs in chickens are general weakness, depression, diarrhea, and sudden death. In laying chickens, egg production may be decreased. However, Kilian et al. (44) reported no immediate drop in egg production in laying pullets, although signs were evident; later there was about a 50–70% drop. Affected ducks, geese, pheasant, and quail generally are depressed, have diarrhea, and die suddenly.

Morbidity and Mortality. Morbidity and mortality are frequently about the same in unvaccinated turkeys. In other species of poultry, morbidity and mortality rates are also approximately equal since most sick birds die. In immunized flocks, however, some birds may be depressed and recover. Both morbidity and mortality vary, ranging from sickness or death of occasional birds in good condition to sudden loss of several within 24–48 hr. Mortality ranges from much less than 1% to as high as 25–50% of a given group, though adjacent groups may not be affected. Mortality ranges could vary due to prior immunization or early treatment. Mortality rates vary among different avian species.

Gross Lesions. In naturally occurring outbreaks, the lesions are suggestive of a generalized septicemia and the following lesions have been observed in different outbreaks in turkeys. There is generalized congestion; degeneration of fat on the anterior edge of the thigh; degeneration and hemorrhage in pericardial fat; petechial hemorrhage in abdominal fat; hemorrhage in heart muscle; and a friable, enlarged, and possibly mottled liver, spleen, and usually kidney. Other gross lesions may be fibrinopurulent exudate in joints and pericardial sac, fibrin plaques on heart muscle, thickening of the proventriculus and gizzard wall with ulceration, small yellow nodules in ceca, catarrhal or sanguinocatarrhal enteritis, vegetative endocarditis, dark crusty skin lesions, a turgid irregular reddish purple snood in toms, hydropericardium, and distended visceral blood vessels (64). Other lesions noted with varying frequency in field outbreaks were diffuse skin reddening and a dirty brick-red muscle color. Some birds that died had no lesions other than slight catarrhal enteritis and petechiae in the heart fat.

In experimental infections, some of the lesions observed in naturally occurring outbreaks are not uncommon. Endocarditis, except in vaccinated birds, is rare in experimentally infected birds. In some field cases, and in birds vaccinated twice or more with bacterin and intravenously challenged, congestive heart failure with vegetations of the atrioventricular valves (sometimes extending as much as 7 cm into the aorta) have been found. Asymptomatic carrier turkeys are usually free of gross lesions.

In at least two field outbreaks in chicken layers, lesions in endocardium, joints, and skin were not observed (6). In ducks, geese, and pheasant, lesions are similar to those observed in other avian species, with addition of dark congested areas in foot webs of ducks.

Histopathology. Generally, the histopathologic features of acute erysipelas in turkeys reflect rather closely the observed gross findings, and specific cellular alterations are those expected in septicemic infections (5). Vascular changes dominate the histopathologic picture, with generalized engorgement of blood vessels and sinusoidal channels in virtually all organs. While there may be a strong central (cardiac or vasomotor) basis for vascular congestion, there is also evidence of direct vascular damage. Intravascular aggregations of bacteria accompanied by fibrin thrombi are frequent in capillaries, sinusoids, and venules. Overt hyalinization of walls of affected vessels is not uncommon. Edema and hemorrhage, especially prominent in lung and heart (Fig. 14.7), are further evidence of severe vascular damage. In addition, rounding up of vascular endothelial cells or reticuloendothelial (RE) cells of sinusoids is a consistent histologic finding, and engulfed bacteria are readily demonstrated in RE cells in liver and spleen.

Damage to parenchymal cells is generalized in acute erysipelas and especially obvious in liver, spleen, and kidney. Degenerative changes in hepatic cells vary from cloudy swelling with cellular dissociation to overt coagulative necrosis. Focal or massive necrosis apparently related to thrombosis of major portal vessels is seen occasionally, but diffuse degenerative changes are much commoner (Fig. 14.8). In spleen, the earliest observable change is necrosis and lysis of lymphoid elements. This progresses to nearly total loss of lymphocytes, with hyalinization of sheathed arteries of white pulp and surrounding reticular elements (Fig. 14.9). The epithelium of proximal tubules undergoes early degenerative change in affected turkeys. Swelling, dissociation, and separation from the basement membrane are frequent and prominent changes are seen in renal epithelial cells; overt coagulative necrosis is rare. Certain of these pathologic changes in kidney have also been reported by others (82). It is not unusual to find degenerative changes or necrosis in a variety of other organs such as lung, heart, pancreas, gastrointestinal tract, skeletal mus-

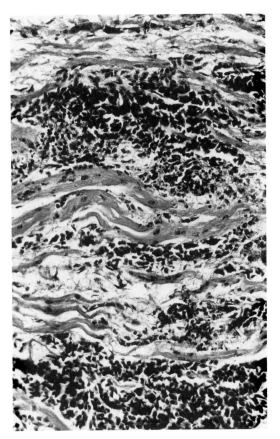

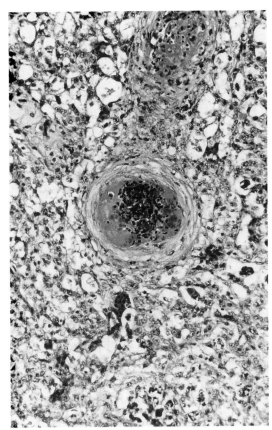

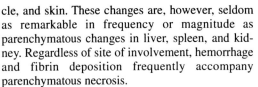

14.7. Acute erysipelas, turkey heart. Interstitial hemorrhages and separation of myocardial fibers (edema). H & E, ×100.

14.8. Acute erysipelas, turkey liver. Fibrin thrombus containing bacterial aggregates in the central portal blood vessel. Severe vacuolar degeneration of surrounding hepatocytes and several large basophilic sinusoidal, reticuloendothelial (Kupffer) cells are evident. H & E, ×100.

cle, and skin. These changes are, however, seldom as remarkable in frequency or magnitude as parenchymatous changes in liver, spleen, and kidney. Regardless of site of involvement, hemorrhage and fibrin deposition frequently accompany parenchymatous necrosis.

The cellular inflammatory component of peracute or acute erysipelas lesions is minimal. In scarified skin of turkeys infected by this route, there may be extensive heterophil infiltration, congestion, edema, and necrosis. Cellular inflammatory response as judged from examination of field cases is more prominent in turkeys with subacute or chronic disease. Heterophil and mononuclear leukocytic infiltration as well as proliferation of RE cells can be found around necrotizing lesions in liver and spleen as well as in heart valves and synovial membranes of joints. The pathology of experimentally induced subacute or chronic erysipelas in turkeys has not been reported.

In a study of acute erysipelas outbreaks in chick-

ens (6), histopathologic alterations very similar to those described in turkeys were reported.

Immunity

ACTIVE. Birds recovered from acute infections have a high degree of resistance to reinfection and death. Killed bacterins, the current commercially available immunoprophylactic agent for the immunization of turkeys against erysipelas, will prevent disease under both experimental and field conditions. Bacterin in conjunction with penicillin at the beginning of an outbreak will usually control losses. Long-lasting immunity is not produced by only one bacterin injection in turkeys. The immune response is more effective from two or more doses at intervals of at least 2–4 wk. Experiments with 4- to 7-wk-old turkeys have shown that protective immunity begins to decline between 4 and 5 wk postvaccination.

Krasnodebska-Depta and Janowska (46) reported

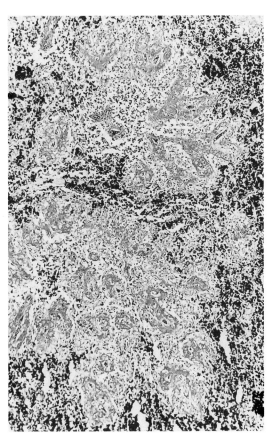

14.9. Acute erysipelas, turkey spleen. Hyalinized sheathed arteries within two malpighian corpuscles and nearly total depletion of lymphocytes are evident. Surrounding sinusoids are engorged with erythrocytes. H & E, ×100.

that 28- and 30-wk-old turkeys vaccinated with a bacterin made for swine were resistant to challenge 2 mo postvaccination. Aerosol immunization of ducks with an erysipelas vaccine has been reported to be very effective in eliminating the disease.

Osebold (58) reported limited protection with a live vaccine strain when administered SC to turkeys followed by subsequent challenge with a virulent strain. Bricker and Saif (11) reported on an effective level of protection in turkeys vaccinated through the drinking water with a live serotype 1a strain of *E. rhusiopathiae* followed by challenge with the homologous serotype. Two vaccine doses administered 2–3 wk apart were necessary to induce a sufficient protective response that lasted at least 3 wk following administration of the second vaccine dose. Administration of this live vaccine directly into the esophagus of turkeys did not induce a protective immune response. It is speculated that lymphoid tissue in the pharyngeal region plays a role in induction of an immune response to organisms introduced by the drinking water route.

PASSIVE. Treatment with swine erysipelas antiserum (horse origin) alone is said to be of some value if administered very early, but it is not practical because of expense and lack of uniform efficacy. Antiserum and penicillin have been successfully used in ducks (63).

DIAGNOSIS

Isolation and Identification of Causative Agent. Since gross lesions of dead birds indicate septicemia, diagnosis depends on demonstration and identification of *E. rhusiopathiae*. Rapid presumptive diagnosis is provided by the presence in liver, spleen, heart blood, or bone marrow smears of clumps and segregated gram-positive, beaded, slender, pleomorphic rods. Particularly helpful with decomposed specimens are bone marrow culture and smear.

Isolation of *E. rhusiopathiae* from sick birds that are killed and then cultured is neither as easy nor as frequently positive as culturing from birds dead of the disease. Detecting the organism from a carrier requires multiple samples from various tissues. Isolation from endocardial tissues is facilitated by finely mincing before inoculating enrichment broth. With birds dead from the infection, however, liver, spleen or bone marrow will suffice. Useful inhibitory media are the sodium azide–crystal violet medium described by Packer (59) and the tryptose phosphate broth medium with 5% horse serum plus kanamycin, neomycin, vancomycin, and novobiocin described by Wood (90). These media are the most satisfactory, though they do not completely prevent growth of other organisms (particularly with samples of intestinal contents) and may inhibit growth of some strains of *E. rhusiopathiae* (10). For primary isolation, recovery is favored by inoculating biplates containing 5% blood agar and Packer's medium followed by incubation in an atmosphere of 5–10% CO_2 or reduced oxygen. Ordinary atmosphere is suitable after a few passages on artificial media. Typical colonies composed of gram-positive rods are selected and placed in TSI medium or Kligler's lead acetate medium and incubated for 24 hr at 37 C. An excellent presumptive test for *E. rhusiopathiae* is a blackening (due to H_2S production) before there is a very noticeable change in the medium color.

The mouse, pigeon, or budgerigar may be used for a confirmatory protection test using erysipelas antiserum (the *E. rhusiopathiae* isolate, however, must be pathogenic for the test species chosen). One group of experimental animals is inoculated parenterally with a 24-hr culture of the isolate; another is inoculated with *E. rhusiopathiae* antiserum and immediately thereafter with the isolate. The unprotected group should die within 4 days, whereas animals receiving antiserum will live. *E. rhusiopathiae* may be detected in tissues using the fluorescent antibody technique (53, 56), which may also be used as a confirmatory test in diagnosis (17).

Sudden losses of adolescent turkeys in good flesh but with septicemic lesions, IM and subpleural ecchymotic and suffusion hemorrhages, and erysipeloid swelling of the snood point toward erysipelas. Also significant is a marked hemorrhagic condition of skin and facial and muscular tissues of the breast. In many cases, predominant losses will be in males, but in breeding flocks, sudden losses in hens with peritonitis, SC, and cutaneous discoloration, and a history of insemination just prior to this suggest *E. rhusiopathiae* infection. Diagnosis is further validated by procedures described above and in more detail by Corstvet (17). Recently, Makino et al. (51) described a direct, rapid, and sensitive detection test using the polymerase chain reaction methodology. The test detects both *E. rhusiopathiae* and *E. tonsillarum.*

Serology. Information regarding the nature of immunity induced in turkeys following natural exposure to *E. rhusiopathiae* or to erysipelas vaccines is scarce. Infected birds that recover appear to be solidly immune. Plate, tube, and microagglutination tests, in addition to passive hemagglutination, hemagglutination-inhibition, complement-fixation, growth agglutination, and growth inhibition tests, have been used in swine erysipelas research, but their usefulness for avian erysipelas studies have not been fully evaluated. Agglutination titers have been reported to be usually 160 or higher in antibiotic-treated recovered turkeys and turkeys that are carriers for the organism. Sikes and Tumlin (70), however, suggested that titers of 40 or greater are indicative of *E. rhusiopathiae* infection in turkeys. Currently, it is not known whether one particular serotype or strain of the organism is effective in detecting antibodies to other serologic types or strains of *E. rhusiopathiae*. At present, these tests are mainly useful for research studies only.

Differential Diagnosis. Fowl cholera, *Escherichia coli* infections, salmonellosis, and peracute Newcastle disease might be confused with the acute septicemic form of the disease (17). The less common forms of the disease (urticaria and endocarditis) may be caused by other miscellaneous bacterial agents or possibly fungal pathogens. All of these agents are easily differentiated from *E. rhusiopathiae* by gram staining or biochemical activity. *Lactobacillus* sp., which may occasionally be isolated from intestinal tracts or livers of poultry and is biochemically similar to *Erysipelothrix,* may be differentiated using the highly selective Packer's medium containing sodium azide and crystal violet. Gram staining, growth on Packer's medium, and the typical reaction pattern in TSI medium or Kligler's lead acetate medium are excellent presumptive tests. Confirmatory diagnosis is by fluorescent antibody test or animal pathogenicity tests.

TREATMENT. The antibiotic of choice for an outbreak in market or breeder turkeys is a rapid-acting form of penicillin. Any antibiotic should be used under veterinary supervision according to current treatment procedure. Label directions should be followed carefully. As soon as diagnosis is definitely established, potassium or sodium penicillin should be administered IM at the rate of about 10,000 U/lb body weight (200,000–300,000 U) simultaneously with a full dose of erysipelas bacterin. Control has usually been attained by giving penicillin (1,000,000 U/gal) in drinking water for 4 or 5 days to all birds in the flock when a presumptive diagnosis is made. All birds in the affected flock should be treated. Some recommendations suggest use of procaine penicillin or other longer-acting derivatives; under certain circumstances, these may be used successfully, but in outbreaks, rapid-acting formulations are almost mandatory. A combination of longer-acting and rapid-acting antibiotic formulations may provide best control if individual SC or IM injection is feasible and cost effective. Especially in meat-bird flocks, however, catching and handling each bird may be impractical or even harmful. Sterile abscesses and downgrading may follow IM injections. Care should be taken to observe the required withdrawal periods for the antibiotic used. Turkeys and possibly other birds with advanced signs of the disease at treatment time often will not recover. Experimental use of certain antibiotics including penicillin will control the infection but will not eliminate carriers. Antibiotics other than penicillin may increase the carrier rate in a flock of turkeys (19).

Comparative studies are lacking on efficacy of various antibiotics for controlling *E. rhusiopathiae* infection in avian populations. Erythromycin and broad-spectrum antibiotics have been found effective. In vitro studies have shown the organism to be resistant to neomycin (27). Sulfonamides and oral oxytetracycline are not effective treatments.

Beneficial management practices in handling an outbreak of erysipelas in turkeys include thorough decontamination of equipment, prompt removal of dead birds and other carrion from premises, encouraging adequate feed and water intake, and handling birds as little and as gently as possible or practical. If unlimited range is available, it might be desirable to move the flock to clean ground, but such a practice may contaminate the new range.

PREVENTION AND CONTROL

Management Procedures. It has been suggested, though not established, that various environmental factors may make avian species more susceptible to *E. rhusiopathiae* infection. Early field observations indicated that the beginning of rainy, cold weather, which frequently coincided with sexual maturity, was related to outbreaks of erysipelas in turkeys on the range. This may apply to flocks of other avian species. Source of the organism may be contaminated feed, soil, or decaying matter; infected carrier birds in the flock; or infected rodents. Apparently, the relationship between environmental factors and disease does not apply to cases involving individually confined birds, as in a zoo.

It is not possible to make clear-cut and specific recommendations for preventive or control management. A general suggestion is to use clean disinfected equipment and rotate turkey ranges away from previously contaminated areas. Certain disinfectants, notably 1–2% sodium hydroxide (lye) solutions, are effective against *E. rhusiopathiae*; phenols, cresols and related disinfectants, iodine, and certain household soaps are moderately effective (37).

With no specific and effective recommendations for management control of this disease in turkeys, it is suggested that birds be properly immunized in areas where erysipelas is known to be a problem.

Immunization.   The most widely used products for the immunization of turkeys against erysipelas are the formalin-inactivated, aluminum hydroxide-adsorbed whole-cell *E. rhusiopathiae* bacterins. These bacterins were initially developed for use in swine and were shown to be effective in preventing erysipelas in turkeys (1, 2, 15). Only certain strains of *E. rhusiopathiae* belonging to serotype 2, however, have been effective for use in bacterins. These strains are highly immunogenic because of the production of a "soluble immunizing substance" that is released into the culture medium when the organism is grown in a complex medium containing serum (81). This soluble immunizing substance is adsorbed and precipitated by aluminum hydroxide, which also adsorbs the whole cells. The presence of this soluble substance is considered necessary for the production of an effective bacterin.

Various investigators have employed different approaches in attempts to characterize a protective antigen (65, 80, 89). Galan and Timoney (28) described a protective antigen which was cloned and expressed as a fusion protein in a heterologous vector. Protection against challenge, however, was low in mice that were vaccinated with the fusion protein. Groschup et al. (35) described a 64,000- to 66,000-MW protein that was protective for mice. This antigen could be extracted with 10-mM NaOH and was hydrophobic.

A regimen of immunization can be suggested for meat turkeys as well as those kept for hatching egg production. Since the disease in other avian species is so sporadic, immunization other than in turkeys is

not generally recommended. It is also important to remember that effective immunization of mice or swine is not an adequate demonstration of the ability of a bacterin to protect turkeys. Cultures avirulent for turkeys and without immunogenicity for them may kill mice or provide protection. Immunizing capacity for turkeys can be properly assessed only with challenge of vaccinated turkeys.

Suggested for meat turkeys in areas of high risk is a single dose of the bacterin inoculated SC at the dorsal surface of the neck behind the atlas. The original investigation and demonstration of efficacy were based on IM injection of bacterin; however, because of the possibility of sterile abscesses (with downgrading at slaughter), SC inoculation is now used.

For turkeys kept as breeders, at least two doses of bacterin given at a 4-wk interval, should be administered prior to onset of egg production. The first dose may be given at 16–20 wk of age (at selection time) and an additional dose (2 mL/hen, 4 mL/tom) just prior to beginning of lay.

Though live erysipelas vaccines for swine have been around for over 30 yr, only recently have live vaccines become available for use in turkeys. Historically, Osebold (58) reported limited success after administration of a live culture vaccine SC to 9-mo-old turkeys followed by challenge with a virulent *E. rhusiopathiae* isolate 3 mo later. Experimentally, Bricker and Saif (11) demonstrated protection in turkeys vaccinated via the drinking water with a live type 1a erysipelas vaccine licensed for use in swine. At least two vaccine treatments, consisting of two doses each (4×10^9 organisms/dose) administered 2–3 wk apart induced significant protection in vaccinates following challenge with the homologous serotype. Improved vaccines properly used, adequate testing of the biologicals, planned immunization programs based on flock and premise history, and proper diagnosis of disease outbreaks as a basis for prompt treatment must be combined for effective prevention of erysipelas.

REFERENCES
1. Adler, H.E., and M.A. Nilson. 1952. Immunization of turkeys against swine erysipelas with several types of bacterins. Can J Comp Med 16:390–393.
2. Adler, H.E., and G.R. Spencer. 1952. Immunization of turkeys and pigs with an erysipelas bacterin. Cornell Vet 42:238–246.
3. Barber, M. 1939. A comparative study of Listerella and Erysipelothrix. J Pathol Bacteriol 48:11–23.
4. Beaudette, F.R., and C.B. Hudson. 1936. An outbreak of acute swine erysipelas infection in turkeys. J Am Vet Med Assoc 88:475–488.
5. Bickford, A.A., R.E. Corstvet, and A.S. Rosenwald. 1978. Pathology of experimental erysipelas in turkeys. Avian Dis 22:503–518.
6. Bisgaard, M., and P. Olsen. 1975. Erysipelas in egg-laying chickens: Clinical, pathological, and bacteriological investigations. Avian Pathol 4:59–71.
7. Bisgaard, M., V. Norrung, and N. Tornoe. 1980. Erysipelas in poultry. Prevalence of serotypes and epidemiological investigations. Avian Pathol 9:355–362.

8. Blackmore, D.K., and G.L. Gallagher. 1964. An outbreak of erysipelas in captive wild birds and mammals. Vet Rec 76:1161–1164.

9. Boyer, C.I., and J.A. Brown. 1957. Studies on erysipelas in turkeys. Avian Dis 1:42–52.

10. Bratberg, M. 1981. Observations on the utilization of a selective medium for the isolation of Erysipelothrix rhusiopathiae. Acta Vet Scand 22:55–59.

11. Bricker, J.M., and Y.M. Saif. 1988. Use of a live oral vaccine to immunize turkeys against erysipelas. Avian Dis 32:668–673.

12. Buchanan, R.E., and N.E. Gibbons. 1974. Bergey's Manual of Determinative Bacteriology, 8th ed. Williams and Wilkins. Baltimore, MD, p. 597.

13. Butcher, G., and B. Panigrahy. 1985. An outbreak of erysipelas in chukars. Avian Dis 29:843–845.

14. Chooromoney, K.N., D.J. Hampson, G.J. Eamens, and M.J. Turner. 1994. Analysis of Erysipelothrix rhusiopathiae and Erysipelothrix tonsillarum by multilocus enzyme electrophoresis. J Clin Microbiol 32:371–376.

15. Cooper, M.S., G.R. Personeus, and B.R. Choman. 1954. Laboratory studies on the vaccination of mice and turkeys with an Erysipelothrix rhusiopathiae vaccine. Can J Comp Med 18:83–92.

16. Corstvet, R.E. 1967. Pathogenesis of Erysipelothrix insidiosa in the turkey [abst]. Poult Sci 46:1247.

17. Corstvet, R.E. 1980. Erysipelas. In S.B. Hitchner, C.H. Domermuth, H.G. Purchase, and J.E. Williams (eds.). Isolation and Identification of Avian Pathogens. American Association of Avian Pathologists, Kennett Square, PA.

18. Corstvet, R.E., and C.H. Holmberg. 1968. The carrier state of Erysipelothrix insidiosa in turkeys. Poult Sci 47:1662.

19. Corstvet, R.E., and C. Howard. 1974. Evaluation of certain antibiotics in relation to the carrier state of Erysipelothrix rhusiopathiae (insidiosa) in turkeys [Abstr]. J Am Vet Med 165:744.

20. Corstvet, R.E., C.A. Holmberg, and J.K. Riley. 1970. 14th Congr Mund Avic, Madrid, Spain. Commun Sci 3:149–158.

21. Cross, G.M.J., and P.D. Claxton. 1979. Serological classification of Australian strains of Erysipelothrix rhusiopathiae isolated from pigs, sheep, turkeys and man. Aust Vet J 55:77–81.

22. Dhillon, A.S., R.W. Winterfield, H.L. Thacker, and J.A. Richardson. 1980. Erysipelas in domestic white pekin ducks. Avian Dis 24:784–787.

23. Dickinson, E.M., A.C. Jerstad, H.E. Adler, M. Cooper, W.E. Babcock, E.E. Johns, and C.A. Bottorff. 1953. The use of an Erysipelothrix rhusiopathiae bacterin for the control of erysipelas in turkeys. Proc 90th Ann Meet Am Vet Med Assoc, pp. 370–375.

24. Eamens, G.J., M.J. Turner, and R.E. Catt. 1988. Serotypes of Erysipelothrix rhusiopathiae in Australian pigs, small ruminants, poultry, and captive wild birds and animals. Aust Vet J 65:249–252.

25. Enoe, C. and V. Norrung. 1992. Experimental infection of pigs with serotypes of Erysipelothrix rhusiopathiae. Proc Int Pig Vet Soc Conf, p. 345.

26. Faddoul, G.P., G.W. Fellows, and J. Baird. 1968. Erysipelothrix infection in starlings. Avian Dis 12:61–66.

27. Fuzi, M. 1963. A neomycin sensitivity test for the rapid differentiation of Listeria monocytogenes and Erysipelothrix rhusiopathiae. J Pathol Bacteriol 85:524–525.

28. Galan, J.E. and J.F. Timoney. 1990. Cloning and expression in Escherichia coli of a protective antigen of Erysipelothrix rhusiopathiae. Infect Immun 58:3116–3121.

29. Geissinger, H.D. 1968. Acute and chronic Erysipelothrix rhusiopathiae infection in rats. Zentralbl Veterinaermed [B] 15:392–405.

30. Geissinger, H.D. 1968. Acute and chronic Erysipelothrix rhusiopathiae infection in white mice. J Comp Pathol 78:79–88.

31. Geraci, J.R., R.M. Sauer, and W. Medway. 1966. Erysipelas in dolphins. Am J Vet Res 27:597–606.

32. Graham, R., N.D. Levine, and H.R. Hester. 1939. Erysipelothrix rhusiopathiae associated with a fatal disease in ducks. J Am Vet Med Assoc 95:211–216.

33. Grenci, C.M. 1943. The isolation of Erysipelothrix rhusiopathiae and experimental infection of turkeys. Cornell Vet 33:56–60.

34. Griffiths, G.L. and N. Buller. 1991. Erysipelothrix rhusiopathiae infection in semi-intensively farmed emus. Aust Vet J 68:121–122.

35. Groschup, M.H., K. Cussler, R. Weiss, and J.F. Timoney. 1991. Characterization of a protective protein antigen of Erysipelothrix rhusiopathiae. Epidemiol Infect 107:637–649.

36. Hall, S.A. 1963. A disease in pullets due to Erysipelothrix rhusiopathiae. Vet Rec 75:333–334.

37. Hinshaw, W.R. 1965. Erysipelas. In H.E. Biester, and L.H. Schwarte (eds.). Diseases of Poultry, 5th ed. Iowa State University Press, Ames, IA, pp. 1271–76.

38. Hudson, C.B. 1949. Erysipelothrix rhusiopathiae infection in fowl. J Am Vet Med Assoc 115:36–39.

39. Hudson, C.B., J.J. Black, J.A. Bivins, and D.C. Tudor. 1952. Outbreaks of Erysipelothrix rhusiopathiae infection in fowl. J Am Vet Med Assoc 121:278–284.

40. Iliadis, V.N., T. Tsangaris, H. Kaldrymidou, and S. Lekas. 1983. Experimentelle infektion mit Erysipelothrix insidiosa bei puten und tauben. Weiner Tierarz Monatsh 70:282–285.

41. Jasmin, A.M., and J. Baucom. 1967. Erysipelothrix insidiosa infections in the caiman (Caiman crocodilus) and the American crocodile (Crocodilus acutus). Am J Vet Clin Pathol 1:173–177.

42. Jensen, W.I., and S.E. Cotter. 1976. An outbreak of erysipelas in eared grebes (Podiceps nigricollis). J Wildl Dis 12:583–86.

43. Kalf, G.F. and T.G. White. 1963. The antigenic components of Erysipelothrix rhusiopathiae. II. Purification and chemical characterization of a type-specific antigen. Arch Biochem Biophys 102:39–47.

44. Kilian, J.G., W.E. Babcock, and E.M. Dickinson. 1958. Two cases of Erysipelothrix rhusiopathiae infection in chickens. J Am Vet Med Assoc 133:560–562.

45. Krasemann, C. and H.E. Muller. 1975. The virulence of Erysipelothrix rhusiopathiae strains and their neuraminidase production. Zentralbl Backteriol [Orig A] 231:206–213.

46. Krasnodebska-Depta, A., and I. Janowska. 1980. Wlasciwodsci immunogenne niektorych szczepow wloskowca rozycy dla indikow. Med Weter 36:331–33. (Abstr Vet Bull 51:81)

47. Kuscera, G. 1973. Proposal for standardization of the designations used for serotypes of Erysipelothrix rhusiopathiae (Migula) Buchanan. Int J Syst Bacteriol 23:184–188.

48. Lachmann, P.G., H. Deicher. 1986. Solubilization and characterization of surface antigenic components of Erysipelothrix rhusiopathiae T28. Infect Immun 52:818–822.

49. Levine, N.D. 1965. Erysipelas. In H.E. Biester and L.H. Schwarte (eds.). Diseases of Poultry, 5th ed. Iowa State University Press, Ames, IA, pp. 461–469.

50. Madsen, D.E. 1937. An erysipelas outbreak in turkeys. J Am Vet Med Assoc 91:206–208.

51. Makino, S., Y. Okada, T. Maruyama, K. Ishikawa, T. Takahashi, M. Nakamura, T. Ezaki, H. Morita. 1994. Direct and rapid detection of Erysipelothrix rhusiopathiae DNA in animals by PCR. J Clin Microbiol 32:1526–1531.

52. Malik, Z. 1962. Pokusy s experimentalnou vnimavostou kurciat voci mikrobu Erysipelothrix rhusiopathiae. Vet Cas 11:89–94.

53. Marshall, J.D., W.C. Eveland, and C.W. Smith. 1959. The identification of viable and nonviable Erysipelothrix insidiosa with fluorescent antibody. Am J Vet Res 20:1077–1080.

54. Muller, H. E. 1981. Neuraminidase and other enzymes of Erysipelothrix rhusiopathiae as possible pathogenic factors. In H. Deicher (ed.). Arthritis: Models and Mechanisms. Berlin, Springer-Verlag, p. 58.

55. Murase N., K. Suzuki, and T. Nakahara. 1959. Studies on the typing of Erysipelothrix rhusiopathiae. II. Serological behaviours of the strains isolated from fowls including those from cattle and humans. Jpn J Vet Sci 21:177–181.

56. Nelson, J.D., and S. Shelton. 1963. Immunofluorescent studies of Listeria monocytogenes and Erysipelothrix insidiosa. Application to clinical diagnosis. J Lab Clin Med 62:935–942.

57. Norrung, V. 1970. Studies on Erysipelothrix insidiosa s. rhusiopathiae. I. Morphology, cultural features, biochemical reactions and virulence. Acta Vet Scand 11:577–585.

58. Osebold, J.W., E.M. Dickinson, and W.E. Babcock. 1950. Immunization of turkeys against Erysipelothrix rhusiopathiae with avirulent live culture. Cornell Vet 40:387–391.

59. Packer, R.A. 1943. The use of sodium azide (NaN$_3$) and crystal violet in a selective medium for streptococci and Erysipelothrix rhusiopathiae. J Bacteriol 46:343–349.

60. Partridge, J., J. King, J. Krska, D. Rockabrand, and P. Blum. 1993. Cloning, heterologous expression, and characterization of the Erysipelothrix rhusiopathiae DnaK protein. Infect Immun 61:411–417.

61. Polner, T., G. Cajdacs, F. Kemenes, G. Kucsera, and J. Durst. 1984. Stress effect of plucking as modulation of host's defense in birds. Ann Immunol Hung 23:211–224.

62. Reboli, A.C. and W.E. Farrar. 1989. Erysipelothrix rhusiopathiae: an occupational pathogen. Clin Microbiol Rev 2:354–359.

63. Reetz, G., and L. Schulze. 1978. Rotlaufinfektion bei mastenten. Monatsh Veterinaermed 33:170–173.

64. Rosenwald, A.S., and E.M. Dickinson. 1941. A report of swine erysipelas in turkeys. Am J Vet Res 2:202–213.

65. Rothe, F. 1982. Das protektive antigen des rotlaufbakteriums (Erysipelothrix rhusiopathiae). II. Mitteilung: die weitere charakterisierung des protektiven antigens. Arch Exp Vet Med 36:255–267.

66. Sadler, W.W. and R.E. Corstvet. 1965. The effect of Erysipelothrix insidiosa infection on wholesomeness of market turkeys. Am J Vet Res 26:1429–1436.

67. Saif, Y.M., K.E. Nestor, R.N. Dearth, and P.A. Renner. 1984. Possible genetic variation in resistance of turkeys to erysipelas and fowl cholera. Avian Dis 28:770–773.

68. Sawada, T. and T. Takahashi. 1987. Cross protection of mice and swine inoculated with culture filtrate of attenuated Erysipelothrix rhusiopathiae and challenge exposed to strains of various serovars. Am J Vet Res 48:239–242.

69. Shimoji, Y., Y. Yokomizo, T. Sekizaki, Y. Mori, and M. Kubo. 1994. Presence of a capsule in Erysipelothrix rhusiopathiae and its relationship to virulence for mice. Infect Immun 62:2806–2810.

70. Sikes, D., and T.J. Tumlin. 1967. Further studies on the Erysipelothrix insidiosa tube agglutination test. Am J Vet Res 28:1177–1181.

71. Silberstein, E.B. 1965. Erysipelothrix endocarditis. Report of a case with cerebral manifestations. J Am Med Assoc 191:158-160.

72. Smith, T. 1885. Second Annual Report of the Bureau of Animal Industry. Washington, DC, U.S. Department of Agriculture, p. 187.

73. Takahashi, T., M. Takagi, T. Sawada. 1984. Cross protection in mice and swine immunized with live erysipelas vaccine to challenge exposure with strains of Erysipelothrix rhusiopathiae of various serotypes. Am J Vet Res 45:2115–2118.

74. Takahashi, T., N. Hirayama, T. Sawada, Y. Tamura, and M Muramatsu. 1987. Correlation between adherence of Erysipelothrix rhusiopathiae strains of serovar 1a to tissue culture cells originated from porcine kidney and their pathogenicity in mice and swine. Vet Microbiol 13:57–64.

75. Takahashi, T., T. Fujisawa, Y. Benno, Y. Tamura, T. Sawada, S. Suzuki, M. Muramatsu, and T. Mitsuoka. 1987. Erysipelothrix tonsillarum sp. nov. isolated from tonsils of apparently healthy pigs. Int J Syst Bacteriol 37:166–168.

76. Takahashi, T., T. Fujisawa, Y. Tamura, S. Suzuki, M. Muramatsu, T. Sawada, Y. Benno, and T. Mitsuoka. 1992. DNA relatedness among Erysipelothrix rhusiopathiae strains representing all twenty-three serovars and Erysipelothrix tonsillarum. Int J Syst Bacteriol 42:469–473.

77. Takahashi, T., M. Takagi, R. Yamaoka, K. Ohishi, M. Norimatsu, Y. Tamura, and M. Nakamura. 1994. Comparison of the pathogenicity for chickens of Erysipelothrix rhusiopathiae and Erysipelothrix tonsillarum. Avian Pathol 23:237–245.

78. Timoney, J. 1969. The inactivation of Erysipelothrix rhusiopathiae in macrophages from normal and immune mice. Res Vet Sci 10:301–302.

79. Timoney, J. 1970. The inactivation of Erysipelothrix rhusiopathiae in pig buffy-coat leucocytes. Res Vet Sci 11:189–190.

80. Timoney, J.F. and M.M. Groschup. 1993. Properties of a protective protein antigen of Erysipelothrix rhusiopathiae. Vet Microbiol 37:381–387.

81. Traub, F. 1947. Immunisierung gegen schweinerotlauf mit konzentrierten adsorbatimpfstoffen. Monatsh Veterinaermed 10:165–172.

82. Tsangaris, R., N. Iliadis, E. Kaldrymidou, T. Lekkas, E. Tsiroyannis, and E. Artopios. 1980. Experimentaller rotlauf der tuten nach sintroavenoser infection mit E. insidia I elecktronen mikroskopische befunde inden nieren. Zentralbl Veterinaermed [B] 27:705–13.

83. Vaissaire, J., P. Desmettre, G. Paille, G. Mirial, and M. Laroche. 1985. Erysipelothrix rhusiopathiae: agent du rouget dans les differentes especes animales. Donnees actuelles. Bull Acad Vet France 58:259–265.

84. Vallee, M. 1930. Sur l'etiologie du rouget. Rev Pathol Comp [abst] 30:857–858.

85. Van Es, L. and C.B. McGrath. 1936. Swine erysipelas. Neb Agric Exp Stn Res Bull 84:1–47.

86. Wellmann, G. 1950. The transmission of swine erysipelas by a variety of blood-sucking insects to pigeons. Zentr Bakteriol Parasitenk Abt I Orig 155:109–115.

87. White, T.G., and G.F. Kalf. 1961. The antigenic components of Erysipelothrix rhusiopathiae. I. Isolation and serological identification. Arch Biochem Biophys 95:458–463.

88. White, T.G., and R.D. Shuman. 1961. Fermentation reactions of Erysipelothrix rhusiopathiae. J Bacteriol 82:595–599.

89. White, R.R., and W.F. Verwey. 1970. Isolation and characterization of a protective antigen-containing particle from culture supernatant fluids of Erysipelothrix rhusiopathiae. Infect Immun 1:380–386.

90. Wood, R.L. 1965. A selective liquid medium utilizing antibiotics for isolation of Erysipelothrix insidiosa. Am J Vet Res 26:1303–1308.

91. Wood, R.L. 1973. Survival of Erysipelothrix rhusiopathiae in soil under various environmental conditions. Cornell Vet 63:390–410.

92. Wood, R.L. 1979. Specificity in response of vaccinated swine and mice to challenge exposure with strains of Erysipelothrix rhusiopathiae of various serotypes. Am J Vet Res 40:795–801.

93. Wood, R.L. 1986. Erysipelas. In A.D. Leman, R. Straw, R.D. Glock, W.L. Mengeling, R.H.C. Penny, and E. Scholl (eds.). Diseases of Swine, 7th ed.. Iowa State University Press, Ames, IA, pp. 475–486.

94. Woodbine, M. 1950. Erysipelothrix rhusiopathiae. Bacteriology and chemotherapy. Bacteriol Rev 14:161–178.

95. Xu, K.Q., X.F. Hu, C.H. Gao, Q.Y. Lu, and J.H. Wu. 1984. Studies on the serotypes and pathogenicity of Erysipelothrix rhusiopathiae isolated from swine and poultry. Chin J Vet Med 10:9–11.

PSEUDOTUBERCULOSIS

Richard B. Rimler and J. R. Glisson

INTRODUCTION. Avian pseudotuberculosis (AP) is a contagious disease of domesticated and wild birds. It is characterized by an acute septicemia of short duration, followed by chronic focal infections that result in caseous nodules resembling the tubercles of tuberculosis. Research on this disease has been limited, and most publications on this disease are case reports.

HISTORY AND DISTRIBUTION. The causative agent, *Yersinia pseudotuberculosis,* was first isolated from a guinea pig inoculated with material from a subcutaneous tubercular lesion on the forearm of a child (13). Since then, the organism has been isolated from many species of mammals and birds. In describing a case of AP in a blackbird, Beaudette (2) gave an extensive review of the disease in birds. He credited Riech in 1889 and Kinyoun in 1906 with making the first isolation from birds in Europe and the United States, respectively.

Avian pseudotuberculosis has been reported in many countries and probably occurs throughout the world. It occurs sporadically in domestic poultry and occasionally causes severe losses in turkeys. Because of its minor economic importance, however, AP has received little research attention.

ETIOLOGY

Classification. The bacterium, *Y. pseudotuberculosis,* has been given many names (3, 16): *Bacillus pseudotuberculosis,* 1889; *Bacterium pseudotuberculosis* 1900; *Streptobacillus pseudotuberculosis-rodentium,* 1894; *Bacterium pseudotuberculosis-rodentium,* 1896; *Corynebacterium pseudotuberculosis,* 1925; *Pasteurella pseudotuberculosis,* 1929; *C. rodentium,* 1932; *C. pseudotuberculosis-rodentium,* 1933; *Malleomyces pseudotuberculosis-rodentium,* 1933; *Shigella pseudotuberculosis,* 1935; *Y. rodentium,* 1944; *P. rodentium,* 1944; *P. pseudotuberculosis-rodentium,* 1947; *Cillopasteurella pseudotuberculosis-rodentium,* 1953; and *Y. pseudotuberculosis,* 1974.

Morphology and Staining. *Y. pseudotuberculosis* is a gram-negative rod, 0.5 × 0.8–5.0 μm. Coccoid and long filamentous forms also occur. The coccoid forms usually show some bipolar staining. According to Cook (7), it is slightly acid-fast, which can be demonstrated in imprint smears using a modified Ziehl-Nielsen staining method. Neither spores nor visible capsules are formed, although at 22 C an envelope may be seen in India ink preparations. Single rods occasionally show peritrichous flagellae, which develop at temperatures between 20 and 30 C.

Growth Requirements and Colonial Morphology. *Y. pseudotuberculosis* grows in the presence or absence of oxygen; optimal temperature is 30 C. Burrows and Gillett (4) studied seven strains of various serotypes and observed that some grown at 28 C required thiamine or pantothenate. At 37 C, most strains could grow with the addition of any three of four factors—glutamic acid, thiamine, cystine, and pantothenate; other strains required all four factors and nicotinamide.

Good growth occurs in peptone broth. Growth at 22 C is diffuse, with some clumped masses and occasionally ring and pellicle formation. Cultivation at 37 C, especially in acid media, accelerates dissociation. On peptone or infusion agar media, it forms colonies that are smooth to slimy, granular, translucent, grayish yellow, butyrous, and 0.5–1 mm in diameter. On agar medium containing blood, colonies grow to 2–3 mm in diameter by the 2nd day. At 37 C, colonies are thin, dry, and irregular, with rough edges. Growth occurs on MacConkey agar. *Y. pseudotuberculosis* is motile at 25 C but not at 37 C. Motility is best demonstrated in semisolid medium.

Physiologic Properties. *Y. pseudotuberculosis* metabolizes many compounds without producing gas. The following properties are characteristic of *Y. pseudotuberculosis*:

Arabinose	fermented
Dextrin	fermented
Fructose	fermented
Glucose	fermented
Glycerol	fermented
Maltose	fermented
Mannitol	fermented
Mannose	fermented
Melibiose	fermented
Rhamnose	fermented
Trehalose	fermented
Xylose	usually fermented
Salicin	usually fermented
Sucrose	not fermented
Dulcitol	not fermented
Inositol	not fermented
Lactose	not fermented
Raffinose	not fermented
Sorbitol	not fermented
Urease	produced
Catalase	produced

Ammonia	produced
Hydrogen sulfide	usually not produced
Nitrates	reduced
Methylene blue	reduced
Blood	not hemolyzed
Indole	not produced
Gelatin	not liquified
MacConkey agar	usually growth

Resistance to Chemical and Physical Agents. *Y. pseudotuberculosis* is easily destroyed by sunlight, drying, heat, or ordinary disinfectants. It remains viable for years on sealed agar slants or when lyophilized.

Antigenic Structure. Somatic and flagellar antigens are used to characterize strains of *Y. pseudotuberculosis*. Fifteen somatic antigens are demonstrable by agglutination and agglutination-adsorption serologic tests. These heat-stable somatic antigens are used to differentiate six serotypes; four of which have two subtypes each (16). Five heat-labile flagellar antigens are recognized, but they are infrequently used for antigenic characterization. Antigens and serotypes are indicated in Table 14.2.

Additional serotypes VII and VIII, and an additional subtype, IIC, have been proposed (21). Among strains isolated from birds, serotype I is most common, followed by II and IV. Serotype III is rare and V and VI have not been reported from birds (19).

Thal (20) studied 186 strains of *Y. pseudotuberculosis*; of these, 33 were isolated from eight species of birds. All were biochemically identical; there were five serologically distinct groups. Most strains in group III produced thermolabile exotoxins that were convertible to toxoids. Experimentally, antiinfection immunity was produced with live avirulent strains, thus protecting against infection with atoxic strains and subtoxic culture doses of toxic strains. Antitoxic immunity protected against toxin and, to a degree, against infection with toxic strains but not against infection with atoxic strains.

Mair (12) studied the type distribution of *Y. pseudotuberculosis* in Great Britain during 1961–64; 177 strains were isolated from 39 different species of mammals and birds. Sixty-five isolates were from 26 species of birds; 39 of these were type IA, 16 type IB, 6 type IIA, 2 type IIB, and 2 type IV. Of 17 isolates from turkeys, 9 were type IA and 8 were type IB. In studies of 22 strains isolated from birds in New Zealand, 7 were serotype I and 15 were serotype II (9).

PATHOGENESIS AND EPIZOOTIOLOGY

Natural and Experimental Hosts. Avian pseudotuberculosis has been reported in turkeys, ducks, geese, chickens, guinea fowl, companion birds, and wild birds. It has also been reported in many species of mammals. Of the laboratory animals, guinea pigs, rabbits, mice, monkeys, and baboons are quite susceptible; white rats and hamsters are refractory. Ground squirrels can become infected and may play a role in transmission to turkeys (22).

Avian pseudotuberculosis occurs occasionally in turkeys; losses have been as high as 80% (1, 10, 15, 18, 22, 23).

Avian pseudotuberculosis among stock doves in Hampshire, England, was observed by Clapham (5). In a search for the source of infection, *Y. pseudotuberculosis* was isolated from a lark, wood pigeon, jackdaw, rook, and hare. This author also isolated the organism from gray partridge, pheasants, and bobwhite quail. Outbreaks in Denmark affected pigeons, canaries, snow buntings, waxwings, and a turkey (14). An epornitic of AP in common grackles (*Quiscalus quiscula*) occurred at a major winter roost in Maryland (6). Mortality and morbidity were extensive and continued for several weeks until spring roost breakup. Occurrence of extensive infection in a large migratory bird population has major epizootiologic significance.

Transmission, Pathogenesis, and Incubation Period. Body excretions of diseased birds or mammals may contaminate soil, food, or water and are important factors in dissemination of AP. Predisposing causes are apparently important; as a rule, the only birds affected are those whose resistance has been lowered by inadequate feeding, exposure to cold, or worm infection. Very young birds are particularly susceptible. During cold and wet weather in the fall, considerable losses may occur among young turkeys. In susceptible birds, the organism gains entrance to the bloodstream through breaks in the skin or through the mucous membranes, perhaps mostly in the digestive tract. Thus a bacteremia is established. Usually, the bacteremic

Table 14.2. Serotypes and antigens of *Yersinia pseudotuberculosis*.

Serotype	Subtype	O antigens	H antigens
I	A	1, 2, 3	a, c
	B	1, 2, 4	a, c
II	A	1, 5, 6	a, d
	B	1, 5, 7	a, d
III	–	1, 8	a
IV	A	1, 9, 11	a, b;b
	B	1, 9, 12	a, b, d
V	A	1, 10, 14	a;a, b, e
	B	1, 10, 15	a
VI	–	1, 13	a

condition is of short duration, but the bacteria are not all destroyed. Some establish foci of infection in one or more organs such as liver, spleen, lungs, or intestines, giving rise to tuberculelike lesions. Such lesions have also been found in the mesentery and breast muscles.

The incubation period of artificial infection varies considerably and depends on the virulence of the organism, amount of inoculum, avenue of introduction, and host species. Sparrows and canaries were very susceptible and may die in 1–3 days from small doses of organisms injected subcutaneously, intramuscularly, or intraperitoneally. Feeding of cultures is usually ineffective unless some intestinal inflammation is present to act as a predisposing influence. Canaries fed mustard seed to cause intestinal irritation sickened 5 days after being given cultures by mouth; death resulted 2 days later. Judging from various reports, the incubation period may vary from 3 to 6 days in acute attacks and 2 or more weeks in chronic cases.

Signs.   Signs vary considerably. In very acute cases, birds may die suddenly without clinical signs

or may live a few hours or days after showing the first signs. Such cases are usually marked by sudden appearance of diarrhea and manifestations of acute septicemia. More often, however, the course of this disease extends over 2 or more wk, in which case the signs appear 2–4 days before death. In such cases, birds will show weakness, dull and ruffled feathers, and difficult breathing. Diarrhea is also a common sign. Occasionally, the disease will run a more protracted course, and emaciation and extreme weakness or paralysis may be evident. Such manifestations as stiffness, difficulty in walking, droopiness, somnolence, constipation, and discoloration of the skin have also been observed. In early stages of the chronic form of the disease, birds may eat normally, but the appetite is usually completely lost 1 or 2 days before death.

Lesions.   When deaths occur early in the septicemic stage of the disease, enteritis and enlarged livers and spleens may be the only lesions. Later, miliary necrotic foci become evident in visceral organs, particularly livers and spleens (Fig. 14.10) and in muscle. Enteritis, varying in severity from

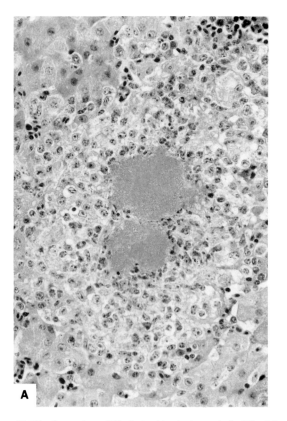

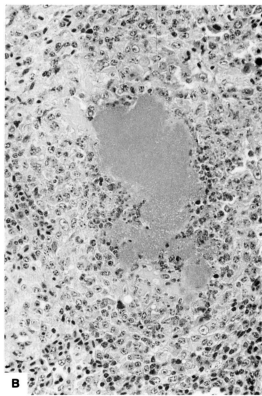

14.10.   Large, basophilic, botryoid colonies typical of *Yersinia pseudotuberculosis* infection in the liver *(A)* and spleen *(B)* of an experimentally infected bird. Colonies are surrounded by fibrin and an infiltration of inflammatory cells primarily composed of macrophages and occasional heterophils. (De Herdt, Haaesebrouck, Barnes)

catarrhal to hemorrhagic, is common. Serous cavities sometimes contain an increased amount of fluid. Osteomyelitis sometimes occurs in affected turkey flocks (22, 23), causing caseous necrotic foci near the growth plates of long bones in some cases (22). Degenerative myopathy has also been observed in affected turkey flocks with locomotor difficulties (8).

DIAGNOSIS. A definitive diagnosis can be established only by isolation and identification of the organism, since the signs and lesions are very similar to those of several other diseases such as fowl cholera, fowl typhoid, paratyphoid, spirochetosis, tuberculosis, and certain neoplastic diseases.

Isolation and Identification. Primary isolation is made by streaking specimens from affected tissues on blood or trypticase soy agar or by inoculating trypticase soy broth, followed by streaking onto agar after 3–5 hr incubation at 37 C. The medium of Patterson and Cook (17) is recommended for isolation of *Y. pseudotuberculosis* from feces. The surface of the agar is inoculated by streaking a suspension of 10% feces in phosphate buffer (pH 7.6) and incubating at 37 C for 24–48 hr. Identification is based primarily on physiologic characteristics as described in the section on physiologic properties.

Differential Diagnosis. The bacterium *Y. pseudotuberculosis* is quite similar in many respects to *Y. pestis* and *Y. enterocolitica*. Although these two organisms are not likely to be encountered in poultry, they may be carried by rodents having access to the poultry area. A summary of differential tests of *Y. pseudotuberculosis*, *Y. pestis*, and *Y. enterocolitica* is shown in Table 14.3.

An unusual strain of *Y. pseudotuberculosis* with similarities to *Salmonella pullorum* was isolated from turkey hens by Kiliam et al. (11). It resembled *S. pullorum* on brilliant green agar; was agglutinated by *S. pullorum* antiserum; produced acid but not gas from glucose and mannitol; and did not ferment lactose, sucrose, maltose, dulcitol, or salicin. Antiserum from sensitized guinea pigs, chickens, and turkeys, which agglutinated homologous antigen, failed to agglutinate either *S. pullorum* or *S. typhimurium*.

TREATMENT AND PREVENTION. Little current information is available on the use of chemotherapeutic agents for treatment of pseudotuberculosis in birds. In one case, treatment of affected turkeys with chloramphenicol and streptomycin sulfate (0.6 g and 0.5 g/L, respectively) in drinking water for 2 days, followed by tetracycline (0.5 g/L) for 4 days resulted in decreased death losses; no relapse occurred (8). In another case, treatment with high levels of tetracycline in the feed seemed to arrest the disease, but surviving turkeys were later condemned at processing because of lesions of a septicemia (22). Vaccines are not available for use in preventing avian pseudotuberculosis; therefore, prevention is limited to use of good management procedures (see Chapter 1).

REFERENCES
1. Adamec, Z., and K. Matousek. 1965. Pseudotuberculosis in turkeys. Veter 15:158–160.
2. Beaudette, F.R. 1940. A case of pseudotuberculosis in a blackbird. J Am Vet Med Assoc 97:151–157.
3. Buchanan, R.E., J.G. Holt, and E.F. Lessel. 1966. Index Bergeyana. Williams & Wilkins, Baltimore.
4. Burrows, T.W., and W.A. Gillett. 1966. The nutritional requirements of some Pasteurella species. J Gen Microbiol 45:333–345.
5. Clapham, P.A. 1953. Pseudotuberculosis among stock-doves in Hampshire. Nature 172:353.
6. Clark, M.C., and L.N. Locke. 1962. Case report: Observations on pseudotuberculosis in common grackles. Avian Dis 6:506–510.
7. Cook, R. 1952. A method of demonstrating Pasteurella pseudotuberculosis in smears from animal lesions. J Pathol Bacteriol 64:228–229.
8. Hinz, K.H., E.F. Kaleta, B. Stiburek, G. Glunder, and K. Tessler. 1981. Eine durch Yersinia pseudotuberculosis bei Mastputen verursachte Myopathie. Dtsch Tieraerztl Wochenschr 88:352–354.
9. Hodges, R.T., M.G. Carman, and W.J. Mortimer. 1984. Serotypes of Yersinia pseudotuberculosis recovered from domestic livestock. N Z Vet J 32:11–13.
10. Karlsson, K.F. 1945. Pseudotuberkulos hos honsfaglar. Scand Vet Tidskr 35:673–687.
11. Kiliam, J.G., R. Yamamoto, W.E. Babcock, and E.M. Dickenson. 1962. An unusual aspect of Pasteurella pseudotuberculosis in turkeys. Avian Dis 6:403–405.
12. Mair, N.S. 1965. Sources and serological classification of 177 strains of Pasteurella psuedotuberculosis isolated in Great Britain. J Pathol Bacteriol 90:275–278.
13. Malassez, L., and W. Vignal. 1883. Tuberculose zoologique (forme on espice de tuberculose sans bacillis). Arch Physiol Norm Pathol Ser 3, 2:369–412.
14. Marthedal, H.E., and G. Velling. 1954. Pasteurellosis and pseudotuberculosis among fowls in Denmark. Nord Vet Med 6:651–665.

Table 14.3. Differential characteristics of *Yersinia pseudotuberculosis*, *Y. pestis*, and *Y. enterocolitica*

Test	*Y. pseudotuberculosis*	*Y. pestis*	*Y. enterocolitica*
Urease	+	−	+
Ornithine decarboxylase	−	−	+
Adonitol	+	−	−
Cellobiose	−	−	+
Motility at 22 C	+	−	+

15. Mathey, W.J., Fr., and P.J. Siddle. 1954. Isolation of Pasteurella pseudotuberculosis from a California turkey. J Am Vet Med Assoc 125:482–483.

16. Mollaret, H.H. and E. Thal. 1974. Yersinia. In R.E. Buchanan and N.E. Gibbons (eds.). Bergey's Manual of Determinative Bacteriology. Williams and Wilkins Co, Baltimore, pp. 330–332.

17. Paterson, J.S., and R. Cook. 1963. A method for the recovery of Pasteurella pseudotuberculosis from faeces. J Pathol Bacteriol 85:241–242.

18. Rosenwald, A.S., and F.M. Dickinson. 1944. A report on Pasteurella pseudotuberculosis infection in turkeys. Am J Vet Res 5:246–249.

19. Stovell, P.L. 1980. Pseudotubercular yersiniosis. In J. H. Steele, H. Stoenner, W. Kaplan and M. Torten (eds.). CRC Handbook Series in Zoonoses, sect A, vol II. CRC Press, Inc., Boca Raton, FL, pp. 209–256.

20. Thal, E. 1954. Untersuchungen ueber Pasteurella pseudotuberculosis unter besonder Beruecksichtigun ihres immunologischen Verhaltens. Thesis. Berlingska Boktryckeriet, Lund, Sweden.

21. Tsubokura, M., K. Otsuki, Y. Kawasoka, H. Fukushima, K. Ikemure, and K. Kanazawa. 1984. Addition of new serogroups and improvement of the antigenic designs of Yersinia pseudotuberculosis. Curr Microbiol 11:89–92.

22. Wallner-Pendleton, E., and G. Cooper. 1983. Several outbreaks of Yersinia pseudotuberculosis in California turkey flocks. Avian Dis 27:524–526.

23. Wise, D.R., and P.K. Uppal. 1972. Osteomyelitis in turkeys caused by Yersinia pseudotuberculosis. J Med Microbiol 5:128–130.

SPIROCHETOSIS (BORRELIOSIS)

H. John Barnes

INTRODUCTION. Spirochetosis is a nonrelapsing, tick-borne borreliosis of avian species caused by the spirochete *Borrelia anserina*. It is usually an acute, septicemic disease characterized by marked illness, variable morbidity, and high mortality. In endemic areas, spirochetosis causes significant economic losses (69). Although closely related to *Borrelia* spp., causing disease in humans (6, 36), *B. anserina* is not known to infect humans or be of public health significance. However, birds may be important in the spread of Lyme disease (4), a borreliosis of humans caused by *B. burgdorferi*; mallards and bobwhite quail can be experimentally infected and shed this spirochete (7, 10). *B. burgdorferi* appears to be unique among borreliae in its ability to infect by natural means both mammals and birds. *B. anserina* and *B. burgdorferi* share common flagellar antigens, suggesting they are closely related to each other (74).

HISTORY. Spirochetosis was first described in 1891 (65) as a severe, septicemic disease of geese in Russia. In 1903, the disease was recognized in fowl in Brazil, and the role of fowl ticks as primary vectors was identified (46). Subsequently, spirochetosis was recognized in many countries, often associated with ticks, which were considered the primary means of introduction. Many names for the spirochete were published by various authors, resulting in numerous synonyms; and confusion with another tick-borne avian pathogen, *Aegyptianella pullorum*, led to considerable controversy about the spirochete's life cycle. Spirochetosis was first described in the United States among turkeys in California in 1946 (33). Although occasional additional outbreaks have been identified in the southwestern United States in fowls, turkeys, and pheasants, the disease has never been common. Recently, spirochetosis was diagnosed in a flock of game chickens in California (14).

INCIDENCE AND DISTRIBUTION. Spirochetosis occurs worldwide, most frequently in tropical and subtropical parts of the world where fowl ticks are common, and in extensive, free-range husbandry systems; occurrence in temperate areas or intensively managed flocks is uncommon (39, 64). Sporadic outbreaks of relatively mild disease occur in the southwestern United States.

ETIOLOGY. The causative organism is *B. anserina*. Synonyms include *Spirochaeta anserina* (65), *S. gallinarum, S. anatis,* and *Treponema anserinum.* The organism belongs in the order Spirochaetales and family Spirochaetaceae (6). For additional information on the genus *Borrelia*, see (6, 9).

Morphology and Staining. *B. anserina* is a highly motile, helical bacterium, with 5–8 spirals (Fig. 14.11) measuring about 6–30 × 0.3 μm. It will pass through a 0.45-μm filter (8). Borreliae have 15–22 flagella that are in the periplasmic space beneath the outer cell membrane and are attached subterminally near the ends of and overlap (30–44 flagella) at the middle of the spirochete. Borreliae differ from treponemes and leptospires, staining readily with ordinary aniline dyes in addition to Romanowsky-type stains and silver impregnation (6). Spirochetes can be readily identified in wet smears of blood or tissues by dark-field or phase microscopy (Fig. 14.12).

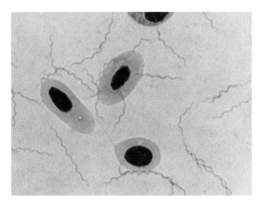

14.11. *Borrelia anserina* in blood film during acute stage of infection. Giemsa, ×1200.

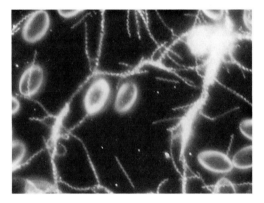

14.12. *Borrelia anserina* in plasma from infected chicken during terminal stages of spirochetosis. Note agglomeration of organisms. Dark-field,

Growth Requirements. Borreliae are microaerophilic, reproduce by binary fission, produce acid from glucose, and cannot be cultured on ordinary bacteriologic media. Recently, *B. anserina* has been successfully grown in Barbour–Stoenner–Kelly medium, but the organism lost its virulence within 12 passages (45). *B. anserina* is usually maintained in infected ticks, serially passaged by transfer of blood by any of several routes at 3- to 5-day intervals in chicks, or propagated in chicken (48) or turkey (49) embryos by yolk sac inoculation. Spirochetes are most numerous in embryo tissues, especially liver, blood, and membranes, with only few organisms in extraembryonic fluids uncontaminated by blood.

Resistance to Chemical and Physical Agents. *B. anserina* is not resistant outside the host. Fowl ticks serve as the reservoir for the or-

ganism. The spirochete can survive in carcasses for up to 31 days at 0 C (49) and can be stored for as long as 3–4 wk in serum at 4 C. Strains can be maintained for extended periods at -70 C, especially if 10–15% glycerol or dimethylsulfoxide is added to infective blood (28).

Strain Classification. Immunologically distinct strains of *B. anserina* exist, but no formal serotype classification scheme has been developed (15, 21, 40, 68). Multiple serotypes can often be identified in a given area, suggesting antigenic diversity may be considerable (72). Strains also differ considerably in virulence (14, 15, 16).

Pathogenicity. *B. anserina* is pathogenic for birds. Mammals except for rabbits and mice, which may have transient infections, are resistant to infection. Attempts to adapt *B. anserina* to intact or splenectomized mice failed after the 3rd passage (58). In chicks, intravenous (IV), intramuscular (IM), and subcutaneous inoculation give the shortest incubation periods and highest mortality (49). However, infection can be established by other routes including oral, ocular, nasal, and cloacal. Virulent strains are capable of penetrating unbroken skin (38).

PATHOGENESIS AND EPIZOOTIOLOGY

Natural and Experimental Hosts. Chickens, turkeys, pheasants, ducks, geese, and canaries have been naturally infected with *B. anserina* (41, 47). Local breeds of chickens are usually more resistant than are commercial strains (59). A gray parrot (*Psittacus erithacus*) developed spirochetosis and died shortly after being imported from Ghana (23), and a *Borrelia* sp. was recovered from ticks collected from egret rookeries in South Africa (29). A wide variety of birds can be experimentally infected (17, 49). Pigeons and, to a lesser degree, guinea fowl are relatively resistant to experimental infection (41), although 3.26% of urban pigeons in Italy were found to have *B. anserina* antibodies (25). Chicks <3 wk old are most susceptible; older birds tend to be more resistant (16). Infected day-old chicks experience a milder disease, lower mortality, and prolonged spirochetemia lasting 2–3 wk as compared with 3–5 days in older birds (13).

Transmission, Vectors, and Carriers. Spirochetosis can be transmitted by virtually any means whereby blood, excreta, or tissues from an infected live or recently dead bird comes in contact with a susceptible bird. Cannibalism, ingestion of blood or droppings, either directly or indirectly via contaminated feed and water, or use of syringes and needles for inoculating or sampling multiple birds are all means by which the disease can be transmitted. A severe outbreak occurred in goslings injected with contaminated antiserum prepared for passive protection against viral hepatitis, even though the serum had been filtered to remove bacteria (8).

Ornithophilic biting arthropods including mosquitoes (61, 63, 77) and fowl mites (*Dermanyssus*) (35) are capable of transmitting the spirochete.

Although a frequent means of spirochete transmission, especially among different groups of birds, soft ticks of the genus *Argas* serve in a much more important way as the main reservoirs of the organism (29). *B. anserina* is incapable of surviving in either the bird or environment for long periods; the organism must rely on the tick for its continued existence. Not all species of *Argas* function equally as well as biologic vectors of the spirochete; references to *A. persicus* in earlier literature may or may not have been that species (18). *A. sanchezi* and *A. arboreus* are other tick species known to transmit *B. anserina* (15, 18).

A. persicus is an important vector. After it feeds on a heavily infected chicken, spirochetes are numerous in the gut lumen initially, decline in numbers during the next week, became immobile by days 15–20, and die by day 20. Within 2 hr of feeding, spirochetes penetrate the gut wall and are present in hemolymph, where they increase in numbers during the next 7 days. By day 7, organisms can be found in the tick's tissues, particularly the central nerve mass, salivary glands, and gonads, where they remain at least 60 days (18). *B. anserina* survives transstadial molting from larva to adult and is transmitted transovarially from one generation to the next by suitable tick species (76). Infection rates in larvae from infected female ticks may be as high as 100% (76).

Ticks become infective 6–7 days after biting a host and can remain infective up to 488 days (41). Larval ticks ("seed ticks," "fleas") remain attached to the bird and feed for 4–5 days, in contrast to nymphs and adults, which are intermittent, nocturnal feeders that spend most of their time in cracks and crevices in the poultry house or environment. Each stage can survive for months to years without feeding. Tick activity increases with increasing temperature and humidity, and the spirochete develops most rapidly when ambient temperatures are >35 C. Although spirochete outbreaks are possible throughout the year, they are most common during warm, humid seasons. Birds can become infected from saliva introduced by the tick when bitten, or by ingesting infected ticks or ova (41).

Recovered birds are not carriers (19, 41). Organisms disappear from tissues at or shortly after they disappear from the circulation (20).

Incubation Period.   Incubation period depends on method of exposure, number of organisms in inoculum, and virulence of the *B. anserina* strain. Natural exposure via either tick bites or ingestion of infective blood or infected tick ova results in an incubation period of 3–12 days with 33–77% mortality. After IM or IV inoculation, it may be as short as 24 hr with 100% mortality (41).

Signs.   Birds infected with virulent strains of *B. anserina* are visibly sick, with cyanosis or pallor, especially of comb and wattles; ruffled feathers; droopy, huddled-up appearance; and greenish diarrhea, and are inactive and anorexic. Characteristic findings in spirochetosis are an abrupt, marked elevation in body temperature beginning shortly after infection, which, in turkeys, may reach or exceed 43 C (49), and a rapid loss of body weight that can exceed 20% during a 4–5 day course of illness. Body temperatures are elevated when spirochetes are in the circulation, even if their numbers are too low to detect by conventional methods. Affected birds pass fluid, green droppings containing excess bile and urates, probably resulting from anorexia, and have increased water consumption. Late in the disease, birds develop paresis or paralysis, become anemic, and are somnolent to comatose. Body temperatures are subnormal just prior to death. Birds recovering from the disease are often emaciated and have a temporary residual weakness or paralysis of one or both wings or legs. Infection with low virulent strains may be inapparent (16).

Clinical Pathology.   Anemia without intravascular hemolysis is a prominent and consistent finding in spirochetosis. Marked reductions in erythrocyte numbers, packed cell volumes, and hemoglobin, along with an increased erythrocyte sedimentation rate occur. Peak anemia occurs after spirochetes have disappeared from the circulation. There are significant differences between infected normal and dwarf chickens in degree of anemia, its development, and erythrocyte fragility (37). Both cold agglutinins (42) and soluble immune complexes (43) have been identified and associated with anemia. It is postulated that these adhere to erythrocytes, enhancing their phagocytosis by macrophages in tissues, especially spleen.

Slight leucocytosis with increased mononuclear cells and decreased granulocytes, and an increase in coagulation time, have been found in chickens with experimental spirochetosis (66). Both qualitative and quantitative changes in serum proteins also occur (52, 53). Alterations in serum chemistries of chickens with spirochetosis include increases in total protein, globulins, uric acid, glutamate-oxalacetate transaminase, creatinine, creatine, urea, and bilirubin; and decreases in alkaline phosphatase, albumin, total lipids, cholesterol, inorganic phosphorus (slight), chloride, and iron. Blood glucose is either unchanged or decreased, and acid phosphatase is unchanged (60, 66). Changes in the composition of blood from naturally infected ducks are similar to those of chickens (67).

Morbidity and Mortality. Morbidity and mortality are highly variable, ranging from 1–2% to 100%. Lowest rates occur in closed flocks with constant exposure to infected ticks. Adults possess high immunity that is passively transferred to their progeny. When these chicks become exposed at a time when their resistance allows an attenuated infection, they subsequently develop active immunity, which is continually boosted, protecting them from clinical disease. Highest rates occur either when susceptible birds are mixed with birds or are placed in an environment infested with infected ticks, or when tick-infested birds or equipment are mixed with susceptible birds. In either situation, explosive outbreaks may occur with high morbidity and mortality.

Gross Lesions. Marked enlargement and mottling of the spleen is the most characteristic lesion found in spirochetosis (Fig. 14.13). Splenomegaly, however, may not be as evident when birds are infected with low virulent strains or early in the disease (14). The liver may be enlarged and contain small hemorrhages and pale foci. Occasionally, marginal liver infarcts may be observed. Kidneys are swollen and pale with urates visible in ureters. Green, mucoid intestinal contents are usually present, and there is often variable amounts of hemor-

rhage, especially at the proventriculus–ventriculus junction. Occasionally, there is mild, fibrinous pericarditis, but other serous membranes are not involved (49). Extensive hemorrhage and muscle necrosis occurred in naturally infected pheasants (47).

Histopathology. Splenic lesions result from an inflammatory reaction characterized by exaggerated macrophage response, mononuclear–phagocyte system (MPS) hyperplasia, erythrophagocytosis, and hemosiderin deposits (5). Central areas of MPS foci undergo hyalinization at times. Massive areas of hemorrhage may be present in some birds. Diffuse lymphatic tissue undergoes rapid growth. Cells consist of young large and medium-sized lymphocytes and hemocytoblasts. Numerous mitotic figures are present. In poults, spirochetes occur in foci throughout the spleen but do not appear to be phagocytized by MPS cells. The liver is congested with increased periportal infiltrates of mixed lymphocytes, hemocytoblasts, and phagocytic cells with vacuolated cytoplasm. Erythrophagocytosis and hemosiderin is seen in Kupffer cells. Extramedullary hematopoiesis may be present. Silver stains reveal spirochetes in intercellular spaces and bile canaliculi. Organisms within hepatocytes are often fragmented or coiled, forming small rings. Lymphoplasmacytic infiltrates may be found in kidneys and intestinal lamina propria (14). A mild to moderate lymphocytic meningoencephalitis is occasionally present (49).

Immunity. Long-lasting active immunity follows recovery from disease or immunization (24, 69). Active immunity is serotype-specific; infection with other *B. anserina* serotypes can occur in recovered or vaccinated birds (50). Passive maternal immunity capable of providing resistance to spirochetosis for as long as 5–6 wk was recognized as early as 1906 (44). Hyperimmune serum prepared in chickens or goats protects birds against challenge for up to 3 wk (51). Prior inoculation of chickens with *B. theileri,* a spirochete of ruminants, did not provide protection against *B. anserina* infection (75).

DIAGNOSIS. A clinical diagnosis of spirochetosis can be made on finding characteristic lesions in birds with signs consistent with the disease. Presence of larval ticks, most often found on the underneath side of wing webs; presence of punctate hemorrhages from tick bites, especially on the shanks; or presence of ticks in the bird's environment increases the likelihood of spirochetosis in severely ill birds (64).

Confirmation of spirochetosis requires demonstration of *B. anserina* or its antigen. During clini-

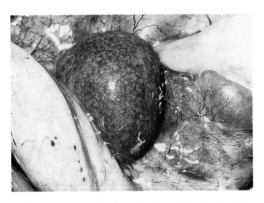

14.13. Mottled spleen in a chicken with spirochetosis. This lesion is characteristic of the disease caused by highly virulent strains of *Borrelia anserina* but may be absent when infection is with low virulent spirochetes. Splenic changes also occur in other avian species but may appear different from those in chickens depending on amount of necrosis and hemorrhage. There are also a few serosal hemorrhages on the proventriculus of this bird.

cal illness, spirochetes can be found in stained blood or organ smears, wet mounts examined by dark-field or phase microscopy or by immunofluorescence. Stained blood smears are best used when only a small quantity of blood is available, time between blood collection and examination will be long, specialized equipment and reagents for dark-field or fluorescent microscopy are unavailable, or a permanent specimen of the sample is needed. Giemsa stain is most often used, but the organism stains readily with most aniline and Romanowsky dyes. For demonstrating spirochetes in tissue sections, silver impregnation procedures are used (14, 26).

Dark-field microscopy is the diagnostic method of choice because of its ease, rapidity, and accuracy. Autolysis produces background staining in tissue smears, which may obscure spirochetes, making wet mounts preferable for identifying the organism from carcasses. Early in the disease, spirochetemia may be so low that detection of the organism is difficult. *B. anserina* can be concentrated in the buffy coat (32, 47). Examination of buffy coat smears is useful in epidemiologic studies to identify early infections or infection with low virulent strains. A simple procedure used by the author is the following: fill microhematocrit tubes with blood, centrifuge for 5 min in a microhematocrit centrifuge, score tubes between packed red cells and buffy coat with a diamond-tipped pen, break the tube, expel buffy coat and plasma onto a slide leaving buffy coat intact, place cover slip on wet mount and gently press it over buffy coat pellet to spread pellet to about twice its original size, allow slide to sit at room temperature for at least 5 min, examine periphery of buffy coat for spirochetes using dark-field microscopy. If present, organisms move into the plasma from the buffy coat pellet and are easily recognized.

Spirochetes undergo agglomeration followed by lysis in the terminal stages of the disease and may no longer be recognizable in blood or tissues. In these cases, spirochetal antigens can often be identified in liver or spleen by serologic tests (1, 2, 70) or immunofluorescence (30, 73).

Spirochetes can be cultured by inoculating embryos or chicks with infective blood or organ suspensions. Six-day-old embryonated eggs from spirochete-free hens inoculated via the yolk sac are preferred for embryo culture. Live embryos are examined 6 days after inoculation. Bleeding into chorioallantoic fluids is essential if spirochetes are to be found (48). Chicks free of spirochetal antibodies less than 3 wk are most susceptible to infection. Bursectomy or dexamethasone treatment may be necessary for low virulent strains to grow to detectable numbers (16).

Serology. Several serologic tests have been developed to identify antibodies in immune birds including serum plate agglutination test (27), slide agglutination and immobilization tests (71), agar gel precipitin test (11), and indirect fluorescent antibody test (55). Plate agglutination, tube agglutination, and spirochete immobilization tests have equal sensitivity when used for both hyperimmune and convalescent serums (12). Spirochetal antibodies can be readily detected in yolk of eggs laid by immune hens (3, 22).

Differential Diagnosis. Spirochetosis can resemble other poultry diseases characterized by acute septicemia including fowl typhoid, fowl cholera, and colisepticemia; acute viral diseases including viscerotropic, velogenic Newcastle disease, highly virulent influenza, and Marek's disease. The characteristic lesions of spirochetosis; inability to culture *Salmonella, Pasteurella,* or *Escherichia coli*; absence of respiratory disease and extensive hemorrhages in gastrointestinal tract and other tissues typical of virulent Newcastle disease and influenza infections; and absence of ocular, neural, or visceral tumors should allow distinction of spirochetosis from similar diseases.

TREATMENT. Initially a variety of arsenicals were used to treat birds affected with spirochetosis; antibiotics have superseded arsenicals as the treatment of choice. *B. anserina* is sensitive to most antibiotics including penicillin, chloramphenicol, kanamycin, streptomycin, tylosin, and tetracyclines (8, 34, 54). In addition, numerous reports have been published concerning the value of locally available or experimental antimicrobials. Intramuscular injections of penicillin at 20,000 IU/bird given 3 times in 24 hr or 20 mg oxytetracycline given for 2 days represent currently used treatment regimens (69). Placing affected flocks on water containing approximately 1 g oxytetracycline/gal drinking water for 3 days and treating severely affected birds with an intracrop gavage of 5 mg oxytetracycline in 5% glucose were found to be highly effective by the author.

PREVENTION AND CONTROL. Spirochetosis is best prevented in endemic areas by not introducing tick-infested birds into clean flocks nor introducing susceptible birds into infested flocks or housing where infected birds were once kept. Adult ticks can remain alive without feeding and carry the spirochete for as long as 3 yr.

Once the tick is present, it is extremely difficult to eradicate. The only complete success had by the author resulted when houses were depopulated and burned. Larval ticks can be controlled on birds by dipping them in 0.5% malathion. Dipping is more effective than using insecticide dusts. Dusts are helpful when used in dusting baths. High-pressure spraying of the house and environment, paying particular attention to cracks, crevices, and other places where ticks hide, with 3% malathion at monthly intervals helps keep ticks at low levels. Insecticide laced "paints" and "pastes" can control ticks if vigorously used (62). Attempts to "tick-proof" roosts by suspending them from wire and keeping grease spread on the wire, or by placing roost legs in oil-filled containers, require almost constant attention to be effective. The same is true for "tick-proof" houses surrounded by an oil-filled moat. If affected birds are roosting in trees, cutting and burning the trees and simultaneously dipping birds may be successful.

Immunization. Vaccination is practiced in areas where spirochetosis is prevalent. They are best prepared from local strains where they are to be used (69). Birds are usually inoculated at 8–10 wk of age (69). Vaccines are inactivated with formalin or phenol and prepared from lysates of blood, tissues, or embryos infected with *B. anserina* (31, 56, 57). Both lyophilized and liquid products are available. Immunity is type-specific; an autogenous or polyvalent vaccine containing multiple serotypes occurring in a given area may be necessary to provide full protection (72). Deliberate infection followed by antibiotic treatment 3 days later has also been used to induce immunity (54).

REFERENCES

1. Al-Attar, M.A., and F.M. Jahanly. 1974. Demonstration by immunodiffusion agar-gel test of Borrelia anserina antigens in the organs of infected chickens. Avian Dis 18:463–466.

2. Al-Hilly, J.N.A. 1969. Immunodiffusion agar-gel test for demonstration of Borrelia anserina antigen produced by liver of infected chickens. Am J Vet Res 30:1877–1880.

3. Al-Hilly, J.N.A. 1971. Immobilization and immunodiffusion tests for determination of antibodies against spirochetosis in the yolk of convalescent fowls. Avian Dis 15:419–421.

4. Anderson, J.F., R.C. Johnson, L.A. Magnarelli, and F.W. Hyde. 1986. Involvement of birds in the epidemiology of the Lyme disease agent Borrelia burgdorferi. Infect Immun 51:394–396.

5. Bandopadhyay, A.C., and J.L. Vegad. 1983. Observations on the pathology of experimental avian spirochaetosis. Res Vet Sci 35:138–144.

6. Barbour, A.G., and S.F. Hayes. 1986. Biology of Borrelia species. Microbiol Rev 50:381–400.

7. Bishop, K.L., M.I. Khan, and S.W. Nielsen. 1994. Experimental infection of northern bobwhite quail with Borrelia burgdorferi. J Wildl Dis 30:506–513.

8. Bok, R., Y. Samberg, M. Rubina, and A. Hadani. 1975. Studies on fowl spirochaetosis—survival of Borrelia anserina at various temperatures and its sensitivity to antibiotics. Refu Vet 32:147–153.

9. Burgdorfer, W., and T.G. Schwan. 1991. Borrelia. In A. Balows, W.J. Hausler, Jr., K.L. Herrmann, H.D. Isenberg, and H.J. Shadomy (eds.). Manual of Clinical Microbiology, 5th ed. American Society of Microbiology, Washington, DC, pp. 560–566.

10. Burgess, E.C. 1989. Experimental inoculation of mallard ducks (Anas platyrhynchos platyrhynchos) with Borrelia burgdorferi. J Wildl Dis 25:99–102.

11. Chatterjee, A., and A.N. Sawhney. 1971. Diagnosis of fowl spirochaetosis by agar-gel-precipitation test. Indian J Anim Sci 41:727–730.

12. Chatterjee, A., and A.N. Sawhney. 1971. Serological studies on experimental fowl spirochaetosis. Indian J Anim Sci 41:1151–1153.

13. Choudhary, C.R., and K.N.P. Rao. 1985. Studies on clinicopathological changes in fowl spirochaetosis in young chicks. Indian Vet J 62:465–468.

14. Cooper, G.L., and A.A. Bickford. 1993. Spirochetosis in California game chickens. Avian Dis 37:1167–1171.

15. DaMassa, A.J., and H.E. Adler. 1978. Avian spirochetosis: natural transmission by Argas (Persicargas) sanchezi (Ixodoidea:Argasidae) and existence of different serologic and immunologic types of Borrelia anserina in the United States. Am J Vet Res 40:154–157.

16. DaMassa, A.J., and H.E. Adler. 1979. Avian spirochaetosis: enhanced recognition of mild strains of Borrelia anserina with bursectomized and dexamethasone-treated chickens. J Comp Pathol 89:413–420.

17. DaMassa, A.J., and H.E. Adler. 1980. Avian spirochetosis: general comments and preliminary data on the experimental disease in budgerigars. Proc 29th West Poult Dis Conf, pp. 83–85.

18. Diab, F.M., and Z.R. Soliman. 1977. An experimental study of Borrelia anserina in four species of Argas ticks. 1. Spirochete localization and densities. Z Parasitenkd 53:201–212.

19. Dickie, C.W., and J. Barrera. 1964. A study of the carrier state of avian spirochetosis in the chicken. Avian Dis 8:191–195.

20. Djankov, I., I. Soumrov, T. Lozeva, and P. Penev. 1970. Persistence and excretion of Treponema anserinum (Sakharoff, 1891) in hens. Zentralbl Veterinaermed [B] 17:544–548.

21. Djankov, I., I. Soumrov, and T. Lozeva. 1972. Use of the immunofluorescence method for the serotype identification of Borrelia anserina (Sakharoff, 1891) strains. Zentralbl Veterinaermed [B] 19:221–225.

22. Dutta, G.N., M.L. Mehta, and A.R. Muley. 1977. Studies on immunity in fowl spirochaetosis. Indian J Anim Sci 47:554–558.

23. Ehrsam, H. von. 1977. Borreliose (spirochaetose) bei einem graupapagei (Psittacus erithacus). Schweiz Arch Tierheilkd 119:41–43.

24. El Dardiry, A.H. 1945. Studies on avian spirochetosis in Egypt. Min Agric Tech Sci Serv Bull 243:1–78.

25. Fabbi, M., V. Sambri, A. Marangoni, S. Magnino, F.S. Basano, R. Cevenini, and C. Genchi. 1995. Borrelia in pigeons: no serological evidence of Borrelia burgdorferi infection. J Vet Med [B] 42:503–507.

26. Felsenfeld, O. 1971. Borrelia Strains, Vectors, Human and Animal Borreliosis. Warren H. Green, Inc., St. Louis, MO.

27. Garg, R.R., and O.P. Gautam. 1971. Serological diagnosis of fowl spirochetosis. Avian Dis 15:1–6.

28. Ginawi, M.A., and A.M. Shommein. 1980. Preservation of Borrelia anserina at different temperatures. Bull Anim Health Prod Afr 28:221–223.

29. Gothe, R., and W. Schrecke. 1972. Zur epizootiologishen bedeutung von Persicarges-zecken der huhner in Transvaal. Berl Munch Tierarztl Woshenschr 85:9–11.

30. Gross, W.M., and M.R. Ball. 1964. Use of fluorescein-labeled antibody to study Borrelia anserina infection (avian spirochetosis) in the chicken. Am J Vet Res 25:1734–1739.

31. Hart, L. 1963. Spirochaetosis in fowls: studies on immunity. Aust Vet J 39:187–191.

32. Higgins, A.R. 1986. Demonstrating Borellia [sic] anserina: "A can of worms." Vet Rec 119:120.

33. Hoffman, H.A., and T.W. Jackson. 1946. Spirochetosis in turkeys. J Am Vet Med Assoc 109:481–486.

34. Hsiang, C.M., and A. Packchanian. 1951. A comparison of eleven antibiotics in the treatment of Borrelia anserina infection (spirochetosis) in young chicks. Tex Rep Biol Med 9:34–45.

35. Hungerford, T.G., and L. Hart. 1937. Fowl tick fever

(spirochaetosis) also transmitted by common red mite. Agric Gaz 48:591–592.

36. Hyde, F.W. and R.C. Johnson. 1986. Genetic analysis of Borrelia. Zentralbl Bakteriol Hyg Abt 263:119–122.

37. Joshi, A.G., J.L. Soni, and A.G. Khan. 1980. Spirochaetosis anaemia and its influence on erythrocyte size in normal and dwarf chickens. Indian J Anim Sci 50:753–756.

38. Kapur, H.R. 1940. Transmission of spirochaetosis through agents other than Argas persicus. Indian J Vet Sci Anim Husb 10:354–360.

39. Kaschula, V.R. 1961. A comparison of the spectrum of disease in village and in modern poultry flocks in Nigeria. Bull Epizoot Dis Afr 9:397–407.

40. Kligler, I.J., D. Hermoni, and M. Perek. 1938. Studies on fowl spirochetosis. II. Presence of serologically differentiated types of spirochetes. J Comp Pathol Ther 51:206–212.

41. Knowles, R., B.M. Das Gupta, and B.C. Basu. 1932. Studies in avian spirochaetosis. Indian Med Res Mem 22:1–113.

42. Lad, P.L., and J.L. Soni. 1983. Role of cold agglutinin (CA) in anaemia production in acute avian spirochaetosis. Indian J Anim Sci 53:937–943.

43. Lad, P.L., and J.L. Soni. 1983. Soluble spirochaete antigen-antibody immune complex in plasma of Borrelia anserina-infected chickens. Indian J Anim Sci 53:538–541.

44. Levaditi, C. 1906. La spirillose des embryons de poulet dans ses rapports avec la treponemose hereditaire de l'homme. Ann Inst Pasteur 20:924.

45. Levine, J.F., M.J. Dykstra, W.L. Nicholson, R.L. Walker, and G. Massey. 1990. Attenuation of Borrelia anserina by serial passage in liquid medium. Res Vet Sci 48:64–69.

46. Marchoux, E., and A. Salimbeni. 1903. La spirillose des poules. Ann Inst Pasteur 17:569–580.

47. Mathey, W.J., Jr., and P.J. Siddle. 1955. Spirochetosis in pheasants. J Am Vet Med Assoc 126:123–126.

48. McKercher, D.G. 1950. The propagation of Borrelia anserina in embryonated eggs employing the yolk sac technique. J Bacteriol 59:446–447.

49. McNeil, E., W.R. Hinshaw, and R.E. Kissling. 1949. A study of Borrelia anserina infection (spirochetosis) in turkeys. J Bacteriol 57:191–206.

50. Mehta, M.L., and A.R. Muley. 1969. Efficacy of spirochaetosis vaccine prepared from the local (Jabalpur) strain of Borrelia gallinarum. Indian J Anim Sci 39:225–230.

51. Morcos, Z., O.A. Zaki, and R. Zaki. 1946. A concise investigation of fowl spirochetosis in Egypt. J Am Vet Med Assoc 109:112–116.

52. Pavlow, P., Y. Dumanov, Y. Denev, M. Kolev, R. Stoyanova, T. Loseva, and I. Djankov. 1973. A study of parasite-host immunological interrelations. IV. Investigation of the protein profiles in lambs, cats and birds in experimental spirochetosis and leptospirosis. Zentralbl Veterinaermed [B] 20:230–240.

53. Perk, K., and I. Hort. 1966. Paper electrophoretic studies of the serum proteins of chicks during experimental spirochetosis. Avian Dis 10:208–215.

54. Phulan, M.S., A.N. Sokolov, S.N. Buriro, W.M. Bhatti, and I.A. Soomro. 1988. Formation of immunity with tylan against spirochaetosis in poultry. Pakistan Vet J 8:42–43.

55. Prudovsky, S., A. Hadani, M. Rubina, and A. Sklair. 1978. The use of the indirect fluorescent antibody technique in avian spirochaetosis. Avian Pathol 7:421–425.

56. Rao, S.B.V. 1958. Spirochaetosis in Poultry. Indian Council on Agricultural Research, New Delhi, Research Series No. 18.

57. Rao, M.L.V., and J.L. Soni. 1982. Augmentation of haemo-tissue vaccine doses out-turn through blood transfusion in Borrelia anserina infected chickens. Zentralbl Veterinaermed [B] 29:408–410.

58. Rao, M.L.V., and J.L. Soni. 1986. Preliminary studies on murinization of Borrelia anserina. Indian J Anim Sci 56:1187–1189.

59. Rashid, J., and A. Ali. 1991. Comparative study of pathogenicity of experimentally produced Borrelia anserina infection in commercial broiler and desi chicks. Pakistan J Zool 23:361–362.

60. Rivetz, B., E. Bogin, Y. Weisman, J. Avidar, and A. Hadani. 1977. Changes in the biochemical composition of blood in chickens infected with Borrelia anserina. Avian Pathol 6:343–351.

61. Roberts, J.A. 1961. Experimental transmission of Borrelia anserina (Sakharoff 1891) by Aedes aegypti. Nature 191:1225.

62. Rodey, M.V., and J.L. Soni. 1977. Epidemiology of spirochaetosis in chickens: effective measures for control of ticks—Argas persicus. Poult Guide 14:35–37.

63. Rubina, M., Y. Braverman, and M. Malkinson. 1975. On the possible transmission of Borrelia anserina (Sakharoff 1891) by mosquitoes. Refu Vet 32:16–18.

64. Sa'idu, L., R.I.S. Agbede, and A.P. Abdu. 1995. Prevalence of avian spirochaetosis in Zaria (1980–1989). Isr J Vet Med 50:39–40.

65. Sakharoff, M.N. 1891. Spirochaeta anserina et la septicemie des oies. Ann Inst Pasteur 5:564–566.

66. Soliman, M.K., A.A.S. Ahmed, S. El Amrousi, and I.H. Moustafa. 1966. Cytological and biochemical studies on the blood constituents of normal and spirochete-infected chickens. Avian Dis 10:394–400.

67. Soliman, M.K., S. El Amrousi, and A.A.S. Ahmed. 1966. Cytological and biochemical studies of the blood of normal and spirochaete-infected ducks. Zentralbl Veterinaermed [B] 13:82.

68. Soni, J.L., and A.G. Joshi. 1980. A note on strain variation in Akola and Jabalpur strains of Borrelia anserina. Zentralbl Veterinaermed [B] 27:70–72.

69. Supekar, P.G. 1989. Avian spirochaetosis is a perpetuating menace. Poultry 5:40–41.

70. Verma, K.C., and B.S. Malik. 1968. Diagnosis of spirochaetosis of poultry by gel diffusion test. Indian Vet J 45:460–462.

71. Verma, K.C., and B.S. Malik. 1968. Diagnosis of spirochaetosis of poultry by slide agglutination and spirochaete immobilization tests. Curr Sci 37:170–171.

72. Verma, R.K., A.R. Muley, and K.N.P. Rao. 1991. Some observations on the strain variation of Borrelia anserina. Indian Vet J 68:818–821.

73. Wadalkar, B.G., and J.L. Soni. 1982. Use of fluorescent antibody technique for the detection of spirochaete antigen in prepatent, peak and post-spirochaetemic phase organs. Indian J Anim Sci 52:776–781.

74. Walker, R.L., R.T. Greene, W.L. Nicholson, and J.F. Levine. 1989. Shared flagellar epitopes of Borrelia burgdorferi and Borrelia anserina. Vet Microbiol 19:361–371.

75. Wouda, W., Tj.W. Schillhorn van Veen, and H.J. Barnes. 1975. Borrelia anserina in chickens previously exposed to Borrelia theileri. Avian Dis 19:209–210.

76. Zaher, M.A., Z.R. Soliman, and F.M. Diab. 1977. An experimental study of Borrelia anserina in four species of Argas ticks. 2. Transstadial survival and transovarial transmission. Z Parasitenkd 53:213–223.

77. Zuelzer, M. 1936. Culex, a new vector of Spirochaeta gallinarum. J Trop Med Hyg 39:204.

AVIAN INTESTINAL SPIROCHETOSIS

David E. Swayne

INTRODUCTION. Avian intestinal spirochetosis (AIS) is a subacute to chronic, nonsepticemic intestinal disease characterized by spirochetes in the cecum and/or rectum, and variable clinical illness, morbidity, and mortality. *Borrelia anserina* is the spirochetal etiology of nonrelapsing, tick-borne, acute septicemic borreliosis and is related to, but distinct from, avian intestinal spirochetes (see preceding section in this chapter on spirochetosis).

Intestinal spirochetes are a heterogenous group of spiral bacteria that colonize the large intestine of a variety of mammalian and avian hosts including swine, humans, and poultry. Colonization may be part of the normal intestinal flora or can be associated with, or the cause of, significant clinical disease (8, 45, 52, 57, 59, 61). Avian intestinal spirochetosis has clinical signs, gross lesions, and histopathology to intestinal spirochetosis similar to those of mammals. Infection of 1-day-old chicks with swine and human intestinal spirochetes has been used in comparative studies to determine mechanisms of colonization and pathogenicity of intestinal spirochetes, including those from poultry (2, 13, 54, 55, 56).

HISTORY. Spiral bacteria have been identified by light microscopy in the digestive tracts of humans and animals since 1884, but it was not until development of the electron microscope, indirect fluorescent antibody tests, and specific culture techniques that spirochetes were consistently and definitively distinguished from other spiral-shaped bacteria, e.g., *Campylobacter* spp. and *Helicobacter* spp. (21). Swine dysentery, a mucohemorrhagic diarrheal disease of young pigs caused by *Serpulina* (*Treponema*) *hyodysenteriae,* has been the most extensively and thoroughly studied of all intestinal spirochetal diseases (22). Intestinal spirochetal infections of birds, except for three early reports (16, 24, 37), is of more recent description (8, 17, 59).

In 1910, Fantham (16) described "*Spirochaeta lovati*" as an intestinal spirochete in the cecal lumina of normal young and adult grouse in Great Britain. Spirochetes of three morphologic types were visualized in cecal droppings from both clinically normal and sick chickens obtained from Baltimore live-poultry markets in 1930 (24). Subsequently, large caseous nodules with associated spirochetes were sporadically identified in cecal walls of turkeys, chickens, and pheasants in the United States (37).

Since 1986, AIS has been reported in commercial laying chickens in the Netherlands (8), England (17), and the United States (59). In 1990, AIS with severe cecal lesions (necrotizing typhlitis) causing high mortality was identified in common rheas (*Rhea americana*) in the United States (45). Sporadic cases of AIS also have been identified in domestic turkeys, broilers (11), and broiler breeders in recent years.

INCIDENCE AND DISTRIBUTION. Spirochetes infect the ceca and rectum of a variety of avian species throughout the world. In poultry, cases of AIS have been identified on three continents: Europe, North America, and Australia. Necrotizing typhlitis in rheas is widespread in the United States; affected birds have been identified in Arkansas, Alabama, California, Missouri, Nebraska, Ohio, Oregon, South Carolina, and Texas (20, 58).

The incidence of intestinal spirochete infection and disease varies with the avian species and methods used for demonstrating spirochetes. The incidence of AIS in poultry in the United States is unknown, but the disease is routinely diagnosed in Europe (46). In a European survey, 27.6% of chicken flocks with intestinal disorders were positive for intestinal spirochetes, while only 4.4% of flocks without enteric signs were positive (10). In a zoologic survey of various bird species in the United States, the highest infection rates were found in common rheas (32%) and birds of the order Anseriformes (46%) (53).

ETIOLOGY

Classification. Historically, spirochetes were taxonomically classified based on morphologic characteristics, motility, host species, and anatomic location of colonization. Avian isolates of the early 1900's such as *Spirochaeta gallinarum, Spirochaeta lovati, Treponema caeci-gallorum, Spironema caeci-gallorum,* and *Fusi-spirochaeta caeci-gallorum* (24, 37) were classified and named based on these historical criteria. With the recent development of more sophisticated and discriminating methods that analyze basic genetic and phenotypic information such as DNA, RNA, and cytosol isoenzymes, the historical method of classification has come under increased scrutiny. Although most avian and mammalian intestinal spirochetes still remain unclassified, genotypic and phenotypic information has enabled determination of the relatedness between classified and unclassified spirochetes, forming the foundation for future taxonomy.

Spirochetes are classified into a single order (Spirochaetes), two families (Spirochaetaceae and Leptospiraceae), and eight genera (6, 44, 50). Seven of the genera can colonize animal hosts. The family Leptosiraceae has two genera, *Leptonema* and *Leptospira*; only the latter contains pathogenic species. The family Spirochaetaceae has six genera, of which *Borrelia, Serpulina,* and *Treponema* have species pathogenic for animals, whereas *Brachyspira, Christispira* and *Spirochaeta* do not. Spirochetes that infect the large intestines of avian species are a heterogenous group. Based on rRNA gene restriction analysis, multilocus enzyme electrophoresis (MEE), and 16s rRNA sequencing, one avian intestinal spirochete has been taxonomically classified as *S. hyodysenteriae* (29). The remaining avian intestinal spirochetes are unclassified but have morphologic and biochemical features that indicate placement in either the genus *Serpulina* or *Treponema* (44, 51, 50, 61).

Current comparative MEE data for human-, swine-, and avian-origin intestinal spirochetes suggests occurrence of seven groups (32, 33, 34, 41, 61). Five groups either have approved classifications or provisional designations. Avian spirochetes have been identified in four groups (Table 14.4); *S. hyodysenteriae,* "*S. intermedius,*" *S. pilosicoli* ("*Angullina coli,*") and an unnamed group of chicken spirochetes (91-1207/c1 and 91-1207/c2) with characteristics intermediate between *S. innocens* and "*S. murdochii*" (38, 39, 61). Ribosomal RNA gene restriction analysis confirmed that chicken C1 and C2 spirochetes were different from *S. hyodysenteriae, S. innocens,* and six other porcine spirochetes (39, 61).

Morphology and Staining. Intestinal spirochetes of poultry are gram-negative, helix-shaped bacteria with diameters ranging from 0.25 to 0.6 µm, lengths from 7 to 19 µm, amplitudes from 0.45 to 0.79 µm, and wavelengths from 2.7 to 3.7 µm (8, 52, 61). They stain brown with silver-impregnation staining techniques, blue with Wright's-Giemsa stains, and are readily identified in wet mounts by dark-field microscopy. Each spirochete cell contains a central protoplasmic cylinder, multiple periplasmic flagella (axial filaments), and an outer envelope (outer sheath) (Fig. 14.14) (6). The periplasmic flagella are endocellular and divided into two equal sets. Each set originates from opposite poles of the protoplasmic cylinder and overlaps with the other set in the middle of the cell. This unique anatomic feature is responsible for numeric variations in periplasmic flagella reported for each spirochete species, especially if counts are based on transverse ultrathin sections of bacterial cells. Optimally, periplasmic flagellar numbers should be reported as a ratio between end:middle:end numbers determined from negative-stained, transmission electron–microscope preparations. For avian spirochetes, the periplasmic flagella ratios are most commonly either 8:16:8 or 5:10:5 (Table 14.4).

Rotation of periplasmic flagella between the outer membrane and protoplasmic cylinder results in movement of spirochete cells (3, 7). These morphologic features and type of motility permit spirochetes to traverse highly viscous liquids, such as mucus, that would immobilize externally flagellated (e.g., *Escherichia coli, Salmonella typhimurium*) and nonflagellated bacteria (7).

Growth Requirements. Avian intestinal spirochetes are anaerobic (61). Primary isolation has been accomplished on various solid media systems used to isolate swine intestinal spirochetes (1, 8, 17, 27, 31, 49, 59, 65). Typically, media contain

Table 14.4. Morphologic and biochemical properties of avian intestinal spirochetes

Characteristic	Species or provisional designation			
	Serpulina hyodysenteriae	"*Serpulina intermedius*"	"*Angullina coli*"	Unclassified poultry isolates
Host origin	Common rheas	Chickens	Chickens, wild ducks	Chickens
Continent	North America	Europe, Australia	North America	North America
Pathogenicity	Severe	Moderate	Mild to apathogenic	Mild to apathogenic
Colonization of cecal epithelial surface	Random	Random	Right angles	Random
Periplasmic flagellar ratio	8:16:8	8:16:8	5:10:5	8:16:8
Hemolysis pattern	Strong	Intermediate	Weak	Weak
Indole production	+	?	−	−
Cytosolic enzymes				
α-galactosidase	−	?	+	+
α-glucosidase	+	+	+	−
API ZYM profile	14.0.4.10.1	?	14.0.4.11.1	14.0.4.3.1

Sources: (8, 33, 38, 52, 61, 65)

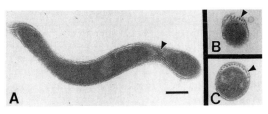

14.14. Unclassified C1 chicken spirochete. Spirochete cell is helically shaped on longitudinal orientation (*A*). On transverse sections, an end (*B*) and the middle (*C*) of spirochete cells have 8 and 16 periplasmic flagella (*arrows*), respectively. (*Infection and Immunity*)

a blood agar base, such as trypticase soy agar with 5–10% sheep blood, and one to five selective antibiotics (i.e., spectinomycin, rifampin, spiramycin, vancomycin, and/or colistin). Antibiotics inhibit growth of nonspirochete enteric anaerobes. Incubation is at 37–42 C for a minimum of 10 days; however, growth usually occurs in 2–5 days.

Colony Morphology. Because of the vigorous motility, spirochetes spread rapidly over agar plates; discrete colonies do not form. With some isolates, growth is detectible by hemolysis of blood agar. With nonhemolytic or slow-growing weakly ß-hemolytic spirochetes, however, areas of growth are evident as a dull sheen on the agar surface. Bacterial growth should be confirmed as spirochetes by characteristic motility on wet mounts using darkfield microscopy or morphology as visualized in Wright's-Giemsa or Gram's stained smears.

Biochemical Properties. Avian intestinal spirochetes contain alkaline and acid phosphatases, esterase, esterase lipase, ß-galactosidase, and phosphorylase (52). Differences in hemolysis patterns, indole production, and presence or absence of α-galactosidase and α-glucosidase activities are used to categorize avian and mammalian intestinal spirochete isolates and to predict their potential for causing disease (Table 14.4). Use of an API ZYM system and numerical five-digit coding system has been useful in categorizing avian and mammalian isolates (26, 52).

Resistance to Chemical and Physical Agents. *S. hyodysenteriae* survives in feces for 60 days, especially in waste pits. Warm temperatures above 15 C decrease survival time of spirochetes in contaminated soils. Most disinfectants are efficacious against spirochetes if surfaces are first cleaned to remove protective organic materials (22).

Antigenic Structure and Potential Virulence Factors. Mechanisms of pathogenicity from intestinal spirochetes are incompletely understood, but virulence factors are important determinants of colonization, lesion development, and disease production. Development of AIS probably requires multiple virulence factors as has been shown in mammalian intestinal spirochetosis. The hemolysin group of proteins are a major virulence factor involved in pathogenicity of *S. hyodysenteriae*. Hemolysins induce epithelial cell degeneration and necrosis (36). Other potential toxins include lipopolysaccharide (36, 42), an uncharacterized inhibitor of sodium and chloride transport across enterocyte cell membranes, and a trypsinlike protease (62). In addition to toxins, the vigorous motility of spirochetes in the mucus gel of the large bowel may give them an advantage in survival and proliferation. Furthermore, proliferating spirochetes secrete waste products that inhibit growth of some and enhance growth of other flora. Such changes in ecologic balance of bacteria may result in alterations of fluid absorption by changing the content of organic ions that are excreted and/or absorbed.

Pathogenicity. Based on experimental studies and naturally occurring infections, avian intestinal spirochetes can be divided into three pathotypes: 1) severely pathogenic, 2) mildly to moderately pathogenic, and 3) subclinical or apathogenic (Table 14.4). In vivo testing in 1-day-old chickens has been used to study the pathogenesis of swine-origin *S. hyodysenteriae* infections (2, 54, 56). This also may be a useful method for determining the potential of avian intestinal spirochetes to produce disease (60, 61). Pathogenicity of avian and mammalian intestinal spirochetes varies with spirochete species, route of inoculation, age of host, host species, environmental stressors, and presence of certain bacterial microflora in the intestines (57, 59). Experimentally, pathogenicity of avian intestinal spirochetes is greatest when given via crop gavage to 1-day-old birds (57, 61). Pathogenicity of *S. hyodysenteriae* is greater for rheas than it is for chickens or turkeys (57). Environmental stressors such as molting and poor diets increase severity of avian intestinal spirochete infections (59). Presence of other anaerobic bacteria in the large intestine has been shown to be a prerequisite for full expression of *S. hyodysenteriae* pathogenicity (23, 57, 67).

PATHOGENESIS AND EPIZOOTOLOGY

Natural and Experimental Hosts. Intestinal spirochetes have been shown to infect a variety of avian species including chickens (24, 59), common rheas (45), grouse (16), pheasants (37), turkeys

(37), and wild birds (53). Experimental studies have shown that intestinal spirochetes isolated from wild birds can infect chickens, turkeys, and ducks (4, 52). Swine-origin and rhea-origin *S. hyodysenteriae* can experimentally infect poultry (2, 54, 56, 57), but no cases of naturally occurring disease or infection of poultry, except rheas, have been confirmed. Intestinal spirochete infections have not been reported in ostriches.

Transmission, Carriers, and Vectors. Intestinal spirochetes are transmitted by the fecal–oral route. Ticks and biting insects are not transmission vectors. In fact, parenteral inoculation of *S. hyodysenteriae* into chickens does not result in systemic or intestinal infections (57). Rats, mice, flies, or other animal species can serve as mechanical vectors.

Incubation Period. The incubation period of AIS is variable. Dose of organism and secondary environmental factors have a profound influence on incubation time. Experimentally, disease signs can occur in chickens as early as 5 days after inoculation (61).

Pathobiology of Avian Intestinal Spirochetes. Intestinal spirochetes are most frequently identified in the ceca, but they occasionally can be found in the rectum and ileum. Duodenum and jejunum are not sites of colonization. In ceca, spirochetes primarily are found in crypt lumina and, to a lesser extent, the cecal contents adjacent to villous epithelium. Spirochetes can persistently infect ceca (12, 14). In one experimental study, spirochetes were detected in cecal droppings until termination of the experiment at 23 wk postinfection (15).

Naturally occurring or experimental infections of birds with intestinal spirochetes can result in 1) subclinical infection, 2) mild-to-moderate clinical disease, or 3) severe clinical disease.

SUBCLINICAL DISEASE. Most spirochetes identified in ceca of wild birds, especially waterfowl, are not associated with enteric disease in the original host species and are considered apathogenic. In addition, cecal spirochetes have been identified in clinically normal chickens (24). However, inoculation of 1-day-old chickens with some apathogenic wild bird isolates has resulted in mild transient diarrhea and yellowish green, frothy cecal contents (60, 52).

MILD-TO-MODERATE DISEASE. Layer chickens with AIS have wet feces, increased crude fat content of feces, diarrhea, pasty vents, retarded growth rates, delayed onset of laying, production of dirty, fecal-stained eggshells, reduced mean egg weights, and reduced egg carotenoid content (8, 12, 14, 15, 17, 59). Within individual houses, clinical diarrhea may be evident in 5–25% of chickens (59, 65). Increased mortality is uncommon (59, 65). Features of AIS in turkeys, broilers, and broiler breeders are similar to those in layers, except that growth retardation is most severe in broilers (12, 15). Initiation and severity of clinical disease is influenced by husbandry, nutrition, environment, and genetics (30); factors include molting, onset of egg production, poor feed quality, floor housing, and light-laying breeds (30, 59).

Infected chickens have slimy to frothy, yellowish to brown, fluid-filled ceca, and either lack inflammation or have mild lymphocytic typhlitis (Fig. 14.15) (11, 12, 17, 59, 61). Penetration of spirochetes between and below cecal epithelial cells or cecal epithelial cell erosions/necrosis are frequent with infections of European "*S. intermedius*" isolates (8, 11, 14), but rare with U.S. *Serpulins pilosicoli* ("*Angullina coli*") and unclassified poultry isolates (59, 61, 65). Spirochetes are randomly oriented on the cecal epithelial luminal surface (Fig. 14.16) (61) or are oriented at right angles to the surface epithelium (Fig. 14.17, Table 14.4) (65). In broiler chickens, serum concentrations of protein, lipid, carotenoids, and bilirubin are decreased, but growth weights are not consistently affected (12).

SEVERE DISEASE. Infection of juvenile common rheas with intestinal spirochetes produces necrotizing typhlitis (45, 58) with mortality rates that can range from 25 to 80% (45, 58). Most clinically affected rheas are more than 6 mo of age (5), and most cases occur from July through October (58).

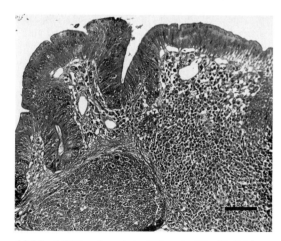

14.15. Mild lymphocytic typhlitis and mild epithelial hyperplasia in a chicken infected with unclassified C1 spirochete. Bar = 50 μm. (*Infection and Immunity*)

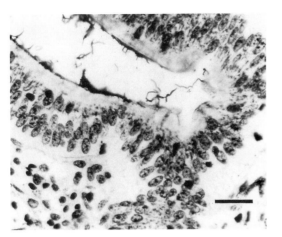

14.16. Randomly oriented unclassified C1 chicken spirochetes on the villous surface epithelium in the cecum. Warthin-Starry silver stain. Bar = 20 μm.

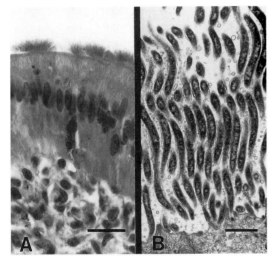

14.17. Tight association of *Serpulina pilosicoli* ("*Angullina coli*") with the luminal surface of cecal epithelium (*A*). The orientation is at right angles to the epithelial cells (*B*).

Adult birds can be affected, but these cases usually involve concurrent stress such as recent shipping.

Clinically, 1–2 days prior to death a few birds may show depression, have reduced body weights, and pass watery feces with caseous cores (57); however, rheas most often die suddenly without clinical signs (45). Ceca are dilated and have thickened walls with ulcerations and lumina containing thick pseudomembranes (Fig. 14.18) (45, 57). Histologically, cecal walls have severe mucosal necrosis, crypt elongation, glandular epithelial and goblet

cell hyperplasia, and cecal lumina containing mucus, colonies of spirochetes and bacilli, and fibrinonecrotic debris (Fig. 14.19). Experimental inoculation of 1-day-old chickens and turkeys with intestinal spirochetes from rheas will produce similar, but less severe, lesions (29).

In the original rhea cases, a strongly ß-hemolytic spirochete was isolated and identified as *S. hyodysenteriae* (29). Inoculation of 1-day-old common

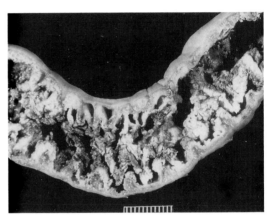

14.18. Thick necrotic pseudomembrane attached to the cecal mucosa of a juvenile common rhea with necrotizing typhlitis.

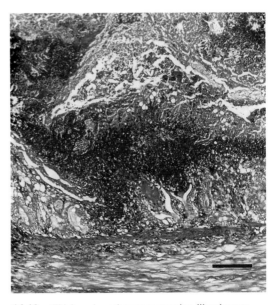

14.19. Thickened cecal mucosa contains dilated crypts filled with mucus. Lumen has a necrotic pseudomembrane composed of necrotic heterophils and sloughed epithelium, bacteria, and mucus. H & E. Bar = 50 μm.

rhea chicks reproduced the gross and histologic lesions within 5–9 days (57). In contrast, weakly ß-hemolytic spirochetes have been isolated from more recent cases (4). These spirochetes are unclassified. In addition to spirochetes, various indigenous anaerobic bacilli can be concurrently recovered with spirochetes from cecal lesions (4). Production of AIS in rheas may require synergism between various spirochetes and nonspirochetal, anaerobic, cecal flora.

Immunity.   Little is known concerning immunity to intestinal spirochetes in birds. Humoral antibodies may or may not be produced following naturally occurring infection. Antibodies can be detected in birds from which spirochetes cannot be isolated, while other birds may yield spirochetes on culture but be serologically negative (52, 53).

DIAGNOSIS

Isolation and Identification of Causative Agent.
Visual demonstration of helix-shaped bacteria in feces or cecal droppings by dark-field or light microscopy is sufficient for tentative identification of spirochetes. Because spirochetes can be normal flora or produce subclinical infections, however, characteristic clinical signs and lesions must be present for a presumptive diagnosis of AIS.

Confirmation of bacteria as spirochetes should be through visualization of distinctive ultrastructural features, demonstration of spirochete antigens, or isolation in culture. Demonstration of organisms with periplasmic flagella in ultrathin sections of cecal mucosa or in negative-stained preparations of clarified cecal contents are diagnostic for spirochetes. Demonstration of spirochete antigens by direct or indirect fluorescent antibody (25) or immunohistochemical methods are easier and more rapid than that by electron microscopy. However, neither ultrastructural morphology nor antigen recognition will distinguish between spirochete groups or species.

Culturing and further characterization is necessary to categorize or classify spirochetes and to confirm a diagnosis of AIS. However, sensitivity of culturing is dependent on the number of organisms and type and condition of the sample (22). Fresh cecal droppings or cecal mucosa are optimal samples. Samples chilled at 4 C for up to 1 wk are acceptable, but frozen samples, especially those stored at -20 C, will have lower isolation rates. Isolated bacteria can be confirmed as spirochetes by transmission electron or immunofluorescent microscopy, but categorization and classification require additional testing such as serotyping (18), growth-inhibition testing (22), biochemical differentiation profiling (26), rRNA restriction pattern analysis (28), or MEE (35). Methods using antibodies to detect membrane specific antigens can differentiate *S. hyodysenteriae* from other intestinal spirochetes (63).

Serology.   Several serologic tests have been developed and used in swine to determine exposure to intestinal spirochetes. Such tests are not based on species-specific antigens and have low specificity and sensitivity. They include enzyme-linked immunosorbent assay, plate and microagglutination tests, agar gel diffusion, passive hemolysis assay, and indirect fluorescent antibody test (22, 48). Similar methods can be used in poultry. An agar gel diffusion test has been used to identify intestinal spirochete infections of birds (53). Its major advantage is the ability to use a single test to screen individuals from diversely different orders and families of birds for spirochete infections (53). The test does not, however, distinguish between different spirochete species and is relatively insensitive.

Differential Diagnosis.   In poultry, spirochetes identified in fecal specimens should be distinguished from other spiral bacteria including *Campylobacter, Arcobacter, Helicobacter,* and *Spirillum.* Many spiral bacteria can be apathogenic indigenous flora of gastrointestinal tracts of birds. In cases of chronic diarrhea or pasty vents, nutritional problems such as excess dietary salt, fats, or soybean meal should be investigated. Other causes of chronic diarrhea include enteric salmonellosis, colibacillosis, and coccidiosis.

In rheas, intestinal spirochetes causing a necrotizing typhlitis must be distinguished from other potential causes including *Salmonella,* especially group B serotypes, *Clostridium difficile, C. perfringens, C. sordelli,* and *Histomonas meleagridis* (9, 40, 47). Furthermore, cecal lesions of eastern equine encephalitis virus (EEEV) infection could be confused with AIS, but EEEV also produces copious small intestinal hemorrhages and necrosis, and widespread petechiation and necrosis in visceral organs (66).

TREATMENT.   In the United States, no chemotherapeutic compound has Food and Drug Administration approval for treatment or prevention of AIS, but compounds used to treat or prevent swine dysentery would have similar efficacy (22). Elsewhere, use of 5-nitroimidazole in water at a concentration of 120 ppm for 6 days is generally effective, although retreatment after 4–8 wk may be necessary. For rheas, extralabel use of dimetridazole (25–50 mg/kg body weight once or twice daily), lincomycin (25 mg/kg twice daily), or erythromycin (15–25 mg/kg once daily) for 5–7 days has been successful as treatments to reduce illness and deaths (20). Concurrent increases in dietary fiber facilitate recovery from clinical disease either through stimulating peristalsis or altering cecal pH.

Following treatment with chemotherapeutics, rheas should receive a probiotic to replace lost normal enteric flora. Cleaning and disinfection are necessary to prevent environmental survival of spirochetes and reinfection of birds.

For intestinal spirochetes of commercial poultry and rheas, efficacy of chemotherapeutics is variable among different isolates. In some field cases in chickens, neomycin has produced clinical improvement (64).

PREVENTION AND CONTROL.
Avian intestinal spirochetosis in chickens is a mild disease, but prevention is still more economical than is treatment. Measures to prevent AIS in commercial poultry operations include decreasing contact with feces by raising birds off floors, frequent changing of litter or manure removal, good rodent and insect control programs, minimizing dietary and molting stress, provision of high-quality feed ingredients, and use of biosecurity measures to prevent introduction of spirochetes on contaminated shoes and clothing following visits to other operations (see Chapter 1).

The seriousness of AIS in rheas warrants the prevention of introduction of *S. hyodysenteriae* into an established flock. Raising of swine on the same farm or having contact with swine should be avoided. Visiting other rhea farms should be discouraged. Proper cleaning and disinfection of clothing, shoes, and equipment should be done before returning to the home flock following visits to rhea shows, rhea farms, or swine operations. All introductions of new rhea stocks should follow a minimum 60 days of quarantine and take place after two to three negative cloacal cultures for *S. hyodysenteriae*. Birds should be segregated into age groups and strict biosecurity measures should be implemented to minimize potential transmission of *S. hyodysenteriae* from asymptomatic adolescent or adult birds to susceptible rhea chicks.

No vaccines are available to prevent AIS. Experimental and commercial killed vaccines developed for prevention of swine dysentery have had either deleterious consequences (43) or have provided inconsistent protection (19, 22).

REFERENCES
1. Achacha, M., and S. Messier. 1992. Comparison of six different culture media for isolation of Treponema hyodysenteriae. J Clin Microbiol 30:249–251.
2. Adachi, Y., M. Sueyoshi, E. Miyagawa, H. Minato, S. and Shoya. 1985. Experimental infection of young broiler chicks with Treponema hyodysenteriae. Microbiol Immunol 29:683–688.
3. Berg, H.C. 1976. How spirochetes may swim. J Theor Biol 56:269–273.
4. Buckles, E.L. 1995. Avian Intestinal Spirochetes. M.S. thesis, Ohio State University, Columbus, OH.
5. Buckles, E.L., D.E. Swayne, and K.A. Eaton. 1994. Cases of a necrotizing typhlitis associated with a cecal spirochete in common rheas (Rhea americana). Vet Pathol 31:612.
6. Canale-Parola, E. 1984. Order I. Spirochaetales Buchanan 1917. In N.R. Krieg (ed.). Bergey's Manual of Systematic Bacteriology, vol 1. Williams and Wilkins, Baltimore, MD, pp. 38–70.
7. Charon, N.W., E.P. Greenberg, M.B.H. Koopman, and R.J. Limberger. 1992. Spirochete chemotaxis, motility, and the structure of the spirochetal periplasmic flagella. Res Microbiol 143:597–603.
8. Davelaar, F.G., H.F. Smit, K. Hovind-Hougen, R.M. Dwars, and P.C. van der Valk. 1986. Infectious typhlitis in chickens caused by spirochetes. Avian Pathol 15:247–258.
9. Dhillon, A.S. 1983. Histomoniasis in a captive great rhea (Rhea americana). J Wildl Dis 19:274-275
10. Dwars, R.M., H.F. Smit, F.G. Davelaar, and W. van T Veer. 1989. Incidence of spirochaetal infections in cases of intestinal disorder in chickens. Avian Pathol 18:591–595.
11. Dwars, R.M., H.F. Smit, and F.G. Davelaar. 1990. Observations on avian intestinal spirochaetosis. Vet Q 12:51–55.
12. Dwars, R.M., F.G. Davelaar, and H.F. Smit. 1992. Spirochaetosis in broilers. Avian Pathol 21:261–273.
13. Dwars, R.M., F.G. Davelaar, and H.F. Smit. 1992. Infection of broiler chicks (Gallus domesticus) with human intestinal spirochetes. Avian Pathol 21:559–568.
14. Dwars, R.M., H.F. Smit, and F.G. Davelaar. 1992. Influence of infection with avian intestinal spirochetes on the faeces of laying hens. Avian Pathol 21:513–515.
15. Dwars, R.M., F.G. Davelaar, and H.F. Smit. 1993. Infection of broiler parent hens with avian intestinal spirochetes: Effects on egg production and chick quality. Avian Pathol 22:693–701.
16. Fantham, H.B. 1910. Observations on the parasitic protozoa of the red grouse (Lagopus scoticus), with a note on the grouse fly. Proc Zoolog Soc Lond May:692–708.
17. Griffiths, I.B., B.W. Hunt, S.A. Lister, and M.H. Lamont. 1987. Retarded growth rate and delayed onset of egg production associated with spirochaete infection in pullets. Vet Rec 121:35–37.
18. Hampson, D.J. 1991. Slide-agglutination for rapid serological typing of Treponema hyodysenteriae. Epidemiol Infect 106:541–547.
19. Hampson, D.J., I.D. Robertson, and J.R.L. Mhoma. 1993. Experiences with a vaccine being developed for the control of swine dysentery. Aust Vet J 70:18–20.
20. Hanley, R.S., L.W. Woods, D.J. Stillian, and G.A. Dumonceaux. 1994. Serpulina-like spirochetes and flagellated protozoa associated with necrotizing typhlitis in the rheas (Rhea americana). Proc Annu Meet Assoc Avian Vet 1994:157–162.
21. Harris, D.L., and J.M. Kinyon. 1974. Significance of anaerobic spirochetes in the intestines of animals. Am J Clin Nutr 27:1297–1304.
22. Harris, D.L., and R.J. Lysons. 1992. Swine dysentery. In A.D. Leman, B.E. Straw, W.L. Mengling, S. D'Allaire, and D.J. Taylor (eds.). Diseases of Swine, 7th ed. Iowa State University Press, Ames, IA, pp. 599–616.
23. Harris, D.L., T.J.L. Alexander, S.C. Whipp, I.M. Robinson, R.D. Glock, and P.J. Matthews. 1978. Swine dysentery: Studies of gnotobiotic pigs inoculated with Treponema hyodysenteriae, Bacteroides vulgatus, and Fusobacterium necrophorum. J Am Vet Med Assoc 172:468–471.
24. Harris, M.B.K. 1930. A study of spirochetes in chickens with special reference to those of the intestinal tract. Am J Hyg 12:537–569.
25. Hunter, D., and A. Clark. 1975. The direct fluorescent antibody test for the detection of Treponema hyodysenteriae in pigs. Res Vet Sci 19:98–99.
26. Hunter, D., and T. Wood. 1979. An evaluation of the API ZYM system as a means of classifying spirochaetes associated with swine dysentery. Vet Rec 104:383–384.
27. Jenkinson, S.R., and C.R. Wingar. 1981. Selective medium for the isolation of Treponema hyodysenteriae. Vet Rec 109:384–385.

28. Jensen, N.S., T.A. Casey, and T.B. Stanton. 1992. Characterization of Serpulina (Treponema) hyodysenteriae and related intestinal spirochetes by ribosomal RNA gene restriction patterns. FEMS Microbiol Lett 93:235–242.

29. Jensen, N.S., T.B. Stanton, and D.E. Swayne. 1995. Identification of the swine pathogen Serpulina hyodysenteriae in rheas (Rhea americana). Vet Microbiol 52:259–269.

30. Kouwenhoven, B. 1993. Environment, husbandry, genetics and nutritional interactions in infectious diseases in poultry. In J. York (ed.). Proc Xth Int Cong World Vet Poult Assoc. Australian Veterinary Poultry Association, Sydney, Australia, pp. 113–126.

31. Kunkle, R.A., Harris, D.L., and Kinyon, J.M. 1986. Autoclaved liquid medium for propagation of Treponema hyodysenteriae. J Clin Microbiol 24:669–671.

32. Lee, J.I., and D.J. Hampson. 1994. Genetic characterisation of intestinal spirochaetes and their association with disease. J Med Microbiol 40:365–371.

33. Lee, J.I., D.J. Hampson, A.J. Lymbery, and S.J. Harders. 1993. The porcine intestinal spirochaetes: Identification of new genetic groups. Vet Microbiol 34:273–285.

34. Lee, J.I., A.J. McLaren, A.J. Lymbery, and D.J. Hampson. 1993. Human intestinal spirochetes are distinct from Serpulina hyodysenteriae. J Clin Microbiol 31:16–21.

35. Lymbery, A.J., D.J. Hampson, R.M. Hopkins, B. Combs, and J.R.L. Mhoma. 1990. Multilocus enzyme electrophoresis for identification and typing of Treponema hyodysenteriae and related spirochetes. Vet Microbiol 22:89–99.

36. Lysons, R.J., K.A. Kent, A.P. Bland, R. Sellwood, W.F. Robinson, and A.J. Frost. 1991. A cytotoxic haemolysin from Treponema hyodysenteriae—a probable virulence determinant in swine dysentery. J Med Microbiol 34:97–102.

37. Mathey, W.J., and D.V. Zander. 1955. Spirochetes and cecal nodules in poultry. J Am Vet Med Assoc 126:475–477.

38. McLaren, A.J., D.J. Trott, D.E. Swayne, J.W. Stoutenburg, and D.J. Hampson. 1994. Characterisation of avian intestinal spirochetes. Proc North Central Avian Dis Conf 45:66–67.

39. McLaren, A.J., D.J. Trott, D.E. Swayne, S.L. Oxberry, and D.J. Hampson. 1996. Genetic and phenotypic characterization of intestinal spirochetes colonizing chickens, and association with disease of known pathogenic isolates to three distinct genetic groups. J Clin Microbiol (in press).

40. McMillan, E.G., and G. Zellen. 1991. Histomoniasis in a rhea. Can Vet J 32:244.

41. Neef, N.A., R.J. Lysons, D.J. Trott, D.J. Hampson, P.W. Jones, and J.H. Morgan. 1994. Pathogenicity of porcine intestinal spirochetes in gnotobiotic pigs. Infect Immun 62:2395–2403.

42. Nuessen, M.E., L.A. Joens, and R.D Glock. 1983. Involvement of lipopolysaccharide in the pathogenicity of Treponema hyodysenteriae. J Immunol 131:997–999.

43. Olson, L.D., I.I. Dayalu, and G.T. Schlink. 1994. Exacerbated onset of dysentery in swine vaccinated with inactivated adjuvanted Serpulina hyodysenteriae. Am J Vet Res 55:67–71.

44. Paster, B.J., F.E. Dewhirst, W.G. Weisburg, L.A. Tordoff, G.J. Fraser, R.B. Hespell, T.B. Stanton, L. Zablen, L. Mandelco, and C.R. Woese. 1991. Phylogenetic analysis of the spirochetes. J Bacteriol 173:6101–6109.

45. Sagartz, J.E., D.E. Swayne, K.A. Eaton, J.R. Hayes, K.D. Amass, R. Wack, and L. Kramer. 1992. Necrotizing typhlocolitis associated with a spirochete in rheas (Rhea americana). Avian Dis 36:282–289.

46. Smit, H.F. 1996. Personal communication.

47. Smith, J.A., J.R. Glisson, R.K. Page, and G.N. Rowland. 1991. Necrotic enteritis and colitis in ratite birds. Proc West Poult Dis Conf 40:258–260.

48. Smith, S.E., L.M. Barrett, T. Muir, W.L. Christopher, and P.J. Coloe. 1991. Application and evaluation of enzyme-linked immunosorbent assay and immunoblotting for detec-

tion of antibodies to Treponema hyodysenteriae in swine. Epidemiol Infect 107:285–296.

49. Songer, J.G., J.M. Kinyon, and D.L. Harris. 1976. Selection medium for isolation of Treponema hyodysenteriae. J Clin Microbiol 4:57–60.

50. Stanton, T.B. 1992. Proposal to change the genus designation Serpula to Serpulina gen. nov. containing the species Serpulina hyodysenteriae comb. nov. and Serpulina innocens comb. nov. Int J Sys Bacteriol 42:189–190.

51. Stanton, T.B. N.S. Jensen, T.A. Casey, L.A. Tordoff, F.E. Dewhirst, and B.J. Paster. 1991. Reclassification of Treponema hyodysenteriae and Treponema innocens in a new genus, Serpula gen. nov., as Serpula hyodysenteriae comb. nov. and Serpula innocens comb. nov. Int J Sys Bacteriol 41:50–58.

52. Stoutenburg, J.W. 1993. Studies of intestinal spirochetes in avian species, M.S. thesis, Ohio State University, Columbus, OH.

53. Stoutenburg, J.W., D.E. Swayne, T.M. Hoepf, R. Wack, and L. Kramer. 1995. Frequency of intestinal spirochetes in avian species from a zoologic collection and private rhea farms in Ohio. J Zoolog Wildl Med 26:272–278.

54. Sueyoshi, M., and Y. Adachi. 1990. Diarrhea induced by Treponema hyodysenteriae: a young chick cecal model of swine dysentery. Infect Immun 58:3348–3362.

55. Sueyoshi, M., Y. Adachi, S. Shoya, E. Miyagawa, and H. Minato. 1986. Investigations into location of Treponema hyodysenteriae in the cecum of experimentally infected young broiler chicks by light- and electron microscopy. Zentralbl Bakteriol Hyg Abt 261:447–453.

56. Sueyoshi, M., Y. Adachi, and S. Shoya. 1987. Enteropathogenicity of Treponema hyodysenteriae in young chicks. Zentralbl Bakteriol Hyg Abt 266:469–477.

57. Swayne, D.E. 1994. Pathobiology of intestinal spirochetosis in mammals and birds. Proc Annu Meet Am Coll Vet Pathol 45:224–238.

58. Swayne, D.E., and E. Buckles. 1993. Update on spirochete-associated typhlitis of common rheas (Rhea americana) in the U.S.A.. Proc North Central Avian Dis Conf 44:89–90.

59. Swayne, D.E., A.J. Bermudez, J.E. Sagartz, K.A. Eaton, K.A., J.D. Monfort, J.W. Stoutenburg, and J.R. Hayes. 1992. Association of cecal spirochetes with pasty vents and dirty eggshells in layers. Avian Dis 36:776–781.

60. Swayne, D.E., K.A. Eaton, J.W. Stoutenburg, and E.L. Buckles. 1993. Comparison of the ability of orally inoculated avian-, pig-, and rat-origin spirochetes to produce enteric disease in 1-day-old chickens. Proc Annu Meet Am Vet Med Assoc 130:155.

61. Swayne, D.E., K.A.Eaton, J.W. Stoutenburg, D.J. Trott, D.J. Hampson, and N.S. Jensen. 1995. Identification of a new intestinal spirochete with pathogenicity for chickens. Infect Immun 63:430–436.

62. Terhuurne, A.A.H.M., S. Muir, M. Vanhouten, M.B.H. Koopman, J.G. Kusters, B.A.M. Vanderzeijst, and W. Gaastr. 1993. The role of hemolysin(s) in the pathogenesis of Serpulina-hyodysenteriae. Zentralbl Bakteriol 278:316–325.

63. Thomas, W., and R. Sellwood. 1992. Monoclonal antibodies to a 16-kDa antigen of Serpulina (Treponema) hyodysenteriae. J Med Microbiol 37:214–220.

64. Trampel, D.W. 1996. Personal communication.

65. Trampel, D.W., N.S. Jensen, and L.J. Hoffman. 1994. Cecal spirochetosis in commercial laying hens. Avian Dis 38:895–898.

66. Veazey, R.S., C.C. Vice, D.Y. Cho, T.N. Tully, and S.M. Shane. 1994. Pathology of eastern equine encephalitis in emus (Dromaius novaehollandiae). Vet Pathol 31:109–111.

67. Whipp, S.C., I.M. Robinson, D.L. Harris, R.D. Glock, P.J. Matthews, and T.J.L. Alexander. 1979. Pathogenic synergism between Treponema hyodysenteriae and other selected anaerobes in gnotobiotic pigs. Infect Immun 26:1042–1047.

15 Chlamydiosis (Psittacosis, Ornithosis)

Arthur A. Andersen, James E. Grimes, and Priscilla B. Wyrick

INTRODUCTION. Avian chlamydiosis is caused by the bacterium *Chlamydia psittaci*. The disease in birds and humans was originally called psittacosis or parrot fever (55), as it was first recognized in psittacine birds and in humans associated with psittacine birds. *Ornithosis* is a term introduced in 1941 by Meyer (50) to differentiate the disease in or contracted from domestic and wild fowl from the disease in or contracted from psittacine birds. The two syndromes are currently considered to be the same (67). Their earlier separation was based on the assumption that in humans, ornithosis is a milder disease than psittacosis. However, it should be noted that the disease in humans contracted from turkeys is often more severe than that from psittacine birds.

The serotypes of *C. psittaci* that naturally infect birds are distinct from those associated with chlamydiosis in mammals. Currently, six serotypes of *C. psittaci* are known to infect birds. Each serotype appears to be associated with a different group or order of birds (2, 86).

Avian chlamydiosis in birds is usually systemic and occasionally fatal. The clinical signs vary greatly in severity and depend on the species and age of the bird and on the strain of chlamydia. Avian chlamydiosis can produce lethargy, hyperthermia, abnormal excretions, nasal and eye discharges, and reduced egg production. Mortality rates range up to 30%. In pet birds, the most frequent clinical signs are anorexia and weight loss, diarrhea, yellowish droppings, sinusitis, and respiratory distress (54). Many birds, especially older psittacine birds, may show no clinical signs; nevertheless, they will often shed the agent for extended periods. Necropsy of infected birds will often reveal spleen and liver enlargement, fibrinous airsacculitis, pericarditis, and peritonitis (60, 80).

The avian strains of *C. psittaci* can infect humans, and precautions should be taken when handling infected birds or contaminated materials. Human infections are common following handling or processing of infected turkeys or ducks. Most infections are through inhalation of infectious aerosols; therefore, processing plant employees are especially at risk. Also at risk are farm workers and poultry inspectors at processing plants. Personnel who are employed to process turkey meat further have also become infected. Pigeons also may pose public health threats, mainly to their producers. Chickens and pheasants are of lesser importance as potential public health hazards.

In humans, the incubation period of avian chlamydiosis is usually 5–14 days; however, longer periods have been known to occur. Infections vary from inapparent to severe systemic disease with pneumonia. Because the disease is rarely fatal in properly treated patients, awareness of the danger and early diagnosis are important. Infected humans typically develop headache, chills, malaise, and myalgia, with or without signs of respiratory involvement. While pulmonary involvement is common, auscultatory findings may appear normal or underestimate the extent of involvement.

A human chlamydial strain (*C. pneumonia* strain TWAR) produces similar disease symptoms in humans (19, 21). The recommended therapy for it is the same as for the avian strain, so a differential diagnosis is not required. If a differential diagnosis is desired, however, it can be done by specialized laboratories by either identifying the agent if an isolate was obtained, or by serologic testing using the microimmunofluorescence (MIF) assay. The differential diagnosis should be considered if the patient has not been exposed to infected birds, and the source of infection is unknown.

This chapter primarily covers avian chlamydiosis, as it occurs in birds raised commercially for meat and egg production—turkeys, ducks, and pigeons. It should be noted that the disease in pet birds is quite similar and the disease characteristics, transmission, and diagnosis are essentially the same. A summary of the disease and control procedures for chlamydiosis in companion birds has been published (75). Public health and other factors relating to avian chlamydiosis as a zoonotic infection have been summarized by Grimes (24).

HISTORY. Avian chlamydiosis gained world prominence during a pandemic in 1929 to 1930 that involved at least 12 countries. In the United States, the disease was attributed to the importation of green Amazon parrots from South America. In 1931, strict regulations were placed on the importation of parrots from tropical countries, as the pandemic was being curbed in other countries by restrictions on the importations of parrots. Leventhal, Cole, and Lillie (cited in 51) independently observed very small basophilic bodies in the tissues of infected birds and humans and suggested that they were the causative agent. The etiologic relationship between basophilic bodies and disease was soon established conclusively by Bedson and Bland (cited in 51).

During the next 20 yr, it became clear that chlamydiae were not limited to psittacine birds, were widespread in almost all avian species, and that chlamydia from other avian species was transmissible to humans. In 1939, chlamydiae were isolated from two pigeons sent to the diagnostic laboratory in South Africa by a pigeon fancier who was losing a few birds from his flocks. Isolates were soon recovered from racing and carrier pigeons in California, and infections in two humans in New York were attributed to contact with feral pigeons. In 1942, serologic evidence showed that ducks and turkeys could be infected naturally. Within 3 yr, human infections due to contact with ducks were reported in California and New York. It was not until the early 1950s, however, that isolates were made both from turkeys and from humans in contact with the turkeys (51). The list of avian species in which naturally occurring chlamydial infections were identified increased rapidly: 130 species of birds belonging to 12 orders were on a list compiled by Meyer (52).

The chlamydiosis pandemic of the early 1930s was of high virulence, causing significant economic losses and many human infections. Public concern led to increased research. These studies formed the basis for recommendations and reforms in management of birds in areas of high incidence of avian chlamydiae, and for treatment, handling, and processing of birds suspected of having the disease.

During the 1960s, the incidence of severe epidemics in poultry in the United States and Europe declined, although occasional outbreaks and serologic evidence show that avian chlamydia is a continuing threat both to birds and to humans in contact with them. Outbreaks in turkeys were reported in the United States during the 1980s (30) and more recently in Europe (73, 87). An increase in the number of outbreaks due to chlamydia in ducks has been reported in recent years. Human infections were associated with a number of these outbreaks (8, 43, 48, 59).

INCIDENCE AND DISTRIBUTION. Avian chlamydiosis occurs worldwide, with the incidence and distribution varying greatly with the species of bird and the serotype of the chlamydial organism. The psittacine birds harbor primarily one serotype of chlamydia that is endemic, and many psittacine birds are chronically infected. When under stress, chronically infected birds may become clinically ill or shed the organism. At these times, humans may become infected. The economic losses and the human infections usually follow a sporadic pattern; however, there are reports of outbreaks following introduction of infected birds into pet stores or into homes. In recent years, antibiotics have been used extensively to control the spread of the disease and to reduce the risk to humans. The pattern in pigeons appears to be similar, with at least two different serotypes being involved.

The disease pattern in turkeys is different: Most outbreaks are explosive, involving one or more flocks. In the past, chlamydia in turkeys was thought to be limited to the United States and to free-ranging flocks. A recent outbreak in the Netherlands involving confinement-raised commercial broiler turkeys was found to be caused by the same serotype of *C. psittaci* that had caused large outbreaks in the United States (87). In the past, reports of chlamydia in turkeys in Europe were always discounted, as human cases had not been associated with them.

Isolates from a number of turkey outbreaks that occurred during the last 40 yr in the United States have been serotyped. Almost all of these isolates are of either serotype D (virulent turkey) or serotype B (pigeon), which is less virulent in the turkey (2). There is no indication that either of these serotypes is endemic in turkeys. This would indicate that the chlamydial agent must be introduced into turkeys from the outside, which would help explain the explosive nature of the outbreaks. The increase in confinement-rearing of turkeys and the prevention of commingling of free-flying birds with turkeys would contribute to the decreased incidence seen in later years.

Information on the epidemiology of chlamydia in ducks is more limited. In the United States, it has not been a significant problem. In Europe, there have been a number of outbreaks, some of which have occurred in recent years. Isolates from only a few European outbreaks have been serotyped, and these have all been of serotype C (86). This serotype has also been recovered from geese and swans. This research indicates that serotype C of *C. psittaci* is endemic in the duck population; however, no further information is available on whether the agent establishes chronic infection similar to that that occurs in the psittacine bird, or whether it can be passed vertically through the egg.

Chlamydial strains from mammals are not a problem for the poultry producer. Recent advances in serotyping using monoclonal antibodies and in strain identification using polymerase chain reaction–restriction fragment length polymorphism (PCR–RFLP) demonstrate that the strains occurring naturally in birds are distinct from those in mammals (1, 2). Attempts to infect birds with mammalian strains usually result in aborted or asymptomatic infections (45, 80). Avian strains will infect humans and may produce a severe pneumonia; however, the infections are usually self-limiting without secondary spread.

ETIOLOGY

Classification.   Most chlamydial strains are host and disease specific. Knowing the classification of chlamydiae is important in understanding what diseases they can cause and their epidemiology.

The genus chlamydia was originally classified into two species, *C. trachomatis* and *C. psittaci*. *C. trachomatis* strains were separated by their susceptibility to sulfadiazine, accumulation of glycogen in their inclusions, and production of oval-vacuolar inclusions (63). This effectively classified all human isolates as *C. trachomatis* and all animal isolates as *C. psittaci*, with a few exceptions. Currently, there are 18 human strains of *C. trachomatis* in two biovars, lymphogranuloma verenum (LGV) and trachoma (89). Two nonhuman *C. trachomatis* strains have been isolated: One is a mouse strain that was an early isolate, and the other is a recently reported isolate from swine (46). The remaining chlamydial isolates were all placed in the species *C. psittaci* until recently. A human respiratory isolate (TWAR), identified in the 1980s, was placed in a separate species (*C. pneumoniae*) represented by a single strain (20). A fourth species (*C. pecorum*) has been proposed to include strains from cattle and sheep that cause polyarthritis, pneumonia, encephalomyelitis, and enteritis (16). Early studies indicate that *C. pecorum* will also include a number of swine strains (46).

The remaining *C. psittaci* isolates are still a heterologous group (39), and further division will likely be made when more information becomes available. Currently, there are six known avian serovars and eight to 10 mammalian serovars (2, 69).

Morphology and Biochemical Properties.
There are two morphologically distinct forms of chlamydia, termed elementary body (EB) and reticulate body (RB) (Fig. 15.1). The EB is a small, dense, spherical body, about 0.2–0.3 µm in diameter, which rivals mycoplasma for the smallest of the prokaryotes. The EB is the infectious form of the organism, which attaches to target columnar epithelial cells and gains entry. Rigidity of the EB membrane is believed to be due more to disulfide bond cross-linking among the major outer membrane proteins than to an extensively cross-linked classic peptidoglycan matrix, since muramic acid is absent. The distribution of amino acids in chlamydial cell walls is similar to that of the cell walls of *Escherichia coli*, the wall content being largely protein (70%) and lipid (5.1%), with the remainder presumably carbohydrate (47). The EBs are nonmotile, lacking flagella, and nonpiliated.

The RB is the intracellular, metabolically active form and divides by binary fission. It is larger than the EB, about 0.6–1.5 µm in diameter, and is osmotically fragile. While DNA and RNA are found in both the EB and the RB, the ratio of RNA to DNA is greater in the RB. The RB forms synthesize their own DNA, RNA, and protein, but some of their metabolic capabilities are limited when compared with free-living, colonizing bacteria. For example, they cannot complete the pentose cycle and do not utilize pyruvate by way of the tricarboxylic acid cycle. They can, however, catabolize pyruvic, aspartic, and glutamic acids, generating CO_2 and 2- and 4-carbon residues.

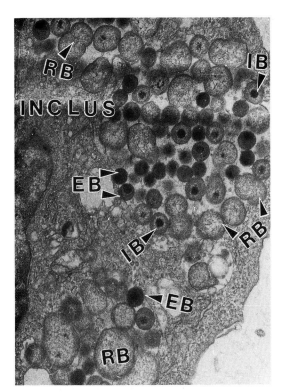

15.1.   Transmission electron photomicrograph of a *Chlamydia psittaci* inclusion (*INCLUS*) in infected L929 cells. The various morphologic forms of chlamydiae are present: elementary body (*EB*), reticulate body (*RB*), and intermediate body (*IB*). ×15,000

The chlamydial genome is a closed circular DNA molecule with a molecular weight of 6.6×10^8. A molecule of this size can provide information for about 600 different proteins, which is about one-fourth the amount provided by the *E. coli* genome. All strains of *C. trachomatis* and some strains of *C. psittaci* also possess plasmids, but their function has yet to be determined (38).

Developmental Cycle. An unusual developmental cycle characterizes the growth of these obligate intracellular bacteria in their eukaryotic host cells. The cycle consists of essentially five major phases: 1) attachment and penetration by the EB, 2) transition of the metabolically inert EB into the metabolically active RB, 3) multiplication of the RB by binary fission, producing many progeny, 4) maturation of the noninfectious RBs into infectious EBs, and 5) release of EBs from the host cell (57, 77).

The initial event in the infectious process begins with attachment of *C. psittaci* EBs to microvilli at the apical surface of a susceptible columnar epithelial cell. The EB travels down the microvilli and locates in indentions of the eukaryotic plasma membrane, some of which resemble coated pits (44). The EBs are subsequently internalized in invaginations of the plasma membrane. Thus uptake is akin to an endocytosislike process. The *C. psittaci*-containing endocytic vesicles escape interaction with lysosomes and proceed to the nuclear hof area. The chlamydia remain surrounded and protected by the endosome membrane throughout their intracellular development.

Alterations in the EB cell wall occur, and result in a conversion of the EB to the RB form. These changes primarily involve reduction in disulfide bond cross-linking among the outer-membrane proteins (37, 58). Synthesis of DNA, RNA, and protein is initiated, permitting growth of the RB and division by binary fission. The RBs, however, cannot generate high-energy phosphate bonds. Thus, their adaptation to an intracellular habitat is due to their dependency on eukaryotic cells for energy. At some point, host-cell mitochondria are positioned against the enlarging chlamydial endosome, enabling the RB to parasitize mitochondrial ATP via a chlamydial ATP–ADP translocase. The ATP is broken down to ADP by a specific RB ATPase, and the resultant proton motive force helps drive the transport of nutrients (36). The chlamydiae possess unusual cylindrical surface projections, averaging 18 in number and arranged in a hexagonal array. These projections are anchored in the cytoplasmic membrane and protrude through holes in the envelope. Evidence suggests that the projections penetrate the endosome membrane, which surrounds the developing chlamydial microcolony, permitting uptake of nutrients from the host cytoplasm (49).

The developing chlamydial microcolony is termed an "inclusion" and may contain anywhere from 100 to 500 progeny, depending on the species of chlamydia. In some cases, multiple inclusions appear in *C. psittaci*-infected cells (Fig. 15.2). In contrast, *C. trachomatis*-containing endosomes seem to fuse with one another early in the developmental cycle, resulting in the eventual appearance of usually only one inclusion. By 48 hr, there is a marked increase in glycogen accumulation in the *C. trachomatis* inclusion. Presumably, when the nutrients have been depleted, the RB progeny mature and condense into EBs and are released. With most strains of chlamydiae, the host cell is usually severely damaged by 48 hr and release of chlamydiae is by lysis. Exocytosis of the inclusions, followed by a "healing" or closing of the open-cavern structures where the inclusions had existed, has been reported (84).

The pathology associated with human psittacosis includes inflammatory exudate within the alveoli in which polymorphonuclear leukocytes, and subsequently mononuclear phagocytes, are prominent. Opsonized EBs are rapidly engulfed by these cells and destroyed in the phagolysosomes. However, if the EBs are not coated by antibody and/or complement, they are still efficiently internalized by the professionally phagocytic cells, but their fate is different. The majority of the chlamydiae do not survive in the short-lived polymorphonuclear leukocytes, but *C. psittaci* do survive and grow in macrophages (71).

Chlamydia-specific lipopolysaccharide is exported to the surface of the infected eukaryotic host cell concomitant with active RB growth (72). The exoglycolipid is postulated to reduce plasma membrane fluidity, thereby protecting the chlamydiae from cytotoxic T-cell onslaught. Whether or not this

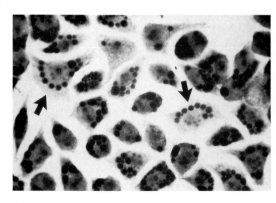

15.2. Multiple *Chlamydia psittaci* (Cal 10) inclusions in 24-hr infected L929 cells. ×450. (Hodinka, Infect Immun)

highly antigenic lipopolysaccharide plays a role in the perpetuation of disabling chlamydial disease via prolonged inflammatory response and immune-mediated pathology is at present a controversial issue (81, 82).

Staining Characteristics. Chlamydiae are large enough that they can be seen either with a light microscope using special optics or with selective stains. Staining has the advantage that some stains differentiate species and serovars. In wet mounts of impression smears of infected tissues or exudates, intracellular chlamydiae are large enough to be seen at magnifications of ×800 or more in phase contrast microscopes (Fig. 15.3A). They are readily seen by dark-field illumination (Fig. 15.3B). With either technique, however, they cannot be distinguished from contaminating intracellular mycoplasma organisms. When only bright-field optics are available, chlamydiae may be seen in touch impressions of infected tissues by staining them with Giemsa, Castaneda, Macchiavello, or Gimenez methods after appropriate fixation. They appear dark purple with Giemsa, blue with Castaneda, and red with Macciavello and Gimenez stains against contrasting backgrounds. The Gimenez method (18) is preferred for staining chlamydiae in touch impressions of yolk sacs of infected chicken embryos, and has proved very useful in obtaining presumptive diagnoses in microscopic examination of touch impressions of diseased air sacs, spleens, and pericardia of naturally infected birds (22).

In recent years, monoclonal antibodies (MAbs) have been developed and are available to detect chlamydiae in clinical specimens. While the antigen-detection approach is slightly less sensitive than culture, it is faster and less expensive. The specificity of the staining depends greatly on the monoclonal antibodies or antisera used, as some will cross-react with other gram-negative organisms. Laboratories are now developing serovar-specific monoclonal antibodies that can be used to differentiate the species and strains of chlamydiae. The use of these monoclonal antibodies is replacing iodine staining for the identification of the human *C. trachomatis* strains.

In infected cell cultures chlamydiae stain well with Giemsa (Figs. 15.4E,F), Gimenez (Fig. 15.4D), and immunofluorescence (IF) (Fig. 15.4 G) methods. All chlamydiae are gram-negative, but the Gram stain is of no practical value in identifying intracellular organisms.

Antibiotic Susceptibility. Multiplication of all strains of chlamydiae (except for experimental mutants) is strongly inhibited by appropriate concentrations of tetracyclines, chloramphenicol, and erythromycin, and less so by penicillin. Some strains are inhibited by D-cycloserine. All strains of *C. trachomatis* are inhibited by sodium sulfadiazine. Tetracyclines, chloramphenicol, and erythromycin inhibit synthesis of protein on chlamydial ribosomes by varied mechanisms. Penicillin interferes with chlamydial cell wall synthesis, resulting in the interruption of RB binary fission and thus the formation of abnormally large RBs, which cannot mature into EBs; it does not prevent infection of cells by EBs, conversion of EBs to RBs, or metabolism of RBs. D-cycloserine acts similarly, but the drug's action can be reversed by the addition of alanine. Inhibition of multiplication by sodium sulfadiazine reflects the organism's ability to produce folic acid. This inhibition can be reversed by the addition of *p*-aminobenzoic acid. Certain antibiotics have little or no effect on the growth of chlamydiae and this fact can be useful in selecting for viable chlamydiae in suspensions containing contaminating bacteria. Concentrations of 1 mg/mL of streptomycin sulfate, vancomycin, and kanamycin sulfate may be used for this purpose.

A
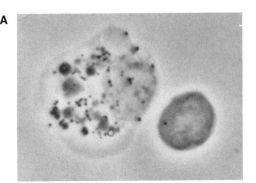

B
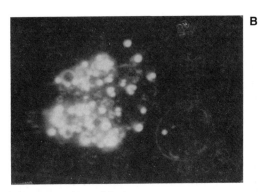

15.3. *A.* Phase contrast photomicrograph of chlamydiae-laden mononuclear cell in air sac exudate of turkey infected with *Chlamydia psittaci. B.* Dark-field photomicrograph of mononuclear cell in A. ×4000 (Page)

Chlamydiae are also unaffected by bacitracin, gentamicin, and neomycin.

Resistance to Chemical and Physical Agents.

Chlamydiae are very susceptible to chemicals that affect their lipid content or the integrity of their cell walls. Even in a milieu of tissue debris, they are rapidly inactivated by surface-active compounds such as quaternary ammonium compounds (Roccal) and lipid solvents. They are somewhat less susceptible to dilute solutions of protein denaturants, acids, and alkalies (methanol, ethanol, ammonium or zinc sulfate, phenol, hydrochloric acid, or sodium hydroxide). Infectivity is destroyed within minutes, however, by exposure to common disinfectants such as benzalkonium chloride, alcoholic iodine solution, 70% ethanol, 3% hydrogen peroxide, and silver nitrate; but they are resistant to cresol compounds and lime (79). Dilute suspensions (20%) of infectious tissue homogenates are inactivated by incubation for 5 min at 56 C, 48 hr at 37 C, 12 days at 22 C, and 50 days at 4 C (61).

Infectious dense forms of the organisms in yolk sac membranes or mouse tissues may be preserved indefinitely at -20 C or below, although the initial freezing and subsequent thawing incurs a titer loss of 1–2 $\log_{10}$. Infectivity of the suspension is destroyed after six freeze–thaw cycles (61). Thin-walled, large forms of the organism are inactivated at -70 C. Cell walls of the dense forms are disrupted by ultrasonification at frequencies above 100 KC or by treatment of intact organisms with sodium deoxycholate.

Antigenic Structure and Toxins.

Chlamydiae are antigenically complex, consisting primarily of the immunodominant genus-specific lipopolysaccharide (LPS) and numerous proteins. The LPS is a major surface- or group-reactive antigen and may play a role in pathogenesis; however, there is no evidence that antibody to the LPS is protective. It is chemically and serologically related to the LPS of enterobacterial Re-mutants. Chlamydial LPS possesses at least three antigenic epitopes. One of these is a genus-specific epitope that has not been detected in any other bacterium. This epitope is composed of a trisaccharide of 3-deoxy-D-manno-octulosonic acid (KDO). It is surface exposed on the EBs and RBs and is immunoaccessible. Chlamydial LPS also contains at least two additional epitopes that are shared with LPS epitopes in some gram-negative bacteria. These may explain some of the cross-reactions often seen with some enzyme-linked immunosorbent assay (ELISA) tests and may also be a factor in low level complement-fixation (CF) titers.

The number of proteins that chlamydiae produce is unknown and only a limited number have been studied for their antigenic importance. The major outer membrane protein (MOMP) has a molecular mass of approximately 40,000 daltons (40 kD). It accounts for approximately 60% of the outer-membrane protein mass and is assumed to be of importance in the immune response. Serovar-specific MAbs often neutralize the infectivity of chlamydiae. These MAbs are thought to be against the MOMP, as serovar specificity correlates with changes in the MOMP as measured by PCR–RFLP. However, these MAbs are nonreactive in the standard sulfate–polyacrylamide gel electrophoresis (SDS–PAGE) analysis. These neutralizing MAbs may recognize a trimer of the MOMP (41). Conformational epitopes would explain these reaction patterns. This finding should advance vaccine development.

A 60-kD protein has also received extensive attention in *C. trachomatis* infections. The protein is a heat shock protein similar to groEL heat shock protein in gram-negative organisms (10, 56). This protein has been associated with the hypersensitivity often seen in repeated chlamydial infections. It is thought to play a major role in the scar formation seen in eye and reproductive sequelae following repeated chlamydial infections.

Toxigenicity of chlamydiae can be demonstrated by intravenous inoculation of mice with freshly harvested yolk sac cultures. Toxigenicity appears to be associated with cell wall components and is neutralizable by specific antiserum. Many cross-reactions have been demonstrated among the toxins of chlamydia from various birds and mammals.

Strain Classification.

For years, it has been recognized that *C. psittaci* is a collection of genetically heterogenous strains. Numerous attempts have been made to classify these strains including biotyping, conventional sera, monoclonal antibodies, and genetic diversity (39). A panel of serovar-specific MAbs to 12 avian and mammalian strains has been used successfully to serotype over 200 avian isolates (2, 86). The avian isolates all fell into six serotypes. It has been suggested that the first four serovars be labeled A through D (86) and since then, two additional serovars have been identified. The serovars and the avian species that they are primarily associated with are given in Table 15.1. It is

Table 15.1. Serotypes of avian strains of chlamydia

Serotype	Representative chlamydial isolate	Birds primarily infected
A	VS1	Psittacines
B	CP3	Pigeons, doves
C	GR9	Ducks, geese
D	NJ1	Turkeys
E	MN	Pigeons, turkeys
F	VS225	Psittacines

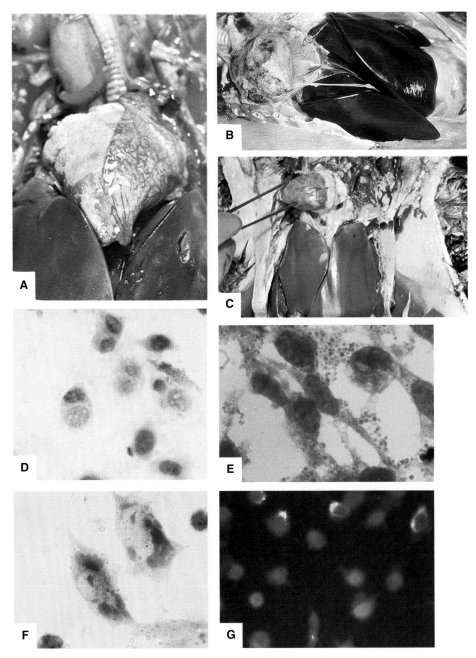

15.4. *A.* Gross lesions of acutely fatal chlamydiosis in young turkey infected by airborne route. Thickened, congested pericardial membrane has been partially removed to show severe pericarditis and epicardial encrustation. Cardiomegaly and hepatomegaly also are evident. (Page) *B.* Gross lesions in turkey infected with virulent *Chlamydia psittaci* strain isolated from turkeys in South Carolina in 1973. Enlargement of heart and liver and severe pericarditis are the most prominent lesions. (Page) *C.* Field case of chlamydiosis caused by *C. psittaci* of low virulence. *Arrows* point to fibrin plaques on heart and the enlarged liver. (Page) *D–G.* Light photomicrographs of *Chlamydia* spp. inclusions in L929 cells. (Winsor, Nettum, and Grimes). *D.* Gimenez-stained *C. psittaci,* ×1600. *E.* Giemsa-stained *C. trachomatis,* ×4000. *F.* Giemsa-stained *C. psittaci,* ×4000; *G.* Immunofluorescence-stained *C. psittaci,* ×1600.

expected that other avian strains will be added to this list when better methods to isolate and grow chlamydiae are available and as isolates are recovered from additional avian species.

Polymerase chain reaction–restriction fragment length polymorphism of the MOMP genome using the Alu I restriction enzyme has also been used for classification. There are published comparisons using it for *C. trachomatis* and some *C. psittaci* strains. We have used it with representative avian strains with complete agreement with the MAb serotype results. The method of choice will depend on the laboratory, as either can be used readily to classify the avian chlamydial isolates.

Pathogenicity.

Based on natural pathogenicity for domestic fowl, strains of *C. psittaci* isolated from these birds fall into two general categories: 1) Highly virulent strains that cause acute epidemics in which 5–30% of affected birds die and 2) less virulent strains that cause slowly progressive epidemics. Strains of both high and low virulence appear to have equal ability to spread rapidly through a flock, as evidenced by serologic test results. Such studies show that more than 90% of birds in any one enclosure develop antibodies to the chlamydial group antigen by the time clinical signs of disease appear in the flock. Highly virulent strains are isolated most often from turkeys and occasionally from unaffected wild birds. The isolates serotyped from some of the earlier outbreaks with high mortality have been of serotype D (2, 90). These strains are also labeled "toxigenic," because in natural and experimental hosts they produce rapidly fatal disease with lesions characterized by extensive vascular congestion and inflammation of vital organs. Toxigenic strains have a broad spectrum of pathogenicity for laboratory animals and can cause serious human infections (some fatal) in poultry handlers and laboratory research workers. Strains of low virulence cause slowly progressive epidemics with a mortality rate of less than 5% when uncomplicated by secondary bacterial or parasitic infection. Strains of this category are routinely isolated from pigeons and ducks and occasionally from turkeys, sparrows, and other wild birds. The turkey isolates from outbreaks with low mortality have been of serotype B or E. Birds infected with these strains usually do not develop the severe vascular damage typical in birds infected with the virulent toxigenic strains, nor do they have the severe clinical signs (80). Unless unusually high levels of exposure alter the balance between infection and resistance, humans are less susceptible to the strains commonly found in pigeons and ducks.

Chlamydiosis in pigeons, ducks, and some psittacine birds often is accompanied by concurrent infection with salmonellae. In such cases, the mortality rate among birds is high; and chlamydiae are shed in very large numbers, and susceptible hosts in the immediate environment of infected birds are exposed to doses that can result in clinical disease.

PATHOGENESIS AND EPIDEMIOLOGY

Natural and Experimental Hosts.

In addition to the naturally occurring chlamydial infections in domesticated birds, Meyer (52) has listed over 130 wild avian species that are either transient or long-term hosts. Common reservoirs of chlamydia in the United States include wild and feral birds such as sea gulls, ducks, herons, egrets, pigeons, blackbirds, grackles, house sparrows, and killdeer, all of which freely intermingle with domestic birds. Highly virulent strains of *C. psittaci* can be carried by and excreted in large numbers by sea gulls and egrets without any apparent effect on these hosts.

Experimental hosts of avian chlamydia can include virtually any species of bird. However, different species may vary in susceptibility with some being more or less refractory, whereas infections may be easily established in others. The duration of shedding and the numbers of chlamydiae shed may vary considerably depending upon the avian species. Antibody production as a consequence of a chlamydial infection also may vary.

Mammalian laboratory hosts used for avian chlamydia are principally mice and occasionally guinea pigs. Both of these hosts can have naturally occurring chlamydial infections. Therefore, investigators using these animals should determine the chlamydial status of the breeding stock. Rabbits are refractory to clinical disease caused by avian chlamydiae, but they may be used to produce polyclonal antibodies (90).

Cell culture lines such as McCoy, mouse L cells, HeLa, Vero, BHK 21, BGM, and others may be used to propagate chlamydiae. Some avian strains are more infectious for mouse L cells (90), whereas Vero cells are reported to be superior for growing other strains (83). The BGM cell cultures have been shown to be equally as sensitive as embryonated eggs for isolation of *C. psittaci* from birds (85).

Younger domestic birds are generally more susceptible than older birds to infection, clinical disease, and mortality. Infection in old turkeys such as spent breeder hens can go unnoticed unless birds are subjected to stressful conditions such as shipment to market on crowded trucks. Turkey toms may have a higher mortality rate than turkey hens.

Transmission, Carriers, and Vectors.

The development of methods to serotype readily *C. psittaci* isolates is increasing the understanding of the epidemiology of the disease in birds. It is apparent that certain serovars of *C. psittaci* are usually associated with a given type of bird (e.g., psittacines) and that some of these serovars have a parasitic-like relationship with a given host. That is, infection with *C. psittaci* will result in an inapparently infected carrier that under certain conditions such as stress will shed the organism. The problem of *C. psittaci* carrier status has been known for years with pigeons and psittacine birds and likely occurs with other birds. Chlamydia recovered from psittacine birds is almost always serovar A and, from pigeons and doves, serovar B or serovar E (2, 86).

In turkeys, it does not appear that the serovars associated with disease are endemic, but that they are introduced from feral birds. Isolates from large chlamydial outbreaks in turkeys are generally serovar B or serovar D (2, 86). Serovar B is common in pigeons and has been isolated from clinically normal pigeons. It has been recovered from a number of outbreaks with low mortality in turkeys. Serovar D, which is usually found in high mortality outbreaks, has never been consistently associated with any avian species except turkeys; however, because of the methods used to raise turkeys and the time between outbreaks, it is doubtful that it is endogenous in the turkey population. If it is endogenous in turkeys, an occasional major change in virulence would be required to explain the sporadic nature of the outbreaks. Therefore, it is likely endogenous in some other species of bird that occasionally commingles with turkeys. The source or reservoir of this serovar is not known.

Chlamydial isolates of the serovar C have been isolated from ducks and swans in Europe (86). The number of isolates that have been serotyped are too few to determine whether it is primarily a strain from ducks and other anseriformes type of birds. It is interesting that this serovar has not been identified from other birds. In recent years, a few chlamydial isolates have been made from fatal cases in ratites. These isolates have usually been of serovar E, indicating that the ratites may be contracting it from pigeons or doves (3, 28).

Transmission of chlamydiae is probably by inhalation or ingestion of contaminated material. Large numbers of chlamydiae can be in respiratory tract exudate and fecal material of infected birds. The importance of the respiratory exudate has become more apparent: in turkeys, the lateral nasal glands become infected early and remain infected for over 60 days (80). Cloanal/oropharyngeal swabs are more consistent for isolation of the agent than fecal swabs, especially during early stages of infection. Direct transmission through aerosolization of respiratory exudate must be considered as the primary method of transmission during outbreaks.

The role of arthropods in the transmission of chlamydiae is uncertain. Mites from turkey nests can contain chlamydiae (15), and during an epidemic in turkeys in South Carolina, simulid flies were suspected as a possible method of transfer (68). Vertical transmission through the egg was not documented in turkeys (14, 66), but a recent experiment on chickens did indicate this possibility (91).

Incubation Period, Pathogenesis, Signs, Morbidity and Mortality, Gross Lesions, and Histopathology

TURKEYS. Page (60) described the pathogenesis of experimental chlamydiosis when susceptible turkeys were exposed by the airborne route. Within 4 hr, small numbers of organisms had penetrated the abdominal air sacs and mesentery, with larger numbers present in the lungs and thoracic air sacs. Organisms had multiplied extensively by 24 hr and within 48 hr, low numbers of chlamydiae were present in blood, spleen, and kidney. At 72 hr, large numbers of chlamydia were present in the turbinates and colon contents. By 4 days, large numbers were present on the heart. As organisms multiplied in the lung, air sacs, and pericardial membranes, they were released into the bloodstream and filtered out in the spleen, liver, and kidney, or were returned to the environment via nasal and intestinal secretions. When birds had succumbed to acute chlamydiosis, these tissues were found to contain greater than 10^8 organisms per gram.

The incubation period of chlamydiosis in naturally infected birds varies, depending upon the numbers of chlamydiae inhaled and the virulence (toxigenicity) of the infecting strain for that host species. Experimentally, definitive disease signs in young turkeys receiving a virulent strain may be evident in 5–10 days. In birds naturally exposed to smaller doses or in older birds receiving greater exposures, the period may be longer. Strains of lower virulence, which cause less severe signs, may have indefinite incubation periods. Therefore, it may be 2–8 wk after exposure before signs are noticeable.

Signs of chlamydiosis in turkeys infected with virulent strains are cachexia, anorexia, and elevated body temperature. The birds excrete yellow-green, gelatinous droppings. Egg production of severely affected hens declines rapidly (60% production down to 10–20%) and may temporarily cease or remain at a very low rate until complete recovery. Disease signs in a flock infected with strains of low virulence are usually anorexia, and loose, green droppings in some birds, with less effects on egg production.

At the peak of disease in a flock infected with a virulent strain, 50–80% of the birds will show clinical signs, whereas morbidity from less virulent strains is only 5–20%. Mortality caused by virulent chlamydia ranges from 10 to 30% and is only 1–4% with less virulent strains.

The less virulent strains cause gross lesions that are similar to those caused by virulent strains, only less severe and extensive. In overwhelming infections with virulent strains, lungs show diffuse congestion and the pleural cavity may contain fibrinous exudate. In fatal cases, a dark transudate may fill the thoracic cavity. The pericardial membrane is thickened, congested, and coated with fibrinous exudate. The heart may be enlarged and its surface may be covered with thick fibrin plaques or encrusted with yellowish, flaky exudate (Fig. 15.4A,B). Severe damage to the lungs and heart undoubtedly is a major cause of death. The liver is enlarged and discolored and may be coated with thick fibrin. Air sacs are thickened and heavily coated with fibrinous exudate. The spleen is enlarged, dark, and soft and may be covered with gray-white spots representing areas of focal cellular proliferation. The peritoneal serosa and mesentery show vascular congestion and may be coated with foamy, white fibrinous exudate. All of these exudates contain large numbers of mononuclear cells in which numerous microcolonies of chlamydial RBs may be seen. Fibrinous exudates, found on all organs and tissues of the thoracic and peritoneal cavities, reflect vascular damage as well as increasing inflammatory response caused by the continued multiplication of the organisms.

In birds that survive infection with a strain of low virulence, the lungs may not be seriously affected. However, multiplication of organisms on the epicardium may result in the formation of one or more fibrin plaques on the heart (Fig. 15.4C).

Histopathologic changes occurring in turkeys of various ages injected intratracheally with the virulent TT strain of *C. psittaci* were described by Beasley et al. (11). They observed both necrotizing and proliferative changes comparable to those caused by other chlamydial strains in other species (with the exception of focal necrosis of the liver, which is prominent in parrots and mice). Specific cellular changes and corresponding organ damage were decidedly more severe and extensive in young turkeys than in older ones. A majority of the birds examined had tracheitis characterized by extensive infiltration of mononuclear cells, lymphocytes, and heterophils in the lamina propria and submucosa. Cilia were absent in severely affected areas. This extensive tracheal damage is not necessarily characteristic of naturally infected birds and may be a result of intratracheal inoculation of large numbers of organisms. Epithelioid pneumonitis in varying degrees was found in 80–100% of 10-wk-old birds, but less often (10–20%) in mature birds. Lungs of severely affected birds were congested and had extensive infiltration of the tertiary bronchi and respiratory tubules with large mononuclear cells and fibrin. There was necrosis of individual cells and large

areas of tissue; the parenchyma and stroma were equally affected.

Fibrinous to fibrinopurulent inflammatory exudates were present on respiratory and peritoneal surfaces and on the epicardium in a majority of infected turkeys. The pericardium and epicardium were thickened by swelling of congested vessels and an inflammatory exudate containing fibrin, large mononuclear cells, and varying numbers of lymphocytes and heterophils.

Infectious myocarditis was observed in more than half the infected birds, but arteritis was present in only 8%. Hepatitis was present in over 90% of the birds, and in severely affected individuals, there was a diffuse dilation of sinusoids with infiltration of mononuclear cells, lymphocytes, and heterophils. Proliferated and swollen Kupffer cells were filled with debris and a yellowish pigment thought to be hemosiderin. Necrotic hepatic cells were scattered throughout the organ with little focal necrosis. Acutely sick turkeys had a catarrhal enteritis. Spleens of a majority of birds were altered with cellular proliferation and necrosis causing the enlarged and mottled appearance, which was more marked in younger than in older birds.

The organisms also caused orchitis and epididymitis, seeming to have an affinity for the active germinal epithelium (12). Fibrin and inflammatory cells appeared in association with the desquamated and necrotic epithelium, filling the seminiferous tubules with eosinophilic exudate. It was also observed that often the immediate cause of death in adult males was rupture of testicular blood vessels followed by massive internal bleeding. The brains of six infected birds examined were without significant changes.

The less virulent strains of *C. psittaci* also cause cellular proliferation, necrosis of major organs, and vascular congestion in turkeys, but lesions are less extensive and severe (except in the air sacs) than those caused by more virulent strains. Pneumonitis is seen only in birds that succumb to the disease. Infections with strains of low virulence tend to produce chronic long-lasting infections with low mortality (17).

DUCKS. Chlamydiosis in domestic ducks is not an important disease in the United States, but it is important both economically and as a public health hazard in Europe. Severe epidemics occurred in Czechoslovakia between 1949 and 1963 and have been reviewed in detail by Strauss (78). Chlamydiosis in ducks is usually a severe, debilitating, often fatal disease in which young ducks develop trembling, imbalanced gait, and cachexia. They become anorexic with green, watery intestinal contents. They develop a serous or purulent discharge from the eyes and nostrils causing the feathers on the head to become encrusted with exudate. As the disease progresses, the ducks become emaciated and die in convulsions. Morbidity ranges from 10 to 80% and mortality varies from 0 to 30% depending on age and the presence of concurrent infection with salmonellae.

In recent years, a number of outbreaks occurred in ducks in Europe and Australia in which the disease signs in some outbreaks were minimal or absent (8, 43, 48, 59). Deaths and/or clinical signs were associated with stress of handling or with infection by other disease agents. The apparent change in pathogenicity could be attributed to either a change in virulence of the chlamydial agent or improved control of other, synergistic disease agents. Despite this change in pathogenicity, chlamydiae in ducks has remained a public health problem, as a large number of workers became clinically ill and two deaths were reported.

PIGEONS.   The incubation period for chlamydiosis in pigeons is not known. Infection is endemic and is believed to be perpetuated primarily by a parent-to-nestling transmission cycle (13, 53).

Signs of uncomplicated chlamydiosis in pigeons are variable, but those that develop acute disease are anorexic, unthrifty, and diarrhetic. Some develop conjunctivitis, swollen eyelids, and rhinitis (Fig. 15.5). Respiratory difficulty is accompanied by rattling sounds. As disease progresses, birds become weak and emaciated. Recovered birds become carriers without signs of disease. Some birds progress through an infection showing no signs or, at the most, transient diarrhea before becoming carriers. Salmonellosis or trichomoniasis exacerbates the illness in chlamydia-infected carrier birds, inducing signs and lesions of acute disease. Serologic surveys indicate that 30–90% of pigeons experience chlamydial infection with an active infection rate of 19.9% (51).

Gross lesions of uncomplicated chlamydiosis in pigeons are fibrinous exudates on thickened air sacs, the peritoneal serosa, and occasionally the epicardium. The liver is usually swollen, soft, and discolored. The spleen may be enlarged, soft, and dark. Higher than normal amounts of urates are seen in cloacal contents if catarrhal enteritis occurs. Less severe infections may involve only the liver or air sacs. Some heavily infected shedders have no lesions whatsoever (66).

CHICKENS.   Epidemiologic and laboratory evidence indicates that chickens appear to be relatively resistant to disease caused by *C. psittaci*. Acute infection progresses to disease and mortality only in young birds, and the incidence of actual epidemics is very low. Experimentally, even young birds are resistant to many strains of *C. psittaci*. In acute cases, birds have fibrinous pericarditis and he-

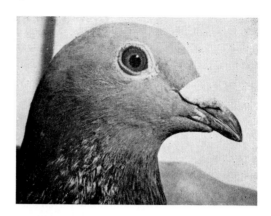

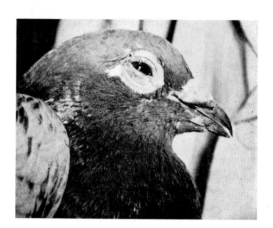

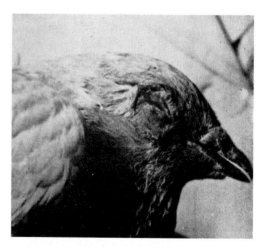

15.5.   Pigeons with no signs of chlamydial infection (*top*); moderate chlamydial conjunctivitis (*middle*); and severe chlamydial conjunctivitis (*bottom*). (Jansen)

patomegaly. Most naturally occurring infections in chickens are inapparent and transient; however, clinical cases with conjunctivitis, pericarditis, perihepatitis and airsacculitis have been reported (7, 9).

GEESE. Incidental to studies of chlamydiosis in ducks, several investigators have observed the disease in geese and have isolated *C. psittaci* from diseased tissues (78). Clinical disease and necropsy findings were similar to those in ducks.

PHEASANTS. Chlamydiae of low virulence have been isolated from tissues of sick pheasants raised on pheasant farms, but no large-scale epidemics of chlamydiosis in this species have been reported (51). Serologic surveys of both wild and commercially raised pheasants in Illinois (51) and Iowa (30) indicate that incidence of infection with chlamydia is very low in the Midwest. Strauss (78), however, reported that humans have contracted psittacosis after contact with pheasants. It seems likely that both wild and domestic pheasants occasionally would be exposed to infectious chlamydia excreted by other hosts, but factors accounting for the lack of acute chlamydiosis in this species are not known.

Immunity. Immunity to chlamydia is generally poor and short-lived. As birds become older, however, they become more resistant to clinical disease, even though infection may occur. Indeed, some birds, notably pigeons, are refractory to disease-producing infection even with highly virulent strains.

In turkeys, a moderate degree of resistance to organ damage is present by 15 wk of age (12) and it probably increases slightly with further aging. The degree of active immunity to reinfection induced in turkeys by naturally occurring infection has not been tested, nor has the resistance induced by experimental infection with organisms of low virulence been determined. That some postinfection immunity occurs in turkeys, however, was implied in experiments of Page (66). The progress of infection initiated by an oral dose of chlamydiae and then spread by natural means through a group of 19 turkeys was followed by isolation attempts from blood and clinical observations. At varying times over a period of 47 days, each bird developed chlamydemia, hyperthermia, and mild anorexia. The chlamydemia lasted up to 10 days in each bird, but was followed by clinical normalcy and apparent resistance to further bloodstream infection in spite of environmental contamination sufficient to infect all unexposed birds.

In ducks, resistance and immunity has not been sufficiently studied. Pigeons are apparently resistant to many avian strains of *C. psittaci,* even the highly toxigenic ones, but they are very susceptible to isolates from pigeons and sparrows (51, 62).

Both antibodies and cell-mediated immunity are likely to be important in resistance to reinfection with chlamydia. One recent study of immunity to *C. trachomatis* in a guinea pig model indicates that serum IgG, secretory IgA, and cell-mediated immunity begin to wane by 30 days after infection, and that reinfection can readily occur (70). Additionally, complete immunity to a third infection was not increased in duration after animals had recovered from two previous infections.

DIAGNOSIS

Specimen Collection and Direct Examination.
The methods used to diagnose avian chlamydiosis vary greatly among laboratories. The preferred method is the isolation and identification of the organism. Because of the time involved, the need for high-quality samples, and the hazard to laboratory personnel, other techniques are often used. These include histochemical staining of exudate, fecal smears, or impression smears, and the immunochemical staining of smears and histologic preparations. Recently, ELISA and PCR techniques have been used; however, the sensitivity and specificity of these tests have not been established at this time.

The samples to be collected will depend on the disease signs, as chlamydia in a bird is often systemic. Samples must be collected aseptically, especially for isolation, as contaminant bacteria can interfere with test results. At necropsy, the tissues of choice are air sacs, spleen, pericardium, heart, liver, and kidney. From live birds, cloanal/oropharyngeal swabs and cloacal swabs are the first choices (5, 6). Feces should not be collected for isolation attempts unless there is no alternative choice. Heparinized blood, conjunctival scrapings, and peritoneal fluids can be collected if indicated by the disease signs.

If the samples are for isolation, proper handling is necessary to prevent loss of infectivity of chlamydiae during shipment and handling. A transport medium consisting of sucrose–phosphate–glutamate (SPG) developed for Rickettsia is satisfactory for chlamydiae. The medium as recommended for chlamydiae consists of SPG buffer (sucrose 74.6 g/L; KH_2PO_4, 0.512 g/L; K_2HPO_4, 1.237 g/L; and L-glutamic acid 0.721 g/L), and can be autoclaved or filtered (76). To this is added 10% fetal calf serum and antibiotics. The transport medium can be used as a diluent for freezing of chlamydia. The samples should not be frozen if they can be processed in 2–3 days. Similarly, a sucrose, albumin (bovine), phosphate solution, pH 7.2, with antibiotics has been satisfactory for maintaining chlamydial infectivity (29).

HISTOCHEMICAL STAINING. Chlamydiae can be detected in smears and paraffin-embedded tissue sections by a number of techniques. The Gimenez- and the Giemsa-staining techniques are commonly used. A modified Gimenez technique or PVK stain as routinely used by a number of laboratories is published (4). The chlamydial EBs in this test will appear red against a green background.

IMMUNOHISTOCHEMICAL STAINING. Immunohistochemical staining is another method for detection of chlamydiae in cytologic and histologic preparations. This technique is more sensitive, but interpretation of the results requires experience. The staining can be done either by IF or immunoperoxide techniques. A number of procedures have been published (4, 88). It should be noted that some monoclonal antibodies do not readily detect formalin-fixed chlamydia. Some monoclonal antibodies to the LPS and polyclonal sera may react with some gram-negative bacteria strains. This usually is not a problem for those laboratory personnel with experience with chlamydiae.

The ELISA is a relatively new technique and may have potential for the future. The ELISA test kits produced for human use have been tried for detection of chlamydia in birds (88). These test kits detect the LPS or genus-specific antigen and will react with *C. psittaci* isolates from birds. One problem with some of the kits is that the chlamydial LPS shares some antigenic epitopes with other gram-negative bacteria, and these epitopes can cross-react, resulting in a high number of false-positives. Cross-reactions have been reduced or eliminated in recently designed kits by more careful selection of the monoclonal antibodies. However, these kits still lack sensitivity: most require 500 or more organisms to give a positive reaction. Good culture techniques will outperform them for sensitivity. It is generally felt that these tests can be relied on if there is a positive result from a bird with signs of chlamydia. However, negative reactions from sick birds or positive reactions from normal birds must be questioned.

The newer technique, PCR, has been used to detect chlamydiae in birds (42). This is a new area of research, and comparison studies with isolations are not yet available. The PCR tests developed for use in humans are highly specific and sensitive; however, they will only detect the human *C. trachomatis* strains.

SPECIMEN PREPARATION AND INOCULATION. Isolation attempts may be made by the inoculation of properly processed specimens onto cell culture monolayers, into the yolk sac of 7-day-old chicken embryos, or into mice by the intraperitoneal route. A 20% (w/v) suspension of an appropriate specimen is made in a suitable diluent containing antibiotics that will control ordinary bacteria without effect on chlamydia (see Antibiotic Susceptibility). Specimen suspensions are centrifuged lightly (less than $800 \times g$) for 15–20 min prior to inoculation of the desired host system.

Isolation. Cell cultures are the most convenient method for isolating the avian strains of *C. psittaci*. McCoy, HeLa, Vero, and L929 are the most commonly used cell lines, although a number of other cell cultures can be used. Standard tissue culture media and procedures, with a few modifications, are used. The laboratory equipment and supplies must be suitable to 1) stain and examine for chlamydial inclusions by direct IF or other appropriate staining techniques, 2) permit centrifugation of the inoculum onto the cell monolayer at 37 C or as near as possible, 3) permit staining and examination at 2–3 times during a passage, 4) permit blind passage at 6–7 days, and 5) provide protection of humans against possible infection. Small flat bottom vials (1 dram shell vials) or 24-well multiwell culture plates with 12-mm diameter glass cover slips will meet these requirements and are often used (4, 22). Usually three to four vials are inoculated to permit both the examination of the culture at various times and the repassage of negative samples 6 days after inoculation.

It is common to suppress cell division in order to increase nutrients for the growth of the chlamydiae and to permit longer observation of the infected cell cultures. The host cells can be suppressed by irradiation or by cytotoxic chemicals. Cytotoxic chemicals include 5-iodo-2-deoxygiodine, cytochalasin B, cycloheximide, and emetine hydrochloride (40). Cycloheximide is the most commonly used and is added to medium at a rate of 0.5–2.0 µg/mL at the time of inoculation of the monolayer. Emetine may have an advantage in some operations because it is removed following treatment of the cells for 5 min with 0.5 µg/mL. After treatment and removal of the emetine, the cells can be infected and overlayered as normal. The effects of these drugs on replication of the chlamydiae can be variable; however, they appear to have no effect or a possible enhancing effect on the growth of the avian chlamydial strains.

Another method used to enhance the infection rate is to centrifuge the inoculum onto the cell monolayer. Centrifugation is routinely done at 500–$1500 \times g$ for 30 to 90 min. Temperatures near 37 C are preferred. Following centrifugation, the inoculum is removed and replaced with tissue culture medium containing the proper cell division inhibitor and then incubated at 37–39 C.

Monolayers are stained and examined for inclusions on day 2 or 3 and on day 5 or 6 postinfection. Before staining, the monolayers are first fixed with acetone or an acetone–methyl alcohol mixture, depending on the cell culture vessel.

The preferred method to demonstrate the chlamydial inclusion is by direct IF (4). The inclusion can also be demonstrated by indirect IF immunohistochemical or histochemical, especially Gimenez, Giemsa, or Macchiavello, techniques.

CHICKEN EMBRYO INOCULATION. Fertile chicken eggs incubated 6 or 7 days at 39 C are inoculated with 0.2–0.5 mL/embryo via the yolk sac. Eggs for this use must be from chickens that are not consuming chlamydiastatic antibiotics in their feed. Inoculated embryos should be incubated at 39 C because that temperature significantly accelerates chlamydial growth (64). Vascular congestion in the yolk sac is the predominant lesion seen in embryos dying from *C. psittaci* infection. The yolk sacs are harvested from embryos that die from 3 to 10 days after inoculation. If no embryos die, one or two blind passages should be performed. Touch impressions are prepared for staining and microscopic examination, or the yolk sac harvest is inoculated onto tissue culture monolayers and later identified with chlamydia specific MAbs.

Identification. To be identified as *C. psittaci*, a pure chlamydial isolate must have microcolonies (inclusions) that are dense and of variable shape. This is readily demonstrated in infected cell cultures that have been stained by Gimenez or other histochemical methods. Inclusions must not contain glycogen, which is detectable by appropriate iodine staining of organisms in cell cultures. Additionally, growth of the isolate must not be inhibited more than 10-fold (LD_{50}) in chicken embryos, which are also inoculated with 1 mg of sodium sulfadiazine/embryo when compared with embryos without the drug.

The presence of *Chlamydia* (genus-specific) antigen in infected cell cultures, chicken embryo yolk sacs, or mouse tissues or exudates also may be detected by appropriate complement-fixing antibodies to identify further the agent as a chlamydial isolate. Direct or indirect immunofluorescence, with appropriate fluorescein isothiocyanate-conjugated immunoglobulins, may be used for the same purpose, as can direct or indirect ELISA methods with appropriate enzyme-conjugated immunoglobulins.

Serology. The various serologic methods for detecting chlamydial antibodies have been reviewed recently (23). Therefore, only the most commonly used methods are discussed here; newer methods currently being evaluated receive less discussion.

Complement fixation (CF) is a widely used method for detecting chlamydial antibodies. This is partly because the immunodominant carbohydrate-containing antigen of chlamydia readily induces complement-fixing antibodies. Such antibodies are no indication of immunity to reinfection with chlamydiae. They are useful, however, in detecting chlamydial infection, especially in a flock of birds. Generally, higher titers (≥64 in poultry) are indicative of a current or recent infection. If low titers are obtained, it may be necessary to retest in about 10–14 days to detect any change in titer. A fourfold or greater increase is considered to be diagnostic of a current chlamydial infection. Guinea pig serum as a source of complement for the test must come from chlamydia-free animals.

DIRECT COMPLEMENT FIXATION. Antigen prepared from cell culture-propagated chlamydiae (31) has been used in a microprocedure to detect chlamydial antibodies in turkey serum (35), in wild bird sera (29), and in psittacine bird sera (22). Direct CF is a relatively sensitive method for detecting chlamydial antibody. Details of the microprocedure and for the method of antigen production are published (32).

MODIFIED DIRECT COMPLEMENT FIXATION. By the addition of fresh normal chicken serum at a level of 5% (v/v) to the complement, the sensitivity of the CF procedure is increased (29), so that the procedure can be used to test sera from avian species whose antibodies do not normally fix guinea pig complement.

LATEX AGGLUTINATION AND ELEMENTARY BODY AGGLUTINATION. These methods were developed for use with psittacine bird sera. It also has been shown, however, that the latex agglutination (LA) test is useful for screening turkey serum for antibodies (25) and for testing pigeon and dove sera (26). Its usefulness for testing sera of ducks and geese is not known. The LA method predominantly detects IgG, but will detect IgM (33). Its main disadvantage is that it is not as sensitive as direct CF, which detects only IgG activity in avian serum (33), nor as sensitive as the more recently described elementary body agglutination (EBA) test, which detects only IgM activity (27, 34). The EBA test has been evaluated and is currently being used for detecting antibody activity in various types of birds. It should have value in detecting current or recent infections as it detects IgM activity.

INDIRECT MICROIMMUNOFLUORESCENCE AND INDIRECT IMMUNOFLUORESCENCE. The indirect MIF and indirect IF (IIF) tests have been used extensively for serotyping of *C. trachomatis* in humans and more recently for identifying whether an immune response in humans is to *C. trachomatis, C. pneumonia,* or *C. psittaci*. The principles of the tests are similar in that both are an indirect IF test, with the IIF test detecting reactions to inclusions in infected cell culture and the MIF test detecting the EBs attached to a microscope slide. A report (74) compared these tests to the CF and the ELISA for measuring antibody in pigeon sera, and found the IIF and MIF tests to be highly specific and efficient. The tests are used in serotyping avian isolates (2, 86) and have potential as a serologic test. Older serologic methods that are not widely used, e.g., rapid plate (or slide) and capillary tube agglutination, indirect CF inhibition, passive hemagglutination, immunodiffusion, and others, are described elsewhere (23).

Newer methods such as indirect ELISA and indirect IF are being used but they need to be thoroughly researched and evaluated to ascertain their usefulness. A competitive-inhibition (also termed "blocking") ELISA was developed and widely used in Germany (75), but it has been discontinued.

Differential Diagnosis.

Suspected chlamydiosis may have to be differentiated from pasteurellosis, particularly in turkeys in which some signs and lesions may be similar. Pasteurellosis can be ruled out by appropriate culture procedures. Because of some similar signs and lesions, mycoplasmosis may need to be ruled out in turkeys suspected of having chlamydiosis. That can be accomplished by culturing and serologic testing for mycoplasmosis. Colibacillosis may mimic chlamydiosis to some extent; it can be excluded by the use of the appropriate coliform culturing procedures. Avian influenza may have to be ruled out in suspected chlamydiosis by virus isolation attempts and by serologic testing.

TREATMENT.

Turkeys should be treated with chlortetracycline (CTC) at a concentration of 400 g/ton of pelleted feed. Care must be taken so that heat produced during the pelleting process does not destroy CTC and lower the concentration below an effective level. The CTC-medicated feed must be given for 2 wk and then replaced by nonmedicated feed for 2 days prior to the birds being slaughtered for meat for human consumption. Calcium supplement should not be added to CTC-medicated pellets because calcium ions chelate CTC and diminish its effectiveness. It is recommended that all turkeys on an infected premise be treated and sent for slaughter. Reinfection can recur readily since resident wild birds may continue to harbor chlamydiae, or the treatment outlined may not rid all birds of chlamydia. Further discussion of treatment with CTC is discussed in Page and Grimes (67). Prior to turkeys being marketed, they should be examined by a veterinarian and 1–2% should be tested serologically. It may be advisable to also attempt isolations on tissues from birds randomly selected from those tested serologically.

Essentially the same treatment methods are used to treat other fowl infected with *C. psittaci.* In other birds, salmonellosis may often be a complicating factor, so it may be necessary to use a combination of antibiotics.

Pigeons should be treated with CTC-medicated feed, but the treatment may not be effective in eliminating the carrier state. Alternating periods of treatment with periods of no treatment may eventually clear the chronic infection (51).

PREVENTION AND CONTROL

Management Procedures.

Ideally birds should be reared in confinement without any contact with potentially contaminated equipment or premises. Contact with potential reservoirs or vectors such as wild and feral birds should also be prevented. General sanitation must be practiced diligently. Movement of people should be restricted so that visitors do not have free access to premises holding birds. This is easier to accomplish if birds are confined in houses.

Immunization.

There are no commercial chlamydial vaccines that induce long-lasting protective immunity against chlamydia. In birds, Page (65) was successful in eliciting a cell-mediated response that protected 90% of turkeys against severe challenge. There was virtually no detectable humoral antibody response and two doses of vaccine had to be given 8 wk apart for best results. Additional discussion on vaccination and vaccines is given by Page and Grimes (67). The practicality of immunizing large numbers of birds that experience occasional epidemics of chlamydial infections is questionable.

State and Federal Regulations.

State regulatory agencies may impose quarantine on intrastate movement of diseased flocks and may require antibiotic treatment of the flock prior to slaughter. Because regulations may vary from state to state, the appropriate public health and/or animal health agencies should be consulted as necessary.

According to United States Department of Agriculture (USDA) regulations, movement of poultry, carcasses, or offal from any premise is prohibited where the existence of chlamydiosis has been proven by isolation of a chlamydial agent. The Animal and Plant Health Inspection Service of the USDA and the U.S. Department of Health and Human Services forbid interstate movement of birds from infected flocks, but there is no restriction of movement of eggs from such flocks.

REFERENCES

1. Andersen, A.A. 1991. Comparison of avian Chlamydia psittaci isolates by restriction endonuclease analysis

and serovar-specific monoclonal antibodies. J Clin Microbiol 29:244-249.

2. Andersen, A.A. 1991. Serotyping of Chlamydia psittaci isolates using serovar–specific monoclonal antibodies with the microimmunofluorescence test. J Clin Microbiol 29:707–711.

3. Andersen, A.A. 1995. Unpublished data.

4. Andersen, A.A., and J.P. Tappe. 1989. Chlamydiosis. In H.G. Purchase, L.H. Arp, C.H. Domermuth, J.E. Pearson, (eds.). A Laboratory Manual for the Isolation and Identification of Avian Pathogens, 3rd ed. Kendall/Hunt Publishing Co., Dubuque, IA, pp. 68–74.

5. Andersen, A.A., T.P. Sanderson, and J.P. Tappe. 1988. Comparison of fecal, cloacal, and oral samples for the Diagnosis of Chlamydiosis. Proc 31st Annu Meet Am Assoc Vet Lab Diagn, p. 55.

6. Arizmendi, F., and J.E. Grimes. 1995. Comparison of the Gimenez staining method and antigen detection ELISA with culture for detecting chlamydiae in birds. J Vet Diagn Invest 7:400-401.

7. Arzey, G.G., and K.E. Arzey. 1990. Chlamydiosis in layer chickens. Aust Vet J 67:461.

8. Arzey, K.E., G.G. Arzey, and R.L. Reece. 1990. Chlamydiosis in commercial ducks. Australian Vet J 67:333–334.

9. Barr, D.A., P.C. Scott, M.D. O'Rourke, and R.J. Coulter. 1986. Isolation of Chlamydia psittaci from commercial broiler chickens. Aust Vet J 63:377–378.

10. Baviol, P., R.S. Stephens, and S. Falkow. 1990. A soluble 60,000 M.W. antigen of chlamydia spp. is a homolog of Escheria coli GroEL. Mol Microbiol 4:461–469.

11. Beasley, J.N., D.E. Davis, and L.C. Grumbles. 1959. Preliminary studies on the histopathology of experimental ornithosis in turkeys. Am J Vet Res 20:341–349.

12. Beasley, J.N., R.W. Moore, and J.R. Watkins. 1961. The histopathologic characteristics of disease producing inflammation of the air sacs in turkeys: A comparative study of pleuropneumonia-like organisms and ornithosis in pure and mixed infections. Am J Vet Res 22:85–92.

13. Davis, D.J. 1955. Psittacosis in pigeons. In F.R. Beaudett (ed.). Psittacosis: Diagnosis, Epidemiology, and Control, pp. 66–73. Rutgers University Press, New Brunswick, NJ.

14. Davis, D.E., J.P. Delaplane, and J.R. Watkins. 1957. The role of turkey eggs in the transmission of ornithosis. Am J Vet Res 18:409–413.

15. Eddie, B., K.F. Meyer, F.L. Lambrecht, and D.P. Furman. 1962. Isolation of ornithosis bedsoniae from mites collected in turkey quarters and from chicken lice. J Infect Dis 110:231–237.

16. Fukushi, H., and K. Hirai. 1992. Proposal of Chlamydia pecorum sp. Nov. for Chlamydia strains derived from ruminants. Int J Syst Bacteriol 42:306–308.

17. Gale, C., V.L. Sanger, and B.S. Pomeroy. 1960. The gross and microscopic pathology of an ornithosis virus of low virulence for turkeys. Am J Vet Res 21:491–497.

18. Gimenez, J.F. 1964. Staining rickettsiae in yolk sac cultures. Stain Technol 39:135–140.

19. Grayston, J.T. 1992. Chlamydia pneumoniae, strain TWAR pneumonia. Annu Rev Med 43:317–323.

20. Grayston, J.T., C.-C. Kuo, L.A. Campbell, and S.-P. Wang. 1989. Chlamydia pneumoniae sp. Nov. for Chlamydia sp. strain TWAR. Int J Syst Bacteriol 39:88–90.

21. Grayston, J.T., L.A. Campbell, C.-C. Kuo, C.H. Mordhorst, P. Saikku, D.H. Thom, and S.-P. Wang. 1990. A new respiratory tract pathogen: Chlamydia pneumoniae strain TWAR. J Infect Dis 161:618–625.

22. Grimes, J.E. 1985. Enigmatic psittacine chlamydiosis: Results of serotesting and isolation attempts, 1978 through 1983, and considerations for the future. Am J Vet Med Assoc 186:1075–1079.

23. Grimes, J.E. 1989. Serodiagnosis of avian chlamydia infection. J Am Vet Med Assoc 195:1561–1564.

24. Grimes, J.E. 1994. Avian Chlamydiosis. In G.W. Beran and J.H. Steele (eds.). Handbook of Zoonoses, 2nd ed. CRC Press, Boca Raton, FL, pp. 389–402.

25. Grimes, J.E. 1995. Unpublished data.

26. Grimes, J.E., and F. Arizmendi. 1992. Bases for interpretation of chlamydia serology results. Proc 1992 Annu Conf Assoc Avian Vet, pp. 59–71.

27. Grimes, J.E., and F. Arizmendi. 1993. Elementary body agglutination: A rapid clinical diagnostic aid for avian chlamydiosis. Proc 1993 Annu Conf Assoc Avian Vet, pp. 30–40.

28. Grimes, J.E., and F. Arizmendi. 1994. Case reports of ratite chlamydiosis and update on the chlamydias. Proc 1994 Annu Conf Assoc Avian Vet, pp. 133–140.

29. Grimes, J.E., and L.A. Page. 1978. Comparison of direct and modified direct complement-fixation and agar-gel precipitin methods in detecting chlamydial antibody in wild birds. Avian Dis 22:422–430.

30. Grimes, J.E., and P.B. Wyrick. 1991. Chlamydiosis (Ornithosis). In B.W. Calnek, H.J. Barnes, C.W. Beard, W.M. Reid, and H.W. Yoder, Jr. (eds.). Diseases of Poultry, 9th ed. Iowa State University Press, Ames, IA, pp. 311–325.

31. Grimes, J.E., L.C. Grumbles, and R.W. Moore. 1970. Complement-fixation and hemagglutination antigens from a chlamydial (ornithosis) agent grown in cell cultures. Can J Comp Med 34:256–260.

32. Grimes, J.E., B.E. Daft, L.C. Grumbles, J.E. Pearson, and T.E. Vice. 1987. A manual of methods for laboratory diagnosis of avian chlamydiosis. American Association of Avian Pathologists, Kennett Square, PA.

33. Grimes, J.E., D.N. Phalen, and F. Arizmendi. 1993. Chlamydia latex agglutination antigen and protocol improvement and psittacine bird anti-chlamydia immunoglobulin reactivity. Avian Dis 37:817–824.

34. Grimes, J.E., T.N. Tully, Jr., F. Arizmendi, and D.N. Phalen. 1994. Elementary body agglutination for rapidly demonstrating chlamydial agglutins in avian serum with emphasis on testing cockatiels. Avian Dis 38:822–831.

35. Hall, C.F., S.E. Glass, J.E. Grimes, and R.W. Moore. 1975. An epidemic of ornithosis in Texas turkeys in 1974. Southwest Vet 28:19–21.

36. Hatch, T.P., E. Al-Hossainy, and J.A. Silverman. 1982. Adenine nucleotide and lysine transport in C. psittaci. J Bacteriol 150:622–670.

37. Hatch, T.P., I. Allan, and J.H. Pearce. 1984. Structural and polypeptide differences between envelopes of infective and reproductive life cycle forms of Chlamydia spp. J Bacteriol 157:13–20.

38. Hatt, C., M.E. Ward, and I.N. Clark. 1988. Analysis of the entire nucleotide sequence of the cryptic plasmid of Chlamydia trachomatis serovar L1: evidence for involvement in DNA replication. Nucleic Acids Res 16:4053–4067.

39. Herring, A.J. 1993. Typing Chlamydia psittaci—A review of methods and recent findings. Br Vet J 149:455–475.

40. Herring, A.J., M. McClenaghan, and I.D. Aitken. 1986. Nucleic acid techniques for strain differentiations and detection of Chlamydia psittaci. In D. Oriel, G. Ridgeway, J. Schachter, D. Taylor-Robinson, and M. Ward (eds.). Chlamydial Infections. Cambridge University Press, Cambridge, United Kingdom, pp. 578–580.

41. Herring, A.J., M.C. McCafferty, G.E. Jones, S. Dunbar, and A.A. Andersen. 1994. Vaccination against chlamydial abortion in sheep: Problems and progress with a recombinant vaccine. In J. Orfila, G.I. Byrne, M.A. Chernesky, J.T. Grayston, R.B. Jones, G.L. Ridgway, P. Saikku, J. Schachter, W.E. Stamm, and R.S. Stephens (eds.). Chlamydial Infections. Proceedings of the Eighth International Symposium on Human Chlamydial Infections, Chateau de Montvillargenne, Gouvieux-Chantilly, France, pp. 118–121.

42. Hewinson, R.G., S.E.S. Rankin, B.J. Bevan, M. Field, and M.J. Woodward. 1991. Detection of Chlamydia psittaci

from avian field samples using the PCR. Vet Rec 128:129–130.

43. Hinton, D.G., A. Shipley, J.W. Galvin, J.T. Harkin, and R.A. Brunton. 1993. Chlamydiosis in workers at a duck farm and processing plant. Aust Vet J 70:174–176.

44. Hodinka, R.L., and P.B. Wyrick. 1986. Ultrastructural study of mode of entry of C. psittaci into 929 cells. Infect Immun 54:855–863.

45. Johnson, M.C., and J.E. Grimes. 1983. Resistance of wild birds to infection by Chlamydia psittaci of mammalian origin. J Infect Dis 147:162.

46. Kaltenboeck, B., and J. Storz. 1992. Biological properties and genetic analysis of the ompA locus in chlamydiae isolated from swine. Am J Vet Res 53:1482–1487.

47. Manire, G.P., and A. Tamura. 1967. Preparation and chemical composition of the cell walls of mature infectious dense forms of meningopneumonitis organisms. J Bacteriol 94:1178–1183.

48. Martinov, S.P., and G.V. Popov. 1992. Recent outbreaks of ornithosis in ducks and humans in Bulgaria. In P.A. Mardh, M. La Placa, and M. Ward, (eds.). Proceedings of the European Society for Chlamydia Research. Uppsala University Centre for STD Research, Uppsala, Sweden, pp. 203.

49. Matsumoto, A. 1981. Isolation and electron microscopic observations of intracyoplasmic inclusions containing C. psittaci. J Bacteriol 145:605–612.

50. Meyer, K.F. 1941. Phagocytosis and immunity in psittacosis. Schweiz Med Wochenschr 71:436–438.

51. Meyer, K.F. 1965. Ornithosis. In H.E. Biester and L.H. Schwarte (eds.). Diseases of Poultry, 5th ed. Iowa State University Press, Ames, IA, pp. 675–770.

52. Meyer, K.F. 1967. The host spectrum of psittacosis-lymphogranuloma venereum (PL) agents. Am J Ophthamol 63:1225–1246.

53. Meyer, K.F., B. Eddie, and H.Y. Yanamura. 1942. Ornithosis (psittacosis) in pigeons and its relation to human pneumonitis. Proc Soc Exp Biol Med 49:609–615.

54. Mohan, R. 1984. Epidemiologic and laboratory observations of Chlamydia psittaci infection in pet birds. J Am Vet Med Assoc 184:1372–1374.

55. Morange, A. 1895. De la psittacose, ou infection speciale determinee par des perruches. These, Academie de Paris.

56. Morrison, R.P., K. Lyung, and H.D. Caldwell. 1989. Chlamydial disease pathogens: Ocular delayed hypersensitivity elicited by a genus specific 57 kD protein. J Exp Med 169:663–675.

57. Moulder, J.W. 1985. Comparative biology of intra-cellular parasitism. Microbiol Rev 49:298–337.

58. Newhall, W.J.V., and R.E. Jones. 1983. Disulfide-linked oligomers of MOMP of Chlamydia. J Bacteriol 154:998–1001.

59. Newman, C.P.St. J., S.R. Palmer, F.D. Kirby, and E.O. Caul. 1992. A prolonged outbreak of ornithosis in duck processors. Epidemiol Infect 108:203–210.

60. Page, L.A. 1959. Experimental ornithosis in turkeys. Avian Dis 3:51–66.

61. Page, L.A. 1959. Thermal inactivation studies on a turkey ornithosis virus. Avian Dis 3:67–79.

62. Page, L.A. 1967. Comparison of "pathotypes" among chlamydial (psittacosis) strains recovered from diseased birds and mammals. Bull Wildl Dis Assoc 3:166–175.

63. Page, L.A. 1968. Proposal for the recognition of two species in the genus Chlamydia Jones, Rake, and Stearns, 1945. Int J Syst Bacteriol 18:51–66.

64. Page, L.A. 1971. The influence of temperature upon the multiplication of chlamydiae in chicken embryos. Excerpta Med Proc Trachoma Conf, Int Conf, Ser 223, pp. 40–41.

65. Page, L.A. 1975. Stimulation of cell-mediated immunity to chlamydiosis in turkeys by inoculation of chlamydial bacterin. Am J Vet Res 39:473–480.

66. Page, L.A., and R.A. Bankowski. 1959. Investigation of a recent ornithosis epornitic in California turkeys. Am J Vet Res 20:941–945.

67. Page, L.A., and J.E. Grimes. 1984. Avian Chlamydiosis (Ornithosis). In M.S. Hofstad, H.J. Barnes, B.W. Calnek, W.M. Reid, and H.W. Yoder, Jr. (eds.). Diseases of Poultry, 8th ed. Iowa State University Press, Ames, IA, pp. 283–308.

68. Page, L.A., W.T. Derieux, and R.C. Cutlip. 1975. An epornitic of fatal chlamydiosis (ornithosis in South Carolina turkeys. J Am Vet Med Assoc 166:175–178.

69. Perez-Martinez, J.A., and J. Storz. 1985. Antigenic diversity of Chlamydia psittaci of mammalian origin determined by microimmunofluorescence. Infect Immun 50:905–910.

70. Rank, R.G., B.E. Batteiger, and L.S.F. Soderberg. 1988. Susceptibility to reinfection after a primary chlamydial genital infection. Infect Immun 56:2243–2249.

71. Register, K.B., P.A. Morgan, and P.B. Wyrick. 1986. Interaction between Chlamydia spp. and human polymorphonuclear leukocytes in vitro. Infect Immun 52:664–670.

72. Richmond, S.K., and P. Stirling. 1981. Localization of Chlamydial group antigen in McCoy cell monolayers infected with C. trachomatis or C. psittaci. Infect Immun 34:561–570.

73. Ryll, M., K.-H. Hinz, U. Neumann, and K.-P. Behr. 1994. Pilotstudie uber das vorkommen von Chlamydia psittaci-infectionen in kommerzillen putenherden niedersachsens. Dtsch Tierarztl Wochenschr 101:163–165.

74. Salinas, J., M.R. Caro, and F. Cuello. 1993. Comparison of different serological methods for the determination of antibodies to chlamydia psittaci in pigeon sera. J Vet Med B 40:239–244.

75. Satalowich, F.T., L. Barrett, C. Sinclair, K. Smith, and L.P. Williams (National Association of State Public Health Veterinarians Compendium Committee). 1993. Compendium of chlamydiosis (psittacosis) control, 1994. J Am Vet Med Assoc 203:1673–1680.

76. Spencer, W.N., and F.W.A. Johnson. 1983. Simple transport medium for the isolation of Chlamydia psittaci from clinical material. Vet Rec 113:535–536.

77. Storz, J., and P. Spears. 1977. Chlamydiales: Properties, cycle of development and effect on eukaryotic host cells. Curr Top Microbiol Immunol 76:167–214.

78. Strauss, J. 1967. Microbiologic and epidemiologic aspects of duck ornithosis in Czechoslovakia. Am J Ophthalmol 63:1246–1259.

79. Tam, M.R., W.E. Stamm, H.H. Handsfield, R. Stephens, K.K. Holmes, K. Ditzenberger, M. Crieger, and R.C. Nowiniski. 1984. Culture-independent diagnosis of Chlamydia trachomatis using monoclonal antibodies. N Engl J Med 310:1146–1150.

80. Tappe, J.P., A.A. Andersen, and N.F. Cheville. 1989. Respiratory and pericardial lesions in turkeys infected with avian or mammalian strains of Chlamydia psittaci. Vet Pathol 26:386–395.

81. Taylor, H.R., and R.A. Pendergrast. 1987. Attempted oral immunization with chlamydial lipopolysaccharide subunit vaccine. Invest Ophthal Visual Sci 28:1722–1726.

82. Taylor, H.R., J. Schachter, and H.D. Caldwell. 1987. Pathogenesis of trachoma: The stimulus for inflammation. J Immunol 138:3023–3027.

83. Tessler, J. 1984. Growth of several strains of Chlamydia psittaci in Vero and McCoy cells in the presence of cytochalasin and cortisone. Can J Comp Med 48:290–293.

84. Todd, W.J., and H.D. Caldwell. 1985. The interaction of Chlamydia trachomatis with host cells: Ultrastructural studies of the mechanism of release of a biovar II strain from Hela 220 cells. J Infect Dis 151:1037–1044.

85. Vanrompay, D., R. Ducatelle, and F. Haesebrouck. 1992. Diagnosis of avian chlamydiosis: Specificity of the Modified Gimenez staining on smears and comparison of the sensitivity of isolation in eggs and three different cell cultures. J Vet Med B 39:105–112.

86. Vanrompay, D., A.A. Andersen, R. Ducatelle, and F.

Haesebrouck. 1993. Serotyping of European isolates of Chlamydia psittaci from poultry and other birds. J Clin Microbiol Jan:134–137.

87. Vanrompay D., R. Ducatelle, F. Haesebrouck, and W. Hendrickx. 1993. Primary pathogenicity of an European isolate of Chlamydia psittaci from turkey poults. Vet Microbiol 38:103–113.

88. Vanrompay, D., A. Van Nerom, R. Ducatelle, and F. Haesebrouck. 1994. Evaluation of five immunoassays for detection of Chlamydia psittaci in cloacal and conjunctival specimens from turkeys. J Clin Microbiol 32:1470–1474.

89. Wang, S.-P., and J.T. Grayston. 1991. Three new serovars of chlamydia trachomatis: Da, Ia, and L₂a. J Infect Dis 163:403–405.

90. Winsor, D.K., Jr., and J.E. Grimes. 1988. Relationship between infectivity and cytopathology for L-929 cells, membrane proteins, and antigenicity of avian isolates of Chlamydia psittaci. Avian Dis 35:421–431.

91. Wittenbrink, M.M., M. Mrozek, and W. Bisping. 1993. Isolation of Chlamydia psittaci from a chicken egg: Evidence of egg transmission. J Vet Med B 40:451–452.

16 Fungal Infections

INTRODUCTION
Harold L. Chute and John L. Richard

Advances and discoveries in the control and treatment of bacterial and virus diseases of birds have been outstanding in recent years. However, less progress has been made in the control of fungal infections in birds. Fungal infections, while not the most economically important of the various poultry diseases, still have an impact on the health of birds.

Much research has transpired in relation to the growth and metabolism of the specific fungi, but no one has consolidated this data for the benefit of healthier flocks. Newer research has led to the recognition that toxins associated with some fungal isolates can be important in the pathogenesis of the associated fungal disease.

Fungal infections such as histoplasmosis and cryptococcosis are not common pathogens of domestic poultry but are included because they are of public health significance. These pathogens occur widely in the environment and are more common in exotic birds. For information on favus, and some of the older literature references on all fungal infections, please refer to the 8th edition of this book.

ASPERGILLOSIS
John L. Richard

INTRODUCTION. Aspergillosis is defined as any disease condition caused by a member of the fungal genus *Aspergillus*. When avian aspergillosis is mentioned, however, it is usually in the context of pulmonary aspergillosis. Thus, synonyms such as mycotic pneumonia and brooder pneumonia will often appear in the literature. Although the primary target of the agent is the pulmonary system, other disease manifestations also occur in poultry.

HISTORY. Molds, likely belonging to the genus *Aspergillus,* were described in wild birds in the early 1800s occurring in such species as the Scaup duck, jay, and swans (6, 61). The first time that an *Aspergillus* was described in a lesion, however, was in 1842 when Rayer and Montagne (57) identified *A. candidus* from the air sac of a bullfinch. *Aspergillus fumigatus,* the most frequently observed agent of avian aspergillosis, was first found in the lungs of a bustard (*Otis tardaga*) in 1863 and the species name was attributed to Fresenius (14). He also applied the term *aspergillosis* to this respiratory disease. Interestingly, early investigators believed that fungi found in lesions of avian species were growing saprophytically on "morbid products" in the body (6). Aspergillosis is common in turkey poults, having been described by Lignieres and Petit (44). Hinshaw (34) described the disease in adult turkeys.

INCIDENCE AND DISTRIBUTION. Primarily two forms of aspergillosis occur in poultry. Acute aspergillosis is usually characterized by severe outbreaks in young birds and high morbidity and high mortality. Chronic aspergillosis occurs in adult breeder birds (particularly turkeys) or occasionally in birds in an adult flock or aviary. The incidence of chronic disease is not as great, but in commercial poultry flocks there are significant economic losses when adult birds succumb to this disease. Aspergillosis appears to be more significant in confinement situations where stress factors may be involved or where moldy litter or grain is present.

Contaminated poultry litter is often the source of *Aspergillus* conidia (23). Pinello et al. (55) isolated 73 species of fungi from air, litter, and tissues in a confinement turkey house and *Aspergillus* was among the four major genera found. *Aspergillus* spp. were among the most common fungi found in other studies of air or litter flora of poultry houses (42, 45, 72, 77). Air flora density of the four major genera within the poultry house decreased when the windows were opened during the spring (67). Reducing the dust in poultry houses and improving ventilation resulted in a 75% decrease in the incidence of fungal disease (59). Elimination of moldy feed from the diet and environment, along with proper management of the sawdust litter, prevented reoccurrences of fungal ophthalmitis in poultry houses where there was a history of such problems (9).

Outbreaks occur when the organism is present in sufficient quantities to establish disease or when the bird's resistance is impaired by factors such as environmental stresses, immunosuppressive compounds, or inadequate nutrition.

Chute et al. (17) observed that *A. fumigatus* is found frequently and is not always pathogenic in young broiler chicks. Sixteen isolates of *A. fumigatus* were compared for pathogenicity by air sac inoculation of turkey poults. Mortalities were not influenced by the number of conidia given or the source of the isolates, although a single environmental isolate produced no mortality (53). Chute and coworkers (17) found the following genera in lungs and air sacs: *Aspergillus, Penicillium, Paecilomyces, Cephalosporium, Trichoderma, Scopulariopsis,* and *Mucor.*

Aspergillosis can be one of the most frequently reported diseases and a source of considerable monetary loss in turkeys (52).

ETIOLOGY. The two major agents causing aspergillosis of poultry are *A. fumigatus* and *A. flavus.* Other organisms that may be involved are *A. terreus, A. glaucus, A. nidulans, A. niger, A. amstelodami,* and *A. nigrescens.* Both major organisms lack a sexual stage and therefore are classified in the Form Family Moniliaceae, Form Order Moniliales, and Form Class Fungi Imperfecti. These organisms are ubiquitous, commonly occurring in decaying vegetative matter, soil, and feed grains. Therefore, their reproductive structures (conidia) occur in the air flora of most environments. The organisms grow readily on most common laboratory media and the characteristics given below generally are obtained when *A. fumigatus* or *A. flavus* are grown on any of the three media mentioned.

A. FUMIGATUS FRESENIUS 1850

Colony Morphology. The organism grows rapidly on Sabouraud dextrose, Czapek's solution, or potato dextrose agar (25–37 C) with colonies having a diameter of approximately 3–4 cm in 7 days. The flat colonies are white at first, then bluish

green as conidia begin to mature, especially near the center of the colony. As the colony matures, the conidial masses become gray-green while the colony edge remains white. The colony surface varies slightly among isolates being either smooth and velvety to slightly floccose or folded. The colony reverse is usually colorless. A distinctive feature of *A. fumigatus* is the development of columnar masses of chains of conidia arising from the vesicle. The conidial chains may attain a length of up to 400 µm.

The organism is quite thermotolerant growing well at 45 C. The description presented here includes the most typical characteristics, but variations occur in colony color, both surface and reverse, and colony morphology.

Microscopic Morphology. The conidiophores of *A. fumigatus* are smooth, colorless to light green near the vesicle, up to 300 µm in length, and 5–8 µm in diameter (Fig. 16.1). The conidiophore gradually enlarges distally to form a flask-shaped vesicle. The vesicle is 20–30 µm in diameter with a single series of phialides (conidiogenous cells) over the distal half. The phialides (6–8 µm in length) are arranged upward paralleling the axis of the conidiophore. The conidia, green in mass, are echinulate, globose to subglobose, with a diameter of 2–3 µm.

A. FLAVUS LINK 1809

Colony Morphology. The organism grows very rapidly, obtaining a colony diameter of 6–7 cm in 10 days at 25 C on Sabouraud dextrose, Czapek's solution, or potato dextrose agar. Some isolates may be slower growing. The colonies begin as white, close-textured mycelium, turning yellowish to yellow-green with a white colony edge as conidia develop. Mature colonies may become somewhat olive-green. The colony may be radially furrowed or flat. Brownish to black-brown sclerotia, which begin as white tufts of mycelium, may be more evident than conidial development in some isolates. The colony reverse varies from colorless to pinkish drab to brownish in sclerotial strains. The conidial heads of *A. flavus* are radiate with the chains of conidia splitting to form loose columns.

Microscopic Morphology. The conidiophores (up to 100-µm long and 10–65 µm in diameter) of *A. flavus* are thick-walled, rough, and colorless. The vesicles, although more elongated when young, are globose to subglobose (10–65 µm in diameter) with phialides usually in two series (biseriate or two-layered) on the entire surface of the vesicle (Fig. 16.2). Phialides may be one series (uniseriate) or, more rarely, each condition may be

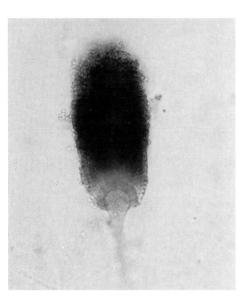

16.1. Conidiophore with flask-shaped vesicle, phialides and columnar mass of chains of conidia of *Aspergillus fumigatus.* ×250.

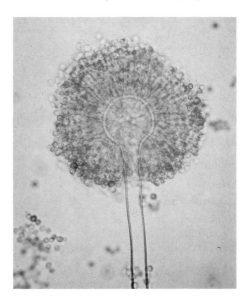

16.2. Conidiophore with globose vesicle, phialides and radiate chains of conidia of *Aspergillus flavus.* ×250.

present in a single head. The conidia are globose to subglobose, echinulate and are between 3 and 6 μm in diameter (usually 3.5–4.5 μm).

Isolates vary considerably in color and number of sclerotia, if any are present. Because the majority of the fungi are identified using morphologic criteria, biochemical properties are not used for this purpose. Some species of the genus *Aspergillus* appear to be quite resistant to chemical agents and have been known to occur in "sanitizing" fluids, sulfuric acid, copper sulfate plating baths, and formalinized tissues for museum specimens (70).

Antigens prepared from *A. fumigatus* and *A. flavus* have been used in the detection of antibodies in experimentally exposed turkey poults (65). These were culture filtrate antigens produced on either a neopeptone dialysate medium or on Dorsett's medium (78).

Japanese workers (5) studied an allergic skin reaction in avian species against an alcoholic precipitate from a mycelial extract of *A. fumigatus*. Penguins showed severe and prolonged skin sensitivity, whereas pigeons and ducks were quite resistant. Zoo penguins frequently die from *A. fumigatus* infections.

TOXINS. *Aspergillus* spp. are among the three most common mycotoxigenic genera. Aflatoxins, along with other mycotoxins are discussed in detail in Chapter 36.

Numerous experimental studies have demonstrated that toxins consumed by poultry can interfere with resistance to various infections. A concept that is not well-recognized, however, is that the pathogenic species of *Aspergillus*, particularly *A. flavus* and *A. fumigatus,* produce toxins that could be involved in the pathogenesis of aspergillosis in poultry. Richard et al. (65) found no enhanced pathogenicity of aflatoxigenic strains of *A. flavus* in turkey poults. On the other hand, *A. fumigatus* conidia caused approximately 50% mortality and induced antibodies in poults exposed by aerosol, whereas *A. flavus* conidia caused neither mortality nor antibody production (65). Some authors had considered previously that a toxin was involved in avian aspergillosis caused by *A. fumigatus* (75). Extensive necrotic lesions (65) and torticollis observed in turkey poults in the absence of brain lesions (66) were reasons for consideration of toxin involvement in aspergillosis caused by *A. fumigatus* (69).

Gliotoxin is one of several toxins produced by various isolates of *A. fumigatus*; it was found to be produced by most of the isolates obtained in an outbreak of aspergillosis of turkeys (62). Turkeys are quite sensitive to oral doses of the toxin, which is quite necrotizing. Gliotoxin also is immunosuppressive; it is cytotoxic to, and inhibits transformation of, turkey peripheral blood lymphocytes (68). Richard and DeBey (63) found that gliotoxin was produced in excess of 6 ppm in some infected tissues in turkey poults. Because of the pathologic changes observed in turkey poults with aspergillosis, and the production of gliotoxin during the pathogenic state in turkey poults, they concluded that gliotoxin could likely be involved in the disease.

PATHOGENESIS AND EPIZOOTIOLOGY

Disease Manifestations

PULMONARY ASPERGILLOSIS. Experimental pulmonary aspergillosis was readily produced by intrathoracic injection of fungal conidia as early as 1884 (79). In 1935, Durant and Tucker (22) produced the disease in a poult by feeding mash contaminated with *A. fumigatus*. Ghori and Edgar (29) found differences in susceptibility to *A. fumigatus* among Japanese quail, turkeys, and chickens, and also strain differences among three strains of chickens (30). Inbred strains were more susceptible than crossbred or outbred strains during an outbreak of aspergillosis in hatchery chicks (11).

Penguins appear to be extremely susceptible to aspergillosis (3), but the disease is significant primarily in captive penguins (41, 50).

The disease is known to occur in a wide variety of avian species, and perhaps all birds, captive and free, domesticated and wild, should be considered as potential hosts susceptible to *Aspergillus* infection (1). Interestingly, 3- to 8-wk-old ostriches in Israel were found to have pulmonary aspergillosis as a dual infection with *A. flavus* and *A. niger* (54). These two organisms were isolated from all samples of affected lungs.

Vigorous healthy birds apparently can withstand considerable exposure to *Aspergillus* conidia under natural conditions. Inhalation of large numbers may occur when litter or feed is heavily contaminated with the organisms, and infections may ensue. Approximately 50% of turkey poults died following a 10-min aerosol exposure to conidia of *A. fumigatus* resulting in 5×10^5 colony-forming units/g of lung tissue (65). No deaths occurred in turkey poults similarly exposed to *A. flavus,* perhaps because the size of *A. flavus* conidia (3–6 µm) is considerably greater than that of *A. fumigatus* (2–3 µm) and, thus, they would not reach as deeply into the respiratory tract. Walker (81) reported that 5- to 7-day-old ostriches succumbed in 2–8 days from pulmonary aspergillosis after conidia were aerosolized into the trachea. Turkey poults aerosol-exposed to 2.2×10^6 viable units of *A. fumigatus*/g of lung tissue all died by day 5; lower doses (5.2×10^5 viable units) delayed and reduced mortality. Deaths began by 3–4 days postexposure.

Julian and Goryo (39) described ascites as a frequent sequela to pulmonary aspergillosis caused by *A. fumigatus*. They determined that the cause could be due to right ventricular failure resulting from pulmonary hypertension secondary to lung damage.

SYSTEMIC ASPERGILLOSIS. Systemic aspergillosis in poults was reported by Witter and Chute (83). Chute et al. (16) also reported systemic aspergillosis infection in caponized 5-wk-old cockerels. The

authors concluded that this resulted from a caponizing infection. An outbreak of *A. flavus*-induced systemic aspergillosis in turkey poults with sternal bone involvement was described by Ghazikhanian (28).

DERMATITIS. Necrotic granulomatous dermatitis was described in chickens and *A. fumigatus* was isolated from infected tissue (86). Lahaye (43) discussed cutaneous aspergillosis of pigeons. Otherwise cutaneous lesions as a manifestation of aspergillosis are rare in avian species.

OSTEOMYCOSIS. *A. fumigatus* infection in bone caused deformed vertebrae resulting in partial paralysis of young chickens (10). Presumably, the infections were sequelae to lung disease with hematogenous dissemination of the organism. Note that the outbreak of systemic aspergillosis described above (28) included involvement of the sternal bone and was caused by *A. flavus*.

OPHTHALMITIS. Ophthalmic lesions in birds due to *Aspergillus* (Fig. 16.3A) have been reported since 1940 when Reis (60) recognized aspergillosis in the chicken eye. Similar lesions were described by Hudson (35) in young chicks and by Moore (49) in turkey poults. While these cases of ophthalmitis in avian species were similar in that the infection was unilateral, an important difference occurred in these early reported cases. The first two cases had involvement primarily of the conjunctiva and external surfaces of the eye with the development of a cheesy exudate or plaque forming beneath the nictitating membrane. The fungus could be isolated readily from cultured plaque material. The eye infection described by Moore (49) involved turkey poults that had respiratory aspergillosis and the cornea of the eye was not involved. Most of the pathologic changes occurred in the posterior eye involving the vitreous humor and extending into adjacent tissue. Thus, the pathogenesis of the two conditions was apparently quite different; the keratitis and superficial infection probably resulted from exposure of conjunctival surfaces to viable fungal elements from environmental sources. The fungal ophthalmitis involving the posterior eye, however, may have resulted from a hematogenous or lymph dissemination of the organism from a primary respiratory infection. Although not a frequent occurrence, the latter type of eye infection usually is apparent in birds with respiratory involvement. Reis (60) was able to reproduce a superficial eye infection in chickens by introducing conidia of *A. fumigatus* into the eye. The yellow caseous plaque can become adherent to the cornea in the superficial type of infection (37). Because of swelling, this infection may resemble coryza or vitamin A deficiency in chicks (76). After Chute and O'Meara

(15) injected conidia of *A. fumigatus* into the abdominal air sacs of chickens, one bird developed a plaque on the surface of one eye. They did not speculate concerning the route of infection.

Recently, Beckman and coworkers (9) described a somewhat different fungal ophthalmitis in a group of chicks from a breeder farm that had recurring problems with similar eye infections. The causative agent was *A. fumigatus*, but in addition to exudate within the conjunctival sac, there was histopathologic evidence of fungal invasion of the anterior chamber and cornea similar to that described by Moore (49). Although the chicks had respiratory lesions, the authors did not consider the route of infection to be hematogenous from the respiratory lesions because there was no involvement of intraocular structures.

Occasionally, turkeys experimentally exposed to aerosols of conidia developed a cloudy eye with retinitis, iridocyclitis, and secondary involvement of the remainder of the eye (67). There was a cellular infiltration of heterophils and macrophages, and cellular debris and fungal elements were present in the chambers and retina. The pecten was severely involved with edema, heterophils, mononuclear cells, and fungal elements present. In some turkeys, the pecten contained granulomas.

Conidia of *A. fumigatus* may be disseminated by the hematogenous route. Richard and Thurston (64) isolated *A. fumigatus* from the blood of turkeys immediately after a 15-min aerosol exposure of conidia. At this time, respiratory macrophages contained numerous ingested conidia. This may be the route of dissemination resulting in the eye and brain lesions (67). Usually, by 24 hr postexposure the organism was cleared from the bloodstream.

Following oculonasal vaccination against Newcastle disease, mortalities increased rapidly in chickens that had contracted superficial ocular aspergillosis in the hatchery (47). This type of ocular involvement was described by Moore (49) and occurred in five widely separated flocks of young poults and in three breeding flocks.

ENCEPHALITIS. Numerous reports have described encephalitic or meningoencephalitic aspergillosis in a variety of avian species. In turkeys, necrotic foci in the cerebrum or cerebellum were found to occur naturally (56). Richard et al. (66) found such foci in turkey poults experimentally exposed to aerosols of *A. fumigatus* conidia. Outbreaks of meningoencephalitis have occurred in turkey poults, eider ducklings, and chickens (87). Others have described encephalitic aspergillosis in turkey poults and chickens occurring as caseous necrotic lesions of the cerebrum and cerebellum or as granulomatous encephalitis (2, 31).

Jungherr and Gifford (40) found fungal hyphae in the cerebellum of a poult that had exhibited nervous

symptoms. In another outbreak in poults with pneumomycosis and nervous manifestations, they recovered *A. fumigatus*, *A. niger*, and *Penicillium varioti* from internal organs. *P. varioti* was also isolated from the brain of one poult, but since fungal hyphae could not be demonstrated and the culture proved nonpathogenic, it was concluded that the symptoms and brain lesions had a toxigenic origin. Bullis (12) recovered *A. fumigatus*, and later *Diplococcium* spp., from cerebrums of poults that showed incoordination. In most cases, there was concurrent infection of the lungs and air sacs, and often the kidney and liver were involved.

Richard et al. (67) speculated that the brain lesions found after experimental aerosol exposure of turkeys may be the result of hematogenous dissemination as has been described in humans (71). Some experimentally exposed turkeys had a notable torticollis, and brain lesions were found at necropsy. Torticollis occurs also in naturally occurring infections of *A. fumigatus* in turkeys, geese, and chickens (80).

Transmission.   A case of egg-borne aspergillosis was reported by Eggert and Barnhart (24). They suggested that the fungus had penetrated through the eggshell during incubation and recently hatched chicks were infected. Clark et al. (18) reported on other cases of aspergillosis that originated in hatcheries. From 21 ranches where 210,000 chicks were involved, there was mortality of 1–10%. Infection could not be traced to hatching eggs but was readily found in incubators, hatchers, incubator rooms, and intake ducts. Signs and lesions were noted in some day-old chicks, but generally, classic lesions were observed in chicks 5 days of age.

O'Meara and Chute (51) found that hatching chicks and up to 2-day-old chicks were easily infected with *A. fumigatus* spores by contaminating the forced-draft incubator with wheat seeded with *A. fumigatus*. Chicks older than 3 days were resistant to infection.

Egg embryos are quite susceptible to infection by *A. fumigatus* during incubation. Embryo contamination occurred when a petroleum jelly suspension of *A. fumigatus* conidia was applied to the surface of incubating eggs (84), and infections increased when the incubating eggs were dusted with *A. fumigatus* conidia (85). Within 8 days after the dusting application, the organism had penetrated the eggshell.

Signs.   Dyspnea, gasping, and accelerated breathing may be present. When these signs are associated with other respiratory diseases such as infectious bronchitis and infectious laryngotracheitis, they are often accompanied by gurgling and rattling noises, whereas in aspergillosis there usually is no sound. Guberlet (32) ascribed somnolence, inappetence, emaciation, increased thirst, and pyrexia to aspergillosis. Cases under his observation emaciated rapidly and showed diarrhea in the later stages. Dysphagia was noted in cases in which esophageal mucosa was involved. Mortality was as high as 50% in confined birds on some farms, whereas birds running outdoors were more resistant or escaped infection entirely. According to Van Heelsbergen (79), some workers reported serous excretions from nasal and ocular mucosa. Extreme dyspnea was recorded in canaries by De Jong (20). Onset of signs did not occur before 48 hr in turkey poults experimentally infected with high doses of *A. fumigatus* or *A. flavus* (67). In an outbreak in captive wild poults, mortality totaling 75% began at 5 days, reached a peak at 15 days, and subsided at 3 wk of age (22). Some affected poults died in convulsions within 24 hr. Gauger (27) reported an outbreak in adult chickens in which about 10% of the flock had signs characteristic of laryngotracheitis and in which there was no abnormal mortality, but egg production was temporarily lowered.

Because torticollis and/or lack of equilibrium occurs in both experimental (66) and in naturally occurring infections by *Aspergillus* spp. (56, 80), this should be considered as a sign of avian aspergillosis. However, other infectious agents, including other genera of fungi, can cause similar signs.

Gross Lesions. Early lesions in experimental infection in turkey poults consisted of small white caseous nodules (approximately 1 mm in diameter) scattered throughout lung tissue (Fig. 16.3B), usually accompanied by similar sized caseous plaques on thickened air sac membranes (67, 74) (Fig. 16.3C). The caseous nodules consisted of inflammatory exudate and fungus tissue. Occasionally, red-tinged ascites was present. In more advanced cases, the plaques were larger and more numerous on greatly thickened air sac membranes; the plaques often coalesced to form aggregate lesions (67). In advanced cases of aspergillosis, the organism often sporulates on the surface of the caseous lesions and on the walls of the thickened air sacs (67, 74) as evidenced by visible greenish-gray mold growth. Durant and Tucker (22) observed yellowish-white nodules up to 5 × 8 mm in lungs of wild poults reared in captivity. Hyphae of the fungus also penetrated lung tissue, and there was involvement of adjacent air sacs.

In an outbreak of aspergillosis in chicks, no evidence of yellowish foci was found, but the lungs were a diffuse grayish yellow (73). Mohler and Buckley (48) described lesions in a flamingo consisting of membranous masses of mycelia covering the bronchial mucosa in addition to lung nodules. Similarly, bronchiolar lesions of microcolonies of fungus were described in an ostrich (4). In another

case in an ostrich, the lungs were covered with miliary foci (38).

Caseous exudate and mycelia, sometimes with mucopurulent to gelatinous exudate, may be present in the syrinx in infected birds (Fig. 16.3D). Variations in lesions depend on the location. Localized tracheal aspergillosis caused by *A. flavus,* described by Barton and coworkers (8), was characterized by grossly visible yellow caseous plaques adherent to the mucosal surface that sometimes occluded the lumina. The tracheal walls were reddened as well.

Lesions in brain tissue were described by Richard et al. (67) as white to yellow circumscribed areas (Fig. 16.3E), usually visible on the brain surface. They were present either in the cerebellum or cerebrum or less frequently in both.

In canaries observed by De Jong (20), there were small, whitish-yellow, crusty coatings on the tongue, palate, and aditus laryngis, and in the trachea and syrinx. Caseous foci in lungs and caseous coatings on the pleura and peritoneum were also observed. Lahaye (43) stated that *A. glaucus* may be the cause of a skin disease in pigeons, particularly in young birds, and that any part of the body may be affected with yellow scaly spots. Feathers in the affected areas were dry and easily broken.

Histopathology. Examination of lung tissues from turkey poults revealed no differences in histopathologic lesions caused by *A. fumigatus* or *A. flavus* (65). Early lesions were characterized by focal accumulations of lymphocytes, some macrophages, and a few giant cells. Later, lesions

16.3. Aspergillosis (*A-G*). Thrush (*H*). A. Ocular aspergillosis. This form is characterized by extensive keratoconjunctivitis. Panophthalmitis is another form of ocular aspergillosis in which internal structures, especially those in the posterior chamber of the eye are affected. The latter is considered to result from hematogenous spread. B. Respiratory aspergillosis in the lung showing large and extensive caseous nodules. (Peckham) C. Caseous nodules due to aspergillosis in the air sac. D. Caseous exudate in the syrinx of a bird affected with aspergillosis. (Peckham) E. Mycotic encephalitis. Focal lesions in the brain can be extensive. F. Experimentally induced granulomatous lesion in the air sac due to aspergillosis. A central caseous core is bordered by a narrow, uniform palisade of macrophages and small giant cells surrounded by a less distinct broad zone of predominantly macrophages and scattered heterophils. ×90. (Kunkle and Barnes) G. Gomori's methenamine silver stained-section of (*F*) demonstrating extensive black-staining fungus. ×90. (Kunkle and Barnes) H. Candidiasis (crop mycosis). Crop is markedly thickened by a soft, yellow-white to gray irregular pseudomembrane, which has a curdlike appearance. (Peckham)

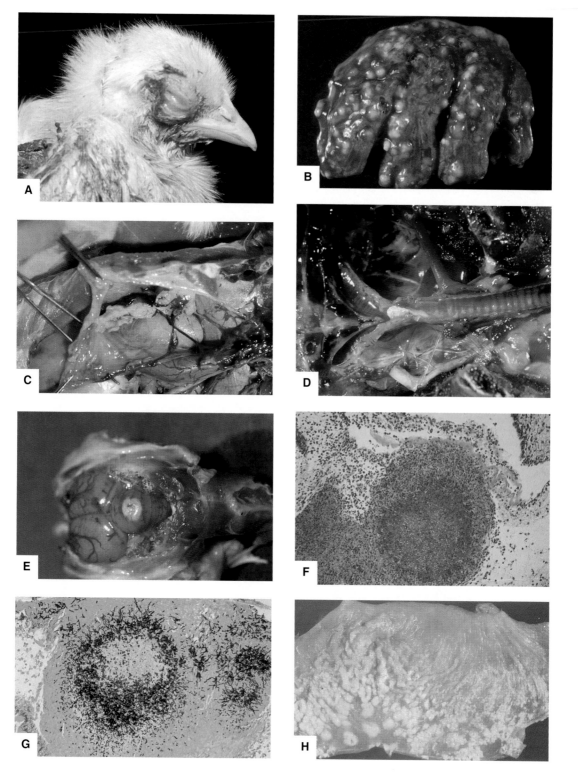

consisted of granulomas with a central area of necrosis containing heterophils surrounded by macrophages, giant cells, lymphocytes, and some fibrous tissue. By 8 wk postexposure, surviving poults had late granulomatous lesions consisting of a necrotic center surrounded by giant cells and a thick layer of fibrous tissue containing a few scattered heterophils (Fig. 16.3F). Using special stains for fungi, the organisms can be seen within the necrotic areas of the lesions (Fig. 16.3G). In tissue sections of the well-oxygenated bronchi, bronchioles, and air sacs, the organism was sporulating asexually.

Brain lesions consisted of solitary abscesses with necrotic centers infiltrated with heterophils and surrounded by giant cells. Hyphae were seen in the central area of some lesions.

Eye lesions were characterized by edema of the pecten, which was heavily infiltrated with heterophils and mononuclear cells. Typical granulomas were found in the pecten. Fungal hyphae, heterophils, macrophages, and cellular debris were found in the chambers and retina of the eye. Edema and some heterophils were found in the sclera and surrounding tissues. In cases of ophthalmitis in turkeys described by Moore (49), primary involvement was in the vitreous humor and adjoining tissues. In one turkey, he observed hyphae in the crystalline lens.

In tracheal lesions, occlusions consisted of fungal mycelia and pyogranulomatous exudate, while the mucosa was necrotic and infiltrated with macrophages and fibroplasia was evident in the subadjacent tracheal wall (8).

DIAGNOSIS

Isolation and Identification of Causative Agent.
Aspergillosis is usually diagnosed at postmortem examination, often based upon observation of white caseous nodules in the lungs or air sacs of affected birds. Bronchoscopy was used, however, in observation of plaques in the bronchi and trachea of an ostrich, and biopsy specimens of infected material were obtained for histologic evaluation and bacterial and fungal examination and culture (46). Although it is sometimes possible to observe fungal growth and sporulation on the caseous nodules or plaques, especially in the air sacs, confirmation should be made by cultural isolation and identification of the causative fungus. Although *A. fumigatus* is the most likely agent of avian aspergillosis, other species of fungi can cause the disease. Therefore, isolates should be identified.

Because most agents of the mycoses are ubiquitous saprophytes, diagnostic samples should be carefully collected using aseptic technique. Samples so collected can be examined microscopically by placing a small portion of the nodule in 20%

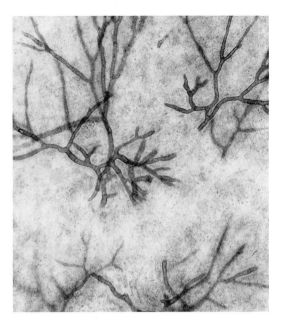

16.4. Hyphae of *Aspergillus fumigatus* in lesion material prepared as a wet mount in 20% KOH and ink dye. ×450.

KOH on a microscope slide, teasing the material apart, and covering it with a glass coverslip. Following gentle heating of the slide over a flame, the specimen can be examined for presence of hyphae within the exudate. If the preparation is too thick, the slide should be incubated 12–24 hr in a moist chamber and re-examined. To aid in elucidating the fungus, the KOH can be mixed with ink dye (Ink blue pp or asb, Parker Pen Co., Janesville, WI). Hyphae of *Aspergillus* stained with the ink dye appear as blue-stained, septate, dichotomously branched structures 2–4 μm in diameter with hyphal walls generally parallel (Fig. 16.4).

Aseptically obtained specimens can be plated directly onto appropriate mycologic media. Alternatively, specimens can be placed in saline solution, minced briefly in a tissue grinder, and then streaked onto the surfaces of mycologic media. Replicate plates should be incubated at both 27 and 37 C. Collected fluids can be centrifuged and the sediment can be examined microscopically or cultured as above.

Satisfactory media for isolation and identification of most isolates from cases of aspergillosis include Sabouraud dextrose agar, Czapek's solution agar, and potato dextrose agar. All cultures should be examined daily and portions of fungal colonies should be transferred to fresh media.

For light microscopic examination, a small portion of the colony containing reproductive structures can be placed in a drop of suitable mounting medium (e.g., lactophenol blue) on a clear glass slide, teased apart, covered with a coverslip and examined.

Although an indirect histochemical technique was used to diagnose aspergillosis in a lovebird (13) the major pathogens of aspergillosis can be identified based on specific characteristics of *A. fumigatus* or *A. flavus* (see Etiology).

Serology. Serologic tests are of limited value due to the nonspecific nature of the antigens. Agar gel precipitin tests were used by Richard et al. (65) in comparisons of *A. fumigatus* and *A. flavus* infections in turkey poults. While most of the *A. fumigatus*-infected poults were positive for precipitating antibodies, poults infected with *A. flavus* were not. A direct enzyme-linked immunosorbent assay (ELISA) technique has been used in turkeys with a correlation occurring between exposure level and ELISA optical density (58). Perhaps the use of serologic methods for identifying poults with aspergillosis for culling procedures would be advantageous, but presently there is no legal or effective therapy for treating positive birds.

PREVENTION AND CONTROL. *Aspergillus fumigatus* infection in young chicks and poults has been somewhat controlled by hatchery sanitation. Sophisticated sampling equipment and media are available to monitor air in hatcheries. Moldy litter or feed and access to musty, moldy strawstacks should be avoided to prevent outbreaks of aspergillosis. Examination of premises or materials used for feed or litter will usually reveal the source of infection.

Areas around feed hoppers and watering places are fertile areas for growth of molds. Unless a permanent yard system is used, frequent moving of feed troughs and watering places is advisable. Placing feed containers and watering fountains on screened, elevated platforms helps to prevent turkeys from picking up molds that develop in such places. Drainage is advisable for areas where water is likely to stand after rains.

Daily cleaning and disinfection of feed and water utensils will aid in eliminating infection. Spraying the ground around containers with chemical solutions may be advisable if it is impossible to change feeding areas frequently. In outbreaks, a 1:2000 aqueous solution of copper sulfate for all drinking water may be used to aid in preventing the spread, though it should not be relied upon as a method to be used continually. Dyar et al. (23) reduced the mold count of contaminated litter and the mortalities of turkeys due to aspergillosis by treating the litter with nystatin and copper sulfate. A thiabendazole solution sprayed on green oak wood shaving litter was efficacious in reducing mold spore counts in the litter and there were reductions in pulmonary lesions of aspergillosis in turkeys raised on that litter (25).

Wawrzkiewicz and Cygan (82) studied 64 strains of fungi of *Aspergillus,* 26 of *Rhizopus,* and 2 of *Mucor* from 56 lung tissue samples of poultry with aspergillosis. The most active fungistats against these in vitro were nystatin, amphotericin B, crystal violet, and brilliant green.

Evidently, increased ventilation within poultry rearing houses reduces the airborne mycoflora (67) suggesting that this could be used as a preventive measure in controlling aspergillosis. Natural ventilation appeared to be better than forced-air ventilation. A significant effect of the type of natural ventilation design (curtain or sliding door), however, was not evident in studies evaluating turkey performance using mortality, average daily gain, feed conversion, condemnations at slaughter, or average individual bird weight as measures of production (19).

Generally, an effective means of therapy for avian aspergillosis is not available. While certain drugs (some are quite new) have been used for treatment of mammalian aspergillosis, they are apparently not cost-effective for poultry. Prevention is currently the preferred means of control. This usually involves eliminating the source of the organism, such as moldy feed and litter, and treating the poultry houses and litter with antifungal compounds. In spite of precautions and preventive measures, outbreaks of aspergillosis frequently occur in some houses and at certain times of the year, particularly during the winter in closed rearing houses. Vaccines could be used; however, none are commercially available. Richard et al. (67) has reduced mortalities by 50% in turkey poults vaccinated with a germling (germinated conidia) vaccine prepared from *A. fumigatus* and subsequently challenge-exposed to aerosols of *A. fumigatus* conidia. Viable spores of *A. fumigatus* administered to ducks provided some protection from death following challenge exposure (5). Hamycin in the drinking water was reportedly successful in controlling an outbreak of aspergillosis in young chicks (7). Miconazole was used successfully in the treatment of raptors with clinical aspergillosis (26). Infections in chick embryos have been controlled by use of amphotericin B (36) and phenylmercuric dinaphthylmethane disulfonate (33). Dimethyldithiocarbamate, injected subcutaneously, was effective against *A. fumigatus* infection in 5- and 10-wk-old chickens. The drug significantly reduced the lesion size and the rate of isolation of the organism from tissues in comparisons between treated and untreated infected birds (21).

REFERENCES

1. Ainsworth, G.C., and P.K. Austwick. 1973. Fungal Diseases of Animals. Farnham Royal, Slough, England.

2. Alexandrov, M., and A. Vesselinova. 1973. Durch Aspergillus fumigatus Fresenius bei truthuhnern verursachte meningoenzephalitis. Zentralbl Vetarinarmed [B] 20:204–309.

3. Appleby, E.C. 1962. Mycosis of the respiratory tract in penquins. Proc Zool Soc Lond 139:395–402.

4. Archibald, R.G. 1913. Aspergillosis in the Suda ostrich. J Comp Pathol Ther 26:171–173.

5. Asakura, A., S. Nakagawa, M. Masui, and J. Yasuda. 1962. Immunological studies of aspergillosis in birds. Mycopathol 18:249–256.

6. Austwick, P.K.C. 1965. Pathogenicity. In Raper, K.B., and D.I. Fennell (eds.). The Genus Aspergillus. Williams and Wilkins Co., Baltimore, MD, pp. 82–126,.

7. Babras, M.A. and C.V. Radhakrishnan. 1967. Aspergillosis in chicks and trial of hamycin in an outbreak. Hind Antibiot Bull 9:244–245.

8. Barton, J.T., B.M. Daft, D.H. Read, H. Kinde, and A.A. Bickford. 1992. Tracheal aspergillosis in 6 1/2-week-old chickens caused by Aspergillus flavus. Avian Dis 36:1081–1085.

9. Beckman, B.J., C.W. Howe, D.W. Trampel, M.C. DeBey, J.L. Richard, and Y. Niyo. 1994. Aspergillus fumigatus keratitis with intraocular invasion in 15-day-old chicks. Avian Dis 38:660–665.

10. Bergmann, V., G. Heider, and K. Vogel. 1980. Mycotic spondylitis as a cause of locomotor disorders in broiler chicken. Monatsh Veterinarmed 35:349–351.

11. Brooksbank, N.H., and P.K. Austwick. 1955. Susceptibility of inbred and outbred chicks to aspergillosis. Br Vet J 111:64–67.

12. Bullis, K.L. 1950. Poultry disease control service. Univ Mass Agric Exp Sta Annu Rep 459:85.

13. Carrasco, L, M.J. Bautista, J.M. de las Mulas, and H.E. Jensen. 1993. Application of enzyme-immunohistochemistry for the diagnosis of aspergillosis, candidiasis and zygomycosis in three lovebirds. Avian Dis 37:923–927.

14. Castellani, A. 1928. Bronchomoniliasis fungi and fungus disease. Arch Dermatol Syph 17:61–97.

15. Chute, H.L., and D.C. O'Meara. 1958. Experimental fungous infections in chickens. Avian Dis 2:154–166.

16. Chute, H.L., J.F. Witter, J.L. Rountree, and D.C. O'Meara. 1955. The pathology of a fungous infection associated with a caponizing injury. J Am Vet Med Assoc 127:250–254.

17. Chute, H.L., D.C. O'Meara, H.D. Tresner, and E. Lacombe. 1956. The fungous flora of chickens with infections of the respiratory tract. Am J Vet Res 17:763–765.

18. Clark, D.S., E.E. Jones, W.B. Crowl, and F.K. Ross. 1954. Aspergillosis in newly hatched chicks. J Am Vet Med Assoc 124:116–117.

19. DeBey, M.C., D.W. Trampel, J.L. Richard, D.S. Bundy, L.J. Hoffman, V.M. Meyer, and D.F. Cox. 1994. Effect of building ventilation design on environment and performance of turkeys. Am J Vet Res 55:216–220.

20. De Jong, D.A. 1912. Aspergillosis der Kanarienvögel (Aspergillosis in canaries). Zentralbl Bakteriol I Orig 66:390–393.

21. Delap, S.K., J.K. Skeeles, J.N. Beasley, D.L. Kreider, C.E. Whitfill, G.E. Houghten, E.M. Walker, D.J. Cannon, and P.L. Earls. 1989. In vivo studies with dimethyldithiocarbamate, a possible new antimicrobial for use against Aspergillus fumigatus in poultry. Avian Dis 33:497–501.

22. Durant, A.J., and C.M. Tucker. 1935. Aspergillosis of wild turkeys reared in captivity. J Am Vet Med Assoc 86:781–784.

23. Dyar, P.M., O.J. Fletcher, and R.K. Page. 1984. Aspergillosis in turkeys associated with use of contaminated litter. Avian Dis 28:250–255.

24. Eggert, M.J., and J.V. Barnhart. 1953. A case of eggborne aspergillosis. J Am Vet Med Assoc 122:225.

25. Fate, M.A., J.K. Skeeles, J.N. Beasley, M.F. Slavik, N.A. Lapp, and J.W. Shriver. 1987. Efficacy of thiabendazole (Mertect 340-F) in controlling mold in turkey confinement housing. Avian Dis 31:145–148.

26. Furley, C.W., and A.G. Greenwood. 1982. Treatment of aspergillosis in raptors (order Falconiformes) with miconazole. Vet Rec 111:584–585.

27. Gauger, H.C. 1941. Aspergillus fumigatus infection in adult chickens. Poult Sci 20:445–446.

28. Ghazikhanian, G.Y. 1989. An outbreak of systemic aspergillosis caused by Aspergillus flavus in turkey poults [abst]. J Am Vet Med Assoc 194:1798.

29. Ghori, H.M., and S.A. Edgar. 1973. Comparative susceptibility of chickens, turkeys and Coturnix quail to aspergillosis. Poult Sci 52:2311–2315.

30. Ghori, H.M., and S.A. Edgar. 1979. Comparative susceptibility and effect of mild Aspergillus fumigatus infection on three strains of chickens. Poult Sci 58:14–17.

31. Guarda, F. 1974. Aspergillosi encefalica nei polli. Schweiz Arch Tierheilkd 116:467–476.

32. Guberlet, J.E. 1923. An epizootic of aspergillosis in chickens. J Am Vet Med Assoc 63:612–622.

33. Harry, E.G., and D.M. Cooper. 1970. The treatment of hatching eggs for the control of egg transmitted aspergillosis. Br Poult Sci 11:269–272.

34. Hinshaw, W.R. 1937. Diseases of turkeys. Calif Agric Exp Sta Bull 613.

35. Hudson, C.B. 1947. Aspergillus fumigatus infection in the eyes of baby chicks. Poult Sci 26:192–193.

36. Huhtanen, C.N., and J.M. Pensack. 1967. Effect of antifungal compounds on aspergillosis in hatching chick embryos. Appl Microbiol 15:102–109.

37. Itakura, C., and M. Goto. 1973. Pathological observation of fungal (Aspergillus fumigatus) ophthalmitis in chicks. Jpn J Vet Sci 35:473–479.

38. Jowett, W. 1913. Pulmonary mycosis in the ostrich. J Comp Pathol Ther 26:253–257.

39. Julian, R.J., and M. Goryo. 1990. Pulmonary aspergillosis causing right ventricular failure and ascites in meat-type chickens. Avian Pathol 19:643–654.

40. Jungherr, E., and R. Gifford. 1944. Three hitherto unreported turkey diseases in Conn.: Erysipelas, hexamitiasis, mycotic encephalomalacia. Cornell Vet 34:214–226.

41. Kageruka, P. 1967. The mycotic flora of Antarctic Emperor and Adelia penguins. Acta Zool 44:87–99.

42. Katoch, R.C., K.B. Bhowmik, and B.S. Katoch. 1975. Preliminary studies on mycoflora of poultry feed and litter. Indian Vet J 52:759–762.

43. Lahaye, J. 1928. Maladies des Pigeons et des Poules, des Oiseaux de Basee-Cour et de Voliere (Diseases of Pigeons and Chickens, of Birds in the Farmyard and Pigeon Loft: Anatomy, Hygiene, Nutrition). Imprimerie Steinmetz-Haenen, Remouchamps.

44. Lignieres, J., and G. Petit. 1898. Péritonite aspergillaire des dindons (Aspergillus peritonitis of turkey toms). Rec Med Vet 5:145–148.

45. Lovett, J., J.W. Messer, and R.B. Read. 1971. The microflora of southern Ohio poultry litter. Poult Sci 50:746–751.

46. Marks, S.L., E.H. Stauber, and S.B. Ernstrom. 1994. Aspergillosis in an ostrich. J Am Vet Med Assoc 204:784–785.

47. Milakovic-Novak, L., A. Nemanic, and A. Kostanjevac. 1977. Ocular aspergillosis in chicken (Aspergiloza ociju u pilica). Vet Arh 47:213–215.

48. Mohler, J.R., and J.S. Buckley. 1904. Pulmonary mycosis of birds with report of a case in a flamingo. USDA BAI Circ 58:122–136.

49. Moore, E.N. 1953. Aspergillus fumigatus as a cause of ophthalmitis in turkeys. Poult Sci 32:796–799.

50. Obendorf, D.L., and K. McColl. 1980. Mortality in little penguins (Eudyptula minor) along the coast of Victoria, Australia. J Wildl Dis 16:251–259.

51. O'Meara, D.C., and H.L. Chute. 1959. Aspergillosis

experimentally produced in hatching chicks. Avian Dis 3:404–406.

52. Owings, W.J. 1986. Turkey health surveys, air quality study. Poultry Newsletter (Cooperative Extension Service, Iowa State University, Summer, 1986), pp. 1–10.

53. Peden, M.W., and K.R. Rhoades. 1992. Pathogenicity differences of multiple isolates of Aspergillus fumigatus in turkeys. Avian Dis 36:537–542.

54. Perelman B., and E.S. Kuttin. 1992. Aspergillosis in ostriches. Avian Pathol 21:159–163.

55. Pinello, C.B., J.L. Richard, and L.H. Tiffany. 1977. Mycoflora of a turkey confinement brooder house. Poult Sci 56:1920–1926.

56. Raines, T.V., C.D. Kuzdas, F.H. Winkel, and B.S. Johnson. 1956. Encephalitic aspergillosis in turkeys: a case report. J Am Vet Med Assoc 129:435–436.

57. Rayer and Montagne. 1842. Mycose aspergillaire dans les poches aeriennes d'un bouvreuil. J Inst Paris Muller's Arch 270 (cited in Austwick, 1965).

58. Redig, P.T., G. Post, T. Concannon, and J. Dunnette. 1986. A direct ELISA for diagnosis of aspergillosis in turkeys [abst]. Proc Conf Res Workers Anim Dis, 67th Meeting. Chicago, IL, p. 30.

59. Reece, R.L., K. Taylor, D.B. Dickson, and P.J. Kerr. 1986. Mycosis of commercial japanese quail, ducks and turkeys. Aust Vet J 63:196–197.

60. Reis, J. 1940. Queratomicose aspergilica epizootica em pintos. Arch Inst Biol Sao Paulo 11:437–462.

61. Richard, J.L. 1975. Aspergillosis. In W.T. Hubbert, W.F. MaCulloch, and P.R. Schnurrenberger (eds.). Diseases Transmitted from Animals to Man. Charles C. Thomas, Springfield, IL, pp. 529–532.

62. Richard, J.L. 1990. Additional mycotoxins of potential importance to human and animal health. Vet Hum Toxicol 32(suppl):63–69.

63. Richard, J.L., and M.C. DeBey. 1995. Production of gliotoxin during the pathogenic state in turkey poults by Aspergillus fumigatus Fresenius. Mycopathologia 129:111-115.

64. Richard, J.L., and J.R. Thurston. 1983. Rapid hematogenous dissemination of Aspergillus fumigatus and A. flavus spores in turkey poults following aerosol exposure. Avian Dis 27:1025–1033.

65. Richard, J.L., R.C. Cutlip, J.R. Thurston, and J. Songer. 1981. Response of turkey poults to aerosolized spores of Aspergillus fumigatus and aflatoxigenic and non-aflatoxigenic strains of Aspergillus flavus. Avian Dis 25:53–67.

66. Richard, J.L., J.R. Thurston, R.C. Cutlip, and A.C. Pier. 1982. Vaccination studies of aspergillosis in turkeys: Subcutaneous inoculation with several vaccine preparations followed by aerosol challenge exposure. Am J Vet Res 43:488–492.

67. Richard, J.L., J.R. Thurston, W.M. Peden, and C. Pinello. 1984. Recent studies on aspergillosis in turkey poults. Mycopathologia 87:3–11.

68. Richard, J.L., W.M. Peden, and P.P. Williams. 1994. Gliotoxin inhibits transformation and its cytotoxic to turkey peripheral blood lymphocytes. Mycopathologia 126:109–114.

69. Richard, J.L., M.C. DeBey, R. Chermette, A.C. Pier, A. Hasegawa, A. Lund, A.M. Bratberg, A.A. Padhye, and M.D. Connole. 1995. Advances in veterinary mycology. J Med Vet Mycol 32:(suppl 1):169–187.

70. Rippon, J.W. 1982. Medical Mycology, the Pathogenic Fungi and the Pathogenic Actinomyctes. W.B. Saunders Co., Philadelphia.

71. Saravia-Gomez, J. 1978. Aspergillosis of the central nervous system. Handbook Clin Neurol 35:395–400.

72. Sauter, E.A., C.F. Peterson, E.E. Steele, J.F. Parkinson, J.E. Dixon, and R.C. Stroh. 1981. The airborne microflora of poultry houses. Poult Sci 60:569–574.

73. Savage, A., and J.M. Isa. 1933. A note on mycotic pneumonia of chickens. Sci Agric 13:341.

74. Schlegel, M. 1918. Aspergillosis (pneumonomycosis aspergillina) bei Truthennen und Hühnern. Z Infektionskr Parasit Kr Hyg Houstiere 19:333–334.

75. Skinner, C.E., C.W. Emmons, and H.M. Tsuchiya. 1947. Henrici's Molds, Yeasts, and Actinomycetes, 2nd ed. John Wiley and Sons, Inc., New York.

76. Sperling, F.G. 1953. Ophthalmic aspergillosis in chickens. Proc 25th Northeast Conf Laboratory Workers Pullorum Dis Control, University of Massachusetts, Amherst, pp. 67-68.

77. Thi So, D., J.W. Dick, K.A. Holleman, and P. Labosky. 1978. Mold spore populations in bark residues used as broiler litter. Poult Sci 57:870–874.

78. Thurston, J.R., J.L. Richard, S.J. Cysewski, and R.E. Fichtner. 1975. Antibody formation in rabbits exposed to aerosols containing spores of Aspergillus fumigatus. Am J Vet Res 36:899–901.

79. Van Heelsbergen, T. 1929. Handbuch der Gelflüegelkrankheiten und der Gelflüegelzucht. Ferdinand Enke, Stuttgart, pp. 312–322.

80. Veen, P.J. 1973. Torticollis and disease of the respiratory tract, caused by Aspergillus fumigatus in fowl. Neth J Vet Sci 5:132–133.

81. Walker, J. 1915. Aspergillosis in the ostrich chick. Union S Afr Dep Agric Annu Rep 3–4:535–574.

82. Wawrzkiewicz, K., and Z. Cygan. 1974. Wrazliwosc in vitro grzybow wyosobnionych z przypadkow grzybic ukladu oddechowego ptakow na fungistatyki. Pol Arch Weter 17:211–224.

83. Witter, J.F., and H.L. Chute. 1952. Aspergillosis in turkeys. J Am Vet Med Assoc 121:387–388.

84. Wright, M.L., G.W. Anderson, and N.A. Epps. 1960. Hatchery sanitation as a control measure for aspergillosis in fowl. Avian Dis 4:369–379.

85. Wright, M.L., G.W. Anderson, and J.D. McConachie. 1961. Transmission of aspergillosis during incubation. Poult Sci 40:727–731.

86. Yamada, S., S. Kamikawa, Y. Uchinuno, A. Tominaga, K. Matsuo, H. Fujikawa, and K. Takeuchi. 1977. Avian dermatitis caused by Aspergillus fumigatus. J Jpn Vet Med Assoc 30:200–202.

87. Zook, B.C., and G. Migaki. 1985. Aspergillosis in Animals. In Y. Al-Doory, and G.E. Wagner (eds.). Aspergillosis. Charles C. Thomas, Springfield, IL, pp. 207–256.

THRUSH (MYCOSIS OF THE DIGESTIVE TRACT)

Harold L. Chute

Stomatitis oidica, muguet, soor, moniliasis, oidiomycosis, candidiasis, and *sour crop* are other terms applied to mycotic infections of the digestive tract.

INCIDENCE. Mycosis of the digestive tract probably occurs rather frequently, but in many cases does not appear to be of sufficient significance to be considered seriously. Numerous general discussions of poultry diseases fail to mention this disorder, and the paucity of diagnoses in reports from diagnostic laboratories suggests that it may not be of great consequence. Serious outbreaks have been reported, however, in many species of birds. Animals and humans are also affected. Thrush has been observed in chickens, pigeons, geese, turkeys, pheasants, ruffed grouse, quail, peacocks, and parakeets.

Gierke (4) reported an outbreak of a thrushlike disease occurring in turkeys in California. Hart (5) reported the disease in turkeys and other fowl in New South Wales. A soluble endotoxin, toxic for mice, has been isolated from *Candida albicans*. A review of the disease in turkeys and chickens in California was recorded by Mayeda (13).

ETIOLOGY. The etiologic significance of yeast-like fungi in infections of the digestive tract of humans was recognized by Langenbeck in 1839. Questions relating to the validity of species described and their generic nomenclature have retarded proper understanding of this type of disease. Jungherr (8, 9) found *Monilia albicans, M. krusei,* and *Oidium pullorum* sp. n. to be associated with cases of thrush but considered *M. krusei* to be of no etiologic significance. *Mucor* spp. and aspergillae were also found in association with some cases. Hinshaw (6) reported *M. albicans* to be found in most cases of thrush in turkeys and chickens that came to his attention. Both investigators noted that the mycotic infections were apt to be associated with unhygienic conditions.

Studies of Benham (1), Worley and Stovall (19), Martin et al. (12), and others indicated the complexity of the problem. Stovall (14) presented a means of improving the present uncertain status, suggesting a specific set of environmental conditions under which biologic characteristics of the organism were constant and could be demonstrated. Jungherr (9) stated that *M. albicans* is of widespread occurrence in gallinaceous birds, pathogenic to birds and also to rabbits on intravenous (IV) injection, and indistinguishable from strains isolated

from human sources. On Sabouraud dextrose agar it produces a whitish, creamy, high-convex colony after incubation for 24–48 hr at 37 C. Young cultures consist of oval budding yeast cells about 5.5×3.5 μm. Older cultures show septate hyphae and occasionally spherical, swollen cells with thickened membrane, the so-called chlamydospores. In Dunham's peptone water containing 1% fermentable substance and 1% Andrade's indicator, the organism produces acid and gas in dextrose, levulose, maltose, and mannose; slight acid in galactose and sucrose; and does not attack dextrin (variable according to brand), inulin, lactose, and raffinose. Gelatin stab cultures show short villous to arborescent outgrowths without liquefaction of the medium.

The term *medical monilias* is frequently used in connection with the generic term *Monilia*, which is also used for a separate group of fungi. Most workers have accepted the decision of an informal group meeting at the Third International Microbiological Congress in 1939 and use *Candida* as a generic name to replace the familiar but invalid *Monilia. C. albicans* is the most frequently isolated etiologic agent associated with the disturbance commonly referred to as moniliasis.

PATHOGENESIS AND EPIZOOTIOLOGY

Signs and Lesions. Signs are not particularly characteristic. Affected chicks show unsatisfactory growth, stunted appearance, listlessness, and roughness of feathers. Lesions occur most frequently in the crop and consist of thickening of the mucosa with whitish, circular, raised ulcer formations (Fig. 16.3H [*Note*: Figure 16.3 can be found in the section entitled Aspergillosis in this chapter]), the surfaces of which tend to scale off. Pseudomembranous patches and easily removed necrotic material over the mucosa are not uncommon. The mouth and esophagus may show ulcerlike patches. When the proventriculus is involved, it is swollen, the serosa has a glossy appearance, and the mucosa is hemorrhagic and may be covered with catarrhal or necrotic exudate. Histologically, Jungherr (7) reported that crops showed extensive destruction of the stratified epithelium deep in the malpighian layer, and quite often walled-off ulcers or extensive diphtheroid to diphtheritic membranes were present. Lesions were characterized by absence of inflammatory reaction. Periportal focal necrosis in the liver in some cases suggested toxic action upon the system.

The frequent association of mycosis of the digestive tract with other debilitating conditions such as gizzard erosions and intestinal coccidiosis must be considered. Gizzard erosions, as such, probably are not directly related to thrush. Likewise, the thickened intestine with watery contents frequently noted in cases of thrush is probably due to coccidiosis or other protozoan infections.

In the case of thrush, the esophagus, crop, and proventriculus show an ulcerated and scaly condition. Spores and hyphae of what is termed *O. albicans* can readily be demonstrated in lesions. Diphtheroid lesions are noted in the proventriculus and small intestine. Abscess formations are present under pulpy, soft, grayish-white to brownish-red necrotic masses. Hinshaw (6) reported thrush in 12 flocks of turkeys, with lesions similar to those noted in chickens. Blaxland and Fincham (2) studied five serious outbreaks in young turkeys. Their observations supported previous conclusions that moniliasis is likely to be associated with unhygienic surroundings and other debilitating conditions, but spread of infection appeared definite in many instances. The disease has been described in pigeons and geese.

Tripathy (15) considered that vascular damage in infected turkeys may be associated with candida endotoxin. Atheromatous lesions were present on the intimal surface of the abdominal aorta in more than 50% of turkeys exposed to *C. albicans,* whereas there was only a 12.5% incidence of similar lesions in uninfected controls.

Young birds are more susceptible than older birds to mycosis of the digestive tract. Thus, as infected birds grow older they tend to overcome the infection. Jungherr (7) observed an outbreak in which losses amounted to 10,000 chicks out of 50,000 that were less than 60 days of age. He also reported (9) that turkeys under 4 wk of age succumbed rapidly to infection, but that outbreaks in birds 3 mo of age resulted in a high percentage of recoveries.

Wyatt et al. (20) induced systemic candidiasis in 14-day-old broiler chickens with an intravenous injection of a suspension of *C. albicans* cells. Growth was severely retarded, with reddened livers and kidneys, pancreatitis, and neural disturbances.

DIAGNOSIS. Observation of characteristic proliferative, relatively noninflammatory lesions, with resultant heavy growth on primary cultures, serves to diagnose thrush. Because of the possibility of cultivation of *C. albicans* from apparently normal tissues, an original heavy growth is considered essential for diagnosis. Recognition of spores and more especially hyphae in fresh smear preparations is attended with some difficulty. Miliary abscesses are produced in kidneys of rabbits injected intravenously (1).

Underwood (16) described an instrument known as McCarthy's foroblique panendoscope that was used to diagnose experimental crop moniliasis. This instrument was equipped with a viewing lens and an independent light source. Birds were starved for 12 hr to empty the crop to allow a clear view of the mucosa. A normal crop appeared to be light pink, with a glistening smooth surface having numerous shallow convolutions, whereas a fungus-infected crop showed severe corrugations to mild whitish streaks, erosions or diphtheritic formations, and a deep red surrounding mucosa.

TREATMENT AND CONTROL. Since mycosis of the digestive tract is apt to be related to unhygienic, unsanitary, overcrowded conditions, they should not be allowed to exist or should be corrected. Jungherr (8) found that denatured alcohol and coal-tar derivatives were ineffective as disinfectants and suggested that iodine preparations be used. As a treatment, he recommended that following an Epsom salt flush, 1 level teaspoon powdered bluestone ($CuSO_4$) be added to each 2 gal drinking water in nonmetal containers every other day for 1 wk. Hinshaw recommended that a 1:2000 solution of $CuSO_4$ for turkeys be used as the sole source of drinking water during the course of the outbreak. On the other hand, Underwood et al. (17) found $CuSO_4$ to be ineffective for treating or preventing the disease in chicks and poults with experimentally produced moniliasis. Affected birds should be segregated. Lesions in the mouth can be treated by local application of a suitable antiseptic. Appearance of the disease in very young chicks suggests the surface of the egg as a source of infection. Such a possibility could be removed by dipping eggs in an iodine preparation prior to incubation.

Kostin (11) found that *C. albicans* organisms mixed with poultry droppings and applied to wooden boards could be killed by exposure to 2% formaldehyde or 1% sodium hydroxide solution for 1 hr. Treatment with a 5% solution of iodine monochloride in hydrochloric acid for 3 hr was also successful in disinfection.

Nystatin has been studied by Gentry et al. (3) and Kahn and Weisblatt (10). One group reported that 220 mg nystatin/kg diet was effective in eliminating moniliasis in a flock of turkeys. The other group found that in experimental infections with *C. albicans* in both chickens and turkeys, crop lesion severity appeared to be significantly reduced in the group fed the lowest level of nystatin (11 mg/kg). The highest level (110 mg/kg) showed very significant protection against mycotic infection.

Yacowitz et al. (21) reported successful prevention of candidiasis in chickens by addition of nystatin at a minimum level of 142 mg/kg ration for 4 wk. Kahn and Weisblatt (10) obtained similar results. Wind and Yacowitz (18) successfully treated crop mycosis with nystatin by dispersing it in drinking water at levels of 62.5–250 mg/L with sodium lauryl sulfate (7.8–25 mg/L) for 5 days.

Tripathy (15) found that addition of chlortetracycline (500 g/ton) to a vitamin A–deficient ration had no effect on incidence or severity of crop candidiasis, but increased the cells being shed in feces. Turkeys fed nystatin (100 g/ton) had a higher average weight and milder crop lesions than untreated controls.

REFERENCES

1. Benham, R.W. 1931. Certain molilias parasitic on man. J Infect Dis 49:183–215.
2. Blaxland, J.D., and I.H. Fincham. 1950. Mycosis of the crop (moniliasis) in poultry, with particular reference to serious mortality occurring in young turkeys. Br Vet J 106:221–231.
3. Gentry, R.F., G.R. Bubash, and H.L. Chute. 1960. Candida albicans in turkeys. 1. Treatment of crop infections with mycostatin. Poult Sci 39:1252.
4. Gierke, A.G. 1932. A preliminary report on a mycosis of turkeys, Calif Dept Agric Monthly Bull 21:229–231.
5. Hart, L. 1947. Moniliasis in turkeys and fowls in New South Wales. Aust Vet J 23:191–192.
6. Hinshaw, W.R. 1933. Moniliasis (thrush) in turkeys and chickens. Proc 5th World's Poult Congr 3:190.
7. Jungherr, E.L. 1933. Observations on a severe outbreak of mycosis in chicks. J Agric 2:169–178.
8. Jungherr, E.L. 1933. Studies on yeast-like fungi from gallinaceous birds. Storrs Agric Exp Stn Bull 188.
9. Jungherr, E.L. 1934. Mycosis in fowl caused by yeast-like fungi. J Am Vet Med Assoc 3:500–506.
10. Kahn, S.G., and H. Weisblatt. 1963. A comparison of nystatin and copper sulfate in experimental moniliasis of chickens and turkeys. Avian Dis 3:304–309.
11. Kostin, V.V. 1966. Razrabotka rezhimov dezinfektsii pri kandidamikose Pt ts. (Development of method for disinfection in candidiasis of fowls.). Trudy Vses Inst Vet Sanit 26:157–162.
12. Martin, D.S., C.P. Jones, K.F. Yao, and L.E. Lee, Jr. 1937. A practical classification of the monilias. J Bacteriol 34:99.
13. Mayeda, B. 1961. Candidiasis in turkeys and chickens in the Sacramento Valley of California. Avian Dis 3:232–243.
14. Stovall, W.D. 1939. Classification and pathogenicity of species of Monilia. Microbiol 3rd Int Congr, p. 202.
15. Tripathy, S.B. 1965. Observations of changes in turkeys exposed to Candida albicans. Diss Abstr 6:3187.
16. Underwood, P.C. 1955. Detection of crop mycosis (moniliasis) in chickens and turkeys with a panendoscope. J Am Vet Med Assoc 127:229–231.
17. Underwood, P.C., J.H. Collins, C.G. Durgin, F.A. Hodges, and H.E. Zimmerman, Jr. 1956. Critical tests with copper sulphate for experimental moniliasis (crop mycosis) of chickens and turkeys. Poult Sci 3:599–605.
18. Wind, S., and H. Yacowitz. 1960. Use of mycostatin in the drinking water for the treatment of crop mycosis in turkeys. Poult Sci 39:904–905.
19. Worley, G., and N.D. Stovall. 1937. A study of milk coagulation by Monilia species. J Infect Dis 2:134.
20. Wyatt, R.D., D.C. Simmons, and P.B. Hamilton. 1975. Induced systemic candidiosis in young broiler chickens. Avian Dis 19:533–543.
21. Yacowitz, H., S. Wind, W.P. Jambor, N.P. Willett, and J.F. Pagano. 1959. Use of mycostatin for the prevention of moniliasis (crop mycosis) in chicks and turkeys. Poult Sci 3:653–660.

MISCELLANEOUS FUNGAL INFECTIONS

Harold L. Chute

A number of rare fungal isolations from birds have been reported. These may not be of economic significance to the poultry industry, but should be noted for diagnosticians and researchers.

HISTOPLASMOSIS

Histoplasmosis is an infectious, but not contagious, mycotic disease of human and lower animals. It has been reported commonly in zoo birds, and occasionally, in chicken and turkey populations. It occurs worldwide, especially in areas in the United States bordering the Missouri, Ohio, and Mississippi rivers where the disease appears to be indigenous.

The *Histoplasma capsulatum* organism grows readily in culture media and soil as a white to brown mold that bears spores of two types: 1) spherical, minutely spiny microconidia 3–4 µm in diameter and 2) spherical, or rarely clavate, macroconidia 8–12 µm in diameter, with evenly spaced fingerlike projections. The organism grows in the yeastlike phase, but with difficulty. It requires a temperature of 37 C, a medium rich in protein, preferably blood, and high levels of humidity and carbon dioxide.

The mycelial phase grows on Sabouraud's medium, dextrose agar, potato, gelatin, or bread at any temperature. Colonies appear as white to brownish after 2 wk. The segmented branched hyphae are 2.5-μm wide and give rise to chlamydospores, often in chains with large round cells 20 μm in diameter.

Dodge (1) found the organism in samples from a starling roost in Italy and in soil samples from a schoolyard; a high proportion of the school children were histoplasmin-positive.

Diagnosis is based on three criteria: culture of the organism, histopathology, and histoplasmin sensitivity. The characteristic histopathology is an extensive proliferation of reticuloendothelial cells, many of which contain yeast forms.

Recognized cases of histoplasmosis in humans and animals have not been successfully treated. There is some evidence that the disease occurs in animals in a mild unrecognized form.

REFERENCES

1. Dodge, H.J. 1965. The association of a bird-roosting site with infection of school children by Histoplasma capsulatum. Am J Publ Health 55:1203–1211.

CRYPTOCOCCOSIS

Cryptococcosis is a disease of humans and animals. In humans, it is characterized by a meningitis. Synonyms are torulosis, torula, yeast meningitis and European blastomycosis.

An encapsulated yeast-like fungus in human lesions was reported in 1894. Although it has not been diagnosed as a pathogen in birds, and epizootics have not occurred, its importance to public health and its occurrence in bird's environments warrant discussion.

The disease is widely distributed around the world and although not of economic significance in poultry, there are many sporadic reports from zoo birds.

The fungus belongs to the imperfect yeast group under the name of *Cryptococcus neoformans*. It reproduces by budding; cells are perfectly spherical and surrounded by a thick mucilaginous capsule. Cell diameter is 4–6 μm and the capsule is 1–2 μm thick. It grows well within 48 hr at 30 C on glucose agar.

Bisbocci (1) isolated cryptococci from a pheasant with enterohepatitis. Chickens were experimentally infected and developed the disease. Lesions consisted of granulomas and necrotic processes in liver, intestines, lungs, and spleen.

Emmons (3) shocked the public health world by isolating *C. neoformans* from 16 of 19 premises and 63 of 111 specimens of pigeon droppings. The organism was found in the dropping sites but was not isolated from 20 pigeons examined. It appeared to grow as a saprophyte. Bishop et al. (2) confirmed those findings by isolating *C. neoformans* from 6 of 13 samples of pigeon nests and droppings.

Staib (5) isolated cryptococci from 28 fecal samples obtained from 201 species of birds at zoological gardens and pet shops in Germany. Twelve isolates were from canaries, one was from a wild pigeon, and the remainder were from psittacine and other birds. Fragner (4) isolated cryptococci from feces of 48 pigeons, 13 fowl, 7 pheasants, 10 house martins, 4 jackdaws and 3 chaffinches.

Infections can be diagnosed by culturing the organism. Histopathology has proved extremely useful in diagnosis of cases in mammals. A significant feature is absence of an inflammatory reaction except in late stages, when compression effects end and a chronic inflammatory reaction is produced. Mucicarmine stain is specific; it shows many budding spores, with the thick capsule being darkly stained.

Prognosis is very grave for infected mammals, and no satisfactory treatment is known.

REFERENCES

1. Bisbocci, G. 1938. Infectious entero-hepatitis in fowls due to a cryptococcus. Nouvo Ercolani 43:290–314.

2. Bishop, R.H., R.K. Hamilton, and J.M. Slack. 1960. The isolation of cryptococcus neoformans from pigeon nests. Abstr W Va Bull 26:31–32.

3. Emmons, C.W. 1955. Saprophytic sources of cryptococcus neoformans associated with the pigeon (Columba livia). Am J Hyg 62:227–232.

4. Fragner, P. 1962. Isolation of cryptococcus from bird feces. Csl Epidem Mikrobiol Immunol 11:135–139.

5. Staib, F. 1961. C. neoformans in bird feces. Zbl Bakt 1, (orig.) 182:562–563.

OTHER FUNGAL INFECTIONS

Over the years there have been numerous reports of individual fungal isolations from all classes of birds. Many of these may have been opportunist infections. The most complete review of many of these infections is in a partially annotated bibliography of avian mycosis by Barden et al. (1). In another review (5), Wobeser and Saunders reported several cases of pulmonary oxalosis in humans and animals from an infection with *Aspergillus niger*. This fungus produced appreciable quantities of oxalix acid, which in turn caused tissue necrosis adjacent to the mycelial growth. A detailed description was given for a case in a great horned owl (*Bubo virginianus*).

Ranck et al. (3) described dactylariosis, a new fungal disease of chickens. A fatal encephalitis resulted from the thermophilic fungus *Dactylaria gallopava* in 200 birds from a flock of 65,000. The disease was experimentally reproduced by a spore suspension injected into the left posterior thoracic air-sac, left maxillary sinus, and cerebrum. Brain lesions similar to those in the natural outbreak resulted. Georg et al. (2) described this thermophilic dematiaceous hyphomycete as the casual agent of encephalitis in poults, and Waldrip (4) reported an outbreak in 60,000 birds with a mortality rate of 3–5%. In the latter case, the organism was also isolated from litter samples of broiler houses. It was suggested that wood chips and sawdust litter might have introduced the organism.

Other rare fungal infections have included *Paecilomyces variota*, *Geotrichum candidum*, and *Trichophyton verrucosum*.

Although apparently unimportant and rare, such cases should be reported. The diagnosis of fungal diseases is becoming very complex, particularly as it relates to mycotoxic effects on growth of birds.

REFERENCES

1. Barden, E.S., H.L. Chute, D.C. O'Meara, and H.T. Wheelwright. 1971. A bibliography of avian mycosis (partially annotated). College of Life Sciences and Agriculture. University of Maine, Orono, pp. 1–193.

2. Georg, L.K., B.W. Bierer, and W.B. Cooke. 1964. Encephalitis in turkey poults due to a new fungus species. Sabouraudia 3:239–244.

3. Ranck, F.M., Jr., K. Georg, and H. Wallace. 1974. Dactylariosis a newly recognized fungus disease of chickens. Avian Dis 18:4–20.

4. Waldrip, D.W., A.A. Padhye, L. Ajello, and M. Ajello. 1974. Isolation of Dactylaria gallopava from broiler-house litter. Avian Dis 18:445–451.

5. Wobeser, G., and J.R. Saunders. 1975. Pulmonary oxalosis in association with Aspergillus niger infection in a great horned owl. (Bubo virginianus). Avian Dis 19:388–392.

17 Neoplastic Diseases

INTRODUCTION

B. W. CALNEK

This chapter deals with a variety of related and unrelated conditions possessing a single common denominator: neoplastic character. Some have been extensively studied because of their considerable economic importance. Others have served as highly suitable models for studying various phenomena of neoplasia; indeed, medical research has found avian oncology an abundant resource. For this chapter, neoplasms are divided into two main categories, depending on whether the etiologic agent is known.

Virus-induced tumors are principally of mesodermal origin and are transmissible. Five diseases or disease complexes are described, each in a separate section because of its etiologic distinctness. One, Marek's disease (MD), is a lymphoproliferative disease affecting the peripheral nervous system and, to a greater or lesser degree, other tissues and visceral organs. MD is caused by a herpesvirus.

Second is a group of leukoses, sarcomas, and related neoplasms induced by a number of closely related RNA retroviruses (now called the leukosis/sarcoma group). Prominent in this group is lymphoid leukosis, another lymphoproliferative disease, affecting primarily the bursa of Fabricius and visceral organs. Also included are other neoplasms of hematopoietic origin (erythroblastosis, myeloblastosis, myelocytomatosis, and certain related neoplasms such as nephroblastoma and osteopetrosis). These conditions, along with sarcomas and other connective tissue tumors, are etiologically related and are discussed as a group.

A third section describes conditions associated with the reticuloendotheliosis virus (REV) group. Some members of this antigenically related group of RNA-containing retroviruses (unrelated to the leukosis/sarcoma group) cause nonneoplastic conditions in ducks, others apparently are the cause of lymphoid neoplasms in turkeys, and certain isolates induce reticuloendotheliosis or lymphomas of either B- or T-cell origin in experimentally infected chickens.

The fourth section briefly describes a condition in turkeys called lymphoproliferative disease, which apparently is caused by yet another RNA retrovirus that is distinct from both the REV and leukosis/sarcoma groups.

Tumors of unknown etiology of necessity are described only on the basis of morphologic characteristics and are discussed in the final section. Included are a wide variety of benign and malignant neoplasms derived from muscle, epithelial, and nerve tissues; serous membranes; and pigmented cells.

Classification and nomenclature of the known transmissible neoplasms present a problem. The dilemma is largely due to two factors. First, many virus strains appear to have multipotent characteristics; i.e., they can sometimes induce a variety of neoplasms. Second, certain of the viruses induce some pathologic lesions difficult to distinguish from those induced by another unrelated virus. The two prevalent lymphomatotic diseases, now called lymphoid leukosis and Marek's disease, are particularly confusing with regard to the latter point, and, although REV-induced lymphoid tumors are observed only infrequently, or only under experimental conditions, they may add to the confusion. The problem is compounded by the fact that most flocks and many birds (sometimes including those employed for experimental purposes) are infected with more than one agent, and it is virtually impossible to examine one virus strain without often also observing effects of a second unrelated tumor virus. Prevalence of various unrelated (and related, but different) viruses in experimental birds used for passage of a given virus strain undoubtedly resulted in mixed virus populations in most cases (especially in earlier studies), a factor that must be considered in arguments of the multipotent character of some viruses.

Choice of terminology for this chapter (Table 17.1) is based on that originally adopted by the World Veterinary Poultry Association (2) and includes modifications in current use. The classification system accompanying this nomenclature is especially suited to the mode of presentation that follows, i.e., categorization of diseases or disease complexes by agent type instead of pathologic manifestation. Subdivision within agent-type diseases

Table 17.1.   Transmissible neoplasms

Virus type	Nucleic acid type	Virus classification of etiologic agent	Neoplastic diseases

Retrovirus	RNA	Leukosis/sarcoma group	Leukoses
			    Lymphoid leukosis
			Erythroblastosis
			Myeloblastosis
			Sarcomas and other connective tissue tumors
			    Fibrosarcoma, fibroma
			    Myxosarcoma, myxoma
			    Osteogenic sarcoma, osteoma
			    Histiocytic sarcoma
			Related neoplasms
			    Hemangioma
			    Nephroblastoma
			    Hepatocarcinoma
			    Osteopetrosis

		Reticuloendotheliosis group	Reticuloendotheliosis Lymphoid leukosis
Herpesvirus	DNA	Marek's disease virus	Marek's disease

by pathologic expression has been employed where it seemed appropriate.

Incidence and importance of neoplasms in poultry can only be generally estimated. Feldman and Olson (3) quoted reports (1915–55) in which the incidence of tumors, except neurolymphomatosis and osteopetrosis, varied from 3 to 19%. More recently, we have had the advantage of data accumulated by the United States Department of Agriculture (USDA) from federally inspected slaughtered poultry. These data showed that incidence of "leukosis" in young chickens (probably nearly all MD) increased dramatically during a 10-yr period beginning in 1961.

There was a gradual rise in leukosis condemnations in young chickens from about 0.1% in 1961 to over 1.5% in 1968–70 (see 5). After 1970, the trend was reversed and condemnations of young birds returned to 1961 levels, undoubtedly the result of MD vaccination of broilers. During peak years, however, over 40 million young birds (nearly 50% of all condemnations) were condemned for leukosis, and it was conceded that it was one of the most serious problems confronting the poultry industry.

Condemnations due to leukosis in mature birds were fairly consistent and much lower (less than 0.5 million birds, usually less than 10% of all condemnations). Condemnation rates with other tumors, many of which were leiomyomas of the mesosalpinx, were actually much higher (up to five times) than those from leukosis. Because most losses from leukotic diseases occur during growing and productive periods of layers, presence of gross lesions at slaughter is a poor index of their true incidence and importance.

Annual losses in the United States were placed at more than $150 million in 1967, prior to the introduction of MD vaccines (1). In 1985, Purchase (5) estimated that benefits derived by the poultry industry in the United States as a result of MD vaccine totaled nearly $170 million annually. This included increased egg production and decreased losses from non-MD causes as indirect benefits as well as the direct effect of lowered MD mortality and condemnations. Lymphoid leukosis losses may be significant in some flocks, but mortality probably constitutes only a small portion of the economic loss from that disease. Studies by Gavora et al. (4) and Spencer et al. (6) have shown that lowered egg production and increased mortality from causes other than lymphoid leukosis are associated with infection by lymphoid leukosis virus, and the total economic impact from these could be extremely significant. Present efforts to reduce the infection rate or to eradicate infection could markedly lower this impact. Incidence of neoplasms other than lymphoid tumors appears to be low and of questionable economic significance.

REFERENCES

1. AAAP. 1967. Report of the AAAP-Sponsored Leukosis Workshop. Avian Dis 11:694–702.

2. Biggs, P.M. 1962. Some observations on the properties of cells from the lesions of Marek's disease and lymphoid leukosis. Proc 13th Symp Colston Res Soc, pp. 83–99.

3. Feldman, W.H. and C. Olson. 1965. Neoplastic diseases of the chicken. In H.E. Biester and L.H. Schwarte (eds.). Diseases of Poultry, 5th ed. Iowa State University Press, Ames, IA, pp. 863–924.

4. Gavora, J.S., J.L. Spencer, R.S. Gowe, and D.L. Harris. 1980. Lymphoid leukosis virus infection: Effects on production and mortality and consequences in selection for high egg production. Poult Sci 59:2165–2178.

5. Purchase, H.G. 1985. Clinical disease and its economic impact. In L.N. Payne (ed.). Marek's Disease: Developments in Veterinary Virology. Martinus Nijhoff Publishing, Boston, pp. 17–42.

6. Spencer, J.L., J.S. Gavora, and R.S. Gowe. 1980. Lymphoid leukosis virus: Natural transmission and nonneoplastic effects. Cold Spring Harb Conf Cell Prolif 7:553–564.

MAREK'S DISEASE

B. W. Calnek and R. L. Witter

INTRODUCTION. The most common of the lymphoproliferative diseases of chickens is Marek's disease (MD), which is characterized by a mononuclear infiltration of one or more of the following: peripheral nerves, gonad, iris, various viscera, muscle, and skin. Marek's disease is caused by a herpesvirus, is transmissible, and can be distinguished etiologically from other lymphoid neoplasms of birds.

Terminology has been confusing. The wide variety of clinical signs and pathologic expressions, depending primarily on the location of lesions, led to promulgation of an equally wide variety of terms to identify the conditions. Mononuclear infiltration of peripheral nerves results in gross enlargement and causes paralysis. The inflammatory character of some of the peripheral nerve lesions prompted Marek (273) to identify the disease as *polyneuritis*. Synonyms subsequently employed include *neuritis, neurolymphomatosis gallinarum,* and *range paralysis*. Mononuclear infiltration of the iris, which causes changes ranging from depigmentation to grayish opacity, is the basis for terms such as *blindness, gray eye, iritis, uveitis,* and *ocular lymphomatosis*. Leukotic lesions in various visceral organs and muscles were often referred to simply as visceral lymphomatosis, and those in the skin as skin leukosis. In 1961, Biggs (22) promoted the use of the term *Marek's disease* to distinguish the condition clearly from etiologically different lymphoproliferative diseases. This term is in common use.

Prior to use of vaccines, MD constituted a serious economic threat to the poultry industry because of heavy annual losses. Since vaccines are not 100% effective, losses still occur, but they are no longer as serious a problem. Purchase (371) estimated that mortality and condemnation losses due to MD totaled about $12 million in the United States in 1984. When combined with economic loss from cost of vaccine and application, and reduced egg production, however, the total was about $169 million in the United States and $943 million worldwide.

Purchase and Witter (375) have made a comprehensive review of the literature related to Marek's disease and human health concerns, particularly human cancer. They cite numerous reports of virologic, pathologic, serologic, and epidemiologic studies that support a conclusion that there is no etiologic relationship between MD virus (MDV) or any of the MD vaccine viruses and human cancer.

The literature on MD is voluminous and growing. Because it is increasingly difficult to cite all relevant publications, and because a number of very comprehensive reviews on various aspects of MD are now available, literature citations for this chapter are somewhat more selective than in previous editions. This is especially true of older literature. Where possible, reference to reviews substitutes for many of the possible individual citations. A particularly useful source of information on Marek's disease is the multiauthored book *Marek's Disease, Scientific Basis and Methods of Control,* edited by L. N. Payne (332). Also, the proceedings from several international symposia on Marek's disease (366, 367, 368) offer reviews on various aspects of the disease.

HISTORY. Marek's 1907 report (273) of paresis in roosters owing to mononuclear infiltration of peripheral nerves and spinal nerve roots is probably the first account of the disease. Outbreaks dating to 1914 were reported in the United States; subsequent observations of the disease came from The Netherlands, Great Britain, and many other countries (citations in 24).

As observations were added to Marek's early description, it became apparent that lesions were not restricted to the spinal cord and peripheral nerves. It was learned that blindness was frequently accompanied by paralysis and that extraneural lesions included visceral lymphomas, particularly in the ovary, and infiltration of the iris and brain. Outbreaks of so-called acute MD with unusually high mortality and a preponderance of visceral lymphomas have been observed at least since 1949 (21) and became quite common between 1960 and 1970.

Attempts to transmit the disease, often unsuccessful (citations in 318), along with descriptions of gross and microscopic lesions, accounted for much of the research effort during the 1920s and 1930s.

The importance of genetic constitution as it affected susceptibility to the disease was brought out by the classic work of Hutt and Cole (191). Their studies, which began in the 1930s, laid the foundation for efforts to control losses through genetic selection of breeding stocks.

During a 10-yr period beginning in the early 1960s, there was an exceptional succession of research findings that had a very profound effect on MD and, indeed, on cancer research in all species including humans. The first major breakthrough was the successful and regular experimental transmission of the disease (29, 422). The avid cell association of the agent (30) made identity of the agent elusive. It was not until 1967 that nearly simultaneous, but independent, research in Great Britain (32,

107) and the United States (301, 456) uncovered a herpesvirus as the etiologic agent, following its successful propagation in cell cultures.

Virus culture and identification were followed by a veritable flood of data in which epizootiology, much of the pathogenesis, and many immunologic aspects of the disease were unraveled. A historic account of this work, which came from many laboratories, was provided by Witter (492). Perhaps the most important practical development was the attenuation of virus and its successful application as a vaccine against MD (109, 110). Although superseded by other vaccines, it nonetheless was the first practical effective cancer vaccine in any species and should be recognized as a major advance in medical science.

The findings by Fabricant and coworkers (citations in 142) that MDV infection may lead to arteriosclerosis in chickens have profound implications as a model for the same condition in humans. This discovery, along with continuing studies on the oncogenic and immunologic features of MD as a model of oncogenic herpesvirus infection in other species and the need to develop alternative vaccines or other control methods for flocks with apparent vaccine failures, guarantees that research into the disease will continue. As with most infectious diseases, the preponderance of contemporary work on MD is founded on molecular studies.

Additional historical details can be found in a review by Payne (330).

INCIDENCE AND DISTRIBUTION.
Marek's disease exists in poultry-producing countries throughout the world, as reviewed by Purchase (371). Quite probably every flock of chickens raised in areas where poultry is prevalent experiences some loss, but reporting systems vary and it is difficult to determine the true incidence.

In the United States, the incidence prior to the availability of vaccines was not uniform, largely because of repetitive, acute explosive outbreaks in certain geographic areas. Losses were especially high in areas where poultry (broiler) raising was intensive. Such areas probably continue to have the greatest risk even in the face of vaccination. This uneven distribution may represent existence of a more virulent form of the disease that can occur as an epizootic in certain areas (23). Several reports lend credence to the implication of exceptionally virulent MDV isolates in vaccine failures on certain premises or in some areas (136, 351, 406, 524; additional citations in 497).

Purchase (371) noted that there is a seasonal incidence in broiler flocks with losses higher during winter months, presumably because of lowered air circulation.

Condemnation data from the USDA offer the most definitive information on the variable and in-

consistent incidence of the disease within and between areas; examples are illustrated in Figure 17.1.

ETIOLOGY

Classification. Marek's disease virus is a cell-associated herpesvirus (32, 107, 301, 456, 515) with lymphotropic properties similar to those of gamma herpesviruses. However, its molecular structure and genomic organization are similar to those of alpha herpesviruses (48). Marek's disease virus is the prototype virus of the MDV group, and is designated as serotype 1.

Two additional groups of nononcogenic herpesviruses isolated from turkeys (230, 516) and chickens (28, 101), respectively, also are considered part of the MDV group and, therefore, are included in this chapter. The nononcogenic chicken isolates are designated as serotype 2 MDVs and the turkey herpesviruses, called HVTs based on earlier terminology (516), are designated as serotype 3 viruses. The serotypic classification for MDV and HVT strains (51, 52) is based on the recognition of common and distinct antigenic epitopes for each serotype. Except where otherwise indicated, MDV indicates serotype 1 viruses.

Morphology and Morphogenesis. The morphology and morphogenesis of MDV have been reviewed by Kato and Hirai (227) and Schat (397). In general, viral particles are typical of those described for other herpesviruses. Virions are commonly seen in the nucleus and more rarely in the cytoplasm or extracellular spaces. Hexagonal naked particles or nucleocapsids 85–100 nm in diameter and enveloped particles 150–160 nm in diameter may be seen in thin sections of infected cell cultures. Virus particles observed in negatively stained preparations of lysed feather follicle epithelium (FFE) had envelopes measuring 273–400 nm and appeared as irregular amorphous structures (72). Thin-section preparations of the FFE revealed large numbers of cytoplasmic enveloped herpesvirus particles in keratinizing cells.

In general, morphology of HVT resembles that of MDV. In thin sections, however, nucleocapsids of HVT commonly show a unique crossed appearance (302).

The morphology of serotype 2 MDV has not been studied in detail, but typical particles have been visualized (402).

The morphology of MDV and HVT virions is shown in Figure 17.2.

Viral DNA

PHYSICAL PROPERTIES. The DNA of MDV is a linear, double-stranded molecule that has a buoyant density of 1.706 g/mL, a base composition of 46%

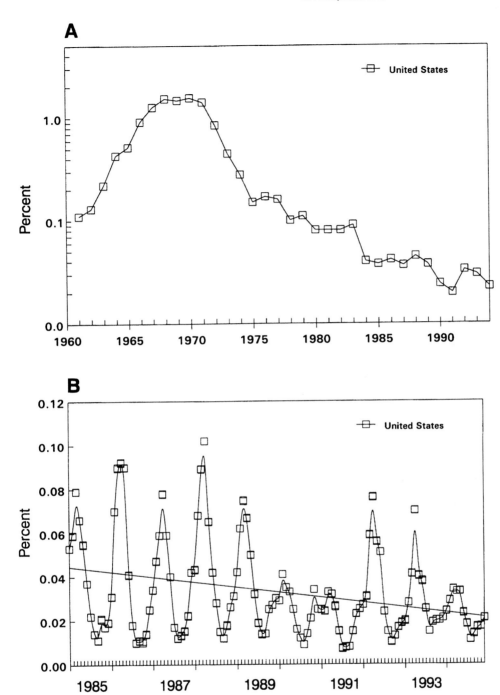

17.1. Marek's disease condemnations in young broilers in the United States. *A.* Annual averages 1960–1994. *B.* Monthly averages 1985-1994. (Data from National Agricultural Statistics Service)

guanine plus cytosine ratio and a molecular weight of 108–120 × 10^6 d (93, 179, 251), which is equivalent to a size of 166–184 kb. The buoyant density and guanine plus cytosine ratio of HVT DNA is generally similar to that of MDV DNA (252); both are difficult to separate from host cell DNA, but

preparative techniques have been described (220). Infectivity of MDV DNA has been demonstrated both in vitro and in vivo (218).

STRUCTURAL ORGANIZATION. All three serotypes have genome structures consisting of a long

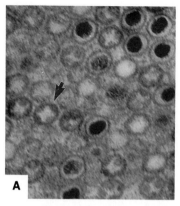 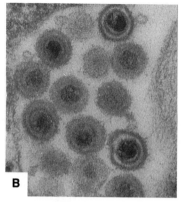 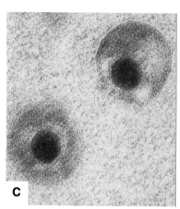

17.2. Electron micrographs of Marek's disease virus (MDV) and turkey herpesviruses (HVT). *A.* Thin section of cultured duck embryo fibroblast infected with HVT. Many nucleocapsids are seen with the typical cross-shaped internal structure (*arrow*). ×70,000. *B.* Thin section of cultured duck embryo fibroblast infected with MDV, showing enveloped virions in a nuclear vesicle. ×60,000. *C.* Thin section of feather follicle epithelium (FFE) of chicken infected with MDV showing enveloped virions within the cytoplasmic inclusions. Note difference in morphology compared with (*B*). ×70,000. (Nazerian)

unique region and a short unique region, each bounded by inverted repeats (93). Physical maps of restriction endonuclease fragments have been constructed for MDV (153), serotype 2 MDV (320), and HVT (193). Based on cross hybridization of cloned DNA fragments, the genomes of all three serotypes are similarly organized, or collinear (193, 320). However, minor but potentially important differences in the genomes have been observed. The genome sizes differ; MDV is largest, HVT is smallest, and serotype 2 MDV is intermediate (93, 179). All three serotypes differ substantially in their restriction endonuclease digestion patterns (157, 179, 391, 448), but share significant homology at the DNA level, particularly with certain individual genes such as gB, gC, gD, and gH (116, 417, 533, 539). The size and structural organization of the genomes of the three viral serotypes are illustrated in Figure 17.3.

VIRAL GENES AND ANTIGEN. Efforts to identify and localize the 70–80 specific genes or genomic regions associated with certain biologic functions in the three serotypes continue to yield useful information, and knowledge is accumulating, particularly with MDV. The approximate locations of identified genes for each serotype are indicated in Figure 17.3.

Although as many as 46 virus-specific polypeptides have been identified by immunoprecipitation from extracts of cells infected with MDV or HVT (194, 479, 480), only a few of these (A antigen, B antigen, and pp38) are thus far known to have important antigenic or functional properties. Specific monoclonal antibodies such as M26 for A antigen (197), IAN86 for B antigen (449), and H19 for pp38

(258) are critical for most detection methods.

The known genes of MDV may be grouped into the following categories: oncogenicity related, glycoprotein, and other. The major genes, gene products, and their putative functions are listed in Table 17.2 and some of these are also discussed below.

Oncogenicity-related genes. Three genes or DNA sequences that may be associated with oncogenicity of serotype 1 MDV include genes flanking the 132 base pair repeats, pp38 and meq. A heterogenous expansion region containing multiple, tandem 132 base pair repeats (bpr) has been identified in attenuated MDV and mapped to the inverted repeat region flanking the unique long portion of the genome (154, 272, 450). This region has been identified as a gene family containing three exons (42, 241). Usually, virulent strains have few copies and attenuated strains have multiple copies of the 132 bpr (223, 389), a distinction that forms the basis of differentiation by polymerase chain reaction (PCR) assays (20, 447, 542). The function of this region requires further study, but the finding that oligonucleotides complementary (antisense) to 132-bpr transcripts inhibited proliferation of lymphoblastoid cell lines (231) may provide an initial insight.

The pp38 gene has been cloned and sequenced (119, 120). It is of interest because its product, a 38-kD phosphoprotein, is variably expressed in tumors and cell lines (293, 294) and because no homologue exists in mammalian herpesviruses (120). Homologues of pp38 also occur in serotype 2 MDV (321) and HVT (452) but neither gene appears closely related to MDV pp38.

The pp38 antigen is a virus-specific phosphorylated protein complex containing polypeptides of

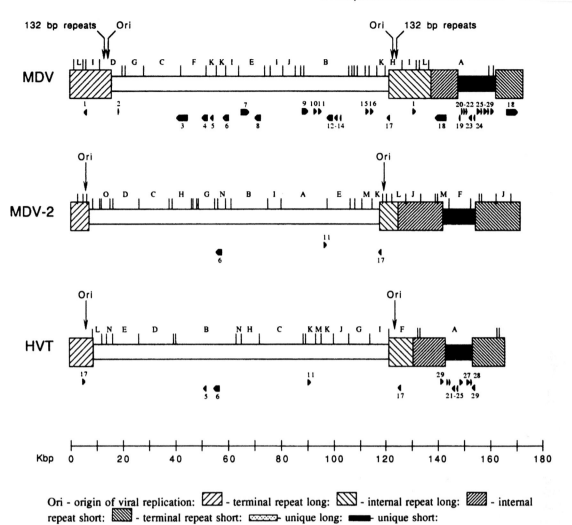

Ori - origin of viral replication: ▨ - terminal repeat long: ▧ - internal repeat long: ▨ - internal repeat short: ▨ - terminal repeat short: ▭ - unique long: ▬ unique short:

17.3.   Structural diagram of the genomes of the three Marek's disease virus (MDV) serotypes. Below each genome, the location and direction of transcription of major viral genes are indicated with *solid arrows* (see Table 17.2 for gene codes). Above each genome, BamH1 restriction sites and letter designations for major fragments are indicated. (Prepared by R.F. Silva)

39–36 kD and 24 kD, which was demonstrated in the cytoplasm of MDV-transformed, latently infected lymphocytes as well as productively infected cells including the FFE (199, 293, 294). This antigen can be demonstrated in latently infected cells and MD tumor cells (119, 199) as well as cells productively infected with serotype 1 MDVs except, curiously, the CVI988 strain and its derivatives (527). Expression of pp38 is variable (or inconsistent) but may be enhanced by treatment with IUdR (202) or transfection with the ICP4 gene (365). The pp38 antigen may have diagnostic value when present in tumor cells.

Meq (Marek's EcoQ) is expressed in transformed cells (214). This gene has homology to the leucine-zipper class of oncogenes and also codes for a proline-rich domain characteristic of another class of transcription factors (214). A promoter region of this gene contains sequences that resemble a heat-shock element (213). The protein product of meq has not been characterized.

All three potential oncogenicity-related genes map close together in the repeat regions of the MDV genome. In MD lymphomas, gene expression, as measured by transcription, is largely limited to a similar area of the genome located in or near the repeat regions (477, 411, 465) and another region near the ICP4 gene (316). Further research will be needed to establish a causal relationship between any of these genes and oncogenicity.

Table 17.2. Important genes and gene products

Code	Gene	Gene Product Name	MW (Kd)	Present in Serotype	Comment
1	meq	meq	40	1	Resembles *jun/fos* oncogene
2	UL1	gL	25	1	
3	UL19	MCP	150	1	
4	UL22	gH	91	1	
5	TK	TK	39	1, 3	
6	gB	gB, B antigen	49,60,100	1, 2, 3	Immune protection
7	UL30	DNA poly-merase	130	1	
8	UL32	gp82	82	1	
9	UL39	RR$_1$	92	1, 2, 3	
10	UL40	RR$_2$	38	1, 2, 3	
11	UL44	gC, C antigen	57-65	1, 2, 3	Stimulates AGP antibodies
12	UL47		92	1	
13	UL48	VP16	49	1	
14	UL49		28	1	
15	UL53	gK	40	1	
16	UL54	ICP27	55	1	
17	pp38	pp38	38	1, 2, 3	Expressed in cell lines and some tumors
18	ICP4	ICP4	155	1	
19	SORF1		10	1	
20	SORF2		20	1	Homology with fowlpox virus
21	US1	ICP22	20	1, 3	
22	US10	VP22	24	1, 3	
23	SORF3		41	1, 3	
24	US2		30	1, 3	
25	US3	Protein kinase	45	1, 3	
26	SORF4		17	1	
27	US6	gD	43	1, 3	
28	US7	gI	38	1, 3	
29	US8	gE	54	1, 3	

g(gp), glycoprotein; ICP, intracellular protein; Kd, kilodalton; MCP, major capsid protein; meq, Marek's EcoQ; pp, phospho-protein; RR, ribonucleotide reductase; SORF, MDV specific U$_s$ open reading frame; TK, thymidine kinase; UL, unique long; US, unique short; VP, virion protein. Names of genes and gene products are based on HSV homologues.

Table prepared by L.F. Lee.

Glycoprotein genes. The gC gene encodes the gly-coprotein known as A antigen (117) and is of inter-est because of its extensive expression in produc-tively infected cells.

The A antigen, originally identified in super-natant fluids of infected cell cultures by agar gel precipitation (AGP) tests (109) has been character-ized as a 57–65 kD glycoprotein (gp57/65) (116, 200, 206, 207). It is demonstrated on the cell sur-face and in the cytoplasm of productively infected cells, is actively secreted by infected cells, does not appear related to oncogenicity, and is probably the antigen most responsible for antibodies detected in convalescent antisera by the AGP test. Production of A antigen decreases with serial passage of MDV in cell culture (109, 196), probably due to reduced transcription of the A antigen gene (491).

The gB gene (392), which encodes the B antigen, is of interest because its protein product has been

associated with protective immune responses (305, 319, 393).

The B antigen, also identified originally by AGP tests as a nonsecreted antigen (109), is a complex of three glycoproteins with molecular weights of 100 kD, 60 kD, and 49 kD (gp100, gp60, gp49) (95, 198, 205, 312, 449). The antigen is located on the cell surface and in the cytoplasm of productively in-fected cells (227). It induces neutralizing antibodies (123, 319). Differences among the B antigens of the three viral serotypes have been noted (533). Multi-ple epitopes on B antigen have been detected (260, 271).

gD (388) is not expressed in vitro (47), although the presence of anti-gD antibodies in convalescent sera (539) argues for at least limited expression in vivo. Deficiencies in expression of gD may be linked to the failure of MDV to produce infectious virions, explaining the cell-associated nature of the virus (47). Deletion of gD, however, did not abrogate the ability of MDV to infect chickens and spread by contact (287).

Other glycoprotein genes thus far characterized include gE (45, 47, 417, 540), gH (417), gI (45, 47, 388, 540), gK (381), and gL (532).

Other genes. A number of other genes have been identified and some functions have been established or can be inferred by comparisons to homologues in other herpesviruses. Several genes encoding enzymes that may be involved in replication have been identified, e.g., thymidine kinase, ribonucleotide reductase, and DNA polymerase (249, 275, 416, 466). Genes predicted to encode tegument proteins include UL49, UL48, UL47, and UL46 (531). The UL48 may code for the homologue of VP16 (242), which in other herpesviruses is involved with the *trans*-activation of immediate–early genes. Other immediate–early genes encoding proteins that presumably regulate events involved with viral replication include ICP4 and ICP27 (7, 381). Antisense transcripts of the ICP4 gene may be associated with latency (90). Origins of replication have been identified in all three serotypes (42, 89, 452). Although many MDV gene sequences represent homologues of herpes simplex virus, unique sequences have also been identified, e.g., SORF1, SORF2, and SORF3 (46). Since no attempt has been made to discuss every gene or putative gene sequence thus far described, and since the list of known genes is rapidly expanding, the reader must review the contemporary literature for additional information.

Viral membrane antigens (94, 204, 280, 282, 529) and viral internal antigens (69, 369, 461) of unspecified molecular characteristics have been demonstrated by fluorescent antibody (FA) tests with convalescent sera. Both types of antigens are probably mixtures of antigens coordinately produced in productively infected cells. Although poorly defined, these antigens contributed to many early studies and still have value as indicators of viral infection. The pp40 antigen, detectable by monoclonal antibody 2BN90 in the nucleus of infected cells (248), was found in all serotype 1 MDVs tested including several CVI988 strains; the gene for this antigen has not yet been identified.

VIRAL VECTORS. The use of all three MDV serotypes as viral expression vectors for foreign genes (148, 457) is an emerging strategy for poultry vaccines. Such vectors have expressed genes from other organisms such as Newcastle disease or *Escherichia coli,* or from other MDV serotypes (274, 288, 289, 295, 393). One advantage of MDV herpesvirus-vectored vaccines is their ability to induce immunity against MD as well as the foreign gene product (289).

RECOMBINATION AND MUTATION. Spontaneous recombination among the three MDV serotypes has not yet been demonstrated and is probably not common, despite the frequency of concomitant infections in the same tissue (99) or cell (310). All three serotypes, however, quickly develop altered molecular and biologic characteristics upon serial passage in vitro (109, 448, 509, 528), indicating that spontaneous mutations may have occurred. A temperature-sensitive mutant of MDV (509) and a mutant of HVT that was resistant to inhibition by phosphonoacetate (255) have been described. The gradual evolution of pathotypes toward greater virulence and the changes in biologic properties of MDV during in vivo backpassage (499) further support the mutability of MDVs. Cocultivation of MDV with avian retroviruses in vitro resulted in spontaneous insertion of LTRs of the retroviral provirus in the MDV genome, often at preferred sites (208, 215).

VIRUS REPLICATION. Replication of MDV, serotype 2 MDV, and HVT is typical of other cell-associated herpesviruses, and has been reviewed by Kato and Hirai (227) and Ross (387). For initial infection of cultures or chickens by cell-free virus, enveloped virions enter susceptible cells by conventional absorption and penetration, which, in cell cultures, occurs within 1 hr. The process is enhanced by chelators such as ethylenediaminetetraacetic acid (EDTA) in the case of MDV (1). Initial infection by cell-associated virus, and spread of infection initiated by either cell-free or cell-associated virus, occur by direct contact with infected cells. Cell-to-cell transfer of infection in vitro is enhanced by cell fusion (182), is normally accomplished through formation of intracellular bridges (222), and is presumed to be the principal mode of virus spread both in vitro and in vivo. Viral DNA replication occurs during the S phase of cell replication (245). Replication rates vary with serotype and passage level of the virus strain.

Three general types of virus–cell interactions are recognized: productive, latent, and transforming.

PRODUCTIVE INFECTION. In productive infection, replication of viral DNA occurs, antigens are synthesized, and in some cases, virus particles are produced. The number of genome copies per cell can exceed 1200 (225). There are two types of productive infection. Fully productive infection with MDV in the FFE of chickens results in development of large numbers of enveloped, fully infectious virions (72). In productive-restrictive infection antigens are produced, but most of the virions produced are nonenveloped and thus noninfectious. A variable number of the virions in cultured cells may be enveloped, however, and these can be recovered cell free and infectious by disruption of cells in distilled water (114) or an appropriate stabilizer (73,

100). A variant strain of HVT that releases large quantities of cell-free virus into the medium of infected cell cultures has been described (530).

In all types of cells, productive infection is lytic and leads to intranuclear inclusion body formation, cell destruction, and in the chicken, frank necrobiotic lesion formation. Because of this, productive infection has been termed cytolytic and the terms are used synonymously (66). Polykaryocytosis is seen in cultured fibroblasts and is a major component of the viral plaques or foci frequently used as a marker in virus assays.

Antigens present in productively infected cells, at least in fully productive infections in which enveloped virions are produced, probably represent the products of a number of expressed viral genes.

In productively infected fibroblasts, most of the MDV genome is transcribed (387, 451). Transcribed viral RNA can be detected in both nucleus and cytoplasm (387). Differences in transcripts between productive infection with virulent and attenuated serotype 1 strains (38, 42) have been described.

Productive infection in cell cultures is influenced by several factors. Arginine is required (281). The replicative process requires synthesis of a DNA polymerase (41) that can be inhibited by phosphonoacetate (254) and phosphonoformate (383). The effect of other inhibitors of MDV replication has been reviewed by Ross (387). Plaque size was increased or decreased by different doses of dimethylsulfoxide in the culture medium (279). Although interferon may be produced by at least some MDV and HVT strains (188, 221), its effect on virus replication appears slight (9). Growth rate of MDV and HVT in vitro is also influenced by culture temperature and cell type.

LATENT INFECTION. Latent infections are nonproductive and can be detected only by hybridization with DNA probes or methods designed to activate the viral genome such as in vitro cultivation. Only about five copies of the viral genome are present (387). Although some genes may be transcribed (465), translation does not occur and normally no virus- or tumor-associated antigens are found (78, 426). In vitro cultivation, however, results in production of viral antigens and virus particles (78, 88, 92), representing a release from latency. At least two cytokines produced by concanavalin A-stimulated spleen cell cultures can help maintain latency in cultured lymphocytes (56). One of these has been definitely identified as interferon, which was shown to suppress production of immediate–early, early, and late viral antigens in latently infected lymphocytes (487). Curiously, interferon was more effective in suppression of viral genes in later stages of latency than during early stages. Latent infection has been demonstrated following infection of

chickens with serotype 2 and 3 viruses (442). Holland et al. (186) has reported low levels of gB expression in lymphoid tissues latently infected with HVT, but this may indicate viral reactivation in selected cells rather than latency. Indeed, selective reactivation of latently infected cells can be induced by treatment with cyclosporin or betamethazone (57), but not by infection with immunodepressive viruses such as infectious bursal disease or reticuloendotheliosis (58).

TRANSFORMING INFECTION. Transforming infection occurs, by definition, in cells transformed by serotype 1 MDV. Unlike latent infection, in which the viral genome is present but is expressed only to a very limited degree, the transformed phenotype is characterized by more extensive expression of the MDV genome, occasionally resulting in antigen production. Transformed cells contain about 5–15 copies of viral genome (387) although the mean number varies in different cell lines under different conditions, perhaps in relation to the proportion of productively infected cells in the population (253, 180, 303). The viral DNA of transformed cells is highly methylated, whereas methylation was not detected in viral DNA from productively infected cells (224).

A portion of the viral genome may be transcribed (451), and a number of transcripts in transformed cells have been identified and mapped. Some (181, 477), but not all (187), of these transcripts differ from those in productively infected cells. Of the several viral antigens, only pp38 has been detected in transformed cells (202, 294), but the frequency of pp38-expressing cells is variable. The pp40 antigen has also been detected in lymphoblastoid cell lines (248). No antigens are detected in cells of lymphomas or lymphoblastoid cell lines by FA tests with convalescent serum except for occasional cells that have probably converted to a productive infection (4, 75) and, by definition, are no longer transformed.

Some transformed lymphocytes can be induced to produce viral antigens by treatment with iododeoxyuridine (79, 134, 248) or by culture at suboptimal temperatures (8, 79).

An MD tumor–associated surface antigen (MATSA) was detected on cells from MD lymphomas and lymphoblastoid cell lines derived from lymphomas (355, 521). This antigen was not detected on the surface of productively infected cells (521). Although initially it did not appear to be associated with most latently infected lymphocytes (78, 426), MATSA was also detected on lymphocytes from chickens vaccinated with HVT or nononcogenic strains of MDV (237, 352, 404), and subsequent studies with monoclonal antibodies (259, 266) revealed MATSA to be present on activated T cells from uninfected chickens (278). Thus,

MATSA is now considered to be a host antigen and is clearly not tumor specific. However, it still has importance in the differential diagnosis of MD.

INTEGRATION OF VIRAL DNA. The extent to which viral DNA is integrated into the host cell genome during productive, latent, or transforming infections has been difficult to determine. Initial reports indicated an absence of integration (471) or a mixture of integrated and episomal DNA (226, 395). Viral DNA was associated with chromosomes of two size classes separated by density gradient centrifugation (190) and with chromosomes numbers 2 and 4 by in situ hybridization (227), further supporting the idea that some integration occurs. More recently, viral DNA was shown by fluorescent in situ hybridization to be integrated at two to 12 sites in chromosomes, although integration patterns differed among cell lines (127). In primary lymphoma cells, integration occurred randomly at multiple sites, but extrachromosomal, circular MDV genomes and linear virion DNA were not detected (128). These data also suggest that MD lymphomas have a clonal origin (127, 128), a novel observation with important implications for mechanisms of oncogenesis.

DIFFERENCES BETWEEN SEROTYPES. In most reports, replication of MDV and HVT is similar. All three serotypes induce productive infection in permissive fibroblast cultures. Latent infection also occurs with all viruses. However, transforming infection has only been demonstrated with virulent MDV. Since HVT and serotype 2 MDV are nononcogenic (402, 516), no cell lines have been developed equivalent to those derived from MD lymphomas. However, a cell line has been derived from spleen cells of a chicken vaccinated with HVT (238) that has genomes of both MDV and HVT (180). The virus responsible for transformation is not clear, but the ability of both genomes to coexist in a single cell is of interest. Calnek et al. (75) also recovered infectious HVT and MDV from a single cell line.

VIRUS STOCK PRODUCTION. Productively infected cell cultures have been a common source of cell-associated virus stocks for all three viral serotypes and for cell-free HVT stocks. Cell-free virus from serotypes 1 and 2 is best obtained from FFE (low passage virus) or infected cell cultures (high passage virus), although small quantities of low passage virus can be obtained from lysed infected cells in vitro. Techniques for the production and cryopreservation of both cell-free and cell-associated virus stocks have been described (30, 73, 460).

Stability and Disinfection. Marek's disease virus and HVT exist in either cell-associated or cell-free states, which have greatly different survival properties.

Cell-associated stocks of MDV or HVT may be cryopreserved by standard methods and stored at −196 C (460). The infectivity of such stocks, however, is directly related to viability of the cells contained in these preparations. Under ideal conditions the half-life of diluted, cell-associated vaccines may be 2–6 hr (475).

Cell-free preparations of MDV obtained from skin of infected chickens were inactivated when treated for 10 min at pH 3 or 11 and stored for 2 wk at 4 C, 4 days at 25 C, 18 hr at 37 C, 30 min at 56 C, or 10 min at 60 C (68). Cell-free MDV from skin and either MDV or HVT from infected cultured cells can be stored at -70 C or lyophilized (73). Dander, litter, and feathers from infected chickens are infectious and presumably contain cell-free virus from the FFE bound to cellular debris. The infectivity of such materials was retained for 4–8 mo at room temperature (184, 513) and for at least 10 yr at 4 C (62), but infectivity was inactivated by a variety of common chemical disinfectants within a 10-min treatment period (70, 185). Survival of virus in litter may be adversely affected by increased humidity (513).

Potency of both cell-associated and cell-free vaccines can be adversely affected by storage temperature, reconstitution technique, choice of diluent, and holding time and temperature after reconstitution (167, 308, 327, 446).

Strain Classification

SEROTYPES. Bülow and Biggs (51, 52) classified the MDV herpesvirus group into three distinct virus groups that correlated with biologic properties (see previous section). Type-specific monoclonal antibodies (195, 258) are normally used to determine virus serotype.

Although distinguishable by serologic tests, the three serotypes also share many common antigens. Thus, sera against one serotype will usually react with antigens of other serotypes, although somewhat less vigorously than with homologous antigens (52).

A number of biologic characteristics are associated with viral serotype (28, 397). Low-passage serotype 1 viruses grow best in duck embryo fibroblast or chicken kidney cell cultures, grow slowly, and produce small plaques. Serotype 2 viruses grow best in chicken embryo fibroblasts, grow slowly, and produce medium plaques with some large syncytia. Serotype 3 viruses (HVT) grow best in chicken embryo fibroblasts, grow rapidly, and produce large plaques. More infectious virus can be extracted from HVT-infected cells than from cells infected with serotype 1 or 2 viruses.

PATHOTYPES. Virulence or oncogenicity is associated only with serotype 1 MDVs. Within this group, however, a wide variation in pathogenic potential is recognized and undoubtedly represents a continuum from nearly avirulent to maximally virulent. A pathotypic classification was proposed (495, 496) in which three classes of viruses and associated acronyms are designated as mild (mMDV), virulent (vMDV), or very virulent (vvMDV). Pathotyping of virus isolates involves pathogenicity tests in vaccinated or unvaccinated chickens (500). No in vitro methods have yet been developed. Prototypes are the CU2 (453) strain of mMDV, the JM (422), GA (135) and HPRS-16 (372) strains of vMDVs, and the Md5 (524) and RB1B (408) strains of vvMDVs. Pathotypes that exceed the virulence of vvMDVs have been suspected or postulated, and at least one such strain, 584A (504), has been reported.

A pattern of evolution in the virulence of MDV strains is recognized. For many years, MD was a classic disease induced by viruses of the mMDV pathotype. A more virulent form of MD was first noted in the late 1940s (21) associated with viruses of the vMDV pathotype, which became the dominant pathotype during the 1960s. The vvMDV pathotype virus strains were first noted in the late l970s (136), mainly in HVT-vaccinated flocks with excessive MD losses, and now appear to be the dominant type.

Certain biologic characteristics are also associated with pathotypes of serotype 1 MDVs, but are most pronounced between low-passage and high-passage (attenuated) strains. Serial passage in vitro (30–70 passages normally required) results in attenuation of virulent isolates (109, 385, 494). Attenuated strains grow more readily in vitro, but produce lower viremia titers in vivo (508), which may be associated with a marked decrease in ability to infect and/or replicate in lymphocytes (410). The production of A antigen is reduced or absent (109). Attenuated strains do not spread well among chickens by contact (125, 499). Some strains are incompletely attenuated and induce minor lesions in susceptible chickens (50, 344, 499). Overattenuated strains do not replicate in or protect chickens (240, 509). The in vivo growth potential of attenuated serotype 1 isolates has been improved by backpassage in chickens (126, 499), although in one case virulence was also increased (499).

The incidence of tumors induced by low-virulence strains of serotype 1 MDV is increased by infection in ovo or by immunosuppression (74, 77). Viruses of serotype 2 and 3 remained nononcogenic following similar treatments (77, 402).

Laboratory Host Systems. Marek's disease virus is normally propagated and assayed in newly hatched chicks, tissue cultures, and embryonated eggs. Lymphoblastoid cell lines from MD lymphomas are also an important laboratory host system.

CHICKENS. Newly hatched chicks inoculated with virulent, serotype 1 MDV develop lesions that can be detected histologically in ganglia, nerves, and certain viscera after 2–4 wk. Response is greatly dependent on genetic susceptibility of the chicken and virulence of the MDV isolate. Presence of virus or antibody, which can be detected by in vitro tests, or presence of virus-associated antigen detected by FA tests on tissues are also specific host responses of inoculated chickens to MD infection. All these responses are markedly enhanced in chicks lacking maternal antibodies against MDV (59). The induction of virus-specific lesions in the wing web (87) or the feather pulp (290) constitutes alternate host systems that provide direct access to the site of lesion development.

CELL CULTURES. Cultured duck embryo fibroblasts or chicken kidney cells are suitable for propagation of low-passage MDV isolates (107, 456). Attenuated MDV and serotype 2 and 3 viruses all grow well on chicken embryo fibroblast cultures (28, 402). Infected cultures usually develop discrete focal lesions, which consist of clusters of rounded, refractile degenerating cells when mature. These lesions are called foci or plaques (Fig. 17.4). Lesions are usually less than 1 mm in diameter and of variable cell density. Affected cells may contain two to several hundred nuclei, and type A intranuclear inclusion bodies are commonly seen. Despite release of rounded cells into the medium as plaques mature, large areas of cell lysis are not seen.

Serotype 1 plaques develop in 5–14 days on primary isolation and in 3–7 days after adaptation to culture, and are usually enumerated by microscopic examination. Differences in development and morphology of serotype 1 plaques in chick and duck cells (458, 514) and in plaques induced by the three viral serotypes (28, 397) have been described. Other cell culture systems such as chick embryo skin (361) or tracheal explants (379) have been also used.

Serotype 1, but not serotype 2, MDVs can also be grown in chicken splenic lymphocytes in vitro (80). Passages are made by the addition of fresh spleen cells to the suspension cell cultures every 2 days, and infection is monitored by immunofluorescence. Turkey herpesviruses may be similarly grown in turkey spleen cell cultures, but viral antigen is seen rarely, if at all.

EMBRYOS. Virus pocks (Fig. 17.5) develop on the chorioallantoic membrane (CAM) of chicken em-

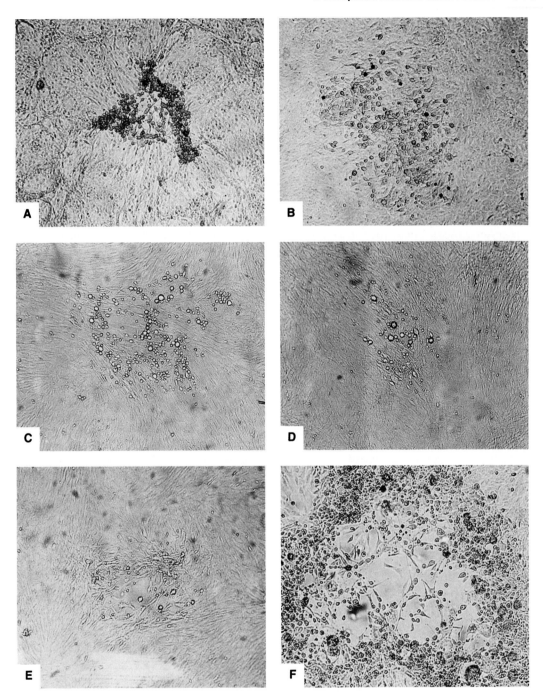

17.4. Focal lesions in cultured cells infected with various Marek's disease virus (MDV) serotypes. *A.* Low-passage serotype 1 MDV in chicken kidney cells cultured from an infected chicken, 9 days. *B.* Low-passage serotype 1 MDV in duck embryo fibroblasts (DEF), 5 days. *C.* High-passage, attenuated serotype 1 MDV in chicken embryo fibroblasts (CEF), 5 days. *D.* Low-passage serotype 2 MDV in CEF, 8 days. *E.* Low-passage HVT (serotype 3) in CEF, 4 days. *F.* Low-passage turkey herpesviruses (HVT) in DEF, 12 days. All photos unstained, about ×40.

bryos following yolk sac inoculation with cellular MDV preparations (27, 49). Embryos have also been used for MD vaccine evaluation, since in ovo vaccination is becoming increasingly common in the field. In this case, embryos are normally inoculated with vaccine viruses in the amnionic sac on the 18th day (431). The growth potential of serotype 1 MDV is less than for serotypes 2 and 3 in 18-day embryos (428).

LYMPHOBLASTOID CELL LINES. Lymphoblastoid cell lines developed from MD lymphomas (4, 67, 78, 298, 339) grow continuously in cell culture without attachment to the culture vessel. Lymphoblastoid cell lines can also be established from lymphocytes harvested from early (4–6 days postinfection [PI]) lesions induced in the wing-web or pectoral muscle by injection of a mixture of MDV and allogeneic kidney cells. All lines from either chicken lymphomas or early local lesions have T-cell markers; those from lymphomas are usually CD4+/CD8-, whereas those from early lesions may be CD4+/CD8-, CD4-/CD8+, or CD4-/CD8- (412). Most can be termed "producer" lines, since a small proportion (1–2%) of the cells enter into productive infection (355). Virus can be readily recovered from most cell lines, although several nonproducer cell lines have been developed in which evidence of genome expression is limited or lacking (304, 339, 471). In one such line (MDCC-RP1), the MDV genome may be incomplete because no virus can be rescued by in vitro or in vivo assays (304). Prolonged culture can result in reduced expression of

the MDV genome (277). Most, but not all, MD cell lines established from lymphomas were found to display a chromosomal aberration in which an amplification of DNA resulted in an extra G-band and interband in the short arm of one homologue of chromosome 1 (40, 285). The aberration was found only infrequently in MD lines established from local MD lesions (286), and it remains to be determined whether there is any relationship between this change and neoplastic transformation.

Success rates for establishing cell lines from MD lymphomas have improved because of better methodology (79, 339). One cell line generated from in vitro infection has been reported (201). Many cell lines are now available (298) including several from MD lymphomas in turkeys. Cells of the MDCC-RP1 line are illustrated in Fig. 17.6.

PATHOGENESIS AND EPIZOOTIOLOGY

Natural and Experimental Hosts. Chickens are by far the most important natural host for MD; the disease is very rare and probably of no real importance in other species (citations in 71), with the possible exception of quail.

Marek's disease viruses isolated from either chickens or Japanese quail have been used to reproduce the MD in both quail and chickens (235, 358, 359). However, quail-origin MDV appeared be more pathogenic than chicken-origin MDV for quail (203). Furthermore, the pathogenesis of infection was somewhat different (203) and turkey herpesvirus MD vaccine failed to protect quail against MDV challenge (228). Powell and Rennie (353) found chicken-quail hybrids to be susceptible to MD.

Some genera of the order Galliformes (especially *Gallus*), including red and Ceylon jungle fowl, have

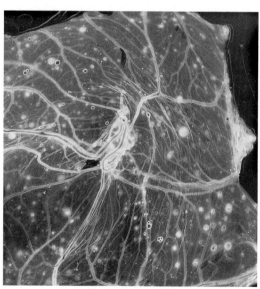

17.5. Chorioallantoic membrane (CAM) from 19-day-old chicken embryo inoculated via yolk sac at 4 days with blood from chickens infected with JM isolate.

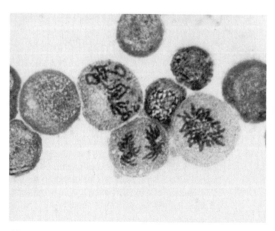

17.6. Smear from the MDCC-RP1 cell line. Note the characteristic lymphoblastoid morphology and the mitotic figures. Giemsa, ×1500. (Nazerian)

virologic or serologic evidence of infection with MDV (102, 488), but several other avian species in which lesions suggestive of MD have been reported failed to have a confirmatory etiologic relationship established (citations in 71).

Experimental transmission of MD was claimed for pheasants (171, 212). Sparrows were refractory to infection (235), whereas ducks became infected but without disease after MDV inoculation (18). Various mammalian species including hamsters, rats, marmosets, and monkeys (cynomolgus, rhesus, bonnet) were refractory to infection with virulent MDV (108, 183, 385, 436, 438).

Transmission. Direct or indirect contact between birds affects virus spread, apparently by the airborne route (citations in 26). Epithelial cells in the keratinizing layer of the feather follicle replicate fully infectious virus (72), and these cells serve as a source of contamination to the environment. Virus associated with feathers and dander is infectious (19, 72), and contaminated poultry house dust remains infectious for at least several months at 20–25 C and for years at 4 C (citations in 63).

Many apparently normal birds are carriers that can transmit the infection (235). Infection probably persists indefinitely (518). Continual shedding of virus by infected birds and hardiness of the virus (see Etiology) make prevalence of infection easy to understand.

Studies relating to transfer hosts for MDV were reviewed by Witter (493). Darkling beetles (*Alphitobius diaperinus*) were shown to passively carry the virus; however, free-living litter mites, mosquitoes, and coccidial oocysts could not be associated with transmission.

Apparently, there is no vertical transmission of MDV (511), and transmission from dam to progeny as the result of external egg contamination is also unlikely because of poor virus survival at temperature and humidity levels employed for incubation (70).

Experimental transmission is effected most consistently by inoculation of day-old, genetically susceptible chicks with blood, tumor suspensions, or cell-free virus or by direct or indirect contact with infected birds. Intratracheal instillation or inhalation exposure using cell-free virus is also effective for experimental transmission. With inoculation of tumor cell suspensions there is always the hazard of inducing tumors by cell transplantation; however, transplantation is not the usual cause of lesions in experimental birds (323).

The transmission of serotype 2 and 3 viruses is discussed under Turkey and Chicken Herpesviruses.

Incubation Period. The incubation period for experimentally induced MD is rather well estab-

lished (see reviews 63, 337, 371). Chicks inoculated at 1 day of age excrete virus beginning about 2 wk PI (234), with maximal shedding occurring between the 3rd and 5th wk (493). Cytolytic infections at 3–6 days PI are followed by degenerative lesions in lymphoid organs within 6–8 days PI. Mononuclear infiltrations may be found in nerves and other organs after about 2 wk (334). Clinical signs and gross lesions, however, generally do not appear until between the 3rd and 4th wk (333, 422).

While these figures represent the shortest incubation, there can be considerable variation. The same factors that influence incidence of disease also affect incubation period. These include virus strain, dosage, maternal antibody status, and route of infection as well as age, genetic strain, and sex of the host. Induction of tumors within 10–14 days after inoculation of cellular material is suggestive of a transplantation response, although death from an "early mortality syndrome" may occur as early as 8–12 days PI (524).

It is difficult to determine the incubation period of the disease under field conditions. While outbreaks sometimes occur in birds as young as 3–4 wk, most serious cases begin after the 8th or 9th wk, and it is usually impossible to determine the time and conditions of exposure. Purchase (371) noted that clinical signs in egg-type flocks are often not seen until 16–20 wk and occur as late as 24–30 wk. Nicholls (309) noted one outbreak as late as 60 wk. The transient paralysis that occasionally affects birds occurs at about 6–10 wk.

Signs. Signs associated with MD have been described by numerous workers as reviewed by Biggs (24). In general, they are those associated with asymmetric progressive paresis and, later, complete paralysis of one or more of the extremities. Since any one or several nerves may be affected, signs vary from bird to bird. Wing involvement is characterized by drooping of the limb. If nerves controlling neck muscles are affected, the head may be held low and there may be some torticollis. Vagal involvement can result in paralysis and dilation of the crop and/or gasping. Because locomotory disturbances are easily recognized, incoordination or stilted gait may be the first observed sign. A particularly characteristic attitude is that in which the bird has one leg stretched forward and the other back as a result of unilateral paresis or paralysis of the leg.

A transient paralysis syndrome associated with MD has been described and reproduced (citations in 418), although it has been observed infrequently since vaccination has been practiced. Affected birds display varying degrees of ataxia and partial or whole body paralysis beginning 8–12 days after virus inoculation and lasting 1–2 days. Many affected birds may recover only to succumb a few weeks later from clinical MD. The syndrome appears to be the result of vasogenic brain edema (243, 467, 468).

With acute outbreaks of MD, the syndrome is much more explosive and initially is characterized by a high proportion of birds with severe depression. A few days later, some but not all birds develop ataxia and subsequent unilateral or bilateral paralysis of extremities. Others may die without extensive clinical disease. Many birds become dehydrated, emaciated, and comatose.

Blindness may result from involvement of the iris. Affected eyes gradually lose their ability to accommodate to light intensity. Clinical examination also reveals changes varying from concentric annular or spotty depigmentation or diffuse bluish fading to diffuse grayish opacity of the iris (see Fig. 17.16C). The pupil at first becomes irregular and at advanced stages is only a small pinpoint opening.

Nonspecific signs such as weight loss, paleness, anorexia, and diarrhea may be observed, especially in birds in which the course is prolonged. Under commercial conditions, death often results from starvation and dehydration because of inability to reach food and water or, in many cases, from trampling by penmates.

Morbidity and Mortality. Incidence of MD is quite variable. A few birds that develop signs may recover from the clinical disease (30), but in general, mortality is nearly equal to morbidity. Prior to use of vaccines, losses in affected flocks were estimated to range from a few birds to 25 or 30% and occasionally as high as 60%. Presently between 95 and 100% of egg-type chickens are vaccinated against MD, and this has reduced losses to less than 5% in most countries (371). Broiler flocks, which are vaccinated in some but not all countries, may experience losses of 0.1 to 0.5% and condemnations of 0.2% or more (371), although the average condemnation rate in the United States has been much lower, reaching less than 0.04% in 1994 (see Fig. 17.1).

After the disease appears, mortality builds gradually and generally persists for 4–10 wk. Outbreaks occur in isolated flocks, or occasionally in several flocks in a region or in succeeding flocks on a farm.

A number of factors influence the extent of losses in affected flocks. These deal with either the infective agent or host. Those specifically related to the agent are virus strain, dosage, and route of exposure. Strains of virus associated with acute outbreaks of MD are more virulent and cause a higher disease incidence and more visceral lymphomas than those associated with the so-called classic form of the disease (31, 372, 397). In some outbreaks, a high incidence of ocular lesions appears to be related to the virus strain(s) (147, 463). The degree of pathogenicity (morbidity and mortality) and lesion spectrum thus depends in part on the virus

strain. Virulence of a given strain, however, in turn depends in part on genetic constitution of the host (406, 454).

Dosage may be a factor under natural conditions, although the MD response in genetically susceptible birds given virulent virus was found to be maximal even when a limiting dilution of virus was inoculated (454). Dosage may be more significant in immunologically competent hosts (genetically resistant birds that have acquired age resistance), in vaccinated birds, or with viruses of lower virulence. Route of exposure probably functions in the same manner; less efficient routes may effectively decrease the dose to the bird.

Influential host factors include sex, passive antibody, genetic constitution, and age. Biggs (25) cited several studies in which it was observed that females experienced higher losses than males; their greater susceptibility was manifested in a shorter latent period. The difference was apparently not due to sex hormones, varied with the genetic strain, being most pronounced with susceptible strains of chickens, and was apparent only in the case of infection with the more virulent virus isolates (vMDVs).

Passive antibody (see Immunity) reduces MD mortality (106), clinical signs of transient paralysis, and early mortality syndrome (326), probably by limiting spread of virus in tissues during the first few days postexposure (61).

Both genetic factors (see Prevention and Control) and age are important in determining the level of morbidity and mortality (see reviews 64, 112). It seems probable that host immune response to infection is the most significant event and that this forms a common basis to what has been called "genetic resistance" or "age resistance." Indeed, these two types are probably the same, since resistance associated with age could generally be associated with genetically resistant strains and, to a much lesser degree, with susceptible strains (5, 25, 61, 484, 520).

In studies comparing genetic strains (see reviews 63, 64, 348, 349, 418), resistance correlated with development of virus-neutralizing antibody (60, 433) and retention of cell-mediated immune functions (257, 405). This resulted from a sparing of immune competence in the case of resistant birds, rather than from an inherent difference between strains (176, 177, 453). Lesion regression has been identified as the basis for age-related resistance (437); success of thymectomy and X-irradiation (437) but failure of bursectomy (434) to circumvent resistance points to cellular immunity as the mediating factor.

Other resistance mechanisms that might conceivably influence incidence of MD morbidity and mortality include interferon production and natural killer (NK) cell activity (see Immunity). Variations in the level of MD not explained by other mechanisms could be due to the fact that some flocks experience naturally occurring infections with serotype 2 MDV, and thus are afforded protection against oncogenic strains (209).

Various environmental or other factors, and concurrent infections, have been claimed to affect incidence of MD. Gross (161) observed increased incidence among chickens subjected to a high degree of social stress (or selected for high concentrations of plasma corticosterone), and Powell and Davison (350) showed that administration of corticosteroids to latently infected chickens precipitated the appearance of clinical MD. This could be related to a reactivation of infection, which has been shown to occur following immunosuppression (57). Reduced feed intake delayed and reduced incidence, and selection of chickens for fast growth rate seemed to correlate with increased susceptibility (168, 169). Concurrent infection with cryptosporidia (292) or immunosuppressive viruses, e.g., chicken infectious anemia virus (211), may also increase the severity of MD.

Gross Lesions. Pathologic changes in MD have been well summarized and reviewed (331, 337). Nerve lesions are a frequent finding in affected birds. Macroscopic changes are not seen in the brain, but gross lesions can usually be found in one or more peripheral nerves and in spinal roots and root ganglia. Lesion distribution appears to be similar for naturally occurring and experimental diseases (325, 333). Goodchild (159) made detailed macroscopic examinations of 502 birds with MD and found that certain autonomic nerves, as well as the more obvious nerves and plexuses, were commonly affected. Ninety-nine percent of the cases could have been diagnosed by examining only the following: celiac, cranial mesenteric, brachial, and sciatic plexuses; nerve of Remak; and greater splanchnic nerve. The celiac plexus was most commonly involved; it was positive in 78% of the birds. Usually, plexuses of the sciatic and brachial nerves are more enlarged than the respective trunks. Witter (506) has found the cervical vagus to be of particular diagnostic importance. Sevoian et al. (422) found that dorsal root ganglia were consistently affected in chicks inoculated with JM strain.

Affected peripheral nerves are characterized by loss of cross-striations, gray or yellow discoloration, and sometimes an edematous appearance. Localized or diffuse enlargement causes the affected portion to be two to three times normal size, in some cases much more. Because lesions are often unilateral, it is especially helpful to compare opposite nerves in the case of slight changes. Careful examination of the various nerve ramifications may be necessary to expose gross lesions in some birds, since enlargement can vary in degree from one portion of an affected nerve to another. Fig. 17.7 illustrates characteristic gross changes in nerves.

Pappenheimer et al. (325) described affected spinal root ganglia as enlarged, somewhat translucent, and of slightly yellowish tinge. Enlargement was rarely symmetric and lesions often extended into contiguous tissue of the spinal cord. Ganglia may be exposed by removal of the dorsal part of the vertebral column.

Lymphoid tumors may occur in one or more of a variety of organs. Lymphomatous lesions can be found in the gonad (especially the ovary), lung, heart, mesentery, kidney, liver, spleen, bursa, thymus, adrenal gland, pancreas, proventriculus, intestine, iris, skeletal muscle, and skin. Probably no site is without occasional involvement.

Both the genetic strain and the virus strain can influence the location of lesions. Visceral tumors are especially common in more acute forms of the disease and may be found in the absence of gross nerve lesions. Virus isolates from severe outbreaks tested by Purchase and Biggs (372) induced visceral lesions in 62–89% of inoculated birds. In contrast, an isolate from a milder (classic) case of MD caused visceral lymphomata in only 5–7% of inoculated birds.

Macroscopic changes in affected viscera, with the possible exception of the bursa of Fabricius, are indistinguishable from leukotic lesions induced by other agents (e.g., lymphoid leukosis virus). Enlargement of the organ, sometimes to several times normal size, is evident, and there is diffuse grayish discoloration. In some birds, nodular tumorlike growths are found within and extending from the parenchyma of the organ. These are firm and smooth on cutting. Involvement of the lung results in solidification (see Fig. 17.16E).

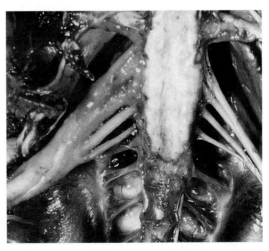

17.7. Leukotic sciatic plexus (*left*) and normal plexus (*right*). (Peckham)

Diffuse infiltration of the liver causes loss of normal lobule architecture and often gives the surface a coarse granular appearance. Nodular tumors may also be seen in the liver. Lesions in the nonproducing ovary are observed as small to large grayish translucent areas (see Fig. 17.16B). With large tumors, the normal foliated appearance of the ovary is obliterated. Mature ovaries may retain function even though some follicles are tumorous. Marked involvement is indicated by a cauliflowerlike appearance. The proventriculus becomes thickened and firm as a result of small to large leukotic areas within and between the glands. These areas may be seen through the serosal surface or on section. Affected hearts are pale from diffuse infiltration or have single or multiple nodular tumors in the myocardium (see Fig. 17.16F), or pinpoint foci may be seen in the epicardium. Skin lesions are usually associated with, but not limited to, feather follicles. They may coalesce. Distinct whitish nodules (see Fig. 17.16A), especially evident in the dressed carcass, may become scablike with brownish crust formation in extreme cases (21). Lapen and Kenzy (244) found lesions in certain feather tracts more frequently than in others; the highest incidences were in external and internal crural and dorsal cervical tracts. Muscle lesions may be in both superficial and deep layers and, according to Benton and Cover (21), are most common in pectoral muscles. Gross changes vary from tiny whitish streaks to nodular tumors. Affected areas are a lusterless whitish gray or may have a definite yellow-orange color (probably associated with necrosis). Muscle lesions can also include atrophic changes of neurogenic origin when nerve trunks are severely affected (270, 490).

Gross ocular changes include loss of pigmentation in the iris ("gray eye") and irregularity of the pupil, both the result of mononuclear infiltration of the iris (see Fig. 17.16C). Ficken et al. (147) described cases in which conjunctivitis, occasionally with multifocal hemorrhages, and corneal edema were observed.

The bursa of Fabricius, while usually atrophic when affected (372), may (rarely) develop tumors that appear as diffuse thickening owing to interfollicular distribution of tumor cells. This lesion differs from the nodular tumor characteristic of lymphoid leukosis and may be easily differentiated histologically.

Nonneoplastic lesions of MD include severe atrophy of the bursa of Fabricius and thymus as well as degenerative lesions in the bone marrow and various visceral organs (210, 524). These are the result of intense cytolytic infections and they can result in death of chickens at an early age before lymphomas develop.

A discussion of MD pathology must include oc-clusive atherosclerosis following the discovery by Fabricant et al. (143) that such lesions may result from infection with MDV. Susceptible P-line chickens inoculated with the CU2 isolate of MDV developed grossly visible fatty atheromatous lesions in large coronary arteries, aortas and major aortic branches, and other arteries (see Fig. 17.16D). These lesions were reputed as closely resembling those of chronic atherosclerosis in humans (284). A possible association between MDV and cholesterol-induced atherosclerosis in a susceptible strain of Japanese quail was reported by Shih et al. (444). They found DNA sequences complimentary to MDV DNA in the germline, and suggested that there may be an interaction between the gene(s) and cholesterol in pathogenesis of atherosclerosis in the susceptible strain.

Experimentalists often are faced with the need for criteria of a positive response to infection with MDV in the course of determining relative virulence of isolates or efficacy of vaccines or other treatments in preventing the disease. In addition to the more usual gross and microscopic evidence of inflammatory and lymphoproliferative lesions described for nerves, viscera, and other tissues, the spectrum of lesions that must be considered includes: 1) those of the early mortality syndrome (with care to consider other causes such as infection with chicken infectious anemia virus); 2) transient paralysis; and 3) later occurring degenerative lesions in lymphoid organs.

Histopathology.   Histopathologic changes associated with MD have been described by numerous workers who were in general agreement about types of histologic lesions and cells involved (329, 337).

There are two main types of lesions in peripheral nerves. One is interpreted as neoplastic in character, consisting of masses of proliferating lymphoblastic cells; in some cases, demyelination and Schwann cell proliferation are associated with this lesion. The other lesion is essentially inflammatory in character and is characterized by diffuse, light-to-moderate infiltration by small lymphocytes and plasma cells, usually with edema, and sometimes, with demyelination and Schwann cell proliferation. A few macrophages may be found. Payne and Biggs (333) referred to these responses as types A and B, respectively, and noted that the two types may be observed in different nerves of the same bird or even in different areas of the same nerve.

In a chronologic study of ultrastructural changes in nerves in MD, Lawn and Payne (246) observed cellular infiltrations as early as 5 days, which gradually increased in intensity until 3 wk when severe proliferative lesions were seen in the absence of paralysis or demyelination. Coincident with initial

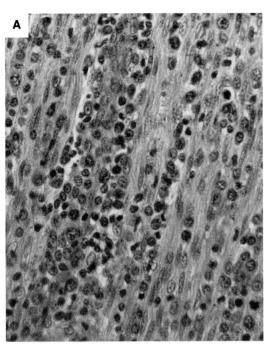 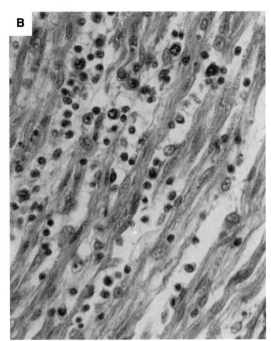

17.8. Microscopic lesions of Marek's disease (MD) in peripheral nerves. *A.* Type A lesion characterized by marked cellular infiltration, numerous proliferating lymphoblastic cells, and no edema. H & E, ×530. *B.* Type B lesion with edema, scattered infiltrating small and medium lymphocytes, plasma cells, and an occasional lymphoblast. H & E, ×530.

neurologic signs seen at 4 wk postinoculation, areas of widespread demyelination could be found within the proliferative lesions. Finally, characteristic inflammatory lesions (edema, sparse infiltrations) appeared. Characteristic changes in nerves are illustrated in Figure 17.8.

Pappenheimer et al. (325) described brain lesions as always focal in distribution, consisting of either compact perivascular cuffs of small densely staining lymphocytes (Fig. 17.9) or submiliary nodules composed of lymphocytes and paler elements. Jungherr and Hughes (217) stated that the latter were probably of glial origin. The spinal cord had, in addition to regional infiltrations, focal accumulations in white matter and occasionally in central gray matter. Root ganglia were intensely infiltrated but ganglion cells were intact. Wight (489) found the central nervous system (CNS) of affected birds was often histologically normal or with only minimal lesions, and concluded that MD is essentially a disease of peripheral nerves.

In studies on transient paralysis, Swayne et al. (468, 469, 470) described a vasculitis leading to vasogenic edema. There was leakage of immunoglobulin G (IgG) and albumin. Lesions were most consistently seen in the cerebellum. Ultrastructural changes did not include demyelination (243, 470).

According to Jungherr and Hughes (217), the

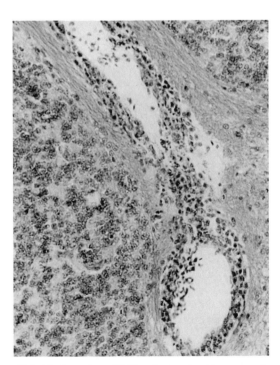

17.9. Perivascular cuff of lymphocytes in white matter of cerebellum of Marek's disease virus (MDV)-infected chicken. H & E, ×250. (Helmboldt)

most constant change in the eye is mononuclear infiltration of the iris (Fig. 17.10), but infiltrates may also be found in eye muscles, especially in rectus lateralis and ciliaris. Granular or amorphous material is sometimes present in the anterior chamber. Other, but more rarely, observed lesions involve the cornea (near Schlemm's canal), bulbar conjunctiva, pecten, and optic nerve. Ficken et al. (147) found that uveal changes invariably included increased aqueous humor protein, and that changes in the iris ranged from vascular engorgement and mild hyperemia to severe swelling. Sevoian and Chamberlain (419) and Smith et al. (455) reproduced ocular lesions experimentally. The latter reported that sequential changes included infiltration of proliferating lymphoreticular cells in optic and ciliary nerves and uvea followed by similar infiltrations throughout the eye. Dukes and Petit (133) found cataracts present in 7 of 18 spontaneous cases of ocular MD.

Lymphomatous lesions in visceral organs are more uniformly proliferative in nature (Fig. 17.11). Cellular composition is much like the proliferative lesions described for nerves, consisting of diffusely proliferating small-to-medium lymphocytes, lymphoblasts, and activated and primitive reticulum cells (333) (Fig. 17.12). Plasma cells are rarely present (372). The cellular composition of tumors is the same from one organ to another even though the gross pattern of involvement may vary. Ultrastructural features of tumor cells have been described by several workers (130, 150).

Lesions in the skin appear largely inflammatory, but may also be lymphomatous. They are localized

around infected feather follicles (Fig. 17.13). In addition to the sometimes massive accumulations of mononuclear cells around feather follicles, compact aggregates of proliferating cells, often perivascular, and a few plasma cells and histocytes are seen in the dermis (174, 333). With small lesions, the architectural integrity of skin is maintained, but massive proliferative lesions may cause disruption of the epidermis, resulting in an ulcer. Moriguchi et al. (290) described both inflammatory and lymphoproliferative lesions in the feather pulp; the latter were closely related to the incidence of MD. An unusual involvement of the comb was reported by Ekperigin et al. (137).

Pradhan et al. (360) found immune complexes in the kidney, leading to glomerulopathy, in MDV-infected chickens. They suggested that these lesions might be one of the major causes of death in MD.

Productive herpesvirus replication in the bursa of Fabricius and thymus results in degenerative changes in these organs (citations in 63, 337). In experimental infections, bursal lesions consisted of cortical and medullary atrophy, necrosis, cyst formation, and interfollicular lymphoid infiltration (Fig. 17.14). Atrophy of the thymus was sometimes severe and involved both cortex and medulla. In some cases, there were areas of lymphoid proliferation in the thymus. Cowdry's type A intranuclear inclusions can sometimes be found in cells associated with degenerative lesions. Chicks infected in the absence of maternal antibody may have aplastic bone marrow with accompanying anemia, along with focal or generalized necrosis in a variety of organs, including the kidney (59, 149, 210).

Blood leukocytes may be elevated, largely because of increased numbers of large lymphocytes and lymphoblasts (141). Payne et al. (336) identified the majority of leukemic cells as T cells. The leukemic response is not consistent and may be absent or there may be only a mild leukocytosis (217, 420). Bone marrow changes in MD have variously been reported to include multiple tumor nodules (420) or aplasia (210), or changes were not observed (372). Productive viral infection of hematopoietic cells in bone marrow is the probable cause of anemia seen in some birds (141, 210), although the possibility of concurrent infection with chicken anemia agent (see Chapter 30, Chicken Infectious Anemia) would have to be considered.

Arterial lesions reported to be associated with MDV-induced atherosclerosis include proliferative and fatty-proliferative changes in aortic, coronary, celiac, gastric, and mesenteric arteries (143, 284) (Fig. 17.15). Internal and medial foam cells, extracellular lipid, cholesterol clefts, and calcium deposits characterized the fatty-proliferative lesions. Also, MD viral antigens could be detected by immunofluorescence adjacent to the arterial lesions. An altered lipid metabolism is suggested by the

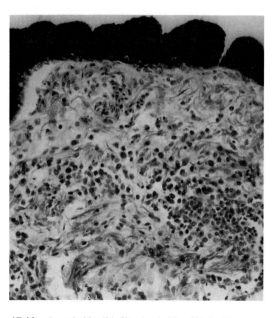

17.10. Lymphoid cell infiltration in iris of bird with ocular lesions of MD. H & E, ×250. (Helmboldt)

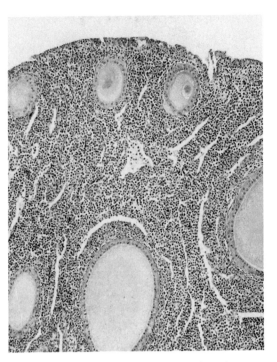

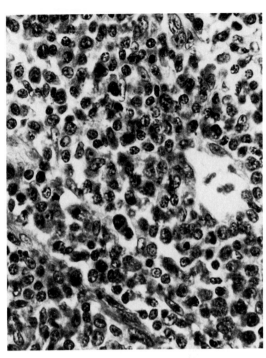

17.11. Lymphoid cell infiltration of ovary. Organ is largely composed of tumor cells, but a few ovarian follicles can be seen. H & E, ×116

17.12. Higher magnification of ovarian lymphoma showing pleomorphic tumor cells. H & E, ×640 (Payne)

finding of Fabricant et al. (144) that MDV infection of arterial smooth muscle cells in vitro induced accumulation of phospholipids, free fatty acid, cholesterol, and cholesterol esters. In vivo studies supported this conclusion; Hajjar et al. (165) found that lipid accumulations in aortas resulted, in part, from altered cholesterol/cholesteryl ester metabolism during early stages of the disease.

Pathogenesis.   Sequential events of MD have been extensively studied in many laboratories. Several comprehensive reviews have been published (25, 63, 65, 66, 297, 329, 337, 370, 398, 418); these should be consulted for details of the large number of contributions that provide our current understanding of MD. Also, Venugopal and Payne (482) recently provided an excellent review relating some of the pathogenetic events to molecular biology features of infection.

Four phases of infection in vivo can be delineated: 1) early productive-restrictive virus infection causing primarily degenerative changes, 2) latent infection, 3) a second phase of cytolytic, productive-restrictive infection coincident with permanent immunosuppression, and 4) a proliferative phase involving nonproductively infected lymphoid cells that may or may not progress to the point of lymphoma formation.

The virus gains entrance via the respiratory tract,

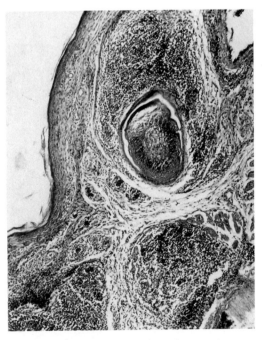

17.13. Dermal focal accumulations of mononuclear cells; note that one mass surrounds a feather shaft. H & E. ×100.

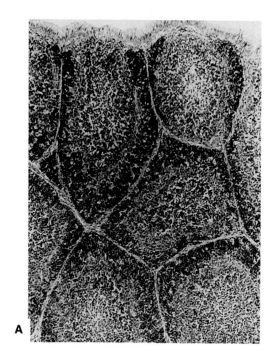
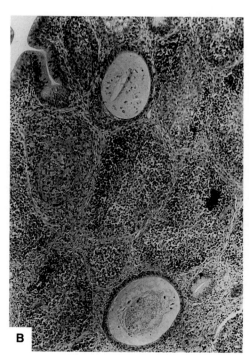

17.14. Changes in bursa of Fabricius associated with Marek's disease (MD). *A.* Normal bursal follicles in chicken killed at 15 days of age. Note uniform architecture. *B.* Cystic and necrotic follicles in atrophied bursa from chicken killed 28 days postinoculation with HPRS-16 isolate of Marek's disease virus (MDV). H & E, ×50. (Purchase and Blackwell Scientific Publications)

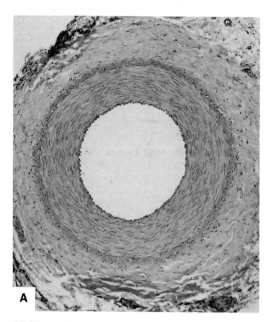
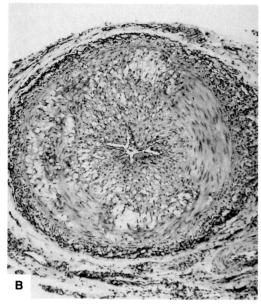

17.15. *A.* Gastric artery of normal chicken. *B.* Atherosclerotic artery in gizzard of chicken infected with CU2 isolate of Marek's disease virus (MDV). Lumen is occluded by thickened intima and there are atheromatous changes deep in the intima and media. H & E, ×24. (C. Fabricant)

where it is probably picked up by phagocytic cells. Shortly thereafter, cytolytic infection can be detected in the spleen, bursa of Fabricius, and thymus, peaking at 3–6 days. Shek et al. discovered that the primary target cells in all three organs are B cells, although some activated T cells become infected and undergo degeneration as well (443). Resting T cells are refractory to infection (84). The necrotizing effects of this early infection provoke an acute inflammatory reaction with infiltration of various cells including macrophages, granulocytes, and both immunologically committed and uncommitted lymphocytes (335). A hyperplastic response in the spleen can follow, and at about 7 days, a transient immunosuppression may occur due to the presence of suppressor macrophages (see Immunity). Ultimately, there can be atrophy of the bursa and thymus. Chickens of susceptible and resistant strains of differing ages are equally susceptible to infection (61, 423, 520), and the level of infection in all birds is equally high in all cases during the early cytolytic period (145). However, the pathogenicity of the virus strain may affect the severity of early infection. Witter et al. (524) reported that more highly oncogenic MDV strains, such as Md5, can cause more severe lymphoid organ atrophy than do less oncogenic strains and can cause an early death syndrome as the result of an especially marked cytolytic infection.

At about 6–7 days, the infection switches to latency coincident with the development of immune responses. Cell-mediated immunity (CMI) has been shown to be important in the switch (57), perhaps through a soluble mediator (56). Most latently infected cells are activated T cells, although B cells can also be involved (83, 443). The latent infection is persistent and can last for the lifetime of the bird (518). The extent to which nonlymphoid cells also are latently infected is not known, although apparent latent infection has been observed in Schwann cells and satellite cells in spinal ganglia (341).

Infection in genetically resistant birds often does not progress past the second phase (latency) aside from a persistent low-grade productive infection in the FFE (61, 69, 257, 461). Susceptible birds, however, develop a second wave of cytolytic infections after the 2nd or 3rd wk coincident with permanent immunosuppression. The lymphoid organs are again involved and localized foci of infection can be found in tissues of epithelial origin in various visceral organs (e.g., kidney, pancreas, adrenal gland, proventriculus, etc.) and especially in the skin, where a striking infection of the feather follicle epithelium occurs. The latter is unique in that it is the only known site of complete virus replication. There is focal necrosis, and inflammatory reactions develop around affected areas. The extent of infection during this phase (unlike that in the earlier phase in lymphoid organs) depends on factors known to govern incidence of tumors; the most susceptible birds develop the most widespread and intense infections.

The cause of inflammatory CNS lesions associated with MDV-induced transient paralysis is not clear, but it is known that the syndrome is under the control of genes of the major histocompatibility complex and that B cells are required for its induction (326, 414).

Lymphoproliferative changes constituting the ultimate response in the disease may progress to tumor development, although regression of lesions can and commonly does occur either before or after frank lymphomas are apparent (437). Death from lymphomas may occur at any time from about 3 wk onward.

The composition of lymphomas is complex, consisting of a mixture of neoplastic, inflammatory, and immunologically active cells. Both T and B cells are present, although the former predominate (189, 394).

The usual target cells for transformation are CD4+, activated T cells, presumably T-helper cells (413). If the conditions of infection are modified experimentally (87), however, it is possible to show that a variety of T-cell subsets, including CD4+, CD8+, and CD4-/CD8- cells, are transformable (413), and both B-cell and T-cell MD tumors from turkeys have been reported (300, 357). Although the usual transformed cell appears to be a T-helper cell, tumor cells have the ability to suppress certain in vitro tests of CMI competence such as mitogenic stimulation of spleen cells and NK cell activity (54, 173, 378, 473). The infection in transformed cells is mostly, but not entirely, nonproductive in vivo and in vitro. A normal antigen (MATSA, see Etiology) found on some populations of noninfected, activated T cells (278) may be a marker expressed on transformation targets, since it is present on MD tumor cells. Marek's disease lymphomas in some, but not all, chicken strains contain cells expressing chicken fetal antigen, indicating that the degree of dedifferentiation of tumor cells varies among strains (356). Some turkey MD lymphoblastoid cell lines (300) have been identified as B cells, others (357) as T cells. Further description of transformed cells can be found in the Etiology section.

The possibility that MD tumors are of clonal origin has been proposed based on observations of random MDV DNA integration into the genomes of lymphoma cells (127, 128). Although integration was random, the pattern of integration sites among cells from a given lymphoma or a given lymphoma-derived cell line was consistent. This work has fundamental implications regarding the pathogenesis of MD, but awaits confirmation and further definition. Earlier studies by Schat et al. (413), on the other hand, clearly showed that different lymphomas in the same bird could yield cell lines representing different T-cell phenotypes based on surface CD and T-cell–receptor markers.

Studies of graft-versus-host reactions in different genetic strains led Longenecker et al. (267) and Pazderka et al. (340) to suggest that low alloimmune competence and resistance to MD are very closely related through genetic linkage or functional dependence. That prompted speculation by Schat et al. (407) and Calnek (66) that the activation of T cells in response to the necrotizing infection of B cells acts as a very significant event in pathogenesis by providing an abundant supply of cells that are the usual target cells for transformation. This has been borne out by studies by Calnek showing that tumor induction at the site of inoculation with MDV is enhanced by provoking a CMI reaction against allogeneic cells at the site (86, 87). It is plausible that transformation requires 1) susceptibility to infection, 2) intrinsic or extrinsic control of virus replication (latency), 3) cell division to integrate virus genome, and 4) expression of viral oncogenes or activation of cellular oncogenes. Activated T cells infected at the time CMI responses cause a switch to latency could fit this model. Interestingly, cells present as early as 4 days after inoculation of MDV-infected allogeneic kidney cells can be grown in vitro as MD cell lines (86, 87). Thus, transformed cells, or at least transformation target cells, are present even during the early cytolytic phase of MD.

The pathogenesis of infection with oncogenic MDV that has become attenuated by passage in vitro has been studied by Bradley, Frazier, and Payne (quoted in 337) and by Schat et al. (410). Both groups found that attenuated virus failed to cause cytolytic infection of lymphoid organs and that cell-associated viremia levels were low. The latter authors further learned that attenuated virus was not infectious for lymphocytes in vitro, perhaps explaining the in vivo observations.

Vaccination alters the pathogenesis of MDV infection by severely curtailing or eliminating the early cytolytic phase (77, 454). Also, the level of latent infection with MDV is markedly reduced, and neither late cytolytic infection nor immunosuppression occurs.

The actual mechanism(s) by which pathogenesis is altered in the case of host resistance is not clear. CMI is probably involved, however, and there is evidence (see Immunity) to suggest that immune responses of the host may be directed against either the early virologic events or the later proliferative phase, and that an effective response at either stage might reduce the chance of overt disease. Both age and genetic resistance are dependent on immunologic competence (61, 439). The availability of appropriate target cells is probably also important. If the hypothesis is correct that tumor development is enhanced by a strong T-cell response against the

early cytolytic infection of B cells, then factors that limit that response should reduce tumor incidence. Vaccinal immunity and embryonal bursectomy both suppress the active viral infection (77, 408, 454), thereby obviating an inflammatory response, and both reduce the incidence of tumors. Also, at least one genetic strain (line 6) is thought to be resistant to MD because of a paucity of T-cell targets (257). Interestingly, there is evidence (citations in 64, 85) that some genetic strains that have unusually strong CMI responses are especially susceptible to MD, although this is not true in all cases.

Virus strains differ in oncogenicity, but differences in pathogenesis associated with the strains are not well defined. All cause similar early cytolytic infections. Both the genetic strain and the virus strain are involved in determining the distribution as well as the incidence of lymphomas.

The immune response itself may be responsible for some lesions characteristic of MD. Nerve lesions have some characteristics suggestive of an autoimmune disease (384), and MD has been identified as a model for the Landry-Guillain-Barré syndrome (341). Additional evidence supporting an autoimmune component for MD comes from studies showing immune complexes in the kidneys of MDV-infected chickens and quail (229, 360).

The pathogenesis of atherosclerotic lesions is unknown.

Immunity. Importance of the immune response in MD cannot be overemphasized. The concern is fourfold: 1) MD can be immunosuppressive, 2) immunologic response is probably the basis to resistance in MD, 3) vaccinal immunity is the prime means of control, and 4) immunologic response may contribute to the cellular mass of the lymphoma (see Pathogenesis).

Immune responses and immunosuppressive features of MD have been well documented and reviewed. For details, the various reviews (63, 337, 347, 348, 349, 398, 399, 400, 401, 418, 424) should be consulted.

IMMUNOSUPPRESSION. Impairment of the immune response might result directly from MDV infection through lytic infection of lymphocytes (citations in 337), or indirectly from activity of suppressor cell populations (256, 472). Probably both are important. In vitro studies (54, 173, 378, 473) suggest that the MD tumor cells themselves might have suppressor activity. This could be because they are true suppressor T cells or, perhaps, because they express chicken fetal antigen, which has been shown to have suppressor activity (315). Studies by Schat et al. (413) showing tumor cell lines to carry CD4 antigen, a marker for helper T cells, argues against the former, but direct evidence either way is lacking. Permanent immunosuppression tends to correlate with eventual tumor development (405) and may only be seen in birds that have already developed neoplasms (474); thus it is difficult to distinguish between cause and effect. Generally, the first appearance of permanent immunosuppression coincides with the second phase of cytolytic infection (see Pathogenesis). Because immunocompetence is required for latency to be maintained (57), it might be that immunosuppression associated with the appearance of transformed lymphoblasts results in the loss of additional B and T cells through cytolytic infection, thus compounding the situation and resulting in the bursal and thymic atrophy seen in birds destined to succumb to MD. A possible association between immunosuppression, reactivation of cytolytic infection, and MD breaks during the laying cycle should be considered.

Both humoral immunity and cell-mediated immunity can be depressed by MD; these are reflected by reduced antibody response to a variety of antigens and by alterations in T-cell functions such as skin graft rejection, mitogen stimulation of lymphocytes, delayed hypersensitivity, reduced NK cell activity, and impaired Rous sarcoma regression (citations in 337). Marek's disease virus infection can increase susceptibility to primary and secondary infection with coccidia (33). It should be emphasized that while there may be depression, there is not a total loss of function.

A transient depression in cellular immunity, as measured by in vitro responsiveness to mitogens, is seen at about 7 days PI regardless of genetic constitution or virulence of the virus strain (citations in 399). This is apparently due to a population of suppressor macrophages (256).

IMMUNE RESPONSES. Both humoral and cell-mediated immunity develop in competent birds after infection with MDV. These can involve several types of responses and be directed against a variety of antigens.

Payne (329) speculated that MD immunity could be either early against virus infection or later against transformed and proliferating lymphoid cells. Indeed, inactivated viral or tumor antigens can be used to immunize against MD (219, 250, 262, 291, 345, 354). Inactivated antiviral vaccines protect against early cytolytic infections, latent infections, and tumor formation, whereas killed tumor cell vaccines only prevent the latter. An exception was an oil-emulsion inactivated MDV reported to induce non–virus-neutralizing antibodies, which could passively immunize chicks against early viral-related effects of MDV infection, but not against later tumor development (250).

Humoral Immunity. Precipitating and virus-neutralizing (VN) antibodies can be detected within 1–2 wk; a transient immunoglobulin M (IgM) response is replaced by IgG (177). These antibodies generally persist throughout the life of the bird. Virus-neutralizing, but not precipitating, antibodies correlate with survival of infected birds (60, 433). Probably, this is an effect rather than a cause and may result from sparing of the bursa-dependent system in resistant birds (176, 177, 453).

A protective role for passively acquired humoral antibody has been observed in chicks (16, 105, and others); the effect of antibody is not to exclude, but to reduce, the level of infection, perhaps by impeding spread. In vivo VN can occur (55); however, the exact mechanism is unknown. A humoral antibody response is not required for resistance to MD, since bursectomized birds may survive infection (434), but this does not preclude a role for early antibody in suppressing destructive infection of immunologic organs required for subsequent resistance.

Cell-Mediated Immunity. Since antibodies are not a required component of immune resistance to MD, it can be presumed that CMI is important. This conclusion is bolstered by the observation that functional T cells are required for resistance (74, 439) as well as vaccinal immunity (338).

Few specific antigens involved in either humoral or cell-mediated immunity have been identified. Virus-neutralizing antibodies in infected birds are probably directed against glycoprotein B (gB) (see Etiology), and monospecific antibodies against gB neutralized cell-free virus (123). Furthermore, either gB alone (319), or recombinant fowl poxvirus vaccine (FPV), or HVT vaccine expressing the MDV gB gene (305, 393) protected birds against MDV challenge. Glycoprotein A, expressed by a baculovirus vector (311), induced antibodies in chickens, but protection studies have not been reported. Antigen produced by serotype 1 MDV seems to provide more effective protection than that from other serotypes (299). A recombinant FPV expressing the phosphoprotein pp38 was nonprotective (305), although Pratt et al. (364) found lymphoblastoid cell lines expressing pp38 to be targets for major histocompatibility complex (MHC)-restricted lysis by cytotoxic T lymphocytes (CTL) induced by all three serotypes of MDV. The pp38 antigen is of special interest because it occurs on both productively infected chick kidney cells and non–virus-producer MD cell lines (199, 202, 294). The approach used by Pratt et al., i.e., transfection of MDV genes into reticuloendotheliosis-transformed cell lines that can serve as syngeneic targets for CTL in a chromium-release assay (CRA), should help identify other antigens important in CMI. Other CRA studies have used MD cell lines as targets, but alloantigens were involved and thus the effector cells were not CTL (409).

The possibility that a surface antigen found on

MDV-transformed cells could be involved in immunity was raised by studies in which anti-idiotype antibodies against MATSA (see Etiology) were shown to immunize chickens against challenge with virulent MDV (121).

Vaccinal Immunity. Vaccinal immunity is almost certainly immunologic in nature. Not only does the protective effect of inactivated vaccines rule out the alternate possibility of viral interference, but vaccinal immunity can be abrogated by immunosuppressive treatments affecting CMI, such as cyclophosphamide treatment (374), or by infection with the immunosuppressive chicken infectious anemia virus (322). Deletion of humoral immunity by bursectomy and X-irradiation has no effect on protection conferred by attenuated MDV (140), although a similar treatment partially impairs vaccinal immunity from HVT (382).

Immunity from live virus vaccines including HVT, attenuated MDV, and serotype 2 MDV appears to be directed largely against viral antigens but possibly also against tumor antigens. All protect against early replication of virulent viruses in the lymphoid organs of challenged birds and reduce the level of latent infection (77, 354, 377, 408, 454). Evidence suggesting antitumor immunity comes from reports that lymphoblastoid cells may induce MHC-restricted immunity in birds challenged with transplantable MD lymphomas (129), and that attenuated MDV, HVT, and SB-1 can all immunize against transplantable MD tumors including the JMV transplant (276, 421, and others). None of the transplantable cells or the cell lines used in these studies express any of the usual virus-associated antigens. The phosphoprotein, pp38, noted above, however, could account for the ability of some MD vaccines to immunize against challenge with transplantable MD tumor cells and, conversely, for the ability of nonproducer cells such as JMV to induce immunity against MDV challenge. Other, yet undiscovered, immunogens may also be shared by tumor cells and productively infected cells. The existence of such a viral antigen(s) in transformed cells was predicted by Powell (346).

OTHER RESISTANCE MECHANISMS. Macrophages may be involved in resistance by restricting virus replication directly (163, 178) or in concert with antibody (239, 247). Immune B cells and macrophages can interact to inactivate cell-free virus (403). Activation of macrophages by injection of thioglycollate broth into the peritoneal cavity markedly reduced the incidence of MD in challenged birds (162). Macrophages are also apparently involved in early transient immunosuppression following MDV infection (256, 261) and can inhibit DNA synthesis and proliferation by MD lymphoblastoid cell lines in vitro (256, 324, 425).

Various cytokines may be important in MD. Settnes (418) reviewed possible effects of interferon, and noted that levels of this cytokine, as an early response to MDV infection, may be higher in resistant, than susceptible, birds (188). Interferon protects against the transplantable JMV tumor (481), and it appears that it is one of the cytokines important to the development and maintenance of latency with MDV (57, 487).

Innate resistance in the form of NK cells could also be important (see reviews 348, 399). Natural killer cells are cytotoxic for MD tumor cells, and there may be a relationship between these cells and age-related, and perhaps also genetic, resistance. There is increased NK cell activity after vaccination with HVT or SB-1, and elevated levels of NK cells in regressive, but not progressive, tumors could indicate a role for intratumoral immunity in tumor regression. Interestingly, supernatant fluid from cultures of the JMV-1 lymphoblastoid cell line is protective when used as a treatment prior to challenge with MDV (232), apparently due in part to lymphokine activation of NK cells (233).

DIAGNOSIS

Virus Isolation. Although not especially helpful in establishing a diagnosis of MD, techniques for virus isolation have value in epizootiologic and other virus characterization studies. Related techniques are used for the titration of MDV and its related vaccine viruses. Procedures have been reviewed by Sharma (430).

SOURCE OF VIRUS. Marek's disease virus can be isolated as early as 1 or 2 days postinoculation (342) or 5 days after contact exposure (2) and throughout the life of the chicken. Intact viable cells are the preferred inoculum because, in most cases, infectivity is avidly cell-associated, although cell-free preparations from skin, dander, or feather tips of infected chickens may contain the virus (72). In-

17.16. *A.* Leukotic tumors involving feather follicles (skin leukosis). (Peckham) *B.* Experimentally induced Marek's disease (MD) lymphoma in immature ovary (*bottom*) compared with normal ovary (*top*). *C.* Ocular lesions of MD. Note that normal eye (*left*) has a sharply defined pupil and well-pigmented iris. Affected eye (*right*) has a discolored iris and very irregular pupil as a result of mononuclear cell infiltration. (Peckham) *D.* Gizzard from a chicken infected with CU-2 isolate of MDV. Note the grossly obvious atherosclerotic change in the arteries. (C. Fabricant) Microscopic changes from similar arteries are shown in Fig. 16.16B. (Shivaprasad) *E.* Multiple lymphomas in lungs. *F.* Multiple lymphomas in heart. (Shivaprasad)

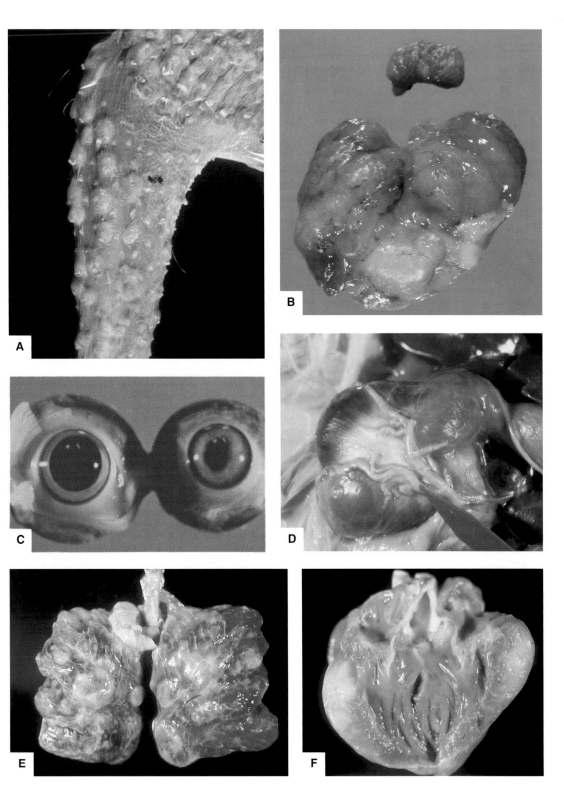

ocula may consist of blood lymphocytes, heparinized whole blood, splenocytes, or isolated tumor cells. The virus can often be recovered from infected cell suspensions following storage for 24 hr at 4 C, thus facilitating transport of samples (525).

CELL CULTURE TECHNIQUES. Probably the most widely used method for primary isolation of MDV is inoculation of susceptible tissue cultures with blood lymphocytes or single-cell suspensions from lymphoid tissues of infected chickens. Chicken kidney cell and duck embryo fibroblast cultures are preferred substrates for isolation of serotype 1 MDV, whereas chicken embryo fibroblasts are normally used for isolation of viruses of serotypes 2 and 3. Cultures are inoculated with 10^6 to 10^7 cells although some inhibition of viral plaque formation may be encountered with doses over 8×10^6 cells for some viruses (81). After 24–48 hr, the inoculum is washed off and the culture maintained under liquid or agar medium, usually without subculture.

Development of typical plaques (see Fig. 17.4) in inoculated cultures within 5–14 days, and absence of such changes in comparable uninoculated (or sham inoculated) control cultures, are evidence for isolation of MDV. The plaques induced by serotype 1, 2, and 3 viruses can be distinguished, with practice, by morphologic criteria (397, 495), but immunofluorescent staining with serotype-specific monoclonal antibodies provides a more accurate differentiation. Optimal time for observation of plaques varies with the cell substrate and serotype of the virus. Known virus-infected inoculum may be used to determine susceptibility of the test cultures.

Marek's disease virus has been isolated by direct cultivation of kidney cells from infected chickens (514). The short-term lymphocyte culture technique followed by an FA test is an especially useful method to demonstrate virus (78), and presumably could also be used to recover virus if antigen-positive cultured lymphocytes were transferred to susceptible monolayer cultures. Marek's disease virus has also been isolated from explants of various tissues, including nerves and ganglia, on chicken embryo fibroblast monolayers (341).

ISOLATE IDENTIFICATION. The identity and purity of a suspect isolate must be carefully ascertained. All three viral serotypes may coexist in the same chicken and are frequently isolated simultaneously. Procedures helpful in deriving serotypically pure MDV isolates include the use of inocula from nonvaccinated sentinel chickens placed in suspect flocks (to avoid contamination with serotype 3 viruses, which spread poorly by contact), the plaque purification or cloning of the isolate at the earliest possible passage, and the selective use of cell substrates (chicken and duck fibroblasts are relatively

resistant to serotype 1 and 2 isolates, respectively) (500). Serotype identity and purity can be confirmed by immunofluorescent staining with serotype-specific monoclonal antibodies (258). Pathotyping of serotype 1 MDVs may be accomplished by inoculation of nonvaccinated chickens as well as chickens vaccinated with HVT or bivalent vaccines (500) (see Etiology). Freedom from other viruses is also critical, since contamination may alter the apparent pathogenicity of the isolate (53, 211). Propagation of MDV isolates for up to six passages in chicken embryo fibroblasts or chicken kidney cell cultures will exclude contaminants such as chicken anemia virus (534) and permit preparation of seed and working stocks, which can be more easily standardized and titrated. Although the possibility of attenuation must be considered, this usually requires 20 or more cell-culture passages (109) and occurs more gradually in chicken kidney cells or duck embryo fibroblasts compared with chicken embryo fibroblasts.

VIRUS ASSAY AND TITRATION. Viruses of serotypes 1, 2, and 3 can be quantitated by in vitro techniques similar to those described for virus isolation. Methods differ for different serotypes, but all rely on plaque induction in susceptible cell cultures. Enumeration should be done as soon as plaques become mature (time varies with isolate), since secondary plaques may occur when cultures are maintained with liquid medium. Agar overlay methods have been described (459) but are not commonly used, probably because plaque formation is often delayed under agar and because secondary plaque formation under liquid medium has not been considered a significant problem. Procedures for titration of vaccine viruses have been reviewed (475) and are not fundamentally different from those for pathogenic isolates.

Viral Markers in Tissues. It is often desirable to detect the presence of viral infection in chickens without isolating the virus in culture. Such infection markers also have value for the identification of putative MDV isolates in cell cultures.

ANTIGEN DETECTION. Although polyclonal antibodies obtained from MDV-infected chickens have been applied to the detection of antigens in tissues, the availability of monoclonal antibodies directed to specific antigens or epitopes has greatly facilitated many of these tests. Monoclonal antibodies have been prepared against type-common and type-specific epitopes of all three MDV serotypes (258). Viral antigens can be detected in feather tips and FFE, cytolytically infected lymphoid tissues, or infected cell cultures with appropriate antibodies by FA tests (461), immunoperoxidase tests (91), AGP tests (164, 263), and enzyme-linked immunosorbent assays (ELISA) (122, 415). Marek's disease virus antigen–containing cells are rare in lymphomas and latently infected tissues, but antigens can be induced in some cells by short-term lymphocyte culture (78).

POLYMERASE CHAIN REACTION ASSAYS. Primers designed to amplify 132-bpr sequences specific to MDVs of serotype 1 have been described (20, 447, 542). This assay can discriminate between attenuated and wild-type strains and has the potential to detect viral DNA in lymphomas (124), but may not be sensitive enough to detect latently infected tissues, probably due to the lower frequency of positive cells and lower number of viral genomes per cell. A PCR assay has also been used to amplify the gC gene of MDV and HVT (541).

DNA PROBES. Methods utilizing DNA–DNA dot-blot hybridization with DNA probes for the detection of MDV DNA in feather tip extracts have been described (122). Furthermore, the localization of virus-infected cells has been accomplished by in situ hybridization for both MDV (390) and HVT (186).

ELECTRON MICROSCOPY. Herpesvirus particles can be detected in the FFE and other tissues of infected chickens and in productively infected cells in vitro (72, 296, 478).

Antibody Demonstration. Tests for identifying the presence of specific antibodies in chicken sera are useful in studies of viral pathogenesis and for monitoring specific-pathogen–free flocks. A number of procedures including AGP, FA, ELISA, and VN are in common use; methods have been described (430). At this time, commercial reagents are available only for the AGP test, which is the least sensitive test but is adequate to detect serologic responses in infected or vaccinated chicken flocks. None of these tests, however, is capable of determining antibodies to a specific viral serotype in chickens exposed to multiple viral serotypes. Antigenic differences between serotypes have been reported (51, 52), but common antigens also appear to exist. The biologic significance of antibodies detected by different methods may vary (60).

Differential Diagnosis. Despite established guidelines (373, 445), the clinical diagnosis of MD has been considered difficult in practice, probably because there is no truly pathognomonic gross lesion and because MD lesions can closely resemble those of lymphoid leukosis (LL), which continues to be common, or reticuloendotheliosis (RE), which recently has become common in the Middle East. The RE virus (REV) is widespread in the United States and can induce experimental lesions (nerve

enlargements and lymphomas) that resemble MD even more closely than those induced by avian leukosis viruses (ALV) (see Reticuloendotheliosis).

INFECTION CRITERIA. Marek's disease virus is highly contagious and virtually ubiquitous among chickens. Only a small percentage of infected chickens develop clinical MD. Because of these factors, indicators of virus infection are normally considered to have limited value in diagnosis of the disease. Diagnoses, therefore, have traditionally been based on disease-specific criteria such as epidemiology, pathology, and tumor-specific markers.

The availability of PCR and immunohistochemical assays, however, has expanded the role of infection criteria in differential diagnosis. The PCR assays, as discussed earlier, may detect serotype 1-specific viral DNA in MD tumors. Immunohistochemical staining with appropriate antibodies may detect MDV antigens (such as pp38) expressed in a proportion of MD transformed cells, and will detect REV or ALV antigens in virtually every transformed cell in LL or REV lymphomas. Exclusion of ALV or REV, where possible, through negative PCR or histochemical assays on tumor tissue, may provide strong support for a diagnosis of MD when other MD-related criteria are positive. Although the practical value of such tests is still under evaluation, it seems likely that PCR or histochemical assays for all three tumor viruses will help provide definitive diagnoses of MD.

GROSS PATHOLOGY. Although enlarged peripheral nerves and visceral lymphomas are common in MD, neither lesion occurs consistently or is pathognomonic. Thus, other criteria such as age and lesion distribution must be considered in the postmortem diagnosis of MD. Historically, chickens have been diagnosed positive for MD on the basis of gross pathology and age if at least one of the following conditions is met: (1) leukotic enlargement of peripheral nerves; (2) lymphoid tumors in various tissues (liver, heart, gonad, skin, muscle, proventriculus) in birds under 16 wk of age; (3) visceral lymphoid tumors in birds 16 wk or older that lack neoplastic involvement of the bursa of Fabricius; or (4) iris discoloration and pupil irregularity, as in Fig. 17.16C.

Some critical assumptions are the absence of bursal tumors in cases of MD in birds older than 16 wk, the consistent presence of gross bursal tumors in cases of LL, and the occurrence of LL or other unrelated tumors only in birds older than 16 wk. Another assumption is that REV infection only rarely induces nerve enlargements or lymphomas in the absence of bursal involvement in commercial chickens. Although these assumptions may not be invariably correct, diagnostic errors on a flock basis are expected to be infrequent if necropsies are done with care and several birds are examined. Proper examination of the bursa is particularly important and requires incision of the organ with close inspection of the epithelial surface. However, diagnoses based only on gross pathologic criteria can no longer be considered definitive.

HISTOLOGY AND CYTOLOGY. Diagnostic accuracy may be enhanced by employment of histologic or cytologic procedures. A mixed population of small to large lymphocytes, lymphoblasts, plasma cells, and MD cells are found in MD tumors. These diagnostic features may be seen in routine histologic sections stained with hematoxylin and eosin. However, examination of touch preparations taken directly from lesions of freshly killed birds and stained with methyl green pyronin or Shorr's stain gives better cytologic detail and can be prepared in a few minutes. Pyroninophilia is observed infrequently in cells of MD tumors (445). Even these procedures, however, cannot always differentiate MD lesions from nonbursal lymphomas or nerve lesions induced by REV infection.

TUMOR-ASSOCIATED MARKERS. Even though MATSA is recognized as a host antigen associated with activated T cells (278), this and other host cell markers have diagnostic value. Membrane immunofluorescent staining for MATSA and IgM has proved particularly useful for the diagnosis of MD (131, 306, 307): MD lymphomas have 5–40% of cells positive for MATSA, whereas IgM is present on less than 5% of cells from MD lymphomas. Positive immunohistochemical staining for pp38 antigen, which is expressed in a small but variable proportion of MD lymphoma cells (199, 293), should be diagnostic for MD. Detection of cell surface markers such as Ia (MHC class II) and CD4/CD8 antigens may also help differentiate MD lymphomas from those caused by REV. Marek's disease lymphoma cells are positive for Ia antigen and most cells express CD4 antigen (413), whereas cells from nonbursal RE lymphomas are negative for Ia and predominantly stain for CD8 antigen (115). Further development of this technology for differential diagnosis of avian tumors is in progress.

DIFFERENTIATION FROM OTHER DISEASES. Lymphoid leukosis is still the principal disease to be considered in differential diagnosis of MD; however, LL can usually be differentiated from MD by its common involvement of the bursa of Fabricius, uniform blast morphology, pyroninophilia, presence of B-cell markers, presence of ALV genomes or antigens, and absence of MATSA on tumor cells.

Accidental or experimental inoculation of chickens with nondefective REV has caused clinical disease characterized by enlarged nerves, runting, and both bursal and nonbursal visceral lymphomas.

Two types of REV-induced pathology closely resemble MD: nonbursal lymphomas that occur as early as 6 wk of age (526), and enlargements of peripheral nerves that occur both alone (517) and in groups where some individual chickens also have lymphomas (526). Such lesions can best be distinguished from MD by infection-related criteria (see Reticuloendotheliosis). These lesions are not commonly recognized in the field, but potentially may become more prevalent as evidence of REV infection is increasing.

Other diseases that may present confusing gross lesions or paralytic signs are myeloblastosis, erythroblastosis, carcinoma of the ovary, other neoplasms, riboflavin deficiency, tuberculosis, histomoniasis, genetic gray eye, Newcastle disease, avian encephalomyelitis, and joint infections or injuries.

A peripheral neuropathy, similar to that reported in specific-pathogen chickens (37), has recently been recognized as common in commercial chickens in the United States (216). This lesion is characterized by edema and limited cellular infiltration of peripheral nerves and is associated with clinical lameness leading to mortality. The incidence of lesions varies with MHC haplotype (12). It is differentiated from MD by the absence of visceral lymphomas, the paucity of lymphocytes in nerve lesions, and the failure to demonstrate MDV by PCR and virus isolation (13).

TREATMENT. There is no effective practical treatment for MD in either flocks or individual chickens. Some birds showing clinical signs of MD, however, spontaneously regress their lesions and recover under certain circumstances (333, 341, 437).

PREVENTION AND CONTROL. Development of successful vaccines for control of MD (110, 317, 385) is a significant achievement both in agriculture (since MD prior to vaccination had become the most costly poultry disease) and basic cancer research (since this was the first time an important neoplastic disease had been so controlled in any species). Vaccination represents, for now and the foreseeable future, the central strategy for the prevention and control of MD. Genetic resistance and biosecurity, however, are important as adjuncts to vaccination and may assume greater significance as the limitations of vaccination are more widely recognized. Detailed reviews are available (327, 496).

Vaccination

TYPES OF VACCINES. Vaccines based on all three viral serotypes, mixtures of serotypes, and recombinant DNA vaccines are all capable of protecting chickens against MD. Monovalent vaccines include attenuated serotype 1 MDV (110, 385) and HVT (317). The naturally avirulent isolates of serotype 2 (402, 537) are usually combined with HVT to take advantage of the synergistic activity documented between serotypes 2 and 3 (494). In addition, many other combinations of viral serotypes are in common use. Experimental vaccines based on recombinant DNA technology have been developed, but are not yet licensed for use. Although all vaccine types are protective, HVT has been most extensively used because it is economical to produce and cell-free virus extracted from infected cells may be lyophilized (73) for more convenient storage and handling. A cell-associated form of HVT requiring storage in liquid nitrogen has been most widely used, probably because it is more effective than cell-free virus in the presence of maternal antibodies (507). Only cell-associated vaccines of serotypes 1 and 2 are presently available.

FACTORS AFFECTING EFFICACY. Vaccine is usually administered at hatching. Both cell-associated and cell-free vaccines are given by parenteral inoculation at a dose usually in excess of 1000 plaque-forming units (PFU)/chick. The intramuscular route may be slightly more effective than the subcutaneous route (314), but this advantage was not observed by all workers (483).

Sharma and Burmester (431) found that vaccination of 18-day-old embryos accelerated development of protective immunity by several days, and proposed this technique for controlling detrimental effects of early exposure to virulent MDV. Embryo vaccination was advantageous even in the presence of maternal antibodies (432) and with several types of MD vaccines (435). This procedure has been automated and is now used in over 50% of commercial broilers in the United States. Embryo vaccination has resulted in reduced labor costs and greater precision of vaccine administration, but, in contrast to the early laboratory data, no significant reduction in MD losses has yet been recognized in the field (283, 396).

The adjuvant, acemannan, has been reported to increase the effectiveness of HVT and other MD vaccines, especially when challenge is given at 2 days postvaccination (313). This product is in commercial use, but the extent to which its use has decreased MD losses remains to be established.

The shorter the interval between vaccination and exposure to the virulent field virus, the poorer the level of protection (317). Early exposure is undoubtedly one of the most important causes of excessive MD in vaccinated flocks, since up to 7 days is required for a solid immunity to be established (17) and since field exposure usually occurs very soon after placement of chickens (516). Severe MD losses have been associated with multiage layer operations, where there is little opportunity to prevent early exposure.

The strain of chicken is also an important factor in MD vaccinal immunity (see Genetic Resistance). Schat et al. (408) found that HVT vaccine in a genetically resistant chicken provided better immunity than did the bivalent (HVT + SB-1) vaccine in a susceptible chicken.

In an effort to improve efficacy, increased vaccine doses (136, 495) or double vaccination (15) were tried with little or no success; however, in response to a perceived need, vaccine manufacturers have continued to increase recommended dosages. Many layer and breeder chickens now receive up to 10,000 PFU of HVT at hatching. Double vaccination has become popular in Europe and is occasionally used in the United States, but there is no convincing evidence of its effectiveness.

Stress has long been suspected to interfere with the maintenance of vaccinal immunity. Apparent confirmation has been provided by Powell and Davison (350), who induced MD lesions and mortality by immunosuppressive treatment at 10 wk of age of vaccinated and previously challenged chickens. An attempt to confirm this observation was unsuccessful (429), but the possibility that immunosuppressive stress may play an important role in MD losses, especially those that occur after the onset of egg production, deserves consideration.

Despite field observations to the contrary, there is no direct evidence that the late onset of MD losses in vaccinated chickens is the result of recent or late exposure to a "new" viral strain. In fact, this possibility seems unlikely given the natural resistance of older chickens to MD infection (5, 30, 520) and the probability that this resistance is augmented by prior vaccination and exposure to other field strains.

Various other infections, including infectious bursal disease (427), REV (523), reovirus (386), and chicken anemia agent (322, 535), have been reported to interfere with the induction of vaccinal immunity, although very specific conditions are sometimes required.

Naturally occurring infection with avirulent serotype 2 or low virulence serotype 1 isolates may provide protection against subsequent exposure to virulent isolates (35, 36, 209, 454) and may be an adjunct to vaccination. However, carryover of spreading vaccines from previous flocks has not been easy to demonstrate, even when placement of new chicks occurred within 2 wk on the same litter used by previous SB-1–vaccinated chickens (525). A role for natural exposure to virulent MDV strains in the maintenance of vaccinal immunity for long periods has also been proposed (483).

Proper handling of vaccine during thawing and reconstitution is crucial (167). Also, vaccination of breeders with a serotype 1 or 2 virus rather than

HVT leaves progeny more responsive to vaccination with HVT (236); this technique to reduce the detrimental effect of homologous maternal antibody is in use in several parts of the world and, following the availability of highly effective serotype 1 vaccines for breeder vaccination, is now being evaluated in the United States.

Outbreaks associated with vvMDV strains in flocks vaccinated with HVT can often be controlled by vaccination with polyvalent vaccines composed of all three viral serotypes, or of serotypes 2 and 3 (82, 494, 508). The improved efficacy of a bivalent vaccine against challenge with very virulent MDV strains was confirmed by Schat et al. (408) and others (485).

Synergism among vaccine viruses is best demonstrated with viruses of serotypes 2 and 3 (499, 501, 504). Bivalent vaccines composed of the FC126 strain of HVT coupled with either the SB-1 (408) or 301B/1 (499) strains of serotype 2 MDV have provided excellent protection and are widely used. A variety of other combinations are also used, including bivalent vaccines with serotypes 1 and 3 or trivalent vaccines with all three serotypes. Although the advantage of these polyvalent vaccines compared with simpler combinations has not been demonstrated, no negative consequences of their use is apparent.

VACCINATION STRATEGIES. Marek's disease vaccines are unusually effective, often achieving over 90% protection under commercial conditions (497, 502). However, attention is often focused on an increasing number of flocks in which MD losses are perceived to be excessive (538). Causes for such "vaccine failures" are difficult to ascertain by retrospective analysis (496), although early exposure and emergence of new MDV strains with increased virulence may be important.

As the menu of available MD vaccines has expanded, selection of the appropriate vaccine has become more difficult. As of 1995, seven vaccine strains were licensed for use in the United States. A brief description of each follows.

HVT (317) continues to be widely used as a monovalent product in many countries, probably because of its low cost, availability as cell-associated and cell-free forms, and effectiveness where field exposure is not too severe.

HVT + SB-1 (bivalent) vaccine (408, 494) was the first commercial vaccine based on synergism between serotype 2 and 3 viruses. It is widely used in the United States for layer, breeder, and some broiler flocks. HVT + 301B/1 (499) is another bivalent vaccine utilizing a different serotype 2 MDV component.

R2/23 (503) is an attenuated serotype 1 strain derived from the Md11 strain of vvMDV isolated in the United States. This strain is also identified as Md11/75C or Md11.75C/R2/23.

CVI988 was derived from a virus of unclassified pathogenicity (probably mild) isolated in The Netherlands (385). Three CVI988-derived vaccines are in use in the United States. Although each is sometimes given the name "Rispens" (commemorating the person who first isolated the strain), the vaccines have very different properties. The original CVI988 strain, used successfully in Europe and other countries since the early 1970s (268), has been available in the United States only since 1994. CVI988/C is a derivative cloned from higher passages of CVI988 in cell culture; it was also back-passaged in chickens to yield CVI988/C/R6, which is claimed to provide greater protection than CVI988/C (126).

In practice, a number of other combinations of these vaccines are used, including serotypes 1+3 and serotypes 1+2+3. However, evidence for synergism between serotype 1 and other serotypes is lacking (501, 504).

Much current research directed to development of improved vaccines employs recombinant DNA approaches. Recombinant fowl pox (305) or HVT (393) vaccines expressing the gB gene of serotype 1 MDV have shown some protective efficacy. It remains to be determined, however, whether these or other vaccine types will be more efficacious than existing products.

Efficacy data that compare certain groups of vaccines are available (citations in 496), but no systematic evaluation of licensed strains in their various combinations has been published. Although HVT and CVI988/C are effective, bivalent serotype 2+3 vaccines and the remaining serotype 1 vaccines are probably more effective (499). In one series of trials in which protective efficacy was determined for most of the principal vaccines (except CVI988/C/R6), the original CVI988 vaccine provided the highest levels of protection (505), a result consistent with earlier reports from Europe (486). Efficacy rankings of vaccines, however, have not always been reproducible when performed under different conditions in different laboratories, and thus should be interpreted with caution.

The emergence of increasingly virulent viral strains, coupled with an apparent reduction of vaccine efficacy during the past 20 years, has prompted justifiable concern. This suggests that vaccination by itself does not provide a complete control program and certainly is not the ultimate solution for MD. Strict biosecurity procedures to reduce early exposure, and the presence of genetic resistance, are essential adjuncts to a successful vaccination program (see next sections).

Genetic Resistance. Genetically controlled

differences in MD susceptibility among lines of chickens has been reviewed by Calnek (64). Lines of chickens with genetic resistance to MD have been selected and maintained experimentally (111, 192, 464) and commercially. Marek's disease resistance appeared independent of genetic factors that control production traits (34), and variation of MD susceptibility in single-sire families indicated that there was sufficient heterogeneity to warrant selection for resistance in commercial chickens (34, 111). Resistance has been traditionally measured by challenge of unvaccinated chickens with virulent MDV, but recent studies (11) conclude that resistance may better be determined in vaccinated stocks (see later section).

SELECTION METHODS. Selection programs for resistance have historically been based on progeny testing (111) or reproduction from survivors of exposed breeding flocks (269).

Selection based on blood typing relies on the close relationship between MD resistance and alleles of the B-F region of the MHC, especially B^{21} (43, 44, 170, 267). Other B alleles are associated with susceptibility or with lesser degrees of resistance (10, 175). Such a selection procedure may simplify production of resistant stocks in populations containing a specific allele for resistance, although the possibility of negative associations with productivity traits needs to be measured (158). Furthermore, the value of selection for MHC-associated markers may vary considerably among commercial lines and crosses (39, 172).

Evidence that non-MHC genes may also be involved in resistance is provided by the observation that RPL line 6 and 7 chickens, which are both homozygous at the B locus for the B^2 allele, differ markedly in MD susceptibility (118). Furthermore, non-MHC effects were considered more important than MHC effects in studies on several commercial lines (160). Studies to identify and map such genes, currently in progress, may provide new tools to enhance selection programs for MD resistance. Resistance has been considered dominant, although this varies to some extent (175) and, in most cases, resistance of crosses has been intermediate to that of the parent strains (39, 64).

The mechanism(s) by which genetic constitution influences the incidence of MD is discussed elsewhere (see Pathogenesis).

APPLICATIONS. Since Spencer et al. (462) found genetically resistant chickens were protected by vaccination to a greater extent than more susceptible ones, breeding for genetic resistance is considered to be a valuable adjunct to immunization for control of MD. Furthermore, evidence suggests that genetic resistance might reduce the need for biva-

lent or serotype 1 vaccination, now used to control challenge with very virulent strains (408). However, resistance of vaccinated and nonvaccinated chickens may sometimes (156), but not always, vary in parallel (11), suggesting that selection should be performed in vaccinated stocks (10). Bacon and Witter (12) found that the ranking of chicken lines for MD resistance varied depending on which serotype of vaccine was used.

In light of the selection tools available, the virtual absence of negative correlations, and the major benefits to be derived, it is not surprising that breeders are beginning to place a higher priority on this approach.

Biosecurity. Because embryo transmission is unimportant in MD, isolation rearing and environmental sanitation constitute a primary control method that is successful and widely used for specific-pathogen–free flocks (483). The use of filtered-air, positive-pressure houses is generally required (6, 132).

Strict biosecurity practices to limit the extent of early MDV exposure, while impractical as a primary control procedure, are a crucial and cost-effective adjunct to vaccination. Unfortunately, modern poultry management too often places replacement flocks of different ages in close proximity to each other, or requires the reuse of litter from a previous broiler flock. The failure to prevent early exposure is perhaps the most important single cause of vaccine failures. Improved hygiene has often appeared to play a key and cost-effective role in the elimination of excessive MD losses in vaccinated flocks. Relevant sanitation principles have been reviewed (26, 327).

NONONCOGENIC TURKEY AND CHICK-EN HERPESVIRUSES. Turkey herpesviruses and serotype 2 MDV are not recognized as pathogens in avian hosts. Interest in these viruses derives mainly from their use to immunize chickens against MD, reference to which is made earlier. Both are naturally occurring viruses, however, and it seems appropriate to also consider some aspects of their epizootiology and pathogenesis in their natural or alternate avian hosts, since this has not been discussed elsewhere.

Turkey Herpesvirus. Turkey herpesvirus was isolated from normal turkeys by Kawamura et al. (230) and Witter et al. (516). The virus is ubiquitous in domestic turkeys (418, 510) and isolations have also been reported from wild turkeys (113). In chickens, the virus has also become ubiquitous because of its widespread administration to day-old chickens to prevent MD.

In turkeys, the virus spreads rapidly through exposed flocks, presumably by contact exposure; virtually all individual turkeys become viremic and develop antibody within a few weeks (510). The virus appears to mature in the FFE, since cell-free skin extracts are infectious (519), although viral antigen was found only infrequently and at low levels in the FFE of infected turkeys (146). No vertical transmission has been demonstrated (328, 510). The virus may be transmitted from turkeys to chickens under experimental conditions (512), but such transmission is probably rare in the field. There is limited contact spread among chickens (103, 104), presumably because of maturation of virus in the FFE (96, 543). The virus appears to replicate less efficiently than MDV in skin (362), although increased levels of HVT DNA were observed in FFE of HVT-vaccinated chickens after MDV challenge (264).

Fabricant et al. (146) compared early pathogenesis of HVT infection in chickens and turkeys. Chickens had no cytolytic infections in lymphoid organs. In contrast, turkeys infected with HVT did have some viral antigen-positive cells at 4–14 days postexposure but no cytolytic infections in bursa or thymus were seen. In chickens, there was no depression of bursa or thymus size, and NK cell activity was stimulated through at least 8 wk postinoculation (441). No adrenal-mediated stress response was detected through 3 wk postinoculation (151).

The virus is apparently nononcogenic in turkeys (512, 516), but the possibility of fertility problems in HVT-infected toms has been raised (3, 476). Evaluation of the effect of HVT on production characteristics of turkeys has been hampered by the difficulty in maintaining infection-free control flocks for long periods, but this deserves further study.

The virus generally causes no clinical disease in intact or immunodepressed chickens (440, 516) and is not normally detrimental to the immune response (152), although atrophy of the bursa and thymus was noted following administration of high doses (166). In contrast, when chickens were infected with HVT in ovo and then hatched and raised, up to 19% developed clinical paralysis (77), and gross nerve enlargement due to inflammatory type lesions was observed. Turkey herpesvirus can be recovered from infected chickens for long periods and antibodies persist for life (376, 522).

No protection by HVT was noted in turkeys or quail against MD lymphoma induction following challenge with oncogenic MDV (139, 228, 300).

Serotype 2 Marek's Disease Virus.
Viruses isolated from clinically normal chickens and originally described as apathogenic or low pathogenic strains of MDV (28, 101) were subsequently grouped in a separate serotype on the basis of FA

and AGP tests (51, 52). The protective ability of such strains against MD challenge was recognized early (28, 537). Other unique features of this virus group were further elucidated following the isolation of the SB-1 strain (402).

Epidemiologic studies are meager, probably because virus isolation is more difficult than for other serotypes, and antibodies are usually masked by those of other serotypes. Witter (498) isolated serotype 2 virus from 34% of chicken flocks in seven states, suggesting the virus was reasonably prevalent, but perhaps less so than serotype 1. The prevalence is further supported by early studies where 8 of 25 random MDV isolates were typed as avirulent (28). Similar viruses were considered prevalent in Australia (363).

The epidemiology in chickens has been complicated by the artificial distribution of the virus in the United States through a seeder chick program (536, 537) or through inoculation as a vaccine (82, 525). The virus must now be considered ubiquitous in chickens. Several prevaccine field strains showed only limited differences (528).

Chickens appear to be the only natural host, although apathogenic isolates that resembled the HN strain were isolated from Japanese silkies, red jungle fowl, and Ceylon jungle fowl reared in a zoo (98).

Viruses of this group spread readily by contact (402, 527) and are shed in the FFE (99), although perhaps at lower levels than serotype 1 MDV (380). Following inoculation of day-old chickens, the virus can be first isolated 5–6 days postinoculation (76). The virus reaches peak titers at 2–4 wk and persists for long periods (76, 527). Antibodies are induced readily and persist.

The SB-1 strain produced no neoplastic lesions in immunocompetent or immunosuppressed chickens, but because some cytolytic lesions were noted in immunosuppressed chickens, the virus was designated nononcogenic rather than apathogenic (402). Also, a variety of lesions were induced by in ovo inoculation of SB-1, but none were neoplastic (77, 528). The absence of gross neoplastic lesions has been noted by other workers (28, 97, 527), but Pol et al. (343) described endoneural and visceral lymphomas in 2 of 48 chickens inoculated with the HPRS-24 strain.

A distinct splenomegaly was induced between 4–12 days after inoculation of chicks with SB-1 (76). No bursal atrophy and only occasional thymic atrophy was seen and there was no cytolytic infection of lymphoid organs. In contrast, Lin et al. (265) found that viral antigens were expressed in spleen and bursal tissues 5–14 days after infection, primarily in B cells, but no gross or microscopic changes were observed. SB-1 did not cause suppression of humoral immunity (138) and is not normally considered immunosuppressive, although Friedman et al. (152) found a diminished response to a B-lymphocyte–specific mitogen and decreased antibody responses to bovine serum albumen in chickens vaccinated with the SB-1 strain in combination with HVT.

Vaccination with serotype 2 viruses causes a pronounced enhancement of LL in certain genetic strains of chickens exposed to avian leukosis virus at an early age (14). Apparently, the subpopulation of B-cells susceptible to transformation by ALV is also uniquely susceptible to infection by serotype 2 MDVs, but not by HVT (155). Because few commercial strains are susceptible to this phenomenon and because ALV has now been eradicated from most of the susceptible strains, problems in the field are relatively rare (see subchapter, Leukosis/Sarcoma Group).

REFERENCES

1. Adldinger, H.K., and B.W. Calnek. 1972. Effect of chelators on the in vitro infection with Marek's disease virus. In P.M. Biggs, G. de Thé, and L.N. Payne (eds.). Oncogenesis and Herpesviruses. IARC, Lyon, France, pp. 99–105.

2. Adldinger, H.K., and B.W. Calnek. 1973. Pathogenesis of Marek's disease: Early distribution of virus and viral antigens in infected chickens. J Natl Cancer Inst 50:1287–1298.

3. Adldinger, H.K., R.J. Thurston, R.F. Solorzano, and H.V. Biellier. 1974. Herpesvirus: A possible cause of low fertility in male turkeys. Arch Gesamte Virusforsch 46:370–376.

4. Akiyama, Y., and S. Kato. 1974. Two cell lines from lymphomas of Marek's disease. Biken J 17:105–116.

5. Anderson, D.P., C.S. Eidson, and D.J. Richey. 1971. Age susceptibility of chickens to Marek's disease. Am J Vet Res 32:935–938.

6. Anderson, D.P., D.D. King, C.S. Eidson, and S.H. Kleven. 1972. Filtered-air positive-pressure (FAPP) brooding of broiler chickens. Avian Dis 16:20–26.

7. Anderson, A.S., A. Francesconi, and R.W. Morgan. 1992. Complete nucleotide sequence of the Marek's disease virus ICP4 gene. Virology 189:657–667.

8. Arita, K., and S. Nii. 1979. Short communication—Effect of culture temperature on the production of Marek's disease virus antigens in a chicken lymphoblastoid cell line. Biken J 22:31–34.

9. Ash, R.J., and J.D. Ware. 1972. Growth characteristics of a herpesvirus of turkeys. Appl Microbiol 24:943–946.

10. Bacon, L. 1987. Influence of the major histocompatability complex on disease resistance and productivity. Poult Sci 66:802–811.

11. Bacon, L.D., and R.L. Witter. 1992. Influence of turkey herpesvirus vaccination on the B-haplotype effect on Marek's disease resistance in 15.B-congenic chickens. Avian Dis 36:378–385.

12. Bacon, L.D., and R.L. Witter. 1994. B haplotype influence on the relative efficacy of Marek's disease vaccines in commercial chickens. Poult Sci 73:481–487.

13. Bacon, L.D., and R.L. Witter. 1995. Personal communication.

14. Bacon, L.D., R.L. Witter, and A.M. Fadly. 1989. Augmentation of retrovirus-induced lymphoid leukosis by Marek's disease herpesviruses in white leghorn chickens. J Virol 63:504–512.

15. Ball, R.F., and J.F. Lyman. 1977. Revaccination of chicks for Marek's disease at twenty-one days old. Avian Dis 21:440–444.

16. Ball, R.F., J.F. Hill, J. Lyman, and A. Wyatt. 1971. The resistance to Marek's disease of chicks from immunized breeders. Poult Sci 50:1084–1090.

17. Basarab, O., and T. Hall. 1976. Comparisons of cell-free and cell-associated Marek's disease vaccines in maternally immune chicks. Vet Rec 99:4–6.

18. Baxendale, W. 1969. Preliminary observations on Marek's disease in ducks and other avian species. Vet Rec 85:341–342.

19. Beasley, J.N., L.T. Patterson, and D.H. McWade. 1970. Transmission of Marek's disease by poultry house dust and chicken dander. Am J Vet Res 31:339–344.

20. Becker, Y., Y. Asher, E. Tabor, I. Davidson, M. Malkinson, and Y. Weisman. 1992. Polymerase chain reaction for differentiation between pathogenic and non-pathogenic serotype 1 Marek's disease viruses (MDV) and vaccine viruses of MDV-serotypes 2 and 3. J Virol Meth 40:307–322.

21. Benton, W.J., and M.S. Cover. 1957. The increased incidence of visceral lymphomatosis in broiler and replacement birds. Avian Dis 1:320–327.

22. Biggs, P.M. 1961. A discussion on the classification of the avian leucosis complex and fowl paralysis. Br Vet J 117:326–334.

23. Biggs, P.M. 1967. Marek's disease. Vet Rec 81:583–592.

24. Biggs, P.M. 1968. Marek's disease—Current state of knowledge. Curr Top Microbiol Immunol 43:93–125.

25. Biggs, P.M. 1973. Marek's disease. In A.S. Kaplan (ed.). The Herpesviruses. Academic Press, New York, pp. 557–594.

26. Biggs, P.M. 1985. Spread of Marek's disease. In L.N. Payne (ed.). Marek's Disease. Martinus Nijhoff, Boston, MA, pp. 329–340.

27. Biggs, P.M., and B.S. Milne. 1971. Use of the embryonating egg in studies on Marek's disease. Am J Vet Res 32:1795–1809.

28. Biggs, P.M., and B.S. Milne. 1972. Biological properties of a number of Marek's disease virus isolates. In P.M. Biggs, G. de Thé, and L.N. Payne (eds.). Oncogenesis and Herpesviruses. IARC, Lyon, France, pp. 88–94.

29. Biggs, P.M., and L.N. Payne. 1963. Transmission experiments with Marek's disease (fowl paralysis). Vet Rec 75:177–179.

30. Biggs, P.M., and L.N. Payne. 1967. Studies on Marek's disease. I. Experimental transmission. J Natl Cancer Inst 39:267–280.

31. Biggs, P.M., H.G. Purchase, B.R. Bee, and P.J. Dalton. 1965. Preliminary report on acute Marek's disease (fowl paralysis) in Great Britain. Vet Rec 77:1339–1340.

32. Biggs, P.M., P.L. Long, S.G. Kenzy, and D.G. Rootes. 1968. Relationship between Marek's disease and coccidiosis. II. The effect of Marek's disease on the susceptibility of chickens to coccidial infection. Vet Rec 83:284–289.

33. Biggs, P.M., R.J. Thorpe, and L.N. Payne. 1968. Studies on genetic resistance to Marek's disease in the domestic chicken. Br Poult Sci 9:37–52.

34. Biggs, P.M., A.E. Churchill, D.G. Rootes, R.C. Chubb. 1968. The etiology of Marek's disease virus—an oncogenic herpes-type virus. In Morris Pollard (ed.). Perspectives In Virology. VI. Virus-Induced Immunopathology. Academic Press, New York, pp. 211–237.

35. Biggs, P.M., D.G. Powell, A.E. Churchill, and R.C. Chubb. 1972. The epizootiology of Marek's disease. I. Incidence of antibody, viraemia and Marek's disease in six flocks. Avian Pathol 1:5–25.

36. Biggs, P.M., C.A.W. Jackson, and D.G. Powell. 1973. The epizootiology of Marek's disease. II. The effect of supply flock, rearing house, and production house on the incidence of Marek's disease. Avian Pathol 2·127–134.

37. Biggs, P.M., R.F.W. Shilleto, A.M. Lawn, and D.M. Cooper. 1982. Idiopathic polyneuritis in SPF chickens. Avian Dis 11:163–178.

38. Binns, M.M., K.A. Schat, C.A. Sutton, P.A. Kitchen, and L.J.N. Ross. 1988. Personal communication.

39. Blankert, J.J., G.A.A. Albers, W.E. Briles, M. Vrielink-van Ginkel, A.J.C. Groot, G.P. Te Winkel, M.G.J. Tilanus, and A.J. van der Zijpp. 1990. The effect of serologically defined major histocompatibility complex haplotypes of Marek's disease resistance in commercially bred white leghorn chickens. Avian Dis 34:818–823.

40. Bloom, S.E. 1981. Detection of normal and aberrant chromosomes in chicken embryos and in tumor cells. Poult Sci 60:1355–1361.

41. Boezi, J.A., L.F. Lee, R.W. Blakesley, M. Koenig, and H.C. Towle. 1974. Marek's disease herpesvirus-induced DNA polymerase. J Virol 14:1209–1219.

42. Bradley, G., M. Hayashi, G. Lancz, A. Tanaka, and M. Nonoyama. 1989. Structure of the Marek's disease virus BamHI-H gene family: Genes of putative importance for tumor induction. J Virol 63:2534–2542.

43. Briles, W.E., H.A. Stone, and R.K. Cole. 1977. Marek's disease: Effects of B histocompatibility alloalleles in resistant and susceptible chicken lines. Science 195:193–195.

44. Briles, W.E., R.W. Briles, R.E. Taffs, and H.A. Stone. 1983. Resistance to a malignant lymphoma in chickens is mapped to subregion of major histocompatibility (B) complex. Science 219:977–979.

45. Brunovskis, P., and L.F. Velicer. 1992. Genetic organization of the Marek's disease virus unique short region and identification of Us-encoded polypeptides. In G. de Boer and S.H.M Jerissen (eds.). Proc 4th Int Symp Marek's Dis. Ponsen & Looijen, Wageningen, Amsterdam, The Netherlands, pp. 74–78.

46. Brunovskis, P., and L.F. Velicer. 1995. The Marek's disease virus (MDV) unique short region; alphaherpesvirus-homologous, fowlpox virus-homologous, and MDV-specific genes. Virology 206:324–338.

47. Brunovskis, P., X. Chen, and L.F. Velicer. 1992. Analysis of Marek's disease virus glycoproteins D, I and E. In G. de Boer and S.H.M Jerissen (eds.). Proc 4th Int Symp Marek's Dis. Ponsen & Looijen, Wageningen, Amsterdam, The Netherlands, pp. 118–122.

48. Buckmaster, A.E., S.D. Scott, M.J. Sanderson, M.E.G. Boursnell, L.J.N. Ross, and M.M. Binns. 1988. Gene sequence and mapping data from Marek's disease virus and herpesvirus of turkeys—implications for herpesvirus classification. J Gen Virol 69:2033–2042.

49. Bülow, V.v. 1971. Diagnosis and certain biological properties of the virus of Marek's disease. Am J Vet Res 32:1275–1288.

50. Bülow, V.v. 1977. Further characterisation of the CVI 988 strain of Marek's disease virus. Avian Pathol 6:395–403.

51. Bülow, V.v., and P.M. Biggs. 1975. Differentiation between strains of Marek's disease virus and turkey herpesvirus by immunofluorescence assays. Avian Pathol 4:133–146.

52. Bülow, V.v., and P.M. Biggs 1975. Precipitating antigens associated with Marek's disease viruses and a herpesvirus of turkeys. Avian Pathol 4:147–162.

53. Bülow, V.v., B. Fuchs, E. Vielitz, and H. Landgraf. 1983. Fruhsterblichkeitssyndrom bei Küken nach Doppelinfektion mit dem Virus der Marekshen Krankheit (MDV) und einem Anämie-Erreger (CAA). Zentralbl Veterinaermed Reihe B 30:742–750.

54. Bumstead, J.M., and L.N. Payne. 1987. Production of an immune suppressor factor by Marek's disease lymphoblastoid cell lines. Vet Immunol Immunopathol 16:47–66.

55. Burgoyne, G.H., and R.L. Witter. 1973. Effect of passively transferred immunoglobulins on Marek's disease. Avian Dis 17:824–837.

56. Buscaglia, C., and B.W. Calnek. 1988. Maintenance of Marek's disease herpesvirus latency in vitro by a factor found in conditioned medium. J Gen Virol 69:2809–2818.

57. Buscaglia, C., B.W. Calnek, and K.A. Schat. 1988. Effect of immunocompetence on the establishment and maintenance of latency with Marek's disease herpesvirus. J Gen Virol 69:1067–1077.

58. Buscaglia, C., B.W. Calnek, and K.A. Schat. 1989. Effect of reticuloendotheliosis virus and infectious bursal disease virus on Marek's disease herpesvirus latency. Avian Pathol 18:265–281.

59. Calnek, B.W. 1972. Effects of passive antibody on early pathogenesis of Marek's disease. Infect Immun 6:193–198.

60. Calnek, B.W. 1972. Antibody development in chickens exposed to Marek's disease virus. In P.M. Biggs, G. de Thé, and L.N. Payne (eds.). Oncogenesis and and Herpesviruses. IARC, Lyon, France, pp. 129–136.

61. Calnek, B.W. 1973. Influence of age at exposure on the pathogenesis of Marek's disease. J Natl Cancer Inst 51:929–939.

62. Calnek, B.W. 1979. Unpublished data.

63. Calnek, B.W. 1980. Marek's disease virus and lymphoma. In F. Rapp (ed.). Oncogenic Herpesviruses. CRC Press, Boca Raton, FL, pp. 103–143.

64. Calnek, B.W. 1985. Genetic Resistance. In L.N. Payne (ed.). Marek's Disease. Martinus Nijhoff, Boston, MA, pp. 293–328.

65. Calnek, B.W. 1985. Pathogenesis of Marek's disease: A review. In B.W. Calnek and J.L. Spencer (eds.). Proc Int Symp Marek's Dis. American Association of Avian Pathologists, Kennett Square, PA, pp. 374–390.

66. Calnek, B.W. 1986. Marek's disease: a model for herpesvirus oncology. CRC Crit Rev Microbiol 12:293–320.

67. Calnek, B.W. 1987. Established cell lines of avian lymphocytes and their use. In A. Toivanen and P. Toivanen (eds.). Avian Immunology Basis and Practice, vol. II. CRC Press, Boca Raton, FL, pp. 57–70.

68. Calnek, B.W., and H.K. Adldinger. 1971. Some characteristics of cell-free preparations of Marek's disease virus. Avian Dis 15:508–517.

69. Calnek, B.W., and S.B. Hitchner. 1969. Localization of viral antigen in chickens infected with Marek's disease herpesvirus. J Natl Cancer Inst 43:935–949.

70. Calnek, B.W., and S.B. Hitchner. 1973. Survival and disinfection of Marek's disease virus and the effectiveness of filters in preventing airborne dissemination. Poult Sci 52:35–43.

71. Calnek, B.W., and R.L. Witter. 1991. Marek's disease. In B.W. Calnek, H.J. Barnes, C.W. Beard, W.M. Reid, and H.W. Yoder, Jr. (eds.). Diseases of Poultry, 9th ed. Iowa State University Press, Ames, IA, pp. 342–385.

72. Calnek, B.W., H.K. Adldinger, and D.E. Kahn. 1970. Feather follicle epithelium: A source of enveloped and infectious cell-free herpesvirus from Marek's disease. Avian Dis 14:219–233.

73. Calnek, B.W., S.B. Hitchner, and H.K. Adldinger. 1970. Lyophilization of cell-free Marek's disease herpesvirus and a herpesvirus from turkeys. Appl Microbiol 20:723–726.

74. Calnek, B.W., J. Fabricant, K.A. Schat, and K.K. Murthy. 1977. Pathogenicity of low-virulence Marek's disease viruses in normal versus immunologically compromised chickens. Avian Dis 21:346–358.

75. Calnek, B.W., K.K. Murthy, and K.A. Schat. 1978. Establishment of Marek's disease lymphoblastoid cell lines from transplantable versus primary lymphomas. Int J Cancer 21:100–107.

76. Calnek, B.W., J.C. Carlisle, J. Fabricant, K.K. Murthy, and K.A. Schat. 1979. Comparative pathogenesis studies with oncogenic and nononcogenic Marek's disease viruses and turkey herpesvirus. Am J Vet Res 40:541–548.

77. Calnek, B.W., K.A. Schat, and J. Fabricant. 1980. Modification of Marek's disease pathogenesis by in ovo infection or prior vaccination. In M. Essex, G. Todaro, and H. zur Hausen (eds.). Viruses in Naturally Occurring Cancers, vol. 7, pp. 185–197. Cold Spring Harbor, New York.

78. Calnek, B.W., W.R. Shek, and K.A. Schat. 1981. Latent infections with Marek's disease virus and turkey herpesvirus. J Natl Cancer Inst 66:585–590.

79. Calnek, B.W., W.R. Shek, and K.A. Schat. 1981. Spontaneous and induced herpesvirus genome expression in

Marek's disease tumor cell lines. Infect Immun 34:483–491.

80. Calnek, B.W., K.A. Schat, W.R. Shek, and C.-L.H. Chen. 1982. In vitro infection of lymphocytes with Marek's disease virus. J Natl Cancer Inst 69:709–713.

81. Calnek, B.W., W.R. Shek, K.A. Schat, and J. Fabricant. 1982. Dose-dependent inhibition of virus rescue from lymphocytes latently infected with turkey herpesvirus or Marek's disease virus. Avian Dis 26:321–331.

82. Calnek, B.W., K.A. Schat, M.C. Peckham, and J. Fabricant. 1983. Research note—Field trials with a bivalent vaccine (HVT and SB-1) against Marek's disease. Avian Dis 27:844–849.

83. Calnek, B.W., K.A. Schat, L.J.N. Ross, W.R. Shek, and C.-L.H. Chen. 1984. Further characterization of Marek's disease virus-infected lymphocytes. I. In vivo infection. Int J Cancer 33:289–398.

84. Calnek, B.W., K.A. Schat, E.D. Heller, and C. Buscaglia. 1985. In vitro infection of T-lymphoblasts with Marek's disease virus. In B.W. Calnek and J.L. Spencer (eds.). Proc Int Symp Marek's Dis. American Association of Avian Pathologists, Kennett Square, PA, pp. 173–187.

85. Calnek, B.W., D.F. Adene, K.A. Schat, and H. Abplanalp. 1988. Immune response versus susceptibility to Marek's disease. Poult Sci 68:17–26.

86. Calnek, B.W., B. Lucio, and K.A. Schat. 1989. Pathogenesis of Marek's disease virus-induced local lesions. 2. Influence of virus strain and host genotype. In S. Kato, T. Horiuchi, T. Mikami, and K. Hirai (eds.). Advances in Marek's Disease Research. Japanese Association on Marek's Disease, Osaka, Japan, pp. 324–330.

87. Calnek, B.W., B. Lucio, K.A. Schat, and H.S. Lillehoj. 1989. Pathogenesis of Marek's disease virus-induced local lesions. 1. Lesion characterization and cell line establishment. Avian Dis 33:291–302.

88. Campbell, J.G., and G.N. Woode. 1969. Demonstration of a herpes-type virus in short-term cultured blood lymphocytes associated with Marek's disease. J Med Microbiol 3:463–473.

89. Camp, H.S., P.M. Coussens, and R.F. Silva. 1991. Cloning, sequencing, and functional analysis of a Marek's disease virus origin of DNA replication. J Virol 65:6320–6324.

90. Cantello, J.L., A.S. Anderson, and R.W. Morgan. 1994. Identification of latency-associated transcripts that map antisense to the ICP4 homolog gene of Marek's disease virus. J Virol 68:6280–6290.

91. Cauchy, L. 1974. The detection of viral antigens in Marek's disease by immunoperoxidase. In E. Krustak and R. Morisett (eds.). Viral Immunodiagnosis. Academic Press, New York, pp. 77–78.

92. Cauchy, L., and F. Coudert. 1972. Virologie - Particules de type Herpès de la maladie de Marek dans les lymphocytes infectes et maintenus in vitro. C R Acad Sci Paris 274:1864–1866.

93. Cebrian, J., C. Kaschka-Dierich, N. Berthelot, and P. Sheldrick. 1982. Inverted repeat nucleotide sequences in the genomes of Marek's disease virus and the herpesvirus of the turkey. Proc Natl Acad Sci USA 79:555–558.

94. Chen, J.H., and H.G. Purchase. 1970. Surface antigen on chick kidney cells infected with the herpesvirus of Marek's disease. Virology 40:410–412.

95. Chen, X.-B., and L.F. Velicer. 1992. Expression of the Marek's disease virus homolog of herpes simplex virus glycoprotein B in Escherichia coli and its identification as B antigen. J Virol 66:4390–4398.

96. Cho, B.R. 1975. Horizontal transmission of turkey herpesvirus to chickens. IV. Viral maturation in the feather follicle epithelium. Avian Dis 19:136–141.

97. Cho, B.R. 1976. A possible association between plaque type and pathogenicity of Marek's disease herpesvirus. Avian Dis 20:324–331.

98. Cho, B.R. 1976. In vitro biological differences between the pathogenic and apathogenic Marek's disease her-

pesvirus. Avian Dis 20:242–252.

99. Cho, B.R. 1977. Dual virus maturation of both pathogenic and apathogenic Marek's disease herpesvirus (MDHV) in the feather follicles of dually infected chickens. Avian Dis 21:501–507.

100. Cho, B.R. 1978. An improved method for extracting cell-free herpesviruses of Marek's disease and turkeys from infected cell cultures. Avian Dis 22:170–176.

101. Cho, B.R., and S.G. Kenzy. 1972. Isolation and characterization of an isolate (HN) of Marek's disease virus with low pathogenicity. Appl Microbiol 24:299–306.

102. Cho, B.R., and S.G. Kenzy. 1975. Virologic and serologic studies of zoo birds for Marek's disease virus infection. Infect Immun 11:809–814.

103. Cho, B.R., and S.G. Kenzy. 1975. Horizontal transmission of turkey herpesvirus to chickens. 3. Transmission in three different lines of chickens. Poult Sci 54:109–115.

104. Cho, B.R., S.G. Kenzy, and S.A. Haider. 1971. Horizontal transmission of turkey herpesvirus to chickens. 1. Preliminary observation. Poult Sci 50:881–887.

105. Chubb, R.C., and A.E. Churchill. 1968. Precipitating antibodies associated with Marek's disease. Vet Rec 83:4–7.

106. Chubb, R.C., and A.E. Churchill. 1969. Effect of maternal antibody on Marek's disease. Vet Rec 85:303–305.

107. Churchill, A.E., and P.M. Biggs. 1967. Agent of Marek's disease in tissue culture. Nature 215:528–530.

108. Churchill, A.E., and P.M. Biggs. 1968. Herpes-type virus isolated in cell culture from tumors of chickens with Marek's disease. II. Studies in vivo. J Natl Cancer Inst 41:951–956.

109. Churchill, A.E., R.C. Chubb, and W. Baxendale. 1969. The attenuation, with loss of oncogenicity of the herpes-type virus of Marek's disease (strain HPRS-16) on passage in cell culture. J Gen Virol 4:557–564.

110. Churchill, A.E., L.N. Payne, and R.C. Chubb. 1969. Immunization against Marek's disease using a live attenuated virus. Nature 221:744–747.

111. Cole, R.K. 1968. Studies on genetic resistance to Marek's disease. Avian Dis 12:9–28.

112. Cole, R.K. 1985. Natural resistance to Marek's disease: A review. In B.W. Calnek and J.L. Spencer (eds.). Proc Int Symp Marek's Dis. American Association of Avian Pathologists, Kennett Square, PA, pp. 318–329.

113. Colwell, W.M., C.F. Simpson, L.E. Williams, Jr., and D.J. Forrester. 1973. Isolation of a herpesvirus from wild turkeys in Florida. Avian Dis 17:1–11.

114. Cook, M.K., and J.F. Sears. 1970. Preparation of infectious cell-free herpes-type virus associated with Marek's disease. J Virol 5:258–261.

115. Cooper, M.D., C.-L.H. Chen, R.P. Bucy, and C.B. Thompson. 1991. Avian T-cell ontogeny. Adv Immunol 50:87–117.

116. Coussens, P.M., and L.F. Velicer. 1988. Structure and complete nucleotide sequence of the Marek's disease herpesvirus gp57-65 gene. J Virol 62:2373–2379.

117. Coussens, P.M., M.R. Wilson, H. Roehl, R.J. Isfort, and L.F. Velicer. 1989. Nucleotide sequence analysis of the MDHV strain GA and HVT strain FC126 gp 57-65 (A antigen) genes. In S. Kato, T. Horiuchi, T. Mikami, and K. Hirai (eds.). Advances in Marek's Disease Research. Japanese Association on Marek's Disease, Osaka, Japan, pp. 99–106.

118. Crittenden, L.B., R. Muhm, and B.R. Burmester. 1972. Genetic control of susceptibility to the avian leukosis complex. Poult Sci 51:261–267.

119. Cui, Z.-Z., Y. Ding, and L.F. Lee. 1990. Marek's disease virus gene clones encoding virus-specific phosphorylated polypeptides and serological characterization of fusion proteins. Virus Genes 3:309–322.

120. Cui, Z.-Z., L.F. Lee, J.-L. Liu, and H.-J. Kung. 1991. Structural analysis and transcriptional mapping of the Marek's disease virus gene encoding pp38, an antigen associated with transformed cells. J Virol 65:6509–6515.

121. Dandapat, S., H.K. Pradhan, and G.C. Mohanty.

1994. Anti-idiotype antibodies to Marek's disease-associated tumour surface antigen in protection against Marek's disease. Vet Immunol Immunopathol 40:353–366.

122. Davidson, I., M. Malkinson, C. Strenger, and Y. Becker. 1988. An improved ELISA method, using a streptavidin-biotin complex, for detecting Marek's disease virus antigens in feather-tips of infected chickens. J Virol Methods 14:237–241.

123. Davidson, I., Y. Becker, and M. Malkinson. 1991. Monospecific antibodies to Marek's disease virus antigen B dimer (200 kDa) and monomer (130 and 60 kDa) glycoproteins neutralize virus infectivity and detect the antigen B proteins in infected cell membranes. Arch Virol 121:125–139.

124. Davidson, I., A. Borovskaya, S. Perl, and M. Malkinson. 1995. Use of the polymerase chain reaction for the diagnosis of natural infection of chickens and turkeys with Marek's disease virus and reticuloendotheliosis virus. Avian Pathol 24:69–94.

125. de Boer, G.F., J. Pol, and H. Oei. 1987. Biological characteristics of Marek's disease vaccine CVI-988 clone Cl. Vet Q 9:16S–28S.

126. de Boer, G.F., J.M.A. Pol, and S.H.M. Jeurissen. 1989. Marek's disease vaccination strategies using vaccines made from three avian herpesvirus serotypes. In S. Kato, T. Horiuchi, T. Mikami, and K. Hirai (eds.). Advances in Marek's Disease Research. Japanese Association on Marek's Disease, Osaka, Japan, pp. 405–413.

127. Delecluse, H-J., and W. Hammerschmidt. 1993. Status of Marek's disease virus in established lymphoma cell lines: Herpesvirus integration is common. J Virol 67:82–92.

128. Delecluse, H-J., S. Schüller, and W. Hammerschmidt. 1993. Latent Marek's disease virus can be activated from its chromosomally integrated state in herpesvirus-transformed lymphoma cells. Eur Mol Biol Organ J 12:3277–3286.

129. DiFronzo, N.L., and L.W. Schierman. 1989. Transplantable Marek's disease lymphomas. III. Induction of MHC-restricted tumor immunity by lymphoblastoid cells in F1 hosts. Int J Cancer 44:474–476.

130. Doak, R.L., J.F. Munnell, and W.L. Ragland. 1973. Ultrastructure of tumor cells in Marek's disease virus-infected chickens. Am J Vet Res 34:1063–1069.

131. Dren, C.N., and I. Nemeth. 1985. Differential diagnosis of Marek's disease and lymphoid leukosis on the basis of cell-surface antigens. In B.W. Calnek and J.L. Spencer (eds.). Proc Int Symp Marek's Dis. American Association of Avian Pathologists, Kennett Square, PA, pp. 196–213.

132. Drury, L.N., W.C. Patterson, and C.W. Beard. 1969. Ventilating poultry houses with filtered air under positive pressure to prevent airborne diseases. Poult Sci 48:1640–1646.

133. Dukes, T.W., and J.R. Pettit. 1983. Avian ocular neoplasia—A description of spontaneously occurring cases. Can J Comp Med 47:33–36.

134. Dunn, K., and K. Nazerian. 1977. Induction of Marek's disease virus antigens by IdUrd in a chicken lymphoblastoid cell line. J Gen Virol 34:413–419.

135. Eidson, C.S., and S.C. Schmittle. 1968. Studies on acute Marek's disease. I. Characteristics of isolate GA in chickens. Avian Dis 12:467–476.

136. Eidson, C.S., R.K. Page, and S.H. Kleven. 1978. Effectiveness of cell-free or cell-associated turkey herpesvirus vaccine against Marek's disease in chickens as influenced by maternal antibody, vaccine dose, and time of exposure to Marek's disease virus. Avian Dis 22:583–597.

137. Ekperigin, H.E., A.M. Fadly, L.F. Lee, X. Liu, and R.H. McCapes. 1983. Comb lesions and mortality patterns in white leghorn layers affected by Marek's disease. Avian Dis 27:503–512.

138. Ellis, M.N., C.S. Eidson, J. Brown, O.J. Fletcher, and S.H. Kleven. 1981. Serological responses to mycoplasma synoviae in chickens infected with virulent or avirulent strains of Marek's disease virus. Poult Sci 60:1344–1347.

139. Elmubarak, A.K., J.M. Sharma, R.L. Witter, and V.L. Sanger. 1982. Marek's disease in turkeys: Lack of protection by vaccination. Am J Vet Res 43:740–742.

140. Else, R.W. 1974. Vaccinal immunity to Marek's disease in bursectomized chickens. Vet Rec 95:182–187.

141. Evans, D.L., and L.T. Patterson. 1971. Serum lysozyme determinations in Marek's disease-infected chickens. Poult Sci 50:1575. (Abstr)

142. Fabricant, C.G. 1985. Atherosclerosis: The consequence of infection with a herpesvirus. Adv Vet Sci Comp Med 30:39–66.

143. Fabricant, C.G., J. Fabricant, M.M. Litrenta, and C.R. Minick. 1978. Virus-induced atherosclerosis. J Exp Med 148:335–340.

144. Fabricant, C.G., D.P. Hajjar, C.R. Minick, and J. Fabricant. 1981. Herpesvirus infection enhances cholesterol and cholesteryl ester accumulation in cultured arterial smooth muscle cells. Am J Pathol 105:176–184.

145. Fabricant, J., M. Ianconescu, and B.W. Calnek. 1977. Comparative effects of host and viral factors on early pathogenesis of Marek's disease. Infect Immun 16:136–144.

146. Fabricant, J., B.W. Calnek, and K.A. Schat. 1982. The early pathogenesis of turkey herpesvirus infection in chickens and turkeys. Avian Dis 26:257–264.

147. Ficken, M.D., M.P. Nasisse, G.D. Boggan, J.S. Guy, D.P. Wages, R.L. Witter, J.K. Rosenberger, and R.M. Nordgren. 1991. Marek's disease virus isolates with unusual tropism and virulence for ocular tissues: Clinical findings, challenge studies and pathological features. Avian Pathol 20:461–474.

148. Finkelstein, A., and R.F. Silva. 1989. Live recombinant vaccines for poultry. Trends Biotechnol 7:273–277.

149. Fletcher, O.J., Jr., C.S. Eidson, and R.K. Page. 1971. Pathogenesis of Marek's disease induced in chickens by contact exposure to GA isolate. Am J Vet Res 32:1407–1416.

150. Frazier, J.A. 1974. Ultrastructure of lymphoid tissue from chicks infected with Marek's disease virus. J Natl Cancer Inst 52:829–837.

151. Freeman, B.M., A.C.C. Manning, and R.S. Phillips. 1984. Failure to induce stress reactions following vaccination against Marek's disease or Newcastle disease. Res Vet Sci 36:247–250.

152. Friedman, A., E. Shalem-Meilin, and E.D. Heller. 1992. Marek's disease vaccines cause temporary B-lymphocyte dysfunction and reduced resistance to infection in chicks. Avian Pathol 21:621–631.

153. Fukuchi, K., M. Sudo, Y.S. Lee, A. Tanaka, and M. Nonoyama. 1984. Structure of Marek's disease virus DNA: Detailed restriction enzyme map. J Virol 51:102–109.

154. Fukuchi, K., M. Sudo, A. Tanaka, and M. Nonoyama. 1985. Map location of homologous regions between Marek's disease virus and herpesvirus of turkey and the absence of detectable homology in the putative tumor-inducing gene. J Virol 53:994–997.

155. Fynan, E., T.M. Block, J. DuHadaway, W. Olson, and D.L. Ewert. 1992. Persistence of Marek's disease virus in a subpopulation of B cells that is transformed by Avian Leukosis virus, but not in normal bursal B cells. J Virol 66:5860–5866.

156. Gavora, J.S., J.L. Spencer, I. Okada, A.A. Grunder, P.S. Griffin, and E. Sally. 1990. Correlations of genetic resistance of chickens to Marek's disease viruses with vaccination protection and in vivo response to phytohemagglutinin. Genet Sel Evol 22:457–469.

157. Gibbs, C.P., K. Nazerian, L. Velicer, and H.J. Kung. 1983. Extensive homology exists between Marek's disease herpesvirus and its vaccine virus, herpesvirus of turkeys. Proc Natl Acad Sci USA 81:3365–3369.

158. Gomez, V.M.J.E., R. Preisinger, E. Kalm, D.K. Flock, and E. Vielitz. 1991. Marek's disease (MD): possibilities and problems to improve disease resistance by breeding. Arch Geflügelkd 55:207–212.

159. Goodchild, W.M. 1969. Some observations on Marek's disease (fowl paralysis). Vet Rec 84:87–89.

160. Groot, A.J.C., and G.A.A. Albers. 1992. The effect of MHC on resistance to Marek's disease in White Leghorn crosses. In G. de Boer and S.H.M Jerissen (eds.). Proc 4th Int Symp Marek's disease. Ponsen & Looijen, Wageningen, Amsterdam, The Netherlands, pp. 185–188.

161. Gross, W.B. 1972. Effect of social stress on occurrence of Marek's disease in chickens. Am J Vet Res 33:2275–2279.

162. Gupta, M.K., H.V.S. Chauhan, G.J. Jha, and K.K. Singh. 1989. The role of the reticuloendothelial system in the immunopathology of Marek's disease. Vet Microbiol 20:223–234.

163. Haffer, K., M. Sevoian, and M. Wilder. 1979. The role of the macrophage in Marek's disease: In vitro and in vivo studies. Int J Cancer 23:648–656.

164. Haider, S.A., R.F. Lapen, and S.G. Kenzy. 1970. Use of feathers in a gel precipitation test for Marek's disease. Poult Sci 49:1654–1657.

165. Hajjar, D.P., C.G. Fabricant, C.R. Minick, and J. Fabricant. 1986. Virus-induced atherosclerosis. Am J Pathol 122:62–70.

166. Halouzka, R., and V. Jurajda. 1992. Pathological lesions in the organs of chicks after infection with turkey herpesvirus THV-BI0-I. Vet Med (Praha) 37:463–470.

167. Halvorson, D.A., and D.O Mitchell. 1979. Loss of cell-associated Marek's disease vaccine titer during thawing, reconstitution and use. Avian Dis 23:848–853.

168. Han, P.F.S., and J.R. Smyth, Jr. 1972. The influence of restricted feed intake on the response of chickens to Marek's disease. Poult Sci 51:986–991.

169. Han, P.F.S., and J.R. Smyth, Jr. 1972. The influence of growth rate on the development of Marek's disease. Poult Sci 51:975–985.

170. Hansen, M.P., J.N. Van Zandt, and G.R.J. Law. 1967. Differences in susceptibility to Marek's disease in chickens carrying two different B locus blood group alleles [abst]. Poult Sci 46:1268.

171. Harriss, S.T. 1939. Lymphomatosis (fowl paralysis) in the pheasant. Vet J 95:104–106.

172. Hartmann, W., K. Hala, and G. Heil. 1992. The B blood group system of the chicken and resistance to Marek's disease: Effect of B blood group genotypes in leghorn crosses. Arch Tierz 35:169–180.

173. Heller, E.D., and K.A. Schat. 1985. Inhibition of natural killer activity in chickens by Marek's disease virus-transformed cell lines. In B.W. Calnek and J.L. Spencer (eds.). Proc Int Symp Marek's Dis. American Association of Avian Pathologists, Kennett Square, PA, pp. 286–294.

174. Helmboldt, C.F., F.K. Wills, and M.N. Frazier. 1963. Field observations of the pathology of skin leukosis in Gallus gallus. Avian Dis 7:402–411.

175. Hepkema, B.G., J.J. Blankert, G.A.A. Albers. M.G.J. Tilanus, E. Egberts, A.J. van der Zijpp, and E.J. Hensen. 1993. Mapping of susceptibility to Marek's disease within the major histocompatibility (B)-complex by refined typing of white leghorn chickens. Anim Genet 24:283–287.

176. Higgins, D.A., and B.W. Calnek. 1975. Fowl immunoglobulins: Quantitation in birds genetically resistant and susceptible to Marek's disease. Infect Immun 12:360–363.

177. Higgins, D.A., and B.W. Calnek. 1975. Fowl immunoglobulins: Quantitation and antibody activity during Marek's disease in genetically resistant and susceptible birds. Infect Immun 11:33–41.

178. Higgins, D.A., and B.W. Calnek. 1976. Some effects of silica treatment on Marek's disease. Infect Immun 13:1054–1060.

179. Hirai, K., K. Ikuta, and S. Kato. 1979. Comparative studies on Marek's disease virus and herpesvirus of turkey DNAs. J Gen Virol 45:119–131.

180. Hirai, K., K. Ikuta, N. Kitamoto, and S. Kato. 1981. Latency of herpesvirus of turkey and Marek's disease virus genomes in a chicken T-lymphoblastoid cell line. J Gen Virol 53:133–143.

181. Hirai, K., A. Kanamori, M. Niikura, K. Ikuta, and S. Kato. 1989. RNA transcribed from Marek's disease virus genomes in productively and latently infected cells. In S. Kato, T. Horiuchi, T. Mikami, and K. Hirai (eds.). Advances in Marek's Disease Research. Japanese Association on Marek's Disease, Osaka, Japan, pp. 140–147.

182. Hlozanek, I. 1970. The influence of ultraviolet-inactivated Sendai virus on Marek's disease virus infection in tissue culture. J Gen Virol 9:45–50.

183. Hlozanek, I., and V. Sovova. 1974. Lack of pathogenicity of Marek's disease herpesvirus and herpesvirus of turkeys for mammalian hosts and mammalian cell cultures. Folia Biol 20:51–58.

184. Hlozanek, I., O. Mach, and V. Jurajda. 1973. Cell-free preparations of Marek's disease virus from poultry dust (persisting infectivity/induction of tumours/temperature dependence/sucrose-density gradient and electron-microscopic characteristics). Folia Biol 19:118–123.

185. Hlozanek, I., V. Jurajda, and V. Benda. 1977. Disinfection of Marek's disease virus in poultry dust. Avian Pathol 6:241–250.

186. Holland, M.S., R.F. Silva, C.D. Mackenzie, R.W. Bull, and R.W. Witter. 1994. Identification and localization of glycoprotein B expression in lymphoid tissues of chickens infected with turkey herpesvirus. Avian Dis 38:446–453.

187. Hong, Y., and P.M. Coussens. 1994. Identification of an immediate-early gene in the Marek's disease virus long internal repeat region which encodes a unique 14-kilodalton polypeptide. J Virol 68:3593–3603.

188. Hong, C.C., and M. Sevoian. 1971. Interferon production and host resistance to type II avian (Marek's) leukosis virus (JM strain). Appl Microbiol 22:818–820.

189. Hudson, L., and L.N. Payne. 1973. An analysis of the T and B cells of Marek's disease lymphomas of the chicken. Nature (New Biol) 241:52–53.

190. Hughes, S.K., E. Stubblefield, K. Nazerian, and H.E. Varmus. 1980. DNA of a chicken herpesvirus is associated with at least two chromosomes in a chicken lymphoblastoid cell line. Virology 105:234–240.

191. Hutt, F.B., and R.K. Cole. 1947. Genetic control of lymphomatosis in the fowl. Science 106:379–384.

192. Hutt, F.B., and R.K. Cole. 1948. The development of strains genetically resistant to avian lymphomatosis. Proc 8th World's Poult Congr, pp. 719–725.

193. Igarashi, T., M. Takagashi, J. Donovan, J. Jessip, M. Smith, K. Hirai, A. Tanaka, and M. Nonoyama. 1987. Restriction enzyme map of herpesvirus of turkey DNA and its collinear relationship with Marek's disease virus DNA. Virology 157:351–358.

194. Ikuta, K., Y. Nishi, S. Kato, and K. Hirai. 1981. Immunoprecipitation of Marek's disease virus-specific polypeptides with chicken antibodies purified by affinity chromatography. Virology 114:277–281.

195. Ikuta, K., H. Honma, K. Maotani, S. Ueda, S. Kato, and K. Hirai. 1982. Monoclonal antibodies specific to and cross-reactive with Marek's disease virus and herpesvirus of turkeys. Biken J 25:171–175.

196. Ikuta, K., S. Ueda, S. Kato, and K. Hirai. 1983. Most virus-specific polypeptides in cells productively infected with Marek's disease virus or herpesvirus of turkeys possess cross-reactive determinants. J Gen Virol 64:961–965.

197. Ikuta, K., S. Ueda, S. Kato, and K. Hirai. 1983. Monoclonal antibodies reactive with the surface and secreted glycoproteins of Marek's disease virus and herpesvirus of turkeys. J Gen Virol 64:2597–2610.

198. Ikuta, K., S. Ueda, S. Kato, and K. Hirai. 1984. Processing of glycoprotein gB related to neutralization of Marek's disease virus and herpesvirus of turkeys. Microbiol Immunol 28:923–933.

199. Ikuta, K., S. Ueda, S. Kato, K. Ono, S. Osafune, I. Yoshida, T. Naito, M. Naito, and K. Hirai. 1985. Identification of Marek's disease virus-specific antigens in Marek's disease lymphoblastoid cell lines using monoclonal antibody

against virus-specific phosphorylated polypeptides. Int J Cancer 35:257–264.

200. Ikuta, K., K. Nakajima, S. Ueda, S. Kato, and K. Hirai. 1985. Differences in the processing of secreted glycoprotein A induced by Marek's disease virus and herpesvirus of turkeys. J Gen Virol 66:1131–1137.

201. Ikuta, K., K. Nakajima, A. Kanamori, K. Maotani, J.S. Mah, S. Ueda, S. Kato, M. Yoshida, S. Nii, M. Naito, C. Nishida-Umehara, M. Saski, and K. Hirai. 1987. Establishment and characterization of a T-lymphoblastoid cell line MDCC-MTB1 derived from chick lymphocytes infected in vitro with Marek's disease serotype 1. Int J Cancer 39:514–520.

202. Ikuta, K., K. Nakajima, M. Naito, A. Kanamori, K. Hirai, and S. Kato. 1989. Expression of the antigen related to Marek's disease virus serotype 1-specific phosphorylated polypeptides in in vitro transformed cell line, MDCC-MTB-1. In S. Kato, T. Horiuchi, T. Mikami, and K. Hirai (eds.). Advances in Marek's Disease Research. Japanese Association on Marek's Disease, Osaka, Japan, pp. 135–139.

203. Imai, K., N. Yuasa, K. Furuta, M. Narita, H. Banba, S. Kobayashi, and T. Horiuchi. 1991. Comparative studies on pathogenical, virological and serological properties of Marek's disease virus isolated from Japanese quail and chicken. Avian Pathol 20:57–65.

204. Inoue, M., T. Mikami, H. Kodama, M. Onuma, and H. Izawa. 1980. Antigenic difference between intracellular and membrane antigens induced by herpesvirus of turkeys. Arch Virol 63:23–30.

205. Isfort, R.J., I. Sithole, H.J. Kung, and L.F. Velicer. 1986. Molecular characterization of the Marek's disease herpesvirus B antigen. J Virol 59:411–419.

206. Isfort, R.J., R.A. Stringer, H.-J. Kung, and L.F. Velicer. 1986. Synthesis, processing, and secretion of the Marek's disease herpesvirus A antigen glycoprotein. J Virol 57:464–474.

207. Isfort, R., H. Kung, and L. Velicer. 1987. Identification of the gene encoding Marek's disease herpesvirus A antigen. J Virol 61:2614–2620.

208. Isfort, R.J., Z. Qian, D. Jones, R.F. Silva, R. Witter, and H. Kung. 1994. Integration of multiple chicken retroviruses into multiple chicken herpesviruses: Herpesviral gD as a common target of integration. Virology 203:125–133.

209. Jackson, C.A.W., P.M. Biggs, R.A. Bell, F.M. Lancaster, and B.S. Milne. 1976. The epizootiology of Marek's disease. 3. The inter-relationship of virus pathogenicity, antibody and the incidence of Marek's disease. Avian Pathol 5:105–123.

210. Jakowski, R.M., T.N. Fredrickson, T.W. Chomiak, and R.E. Luginbuhl. 1970. Hematopoietic destruction in Marek's disease. Avian Dis 14:374–385.

211. Jeurissen, S.H.M., and G.F. de Boer. 1993. Chicken anaemia virus influences the pathogenesis of Marek's disease in experimental infections depending on the dose of Marek's disease virus. Vet Q 14:81–84.

212. Johnson, E.P. 1941. Fowl leukosis—Manifestations, transmission, and etiological relationship of various forms. VA Agric Exp Stn Tech Bull 76.

213. Jones, D., and H.J. Kung. 1992. A heat-shock-like sequence in the meq gene promoter binds a factor in MDV lymphoblastoid cells. In G. de Boer and S.H.M Jerissen (eds.). Proc 4th Int Symp Marek's Dis. Ponsen & Looijen, Wageningen, Amsterdam, The Netherlands, pp. 58–61.

214. Jones, D., L. Lee, J.L. Liu, H.J. Kung, and J.K. Tillotson. 1992. Marek's Disease virus encodes a basic-Leucine Zipper gene resembling the fos/jun oncogenes that is highly expressed in lymphoblastoid tumors. Proc Natl Acad Sci USA 89:4042–4046.

215. Jones, D., R. Isfort, R. Witter, R. Kost, and H-J. Kung. 1993. Retroviral insertions into a herpesvirus are clustered at the junctions of the short repeat and short unique sequences. Proc Natl Acad Sci USA 90:3855–3859.

216. Julian, R.J. 1992. Peripheral neuropathy causing "range paralysis" in Leghorn pullets [abst]. Proc 129th Annu Meet Am Vet Med Assoc, p. 130.

217. Jungherr, E.L., and W.F. Hughes. 1965. The avian leukosis complex. In H.E. Biester and L.H. Schwarte (eds.). Diseases of Poultry, 5th ed. Iowa State University Press, Ames, IA, pp. 512–567.

218. Kaaden, O.R. 1978. Transfection studies in vitro and in vivo with isolated Marek's disease virus DNA. In G. de Thé, W. Henle, F. Rapp (eds.). Oncogenesis and Herpesviruses III. IARC, Lyon, France, pp. 627–634.

219. Kaaden, O.R., B. Dietzschold, and S. Uberschar. 1974. Vaccination against Marek's disease: Immunizing effect of purified turkey herpesvirus and cellular membranes from infected cells. Med Microbiol Immunol 159:261–269.

220. Kaaden, O.R., A. Scholtz, A. BenZeev, and Y. Becker. 1977. Isolation of Marek's disease virus DNA from infected cells by electrophoresis on polyacrylamide gels. Arch Virol 54:75–84.

221. Kaleta, E.F., and R.A. Bankowski. 1972. Production of interferon by the Cal-l and turkey herpesvirus strains associated with Marek's disease. Am J Vet Res 33:567–571.

222. Kaleta, E.F., and U. Neumann. 1977. Investigations on the mode of transmission of the herpesvirus of turkeys in vitro. Avian Pathol 6:33–39.

223. Kanamori, A., K. Nakajima, K. Ikuta, S. Ueda, S. Kato, and K. Hirai. 1986. Copy number of tandem direct repeats within the inverted repeats of Marek's disease virus DNA. Biken J 29:83–89.

224. Kanamori, A., K. Ikuta, S. Ueda, S. Kato, and K. Hirai. 1987. Methylation of Marek's disease virus DNA in chicken T-lymphoblastoid cell lines. J Gen Virol 68:1485–1490.

225. Kaschka-Dierich, C., and R. Thomssen. 1979. Studies on the temperature-dependent DNA replication of the herpesvirus of the turkey in chicken embryo fibroblasts. J Gen Virol 45:253–261.

226. Kaschka-Dierich, C., K. Nazerian, and R. Thomssen. 1979. Intracellular state of Marek's disease virus DNA in two tumor-derived chicken cell lines. J Gen Virol 44:271–280.

227. Kato, S., and K. Hirai. 1985. Marek's disease virus. Adv Virus Res 30:225–277.

228. Kaul, L., and H.K. Pradhan. 1991. Vaccination trial of quail with herpes virus of turkey. Prev Vet Med 11:69–73.

229. Kaul, L., and H.K. Pradhan. 1991. Immunopathology of Marek's disease in quails: Presence of antinuclear antibody and immune complex. Vet Immunol and Immunopathol 28:89–96.

230. Kawamura, H., D.J. King, Jr., and D.P. Anderson. 1969. A herpesvirus isolated from kidney cell culture of normal turkeys. Avian Dis 13:853–863.

231. Kawamura, M., M. Hayashi, T. Furuichi, M. Nonoyama, E. Isogai, and S. Namioka. 1991. The inhibitory effects of oligonucleotides, complementary to Marek's Disease virus mRNA transcribed from the BamHI-H region, on the proliferation of transformed lymphoblastoid cells, MDCC-MSB1. J Gen Virol 72:1105–1111.

232. Keller, L.H., K.A. Belden, and M. Sevoian. 1987. Immunization of chickens against Marek's disease with cell free supernatant from the JMV-1 lymphoblastoid cell line. In W.T Weber and D.L. Ewert (eds.). Avian Immunology. Alan Liss, New York, pp. 265–279.

233. Keller, L.H., H.S. Lillehoj, and J.M. Solnosky. 1992. JMV-1 stimulation of avian natural killer cell activity. Avian Pathol 21:239–250.

234. Kenzy, S.G., and P.M. Biggs. 1967. Excretion of the Marek's disease agent by infected chickens. Vet Rec 80:565–568.

235. Kenzy, S.G., and B.R. Cho. 1969. Transmission of classical Marek's disease by affected and carrier birds. Avian Dis 13:211–214.

236. King, D., D. Page, K.A. Schat, and B.W. Calnek. 1981. Difference between influences of homologous and heterologous maternal antibodies on response to serotype-2 and

serotype-3 Marek's disease vaccines. Avian Dis 25:74–81.

237. Kitamoto, N., K. Ikuta, S. Kato, and K. Wataki. 1979. Demonstration of cells with Marek's disease tumor-associated surface antigen in chicks infected with herpesvirus of turkey, 01 strain. Biken J 22:137–142.

238. Kitamoto, N., K. Ikuta, and S. Kato. 1980. Persistence of genomes of both herpesvirus of turkeys and Marek's disease virus in a chicken T-lymphoblastoid cell line. Biken J 23:1–8.

239. Kodama, H., T. Mikami, M. Inoue, and H. Izawa. 1979. Inhibitory effects of macrophages against Marek's disease virus plaque formation in chicken kidney cell cultures. J Natl Cancer Inst 63:1267–1271.

240. Konobe, T., T. Ishikawa, K. Takaku, K. Ikuta, N. Kitamoto, and S. Kato. 1979. Marek's disease virus and herpesvirus of turkey noninfective to chickens, obtained by repeated in vitro passages. Biken J 22:103–107.

241. Kopáček, J., L.J.N. Ross, V. Zelnik, and J. Pastorek. 1992. RNA transcripts from 1.8 kb family of MDCC-MSB1 contain 132 bp repeats. In G. de Boer and S.H.M Jerissen (eds.). Proc 4th Int Symp Marek's Dis. Ponsen & Looijen, Wageningen, Amsterdam, The Netherlands, pp. 80–83.

242. Koptidesová, D., J. Kopáček, V. Zelnik, L.J.N. Ross, S. Pastoreková, and J. Pastorek. 1995. Identification and characterization of a cDNA clone derived from the Marek's disease tumour cell line RPL1 encoding a homolog of Alpha-transinducing factor (VP16) of HSV-1. Arch Virol 140:355–362.

243. Kornegay, J.N., E.J. Gorgacz, M.A. Parker, J. Brown, and L.W. Schierman. 1983. Marek's disease virus-induced transient paralysis: Clinical and electrophysiologic findings in susceptible and resistant lines of chickens. Am J Vet Res 44:1541–1544.

244. Lapen, R.F., and S.G. Kenzy. 1972. Distribution of gross cutaneous Marek's disease lesions. Poult Sci 51:334–336.

245. Lau, R.Y., and M. Nonoyama. 1980. Replication of the resident Marek's disease virus genome in synchronized nonproducer MKT-1 cells. J Virol 33:912–914.

246. Lawn, A.M., and L.N. Payne. 1979. Chronological study of ultrastructural changes in the peripheral nerves in Marek's disease. Neuropathol Appl Neurobiol 5:485–497.

247. Lee, L.F. 1979. Macrophage restriction of Marek's disease virus replication and lymphoma cell proliferation. J Immunol 123:1088–1091.

248. Lee, L.F. 1993. Characterization of a monoclonal antibody against a nuclear antigen associated with serotype-1 Marek's disease virus-infected and transformed cells. Avian Dis 37:561–567.

249. Lee, L.F. 1996. Ribonucleotide reductase gene in Marek's disease. Proc 5th Int Symp Marek's Dis (in press).

250. Lee, L.F., and R.L. Witter. 1991. Humoral immune responses to inactivated oil-emulsified Marek's disease vaccine. Avian Dis 35:452–459.

251. Lee, L.F., E.D. Kieff, S.L. Bachenheimer, B. Roizman, P.G. Spear, B.R. Burmester, and K. Nazerian. 1971. Size and composition of Marek's disease virus deoxyribonucleic acid. J Virol 7:289–294.

252. Lee, L.F., R.L. Armstrong, and K. Nazerian. 1972. Comparative studies of six avian herpesviruses. Avian Dis 16:799–805.

253. Lee, L.F., K. Nazerian, and J.A. Boezi. 1975. Marek's disease virus DNA in a chicken lymphoblastoid cell line (MSB-1) and in virus-induced tumours. In G. de Thé, M.A. Epstein, and H. zur Hausen (eds.). Oncogenesis and Herpesviruses II. IARC, Lyon, France, pp. 199–204.

254. Lee, L.F., K. Nazerian, S.S. Leinbach, J.M. Reno, and J.A. Boezi. 1976. Effect of phosphonoacetate on Marek's disease virus replication. J Natl Cancer Inst 56:823–827.

255. Lee, L.F., K. Nazerian, R.L. Witter, S.S. Leinbach, and J.A. Boezi. 1978. A phosphonoacetate-resistant mutant of herpesvirus of turkeys. J Natl Cancer Inst 60:1141–1146.

256. Lee, L.F., J.M. Sharma, K. Nazerian, and R.L. Witter. 1978. Suppression of mitogen-induced proliferation of normal spleen cells by macrophages from chickens inoculated with Marek's disease virus. J Immunol 120:1554–1559.

257. Lee, L.F., P.C. Powell, M. Rennie, L.J.N. Ross, and L.N. Payne. 1981. Nature of genetic resistance to Marek's disease in chickens. J Natl Cancer Inst 66:789–796.

258. Lee, L.F., X. Liu, and R.L. Witter. 1983. Monoclonal antibodies with specificity for three different serotypes of Marek's disease viruses in chickens. J Immunol 130:1003–1006.

259. Lee, L.F., X. Liu, J.M. Sharma, K. Nazerian, and L.D. Bacon. 1983. A monoclonal antibody reactive with Marek's disease tumor-associated surface antigen. J Immunol 130:1007–1011.

260. Lee, L.F., Y. Li, D. Sui, and J.D. Reilly. 1992. Conservation of antigenic epitopes of Marek's disease virus and herpes simplex virus glycoprotein B (gB). In G. de Boer and S.H.M Jerissen (eds.). Proc 4th Int Symp Marek's Dis. Ponsen & Looijen, Wageningen, Amsterdam, The Netherlands, pp. 93–96.

261. Lee, Y-S., A. Tanaka, S. Silver, M. Smith, and M. Nonoyama. 1979. Minor DNA homology between herpesvirus of turkey and Marek's disease virus? Virology 93:277–280.

262. Lesnik, F., and L.J.N. Ross. 1975. Immunization against Marek's disease using Marek's disease virus-specific antigens free from infectious virus. Int J Cancer 16:153–163.

263. Lesnik, F., D. Chudy, J. Bogdan, O.J. Vrtiak, and M. Rudic. 1978. Testing the immunogenicity of the dermal antigen of Marek's disease virus. Vet Med (Praha) 23:421–430.

264. Levy, H., T. Maray, I. Davidson, M. Malkinson, and Y. Becker. 1991. Replication of Marek's disease virus in chicken feather tips containing vaccinal turkey herpesvirus DNA. Avian Pathol 20:35–44.

265. Lin, J.A., H. Kodama, M. Onuma, and T. Mikami. 1991. The early pathogenesis in chickens inoculated with non-pathogenic serotype 2 Marek's disease virus. J Vet Med Sci 53:269–273.

266. Liu, X., and L.F. Lee. 1983. Development and characterization of monoclonal antibodies to Marek's disease tumor-associated surface antigen. Infect Immun 31:851–854.

267. Longenecker, B.M., F. Pazderka, J.S. Gavora, J.L. Spencer, and R.F. Ruth. 1976. Lymphoma induced by herpesvirus: Resistance associated with a major histocompatibility gene. Immunogenetics 3:401–407.

268. Maas, H.J.L., B.H. Rispens, and J.E. Groenendal. 1974. Control of Marek's disease in the Netherlands: Large scale field trials with the avirulent cell-associated Marek's disease vaccine virus (strain CVI988). Tijdschr Diergeneeskd 99:1273–1288.

269. Maas, H.J.L., H.W. Antonisse, Van Der A.J. Zypp, J.E. Groenendal, and G.L. Kok. 1981. The development of two white plymouth rock lines resistant to Marek's disease by breeding from survivors. Avian Pathol 10:137–150.

270. Madarame, H., Y. Fujimoto, and R. Moriguchi. 1986. Ultrastructural studies on muscular atrophy in Marek's disease. II. Muscular lesions in spontaneous cases. Jpn J Vet Res 34:51–75.

271. Malkinson, M., I. Davidson, and Y. Becker. 1992. Antigen-B of the vaccine strains of Marek's disease virus and herpesvirus of turkeys presents heat-labile group and serotype specific epitopes. Arch Virol 127:169–184.

272. Maotani, K., A. Kanamori, K. Ikuta, S. Ueda, S. Kato, and K. Hirai. 1986. Amplification of a tandem direct repeat within inverted repeats of Marek's disease virus DNA during serial in vitro passage. J Virol 58:657–660.

273. Marek, J. 1907. Multiple Nervenentzuendung (Polyneuritis) bei Huehnern. Dtsch Tierarztl Wochenschr 15:417–421.

274. Marshall, D.R., J.D. Reilly, X. Liu, and R.F. Silva. 1993. Selection of Marek's disease virus recombinants ex-

pressing the Escherichia coli gpt gene. Virology 195:638–648.

275. Martin, S.L., D.I. Aparisio, and P.K. Bandyopadhyay. 1989. Genetic and biochemical characterization of the thymidine kinase gene from herpesvirus of turkeys. J Virol 63:2847–2852.

276. Mason, R.J., and K.E. Jensen. 1971. Marek's disease: Resistance of turkey herpesvirus-infected chicks against lethal JM-V agent. Am J Vet Res 32:1625–1627.

277. McColl, K. 1988. Cellular and molecular studies on transformed cells in Marek's disease. Ph.D. Thesis, Cornell University, Ithaca, NY.

278. McColl, K., B.W. Calnek, W.V. Harris, K.A. Schat, and L.F. Lee. 1987. Expression of a putative tumor-associated antigen on normal versus Marek's disease virus-transformed lymphocytes. J Natl Cancer Inst 79:991–1000.

279. Mikami, T., and R.A. Bankowski. 1971. Pathogenic and serologic studies of type 1 and type 2 plaque-producing agents derived from Cal-1 strain of Marek's disease virus. Am J Vet Res 32:303–317.

280. Mikami, T., M. Onuma, and T.T.A. Hayashi. 1973. Membrane antigens in arginine-deprived cultures infected with Marek's disease herpesvirus. Nature 246:211–212.

281. Mikami, T., M. Onuma, and T.T.A. Hayashi. 1974. Requirement of arginine for the replication of Marek's disease herpesvirus. J Gen Virol 22:115–128.

282. Mikami, T., M. Inoue, H. Kodama, F. Inage, M. Onuma, and H. Izawa. 1980. Relation between the neutralization of herpesvirus of turkeys and the antibody to late-appearing membrane antigen induced by the virus. J Gen Virol 47:221–226.

283. Miles, A.M., C.J. Williams, C.L. Womack, D.L. Murray, and R.P. Gildersleeve. 1992. Commercial broiler studies of Marek's disease vaccination in ovo. In G. de Boer and S.H.M Jerissen (eds.). Proc 4th Int Symp Marek's Dis. Ponsen & Looijen, Wageningen, Amsterdam, The Netherlands, pp. 320–322.

284. Minick, C.R., C.G. Fabricant, J. Fabricant, and M.M. Litrenta. 1979. Atheroarteriosclerosis induced by infection with a herpesvirus. Am J Pathol 96:673–706.

285. Moore, F.R., K.A. Schat, N. Hutchison, C. LeCiel, and S.E. Bloom. 1993. Consistent chromosomal aberration in cell lines transformed with Marek's disease herpesvirus: Evidence for genomic DNA amplification. Int J Cancer 54:685–692.

286. Moore, F.R., B.W. Calnek, and S.E. Bloom. 1994. Cytogenetic studies of cell lines derived from Marek's disease virus-induced local lesions. Avian Dis 38:797–799.

287. Morgan, R.W. 1995. Personal Communication.

288. Morgan, R.W., J. Gelb, Jr., C.S. Schreurs, D. Lutticken, J.K. Rosenberger, and P.J.A. Sondermeijer. 1992. Protection of chickens from Newcastle and Marek's disease with a recombinant herpesvirus of turkeys vaccine expressing the Newcastle disease virus fusion protein. Avian Dis 36:858–870.

289. Morgan, R.W., J. Gelb, Jr., C.R. Pope, and P.J.A. Sondermeijer. 1993. Efficacy in chickens of a herpesvirus of turkeys recombinant vaccine containing the fusion gene of Newcastle disease virus: Onset of protection and effect of maternal antibodies. Avian Dis 37:1032–1040.

290. Moriguchi, R., M. Oshima, F. Mori, I. Umezawa, and C. Itakura. 1989. Chronological change of feather pulp lesions during the course of Marek's disease virus-induced lymphoma formation in field chickens. In S. Kato, T. Horiuchi, T. Mikami, and K. Hirai (eds.). Advances in Marek's Disease Research. Japanese Association on Marek's Disease, Osaka, Japan, pp. 338–343.

291. Murthy, K.K., and B.W. Calnek. 1979. Pathogenesis of Marek's disease: Effect of immunization with inactivated viral and tumor-associated antigens. Infect Immun 26:547–553.

292. Naciri, M., O. Mazzella, and F. Coudert. 1989. Inter-

actions of cryptosporidia and savage or vaccinal virus in Marek's diseases in chickens. Rec Med Vet 165:383–387.

293. Naito, M., K. Nakajima, N. Iwa, K. Ono, I. Yoshida, T. Konobe, K. Ikuta, S. Ueda, S. Kato, and K. Hirai. 1986. Demonstration of a Marek's disease virus-specific antigen in tumour lesions of chickens with Marek's disease using monoclonal antibody against a virus phosphorylated protein. Avian Pathol 15:503–510.

294. Nakajima, K., M. Ikuta, S. Naito, S. Ueda, S. Kato, and K. Hirai. 1987. Analysis of Marek's disease virus serotype-1 specific phosphorylated polypeptides in virus-infected cells and Marek's disease lymphoblastoid cells. J Gen Virol 68:1379–1390.

295. Nakamura, H., M. Sakaguchi, Y. Hirayama, N. Miki, M. Yamamota, and K. Hirai. 1992. Protection against Newcastle Disease by recombinant Marek's disease virus serotype-1 expressing the fusion protein of Newcastle Disease virus. In G. de Boer and S.H.M Jerissen (eds.). Proc 4th Int Symp Marek's Dis. Ponsen & Looijen, Wageningen, Amsterdam, The Netherlands, pp. 332–335.

296. Nazerian, K. 1971. Further studies on the replication of Marek's disease virus in the chicken and in cell culture. J Natl Cancer Inst 47:207–217.

297. Nazerian, K. 1979. Marek's disease lymphoma of chicken and its causative herpesvirus. Biochim Biophys Acta 560:375–395.

298. Nazerian, K. 1987. An updated list of avian cell lines and transplantable tumours. Avian Pathol 16:527–544.

299. Nazerian, K. 1995. Personal communication.

300. Nazerian, K., and J.M. Sharma. 1985. Pathogenesis of Marek's disease in turkeys. In B.W. Calnek and J.L. Spencer (eds.). Proc Int Symp Marek's Dis. American Association of Avian Pathologists, Kennett Square, PA, pp. 262–267.

301. Nazerian, K., J.J. Solomon, R.L. Witter, and B.R. Burmester. 1968. Studies on the etiology of Marek's disease. II. Finding of a herpesvirus in cell culture. Proc Soc Exp Biol Med 127:177–182.

302. Nazerian, K., L.F. Lee, R.L. Witter, and B.R. Burmester. 1970. Ultrastructural studies of a herpesvirus of turkeys antigenically related to Marek's disease virus. Virology 43:442–452.

303. Nazerian, K., T. Lindahl, G. Klein, and L.F. Lee. 1973. Deoxyribonucleic acid of Marek's disease virus in virus-induced tumors. J Virol 12:841–846.

304. Nazerian, K., E.A. Stephens, J.M. Sharma, L.F. Lee, M. Gailitis, and R.L. Witter. 1977. A nonproducer T lymphoblastoid cell line from Marek's disease transplantable tumor (JMV). Avian Dis 21:69–76.

305. Nazerian, K., L.F. Lee, N. Yanagida, and R. Ogawa. 1992. Protection against Marek's disease by a fowlpox virus recombinant expressing the glycoprotein B of Marek's disease virus. J Virol 66:1409–1413.

306. Neumann, U., and R.L. Witter. 1978. Differential diagnosis of lymphoid leukosis and Marek's disease by tumor-specific criteria. I. Studies on experimentally infected chickens. Avian Dis 23:417–425.

307. Neumann, U., and R.L. Witter. 1978. Differential diagnosis of lymphoid leukosis and Marek's disease by tumor-specific criteria. II. Studies on field cases. Avian Dis 23:426–433.

308. Nicholas, R.A.J., J.C. Muskett, and D.H. Thornton. 1979. A comparison of titration methods for Marek's disease vaccines. J Biol Stand 7:43–51.

309. Nicholls, T.J. 1984. Marek's disease in sixty week-old laying chickens. Aust Vet J 61:243.

310. Nii, S., M. Yamada, M. Yoshida, Y. Arao, F. Uno, T. Ishikawa, M. Hayashi, K. Ono, and K. Hirai. 1989. Growth of MDV II in MDCC-MSB1-41C. In S. Kato, T. Horiuchi, T. Mikami, and K. Hirai (eds.). Advances in Marek's Disease Research. Japanese Association of Marek's Disease, Osaka, Japan, pp. 197–203.

311. Niikura, M. Y. Matsuura, M. Hattori, M. Onuma, and T. Mikami. 1991. Expression of the A antigen (gp57-65) of Marek's disease virus by a recombinant baculovirus. J Gen Virol 72:1099–1104.

312. Niikura, M., Y. Matsuura, D. Endoh, M. Onuma, and T. Mikami. 1992. Expression of the Marek's Disease Virus (MDV) homolog of glycoprotein B of herpes simplex virus by a recombinant baculovirus and its identification as the B antigen (gp100, gp60, gp49) of MDV. J Virol 66:2631–2638.

313. Nordgren, R.M., B. Stewart-Brown, and J.H. Rodenberg. 1992. The role of acemannan as an adjuvant for Marek's disease vaccine. In G. de Boer and S.H.M Jerissen (eds.). Proc 4th Int Symp Marek's Dis. Ponsen & Looijen, Wageningen, Amsterdam, The Netherlands, pp. 165–169.

314. Oei, H.L., and G.F. de Boer. 1986. Comparison of intramuscular and subcutaneous administration of Marek's disease vaccine. Avian Pathol 15:569–579.

315. Ohashi, K., T. Mikami, H. Kodama, and H. Izawa. 1987. Suppression of NK activity of spleen cells by chicken fetal antigen present on Marek's disease lymphoblastoid cell line cells. Int J Cancer 40:378–382.

316. Ohashi, K., P.H. O'Connell, and K.A. Schat. 1994. Characterization of Marek's disease virus BamHI-A-specific cDNA clones obtained from a Marek's disease lymphoblastoid cell line. Virology 199:275–283.

317. Okazaki, W., H.G. Purchase, and B.R. Burmester. 1970. Protection against Marek's disease by vaccination with a herpesvirus of turkeys. Avian Dis 14:413–429.

318. Olson, C. 1940. Transmissible fowl leukosis. A review of the literature. Mass Agric Exp Stn Bull 370.

319. Ono, K., M. Takashima, T. Ishikawa, M. Hayashi, I. Yoshida, T. Konobe, K. Ikuta, K. Nakajima, S. Ueda, S. Kato, and K. Hirai. 1985. Partial protection against Marek's disease in chickens immunized with glycoproteins gB purified from turkey-herpesvirus-infected cells by affinity chromatography coupled with monoclonal antibodies. Avian Dis 29:533–539.

320. Ono, M., R. Katsuragi-lwanaga, T. Kitazawa, N. Kamiya, T. Horimoto, M. Niikura, C. Kai, K. Hirai, and T. Mikami. 1992. The restriction endonuclease map of Marek's disease virus (MDV) serotype 2 and collinear relationship among three serotypes of MDV. Virology 191:459–463.

321. Ono, M., Y. Kawaguchi, K. Maeda, N. Kamiya, Y. Tohya, C. Kai, M. Niikura, and T. Mikami. 1994. Nucleotide sequence analysis of Marek's disease virus (MDV) serotype 2 homolog of MDV serotype 1 p38, an antigen associated with transformed cells. Virology 201:142–146.

322. Otaki, Y., T. Nunoya, M. Tajima, A. Kato, and Y. Nomura. 1988. Depression of vaccinal immunity to Marek's disease by infection with chicken anaemia agent. Avian Pathol 17:333–347.

323. Owen, J.J.T., M.A.S. Moore, and P.M. Biggs. 1966. Chromosome studies in Marek's disease. J Natl Cancer Inst 37:199–209.

324. Ozaki, K., H. Kodama, M. Onuma, H. Izawa, and T. Mikami. 1983. In vitro suppression of proliferation of Marek's disease lymphoma cell line (MDCC-MSB1) by peritoneal exudate cells from chickens infected with MDV or HVT. Zentralbl Vet Med [B] 30:223–231.

325. Pappenheimer, A.M., L.C. Dunn, and V. Cone. 1926. A study of fowl paralysis (neuro-lymphomatosis gallinarum). Storrs Agric Exp Stn Bull 143:187–290.

326. Parker, M.A., and L.W. Schierman. 1983. Suppression of humoral immunity in chickens prevents transient paralysis caused by a herpesvirus. J Immunol 130:2000–2001.

327. Pattison, M. 1985. Control of Marek's disease by the poultry industry: Practical considerations. In L.N. Payne (ed.). Marek's Disease. Martinus Nijhoff, Boston, MA, pp. 341–349.

328. Paul, P., C.T. Larsen, M.C. Kumar, and B.S. Pomeroy. 1972. Preliminary observations on egg transmission of turkey herpesvirus (HVT) in turkeys. Avian Dis 16:27–33.

329. Payne, L.N. 1972. Pathogenesis of Marek's disease—A review. In P.M. Biggs, G. de Thé, and L.N. Payne (eds.). Oncogenesis and Herpesviruses. IARC, Lyon, France, pp. 21–37.

330. Payne, L.N. 1985. Historical review. In L.N. Payne (ed.). Marek's Disease. Martinus Nijhoff, Boston, MA, pp. 1–15.

331. Payne, L.N. 1985. Pathology. In L.N. Payne (ed.). Marek's Disease. Martinus Nijhoff, Boston, MA, pp. 43–75.

332. Payne, L.N. 1985. Marek's Disease: Scientific Basis and Methods of Control, Martinus Nijhoff, Boston, MA.

333. Payne, L.N., and P.M. Biggs. 1967. Studies on Marek's disease. II. Pathogenesis. J Natl Cancer Inst 39:281–302.

334. Payne, L.N., and M. Rennie. 1973. Pathogenesis of Marek's disease in chicks with and without maternal antibody. J Natl Cancer Inst 51:1559–1573.

335. Payne, L.N., and J. Roszkowski. 1973. The presence of immunologically uncommitted bursa and thymus dependent lymphoid cells in the lymphomas of Marek's disease. Avian Pathol 1:27–34.

336. Payne, L.N., P.C. Powell, and M. Rennie. 1974. Response of B and T lymphocytes and other blood leukocytes in chickens with Marek's disease. Cold Spring Harb Symp Quant Biol 39:817–826.

337. Payne, L.N., J.A. Frazier, and P.C. Powell. 1976. Pathogenesis of Marek's disease. Int Rev Exp Pathol 16:59–154.

338. Payne, L.N., M. Rennie, P.C. Powell, and J.G. Rowell. 1978. Transient effect of cyclophosphamide on vaccinal immunity to Marek's disease. Avian Pathol 7:295–304.

339. Payne, L.N., K. Howes, M. Rennie, J.M. Bumstead, and A.W. Kidd. 1981. Use of an agar culture technique for establishing lymphoid cell lines from Marek's disease lymphomas. Int J Cancer 28:757–766.

340. Pazderka, F., B.M. Longenecker, G.R.J. Law, H.A. Stone, W.E. Briles, and R.F. Ruth. 1974. Detection of identical B alleles in different strains of chickens: Association with resistance to Marek's disease. Anim Blood Groups Biochem Genet 5:18.

341. Pepose, J.S., J.G. Stevens, M.L. Cook, and P.W. Lampert. 1981. Marek's disease as a model for the Landry-Guillain-Barré Syndrome: Latent viral infection in nonneuronal cells is accompanied by specific immune responses to peripheral nerve and myelin. Am J Pathol 103:309–320.

342. Phillips, P.A., and P.M. Biggs. 1972. Course of infection in tissues of susceptible chickens after exposure to strains of Marek's disease virus and turkey herpesvirus. J Natl Cancer Inst 49:1367–1373.

343. Pol, J.M.A., Kok, G.L., and G.F. de Boer. 1985. Studies on the oncogenic properties of various Marek's disease virus strains. In B.W. Calnek and J.L. Spencer (eds.). Proc Int Symp Marek's Dis. American Association of Avian Pathologists, Kennett Square, PA, pp. 469–479.

344. Pol, J.M.A., Kok, G.L., Oei, H.L., and G.F. de Boer. 1986. Pathogenicity studies with plaque-purified preparations of Marek's disease virus strain CVI-988. Avian Dis 30:271–275.

345. Powell, P.C. 1975. Immunity to Marek's disease induced by glutaraldehyde-treated cells of Marek's disease lymphoblastoid cell lines. Nature 257:684–685.

346. Powell, P.C. 1978. Protection against the JMV Marek's disease-derived transplantable tumour by Marek's disease virus-specific antigens. Avian Pathol 7:305–309.

347. Powell, P.C. 1981. Immunity to Marek's disease. In M.E. Rose, L.N. Payne, and B.M. Freeman (eds.). Avian Immunology. Br Poult Sci, Edinburgh, Scotland, pp. 263–283.

348. Powell, P.C. 1985. Immunity. In L.N. Payne (ed.). Marek's Disease. Martinus Nijhoff, Boston, MA, pp. 177–201.

349. Powell, P.C. 1985. Host resistance factors: Immune responses—A review. In B.W. Calnek and J.L. Spencer (eds.). Proc Int Symp Marek's Dis. American Association of

Avian Pathologists, Kennett Square, PA, pp. 238–261.

350. Powell, P.C., and T.F. Davison. 1986. Induction of Marek's disease in vaccinated chickens by treatment with betamethasone or corticosterone. Isr J Vet Med 42:73–78.

351. Powell, P.C., and F. Lombardini. 1986. Isolation of very virulent pathotypes of Marek's disease virus from vaccinated chickens in Europe. Vet Rec 118:688–691.

352. Powell, P.C., and M. Rennie. 1980. Failure of attenuated Marek's disease virus and herpesvirus of turkey antigens to protect against the JMV Marek's disease derived transplantable tumour. Avian Pathol 9:193–200.

353. Powell, P.C., and M. Rennie. 1984. The expression of Marek's disease tumor-associated surface antigen in various avian species. Avian Pathol 13:345–349.

354. Powell, P.C., and J.G. Rowell. 1977. Dissociation of antiviral and antitumor immunity in resistance to Marek's disease. J Natl Cancer Inst 59:919–924.

355. Powell, P.C., L.N. Payne, J.A. Frazier, and M. Rennie. 1974. T lymphoblastoid cell lines from Marek's disease lymphomas. Nature 251:79–80.

356. Powell, P.C., K.J. Hartley, B.M. Mustill, and M. Rennie. 1983. The occurrence of chicken foetal antigen after infection with Marek's disease virus in three strains of chicken. Oncodev Biol Med 4:261–271.

357. Powell, P.C., K. Howes, A.M. Lawn, B.M. Mustill, L.N. Payne, M. Rennie, and M.A. Thompson. 1984. Marek's disease in turkeys: The induction of lesions and the establishment of lymphoid cell lines. Avian Pathol 13:201–214.

358. Pradhan, H.K., G.C. Mohanty, and A. Mukit. 1985. Marek's disease in Japanese quails (Coturnix coturnix japonica): A study of natural cases. Avian Dis 29:575–582.

359. Pradhan, H.K., C.G. Mohanty, A. Mukit, and B. Paatnaik. 1987. Experimental studies on Marek's disease in Japanese quail (Coturnix coturnix japonica). Avian Dis 31:225–233.

360. Pradhan, H.K., G.C. Mohanty, W.Y. Lee, L. Kaul, and J.M. Kataria. 1988. Immune complex-mediated glomerulopathy in Marek's disease. Vet Immunol Immunopathol 19:165–171.

361. Prasad, L.B.M., and P.B. Spradbrow. 1977. Multiplication of turkey herpes virus and Marek's disease virus in chick embryo skin cell cultures. J Comp Pathol 87:515–520.

362. Prasad, L.M.B., and P.B. Spradbrow. 1980. Ultrastructure and infectivity of tissue from normal and immunodepressed chickens inoculated with turkey herpesvirus. J Comp Pathol 90:47–56.

363. Prasad, L.B.M., Scott, J., and P.B. Spradbrow. 1977. Isolation of Marek's disease herpesvirus of low pathogenicity from commercial chickens. Aust Vet J 53:405–406.

364. Pratt, W.D., R.W. Morgan, and K.A. Schat. 1992. Characterization of reticuloendotheliosis virus-transformed avian T-lymphoblastoid cell lines infected with Marek's disease virus. J Virol 66:7239–7244.

365. Pratt, W.D., J. Cantello, R.W. Morgan, and K.A. Schat. 1994. Enhanced expression of the Marek's disease virus-specific phosphoproteins after stable transfection of MSB-1 cells with the Marek's disease virus homolog of ICP4. Virology 201:132–136.

366. Proc. Internat. Symp. on Marek's Disease. 1985. B.W. Calnek and J.L. Spencer (eds.). American Association of Avian Pathologists, Kennett Square, PA.

367. Proc. 3rd Internat. Symp. on Marek's Disease. 1988. S. Kato, T. Horiuchi, T. Mikami and K. Hirai (eds.). Advances in Marek's Disease Research. Japanese Association on Marek's Disease, Osaka, Japan.

368. Proc. 19th World's Poultry Congress, Amsterdam. 1992. Ponsen & Looijen, Wageningen, Wageningen, Amsterdam, The Netherlands, vol. 1.

369. Purchase, H.G. 1969. Immunofluorescence in the study of Marek's disease. I. Detection of antigen in cell culture and an antigenic comparison of 8 isolates. J Virol 3:557–565.

370. Purchase, H.G. 1972. Recent advances in the knowledge of Marek's disease. Adv Vet Sci Comp Med 16:223–258.

371. Purchase, H.G. 1985. Clinical disease and its economic impact. In L.N. Payne (ed.). Marek's Disease. Martinus Nijhoff, Boston, MA, pp. 17–24.

372. Purchase, H.G., and P.M. Biggs. 1967. Characterization of five isolates of Marek's disease. Res Vet Sci 8:440–449.

373. Purchase, H.G., and J.M. Sharma. 1970. The differential diagnosis of lymphoid leukosis and Marek's disease [slide study set]. American Association of Avian Pathologists, Kennett Square, PA.

374. Purchase, H.G., and J.M. Sharma. 1974. Amelioration of Marek's disease and absence of vaccine protection in immunologically deficient chickens. Nature 248:419–421.

375. Purchase, H.G., and R.L. Witter. 1986. Public health concerns from human exposure to oncogenic avian herpesviruses. J Am Vet Med Assoc 189:1430–1436.

376. Purchase, H.G., W. Okazaki, and B.R. Burmester. 1972. Long term field trials with the herpesvirus of turkeys vaccine against Marek's disease. Avian Dis 16:57–71.

377. Purchase, H.G., W. Okazaki, and B.R. Burmester. 1972. The minimum protective dose of the herpesvirus turkeys vaccine against Marek's disease. Vet Rec 91:79–84.

378. Quere, P. 1992. Suppression mediated in vitro by Marek's disease virus-transformed T-lymphoblastoid cell lines: Effect on lymphoproliferation. Vet Immunol Immunopathol 32:149–164.

379. Ramachandra, R.N., R. Raghavan, and B.S. Keshavamurthy. 1978. Propagation of Marek's disease virus in chicken tracheal explants. Indian J Anim Sci 48:525–528.

380. Rangga-Tabbu, C., and B.R. Cho. 1982. Marek's disease virus (MDV) antigens in the feather follicle epithelium: Difference between oncogenic and nononcogenic MDV. Avian Dis 26:907–917.

381. Ren, D., L.F. Lee, and P.M. Coussens. 1994. Identification and characterization of Marek's disease virus genes homologous to ICP27 and glycoprotein K of herpes simplex virus-1. Virology 204:242–250.

382. Rennie, M., P.C. Powell, and B.M. Mustill. 1980. The effect of bursectomy on vaccination against Marek's disease with the herpesvirus of turkeys. Avian Pathol 9:557–566.

383. Reno, J.M., L.F. Lee, and J.A. Boezi. 1978. Inhibition of herpesvirus replication and herpesvirus-induced deoxyribonucleic acid polymerase by phosphonoformate. Antimicrob Agents Chemother 13:188–192.

384. Ringen, L.M., and A.S. Akhtar. 1968. Electrophoretic analysis of serum proteins from paralyzed and unparalyzed chickens exposed to Marek's disease. Avian Dis 12:4–9.

385. Rispens, B.H., H.J. VanVloten, N. Mastenbroek, H.J.L. Maas, and K.A. Schat. 1972. Control of Marek's disease in the Netherlands. I. Isolation of an avirulent Marek's disease virus (strain CVI988) and its use in laboratory vaccination trials. Avian Dis 16:108–125.

386. Rosenberger, J.K. 1983. Reovirus interference with Marek's disease vaccination. Proc 32nd West Poult Dis Conf, pp. 50–51.

387. Ross, L.J.N. 1985. Molecular biology of the virus. In L.N. Payne (ed.). Marek's Disease. Martinus Nijhoff, Boston, MA, pp. 113–150.

388. Ross, L.J.N., and M.M. Binns. 1991. Properties and evolutionary relationships of the Marek's disease virus homologs of protein kinase, glycoprotein D and glycoprotein I of herpes simplex virus. J Gen Virol 72:939–947.

389. Ross, N., and B. Milne. 1989. Manipulation of the genomes of MDV and HVT. In S. Kato, T. Horiuchi, T. Mikami, and K. Hirai (eds.). Advances in Marek's Disease Research. Japanese Association on Marek's Disease, Osaka, Japan, pp. 43–49.

390. Ross, L.J.N., W. Delorbe, H.E. Varmus, J.M. Bishop, and M. Brahic. 1981. Persistence and expression of Marek's disease virus DNA in tumour cells and peripheral nerves studied by in situ hybridization. J Gen Virol 57:285–296.

391. Ross, L.J.N., B. Milne, and P.M. Biggs. 1983. Restriction endonuclease analysis of Marek's disease virus DNA and homology between strains. J Gen Virol 64:2785–2790.

392. Ross, L.J.N., M. Sanderson, S.D. Scott, M.M. Binns, T. Doel, and B. Milne. 1989. Nucleotide sequence and characterization of the Marek's disease virus homolog of glycoprotein B of herpes simplex virus. J Gen Virol 70:1789–1804.

393. Ross, L.J.N., M.M. Binns, P. Tyers, J. Pastorek, V. Zelnik, and S. Scott. 1993. Construction and properties of a turkey herpesvirus recombinant expressing the Marek's disease virus homolog of glycoprotein B of herpes simplex virus. J Gen Virol 74:371–377.

394. Rouse, B.T., R.J.H. Wells, and H.L. Warner. 1973. Proportion of T and B lymphocytes in lesions of Marek's disease: Theoretical implications for pathogenesis. J Immunol 110:534–539.

395. Rziha, H.J., and B. Bauer. 1982. Circular forms of viral DNA in Marek's disease virus-transformed lymphoblastoid cells. Arch Virol 72:211–216.

396. Sarma, G., W. Greer, R.P. Gildersleeve, D.L. Murray, and A.M. Miles. 1995. Field safety and efficacy of in ovo administration of HVT and SB-1 bivalent Marek's disease vaccine in commercial broilers. Avian Dis 39:211–217.

397. Schat, K.A. 1985. Characteristics of the virus. In L.N. Payne (ed.). Marek's Disease. Martinus Nijhoff, Boston, MA, pp. 77–112.

398. Schat, K.A. 1987. Marek's disease: A model for protection against herpesvirus-induced tumours. Cancer Surveys 6:1–37.

399. Schat, K.A. 1987. Immunity in Marek's disease and other tumors. In A. Toivanen and P. Toivanen (eds.). Avian Immunology: Basis and Practice. CRC Press, Boca Raton, FL, pp. 101–128.

400. Schat, K.A. 1991. Importance of cell-mediated immunity in Marek's disease and other viral tumor diseases. Poult Sci 70:1165–1175.

401. Schat, K.A. 1992. Immune responses against Marek's disease virus. In G. de Boer and S.H.M. Jerissen (eds.). Proc 4th Int Symp Marek's Dis. Ponsen & Looijen, Wageningen, Amsterdam, The Netherlands, pp. 233–238.

402. Schat, K.A., and B.W. Calnek. 1978. Characterization of an apparently nononcogenic Marek's disease virus. J Natl Cancer Inst 60:1075–1082.

403. Schat, K.A., and B.W. Calnek. 1978. In vitro inactivation of cell-free Marek's disease herpesvirus by immune peripheral blood lymphocytes. Avian Dis 22:693–697.

404. Schat, K.A., and B.W. Calnek. 1978. Demonstration of Marek's disease tumor-associated surface antigen in chickens infected with nononcogenic Marek's disease virus and herpesvirus of turkeys. J Natl Cancer Inst 61:855–857.

405. Schat, K.A., R.D. Schultz, and B.W. Calnek. 1978. Marek's disease: Effect of virus pathogenicity and genetic susceptibility on response of peripheral blood lymphocytes to concanavalin-A. In P. Bentvelzen, J. Hilgers, and D.S. Yohn (eds.). Advances Comparative Leukosis Research. Elsevier, Amsterdam, The Netherlands, pp. 183–185.

406. Schat, K.A., B.W. Calnek, and J. Fabricant. 1981. Influence of oncogenicity of Marek's disease virus on evaluation of genetic resistance. Poult Sci 60:2559–2566.

407. Schat, K.A., C.-L.H. Chen, W.R. Shek, and B.W. Calnek. 1982. Surface antigens on Marek's disease lymphoblastoid tumor cell lines. J Natl Cancer Inst 69:715–720.

408. Schat, K.A., B.W. Calnek, and J. Fabricant. 1982. Characterisation of two highly oncogenic strains of Marek's disease virus. Avian Pathol 11:593–605.

409. Schat, K.A., W.R. Shek, B.W. Calnek, and H. Abplanalp. 1982. Syngeneic and allogeneic cell-mediated cytotoxicity against Marek's disease lymphoblastoid tumor cell lines. Int J Cancer 29:187–194.

410. Schat, K.A., B.W. Calnek, J. Fabricant, and D.L. Graham. 1985. Pathogenesis of infection with attenuated Marek's disease virus strains. Avian Pathol 14:127–146.

411. Schat, K.A., A. Buckmaster, and L.J.N. Ross. 1989. Partial transcription map of Marek's disease herpesvirus in lytically infected cells and lymphoblastoid cell lines. Int J Cancer 44:101–109.

412. Schat, K.A., C.-L.H. Chen, H. Lillehoj, B.W. Calnek, and D. Weinstock. 1989. Characterization of Marek's disease cell lines with monoclonal antibodies specific for cytotoxic and helper T cells. In S. Kato, T. Horiuchi, T. Mikami, and K. Hirai (eds.). Advances in Marek's Disease Research. Japanese Association on Marek's Disease, Osaka, Japan, pp. 220–226.

413. Schat, K.A., C-L.H. Chen, B.W. Calnek, and D. Char. 1991. Transformation of T-lymphocyte subsets by Marek's disease herpesvirus. J Virol 65:1408–1413.

414. Schierman, L.W., and O.J. Fletcher. 1980. Genetic control of Marek's disease virus-induced transient paralysis: Association with the major histocompatibility complex. In P.M. Biggs (ed.). Resistance and Immunity to Marek's Disease. Commission European Communities, Luxembourg, pp. 429–442.

415. Scholten, R., L.A.Th. Hilgers, S.H.M. Jeurissen, and M.W. Weststrate. 1990. Detection of Marek's disease virus antigen in chicken by a novel immunoassay. J Virol Methods 27:221–226.

416. Scott, S.D., L.J.N. Ross, and M.M. Binns. 1989. Nucleotide and predicted amino acid sequences of the Marek's disease virus and turkey herpesvirus thymidine kinase genes; comparison with thymidine kinase genes of other herpesviruses. J Gen Virol 70:3055–3065.

417. Scott, S.D., G.D. Smith, L.J.N. Ross, and M.M. Binns. 1993. Identification and sequence analysis of the homologs of the herpes simplex virus type 1 glycoprotein H in Marek's disease virus and the herpesvirus of turkeys. J Gen Virol 74:1185–1190.

418. Settnes, O.P. 1982. Marek's disease—A common naturally herpesvirus-induced lymphoma of the chicken. Nord Veterinaermed Suppl:11–132.

419. Sevoian, M., and D.M. Chamberlain. 1962. Avian lymphomatosis. II. Experimental reproduction of the ocular form. Vet Med 57:608–609.

420. Sevoian, M., and D.M. Chamberlain. 1964. Avian lymphomatosis. IV. Pathogenesis. Avian Dis 8:281–308.

421. Sevoian, M., and C.R. Weston. 1972. The effects of JM and JM-V leukosis strains on chicks vaccinated with herpes virus of turkeys (HVT). Poult Sci 51:513–516.

422. Sevoian, M., D.M. Chamberlain, and F.T. Counter. 1962. Avian lymphomatosis. I. Experimental reproduction of the neural and visceral forms. Vet Med 57:500–501.

423. Sharma, J.M. 1973. Lack of a threshold of genetic resistance to Marek's disease and the incidence of humoral antibody. Avian Pathol 2:75–90.

424. Sharma, J.M. 1979. Immunosuppressive effects of lymphoproliferative neoplasms of chickens. Avian Dis 23:315–327.

425. Sharma, J.M. 1980. In vitro suppression of T-cell mitogenic response and tumor cell proliferation by spleen macrophages from normal chickens. Infect Immun 28:914–922.

426. Sharma, J.M. 1981. Fractionation of Marek's disease virus induced lymphoma by velocity sedimentation and association of infectivity with cellular fractions with and without tumor antigen expression. Am Vet Res 42:483–486.

427. Sharma, J.M. 1984. Effect of infectious bursal disease virus on protection against Marek's disease by turkey herpesvirus vaccine. Avian Dis 28:629–640.

428. Sharma, J.M. 1987. Delayed replication of Marek's disease following in ovo inoculation during late stages of embryonal development. Avian Dis 31:570–576.

429. Sharma, J.M. 1987. Personal Communication.

430. Sharma, J.M. 1989. Marek's disease. In H.G. Purchase, L.H. Arp, C.H. Domermuth, and J.E. Pearson (eds.). A

Laboratory Manual for the Isolation and Identification of Avian Pathogens, 3rd ed. American Association of Pathologists, New Bolton Center, PA, pp. 89–94.

431. Sharma, J.M., and B.R. Burmester. 1982. Resistance to Marek's disease at hatching in chickens vaccinated as embryos with the turkey herpesvirus. Avian Dis 26:134–149.

432. Sharma, J.M., and C.K. Graham. 1982. Influence of maternal antibody on efficacy of embryo vaccination with cell-associated and cell-free MD vaccine. Avian Dis 26:860–870.

433. Sharma, J.M., and H.A. Stone. 1972. Genetic resistance to Marek's disease. Delineation of the response of genetically resistant chickens to Marek's disease virus infection. Avian Dis 16:894–906.

434. Sharma, J.M., and R.L. Witter. 1975. The effect of B-cell immunosuppression on age-related resistance of chickens to Marek's disease. Cancer Res 35:711–717.

435. Sharma, J.M., and R.L. Witter. 1983. Embryo vaccination against Marek's disease with serotypes 1, 2 and 3 vaccines administered singly or in combination. Avian Dis 27:453–463.

436. Sharma, J.M., D. Burger, and S.G. Kenzy. 1972. Serological relationships among herpesviruses: Cross-reaction between Marek's disease virus and pseudorabies virus as detected by immunofluorescence. Infect Immun 5:406–411.

437. Sharma, J.M., R.L. Witter, and B.R. Burmester. 1973. Pathogenesis of Marek's disease in old chickens: Lesion regression as the basis for age-related resistance. Infect Immun 81:715–724.

438. Sharma, J.M., R.L. Witter, B.R. Burmester, and J.C. Landon. 1973. Public health implications of Marek's disease virus and herpesvirus of turkeys. Studies on human and subhuman primates. J Natl Cancer Inst 51:1123–1128.

439. Sharma, J.M., R.L. Witter, and H.G. Purchase. 1975. Absence of age-resistance in neonatally thymectomised chickens as evidence for cell-mediated immune surveillance in Marek's disease. Nature 253:477–479.

440. Sharma, J.M., L.F. Lee, and R.L. Witter. 1980. Effect of neonatal thymectomy on pathogenesis of herpesvirus of turkeys in chickens. Am J Vet Res 40:761–764.

441. Sharma, J.M., L.F. Lee, and P.S. Wakenell. 1984. Comparative viral, immunologic, and pathologic responses of chickens inoculated with herpesvirus of turkeys as embryos or a hatch. Am J Vet Res 45:1619–1623.

442. Shek, W.R., K.A. Schat, and B.W. Calnek. 1982. Characterization of nononcogenic Marek's disease virus-infected and turkey herpesvirus infected lymphocytes. J Gen Virol 63:333–341.

443. Shek, W.R., B.W. Calnek, K.A. Schat, and C.-L.H. Chen. 1983. Characterization of Marek's disease virus-infected lymphocytes: Discrimination between cytolytically and latently infected cells. J Natl Cancer Inst 70:485–491.

444. Shih, J.C.H., R. Pyrzak, and J.S. Guy. 1989. Discovery of noninfectious viral genes complementary to Marek's disease herpes virus in quail susceptible to cholesterol-induced atherosclerosis. J Nutr 119:294–298.

445. Siccardi, F.J., and B.R. Burmester. 1970. The differential diagnosis of lymphoid leukosis and Marek's disease. USDA Tech Bull 1412, Washington, DC.

446. Siegmann, O., E.F. Kaleta, and P. Schindler. 1980. Short-and long-term stability studies on four lyophilized and one cell-associated turkey herpesvirus vaccines against Marek's disease of chickens. Avian Pathol 9:21–32.

447. Silva, R.F. 1992. Differentiation of pathogenic and non-pathogenic serotype 1 Marek's disease viruses (MDVs) by the polymerase chain reaction amplification of the tandem direct repeats within the MDV genome. Avian Dis 36:521–528.

448. Silva, R.F., and J.C. Barnett. 1991. Restriction endonuclease analysis of Marek's disease virus DNA: Differentiation of viral strains and determination of passage history. Avian Dis 35:487–495.

449. Silva, R.F., and L.F. Lee. 1984. Monoclonal antibody-mediated immunoprecipitation of proteins from cells infected with Marek's disease virus or turkey herpesvirus. Virology 136:307–320.

450. Silva, R.F., and R.L. Witter. 1985. Genomic expansion of Marek's disease virus DNA is associated with serial in vitro passage. J Virol 54:690–696.

451. Silver, S., A. Tanaka, and M. Nonoyama. 1979. Transcription of the Marek's disease virus genome in a nonproductive chicken lymphoblastoid cell line. Virology 93:127–133.

452. Smith, G.D., V. Zelnik, and L.J.N. Ross. 1995. Gene organization in herpesvirus of turkeys: Identification of a novel open reading frame in the long unique region and a truncated homolog of pp38 in the internal repeat. Virology 207:205–216.

453. Smith, M.W., and B.W. Calnek. 1973. Effect of virus pathogenicity on antibody production in Marek's disease. Avian Dis 17:727–736.

454. Smith, M.W., and B.W. Calnek. 1974. High virulence Marek's disease virus infection in chickens previously infected with low-virulence virus. J Natl Cancer Inst 52:1595–1603.

455. Smith, T.W., D.M. Albert, N. Robinson, B.W. Calnek, and O. Schwabe. 1974. Ocular manifestations of Marek's disease. Invest Ophthalmol 13:586–592.

456. Solomon, J.J., R.L. Witter, K. Nazerian, and B.R. Burmester. 1968. Studies on the etiology of Marek's disease. I. Propagation of the agent in cell culture. Proc Soc Exp Biol Med 127:173–177.

457. Sondermeijer, P.J.A., J.A.J. Claessens, P.E. Jenniskens, A.P.A. Mockett, R.A.J. Thijssen, M.J. Willemse, and R.W. Morgan. 1993. Avian herpesvirus as a live viral vector for the expression of heterologous antigens. Vaccine 11:349–358.

458. Spencer, J.L. 1969. Marek's disease herpesvirus: In vivo and in vitro infection of kidney cells of different genetic strains of chickens. Avian Dis 13:753–761.

459. Spencer, J.L. 1970. Marek's disease herpesvirus: Comparison of foci (macro) in infected duck embryo fibroblasts under agar medium with foci (micro) in chicken cells. Avian Dis 14:565–578.

460. Spencer, J.L., and B.W. Calnek. 1967. Storage of cells infected with Rous sarcoma virus or JM strain of avian lymphomatosis agent. Avian Dis 11:274–287.

461. Spencer, J.L., and B.W. Calnek. 1970. Marek's disease: Application of immunofluorescence for detection of antigen and antibody. Am J Vet Res 31:345–358.

462. Spencer, J.L., J.S. Gavora, A.A. Grunder, A. Robertson, and G.W. Speckman. 1974. Immunization against Marek's disease: Influence of strain of chickens, maternal antibody, and type of vaccine. Avian Dis 18:33–44.

463. Spencer, J.L., F. Gilka, J.S. Gavora, R.J. Hampson, and D.J. Caldwell. 1992. Studies with a Marek's disease virus that caused blindness and high mortality in vaccinated flocks. In G. de Boer and S.H.M. Jerissen (eds.). Proc 4th Int Symp Marek's Dis. Ponsen & Looijen, Wageningen, Amsterdam, The Netherlands, pp. 199–201.

464. Stone, H.A. 1975. The usefulness and application of highly inbred chickens to research programs. USDA Tech Bull 1514, Washington, DC.

465. Sugaya, K., G. Bradley, M. Nonoyama, and A. Tanaka. 1990. Latent transcripts of Marek's disease virus are clustered in the short and long repeat regions. J Virol 64:5773–5782.

466. Sui, D., P. Wu, H.-J. Kung, and L.F. Lee. 1995. Identification and characterization of a Marek's disease virus gene encoding DNA polymerase. Virus Res 36:269–278.

467. Swayne, D.E., O.J. Fletcher, and L.W. Schierman. 1988. Marek's disease virus-induced transient paralysis in chickens: Alterations in brain density. Acta Neuropathol 76:287–291.

468. Swayne, D.E., O.J. Fletcher, and L.W. Schierman. 1989. Marek's disease virus-induced transient paralysis in chickens: Demonstration of vasogenic brain oedema by an immunohistochemical method. J Comp Path 101:451–462.

469. Swayne, D.E., O.J. Fletcher, and L.W. Schierman. 1989. Marek's disease virus-induced transient paralysis in chickens. 1. Time course association between clinical signs and histological brain lesions. Avian Pathol 18:385–396.

470. Swayne, D.E., O.J. Fletcher, and L.W. Schierman. 1989. Marek's disease virus-induced transient paralysis in chickens. 2. Ultrastructure of central nervous system. Avian Pathol 18:397–412.

471. Tanaka, A., S. Silver, and M. Nonoyama. 1978. Biochemical evidence of the nonintegrated status of Marek's disease virus DNA in virus-transformed lymphoblastoid cells of chickens. Virology 88:19–24.

472. Theis, G.A. 1977. Effects of lymphocytes from Marek's disease-infected chickens on mitogen responses of syngeneic normal chicken spleen cells. J Immunol 118:887–894.

473. Theis, G.A. 1981. Subpopulations of suppressor cells in chickens infected with cells of a transplantable lymphoblastic leukemia. Infect Immun 34:526–534.

474. Theis, G.A., R.A. McBride, and L.W. Schierman. 1975. Depression of in vitro responsiveness to phytohemagglutinin in spleen cells cultured from chickens with Marek's disease. J Immunol 115:848–853.

475. Thornton, D.H. 1985. Quality control and standardization of vaccines. In L.N. Payne (ed.). Marek's Disease. Martinus Nijhoff, Boston, MA, pp. 267–291.

476. Thurston, T.J., R.A. Hess, H.K. Adldinger, R.F. Solorzano, and H.V. Biellier. 1975. Ultrastructural studies of semen abnormalities and herpesvirus associated with cultured testis cells from domestic turkeys. J Reprod Fertil 45:507–514.

477. Tillotson, J.K., Lee, L.F., and H.J. Kung. 1989. Accumulation of viral transcripts coding for a DNA binding protein in Marek's disease tumor cells. In S. Kato, T. Horiuchi, T. Mikami, and K. Hirai (eds.). Advances in Marek's Disease Research. Japanese Association on Marek's Disease, Osaka, Japan, pp. 128–134.

478. Ubertini, T., and B.W. Calnek. 1970. Marek's disease herpesvirus in peripheral nerve lesions. J Natl Cancer Inst 45:507–514.

479. Van Zaane, D., J.M.A. Brinkhof, F. Westenbrink, and A.L.J. Gielkens. 1982. Molecular-biological characterization of Marek's disease virus. I. Identification of virus-specific polypeptides in infected cells. Virology 121:116–132.

480. Van Zaane, D., J.M.A. Brinkhof, F. Westenbrink, and A.L.J. Gielkens. 1982. Molecular-biological characterization of Marek's disease virus. II. Differentiation of various MDV and HVT strains. Virology 121:133–146.

481. Vengris, V.E., and C.J. Mare. 1973. Protection of chickens against Marek's disease virus JM-V strain with statolon and exogenous interferon. Avian Dis 17:758–767.

482. Venugopal, K., and L.N. Payne. 1995. Molecular pathogenesis of Marek's disease—Recent developments. Avian Pathol 24:597-609.

483. Vielitz, E. 1987. Recent problems and advances in the control of Marek's disease. Proc 10th Lat Am Poult Congr, Buenos Aires, Argentina, pp. 155–184.

484. Vielitz, E., and H. Landgraf. 1970. Beitrag zur Epidemiologie und Kontrolle der Marek'schen Krankheit. Dtsch Tierarztl Wochenschr 77:357–362.

485. Vielitz, E., and H. Landgraf. 1985. Experiences with monovalent and bivalent Marek's disease vaccines. In B.W. Calnek and J.L. Spencer (eds.). Proc Int Symp Marek's Dis. American Association of Avian Pathologists, Kennett Square, PA, pp. 570–575.

486. Vielitz, E., and H. Landgraf. 1986. Protection against Marek's disease with different vaccines, determination of PD50 and duration of vaccinal immunity. Dtsch Tierarztl Wochenschr 93:53–55.

487. Volpini, L.M., B.W. Calnek, M.J. Sekellick, and P.I. Marcus. 1995. Stages of Marek's disease virus latency defined by variable sensitivity to interferon modulation of viral antigen expression. Vet Microbiol 47:99-109.

488. Weiss, R.A., and P.M. Biggs. 1972. Leukosis and Marek's disease virus of feral red jungle fowl and domestic fowl in Malaya. J Natl Cancer Inst 39:1713–1725.

489. Wight, P.A.L. 1962. The histopathology of the central nervous system in fowl paralysis. J Comp Pathol Ther 72:348–359.

490. Wight, P.A.L. 1966. Histopathology of the skeletal muscles in fowl paralysis (Marek's disease). J Comp Pathol 76:333–339.

491. Wilson, M.R., R.A. Southwick, J.T. Pulaski, V.L. Tieber, Y. Hong, and P.M. Coussens. 1994. Molecular analysis of the glycoprotein C-negative phenotype of attenuated Marek's disease virus. Virology 199:393–402.

492. Witter, R.L. 1971. Marek's disease research—History and perspectives. Poult Sci 50:333–342.

493. Witter, R.L. 1972. Epidemiology of Marek's disease—A review. In P.M. Biggs, G. de Thé, and L.N. Payne (eds.). Oncogenesis and Herpesviruses. IARC, Lyon, France, pp. 111–122.

494. Witter, R.L. 1982. Protection by attenuated and polyvalent vaccines against highly virulent strains of Marek's Disease virus. Avian Pathol 11:49–62.

495. Witter, R.L. 1983. Characteristics of Marek's disease viruses isolated from vaccinated commercial chicken flocks: Association of viral pathotype with lymphoma frequency. Avian Dis 27:113–132.

496. Witter, R.L. 1985. Principles of vaccination. In L.N. Payne (ed.). Marek's Disease. Martinus Nijhoff, Boston, MA, pp. 203–250.

497. Witter, R.L. 1985. Review: Vaccines and vaccination against Marek's disease. In B.W. Calnek and J.L. Spencer (eds.). Proc Int Symp Marek's Dis. American Association of Avian Pathologists, Kennett Square, PA, pp. 482–500.

498. Witter, R.L. 1985. Association in broiler chickens between natural serotype 2 Marek's disease virus infection and leukosis condemnations. In B.W. Calnek and J.L. Spencer (eds.). Proc Int Symp Marek's Dis. American Association of Avian Pathologists, Kennett Square, PA, pp. 545–554.

499. Witter, R.L. 1987. New serotype 2 and attenuated serotype 1 Marek's disease vaccine viruses: Comparative efficacy. Avian Dis 31:752–765.

500. Witter. 1988. Vary virulent Marek's disease viruses: Importance and control. In Proc 18th World's Poult Congress. World's Poultry Congress, Nagoya, Japan, pp. 92–97.

501. Witter, R.L. 1989. Very virulent Marek's disease viruses: Importance and control. World's Poult Sci J 45:60–75.

502. Witter, R.L. 1989. Protective synergism among Marek's disease vaccine viruses. In S. Kato, T. Horiuchi, T. Mikami, and K. Hirai (eds.). Advances in Marek's Disease Research. Japanese Association on Marek's Disease, Osaka, Japan, pp. 398–404.

503. Witter, R.L. 1991. Attenuated revertant serotype 1 Marek's disease viruses: Safety and protective efficacy. Avian Dis 35:877–891.

504. Witter, R.L. 1992. Influence of serotype and virus strain on synergism between Marek's disease vaccine viruses. Avian Pathol 21:601–614.

505. Witter, R.L. 1992. Safety and comparative efficacy of the CVI988/Rispens vaccine strain. In G. de Boer and S.H.M Jerissen (eds.). Proc 4th Int Symp on Marek's disease. Ponsen & Looijen, Wageningen, Amsterdam, The Netherlands, pp. 315–319.

506. Witter, R.L. 1995. Unpublished observations.

507. Witter, R.L., and B.R. Burmester. 1979. Differential

effect of maternal antibodies on efficacy of cellular and cell-free Marek's disease vaccines. Avian Pathol 8:145–156.

508. Witter, R.L., and L.F. Lee. 1984. Polyvalent Marek's disease vaccines: Safety, efficacy and protective synergism in chickens with maternal antibodies. Avian Pathol 13:75–92.

509. Witter, R.L., and L. Offenbecker. 1979. Nonprotective and temperature-sensitive variants of Marek's disease vaccine viruses. J Natl Cancer Inst 62:143–151.

510. Witter, R.L., and J.J. Solomon. 1971. Epidemiology of a herpesvirus of turkeys: Possible sources and spread of infection in turkey flocks. Infect Immun 4:356–361.

511. Witter, R.L., and J.J. Solomon. 1972. Prospects for the control of Marek's disease through isolation rearing. Progr Immunobiol Stand 5:163–168.

512. Witter, R.L., and J.J. Solomon. 1972. Experimental infection of turkeys and chickens with a herpesvirus of turkeys (HVT). Avian Dis 16:34–44.

513. Witter, R.L., G.H. Burgoyne, and B.R. Burmester. 1968. Survival of Marek's disease agent in litter and droppings. Avian Dis 12:522–530.

514. Witter, R.L., J.J. Solomon, and G.H. Burgoyne. 1969. Cell culture techniques for primary isolation of Marek's disease-associated herpesvirus. Avian Dis 13:101–118.

515. Witter, R.L., G.H. Burgoyne, and J.J. Solomon. 1969. Evidence for a herpesvirus as an etiologic agent of Marek's disease. Avian Dis 13:171–184.

516. Witter, R.L., K. Nazerian, H.G. Purchase, and G.H. Burgoyne. 1970. Isolation from turkeys of a cell-associated herpesvirus antigenically related to Marek's disease virus. Am J Vet Res 31:525–538.

517. Witter, R.L., H.G. Purchase, and G.H. Burgoyne. 1970. Peripheral nerve lesions similar to those of Marek's disease in chickens inoculated with reticuloendotheliosis virus. J Natl Cancer Inst 45:567–577.

518. Witter, R.L., J.J. Solomon, L.R. Champion, and K. Nazerian. 1971. Long term studies of Marek's disease infection in individual chickens. Avian Dis 15:346–365.

519. Witter, R.L., K. Nazerian, and J.J. Solomon. 1972. Studies on the in vivo replication of turkey herpesvirus. J Natl Cancer Inst 49:1121–1130.

520. Witter, R.L., J.M. Sharma, J.J. Solomon, and L.R. Champion. 1973. An age-related resistance of chickens to Marek's disease: Some preliminary observations. Avian Pathol 2:43–54.

521. Witter, R.L., E.A. Stephens, J.M. Sharma, and K. Nazerian. 1975. Demonstration of a tumor-associated surface antigen in Marek's disease. J Immunol 115:177–183.

522. Witter, R.L., J.M. Sharma, and L. Offenbecker. 1976. Turkey herpesvirus infection in chickens: Induction of lymphoproliferative lesions and characterization of vaccinal immunity against Marek's disease. Avian Dis 20:676–692.

523. Witter, R.L., B.W. Calnek, S. Kato, and P.C. Powell. 1979. A proposed method for designating avian cell lines and transplantable tumours. Avian Pathol 8:487–498.

524. Witter, R.L., J.M. Sharma, and A.M. Fadly. 1980. Pathogenicity of variant Marek's disease virus isolants in vaccinated and unvaccinated chickens. Avian Dis 24:210–232.

525. Witter, R.L., J.M. Sharma, L.F. Lee, H.M. Opitz, and C.W. Henry. 1984. Field trials to test the efficacy of polyvalent Marek's disease vaccines in broilers. Avian Dis 28:44–60.

526. Witter, R.L., Sharma, J.M., and A.M. Fadly. 1986. Nonbursal lymphomas induced by nondefective reticuloendotheliosis virus. Avian Pathol 15:467–486.

527. Witter, R., R. Silva, and L. Lee. 1987. New serotype 2 and attenuated serotype 1 Marek's disease vaccine viruses: Selected biological and molecular characteristics. Avian Dis 31:829–840.

528. Witter, R.L., L.F. Lee, and J.M. Sharma. 1990. Biological diversity among serotype 2 Marek's disease viruses. Avian Dis 34:944–957.

529. Yachida, S., T. Mikami, M. Onuma, and H. Izawa. 1983. Comparative studies on antigens induced by turkey herpesvirus and Marek's disease virus. II. Immunofluorescent studies. Zentralbl Veterinarmed [B] 30:669–677.

530. Yachida, S., T. Kondo, K. Hirai, H. Izawa, and T. Mikami. 1986. Establishment of a variant type of turkey herpesvirus which releases cell-free virus into the culture medium in large quantities. Arch Virol 91:183–192.

531. Yanagida, N., S. Yoshida, K. Nazerian, and L.F. Lee. 1993. Nucleotide and predicted amino acid sequences of Marek's disease virus homologs of herpes simplex virus major tegument proteins. J Gen Virol 74:1837–1845.

532. Yoshida, S., L.F. Lee, N. Yanagida, and K. Nazerian. 1994. Identification and characterization of a Marek's disease virus gene homologous to glycoprotein L of herpes simplex virus. Virology 204:414–419.

533. Yoshida, S., L.F. Lee, N. Yanagida, and K. Nazerian. 1994. The glycoprotein B genes of Marek's disease virus serotypes 2 and 3: Identification and expression by recombinant fowlpox viruses. Virology 200:484–493.

534. Yuasa, N. 1983. Propagation and infectivity titration of the GIFU-1 strain of chicken anemia agent in a cell line (MDCC-MSB1) derived from Marek's disease lymphoma. Natl Inst Anim Hlth Q 23:13–20.

535. Yuasa, N., and K. Imai. 1988. Efficacy of Marek's disease vaccine, herpesvirus of turkeys, in chickens infected with chicken anemia agent. In S. Kato, T. Horiuchi, T. Mikami, and K. Hirai (eds.). Advances in Marek's Disease Research. Japanese Association on Marek's Disease, Osaka, Japan, pp. 358–363.

536. Zander, D.V., and R.G. Raymond. 1985. Partial flock inoculation with a apathogenic strain (HN-1) of chicken herpesvirus of Marek's disease (MD) to immunize chicken flocks against pathogenic field strains of MD. In B.W. Calnek and J.L. Spencer (eds.). Proc Int Symp Marek's Dis. American Association of Avian Pathologists, Kennett Square, PA, pp. 514–530.

537. Zander, D.V., R.W. Hill, R.G. Raymond, R.K. Balch, R.W. Mitchell, and J.W. Dunsing. 1972. The use of blood from selected chickens as an immunizing agent for Marek's disease. Avian Dis 16:163–178.

538. Zanella, A. 1982. Marek's disease—Survey on vaccination failures. Dev Biol Stand 52:29–37.

539. Zelnik, V., L.J.N. Ross, G.D. Smith, L.A. Ramsay, and J. Pastorek. 1992. Comparison of glycoprotein D (gD) genes of Marek's disease virus and herpesvirus of turkeys. In G. de Boer and S.H.M Jerissen (eds.). Proc 4th Int Symp Marek's Dis. Ponsen & Looijen, Wageningen, Amsterdam, The Netherlands, pp. 114–117.

540. Zelnik, V., L.J.N. Ross, and J. Pastorek. 1994. Characterization of proteins encoded by the short unique region of herpesvirus of turkeys by in vitro expression. J Gen Virol 75:2747–2753.

541. Zerbes, M., G.A. Tannock, R.J. Jenner, and P.L. Young. 1994. Some characteristics of a recent virulent isolate of Marek's disease virus. Aust Vet J 71:21–22.

542. Zhu, G.S., T. Ojima, T. Hironaka, T. Ihara, N. Mizukoshi, A. Kato, S. Ueda, and K. Hirai. 1992. Differentiation of oncogenic and nononcogenic strains of Marek's disease virus type 1 by using polymerase chain reaction DNA amplification. Avian Dis 36:637–645.

543. Zygraich, N., and C. Huygelen. 1972. Inoculation of one-day-old chicks with different strains of turkey herpesvirus. II. Virus replication in tissues of inoculated animals. Avian Dis 16:793–798.

LEUKOSIS/SARCOMA GROUP

L. N. Payne and A. M. Fadly

INTRODUCTION

Definition and Synonyms. The leukosis/sarcoma group of diseases comprises a variety of transmissible benign and malignant neoplasms of chickens caused by members of a genus of avian retroviruses belonging to the family *Retroviridae* (77). Under natural conditions, by far the most common is lymphoid leukosis. The neoplasms and their synonyms are listed in Table 17.3. These avian viruses are characterized, as are all members of the *Retroviridae*, by possession of an enzyme reverse transcriptase, which directs the synthesis of the proviral DNA form of the RNA virus that forms part of the retroviral life cycle, and from which the family name is derived. These avian retroviruses, formerly included in a subgenus termed avian type C oncoviruses (235), are now provisionally termed avian leukosis virus (ALV)-related viruses (77): they have similar physical and molecular characteristics and share a common group-specific antigen.

Because of the relationships between these viruses, they are discussed as a group in most parts of this chapter. Sections reflecting the host response (Incubation Period, Signs, Gross Lesions, Histopathology, Ultrastructure, Hematology, Pathogenesis, Differential Diagnosis) are discussed under the pathologic entities without regard for virologic properties of the inducing agent(s) other than their inclusion in the leukosis/sarcoma group.

Economic and Public Health Significance. Economic losses from the leukosis/sarcoma group of diseases come from two sources. First, mortality from the group commonly amounts to around 1–2% of birds, with occasional losses of up to 20% or more. Second, subclinical infection by ALV, to which most flocks are subject, produces a depressive effect on a number of important performance traits, including especially egg production and quality (166).

Avian leukosis/sarcoma viruses present no apparent public health risk (206).

HISTORY. Leukotic diseases appear to have been recognized for a long time. Roloff (320) reported a case of "lymphosarcomata" in 1868 and Caparini (67) described fowl leukemia in 1896. In 1905, Butterfield (60) made a diagnosis of "aleukemic lymphadenosis" in three hens in the United States. Ellermann (128) described three types of leukemia: erythroid ("intravascular lymphoid leukosis"), myeloid ("myeloic leukosis"), and lymphoid ("lymphatic leukosis"). Comprehensive reviews of the conditions or their agents are those of Beard (25), Temin (368, 369), Hanafusa (187), Weiss (391), Weiss et al. (396, 397), de Boer (109), and Payne (275). Reviews of the history of avian retrovirus research are provided by Burmester and Purchase (51), Dougherty (118), and Payne (275).

LYMPHOID LEUKOSIS. Jung err (207) termed the disease *visceral lymphomatosis,* but this nomenclature was superseded by that of Biggs (31) and Campbell (64), and the disease is now called lymphoid leukosis (LL).

Furth (163) provided evidence for transmission of LL with filtrates, but proof of the filterability of the agent or agents awaited the work of Burmester and his associates (40, 46, 47).

ERYTHROBLASTOSIS. Ellermann and Bang (130) were the first to report experimental transmission of erythroblastosis. Subsequently, numerous strains were established, and the viral etiology and pathologic nature of the disease were characterized (22, 56, 52, 127).

MYELOBLASTOSIS. Myeloblastosis was transmitted by Schmeisser in 1915 (338); since then, Furth (162), Engelbreth Holm and Rothe-Meyer (132), and Nyfeldt (258) have observed myeloblastosis in transmission experiments. Early passages of the BAI strain (BAI-A) virus (185) caused both erythroblastosis and myeloblastosis; however, passages derived by selection and cloning have induced a wide variety of tumors (25).

MYELOCYTOMATOSIS. The distinctive appearance and aleukemic character of this disease were first described by Pentimalli (288); later, Furth (162) described some leukemic cases. Most strains (isolates) causing myelocytoma also caused other neoplasms (25, 242, 284).

CONNECTIVE TISSUE TUMORS. Fibrosarcomas and myxosarcomas were first transmitted with cell-free filtrates by Rous in 1911 (322). Ellermann and Bang (130) noticed this tumor in their early transmission studies.

NEPHROMAS AND NEPHROBLASTOMAS. Several viruses of the leukosis/sarcoma group have

The authors are greatly indebted to B.R. Burmester and H.G. Purchase for their contributions to earlier editions of this chapter.

Table 17.3.   Neoplasms caused by viruses of leukosis/sarcoma group

Neoplasm	Synonyms (Reference Nos.)
Leukoses	
Lymphoid leukosis	Big liver disease, lymphatic leukosis (127), visceral lymphoma (270), lymphocytoma (150), lymphomatosis (163), visceral lymphomatosis (207), lymphoid leukosis (31, 64)
Erythroblastosis	Leukemia (388), intravascular lymphoid leukosis (128), erythroleukosis (129, 162), erythromyelosis (21), erythroblastosis (132), erythroid leukosis (31, 64)
Myeloblastosis	Leukemic myeloid leukosis (128), leukomyelose (218), myelomatosis (163), myeloblastosis (258), granuloblastosis (207), myeloid leukosis (108)
Myelocytoma(tosis)	Myelocytoma (284, 288), aleukemic myeloid leukosis (127), leukochloroma (233), myelomatosis (163)
Connective tissue tumors	
Fibroma and fibrosarcoma	
Myxoma and myxosarcoma	
Histiocytic sarcoma	
Chondroma	
Osteoma and osteogenic sarcoma	
Epithelial tumors	
Nephroblastoma	Embryonal nephroma (151), renal adenocarcinoma (68), adenosarcoma (374), nephroblastoma (204, 286, 386), cystadenoma (242)
Nephroma	Papillary cystadenoma, carcinoma of the kidney (25, 241)
Hepatocarcinoma (25, 241)	
Adenocarcinoma of the pancreas (25)	
Thecoma (25)	
Granulosa cell carcinoma (25, 284)	
Seminoma	Adenocarcinoma of the testis (25)
Squamous cell carcinoma (25)	
Endothelial tumors	
Hemangioma	Hemangiomatosis, endothelioma (163), hemangioblastomas, hemangioendotheliomas
Angiosarcoma (210, 344)	
Endothelioma (242)	
Mesothelioma (25, 71)	
Related tumors	
Osteopetrosis	Marble bone, thick leg disease, sporadic diffuse osteoperiostitis (301), osteopetrosis gallinarum (208)
Meningioma (25)	
Glioma (25)	

been found to induce kidney tumors, including nephromas and nephroblastomas; e.g., BAI-A (myeloblastosis), ES4 strain (erythroblastosis/sarcoma), MH2 strain (reticuloendothelioma), and MC29 and HPRS-103 strains (myelocytomatosis) (25, 56, 68, 69, 242, 284).

OTHER EPITHELIAL TUMORS. Leukosis viruses were shown to cause other epithelial tumors, including hepatocarcinomas (225), adenocarcinomas of the pancreas (241), thecomas and granulosa cell tumors of the ovary, adenocarcinomas of the seminiferous tubules of the testes (seminoma), and squamous cell carcinomas of the skin (25).

ENDOTHELIAL TUMORS. Leukosis viruses were early recognized to cause a variety of tumors of the endothelium (163, 242) and have more recently been found to cause mesotheliomas (25, 71).

OSTEOPETROSIS. It is now apparent that the hypertrophic osteopathies of fowl described in the 1920s were probably osteopetrosis (301). Jungherr and Landauer (208) described the pathologic alterations and suggested the term *osteopetrosis gallinarum*. They were the first to reproduce the disease and call attention to its frequent association with LL. For this reason, they suggested its inclusion in the avian leukosis complex. Burmester and his associates (40, 156) also noticed that osteopetrosis was frequently associated with LL. Others have reproduced the disease without LL (65, 154, 197).

OTHER RELATED TUMORS. Viruses have been shown to cause meningiomas and gliomas in the brain (25).

INCIDENCE AND DISTRIBUTION.

With few exceptions, infection occurs in all chicken flocks; by sexual maturity, most birds have been exposed. Nevertheless, the incidence of clinical disease is generally low.

Incidence of Disease. Lymphoid leukosis only occasionally produces heavy losses, e.g., 23% in commercial breeder flocks (309), although sporadic cases occur in most flocks. De Boer (112) reported LL mortality in the Netherlands as 2.18% of 11,220 white layers and 0.57% of 7920 brown layers, recorded in random sample tests over the period of 1973 to 1979. The incidence of LL in chickens may be reduced by the widespread occurrence of infectious bursal disease virus (94, 304). Lymphoid leukosis has been reported in many species of birds, but there is no assurance that such cases are not other types of lymphoid tumor.

Compared with LL, erythroblastosis occurs infrequently under field conditions (309). Exceptionally, it has been reported to occur in 5-wk-old birds as an epizootic (186). There are very few reports of natural occurrence of myeloblastosis, but cases occur sporadically.

Sporadic cases of myelocytomatosis occur among young adult birds (309). The disease was observed in about 1% of birds in two consecutive broiler flocks on one farm (234). An overall incidence of 27% myelocytomatosis was reported in meat-type chickens inoculated with strain HPRS-103 of subgroup J ALV (284).

Of all tumors other than leukotic tumors, hemangiomas make up 25 and 19%, and nephroblastomas 19 and 3–10%, in broilers (66) and layers (309), respectively. Epizootic outbreaks of hemangiosarcomas have recently occurred in layers in Israel (58).

There is little information on incidence of connective tissue tumors, which are often not the primary cause of death; they make up about 20% of tumors other than leukosis in broilers (66). The incidence of connective tissue tumors in chickens is probably less than 1 in 1000 (309), but epizootics have occurred. Perek (289) reported an outbreak of histiocytic sarcomas in a flock of 600 1-yr-old hens. Tumors were found in 90% of 400 birds examined during a 4-mo period.

Osteopetrosis occurs widely, but much less frequently than LL, and epizootics occur sporadically in broilers. In all types of chicken, males are more frequently affected than females. It occurs very rarely in turkeys.

Incidence of Virus Infection. Leukosis/sarcoma viruses are almost ubiquitous. Subgroup A viruses are encountered more commonly than subgroup B. In one study (62), 1.6–12.5% of the embryos from eight commercial flocks representing a variety of sources contained subgroup A viruses, and there was significant shedding in every flock. Subgroup B viruses were relatively rare and were shed in eggs much less frequently than subgroup A. A similar preponderance of subgroup A viruses has been isolated from field outbreaks of LL. In general, fewer studies of the prevalence of ALV in meat lines have been made compared with those in egg lines. Antibodies to the novel subgroup J ALV were found in three of five meat-type chicken lines, but not in seven layer lines examined in the United Kingdom (283).

Viruses representing subgroups A, B, C, and D have been isolated from commercial flocks in Finland; 5 of 10 flocks surveyed had antibody to all four subgroups (330).

Antibodies to subgroups A and B are common among wildfowl and domestic chickens in Kenya and Malaysia, and there was some evidence of antibody to subgroup D viruses in Kenya. Subgroup F viruses have been found in ring-necked and green pheasants, and subgroup G viruses in Ghinghi, silver, and golden pheasants. Subgroup H virus has been isolated from Hungarian partridges and subgroup I virus from Gambel's quail (see Virus Subgroups). Viruses that do not fit known subgroups have been isolated from Mongolian and Swinhoe pheasants, Chinese quail, and chickens. However, none was found in Japanese quail, pigeons, geese, and Pekin and Muscovy ducks (73).

Endogenous retroviral genomes, inherited in a Mendelian fashion, occur at distinct chromosomal loci in most vertebrate species. DNA sequences related to RAV-0, the endogenous avian retrovirus, occur in the germ lines of most domestic chickens and several species of galliform birds. For example, partridges, true pheasants, grouse, and jungle fowl contain sequences complementary to RAV-0, whereas guinea fowl, quail, peafowl, ruffed pheasants, gallo-pheasants, and turkeys do not (159). The structure, function, and regulation of endogenous retroviruses in the genome of the chicken have been reviewed (86).

ETIOLOGY

Classification. Viruses of the leukosis/sarcoma group have been placed recently in a genus (provisionally termed *ALV-related viruses*) of the family *Retroviridae* (77). Viruses of this family are characterized by possession of the enzyme reverse transcriptase, which is necessary for formation of a DNA provirus during viral replication, and include oncogenic C-type RNA viruses of other animal species.

The avian leukosis/sarcoma viruses are closely

related and cause, depending on their genetic makeup, a variety of neoplasms with short to long clinical latencies. Some, mainly laboratory propagated, strains such as avian myeloblastosis virus (AMV), avian erythroblastosis virus (AEV), and the sarcoma viruses, carry specific viral oncogenes that cause rapid neoplastic transformation and tumor development within a few days or weeks. Other ALVs, especially field isolants, lack transformation genes. They are slowly or weakly transforming, and tumor development takes many weeks or months; transformation is believed to be by viral activation of cellular genes (proto-oncogenes) homologous to virus-transforming genes (79).

VIRUS SUBGROUPS. Avian leukosis/sarcoma viruses that occur in chickens have been divided into 6 subgroups (A, B, C, D, E, and J) on the basis of their host range in chicken embryo fibroblasts of different genetic types, interference patterns with members of the same and different subgroups, and viral envelope antigens identified by virus and serum neutralization tests (396) (Table 17.4). These various properties are a reflection of the envelope glycoproteins present on the virus. Viruses of subgroups A and B occur as common exogenous viruses in the field (62). Subgroups C and D viruses have been reported in the field rarely (244, 330),

and subgroup E viruses include the ubiquitous endogenous leukosis viruses of low pathogenicity (347). Subgroup J viruses were isolated recently from meat-type chickens (283, 284).

Viruses of two additional subgroups (F and G) have been rescued from ring-necked pheasant (189, 160) and golden (160) and Lady Amherst pheasant (190). Subgroup G viruses are believed to belong to a virus species that differs from that of the chicken viruses (190). Endogenous virus of subgroup H was isolated from Hungarian partridge (190) and of subgroup I from Gambel's quail (376).

A number of laboratory strains of avian leukosis/sarcoma viruses are genetically defective and lack the viral envelope (*env*) gene; their subgroup is that of the helper leukosis viruses used for their propagation.

VIRUS TYPES. Viruses within a subgroup cross-neutralize to varying extents, but with the exception of partial cross-neutralization between subgroups B and D, viruses of different subgroups do not. Antiserums raised against a particular strain of virus tend to neutralize the homologous virus more strongly than heterologous viruses of the same subgroup (75); viruses within a subgroup vary in ability to induce immunologic tolerance to other members of the subgroup (238). These findings indicate

Table 17.4. Common laboratory strains of avian leukosis/sarcoma viruses of the chicken classified according to predominant neoplasm induced and virus subgroup

Virus Class According to Neoplasm	Virus Class According to Subgroup						No subgroup (defective viruses)
	A	B	C	D	E	J	
Lymphoid leukosis virus (LLV)	RAV-1 RIF-1 MAV-1 RPL-12 HPRS-F42	RAV-2 RAV-6 MAV-2	RAV-7 RAV-49	RAV-50 CZAV	RAV-60		
Avian erythroblastosis virus (AEV)							AEV-ES4 AEV-R
Avian myeloblastosis virus (AMV)							AMV-BAI-A E26
Avian sarcoma virus (ASV)	SR-RSV-A PR-RSV-A EH-RSV RSV29	SR-RSV-B PR-RSV-B HA-RSV	B77 PR-RSV-C	SR-RSV-D CZ-RSV	SR-RSV-E PR-RSV-E		BH-RSV BS-RSV FuSV PRCII PRCIV ESV Y73 UR1 UR2
Myelocytoma/endo-thelioma virus						HPRS-103	MC29 MH2 CMII OK10
Endogenous virus (EV) (no neoplasm)			RAV-0 ILV	EAV			

occurrence of varying antigenic types within subgroups; in general, subgroup B viruses appear to be more heterogenous than those of subgroup A. Differences in propensity of several subgroup-A viruses to induce tolerance following yolk sac infection have been observed (148).

Morphology

ULTRASTRUCTURE. Viruses of the avian leukosis/sarcoma group cannot be distinguished on the basis of their ultrastructural characteristics. In size, shape, and ultrastructural detail, particles from the various diseases studied are identical and similar to other type C retroviruses (257, 368) (Fig. 17.17). Negatively stained preparations reveal essentially spheroidal particles that are readily distorted under certain conditions of drying (24). Characteristic knobbed spikes about 8 nm in diameter are present on the surface of the particles. The inner nucleoid of the virus appears to be less easily distorted than the outer part. Certain fixatives allow the interior nucleoprotein filaments to be visualized; these are approximately 3–5 nm in diameter, of undetermined length, and are probably in the form of an intricate coil (18, 257). Thin sections reveal an inner, centrally located electron-dense core about 35–45 nm in diameter, an intermediate membrane, and an outer membrane. This appearance typifies the C-type particle morphology. Overall diameter of the particle is 80–120 nm, with an average of 90 nm (24).

SIZE AND DENSITY. By filtration through membranes of graded pore size, ultracentrifugation, and electron microscopy, viruses have a diameter of 80–145 nm. The value of 1.15–1.17 g/mL for the buoyant density in sucrose is characteristic of C-type retroviruses (18, 316).

Chemical Composition.

The overall composition of AMV, which has been studied extensively, is 30–35% lipid, 60–65% protein, 2.2% RNA, and a small amount of DNA, perhaps of cellular origin (18, 22).

VIRAL NUCLEIC ACIDS. The major size classes of RNA sediment at 60-70S, which is the viral genome, and at 4-5S, most of which is host tRNA, are thought to be accidentally included in the virion and to play no role in viral replication. However, a tRNA primer associated with 70S RNA does occur and has a role in the viral life cycle. Small amounts of 18 and 28S ribosomal RNAs, viral and cellular mRNA, and DNA are also present. The 60-70S genomic RNA is a dimer and can be split into two subunits of about 34-38S, which are believed to represent a diploid genome. These subunits of genomic RNA are mRNAs, and their genes have been

mapped for several avian retroviruses. The sequences of the structural genes of avian leukosis virus, from the 5′ end to the 3′ end of the RNA molecule, is *gag/pro–pol–env*; these genes encode, respectively, the proteins of the virion group-specific (gs) antigens and protease, RNA-dependent DNA polymerase (reverse transcriptase, or RT), and envelope glycoproteins. The structural genes are flanked by terminal genomic sequences concerned with organization of the replication and translation of viral RNA (77, 193, 396). The genome is about 7.2 kb in size. Acutely transforming viruses possess additional genomic sequences concerned with oncogenic transformation. Nondefective Rous sarcoma virus (RSV) has the genetic composition *gag/pro–pol–env–src*. The additional gene, *src*, responsible for sarcomatous transformation, was evidently acquired originally from a normal cellular gene, cellular *src*. The inclusion of this gene is responsible for the approximately 35S subunits of RSV being slightly larger than those of slowly transforming leukosis viruses. The gene *src* is an example of a number of host cell genes, termed proto-oncogenes or *onc* genes, concerned with acute transformation (133, 387). Viral and cellular versions of *onc* genes, and of the specific varieties such as *src*, are distinguished by the prefixes v- and c-. Specific v-*onc* genes, with c-*onc* counterparts in normal cells, are present in other acute transforming viruses, e.g., *erbA*, *erbB* (AEV), *myb* (AMV), *myc* (avian myelocytomatosis virus), *fps* (Fujinami and PRCII sarcoma viruses), *yes* (Y73 and Esh sarcoma viruses), *sea* (S13 virus), and *ros* (UR2 virus). MH2 endothelioma virus has two oncogenes, *myc* and *mil*, and E26 has *myb* and *ets*. Slow transformation, as in LL, is believed to be caused by an indirect mechanism independent of a v-*onc*, but dependent on activation of a c-*onc*, namely c-*myc*, in LL (220). Sequenced and cloned viral DNA is now available from many viruses of the leukosis/sarcoma group and a number of viruses have been completely sequenced (397).

VIRAL LIPIDS. Viral lipids occur in the virion envelope and have a composition similar to that of the outer cell membrane from which the virion envelope is derived (18, 35).

VIRAL PROTEINS. The nature, location, and synthesis of proteins that constitute avian retroviruses have been extensively studied (77, 396, 397). The virion core contains five nonglycosylated proteins encoded by the *gag* gene: p27, the major gs antigen (27 kD), which is a capsid antigen (CA) (core shell) component; p19 (matrix, MA) and p12 (nucleocapsid, NC), believed to be involved in RNA processing and packaging; p15, a protease (PR) involved in cleavage of protein precursors, and p10. Other minor polypeptides have also been reported. A variant

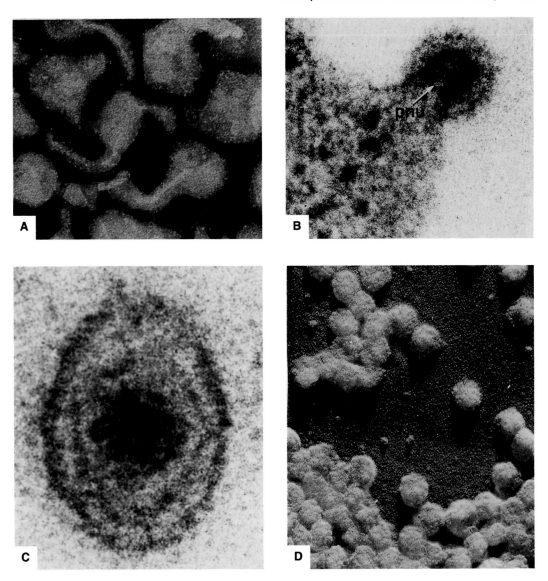

17.17.   Ultrastructure of leukosis/sarcoma viruses. *A.* BAI-A of avian myeloblastosis virus (AMV), unfixed, and negatively stained with neutralized phosphotungstic acid. Peripheral fringe about particles is resolved in some places into discrete "knobs." ×150,000. *B.* Ultrastructure of leukosis/sarcoma virus release. Virus budding at cell membrane of a leukemic myeloblast. Surface of buds and particles peripheral to outer membrane is irregular and indistinct (pnu, dense prenucleoid). ×215,000. *C.* Thin section of BAI-A of AMV sedimented from plasma, fixed in osmium tetroxide, and stained with lead subacetate. Inner and outer membranes and granular character of nucleoid can be seen. Impression of granules might be derived from sectioning of filaments. Some granules appear to be hollow. ×510,000. *D.* Purified BAI-A of AMV fixed and shadowed with chromium. ×50,000. (Bonar and de Thé)

form of p27 has been reported in RAV-0 endogenous virus, but it is not characteristic of all endogenous viruses (201). The virion envelope contains two glycoproteins encoded by the *env* gene: gp85 (SU), the viral surface knoblike structures that determine the subgroup specificity of the avian retroviruses; and gp37 (TM), representing the trans-

membrane structure that attaches the knobs to the envelope. These two envelope proteins are linked to form a dimer, termed virion glycoprotein (VGP).

Virions contain a number of enzymic activities. Reverse transcriptase is present in the core and is encoded by the *pol* gene; it is a complex consisting of the ß subunit (95 kD) and the α subunit (63 kD) derived from it, and has RNA- and DNA-dependent polymerase and DNA:RNA hybrid-specific ribonuclease H activities. Another virus-coded enzyme is p32 (IN) genome, the integrase protein necessary for integration of viral DNA into the host cell. Other enzymatic activities have been detected in virions and are believed to be cellular contaminants (370). Of practical importance is the presence in AMV obtained from blood of infected chickens, or from myeloblast cultures, of adenosine triphosphatase derived from the cell membrane and incorporated into the virus particle envelope during maturation. This enzyme will dephosphorylate adenosine triphosphate, and this activity may be used for virus assay (27). Cells without this enzyme on their surface release virus that is devoid of activity.

Virus Replication.   As with other retroviruses, replication of avian leukosis/sarcoma viruses is characterized by formation of a DNA provirus, under the direction of reverse transcriptase, which becomes linearly integrated into the host cell genome. Subsequently, the proviral genes are transcribed into viral RNAs, which are translated to produce the precursor and mature proteins that constitute the virion. Great effort has been made since the 1970s to elucidate these events, the details of which are discussed by Weiss et al. (396, 397) and Luciw and Leung (229). Only an outline of the main events is provided here.

PENETRATION OF THE HOST CELL.   Although adsorption of the virion to the cell membrane is nonspecific, occurring even in cells resistant to infection (291), penetration of cells is dependent on the occurrence, presumably in the cell membrane, of host gene-encoded receptors specific for each virus subgroup. Dales and Hanafusa (107) observed virions taken into the cell in vacuoles and viral RNA in the nucleus within 120 min of attachment. Recently the gene for the ALV subgroup A receptor has been cloned and the product shown to bind to subgroup A envelope glycoprotein (169, 402). The receptor is related to the low-density lipoprotein receptor (17).

SYNTHESIS AND INTEGRATION OF VIRAL DNA.   The unique features of avian and other retroviruses that characterize viral replication are the formation (under the influence of viral reverse transcriptase) of retroviral DNA from a template of viral RNA, integration of viral DNA (provirus) into the host cell genome, and formation of new viral RNA from the proviral DNA template. Major stages in formation of retroviral DNA are 1) synthesis of the first (minus) strand of viral DNA, forming an RNA:DNA hybrid; 2) removal of RNA from the hybrid by RNase-H and formation on the template of minus-strand DNA of second (plus) strands of viral DNA,

giving rise to linear DNA duplexes (these duplex molecules are detectable in cytoplasm of the cell within a few hours of infection); and 3) migration of linear DNA to the cell nucleus.

Linear viral DNA becomes linearly integrated into the host DNA under the influence of the enzyme integrase. This integration can occur at many sites, and infected cells can contain up to 20 copies of viral DNA. The proviral genes occur in the same order as their RNA copies occur in the virion, and they are flanked on either side by identical sequences of nucleotides—long terminal repeats (LTRs). These are composed of repeated sequences derived from terminal regions of viral RNA and include promoter and enhancer sequences controlling transcription of viral DNA to RNA. The LTR promoters may also cause abnormal transcription of host genes usually downstream of the proviral DNA, leading to oncogenesis.

TRANSCRIPTION.   Formation of new virions in the infected cell is the result of transcription and translation of proviral DNA, the major events being as follows: 1) Transcription of viral RNA on a template of proviral DNA under the influence of a host RNA polymerase. Viral RNA molecules give rise to mRNA in association with polyribosomes, and they also serve as genomic RNA in the newly formed virions. New viral RNA is detectable within 24 hr of infection. 2) mRNA species, bound to polyribosomes, are translated to form the *gag*, *pol*, and *env* gene-coded proteins that compose the virion. The *gag–pol* gene product is a large protein precursor (180 kD) PR180, which is cleaved to give a precursor polyprotein Pr76 (76 kD) from which virion core proteins p19 (MA), p27 (CA), p12 (NC), p15 (PR) and p10 are derived. The Pr180 polyprotein also gives rise to RT (p63 and p95) and integrase (IN) (p32) enzymes. The *env* gene product is a precursor protein (92 kD), gPr92, from which the viral envelope proteins gp85 (SU) and gp37 (TM) are derived. The viral proteins localize at the plasma membrane of the cell, where crescent-shaped structures that develop into virions budded off from the cell may be visualized.

CELL TRANSFORMATION AND TUMOR FORMATION.   Two main types of strategy are involved in oncogenesis by avian retrovirus (79, 133, 220, 275). The acutely transforming viruses carry differing v-*onc* genes (derived from normal cellular sequences), which are responsible for early onset neoplastic transformation (246). Rous sarcoma virus carries the *src* gene, which encodes a transformation-specific phosphoprotein (60 kD), p60, in the infected cell, with protein kinase activity. Phenotypic change associated with high levels of p60 is believed to be responsible for the transformed state

(188, 193). The *onc* genes associated with other acute transforming viruses encode other transformation-associated proteins. In general, oncogene products fall into four classes: growth factors, growth factor receptors, signal transducers, and DNA transcription factors.

Slowly transforming viruses such as those causing lymphoid leukosis (Table 17.4) do not possess a v-*onc* gene, but transform cells indirectly by activation of a cellular c-*onc* gene. Molecular studies indicate that the ALV provirus becomes integrated within the host c-*myc* locus, which is then expressed under the influence of the viral LTR promoter sequence. Genetic deletions are a feature of the integrated provirus in lymphoma induction (174, 317). The enhanced expression of the c-*myc* gene by this "promoter insertion" is believed to initiate the lymphomagenic process, but multistep activation of other transforming genes such as B-*lym* and c-*bic* may be necessary for the full development of LL (4, 79, 192, 193, 220).

DEFECTIVENESS AND PHENOTYPIC MIXING. A number of avian retroviruses have been shown to have defective genomes and arise either spontaneously or as a result of experimental mutagenesis (193, 396, 397). Some acutely transforming viruses, such as certain strains of RSV, have lost their v-*onc* gene and ability to transform rapidly: they are called transformation defective (*td*) mutants and have an oncogenic potential similar to that of nondefective leukosis viruses (33). Other viruses (acute leukemia viruses) are defective for genes required for replication–replication defective (*rd*) mutants. They will transform cells, but require the presence of a helper virus to enable them to replicate; e.g., BH-RSV and AMV lack the *env* gene and AEV and MC29 lack the *pol* and *env* genes. *Td* and *rd* mutants are defective under all conditions (nonconditional mutants). Conditional mutants function under permissive conditions, not under nonpermissive conditions, and are exemplified by the temperature-sensitive (*ts*) mutants.

BH-RSV is the classic example of an *rd* mutant and is of practical importance in the nonproducer (NP) cell activation test for avian leukosis viruses (see Diagnosis). On single infection of chicken embryo fibroblasts, the defective virus genome of BH-RSV functions to bring about replication of viral RNA, transformation of infected cells, and production of gs antigen, but only noninfectious progeny particles are produced, which are unable to enter new host cells because of an alteration in their envelope glycoproteins. The morphologically altered cells are called NP cells. A nondefective leukosis virus added to these cells acts as a helper virus by complementing the defective genome of BH-RSV and causes both infectious RSV and progeny leuko-

sis virus to be produced simultaneously. Thus, the presence of infectious RSV in the NP test denotes presence of leukosis virus in added test material. This RSV has envelope antigens identical to those of the helper virus, which thus determines infectivity and range of infectivity in genetically different cells, interference patterns among and between subgroups, and type-specific antigenicity. Stocks of *rd* mutant RSV must by their existence contain helper viruses; these were originally referred to as Rous-associated viruses (RAVs). Infectious RSVs formed in these circumstances are called pseudotypes, and their designation includes the helper virus when this is identified, e.g., BH-RSV (RAV-1) when RAV-1 strain leukosis helper virus is used. This phenomenon is an example of the phenotypic mixing (PM) (34) that occurs readily when two related viruses infect the same cell, and in which virions with the genome of one virus may possess envelope and other structural proteins of the other parent, or both. The phenomenon of PM is also employed in the PM test for detection of leukosis viruses (see Diagnosis). Genetic recombination, in which exchanges of genes between two viruses (and consequent stable phenotypic changes) occur, are well recognized and must be distinguished from PM (394, 401). Use of defective strains of RSV allows tailor-made RSV to be produced with envelope properties of the helper virus. Determinations of host range, interference pattern, and neutralization can be performed more easily with the appropriate pseudotype than with the leukosis virus, since the former can be readily quantified in cell culture, by inoculation of the CAM of chick embryos, or inoculation of chicks.

These factors notwithstanding, infectious RSV may be generated with BH-RSV and other *rd* mutants following solitary infections in absence of added helper viruses in certain types of chicken cells that carry endogenous leukosis virus genomes (see Endogenous Leukosis Viruses). Such RSV has the subgroup E host range of the endogenous virus, however, and may be distinguished from helper viruses of other subgroups when NP tests are conducted.

Phenotypic mixing may also occur between unrelated viruses, such as vesicular stomatitis virus (VSV) and avian RNA tumor viruses (395), or between reticuloendotheliosis virus and RSV (335). The VSV with avian RNA tumor virus envelope may be used in rapid interference, host range, and neutralization tests because it is rapidly cytopathic.

ENDOGENOUS LEUKOSIS VIRUSES. The normal chicken genome contains several classes or families of avian retroviruslike elements (86). These include the endogenous viral (*ev*) loci, recognized nearly 30 years ago, and the most recently discovered moderately repetitive elements EAV (36, 123) and ART-

CH (256), and also the highly repetitive element CR1 (367). The genetic sequences of the *ev* loci are related to subgroup E ALVs, and are present as either complete or defective genomes in almost all normal chickens (85, 87, 315, 347) (Fig. 17.18). Some *ev* loci have been located on particular chromosomes (373). They occur in somatic and germ line cells and are transmitted genetically in a Mendelian fashion to their progeny by both sexes (1, 99, 277). At least 29 *ev* loci have been identified (183, 347), but many more evidently exist. On average, each chicken carries about 5 *ev* loci (323). The phenotypic expressions of these loci vary, depending on the viral genes present and on poorly understood control mechanisms (Tables 17.5 and 17.6). When the complete endogenous viral genome is present, subgroup E leukosis virus may be produced by the cell, either spontaneously or after induction by chemicals such as bromodeoxyuridine (BUDR). When the endogenous viral genome is incomplete (defective), genes present may be phenotypically expressed in the cells, but infectious virus is not produced because of absence of the complete set of genes needed for infectious virion production; e.g., the defective *ev*3 locus possesses the *gag* and *env* genes of subgroup E virus, and cells carrying this locus contain gs antigen and subgroup E viral envelope glycoproteins. However, the locus has a genetic deletion around the *gag-pol* junction, and infectious virions are not formed. Presence of *ev* genes in such cells is responsible for their positive reactions in the enzyme-linked immunosorbent assay (ELISA) test, the complement-fixation test for avian leukosis viruses (COFAL), and the chick helper factor (chf) test (see Diagnosis), whereby genetic defectiveness in the envelope of BH-RSV is complemented by endogenous envelope proteins resulting in an infectious form of RSV with subgroup E host range and other properties. Genetic characteristics of *ev* loci are described in detail by Weiss et al. (396, 397), Smith (347) and Crittenden (86). Expression of endogenous *ev* genes is responsible for a dominant form of genetic resistance of chicken cells to infection by subgroup E viruses from block of virus receptors by envelope protein (280, 318). Transmission of *ev* genes from parent to offspring has been called genetic transmission of leukosis virus, distinguishing it from vertical (congenital) and horizontal (contact) transmission of viruses in an infectious state. However, fully expressed infectious endogenous virus may sometimes also be transmitted vertically and horizontally (353). Related *ev* loci occur in several species of fowl other than domestic chickens, including red jungle fowl and some strains of pheasants, partridges, and grouse, but the distribution does not support a phylogenetic relationship (158). Rather, it is believed that the leukosis virus

genomes have become incorporated at various loci relatively recently in the history of *Gallus* and independent of integration in other genera. It is not known whether endogenous viruses arise from exogenous ALV of other subgroups, from which they differ genomically at the *env* gene and in the LTR region, or vice versa.

Subgroup E ALV, typified by RAV-0 , has little or no oncogenicity (250), apparently because of the weak promoter activity of the LTR. Persistence of

Table 17.5. Phenotypic expression of representative endogenous viral (*ev*) genes in normal chicken cells

Phenotype	Symbol	*ev* locus
No detectable viral product	gs⁻chf⁻	1, 4, 5
Expression of subgroup E envelope antigen	gs⁻chf⁺	9
Coordinate expression of group-specific and envelope antigens	gs⁺chf⁺	3
Spontaneous production of subgroup E virus	V-E⁺	2

Source: Adapted from Smith (347)

Table 17.6. Phenotypes of endogenous retroviral (*ev*) genes in inbred and commercial lines of white leghorn chickens

ev	Phenotype	Line or Source[a]
1	gs⁻chf⁻	Most lines
2	V-E⁺	RPRL72
3	gs⁺chf⁺	RPRL63
4	gs⁻chf⁻	SPAFAS
5	gs⁻chf⁻	SPAFAS
6	gs⁻chf⁺	RPRL151
7	V-E⁺	RPRL 15B
8	gs⁻chf⁻	K18
9	gs⁻chf⁺	K18
10	V-E⁺	RPRL 15I4
11	V-E⁺	RPRL 15I4
12	V-E⁺	RPRL 151
14	V-E⁺	H & N
15(C)	None	K28 x K16
16(D)	None	K28 x K16
17	gs⁻chf⁻	RC-P
18	V-E⁺	RI
19	V-E⁺(?)[b]	RW
20	V-E⁺(?)[b]	RW
21	V-E⁺	Hyline FP

Note: *Ev*13 is associated with the gs⁻ chf⁻ phenotype, but restriction fragments have not been characterized.

[a]Not exclusive to line or source. K, Kimber; R, Reaseheath; H & N, Heisdorf and Nelson; for references see Smith (347).

[b]The presence of five *ev* loci in Reaseheath line W birds precludes definitive assignment with the V-E⁺ phenotype. Definitive association requires further segregation of *ev* genes. Hyline FP birds also carry *ev*1, *ev*3 and *ev*6.

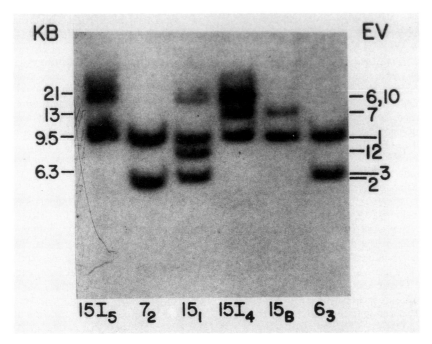

17.18. Endogenous viral (*ev*) loci detected in six inbred lines of white leghorns by restriction fragment polymorphisms generated after Sac-1 endonuclease digestion of red blood cell DNA and hybridized to ^{32}P-labeled RAV-2 genomic sequences. (Smith, Martinus Nijhoff Publishing)

these viral loci suggests that birds carrying them are not at a great disadvantage, and it is possible that they may be beneficial. Thus, Crittenden et al. (101, 103) have shown that presence of *ev*2 or *ev*3 protects birds from a unique nonneoplastic syndrome caused by infection with an exogenous subgroup A ALV. It is possible that endogenous viruses may have either beneficial or detrimental effects, perhaps by their induction of immunity or tolerance to tumor virus antigens, depending on when they are expressed. Embryonic infection with endogenous leukosis virus, RAV-0, caused more persistent viremia and more neoplasms following infection with exogenous ALV, apparently due to tolerant depression of specific humoral immunity (105). Endogenous viruses of the *ev* family are not essential, since it has been possible to produce chickens free of *ev* genes (2). A line of such chickens has been produced, designated line 0 (88), and is of value in research studies where birds or cells free from *ev* loci are needed. Other chickens lacking *ev* loci have been recognized (86) but the great majority have these endogenous sequences.

Of particular importance is the *ev*21 locus, which is tightly linked in White Leghorn stock to the dominant sex-linked gene, *K,* on the Z chromosome, which regulates slow feathering. It is possible that insertion of the *ev* 21 sequence into a feather growth locus is responsible for the slow feathering mutation (86). Some breeders producing feather-sexed crosses have reported reduced egg production and higher leukosis mortality associated with an increased incidence of viremia with exogenous leukosis virus in fast feathering female progeny from dams carrying the *K* gene. It appears that the *ev* 21 gene is expressed as an infectious endogenous virus, EV21, in the dam, which is transmitted congenitally to the progeny, inducing immunologic tolerance and, consequently, increased susceptibility to infection by exogenous leukosis virus (9, 191). Strategies to overcome the *ev*21 locus effect have been studied by Smith et al. (354, 355).

The biologic functions, if any, of the other endogenous elements described, namely CR1, EAV, and ART-CH, remain to be determined. An endogenous EAV-related element, EAV-HP, has very high homology to the *env* gene of the exogenous subgroup J HPRS-103 strain of ALV (11, 12).

Resistance to Chemical and Physical Agents

LIPID SOLVENTS AND DETERGENTS. Avian retroviruses have a high lipid content in the envelope, and their infectivity is abolished by ethyl ether (157). The detergent sodium dodecyl sulfate disrupts the virions and releases RNA and core proteins (316).

THERMAL INACTIVATION. The half-life of various leukosis/sarcoma viruses at 37 C varies from 100 to 540 min (average, around 260 min), depending on the medium in which the virus is suspended, the tissue of origin, and the virus strain (382). Avian tumor viruses are inactivated rapidly at high temperatures; the half-life for RSV at 50 C is 8.5 min and at 60 C, 0.7 min (117).

Thermal lability of infectivity of these viruses is a critical factor in storage. Even at -15 C, the half-life of AMV is less than 1 wk (126); it is only at temperatures below -60 C that avian retroviruses can be stored for several years without loss of infectivity (39). The virus is degraded by freezing and thawing and the gs antigen is released.

pH STABILITY. There is little change in stability of viruses of this group between pH 5 and 9; outside this range, inactivation rates are markedly increased.

ULTRAVIOLET IRRADIATION. Rous sarcoma virus is 10 times more resistant to exposure to ultraviolet light than is Newcastle disease virus, even though these viruses have similar size, structure, RNA content, and sensitivity to X rays (325). Similar resistance has been observed with certain field strains (157).

Strain Classification. Strains of avian leukosis/sarcoma viruses are classified according to the predominant pathologic lesion they induce and the subgroup envelope they possess. Common laboratory strains of avian leukosis/sarcoma viruses are listed in Table 17.4 (396). They are given (by a convention based on common practice) a full and an abbreviated designation on the basis of the predominant neoplasm they induce, with an affix to indicate their origin with an individual, e.g., Rous sarcoma virus (RSV), or location, e.g., Regional Poultry Research Laboratory isolate 12 of LLV (RPL12-LLV). Substrains of RSV are designated according to individuals who studied them, e.g., the high-titer strain of Bryan (BH-RSV), or according to location, e.g., Prague (PR-RSV). Subgroups (e.g., A) may be designated also: PR-RSV-A. The general terms *avian leukosis* (or *leukemia*) *virus* (ALV) and *avian sarcoma virus* (ASV) are widely used to designate members of the group.

Helper viruses isolated from stocks of other viruses, e.g., RAVs, have been designated numerically (e.g. RAV-1). Where a helper virus is used for replication of a defective virus, this is indicated also. Thus, BH-RSV grown with RAV-1 as a helper is designated BH-RSV (RAV-1). Strains of ALV that act as resistance-inducing factors (see Diagno-

sis) were designated RIFs, but this term is now rarely used.

Laboratory Host Systems

CHICK INOCULATION. Rous sarcoma virus and other sarcoma viruses produce tumors when injected by the subcutaneous (SC), intramuscular (IM), or intraabdominal (IA) routes or by contact with inoculated chickens. Subcutaneous injection into the wing web can be used for TD50 assays of stocks of RSV (38), and this route or IM inoculation is used for virus isolation and propagation (243, 307). Intracerebral (IC) inoculation of day-old chicks has been employed for detection of genetic resistance to the virus (182). Following wing-web injection with high doses of virus, tumors are first palpable at about 3 days; in susceptible chickens, these may grow rapidly, ulcerate, and metastasize. With low doses of virus, tumors may occur as late as 35 days postinoculation. There are extensive reviews on methods and interpretation of results (38).

By injecting the RPL12 strain of LLV by the IA route into day-old susceptible line 15I chicks, Burmester and Gentry (49) were able to obtain an LL response in 200–270 days. This procedure was used by Burmester and Fredrickson (48) for initial isolation of virus from field cases. Time required for quantitative assay of certain strains passaged in the laboratory was shortened to 63 days by using the less sensitive erythroblastosis response (42). In these transmission experiments, all sources of virus that caused LL also caused erythroblastosis. Osteopetrosis, hemangiomas, and fibrosarcomas were also observed in chickens of certain strains and passages. The host–virus interrelations were studied in detail by Burmester et al. (55, 57). Avian myeloblastosis virus can be titrated in susceptible chicks by IV inoculation at 1–3 days of age (124, 125); AMV in chicken plasma can be assayed by its adenosine triphosphatase activity. The latter method is useful for routine and large-scale studies (27).

Osteopetrosis-inducing activity of some strains of virus can be examined by IV inoculation of day-old chicks (57) or by IM injection of infective material (198). Guinea fowl are particularly sensitive to osteopetrosis induced by MAV-2(0) (215).

EMBRYO INOCULATION. When RSV and other sarcoma viruses are inoculated onto the chorioallantoic membrane (CAM) of 11-day-old susceptible embryos, tumor pocks develop (Fig. 17.19), which can be counted 8 days later and are linearly related to virus dose (120). This technique is also useful for detecting genetic resistance to infection. Tumors can also be produced by IV inoculation at 10–13 days of incubation and by yolk sac inoculation at 5–8 days' incubation.

Leukosis viruses have been quantitated by their

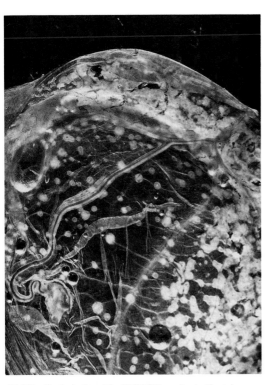

IV inoculation into 11-day-old susceptible chicken embryos. Within 2 wk of hatching, a high incidence of neoplasms occurs (mainly erythroblastosis), although hemorrhages and solid tumors can develop including fibrosarcomas, endothelial tumors, nephroblastomas, and chondromas. When chicks are held for a postinoculation period of 46 days, responses are higher by $1-2 \log_{10}$ dilutions than those following chicken inoculation. Most chickens that survive the acute neoplasms develop LL after 100 days postinoculation (292).

Avian myeloblastosis virus produces a myeloblastosis response within a few weeks when injected IV into susceptible embryos (15).

CELL CULTURE. Rous sarcoma virus and other sarcoma viruses induce rapid neoplastic transformation of cells when inoculated onto monolayer cultures of chicken embryo fibroblasts. The transformed cells proliferate to produce within a few days discrete colonies or foci of transformed cells (Fig. 17.20), which can be used for quantitative assay of virus (371).

Most leukosis viruses replicate in fibroblast culture without producing any obvious cytopathic effect. Their presence can be detected by a variety of tests (see Diagnosis). Leukosis viruses of subgroups B and D may induce cytopathic plaques that may be

17.19. Pocks induced by BH-RSV on chorioallantoic membrane (CAM) of chicken embryo. (Piraino)

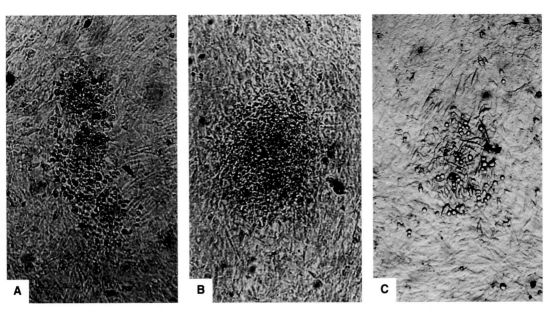

17.20. Foci induced by Rous sarcoma virus (RSV) in cell culture. *A.* Unstained focus of transformed spherical, refractile chicken embryo cells infected 6 days previously with Bryan's standard strain of RSV. ×100. *B.* Unstained focus of transformed, polygonal, opaque Rous sarcoma cells infected 6 days previously with Bryan's high-titer strain. ×100. *C.* Unstained focus of transformed round and fusiform cells infected 6 days previously with Popken's preparation of RSV. ×100.

used for virus assay (175). Morphologic alterations have also been reported after prolonged passage of leukosis virus–infected fibroblasts (61).

Defective leukemia viruses will transform hematopoietic cells in vitro (246). Yolk sac and bone marrow cells in culture are transformed to neoplastic myeloblasts on infection with AMV (248), and bone marrow cells transform to erythroblasts with AEV (176). Transformation of hematopoietic cells by MH2, MC29, and OK10 viruses was observed by Graf and Beug (177). Such acutely transforming ALVs have been extensively used to study avian hematopoietic cell lineages and differentiation (30, 237). In vitro transformation of B lymphocytes by nondefective ALV has not yet been reported.

Tumor cell lines derived from tumors induced in vivo by the avian retroviruses have been developed, including LL (261, 343), myeloblastosis (224), erythroblastosis (178), and myelocytoma (223).

The properties of leukosis/sarcoma viruses in cell culture are described in more detail under Diagnosis.

Pathogenicity. Most strains of avian tumor virus under study were isolated from various types of neoplasms many years ago and have subsequently been passaged experimentally many times in chickens or cell culture. The strains may produce more than one type of neoplasm (Fig. 17.21). The oncogenic spectrum of each strain tends to be characteristic, but often overlaps with responses to other strains, e.g., the RPL12 strain of ALV produces LL, erythroblastosis, fibrosarcomas, hemangiomas, and osteopetrosis; the BAI-A strain of AMV produces myeloblastosis, sarcomas, osteopetrosis, hemangiomas, LL, nephroblastomas, thecomas, granulosa cell tumors, and epitheliomas (Fig. 17.21). As discussed below, the oncogenic patterns of different virus strains are influenced by viral and host factors such as origin; dose; route of inoculation; and age, genotype, and sex of the host. Most studies have been conducted with strains of virus that were not genetically purified, and an important question has been whether ability of a particular strain to cause several neoplasms was a result of presence in virus stocks of a mixture of virus types with differing oncogenic potentials or of pluripotential properties of a single genetic type. Studies show that both explanations can apply. Clone-purified strains of ALV can cause a variety of neoplasms in addition to LL, including erythroblastosis, osteopetrosis, and nephroblastomas (311). Other strains of virus consist of mixtures. This is best exemplified by the defective acute leukemia viruses, which require a nondefective helper virus for their replication. In this situation, oncogenic properties may originate from either the defective or helper virus. Even so, clone-

purified strains of AEV can induce both erythroblastosis and sarcomas, irrespective of the helper virus (179). Varying degrees of relatedness between different pure strains of virus may be demonstrated by nucleic acid hybridization techniques, and the differences can be related to oncogenic properties. These differences may lie in the particular v-*onc* gene present in acute transforming viruses or in other parts of the viral genome in the slowly transforming viruses (193).

ORIGIN OF VIRUS. The strain of virus has a profound effect on the tumor response obtained. The tumor spectrum tends to be characteristic of the strain when it is handled under identical conditions, but may be modified by changes in these conditions. Such differences are also seen in virus strains newly isolated from the field, as exemplified by tumor spectrums of RPL26, RPL27, and RPL28 isolates of ALV (156).

Within a particular strain, differences may be obtained that depend on type of neoplasm used for virus isolation. Thus, using viruses isolated from field cases, Fredrickson et al. (156) observed that serial transfer from donors with LL resulted primarily in LL, whereas virus from donors with erythroblastosis predominantly caused erythroblastosis. In another instance, selection of virus donors with hemangiomas resulted in a larger proportion of virus with this tumor than in the previous passage (55). In some situations, such events may be due to a virus–dose effect, but in other instances, an acutely transforming ALV with a transduced oncogene may have been generated (196).

VIRUS SUBGROUP. Usually no relationship has been observed between virus subgroup and oncogenicity except for endogenous E subgroup LLVs, such as RAV-0, which have little or no oncogenicity (250). However, the low oncogenicity of RAV-0 is believed to be related to differences in the LTR region of the genome and not to the *env* gene. The subgroup J ALV, HPRS-103, induces myelocytomatosis (284), but the viral genetic sequence responsible is not yet known.

VIRUS DOSE. High doses of RPL12-ALV mainly induced erythroblastosis, whereas doses close to the endpoint predominantly induced LL (55). Sarcomas, endotheliomas, and hemorrhages were also more common with high virus doses. Occurrence of osteopetrosis showed no dependency on dose (155).

ROUTE OF INOCULATION. Responses obtained after virus administration by less efficient portals of entry into the host apparently reflect the decreased effective dose. Thus, exposure of susceptible birds by contact with birds inoculated with a high dose of

	Prototype strains and characterizing neoplasms					
Embryonic layer	RPL 12	BAI A	MC 29	R	MH2	RSV, OCS VII
Mesoderm						
Mesenchyme						
Sarcoma	▬	▬	▬	▬	▬	▬
Chondroma			▬			▬
Osteochondrosarcoma						▬
Osteopetrosis	▬	▬		▬		
Endothelioma			▬		▬	
Mesothelioma			▬			
Meningioma						▬
Hemangioma	▬	▬	▬	▬	▬	▬
Hemopoietic tissue						
Erythroblastosis	▬		▬	▬		
Myeloblastosis		▬				
Myelocytomatosis			▬			
Monocytosis (?)					▬	
Lymphomatosis	▬	▬	▬	▬	▬	
Kidney						
Nephroblastoma		▬				
Adenocarcinoma			▬	▬	▬	
Ovary						
Thecoma		▬				
Granulosa cell		▬				
Testis						
Carcinoma					▬	
Endoderm						
Liver						
Hepatocytoma			▬		▬	
Pancreas					▬	
Ectoderm						
Epithelioma		▬	▬		▬	
Glioma						▬

17.21. Oncogenic spectrum of selected avian leukosis viruses. *Black bars* represent a response of that type. (Beard, Raven Press).

RPL12 virus resulted in an LL response similar to that expected with 1/1000 of the inoculated dose (55). Intramuscular inoculation of RPL26 virus favored sarcoma induction, whereas IV inoculation mainly produced erythroblastosis and hemorrhages (155). These differences may reflect variations in amounts of virus that reach the target cells by different routes.

AGE OF HOST. In general, resistance of birds to development of neoplasms of all types increases with age, the rate varying with route of inoculation. Resistance increases rapidly between 1 and 21 days of age with oral or nasal administration, but relatively slowly when virus is inoculated intravenously (57). Types of tumors produced also reflect the decreased effective dose (55). However, the incidence of some tumors decreases more rapidly than expected from the dose effect alone; e.g., certain RPL12 virus preparations given intravenously at 1 day of age caused a high incidence of osteopetrosis; the proportion of chickens inoculated at 3 wk of age and developing osteopetrosis was only one-tenth that of chickens inoculated at 1 day of age (57).

An interesting exception is that very young birds are somewhat less susceptible to strain R of the AEV than older birds (28).

GENOTYPE AND SEX OF HOST. The genetic constitution of the host has a strong influence on response to leukosis/sarcoma viruses (see Pathogenesis and Epizootiology). Females are more susceptible to LL than males. Castration of both sexes increases incidence of this disease, and testosterone increases resistance of males and capons (50). These effects are probably a consequence of hormonal effects influencing regression and, hence, target cell numbers in the bursa of Fabricius.

Homotransplantation.   Many of the tumors induced by viruses of the leukosis/sarcoma group are homotransplantable. In some instances, transplanted tumors can be readily differentiated from primary virus-induced tumors. Thus, transplanted LL tumors grow to a palpable size within 5–10 days and result in death shortly thereafter, whereas primary virus-induced tumors develop 4 mo after inoculation of day-old chicks. Other transplantable tumors also have a shorter incubation period than their virus-induced counterparts. Transplanted LL tumors and nephroblastomas generally appear at the site of inoculation instead of in their originating organs; e.g., in LL tumor transplants, there is usually no bursal tumor (Fig. 17.22). Histologically, transplanted tumors are generally more uniform and more anaplastic than the tumors from which they originate (compare Figs. 17.23 and 17.27). Thus

transplanted LL tumors are composed almost exclusively of large anaplastic lymphoblasts with a vesicular nucleus and several large nucleoli (Fig. 17.23).

Rous sarcomas can be serially transplanted; however, by the second generation only 0.05% of these cells are of donor origin. Even in histocompatible chickens, the proportion of donor cells falls rapidly until there are no mitotic donor cells 6 days after cell inoculation (296). Thus Rous sarcoma cells do not survive long in the recipient, and tumors in the recipient are formed largely from recruited virus-infected cells.

Leukemic myeloblasts from donor birds inoculated with AMV (BAI-A) failed to persist in the recipient when transplanted, and the leukemic cells had the karyotype of the recipient (13).

Erythroblasts from donor birds inoculated with strain R, on the other hand, persisted for longer periods in the recipient: in highly inbred chickens, up to the fifth transplant generation (295).

Lymphoid cells from some LL tumors can be transplanted indefinitely. This is certainly true for the tumor from which the RPL12 strain of virus originated, and for many other virus-induced LL tu-

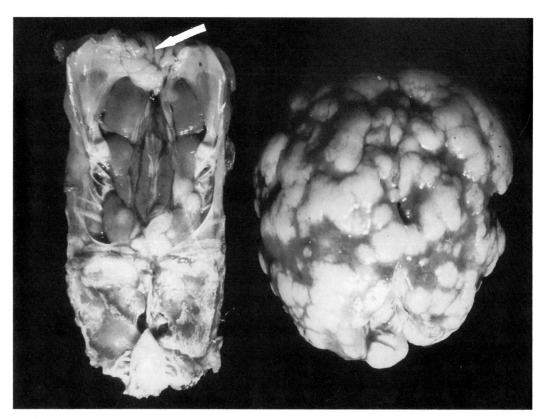

17.22.   Lymphoid leukosis (LL) transplant. Bird died 14 days after inoculation at 1 day of age with suspension from LL tumor induced by HPRS-2 Rous-associated leukosis virus. A lymphoid tumor was also present in abdominal muscle at site of inoculation. Note metastases in liver, lung, and kidney and absence of tumor in bursa (*arrow*).

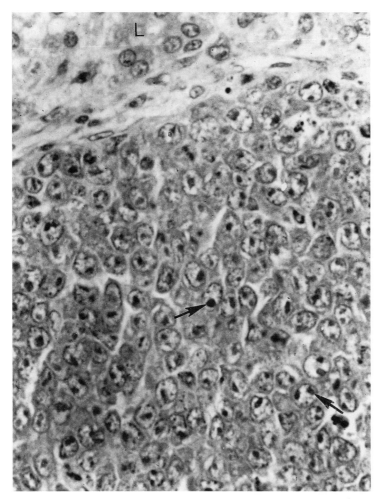

17.23. Microscopic appearance of tumor in Fig. 17.22. Note homogenous large anaplastic lymphoblasts with prominent nucleoli (*arrows*) compressing the liver cells (L). Compare these cells with those in Fig. 17.28 that resulted from infection with virus rather than cells. Cells from bird in Fig. 17.28 were transplanted to induce tumors shown in Figs. 17.22 and 17.23. ×700.

mors. However, some tumors are converted into neoplasms dominated by cells of recipient origin (297).

Several new LL transplantable tumors were described by Okazaki et al. (261).

Nephroblastomas induced by AMV (BAI-A) have been homotransplanted to the breast muscle (204, 386). In addition to tumors at the site of inoculation, recipients have metastatic tumors in the viscera and secondary tumors such as myeloblastosis and LL. Since typical renal growths occurred at the site of inoculation, there is not much doubt that these tumors were of donor origin. However, it is likely that the secondary neoplasms were induced by virus elaborated by the transplant.

Hepatomas induced by MC29 virus are readily transplantable (225, 226). A transplantable epithe-

lial cell line was developed from a liver tumor of a bird infected with MC29 (223).

Investigations of tumor transplants have been of limited assistance in understanding virus-induced tumors; e.g., immunity and genetic resistance to tumors resulting directly from transplantation of neoplastic cells may have no relation to immunity or genetic resistance to virus infection or induction of tumors by virus.

PATHOGENESIS AND EPIZOOTIOLOGY

Natural and Experimental Hosts. Chickens are the natural hosts for all viruses of this group (274), and they have not been isolated from other avian species except pheasants, partridges, and quail, as described under Virus Subgroups. Experimentally, however, some viruses have a wide host range and can be adapted to grow in unusual hosts by passage in very young animals or induction of immunologic tolerance prior to inoculation of the virus. Rous sarcoma virus has the widest host range. It will cause tumors in chickens, pheasants, guinea fowl, ducks, pigeons, Japanese quail, turkeys, and rock partridges. Nehyba et al. (252) found that ALV persisted for at least 3 yr in tissues of ducks embryonally inoculated with ALV in spite of lack of viremia and development of neutralizing antibodies. Some strains of sarcoma virus induce tumors in mammals (382), including monkeys (219). Osteopetrosis can be produced in turkeys by inoculation of fresh whole blood from affected chickens (198). RPL12 strain of ALV did not produce LL or erythroblastosis in Japanese quail (92, 312), and the virus did not multiply in quail. These birds are, however, susceptible to myeloblastosis.

Transmission. Exogenous ALVs are transmitted in two ways: vertically from hen to progeny through the egg, and horizontally from bird to bird by direct or indirect contact (82, 327, 328) (Fig. 17.24). Although usually only a small minority of

chicks are infected vertically, this route of transmission is important epizootiologically because it affords a means of maintaining the infection from one generation to the next. Most chickens become infected by close contact with congenitally infected birds. Although vertical transmission is important in maintenance of the infection, horizontal infection may also be necessary to maintain a rate of vertical transmission sufficient to prevent the infection from dying out (276). The infection does not spread readily from infected birds to birds in indirect contact (in separate pens or cages), probably because of the relatively short life of the virus outside the birds (see Thermal Inactivation).

Four serologic classes occur in mature chickens in relation to ALV infection: 1) no viremia, no antibody (V-A-); 2) no viremia, with antibody (V-A+); 3) with viremia, with antibody (V+A+); 4) with viremia, no antibody (V+A-) (327, 328). Birds in an infection-free flock and genetically resistant birds in a susceptible flock fall into the category V-A-. Genetically susceptible birds in an infected flock fall into one of the other three categories. Most are V-A+, and a minority, usually less than 10%, are V+A-. Most V+A- hens transmit ALV to a varying

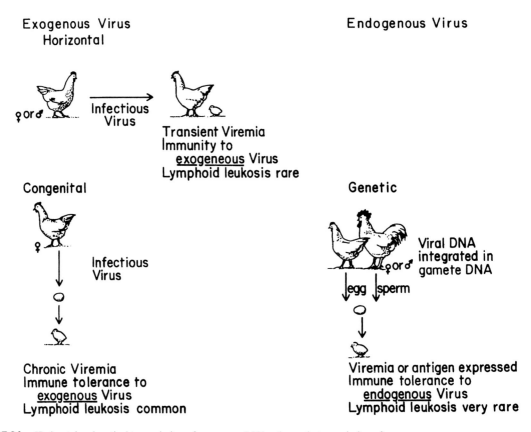

17.24. Horizontal and vertical transmission of exogenous LLV and genetic transmission of endogenous virus. (Crittenden, Avian Pathol)

but relatively high proportion of their progeny (281, 328). A small proportion of V-A+ hens transmit the virus congenitally and do so more intermittently; the tendency for congenital transmission of ALV in this category was found to be more frequent in hens with low antibody titer (380). Congenitally infected embryos develop immunologic tolerance to the virus and after hatching make up the V+A- class, with high levels of virus in the blood and tissues and an absence of antibodies. Older hens (2 or 3 yr of age) transmit virus in their eggs less consistently and at a lower level than birds under 18 mo (53). Infection of the cock apparently does not influence rate of congenital infection of progeny (327, 362). The genetics of the host and the strain of ALV influence shedding and congenital transmission after horizontal infection (103). With electron microscopy, virus budding has been seen on all structures of reproductive organs of cocks except germinal cells (115), indicating that the virus does not multiply in germ cells. The cock, therefore, acts only as a virus carrier and source of contact or venereal infection to other birds (340, 349, 362). Congenital infection of embryos is strongly associated with shedding by the hen of leukosis virus into egg albumen and with presence of virus in the vagina of hens (281, 361). These traits are also highly correlated with viremia.

Shedding of virus into egg albumen and transmission to the embryo is a consequence of virus production by albumen-secreting glands of the oviduct. In most hens congenitally transmitting ALV, the highest titers of virus were found in the ampulla of the oviducts, suggesting that embryo infection is closely related with ALV produced at the oviduct but not with ALV transferred from other parts of the body (378). Electron microscopy studies have revealed a high degree of virus replication in the magnum of the oviduct (114). Virus budding also occurs in various cell types in the ovary, but not in the follicular cells or ovum, and transovarial infection does not seem to be important (281). Not all eggs that have ALV in the albumen give rise to infected embryos or chicks; in the studies of Spencer et al. (361), Payne et al. (281), and Tsukamoto et al. (380) only about one-half to one-eighth of embryos were infected from eggs with virus in the albumen. This intermittent congenital transmission may be a consequence of neutralization of virus by antibody in the yolk and of loss because of thermal inactivation. Congenital transmission of ALV has been found in the absence of detectable shedding of group-specific antigen (202).

Electron microscopy has revealed virus particles in many organs from infected chicken embryos, and virus has been observed to bud and accumulate in large amounts in pancreatic acinar cells of embryos (404). These particles, which are highly infectious,

are shed in droppings of newly hatched chicks (43). Infectious virus is also present in saliva and feces of older birds that provide a source of horizontal infection to other birds (43).

Usually, only a minority of ALV-infected birds develop LL; the others remain as carriers and shedders. Viremic-tolerant (V+A-) birds are reported to be several times more likely to die of LL than those with antibody (V-A+) (327). Incidence of leukosis decreases rapidly if infection by natural routes occurs after the 1st few weeks of age (57); there are well-established genetic differences in susceptibility to LL development in chickens that are equally susceptible to virus infection (97).

Endogenous ALVs (see Etiology) are usually transmitted genetically in germ cells of both sexes (Fig. 17.24). Many are genetically defective and incapable of giving rise to infectious virions, but some are not and may be expressed in an infectious form in either embryos or hatched birds. In this form, they are then transmitted similarly to exogenous viruses, although most chickens are genetically resistant to such exogenous infection. Endogenous viruses have little or no oncogenicity (250) but may influence response of the bird to infection by exogenous ALV (101). Immunodepression induced by infectious bursal disease virus increased the rate of shedding of ALV (147).

Pathology. One or more specific neoplasms induced by leukosis/sarcoma group viruses may occur in a given flock of chickens. Presence of a tumor similar to that produced under experimental conditions is only provisional evidence that the bird was infected with a virus of this group. Some tumors do not yield virus, so it has not been possible to show that all tumors of a given type are caused by a virus of this group. In this section, the pathology of the different neoplasms is discussed without regard for virologic properties of the inducing agent(s). Only entities that have been reproduced with viruses of the leukosis/sarcoma group are described. The strong promoters of gene expression in leukosis/sarcoma viruses can be integrated in many places in the host genome. They then have the capacity to increase expression of genes downstream of them. Depending on where they integrate, they can cause a whole variety of neoplasms and neoplastic processes or disturbances in the normal physiology of the host. Some viruses integrate more frequently in one location than another, and thus tend to induce a particular neoplasm or physiologic disturbance more frequently than other neoplasms or disturbances.

NONNEOPLASTIC CONDITIONS. Chickens, turkeys and jungle fowl exposed to certain leukosis viruses (RAV-1, RAV-60, MAV-2[0], and viruses of subgroups B and D) when young develop anemia, hepatitis, immunodepression, and wasting; some may die (101, 356, 393). A myocarditis and chronic circulatory syndrome was reported in chickens inoculated with RAV-1 ALV (173). Chickens inoculated with RAV-7 develop neurologic signs including ataxia, lethargy, and imbalance resulting from a nonsuppurative meningoencephalomyelitis (398). A persistent infection of the central nervous system, with inflammatory lesions and clinical signs, followed in ovo infection by RAV-1 (136). Anemia is due to an aplastic crisis in the bone marrow in which erythrocytes fail to incorporate iron into hemoglobin and exhibit a decreased survival time (106). Administration of antiviral antibody will prevent anemia (300). The immunodepression may involve atrophy or aplasia of lymphoid organs, hypergammaglobulinemia, decreased mitogen-induced blastogenesis, and decreased antibody response (356). The changes in the immune system are likely due to cessation of B-cell maturation and a block in development of suppressor T cells, possibly due to interference with the synthesis of functional interleukin-2 (197, 221). In addition to stunting and atrophy of the lymphoid organs, RAV-7 causes obesity, high triglyceride and cholesterol levels, reduced thyroxine levels (hypothyroidism), and increased insulin levels (70). The frequent occurrence of stunting may relate to the virus's suppression of thyroid function. Although not examined extensively, leukosis viruses are likely to have similar physiologic effects in the field. Subclinical physiologic effects are likely to contribute to the decreased productivity described below.

Viral infection in the absence of overt disease can adversely affect productivity of egg-laying chickens. Hens that shed virus produced 20–35 fewer eggs per hen housed to 497 days of age; matured later sexually; and produced smaller eggs, at a lower rate, and with thinner shells compared with nonshedders. Mortality from causes other than neoplasms was 5–15% higher, fertility was 2.4% lower, and hatchability was 12.4% lower in shedders than nonshedders (166). These viruses have similar effects on broiler breeders, and also caused a consistent though small (up to 5%) reduction in broiler growth rate (102, 167). Other studies on reduced productivity in chickens with ALV infections, and the genetic consequences, have been reviewed (165, 203, 359). The presence of ALV in semen was not associated with reduced semen production, but there is some evidence for an effect on semen quality and fertility (340).

LYMPHOID LEUKOSIS

Incubation Period. After the inoculation of susceptible embryos or 1- to 14-day-old susceptible chicks (e.g., line 15I) with a standard strain of virus-RPL12 (55), B15, F42 (32), or RAV-1, LL ap-

pears between the 14th and 30th wk of age. Very rarely do cases occur in chickens under 14 wk. Certain laboratory recombinant viruses have been shown to cause lymphoid leukosis within 5–7 wk (210), though such short incubation periods are not found in field outbreaks. In field outbreaks, cases can occur any time after 14 wk of age; however, incidence is usually highest at about sexual maturity.

Signs. Outward signs of disease are not specific. The comb may be pale, shriveled, and occasionally cyanotic. Inappetence, emaciation, and weakness occur frequently. The abdomen is often enlarged and feathers are sometimes spotted with urates and bile pigments. Enlargement of liver, bursa of Fabricius, and/or kidneys can often be detected on palpation, and the nodular nature of liver tumors can at times be detected. Once clinical signs begin to develop, the course is usually rapid.

Gross Lesions. Grossly visible tumors almost invariably involve liver (Fig. 17.25; see also Fig. 17.30A), spleen, and bursa of Fabricius (Figs. 17.26 and 17.30G). Size of tumors is highly variable as are number of organs affected, which may include (in addition to liver and spleen) kidney, lung, gonad, heart, bone marrow, and mesentery.

Tumors are soft, smooth, and glistening; a cut surface appears slightly grayish to creamy white and seldom has areas of necrosis. Growth may be nodular (Fig. 17.25), miliary, or diffuse (see Fig. 17.30A), or a combination of these forms. In the nodular form, lymphoid tumors vary from 0.5 mm to 5 cm in diameter and may occur singly or in large numbers. They are generally spherical but may be flattened when they are close to the surface of an organ. The granular or miliary form, which is most obvious in the liver, consists of numerous small nodules less than 2 mm in diameter and uniformly distributed throughout the parenchyma. In the diffuse form, the organ is uniformly enlarged, slightly grayish in color, and usually very friable. Occasionally, the liver is firm, fibrous, and almost gritty.

Histopathology. Microscopically all tumors are focal and multicentric in origin. Even in organs appearing diffusely involved when examined grossly, the microscopic pattern is one of coalescing foci. As tumor cells proliferate, they displace and compress cells of the organ rather than infiltrate between them (Fig. 17.27). Nodules in the liver are usually surrounded by a band of fibroblastlike cells that have been shown to be remnants of sinusoidal endothelial cells (181).

Tumors consist of aggregates of large lymphoid cells that may vary slightly in size but are all at the same primitive developmental stage. They have a poorly defined cytoplasmic membrane, much basophilic cytoplasm, and a vesicular nucleus in

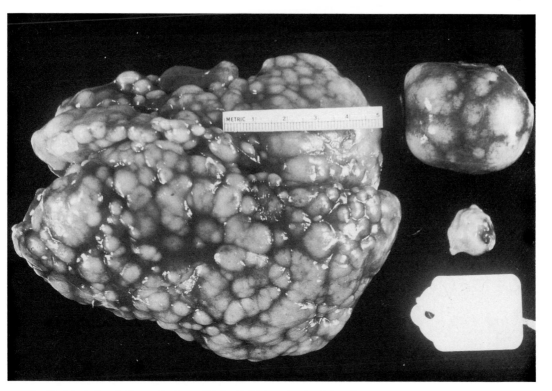

17.25. Nodular lesions in liver and spleen of bird with LL inoculated at 1 day of age with RPL12 virus. Bursa also has a small tumor.

which there is margination and clumping of the chromatin and one or more conspicuous acidophilic nucleoli.

The cytoplasm of most tumor cells contains a large amount of RNA, which stains red with methyl green pyronin, indicating that the cells are immature and rapidly dividing (80). The predominant cell is a lymphoblast. Characteristic features of the cell can best be seen in wet-fixed smears of fresh specimens that have been stained with May-Grünwald-Giemsa, methyl green pyronin, or other cytologic stains.

ULTRASTRUCTURE. Vacuoles are found infrequently in lymphoid cells of birds with LL, but some virus particles have been observed budding from the plasma membranes of lymphoblasts (116, 119). Intracytoplasmic viral matrix inclusion bodies have been observed in the myocardium of ALV-infected adult chickens (171, 251).

HEMATOLOGY. There are no consistent or significant changes in cellular elements of circulating blood. Rarely are there frank leukemic cases in which lymphoblasts predominate. Lymphoblasts are characterized by their large size, large eccentric nucleus with spongy chromatin, and moderate amount of intensely basophilic cytoplasm.

Pathogenesis. Calnek (63) infected day-old chicks and examined them 4–10 wk later. He observed no clinical signs of disease, but found gross lesions in spleen, heart, and testis, and microscopic lesions in liver and other visceral organs as well as dorsal root ganglia. The spleen was slightly or moderately enlarged and usually mottled; the testis and heart had one or more small (up to 1 mm diameter), grayish translucent areas. Microscopically, lesions were either small discrete foci or larger diffuse areas of lymphoblasts (Fig. 17.28). These lesions were transitory, since they were not grossly visible in birds over 10 wk of age, and microscopic accumulations were also markedly reduced. These lesions are most likely inflammatory and may relate to other nonneoplastic disease processes caused by ALVs, e.g. anemia, hepatitis, and wasting (357, 393). Similar early lesions have been reported in ALV-infected turkeys (131).

Three lines of evidence indicate that LL is a malignancy of the bursa-dependent lymphoid system. The first is that removal of the bursa prevents LL, and that it occurs in birds chemically bursectomized and transplanted with viable cells (306) from genetically susceptible chickens, but not from chickens genetically resistant to tumor development (310). The following treatments applied to ALV-infected birds effectively destroy the bursa of Fabricius and

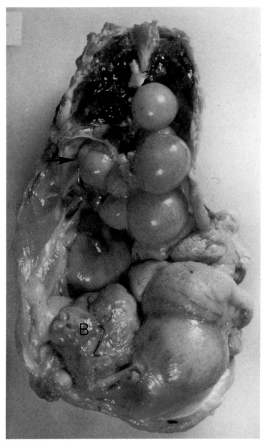

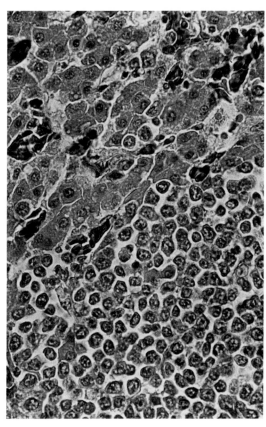

17.27.   Liver tumor from a 20-wk-old chicken inoculated at 1 day of age with RAV-1 ALV. Note displacement and compression of hepatic parenchyma. ×700. (Martinus Nijhoff)

17.26.   Large tumor of bursa of Fabricius (*B*) and kidneys (*arrow*) in naturally occurring case of lymphoid leukosis in adult hen.

eliminate LL: surgical bursectomy between 1 day and 5 mo of age (290), treatment of embryos or hatched chicks with androgens either by inoculation or in feed (45), feeding of androgen analogues (Mibolerone) that have little or no androgenic effect (209, 321), chemical bursectomy with cyclophosphamide (306), and infection with infectious bursal disease virus at 2 or 8 wk (74, 304). Thymectomy has no effect on the course of the disease.

Histopathologic examination of the bursa has provided the second line of evidence. Changes in isolated bursa follicles can be observed as early as 2 wk of age; by 7 wk, abnormal follicles are present in the bursas of most infected chickens (Fig. 17.29) (4, 253, 303). Most tumor nodules originate from transformation of a limited number of cells; i.e., they are clonal (89, 253). As transformed cells proliferate, affected follicles become engorged with uniform blastlike cells with a pyroninophilic cytoplasm, and there is a loss of distinction between the cortex and medulla. Abnormal follicles expand and displace adjacent normal bursal follicles until, by 16–24 wk of age at the earliest, a gross tumor of the

bursa is visible. Constituent cells of abnormal follicles are similar to those in LL tumors of the bursa and other visceral organs. Metastatic tumors in the viscera usually have the same DNA fragments as bursal tumors from the same birds, supporting the idea that they were of bursal origin (89). Autopsies performed on chickens dying with LL have revealed macroscopic tumors of the bursa in almost every case (45, 80, 113).

Immunofluorescence studies provide the third line of evidence. Cells of LL tumors, transplantable tumors, and lymphoid cell lines cultured in vitro have B-cell markers (81, 279) and IgM on their surface (254).

Although target cells may be transformed in the bursa of most birds, only a few develop LL (80). Thus, some early tumors must regress. Other tumors enlarge, and cells burst into the vascular system and initiate metastatic foci in other visceral organs. At about the time of sexual maturity (16–24 wk of age), tumor involvement is so extensive that birds succumb.

Thus even though ALVs multiply in most tissues

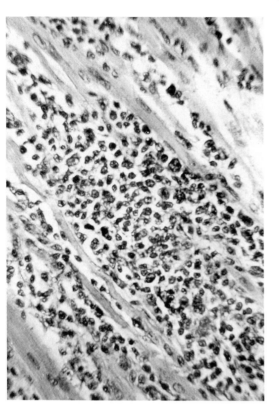

17.28. Lesions in young chickens induced by leukosis virus. Heart from 4-wk-old RIF3-infected chick. Diffuse accumulations of lymphoid cells among myocardial fibers. ×430. (Calnek)

and organs of the body (119, 319), the infection persists longer in bursal lymphocytes than in other hematopoietic tissues (5), and cells of the bursa of Fabricius are the target cells that neoplastically transform. Medullary macrophages may be important in transmitting infection to the lymphoid cells (172). The target cells must have differentiated to some extent (i.e., they are not stem cells) because partial chemical bursectomy will destroy LL target cells before stem cells for the immune response (306). Target cells must be resident in the bursa, however, because bursectomy up to 5 mo of age will eliminate the disease (290).

Molecular biology studies indicate that a viral promoter gene activates a host c-*myc* gene in B cells and results simultaneously in neoplastic transformation and interference with the normal intraclonal switch of B-cell immunoglobulin production from IgM to IgG (89). The c-*myc* host gene is present in all animals and is the cell counterpart of a gene identified first in myelocytomatosis virus MC29. However, experimental inoculation of RAV-1 ALV in 9- to 13-day-old chicken embryos can cause rapid development of LL in which proviral insertion activated the expression of the c-*myb* gene (293,

294). Promotion may be induced by other viruses such as reticuloendotheliosis viruses (see Reticuloendotheliosis) or occur spontaneously in certain virus-free flocks (89). Thus LL tumor cells have IgM on their surface and not IgG or IgA (81). The IgM may be heterogeneous and produced in excessive amounts, particularly late in the disease (351). In addition, subgroup B (but not subgroup A) viruses tested caused T-cell immunosuppression (329).

Serotype 2 MDV was found to enhance the development of LL in certain lines of chickens following exposure to ALV after hatch (10, 140, 141, 142). Molecular and in situ hybridization analysis of the bursa from chickens coinfected with ALV and serotype 2 MDV proved that MDV was closely associated with transformed, but not with nontransformed, bursa cells (164, 232). Recent in vitro studies also showed that serotype 2 MDV can increase ALV as well as RSV gene expression (16, 302, 375).

ERYTHROBLASTOSIS

Incubation Period. The incubation period is influenced by the virus source and strain, dose, route of inoculation, and age and genetic constitution of the host. A major determining factor is likely to be whether the virus strain lacks a viral oncogene, inducing erythroblastosis by promoter insertion activation of the cellular oncogene, c-*erb*B, usually with a long latent period (161, 220), or whether the virus is an acutely transforming strain possessing viral oncogenes. After IA inoculation of the slowly transforming RPL12 strain virus into susceptible day-old chicks, the incubation period varies from 21 to 110 days (55). On IV inoculation of 11-day-old embryos, chicks have occasionally been found to have erythroblastosis on hatching. Strain R virus produces a much more rapid response, and in some experiments, birds inoculated with high doses have all died between 7 and 12 days postinoculation (22). Field strains and viruses passaged in cell culture induce erythroblastosis after a longer incubation period (48). Passage from donors with erythroblastosis greatly shortens the incubation period (156).

Other strains of virus that produce erythroblastosis include F42 (32), ES4, and strain 13 (22). Field cases usually occur in birds over 3 mo of age. Viruses such as RPL12 and F42 are nondefective and slowly transforming, whereas ES4 and R are defective and acutely transforming (177).

Signs. The earliest signs are lethargy, general weakness, and either slight paleness or cyanosis of the comb; as the condition advances, the paleness or cyanosis may increase. There is usually weakness, emaciation, and diarrhea, and there may be profuse

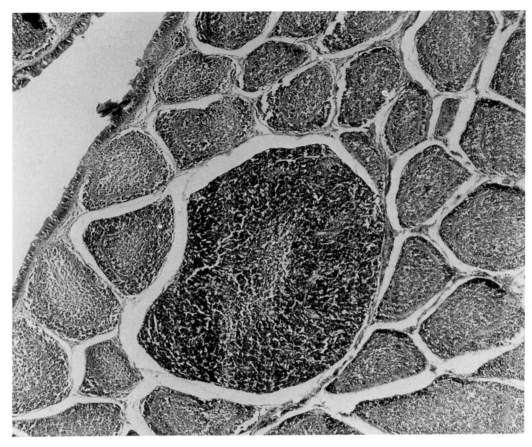

17.29. Lymphoblastic transformation in single bursal follicle in chicken with lymphoma leukosis (LL). All surrounding follicles are histologically normal in this and other sections from 16-day-old chicken infected with RPL12 virus at hatching. Methyl green pyronin, ×40. (Dent, J Natl Cancer Inst)

hemorrhage from one or more feather follicles. The course varies from a few days to several months. With severe anemia, combs may become light yellow to almost white.

Gross Lesions. In birds that die with either form of the disease, there is usually a general anemia often accompanied by petechial hemorrhages in various organs such as muscles, subcutis, and viscera. Thrombosis, infarction, and rupture of the liver or spleen may be observed. There may be subcutaneous edema of lungs, hydropericardium, and ascites, and a fibrinous clot on the ventral surface of the liver (Fig. 17.30B).

The most characteristic gross alteration is diffuse enlargement of liver and spleen and to a lesser extent kidneys. These organs are usually cherry red to dark mahogany (Fig. 17.30B) and are soft and friable. The liver may be finely mottled from degeneration around the central veins of the lobules. The

17.30. Comparison of leukoses. *A.* Lymphoid leukosis (LL). Diffuse form affecting the liver. Lesion is grossly indistinguishable from those in Marek's disease. *B.* Erythroblastosis. Enlarged cherry red liver and spleen. Note the fibrinous exudate. *C.* Myeloblastosis. Note enlarged gray-red liver. *D.* Erythroblastosis. Note basophilic cytoplasm and perinuclear halo. Blood smear, Giemsa, ×975. *E.* Myeloblastosis. Myeloblasts are slightly smaller than erythroblasts; cytoplasm is not as basophilic, nucleus is less vesicular, and nucleoli are not as frequent or conspicuous. Blood smear, Giemsa, ×975. *F.* Myelocytomatosis. Note myelocytes packed with acidophilic granules. Section of tumor, Giemsa, ×975. (Beard) *G.* LL tumors in the bursa of Fabricius (from the same bird as the liver shown in (*A*). *H.* Myeloid leukosis tumor on the surface of the skull. (Peckham)

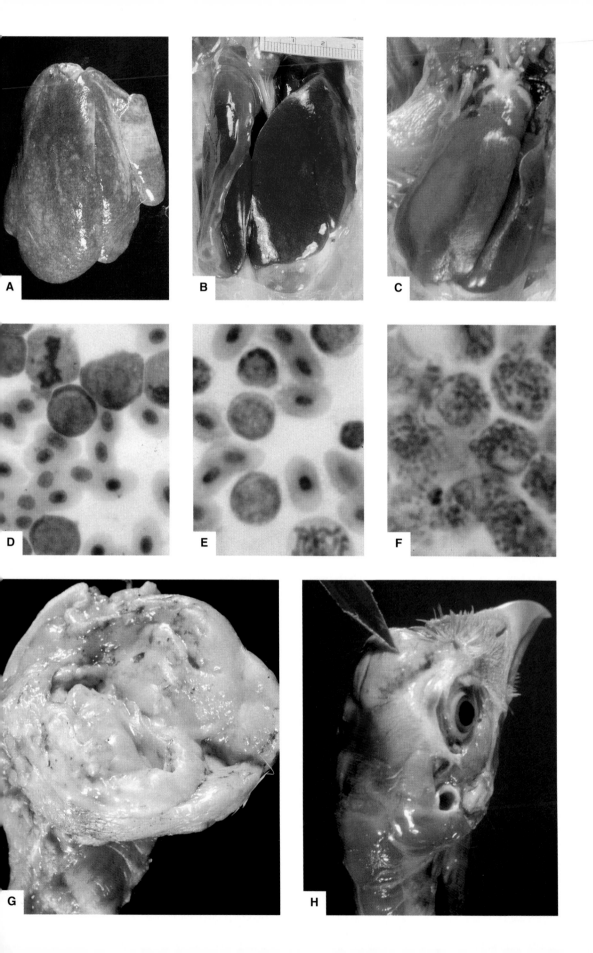

marrow is hyperplastic, very soft or watery, dark blood red or cherry red, and often has hemorrhages.

With severe anemia, visceral organs and organs of the immune system, particularly the spleen, usually atrophy.

Histopathology. Microscopic examination of the marrow in early cases reveals blood sinusoids filled with rapidly proliferating erythroblasts that fail to mature. In advanced cases, marrow consists of sheets of homogeneous erythroblasts with small islands of myelopoietic activity and little or no adipose tissue. With concurrent anemia, the number of erythropoietic cells may be reduced.

Alterations in visceral organs are primarily due to hemostasis resulting in an accumulation of erythroblasts in the blood sinusoids and capillaries (Fig. 17.31). This results in dilation of the sinusoids, which is particularly evident in liver, spleen, and bone marrow. As this process continues, the sinusoids become greatly distended, resulting in pressure atrophy of the parenchyma. In the liver, there may also be a terminal degeneration and even a necrosis of the hepatic cells around the central veins caused by local anoxia. Even though accumulations of erythroblasts may be very extensive, they always remain entirely intravascular, unlike those in LL and myeloblastosis.

Varying degrees of anemia may occur. Sometimes there is no erythroblastosis and there may only be a severe anemia. Extramedullary erythropoiesis is common.

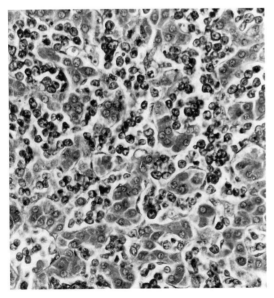

17.31. Erythroblastosis. Liver sinuses permeated with erythroblasts in bird 40 days after inoculation with strain MC29 leukosis virus. ×280. (Beard)

The primary cell involved is the erythroblast. The cell has a large round nucleus with a very fine chromatin and one or two nucleoli and a large amount of cytoplasm that is basophilic. A perinuclear halo, vacuoles, and occasionally fine granules are present. The cell is irregular in shape and often has pseudopodia. Erythroblasts have physiologic markers that identify them as members of the erythrocytic series (see Differential Diagnosis).

ULTRASTRUCTURE. Numerous studies have been made of the primitive cells in erythroblastosis induced by different strains of virus including R (22, 23) and RPL12 (116). Neoplastic erythroblasts in tissues, spleen, and bone marrow are for the most part indistinguishable from corresponding cells of the normal bird, except that virus particles may be present in extracellular spaces and within vacuoles inside cells. In erythoblasts in the circulating blood, as in cell culture, there is a great increase in membrane activity, with vacuolization of the cytoplasm and budding of virus particles from the cell membrane. Only occasionally are aberrant structures seen in erythroblasts (116).

HEMATOLOGY. Changes in the blood reflect those occurring in other organs such as liver, spleen, and bone marrow and depend largely on the extent of anemia or leukemia. When there is severe anemia, the blood is watery and light red and clots slowly. In contrast, acute cases may show no grossly apparent changes, though usually the blood appears dark red with a smoky overcast. Stained blood smears reveal a variable number of erythroblasts (see Fig. 17.30D). These vary in maturity from the early erythroblast, which is the predominant cell, to the various stages of polychrome erythrocytes. The more mature cells often appear early in the course of the disease or during remission, if and when it occurs.

The thrombocytic series of cells may be somewhat increased in number and immaturity. Similarly, in most naturally occurring cases, immature cells of the myelocytic series appear in the peripheral circulation. Occasionally, they are as prominent as the erythroblasts.

Pathogenesis. Acutely transforming erythroblastosis viruses contain the transforming *erbB* gene specific for erythroblastosis viruses (v-*erbB*) and some strains also contain a second gene, v-*erbA,* which blocks erythroid precursor cell differentiation (89, 177, 180).

Slowly transforming ALVs lacking a viral oncogene induce erythroblastosis by inserting a promoter gene adjacent to the cellular oncogene c-*erbB* (161, 220). During the induction of erythroblastosis in this way, new erythroblastosis virus possessing viral *erb* genes may be generated by recombination of host cell genes and ALV genes (196).

Many leukosis viruses, particularly those of subgroups B and D, may induce an anemia that may be independent of neoplasia; i.e., it may occur in the absence of or concurrent with neoplastic proliferation (357). There is evidence that the anemia-inducing potential of these viruses is due to the nondefective helper viruses (180).

When birds are artificially exposed to a strain causing erythroblastosis, the first alterations are found in 3 days as foci of proliferating erythroblasts in bone marrow sinusoids. By the 7th day the primitive cells reach the circulating blood, and some foci of erythropoiesis are present in sinusoids of the liver and spleen. Erythroblasts continue to accumulate in hepatic sinusoids until death of the host. This may occur within a few days of appearance of erythroblasts in the blood, although in most naturally occurring cases, the disease proceeds much more slowly (298).

MYELOBLASTOSIS

Incubation Period.
The most studied strain of virus that induces myeloblastosis predominantly is BAI-A. Virus stocks are defective and contain helper viruses of both A and B subgroups (205). After inoculation of susceptible day-old chicks with large doses of virus, changes in the blood can be observed in 10 days, and birds die a few days thereafter. Mortality continues for about 1 mo, and only a few deaths occur after this (56, 125). The virus E26 (177) also predominantly induces myeloblastosis.

Signs.
Signs are similar to those of erythroblastosis. At first there is lethargy, general weakness, and slight paleness of comb. As the condition develops, these signs become marked, and inappetence, pronounced dehydration, emaciation, and diarrhea are seen. There may be hemorrhage from one or more of the feather follicles caused by blood-clotting deficiency. The course is highly variable, but is generally longer than that for erythroblastosis.

Gross Lesions.
There is usually an anemia. The parenchymatous organs are enlarged and friable, but in chronic cases the liver may be firm. Gray diffuse tumor nodules may occur in the liver and occasionally in other visceral organs. Bone marrow is usually firm and reddish gray to gray. In advanced cases, liver, spleen, and kidneys have grayish infiltrations that are usually diffuse but often give the organ a mottled or even granular appearance (see Fig. 17.30C).

Histopathology.
Microscopic examination of parenchymatous organs reveals massive intravascular and extravascular accumulations of myeloblasts with a variable proportion of promyelocytes (Fig. 17.32). Infiltration and proliferation are particularly extensive outside the sinusoids and around the portal tracts in the liver lobules. There is, therefore, a marked replacement of original tissues by pathologic cells in contrast to the fairly uniform intravascular leukostasis encountered in erythroblastosis. Intensive myeloblastic activity in bone marrow is confined to extrasinusoidal areas.

Pathologic and hematologic features of both erythroblastosis and myeloblastosis overlap in many naturally occurring cases.

ULTRASTRUCTURE.
In circulating myeloblasts from birds with myeloblastosis induced by BAI-A, virus particles are only rarely found, and then in small numbers in clear vacuoles (22, 116). However, reticular and phagocytic elements of the spleen and bone marrow are frequently packed with virus particles. When myeloblasts are transferred to cell culture, large numbers of lysosomes appear in the cytoplasm. After some time in cell culture, virus particles can be seen in lysosomes, in vacuoles, and budding at the cell membrane. No other changes can be observed in these cells.

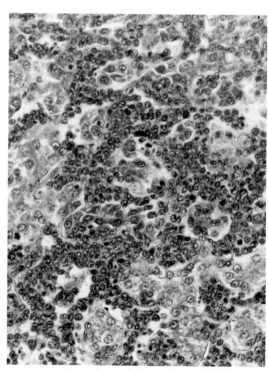

17.32. Myeloblastosis. Distribution of myeloblasts in liver of bird with myeloblastic leukemia 19 days after inoculation with BAI-A virus. ×280. (Langlois)

HEMATOLOGY. Myeloblastosis is characterized by a spectacular leukemia (see Fig. 17.30E). Up to 2 million myeloblasts/mm³ may be found in the peripheral blood. They may compose 75% of all blood cells; thus, on centrifugation, there may be more "buffy coat" than red cells. Myeloblasts are large cells with slightly basophilic clear cytoplasm and a large nucleus containing 1–4 acidophilic nucleoli, which do not usually stain prominently. Often promyelocytes and myelocytes are also present; they can easily be identified by their specific granulation, which in the early forms is primarily basophilic.

The disease may result in a secondary anemia. When this occurs, polychrome erythrocytes and reticulocytes are usually present. Such a secondary anemia is easily distinguished from the conditions in which erythroblastosis and myeloblastosis occur together, since in the latter case, blast forms of both cell series are in the circulating blood.

Pathogenesis. The v-*myb* gene of the virus plays a role in myeloblastosis similar to the role of the v-*erbB* gene in erythroblastosis described earlier (133, 246). The target organ of the causative virus is bone marrow, and the first neoplastic alteration is in the form of multiple foci of proliferating myeloblasts in extrasinusoidal areas. These grow rapidly, overtake normal bone marrow elements, and spill over into the sinusoids. This is followed, perhaps within 1 day, by a leukemia and invasion of other organs by myeloblasts (222). In vitro studies have confirmed the myeloblast as the target cell for transformation by the BAI-A strain of AMV (30).

MYELOCYTOMATOSIS

Incubation Period. Virus-induced myelocytomatosis generally has a longer incubation period than erythroblastosis and myeloblastosis induced by the acutely transforming virus strains, but shorter than LL. On IV injection of MC29 into young chicks, myelocytomas were obtained in 3–11 wk (242). The incubation period in field cases is unknown, but most cases are observed in immature birds. Mathey (234) observed an outbreak in a 6-wk-old broiler flock. The virus CMII also induces myelocytomas (177). Myelocytomatosis induced by the HPRS-103 strain of ALV, which lacks a viral oncogene, had a long latent period (median time to death was 20 wk) (12, 284). However, median time to death with the acutely transforming 879 strain variant of HPRS-103, believed to carry a viral oncogene, was 9 wk (286).

Signs. General signs are similar to those of myeloblastosis. In addition, skeletal growth of myelocytes may result in abnormal protuberances of the head, thorax, and shank. The course is highly variable and usually prolonged.

Gross Lesions. Tumors are distinctive and can be recognized on gross examination with some degree of certainty. Characteristically they occur on the surface of bones in association with the periosteum and near cartilage, though any tissue or organ may be affected. Tumors often develop at the costochondral junctions of the ribs, inner sternum, and cartilaginous bones of the mandible and nares. Flat bones of the skull are also often affected (Fig. 17.30H). Myelocytomas are dull, yellow-white, soft and friable or cheesy, and diffuse or nodular. They sometimes have a thin layer of bone over them, which is easily broken. Multiple tumors are common and are usually bilaterally symmetrical.

Histopathology. Tumors consist of compact masses of strikingly uniform myelocytes with very little stroma (see Fig. 17.30F). Tumor cells are similar to the normal myelocytes found in bone marrow. Their nuclei are large, vesicular, and usually eccentrically located, and a distinct nucleolus is commonly present. The cytoplasm is tightly packed with acidophilic granules, which are usually spherical. When imprint preparations of fresh tumors are stained with May-Grünwald-Giemsa, granules appear brilliant red (see Fig. 17.30F) (242). In the liver, myelocytes crowd the sinuses, invade the acinar cords, and destroy and replace the hepatocytes. A principal attribute of the neoplastic myelocytes is formation of cohesive, organized, and invasive growths in parenchymatous organs (25).

ULTRASTRUCTURE. Ultrastructural features of myelocytoma and myelocytomatosis cells (242) vary from those of well-differentiated myelocytes to those of undifferentiated, nongranulated myelocytes. Myelocytes with granules staining red with May-Grünwald-Giemsa do not differ notably in ultrastructure from their normal myelocyte counterparts. Cells without granules exhibit primitive structure similar but not identical to that of the myeloid progenitor cells. These myelocytes are essentially identical with cells originating in cultures of bone marrow treated with virus strain MC29. Principal features are a singular grainy appearance of the cytoplasm related to high ribosome, polysome, and protein content; sparse rough endoplasmic reticulum; relatively small nucleus with nucleoplasm containing some (but not predominantly) diffuse and dispersed chromatin; and a greatly enlarged nucleolus of usual structure. In structure and behavior, these cells are very different from the myeloblasts induced by BAI-A virus.

HEMATOLOGY. The disease is usually aleukemic, but occasionally is associated with erythroblastosis.

In some birds, especially in the laboratory disease, there may be a distinct leukemia of granulated or nongranulated myeloid cells (Fig. 17.33).

Pathogenesis. The v-*myc* gene of the virus plays a role in myelocytomatosis similar to those of v-*erbB* and v-*myb* genes in erythroblastosis and myeloblastosis (133, 246). The earliest alterations occur in bone marrow in which there is crowding of intersinusoidal spaces, principally by myelocytes, and destruction of the sinusoid walls. Whereas in the normal bird the intersinusoidal spaces contain myeloid series cells in different stages of development, in myelocytomatosis the spaces contain essentially only two types of cells—the primitive hemocytoblastlike cell (myeloid stem cell) and the neoplastic cell (the myelocyte). The latter appears to arise directly from the stem cell, and differentiation is arrested most often at the nongranulated but also at the granulated myelocyte level (242). Nongranulated myelocytes are distinctly different from myeloblasts in morphology and in vitro growth potentials; myeloblasts proliferate enduringly in culture, but myelocytes persist only a few days. (Neoplasms composed of nongranulated cells may be derived from neoplastic transformation of the common stem cell, which gives rise to granulocytes and macrophages; i.e., they may more accurately be called histiocytic sarcomas.) Myelocytes proliferate and soon overgrow the bone marrow. Tumors form by expansion of marrow growths, so that in some cases large neoplasms may crowd through the bone and extend through the periosteum. Extramedullary tumors may arise by metastasis. A transplantable myelocytoma has been developed (223).

HEMANGIOMA

Incubation Period. After experimental inoculation of young chicks with field strains of virus (156), hemangiomas appeared in 3 wk to 4 mo. Most isolates or virus strains have been found to cause hemangiomas (40, 155). These tumors have been found in birds of various ages. In naturally occurring outbreaks, most mortality from hemangiosarcomas occurred at 6–9 mo (58). Induction of lung angiosarcomas by subgroup F ALVs is reported (220, 344).

Signs. Hemangiomas usually occur singly in the skin, though primary multiplicity is not uncommon. When the wall ruptures, profuse hemorrhage ensues. Feathers near the tumor are blood-stained, and the bird may become pale and die of exsanguination.

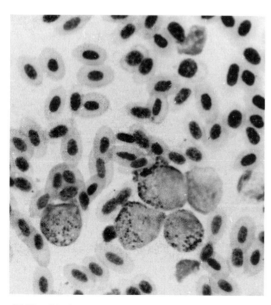

17.33. Myelocytomatosis. Granulated myelocytes in blood smear from bird 23 days after inoculation with strain MC29 leukosis virus. ×750. (Beard)

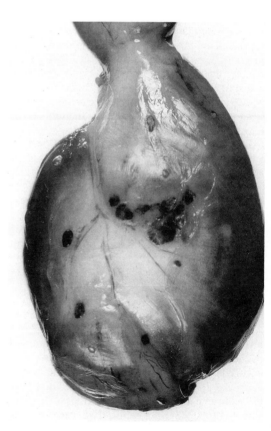

17.34. Hemangioma of gizzard serosa of RPL12 virus-inoculated bird. Note dark circumscribed and raised tumor nodules. (Gross, J Natl Cancer Inst)

Gross Lesions. Hemangiomas in the skin or on the surface of visceral organs can best be described as "blood blisters" (Fig. 17.34). Chickens with ruptured hemangiomas of the skin may be severely anemic. Blood clots are often found in visceral tumors.

Histopathology. The cavernous form is characterized by greatly distended blood spaces with thin walls composed of endothelial cells (Fig. 17.35). Capillary hemangiomas are solid masses varying from gray-pink to red. The endothelium may proliferate into dense masses (hemangioendothelioma), leaving mere clefts for blood channels (Fig. 17.36); develop into a lattice with capillary spaces; or grow into collagen-supported cords with larger interspersed blood spaces. In general, skin tumors are more encapsulated and have more trabeculae than visceral tumors.

ULTRASTRUCTURE. There have been no reports of electron microscopy studies of hemangiomas.

HEMATOLOGY. The blood picture is normal in uncomplicated cases. When the tumor has ruptured, there may be signs of anemia. Hemangiomas often occur in conjunction with erythroblastosis and myeloblastosis.

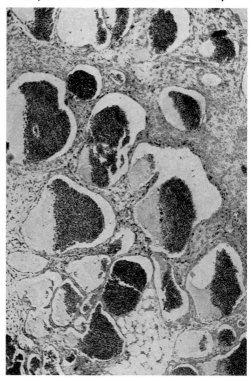

17.35. Cavernous hemangioendothelioma of mesentery. (Feldman and Olson)

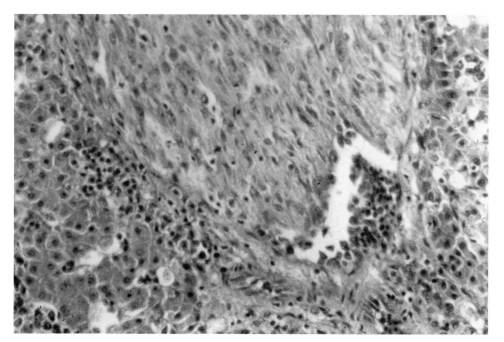

17.36. Endothelioma in liver of bird inoculated with RPL30 leukosis virus. Occlusion of portal vein by inward-growing spindle cells from blood vessel. ×250. (Fredrickson and J Natl Cancer Inst)

Pathogenesis. Hemangiomas are tumors of the vascular system and as such usually involve all layers of blood vessels. In some instances, the endothelium may proliferate more than the supporting tissue. Occasionally, the primitive anaplastic cells may differentiate to hemocytoblasts, so considerable erythropoiesis can occur in these growths. Sequence analysis of an avian hemangioma-inducing virus isolated from layer hens revealed unique elements in both *env* gene and LTR that are probably responsible for its biologic and pathogenic characteristics (59).

NEPHROMA AND NEPHROBLASTOMA. Leukosis virus–induced tumors of the kidney are of two distinct kinds: nephroblastoma of the complex Wilm's tumor type, and adenomatous or carcinomatous growths of widely varied morphology. In studies thus far described, nephroblastomas have been produced experimentally only by BAI-A myeloblastosis virus (25, 56), myeloblastosis-associated virus, MAV-2(N) (390), and virus strain 1911 (286), whereas only the relatively simple though extensive adenomatous or carcinomatous growths are associated with infection by all other virus strains: MC29 (25), ES4 (68), MH2 sarcoma virus (69), Murray-Begg sarcoma virus, HPRS-103 (284), and various field isolates (155).

Incubation Period. Tumors are usually found at necropsy in birds dying or killed because of general aspects of disease. In the field, renal tumors are rarely seen in chickens older than 5 wk. Nephroblastomas induced by BAI-A may reach an incidence of 60–85% in birds not dying of myeloblastosis (56). Most cases are seen in birds between 2 and 6 mo of age.

Carcinomatous growths such as those produced by strain MC29 are found as soon as 18 days or as late as 7 wk after virus inoculation. Incidence in inoculated chickens may be 60% or more, but incidence in field flocks is not known.

Signs. In uncomplicated cases, there are no signs while the tumors are small. As the tumor increases in size, emaciation and general debility are usually seen. Paralysis may result, when the tumor exerts pressure on the sciatic nerve.

Gross Lesions. Nephroblastomas vary from small, pinkish gray nodules embedded in the kidney parenchyma to large, yellowish gray lobulated masses that replace most of the kidney tissue (Fig. 17.37). Tumors are often pedunculated and may be connected to the kidney by only a thin fibrous vascular stalk. Large tumors are often cystic and may involve both kidneys.

Histopathology. In nephroblastomas, the his-

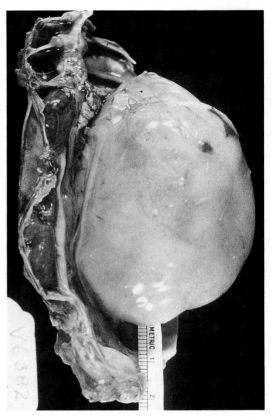

17.37. Nephroblastoma. Bird was inoculated at 1 day of age with avian myeloblastosis virus (AMV) (BAI-A).

tologic variation between different tumors or areas of the same tumor is striking (Fig. 17.38). There is usually neoplastic proliferation of both epithelial and mesenchymal elements, though their proportion and differentiation vary widely. Epithelial structures vary from enlarged tubules with invaginated epithelium and malformed glomeruli; through irregular masses of distorted tubules; to groups of large, irregular, cuboidal, undifferentiated cells with little tubular organization. Particularly in tumors induced by BAI-A AMV, epithelial growths may be embedded in loose mesenchyme or frank sarcomatous stroma. There may be islands of keratinizing stratified squamous epithelial structures (pearls), cartilage, or bone (204). Primary multiplicity of tumors may occur, but metastases are rare.

Adenomatous and carcinomatous growths or nephromas frequently involve both kidneys. Many are enveloped in single or multiple and massive cysts. They vary from a few small nodules to dozens of growths involving the entire organ.

Tumors also vary greatly in microscopic appearance. In tubular adenocarcinomas, primitive abnormal glomeruli frequently occur in large numbers

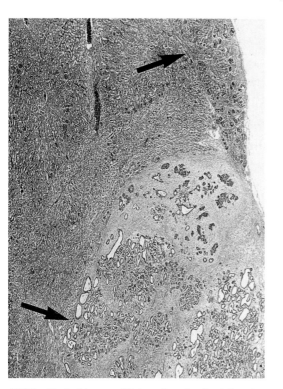

17.38. Nephroblastoma. Bird was inoculated at 1 day of age with cloned preparation of avian myeloblastosis virus (AMV) (BAI-A). Note primary multiplicity of tumors of two distinct types in different areas (*arrows*). ×20

among abnormal tubules. Papillary cyst adenocarcinomas are frequent. At times, solid carcinomatous neoplasms with little evidence of renal tubules develop (26, 242). Rarely is there cartilage, and never are there other mesenchymal tumor tissues. Hemangiomas and endotheliomas sometimes occur in nephromas.

ULTRASTRUCTURE. In the epithelial nephronic elements of nephroblastomas induced by BAI-A virus (22), cytoplasmic aberrant structures are occasionally seen in large or small aggregates. Virus particles bud from cell membranes of epithelial cells, fibroblastic elements of the stroma, and chondrocytes. Sarcomatous elements consist of cells similar in morphology to those in other avian sarcomas. Virus particles have been observed budding from epithelial cells in cystadenomas and adenocarcinomas induced by strain MC29 myelocytomatosis virus (242). Large accumulations of particles in spaces in the cysts and tubules were probably related to lack of tubule and glomerular drainage.

HEMATOLOGY. Uncomplicated cases are aleukemic.

Pathogenesis. Nephroblastomas originate from embryonic rests or nephrogenic buds in kidneys (204). These epithelial structures enlarge and become neoplastic. The supporting stroma of mesenchymal elements also proliferates and in turn may be altered. There is an extensive multiplication of tumor cells (usually convoluted tubules and/or stroma) and varying degrees of differentiation, some abnormal. In the most differentiated form, nephrogenic cells form glomeruli, tubules, or keratinized epithelium, whereas cells of the stroma form sarcomas, cartilage, and bone. Anaplasia of kidney cells can result in sheets of large epithelioid cells with almost no tubular organization. Malformed and blocked tubules result in cysts.

Carcinomatous growths originate only from the epithelial part of the embryonic rests and not from mesenchymal elements. Cartilage that occurs in a few growths originates from morphologically altered epithelial cells. Depending on degree of anaplasia of epithelial elements, tumors formed may be adenomas, adenocarcinomas, or solid carcinomas (26).

HEPATOCARCINOMA. In 18–100 days, the MC29 strain of leukosis virus (25, 225) caused a high incidence of primary tumors of the liver that arose by alteration of hepatocytes, principally in the portal regions. MH2 can also cause liver tumors, but of a different type.

Tumors were elevated above the surface of the liver; varied in diameter from 0.5 to 10 mm or more; yellow-white, gray or reddish tan; and well circumscribed with scant stromal reaction.

Microscopic study revealed several distinct tumor patterns: trabecular, varying in structure from almost normal to markedly disarrayed cell masses; adenomatous or tubular; mosaic and giant cell arrays; hemorrhagic carcinoma complexes; and hepatobiliary cell processes. Within these patterns, there were anaplastic and metaplastic changes, with some cartilage as well as osteoid and spindle-cell tumor formation. Infiltration and invasion of adjacent tissue; penetration of blood vessels; and metastasis to organs such as lung, kidney, and spleen were seen. Prominent features of the tumor cell morphology were very large nuclei of spheroidal and angular contours and large nucleoli ("bird's eye" appearance).

Hepatocarcinomas induced by MH2 are solid structureless masses of large altered liver cells (25) with irregular contours, vesicular nuclei, and large dense nucleoli. Hepatocarcinoma has not been observed under natural conditions.

OTHER EPITHELIAL TUMORS. Thecomas and granulosa cell growths of the ovary have been induced by BAI-A virus (25) and HPRS-103 (284). A seminoma in the testes occurred in one bird inoculated with MH2. This tumor was an adenocarcinomatous growth of seminiferous tubules in which interstitial cells were not involved.

Adenocarcinomas of the pancreas have been induced in chickens by MC29, MH2 and HPRS-103 viruses (25, 241, 284). The Pts-56 strain of osteopetrosis virus produced pancreatic adenomas and adenocarcinomas, and duodenal papillomas in guinea fowl (214, 216, 217). Spontaneous occurrence in nature is very rare.

Squamous cell carcinomas have been observed in a few chicks diseased with MC29 or MH2 (25).

OSTEOPETROSIS

Incubation Period.   After experimental inoculation of day-old chicks with RPL12-L29 (332) or other viruses (197, 198, 300), osteopetrosis may develop anytime after 1 mo of age. It is most commonly seen in birds 8–12 wk of age. The disease probably has a similar incubation period in the field. MAV-2(0) virus will induce palpable osteopetrosis 7–10 days after hatching in chicks inoculated at 1 day of age or as 11- to 12-day-old embryos (154).

Signs.   Long bones of the limbs are most commonly affected (Figs. 17.39, 17.40). There is uniform or irregular thickening of the diaphyseal or metaphyseal regions that can be detected by inspection or palpation. In active cases, the affected areas are unusually warm. Birds with advanced disease have characteristic "bootlike" shanks. Affected chickens are usually stunted and pale and walk with a stilted gait or limp.

Gross Lesions.   The first grossly visible changes occur in the diaphysis of the tibia and/or tarsometatarsus. Alterations soon are seen in other long bones and bones of the pelvis, shoulder girdle, and ribs, but not the digits. Lesions are usually bilaterally symmetric; they first appear as distinct pale yellow foci against the gray-white translucent normal bone. The periosteum is thickened and the abnormal bone is spongy and at first easily cut. The lesion is commonly circumferential and advances to the metaphysis, giving the bone a fusiform appearance (Fig. 17.40). Occasionally, the lesion remains focal or is eccentric. Severity of the lesion varies from a slight exostosis to a massive asymmetric enlargement with almost complete obliteration of the marrow cavity. In long-standing cases, the periosteum is not as thickened as it was earlier; when it is removed, the porous irregular surface of the very hard osteopetrotic bone is revealed.

Osteopetrosis and LL frequently occur together in the same bird. Other tumors have also been described (64). There is an initial slight enlargement of the spleen followed, in birds not simultaneously affected with LL, with splenic atrophy that becomes very severe. There is also a premature atrophy of the bursa and thymus. Many of the other nonneoplastic conditions associated with leukosis/sarcoma viruses occur commonly in birds with osteopetrosis.

Histopathology.   Microscopically, periosteum over the lesion is greatly thickened from an increase in number and size of basophilic osteoblasts. The number of osteoclasts per tibia increases, but the density of osteoclasts (i.e., the number per unit volume of bone) decreases (339). Affected bones differ from normal bones in the following ways. Spongy bone converges centripetally toward the center of the shaft (Fig. 17.41). There is an increase in size and irregularity of the haversian canals, and an increase in number and size, and an alteration in position, of lacunae. Osteocytes are more numerous, large, and eosinophilic; the new bone is basophilic and fibrous.

ULTRASTRUCTURE.   Virus particles bud transiently from osteoblasts and continuously from osteocytes, and accumulate in the periosteocytic space. With calcification of the bone, the particles become incorporated in the bone trabeculae. No virus production is observed from osteoclasts (153).

HEMATOLOGY.   The blood picture is ordinarily aleukemic and there is often a secondary anemia. There may be active erythropoiesis in remaining bone marrow and sometimes in focal areas of the liver, but immature stages are not observed in the peripheral blood. Experimentally, viruses that cause osteopetrosis can induce an aplastic anemia and an increased corpuscular fragility (197, 300).

Pathogenesis.   Avian leukosis virus–induced osteopetrosis is a polyclonal disease of the bone and is thought to be caused by high levels of virus infection perturbing the growth and differentiation of osteoblasts. Recently, much higher levels of virus infection were found in diseased bones than in cultured osteoblasts infected with the Br21 strain of an osteopetrosis-inducing ALV (152). Severe cases of osteopetrosis contained 10 times more viral DNA, 30 times more mature capsid protein, 5 to 10 times more gag precursor protein, and 2 to 3 times more *env* protein than the infected osteoblast cultures. Apparently, the infected cultures lacked aspects of the bone environment that support both the high levels of infection and the aberrant function of osteoblasts characteristic of ALV-induced osteopetrosis. The osteopetrotic lesion is basically proliferative or hypertrophic (64, 332) and may be neoplastic (37, 339). Lesions of the lymphoid organs and bone marrow are degenerative or anaplastic (197). According to Shank et al. (341), the propensity for certain ALVs to induce osteopetrosis

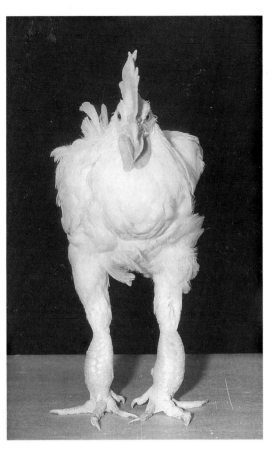

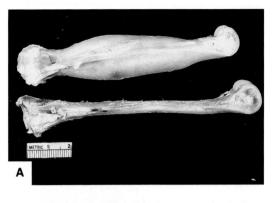

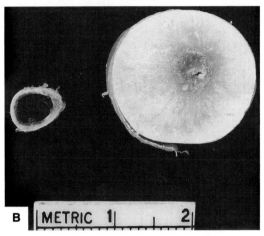

17.39. Osteopetrosis. A 24-wk-old chicken, injected with RPL12 at 1 day of age, with advanced osteopetrotic lesions of the shanks. (Sanger)

17.40. Osteopetrosis of tibia in 10-wk-old chicken.
A. Shorter length of bone is due to reduced growth. Lower tibia is from control bird of same age.
B. Cross section of middle of shaft of bones in *A.* (Sanger, Can J Comp Med Vet Sci)

depends on sequences in the *gag–pol* region of the viral genome.

CONNECTIVE TISSUE TUMORS. This section deals with connective tissue tumors for which there is some evidence of transmissibility and viral etiology. They include fibroma and fibrosarcoma, myxoma and myxosarcoma, histiocytic sarcoma, osteoma and osteogenic sarcoma, and chondrosarcoma. All tumors of this group may occur as either benign or malignant growths. Benign tumors grow slowly, never invade surrounding tissues, and remain almost indefinitely strictly localized processes. Malignant forms grow more rapidly, infiltrate, and are capable of metastasis.

Most virus strains or isolates that induce tumors of the connective tissue are multipotent; i.e., they induce a variety of tumors. Examples are RSV (52) and ES4 (22), which also induce erythroblastosis and LL. Most strains of leukosis virus such as RPL12 (erythroblastosis and LL), BAI-A

(myeloblastosis), and strain R (erythroblastosis) also cause one or more of the solid tumors listed above. Even viruses isolated directly from field cases of LL have produced fibrosarcomas, myxosarcomas, and histiocytic sarcomas as well as hemangiomas and nephroblastomas (155, 156). For review and references, see Beard (22, 25) and Vogt (382).

Incubation Period. Tumors develop readily and are palpable within 3 days after inoculation of chicks with high doses of RSV. With leukosis viruses, sarcomas may occur anytime after inoculation, but are most frequently observed in the first 2–3 mo. In field flocks, connective tissue tumors may occur in birds at any age.

Signs. Until tumors become extremely large, affect the function of an organ, ulcerate, or metastasize, they do not affect the well-being of the host. Some tumors of visceral organs and most of those

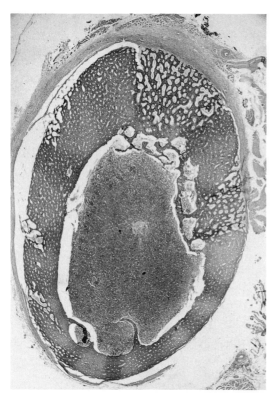

17.41. Osteopetrosis. Cross section of humerus from 8-wk-old chicken. Six separate osteopetrotic foci are present, two of which extend from endosteum to periosteum. ×18. (Sanger, Am J Vet Res)

affecting muscles or integument are palpable. Death may be from secondary bacterial infection, toxemia, hemorrhage, or dysfunction of an organ affected by the tumor. Benign tumors may never cause death, whereas malignant ones may follow a very rapid course, resulting in death within a few days.

Gross Lesions and Histopathology. The different connective tissues distributed throughout the body provide potential sources for a variety of tumors. Fibromas, myxomas, and sarcomas are most likely to arise in the integument or muscles; tumors composed of cartilage or bone or a mixture of these arise where the two tissues are normally found. Sometimes multipotent mesenchymal cells give rise to cartilage and bone where these tissues are not ordinarily present. Of all the connective tissue tumors, histiocytic sarcoma is capable of the widest distribution. Secondary metastatic foci of malignant tumors occur most frequently in lungs, liver, spleen, and intestinal serosa. Primary multiplicity may occur in both benign and malignant tumors; it is characteristic of histiocytic sarcomas.

Fibromas and fibrosarcomas are first noticed as firm lumps attached to the skin, in subcutaneous tissue, muscles, or occasionally other organs. As they grow, the overlying skin often undergoes necrosis and, thus, results in ulceration and secondary infection. When they are cut, their fibrous nature is apparent.

Fibromas in their simplest form consist of mature fibroblasts interspersed with collagen fibers arranged in wavy parallel bands or whorls. Slow-growing tumors are more differentiated and contain more collagen and fewer cells than those growing more rapidly. Some fibromas may have edematous areas and should not be confused with myxomas and myxosarcomas. If necrosis, ulceration, and secondary infection have occurred, various inflammatory and necrotic alterations may be observed in the tumor. Inflammatory changes may be so prominent that the tumor may be confused with a granuloma.

Fibrosarcomas are characterized by aggressive and destructive growth, their cellular composition, and the immaturity of constituent cells (Fig. 17.42). Large irregular and hyperchromic fibroblasts are abundant and mitosis is common. Tumors contain less collagen than fibromas, and this is concentrated in and near irregular septa that subdivide the tumor. Regions of necrosis often occur in rapidly growing tumors. Edema is sometimes present.

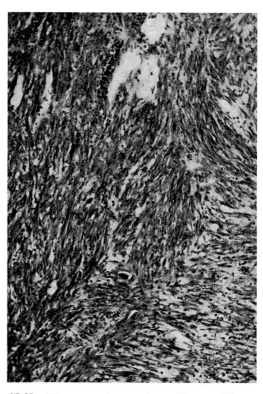

17.42. Fibrosarcoma in musculature of breast. ×120. (Feldman and Olson)

Myxomas and myxosarcomas are softer than fibromas and fibrosarcomas. They contain characteristic tenacious slimy material that pulls out into long strings.

Myxomas consist of stellate or spindle-shaped cells surrounded by a homogeneous, slightly basophilic, mucinous matrix. Long cytoplasmic processes may extend from stellate cells and become fused with sparse collagen fibrils. In the malignant form (myxosarcoma), the mucinous matrix is less abundant and fibroblasts are proportionately more numerous and more immature than in myxomas (Fig. 17.43). Histogenesis and structure of primary myxosarcomatous tumors are similar to those of fibroblastic tumors. The essential difference is that in myxomatous tumors, the fibroblastic cells are more specialized and capable of producing large amounts of mucin in addition to the usual products (collagen and elastic fibrils).

Histiocytic sarcomas are firm fleshy tumors consisting of a mixture of two or more cell types that, while morphologically dissimilar, are closely related histogenically. The most striking microscopic feature is the highly varied nature of the cellular constituents (Fig. 17.44). The cells may be spindle shaped, usually appearing in groups or bundles as in fibrosarcomas; stellate reticulum-producing ele-

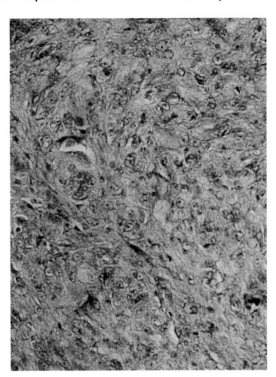

17.44. Histiocytic sarcoma of heart. Note varied character of cellular constituents. ×240. (Helmboldt)

ments (fixed histiocytes); and/or large phagocytic cells or macrophages (free histiocytes). In addition, there usually are numerous transitional forms, many of which are polymorphic. In primary tumors, spindle-shaped cells usually predominate, whereas in metastatic foci primitive histiocytic forms are more numerous.

Osteomas and osteogenic sarcomas are hard tumors that may arise from the periosteum of any bone. Osteomas are structurally similar to bone except that much of the inner histologic details are lacking. They consist of a homogenous acidophilic matrix of osseomucin containing collections of osteoblasts at irregular intervals. Osteogenic sarcomas are usually very cellular infiltrative growths that invade and destroy surrounding tissues. The cells are spindle-shaped, ovoid, or polyhedral, and many are in mitosis. Nuclei are prominent and cytoplasm is basophilic. Multinucleated giant cells may be quite numerous. Although an osteogenic sarcoma is usually a rapidly growing, highly cellular neoplasm of mostly undifferentiated cells, there are usually areas in which there is sufficient differentiation for production of osseomucin. Presence of osseomucin is usually sufficient to identify these tumors.

Chondromas and chondrosarcomas rarely occur in chickens, although cartilage and bone are often found within fibrosarcomas or myxosarcomas.

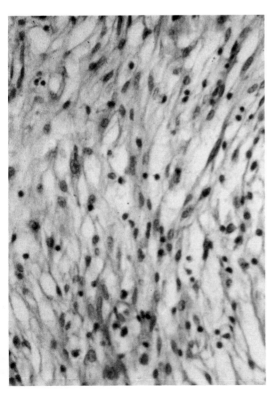

17.43. Myxosarcoma induced by Rous sarcoma virus (RSV). ×240. (Helmboldt)

Such tumors may be designated as fibrochondro-osteosarcomas. Microscopically, chondromas have a typical and unique structure, i.e., groups of two or more chondrocytes lying in a homogeneous matrix of chondromucin. Tumors may be separated into lobules by strands of fibrous connective tissue. In chondrosarcomas there is considerable cellular variation, ranging from the most immature to the fully mature chondrocyte. The former are undifferentiated and spindle shaped, while the latter are spheroidal. Those in the intervening zone are polymorphic.

ULTRASTRUCTURE. Only the sarcomas produced by RSV have been examined in detail. Spindle-shaped cells, macrophagelike cells, and mast cells have been described (22, 184). It is possible that all these forms, as well as those seen in cultures of chick embryo cells treated with RSV, are originally derived from fibroblasts or connective tissue cells. Tumor cells (184) are similar to the cells in culture in showing numerous pseudopodia and pronounced cytoplasmic vacuolization. Some vacuoles may contain virus particles. Structures similar, though not identical, to the gray bodies in myeloblasts have been described, and "clusters" (184) (aberrant structures) may also occur in the cytoplasm. Cartilage and osteoid tissue occasionally occur in nephroblastomas, and their ultrastructure has been described. It is likely that chondrosarcomas and osteosarcomas will have many ultrastructural aspects in common with these tumors.

HEMATOLOGY. Anemia is common when tumors affect bone marrow or when they ulcerate and hemorrhage occurs.

Pathogenesis. Several viral oncogenes have been associated with sarcoma induction, including *src, fps, yes, ros, sea,* and *jun* (133, 231, 246, 345, 387). The product of the v-*src* gene in an infected cell is a phosphoprotein with protein kinase activity that is believed to induce transformation by causing a metabolic imbalance within the cell. Growth of the tumor is by infection and transformation of adjoining cells and proliferation of transformed cells.

Connective tissue tumors probably originate from primitive mesenchymal cells of mesodermal origin. Their diverse structural forms reflect direction and extent of differentiation. Thus frequent occurrence of more than one tissue in a tumor is a reflection of the multipotency of precursor cells; e.g., chondrocytes are derived from primitive mesenchymal cells that have undergone a gradual process of change and maturation. Finally, mature chondrocytes, which produce chondromucin in addition to collagen and elastic fibrils, are evolved. An analogous differentiation occurs during ontogeny of osteoblasts and fibroblasts. The more anaplastic tumors are composed of cells in which maturation has been arrested at an earlier stage.

OTHER TUMORS. By introducing MC29 virus into the peritoneum, Beard (25) induced massive mesotheliomas of serosal cells, which became rounded or pear shaped, often forming solid papillary growths of round cells with large round nuclei and large nucleoli. The mesotheliomas were highly invasive into contiguous structures such as liver, intestine, ovary, and pancreas. Metaplasia to cartilage was common.

Immunity. Under natural conditions, most chicks become infected by exogenous ALV from penmates or their surroundings and, after a transient viremia, develop virus-neutralizing (VN) antibodies that rise to a high titer and persist throughout the life of the bird (328, 358). These antibodies are passed via the yolk to progeny chicks and provide a passive immunity to infection that lasts for 3–4 wk. This passively acquired antibody delays infection by ALV (399), reduces incidence of tumors (41), and reduces the incidence of viremia and shedding of ALV (138). Level and persistence of antibody in the chick is related to the titer of antibody in the dam's serum.

The VN antibodies serve to restrict amounts of virus in the bird, which in turn may limit neoplasia, but they are generally considered to have little direct influence on tumor growth. Cytotoxic lymphocytes directed against viral envelope antigens also occur in birds infected with ALV or RSV (20). Birds infected with leukosis/sarcoma virus also produce antibodies to gs-antigens, but these are apparently not related to resistance to tumor growth (342).

Studies on Rous sarcomas reveal that the tumor-bearing host will also respond to tumor-associated cell surface antigens (TASAs), and this response serves to retard tumor growth or cause regression. The TASAs may be viral structural antigens and be affected by antiviral responses, or they may be neoantigens arising on the tumor cell. Such neoantigens may be virus directed and virus specific or derepressed host antigens, such as embryonic antigens. The TASAs may be designated as tumor-specific transplantation antigens (TSTA) when they induce tumor immunity in vivo or as transformation-specific cell surface antigens (TSSA) when demonstrated in in vitro tests only (19, 272, 384, 385). Little is known about antitumor immunity in LL. Immunosuppression can accompany ALV infection in some circumstances. However, Fadly et al. (145) observed that both B- and T-cell immune functions were normal during early and late stages of infection with RAV-1 ALV.

Genetic Resistance. Two levels of genetic

resistance to leukosis/sarcoma virus-induced tumors are recognized: cellular resistance to virus infection and resistance to tumor development (6, 84, 273).

Inheritance of cellular resistance to infection is of a simple Mendelian type (Table 17.7). Independent autosomal loci control responses to infection by leukosis/sarcoma viruses of subgroups A, B, and C and are designated *tva* (tumor virus A subgroup), *tvb*, and *tvc* respectively. Gene designations given here are those used by Crittenden (86). (A new gene nomenclature system has recently been adopted by the Poultry Committee of the United States Department of Agriculture National Animal Genome Research Program. The new terminology is given alongside the old in Table 17.7.) The *tvb* locus also controls responses to subgroup D virus (266), and linkage occurs between *tva* and *tvc* loci (278). At each *tv* locus, alleles for susceptibility and resistance exist that are designated *tva^s*, *tva^r*; *tvb^s*, *tvb^r*; and *tvc^s*, *tvc^r*, respectively, and the susceptibility alleles are dominant over the resistance alleles. These genes are usually abbreviated to *a^s*, *a^r*, etc. It is probable that multiple alleles occur at each locus, encoding different levels of susceptibility, but this question has not been studied in detail.

Inheritance of resistance to E subgroup virus is more complex, with involvement and interaction of genes at two autosomal loci designated *tve* and *i^e* (280). A dominant resistance gene, *I^e*, acting epistatically, blocks susceptibility conferred by presence of *e^s* allele. It has been reported, however, that susceptibility alleles at the *tvb* locus are required for susceptibility to E subgroup virus, and there is controversy about whether a separate *tve* locus exists (98, 267, 268). Studies suggest that the *i^e* locus is, in fact, an *ev* locus, the ENV glycoproteins of which block the E subgroup receptor (318). Genetic resistance to infection by subgroup J virus has not been

recognized in chickens, although a number of other avian species are resistant (283, 285). Susceptibility genes such as *a^s* code for presence of subgroup-specific virus receptor sites on the cell surface, which interact with viral envelope glycoprotein and allow viral penetration and infection of the cell (392). Progress is being made in identifying the nature of such receptors (see Virus Replication). Cells resistant by virtue of presence of a resistance gene such as *a^r* in the homozygous state are believed to lack the specific receptor sites necessary for infection to occur, although nonspecific adsorption of virus to such cells can occur, but without infection being established.

Cellular susceptibility phenotypes associated with these genes are designated according to a convention that recognizes the virus subgroups to which the chicken (C) cell is resistant (/); e.g., C/AE denotes a cell resistant to A and E subgroups but susceptible to B, C, D, and J subgroups; C/0 denotes a cell resistant to no subgroup, i.e., susceptible to A, B, C, D, E, and J.

Resistance or susceptibility conferred by these genes is expressed by all cells, whether by cells cultured in vitro, such as chicken embryo fibroblasts; by chicken embryo cells, such as those of the CAM; or by chickens after hatching. These responses are applicable to leukosis or sarcoma viruses sharing the same envelope glycoproteins, and thus viral subgroup, but most genetic studies are undertaken with appropriate subgroups of RSV, since infection of the cell is expressed within a few days by visible growth of tumor cells. Thus, the phenotype of an individual may be determined by inoculation of a standard dose of RSV into chicken embryo fibroblasts in culture, with production of foci of transformed cells in susceptible embryo cells but not in resistant cells (326). Similarly, RSV can be inoculated onto the CAM of the chicken embryo, with or

Table 17.7. Genes controlling cellular susceptibility to leukosis/sarcoma viruses

Virus Subgroup	Locus		Alleles		Dominant Trait
	Old	New	Old	New	
A	*tva*	*TVA*	*tva^s*	*TVA*S*	Susceptibility
			tva^r	*TVA*R*	
B and D	*tvb*	*TVB*	*tvb^{s1,s3}*	*TVB*S1,S3*	Susceptibility
			tvb^r	*TVB*R*	
C	*tvc*	*TVC*	*tvc^s*	*TVC*S*	Susceptibility
			tvc^r	*TVC*R*	
E	*tve^d*	*TVE*	*tve^s*	*TVE*S*	Susceptibility
			tve^r	*TVC*R*	
	i^e		*I^e*		Resistance
			i^e		

Note: The old locus designation is adapted from Crittenden (86). The new locus designation is that agreed by the Poultry Committee of the USDA National Animal Genome Research Program, 1994. The allele previously designated *tvb^{s2}* is now considered to be identical to *tvb^{s1}*. The existence of a *tve* locus distinct from the *tvb* locus is not settled. The *i^e* locus is now considered to be an *ev* locus, with blocking of the subgroup E virus receptor by endogenous virus ENV glycoprotein expression.

without production of tumor pocks (95), or intracranially into day-old chicks, with death or survival as the response criterion (389) (see Prevention and Control). The phenotype of individual birds may be determined by culturing fibroblasts from plucked pin feather pulp and challenging these cultures with RSV (96, 282, 364).

Genetically resistant chicks are resistant to infection and tumor induction by leukosis and sarcoma viruses of the subgroups concerned, and they usually fail to develop antibodies (84, 91). Genetic resistance to tumor development has been studied mainly with the Rous sarcoma, regression of which is determined by a dominant gene, *R-RS-1*, that lies within the major histocompatibility complex (MHC locus) of the chicken and located in the B–L region (78, 168, 337). Work of Heinzelmann et al. (194, 195) suggests that progressor birds may have an MHC antigen that cross-reacts with an RSV-induced tumor antigen resulting in immune tolerance. The MHC (*Ea-B*) locus also influences incidence of erythroblastosis and, to a lesser extent, LL (7). Some influence of the lymphocyte antigen *Bu-1* locus on Rous sarcoma regression and of the *Th-1* locus on LL is reported (8).

Genetic resistance to LL tumor development, such as in RPL line 6, is conferred by bursal cells, not by other cellular elements of the immune system such as thymic or thymus-derived cells or non-lymphocytes. It appears as though the intrinsic inability of the bursal target cell to become infected or transformed is the major factor in resistance (310). No obvious difference in the pattern of bursal infection in tumor-susceptible and -resistant lines was detected by Baba and Humphries (3).

DIAGNOSIS

Isolation and Identification of Causative Agent.
Plasma, serum, and tumor are the best materials for virus isolation (305). Virus can also be isolated from most soft organs of the body and from oral washings and feces (43, 327), from albumen of newly laid eggs or the 10-day-old embryo of eggs laid by hens that are transmitting virus vertically (361), from feather pulp (363), and from semen (340). All viruses of this group are very thermolabile and can be preserved for long periods only at temperatures below -60 C.

The first successful procedure developed for virus isolation was inoculation of susceptible chicks (see Laboratory Host Systems). Some viruses (e.g., RSV) produce pocks on the CAM of embryonated eggs. These procedures have been largely superseded by the more rapid and less expensive cell culture techniques described below.

It should be noted that some tests—complement-fixation (CF) and ELISA and possibly nonproducer (NP), PM, R(-)Q cell, and fluorescent antibody (FA)—are suitable for all leukosis and sarcoma viruses. The resistance-inducing factor (RIF) test can be performed only on viruses that are not rapidly cytopathogenic (ALVs). Other tests are specific for certain virus strains. Rapid transformation of fibroblast cultures is produced only by certain sarcoma viruses and of hematopoietic cell cultures only by defective leukemia viruses. The test for adenosine triphosphatase activity is specific for avian myeloblastosis virus. For current procedures for the most widely used tests see Fadly (139) and Spencer (360).

RESISTANCE-INDUCING FACTOR TEST. In general, leukosis viruses do not induce alterations in cultured cells except after prolonged passage (61). When chicken embryo fibroblasts are infected with an ALV, however, they become resistant to superinfection by a sarcoma virus of the same subgroup. Only viruses of the same subgroup interfere with one another in this way. The property of interference has been used for assay of ALVs by the RIF test (324) and also in delineating virus subgroups (383). In the RIF test, known susceptible chicken embryo fibroblast cultures are inoculated with material suspected of containing a leukosis virus. Cells are subcultured at least three times at 3- to 4-day intervals, and at each passage a sample of the cells is tested for susceptibility to RSVs of different subgroups. Alternatively, supernatant fluids may be transferred to new cell cultures every 4 days. In this case, cells may be challenged without subculture 4–6 days postinoculation. Control cultures infected with known ALVs and uninfected cultures are always included to establish validity of the tests. Presence of ALV in a cell culture is indicated by a 10-fold or greater reduction in number of foci produced by a standard stock of RSV when compared with the number of foci on similarly challenged control cells. Several different challenge viruses, one for each subgroup, must be used to detect ALVs belonging to different subgroups; each requires a separate cell culture plate for testing.

TESTS FOR VIRAL-INTERNAL, GROUP-SPECIFIC ANTIGENS. Detection of the major antigen (p27) present in the core of the leukosis/sarcoma viruses forms the basis of several diagnostic tests for virus.

The COFAL test can be used to detect the gs antigen in cultures of fibroblasts that have been inoculated with virus (333). Cells must be susceptible to infection with the virus sought; to obtain a suitable antigen from low-titer inoculate, inoculated fibroblasts must be cultivated for 14 days before they are harvested. The harvested cells are adjusted to a standard concentration, frozen, thawed, and then used as antigen in the test. Various controls are necessary, including uninoculated fibroblasts, because these may contain gs antigen derived from endogenous leukosis virus. Titration of complement-fixing activity of extracts of the control and inoculated cultures allows differentiation between endogenous and exogenous viral antigen, since the titer of the latter is much higher. If available, fibroblasts that do not express endogenous antigen may be used.

Because of the difficulty in distinguishing between gs antigens of endogenous and exogenous viruses, direct CF tests of infected materials, without tissue culture passage, are of limited value. Nevertheless, direct tests may be done in certain circumstances, e.g., on egg albumen (see Eradication).

Complement-fixing antiserum against gs antigen can be obtained from hamsters bearing sarcomas induced by RSV (the Schmidt-Ruppin strain is usually used) (333). Rabbit and other mammalian antiserums prepared against purified gs antigens derived from avian myeloblastosis virus can also be used (346, 365, 366). Antiserums have also been raised in pigeons bearing RSV-induced tumors (334, 336).

Highly sensitive radioimmunoassay (134, 331) and ELISA tests (76, 350) for gs antigens have been developed. They may be used directly for assay of test material or indirectly after culture of cell cultures inoculated with test material. These antigens may also be detected in cells by FA techniques (212, 271). Although serum has recently been identified as an unsuitable test material for detection of exogenous ALV by direct ELISA (287), a variety of samples can be tested for the presence of ALV by ELISA. For detection of exogenous ALV, samples are inoculated on chicken embryo fibroblasts that are genetically resistant to subgroup E ALV. Seven to 9 days later, cell lysates are tested for the presence of ALV gs antigen by ELISA (139, 350). Rabbit anti-p27 antibody that is used to coat ELISA plates and rabbit anti-p27 conjugate, as well as complete kits for running ELISA for detection of ALV gs antigen, are available commercially.

TESTS BASED ON PHENOTYPIC MIXING OF VIRUSES.
Chicken embryo fibroblasts can be infected with envelope-defective strains of RSV (e.g., BH-RSV) to produce transformed cells that are nonproducers of infectious RSV of subgroups A–D. Superinfection of a culture of NP cells by a leukosis helper virus results in production of infectious RSV, which is detectable in supernatant fluid by assays in susceptible chicken embryo fibroblast cultures and forms the basis of the NP cell activation test (313). Several variants of the test are described. Nonproducer cell activation is an example of phenotypic mixing of viruses (see Etiology). Nonproducer cells from embryos with endogenous E sub-

group virus may spontaneously produce an E subgroup RSV from complementation of the defective RSV by E subgroup envelope. In assaying for RSV production following activation, it is then necessary to use fibroblast cultures resistant to subgroup E but susceptible to subgroups A, B, C, D, and J (C/E cells).

A useful modified NP cell activation test uses Japanese quail cells that have been transformed with envelope-defective BH-RSV. Those nonproducing R(-)Q cells can be activated to produce infectious RSV by cocultivation with C/E cells infected with the exogenous LLV under test, thus providing the R(-)Q cell test (100).

Another variant of the NP cell test is the PM test (259, 305), for which cultures of C/O fibroblasts (i.e., cells susceptible to all virus subgroups) pretreated with DEAE dextran are infected heavily with E subgroup RSV (RAV-0), producing RSV-transformed cells. About 24 hr later, the supernatant fluid is discarded and cultures are infected with test material. Cultures are incubated for 7 days and the culture fluid is harvested, frozen, thawed, centrifuged, and assayed for infectious RSV on C/E fibroblasts. Since E subgroup RSV is excluded, presence of RSV foci indicates presence of exogenous ALV in the test material. Various controls must be included in the test.

Variants of these tests have also been developed to detect infectious endogenous E subgroup virus, as well as expression in chick cells of E subgroup envelope glycoprotein termed "chick helper factor" (chf) encoded by the endogenous viral genome (100).

COMPARISON OF TESTS.
In vivo and in vitro tests for detection or assay of exogenous ALVs are compared in Table 17.8.

All five in vitro tests require a standard source of chicken embryos free from exogenous leukosis/sarcoma viruses and of known phenotype for use in cell culture. The following reagents are also required: for the RIF test, stocks of challenge RSV of each subgroup; for the COFAL and ELISA tests, specific antiserum; for the NP test, quantities of NP cells; and for the PM test, stocks of RSV with endogenous helper, RSV(RAV-0). Cells obtained from embryos of unknown genetic origin should not be used in RIF, COFAL, and indirect ELISA tests because the results may be confused by genetic resistance. Both COFAL and indirect ELISA tests require either prolonged maintenance of culture or several subcultures to propagate the virus sufficiently; therefore, much more work is involved than in the NP or PM tests.

The indicator systems are different in the five tests. In the RIF test, the number and appearance of RSV foci after challenge are highly dependent on

Table 17.8. Comparison of methods for assaying exogenous leukosis viruses

Method	Requirements	Response Measured	Additional Requirements for Subgroup Determination	Time Required (days)
In vivo				
Chick inoc 1 day IA	LL susceptible[a]	LL	Genetically resistant chickens	270
Chick inoc 1 day IA	Erythro susceptible[b]	Erythro	Genetically resistant chickens	63
Embryo inoc 11 days IV	Erythro susceptible	Erythro	Genetically resistant chickens	43
Cell culture				
RIF	RSV pseudotypes, C/E cells	Resistance to formation of RSV foci in CC	Challenge virus of known subgroup	12[c] + 6
COFAL	Hamster antiserum, C/E cells	Complement fixation	Genetically resistant cells	14 + 1
ELISA	Enzyme-linked antisera C/E cells	Color change of substrate	Genetically resistant cells	14 + 1
NP	NP cells (chicken or quail)	RSV foci in CC	Genetically resistant cells or RIF test with leukosis virus of known subgroup	8 + 6
PM	RSV(RAV-0), C/0, and C/E cells	RSV foci in CC	Genetically resistant cells or RIF test with leukosis virus of known subgroup	5 + 6

Note: C/E, cells genetically resistant to infection with viruses of E subgroup but susceptible to viruses of other subgroups; C/0, cells phenotypically susceptible to infection by viruses of all subgroups; COFAL, complement fixation for avian leukosis viruses; CC, cell culture; ELISA, enzyme-linked immunosorbent assay; erythro, erythroblastosis; IA, intraabdominal; IV, intravenous; LL, lymphoid leukosis; NP, nonproducer; RIF, resistance-inducing factor; RSV, Rous sarcoma virus; RSV (RAV-0), Rous sarcoma virus with endogenous helper.

[a]Chickens susceptible to infection by the virus and to LL tumor formation, e.g. line 15I chickens.

[b]Chickens susceptible to virus infection and to development of erythroblastosis (or myeloblastosis).

[c]Approximate number of days necessary to cultivate the virus plus the number of days to indicate presence of virus.

the physiologic condition of the cells. Thus, when cell cultures are not in optimal condition, a RIF test cannot be performed. A cell extract is used in the COFAL and ELISA tests, however, and it can be stored frozen and tested on more than one occasion if necessary. Similarly, in the NP and PM tests, the supernatant fluid of cell cultures can be stored and tested for virus by the cell culture technique. Results are usually more clear-cut in the NP and PM tests than in the RIF, COFAL, or ELISA tests. Avian leukosis virus infectivity and titer could be determined by ELISA within 7 days after cultivation, but after 19 days and 3 subcultures by the RIF test (379).

The subgroup of an infecting ALV can be determined by any of the tests. In the RIF test, only RSV belonging to the same subgroup as the ALV is subjected to interference. In COFAL and ELISA tests, genetically resistant cells can be used; thus an ALV of subgroup A will not produce CF antigens in cells of the C/A phenotype (resistant to subgroup A viruses). In the NP test, genetically resistant NP cells can be prepared; and in the PM test, genetically resistant cells can be used in the mixing phase.

In NP and PM tests, supernatant from the activation or mixing phase (which contains RSV of the same subgroup as the ALV) can be placed on genetically resistant cells or embryos or used in an interference test with a leukosis virus of known subgroup.

IMMUNOHISTOCHEMICAL TESTS. Direct (212) and indirect (271) FA tests have been used to detect viral antigen in chicken embryo fibroblast cultures. When mammalian gs antiserums are used and cells are fixed in acetone, the test becomes analogous to the COFAL test. Avian serums are subgroup specific or even type specific (271). Other immunohistochemical techniques have also been described (121, 135, 172, 170).

ENZYME ASSAYS. Avian myeloblastosis virus has on its surface an enzyme (ATPase) that dephosphorylates adenosine triphosphate. This activity can be used as a quantitative assay to determine the amount of virus present in the plasma of infected chickens or in supernatants of myeloblast cultures (27).

All leukosis/sarcoma viruses contain reverse

transcriptase (368). Detection of this enzyme, either directly when the correct template is used (213, 372) or indirectly when the radioimmunoassay is used (265), is an indication of presence of virus.

DETECTION OF VIRAL NUCLEIC ACIDS. Blot-hybridization analysis of viral DNA or RNA in cell extracts is used increasingly for detection of virus in avian tumor virus research (396, 397). A polymerase chain reaction (PCR) specific for ALV subgroup A can be used to detect proviral DNA and viral RNA in various tissues from ALV-infected chickens (381). A PCR using primers based on the proviral LTR sequences in the 3′ (U3) region and those conserved U5 sequences can be used to detect exogenous, but not endogenous, ALVs (348).

HEMATOPOIETIC TRANSFORMATION. Avian myeloblastosis virus will infect cultures of avian hematopoietic tissue and induce focal transformation into myeloblasts. Assays are usually based on a quantal response in which individual cultures are scored as positive or negative (14, 245). Focus assays for myeloblastosis, erythroblastosis, and other defective leukemia viruses have been developed (176, 177, 248). Cultured chicken bone-marrow cells are useful in isolation and propagation of acutely transforming viruses recovered from cases of HPRS-103 ALV-induced myeloid leukosis (286).

TRANSFORMATION OF FIBROBLASTS AND CYTOPATHOLOGY. In sensitive chicken embryo fibroblast cultures, sarcoma viruses produce foci of morphologically transformed cells, which can be seen microscopically after 4–5 days (Fig. 17.20) and grossly after about 10 days (371). The foci consist of rounded refractile cells that become multilayered. Morphology of the transformed cells and shape of the focus produced is characteristic of the infecting virus. Sarcoma viruses also activate NP cells, produce the complement-fixing gs antigen, and can be detected by the FA technique. A number of defective acute leukemia viruses can also transform chick fibroblasts (177).

Leukosis viruses of subgroups B and D induce cytopathic effects in cell culture (175, 211). Because this property is restricted to a few viruses, it cannot be used as an assay for field viruses.

Serology. Plasma, serum, or egg yolk are suitable for antibody determination.

TESTS. Neutralization of a RSV pseudotype is indicative of current or past infection with a leukosis or sarcoma virus of the same subgroup and the same or similar type. A virus of one subgroup will not be neutralized by antibodies provoked by a virus of a different subgroup (383). Usually, a 1:5 dilution of heat-inactivated (56 C for 30 min) serum is mixed

with an equal quantity of a standard preparation of RSV of a known pseudotype; after incubation, the residual virus is quantitated by any one of many procedures, the cell culture assay being most commonly used (328). A microneutralization test using ELISA to assay for residual virus can be used for detection of ALV antibody (149).

More recently, an indirect immunoperoxidase absorbance test (239) and ELISA tests (240, 352, 377) have been described for the detection of antibodies. There are ELISA kits for detection of ALV antibodies available commercially.

SEROTYPES. Viruses of the avian leukosis/sarcoma group occurring in chickens have been divided into six subgroups (A, B, C, D, E, and J) on the basis of host range in genetically susceptible or resistant cells, interference spectrum, and viral envelope antigens (neutralizing antigens) (283, 396).

Viruses of different subgroups can be distinguished by the ability of monovalent antiserums to neutralize them. However, even though there is usually some cross-neutralization between viruses belonging to the same subgroup, the kinetics of neutralization vary and slopes of curves for heterologous systems differ from those of homologous systems. There are no common neutralization antigens among viruses of different subgroups, except for a relationship between subgroups B and D. The diagnosis of infection by serologic means requires that representatives of all serotypes be employed. Leukosis viruses themselves may be used, but more commonly, RSV pseudotypes are employed in the neutralization tests.

Differential Diagnosis

LYMPHOID LEUKOSIS. Lymphoid leukosis and Marek's disease (MD) can be differentiated only with difficulty, because similar lymphoid tumors may occur in both diseases in the same visceral organs during the same age period. Visceral lesions of these two diseases cannot be distinguished by gross examination. Diagnosis is possible in most instances on careful microscopic examination; however, considerable experience is necessary. In coming to a decision, history, signs, gross and microscopic lesions, and cytology should all be considered. This section describes the points that should receive special attention (54, 137, 308).

Ordinarily, LL does not occur before 14 wk of age, and most of the mortality occurs between 24 and 40 wk. On the other hand, MD may occur as early as 4 wk, and the mortality peak varies from 10 to 20 wk. Occasionally, losses continue and may reach a peak after 20 wk.

Nodular tumors of the bursa can often be palpated through the cloaca in birds infected with ALV. Paralysis associated with gross lesions in autonomic and peripheral nervous systems and gross lesions of the iris ("gray eye") are specific for MD.

As stated above, the bursa of Fabricius plays a central role in development of LL. When distinct focal or nodular lymphoid tumors are present in the bursa, a diagnosis of LL can be made. Such tumors are sometimes quite small and may be overlooked. In some birds, MD induces a premature atrophy of the bursa. In others, the bursa may be tumorous, in which case the walls and the plica may be thickened from interfollicular infiltration with pleomorphic lymphocytes. In contrast, intrafollicular tumors of the bursa consisting of uniform large lymphocytes are usual with LL.

Microscopic lymphoid infiltration in nerves, cuffing around small arterioles in white matter of the cerebellum, and feather follicular pattern of lymphoid cell infiltration in the skin, characteristic of MD, are not seen with LL.

Cytologically, LL tumors are generally composed of a homogeneous population of lymphoblasts (see Fig. 17.27). In contrast, tumors of MD usually contain lymphoid cells varying in size and maturity from lymphoblasts to small lymphocytes, and plasma cells may also be present. Special stains such as methyl green pyronin are helpful for cytology. Immature lymphoblasts characteristic of LL tumors are highly pyroninophilic, whereas the medium and small lymphocytes that predominate in tumors of MD do not stain with pyronin.

Lymphoid leukosis tumors are composed almost entirely of B cells and have surface IgM markers, whereas 60–90% of MD tumor cells are T cells that lack IgM markers and only about 3–25% are B cells. In addition, from 0.5 to 35% of MD tumor cells have a tumor-associated cell surface antigen (MATSA), which is absent from LL tumor cells (122, 254, 255, 299).

Other diseases that may be confused with LL are erythroblastosis, myeloblastosis, myelocytomatosis, pullorum disease, tuberculosis, enterohepatitis, Hjarre's disease, and fatty degeneration of the liver.

ERYTHROBLASTOSIS. Although gross lesions of liver, spleen, and bone marrow provide the basis for a presumptive diagnosis, a firm diagnosis must be based on finding large numbers of erythroblasts by microscopic examination of a blood smear and sections or smears of liver and bone marrow. Chickens in early stages of disease or without obvious signs may easily be missed unless microscopic examination is made.

Erythroblastosis with concurrent anemia is often difficult to differentiate from anemia resulting from nonneoplastic causes. In erythroblastosis, there is usually a defect in maturation of erythroblasts, resulting in presence of large numbers of them and very few polychrome erythrocytes. In anemia, the reverse usually occurs. Extramedullary erythropoiesis and stasis of erythroblasts in the sinusoids are usually more prominent in erythroblastosis than in anemia.

Erythroblastosis can be distinguished from myeloblastosis on the following grounds. In myeloblastosis, the liver is usually pale red and the marrow is whitish, whereas in erythroblastosis the liver and marrow are usually cherry red (see Fig. 17.30B,C). In myeloblastosis, the cells accumulate intravascularly and extravascularly, whereas in erythroblastosis they are always intravascular. The erythroblast and myeloblast may be difficult to distinguish. Erythroblasts have a basophilic cytoplasm and perinuclear halo; myeloblasts often have some granules (see Fig. 17.30D,E).

Erythroblasts are cells of the erythropoietic system and can be differentiated from cells of the myelopoietic system on the basis of presence of certain markers. Thus erythroblasts have erythroid markers including hemoglobin, chicken erythrocyte-specific histone H5, and chicken erythrocyte-specific cell surface antigens detected by immunofluorescence. Myeloblasts and myelocytes have myeloid markers including adherence and phagocytic capacity, Fc receptors as determined by rosette formation, macrophage- and granulocyte-specific cell surface antigen as detected by immunofluorescence, and dependence of colony formation on colony-stimulating factor (177, 247).

Erythroblastosis can be distinguished from LL by the nature and distribution of lesions. Microscopically, the cytoplasm of lymphoblasts is somewhat less basophilic than that of erythroblasts, and there is also a larger nuclear-cytoplasmic ratio than in the latter cells. Lymphoblasts are more variable in size and shape than erythroblasts, but they are all at the same primitive developmental stage. Lymphoblasts tend to have an ovoid rather than spherical nucleus and a finer, more delicate-looking chromatin network.

Myelocytomas are easily distinguished from erythroblastosis.

MYELOBLASTOSIS. As in erythroblastosis, a tentative diagnosis may be based on gross lesions; however, these are often so similar to those of lymphoid leukosis that specific diagnosis cannot be made without examination of a blood smear. Examination of liver or bone marrow sections is helpful when identity of the cell type is in doubt. The myeloblast is, on the average, smaller than the erythroblast or lymphoblast; its cytoplasm is more acidophilic and is polygonal or angular. The nucleus is less vesicular; the nucleolus, while present, is not nearly so frequently seen or conspicuous as in the other two leukoses. Myeloblasts also have physiologic markers that identify them as members of the myeloid series (see Differential Diagnosis, Erythroblastosis).

MYELOCYTOMATOSIS. The distinctive character and location of tumor provide the basis for diagnosis, which can be verified by examination of a stained smear or tumor section. Gross tumors must be differentiated from myeloblastosis, LL, osteopetrosis, and necrotic and/or purulent processes occurring in tuberculosis, pullorum disease, and mycotic infections.

HEMANGIOMA. Hemangiomas on the skin should be differentiated from wounds, bleeding feather follicles, and cannibalism. Those in the visceral organs should be differentiated from hemorrhages and sarcomas.

RENAL TUMORS. Renal tumors should be suspected when tumor nodules or large masses are found only in the kidney or are encountered suspended from the lumbar region. Diagnosis can be verified by microscopic examination. Tumors should be differentiated from other causes of kidney enlargement including hematomata, LL, and accumulation of urates.

OSTEOPETROSIS. Bone lesions of advanced cases are sufficiently distinctive to present no difficulty in diagnosis. Cross and longitudinal sectioning of long bones is helpful in detecting slight exostoses and endostoses, particularly in early stages.

Among other osteopathies, rickets and osteoporosis can be differentiated from osteopetrosis by their epiphyseal formation of osteoid or porous bone. In perosis, there is twisting and flattening of the shank while the bone structure itself remains normal.

CONNECTIVE TISSUE TUMORS. These tumors are usually easy to distinguish from the leukoses. They should not be confused with granulomas (Hjarre's disease, tuberculosis, pullorum disease), results of trauma, myelocytomas, or leiomyomas.

TREATMENT. No practical therapeutic measures have been found for treatment of diseases of the avian leukosis complex. In evaluating potentially therapeutic agents, it must be remembered that temporary remissions of clinical signs may occur spontaneously. All attempts to treat virus-induced neoplasia have resulted in negative or nonreproducible results.

PREVENTION AND CONTROL

Eradication. Exogenous ALVs can be eradicated from flocks. Until 1977, eradication was only applicable to experimental or special specific-pathogen–free flocks because methods used were long, complicated, and expensive. Since then, eradication from commercial flocks has become feasible using the techniques of Spencer et al. (361).

Eradication of ALV infection depends on breaking the vertical transmission of virus from dam to progeny. To establish a leukosis-free flock it is necessary to hatch, rear, and maintain in isolation a group of chickens free from congenital infection. To achieve this, embryos must be obtained from dams that are not transmitting virus to their progeny. In earlier work on development of ALV-free flocks, several methods for selecting dams were used or recommended. The dams selected to produce the next and hoped to be virus-free generation were: 1) immune, non–virus shedders. Hens with antibody were selected on the assumption that they were less likely than hens without antibody to shed virus. Chicks were hatched from those that did not transmit virus to their embryos, based on tests on at least three embryos/hen (199). 2) Nonimmune, non–virus shedders. Hens without antibody were selected on the assumption that they had not ever been infected and were less likely than hens with antibody to become intermittent shedders (228). 3) Nonviremic hens regardless of immune status. These were identified and used to provide replacements; however, up to four generations of testing were needed before flocks were free of viremics, and infection of nonviremics was not ruled out (403).

Application of eradication to commercial flocks has depended on associations between virus infections in hens, eggs, embryos, and chicks (361): 1) Egg albumen may contain exogenous ALV and gs antigen, and both are usually present together. 2) There is a strong association between ALV or gs antigen in egg albumen and ALV in vaginal swabs. 3) There is an association between ALV in vaginal swabs or egg albumen and ALV in chicken embryos and newly hatched chicks. Consequently, hens with a low probability of producing infected embryos are hens negative for virus (or gs antigen) by the vaginal swab test, or hens that produce eggs with albumen free from virus or gs antigen. Commonly, virus in vaginal or cloacal swabs may be detected by ELISA, NP, or PM tests, and in egg albumen by ELISA or direct COFAL tests. It is unlikely that a single test will detect all potential shedder hens. A problem that arises in applying the ELISA test to albumen or swabs is the need to differentiate positive reactions due to the presence of gs antigen derived from endogenous ALV or loci from the reactions due to presence of exogenous ALV infection (200). Reactions due to the latter are usually markedly higher, but the setting of the boundary between endogenous and exogenous virus infections is sometimes difficult and somewhat arbitrary. High reactions due to exogenous virus are clearer with albumen samples than with swabs (93). There is a prospect that monoclonal antibodies developed against p27 protein will be used in ELISAs to differentiate between endogenous and exogenous infections (227); also, PCR assays using primers based on the proviral LTR will be useful (348).

A procedure for eradication of ALV involves 1) selection of fertile eggs from hens negative in the egg albumen or vaginal swab test (104, 143, 260, 281); 2) hatching of chicks in isolation in small groups (25–50) in wire-floored cages, avoidance of manual vent sexing (144), and vaccination with a common needle (111) to prevent mechanical spread of any residual infection; 3) testing of chicks for ALV by a biologic assay or PCR on blood, discarding reactors and contact chicks (143, 144, 260, 263, 348); and 4) rearing ALV-free groups in isolation. In practice, selection of hens with a low shedding rate is a simpler requirement to fulfill than the subsequent chick testing and isolation rearing needed to achieve complete eradication. Consequently, some commercial breeder organizations are concentrating only on reduction of infection rate by hen testing. Progress in reducing shedding rates was reported for many lines, although some responded poorly (263). Poor response to selection was not inherent in the lines, but appeared to be related to environmental factors (146). For a review of these and other control methods, see Spencer (359) and de Boer (110).

Chicks are most susceptible to contact infection by ALVs during the period immediately after hatching. Although congenitally infected hatchmates are likely to be the main source of such infection, there are several procedures that can reduce or eliminate infection remaining from previous populations. Incubators, hatchers, brooding houses, and all equipment should be thoroughly cleaned and disinfected between each use. Chick boxes should not be reused, and each farm should ideally have only one age group of chickens. The danger of introducing strains of virus not already present in the population can be eliminated if eggs or chicks from different sources are not mixed and if chicks are reared under isolation conditions that will prevent cross-contamination of flocks.

Vaccination of chickens with virulent ALV at 8 wk of age is reported to prevent virus shedding to eggs and to facilitate eradication of leukosis viruses (314), but this could not be confirmed by Okazaki et al. (262). Reports (230) indicated that while chicks vaccinated at 8 wk of age or older do not usually shed virus to their eggs, they may harbor it, particularly in white blood cells and the spleen.

Selection for Genetic Resistance.

The frequencies of the alleles that encode cellular susceptibility and resistance to infection by exogenous leukosis/sarcoma viruses (see Pathogenesis and Epizootiology) vary greatly among commercial lines of chickens (90, 249). In some lines, high frequencies of a resistant allele may be found naturally. In others, frequencies of the resistant alleles can be increased by artificial selection. In practice, emphasis is placed on resistance to the predominating A subgroup virus and sometimes to B subgroup also.

In artificial selection, genotypes of unknown parents may be determined in a progeny test by mating them to recessive tester birds of the subgroup in question (e.g., $a^r a^r$ for A subgroup virus (269). Depending on the segregation of susceptible and resistant progeny in a particular mating, the genotype of the unknown parent may be determined. The phenotypic identification of progeny in the test may be determined by inoculation of RSV onto the CAM, the embryo being scored as susceptible or resistant on the basis of pock count (95) or intracranial inoculation of RSV into hatched chicks, chicks being scored on the basis of death or survival (389). The former method is preferable and has many advantages.

Crittenden (83, 84) discussed some of the problems raised by this approach. Mutant viruses are more likely to overcome resistance from a single gene than that related to a multiple gene effect, and mutant subgroups may then be favored. In a host population resistant to virus penetration, there can be no effective selection for resistance to development of neoplasms; for this reason mutant viruses may take over. It is probable that past selection for host viability has increased the resistance of infected birds to development of neoplasms. This type of resistance is poorly defined but may be controlled by a number of genes and is, consequently, more difficult to overcome by viral mutation. There is a prospect that it will become possible to control ALV infections by the development of resistant stock by transgenesis (86).

Immunization.

Possible use of antiviral vaccines to increase host resistance is very attractive. In a series of attempts to inactivate leukosis viruses by various means, however, Burmester (44) demonstrated that ability of these virus preparations to induce antibody was destroyed almost concurrently with inactivation. Although some success has been obtained with inactivated virus, the procedures are not suitable for field application. Attempts to produce attenuated strains of virus that do not induce disease have failed (264).

Some success has been obtained in attempts to increase the resistance of the host to RSV by immunization with viral or cellular antigens (29, 272). Similar approaches to study of immunity to lymphoid leukosis are warranted.

Recently, recombinant ALVs expressing subgroup A envelope glycoproteins have been produced that could have potential as vaccines (72, 236, 400).

Congenitally infected chicks are immunologically tolerant, however, and thus cannot be immunized even if a suitable vaccine were available. Unfortunately, these chickens constitute the major source of virus transmission and are the most likely to develop neoplasms.

REFERENCES

1. Astrin, S.M., H.L. Robinson, L.B. Crittenden, E.G. Buss, J. Wyban, and W.S. Hayward. 1979. Ten genetic loci in the chicken that contain structural genes for endogenous avian leukosis viruses. Cold Spring Harb Symp Quant Biol 44:1105–1109.

2. Astrin, S.M., E.G. Buss, and W.S. Hayward. 1979. Endogenous viral genes are non-essential in the chicken. Nature 282:339–341.

3. Baba, T.W., and E.H. Humphries. 1984. Avian leukosis virus infection: Analysis of viremia and DNA integration in susceptible and resistant chicken lines. J Virol 51:123–130.

4. Baba, T.W., and E.H. Humphries. 1985. Formation of a transformed follicle is necessary but not sufficient for development of an avian leukosis virus-induced lymphoma. Proc Natl Acad Sci USA 82:213–216

5. Baba, T.W., and E.H. Humphries. 1986. Selective integration of avian leukosis virus in different hematopoietic tissues. Virology 155:557–566.

6. Bacon, L.D. 1987. Influence of the major histocompatability complex on disease resistance and productivity. Poult Sci 66:802–811.

7. Bacon, L.D., R.L. Witter, L.B. Crittenden, A. Fadly, and J. Motta. 1981. B-haplotype influence on Marek's disease, Rous sarcoma, and lymphoid leukosis virus-induced tumors in chickens. Poult Sci 60:1132–1139.

8. Bacon, L.D., T.L. Fredrickson, D.G. Gilmour, A.M. Fadly, and L.B. Crittenden. 1985. Tests of association of lymphocyte alloantigen genotypes with resistance to viral oncogenesis in chickens. 2. Rous sarcoma and lymphoid leukosis in progeny derived from $6_3 \times 15I$ and 100 x 6_3 crosses. Poult Sci 64:39–47.

9. Bacon, L.D., E.J. Smith, L.B. Crittenden, and G.B. Havenstein. 1988. Association of the slow feathering (K) and an endogenous viral (ev 21) gene on the Z chromosome of chickens. Poult Sci 67:191–197.

10. Bacon, L.D., R.L. Witter, and A.M. Fadly. 1989. Augmentation of retrovirus-induced lymphoid leukosis by Marek's disease herpesviruses in white leghorn chickens. J Virol 63:504–512.

11. Bai, J., K. Howes, L.N. Payne, and M.A. Skinner. 1995. Sequence of host-range determinants in the env gene of a full-length, infectious proviral clone of exogenous avian leukosis virus HPRS-103 confirms that it represents a new subgroup (designated J). J Gen Virol 76:181–187.

12. Bai, J., L.N. Payne, and M.A. Skinner. 1995. HPRS-103 (exogenous avian leukosis virus, subgroup J) has an env gene related to those of endogenous elements EAV-0 and E51 and an E element found previously only in sarcoma viruses. J Virol 69:779–784.

13. Baluda, M.A. 1962. Properties of cells infected with avian myeloblastosis virus. Cold Spring Harb Symp Quant Biol 27:415–425.

14. Baluda, M.A. 1963. Conversion of cells by avian myeloblastosis virus. Perspect Virol 3:118–137.

15. Baluda, M.A., and P.P. Jamieson. 1961. In vivo infectivity studies with avian myeloblastosis virus. Virology 14:33–45.

16. Banders, U.T., and P.M. Coussens. 1994. Interactions between Marek's disease virus encoded or induced factors and the Rous sarcoma virus long terminal repeat promoter. Virology 199:1–10.

17. Bates, P., J.A. Young, and H.E. Varmus. 1993. A receptor for subgroup A Rous sarcoma virus is related to the low density lipoprotein receptor. Cell 74:1043–1051.

18. Bauer, H. 1974. Virion and tumor cell antigens of C-type RNA tumor viruses. Adv Cancer Res 20:275–341.

19. Bauer, H., and B. Fleischer. 1981. Immunobiology of avian RNA tumor virus-induced cell surface antigens. In J.W. Blasecki (ed.). Mechanisms of Immunity to Virus-Induced Tumors. Marcel Dekker, New York, pp. 69–118.

20. Bauer, H., R. Kirth, L. Rohrschneider, and H. Gelderblum. 1976. Immune response to oncornaviruses and tumor-associated antigens in the chicken. Cancer Res 36:598–602.

21. Bayon, H.P. 1929. The pathology of transmissible anaemia (erythromyelosis) in the fowl; its similarity to human hemopathies. Parasitology 21:339–374.

22. Beard, J.W. 1963. Avian virus growths and their etiological agents. Adv Cancer Res 7:1–127.

23. Beard, J.W. 1963. Viral tumors of chickens with particular reference to the leukosis complex. Ann NY Acad Sci 108:1057–1085.

24. Beard, J.W. 1973. Oncornaviruses. I. The avian tumor viruses. In A.J. Dalton and F. Haguenau (eds.). Ultrastructure in Biological Systems, vol. 5. Ultrastructure of Animal Viruses and Bacteriophages. Academic Press, New York, pp. 261–281.

25. Beard, J.W. 1980. Biology of avian oncornaviruses. In G. Klein (ed.). Viral Oncology. Raven Press, New York, pp. 55–87.

26. Beard, J.W., J.F. Chabot, D. Beard, U. Heine, and G.E. Houts. 1976. Renal neoplastic response to leukosis virus strains BAI A (avian myeloblastosis virus) and MC29. Cancer Res 36:339–353.

27. Beaudreau, G.S., and C. Becker. 1958. Virus of avian myeloblastosis. X. Photometric microdetermination of adenosinetriphosphatase activity. J Natl Cancer Inst 20:339–349.

28. Beaudreau, G.S., R.A. Bonar, D. Beard, and J.W. Beard. 1956. Virus of avian erythroblastosis. II. Influence of host age and route of inoculation on dose-response. J Natl Cancer Inst 17:91–100.

29. Bennett, D.D., and S.E. Wright. 1987. Immunization with envelope glycoprotein of an avian RNA tumor virus protects against sarcoma virus tumor induction: Role of subgroup. Virus Res 8:73–77.

30. Beug, H., A. von Kirchbach, G. Döderlein, J-F. Conscience, and T. Graf. 1979. Chicken hematopoietic cells transformed by seven strains of defective avian leukemia virus display three distinct phenotypes. Cell 18:375–390.

31. Biggs, P.M. 1961. A discussion on the classification of the avian leucosis complex and fowl paralysis. Br Vet J 117:326–334.

32. Biggs, P.M., and L.N. Payne. 1964. Relationship of Marek's disease (neural lymphomatosis) to lymphoid leukosis. Natl Cancer Inst Monogr 17:83–98.

33. Biggs, P.M., B.S. Milne, T. Graf, and H. Bauer. 1973. Oncogenicity of non-transforming mutants of avian sarcoma viruses. J Gen Virol 18:399–403.

34. Boettiger, D. 1979. Animal virus pseudotypes. Prog Med Virol 25:37–68.

35. Bolognesi, D.P. 1974. Structural components of RNA tumor viruses. Adv Virus Res 19:315–359.

36. Boyce-Jacino, M.T., K. O'Donoghue, and A.J. Faras. 1992. Multiple complex families of endogenous retroviruses are highly conserved in the genus Gallus. J Virol 66:4919–4929.

37. Boyde, A., A.J. Banes, R.M. Dillaman, and G.L. Mechanic. 1978. Morphological study of an avian bone disorder caused by myeloblastosis-associated virus. Metab Bone Dis Relat Res 1:235–242.

38. Bryan, W.R. 1956. Biological studies on the Rous sarcoma virus. IV. Interpretation of tumour response data involving one inoculation site per chicken. J Natl Cancer Inst 16:843–863.

39. Bryan, W.R., J.B. Moloney, and D. Calnan. 1954. Stable standard preparations of the Rous sarcoma virus preserved by freezing and storage at low temperatures. J Natl Cancer Inst 15:315–329.

40. Burmester, B.R. 1947. Studies on the transmission of avian visceral lymphomatosis. II. Propagation of lymphomatosis with cellular and cell-free preparations. Cancer Res 7:786–797.

41. Burmester, B.R. 1955. Immunity to visceral lymphomatosis in chicks following injection of virus into dams. Proc Soc Exp Biol Med 88:153–155.

42. Burmester, B.R. 1956. Bioassay of the virus of visceral lymphomatosis. I. Use of short experimental period. J Natl Cancer Inst 16:1121–1127.

43. Burmester, B.R. 1956. The shedding of the virus of visceral lymphomatosis in the saliva and feces of individual normal and lymphomatous chickens. Poult Sci 35:1089–1099.

44. Burmester, B.R. 1968. Unpublished data.

45. Burmester, B.R. 1969. The prevention of lymphoid leukosis with androgens. Poult Sci 48:401–408.

46. Burmester, B.R., and G.E. Cottral. 1947. The propagation of filterable agents producing lymphoid tumors and osteopetrosis by serial passage in chickens. Cancer Res 7:669–675.

47. Burmester, B.R., and E.M. Denington. 1947. Studies on the transmission of avian visceral lymphomatosis. I. Variation in transmissibility of naturally occurring cases. Cancer Res 7:779–785.

48. Burmester, B.R., and T.N. Fredrickson. 1964. Transmission of virus from field cases of avian lymphomatosis. I. Isolation of virus in line 15I chickens. J Natl Cancer Inst 32:37–63.

49. Burmester, B.R., and R.F. Gentry. 1956. The response of susceptible chickens to graded doses of the virus of visceral lymphomatosis. Poult Sci 35:17–26.

50. Burmester, B.R., and N.M. Nelson. 1945. The effect of castration and sex hormones upon the incidence of lymphomatosis in chickens. Poult Sci 24:509–515.

51. Burmester, B.R., and Purchase. 1979. The history of avian medicine in the United States. V. Insights into avian tumor virus research. Avian Dis 23:1–29.

52. Burmester, B.R., and W.G. Walter. 1961. Occurrence of visceral lymphomatosis in chickens inoculated with Rous sarcoma virus. J Natl Cancer Inst 26:511–518.

53. Burmester, B.R., and N.F. Waters. 1956. Variation in the presence of the virus of visceral lymphomatosis in the eggs of the same hens. Poult Sci 35:939–944.

54. Burmester, B.R., and Witter, R.L. 1971. An outline of the common neoplastic diseases of the chicken. USDA Prod Res Rep 129, p. 8.

55. Burmester, B.R., M.A. Gross, W.G. Walter, and A.K. Fontes. 1959. Pathogenicity of a viral strain (RPL 12) causing avian visceral lymphomatosis and related neoplasms. II. Host-virus interrelations affecting response. J Natl Cancer Inst 22:103–127.

56. Burmester, B.R., W.G. Walter, M.A. Gross, and A.K. Fontes. 1959. The oncogenic spectrum of two 'pure' strains of avian leukosis. J Natl Cancer Inst 23:277–291.

57. Burmester, B.R., A.K. Fontes, and W.G. Walter. 1960. Pathogenicity of a viral strain (RPL 12) causing avian visceral lymphomatosis and related neoplasms. III. Influence of host age and route of inoculation. J Natl Cancer Inst 24:1423–1442.

58. Burstein, H., M. Gilead, U. Bendheim, and M. Kotler. 1984. Viral aetiology of haemangiosarcoma outbreaks among layer hens. Avian Pathol 13:715–726.

59. Burstein, H., N. Resnick-Rougel, J. Hamburger, G. Arad, M. Malkinson, and M. Kotler. 1990. Unique sequences in the env gene of avian hemangioma retrovirus are responsible for cytotoxicity and endothelial cell perturbation. Virology 179:512–516.

60. Butterfield, E.E. 1905. Aleukaemic lymphadenoid tumors of the hen. Folia Haematol 2:649–657.

61. Calnek, B.W. 1964. Morphological alteration of RIF-infected chick embryo fibroblasts. Natl Cancer Inst Monogr 17:425–447.

62. Calnek, B.W. 1968. Lymphoid leukosis virus: A survey of commercial breeding flocks for genetic resistance and incidence of embryo infection. Avian Dis 12:104–111.

63. Calnek, B.W. 1968. Lesions in young chickens induced by lymphoid leukosis virus. Avian Dis 12:111–129.

64. Campbell, J.G. 1961. A proposed classification of the leucosis complex and fowl paralysis. Br Vet J 117:316–325.

65. Campbell, J.G. 1963. Virus induced tumours in fowls. Proc R Soc Med 56:305–307.

66. Campbell, J.G., and E.C. Appleby. 1966. Tumours in young chickens bred for rapid body growth (broiler chickens): A study of 351 cases. J Pathol Bacteriol 92:77–90.

67. Caparini, U. 1896. Fetati leucemici nei polli. Clin Vet (Milan) 19:433–435.

68. Carr, J.G. 1956. Renal adenocarcinoma induced by fowl leukemia virus. Br J Cancer 10:379–383.

69. Carr, J.G. 1960. Kidney carcinomas of the fowl induced by the MH2 reticuloendothelioma virus. Br J Cancer 14:77–82.

70. Carter, J.K., and R.E. Smith. 1984. Specificity of avian leukosis virus-induced hyperlipidemia. J Virol 50:301–308.

71. Chabot, J.F., D. Beard, A.J. Langlois, and J.W. Beard. 1970. Mesotheliomas of peritoneum, epicardium, and pericardium induced by strain MC29 avian leukosis virus. Cancer Res 30:1287–1308.

72. Chebloune, Y., J. Rukla, F.R. Cosset, S. Valsesia, C. Ronfort, C. Legras, A. Drynda, J. Kuzmak, V.M. Nigon, and G. Verdier. 1991. Immune response and resistance to Rous sarcoma virus challenge of chickens immunized with cell-associated glycoproteins provided with a recombinant avian leukosis virus. J Virol 65:5374–5380.

73. Chen, Y.C., and P.K. Vogt. 1977. Endogenous leukosis viruses in the avian family Phasianidae. Virology 76:740–750.

74. Cheville, N.F., W. Okazaki, P.D. Lukert, and H.G. Purchase, 1978. Prevention of avian lymphoid leukosis by induction of bursal atrophy with infectious bursal disease viruses. Vet Pathol 15:376–382.

75. Chubb, R.C., and P.M. Biggs. 1968. The neutralization of Rous sarcoma virus. J Gen Virol 3:87–96.

76. Clark, D.P., and R.M. Dougherty. 1980. Detection of avian oncovirus group-specific antigens by the enzyme-linked immunosorbent assay. J Gen Virol 47:283–291.

77. Coffin, J.M. 1992. Structure and classification of retroviruses. In J. Levy (ed). The Retroviridae, vol 1. Plenum Press, New York, pp 19–49.

78. Collins, W.H., W.E. Briles, R.M. Zsigray, W.R. Dunlop, A.C. Corbett, K.K. Clark, J.L. Marks, and T.P. McGrail. 1977. The B locus (MHC) in the chicken: Association with the fate of RSV-induced tumors. Immunogenetics 5:333–343.

79. Cooper, G.M. 1982. Cellular transforming genes. Science 217:801–806.

80. Cooper, M.D., L.N. Payne, P.B. Dent, B.R. Burmester, and R.A. Good. 1968. Pathogenesis of avian lymphoid leukosis. I. Histogenesis. J Natl Cancer Inst 41:373–389.

81. Cooper, M.D., H.G. Purchase, D.E. Bockman, and W.E. Gathings. 1974. Studies on the nature of the abnormality of B cell differentiation in avian lymphoid leukosis: Production of heterogeneous IgM by tumor cells. J Immunol 113:1210–1222.

82. Cottral, G.E., B.R. Burmester, and N.F. Waters. 1954.

Egg transmission of avian lymphomatosis. Poult Sci 33:1174–1184.

83. Crittenden, L.B. 1968. Avian tumor viruses: Prospects for control. World's Poult Sci J 24:18–36.

84. Crittenden, L.B. 1975. Two levels of genetic resistance to lymphoid leukosis. Avian Dis 19:281–292.

85. Crittenden, L.B. 1981. Exogenous and endogenous leukosis virus genes—a review. Avian Pathol 10:101–112.

86. Crittenden, L.B. 1991. Retroviral elements in the genome of the chickens: Implications for poultry genetics and breeding. Crit Rev Poultry Biol 3:73–109.

87. Crittenden, L.B., and S.M. Astrin. 1981. Genes, viruses and avian leukosis. Bioscience 31:305–310.

88. Crittenden, L.B., and A.M. Fadly. 1985. Response of chickens lacking or expressing endogenous avian leukosis virus genes to infection with exogenous virus. Poult Sci 64:454–463.

89. Crittenden, L.B., and H.-J. Kung. 1984. Mechanism of induction of lymphoid leukosis and related neoplasms by avian leukosis viruses. In J.M. Goldman and O. Jarrett (eds.). Mechanisms of Viral Leukaemogenesis. Churchill Livingstone, Edinburgh, Scotland, pp. 64–88.

90. Crittenden, L.B., and J.V. Motta. 1969. A survey of genetic resistance to leukosis sarcoma viruses in commercial stocks of chickens. Poult Sci 48:1751–1757.

91. Crittenden, L.B., and W. Okazaki. 1966. Genetic influence of the Rs locus on susceptibility to avian tumor viruses. II. Rous sarcoma virus antibody production after strain RPL12 virus inoculation. J Natl Cancer Inst 36:299–303.

92. Crittenden, L.B., and H.G. Purchase, 1974. Unpublished data.

93. Crittenden, L.B., and Smith, E.J. 1984. A comparison of test materials for differentiating avian leukosis virus group-specific antigens of exogenous and endogenous origin. Avian Dis 28:1057–1070.

94. Crittenden, L.B., and R.L. Witter. 1978. Studies of flocks with high mortality from lymphoid leukosis. Avian Dis 22:16–23.

95. Crittenden, L.B., W. Okazaki, and R. Reamer. 1963. Genetic resistance to Rous sarcoma virus in embryo cell cultures and embryos. Virology 20:541–544.

96. Crittenden, L.B., E.J. Wendel, and D. Ratzsch. 1971. Genetic resistance to the avian leukosis-sarcoma virus group: Determining the phenotype of adult birds. Avian Dis 15:503–507.

97. Crittenden, L.B., H.G. Purchase, J.J. Solomon, W. Okazaki, and B.R. Burmester. 1972. Genetic control of susceptibility to the avian leukosis complex. I. The leukosis-sarcoma virus group. Poult Sci 51:242–267.

98. Crittenden, L.B., E.J. Wendel, and J.V. Motta. 1973. Interaction of genes controlling resistance to RSV(RAV-0). Virology 52:373–384.

99. Crittenden, L.B., J.V. Motta, and E.J. Smith. 1977. Genetic control of RAV-0 production in chickens. Virology 76:90–97.

100. Crittenden, L.B., D.A. Eagen, and F.A. Gulvas. 1979. Assays for endogenous and exogenous lymphoid leukosis viruses and chick helper factor with RSV(-) cell lines. Infect Immun 24:379–386.

101. Crittenden, L.B., A.M. Fadly, and E.J. Smith. 1982. Effect of endogenous leukosis virus genes on response to infection with avian leukosis and reticuloendotheliosis viruses. Avian Dis 26:279–294.

102. Crittenden, L.B., W. Okazaki, and E.J. Smith. 1983. Incidence of avian leukosis virus infection in broiler stocks and its effect on early growth. Poult Sci 62:2383–2386.

103. Crittenden, L.B., E.J. Smith, and A.M. Fadly. 1984. Influence of endogenous viral (ev) gene expression and strain of exogenous avian leukosis virus (ALV) on mortality and ALV infection and shedding in chickens. Avian Dis 28:1037–1056.

104. Crittenden, L.B., E.J. Smith, and W. Okazaki. 1984. Identification of broiler breeders congenitally transmitting avian leukosis virus by enzyme-linked immunosorbent assay. Poult Sci 63:492–496.

105. Crittenden, L.B., S. McMahon, M.S. Halpern, and A.M. Fadly. 1987. Embryonic infection with the endogenous avian leukosis virus Rous-associated virus-0 alters responses to exogenous avian leukosis virus infection. J Virol 612:722–725.

106. Cummins, T.J., and R.E. Smith. 1988. Analysis of hematopoietic and lymphopoietic tissue during a regenerative aplastic crisis induced by avian retrovirus MAV-2(0). Virology 163:452–461.

107. Dales, S., and H. Hanafusa. 1972. Penetration and intracellular release of the genomes of avian RNA tumor viruses. Virology 50:440–458.

108. Darcel, C. le Q. 1957. A note on the classification of the leucotic diseases of the fowl. Can J Comp Med 21:145–159.

109. de Boer, G.F. (ed.). 1987. Avian Leukosis. Martinus Nijhoff, Boston.

110. de Boer, G.F. 1987. Approaches to control of avian lymphoid leukosis. In G.F. de Boer (ed.). Avian Leukosis. Martinus Nijhoff, Boston, MA, pp. 261–286.

111. de Boer, G.F., J van Vloten, and D. van Zaane. 1980. Possible horizontal spread of lymphoid leukosis virus during vaccination against Marek's disease. In P.M. Biggs (ed.). Resistance and Immunity to Marek's Disease. C.E.C. Luxembourg, pp. 552–565.

112. de Boer, G.F., O.J.H. Devos, and H.J.L. Maas. 1981. The incidence of lymphoid leukosis in chickens in the Netherlands. Zootechnica Int 10:32–35.

113. Dent, P.B., M.D. Cooper, L.N. Payne, R.A. Good, and B.R. Burmester. 1967. Characterization of avian lymphoid leukosis as a malignancy of the bursal lymphoid system. Perspect Virol 5:251–265.

114. DiStefano, H.S., and R.M. Dougherty. 1966. Mechanisms for congenital transmission of avian leukosis virus. J Natl Cancer Inst 37:869–883.

115. DiStefano, H.S., and R.M. Dougherty. 1968. Multiplication of avian leukosis virus in the reproductive system of the rooster. J Natl Cancer Inst 41:451–464.

116. Dmochowski, L., C.E. Grey, F. Padgett, P.L. Langford, and B.R. Burmester. 1964. Submicroscopic morphology of avian neoplasms. VI. Comparative studies on Rous sarcoma, visceral lymphomatosis, erythroblastosis, myeloblastosis, and nephroblastoma. Tex Rep Biol Med 22:20–60.

117. Dougherty, R.M. 1961. Heat inactivation of Rous sarcoma virus. Virology 14:371–372.

118. Dougherty, R.M. 1987. A historical review of avian retrovirus research. In G.F. de Boer (ed.). Avian Leukosis. Martinus Nijhoff, Boston, MA, pp. 1–27.

119. Dougherty, R.M., and H.S. DiStefano. 1967. Sites of avian leukosis virus multiplication in congenitally infected chickens. Cancer Res 27:322–332.

120. Dougherty, R.M., J.A. Stewart, and H.R. Morgan. 1960. Quantitative studies of the relationships between infecting dose of Rous sarcoma virus, antiviral immune response, and tumor growth in chickens. Virology 11:349–370.

121. Dougherty, R.M., H.S. DiStefano, and A.A. Marucci. 1974. Application of soluble antigen-antibody complexes to the immune histochemical study of avian leukosis virus antigen. In E. Kurstak and R. Morisset (eds.). Viral Immunodiagnosis. Academic Press, New York, pp. 88–99.

122. Dren, Cs.N., and I. Nemeth. 1987. Demonstration of immunoglobulin M on avian lymphoid leukosis lymphoma cells by the unlabelled antibody peroxidase-antiperoxidase method. Avian Pathol 16:253–268.

123. Dunwiddie, C.T., R. Resnick, M.T. Boyce-Jacino, J.N. Alegre, and A.J. Faras. 1986. Molecular cloning and characterization of gag-, pol-, and env- related gene se-

quences in the ev- chicken. J Virol 59:669–675.

124. Eckert, E.A., D. Beard, and J.W. Beard. 1953. Dose response relations in experimental transmission of avian myeloblastic leukemia. II. Host response to whole blood and to washed primitive cells. J Natl Cancer Inst 13:1167–1184.

125. Eckert, E.A., D. Beard, and J.W. Beard. 1954. Dose-response relations in experimental transmission of avian erythromyeloblastic leukemia III. Titration of the virus. J Natl Cancer Inst 14:1055–1066.

126. Eckert, E.A., I. Green, D.G. Sharp, D. Beard, and J.W. Beard. 1955. Virus of avian erythromyeloblastic leukosis. VII. Thermal stability of virus infectivity; of the virus particle; and of the enzyme dephosphorylating adenosine-triphosphate. J Natl Cancer Inst 16:153–161.

127. Ellermann, V. 1921. Histogenese der uebertragbaren Huehner leukose II. Die intravaskulere lymphoide leukose. Folia Haematol 26:165–175.

128. Ellermann, V. 1921. The Leucosis of Fowls and Leukemia Problems. Gyldendal, London, United Kingdom.

129. Ellermann, V. 1923. Histogenese der uebertragbaren Huehnerleukose. IV. Zusammenfassende Betrachtungen. Folia Haematol 29:203–212.

130. Ellermann, V., and O. Bang. 1908. Experimentelle leukamie bei huhnern. Zentralbl Bakteriol Parasitenkd Infektionskr Hyg Abt I Orig 46:595–609.

131. Elmubarak, A.K., J.M. Sharma, R.L. Witter, L.B. Crittenden, and Sanger, V.L. 1983. Comparative response of turkeys and chickens to avian lymphoid leukosis virus. Avian Pathol 12:235–245.

132. Engelbreth-Holm, J., and A. Rothe-Meyer. 1932. II. Ueber den Zusammenhang zwischen den verschiedenen Huhnerleukoseformen (Anamie-erythroblastose-myelose). Acta Pathol Microbiol Scand 9:312–332.

133. Enrietto, P.J., and M.J. Hayman. 1987. Structure and virus-associated oncogenes of avian sarcoma and leukemia viruses. In G.F. de Boer (ed.). Avian Leukosis. Martinus Nijhoff, Boston, MA, pp. 29–46.

134. Estola, T., K. Sandelin, A. Vaheri, E. Ruoslahti, and J. Suni. 1974. Radioimmunoassay for detecting group-specific avian RNA tumor virus antigens and antibodies. Dev Biol Stand 25:115–118.

135. Ewert, D.L., N. Avdalovic, and C. Goldstein. 1989. Follicular exclusion of retroviruses in the bursa of Fabricius. Virology 170:433–441.

136. Ewert, D.L., I. Steiner, and J. Duttadaway. 1990. In ovo infection with the avian retrovirus RAV-1 leads to persistent infection of the central nervous system. Lab Invest 62:156–162.

137. Fadly, A.M. 1987. Differential diagnosis of lymphoid leukosis. In G.F de Boer (ed.). Avian Leukosis. Martinus Nijhoff, Boston, MA, pp. 197–211.

138. Fadly, A.M. 1988. Avian leukosis virus (ALV) infection, shedding, and tumors in maternal ALV antibody-positive and -negative chickens exposed to virus at hatching. Avian Dis 32:89–95.

139. Fadly, A.M. 1989. Leukosis and sarcoma. In H.G. Purchase, L.H. Arp, C.H. Domermuth, J.E. Pearson (eds). A Laboratory Manual for the Isolation and Identification of Avian Pathogens. American Association of Avian Pathologists, Kennett Square, PA, pp. 135–142.

140. Fadly, A.M. 1992. Some observations on the enhancement of avian leukosis virus-induced lymphomas by serotype 2 Marek's disease virus. Proceedings XIX World's Poultry Congress, Ponsen & Looijen, Wageningen, pp. 281–285.

141. Fadly, A.M., and D.L. Ewert. 1994. Enhancement of avian retrovirus-induced B-cell lymphoma by Marek's disease herpesvirus. World Scientific, Singapore, pp. 1-9.

142. Fadly, A.M., and R.L. Witter. 1993. Effects of age at infection with serotype 2 Marek's disease virus on enhancement of avian leukosis virus-induced lymphomas. Avian Pathol 22: 565–576.

143. Fadly, A.M., W. Okazaki, E.J. Smith, and L.B. Crittenden. 1981. Relative efficiency of test procedures to detect lymphoid leukosis virus infection. Poult Sci 60:2037–2044.

144. Fadly, A.M., W. Okazaki, and R.L. Witter. 1981. Hatchery-related contact transmission and short-term small-group-rearing as related to lymphoid-leukosis-virus-eradication programs. Avian Dis 25:667–677.

145. Fadly, A.M., L.F. Lee, and L.D. Bacon. 1982. Immunocompetence of chickens during early and tumorigenic stages of Rous-associated virus-1 infection. Infect Immun 37:1156–1161.

146. Fadly, A.M., W. Okazaki, and L.B. Crittenden. 1983. Avian leukosis virus infection and congenital transmission in lines of chickens resisting selection for reduced shedding. Avian Dis 27:584–593.

147. Fadly, A.M., R.L. Witter, and L.F. Lee. 1985. Effects of chemically or virus-induced immunodepression on response of chickens to avian leukosis virus. Avian Dis 29:12–25.

148. Fadly, A.M., L.B. Crittenden, and E.J. Smith. 1987. Variation in tolerance induction and oncogenicity due to strain of avian leukosis virus. Avian Pathol 16:665–677.

149. Fadly, A.M., T.F.Davison, L.N. Payne, and K. Howes. 1989. Avian leukosis virus infection and shedding in brown leghorn chickens treated with corticosterone or exposed to various stressors. Avian Pathol 18:283–298.

150. Feldman, W.H. 1932. Neoplasms of Domesticated Animals. W.B. Saunders, Philadelphia.

151. Feldman, W.H., and C. Olson. 1933. Keratinizing embryonal nephroma of the kidneys of the chicken. Am J Cancer 19:47–55.

152. Foster, R.G., J.B. Lian, G. Stein, and H.L. Robinson. 1994. Replication of an osteopetrosis-inducing avian leukosis virus in fibroblasts, osteoblasts, and osteopetrotic bone. Virology 205:179–187.

153. Frank, R.M., and R.M. Franklin. 1982. Electron microscopy of avian osteopetrosis induced by retrovirus MAV.2-0. Calcif Tissue Int 34:382–390.

154. Franklin, R.M., and M.T. Martin. 1980. In ovo tumorigenesis induced by avian osteopetrosis virus. Virology 105:245–249.

155. Fredrickson, T.N., H.G. Purchase, and B.R. Burmester. 1964. Transmission of virus from field cases of avian lymphomatosis. III. Variation in the oncogenic spectra of passaged virus isolates. Natl Cancer Inst Monogr 17:1–29.

156. Fredrickson, T.N., B.R. Burmester, and W. Okazaki. 1965. Transmission of virus from field cases of avian lymphomatosis. II. Development of strains by serial passage in line 15I chickens. Avian Dis 9:82–103.

157. Friesen, B., and H. Rubin. 1961. Some physicochemical and immunological properties of an avian leucosis virus (RIF). Virology 15:387–396.

158. Frisby, D.P., R.A. Weiss, M. Roussel, and D. Stehelin. 1979. The distribution of endogenous chicken retrovirus sequences in the DNA of galliform birds does not coincide with avian phylogenetic relationships. Cell 17:623–634.

159. Frisby, D., R. MacCormick, and R. Weiss. 1980. Origin of RAV-0. The endogenous retrovirus of chickens. Cold Spring Harb Conf Cell Prolifer 7:509–517.

160. Fujita, D.J., Y.C. Chen, R.R. Friis, and P.K. Vogt. 1974. RNA tumor viruses of pheasants: Characterization of avian leukosis subgroups F and G. Virology 60:558–571.

161. Fung, Y.-K.T., W.G. Lewis, L.B. Crittenden, and H.-J. Kung. 1983. Activation of the cellular oncogene c-erbB by LTR insertion: Molecular basis of induction of erythroblastosis by avian leukosis virus. Cell 33:357–368.

162. Furth, J. 1931. Erythroleukosis and the anemias of the fowl. Arch Pathol 12:1–30.

163. Furth, J. 1933. Lymphomatosis, myelomatosis, and endothelioma of chickens caused by a filterable agent. J Exp Med 58:253–275.

164. Fynan, E., T.M. Block, J. DuHadaway, W. Olson, and

D.L. Ewert. 1992. Persistence of Marek's disease virus in a subpopulation of B cells that is transformed by avian leukosis virus, but not in normal bursal B cells. J Virol 66:5860–5866.

165. Gavora, J.S. 1987. Influences of avian leukosis virus infection on production and mortality and the role of genetic selection in the control of lymphoid leukosis. In G.F. de Boer (ed.). Avian Leukosis. Martinus Nijhoff, Boston, MA, pp. 241–260.

166. Gavora, J.S., J.L. Spencer, R.S. Gowe, and D.L. Harris. 1980. Lymphoid leukosis virus infection: Effects on production and mortality and consequences in selection for high egg production. Poult Sci 59:2165–2178.

167. Gavora, J., J. Spencer, and J. Chambers. 1982. Performance of meat-type chickens test-positive and -negative for lymphoid leukosis virus infection. Avian Pathol 11:29–38.

168. Gebriel, G.M., I.Y. Pevzner, and A.W. Nordskog. 1979. Genetic linkage between immune response to GAT and the fate of RSV-induced tumors in chickens. Immunogenetics 9:327–334.

169. Gilbert, J.M., P. Bates, H.E. Varmus, and J.M.White. 1994. The receptor for the subgroup A avian leukosis sarcoma viruses binds to subgroup A but not to subgroup C envelope glycoprotein. J Virol 68:5623–5628.

170. Gilka, F. and J.L. Spencer. 1983. Immunohistochemical identification of group specific antigen in avian leukosis virus infected chickens. Can J Comp Med 48:322–326.

171. Gilka, F., and J.L. Spencer. 1985. Viral matrix inclusion bodies in myocardium of lymphoid leukosis virus-infected chickens. Am J Vet Res 46:1953–1960.

172. Gilka, F., and J.L. Spencer. 1987. Importance of the medullary macrophage in the replication of lymphoid leukosis virus in the bursa of Fabricius of chickens. Am J Vet Res 48:613–620.

173. Gilka, F. and J.L. Spencer. 1990. Chronic myocarditis and circulatory syndrome in a white leghorn strain induced by an avian leukosis virus: light and electron microscopic study. Avian Dis 34:174–184.

174. Goodenow, M.M., and W.S. Hayward. 1987. 5′ long terminal repeats of myc-associated proviruses appear structurally intact but are functionally impaired in tumors induced by avian leukosis viruses. J Virol 61:2489–2498.

175. Graf, T. 1972. A plaque assay for avian RNA tumor viruses. Virology 50:567–578.

176. Graf, T. 1975. In vitro transformation of chicken bone marrow cells with avian erythroblastosis virus. Z. Naturforsch 30:847–849.

177. Graf, T., and H. Beug. 1978. Avian leukemia viruses. Interaction with their target cells in vivo and in vitro. Biochim Biophys Acta 516:269–299.

178. Graf, T., B. Royer-Pokora, G.E. Schubert, and H. Beug. 1976. Evidence for the multiple oncogenic potential of cloned leukemia virus: In vitro and in vivo studies with avian erythroblastosis virus. Virology 71:423–433.

179. Graf, T., D. Fink, H. Beug, and B. Royer-Pokora. 1977. Oncornavirus-induced sarcoma formation obscured by rapid development of lethal leukemia. Cancer Res 37:59–63.

180. Graf, T., H. Beug, M. Roussel, S. Saule, D. Stehelin, and M.J. Hayman. 1980. Avian leukaemia viruses and haematopoietic cell differentiation. Br J Cancer 41:659–661.

181. Gross, M.A., B.R. Burmester, and W.G. Walter. 1959. Pathogenicity of a viral strain (RPL12) causing avian visceral lymphomatosis and related neoplasms. I. Nature of the lesions. J Natl Cancer Inst 22:83–101.

182. Groupé, V., F.J. Rauscher, A.S. Levine, and W.R. Bryan. 1956. The brain of newly hatched chicks as a host-virus system for biological studies on the Rous sarcoma virus (RSV). J Natl Cancer Inst 16:865–876.

183. Gudkov, A.V., E. Korec, M.V. Chernov, A.T. Tikhonenko, I.B. Obukh, and I. Hlozanek. 1986. Genetic structure of the endogenous proviruses and expression of the gag gene in Brown Leghorn chickens. Folia Biol (Praha) 32:65–72.

184. Haguenau, F., and J.W. Beard. 1962. The avian sarcoma-leukosis complex: Its biology and ultrastructure. In A.J. Dalton and F. Haguenau (eds.). Tumors Induced by Viruses. Academic Press, New York, pp. 1–59.

185. Hall, W.J., C.W. Bean, and M. Pollard. 1941. Transmission of fowl leucosis through chick embryos and young chicks. Am J Vet Res 2:272–279.

186. Hamilton, C.M., and C.E. Sawyer, 1939. Transmission of erythroleukosis in young chickens. Poult Sci 18:388–393.

187. Hanafusa, H. 1975. Avian RNA tumor viruses. In F.F. Becker (ed.). Cancer: A Comprehensive Treatise. Vol. 2: Etiology—Viral Carcinogenesis. Plenum, New York, pp. 49–90.

188. Hanafusa, H. 1989. Transformation by Rous sarcoma virus. In H. Hanafusa, A. Pinter, and M.E. Pullman (eds.). Retroviruses and Disease, Academic Press, San Diego, CA, pp 40–56.

189. Hanafusa, T., and H. Hanafusa. 1973. Isolation of leukosis-type virus from pheasant embryo cells: Possible presence of viral genes in cells. Virology 51:247–251.

190. Hanafusa, T., H. Hanafusa, C.E. Metroka, W.S. Hayward, C.W. Rettemier, R.C. Sawyer, R.M. Dougherty, and H.S. DiStefano. 1976. Pheasant virus: New class of ribodeoxyvirus. Proc Natl Acad Sci USA 73:1333–1337.

191. Harris, D.L., V.A. Garwood, P.C. Lowe, P.Y. Hester, L.B. Crittenden, and A.M. Fadly. 1984. Influence of sex-linked feathering phenotypes of parents and progeny upon lymphoid leukosis virus infection status and egg production. Poult Sci 63:401–413.

192. Hayward, W.S. 1989. Multiple stages in avian leukosis virus—induced B cell lymphoma. In H. Hanafusa, A. Pinter and M.E. Pullman (eds.). Retroviruses and Disease. Academic Press, San Diego, CA, pp. 57–65.

193. Hayward, W.S., and B.G. Neel. 1981. Retroviral gene expression. Curr Top Microbiol Immunol 217–276.

194. Heinzelmann, E.W., R.M Zsigray, and W.M. Collins. 1981. Increased growth of RSV-induced tumours in chickens partially tolerant to MHC alloantigens. Immunogenetics 12:275–284.

195. Heinzelmann, E.W., R.M. Zsigray, and W.M. Collins. 1981. Cross-reactivity between RSE-induced tumour antigen and B5 MHC alloantigen in the chicken. Immunogenetics 13:29–37.

196. Hihara, H., H. Yamamoto, H. Shimohira, K. Arai, and T. Shimizu. 1983. Avian erythroblastosis virus isolated from chick erythroblastosis induced by lymphatic leukemia virus subgroup A. J Natl Cancer Inst 70:891–897.

197. Hirota, Y., M.T. Martin, M. Viljanen, P. Toivanen, and R.M. Franklin. 1980. Immunopathology of chickens infected in ovo and at hatching with the avian osteopetrosis virus MAV 2-0. Eur J Immunol 10:929–936.

198. Holmes, J.R. 1964. Avian osteopetrosis. Natl Cancer Inst Monogr 17:63–79.

199. Hughes, W.F., D.H. Watanabe, and H. Rubin. 1963. The development of a chicken flock apparently free of leukosis virus. Avian Dis 7:154–165.

200. Ignjatovic J. 1986. Replication-competent endogenous avian leukosis virus in commercial lines of meat chickens. Avian Dis 30:264–270.

201. Ignjatovic J. 1988. Isolation of a variant endogenous avian leukosis virus: Non-productive exogenous infection with endogenous viruses containing p27 and p27°. J Gen Virol 69:641–649.

202. Ignjatovic, J. 1990. Congenital transmission of avian leukosis virus in the absence of detectable shedding of group specific antigen. Aust Vet J 67:299–301.

203. Ignjatovic J., R.A. Fraser, and T.J. Bagust. 1986. Effect of lymphoid leukosis virus on performance of layer hens and the identification of infected chickens by tests on meconia. Avian Pathol 15:63–74.

204. Ishiguro, H., D. Beard, J.R. Sommer, U. Heine, G. de Thé, and J.W. Beard. 1962. Multiplicity of cell response to

the BAI strain A (myeloblastosis) avian tumor virus. I. Nephroblastoma (Wilms' tumor): Gross and microscopic pathology. J Natl Cancer Inst 29:1–39.

205. Ishizaki, R., A.J. Langlois, and D.P. Bolognesi, 1975. Isolation of two subgroup-specific leukemogenic viruses from standard avian myeloblastosis virus. J Virol 15:906–12.

206. Johnson, E.S. 1994. Poultry oncogenic retroviruses and humans. Cancer Detect Prev 18:9–30.

207. Jungherr, E.L. 1941. Tentative pathologic nomenclature for the disease complex variously designated as fowl leucemia, fowl leucosis, etc. Am J Vet Res 2:116.

208. Jungherr, E.L., and W. Landauer. 1938. Studies on fowl paralysis. III. A condition resembling osteopetrosis (marble bone) in the common fowl. Storrs Agric Exp Stn Bull 222.

209. Kakuk, T.J., F.R. Frank, T.E. Weddon, B.R. Burmester. H.G. Purchase, and C.H. Romero. 1977. Avian lymphoid leukosis prophylaxis with Mibolerone. Avian Dis 21:280–289.

210. Kanter, M.R., R.E. Smith, and W.S. Hayward. 1988. Rapid induction of B-cell lymphomas: Insertional activation of c-myb by avian leukosis virus. J Virol 62:1423–1432.

211. Kawai, S., and H. Hanafusa. 1972. Plaque assay for some strains of avian leukosis virus. Virology 48:126–135.

212. Kelloff, G., and P.K. Vogt. 1966. Localization of avian tumor virus group-specific antigen in cell and virus. Virology 29:377–384.

213. Kelloff, G., M. Hatanaka, and R.V. Gilden. 1972. Assay of C-type virus infectivity by measurement of RNA-dependent DNA polymerase activity. Virology 48:266–269.

214. Kirev, T.T. 1984. Characterization of osteopetrosis induced by viral strain Pts 56 in guinea fowl. Avian Pathol 13:647–656.

215. Kirev, T.T. 1988. Neoplastic response of guinea fowl to osteopetrosis virus strain MAV-2(0). Avian Pathol 17:101–112.

216. Kirev, T.T., T.A. Toshkov, and Z.M. Mladenov. 1986. Virus-induced pancreatic cancer in guinea fowl: a morphological study. J Natl Cancer Inst 77:713–720.

217. Kirev, T.T., T.A. Toshkov, and Z.M. Mladenov. 1987. Virus-induced duodenal adenomas in guinea fowl. J Natl Cancer Inst 79:1117–1121.

218. Kitt, T. 1931. Die leukomyelose der Huehner. Mikrobiol Immunitaetsforsch Exp Ther 12:15–29.

219. Kumanishi, T., F. Ikuta, K. Nishida, K. Ueki, and T. Yamamoto. 1973. Brain tumors induced in adult monkeys by Schmidt-Ruppin strain of Rous sarcoma virus. Gann 64:641–643.

220. Kung, H.-J., and N.J. Maihle. 1987. Molecular basis of oncogenesis by non-acute avian retroviruses. In G.F. de Boer (ed.). Avian Leukosis. Martinus Nijhoff, Boston, MA, pp. 77–99.

221. Labat, M.L. 1986. Retroviruses, immunosuppression and osteopetrosis. Biomed Pharmacother 40:85–90.

222. Lagerlof, B., and P. Sundelin. 1963. The histogenesis and haematology of virus-induced myeloid leukemia in the fowl. Acta Haematol 30:111–122.

223. Langlois, A.J., K. Lapis, R. Ishizaki, J.W. Beard, and D.P. Bolognesi. 1974. Isolation of a transplantable cell line induced by the MC29 avian leukosis virus. Cancer Res 34:1457–1464.

224. Langlois, A.M., R. Ishizaki, G.S. Beaudreau, J.F. Kummer, J.W. Beard, and D.P. Bolognesi. 1976. Virus infected avian cell lines established in vitro. Cancer Res 36:3894–3904.

225. Lapis, K. 1979. Histology and ultrastructural aspects of virus-induced primary liver cancer and transplantable hepatomas of viral origin in chickens. J Toxicol Environ Health 5:469–501.

226. Lapis, K., D. Beard, and J.W. Beard. 1975. Transplantation of hepatomas induced in the avian liver by MC29 leukosis virus. Cancer Res 35:132–138.

227. Lee, L.F., R.F. Silva, Y.-Q. Cheng, E.J. Smith, and

L.B. Crittenden. 1986. Characterisation of monoclonal antibodies to avian leukosis viruses. Avian Dis 30:132–138.

228. Levine, S., and D. Nelsen. 1964. RIF infection in a commercial flock of chickens. Avian Dis 8:358–368.

229. Luciw, P.A. and N.J. Leung. 1992. Mechanisms of retroviral replication. In J. Levy (ed.). The Retroviridae, vol 1, Plenum Press, New York, pp 159–298.

230. Maas, H.J.L., G.F. de Boer, and J.E. Groenendal. 1982. Age related resistance to avian leukosis virus. III. Infectious virus, neutralising antibody, and tumours in chickens inoculated at various ages. Avian Pathol 11:309–327.

231. Maki, Y., T.J. Bos, C. Davis, M. Starbuck, and P.K. Vogt. 1987. Avian sarcoma virus 17 carries the jun oncogene. Proc Natl Acad Sci USA 84: 2848–2852.

232. Marsh, J.D., L.D. Bacon, and A.M. Fadly. 1995. Effect of serotype 2 and 3 Marek's disease virus on the development of avian leukosis virus-induced preneoplastic bursal follicles. Avian Dis 39:743–751.

233. Mathews, F.P. 1929. Leukochloroma in the common fowl. Its relation to myelogenic leukemia and its analogies to chloroma in man. Arch Pathol 7:442–457.

234. Mathey, W.J. 1977. Personal communication.

235. Matthews, R.E.F. 1982. Fourth report of the international committee on taxonomy of viruses. Classification and nomenclature of viruses. Intervirology 17, Nos. 1–3.

236. McBride, M.A.T., and R.M. Shuman. 1988. Immune response of chickens inoculated with a recombinant avian leukosis virus. Avian Dis 32:96–102.

237. McNagny, K.M., F. Lim, S. Grieser, and T. Graf. 1992. Cell surface proteins of chicken hematopoietic progenitors, thrombocytes and eosinophils detected by novel monoclonal antibodies. Leukemia 6:975–984.

238. Meyers, P. 1976. Antibody response to related leukosis viruses induced in chickens tolerant to an avian leukosis virus. J Natl Cancer Inst 56:381–386.

239. Mizuno, Y., and H. Hatakeyama. 1983. Detection of antibodies against avian leukosis virus with indirect immunoperoxidase absorbance test. Jpn J Vet Sci 45:31–37.

240. Mizuno, Y., and S. Itohara. 1986. Enzyme-linked immunosorbent assay to detect subgroup-specific antibodies to avian leukosis viruses. Am J Vet Res 47:551–556.

241. Mladenov, Z. 1980. Comparative pathology of avian leukosis. In D.S. Yohn, B.A. Lapin, and J.R. Blakeslee (eds.). Advances in Comparative Leukemia Research. Elsevier/North Holland Biomedical Press, Amsterdam, The Netherlands, pp. 131–132.

242. Mladenov, Z., U. Heine, D. Beard, and J.W. Beard. 1967. Strain MC29 avian leukosis virus. Myelocytoma, endothelioma, and renal growths: Pathomorphological and ultrastructural aspects. J Natl Cancer Inst 38:251–285.

243. Moloney, J.B. 1956. Biological studies on the Rous sarcoma virus. V. Preparation of improved standard lots of the virus for use in quantitative investigations. J Natl Cancer Inst 16:877–888.

244. Morgan, H.R. 1973. Avian leukosis-sarcoma virus antibodies in wildfowl, domestic chickens, and man in Kenya. Proc Soc Exp Biol Med 144:1–4.

245. Moscovici, C. 1975. Leukemic transformation with avian myeloblastosis virus: Present status. Curr Top Microbiol Immunol 71:79–101.

246. Moscovici, C., and L. Gazzolo. 1987. Virus-cell interactions of avian sarcoma and defective leukemia viruses. In G.F. de Boer (ed.). Avian Leukosis. Martinus Nijhoff, Boston, MA, pp. 151–169.

247. Moscovici, M.G., and C. Moscovici. 1980. AMV-induced transformation of hemopoietic cells: Growth patterns of producers and nonproducers. In G.B. Rossi (ed.). In Vivo and In Vitro Erythropoiesis: The Friend System. Elsevier/North Holland Biomedical Press, Amsterdam, The Netherlands, pp. 503–514.

248. Moscovici, C., L. Gazzolo, and M.G. Moscovici. 1975. Focus assay and defectiveness of avian myeloblastosis virus. Virology 68:173–181.

249. Motta, J.V., L.B. Crittenden, and W.O. Pollard. 1973. The inheritance of resistance to subgroup C leukosis-sarcoma viruses in New Hampshire chickens. Poult Sci 52:578–586.

250. Motta, J.V., L.B. Crittenden, H.G. Purchase, H.A. Stone, and R.L. Witter. 1975. Low oncogenic potential of avian endogenous RNA tumor virus infection or expression. J Natl Cancer Inst 55:685–689.

251. Nakamura, K., F. Abe, H. Hihara, and T. Taniguchi. 1988. Myocardial cytoplasmic inclusions in chickens with haemangioma and lymphoid leukosis. Avian Pathol 17:3–10.

252. Nehyba, J., J. Svoboda, I. Karakoz, and J. Hejnar. 1990. Ducks: a new experimental host system for studying persistent infection with avian leukaemia retroviruses. J Gen Virol 71:1937–1945.

253. Neiman, P.E., L. Jordan, R.A. Weiss, and L.N. Payne. 1980. Malignant lymphoma of the bursa of Fabricius: Analysis of early transformation. Cold Spring Harb Conf Cell Prolifer 7:519–528.

254. Neumann, U., and R.L. Witter. 1979. Differential diagnosis of lymphoid leukosis and Marek's disease by tumor-associated criteria. I. Studies on experimentally infected chickens. Avian Dis 23:417–425.

255. Neumann, U., and R.L. Witter. 1979. Differential diagnosis of lymphoid leukosis and Marek's disease by tumor-associated criteria. II. Studies on field cases. Avian Dis 23:426–433.

256. Nikiforov, M.A., and A.V. Gudkov. 1994. ART-CH: a VL 30 in chickens? J Virol 68:846–853.

257. Nowinski, R.C., E. Fleissner, and N.H. Sarkar. 1973. Structural and serological aspects of the oncornaviruses in vol. 8: Tumor virus infections. Perspect Virol 8:31–60.

258. Nyfeldt, A. 1934. Etude sur les leucoses des poules. I. Une myeloblastose pure. Sang Biol Pathol 8:566–584.

259. Okazaki, W., H.G. Purchase, and B.R. Burmester. 1975. Phenotypic mixing test to detect and assay avian leukosis viruses. Avian Dis 19:311–317.

260. Okazaki, W., B.R. Burmester, A. Fadly, and W.B. Chase. 1979. An evaluation of methods for eradication of avian leukosis virus from a commercial breeder flock. Avian Dis 23:688–697.

261. Okazaki, W., R.L. Witter, C. Romero, K. Nazerian, J.M. Sharma, A. Fadly, and D. Ewert. 1980. Induction of lymphoid leukosis transplantable tumours and the establishment of lymphoblastoid cell lines. Avian Pathol 9:311–329.

262. Okazaki, W., A. Fadly, B.R. Burmester, W.B. Chase, and L.B. Crittenden. 1980. Shedding of lymphoid leukosis virus in chickens following contact exposure and vaccination. Avian Dis 24:474–480.

263. Okazaki, W., A.M. Fadly, L.B. Crittenden, and W.B. Chase. 1982. The effectiveness of selection for reduced avian leukosis virus shedding in different chicken strains. Avian Dis 26:612–617.

264. Okazaki, W., H.G. Purchase, and L.B. Crittenden. 1982. Pathogenicity of avian leukosis viruses. Avian Dis 26:553–559.

265. Panet, A., D. Baltimore, and T. Hanafusa. 1975. Quantitation of avian RNA tumor virus reverse transcriptase by radioimmunoassay. J Virol 16:146–152.

266. Pani, P.K. 1975. Genetic control of resistance of chick embryo cultures to RSV(RAV 50). J Gen Virol 27:163–172.

267. Pani, P.K. 1976. Further studies in genetic resistance of fowl to RSV(RAV-0): Evidence for interaction between independently segregating tumour virus B and tumour virus E genes. J Gen Virol 32:441–453.

268. Pani, P.K. 1977. Evidence for complementary action of tvb and tve genes that control susceptibility to subgroup E RNA tumour virus in chickens. J Gen Virol 37:639–646.

269. Pani, P.K., and P.M. Biggs, 1973. Genetic control of susceptibility to an A subgroup sarcoma virus in commercial chickens. Avian Pathol 2:27–41.

270. Pappenheimer, A.M., L.C. Dunn, and V. Cone. 1926. A study of fowl paralysis (neuro-lymphomatosis gallinarum).

Storrs Agric Exp Stn Bull 143.

271. Payne, F.E., J.J. Solomon, and H.G. Purchase. 1966. Immunofluorescent studies of group-specific antigen of the avian sarcoma-leukosis viruses. Proc Natl Acad Sci USA 55:341–349.

272. Payne, L.N. 1981. Immunity to lymphoid leukosis, Rous sarcoma, and reticuloendotheliosis. In M.E. Rose, L.N. Payne, and B.M. Freeman (eds.). Avian Immunology. British Poultry Science, Edinburgh, Scotland, pp. 285–299.

273. Payne, L.N. 1985. Genetics of cell receptors for avian retroviruses. In W.G. Hill, J.M. Manson, and D. Hewitt (eds.). Poultry Genetics and Breeding. British Poultry Science, Edinburgh, Scotland, pp. 1–16.

274. Payne, L.N. 1987. Epizootiology of avian leukosis virus infections. In G.F. de Boer (ed.). Avian Leukosis. Martinus Nijhoff, Boston, MA, pp. 47–75.

275. Payne, L.N. 1992. Biology of avian retroviruses. In J. Levy (ed.). The Retroviridae, vol 1. Plenum Press, New York, pp 299–404.

276. Payne, L.N., and N. Bumstead. 1982. Theoretical considerations on the relative importance of vertical and horizontal transmission for the maintenance of infection by exogenous avian lymphoid leukosis virus. Avian Pathol 11:547–553.

277. Payne, L.N., and R.C. Chubb. 1968. Studies on the nature and genetic control of an antigen in normal chick embryos which reacts in the COFAL test. J Gen Virol 3:379–391.

278. Payne, L.N., and P.K. Pani. 1971. Evidence of linkage between genetic loci controlling response of fowl to subgroup A and subgroup C sarcoma viruses. J Gen Virol 13:253–259.

279. Payne, L.N., and M. Rennie. 1975. B cell antigen markers on avian lymphoid leukosis tumour cells. Vet Rec 96:454–456.

280. Payne, L.N., P.K. Pani, and R.A. Weiss. 1971. A dominant epistatic gene which inhibits cellular susceptibility to RSV(RAV-0). J Gen Virol 13:455–462.

281. Payne, L.N., A.E. Holmes, K. Howes, M. Pattison, D.L. Pollock, and D.E. Waters. 1982. Further studies on the eradication and epizootiology of lymphoid leukosis virus infection in a commercial strain of chickens. Avian Pathol 11:145–162.

282. Payne, L.N., K. Howes, and D.F. Adene. 1985. A modified feather pulp culture method for determining the genetic susceptibility of adult chickens to leukosis-sarcoma viruses. Avian Pathol 14:261–267.

283. Payne, L.N., S.R. Brown, N. Bumstead, K. Howes, J.A. Frazier, and M.E. Thouless. 1991. A novel subgroup of exogenous avian leukosis virus in chickens. J Gen Virol 72:801–807.

284. Payne, L.N., A.M. Gillespie, and K. Howes. 1992. Myeloid leukaemogenicity and transmission of the HPRS-103 strain of avian leukosis virus. Leukemia 6:1167–1176.

285. Payne, L.N., K. Howes, A.M. Gillespie, and L.M. Smith. 1992. Host range of Rous sarcoma virus pseudotype RSV (HPRS-103) in 12 avian species: support for a new avian retrovirus envelope subgroup, designated J. J Gen Virol 73:2995–2997.

286. Payne, L.N., A.M. Gillespie, and K. Howes. 1993. Recovery of acutely transforming viruses from myeloid leukosis induced by the HPRS-103 strain of avian leukosis virus. Avian Dis 37:438–450.

287. Payne, L.N., A.M. Gillespie, and K. Howes. 1993. Unsuitability of chicken sera for detection of exogenous ALV by the group-specific antigen ELISA. Vet Rec 132:555–557.

288. Pentimalli, F. 1915. Ueber die Geschwuelste bei Huehnern. I. Mitteilung. Allgemeine morphologie der spontanen und der transplantablen Huehnergeschwuelste. Z Krebsforsch 15:111–153.

289. Perek, M. 1960. An epizootic of histiocytic sarcomas in chickens induced by a cell-free agent. Avian Dis 4:85–94.

290. Peterson, R.D.A., H.G. Purchase, B.R. Burmester,

M.D. Cooper, and R.A. Good. 1966. Relationships among visceral lymphomatosis, bursa of Fabricius, and bursa-dependent lymphoid tissue of the chicken. J Natl Cancer Inst 36:585–598.

291. Piraino, F. 1967. The mechanism of genetic resistance of chick embryo cells to infection by Rous sarcoma virus-Bryan strain (BS-RSV). Virology 32:700–707.

292. Piraino, F., W. Okazaki, B.R. Burmester, and T.N. Fredrickson. 1963. Bioassay of fowl leukosis virus in chickens by the inoculation of 11-day-old embryos. Virology 21:396–401.

293. Pizer, E., and E.H. Humphries. 1989. RAV-1 insertional mutagenesis: disruption of the c-myb locus and development of avian B-cell lymphoma. J Virol 63:1630–1640.

294. Pizer, E.S., T.W. Baba, and E.H. Humphries. 1992. Activation of the c-myb locus is insufficient for the rapid induction of disseminated avian B-cell lymphoma. J Virol 66:512–523.

295. Ponten, J. 1962. Transmission in vivo of chicken erythroblastosis by intact cells. J Cell Comp Physiol 60:209–215.

296. Ponten, J. 1964. The in vivo growth mechanism of avian Rous sarcoma. Natl Cancer Inst Monogr 17:131–145.

297. Ponten, J., and B.R. Burmester. 1967. Transplantability of primary tumors of RPL12 virus-induced lymphoid leukosis. J Natl Cancer Inst 38:505–513.

298. Ponten, J., and B. Thorell. 1957. The histogenesis of virus-induced chicken leukemia. J Natl Cancer Inst 18:443–454.

299. Powell, P.C., L.N. Payne, J.A. Frazier, and M. Rennie. 1974. T lymphoblastoid cell lines from Marek's disease lymphomas. Nature 251:79–80.

300. Price, J.A., and R.E. Smith. 1981. Influence of bursectomy on bone growth and anemia induced by avian osteopetrosis viruses. Cancer Res 41:752–759.

301. Pugh, L.P. 1927. Sporadic diffuse osteoperiostitis in fowls. Vet Rev 7:189–190.

302. Pulaski, J.T., V.L. Tieber, and P.M. Coussens. 1992. Marek's disease virus mediated enhancement of avian leukosis virus gene expression and virus production. Virology 186:113–121.

303. Purchase, H.G. 1987. The pathogenesis and pathology of neoplasms caused by avian leukosis viruses. In G.F. de Boer (ed.). Avian Leukosis. Martinus Nijhoff, Boston, MA, pp. 171–196.

304. Purchase, H.G., and N.F. Cheville. 1975. Infectious bursal agent of chickens reduces the incidence of lymphoid leukosis. Avian Pathol 4:239–245.

305. Purchase, H.G., and A.M. Fadly. 1980. Leukosis and sarcomas. In S.B. Hitchner, C.H. Domermuth, H.G. Purchase, and J.E. Williams (eds.). Isolation and Identification of Avian Pathogens. American Association of Avian Pathologists, Kennett Square, PA, pp. 54–58.

306. Purchase, H.G., and D.G. Gilmour. 1975. Lymphoid leukosis in chickens chemically bursectomized and subsequently inoculated with bursa cells. J Natl Cancer Inst 55:851–855.

307. Purchase, H.G., and W. Okazaki. 1964. Morphology of foci produced by standard preparations of Rous sarcoma virus. J Natl Cancer Inst 32:579–589.

308. Purchase, H.G., and J.M. Sharma. 1973. The Differential Diagnosis of Lymphoid Leukosis and Marek's Disease, Slide Study Set 3. American Association of Avian Pathologists, Kennett Square, PA.

309. Purchase, H.G., W. Okazaki, and B.R. Burmester. 1972. Long-term field trials with the herpesvirus of turkeys vaccine against Marek's disease. Avian Dis 16:57–71.

310. Purchase, H.G., D.G. Gilmour, C.H. Romero, and W. Okazaki. 1977. Post infection genetic resistance to avian lymphoid leukosis resides in a B target cell. Nature 270:61–62.

311. Purchase, H.G., W. Okazaki, P.K. Vogt, H. Hanafusa, B.R. Burmester, and L.B. Crittenden. 1977. Oncogenicity of avian leukosis viruses of different subgroups and of mutants of sarcoma viruses. Infect Immun 15:423–428.

312. Rauscher, F.J., J.A. Reyniers, and M.R. Sacksteder. 1964. Response or lack of response of apparently leukosis-free Japanese quail to avian tumor viruses. Natl Cancer Inst Monogr 17:211–229.

313. Rispens, B.H., P.A. Long, W. Okazaki, and B.R. Burmester. 1970. The NP activation test for assay of avian leukosis/sarcoma viruses. Avian Dis 14:738–751.

314. Rispens, B.H., G.F. de Boer, A. Hoogerbrugge, and J. Van Vloten. 1976. A method for the control of lymphoid leukosis in chickens. J Natl Cancer Inst 57:1151–1156.

315. Robinson, H. 1978. Inheritance and expression of chicken genes that are related to avian leukosis sarcoma virus genes. Curr Top Microbiol Immunol 83:1–36.

316. Robinson, W.S., and P.H. Duesberg. 1968. The chemistry of RNA tumor viruses. In H. Fraenkel-Conrat (ed.). Molecular Basis of Virology. Reinhold Book, New York, pp. 306–331.

317. Robinson, H.L., and G.C. Gagnon. 1986. Patterns of proviral insertion in avian leukosis virus induced lymphomas. J Virol 57:28–36.

318. Robinson, H.L., S.M. Astrin, A.M. Senior, and F.H. Salazar. 1981. Host susceptibility to endogenous viruses: Defective, glycoprotein-expressing proviruses interfere with infections. J Virol 40:745–751.

319. Robinson, H.L., L. Ramamoorthy, K. Collart, and D.W. Brown. 1993. Tissue tropism of avian leukosis viruses: analyses for viral DNA and proteins. Virology 193:443–445.

320. Roloff, F. 1868. Mag Ges Thierheilkd 34:190 (cited by Chubb, L.G. and R.F. Gordon. 1957). The avian leukosis complex—a review. Vet Rev Annot 32:97–120.

321. Romero, C.H., H.G. Purchase, F. Frank, L.B. Crittenden, and T.S. Chang. 1978. The prevention of natural and experimental avian lymphoid leukosis with the androgen analogue Mibolerone. Avian Pathol 7:87–103.

322. Rous, P. 1911. A sarcoma of the fowl transmissible by an agent separable from tumor cells. J Exp Med 13:397–411.

323. Rovigatti, V.G., and S.M. Astrin. 1983. Avian endogenous viral genes. Curr Top Microbiol Immunol 103:1–22.

324. Rubin, H. 1960. A virus in chick embryos which induces resistance in vitro to infection with Rous sarcoma virus. Proc Natl Acad Sci USA 46:1105–1119.

325. Rubin, H. 1960. Growth of Rous sarcoma virus in chick embryo cells following irradiation of host cells or free virus. Virology 11:28–47.

326. Rubin, H. 1965. Genetic control of cellular susceptibility to pseudotypes of Rous sarcoma virus. Virology 26:270–276.

327. Rubin, H., A. Cornelius, and L. Fanshier. 1961. The pattern of congenital transmission of an avian leukosis virus. Proc Natl Acad Sci USA 47:1058–1060.

328. Rubin, H., L. Fanshier, A. Cornelius, and W.F. Hughes. 1962. Tolerance and immunity in chickens after congenital and contact infection with an avian leukosis virus. Virology 17:143–156.

329. Rup, B.J., J.D. Hoelzer, and H.R. Bose, Jr. 1982. Helper viruses associated with avian acute leukemia viruses inhibit the cellular immune response. Virology 116:61–71.

330. Sandelin, K., and T. Estola. 1974. Occurrence of different subgroups of avian leukosis virus in Finnish poultry. Avian Pathol 3:159–168.

331. Sandelin, K., T. Estola, S. Ristimaki, E. Ruoslahti, and A. Vaheri. 1974. Radio immunoassays of the group-specific antigen in detection of avian leukosis virus infection. J Gen Virol 25:415–420.

332. Sanger, V.L., T.N. Fredrickson, C.C. Morrill, and B.R. Burmester. 1966. Pathogenesis of osteopetrosis in chick-

ens. Am J Vet Res 27:1735–1744.

333. Sarma, P.S., H.C. Turner, and R.J. Huebner. 1964. An avian leucosis group-specific complement fixation reaction. Application for the detection and assay non-cytopathogenic leucosis viruses. Virology 23:313–321.

334. Sarma, P.S., T.S. Log, R.J. Huebner, and H.C. Turner. 1969. Studies of avian leukosis group-specific complement-fixing serum antibodies in pigeons. Virology 37:480–483.

335. Sawyer, R.C., and H. Hanafusa. 1977. Formation of reticuloendotheliosis virus pseudotypes of Rous sarcoma virus. J Virol 22:634–639.

336. Sazawa, H., T. Sugimori, Y. Miura, and T. Shimizu. 1966. Specific complement fixation test of Rous sarcoma with pigeon serum. Natl Inst Anim Health Q 6:208–215.

337. Schierman, L.W., D.H. Watanabe, and R.A. McBride. 1977. Genetic control of Rous sarcoma regression in chickens: Linkage with the major histocompatibility complex. Immunogenetics 5:325–332.

338. Schmeisser, H.C. 1915. Spontaneous and experimental leukemia of the fowl. J Exp Med 22:820–838.

339. Schmidt, E.V., J.D. Crapo, J.R. Harrelson, and R.L. Smith. 1981. A quantitative histologic study of avian osteopetrotic bone demonstrating normal osteoclast numbers and osteoblastic activity. Lab Invest 44:164–173.

340. Segura, J.C., J.S. Gavora, J.L. Spencer, R.W. Fairfull, R.J. Gowe, and R.B. Buckland. 1988. Semen traits and fertility of White Leghorn males shown to be positive or negative for lymphoid leukosis virus in semen and feather pulp. Br Poult Sci 29:545–553.

341. Shank, P.R., P.J. Schatz, L.M. Jensen, P.N. Tsichlis, J.M. Coffin, and H.L. Robinson. 1985. Sequences in the gag-pol-5'env region of avian leukosis viruses confer the ability to induce osteopetrosis. Virology 145:94–104.

342. Sigel, M.M., P. Meyers, and H.T. Holden. 1971. Resistance to Rous sarcoma elicited by immunization with live virus. Proc Soc Exp Biol Med 137:142–146.

343. Siegfried, L.M., and C. Olson, Jr. 1972. Characteristics of avian transmissible lymphoid tumor cells maintained in culture. J Natl Cancer Inst 48:791–796.

344. Simon, M.C., W.S. Neckameyer, W.S. Hayward, and R.E. Smith 1987. Genetic determinants of neoplastic diseases induced by a subgroup F avian leukosis virus. J Virol 61:1203–1212.

345. Smith, D.R., P.K. Vogt, and M.J. Hayman. 1989. The v-sea oncogene of avian erythroblastosis retrovirus S13: Another member of the protein-tyrosine kinase gene family. Proc Natl Acad Sci USA 86:5291–5295.

346. Smith, E.J. 1977. Preparation of antisera to group-specific antigens of avian leukosis-sarcoma viruses: An alternate approach. Avian Dis 21:290–299.

347. Smith, E.J. 1987. Endogenous avian leukemia viruses. In G.F. DeBoer (ed.). Avian Leukosis. Martinus Nijhoff, Boston, MA, pp. 101–120.

348. Smith, E.J. 1995. Personal communication.

349. Smith, E.J., and A.M. Fadly. 1994. Male-mediated venereal transmission of endogenous avian leukosis virus. Poult Sci 73:488–494.

350. Smith, E.J., A. Fadly, and W. Okazaki. 1979. An enzyme-linked immunosorbent assay for detecting avian leukosis-sarcoma viruses. Avian Dis 23:698–707.

351. Smith, E.J., U. Neumann, and W. Okazaki. 1980. Immune response to avian leukosis virus infection in chickens: Sequential expression of serum immunoglobulins and viral antibodies. Comp Immunol Microbiol Infect Dis 2:519–529.

352. Smith, E.J., A.M. Fadly, and L.B. Crittenden. 1986. Observations on an enzyme-linked immunosorbent assay for the detection of antibodies against avian leukosis-sarcoma viruses. Avian Dis 30:488–493.

353. Smith, E.J., D.W. Salter, R.F. Silva, and L.B. Crittenden. 1986. Selective shedding and congenital transmission of endogenous avian leukosis viruses. J Virol 60:1050–1054.

354. Smith, E.J., A.M. Fadly, and L.B. Crittenden. 1990. Interactions between endogenous virus loci in ev6 and ev21. 1. Immune response to exogenous avian leukosis virus infection. Poult Sci 69:1244–1250.

355. Smith, E.J., A.M. Fadly, and L.B. Crittenden. 1990. Interactions between endogenous virus loci ev 6 and ev 21. 2. Congenital transmission of EV21 viral product to female progeny from slow-feathering dams. Poult Sci 69:1251–1256.

356. Smith, R.E. 1987. Immunology of avian leukosis virus infections. In G.F. de Boer (ed.). Avian Leukosis. Martinus Nijhoff, Boston, MA, pp. 121–129.

357. Smith, R.E., and E.V. Schmidt. 1982. Induction of anemia by avian leukosis viruses of five subgroups. Virology 117:516–518.

358. Solomon, J.J., B.R. Burmester, and R.N. Fredrickson. 1966. Investigations of lymphoid leukosis infection in genetically similar chicken populations. Avian Dis 10:477–484.

359. Spencer, J.L. 1984. Progress towards eradication of lymphoid leukosis viruses—a review. Avian Pathol 13:599–619.

360. Spencer, J.L. 1987. Laboratory diagnostic procedures for detecting avian leukosis virus infections. In G.F. de Boer (ed.). Avian Leukosis. Martinus Nijhoff, Boston, MA, pp. 213–240.

361. Spencer, J.L., L.B. Crittenden, B.R. Burmester. W. Okazaki, and R.L. Witter. 1977. Lymphoid leukosis: Interrelations among virus infections in hens, eggs, embryos, and chicks. Avian Dis 21:331–345.

362. Spencer, J.L., J.S. Gavora, and R.S Gowe. 1980. Lymphoid leukosis virus: Natural transmission and nonneoplastic effects. Cold Spring Harb Conf Cell Prolifer 7:553–564.

363. Spencer, J.L., F. Gilka, and J.S. Gavora. 1983. Detection of lymphoid leukosis virus infected chickens by testing for group specific antigen for virus in feather pulp. Avian Pathol 12:85–99.

364. Spencer, J.L., J.S. Gavora, and F. Gilka. 1987. Feather pulp organ cultures for assessing host resistance to infection with avian leukosis-sarcoma viruses. Avian Pathol 16:425–438.

365. Stephenson, J.R., R.E. Wilsnack, and S.A. Aaronson. 1973. Radioimmunoassay for avian C-type virus group-specific antigen: Detection in normal and virus-transformed cells. J Virol 11:893–899.

366. Stephenson, J.R., E.J. Smith, L.B. Crittenden, and S.A. Aaronson. 1975. Analysis of antigenic determinants of structural polypeptides of avian type C tumor viruses. J Virol 16:27–33.

367. Stumph, W.E., C.P. Hodgson, M.J. Tsai, and B.W. O'Malley. 1984. Genomic structure and possible retroviral origin of the chicken CR1 repetitive DNA sequence family. Proc Natl Acad Sci USA 81:6667–6671.

368. Temin, H.M. 1974. The cellular and molecular biology of RNA tumor viruses, especially avian leukosis-sarcoma viruses, and their relatives. Adv Cancer Res 19:47–104.

369. Temin, H.M. 1974. On the origin of RNA tumor viruses. Annu Rev Genet 8:155–177.

370. Temin, H.M. 1974. The Bertner Foundation Memorial Award Lecture—from proviruses to protoviruses: RNA-directed DNA synthesis by RNA tumor viruses and cells. Molecular Studies in Viral Neoplasia. Williams & Wilkins, Baltimore, MD, pp. 7–38.

371. Temin, H.M., and H. Rubin. 1958. Characteristics of an assay for Rous sarcoma virus and Rous sarcoma cells in tissue culture. Virology 6:669–688.

372. Tereba, A., and K.G. Murti. 1977. A very sensitive biochemical assay for detecting and quantitating avian oncornaviruses. Virology 80:166–176.

373. Tereba, A., L.B. Crittenden, and S.M. Astrin. 1981. Chromosomal localization of three endogenous retrovirus

loci associated with virus production in white leghorn chickens. J Virol 39:282–289.

374. Thorell, B. 1958. Induktion von Nierentumoren durch Leukaemievirus. Zentralbl Allg Pathol Pathol Anat 98:98–314.

375. Tieber, V.L., L.L. Zalinskis, R.F. Silva, A. Finkelstein, and P.M. Coussens. 1990. Transactivation of the Rous sarcoma virus long terminal repeat promoter by Marek's disease virus. Virology 179:719–727.

376. Troesch, C.D., and P.K. Vogt. 1985. An endogenous virus from Lophortyx quail is the prototype for envelope subgroup I of avian retroviruses. Virology 143:595–602.

377. Tsukamoto, K., Y. Kono, and K Arai. 1985. An enzyme linked immunosorbent assay for detection of antibodies to exogenous avian leukosis virus. Avian Dis 29:1118–1129.

378. Tsukamoto, K., M. Hasebe, S. Kakita, H. Hihara, and Y. Kono. 1991. Identification and characterization of hens transmitting avian leukosis virus (ALV) to their embryos by ELISAs for detection infectious ALV, ALV antigens and antibodies to ALV. J Vet Med Sci 53:859–864.

379. Tsukamoto, K., H. Hihara, and Y. Kono. 1991. Detection of avian leukosis virus antigens by the ELISA and its use for detecting infectious virus after cultivation of samples and partial characterization of specific pathogen-free chicken lines maintained at this laboratory. J Vet Med Sci 53:399–408.

380. Tsukamoto, K., M. Hasebe, S. Kakita, Y. Tanigichi, H. Hihara, and Y. Kono. 1992. Sporadic congenital transmission of avian leukosis virus in hens discharging the virus into the oviducts. J Vet Med Sci 54:99–103.

381. Van Woensel, P.A.M., A. van Blaaderen, R.J.M. Mooman, and G.F. de Boer. 1992. Detection of proviral DNA and viral RNA in various tissues early after avian leukosis virus infection. Leukemia 6(Suppl 3):135S–137S.

382. Vogt, P.K. 1965. Avian tumor viruses. Adv Virus Res 11:293–385.

383. Vogt, P.K., and R. Ishizaki. 1966. Criteria for the classification of avian-tumor viruses. In W.J. Burdett (ed.). Viruses Inducing Cancer. University of Utah Press, Salt Lake City, UT, pp. 71–90

384. Wainberg, M.A., and M.S. Halpern. 1987. Avian sarcomas: Immune responsiveness and pathology. In G.F. de Boer (ed.). Avian Leukosis. Martinus Nijhoff, Boston, MA, pp. 131–152.

385. Wainberg, M.A., and E.R. Phillips. 1976. Immunity against avian sarcomas—a review. Isr J Med Sci 12:388–406.

386. Walter, W.G., B.R. Burmester, and C.H. Cunningham. 1962. Studies on the transmission and pathology of a viral-induced avian nephroblastoma (embryonal nephroma). Avian Dis 6:455–477.

387. Wang, L.H., and H. Hanafusa. 1988. Avian sarcoma viruses. Virus Res 9:159–203.

388. Warthin, A.S. 1907. Leukemia of the common fowl. J Infect Dis 4:369–380.

389. Waters, N.F., and B.R. Burmester. 1961. Mode of inheritance of resistance to Rous sarcoma virus in chickens. J Natl Cancer Inst 27:655–661.

390. Watts, S.L., and R.E. Smith. 1980. Pathology of chickens infected with avian nephroblastoma virus MAV-2(N). Infect Immun 27:501–512.

391. Weiss, R.A. 1975. Genetic transmission of RNA tumor viruses. Perspect Virol 9:165–205.

392. Weiss, R.A. 1981. Retrovirus receptors. In K. Longberg-Holm and L. Philipson (eds.). Virus Receptors. Pt. 2: Receptors and Recognition, series B, vol. 8, pp. 187–202. Chapman and Hall, London, United Kingdom.

393. Weiss, R.A., and D.P. Frisby. 1981. Are avian endogenous viruses pathogenic? In D.S. Yohn (ed.). 10th International Symposium for Comparative Research on Leukosis and Related Diseases. Elsevier/North Holland, New York.

394. Weiss, R.A., W.S. Mason, and P.K. Vogt. 1973. Genetic recombinants and heterozygotes derived from endogenous and exogenous avian RNA tumor viruses. Virology 52:535–552.

395. Weiss, R.A., D. Boettiger, and H.M. Murphy. 1977. Pseudotypes of avian sarcoma viruses with the envelope properties of vesicular stomatitis virus. Virology 76:808–825.

396. Weiss, R.A., N. Teich, H. Varmus, and J. Coffin (eds.). 1982. RNA Tumor Viruses, 2nd ed. Cold Spring Harbor Laboratory, Cold Spring Harbor, New York.

397. Weiss, R.A., N. Teich, H. Varmus, and J. Coffin (eds.). 1985. RNA Tumor Viruses, 2nd ed. Supplements and Appendices. Cold Spring Harbor Laboratory, Cold Spring Harbor, New York.

398. Whalen, L.R., D.W. Wheeler, D.H. Gould, S.A. Fiscus, L.C. Boggie, and R.E. Smith. 1988. Functional and structural alterations of the nervous system induced by avian retrovirus RAV-7. Microb Pathog 4:401–416.

399. Witter, R.L., B.W. Calnek, and P.P. Levine. 1966. Influence of naturally occurring parental antibody on visceral lymphomatosis virus infection in chickens. Avian Dis 10:43–56.

400. Wright, S.E. and D.D. Bennett. 1992. Avian retroviral recombinant expressing foreign envelope delays tumour formation of ASV-A-induced sarcoma. Vaccine 10:375–378.

401. Wyke, J.A., J.G. Bell, and J.A. Beamand. 1975. Genetic recombination among temperature-sensitive mutants of Rous sarcoma virus. Cold Spring Harb Symp Quant Biol 39:897–905.

402. Young, J.A., P. Bates, and H.E. Varmus. 1993. Isolation of a chicken gene that confers susceptibility to infection by subgroup A avian leukosis and sarcoma viruses. J Virol 67:1811–1816.

403. Zander, D.V., R.G. Raymond, C.F. McClary, and K. Goodwin. 1975. Eradication of subgroups A and B lymphoid leukosis virus from commercial poultry breeding flocks. Avian Dis 19:408–423.

404. Ziegel, R.F. 1961. Morphological evidence of the association of virus particles with the pancreatic acinar cells of the chick. J Natl Cancer Inst 26:1011–1039.

RETICULOENDOTHELIOSIS

R. L. Witter

INTRODUCTION AND HISTORY. Reticuloendotheliosis (RE) designates a group of pathologic syndromes caused by retroviruses of the reticuloendotheliosis virus (REV) group. The disease syndromes include 1) acute reticulum cell neoplasia, 2) a runting disease syndrome, and 3) chronic neoplasia of lymphoid and other tissues.

The initial REV isolate, strain T, was obtained in 1958 from a turkey with visceral lymphomas and was serially passaged over 300 times in turkeys and chickens (160). Although these authors obtained considerable experimental data on this virus during the period 1958–60, publication was delayed because the unique nature of this viral isolate was not immediately recognized (31). Sevoian obtained this isolate from Twiehaus and found it acutely oncogenic, causing death of young chicks 6–21 days after inoculation (176). Theilen et al. confirmed the acute oncogenicity of strain T for young chickens, turkeys and Japanese quail; these authors were the first to designate the disease as a "reticuloendotheliosis" on the basis of the prominent cell in the neoplastic lesion (200).

Strain T is defective for replication in chicken fibroblast tissue cultures and possesses a unique oncogene of cellular origin (v-*rel*) that is responsible for its acute oncogenicity (76, 77). Stocks of strain T also contain a helper REV that replicates in chicken fibroblast cultures but lacks acute oncogenic properties (76). The helper virus has been variously designated as REV-A (76) or as nondefective strain T (228).

The REV group now includes strain T, chick syncytial virus (47), duck infectious anemia virus (111), spleen necrosis virus (204), and other isolates obtained from turkeys, chickens, ducks, pheasants and geese (see 42).

Replication defectiveness and acute oncogenicity appear to be properties unique to strain T. All other strains thus far characterized, including strain T helper virus, are nondefective (replication competent). The nondefective REVs are responsible for the runting disease and the chronic neoplastic disease, both of which occur in nature. The acute reticulum cell neoplasia is induced only by strain T and is not known to occur in nature. Therefore, although strain T has long been recognized as the prototype REV, it is clearly atypical of the group.

For a variety of reasons, RE has received uncommon attention by researchers, considering that it is not a major economic problem to the poultry industry. The acute and chronic neoplastic diseases represent (with Marek's disease and lymphoid leukosis) a third etiologically distinct group of avian viral neoplasms. The chronic neoplastic disease sporadically appears to cause significant death and condemnation loss in commercial turkey flocks, and more recently, also in chicken flocks in the Middle East. REV is a potential contaminant of poultry vaccines. The various REV-induced neoplastic syndromes in chickens resemble both lymphoid leukosis and Marek's disease and certain other less well-characterized syndromes (74). Reticuloendotheliosis is considered a good model for the study of lymphoid leukosis in chickens and retrovirus-induced neoplastic and immunosuppressive diseases of humans and other mammalian species. REVs have been used as expression vectors to insert foreign genes into chicken and mammalian cells; such vectors may have diverse uses from production of transgenic chickens (24, 181) to gene therapy in humans (56).

No public health hazard has been associated with REVs. The extended host range of REVs, which includes certain mammalian cells (1, 215) and sequence homologies that suggest an evolutionary linkage with mammalian retroviruses (11, 100), has raised concerns (91), but there is no direct evidence supporting a role of REVs in human infection or disease. The lack of public health concerns has been cited (56) in support of REV vectors for human therapeutics.

Other reviews on reticuloendotheliosis may be consulted (6, 22, 56, 150, 123, 146, 152).

INCIDENCE AND DISTRIBUTION. In turkeys, the chronic neoplastic form of RE appears to occur naturally, albeit sporadically. In addition to the original isolation by Robinson and Twiehaus (160), other outbreaks have been described in the United States (142, 187, 223, 225), England (117), and Israel (83). Lymphomas typical of reticuloendotheliosis have also been reported in wild turkeys (75, 106).

In chickens, chronic RE neoplastic disease also has been documented. Histiocytic lymphosarcomas were reported in a laying flock in Australia following administration of an REV-contaminated Marek's disease vaccine (6, 154). Recently, two broiler breeder flocks in the United States developed REV-associated lymphomas associated with use of an REV-contaminated fowl pox vaccine (64). REV-associated lymphomas, not associated with contaminated vaccines, have been observed primarily in the Middle East (53, 83, 120), but cases also have been described in Europe (145) and Africa (140).

Chronic neoplasia associated with REV has also

been observed in ducks (72, 141, 147), quail (35, 170, 209), pheasants (57), and geese (58).

A runting disease characterized by poor growth, abnormal feathering, proventriculitis, and immunodepression has been seen in chickens accidently vaccinated with REV-contaminated vaccines (90, 96, 235), and may have also occurred naturally in association with necrotic dermatitis in chickens (78).

Virus infection is far more prevalent than clinical disease and is widely disseminated among avian species. This was first recognized by Aulisio and Shelokov (4) who found specific antibodies in yolks of eggs from 41 of 92 chicken flocks in the United States. Subsequent studies, summarized by Bagust (6), have confirmed the presence of REV antibodies (or virus) in commercial chicken and turkey flocks in a number of countries, although at varying frequencies. Seropositive flocks were detected in Japan as early as 1964 (211, 233), well prior to the use of REV-contaminated vaccines. Recent studies that document REV antibodies in up to 60–80% of birds in certain flocks in the United States and Japan indicate that the frequency of seropositive flocks may be increasing (59, 167), but the reasons for this apparent increase are not known. Bagust (6) has described the persistence of REV infection on the same production sites over a period of several years.

Thus, on the basis of reported clinical disease, the economic importance of RE in turkeys and chickens is minor. Progeny of seropositive flocks are prohibited from export to certain countries, however, causing economic loss to certain breeders. Significant costs are also incurred by vaccine companies and producers of specific-pathogen–free flocks who must routinely monitor their products for REV contamination. Potential problems such as the possibility of immunodepressive disease from environmental exposure or contaminated vaccines or infection becoming endemic in valuable breeding stock have raised the level of concern.

ETIOLOGY

Classification. REVs are retroviruses immunologically, morphologically, and structurally distinct from the leukosis/sarcoma group of avian retroviruses (see review 150). Within the classification of retroviruses, REVs are a subgenus under the genus murine leukemia virus-related, whereas the avian leukosis/sarcoma group is classified in its own genus (45).

A relationship between REV and various mammalian retroviruses, especially those from old world primates, has been described on the basis of morphology, nucleic acid sequences, amino acid sequences of major polypeptides, and immunologic determinants (see review 123) and receptor inter-

ference patterns (98, 100). Although this may indicate an evolutionary link, no biologic relationships are recognized and the host range of REV, except for certain mammalian cell cultures, remains largely restricted to avian species.

Stability. Cell-free stocks of REV can be prepared from tissues of infected chickens or fluids from infected cell cultures and may be stored without loss of activity for long periods at -70 C. The virus was relatively stable at 4 C, but at 37 C, 50% of the infectivity was lost in 20 min and 99% was lost after 1 hr (34). Infected cells may be stored indefinitely with dimethylsulfoxide at -196 C.

Morphology. Viral particles are about 100 nm in diameter (237), and are covered with surface projections about 6-nm long and 10 nm in diameter (95). Virions have a density of 1.16–1.18 g/mL in sucrose density gradients (16), but can be differentiated from avian leukosis/sarcoma viruses by morphology in thin sections (122, 237) and by density in cesium chloride gradients (114). The morphology of the viral particles is shown in Figure 17.45.

Chemical Composition

NUCLEIC ACID. Genomic single stranded RNA of REVs consists of a 60–70 S complex containing two 30–40 S RNA subunits, each having a size of about 3.9×10^6 d (18, 115). The nondefective REV has a genome of about 9.0 kb, the replication-defective strain T genome is only about 5.7 kb due principally to a large deletion in the *gag-pol* region and a smaller deletion in the *env* region (45). Moreover, the replication-defective strain T genome contains a substitution of 0.8–1.5 kb in the *env* region that represents the transforming gene, identified as v-*rel* (41, 46, 231). The v-*rel* is not present in nondefective REVs or other avian or mammalian retroviruses. Related sequences (c-*rel*), conserved in many vertebrates, are present in the DNA of normal avian cells, including turkey cells from whence the oncogene was most likely transduced (41, 219, 220, 231). Mechanisms by which oncogenes are acquired by retroviruses have been reviewed by Sugden (190). Only limited sequence homology exists between the RNA of nondefective REV and the DNA of normal avian cells (94), and no endogenous REV sequences in host DNA have been recognized. The terminal regions of the viral genome, designated as the long terminal repeats (LTRs), consist of 569 base-pair repeats (180) and are efficient promoters in a variety of cell types (158).

ONCOGENE. The nucleotide sequence of the v-*rel* gene has been determined (188).

The v-*rel* oncogene is transcribed in strain T-transformed lymphoid cells and produces a phos-

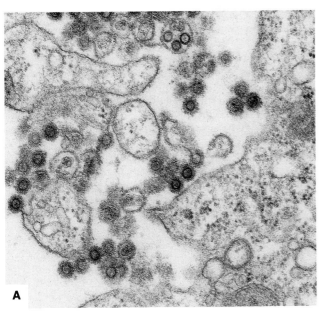
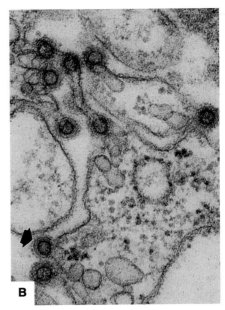

17.45. Electron micrographs of thin sections of chicken embryo fibroblasts infected with REV. *A.* Typical virus particles in the extracellular spaces. ×40,000. *B.* REV particles budding from the plasma membrane of infected cells (*arrow*). ×60,000. (Nazerian)

phoprotein product identified as pp59$^{v\text{-}rel}$. The v-*rel* protein is a member of the rel/dorsal family of proteins, which are related to nuclear factor kappa B and function as DNA-binding transcription factors (21, 163). It differs from the c-*rel* protein both in structure and transforming ability (see 71) and, unlike most other oncogene products, can be detected in both the cytoplasm and nucleus of transformed cells (see 22). The v-rel protein is usually complexed with cellular proteins (99, 109, 189). This protein is responsible for the acute oncogenicity of replication defective strain T, which has been considered the most virulent of all retroviruses (22). The mechanism by which v-rel induced transformation is not yet clear but dominant negative regulation (71, 89) and induction of aberrant transcription (81) have been proposed.

In several cases, REV isolates other than strain T have induced neoplastic disease within very short latent periods (57, 58, 153, 155). Examination of such strains for viral oncogenes of cellular origin may be of interest.

PROTEINS. REVs contain an RNA-directed DNA polymerase (reverse transcriptase) that differs structurally and immunologically from the comparable enzyme of leukosis/sarcoma viruses (15, 122). The preference of the REV-associated enzyme for Mn^{2+} ions is a characteristic by which it can be differentiated from enzymes of other avian retroviruses (122, 173, 234).

A variety of polypeptides have been isolated from REV including two *env* gene–encoded glycoproteins, gp90 and gp20 (205, 207), and five *gag* gene–encoded structural proteins, p12, pp18, pp20, p30, and p10 (206). The C-terminal epitope of gp90 is located on the surface of infected cells (205). The gp90 protein contains both continuous and discontinuous epitopes and was considered the immunodominant protein of the virus (54). The 30-kD (p30) protein constitutes the major group-specific antigen that plays a role in viral particle assembly (216). Mosser et al. (125) located the two glycoproteins and two other proteins on the surface of the virions. Antiserum to p30 cross-reacted with p30 of several other REVs, thus establishing this protein as group specific (116). Earlier reports described similar proteins, although with slightly different molecular weights (115, 232).

Replication

NONDEFECTIVE STRAINS. The cycle of replication is similar to that of other retroviruses and has been reviewed by Dornburg (56). Virus entry involves binding of the envelope glycoprotein to a specific receptor on the cell surface that has not yet been identified. Entry is probably by direct membrane fusion. Expression of viral envelope blocks receptors and results in superinfection interference. Integration of the DNA provirus proceeds by different mechanisms in chicken and D17 cells. Viral RNA transcription and translation are initiated through promoter and enhancer sequences in the

LTR. Two polyproteins are encoded, gag–pol and env; the gag precursor protein is myristylated. The encapsidation sequence is located in the *gag* gene. The final stage is budding of viral particles from the plasma membrane. Virus particle production was first noted at 24 hr (95), and maximum virus production occurred 2–4 days after infection in chicken cells (23, 68, 196).

DEFECTIVE STRAIN. The replication-defective strain T virus requires a nondefective RE helper virus for replication (76). Oncogenicity of this strain is maintained during passage in vivo (160) or during culture of infected hematopoietic cells (76), but is rapidly lost during passage in chicken fibroblast cultures (103, 200, 226) and dog thymus cells (1). Breitman et al. (25) showed this apparent attenuation in chick embryo fibroblast cultures to be due to the loss of the replication-defective, acutely oncogenic virus, which was completely absent after three passages; the helper REV continued to replicate.

CYTOPATHOLOGY. In early studies, cytopathology was not regularly associated with infection of avian fibroblasts in vitro (200). Syncytial cell formation has been noted in infected cultures (47, 144), however, and Temin and Kassner (196) reported that certain strains caused a mild, degenerative cytopathic change in several avian cell types. Temin et al. (198) proposed the following model: Infected cells synthesize unintegrated viral DNA, a part of which is integrated at multiple sites in the cellular genome. Progeny virus then superinfects the already infected cells, leading to an accumulation of unintegrated viral DNA (40, 97, 218). Cells with large amounts of unintegrated DNA die, while those cells able to prevent early superinfection have few copies of unintegrated viral DNA and survive.

The acute phase of cell killing (Fig. 17.46 A,B) lasts 2–10 days after infection and is followed by a state of chronic infection characterized by the disappearance of cytopathology and continued virus production (Fig. 17.46 C) (196, 197). This cytopathic effect is the basis of a plaque assay (32, 124, 196), but the method has not been widely used, perhaps because the cytopathology is somewhat inconsistent. Cho (43, 44) described a plaque assay in the QT35 line of chemically transformed Japanese quail fibroblasts.

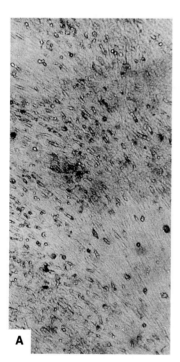 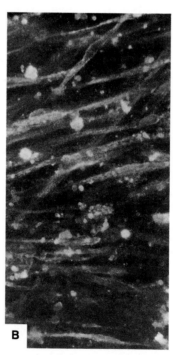 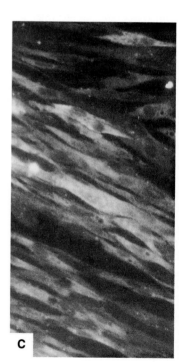

17.46. Acute (cytopathic) and chronic (noncytopathic) infection of chicken embryo fibroblasts inoculated with nondefective REV, strain T. *A*. Mild cytopathic changes 13 days after infection. Unstained, ×55. *B*. Cytopathic changes and viral antigens 13 days after infection demonstrated by indirect immunofluorescent staining. *C*. Chronically infected cultures 48 days after infection showing relatively normal-appearing cells, most of which contain cytoplasmic viral antigens as demonstrated by immunofluorescent staining. ×360.

HOST RANGE. Cells from many or all avian species are susceptible to infection in vitro and are widely used for virus propagation and assay. However, certain mammalian cells support at least limited viral replication. Nondefective REV has been grown in D17 dog sarcoma cells (11, 215), Cf2th dog thymus cells (1, 182), normal rat kidney cells (97), mink lung cells (1), and bovine cells (10). D17 cells are susceptible and constitute a useful host system for virus propagation (214, 215), although REVs require some adaptation before high titers are obtained. Rat and mouse cells were only semipermissive for replication of REV, with blocks at different replication steps (60, 61). Chimeric vector particles containing the REV-A matrix protein infected mammalian cells more efficiently than those containing the matrix protein of spleen necrosis virus strain (39). However, there is no evidence for in vivo replication of REV in nonavian species.

PSEUDOTYPES. The envelope component of nondefective REV forms pseudotypes with Rous sarcoma virus (168, 208) and with vesicular stomatitis virus (93). The pseudotype virus can be neutralized by antiserum to REV; Crittenden et al. (50) has used this principle to detect REV antibodies in test sera.

INSERTIONAL MUTAGENESIS. The ability of REV proviral DNA to integrate into the host cell genome as a necessary part of the replication cycle is well known. Recent studies, however, have also demonstrated the ability of REV proviral DNA to integrate into Marek's disease virus (a DNA virus) when both are cocultivated in the same cells (87). Only a portion of the REV genome, usually the LTR, is present in most insertions (92, 101), but in one case, a full-length REV genome has been detected in turkey herpesvirus (88). This phenomenon is important because of the potential for REV to cause mutations in other organisms and because the packaging of REV in another organism represents a possible novel mechanism for transfer of infection.

Strain Classification.

The different isolates of REV are remarkably uniform in antigenicity, (26, 151, 226) and appear to belong to a single serotype (42). The nondefective strains have similar structural and chemical properties (15, 95); however, differences in pathogenicity have been noted (151).

Definitive evidence for antigenic differences was provided by Cui et al. (51), who developed monoclonal antibodies that reacted with strain T but not with the chick syncytial strain; at least three different epitopes (A, B, and C) were identified. Chen et al. (42) grouped 26 isolates into three subtypes on the basis of neutralization tests and differential reactivity with monoclonal antibodies. Isolates of subtype 1 were considered to possess epitopes A, B, and C, whereas subtype 2 contained epitope B, and

subtype C contained epitopes A and B (42). Viruses of subtype 1 and 2 could not be differentiated by receptor interference (65), thus confirming the absence of major subgroup differences.

Reticulendotheliosis viral isolates differ also in certain biologic properties, including pathogenicity (150), but such differences have not been the basis for strain classification.

Laboratory Host Systems

CELL CULTURES. Fibroblasts from several avian species and certain cell lines, such as QT35 quail sarcoma cells (44, 49) and D17 dog osteosarcoma cells (11, 215), are susceptible to infection with nondefective REVs. In infected cultures, antigens (Fig. 17.46 B,C), virus particles, proviral DNA, cytopathology, and reverse transcriptase may be detected and serve as criteria for virus assay. When the cultures are grown under agar, foci of cells containing immunofluorescent antigens can be localized and used as the basis for a quantitative fluorescent focus assay (151). Duck embryo fibroblasts may be preferred for demonstration of cytopathic effects (6). However, chicken bone marrow-derived macrophages appear resistant to infection (28).

EMBRYOS AND BIRDS. Other laboratory host systems for REV include chicken embryos (177) and a variety of avian species including young chickens, Japanese quail, ducks, geese, turkeys, pheasants, and guinea fowl (153, 200). Embryos and animals may respond to infection by development of specific lesions, viremia, or antibodies.

CELL LINES. Cell lines consisting of cells transformed by REVs are further laboratory host systems of potential value. Lines of hematopoietic cells transformed in vivo or in vitro by the replication-defective strain T have been described; the cell types and surface markers vary based on the strain of helper virus and whether transformation occurred in vivo or in vitro (see 22, 81). A line of transformed chicken embryo fibroblasts has also been developed (67). Nonproducer clones can be isolated that produce pseudotypes when infected with nondefective REV strains (77). The cells possess surface viral antigens that co-cap with antigens of the major histocompatibility complex (112). Cell lines have also been derived from chronic lymphomas induced by nondefective strains of REV (136, 152); one of these lines (RP9) has been widely used in cytotoxicity assays to measure natural killer (NK) cell activity (178). Cell lines induced by in vitro transformation of spleen cells with defective REV can serve as useful expression systems for transfected foreign genes (149, 172) or as substrates for the propagation of other viruses (156).

PATHOGENESIS AND EPIZOOTIOLOGY

Natural and Experimental Hosts. Natural hosts for REV infection include turkeys, chickens, ducks, geese, pheasants, and Japanese quail. Disease is also recognized in chickens following inoculation with vaccines accidently contaminated with nondefective REV. Experimental hosts include all of the above species, as well as guinea fowl. Chickens and turkeys have been most frequently employed as experimental hosts.

Responses to Infection. Epizootiologic studies have detailed some of the virologic and serologic responses of chickens and turkeys to infection with nondefective REVs. Tolerant infection, i.e., persistent viremia in the absence of antibody, is induced readily in chickens by embryo inoculation (83, 228) and by vertical transmission of virus from infected dams (9). Tolerant infection occurs also after inoculation at hatching, but the rate of induction is variable (7, 96, 118, 228, 236) and is influenced by the strain of chicken (63). Some tolerantly infected chickens ultimately develop detectable antibody (128), which may indicate a release from tolerance.

More commonly, inoculated or contact-exposed birds develop a transient viremia followed by the development of antibodies (7, 227). Antibodies have been detected as early as 16–21 days after inoculation in chickens (26, 126), but 6–10 wk may be required in contact-exposed birds (83, 96, 104, 118). Precipitating and immunofluorescent antibodies may decline with age (7, 26, 228), but Mc-Dougall et al. (118) detected neutralizing antibodies at high frequency in experimentally infected turkeys through 40 wk. Maternal antibodies can be detected in newly hatched chickens from exposed dams (224). Bagust and Grimes (7) described the persistence of noninfectious RE viral antigens in the blood for several weeks following the disappearance of infectious virus. Major histocompatibility complex (MHC)–restricted cytotoxicity against lymphoblastoid cell lines transformed with defective REV has been described in chickens within 7 days after inoculation with defective or nondefective RE viral strains (113, 217). This response appears to be mediated by activated (MHC class II+) CD8+ T cells (108). However, NK cells were not activated (169). The induction of cytotoxic T cells by REV has been used as a general indicator of immune response in the study of other avian viruses (156).

Factors influencing the susceptibility of avian hosts to infection have not been thoroughly studied. No genetic cellular resistance has been recognized. However, some differences in the pathologic response of lines or families has been recognized in chickens (63, 175, 179, 230) and quail (199). Although endogenous avian leukosis virus genes had no influence on tumor induction or antibody response following exposure of chickens to the chick syncytial strain, virus was isolated more frequently from chickens with ev2 than from chickens lacking this gene (50). A cellular resistance (interference) due to viral envelope gene expression has been described in cultured D17 cells (55, 65) and suggests that similar resistance might be achieved in chickens modified to express envelope glycoproteins by transgenic technologies. An age-related resistance to clinical disease is apparent. Furthermore, maternal antibodies appear to limit susceptibility to infection (184).

Virus Transmission

HORIZONTAL TRANSMISSION. The virus is transmitted by contact with infected chickens and turkeys (104, 143). Virus has been detected in feces and cloacal swabs (7, 148, 228, 236), as well as other body fluids (9), and in litter from seropositive chicken flocks (224). Viral shedding probably occurs mainly during periods of active viremia. Horizontal transmission may be influenced by the host species (151) and the virus strain (224, 236), and was not detected when chickens were separated by wire mesh (9). Contact infection rarely results in clinical disease (148, 151, 224, 236) except, perhaps, in turkeys in which lymphomas have been observed following contact exposure (118, 119, 143).

The role of insects in the transmission of REV has been studied. Although infection persisted in *Triatoma infestans* for 3 days and in *Ornithodoros moubata* for 7 days, an important role for these and other insects, including mosquitoes, in REV transmission was considered unlikely (201, 202). Attempts to propagate REV in cultures of *Aedes albopictus* were unsuccessful (157). Motha et al. (134), however, isolated virus from 7 of 39 batches of mosquitoes in contact with viremic chickens and demonstrated apparent transmission of the infection to recipient chickens exposed to *Culex annulirostris* that had previously fed on birds with persistent viremia. Mosquito transmission may explain higher infection rates during summer months (134) and/or the high prevalence of infection in Southern states (224, 229) and deserves further study.

The possibility of virus dissemination by needles used to administer Marek's disease vaccines in newly hatched chickens should also be considered (6).

VERTICAL TRANSMISSION. Vertical transmission of REV has been reported in both chickens and turkeys, usually at very low rates. McDougall et al. (118) isolated virus from 2 of 25 embryos from tolerantly infected turkey hens. Similar low rates of viral shedding and transmission were documented for tolerantly infected chickens (7, 9, 210, 228), although Motha and Egerton (132) reported transmission to over 50% of chicks in an experiment in which eggs were incubated within 24 hr of lay. Albumen samples from tolerantly infected hens frequently contained RE viral gs antigen, although at low levels; infectious virus was rarely isolated (228). Vertical transmission from nontolerantly infected chickens is not common, but one exceptional antibody-positive, virus-positive, antigen-negative turkey hen transmitted virus to 6 of 21 progeny (225). Vertical transmission also occurs in ducks, since virus was isolated from embryos derived from tolerantly infected females (127).

Although semen from tolerantly infected turkeys contains infectious virus (118, 225), the role of the tom in vertical transmission is not clear. McDougall et al. (118) found that previously nonexposed turkey hens inseminated with infected semen produced infected progeny, but, in contrast, Witter and Salter (225) found the frequency of vertical transmission was no greater from hens mated with viremic males than with hens mated with nonviremic males; however, the hens were from a previously exposed flock. Furthermore, they found no evidence in parents or congenitally infected progeny of clonal insertions of proviral DNA that would be indicative of genetic transmission (225). Insemination of antibody-negative turkey breeder hens with REV-contaminated semen induced only gradual seroconversion and no infected progeny were detected (164). Male transmission has received less attention in chickens, but Salter et al. (165) found RE proviral DNA in 10 of 820 chicks from matings of viremic males and nonviremic females. Clearly, a role for the male in vertical transmission of REV has not been excluded and needs further study.

The relative role of horizontal and vertical transmission in the maintenance of infection in the field is still poorly understood. Infection is most likely maintained by horizontal transmission from an undetermined natural reservoir of infection.

CONTAMINATED VACCINES. Accidental contamination of virus stocks with REV has been observed on a variety of occasions. The use of REV-contaminated fowl pox (19, 64) or Marek's disease (90, 236) vaccines has been documented, sometimes resulting in major economic consequences. Certain stocks of avian myeloblastosis virus widely distributed as a source of reverse transcriptase for biochemical purposes contained a low level of REV (229). Cross contamination of cultures in the laboratory has been observed. The occurrence of such problems points to a further mechanism for increasing the distribution of this virus in nature.

ACUTE RETICULUM CELL NEOPLASIA

Pathology. The pathology of the acute reticulum cell neoplasia caused by replication-defective strain T virus has been well described (135, 160, 176, 200). The incubation period can be as short as 3 days, but death occurs more commonly 6–21 days after inoculation. Because of the short latent period and high mortality, Bose has referred to defective REV strain T as the most virulent of all retroviruses (22). Inoculation of newly hatched chickens or turkeys results in few clinical signs due to the rapid onset of the disease, and mortality rates often reach 100%.

The affected birds develop large livers and spleens with infiltrative focal or diffuse lesions. Lesions are also common in the pancreas, gonads, heart, and kidney. The blood shows a decrease in heterophils and an increase in lymphocytes (195), leading to a frank leukemia a few hours before death (179). The serum transferrin level is elevated (203) and Shen (179) reported elevated globulin and decreased albumin concentrations.

Histologic changes are generally characterized by the infiltration and proliferation of large vesicular cells, variously described as mononuclear cells of the reticuloendothelial system (200) or primitive mesenchymal cells (160, 176). Some lesions are composed almost solely of such cells, whereas others include also a moderate to heavy population of smaller lymphoid elements, probably indicating a host immunologic response to the primary lesion. Areas of necrosis in association with the neoplastic lesions are also frequent. A typical liver lesion is shown in Fig. 17.47.

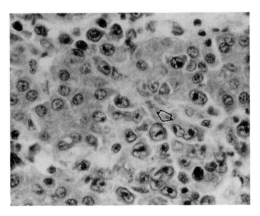

17.47. Microscopic lesions of acute reticulum cell neoplasia (reticuloendotheliosis) in the liver of a chicken inoculated with replication-defective, acutely transforming strain T REV. The liver is infiltrated with large primitive reticular cells (*arrow*).

Transformation.   The identity of the target cell transformed in vivo by defective strain T when associated with REV-A helper has been controversial, but recent studies have shown tumors to be composed of mature cells that express T lymphoid and myeloid markers (14). These cells also express surface MHC class I and II antigens, as well as interleukin-2 receptor (79), and are immunoglobulin M (IgM) negative but vary in expression of CT3 (14). Similar tumors were induced in chemical bursectomized chickens (14). Inoculation directly into the thymus induced thymomas composed of T and B cells (22). On the other hand, defective strain T, when associated with chick syncytial virus helper virus instead of REV-A, induces IgM positive B-cell lymphomas with rearrangements of the heavy- and light-chain immunoglobulin loci (12, 13). Thus, this difference in cell tropism is associated with differential effects of the helper viruses on lymphoid populations.

Neoplastic transformation in acute reticulum cell neoplasia is mediated by the oncogene, v-rel, contained within the replication-defective strain T virus. Transformation does not require the presence of a helper virus (105). Lymphoid cells transformed by strain T in vitro, but which produce no infectious virus, will produce typical RE when transplanted into syngeneic recipients (105, 161).

Immunity.   A protective immune response against the acute neoplasia induced by strain T has been described. Regression of strain T-induced wing-web tumors was partially abrogated by bursectomy, thymectomy, and bursectomy–thymectomy (110). Serum from hyperimmunized chickens was protective against tumor development even after absorption to remove antiviral antibodies (80), thus suggesting the existence of tumor-specific transplantation antigens on RE tumor cells. Chickens immunized with purified or inactivated preparations of nondefective strain T helper virus were resistant to challenge with acutely transforming strain T preparations (17). However, immunization with empty virions (121) did not provide protection.

Runting Disease Syndrome.   The *runting disease syndrome* is a term chosen to designate the several nonneoplastic lesions associated with infection with nondefective REV strains.

Pathology.   The lesions include runting (135, 200, 226), atrophy of the thymus and bursa of Fabricius (135), enlarged peripheral nerves (226), abnormal feather development (102, 103), proventriculitis (90), enteritis (117), anemia (96, 111), and necrosis of the liver and spleen (150, 204). These are often accompanied by depression of cellular and humoral immune responses (26, 36, 83, 96).

Clinically affected birds may be notably stunted and pale. Stunted birds did not consume less food, but had marked reduction of phosphoenolpyruvate carboxykinase, a key gluconeogenic enzyme in the liver (70). Weight depression in infected chicks can be detected as early as 6 days of age (128). Some chickens may have abnormal feather development ("Nakanuke"), i.e., wing feathers with adhesion of the barbs to a localized section of the shaft (102) that is apparently due to REV-induced necrosis of feather-forming cells early after injection (193). Lameness or paralysis is rare even in birds with gross nerve lesions. Affected birds are usually culled prior to death; a culling loss of over 50% between 5 and 8 wk was described in one flock (194). Acute hemorrhagic or chronic ulcerative proventriculitis has been observed (90), but could not be reproduced by Bagust et al. (8) with a similar isolate.

It is still unclear whether the proliferative lesions in enlarged peripheral nerves are neoplastic or inflammatory; however, nerve lesions often occur in the absence of other neoplasms (226). The infiltrating cells are shown in Fig. 17.48. Although lesions of the runting disease syndrome have been most extensively studied in chickens, at least parts of the syndrome occur in ducks inoculated with the spleen necrosis or duck infectious anemia strains of REV, and enlarged nerves (142) of enteritis (117) have been observed in turkeys with RE-related chronic lymphomas. Genetic differences in susceptibility have not yet been described; chicks from lines of different susceptibility to Marek's disease were equally susceptible to the development of nerve lesions following inoculation with REV (226). Virus strain, however, is probably important.

IMMUNODEPRESSION.   Humoral and cellular immune responses are frequently depressed in chickens infected with nondefective REV strains. Depressed antibody responses to Marek's disease virus

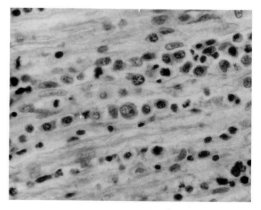

17.48.   Microscopic lesions in a peripheral nerve of a chicken inoculated with nondefective strain T REV. Infiltrating cells consist of mature and immature lymphocytes and plasma cells.

and turkey herpesvirus (26, 96), Newcastle disease virus (83, 235), as well as sheep erythrocytes and *Brucella abortus* (227), are documented. The extent of depression is influenced by the dose and strain of virus, and primary responses are more severely affected than secondary (227). Barth and Humphries (12) found that different strains of nondefective REV varied in ability to induce bursal atrophy and in suppression of B-cell populations available for transformation by v-*rel*. Studies on chimeric viruses derived from REV-A and chick syncytial virus showed that regions in both *gag* and *env* genes were associated with the strong immunodepressive ability of REV-A (66)

Spleen cells from chickens infected with replication-defective strain T were suppressed in their ability to respond to the mitogen, phytohemagglutinin (36, 174). This effect is associated with the nondefective helper virus in strain T stocks (37) and is mediated through a population of suppressor cells (38, 162). The suppressor cells could be demonstrated only through the 3rd wk after infection (161). Other cellular immune responses inhibited by REV infection include mixed lymphocyte reaction and allograft rejection (213).

Witter et al. (227, 228) found depression of humoral responses and mitogen responsiveness was transient following infection with the chick syncytial strain, but persisted through 10–19 wk in chickens tolerantly infected with nondefective strain T. Infected chickens were more susceptible to the development of a Marek's disease tumor transplant (30), to reactions from infectious laryngotracheitis vaccine (126, 183), to natural fowl pox virus infection (133), to infectious bronchitis virus (183), and to mortality induced by *Eimeria tenella* (131) and *Salmonella typhimurium* (130) and may have been more susceptible to necrotic dermatitis (78). No increase in susceptibility to Marek's disease virus was noted (27), but Witter et al. (227) demonstrated interference by REV infection with immunity induced by turkey herpesvirus against Marek's disease in chickens. Humoral immunodepression was also seen in ducks infected with a field RE viral isolate (107).

These immunodepressive effects undoubtedly contribute to the nonneoplastic lesions described earlier and may also enhance the oncogenicity of these viruses. In the field, immunodepression is probably the most important consequence of embryo- or vaccine-derived REV infections. However, immunodepression is much less likely to occur from contact infection (224) and has not commonly been associated with seropositive flocks.

CHRONIC NEOPLASIA

CHICKEN BURSAL LYMPHOMA. Bursal lymphomas constitute the first of two types of chronic neoplastic disease caused by nondefective REV in chickens. Witter and Crittenden (222) found that chickens inoculated with the chick syncytial strain developed a high rate of B-cell lymphomas—involving principally the liver and bursa of Fabricius—that were indistinguishable from lymphoid leukosis (Fig. 17.49). Similar tumors were induced by nondefective strain T (228). A total of 25 lymphomas, 2 sarcomas and 1 adenocarcinoma were induced by the two strains between 17 and 43 wk of age. Interestingly, coinfection of chickens with serotype 2 Marek's disease virus enhanced the incidence of REV bursal lymphomas (2) as had also been reported for lymphoid leukosis (5).

The tumor cells were identified as B cells by IgM and other B-cell specific markers (136, 228). The bursal dependency of this tumor was confirmed by the finding that chemically or surgically bursectomized chickens were refractory to tumor development (62).

Noori-Daloii et al. (139) found in REV-induced lymphomas that the DNA proviral genome of REV was integrated adjacent to c-*myc*, a cellular oncogene important in the induction of lymphoid leukosis by avian leukosis virus. The molecular mechanism by which c-*myc* is activated by insertion of proviral DNA has been studied (69, 159, 191). The proviral insert often contains major deletions that

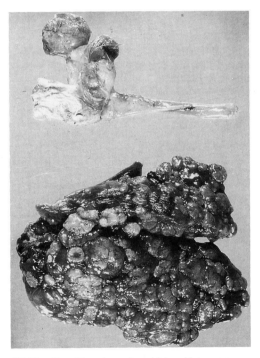

17.49. Bursal lymphoma in a chicken. Note gross lymphomas in the liver and bursa of a chicken 25 wk after inoculation with the nondefective chick syncytial strain of REV.

prevent the expression of infectious virus (192).

Based on pathology, proviral insertional activation of c-*myc*, and enhancement by serotype 2 Marek's disease virus, bursal lymphomas induced by REV and avian leukosis virus appear indistinguishable—a rare case in which the same disease is caused by two unrelated viruses. However, some subtle differences have been noted. For example, chickens of lines resistant and susceptible to lymphoid leukosis were uniformly less susceptible to lymphoma induction by REV than by avian leukosis virus (63), and the REV lymphomas usually require longer latent periods than those induced by avian leukosis virus.

Grimes et al. (73) observed what may be similar lymphomas in two chickens at 22 and 24 wk after inoculation with a field strain of REV, but no bursal involvement was reported. Typical bursal lymphomas were observed in two chicken flocks following administration of an REV-contaminated fowl pox vaccine (64).

CHICKEN NONBURSAL LYMPHOMA. Chronic nonbursal lymphomas have been described in line 6_3 and line 0 chickens following experimental infection with the spleen necrosis or chick syncytial strains of nondefective REV (230). These lymphomas have latent periods as short as 6 wk and involve the thymus, heart, liver, and spleen, but not the bursa of Fabricius (see Fig. 17.50). Nerve enlargements, probably from concomitant expression of the runting disease syndrome, can be seen. Thus, this neoplastic syndrome superficially resembles Marek's disease (230). The cell type has been defined as a T cell on the basis of cell surface markers (48). The molecular mechanism of oncogenesis also involves insertional activation of c-*myc*, but differs from that in bursal lymphomas; the strong tendency for the provirus to be oriented in the same direction as c-*myc* in bursal lymphomas was not observed in nonbursal lymphomas (86). Thus far, T-cell lymphomas have not been documented in the field, but little effort has been made to do so.

TURKEY LYMPHOMA. Naturally occurring infection with REV can result in lymphoma production in turkeys (117, 142) between 15 and 20 wk of age. In transmission studies, similar lymphomas were induced in 10–30% of turkey poults on the first passage after 8–11 wk (143) or 11–12 wk (117). Lesions typically included lymphomas in the liver, intestine, and other visceral organs; Paul et al. (143) and McDougall et al. (117) both described lymphomatous lesions in the bursa, but this lesion was apparently not very common. Critical comparisons between chronic lymphomas in turkeys and chickens have not been made and there is no evidence that a common mechanism of oncogenesis exists.

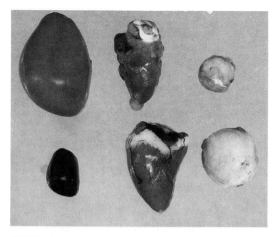

17.50. Nonbursal lymphoma in a chicken 48 days postinoculation with the nondefective spleen necrosis strain of REV. Note enlargement of spleen, nodular lymphomas on heart, and bursal atrophy of infected chicken (*top row*). Organs from age-matched control chicken are shown in the *bottom row*. (Avian Pathol).

OTHER LYMPHOMAS. Chronic lymphomas of the spleen, liver, pancreas, and intestine have been described between 20 and 30 wk in the domestic goose (58); one of four spleen cell preparations when inoculated into chickens and geese induced lymphomas within 11–22 days, whereas the other preparations induced lymphomas after long latent periods. Naturally occurring lymphomas have been described in ducks at 20 wk (72) and at 4–10 wk (141). Perk et al. (147) described an outbreak characterized by generalized leukemia, as well as lymphomas in visceral organs in 6-mo-old ducks. A virus isolate obtained from a duck of unknown age with nodular lymphoid tumors in the liver and spleen produced a high rate of lymphomas and other neoplasms between 8 and 24 wk; the frequency was not affected by age at infection or by embryonal bursectomy (107).

An REV-associated disease in pheasants characterized by cutaneous lesions on the head and mouth and nodular lymphomas in visceral organs occurred between 6 and 12 mo of age (57), and a tumor cell inoculum induced a high rate of lymphomas in pheasant chicks between 2–4 wk postinoculation.

Lymphomas occurring in Japanese quail between 2 and 7 mo of age have been associated with REV infection (35, 170). Lesions included lymphomas of the liver and spleen and nodular tumors of the intestine.

MULTIPLE SYNDROMES. Lesions of the different types can be observed in the same experiment, or even in the same bird. Nondefective REV strains may first induce lesions of the runting disease syndrome and lymphomas may occur later in the survivors, sometimes accompanied by nerve enlargements. Chickens inoculated with replication-defective, acutely transforming strain T, especially those surviving the acute disease, may develop lesions associated with the nondefective strain T helper virus.

DIAGNOSIS. A diagnosis of RE requires not only the presence of typical gross and microscopic lesions, but also the demonstration of REV. This virus, unlike avian leukosis and Marek's disease viruses, is not yet ubiquitous (despite its increasing prevalence). Infectious virus, viral antigens, and proviral DNA are commonly found in tumor cells and their presence has diagnostic value.

Virus Isolation and Identification. Viremia with REV is typically low titered and transient, except following congenital transmission or embryo inoculation that leads to tolerant infection. Birds with lesions are the best source of virus.

Virus may be isolated by inoculation of susceptible tissue cultures with tissue suspensions, whole blood, plasma, or other inocula. In general, cellular inocula are preferred over cell-free inocula, since the former usually contain higher titers of virus than the latter. The tissue cultures should be maintained through at least two blind 7-day passages. Infection may be detected by the presence of cytopathic effects but must be confirmed by detection of antigens by immunofluorescence (226), immunoperoxidase staining (32), complement fixation (186), or enzyme immunoassay (52, 85) using specific antibodies against REV. In comparative studies, enzyme immunoassays were more sensitive than complement fixation tests (52) and indirect immunofluorescence was more sensitive than indirect immunoperoxidase or immunoelectronmicroscopy (137). A convenient and sensitive indirect immunofluorescent assay conducted in 96-well plates (42) has been used for virus isolation from field samples (225). Monoclonal antibodies to REV (51) have been used to detect REV antigens by enzyme immunoassay (52). A commercial test kit based on this procedure is under development.

Virus isolated by this procedure may be identified by reproduction of the typical disease in experimental animals and by further neutralization tests. Virus isolates may be assigned to antigenic subtypes by the differential reactivity of monoclonal antibodies in immunofluorescent assays (42). Subtyping of isolates may have value for epidemiologic studies.

Detection of proviral DNA by polymerase chain reaction (PCR) assays has been described (3). This procedure appears useful for tumor diagnosis (53) and the evaluation of vaccines for possible REV contamination (64). The PCR assay can be used in lieu of antigen detection assays for demonstration of infection in inoculated cell cultures or directly in tissue samples but may not be as well suited as enzyme-linked immunosorbent assay (ELISA) for large-scale testing.

Serology. Confirmation of REV infection by serologic procedures involves the detection of antibodies or antigens in sera from chickens inoculated with suspect isolates or from chickens of field flocks. Antibodies are induced with various frequencies and persist for varied periods. Specific antibody may be detected in the serum or egg yolk from exposed birds by indirect immunofluorescence (4, 226), virus neutralization (118, 151), agar gel precipitin (82, 129), enzyme immunoassay (29, 138, 185) and pseudotype neutralization (50) tests. Enzyme immunoassay kits for antibody detection are commercially available. The agar gel precipitin test may detect viral antigen as well as antibody in sera (83). Antibody tests are particularly useful in ascertaining the absence of viral exposure in specific-pathogen–free breeder flocks or flocks producing progeny for export.

Differential Diagnosis. The differential diagnosis of REV-induced lesions from those of other diseases is difficult due to the lack of lesions pathognomonic for RE, the diverse types of lesions induced, and the similarity of the lesions to those caused by other organisms. As previously stated, diagnoses of RE should be supported by virologic evidence of REV infection. The development of PCR assays for RE (see Virus Isolation) and Marek's disease (see subchapter, Marek's Disease), combined with the pending development of PCR assays for exogenous avian leukosis virus (see subchapter, Leukosis/Sarcoma Group), should assist greatly in the differential diagnosis of RE. Histochemical assays to detect cellular and viral antigens in sections of tumor tissue is another emerging diagnostic technique. These new techniques for differential diagnosis of RE and other avian viral tumors are under current evaluation.

The acute reticulum cell neoplasia syndrome is not known to occur in the field and is unlikely to require differential diagnosis when experimentally reproduced in the laboratory. A new syndrome of broiler chickens characterized by reticuloendothelial proliferation in the spleen and liver, and resulting in condemnation loss at processing, has been confused with RE (74, 212), but can be distinguished by the absence of RE antigens and proviral DNA in the lesions (221).

The runting disease syndrome must be distinguished from Marek's disease in the chicken, especially when nerve lesions are also present. Differences between REV-induced and Marek's disease virus–induced nerve lesions have been discussed (226, 227), but are not consistent. Both types of nerve lesions must be distinguished from spontaneous neuropathy, a probable autoimmune lesion of peripheral nerves (20). Other immunodepressive diseases such as infectious bursal disease and infection with anemia virus may also resemble the runting disease syndrome.

Chronic RE neoplasia in the turkey must be differentiated from lesions of lymphoproliferative disease of turkeys (84); differences in pathology and in properties of the viral reverse transcriptase can be helpful (173, 234). The PCR assays for lymphoproliferative disease (166) and RE (above) should also aid the differentiation of these diseases.

Chronic neoplasia in the chicken where the tumors are of bursal origin cannot usually be differentiated from lymphoid leukosis on pathologic criteria (222); virologic or serologic tests may help providing infection can be established for one virus and excluded for the other. In addition, RE or lymphoid leukosis tumors should contain proviral DNA sequences of the respective virus inserted near the c-*myc* gene, a characteristic that could permit differentiation of tumors by molecular hybridization or PCR.

Chronic neoplasia in the chicken in which bursal tumors are lacking or in which the latent period is too short for that of lymphoid leukosis must be differentiated from Marek's disease. Here too, pathologic criteria are insufficient and virologic assays (including PCR) may be helpful. The pp38 antigen of Marek's disease virus, occasionally expressed in Marek's disease lymphomas (see subchapter, Marek's Disease), is not present in RE lymphomas. Also, MHC class II (Ia) antigens are reported to be present on Marek's disease lymphoma cells (171) but absent on RE nonbursal lymphoma cells (48). In summary, naturally occurring RE lesions can be confused in the chicken with Marek's disease, lymphoid leukosis, and various other lymphoproliferative or immunodepressive conditions, and in the turkey, with lymphoproliferative disease. An increasing awareness of REV-related syndromes, the increasing prevalence of REV infection, and the availability of improved diagnostic techniques should encourage attempts to include RE in the differential diagnosis of avian neoplasms.

TREATMENT. No treatment for RE is known. Since immune responses are mounted to infection, it is possible that some affected birds may recover.

PREVENTION AND CONTROL. No procedures have been applied in commercial practice for the control of RE, mainly because the disease has been sporadic and self-limiting, but also because the necessary techniques and knowledge have not been available. Studies by Witter and Salter (225) on a flock of naturally infected breeder turkeys showed that REV has the potential to be a major economic problem and provided an evaluation of some techniques for identification of shedder hens. Enzyme immunoassays to detect RE viral antigen in albumen samples seems to be the procedure of choice (85, 225). Presumably, it would be necessary to eliminate vertical transmission through removal of potential transmitter hens, and to rear progeny under isolated conditions whereby horizontal infection could be precluded. Many of these principles have been applied to the control of avian leukosis virus in chickens. Compared with avian leukosis virus, however, REV is likely to be vertically transmitted at lower rates, males may warrant greater consideration as potential transmitters, and horizontal infection seems more difficult to control. Such control procedures could be considered if REV infection becomes endemic in valuable breeding stock. Control may also be needed to prevent environmental exposure and seroconversion of breeder flocks where progeny are destined for export. This will be difficult to accomplish, however, until the important natural reservoirs of infection and manner by which infection is introduced are elucidated. Management practices used for specific-pathogen–free flocks appear to limit environmental infection with REV, but are too costly to be generally applicable to commercial breeders.

Although vaccines have not been seriously proposed for control of RE, some candidate vaccines have been described. Vaccination of chickens with a recombinant fowl pox virus expressing the *env* gene of REV (33), or empty REV particles produced by transfected QT35 quail cells (121), provided some protection against the runting disease syndrome.

REFERENCES

1. Allen, P.T., J.A. Mullins, C.L. Harris, A. Hellman, R.F. Garry, and M.R.F. Waite. 1979. Replication of reticuloendotheliosis virus in mammalian cells. Am Soc Microbiol Abst Annual Meet, No. S100, p. 256.
2. Aly, M.M., A.M. Fadly, and R.L. Witter. 1992. Effects of serotype 2 Marek's disease virus on development of viremia, antibody, and lymphoma induced by reticuloendotheliosis virus. In G. de Boer and S.H.M Jerissen (eds.). Proc 4th Int Symp on Marek's disease. Ponsen & Looijen, Wageningen, Amsterdam, The Netherlands, pp. 272–276.
3. Aly, M.M., E.J. Smith, and A.M. Fadly. 1993. Detection of reticuloendotheliosis virus infection using the polymerase chain reaction. Avian Pathol 22:543–554.
4. Aulisio, C.G., and A. Shelokov. 1969. Prevalence of reticuloendotheliosis in chickens: immunofluorescence studies. Proc Soc Exp Biol Med 130:178–181.
5. Bacon, L., R.L. Witter, and A.M. Fadly. 1989. Augmentation of retrovirus-induced lymphoid leukosis by Marek's disease herpesviruses in white leghorn chickens. J Virol 63:504–512.

6. Bagust, T.J. 1993. Reticuloendotheliosis virus. In J.B. McFerran and M.S. McNulty (eds.). Virus Infections of Vertebrates, 4. Virus Infections of Birds. Elsevier Science Publishers B.V. Amsterdam, The Netherlands, pp. 437–454.

7. Bagust, T.J., and T.M. Grimes. 1979. Experimental infection of chickens with an Australian strain of reticuloendotheliosis virus. 2. Serological responses and pathogenesis. Avian Pathol 8:375–389.

8. Bagust, T.J., T.M. Grimes, and D.P. Dennett. 1979. Infection studies on a reticuloendotheliosis virus contaminant of a commercial Marek's disease vaccine. Aust Vet J 55:153–157.

9. Bagust, T.J., T.M. Grimes, and N. Ratnamohan. 1981. Experimental infection of chickens with an Australian strain of reticuloendotheliosis virus. 3. Persistant infection and transmission by the adult hen. Avian Pathol 10:375–385.

10. Ban, J., N.L. First, and H.M. Temin. 1989. Bovine leukemia virus packaging cell line for retrovirus-mediated gene transfer. J Gen Virol 70:1987–1993.

11. Barbacid, M., E. Hunter, and S.A. Aaronson. 1979. Avian reticuloendotheliosis viruses: evolutionary linkages with mammalian type C retroviruses. J Virol 30:508–514.

12. Barth, C.F., and E.H. Humphries. 1988. A nonimmunosuppressive helper virus allows high efficiency induction of B cell lymphomas by reticuloendotheliosis virus strain T. J Exp Med 167:89–108.

13. Barth, C.F., and E.H. Humphries. 1988. Expression of v-rel induces mature B-cell lines that reflect the diversity of avian immunoglobulin heavy- and light-chain rearrangements. Mol Cell Biol 8:5358–5368.

14. Barth, C.F., D.L. Ewert, W.C. Olson, and E.H. Humphries. 1990. Reticuloendotheliosis virus REV-T(REV-A)-induced neoplasia: development of tumors within the T-Lymphoid and myeloid lineages. J Virol 64:6054–6062.

15. Bauer, G., and H.M. Temin. 1980. Specific antigenic relationships between the RNA-dependent DNA polymerases of avian reticuloendotheliosis viruses and mammalian type C retroviruses. J Virol 34:168–177.

16. Baxter-Gabbard, K.L., W.F. Campbell, F. Padgett, A. Raitano-Fenton, and A.S. Levine. 1971. Avian reticuloendotheliosis virus (strain T). II. Biochemical and biophysical properties. Avian Dis 15:850–862.

17. Baxter-Gabbard, K.L., D.A. Peterson, A.S. Levine, P. Meyers, and M.M. Sigel. 1973. Reticuloendotheliosis virus (strain T). VI An immunogen versus reticuloendotheliosis and Rous sarcoma. Avian Dis 17:145–150.

18. Beemon, K.L., A.J. Faras, A.T. Haase, P.H. Duesberg, and J.E. Maisel. 1976. Genomic complexities of murine leukemia and sarcoma, reticuloendotheliosis and visna viruses. J Virol 17:525–537.

19. Bendheim, U. 1973. A neoplastic disease in turkeys following fowl pox vaccination. Refu Vet 30:35–41.

20. Biggs, P.M., R.W. Shilleto, A.M. Lawn, and D.M. Cooper. 1982. Idiopathic polyneuritis in SPF chickens. Avian Pathol 11:163–178.

21. Blank, V., P. Kourilsky, and A. Israel. 1992. NF-kB and related proteins: Rel/dorsal homologies meet ankyrin-like repeats. Trends Biochem Sci 17:135–140.

22. Bose, H.R., Jr. 1992. The rel family: Models for transcriptional regulation and oncogenic transformation. Biochem Biophys Acta 1114:1–17.

23. Bose, H.R., and A.S. Levine. 1967. Replication of the reticuloendotheliosis virus (strain T) in chicken embryo cell culture. J Virol 1:1117–1121.

24. Bosselman, R.A., R.-Y. Hsu, T. Boggs, S. Hu, J. Bruszewski, S. Ou, L.M. Souza, L. Kozar, F. Martin, M. Nicolson, W. Rishell, J.A. Schultz, K.M. Semon, and R.G. Stewart. 1989. Replication-defective vectors of reticuloendotheliosis virus transduce exogenous genes into somatic stem cells of the unincubated chicken embryo. J Virol 63:2680–2689.

25. Breitman, M.L., M.M.C. Lai, and P.K. Vogt. 1980. Attenuation of avian reticuloendotheliosis virus: loss of the defective transforming component during serial passage of oncogenic virus in fibroblasts. Virology 101:304–306.

26. Bülow V. von 1977. Immunological effects of reticuloendotheliosis virus as potential contaminant of Marek's disease vaccines. Avian Pathol 6:383–393.

27. Bülow V. von 1980. Effects of infectious bursal disease virus and reticuloendotheliosis virus infection of chickens on the incidence of Marek's disease and on local tumour development of the non-producer JMV transplant. Avian Pathol 9:109–119.

28. Bülow, V. von, and A. Klasen. 1983. Effects of avian viruses on cultured chicken bone-marrow-derived macrophages. Avian Pathol 12:179–198.

29. Bülow, V. von, and M. Lesjak. 1987. A modified ELISA for the demonstration of antiviral antibodies in chicken sera which included the use of virus-free cellular antigens to control the specificity of assay results. J Vet Med B 34:655–669.

30. Bülow, V. von, and F. Weiland. 1980. Stimulation of local solid tumour development of the nonproducer Marek's disease tumour transplant JMV by virus-induced immunosuppression. Avian Pathol 9:93–108.

31. Burmester, B.R. 1964. Personal communication.

32. Calvert, J.G. and K. Nazerian. 1994. An immunoperoxidase plaque assay for reticuloendotheliosis virus and its application to a sensitive serum neutralization assay. Avian Dis 38:165–171.

33. Calvert, J.G., K. Nazerian, R.L. Witter, and N. Yanagida. 1993. Fowlpox virus recombinants expressing the envelope glycoprotein of an avian reticuloendotheliosis retrovirus induce neutralizing antibodies and reduce viremia in chickens. J Virol 67:3069–3076.

34. Campbell, W.F., K.L. Baxter-Gabbard, and A.S. Levine. 1971. Avian reticuloendotheliosis virus (strain T). I. Virological characterization. Avian Dis 15:837–849.

35. Carlson, H.C., G.L. Seawright, and J.R. Pettit. 1974. Reticuloendotheliosis in Japanese quail. Avian Pathol 3:169–175.

36. Carpenter, C.R., H.R. Bose, and A.S. Rubin. 1977. Contact-mediated suppression of mitogen-induced responsiveness by spleen cells in reticuloendotheliosis virus-induced tumorigenesis. Cell Immunol 33:392–401.

37. Carpenter, C.R., K.E. Kempf, H.R. Bose, and A.S. Rubin. 1978. Characterization of the interaction of reticuloendotheliosis virus with the avian lymphoid system. Cell Immunol 39:307–315.

38. Carpenter, C.R., A.S. Rubin, and H.R. Bose. 1978. Suppression of the mitogen stimulated blastogenic response during reticuloendotheliosis virus-induced tumorigenesis: investigations into the mechanism of action of the suppressor. J Immunol 120:1313–1320.

39. Casella, C.R. and A.T. Panganiban. 1993. The matrix protein is responsible for the differential ability of two retroviruses to function as helpers for vector propagation. Virology 192:458–464.

40. Chen, I.S.Y., and H.M. Temin. 1982. Establishment of infection by spleen necrosis virus: inhibition in stationary cells and the role of secondary infection. J Virol 41:183–191.

41. Chen, I.S.Y., T.W. Mak, J.J. O'Rear, and H.M. Temin. 1981. Characterization of reticuloendotheliosis virus strain T DNA and isolation of a novel variant of reticuloendotheliosis virus strain T by molecular cloning. J Virol 40:800–811.

42. Chen, P-Y., Z. Cui, L.F. Lee, and R.L. Witter. 1987. Serologic differences among non-defective reticuloendotheliosis viruses. Arch Virol 93:233–246.

43. Cho, B.R. 1983. Cytopathic effects and focus formation by reticuloendotheliosis viruses in a quail fibroblast cell line. Avian Dis 27:261–270.

44. Cho, B.R. 1984. Improved focus assay of reticuloendotheliosis in a quail fibroblast cell line (QT35). Avian Dis 28:261–265.

45. Coffin, J.M. 1982. Structure of the retroviral genome. RNA tumor viruses. In R. Weiss, N. Teich, H. Varmus and J. Coffin (eds.). Molecular Biology of Tumor Viruses, 2nd ed. Cold Spring Harbor Laboratory, Cold Spring Harbor, NY, pp. 261–368..

46. Cohen, R.S., T.C. Wong, and M.M.C. Lai. 1981. Characterization of transformation and replication specific sequences of reticuloendotheliosis virus. Virology 113:672–685.

47. Cook, M.K. 1969. Cultivation of a filterable agent associated with Marek's disease. J Natl Cancer Inst 43:203–212.

48. Cooper, M.D., C-L.H. Chen, R.P. Bucy, and C.B. Thompson. 1991. Avian T cell ontogeny. Adv Immunol 50:87–117.

49. Cowen, B.S., and M.O. Braune. 1988. The propagation of avian viruses in a continuous cell line (QT35) of Japanese quail origin. Avian Dis 32:282–297.

50. Crittenden, L.B., A.M. Fadly, and E.J. Smith. 1982. Effect of endogenous leukosis virus genes on response to infection with avian leukosis and reticuloendotheliosis virus. Avian Dis 26:279–294.

51. Cui, Z.-Z., L.F. Lee, R.F. Silva, and R.L. Witter. 1986. Monoclonal antibodies against avian reticuloendotheliosis virus: identification of strain-specific and strain-common epitopes. J Immunol 136:4237–4242.

52. Cui, Z.-Z., L.F. Lee, R.F. Silva, R.L. Witter, and T.S. Chang. 1988. Monoclonal-antibody-mediated enzyme-linked immunosorbent assay for detection of reticuloendotheliosis viruses. Avian Dis 32:32–40.

53. Davidson, I., A. Borovskaya, S. Perl, and M. Malkinson. 1995. Use of the polymerase chain reaction for the diagnosis of natural infection of chickens and turkeys with Marek's disease virus and reticuloendotheliosis virus. Avian Pathol 24:69–94.

54. Davidson, I., H. Yang, R.L. Witter, and M. Malkinson. 1995. The immunodominant proteins of reticuloendotheliosis virus. Vet Microbiol 49:273-284.

55. Delwart, E.L., and A.T. Panganiban. 1989. Role of reticuloendotheliosis virus envelope glycoprotein in superinfection interference. J Virol 63:273–280.

56. Dornburg, R. 1995. Reticuloendotheliosis viruses (REV) and REV derived retroviral vectors. Gene Ther 2:301–310.

57. Dren, C.N., E. Saghy, R. Glavits, F. Ratz, J. Ping, and V. Sztojkov. 1983. Lymphoreticular tumour in pen-raised pheasants associated with a RE-like virus infection. Avian Pathol 12:55–71.

58. Dren, C.N., I. Nemeth, I. Sari, F. Ratz, R. Glavits, and P. Somogyi. 1988. Isolation of a reticuloendotheliosis-like virus from naturally occurring lymphoreticular tumours of domestic goose. Avian Pathol 17:259–277.

59. Eckroade, R.J. 1995. Unpublished data.

60. Embretson, J.E., and H.M. Temin. 1986. Pseudotyped retroviral vectors reveal restrictions to reticuloendotheliosis virus replication in rat cells. J Virol 60:662–668.

61. Embretson, J.E., and H.M. Temin. 1987. Transcription from a spleen necrosis virus 5′ long terminal repeat is suppressed in mouse cells. J Virol 61:3454–3462.

62. Fadly, A.M., and R.L. Witter. 1983. Studies of reticuloendotheliosis virus induced lymphomagenesis in chickens. Avian Dis 27:271–282.

63. Fadly, A.M., and R.L. Witter. 1986. Resistance of Line 63 chickens to reticuloendotheliosis virus-induced bursa-associated lymphomas. Int J Cancer 38:139–143.

64. Fadly, A.M., R.L. Witter, E.J. Smith, R.F. Silva, W.M. Reed, F.J. Hoerr, and M.R. Putnam. 1996. An outbreak of lymphomas in commercial broiler chickens vaccinated with a fowlpox vaccine contaminated with reticuloendotheliosis virus. Avian Pathol 25:35-47.

65. Federspiel, M.J., L.B. Crittenden, and S.H. Hughes. 1989. Expression of avian reticuloendotheliosis virus confers host resistance. Virology 173:167-177.

66. Filardo, E.J., M.F. Lee, and E.H. Humphries. 1994. Structural genes, not the LTRs, are the primary determinants of reticuloendotheliosis virus A-induced runting and bursal atrophy. Virology 202:116–128.

67. Franklin, R.B., C.Y. Kang, K.M.M. Wan, and H.R. Bose. 1977. Transformation of chick embryo fibroblasts by reticuloendotheliosis virus. Virology 83:313–321.

68. Fritsch, E., and H.M. Temin. 1977. Formation and structure of infectious DNA of spleen necrosis virus. J Virol 21:119–130.

69. Fujita, D.J., R.A. Swift, A.A.G. Ridgway, and H.J. Kung. 1984. Reticuloendotheliosis virus induced B lymphomas in chickens characterization of a tumour cell DNA clone containing proviral and c-myc sequences. J Cell Biochem (Suppl 7) Pt B:12.

70. Garry, R.F., G.M. Shackleford, L.F. Berry, and H.R. Bose. 1985. Inhibition of hepatic phosphoenolpyruvate carboxykinase by avian reticuloendotheliosis viruses. Cancer Res 45:5020–5026.

71. Gilmore, T.D. 1992. Role of rel family genes in normal and malignant lymphoid cell growth. Cancer Surv 15:69–87.

72. Grimes, T.M., and H.G. Purchase. 1973. Reticuloendotheliosis in a duck. Aust Vet J 49:466–471.

73. Grimes, T.M., T.J. Bagust, and C.K. Dimmock. 1979. Experimental infection of chickens with an Australian strain of reticuloendotheliosis virus. I. Clinical, pathological and haematological effects. Avian Pathol 8:57–68.

74. Hafner, S., M.A. Goodwin, L.C. Kelley, D.I. Bounous, M. Puette, W.B. Steffens, K.A. Langheinrich, and J. Brown. 1994. Multicentric histiocytosis mimicking reticuloendotheliosis in broiler chickens [abst]. Proc 66th NE Conf Avian Dis, p. 26.

75. Hayes, L.E., K.A. Langheinrich, and R.L. Witter. 1992. Reticuloendotheliosis in a wild turkey (Meleagris gallopavo) from coastal Georgia. J Wildl Dis 28:154–158.

76. Hoelzer, J.D., R.B. Franklin, and H.R. Bose. 1979. Transformation by reticuloendotheliosis virus: development of a focus assay and isolation of a non-transforming virus. J Virol 93:20–30.

77. Hoelzer, J.D., R.B. Lewis, C.R. Wasmuth, and H.R. Bose. 1980. Hematopoietic cell transformation by reticuloendotheliosis virus: characterization of the genetic defect. Virology 100:462–474.

78. Howell, L.J., R. Hunter, and T.J. Bagust. 1982. Necrotic dermatitis in chickens. NZ Vet J 30:87–88.

79. Hrdlickova, R., J. Nehyba, and E.H. Humphries. 1994. v-rel Induces expression of three avian immunoregulatory surface receptors more efficiently than c-rel. J Virol 68:308–319.

80. Hu, C.-P., and T.J. Linna. 1976. Serotherapy of avian reticuloendotheliosis virus-induced tumors. Ann N Y Acad Sci 277:634–646.

81. Humphries, E.H. and G. Zhang. 1992. V-rel and C-rel modulate the expression of both bursal and non-bursal antigens on avian B-cell lymphomas. Curr Top Microbiol Immunol 182:475–483.

82. Iaconescu, M. 1977. Reticuloendotheliosis antigen for the agar gel precipitation test. Avian Pathol 6:259–261.

83. Iaconescu, M., and A. Aharonovici. 1978. Persistent viraemia in chickens, subsequent to in ovo inoculation of reticuloendotheliosis virus. Avian Pathol 7:237–247.

84. Iaconescu, M., K. Perk, A. Zimber, and A. Yaniv. 1979. Reticuloendotheliosis and lymphoproliferative disease of turkeys. Refu Vet 36:2–12.

85. Ignjatovic, J., K.J. Fahey, and T.J. Bagust. 1987. An enzyme-linked immunosorbent assay for detection of reticuloendotheliosis virus infection in chickens. Avian Pathol 16:609–621.

86. Isfort, R., R.L. Witter, and H-J Kung. 1987. C-myc activation in an unusual retrovirus-induced avian T-lymphoma resembling Marek's disease: proviral insertion 5' of exon one enhances the expression of an intron promoter. Oncogene Res 2:81–94.

87. Isfort, R.J., D. Jones, R.G. Kost, R.L. Witter, and H.-J. Kung. 1992. Retrovirus insertion into herpesvirus in vitro and in vivo. Proc Natl Acad Sci USA 89:991–995.

88. Isfort, R.J., Z. Qian, D. Jones, R.F. Silva, R.L. Witter, and H. Kung. 1994. Integration of multiple chicken retroviruses into multiple chicken herpesviruses: Herpesviral gD as a common target of integration. Virology 203:125–133.

89. Ishikawa, H., M. Asano, T. Kanda, S. Kumar, Céline Gélinas and Y. Ito. 1993. Two novel functions associated with the rel oncoproteins: DNA replication and cell-specific transcriptional activation. Oncogene 8(11):2889–2896.

90. Jackson, C.A.W., S.E. Dunn, D.I. Smith, P.T. Gilchrist, and P.A. MacQueen. 1977. Proventriculitis, "Nakanuke" and reticuloendotheliosis in chickens following vaccination with herpesvirus of turkeys (HVT). Aust Vet J 53:457–458.

91. Johnson, E.S. 1994. Poultry oncogenic retroviruses and humans. Cancer Detect Prev 18:9–30.

92. Jones, D., R.J. Isfort, R.L. Witter, R.G. Kost, and H.-J. Kung. 1993. Retroviral insertions into a herpesvirus are clustered at the junctions of the short repeat and short unique sequences. Proc Natl Acad Sci USA 90:3855–3859.

93. Kang, C.-Y., and P. Lambright. 1977. Pseudotypes of vesicular stomatitis virus with the mixed coat of reticuloendotheliosis virus and vesicular stomatitis virus. J Virol 21:1252–1255.

94. Kang, C-Y., and H.M. Temin. 1974. Reticuloendotheliosis virus nucleic acid sequences in cellular DNA. J Virol 14:1179–1188.

95. Kang, C.Y., T.C. Wong, and K.V. Holmes. 1975. Comparative ultrastructural study of four reticuloendotheliosis viruses. J Virol 16:1027–1038.

96. Kawamura, H., T. Wakabayashi, S. Yamaguchi, T. Taniguchi, N. Takayanagi, S. Sato, S. Sekiya, and T. Horiuchi. 1976. Inoculation experiment of Marek's disease vaccine contaminated with reticuloendotheliosis virus. Natl Inst Anim Health Q 16:135–140.

97. Keshet, E., and H.M. Temin. 1979. Cell killing by spleen necrosis virus is correlated with a transient accumulation of spleen necrosis virus DNA. J Virol 31:376–388.

98. Kewalramani, V.N., A.T. Panganiban, and M. Emerman. 1992. Spleen necrosis virus, an avian immunosuppressive retrovirus, shares a receptor with the Type D Simian retroviruses. J Virol 66:3026–3031.

99. Kochel, T. and N.R. Rice. 1992. v-rel- and c-rel- protein complexes bind to the NF-kappaB site in vitro. Oncogene 7:567–572.

100. Koo, H.-M., J. Gu, A. Varela-Echavarria, Y. Ron, and J.P. Dougherty. 1992. Reticuloendotheliosis Type C and primate Type D oncoretroviruses are members of the same receptor interference group. J Virol 66:3448–3454.

101. Kost, R.G., D. Jones, R.J. Isfort, R.L. Witter, and H.-J. Kung. 1992. Retrovirus insertion into Herpesvirus: characterization of a Marek's disease virus harboring a solo LTR. Virology 192:161–169.

102. Koyama, H., Y. Suzuki, Y. Ohwada, and Y. Saito. 1976. Reticuloendotheliosis group virus pathogenic to chicken isolated from material infected with turkey herpesvirus (HVT). Avian Dis 20:429–434.

103. Koyama, H., T. Sasaki, Y. Ohwada, and Y. Saito. 1980. The relationship between feathering abnormalities ("Nakanuke") and tumour production in chickens inoculated with reticuloendotheliosis virus. Avian Pathol 9:331–340.

104. Larose, R.N., and M. Sevoian. 1965. Avian lymphomatosis. IX. Mortality and serological response of chickens of various ages to graded doses of T strain. Avian Dis 9:604–610.

105. Lewis, R.B., J. McClure, B. Rup, D.W. Niesel, R.F. Garry, J. D. Hoelzer, K. Nazerian, and H.R. Bose. 1981. Avian reticuloendotheliosis virus: identification of the hematopoietic target cell for transformation. Cell 25:421–431.

106. Ley, D.H., M.D. Ficken, D.T. Cobb, and R.L. Witter. 1989. Histomoniasis and reticuloendotheliosis in a wild turkey (Meleagris gallopavo) in North Carolina. J Wildl Dis 25:262–265.

107. Li, J., B.W. Calnek, K.A. Schat, and D.L. Graham. 1983. Pathogenesis of reticuloendotheliosis virus infection in ducks. Avian Dis 27:1090–1105.

108. Lillehoj, H.S., E.P. Lillehoj, D. Weinstock, and K.A. Schat. 1988. Functional and biochemical characterizations of avian T lymphocyte antigens identified by monoclonal antibodies. Eur J Immunol 18:2059–2065.

109. Lim, M.Y., N. Davis, J. Zhang, and H.R. Bose, Jr. 1990. The v-rel oncogene product is complexed with cellular proteins including its proto-oncogene product and heat shock protein70. Virology 175:149–160.

110. Linna, T.J., C. Hu, and K.D. Thompson. 1974. Development of systemic and local tumors induced by avian reticuloendotheliosis virus after thymectomy or bursectomy. J Natl Cancer Inst 53:847–854.

111. Ludford, C.G., H.G. Purchase, and H.W. Cox. 1972. Duck infections anemia virus associated with plasmodium louvers. Exp Parasitol 31:29–38.

112. Maccubbin, D., and L. Schierman. 1982. Evidence for association of viral and major histocompatibility complex antigens on reticuloendotheliosis virus transformed cells of chickens. Fed Proc 41:698, No. 2499.

113. Maccubbin, D., and L. Schierman. 1986. MHC-restricted cytotoxic response of chicken T cells: expression, augmentation, and clonal characterization. J Immunol 136:12–16.

114. Maldonado, R.L., and H.R. Bose. 1971. Separation of reticuloendotheliosis virus from avian tumor viruses. J Virol 8:813–815.

115. Maldonado, R.L., and H.R. Bose. 1975. Polypeptide and RNA composition of the reticuloendotheliosis viruses. Intervirology 5:194–204.

116. Maldonado, R.L., and H.R. Bose. 1976. Group-specific antigen shared by the members of the reticuloendotheliosis virus complex. J Virol 17:983–990.

117. McDougall, J.S., P.M. Biggs, and R.W. Shilleto. 1978. A leukosis in turkeys associated with infection with reticuloendotheliosis virus. Avian Pathol 7:557–568.

118. McDougall, J.S., R.W. Shilleto, and P.M. Biggs. 1980. Experimental infection and vertical transmission of reticuloendotheliosis virus in the turkey. Avian Pathol 9:445–454.

119. McDougall, J.S., R.W. Shilleto, and P.M. Biggs. 1981. Further studies on vertical transmission of reticuloendotheliosis virus in turkeys. Avian Pathol 10:163–169.

120. Meroz, M. 1992. Reticuloendotheliosis and "pullet disease" in Israel. Vet Rec 130:107–108.

121. Meyers, N.L. 1993. Antibody response elicited against empty reticuloendotheliosis virus particles in two inbred lines of chicken. Vet Microbiol 36:317–332.

122. Moelling, K., H. Gelderblom, G. Pauli, R. Friis, and H. Bauer. 1975. A comparative study of the avian reticuloendotheliosis virus: relationship to murine leukemia virus and viruses of the avian sarcoma-leukosis complex. Virology 65:546–557.

123. Moore, B.E., and H.R. Bose. 1988. Expression of the v-rel oncogene in reticuloendotheliosis virus-transformed fibroblasts. Virology 162:377–387.

124. Moscovici, C., D. Chi, L. Gazzolo, and M.G. Moscovici. 1976. A study of plaque formation with avian RNA tumor viruses. Virology 73:181–189.

125. Mosser, A.G., R.C. Montelaro, and R.R. Rueckert.

1975. The polypeptide composition of spleen necrosis virus, a reticuloendotheliosis virus. J Virol 15:1088–1095.

126. Motha, M.X.J. 1982. Effects of reticuloendotheliosis virus on the response of chickens to infectious laryngotracheitis virus. Avian Pathol 11:475–486.

127. Motha, M.X.J. 1984. Distribution of virus and tumour formation in ducks experimentally infected with reticuloendotheliosis virus. Avian Pathol 13:303–320.

128. Motha, M.X.J. 1987. Clinical effects, virological and serological responses in chickens following in-ovo inoculation of reticuloendotheliosis virus. Vet Microbiol 14:411–417.

129. Motha, M.X.J. 1987. Demonstration of precipitating antibodies to reticuloendotheliosis virus in egg yolk. Aust Vet J 64:259–260.

130. Motha, M.X.J., and J.R. Egerton. 1983. Effect of reticuloendotheliosis virus on the response of chickens to Salmonella typhimurium infection. Res Vet Sci 34:188–192.

131. Motha, M.X.J., and J.R. Egerton. 1984. Influence of reticuloendotheliosis on the severity of Eimeria tenella infection in broiler chickens. Vet Microbiol 9:121–129.

132. Motha, M.X.J., and J.R. Egerton. 1987. Vertical transmission of reticuloendotheliosis virus in chickens. Avian Pathol 16:141–148.

133. Motha, M.X.J., and J.R. Egerton. 1987. Outbreak of atypical fowlpox in chickens with persistent reticuloendotheliosis viraemia. Avian Pathol 16:177–182.

134. Motha, M.X.J., J.R. Egerton, and A.W. Sweeney. 1984. Some evidence of mechanical transmission of reticuloendotheliosis virus by mosquitoes. Avian Dis 28:858–867.

135. Mussman, H.C., and M.J. Twiehaus. 1971. Pathogenesis of reticuloendotheliosis virus disease in chicks: an acute runting syndrome. Avian Dis 15:483–502.

136. Nazerian, K., R.L. Witter, L.B. Crittenden, M.R. Noori-Daloii, and H.J. Kung. 1982. An IgM-producing B lymphoblastoid cell line established from lymphomas induced by a non-defective reticuloendotheliosis virus. J Gen Virol 58:351–360.

137. Nicholas, R.A.J., and D.H. Thornton. 1983. Relative efficiency of techniques for detecting avian reticuloendotheliosis virus as a vaccine contaminant. Res Vet Sci 34:377–379.

138. Nicholas, R.A.J., and D.H. Thornton. 1987. An enzyme-linked immunosorbent assay for the detection of antibodies to avian reticuloendotheliosis virus using whole cell antigen. Res Vet Sci 43:403–404.

139. Noori-Daloii, M.R., R.A. Swift, H.J. Kung, L.B. Crittenden, and R.L. Witter. 1981. Specific integration of REV proviruses in avian bursal lymphomas. Nature 294:574–576.

140. Okoye, J.O.A., W. Ezema, and J.N. Agoha. 1993. Naturally occurring clinical reticuloendotheliosis in turkeys and chickens. Avian Pathol 22:237–244.

141. Paul, P.S., and R.W. Werdin. 1978. Spontaneously occurring lymphoproliferative disease in ducks (case reports). Avian Dis 22:191–195.

142. Paul, P.S., K.A. Pomeroy, P.S. Sarma, K.H. Johnson, D.M. Barnes, M.C. Kumar, and B.S. Pomeroy. 1976. Brief communication: naturally occurring reticuloendotheliosis in turkeys: transmission. J Natl Cancer Inst 56:419–421.

143. Paul, P.S., K.H. Johnson, K.A. Pomeroy, B.S. Pomeroy, and P.S. Sarma. 1977. Experimental transmission of reticuloendotheliosis in turkeys with the cell-culture-propagated reticuloendotheliosis viruses of turkey origin. J Natl Cancer Inst 58:1819–1824.

144. Paul, P.S., K.A. Pomeroy, C.C. Muscoplat, B.S. Pomeroy, and P.S. Sarma. 1977. Characteristics of two new reticuloendotheliosis virus isolates of turkeys. Am J Vet Res 38:311–316.

145. Paul, I., O. Cotofan, and M. Boisteanu. 1986. The incidence of Marek's disease in anti-MD infected hens. Lucr Stiint Ser Zooteh Med Vet 30:95–96.

146. Payne, L.N. 1992. Biology of avian retroviruses. Retroviridae 1:299–404.

147. Perk, K., M. Malkinson, A. Gazit, A. Yaniv, and A. Zimber. 1981. Reappearance of an acute undifferentiated leukemia in a flock of Muscovy ducks. Proc 10th Int Symp Assoc for Comp Res Leukemia Related Dis, pp. 99–100.

148. Peterson, D.A., and A.S. Levine. 1971. Avian reticuloendotheliosis virus (strain T). IV. Infectivity and transmissibility in day-old cockerels. Avian Dis 15:874–883.

149. Pratt, W.D., R.W. Morgan, and K.A. Schat. 1992. Characterization of reticuloendotheliosis virus-transformed avian T-lymphoblastoid cell lines infected with Marek's disease virus. J Virol 66:7239–7244.

150. Purchase, H.G., and R.L. Witter. 1975. The reticuloendotheliosis viruses. Curr Top Microbiol Immunol 71:103–124.

151. Purchase, H.G., C. Ludford, K. Nazerian, and H.W. Cox. 1973. A new group of oncogenic viruses: reticuloendotheliosis, chick syncytial, duck infectious anemia, and spleen necrosis viruses. J Natl Cancer Inst 51:489–499.

152. Ratnamohan, N. and P.B. Spradbrow. 1982. The reticuloendotheliosis viruses: A review. Pakistan Vet J 2:101–107.

153. Ratnamohan, N., T.J. Bagust, T.M. Grimes, and P.B. Spradbrow. 1979. Transmission of an Australian strain of reticuloendotheliosis virus to adult Japanese quail. Aust Vet J 55:506.

154. Ratnamohan, N., T.M. Grimes, T.J. Bagust, and P.B. Spradbrow. 1980. A transmissible chicken tumour associated with reticuloendotheliosis virus infection. Aust Vet J 56:34.

155. Ratnamohan, N., T. Bagust, and P.B. Spradbrow. 1982. Establishment of a chicken lymphoblastoid cell line infected with reticuloendotheliosis virus. J Comp Pathol 92:527–532.

156. Reddy, S.K., M.J.H. Ratcliffe, and A. Silim. 1993. Flow cytometric analysis of the neutralizing immune response against infectious bursal disease virus using reticuloendotheliosis virus-transformed lymphoblastoid cell lines. J Virol Methods 44:167–178.

157. Rehacek, J., T. Dolan, K. Thompson, R.G. Fischer, Z. Rehacek, and H. Johnson. 1971. Cultivation of oncogenic viruses in mosquito cells in vitro. Curr Top Microbiol Immunol 55:161–164.

158. Ridgway, A.A.G. 1992. Reticuloendotheliosis virus long terminal repeat elements are efficient promoters in cells of various species and tissue origin, including human lymphoid cells. Gene 121:213–218.

159. Ridgway, A.A., R.A. Swift, H.J. Kung, and D.J. Fujita. 1985. In vitro transcription analysis of the viral promoter involved in c-myc activation in chicken lymphomas: detection and mapping for two RNA initiation sites with the reticuloendotheliosis virus long terminal repeat. J Virol 54:161–170.

160. Robinson, F.R., and M.J. Twiehaus. 1974. Isolation of the avian reticuloendothelial virus (strain T). Avian Dis 18:278–288.

161. Rup, B.J., J.L. Spencer, J.D. Hoelzer, R.B. Lewis, C.R. Carpenter, A.S. Rubin, and H.R. Bose. 1979. Immunosuppression induced by avian reticuloendotheliosis virus: mechanism of induction of the suppressor cell. J Immunol 123:1362–1370.

162. Rup, B.J., J.D. Hoelzer, and H.R. Bose. 1982. Helper viruses associated with avian acute leukemia viruses inhibit the cellular immune response. J Virol 116: 61–71.

163. Rushlow, C. and R. Warrior. 1992. The rel family of proteins. Bioessays 14:89–95.

164. Salem, M., L.H. Keller, and R.J. Eckroade. 1990. Venereal exposure of turkey hens to reticuloendotheliosis virus. Proc 39th West Poult Dis Conf, March 4–6, 1990, Sacramento, CA, p. 44.

165. Salter, D.W., E.J. Smith, S.H. Hughes, S.E. Wright, and L.B. Crittenden. 1986. Transgenic chickens: insertion of retroviral genes into the chicken germ line. Virology 157:236–240.

166. Sarid, R., A. Chajut, M. Malkinson, S.R. Tronick, A. Gazit, and A. Yaniv. 1994. Diagnostic test for lymphoproliferative disease virus infection of turkeys, using the polymerase chain reaction. Am J Vet Res 55:769–772.

167. Sasaki, T., S. Sasaki, and H. Koyama. 1993. A survey of an antibody to reticuloendotheliosis virus in sera of chickens and other avian species in Japan. J Vet Med Sci 55:885–888.

168. Sawyer, R.C., and H. Hanafusa. 1977. Formation of reticuloendotheliosis virus pseudotypes of Rous sarcoma virus. J Virol 22:634–639.

169. Schat, K.A. 1991. Importance of cell-mediated immunity in Marek's disease and other viral tumor diseases. Poult Sci 70:1165–1175.

170. Schat, K.A., J. Gonzales, A. Solorzano, E. Avila, and R.L. Witter. 1976. A lymphoproliferative disease in Japanese quail. Avian Dis 20:153–161.

171. Schat, K.A., C.-L. H. Chen, B.W. Calnek, and D. Char. 1991. Transformation of T-lymphocyte subsets by Marek's Disease herpesvirus. J Virol 65:1408–1413.

172. Schat, K.A., W.D. Pratt, R.W. Morgan, D. Weinstock, and B.W. Calnek. 1992. Stable transfection of Reticuloendotheliosis virus- transformed lymphoblastoid cell lines. Avian Dis 36:432–439.

173. Schwarzbard, Z., A. Yaniv, M. Ianconescu, K. Perk, and A. Zimber. 1980. A reverse transcriptase assay for the diagnosis of lymphoproliferative disease. Avian Pathol 9:481–487.

174. Scofield, V.L., and H.R. Bose. 1978. Depression of mitogen response in spleen cells from reticuloendotheliosis virus-infected chickens and their suppressive effect on normal lymphocyte response. J Immunol 120:1321–1325.

175. Scofield, V.L., J.L. Spence, W.E. Briles, and H.R. Bose. 1978. Differential mortality and lesion responses to reticuloendotheliosis virus infection in Marek's disease-resistant and susceptible chicken lines. Immunogenet 7:169–172.

176. Sevoian, M., R.N. Larose, and D.M. Chamberlain. 1964. Avian lymphomatosis. VI. A virus of unusual potency and pathogenicity. Avian Dis 3:336–347.

177. Sevoian, M., R.N. Larose, and D.M. Chamberlain. 1964. Avian lymphomatosis. VIII. Pathological response of the chicken embryo to T virus. J Natl Cancer Inst 17:99–119.

178. Sharma, J.M., and B.D. Coulson. 1979. Presence of natural killer cells in specific-pathogen-free chickens. J Natl Cancer Inst 63:527–531.

179. Shen, P.F.-L. 1981. Immunological, hematogical, pathological, and ultrastructural studies of chickens with reticuloendotheliosis. PhD Dissertation, University of Arkansas.

180. Shimotohno, K., S. Mizutani, and H.M. Temin. 1980. Sequence of retrovirus provirus resembles that of bacterial transposable elements. Nature 285:550–554.

181. Shuman, R.M., and R.N. Shoffner. 1986. Molecular approaches to poultry breeding: gene transfer by avian retroviruses. Poult Sci 65:1437–1444.

182. Simek, S., and N.K. Rice. 1980. Analysis of the nucleic acid components in reticuloendotheliosis virus. J Virol 33:320–329.

183. Sinkovic, B. 1981. In vivo interactions between reticuloendotheliosis virus and some other infectious agents of chickens. Proc 4th Aust Poult Stock Feed Conv, pp. 114–118.

184. Sinkovic, B., and C.O. Choi. 1979. Studies on reticuloendotheliosis maternal antibody. Proc 3rd Aust Poult Stock Feed Conv, pp. 119–122.

185. Smith, E.J., and R.L. Witter. 1983. Detection of antibodies against reticuloendotheliosis viruses by an enzyme-linked immunosorbent assay. Avian Dis 27:225–234.

186. Smith, E.J., J.J. Solomon, and R.L. Witter. 1977. Complement-fixation test for reticuloendotheliosis viruses. Limits of sensitivity in infected avian cells. Avian Dis 21:612–622.

187. Solomon, J.J., R.L. Witter, and K. Nazerian. 1976. Studies on the etiology of lymphomas in turkeys: isolation of reticuloendotheliosis virus. Avian Dis 20:735–747.

188. Stephens, R.M., N.R. Rice, R.R. Hiebsch, H.R. Bose, and R.V. Gilden. 1983. Nucleotide sequence of v-rel: the oncogene of reticuloendotheliosis virus. Proc Natl Acad Sci USA 80:6229–6233.

189. Storms, R.W. and Bose, H.R., Jr. 1992. Alterations within pp59v-rel-containing protein complexes following the stimulation of REV-T-transformed lymphoid cells with zinc. Virology 188:765–777.

190. Sugden, B. 1993. How some retroviruses got their oncogenes. Trends Biochem Sci 18:233–235.

191. Swift, R.A., E. Shaller, R.L. Witter, and H.-J. Kung. 1985. Insertional activation of c-myc by reticuloendotheliosis virus in chicken B lymphoma: nonrandom distribution and orientation of the proviruses. J Virol 54:869–872.

192. Swift, R.A., C. Boerkoel, A. Ridgway, D.J. Fujita, J.B. Dodgson, and H.-J. Kung. 1987. B-lymphoma induction by reticuloendotheliosis virus: characterization of a mutated chicken syncytial virus provirus involved in c-myc activation. J Virol 61:2084–2090.

193. Tajima, M., T. Nunoya, and Y. Otaki. 1977. Pathogenesis of abnormal feathers in chickens inoculated with reticuloendotheliosis virus. Avian Dis 21:77–89.

194. Taniguchi, T., N. Yuasa, S. Sato, and T. Horiuchi. 1977. Pathological changes in chickens inoculated with reticuloendotheliosis-virus-contaminated Marek's disease vaccine. Natl Inst Anim Health Q 17:141–150.

195. Taylor, H.W., and L.D. Olson. 1973. Chronologic study of the T-virus in chicks. II. Development of hematologic changes. Avian Dis 17:794–802.

196. Temin, H.M., and V.K. Kassner. 1974. Replication of reticuloendotheliosis viruses in cell cultures: acute infection. J Virol 13:291–297.

197. Temin, H.M., and V.K. Kassner. 1975. Replication of reticuloendotheliosis viruses in cell culture: chronic infection. J Gen Virol 27:267–274.

198. Temin, H.M., E. Keshet, and S.K. Weller. 1980. Correlation of transient accumulation of linear unintegrated viral DNA and transient cell killing by avian leukosis and reticuloendotheliosis viruses. Cold Spring Harb Symp Quant Biol 44:773–778.

199. Terada, N., T. Kuramoto, and T. Ino. 1977. Comparison of susceptibility to the T-strain of reticuloendotheliosis virus among families of Japanese quail. Jpn Poult Sci 14:259–265.

200. Theilen, G.H., R.F. Zeigel, and M.J. Twiehaus. 1966. Biological studies with REV (strain T) that induces reticuloendotheliosis in turkeys, chickens and Japanese quail. J Natl Cancer Inst 37:731–743.

201. Thompson, K.D., R.G. Fischer, and D.H. Luecke. 1968. Determination of the viremic period of avian reticuloendotheliosis virus (strain T) in chicks and virus viability in Triatoma infestans (KLUG) (Hemiptera:Reduviidae). Avian Dis 12:354–360.

202. Thompson, K.D., R.G. Fischer, and D.H. Luecke. 1971. Quantitative infectivity studies of avian reticuloendotheliosis virus (strain T) in certain hematophagous arthropods. J Med Entomol 8:486–490.

203. Torres-Medina, A., R.C. Mussman, M.B. Rhodes, and M.J. Twiehaus. 1973. Chicken transferrin: high levels in chickens with reticuloendothelial virus disease. Poult Sci 52:747–754.

204. Trager, W. 1959. A new virus of ducks interfering with development of malaria parasite (Plasmodium lophurae). Proc Soc Exp Biol Med 101:578–582.

205. Tsai, W.-P., and S. Oroszlan. 1988. Site-directed cytotoxic antibody against the C-terminal segment of the surface glycoprotein gp90 of avian reticuloendotheliosis virus. Virology 166:608–611.

206. Tsai, W.-P., T.D. Copeland, and S. Oroszlan. 1985. Purification and chemical and immunological characterization of avian reticuloendotheliosis virus gag-gene-encoded structural proteins. Virology 140:289–312.

207. Tsai, W.-P., T.D. Copeland, and S. Oroszlan. 1986. Biosynthesis and chemical and immunological characterization of avian reticuloendotheliosis virus env gene-encoded proteins. Virology 155:567–583.

208. Vogt, P.K., J.L. Spencer, W. Okazaki, R.L. Witter, and L.B. Crittenden. 1977. Phenotypic mixing between reticuloendotheliosis virus and avian sarcoma viruses. Virology 80:127–135.

209. Von dem Hagen, D., and H.A. Loliger. 1978. Studies into epizootiology of quail leukosis. Monatsh Vetinarmed 33:591–593.

210. Wakabayashi, T., and H. Kawamura. 1975. Virus reticuloendotheliosis virus group: persistent infection in chickens and viral transmission to fertile eggs. Proc 79th Annu Meet Jpn World Vet Poult Assoc, pp. 12–13.

211. Wakabayashi, T. and H. Kawamura. 1977. Serological survey of reticuloendotheliosis virus infection among chickens in Japan. Natl Inst Anim Health Q 17:73–74.

212. Waldrip, D.W. 1994. RE-like syndrome [abst]. Proc 29th Natl Meet Poult Health Process, p. 113.

213. Walker, M.H., B.J. Rup, A.S. Rubin, and H.R. Bose. 1983. Specificity in the immunosuppression induced by avian reticuloendotheliosis virus. Infect Immun 40:225–235.

214. Watanabe, S., and H.M. Temin. 1982. Encapsidation sequences for spleen necrosis virus and avian retrovirus are between the 5′ long terminal repeat and the start of the gag gene. Proc Natl Acad Sci USA 79:5986–5990.

215. Watanabe, S., and H.M. Temin. 1983. Construction of a helper cell line for avian reticuloendotheliosis virus cloning vectors. Mol Cell Biol 3:2241–2249.

216. Weaver, T.A., K.J. Talbot, and A.T. Panganiban. 1990. Spleen necrosis virus gag polyprotein is necessary for particle assembly and release but not for proteolytic processing. J Virol 64:2642–2652.

217. Weinstock, D., K.A. Schat, and B.W. Calnek. 1989. Cytotoxic T lymphocytes in reticuloendotheliosis virus-infected chickens. Eur J Immunol 19:267–272.

218. Weller, S.K., and H.M. Temin. 1981. Cell killing by avian leukosis viruses. J Virol 39:713–721.

219. Wilhelmsen, K.C., and H.M. Temin. 1984. Structure and dimorphism of c-rel (turkey), the cellular homolog to the oncogene of reticuloendotheliosis virus strain T. J Virol 49:521–529.

220. Wilhelmsen, K.C., K. Eggleton, and H.M. Temin. 1984. Nucleic acid sequences of the oncogene v-rel in reticuloendotheliosis virus strain T and its cellular homolog the proto-oncogene c-rel. J Virol 52:172–182.

221. Witter, R.L. 1994. Control of Marek's disease. Proc Int Sem Avian Pathol 201–208.

222. Witter, R.L., and L.B. Crittenden. 1979. Lymphomas resembling lymphoid leukosis in chickens inoculated with reticuloendotheliosis virus. Int J Cancer 23:673–678.

223. Witter, R.L., and S.W. Glass. 1984. Reticuloendotheliosis in breeder turkeys. Avian Dis 28:742–750.

224. Witter, R.L., and D.C. Johnson. 1985. Epidemiology of reticuloendotheliosis virus in broiler breeder flocks. Avian Dis 29:1140–1154.

225. Witter, R.L., and D.W. Salter. 1989. Vertical transmission of reticuloendotheliosis virus in breeder turkeys. Avian Dis 33:226–235.

226. Witter, R.L., H.G. Purchase, and G.H. Burgoyne. 1970. Peripheral nerve lesions similar to those of Marek's disease in chickens inoculated with reticuloendotheliosis virus. J Natl Cancer Inst 45:567–577.

227. Witter, R.L., L.F. Lee, L.D. Bacon, and E.J. Smith. 1979. Depression of vaccinal immunity to Marek's disease by infection with reticuloendotheliosis virus. Infect Immun 26:90–98.

228. Witter, R.L., E.J. Smith, and L.B. Crittenden. 1981. Tolerance, viral shedding, and neoplasia in chickens infected with non-defective reticuloendotheliosis viruses. Avian Dis 25:374–394.

229. Witter, R.L., I.L. Peterson, E.J. Smith, and D.C. Johnson. 1982. Serological evidence in commercial chicken and turkey flocks of infection with reticuloendotheliosis virus. Avian Dis 26:753–762.

230. Witter, R.L., J.M. Sharma, and A.M. Fadly. 1986. Nonbursal lymphomas by nondefective reticuloendotheliosis virus. Avian Pathol 15:467–486.

231. Wong, T.C., and M.M.C. Lai. 1981. Avian reticuloendotheliosis virus contains a new class of oncogene of turkey origin. Virology 111:289–293.

232. Wong, T.C., R.B. Lewis, H.R. Bose, Jr., and C.Y. Kang. 1980. Assembly of avian reticuloendotheliosis virus: association of the core precursor polypeptide with the intracellular ribonucleoprotein complex. J Virol 34:484.

233. Yamada, S., S. Kamikawa, Y. Uchinuno, H. Fujikawa, K. Takeuchi, A. Tominaga, and K. Matsua. 1977. Distribution of antibody against reticuloendotheliosis virus and isolation of the virus. J Jap Vet Med Assn 30:387–390.

234. Yaniv, A., A. Gazit, M. Ianconescu, K. Perk, B. Aizenberg, and A. Zimber. 1979. Biochemical characterization of the type C retrovirus associated with lymphoproliferative disease of turkeys. J Virol 30:351–357.

235. Yoshida, I., M. Sakata, K. Fujita, T. Noguchi, and N. Yuasa. 1981. Modification of low virulent Newcastle disease virus infection in chickens infected with reticuloendotheliosis virus. Natl Inst Anim Health Q 21:1–6.

236. Yuasa, N., I. Yoshida, and T. Taniguchi. 1976. Isolation of a reticuloendotheliosis virus from chickens inoculated with Marek's disease vaccine. Natl Inst Anim Health Q 16:141–151.

237. Zeigel, R.F., G.H. Theilen, and M.J. Twiehaus. 1966. Electron microscopic observations on REV (strain T) that induces reticuloendotheliosis in turkeys, chickens, and Japanese quail. J Natl Cancer Inst 37:709-729.

LYMPHOPROLIFERATIVE DISEASE OF TURKEYS

Peter M. Biggs

INTRODUCTION, HISTORY, INCIDENCE, AND DISTRIBUTION. *Lymphoproliferative disease* (LPD) is a term used to describe a lymphoproliferative disorder of turkeys that was first recognized as a disease entity in 1972 in the United Kingdom (2, 3). In the same year, a condition in turkeys described as similar to Marek's disease (MD) and that closely resembled LPD was reported in the Netherlands (30). Since that time, LPD has been reported in Israel (23) and Austria (29) and recognized in several European countries. It probably is not a new disease, because a retrospective examination of sections of tumors submitted for diagnosis in the past revealed a similarity between many of the lesions and those described for LPD (2, 3). In addition, lymphomatosis, leukosis, and MD-like disease have been reported in turkeys over the years (1, 4, 18, 28), and some of these cases could have been LPD. The disease may be endemic or sporadic in occurrence, and some flocks may have a low incidence (3).

ETIOLOGY

Classification. Although Koch's postulates have not been strictly fulfilled for the etiology of LPD because the agent has not been cultivated in vitro, strong circumstantial and experimental evidence indicates that it is a type C oncovirus belonging to the subfamily *Oncovirinae* of the family *Retroviridae*. Type C particles occur in tissues (Fig. 17.51), lesions, and plasma pellets from birds with naturally occurring and experimentally produced disease, and preparations of these materials reproduce the disease when inoculated into poults (3, 17, 24). Type C particles have been described as budding from cells in the proliferative lesions of LPD. The most conclusive evidence comes from the use of a novel in vivo infectivity assay for cloned retroviruses. Gak et al. (8) transfected turkey lymphocytes with cloned provirus prepared from affected turkey tissue and returned the transfected lymphocytes to the same turkeys from which they came. The turkeys developed a retrovirus viremia as well as characteristic lesions of LPD. The inoculation of poults with cell-free plasma collected from the affected turkeys resulted in the development of LPD lesions. The genome of this type C oncovirus (called LPDV) has been fully sequenced and the encoded proteins studied and compared with those of other oncoviruses. Although LPDV has the major characteristics of oncoviruses, it differs suffi-

ciently from other oncoviruses, including the avian leukosis/sarcoma and reticuloendotheliosis viruses, to be considered a representative of a distinct group of avian retroviruses. Of many oncoviruses studied, LPDV is most closely related to the avian leukosis/sarcoma group of viruses (6, 26).

LPDV is not an endogenous virus of turkeys because virus-specific sequences have not been found in the cell genome of normal turkeys (11). There is no oncogene in the genome of LPDV (7), and during replication it integrates into the host cell genome at random sites (5).

Attempts to cultivate the virus in cell culture have been unsuccessful using embryo fibroblasts of chickens, turkeys, ducks and quail, and kidney cells of chicks and turkeys (17).

Morphology. Mature particles measure 90–120 nm and have an electron-dense core with a less dense intermediate layer bounded by an outer envelope. Partially purified virus is infectious after filtration through a membrane filter with a pore diameter of 220 nm, but not when the pore diameter is

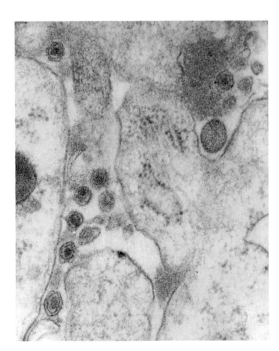

17.51. Electron micrograph of a spleen of a turkey with lymphoproliferative disease showing virus particles. × 73,000

100 nm. Density of infectious particles is 1.16–1.18 g/cm³.

Chemical Composition. The infectivity of partially purified virus is inactivated by lipid solvents.

NUCLEIC ACID. The virus contains high molecular weight RNA, with a sediment coefficient of approximately 70S, and an RNA-dependent DNA polymerase which has a preference for Mg^{2+} over Mn^{2+} in both endogenous and exogenous reactions (27, 31). The LPDV RNA genome is 7143-bp long (26). The proviral genome is bordered by 354-bp long terminal repeats (LTR). The sequence of the LPDV LTR differs significantly from the sequences of avian leukosis/sarcoma group viruses, which have extensive sequence similarity (9).

The genetic organization of LPDV is characteristic of members of the subfamily oncovirus. The viral genome contains three genes coding for the main structural genes, which are in order from the 5′ to the 3′ end of the genome, *gag, pol,* and *env,* but, unlike the avian leukosis/sarcoma group viruses, the protease is not coded for by the *gag* gene but is coded for by a separate fourth open reading frame (ORF). This ORF overlaps the *gag* and *pol* genes. In addition, there are four short ORFs of unknown function (26).

PROTEINS. There has been difficulty in determining the structural polypeptides of LPDV. This is because of the lack of cell cultures susceptible to infection with LPDV and, therefore, an inability to use metabolic labeling techniques.

Virus for study has had to be prepared from plasma collected from viremic turkeys. Preparations of virus from this source seem to be contaminated with host polypeptides, some of which are absorbed to the surface of the virus. The polypeptides of LPDV have been studied by two groups and they seem different from other retroviruses. Gazit et al. (13) described five structural polypeptides with molecular weights of 76, 31, 28, 20, and 15 kD. The 76-kD polypeptide is glycosylated, and these authors suggested that it was a major constituent of the virion envelope. They also suggested that p20 is a constituent of the envelope. They described p31 and p28 as the major structural polypeptides. Patel and Shilleto (21) described three major (p32, p26, and p22/21) and two minor (p41 and p12) structural polypeptides. They also suggested gp76 and a major doublet polypeptide p13.5/13 to be of viral origin. They concluded that gp76 is a surface protein and that p22/21 is probably intramembrane in location, whereas p32, p26, and p13.5/13 are in the viral core, with p13.5/13 likely to be the ribonucleoprotein.

Based on the results of sequencing of the viral genome, the structural proteins have been assigned to their position in the structure of the LPDV particle. These are the 20-kD matrix protein, a 31-kD protein of unknown location in the virion, the 28-kD capsid protein, the nucleocapsid and protease proteins, each of 13-15 kD, and two envelope glycoproteins of 76 kD and 41 kD (10, 26).

PATHOGENESIS AND EPIZOOTIOLOGY

Natural and Experimental Hosts. The disease has been described only in turkeys. Attempts to transmit the infection by parenteral inoculation were successful in turkeys and chickens, but unsuccessful in ducks and geese (16). Gross and microscopic lesions were produced in chickens, but were less severe than in turkeys. The disease occurs naturally in turkeys mainly between 7 and 18 wk of age, although it can occur sporadically in adults (2, 3, 14). Males may be more susceptible to the disease than females. Turkey hybrids differ in susceptibility to development of disease in response to inoculation with infectious material (17), and much of the disease in the field has been restricted to a few commercial hybrids. Lymphoproliferative disease can spread horizontally between poults in contact with one another (17).

An unusual feature of the disease is that poults experimentally infected at 4 wk of age develop a higher incidence of disease than those infected at 1 day (2, 17). It does not appear that this is the result of a change in susceptibility to infection, because poults inoculated at 1 day of age do become infected (15, 17). It is possible that the presence of maternally derived antibody reduces the probability of infection producing disease or, alternatively, that immune competence is required for development of disease. However surgical or chemical bursectomy did not significantly influence the incidence or severity of experimentally produced disease (34).

Incubation Period. The incubation period for the naturally occurring disease is not known. Field observations suggest it can be as short as 7 wk, and experimental transmission studies suggest it could be less than that in some individuals and more in others.

Signs. The clinical course of the disease is rapid, with few, if any, premonitory signs; when clinical signs are noted, they are ruffled feathers, anorexia, and a disinclination to move. Poults showing signs die, and mortality may be as high as 25% of the flock.

Gross Lesions. The most consistent gross lesion is splenomegaly. Affected spleens can be as large as a chicken egg, and usually they are pale pink and marbled in appearance. The liver may be enlarged, but not greatly so, and it may contain miliary gray-white foci. Similar miliary or diffuse lesions may also occur in pancreas, thymus, kidneys, gonads, intestinal wall, lungs, and myocardium. In some birds, peripheral nerves are slightly enlarged (2, 3, 14). Anemia is frequently present; some affected birds have a leukocytosis, others are leukopenic, and elevated immunoglobulin G (IgG) concentration has been recorded (33).

Histopathology.   The characteristic lesion in all organs is lymphoproliferation of pleomorphic cells (Fig. 17.52). Lesions consist of lymphocytes, lymphoblasts, reticulum cells, and plasma cells either scattered throughout the lesion or, in some cases, located around the periphery of small focal lesions. The proliferative lesions may be large and diffuse or small and focal. Rare lesions in peripheral nerves are similar to those of Marek's disease, but they tend to be focal and not diffuse throughout the nerve.

Development of the disease has been studied by McDougall et al. (17) and Zimber et al. (33). Spe-

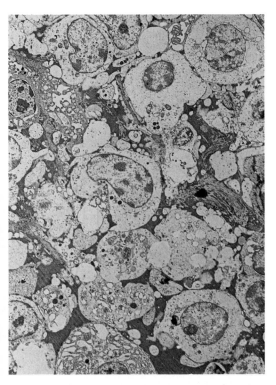

17.52.   Electron micrograph of a lesion of lymphoproliferative disease in the spleen of a turkey showing the pleomorphic cytology characteristic of the disease. × 4000

cific lesions were first recognized in the spleen and thymus 14 days after inoculation of 4-wk-old poults. They referred to these as early lymphoid lesions that were small and consisted mainly of lymphocytes, although lymphoblasts, reticulum cells, and plasma cells were also present (17). In the spleen, these lesions occurred as discrete foci in the red pulp. In the thymus, there was atrophy of the cortex and loss of lymphocytes from the enlarged medulla, which were replaced by lymphoblasts and reticulum and plasma cells. By 21 days postinoculation, the lesions in the spleen had enlarged and obliterated its normal architecture. In the thymus, the cortex was almost completely atrophied. These enlarging lesions contained many mitotic figures and were characteristic of the tumors seen in the naturally occurring disease. At this time, numerous small focal lymphoproliferative lesions were seen in many other organs. A third type of lesion was also noted, which was small and focal and consisted of lymphocytes; many of these lesions contained germinal centers. This type increases in frequency with time after inoculation, which suggests that it is a regressing lesion. These observations are paralleled by appearance of LPD virus-specific RNA sequences (12) and presence of virus particles (17). RNA sequences first appear in bone marrow 3 days postinfection; 2 and 7 days later they are present in the thymus and spleen, and bursa of Fabricius, respectively. By 15 days, RNA sequences appear in many organs but at a lower level than in the lymphoid organs. Five days postinfection there is a viremia that increases in concentration at least until 6 wk postinfection. Over this period, there was an increase in serum IgG (33). Up to 11 wk after infection, a suppression in cell-mediated immunity, but not humoral immunity, has been described (32, 34). Using a competition enzyme-linked immunosorbent assay (ELISA) and radio immunoprecipitation, Patel and Shilleto (19) found that turkeys do not respond to infection by producing antibodies.

DIAGNOSIS.   Virus cannot be cultivated in cell cultures or embryos, and antibodies have not been detected in infected turkeys. For these reasons, the diagnosis of LPD depends on the appearance of signs of the disease in a flock, characteristic gross and microscopic lesions, and application of techniques for the identification of LPDV. The latter include the use of virus-specific antisera in immunofluorescence and indirect ELISA tests, reverse transcriptase assays, and the polymerase chain reaction (PCR).

The reverse transcriptase assay is not specific for LPDV but is useful for diagnostic differentiation between LPD and reticuloendotheliosis (RE). A PCR has been described using oligonucleotide primers that amplify a region of the *gag* gene that is specific to LPDV (25). Not only is this PCR specific for LPDV, but it is more sensitive than the reverse transcriptase assay. It has been difficult to produce virus-specific antibodies because of host components in virus preparations. Treatment with bromelain overcomes this problem, and virus-specific antibodies have been produced in chickens and rabbits using bromelain-treated virus purified from plasma (22). Using such antisera in an indirect immunofluorescence test, LPDV can be demonstrated in buffy coat cells and in frozen sections of spleens for up to 16 mo postinfection (20). An indirect ELISA using antiserum raised against bromelain-digested virus has been described for detecting virus in pellets derived from high-speed centrifugation of plasma from infected turkeys (19). Both tests correlate well with the reverse transcriptase test.

Differential Diagnosis. The main disease with which LPD can be confused is RE. The distinctive features of LPD are the characteristic splenomegaly and pleomorphic nature of the cellular composition of the tumors. A test has been described to aid in differential diagnosis of LPD and RE (27), which takes advantage of the common persistent viremia found in turkeys infected with these viruses, and the difference in the cation requirements for the reverse transcriptase of LPDV and RE virus (REV) (31). Reticuloendotheliosis virus reverse transcriptase prefers Mn^{2+} over Mg^{2+}, whereas the opposite is true for LPDV. The test requires that the exogenous reverse transcriptase test be done using pellets of plasma from the suspect flock in the presence of 0.8 mM magnesium chloride and 0.08 mM manganese chloride (27). The divalent cation requirement index is calculated and defined as the ratio between the reverse transcriptase activity in presence of Mg^{2+} and that in presence of Mn^{2+}. An index above 2.0 is characteristic of LPDV and below 0.5 of REV. Other tests, however, are now available; for RE, virus isolation and serologic tests (see Reticuloendotheliosis) and for LPDV the indirect immunofluorescence test, the indirect ELISA, and the PCR referred to above, which are specific for LPDV and show no cross reactions with REV or avian leukosis viruses (19, 20, 25).

PREVENTION AND CONTROL. There is no information on prevention and control of LPD. Observed differences in susceptibility to LPD in experimental infections suggest that for the long term, a selection for resistance to the disease is a possible approach to prevention. Where serious disease occurs, a change in breed or hybrid of turkey may be beneficial. As with all infectious disease, attention should be paid to management and hygiene procedures.

REFERENCES

1. Andrews, C.H., and R.E. Glover. 1939. A case of neurolymphomatosis in a turkey. Vet Rec 51:934–935.
2. Biggs, P.M., B.S. Milne, J.A. Frazier, J.S. McDougall, and J.C. Stuart. 1974. Lymphoproliferative disease in turkeys. Proc 15th World's Poult Congr, World's Poultry Science Association, Washington, DC, pp 55–56.
3. Biggs, P.M., J.S. McDougall, J.A. Frazier, and B.S. Milne. 1978. Lymphoproliferative disease of turkeys. 1. Clinical aspects. Avian Pathol 7:131–139.
4. Busch, R.H., and L.E. Williams, Jr. 1970. A Marek's disease-like condition in Florida turkeys. Avian Dis 14:550–554.
5. Chajut, A., A. Yaniv, L. Avivi, I. Bar-Am, S.R. Tronick, and A. Gazit. 1991. A novel approach for establishing common or random integration loci for retroviral genomes. Nucleic Acids Res 19:4299.
6. Chajut, A., R. Sarid, A. Yaniv, G.W. Smythers, S.R. Tronick, and A. Gazit. 1992. The lymphoproliferative disease virus of turkeys represents a distinct class of avian type C retrovirus. Gene 122:349–354.
7. Gak, E., A. Yaniv, A. Chajut, M. Ianconescu, S.R. Tronick and A. Gazit. 1989. Molecular cloning of an oncogenic replication-competent virus that causes lymphoproliferative disease in turkeys. J Virol 63:2877–2880.
8. Gak, E., A. Yaniv, M. Ianconescu, S.R. Tronick, and A. Gazit. 1990. An in vivo infectivity assay for cloned retroviruses lacking a susceptible cell culture. J Virol Methods 28:147–154.
9. Gak, E., A. Yaniv, L. Sherman, M. Ianconescu, S.R. Tronick, and A. Gazit. 1991. Lymphoproliferative disease virus of turkeys: sequence analysis and transcriptional activity of the long terminal repeat. Gene 99:157–162.
10. Gazit, A., and A. Yaniv. 1994. Lymphoproliferative disease virus of turkeys. In R.G. Webster and A. Granoff (eds.), Encyclopedia of Virology. Academic Press, London, United Kingdom, pp. 811–814.
11. Gazit, A., A. Yaniv, M. Ianconescu, K. Perk, B. Aizenberg, and Z. Zimber. 1979. Molecular evidence for a type C retrovirus etiology of the lymphoproliferative disease of turkeys. J Virol 31:639–644.
12. Gazit, A., Z. Schwarzbard, A. Yaniv, M. Ianconescu, K. Perk, and A. Zimber. 1982. Organotropism of the lymphoproliferative disease virus (LPDV) of turkeys. Int J Cancer 29:599–604.
13. Gazit, A., R. Basri, M. Ianconescu, K. Perk, A. Zimber, and A. Yaniv. 1986. Analysis of structural polypeptides of the lymphoproliferative disease virus (LPDV) of turkeys. Int J Cancer 37:241–245.
14. Ianconescu, M., K. Perk, A. Zimber, and A. Yaniv. 1979. Reticuloendotheliosis and lymphoproliferative disease of turkeys. Refu Vet 36:2–12.
15. Ianconescu, M., A. Gazit, A. Yaniv, K. Perk, and A. Zimber. 1981. Comparative susceptibility of two turkey strains to lymphoproliferative disease virus. Avian Pathol 10:131–136.
16. Ianconescu, M., A. Yaniv, A. Gazit, K. Perk, and A. Zimber. 1983. Susceptibility of domestic birds to lymphoproliferative disease virus (LPDV) of turkeys. Avian Pathol 12:291–302.
17. McDougall, J.S., P.M. Biggs, R.W. Shilleto, and B.S. Milne. 1978. Lymphoproliferative disease of turkeys. II. Experimental transmission and aetiology. Avian Pathol 7:141–155.
18. McKee, G.S., A.M. Lucas, E.M. Denington, and F.C. Love. 1963. Separation of leukotic and non-leukotic lesions in turkeys on the inspection line. Avian Dis 7:19–30.
19. Patel, J.R., and R.W. Shilleto. 1987. Detection of lymphoproliferative disease virus by an enzyme-linked immunosorbent assay. Epidemiol Infect 99:711–722.
20. Patel, J.R., and R.W. Shilleto. 1987. Diagnosis of lym-

phoproliferative disease virus infection of turkeys by an indirect immunofluorescence test. Avian Pathol 16:367–376.

21. Patel, J.R., and R.W. Shilleto. 1987. Characterization of lymphoproliferative disease virus of turkeys. Structural polypeptides of the C-type particles. Arch Virol 95:159–176.

22. Patel, J.R., and R.W. Shilleto. 1987. Production of virus-specific antisera to lymphoproliferative disease virus of turkeys. Avian Pathol 16:699–705.

23. Perk, K., M. Ianconescu, A. Yaniv, and Z. Zimber. 1978. Lymphoproliferative disease in turkeys—structure, ultrastructure and biochemistry. Refu Vet 35:29.

24. Perk, K., M. Ianconescu, A. Yaniv, and Z. Zimber. 1979. Morphologic characterization of proliferative cells and virus particles in turkeys with lymphoproliferative disease. J Natl Cancer Inst 62:1483–1485.

25. Sarid, R., A. Chajut, M. Malkinson, S.R. Tronick, A. Gazit, and A. Yaniv. 1994. Diagnostic test for lymphoproliferative disease virus infection of turkeys, using the polymerase chain reaction. Am J Vet Res 55:769–772.

26. Sarid, R., A. Chajut, E. Gak, Y. Kim, C.V. Hixson, S. Oroszlan, S.R. Tronick, A. Gazit, and A. Yaniv. 1994. Genome organization of a biologically active molecular clone of the lymphoproliferative disease virus of turkeys. Virology 204:680–691.

27. Schwarzbard, Z., A. Yaniv, M. Ianconescu, K. Perk, and A. Zimber. 1980. A reverse transcriptase assay for the diagnosis of lymphoproliferative disease (LPD) of turkeys. Avian Pathol 9:481–487.

28. Simpson, C.F., D.W. Anthony, and F. Young. 1957. Visceral lymphomatosis in a flock of turkeys. J Am Vet Med Assoc 130:93–96.

29. Tipold von A., G. Loupal, J. Pabst, and L. Vasicek. 1987. Auftreten von Lymphoproliferativer Krankheit in Putenbestanden in Osterreich. Wien Tieraerztl Monatsschr 741:312–318.

30. Voute, E.J., and A.E. Wagenaar-Schaafsma. 1974. Een op de ziekte van Marek lijkende van afwijking bij mestkalkoenen in Nederland. Tijdschr Diergeneeskd 99:166–169.

31. Yaniv, A., A. Gazit, M. Ianconescu, K. Perk, B. Aizenberg, and A. Zimber. 1979. Biochemical characterization of the type C retrovirus associated with lymphoproliferative disease of turkeys. J Virol 30:351–357.

32. Zimber, A., E.D. Heller, K. Perk, M. Ianconescu, and A. Yaniv. 1983. Effect of lymphoproliferative disease virus and of Niridazole on the in vitro blastogenic response of peripheral blood lymphocytes of turkeys. Avian Dis 27:1012–1024.

33. Zimber, A., K. Perk, M. Ianconescu, Y. Yegana, A. Gazit, and A. Yaniv. 1983. Lymphoproliferative disease of turkeys: pathogenesis, viraemia and serum protein analysis following infection. Avian Pathol 12:101–116.

34. Zimber, A., K. Perk, M. Ianconescu, Z. Schwarzbard, and A. Yaniv. 1984. Lymphoproliferative disease of turkeys: effect of chemical and surgical bursectomy on viraemia, pathogenesis and on the humoral immune response. Avian Pathol 13:277–287.

TUMORS OF UNKNOWN ETIOLOGY

Rodney L. Reece

INTRODUCTION. Standard veterinary texts dealing with general pathology or neoplasia rarely mention tumors of poultry, and the most comprehensive description of tumors of the domestic fowl remains that of Campbell (20), even though it is out of print. The purpose of this chapter is to provide an outline of the more commonly encountered tumors of unknown etiology of poultry. In this respect, much is owed to accounts by other veterinary pathologists (see 38, 50, 53, 63, 72, 85). Where relevant, reference is made to tumors in other avian species because their pathogenesis is expected to be similar to that of equivalent tumors in poultry. As with mammalian species, the histologic appearance of avian tumors allows most to be classified according to their cell of origin. More detailed studies involving cytogenetics, immunohistochemistry, and electron microscopy are useful for accurate classification, but such techniques are rarely applied to poultry tumors because of the lack of incentive and resources to investigate what are deemed to be incidental conditions discovered during investigations

of flock problems. Prognosis and treatment are not discussed in this chapter.

In the study of avian tumors, attention has been focused on those of viral etiology, both from the standpoint of their economic importance and as models applicable to cancer in humans (16). Tumors of the reproductive tract of laying hens, keratoacanthomas of broiler chickens (see Dermal Squamous Cell Carcinoma, Chapter 37), and amputation neuromas have been studied to some extent, but little research has been directed to the other neoplastic diseases of poultry. The incidence of nonvirally induced tumors appears to be low, but properly constructed surveys are needed to clarify the situation. In a recent report of cage layers inspected at Irish abattoirs, the condemnation rate was 1.4%, of which one-fifth (0.3%) was due to nodules; 90% of the nodules were tumors and 70% (<0.2%) of these were adenocarcinomas, probably derived from the reproductive tract (114). Caution needs to be exercised in interpreting abattoir findings because early or small tumors are unlikely to be detected, and organs such as the brain and the oviduct lumen are not routinely examined.

The life span of commercially raised chickens

The author gratefully acknowledges the contributions of Dr. T.N. Fredrickson and Dr. C.F. Helmboldt to this chapter.

and turkeys is generally short and may be less than that required for development of most nonvirally induced tumors. The restricted information available on tumor incidence in older birds (the potential life span of chickens is generally considered to be around 15 yr but may be up to 35 yr) comes from several sources. The first is represented by long-term studies of flocks of aged chickens (41). The second is from diagnostic reports by veterinary pathologists, particularly of poultry maintained for periods of time longer than those of poultry kept under intensive conditions (106, 107). The third comes from necropsy reports from zoos where various species of birds often are maintained for natural life spans and are usually necropsied at death (32, 35, 61, 75, 77, 81, 93), and also from studies on other captive and wild birds (14, 28, 94, 99, 104). Reports of neoplastic diseases in the latter category have provided useful information, albeit not directly applicable to poultry. In particular, captive budgerigars (*Melopsittacus undulatus*) have a high incidence of tumors, although there is some evidence of retrovirus infection in this species, which could be partly responsible (51). The incidence of tumors in wild budgerigars is not known.

This chapter includes personal observations of spontaneous neoplasms in a U.S. flock of 466 SPF white leghorn hens, many of which were allowed to live out their natural life span (41); moribund and dead birds from an Australian SPF flock; and field cases submitted for necropsy. The U.S. SPF flock was free of clinical Marek's disease and exogenous avian leukosis virus, and the following tumors were diagnosed: 142 ovarian tumors (adenocarcinomas, granulosa cell tumors, and ovarian Sertoli cell tumors), 40 oviductal tumors (adenocarcinomas and leiomyomas), seven pancreatic adenocarcinomas, and one case each of parabronchial adenocarcinoma, proventricular adenocarcinoma, hepatocellular carcinoma, cholangiocellular carcinoma, and mesothelioma (42). It is not certain, however, how applicable these rates of spontaneous neoplasms are to other breeds and strains of chickens, since this strain had a high incidence of genital tumors for which there is some genetic predisposition (see Reproductive System). The Australian SPF flock was free of Marek's disease virus, exogenous avian leukosis virus, and reticuloendotheliosis virus and the following tumors were identified: two cases each of lymphomas, fibrosarcomas, and metastatic abdominal adenocarcinomas, and one case each of myelocytoma, reticulum cell sarcoma, histiocytic sarcoma, abdominal liposarcoma, subcutaneous lipoma, renal adenocarcinoma, granulosa cell tumor, and adrenocortical adenoma (96). In neither flock were these tumors associated with known oncogenic viruses.

There are reports of lymphoid tumors in SPF chickens (31, 96), which indicates that on occasion, such tumors may be induced by factors besides known transforming viruses. Additionally, lymphomas are a common diagnosis in other avian species (76, 94, 119) in which they are often inappropriately described as Marek's disease or lymphoid leukosis without direct evidence of involvement of transforming viruses. It would be preferable for such cases to be described in morphologic terms rather than ascribing them a name denoting etiology. The older surveys and reports of poultry tumors cited in this review (17, 50, 63, 85) were published prior to the implementation of control programs for Marek's disease and lymphoid leukosis. After allowing for cases likely to have a viral etiology, the prevalence of other tumors was low, with the overwhelming majority being derived from the reproductive tract of adult hens. That situation still appears to prevail.

REPRODUCTIVE SYSTEM

Ovary.   The classification of gonadal tumors of poultry is complex and controversial. It is somewhat complicated because of a tendency for investigators to apply to birds terms used in the diagnosis of mammalian, and particularly human, ovarian tumors. This ignores the dissimilarity between mammalian and avian ovaries in terms of histology, endocrinology, and physiology. All types of ovarian tumors are usually observed in hens more than 1 year of age.

ADENOCARCINOMA.   Early tumors are small, round, white, and firm nodules on the ovarian surface, which may be mistaken for atritic follicles. In advanced cases, these coalesce into a gray-white, firm cauliflowerlike mass. Numerous transcoelomic implants are common at this stage, varying from small pearllike growths to massive nodular tumors on serosal surfaces of the pancreas, oviduct, mesentery, and intestines. Ascites usually develops when such cancerous growth is extensive. The walls of affected intestines are thickened and adhered together, and the intestinal lumina become constricted. Metastatic abdominal adenocarcinomas may originate from either the ovary or the oviduct, and differentiation can be difficult, as in both cases the ovary and the oviduct are involved. Many cases of metastatic abdominal adenocarcinomas are described as ovarian adenocarcinomas without any serious attempt to determine their origin. Failure to detect tumor growth in the mucosal lining of the oviduct indicates that the tumor was not of oviductal origin and, therefore, probably arose from the ovary. For confirmation, frozen tissues can be stained immunohistologically for ovalbumin, which is only present in tumors arising from the magnum of the oviduct (see later). Terminally, hens are extremely thin and assume an upright, penguinlike position. Usually, there are no maturing follicles in advanced cases, and the oviducts are atrophied.

The cell of origin of these tumors remains to be identified but is frequently assumed to be the overlying mesothelium (so-called germinal epithelium) of the ovary or its invaginations into the ovarian cortex; alternatively, they may be derived from thecal glands, interstitial cells, remnants of embryonic sex cords, or the mesonephros. The tumor may start in the theca externa of smaller follicles (Fig. 17.53) in the interfollicular stroma or, occasionally, fairly deep in the ovarian stalk. They are multifocal in origin, but growth is fairly slow over a period of months. Ovarian adenocarcinomas are not associated with excess production of steroidal hormones (41).

Histologically, the commonest structures composing the ovarian adenocarcinoma are acini formed by a single layer of low columnar or cuboidal nonciliated epithelium. These eosinophilic cells with basal, round nuclei are oriented around a lumen of variable size and shape, sometimes containing an intensely eosinophilic, homogeneous material that is periodic acid-Schiff (PAS)-positive

and mucicarmine-negative (Fig. 17.54). Other tumors are more densely cellular, with the acinar structures compressed to give the appearance of islands or sheets of tumor cells, while in another variant, the lumen may be enlarged with infolding of the neoplastic lining forming papillary structures (Fig. 17.55).

The prevalence of mitotic figures varies from scant to abundant, although in most cases they are not prominent. Division of ovarian adenocarcinomas into medullary or scirrhous forms appears unwarranted, as size determines morphology; the acini

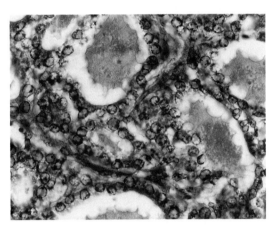

17.54. Acinar structures, typical of ovarian adenocarcinoma filled with eosinophilic material and lined by cuboidal cells containing round nuclei with condensed chromatin and sparse eosinophilic cytoplasm. H&E, ×600.

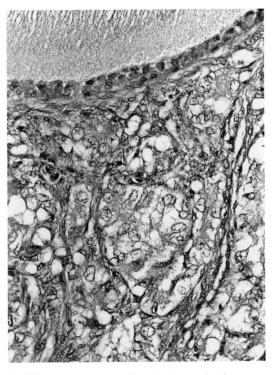

17.53. Ovarian adenocarcinoma in theca region demonstrating delicate trabeculae and round nuclei; note the granulosa cells and yolk of the developing ova (*top*). H&E, ×360.

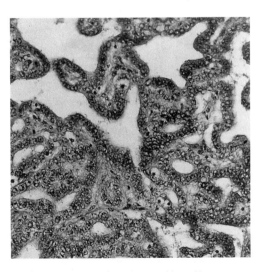

17.55. Ovarian adenocarcinoma with papillary structures projecting into dilated acini. H&E, ×160.

of large tumors are interlaced with dense fibrous tissue (Fig. 17.56), whereas smaller tumors have a lesser component of fibrous tissue. Serosal implants may induce a proliferative response of smooth muscle in the underlying muscularis, but the extent of this varies (83). Ovarian adenocarcinomas similar to those seen in the chicken have been described in mature turkey hens (120).

Occasionally, ovarian adenocarcinomas are found in ovaries covered with grapelike clusters of follicles filled with yellow fluid. In some cases, these cysts are not lined by neoplastic epithelium but appear to be the result of impaired lymphatic drainage, and thus they are not directly comparable to ovarian cystadenocarcinomas of mammals. Cystic ovarian follicles occur in other avian species and are not related to neoplasia (58). Large cystic acini lined by low cuboidal to squamous epithelium may be found in some cases of metastatic abdominal adenocarcinomas, and their lumina contain a PAS-positive mucinous secretion similar to that described above (20, 96). Ovarian myxomas may also be present with tenacious mucinous material exuding from the cut surface, but histologically, they are quite distinctive.

GRANULOSA-THECA CELL TUMOR. This tumor is yellow, round, and lobulated with an extremely friable consistency very different from the firm, cauliflowerlike adenocarcinoma. Granulosa-theca cell tumors are encapsulated within a smooth, glistening membrane, and larger tumors have extensive areas of necrosis and hemorrhage. Tumors that are attached to the ovary only by a thin stalk may grow to enormous size, and metastasis to adjacent viscera occurs occasionally. Histologically, these tumors are composed of pale, eosinophilic, polyhedral to fusiform cells with some cytoplasmic vacuolation (Fig. 17.57). The arrangement of these cells can be very variable even within a single tumor, forming tubular, or less frequently, follicular structures (Fig. 17.58), separated by a delicate vascular stroma. In some cases, there may be elaborate cylindriform or gyriform arrangements (Fig.17.59), or there may be typical rosettes of groups of a dozen or so epithelial cells clustered radially around small central spaces (Fig.17.60). In others the stroma may be prominent. The proportion of mitotic figures varies but tends to be low, and the tumor appears to grow at a slow rate.

The tumor cells have been confirmed as granulosa cells because they have an ultrastructural component called the transosome, which has been identified solely in avian follicular granulosa cells (60). Greatly elevated plasma concentrations of estrogen are found in hens with large granulosa-theca cell tumors (41). It is known that granulosa cells from mature follicles normally produce progesterone, whereas theca cells produce estrogen (88). This, coupled with the observation of numerous theca glands in "granulosa cell tumors," justifies the binomial descriptor granulosa-theca cell tumor. The high concentrations of circulating estrogen result in the oviducts being similar in size to those of laying hens. Comb development is as for hens in lay, but

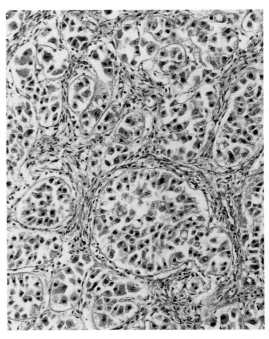

17.57. Lobules of vacuolated epithelial cells separated by moderate trabeculae in a granulosa-theca cell tumor. The central lumina are not as definite as in adenocarcinomas. H&E, ×140

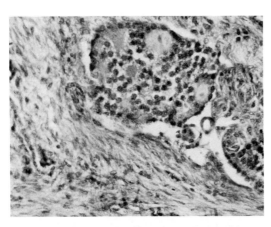

17.56. Another form of ovarian adenocarcinoma with dense bands of stromal cells enclosing clusters of neoplastic acinar cells with intensely basophilic nuclei. H&E, ×160.

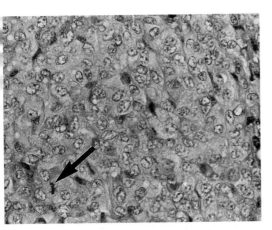

17.58. Granulosa-theca cell tumor composed of a uniform population of tightly packed tumor cells with plentiful, pale eosinophilic cytoplasm and uniform, round vesicular nuclei. Note the mitotic figure (*arrow*). H&E, ×600.

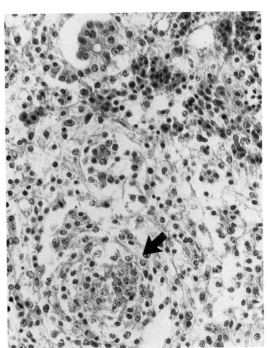

17.60. Granulosa-theca cell tumor showing tubular arrangements and rosettes formed by clusters of cells radiating out from small central lumina. H&E, ×365. (Avian Pathol)

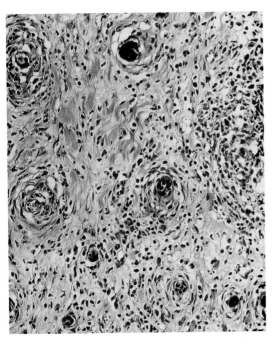

17.59. Gyriform arrangements of cells in one area of an ovary with a granulosa-theca cell tumor. H&E, ×90. (Avian Pathol)

eggs are not produced. The existence of separate ovarian thecal cell tumors such as those described by Campbell (20) must await further study.

ARRHENOBLASTOMA. The terms *arrhenoma* and *arrhenoblastoma* may be applied in a morphologic sense to ovarian tumors with testicular elements, or in a functional sense, to encompass a diverse group of virilizing ovarian tumors. Sex reversal ("virilism") in domestic fowls has been recognized since ancient times (40), but very few of such cases are due to ovarian tumors (20). It must be remembered that in avian species, contrary to the situation in mammals, however, the male is the neutral sex and the female chick is demasculinized by her ovarian hormones (86). In the hen, only the left ovary normally develops, but rudimentary male medullary tissue and primordial cells are present in the normal ovary (46). Surgical removal of the functional ovary leads to hypertrophy of the vestigial right gonad into an organ resembling an ovo-testis or testis, depending upon the age at treatment. The ovo-testis so formed has some areas of immature seminiferous tubules, but spermatogenesis is not normally a feature (15). Destruction of the ovary by a non–steroid-producing tumor or other pathologic processes may result in the formation of an ovo-testis. In studies of sex reversal in the fowl, there is one well-documented case of an adult hen that laid eggs but subsequently developed ovarian pathology, underwent sex reversal, and was able to successfully fertilize eggs. However, this was a case of tubercular oophoritis, not neoplasia (39). The opposite situation of feminization is very poorly documented (see Sertoi Cell Tumor).

In this chapter, the terms *arrhenoma* and *arrhenoblastoma* are reserved for those cases in which there is an ovarian tumor associated with some evidence of sex reversal ("virilism"). There are no reports on hormone production of these tumors in poultry, so it is not known if sex reversal is due to a lack of estrogens or the production of androgens. Arrhenomas are characterized by growth of seminiferous tubules within the ovarian stroma and appear as white solid lobulated masses within atrophic ovaries. They are of uncertain histogenesis and histologically are extremely variable. In the most differentiated form, they are composed of branching cords of columnar epithelium, often two cell layers deep, which resemble immature seminiferous tubules. Spermatogenesis tends to be poor. A loose or compact network of fusiform and epithelial cells arranged as cords, nests, rosettes, or incomplete tubules may be observed in less well-developed forms (Fig. 17.61). The interstitium may be prominent and contain nests of polyhedral lipoidrich cells resembling Leydig cells. The seminiferouslike tubules can be filled with vacuolated cells (55). In large tumors, there may be cystic cavitation and hemorrhage. Experimental induction of masculinizing arrhenoblastomas by injection of radioactive isotopes into the left ovary has been described (121). Arrhenomas may be mistaken for adenocarcinomas. Gynandroblastomas are mixed steroid–producing tumors with estrogens produced by granulosa-theca cell components and androgens produced by arrhenomatous tissue.

OVARIAN SERTOLI CELL TUMORS. In the five cases of ovarian Sertoli cell tumors reported by Fredrickson (41), obvious sex reversal was not apparent, and circulating hormone concentrations were comparable to those of nonlaying hens. Compact masses of tubules developing multifocally under the ovarian capsule were seen histologically. Interstitial cells were variably present, and well-defined tubules were lined by a single layer of columnar epithelial cells with basal nuclei, considered to be Sertoli cells (Fig. 17.62). Some ovarian Sertoli cell tumors appeared to develop within granulosa-theca cell tumors.

DYSGERMINOMA. Wight (123, 124) detected four ovarian tumors in pseudohermaphrodites, and three of these were designated as dysgerminomas, the equivalent of ovarian seminomas. These were not associated with sex reversal, but rather with loss of external morphologic features of hens and acquisition of some male characteristics such as enlarged combs and male-type saddle feathers. These tumors are considered to originate from seminiferous elements within the left ovary or vestigial right gonad. Histologically, they consist of elaborate fibrous tra-

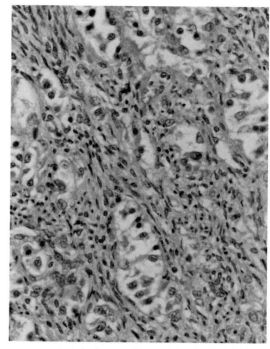

17.61. Arrhenoma from a hen that showed sex reversal. Network of epithelial cells arranged as ill-defined cords and tubules. H&E, ×350. (from a case supplied by C.J. Randall)

beculae surrounding cords or groups of round or polygonal cells and occasional syncytia.

Mesosalpinx

LEIOMYOMA. Leiomyoma of the mesosalpinx is a common tumor in hens. They are usually located centrally in the ventral ligament of the oviduct, an area normally rich in smooth muscle. Occasionally, leiomyomas may be found on the peritoneal surface of the oviduct or growing in the mesentery. They vary from small white nodules to large gray heavily vascularized masses several centimeters in diameter. This tumor is usually a single, sharply circumscribed, encapsulated, solid, round mass with a characteristic white, glistening appearance on the cut surface. They are benign and composed of interlacing bundles of smooth muscle separated into fasciculi by a variable component of fibrous tissue (Fig. 17.63). These tumors may be referred to as leiomyofibromas or fibroleiomyomas, depending upon which tissue predominates. Mitotic figures are rare. They appear to have little effect on the oviduct or its function, although they may predispose to ova escaping into the abdominal cavity. In a recent study (5), the prevalence of this tumor in different strains of SPF and commercial hens varied from 0

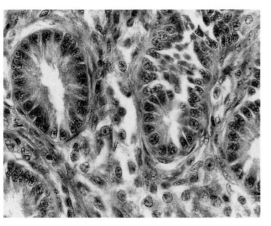

17.62. Ovarian Sertoli cell tumor composed of well-defined seminiferouslike tubules lined by Sertoli cells. Stroma contains interstitial cells. H&E, ×600.

to 60% at the end of their 1st yr of lay. Affected hens had elevated concentrations of circulating 17 ß-estradiol (4) and a high incidence of these tumors was induced in a commercial white leghorn strain by treatment with both diethyl stilbestrol and progesterone, thus confirming a role for these steroid hormones in tumorigenesis (5).

Oviduct

ADENOCARCINOMA. Most adenocarcinomas of the oviduct originate in the upper magnal portion of the oviduct, with occasional cases occurring in the uterus and infundibulum. Large focal and abdomi-

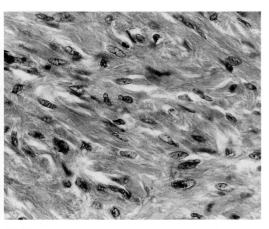

17.63. Leiomyoma of mesosalpinx composed of smooth muscle fibers arranged in compact whorls. Mitoses are absent from this field and the nuclear/cytoplasmic ratio is low. H&E, ×600.

nal metastatic tumors are usually detected in hens more than 1 yr of age. In a survey published in 1969 (47), the prevalence of oviductal adenocarcinomas in end-of-lay hens, determined by examining the mucosa of oviducts, varied from 5 to 81%. A more recent study showed a positive correlation between tumor incidence and mature body weight and egg weight (3). This indicates the possibility of an association with selection for egg laying, but properly constructed surveys need to be carried out. Metastatic abdominal adenocarcinomas observed at necropsy or abattoir inspection are but a small proportion of actual cases of oviductal adenocarcinomas, and some may be of ovarian origin. If the organ of origin is not determined, it would be preferable to refer to them as metastatic abdominal adenocarcinomas of unknown origin.

Studies of magnal tumors in domestic fowls and turkeys revealed a progression from focal dysplasia through sessile clusters to polypoid masses. The earliest lesions are small (2–10 mm in diameter) nodules on the ridges of the glands and may be found in laying hens at 30 wk of age. They are easily overlooked (112). Histologically, these nodules are composed of closely packed columnar cells with secretory granules in the apical cytoplasm and pale nuclei. The cells are oriented concentrically rather than toward the lumen (Fig. 17.64). These lesions are probably pre-neoplastic. Their incidence in commercial poultry is not known.

Individual or clustered sessile adenocarcinomas are gray and firm. They tend to coalesce into large, irregularly shaped tumors protruding into the oviductal lumen. Early lesions are found in hens with active ovaries, whereas abdominal metastases are associated with ascites and loss of bodily condition. In the primary tumor, there is generally a distinct boundary between neoplastic and normal magnal cells (Fig. 17.65). Malignant cells vary in the degree they maintain the normal glandular architecture of the magnum and amount of acidophilic secretory granules within their cytoplasm. Implants of acinar tissue are generally well encapsulated (Fig. 17.66). In some cases, cells are agranular and grow in solid sheets. However, cytologic differences are not reflective of tumor invasiveness, since implants may be found that are composed of well-differentiated cells. The ultrastructural details of these tumors have been described (62).

Magnal adenocarcinomas are extremely malignant. Even when the primary tumor is quite small, it may penetrate through the muscularis and spread through the abdominal cavity via tunnels between the celomic membranes to implant on the intestinal serosa, especially the pancreas and duodenum (66). The muscularis underlying implants on the oviductal or intestinal serosa becomes hyperplastic and hypertrophied. Implants on the intestinal serosa are

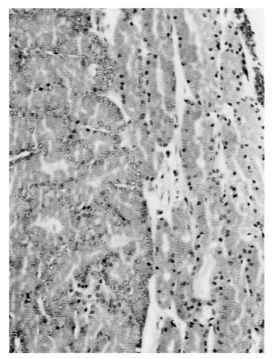

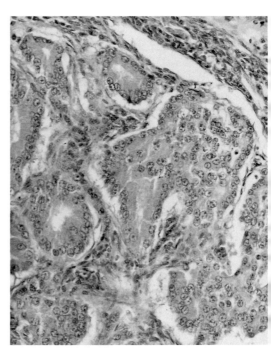

17.64. Dysplastic adenomatous focus in a fold in the magnum showing clear demarcation from surrounding normal glands. The columnar epithelial cells are densely packed and oriented concentrically. H&E, ×175. (Avian Pathol)

17.66. Implant of magnal adenocarcinoma deep in the ovary showing capsule around adenocarcinomatous cells. Despite the apparent aggressiveness of this tumor, mitotic figures are not prominent. H&E, ×200.

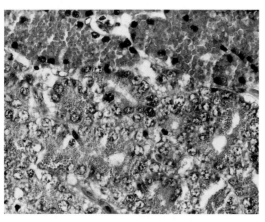

17.65. Magnal adenocarcinoma showing the well-defined margin between normal secretory tissue with cellular cytoplasm containing eosinophilic granules of ovalbumin (*above*) and very lightly granular tumor cells (*below*). H&E, ×600.

generally composed of small islands or acini of fairly anaplastic tumor cells encased in dense fibrous tissue (Fig. 17.67). These are similar, both grossly and histologically, to those produced by ovarian adenocarcinomas, and the ovary itself is a frequent site of implantation. Sometimes metastases may be found quite deep in the ovary. Implants on the oviduct serosa frequently lack intense cirrhosis (Fig. 17.68). Metastasis to the lungs and other viscera occurs via hematogenous emboli (66).

Immunohistochemical studies showed that the tumor cells contained ovalbumin (57) and retained their receptors for estrogen and progesterone (4). Magnal adenocarcinomas were estrogen responsive; their growth was maintained by potent estrogens and suppressed by antiestrogens (3). Oviductal tumors, similar to those found in chickens, also have been described in turkeys (11). Metastatic abdominal adenocarcinomas, probably of oviductal origin, have been reported from many other avian species (94).

Testis

TERATOMA. Teratomas are tumors containing multiple cell types arising from more than one embryonic layer. Involvement of the testes appears to be more common than that of the ovary (20, 59), despite more hens than cockerels being kept to sexual maturity. Teratomas also have been found in a number of other sites including the ovary, kidney, adrenal gland, spinal cord, pineal body, and eye (21,

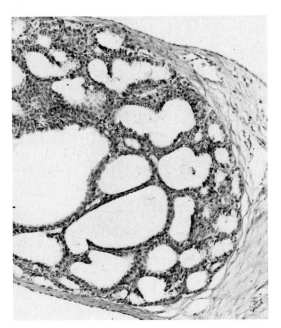

17.68. Magnal adenocarcinoma implanted on the serosa of the isthmus is surrounded by little fibrous tissue. The dilated acinar lumina are lined by cuboidal epithelium. H&E, ×200.

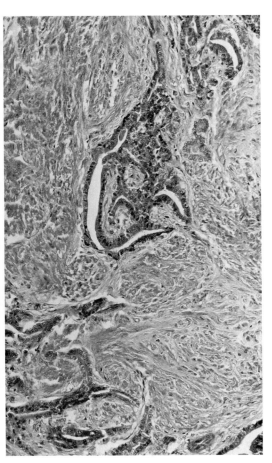

17.67. Compacted acini lined by cuboidal epithelium surrounded by dense drifts of fibrous tissue in this cirrhotic implant in duodenal serosa of a magnal adenocarcinoma. H&E, ×175.

53). They are generally round, yellow to white, encapsulated firm masses that sometimes contain cysts. Histologically, they are composed of bone, cartilage, smooth muscle, nerves, fat, and/or melanocytes. The cysts are often lined with columnar-ciliated epithelium that, along with cartilage and smooth muscle, forms tracheal structures. Additional structures and epithelial pearls formed by squamous epithelium may also be seen. Another type of teratoma presents as a fluid-filled sac containing fully formed feathers (21). They are attached to the spinal column in the lumbar area and resemble dermoid cysts of mammals except for the formation of feathers rather than hair. Histologically, the sac wall is lined by thin keratinized epithelium and fully formed feather follicles, and there are erector pili muscles and nerves in the surrounding tissue. Spontaneous teratomas have been reported in a number of avian species (97) and may be induced experimentally by injection of metallic ions into the testes of young adult cockerels (56).

SERTOLI CELL TUMOR. Sertoli cell tumors have been described in the testes of Japanese quail (49) and budgerigars (94), but they appear to be rare in chickens (20). Grossly they appear as firm, nodular masses with varying degrees of necrosis, hemorrhage, and cyst formation. Histologically, well-defined tumors are characterized by Sertoli-like epithelial cells with a large dense basally situated nucleus and basophilic cytoplasm, arranged in a palisading manner around the central lumina of tubules (Fig. 17.69). In other cases, the tumor cells are arranged as lobules and sheets separated by delicate stroma. Mitotic figures are common. The number of interstitial cells between these tubules and islands is variable, and in some cases such cells may be vacuolated. In mammals, Sertoli cell tumors may be associated with estrogen production and feminization; Siller (105) described a case of feminization in an incompletely surgically castrated cockerel in which a Sertoli cell tumor arose from the gonadal remnants. Additionally, several examples of demasculinization have been reported in budgerigars with Sertoli cell tumors (9). Hormonal studies in poultry have not been reported.

SEMINOMA. Seminomas are large unilateral tumors with a well-defined capsule, and are histologically composed of loose sheets or compact cords interspersed with a delicate stroma (Fig. 17.70). The cells are large and round, containing a round to oval nucleus with prominent nucleoli (19). Occa-

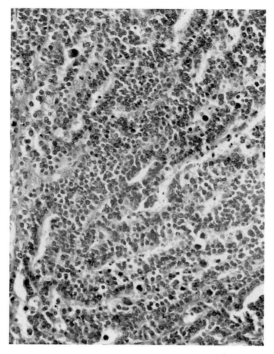

17.69. Sertoli cell tumor in a quail. The tubulelike structures are lined by cells two layers deep. H&E, ×360.

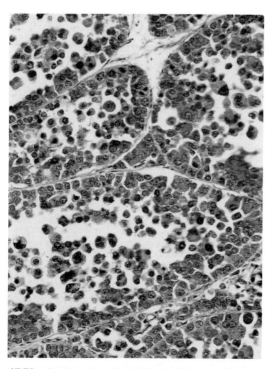

17.70. Seminoma in a duck. Lobules of pleiomorphic polyhedral cells with finely granular cytoplasm: some multinucleated cells. Delicate stroma. H&E, ×180.

sional syncytia are noted and mitotic figures are numerous. Seminomas have also been reported in ducks, quail, and budgerigars (9, 94).

LEYDIG CELL TUMORS. Neoplastic Leydig cells may be a component of a seminoma. Leydig cell tumors are composed of large polygonal cells with eccentrically placed vesicular nuclei and granular acidophilic, sometimes vacuolated, cytoplasm arranged in irregular acini.

DIGESTIVE SYSTEM

Alimentary Tract.   Pharyngeal and esophageal squamous cell carcinomas in chickens have been described (1, 25). A high incidence of this tumor has been reported in chickens from northern China, and humans in the same area also have a high incidence of esophageal carcinoma (22, 90, 103), perhaps indicating a common etiology.

Olson and Bullis (85) reported papillomatouslike growths in the esophagus and crop of chickens, but their etiology and pathogenesis were not known. Proliferative epithelial lesions due to papillomavirus infections are well recognized in passerines and psittacines, and may be found in the gastrointestinal tract (116). However, cloacal papillomas in psittacines consisting of irregular hyperplastic epithelial cells, supported on a connective tissue stalk extending from the lamina propria, are probably not due to papillomaviruses (111). Herpeslike viruses were observed in a cloacal papilloma of a conure (48).

There have been several reports of adenomas of the crop, esophagus, proventriculus, and gizzard of birds (7, 21, 71, 94, 96). Campbell and Appleby (21) described an adenocarcinoma of the gizzard that was similar to tumors seen among broiler chickens in the United States, as shown in Fig. 17.71. Guerin (53) described five epithelial tumors of the small intestine and one of the ileocecal junction, and cited several other reports of intestinal carcinomas in chickens. In these cases, gross examination revealed papillary projections of tumor tissue into the lumen of the affected organ, sometimes with penetration of the muscularis by invading epithelial tissue, which formed acinar or cystic structures containing mucin. Solitary nodular adenocarcinomas of the intestinal mucosa of chickens also have been described (96, 115). Campbell (20) noted that reports of intestinal adenocarcinoma in the chicken should be viewed with caution, as such tumors can be difficult to differentiate from metastatic abdominal adenocarcinomas that arise from the reproductive tract and frequently implant on the intestinal serosa and infiltrate into the underlying mucosa.

Leiomyomas may be found in the muscularis of the gizzard or intestines (see Musculoskeletal Sys-

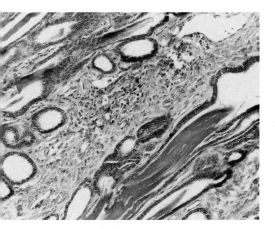

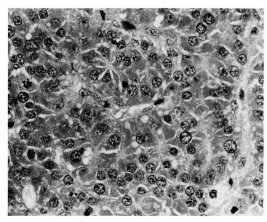

17.71. Adenocarcinoma of gizzard with growth of darkly staining cuboidal tumor cells downward into muscularis. The keratinous product of these cells is shown at *lower right*. H&E, ×200. (from a case supplied by K. Langheinrich)

17.72. Hepatoma composed of large eosinophilic neoplastic cells, some in mitosis forming irregular plates. H&E, ×600.

tem). In pheasants and peafowl, pseudoneoplastic nodules of proliferating fibrous tissue in the cecal wall may be induced by larval stages of *Heterakis isolonche* (52). Enterogenous cysts derived from gastrointestinal tract mucosa have been described in chickens (68).

Liver

HEPATOCELLULAR TUMORS. Spontaneous neoplasms of hepatocytes appear to be rare in chickens, and only occasional reports of either benign trabecular hepatocellular adenomas or anaplastic carcinomas have appeared (20, 26, 85, 96). Typical hepatocellular adenomas grow in the hepatic parenchyma as a large, circumscribed, soft, yellow-gray mass. Microscopically, they are composed of polygonal eosinophilic cells about double the size of normal hepatocytes, forming thick, irregular cords lacking normal hepatic triad structures (Fig. 17.72). Mitotic figures are rare. Hepatocellular carcinomas are often multifocal nodules composed of sheets of basophilic neoplastic cells somewhat smaller than those in hepatomas and with numerous mitoses (91); metastasis to the lung may occur. Such tumors are similar to hepatocellular carcinomas induced with transforming avian retroviruses, most notably avian leukosis virus strain MC29 (10).

Hepatic tumors also have been reported in ducks (18) and appear to be inducible in this species with aflatoxin (24). Additionally, hepatocellular carcinomas in ducks have been associated with duck hepatitis B virus (131). The incidence of hepatic tumors in Chinese ducks is high, ranging from 2 to 15%, with hepatocellular carcinomas being most common (74). The role of genetics, age, diet, and other environmental or virologic factors is not known. Hepatocellular tumors have been described in a variety of other avian species (94, 118).

CHOLANGIOCELLULAR TUMOR. Tumors of the biliary system are not common in chickens. They are generally firm, demarcated from normal hepatic parenchyma, and yellow-gray. The histology varies according to the degree of malignancy. Cholangiomas are composed of clearly recognizable but enlarged tubules resembling distorted bile ducts, interspersed with fibrous connective tissue (21, 42, 96) (Fig. 17.73). In cholangiocarcinomas, duct formation is irregular and the connective tissue is fibroblastic (Fig. 17.74). Infiltration between hepatic

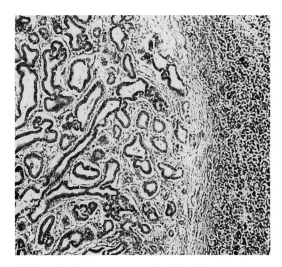

17.73. Cholangioma composed of dilated ducts in a loose fibrocytic stroma. H&E, ×75.

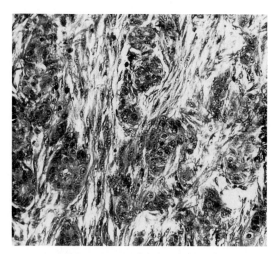

17.74. Cholangiocarcinoma composed of small clusters of epithelial cells in a fibroblastic stroma. H&E, ×190.

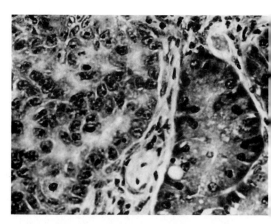

17.75. Pancreatic acinar cell adenocarcinoma with normal exocrine tissue (*right*) and agranular neoplastic cells (*left*). H&E, ×600.

cords is aggressive. Cholangiocellular tumors have been described in pigeons (122) and other birds (89, 118).

Pancreas

ADENOCARCINOMA. Tumors of the pancreas are difficult to differentiate from metastatic abdominal adenocarcinomas derived from the ovary or oviduct, which frequently implant on the pancreatic serosa and invade the organ. There can be absolute certainty of a pancreatic primary tumor only in absence of ovarian or oviductal involvement, as in the case in a male Guinea fowl reported by Okoye and Ilochi (84). In one case observed by Fredrickson and Helmboldt (42), it appeared that the tumor arose from exocrine tissue, rather than ducts, because a clearly defined transitional zone between normal acini and tumor tissue could be distinguished. The large neoplastic cells had extremely vesicular, round nuclei, and cytoplasm contained a variable number of the same deeply eosinophilic granules typical of normal acinar cells (Fig. 17.75). Most pancreatic adenocarcinomas probably originate from ductal epithelium, not acini. They are composed of tubular structures lined by columnar epithelial cells with lightly basophilic cytoplasm (Fig. 17.76). The basal nuclei are round to oval, and mitotic figures are prevalent. Extensive metastatic implants to the serosa of the duodenum and proventriculus and the hepatic capsule can occur, but the ovary is not involved.

Peritoneum

MESOTHELIOMA. Mesotheliomas have been reported in chickens (53, 85), ducks (73), a hawk

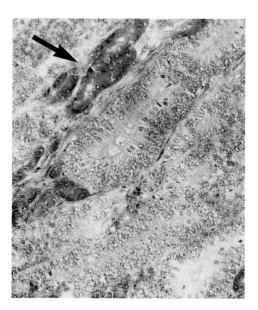

17.76. Pancreatic adenocarcinoma composed of columnar cells forming tubular structures among a few remnant acinar cells (*arrow*). ×160

(29), and ratites (94). In this tumor, both the mesothelial-covering cell and the underlying connective tissue are involved. One case in a SPF hen was described by Fredrickson and Helmboldt (42); the abdominal cavity contained about 200 mL of milky fluid and the serosal surfaces were covered by glistening, gray cystic structures. Histologically, these appeared as papillary outgrowths of peritoneal cells supported by thick connective tissue stroma that formed the walls of the cysts into which the papillary structures projected (Fig. 17.77). Mi-

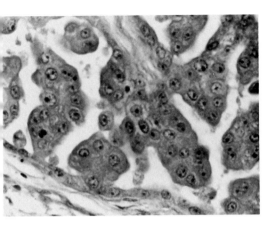

17.77. Mesothelioma with prominent neoplastic epithelial cells supported on a delicate stalk. H&E, ×600.

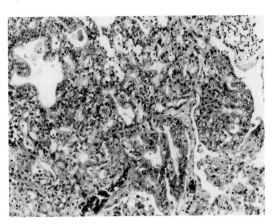

17.78. Adenocarcinoma of lung composed of papillary growth of epithelial cells that have replaced most of the normal lung. H&E, ×200.

totic figures were rare, but tumor growth was extensive.

URINARY SYSTEM. Renal adenocarcinomas (nephromas) and nephroblastomas may occur as spontaneous neoplasms in chickens, but they are inducible with avian leukosis virus and are described elsewhere in this book (see subchapter, Leukosis/Sarcoma Group). Renal adenocarcinomas are common in budgerigars (82), but their etiology is not known.

RESPIRATORY SYSTEM

Lung

ADENOCARCINOMA. Tumors of the respiratory tract of poultry are rare, with Campbell describing only three cases of pulmonary adenocarcinomas in domestic fowls (20). Ducks appear to be more prone than other avian species to pulmonary tumors, as there are several reports of naturally occurring pulmonary adenocarcinomas in ducks (75, 132) and a variety of lung tumors were induced in Pekin ducks given a chemical carcinogen intratracheally (98). Stewart (109) described 20 cases of pulmonary adenocarcinomas or adenomatosis in birds, including 11 in ducks. Most of these cases appeared to originate from the bronchial epithelium. Adenocarcinomas of magnal origin and other tumors (rhabdomyosarcomas, myxosarcomas, and fibrosarcomas) can metastasize to the lungs of domestic fowl (96), and such tumors need to be differentiated from adenocarcinomas arising from within the lungs. The case described by Fredrickson and Helmboldt (42) clearly arose multifocally from parabronchi and resembled papillary adenocarcinomas as described by others (6, 109). Cuboidal epithelium formed distorted bronchial tissue often

containing eosinophilic material (Fig. 17.78). Widespread and distant metastases in the thorax and abdomen attested to the extreme malignancy of this tumor.

NERVOUS SYSTEM

Central Nervous System

ASTROCYTOMA. Sporadic cases of astrocytoma have been described (12, 64, 65, 96), and Wight and Duff (126) investigated a small epizootic affecting 20 birds out of a flock of 1000, of which 13 were examined histologically. Adult birds are usually affected, and all five cases examined by the author (96) were in aged noncommercial hens. Clinical signs include transitory torticollis, retropulsion, and incoordination. Astrocytomas are frequently multiple, unencapsulated, and usually located in the base of the cerebellum or underlying anterior brain stem near the thalmus in the area of the third ventricle. Although each tumor is small, usually no larger than 5 mm in diameter, they may be seen without difficulty, especially in fixed tissues, as sharply delineated whitish masses. There is frequently a marked perivascular reaction of lymphocytes bordering the tumor, but no hemorrhage, giant cells, or areas of pressure necrosis (Fig 17.79). The neoplastic cells vary considerably in morphology, but are mainly polygonal with extended cytoplasmic fibrillar processes (Fig. 17.80), which can be demonstrated with phosphotungstic acid hematoxylin stain. Astrocytomas need to be differentiated from reactive gliosis induced by migrating parasites.

Wight and Campbell (125) reported finding an ependymoma and two meningiomas in chickens. The former was a growth in the lateral ventricle of palisaded or rosette-forming, vacuolated cells, while the meningiomas were the angioblastic vari-

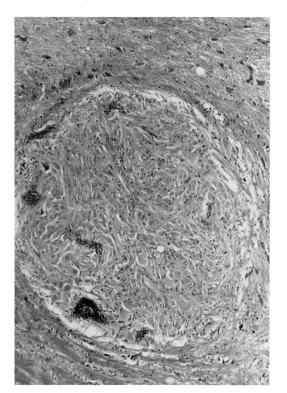

17.79. One of several clearly demarcated but unencapsulated astrocytomas composed of fibrillar astrocytes, in anterior brain stem. There is a significant lymphocytic infiltrate around the blood vessels within the tumor and the adjacent tissue. H&E, ×100. (Avian Pathol)

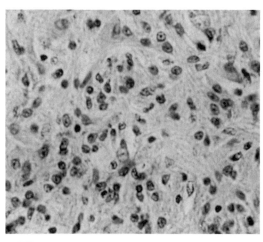

17.80. Astrocytoma composed of uniform astrocytes with extended cytoplasmic processes. H&E, ×190.

ety composed of vascular sinuses lined with plump endothelial cells associated with a dense network of reticulin.

PINEAL BODY TUMOR. There are several reports of avian pineal body tumors (20, 94, 96, 113, 128), but mainly of single cases. Swayne et al. (113) used several criteria to differentiate pineal body tumors from hyperplasia; if tumorous, the pineal body was greatly enlarged, impinged on the adjacent cerebellum, and mitotic figures were present in the epithelial cells. There may be clinical signs such as fine tremors and head pressing, and a large encapsulated mass can be found between the cerebellum and the cerebrum, protruding into the cerebellum. The tumor is composed of lobules of epithelial cells comprising low columnar cells arranged in a palisading manner around a lumen, and there are abundant parafollicular cells with dense nuclei, separated by fine trabeculae (Fig. 17.81).

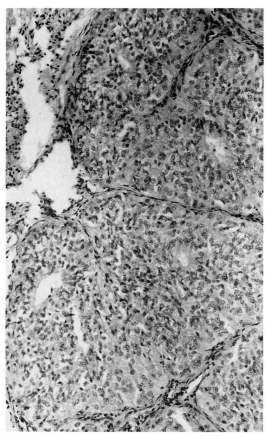

17.81. Lobules of a pineal body tumor separated by fine trabeculae. Palisaded low columnar epithelial cells with large vesicular nuclei are arranged around a small lumen, and these are surrounded by smaller parafollicular cells. H&E, ×200. (Avian Pathol)

Peripheral Nerves

SCHWANNOMA. Tumors of the Schwann cells or perineural cells of peripheral nerves are preferably called Schwannomas, although often they are designated as neurofibromas, neurilemomas, or neurogenic sarcomas; differentiation between these is difficult and they are best considered together. Campbell and Appleby (21) reported 39 tumors of the nerve sheath in broiler chickens and reviewed 17 other cases, some in adult birds. They are generally benign localized tumors forming white nodular or fusiform growths, most often in the region of the dorsal root ganglia. The tumor cells are spindle shaped with a small central nucleus, and usually they form concentric whorls reminiscent of nerve sheaths (Fig. 17.82). Multiple nodular tumors have been reported (2), including a congenital case (21). Tumors described as neurilemomas had cells arranged in a palisading manner with occasional structures resembling Wagner-Meissner tactile corpuscles (20). Tumors resembling Schwannomas should only be so designated if the nerve of origin is identified; otherwise they are best described as fi-brosarcomas to avoid confusion. Some cases of Schwannomas resemble hemangiopericytomas.

NEUROMA. Amputation of the tip of the beak of juvenile chickens and partial amputation of the hallux of male broiler breeders may result in the formation of neuromas (43, 44). There is a nodular or diffuse thickening due to proliferating nerve bundles within a dense collagenous matrix. The pathogenesis is similar to posttraumatic neuromas of domestic mammals and humans where a regenerating nerve stump encounters an obstruction such as dense fibroblastic scar tissue and cannot reinnervate normal dermal tissue so it proliferates as a tangled mass of axons, Schwann cells and associated connective tissue (Fig 17.83). The axons can be identified by staining with Holme's silver method, but they are thinly myelinated. Technically these are an abnormal regeneration rather than neoplasia. Partial beak amputation of young chicks results in looser dermal scar tissue. Compared with chickens, partial beak amputation of turkeys also appeared to be associated with less dense scar tissue and neuromas did not form (45).

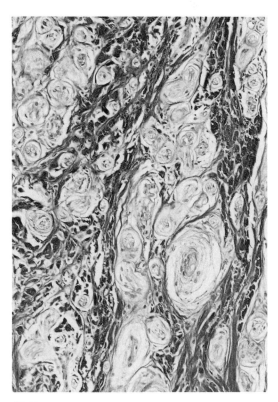

17.82. Schwannoma of the sciatic plexus showing concentric whorling pattern of spindle-shaped cells with central nuclei. Note the mitotic figure (*arrow*). H&E, ×400.

17.83. Posttraumatic neuroma in beak tip showing dense collagenous scar tissue and multiple whorls of nervous tissue composed of poorly myelinated axons, Schwann cells, and associated connective tissue. Martius scarlet blue, ×360. (from a case supplied by C.J. Randall)

MELANOMA. Melanocytes are derived from the neural crest. Thus, melanomas are considered under tumors of neural tissue. Melanosis is common in many avian species, and breeds of chickens such as Silkies have numerous foci of melanocytes especially in gonads, peritoneum, perineurium, and periosteum. Campbell (20) reviewed a number of cases of melanoma and noted that malignant forms may arise in the ovary and metastasize throughout the abdominal cavity. The eye also can be a primary site of melanomas (34). Malignant melanomas have been observed in ducks (32, 94), a great cormorant (95), and budgerigars (101). Amelanotic melanomas occur in the subcutis of racing pigeons (92), and multifocal melanomas have been observed in chickens, but are rare (96). The pleiomorphic fusiform to elongate melanocytes may be arranged as discrete foci or infiltrating into the surrounding tissue. In some cases, the melanocytes may be arranged as small islands of closely packed cells reminiscent of epithelial tissue. Excess melanin can be bleached from sections using various techniques, such as with H_2O_2, to reveal occasional multinucleated cells and numerous mitoses. Melanin granules may be sparse, and in such cases, the brown pigment can be enhanced with ammoniacal silver techniques such as modified Masson-Fontana stain.

SPECIAL SENSES

Eyes. Ocular tumors, besides lymphomas and myelomas, are rare in birds. The avian iris muscle is striated and intraorbital rhabdomyosarcomas were detected in juvenile and subadult chickens (34). Cole (27) described a retinoblastoma, and melanomas and teratomas may involve the eye. Osteosarcomas may originate in the orbit, but these need to be differentiated from intraocular ossification following progressive retinal degeneration (67) or chronic intraocular infections such as toxoplasmosis (117).

ENDOCRINE SYSTEM

Thymus. A few thymomas, as distinct from thymic lymphomas, have been reported in chickens (21, 37, 53, 85), a duck (130), a budgerigar (133), and a Java sparrow (78). They are characterized by replacement of the normal thymic architecture with sheets of large polyhedral epithelial cells interspersed with variable numbers of lymphoid cells. No structural pattern is obvious, although there may be poorly defined lobules. The vesicular nucleus and abundant pale-staining cytoplasm of the epithelial cells contrast with lymphocytic morphology. The borders of the neoplastic cells are indistinct but may show squamous differentiation. The epithelial origin of these cells can be confirmed by immunostaining for cytokeratin (78). Aggregates of cells resembling Hassall's corpuscles are sometimes mixed among the tumor cells.

Pituitary Gland. Pituitary adenomas have been reported in budgerigars (8, 102), and although frequently cited as common, the true incidence in this species is not known. Campbell (20) reported two pituitary adenomas in domestic fowls. None were seen by Fredrickson and Helmboldt, although pituitary glands were examined in several hundred aged hens (42), nor were any seen in the brains of many chickens showing neurologic signs, which were examined histologically by the author (95).

Adrenal Gland. Campbell and Appleby (21) recorded a single case of an adenoma they considered was most likely derived from the adrenal gland, and an adenoma involving the adrenal gland was seen in an adult SPF hen (96). The adenomatous cells were well differentiated with abundant eosinophilic cytoplasm, but there were no particular histologic characteristics that would allow definitive confirmation that these tumors were derived from adrenal tissue. Similar tumors have been described in other avian species (94).

Thyroid and Parathyroid Glands. Guerin (53) described an adenoma arising in the parathyroid gland of a chicken and pointed out that only one other case of parathyroid carcinoma had been reported. Tumors of the thyroid gland in poultry appear to be extremely rare (20, 85). Naturally occurring goiters have been reported in chickens (53), and were induced in chickens and quail by feeding rapeseed meals containing goitrogens (127). Goiters also occur in budgerigars, probably as a consequence of low iodine intake (13, 94). In budgerigars, neoplasia of the thyroid gland may be difficult to differentiate from hyperplasia and dysplasia associated with goiter; however, in the thyroid adenomas reported by Reece (94), there were discrete areas of neoplastic adenomatous tissue. A mixed cell tumor of the thyroid gland was composed of adenomatous tissue and islands of proliferating chondrocytes and fibroblasts.

INTEGUMENT

Subcutis

HEMANGIOPERICYTOMA. Two hemangiopericytomas in the subcutaneous tissue have been reported (106), and four cases were described by Fredrickson and Helmboldt (42). All of these benign tumors occurred as subcutaneous nodules of variable size, usually in the cervical region. The nodules were dense, white, well delineated, and firmly embedded in the subcutis. The histologic appearance was of uniform spindle-shaped cells possessing a fusiform nucleus with diffuse chromatin, and abundant cytoplasm but indistinct cell borders. They were arranged in a concentric manner around central blood vessels, and the intervening reticulin fibers could be readily demonstrated by a silver stain (Fig. 17.84).

LIPOMA AND LIPOSARCOMA. Subcutaneous lipomas are not common in chickens (20), but in mammals they often arise at sites of trauma. Subcutaneous and intraabdominal lipomas are frequently encountered in other avian species, especially psittacines (70, 94). They are generally encapsulated, benign, delicately trabeculated tumors with variable degrees of necrosis and hemorrhage. They are composed of mature adipocytes with large cytoplasmic vacuoles and a displaced pale nucleus. Mitotic figures are rare. Malignant liposarcomas of chickens are rare and may be locally invasive or metastasize (80, 96). They may be similar in histologic appearance to fibrosarcomas except for intracytoplasmic fat vacuoles within tumor cells. In other cases, the tumor may be composed of obviously immature adipocytes. Multifocal liposarcomas have been described in other species (33, 94).

Soft tissue tumors such as fibromas, fibrosarcomas, myxomas, and myxosarcomas are encountered in chickens and may be induced by avian leukosis virus (see subchapter, Leukosis/Sarcoma Group). Occasional cases are reported in SPF poultry and other species. It should be noted that myxomas of the ovary may be mistaken for adenocarcinomas, and both fibrosarcomas and myxosarcomas can occur as metastatic abdominal tumors requiring histologic study to differentiate them from metastatic abdominal adenocarcinomas. Myxomas and fibromas were observed on the rostral extremity of the upper trimmed beaks of hens (96). The etiology of these was not determined.

Cutis

SQUAMOUS CELL CARCINOMA. The tumor of broiler chickens commonly referred to as "dermal squamous cell carcinoma" is probably a keratoacanthoma and is dealt with elsewhere in this book (see Chapter 37, Emerging Diseases and Diseases of Unknown or Complex Etiology). A true squamous cell carcinoma is a malignant tumor of keratinocytes, which form irregular masses or cords that proliferate downward and invade the dermis and subcutis. It is characterized by epithelial cells with intercellular bridges resembling the stratum spinosum, being found on the dermal side of the basal lamina. There is no cushion of basal cells and the epithelial tumor cells lack orderly maturation, although some keratinization usually is found. These tumors are associated with an intense mononuclear inflammatory cell infiltrate and a reactive fibroplasia. Squamous cell carcinomas are locally invasive, but may be slow to metastasize. There are few reports of true dermal squamous cell carcinomas of chickens in the literature and most of these affected the scaly skin of the shanks and lower feet of adults (20, 23, 110). Several cases of squamous cell carcinoma involving the alimentary tract have been reported (see above). Atypical pox lesions of the feathered areas of broiler chickens may mimic dermal squamous cell tumors (36).

FEATHER FOLLICULOMA. Feather folliculomas are usually multiple cystic structures with central lumina containing keratinized debris and feather remnants. They are lined by cuboidal to squamous epithelial cells with abrupt keratinization, and areas of disorganized feather follicle epithelium. There is usually an intense inflammatory cell infiltration into the surrounding dermis and some fibrosis (Fig. 17.85). Feather folliculomas of chickens (96) and turkeys (30) have been described, and they are common in some caged birds such as Norwich canaries (87).

INTRACUTANEOUS KERATINIZING EPITHELIOMA. These are a benign cystic tumor of the facial skin of adult chickens. They present as multiple small well-

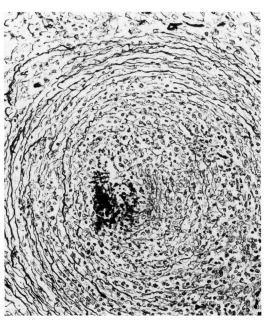

17.84. Hemangiopericytoma with concentric rings of pericytes clearly defined. Silver, ×90.

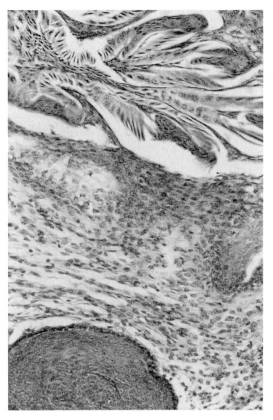

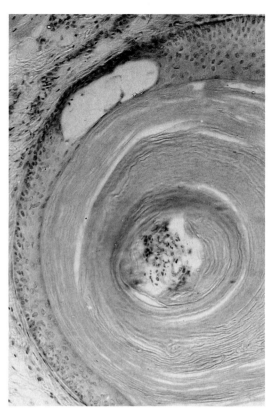

17.85. Edge of a feather folliculoma showing dysplastic specialized feather-forming epithelium and an adjacent cord of basal cells. The lumen was lined by stratified cuboidal to squamous epithelium with abrupt keratinization, and contained keratin and feather remnants. H&E, ×180.

17.86. The lumen of this intracutaneous keratinizing epithelioma contains lamellated keratin. The epithelium shows basal cells aligned on a distinct basal lamina and progression to polyhedral cells with abrupt keratinization. Note the small intraepithelial bulla. H&E, ×190. (Avian Pathol)

encapsulated nodules with a central craterous pore (96). They are lined by well-developed stratified epithelium consisting of basal cells progressing to maturation with prominent intercellular bridges in the stratum spinosum. The lumina contain lamellated keratin but no feather remnants (Fig. 17.86). They are surrounded by a small amount of fibrous tissue and there is little inflammatory cell reaction unless there is rupture of the wall. These tumors are probably derived from keratogenous cysts and are distinct from both keratoacanthomas of broilers and feather folliculomas.

OTHER TUMORS OF THE CUTIS. Hard, horny, papillomatoid tumors of the scale-producing epithelium of the shanks, with heavily keratinized whorls, are acanthomas (20). Adenomas may arise from the preen (uropygeal) gland situated dorsal to the base of the tail in the chicken. Papillomalike lesions on the foot pads of ducks were reported from France but not described in detail, and an association with papillomatous lesions in abattoir workers was postulated (54); their etiology was not determined.

MUSCULOSKELETAL SYSTEM

Leiomyoma and Leiomyosarcoma. Leiomyomas of the ventral ligament of the oviduct are common in laying hens (see Reproductive System). Leiomyomas were observed by the author in the intestinal wall of commercial ducks and freckled ducks (95), in the gizzard musculature of a chicken (96), and attached to the pancreas of pigeons (94). There are a few reports of leiomyosarcomas involving the intestinal wall (2), ovary (63), and tracheal muscle (21) of chickens. Leiomyomas and leiomyosarcomas are rare in other avian species (94, 100, 108).

Rhabdomyosarcoma. Rhabdomyosarcomas tend to be soft, poorly encapsulated and prone to necrosis and hemorrhage. The pectoral and sartorius-gracilis muscles are most commonly involved, but the heart may be affected (21). Metastases to the lung have been reported (69, 96). Histologically, there are irregular bundles of interlacing cells, some of which exhibit a typical racquet or star shape, and multinucleated cells (Fig. 17.87). The cytoplasm is intensely eosinophilic, but cross striations are difficult to detect with either polarized light or phosphotungstic acid stain (20, 85). They also have been described in budgerigars (70, 94).

Osteoma and Osteosarcoma. Osteomas and osteosarcomas are uncommon tumors of poultry (20). Campbell and Appleby (21) described two osteomas, eight osteosarcomas, and one osteoclastoma in broilers, and similar tumors have been reported in other avian species (79, 94). Osteosarcomas may be composed of abundant mineralized trabecular bone, although in some cases there may be a much more cellular tumor composed of spindle-shaped cells and poorly mineralized trabeculae. Even in such cases, some foci of ossification usually can be found. Osteosarcomas may metastasize to the lungs. Multipotent mesenchymal tumors usually occur on the extremities of long bones and contain solid masses of dysplastic bone, islands of cartilage, dense drifts of fibrous tissue and foci of myxomatous tissue. These are frequently described as osteosarcomas. Osteomas are well circumscribed and composed of disorganized bony trabeculae (Fig 17.88).

Chondroma and Chondrosarcoma. Chondromas of poultry are rare. Multifocal chondromas of the plantar aspect of the footpads of nine geese, ducks, and other Anseriformes, and other mesenchymal tumors in the foot pads of four other Anseriformes were described by the author (94). The etiology of these was not determined, but approximately 10% of two flocks of wild mallards

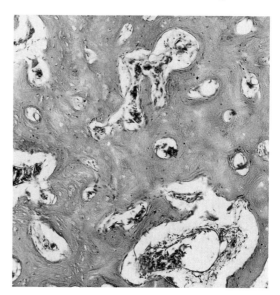

17.88. Osteoma showing thick irregular trabeculae. H&E, ×90. (Avian Pathol)

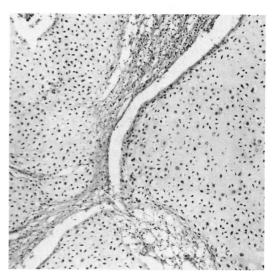

17.89. Multifocal chondroma of the footpad of a goose showing lobules of cartilage separated by fibrovascular trabeculae. H&E, ×75. (Avian Pathol)

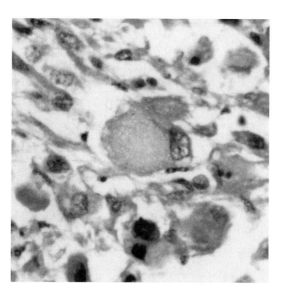

17.87. Rhabdomyosarcoma. Some cells are straplike, whereas others are large and polyhedral: their cytoplasm is eosinophilic. Some cells have multiple nuclei. H&E, ×360. (Avian Pathol)

were affected. The chondromas were characterized by lobules of chondrocytes separated by trabeculae (Fig 17.89). Acanthotic and hyperkeratotic lesions found on the footpad of a duck were associated with herpesviruses (129), but the relationship to other footpad mesenchymal neoplasms is not known.

REFERENCES

1. Anderson, W.I., and H. Steinberg. 1989. Primary glossal squamous-cell carcinoma in a Spanish cochin hen. Avian Dis 33:827–828.

2. Anderson, W.I., P.C. McCaskey, K.A. Langheinrich,

and A.E. Dreesen. 1985. Neurofibrosarcoma and leiomyosarcoma in slaughterhouse broilers. Avian Dis 29:521–527.

3. Anjum, A.D. 1987. Adenocarcinoma of the oviduct of the domestic fowl (Gallus domesticus) and its relationship to steroid sex hormones. PhD Thesis. Royal Veterinary College, London, United Kingdom, pp. 1–356.

4. Anjum, A.D., and L.N. Payne. 1988. Concentration of steroid sex hormones in the plasma of hens in relation to oviduct tumours. Br Poult Sci 29:729–734.

5. Anjum, A.D., L.N. Payne, and E.C. Appleby. 1988. Spontaneous occurrence and experimental induction of leiomyoma of the ventral ligament of the oviduct of the hen. Res Vet Sci 45:341–348.

6. Apperly, F.L. 1935. Primary carcinoma of the lung in the domestic fowl. Am J Cancer 23:556–557.

7. Baker, J.R. 1980. A proventricular adenoma in a Brazilian teal (Amazonetta brasiliensis). Vet Rec 107:63–64.

8. Bauck, L. 1987. Pituitary neoplastic disease in 9 budgies. Proc 1st Int Conf Zoo Avian Med, Oahu, Hawaii. Association of Avian Veterinarians, pp. 87–89.

9. Beach, J.E. 1962. Diseases of budgerigars and other cage birds: A survey of post-mortem findings. Part II. Vet Rec 74:63–68.

10. Beard, J.W., E.A. Hillman, D. Beard, K. Lapis, and U. Heine. 1975. Neoplastic response of the avian liver to host infection with strain MC29 leukosis virus. Cancer Res 35:1603–1627.

11. Beasley, J.N., S. Klopp, and B. Terry. 1986. Neoplasms in the oviducts of turkeys. Avian Dis 30:433–437.

12. Biering-Sorensen, U. 1956. On disseminated, focal gliomatosis ("multiple gliomas") and cerebral calcifications in hens. A study of pathogenesis. Nord Vet Med 8:887–901.

13. Blackmore, D.K. 1963. The incidence and aetiology of thyroid dysplasia in Budgerigars (Melopsittacus undulatus). Vet Rec 75:1068–1072.

14. Blackmore, D.K. 1966. The clinical approach to tumours in cage birds. I. The pathology and incidence of neoplasia in cage birds. J Small Anim Pract 7:217–223.

15. Budras, K.D., M. Hoftmann, and J. Wallenburg. 1979. Umformung des rete ovarii zum rete testis und des epoophoron zum nebenhoden nach experimentellem geschlechtsumkehr bei Gallus domesticus. Acta Anat 104:23–35.

16. Calnek, B.W. 1992. Chicken neoplasia—a model for cancer research. Br Poult Sci 33:3–16.

17. Campbell, J.G. 1945. Neoplastic disease of the fowl with special reference to its history, incidence and seasonal variation. J Comp Pathol 55:908–921.

18. Campbell, J.G. 1949. Spontaneous hepatocellular and cholangiocellular carcinoma in the duck. An experimental study. Br J Cancer 3:198–210.

19. Campbell, J.G. 1951. Some unusual gonadal tumours of the fowl. Br J Cancer 5:69–82.

20. Campbell, J.G. 1969. Tumours of the Fowl. Lippincott, Philadelphia, PA, pp. 1–292.

21. Campbell, J.G., and E.C. Appleby. 1966. Tumours in young chickens bred for rapid body growth (broiler chickens): A study of 351 cases. J Pathol Bacteriol 92:77–90.

22. Cancer Institute, Chinese Academy Medical Sciences. 1973. The epidemiology of esophageal cancer in North China and preliminary results in the investigation of its etiological factors. Acta Zool Sinica 19:309–312.

23. Cardona, C.J., A.A. Bickford, and K. Emanuelson. 1992. Squamous cell carcinoma on the legs of an Aracauna chicken. Avian Dis 36:474–479.

24. Carnaghan, R.B.A. 1965. Hepatic tumours in ducks fed a low level of toxic groundnut meal. Nature (Lond) 208:308.

25. Chin, R.P., and B.C. Barr. 1990. Squamous cell carcinoma of the pharyngeal cavity in a Jersey black giant rooster. Avian Dis 34:775–778.

26. Christopher, J., J.V. Narayana, and G.A. Sastry. 1966. Primary neoplasms of the liver of the domestic fowl. Ceylon Vet J 14:61–64.

27. Cole, R.K. 1946. An avian retinoblastoma. Cornell Vet 36:350–353.

28. Coletti, M., G. Vitellozzi, A. Fioroni, and M.P. Franciosini. 1988. Neoplasie spontanee del piccione domestico (Columba livia). Obiet Doc Vet 9:57–61.

29. Cooper, J.E., and S.L. Pugsley. 1984. A mesothelioma in a ferruginous hawk (Buteo regalis). Avian Pathol 13:797–801.

30. Couvillion, C.E., W.A. Maslin, and R.M. Montgomery. 1990. Multiple feather follicle cysts in a wild turkey. J Wildl Dis 26:122–124.

31. Crittenden, L.B., R.L. Witter, W. Okazaki, and P.E. Neiman. 1979. Lymphoid neoplasms in chicken flocks free of infection with exogenous avian tumor viruses. J Natl Cancer Inst 63:191–200.

32. Dillberger, J.E., S.B. Citino, and N.H. Altman. 1987. Four cases of neoplasia in captive wild birds. Avian Dis 31:206–213.

33. Doster, A.R., J.L. Johnson, G.E. Duhamel, T.W. Bargar, and G. Nason. 1987. Liposarcoma in a Canada goose (Branta canadensis). Avian Dis 31:918–920.

34. Dukes, T.W., and J.R. Pettit. 1983. Avian ocular neoplasia—a description of spontaneously occurring cases. Can J Comp Med 47:33–36.

35. Effron, M., L. Griner, and K. Benirschke. 1977. Nature and rate of neoplasia found in captive wild mammals, birds and reptiles at necropsy. J Natl Cancer Inst 59:185–198.

36. Fallavena, L.C.B., N.C. Rodrigues, W. Scheufler, N.R.S. Martins, A.C. Brage, C.T.P. Salle, and H.L.S. Moraes. 1993. Atypical fowl pox in broiler chickens in southern Brazil. Vet Rec 132:635.

37. Feldman, W.H. 1936. Thymoma in a chicken (Gallus domesticus). Am J Cancer 26:576–580.

38. Feldman, W.H., and C. Olson. 1965. Neoplastic diseases of the chicken. In H.E. Biester and L.H. Schwarte (eds.). Diseases of Poultry, 5th ed. Iowa State University Press, Ames, IA, pp. 863–924.

39. Fell, H.B. 1923. Histologic studies on the gonads of the fowl. I. The histological basis of sex reversal. Br J Exp Biol 1:97–129.

40. Frankenhuis, M.T. 1987. Sex reversal in poultry. Poultry (Misset) 32:46–47.

41. Fredrickson, T.N. 1987. Ovarian tumors of the hen. Environ Health Perspect 73:35–51.

42. Fredrickson, T.N., and C.F. Helmboldt. 1991. Tumors of unknown etiology. In B.W. Calnek, H.J. Barnes, C.W. Beard, W.M. Reid, and H.W. Yoder Jr. (eds.). Diseases of Poultry, 9th ed. Iowa State University Press, Ames, IA, pp. 459–470.

43. Gentle, M.J. 1986. Neuroma formation following partial beak amputation (beak trimming) in the chicken. Res Vet Sci 41:383–85.

44. Gentle, M.J., and L.H. Hunter. 1988. Neural consequences of partial toe amputation in chickens. Res Vet Sci 45:374–376.

45. Gentle, M.J., B.H. Thorp, and B.O. Hughes. 1995. Anatomical consequences of partial beak amputation (beak trimming) in turkeys, Res Vet Sci 58:158–162.

46. Gilbert, A.B. 1979. Female genital organs. In A.S. King and J.M. McLelland (eds.). Form and Function in Birds, vol. 1. Academic Press, London, United Kingdom, pp. 237–360.

47. Goodchild, W.M. 1969. Adenocarcinoma of the oviduct in laying hens. Vet Rec 84:122.

48. Goodwin, M., and E.D. McGee. 1993. Herpes-like virus associated with a cloacal papilloma in an orange-fronted conure (Aratinga canicularis). J Assoc Avian Vet 7:23–25.

49. Gorham, S.L., and M.A. Ottinger. 1986. Sertoli cell tu-

mors in Japanese quail. Avian Dis 30:337–339.

50. Goss, L.J. 1940. The incidence and classification of avian tumors. Cornell Vet 30:75–88.

51. Gould, W.J., P.H. O'Connell, H.L. Shivaprasad, A.E. Yeager, and K.A. Schat. 1993. Detection of retrovirus sequences in budgerigars with tumours. Avian Pathol 22:33–45.

52. Griner, L.A., G. Migaki, L.R. Penner and A.E. McKee Jr. 1977. Heterakidosis and nodular granulomas caused by Heterakis isolonche in the ceca of Gallinaceous birds. Vet Pathol 14:582–590.

53. Guerin, M. 1954. Tumeurs spontanees de la poule. In Tumeurs Spontanees des Animaux de Laboratoire. Legrand, Paris, France, pp. 153–180.

54. Guillet, G., J. Borredon, and M.F. Duboseq. 1987. Prevalence of warts on hands of poultry slaughterers, and poultry warts. Arch Dermatol 123:718–719.

55. Gupta, B.N., and R.F. Langham. 1968. Arrhenoblastoma in an Indian Desi hen. Avian Dis 12:441–444.

56. Guthrie, J. 1967. Specificity of the metallic ion in the experimental induction of teratomas in fowl. Br J Cancer 21:619–622.

57. Haritani, M., H. Kajigaya, T. Akashi, M. Kamemura, N. Tanahara, M. Umeda, M. Sugiyama, M. Isoda, and C. Kato. 1984. A study on the origin of adenocarcinoma in fowls using immunohistological technique. Avian Dis 28:1130–1134.

58. Hasholt, J. 1966. Diseases of the female reproductive organs of pet birds. J Small Anim Pract 7:313–320.

59. Helmboldt, C.F., G. Migaki, K.A. Langheinrich, and R.M. Jakowski. 1974. Teratoma in domestic fowl (Gallus gallus). Avian Dis 18:142–148.

60. Hodges, R.D. 1974. The female reproductive tract. In R.D. Hodges (ed.), The Histology of the Fowl. Academic Press, New York, pp. 326–387.

61. Hubbard, G.B., R.E. Schmidt, and K.C. Fletcher. 1983. Neoplasia in zoo animals. J Zoo Anim Med 14:33–40.

62. Ilchmann, G., and V. Bergmann. 1975. Histologische und elektronenmikroskopische untersuchungen zu adenokarzinomatose der legehennen. Arch Exp Veterinaermed 29:897–907.

63. Jackson, C. 1936. The incidence and pathology of tumors of domesticated animals in South Africa. Onderstepoort J Vet Res 6:1–460.

64. Jackson, C. 1954. Gliomas of the domestic fowl: Their pathology with special reference to histogenesis; and pathogenesis and their relationship to other diseases. Onderstepoort J Vet Res 26:501–592.

65. Jungherr, E.L., and A. Wolf. 1939. Gliomas in animals. A report of two astrocytomas in the common fowl. Am J Cancer 37:493–509.

66. Kajigaya, H., M. Kamemura, N. Tanahara, A. Ohta, H. Suzuki, M. Sugiyama, and M. Isoda. 1987. The influence of celomic membranes and a tunnel between celomic cavities on cancer metastasis in poultry. Avian Dis 31:176–186.

67. Kelley, K.C., R.J. Ulshafer, and E.A. Ellis. 1987. Intraocular ossification in the rd chicken. Avian Pathol 16:189–197.

68. Kelley, L., J. Hill, S. Hafner, and K. Langheinrich. 1993. Enterogenous cysts in chickens. Vet Pathol 30:376–378.

69. Krogh, G. 1953. Two cases of rhabdomyosarcoma in chickens. Nord Vet Med 5:232–236.

70. Latimer, K.S. 1994. Oncology. In Avian Medicine: Principles and Applications. B.W. Ritchie, G.J. Harrison and L.R. Harrison (eds.). Wingers Publications, Lakeworth, FL, pp. 640–668.

71. Leach, M.W., J. Paul-Murphy, and L.J. Lowenstine. 1989. Three cases of gastric neoplasia in psittacines. Avian Dis 33:204–210.

72. Lesbouyries, C. 1941. Les processus tumoraux. In La Pathologie des Oiseaux. Vigot, Paris, France, pp. 143–179.

73. Ling, Y.S., and Y.Q. Guo. 1985. Pathological study of spontaneous mesothelioma in ducks. Chin J Vet Sci Technol 9:15–16.

74. Ling, Y.S., Y.J. Guo, and L.K. Yang. 1993. Pathological observations of hepatic tumours in ducks. Avian Pathol 22:131–140.

75. Lombard, L.S., and E.J. Witte. 1959. Frequency and types of tumors in mammals and birds of the Philadelphia Zoological Garden. Cancer Res 19:127–141.

76. Loupal, G. 1984. Leukosen bei zoo- und wildvogeln. Avian Pathol 13:703–714.

77. Loupal, G., and M. Reifinger. 1986. Tumoren bei zoo-, zier- und wildvogeln. Eine ubersicht uber 25 jahre (1960–1984). J Vet Med A 33:180–192.

78. Maeda, H., K. Ozaki, S. Fukui, and I. Narama. 1994. Thymoma in a Java sparrow (Padda oryzivora). Avian Pathol 23:353–357.

79. Mawdesley-Thomas, L.E., and D.H. Solden. 1967. Osteogenic sarcoma in a domestic goose (Anser anser). Avian Dis 11:365–370.

80. Mohiddin, S.M., and K. Ramakrishna. 1972. Liposarcoma in a fowl. Avian Dis 16:680–684.

81. Montali, R.J. 1980. An overview of tumors in zoo animals. In R.J. Montali and G. Migaki (eds.). Comparative Pathology of Zoo Animals. Smithsonian Institute, Washington, DC, pp. 531–542.

82. Neumann, U., and N. Kummerfeld. 1983. Neoplasms in budgerigars (Melopsittacus undulatus): Clinical, pathomorphological and serological findings with special consideration of kidney tumours. Avian Pathol 12:353–362.

83. Nobel, T.A., F. Neumann, and M.S. Dison. 1964. A histological study of peritoneal carcinomatosis in the laying hen. Avian Dis 8:513–522.

84. Okoye, J.O.A., and C.C. Ilochi. 1993. Pancreatic adenocarcinoma in Guinea fowl. Avian Pathol 22:401–406.

85. Olson, C., and K.L. Bullis. 1942. A survey of spontaneous neoplastic diseases in chickens. Massachusetts Agric Exp Stat Bull 391, pp. 1–25.

86. Ottinger,M.A., E. Adkins-Regan, J. Buntin, M.F. Cheng, T. de Voogd, C. Harding, and H. Opel. 1984. Hormonal mediation of reproductive behaviour. J Exp Zool 232:605–616.

87. Pass, D.A. 1989. The pathology of the avian integument: A review. Avian Pathol 18:1–72.

88. Porter,T.E., B.M. Hargis, J.L. Silsby, and M.E. El-Halawani. 1989. Differential steroid production between theca interna and theca externa cells: A three cell model for follicular steroidogenesis in avian species. Endocrinology 125:109–116.

89. Potter, K., T. Connor, and A.M. Gallina. 1983. Cholangiocarcinoma in a yellow-faced Amazon parrot (Amazona xanthops). Avian Dis 27:556–558.

90. Priester, W.A. 1975. Esophageal cancer in North China; high rates in human and poultry populations in the same areas. Avian Dis 19:213–215.

91. Purvulov, B., and S. Bozhkov. 1984. Pathology of some spontaneous neoplasms of fowls. Obshch i Stravnitelna Patologiya 16:55–58.

92. Randall, C.J. 1992. Personal communication.

93. Ratcliffe, H.L. 1933. Incidence and nature of tumors in captive wild mammals and birds. Am J Cancer 17:116–135.

94. Reece, R.L. 1992. Observations on naturally occurring neoplasms in birds in the state of Victoria, Australia. Avian Pathol 21:3–32.

95. Reece, R.L. 1995. Unpublished observations.

96. Reece, R.L. 1996. Some observations on naturally occurring neoplasms in domestic fowl in the state of Victoria, Australia. Avian Pathol 25:407–447.

97. Reece, R.L., and S.A. Lister. 1993. An abdominal teratoma in a domestic goose (Anseriformes, Anser anser domesticus). Avian Pathol 22:193–196.

98. Rigdon, R.H. 1961. Pulmonary neoplasms produced by methyl cholanthrene in the white Pekin duck. Cancer Res 21:571–574.

99. Rigdon, R.H. 1972. Tumors in the duck (Family Anatidae): A review. J Natl Cancer Inst 49:467–476.

100. Sasipreeyajan, J., J.A. Newman, and P.A. Brown. 1988. Leiomyosarcoma in a Budgerigar (Melopsittacus undulatus). Avian Dis 32:163–165.

101. Saunders, N.C., and G.K. Saunders. 1991. Malignant melanoma in a budgerigar (Melopsittacus undulatus). Avian Dis 35:999–1000.

102. Schlumberger, H.G. 1956. Neoplasia in the parakeet. I. Spontaneous chromophobe pituitary tumors. Cancer Res 14:237–245.

103. She, R.P. 1987. Epidemiology and pathology of oropharyngo-esophageal carcinoma in chickens from different areas in Zhongxian county, Hubei province. Acta Vet Zootech Sinica 18:195–200.

104. Siegfried, L.M. 1983. Neoplasms identified in free-flying birds. Avian Dis 27:86–99.

105. Siller, W.G. 1956. A Sertoli cell tumour causing feminization in a brown leghorn capon. J Endocrinol 14:197–203.

106. Sokkar, S.M., M.A. Mohammed, A.J. Zubaidy, and A. Mutalib. 1979. Study of some non-leukotic avian neoplasms. Avian Pathol 8:69–75.

107. Sriraman, P.K., S.R. Ahmed, N.R.G. Naidu, and P.R. Rao. 1981. Neoplasia in chickens and ducks. Indian J Poult Sci 16:436–437.

108. Steinberg, H. 1988. Leiomyosarcoma of the jejunum in a budgerigar. Avian Dis 32:166–168.

109. Stewart, H.L. 1966. Pulmonary cancer and adenomatosis in captive wild mammals and birds from the Philadelphia Zoo. J Natl Cancer Inst 36:117–138.

110. Sugiyama, M., H. Yamashina, T. Kanbara, H. Kajigaya, K. Konagaya, M. Umeda, M. Isoda, and T. Sakai. 1987. Dermal squamous cell carcinoma in a laying hen. Jpn J Vet Sci 49:1129–1130.

111. Sundberg, J.P, R.E. Junge, M.K. O'Banion, E.J. Basgall, G. Harrison, A.J. Herron, and H.L. Shivaprasad. 1986. Cloacal papillomas in psittacines. Am J Vet Res 47:928–932.

112. Swarbrick, O., J.G. Campbell, and D.M. Berry. 1968. An outbreak of oviduct adenocarcinoma in laying hens. Vet Rec 82:57–59.

113. Swayne, D.E., G.N. Rowland, and O.J. Fletcher. 1986. Pinealoma in a broiler breeder. Avian Dis 30:853–855.

114. Talebi, A., J.D. Collins, and K. Dodd. 1993. An investigation of nodular lesions found in Irish poultry during veterinary inspection at poultry meat plants. Avian Pathol 22:715–724.

115. Turk, J.R., A.L. Forar, and A.M. Gallina. 1980. Intestinal adenocarcinoma in a chicken. Avian Dis 24:507–509.

116. van der Heyden, N. 1988. Psittacine papillomas. Proc Assoc Avian Vet Conf, Houston, Texas. pp 23–26.

117. Vickers, M.C., W.J. Hartley, R.W. Mason, J.P. Dubey, and L. Schollam. 1992. Blindness associated with toxoplasmosis in canaries. J Am Vet Med Assoc 200:1723–1725.

118. Wadsworth, P.F., S.K. Majeed, W.M. Brancker, and D.M. Jones. 1978. Some hepatic neoplasms in non-domesticated birds. Avian Pathol 7:551–555.

119. Wadsworth, P.F., D.M. Jones, and S.L. Pugsley. 1981. Some cases of lymphoid leukosis in captive wild birds. Avian Pathol 10:499–504.

120. Walser, M.M., and P.S. Paul. 1979. Ovarian adenocarcinomas in domestic turkeys. Avian Pathol 8:335–339.

121. Warner, N.E., N.B. Friedman, E.J. Bomze, and F. Masin. 1960. Comparative pathology of experimental and spontaneous androblastomas and gynoblastomas of the gonads. Am J Obstet Gynecol 79:971–988.

122. Webster, W.S., B.C. Bullock, and R.W. Prichard. 1969. A report of three bile duct carcinomas occurring in pigeons. J Am Vet Med Assoc 155:1200–1205.

123. Wight, P.A.L. 1962. Gonadal maldevelopment in a flock of Rhode Island red fowls. J Endocrinol 23:341–349.

124. Wight, P.A.L. 1965. Neoplastic sequelae of gonadal maldevelopment in a flock of domestic fowls. Avian Dis 9:327–335.

125. Wight, P.A.L., and J.G. Campbell. 1976. Three unusual intracranial tumours of the domesticated fowl. Avian Pathol 5:201–214.

126. Wight, P.A.L., and R.H. Duff. 1964. The histopathology of epizootic gliosis and astrocytomata of the domestic fowl. J Comp Pathol 74:373–380.

127. Wight, P.A.L., and D.W.F. Shannon. 1985. The morphology of the thyroid glands of quails and fowls maintained on diets containing rapeseed. Avian Pathol 14:383–399.

128. Wilson, R.B., M.A. Holscher, J.R. Fullerton, and M.D. Johnson. 1988. Pineoblastoma in a cockatiel. Avian Dis 32:591–593.

129. Wojcinski, Z.W., H.S.J. Wojcinski, I.K. Barker, and N.W. King Jr. 1991. Cutaneous herpesvirus infection in a Mallard duck (Anas platyrhynchos). J Wildl Dis 27:129–134.

130. Worms, G., and H.P. Klotz. 1934. Constrution l'etude des tumeurs thymiques. A propos d'un cas d'epitheliome thymique chez un canard. Bull Assoc Fr Etude Cancer 23:420–432.

131. Yokosuka, O., M. Omata, Y.-Z. Zhou, F. Imazeki, and K. Okuda. 1985. Duck hepatitis B virus DNA in liver and serum of Chinese ducks: Integration of viral DNA in a hepatocellular carcinoma. Proc Natl Acad Sci USA 82:5180–5184.

132. Zhang, J.L., F.C. Liang, and Y.J. Chen. 1985. Primary pulmonary tumours in Pekin ducks: Pathological analysis of 16 cases. Chin J Vet Sci Tech 4:32–33.

133. Zubaidy, A.J. 1980. An epithelial thymoma in a budgerigar (Melopsittacus undulatus). Avian Pathol 9:575–581.

18 Infectious Bronchitis

David Cavanagh and Syed A. Naqi

INTRODUCTION

Definition and Synonyms. Infectious bronchitis (IB) is an acute, highly contagious viral respiratory disease of chickens characterized by tracheal rales, coughing, and sneezing. In addition, the disease may affect kidneys, and in laying flocks there is usually a drop in egg production and egg quality. Mortality may occur in young chicks due to respiratory or kidney manifestations of the infection.

Infectious bronchitis is of major economic importance because it is a cause of poor weight gain and feed efficiency, is often a component of mixed infections that produce airsacculitis that may result in condemnations at processing of broilers, and is a cause of egg-production and egg-quality declines. The losses from production inefficiencies are usually of greater concern than losses from mortality. The highly transmissible nature of the disease, and the occurrence of multiple serotypes of IB virus (IBV), have complicated and increased the cost of attempts to prevent the disease by immunization. The disease is also called avian infectious bronchitis.

Economic and Public Health Significance. Infectious bronchitis appears to have no public health significance. Human coronaviruses differ from IBV extensively with respect to protein sequence and antigenicity (17). Serums from individuals who were in contact with chickens by providing direct care or through handling poultry diagnostic accessions were found to have low neutralizing antibody titers against IBV (123), but the significance of the finding remains unknown.

HISTORY. Infectious bronchitis was first observed in the United States in North Dakota in 1930. A report by Schalk and Hawn in 1931 (140) of the clinical signs and preliminary laboratory studies of those cases is recognized as the first report of IB. Initially, IB was recognized as primarily a disease of young chicks; however, it was later observed to be common in semimature and laying flocks. Other manifestations of IB include egg-production declines in laying flocks, noted following the typical respiratory disease in the 1940s, and kidney lesions observed in the 1960s. The prevalence and economic importance of the disease resulted in efforts to prevent IB in laying flocks by controlled exposure of chickens to IBV during the growing stage prior to the onset of egg production. This effort by Van Roekel in 1941, which had some success, was the initial step toward the development of the immunization programs used today (153).

Other early milestones include the establishment of the virus etiology by Beach and Schalm in 1936 (8), the first cultivation of the virus in embryonated chicken eggs by Beaudette and Hudson in 1937 (9), and the report in 1956 by Jungherr et al. (93) that the Connecticut isolate of 1951 and the Massachusetts isolate of 1941 produced similar diseases, but did not cross protect or cross neutralize. The latter report was the first demonstration that the etiology of IB included more than one serotype. Additional historical information can be found in the review by Cunningham (47) and earlier editions of this chapter by Hofstad (79).

INCIDENCE AND DISTRIBUTION. Infectious bronchitis is distributed worldwide. A listing of the reported first identification of IB by country and year through 1966 was included in a review by Estola (63). In the United States, several serotypes in addition to the originally identified Massachusetts (Mass) type of IBV were identified beginning in the 1950s (82, 90). Mass-type strains have been isolated in Europe since the 1940s (19). Many other serotypes, distinct from those in North America, have also been isolated in Europe (19, 27) and Australia (44, 45, 46). Outbreaks of IB still occur, even in vaccinated flocks, and virus strains isolated from those outbreaks are often found to be a serotype distinct from the vaccine type.

ETIOLOGY

Classification. Infectious bronchitis virus is a member of the *Coronaviridae*, which includes two genera, *Coronavirus* and *Torovirus* (23); it is in the genus *Coronavirus*, together with turkey coronavirus (see Chapter 27) and at least nine species in mammals. Infectious bronchitis virus differs extensively with respect to protein sequence and antigenicity from turkey coronavirus, which is more closely related to some mammalian coronaviruses (23). There are no known avian toroviruses.

Morphology. Infectious bronchitis virus is pleomorphic but generally rounded. It possesses an envelope that is approximately 120 nm in diameter with club-shaped surface projections (spikes) about 20 nm in length (Fig. 18.1). The spikes are not packed as closely as the rod-shaped spikes of paramyxoviruses (58). Ribonucleoprotein (RNP, core) structures released from spontaneously disrupted particles could be visualized by shadowing, but not by negative-staining (59). For the most part, the RNP was observed as strands of only 1–2 nm in diameter, but coiled structures of 10–15 nm diameter were occasionally observed (59).

Infectious bronchitis virus strains differ in their density in sucrose gradients, peak density usually being in the range 1.15–1.18 g/mL, but particles of lower (lacking RNP) and higher density can also be obtained. Centrifugation forces of greater than 100,000 g should be avoided, as loss of spikes can occur. Those of IBV-Beaudette appear to be especially unstable; incubation at 37 C sometimes results in the loss of one of the spike components (146).

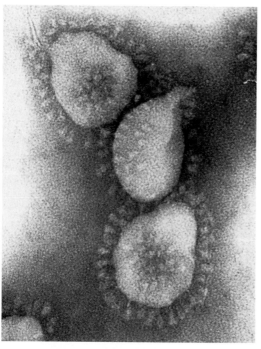

18.1. Virion of avian IBV illustrating club-shaped projections. Preparation negatively stained with phosphotungstic acid. ×300,000. (Berry and Almeida)

Chemical Composition. Several reviews on the composition of coronaviruses are available (23, 142). Infectious bronchitis virus virions contain three major virus-specific proteins; the spike (S) and membrane (M) glycoproteins, and the internal nucleocapsid (N) protein. In addition, a fourth protein (small membrane protein, sM) is believed to be associated with the virion envelope. The S protein comprises two or three copies of each of two glycopolypeptides, S1 and S2 (approximately 520 and 625 amino acids, respectively). Hemagglutination-inhibiting (HI) and most of the virus-neutralizing (VN) antibodies are induced by S1 (20, 94, 97, 104, 132). The structure and biologic properties of S have recently been reviewed (17).

Most of the 225 amino acids of the M protein are either embedded in the virus membrane or at the inner membrane surface; only about 10% of the protein is exposed at the outer virus surface. The N protein is around the single piece of single-stranded, positive sense, RNA genome (to form the RNP) that comprises 27,500 nucleotides, the whole of which has been cloned and sequenced (10). Preparations of purified virus always contain host cell polypeptides (16). The S2 protein can be difficult to detect (16, 18) and some N protein can be missing or degraded.

Virus Replication. Infectious bronchitis virus replicates in the cytoplasm, six messenger RNAs being produced by a discontinuous transcription mechanism that can generate recombinants (110). Virion formation occurs by a budding process at the membranes of the endoplasmic reticulum, not at the cell surface. Although the S protein can migrate through the reticulum to the cell surface (152), the M protein cannot. The virions accumulate in smooth vesicles, but the mechanism of their release from the cell is unknown. New virus starts to appear 3–4 hr after infection, with maximum output per cell being reached within 12 hr at 37 C.

Resistance to Chemical and Physical Agents

THERMOSTABILITY. Most strains of IBV are inactivated after 15 min at 56 C and after 90 min at 45 C (128). Storage of IBV at -20 C should be avoided, but infectious allantoic fluid has remained viable after storage at -30 C for many years. Infected tissues stored in 50% glycerol are well preserved, and tissues in this medium can be shipped to a laboratory for diagnosis without refrigeration (79). Outdoors, survival up to 12 days in spring and 56 days in winter has been reported.

LYOPHILIZATION. Infectious allantoic fluid lyophilized, sealed under vacuum and stored in a refrigerator, has remained viable for at least 30 yr. Ten percent glucose gives a stabilizing effect to IBV in the lyophilized and frozen states (79).

pH STABILITY. Strain variation with respect to stability at pH 3 has been reported (37, 128). In one survey, the reduction in titer following a pH 3 treatment at room temperature for 4 hr varied from 1–2 $\log_{10}$, for most isolates, to 5 $\log_{10}$ for others (37). Infectious bronchitis virus in cell culture was more stable in medium at pH 6.0 and 6.5 than at pH 7.0 to 8.0 (2).

CHEMICAL AGENTS. Infectious bronchitis virus is ether-labile, but some virus survived 20% ether (4 C, 18 hr). All infectivity was destroyed by 50% chloroform (room temperature, 10 min) and 0.1% sodium deoxycholate (4 C, 18 hr) (128). Infectious bronchitis virus is considered to be sensitive to the common disinfectants. Several have been compared for activity against another coronavirus, transmissible gastroenteritis virus of swine (12). Treatment with a final concentration of 0.05 (30) or 0.1% beta-propiolactone (BPL) or 0.1% formalin (98) eliminated IBV infectivity. Only the BPL treatment had no adverse effect on IBV hemagglutination antigen activity.

Strain Classification. Strain classification of IBV is based on features of the S protein. Traditionally, this has focused on VN tests, VN antibody being induced by the S protein. Recent years, however, have seen an increasing use of monoclonal antibodies against S, and analysis of the S gene by sequencing and restriction fragment analysis of DNA copies of the S gene. There is evidence that IBV can undergo recombination during mixed infection (21, 89, 106, 157). This must be taken into account when strains are being classified into groups.

SERUM ANTIBODY ANALYSIS. In the 1960s and 1970s, several serotypes distinct from the well-known Mass serotype were described in the United States (82, 90) and Australia (44, 45, 46). Since then, extensive surveys in The Netherlands (57) and the United Kingdom (28, 29) have revealed many new serotypes of IBV. Virus neutralizing has been performed with chicken tracheal organ cultures (TOCs) (28, 29, 54, 90), chicken kidney (CK) cells using plaque reduction (82), and chicken embryos (57).

Strain classification by HI tests has also been investigated. The HI antibody response following a single exposure and resulting infection can be highly strain specific, even differentiating the Holland from the M41 strains of the same (Mass) serotype (13, 100, 101). The specificity of the early response and the limited cross reactivity are the basis for a procedure for serotyping isolates by HI (101). In contrast, Cook et al. (31) compared the HI test with the VN test in TOCs and concluded that the HI test was subject to high and variable cross-reactions and that IBV strains were more clearly differentiated by the VN test. The reason for the reported differences in cross reactivity is unknown. Both studies based the evaluations on the results from primary sera, since it is known that secondary sera are much more broadly reactive (13, 68).

MONOCLONAL ANTIBODY ANALYSIS. Monoclonal antibodies have been developed against several serotypes of North American origin, including Massachusetts, Connecticut 46, Arkansas 99, Iowa 97 and Gray (94, 97, 104, 132, 155), European isolates of the D274 and D1466 groups (94, 104), and Australian isolates (86). Serotype-specific VN monoclonal antibodies have been used to assign new North American field isolates to one or another classic serotype (97, 126). Many of the anti-D274 monoclonal antibodies are specific for strains known to be closely related on the basis of S1 sequence, and the antibody panel has been used to examine IB outbreaks in The Netherlands. Antigenic groups of Australian isolates defined by monoclonal antibodies correlated better with in vivo cross-protection data than groups defined by antisera (86). The use of monoclonal antibodies to identify isolates is discussed further under Diagnosis.

NUCLEIC ACID ANALYSIS. The S1 gene sequence has been obtained for over 20 isolates of IBV (20, 21, 22, 89; see also 158). Comparison of the deduced S1 amino acid sequences has revealed that many of the serotypes defined by VN tests commonly differ by about 20 to 25%, and occasionally, by as much as 48%; there are, however, exceptions. For example, the Connecticut 46 and Massachusetts 41 strains are in different serotypes, yet their S1 proteins differ by only 7.6% of amino acids (4.6% of nucleotides). Similarly, several isolates which had >97% identity with Dutch isolate D274 were defined in serum VN tests as belonging to different serotypes (22). These findings, and the sequencing of VN-monoclonal-antibody–escape mutants (94), suggest that only a few S1 epitopes induce the major VN antibodies and that a few mutations in these epitopes might result in change to a new serotype. Relationships established by more than one research group using VN tests do not always agree either with each other or with sequence analysis. For example, Johnson and Marquardt (90) considered that Arkansas 99 and Connecticut 46 were different serotypes, consistent with the finding that they differ by 29% in the first 200 S1 residues, whereas Hopkins (82) placed them in the same serotype. Experiments suggest that the degree of cross-protection between strains decreases as the differences between their S1 sequences increase. Nucleic acid analyses are certain to become more useful in IBV strain classification in the future.

Sequencing of genes downstream from the S gene has revealed that some strains have nearly identical downstream genes but extremely different (e.g., 48%) S genes and vice versa. This indicates that some strains have evolved by recombination during mixed infection (21, 89, 107, 157, 158). Thus, it must not be assumed that if two isolates have very similar S proteins, deduced by whatever technique, that they are necessarily very similar in all other genes. Additional aspects of nucleic acid analysis are discussed under Diagnosis.

Laboratory Host Systems

CHICKEN EMBRYOS. Infectious bronchitis virus grows well in the developing chicken embryo. Dwarfing of a few embryos with survival of 90% through the 19th day of incubation is characteristic of IBV field material upon initial inoculation in 10- to 11-day-old embryonated chicken eggs. Embryo mortality and dwarfing increase as the number of serial passages increases, so that by the 10th passage most of the embryos are stunted, and up to 80% may die by the 20th day of incubation.

Characteristic embryo changes are seen several days after inoculation of the virus. Only slight movement of a dwarfed embryo may be observed during candling. Upon opening the air cell end of the egg, the embryo is seen curled into a spherical form with feet deformed and compressed over the head and with the thickened amnion adhered to it (Fig. 18.2).

The yolk sac appears shrunken, and the membrane ruptures easily. An increased volume of usually clear allantoic fluid is present. A consistent internal lesion of the IB-infected embryo is the persistence of the mesonephros containing urates. This lesion appears to be associated with the stunting of the embryo and is not specific for IB infection. Another lesion found in embryonated eggs inoculated with nonlethal isolates of IBV is the thickened amnion and adjacent layer of the allantois covering the stunted embryo. Evidence of this lesion can usually be detected on the 3rd day after inoculation. It likewise is not a pathognomonic lesion, since it can also be observed following inoculation of eggs with lentogenic strains of Newcastle disease virus (NDV) (79).

Microscopic lesions in the embryo infected with IBV-M41 strain have been studied by Loomis et al. (115). They found congestion with perivascular cuffing and some necrosis of the livers by the 6th day after inoculation. All lungs were pneumonic, characterized by congestion, cellular infiltration,

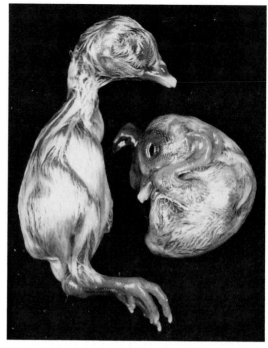

18.2. Comparison of normal 16-day-old embryo (*left*) and curled, dwarfed, infected embryo of the same age (*right*).

and serous exudate in the bronchial sacs. In the kidneys, there was interstitial nephritis with edema and distension of the proximal convoluted tubules with casts. Glomeruli were not altered. The chorioallantoic membrane (CAM) and amniotic membrane were edematous. No inclusion bodies were found.

Optimum age of embryo, temperature, and length of incubation for maximum infectivity titer of IBV-Beaudette following allantoic cavity inoculation have been thoroughly studied and reviewed (92). Following inoculation of approximately 10^7 EID$_{50}$, similar peak titers in allantoic fluid (AF) of embryos inoculated at 10–11 days old were achieved after 12 hr and 24 hr at 37 C and 32 C, respectively. Virus titers of chorioallantoic membranes were higher than those of AFs. Virus-induced embryo death was first observed at 24 hr and 48 hr after incubation at 37 C and 32 C, respectively. Incubation at 42 C resulted in earlier mortality (12 hr) and lower titers. In a different study, a less egg-adapted strain (20–30 embryo passages) attained maximum titers after 24–30 hr at 37 C, irrespective of the inoculum dose (77). In general, inocula of about 10^3 tracheal organ culture infectious doses or 10^4 EID$_{50}$ should give near maximum titers by 36–40 hr at 37 C. Turkey embryos are not normally used for IBV propagation; however, there is evidence that some strains of IBV (Beaudette and M41) have been adapted to grow in turkey embryos (61).

CELL CULTURES. When monolayer cell cultures have been required for IBV studies, chick embryo kidney (CEK) cells and CK cells have been used most successfully. Adaptation of IBV to CEK cells has been examined and reviewed by Gillette (71). The number of passages in CEK required to produce extensive cytopathic effect (CPE), evident in unstained cultures, and maximum titers varied among strains, although plaques, revealed by staining, could be seen after the first passage. Adaptation of some strains to CEK is facilitated by embryo passage. Plaque size and morphology vary among strains; plaque size of most strains was greater at 40 C than at 37 C (71).

The lag phase of IBV in CEK or CK cells is 3–4 hr (53, 117), with maximum titers in the culture medium being at 14–36 hr, depending on the multiplicity of infection (53, 117, 129). Chick embryo liver (CEL) cells produced titers of IBV similar to those from CEK cells (117). Titration of IBV in embryonated eggs gave higher titers (10- to 100-fold) than in CEK or CK cells (53, 117), which in turn were more sensitive than CEL cells (117). Maximum titers of IBV-Beaudette from CK cells were similar over the pH range of 6–9. Virus was released more quickly, but was also inactivated more rapidly, with increasing pH (2). The optimum pH for maximum production of stable virus was pH 6.5.

Infectious bronchitis virus strains that had been passaged in embryos and many times in CK cells replicated in chicken embryo fibroblast cultures, but to titers several $\log_{10}$ less than in CK cells (129). Plaques formed when trypsin was in the culture medium (127). IBV-Beaudette can grow, albeit poorly, in a number of primary kidney and embryo-kidney cultures from various avian and mammalian species (34, 35). IBV-Beaudette (48) and the M41 and Iowa 97 strains (36) have been adapted to the mammalian Vero cell line. Of 10 strains examined, two and none replicated in BHK-21 and HeLa cells, respectively (129).

Chicken kidney cells began to form syncytia 6 hr after inoculation with IBV-Beaudette (2). After 18–24 hr, syncytia contained 20–40 or more nuclei and became vacuolated. The nuclei were pycnotic. Syncytia in CK cultures quickly round up and detach from the substrate, but syncytia in Vero cells infected with Vero cell–adapted IBV-Beaudette contain scores of nuclei and remain on the substrates longer (112).

ORGAN CULTURES. The propagation of IBV in organ cultures of trachea and other tissues has been reviewed by Darbyshire (49). Tracheal rings are prepared from 20-day-old embryos and maintained singly in roller tubes. Following infection with IBV, ciliostasis, easily observed by low-power microscopy, occurs within 3–4 days. Tracheal organ cultures have proved very successful for the isolation, titration, and serotyping of IBV (28, 29) because no adaptation of field strains is required for growth and induction of ciliostasis.

Pathogenicity. Infectious bronchitis virus can replicate in tissues of the respiratory tract, intestinal tract, kidneys, and the oviduct (5, 91, 96, 116). Commonly, IBV isolates, regardless of tissue of origin, readily infect the respiratory tract of chickens and produce characteristic lesions in the trachea. At least one nephropathogenic IBV strain (Australian T strain), however, has been shown to elicit little inflammatory response in the respiratory tract of young chickens (65). In many cases, there is an unremarkable recovery unless the chickens are very young, airsacculitis develops because of a secondary bacterial infection, or kidney disease follows the respiratory phase. Virulent strains of IBV, however, may emerge in the field to induce severe respiratory disease with mortality, e.g., the Delaware 072 strain, which infected broiler flocks in the Northeastern region of the United States in the early 1990s (139). Cumming (45) enumerated some of the management factors that contribute to IB-related kidney disease in Australia. Greater mortality was seen in males, where there was cold stress, in certain breeds, and/or where animal products were the major component of high protein diets. Some of these factors known to exacerbate the clinical disease have been used in experimental models to evaluate the clinical outcome of interaction between such factors and different IBV strains. Chickens fed increased levels of dietary calcium followed by infection with the Gray strain (a nephropathogenic IBV) frequently developed urolithiasis and kidney lesions, but a similar infection introduced 8 wk prior to feeding increased levels of calcium did not induce urolithiasis (72). A combination of cold stress plus *Mycoplasma synoviae* exposure 5 days after an IBV exposure (84) produces an airsacculitis that varies in incidence and severity with the virulence of the IBV strain. A combined intranasal inoculation of different IBV strains and *Escherichia coli* (30) produced mortality in young chickens; neither infection alone was lethal. Mortality ranged from 14 to 82%, with different strains demonstrating that they did differ in virulence.

Other differences in virulence of IBV strains have been noted. Passage of IBV in chicken embryos gradually results in a decrease in virulence. The highly egg-adapted Beaudette strain is apathogenic, causes no detectable damage to the ciliated epithelium of the trachea and replicates predominantly in the subepithelial cells. The immunogenicity of the strain is diminished as well (66). In contrast, the virulent M41 strain destroyed the ciliated epithelium prior to localization in the subepithelium. The Australian T strain is virulent and a known cause of mortality and kidney lesions (1). Viruses of other serotypes that are also known to be nephropathogenic, but of less severity than T strain, include the United States strains Gray and Holte (1), the Mass-Holland 52 strain (119), and the Belgian B1648 isolate (111, 133).

Virulence for the reproductive tract may also differ among IBV strains. Different IBV strains can produce a range of effects in susceptible layers varying from shell pigment changes with no production drop (29) to production drops of 10 to 50% (83). Since the winter of 1990–91, unusual pathology has been observed in the United Kingdom, coincident with the occurrence of infection by a new serotype (793/B) of IBV (74). Broiler breeders exhibited pale and swollen deep pectoral muscle with occasional fascial haemorrhages and a layer of gelatinous edema over the surface of the muscle. Bilateral myopathy affected both deep and superficial pectoral muscles.

PATHOGENESIS AND EPIZOOTIOLOGY

Natural and Experimental Hosts. Although susceptibility to disease varies among breeds or strains of chickens (45, 144), it is generally considered that the chicken is the only bird that is naturally infected by IBV and in which the virus causes disease. Infectious bronchitis virus has been isolated from pheasants, however, in which breeding birds had respiratory signs and an associated depression in egg production and quality, and young birds had considerable respiratory distress (145). The source of the virus was probably a nearby chicken laying unit.

Experimental inoculation of turkeys with IBV by aerosol produced no response, but intravenous inoculation may produce a viremia for varying periods up to 48 hr (79). Ring-neck pheasants and starlings were resistant to intratracheal inoculation with IBV. Bronchial rales were detected in quail inoculated similarly, but no virus was isolated or seroconversion detected (4). Suckling mice are susceptible by intracerebral inoculation to several, but not all, IBV strains (64). The limited host range is not unusual because coronaviruses typically cause clinical disease only in the species from which they are isolated, and they replicate predominantly in cultures derived from that host (159).

AGE OF HOST COMMONLY AFFECTED. All ages are susceptible, but the disease is most severe in baby chicks, causing some mortality (79). As age increases, chickens become more resistant to the nephritogenic effects, oviduct lesions, and mortality due to infection (1, 41, 144).

Transmission, Carriers, Vectors. Infectious bronchitis virus spreads rapidly among chickens in a flock. Susceptible birds placed in a room with infected chickens usually develop signs within 48 hr (47). Virus was isolated consistently from the trachea, lungs, kidneys, and bursae of chickens at 24 hr and through the 7th day after aerosol exposure (80). The frequency of virus isolations declined with time and varied with the infecting strain, but IBV was isolated from the cecal tonsils at 14 wk and from feces 20 wk postinfection (3). Reexcretion of IBV has also been detected from hens that had been virus-negative for several weeks following recovery from inoculation at 1 day of age. Virus was isolated from tracheal and cloacal swabs collected at the point of lay, 19 wk of age (91). While there are reports of virus isolations from eggs up to 43 days after recovery, chickens have been hatched from infected flocks and reared free of IBV (47). The nature of the persistence of IBV infection remains undefined, but reports of extended and intermittent shedding are evidence of the potential risk of flock-to-flock transmission via contamination of personnel or equipment.

The frequency of airborne spread between flocks is unknown, but circumstantial evidence of transmission of IBV over a distance of 1200 yards was reported (46). Vectors do not appear to be a factor in the spread of IBV (79).

Incubation Period. The incubation period of IB is 18–36 hr, depending on dose and route of inoculation. Chickens exposed to an aerosol of undiluted infective egg fluid regularly have tracheal rales within 24 hr. Naturally occurring spread requires about 36 hr or more (79).

Signs. The characteristic respiratory signs of IB in chicks are gasping, coughing, sneezing, tracheal rales, and nasal discharge. Wet eyes may be observed and an occasional chick may have swollen sinuses. The chicks appear depressed, may be seen huddled under a heat source, and feed consumption and weight gain are significantly reduced. In chickens over 6 wk of age and in adult birds, the signs are similar to those in chicks, but nasal discharge does not occur as frequently and the disease may go unnoticed unless the flock is examined carefully by handling the birds or listening to them at night when the birds are normally quiet (47, 79). Some of the field isolates of IBV recovered in the United States and United Kingdom in the early 1990s were unusually pathogenic and produced severe facial swelling, airsacculitis, and varying mortality in semimature and mature chickens (74, 139).

Broiler chickens infected with one of the nephropathic viruses may appear to recover from the typical respiratory phase and then show signs of depression, ruffled feathers, wet droppings, and increased water intake (45, 160). When urolithiasis is associated with IB in layer flocks, there may be increased mortality, but otherwise the flock appears healthy (14, 38).

In laying flocks, declines in egg production and quality are seen in addition to respiratory signs. Infectious bronchitis virus, however, has been isolated from cloacal swabs or cecal tonsil samples from breeder or layer flocks with slight production drops and the production of pale shell eggs, but no respiratory signs (28, 29). The severity of the production declines may vary with the period of lay (62) and with the causative virus strain (29, 83). Six to 8 wk may elapse before production returns to the preinfection level, but in most cases this is never attained (47). In addition to production declines, the number of eggs unacceptable for setting is increased, hatchability is reduced, and soft-shelled, misshapen, and rough-shelled eggs are produced (Fig. 18.3).

Internal quality of eggs, as observed when breaking eggs on a flat surface, may be inferior. The albumen may be thin and watery without definite demarcation between the thick and thin albumen of the normal fresh egg (79) (Fig. 18.4).

Infectious bronchitis virus infection of 1-day-old chicks can produce permanent damage leading to reduced egg production and quality when the chickens come into lay. The severity of oviduct lesions was less in infections of older chickens, and some serotypes failed to produce any pathologic change even in infections of 1-day-old chicks (40, 41, 91).

Morbidity and Mortality. All birds in the flock become infected, but mortality is variable depending on: virulence of the infecting serotype; age; status of immunity, either maternal or active; and stresses such as cold or secondary bacterial infections. Moderate to severe mortality has been noted with some of the respiratory and nephropathogenic strains, such as Delaware 072 and Australian T strain, respectively. Sex, breed, and nutrition are additional factors that contribute to the severity of kidney disease (45). Mortality may be as high as 25% or more in chickens less than 6 wk of age and is usually negligible in chickens over that age (79). Mortality in urolithiasis cases ranged from 0.5 to 1.0% per week (14, 38).

Gross Lesions. Infected chickens have serous, catarrhal, or caseous exudate in the trachea, nasal passages, and sinuses. Air sacs may appear cloudy or contain a yellow caseous exudate. A caseous plug may be found in the lower trachea or bronchi of chicks that die. Small areas of pneumonia may be observed around the large bronchi (79). Nephropathic infections produce swollen and pale kidneys with the tubules and ureters often distended with urates (44, 160) (Fig. 18.5).

Fluid yolk material may be found in the abdominal cavity of chickens that are in production, but this is also seen with other diseases that cause a marked drop in egg production. Permanent lesions in the oviduct may be a consequence of IBV infection of 1-day-old chicks and are a cause of reduced egg production. The middle third of the oviduct is most severely affected and may be nonpatent and hypoglandular (42, 79).

Histopathology. The mucosa of the trachea of chickens with IB is edematous. There is a loss of cilia, rounding and sloughing of epithelial cells, and minor infiltration of heterophils and lymphocytes within 18 hr of infection. Regeneration of the epithelium starts within 48 hr. Hyperplasia is followed by massive infiltration of the lamina propria by

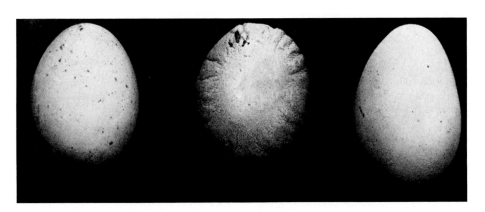

18.3. Thin-shelled, rough, and misshapen eggs laid by hens during an outbreak of IB. (Van Roekel)

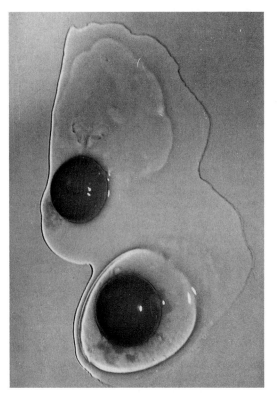

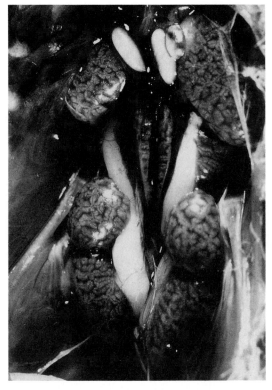

18.4. Contents of two eggs. Normal egg (*bottom*). Egg from chicken exposed to IBV at one day of age (*top*). Note watery albumen with yolk separated from thick albumen. (Hofstad)

18.5. Kidney lesions associated with IB caused by T strain of virus. Note swollen kidneys with tubules and ureters distended with urates. (Cumming)

lymphoid cells and a large number of germinal centers, which may be present after 7 days. If air sac involvement occurs there is edema, epithelial cell desquamation, and some fibrinous exudate within 24 hr. Increased heterophils can be observed later with lymphoid nodules, fibroblast proliferation, and cuboidal epithelial regeneration (137).

The kidney lesions of IB are principally those of an interstitial nephritis. The virus causes granular degeneration, vacuolation and desquamation of the tubular epithelium, and massive infiltration of heterophils in the interstitium in acute stages of the disease. The lesions in tubules are most prominent in the medulla. Focal areas of necrosis may be seen as well as indications of attempted regeneration of the tubular epithelium. During recovery, the inflammatory cell population changes to lymphocytes and plasma cells. In some cases, degenerative changes may persist and result in severe atrophy of one or all of the divisions of the kidneys. In urolithiasis, the ureters associated with atrophied kidneys are distended with urates and often contain large calculi composed mainly of urates (137).

Experimental IB infection of mature hens resulted in decreased height and loss of cilia from ep-ithelial cells, dilation of the tubular glands, infiltration by lymphocytes, mononuclear cells, plasma cells, and heterophils, and edema and fibroplasia of the lamina propria of all regions of the oviduct (137). The histopathology of IB and comparisons with other diseases are given in detail in a book by Riddell (137) and a review of renal pathology by Siller (143).

Immunity

ACTIVE. Both breed- and strain-related genetic resistance to IBV infection has been described in chickens (15, 33, 131, 144). More investigations, however, are warranted to assess the genetic resistance of commercial lines of chickens. Chickens just recovered from the natural disease are resistant to challenge with the same virus (homologous protection), but the extent of protection to challenge with other IBV strains (heterologous protection) varies. Factors that complicate studies of the mechanism and duration of immunity to IB are the multiple serotypes that are recognized (28, 82, 90, 105, 154), the variation in virulence observed among strains (see Pathogenicity), and the different manifestations of IBV infection for which protection may be needed (see Signs).

Respiratory protection is usually evaluated 3–4 wk after an IB infection or immunization, and has been done in several different ways. In most cases, an IBV challenge is given by a respiratory route. The failure to recover IBV from the trachea at 4 to 5 days postchallenge has been used as a single criterion of immunity (78). More comprehensive evaluations have included two or more additional criteria of resistance to challenge including the failure to isolate virus from the kidney and oviduct, no clinical signs of IB, no tracheal lesions, or the presence of tracheal ciliary activity (6, 51, 161). Accumulating scores from the different criteria are used to indicate the range of protection from full to partial or none. An alternative approach is an evaluation of vaccinated chickens for protection against mortality from a challenge with a mixture of IBV and *E. coli*. This method showed evidence of more vaccinal cross protection than found with other assessments of tracheal immunity (30).

Protection against mortality from nephritis is important as evidence of satisfactory vaccinal immunity where nephritis is a major clinical problem, as in Australia (102, 136). The ability to reduce or prevent egg-production declines from a challenge infection is evidence of IB protection in a laying flock (11).

Although there is evidence that the S1 glycopolypeptide is primarily responsible for the induction of VN and HI antibody, and that it plays a major role in the induction of protective immunity (85), the knowledge of the mechanism of protection against clinical disease is incomplete. The local synthesis of neutralizing antibody into nasal secretions might prevent reinfection (81), and there is evidence for a contribution by the Harderian gland in the local response (55). The protective role of antibody is also evident by the fact that chickens immunocompromised by infectious bursal disease virus infection suffer more severe episodes of IBV infection than their immunocompetent counterparts (138, 148). Antibody does not appear to be the only source of resistance, however, as demonstrated in chickens treated with cyclophosphamide, or bursectomized in ovo and then exposed to IBV (24, 32). In those trials, no antibody could be detected, but the chickens resisted IBV challenge. Evidence of cell-mediated immune responses to IBV are lymphocyte transformation assays of live and inactivated virus vaccinates (150, 151), cytotoxic lymphocyte activity (26), delayed type hypersensitivity (27), natural killer cell activity (148), and histologic evidence for significant T-cell (especially CD4+ phenotype) infiltration in the respiratory and kidney tissues of IBV-infected chickens (88). However, the role of these responses in immunity to IBV is not known.

Interferon induction by IBV varies with the virus strain; however, there is no known role of interferon in resistance to IB (130). Immunity to IB and to other poultry diseases has been reviewed (134).

PASSIVE. Maternal antibody can reduce both the severity of vaccinal reaction and the efficacy of the vaccine if the vaccine is of the same type used in the breeder flock immunization (102, 103). Despite this, vaccination of maternally immune 1-day-old commercial chicks is routinely performed without apparent interference by the maternal antibody in the development of active immunity, at least in the respiratory tract. Maternal antibody provided protection against challenge at 1 day and 1 wk, but not at 2 wk of age (124).

DIAGNOSIS. Diagnosis of IBV is based on the clinical history, lesions, seroconversion or rising IBV antibody titers, IBV antigen detection by a number of antibody-based assays (described below), virus isolation, and, more recently, by detection of IBV RNA. The IBV serotype should be identified, if possible, because of the great antigenic variation exhibited by IBV strains and the availability of vaccines designed for different serotypes. Sequencing of the spike protein gene, i.e., genotyping, can also be applied for the same purpose.

Isolation and Identification of the Causative Agent

VIRUS ISOLATION. The trachea is a primary target for IBV and, therefore, is a preferred sampling site. Cecal tonsils collected during postmortem examination, however, can be of particular value in cases in which more than 1 wk may have elapsed since the start of infection. This is because the virus is generally cleared from the trachea sooner than from the intestinal tissues. Samples from the lungs, kidneys, and oviduct should also be considered depending on the clinical history of the disease. Sample selection from extremely large flocks can be a difficult problem. The placement of susceptible sentinel chickens in a problem flock has been successful when direct sampling methods in the flock had failed (69). Sentinels are removed for direct sampling after 1 wk of contact exposure. Procedures for sample collection and processing for IBV isolation have been described in detail (67).

Samples for virus isolation are inoculated into embryonated chicken eggs or tracheal organ cultures. Fluids should be harvested after 48–72 hr from either culture system for blind passage into another set of cultures. Each sample should receive at least four blind passages before being called negative based on failure to cause typical embryo death or lesions or ciliostasis in the organ cultures. Inoculation of susceptible chicks intratracheally with the original samples or first-passage culture fluids will produce typical respiratory signs in 18–36 hr, if IBV is present. No further inoculations are given. Antiserum collected at 4 wk postinoculation should be suitable for use in two-way comparisons to determine the serotype of the isolate.

Isolates from positive cultures should have characteristics typical of a coronavirus as visualized by electron microscopy or determined by other procedures as described below.

CONFIRMATION OF INFECTIOUS BRONCHITIS VIRUS BY ANTIBODY-BASED METHODS. Sections or scrapings of the trachea mucosa and other tissues taken from birds at postmortem can be examined by immunofluorescence or immunoperoxidase assays (25, 67, 76, 125, 162). Since the amount of IBV antigen in infected chicken embryos can sometimes be low, however, sections of the CAM or cells sedimented from the allantoic fluid can be used for immunofluorescence or immunoperoxidase assays (125, 162). Infectious bronchitis virus in allantoic fluid may also be detected and identified as to serotype using monoclonal antibodies in indirect or antigen-capture enzyme-linked immunosorbent assay (ELISA) (94, 97, 104, 126). Serotypic classification of isolates should be done as described under Strain Classification and Diagnosis. This requires that type-specific antisera should be available in the diagnostic laboratory to determine if the isolate is similar to, or different from, any vaccine strains used in the infected flock. The details of identification of IBV isolates from respiratory and egg-production problems (28), urolithiasis (39), and nephritis (118, 122) are described.

CONFIRMATION OF INFECTIOUS BRONCHITIS VIRUS BY NUCLEIC ACID-BASED METHODS. Infectious bronchitis virus RNA has been detected in infected tissues using the reverse-transcriptase/polymerase chain reaction (RT/PCR) method. The RNA can be extracted from tracheal swabs or tissues of live chickens. It is not necessary to have viable IBV on the swabs or in the tissues. The sensitivity of the RT/PCR permitted detection of the virus up to 14 days after experimental infection when it would have been difficult to recover viable virus(108). The presence of IBV in infectious allantoic fluid can be confirmed by extracting RNA directly from a few hundred μL and using some of the RNA in a RT/PCR reaction. The DNA product is visualized by ethidium bromide staining after electrophoresis in agarose or polyacrylamide gels. Universal oligonucleotide primer sets (those that function with a wide range of IBV isolates) corresponding to nucleotide sequences in the S1 gene (109), S2 gene (113, 114), and nucleocapsid gene

(163) have been described. Another oligonucleotide set produced a product from parts of the N and M genes (7, 87).

In addition to demonstrating the presence of IBV, the DNA product can be sequenced or examined by restriction fragment analysis to characterize the strain of IBV (109, 113, 114). Restriction fragment sites believed to be unique to a given serotype permit rapid strain identification, although sequencing is the most accurate, if more demanding, approach.

Serology. Serum antibody assays are routinely used to monitor the vaccinal response and to detect antibody titer increases attributable to field infection. The multiple IBV serotypes and the antigenic variation noted within the described types add complexity to the selection of an appropriate serologic method and the analysis of test results. Antibody is produced to IBV antigens shared by all types, the group-specific antigens, and to the S1 glycopolypeptide, the type-specific antigen. The ELISA, immunofluorescence, or immunodiffusion tests bind antibody to group- as well as type-specific antigens. Because of this dual binding characteristic, IBV types are not differentiated with these tests. Most of the primary antibody response to IBV infection appears to be type specific and functions to differentiate types by VN or HI, which is similar to that reported for another coronavirus (120). As noted in the section on strain classification, however, the secondary response to IBV is more broadly reactive even in VN and HI. Evidence of a broadly reactive serum in those two tests is an extensive reaction to more than one VN or HI antigen. Identification of the infecting strain cannot be determined by serology when such cross reactivity exists, and in such a case, the differentiating capability of a VN or HI test is no better than a group reactive assay.

Routine serology is usually done with either VN, HI, or ELISA. Reviews of the methodologies for several serologic procedures are available (47, 50, 79). Virus-neutralizing tests are done with either a decreasing-virus, constant-serum or constant-virus, decreasing-serum method using embryonated eggs, tracheal organ cultures, or cell culture as the virus assay system. Different HI procedures have been used. A range of 4 to 8 hemagglutination (HA) units antigen in serial dilutions of serum has been used, and the results from the different procedures were compared (99). The treatment of IBV to produce a good HA antigen has recently been reexamined (141). Antibody is detected earlier by HI than VN (73). Optimally, postvaccination serology by VN or HI should be conducted with test antigens homologous with each of the vaccine antigens employed in a flock. The ELISA method is used widely, and kits for conducting the procedure are commercially available. Antibody response can be detected earlier by ELISA than by VN (121). The procedures for immunofluorescence have been either direct (43) or indirect (25, 43). Antibodies detected by the immunodiffusion method have been found to be transient and the method has given variable results (73).

A monoclonal antibody–based blocking or competition ELISA has recently been described for the detection of antibodies to North American serotypes Massachusetts and Arkansas in the sera of experimentally inoculated chickens (95). Chicken serum containing IBV antibodies is added to virus-coated microtiter plates followed by serotype-specific monoclonal antibody. Chicken antibody specific to an IBV serotype blocks binding of monoclonal antibody specific to the same serotype, and the blocking is proportional to the concentration of antibody in chicken serum. Specificity of the blocking ELISA compared well with that of the VN test.

Differential Diagnosis. Infectious bronchitis may resemble other acute respiratory diseases such as Newcastle disease (ND), laryngotracheitis (LT), and infectious coryza (IC). Newcastle disease is generally more severe than IB. Nervous signs may be observed with virulent strains of ND, and in laying flocks, drops in production may be greater than with IB. Laryngotracheitis tends to spread more slowly in a flock, but respiratory signs may be more severe than with IB. Infectious coryza can be differentiated on the basis of facial swelling that only rarely occurs in IB. Production declines and shell quality problems in flocks infected with the egg drop syndrome (EDS) adenovirus are similar to those seen with IB, except that internal egg quality is not affected in the case of EDS (62).

TREATMENT. There is no specific treatment for IB. Provision of additional heat to eliminate cold stress, elimination of overcrowding, and attempts to maintain feed consumption to prevent weight loss are flock management factors that may help reduce losses from IB. Treatment with appropriate antibacterials may be indicated to aid in reducing the losses from airsacculitis. Electrolyte replacers, supplied in the drinking water, are recommended and were used in Australia to compensate for the acute loss of sodium and potassium, and to thereby reduce losses from nephritis. The recommended concentration for treatment is 72 mEq of sodium and/or potassium, with at least one-third in the citrate or bicarbonate salt form (45).

PREVENTION AND CONTROL

Management Procedures. Ideal management includes strict isolation and repopulation with only day-old chicks, following the cleaning and disinfection of the poultry house. Airborne diseases can be prevented by ventilating houses with filtered air under positive pressure (60). Current production methods, which include multiple ages in a house or multiple ages on a farm in a high-density poultry area, make control more difficult and have necessitated the use of immunization to attempt to prevent production losses due to IB. Immunization is also used in isolated single-age laying flocks to prevent the heavy production losses that may result from an IBV infection of a susceptible flock during the laying cycle.

Immunization

TYPES OF VACCINE. Both live and inactivated virus vaccines are used in IB immunization. Live vaccines are used in broilers and for the initial vaccination of breeders and layers. Inactivated oil-emulsion vaccines (11, 147) are used primarily at point of lay in breeders and layers. Infectious bronchitis virus strains used for live vaccines are frequently attenuated by serial passage in embryonated chicken eggs (see Pathogenicity) (102). Extensive passage is avoided to prevent a reduction in immunogenicity as well. The degree and stability of such attenuation probably varies among vaccines. Evidence that some vaccines increased in virulence after back-passage in chickens (84) demonstrates the potential for enhancement of virulence of such vaccines by a cyclic infection in a flock.

Vaccine strains are selected to represent the antigenic spectrum of isolates in a particular country or region. The Massachusetts (M41) strain is used widely because initial isolates from many countries are of that serotype. New types are subsequently included when the prevalence of the new type is established. In the United States, M41, Holland, and Connecticut types are used widely, and other serotypes such as Florida, Arkansas, and JMK are used regionally with special license. In The Netherlands, strains Holland, D274, and D1466 are used; in Australia, strains of their B and C subtypes are used (102, 154).

APPLICATION METHODS. Live vaccine combinations of IBV with NDV are used frequently. If the IBV component is in excess, there may be an interference with the NDV response (75, 149). No similar interference with the IBV response has been reported.

Administration of live vaccine can be individually by eye drop, intratracheal (6), or intranasal. An embryonal injection method has also been used experimentally (156). Mass application methods include coarse spray (6, 56), aerosol, and drinking water (135). Mass administration methods are popular because of convenience, but problems in attaining uniform vaccine application can occur and the aerosol method may cause more severe respiratory reactions. Vaccines applied by the drinking water method are susceptible to inactivation by sanitizers added to control bacterial and fungal contamination of the watering system. Removal of those sanitizers prior to vaccination and the incorporation of powdered skim milk at a 1:400 concentration has been shown to stabilize the virus titer during vaccine administration (70).

Inactivated vaccines require injection of individual birds. These vaccines are usually given after "priming" with live virus and are administered a few weeks before production commences. They may be given in combination with other inactivated vaccines.

Two weeks of age is frequently used as the time for initial immunization (52), but vaccine may be successfully administered at 1 day of age (6, 56). Timing of initial immunization varies due to titer of maternal antibody in chicks and vaccination methods used. Schedules of subsequent immunization at 7–12 or 16–18 wk of age and at point of lay vary with flock management and needs for control of IB as well as other flock diseases. In the United States, many commercial egg-type chickens are vaccinated at 8- to 10-wk intervals throughout the laying cycle with M41 virus administered by drinking water or aerosol.

REFERENCES

1. Albassam, M.A., R.W. Winterfield, and H.L. Thacker. 1986. Comparison of the nephropathogenicity of four strains of infectious bronchitis virus. Avian Dis 30:468–476.

2. Alexander, D.J., and M.S. Collins. 1975. Effect of pH on the growth and cytopathogenicity of avian infectious bronchitis virus in chick kidney cells. Arch Virol 49:339–348.

3. Alexander, D.J., and R.E. Gough. 1977. Isolation of avian infectious bronchitis virus from experimentally infected chickens. Res Vet Sci 23:344–347.

4. Allred, J.N., L.G. Raggi, and G.G. Lee. 1973. Susceptibility and resistance of pheasants, starlings, and quail to three respiratory diseases of chickens. Calif Fish Game 59:161–167.

5. Ambali, A.G., and R.C. Jones. 1990. Early pathogenesis in chicks with an enterotropic strain of infectious bronchitis virus. Avian Dis 34:809–817.

6. Andrade, L.F., P. Villegas, and O.J. Fletcher. 1983. Vaccination of day-old broilers against infectious bronchitis: Effect of vaccine strain and route of administration. Avian Dis 27:178–187.

7. Andreasen, J.R., M.W. Jackwood, and D.A. Hilt. 1991. Polymerase chain reaction amplification of the genome of infectious bronchitis virus. Avian Dis 35:216–220.

8. Beach, J.R., and O.W. Schalm. 1936. A filterable virus, distinct from that of laryngotracheitis, the cause of a respiratory disease of chicks. Poult Sci 15:199–206.

9. Beaudette, F.R., and C.B. Hudson. 1937. Cultivation of the virus of infectious bronchitis. J Am Vet Med Assoc 90:51–60.

10. Boursnell, M.E.G., T.D.K. Brown, I.J. Foulds, P.F. Green, F.M. Tomley, and M.M. Binns. 1987. Completion of the sequence of the genome of the coronavirus avian infectious bronchitis virus. J Gen Virol 68:57–77.

11. Box, P.G., H.C. Holmes, P.M. Finney, and R. Froymann. 1988. Infectious bronchitis in laying hens: The relationship between hemagglutination inhibition antibody levels and resistance to experimental challenge. Avian Pathol 17:349–361.

12. Brown, T.T., Jr. 1981. Laboratory evaluation of selected disinfectants as virucidal agents against porcine parvovirus, psuedorabies virus, and transmissible gastroenteritis virus. Am J Vet Res 42:1033–1036.

13. Brown, A.J., and C.D. Bracewell. 1988. Effect of repeated infections of chickens with infectious bronchitis viruses on the specificity of their antibody responses. Vet Rec 122:207–208.

14. Brown, T.P., J.R. Glisson, G. Rosales, P. Villegas, and R.B. Davis. 1987. Studies of avian urolithiasis associated with an infectious bronchitis virus. Avian Dis 31:629–636.

15. Bumstead, N., M.B. Huggins, and J.K.A. Cook. 1989. Genetic differences in susceptibility to a mixture of avian infectious bronchitis virus and Escherichia coli. Br Poult Sci 30:39–48.

16. Cavanagh, D. 1984. Structural characterization of IBV glycoproteins. Adv Exp Med Biol 173:95–108.

17. Cavanagh, D. 1995. Coronaviruses. In A.Z. Zuckerman, J. E. Banatvala and J.R. Pattison (eds.). Principles and Practice of Clinical Virology, 3rd ed. John Wiley and Sons, Chichester, United Kingdom, pp. 325–336.

18. Cavanagh, D., and P.J. Davis. 1987. Coronavirus IBV: Relationships among recent European isolates studied by limited proteolysis of the virion glycopolypeptides. Avian Pathol 16:1–13.

19. Cavanagh, D., and P.J. Davis. 1992. Sequence analysis of strains of avian infectious bronchitis coronavirus isolated during the 1960s in the U.K. Arch Virol 130:471–6.

20. Cavanagh, D., P.J. Davis, and A.P.A. Mockett. 1988. Amino acids within hypervariable region 1 of avian coronavirus IBV (Massachusetts serotype) spike glycoprotein are associated with neutralization epitopes. Virus Res 11:141–150.

21. Cavanagh, D., P.J. Davis, and J.K.A. Cook. 1992. Infectious bronchitis virus: Evidence for recombination within the Massachusetts serotype. Avian Pathol 21:401–408.

22. Cavanagh, D., P.J. Davis, J.K.A. Cook, D. Li, A. Kant, and G. Koch. 1992. Location of the amino acid differences in the S1 spike glycoprotein subunit of closely related serotypes of infectious bronchitis virus. Avian Pathol 21:33–43.

23. Cavanagh, D., D.A. Brian, M.A. Brinton, L. Enjuanes, K.V. Holmes, M.C. Horzinek, M.M.C. Lai, H. Laude, P.G.W. Plagemann, H., S.G. Siddell, W. Spaan, F. Taguchi, and P.J. Talbot. 1994. Revision of the taxonomy of the Coronavirus, Torovirus and Arterivirus genera. Arch Virol 135:227–237.

24. Chubb, R.C. 1974. The effect of the suppression of circulating antibody on resistance to the Australian avian infectious bronchitis virus. Res Vet Sci 17:169–173.

25. Chubb, R.C. 1986. The detection of antibody to avian infectious bronchitis virus by the use of immunofluorescence with tissue sections of nephritic kidneys. Aust Vet J 63:131–132.

26. Chubb, R.C., V. Huynh, and R. Law. 1987. The detection of cytotoxic lymphocyte activity in chickens infected with infectious bronchitis virus or fowl pox virus. Avian Pathol 16:395–405.

27. Chubb, R.C., V. Huynh, and R. Bradley. 1988. The induction and control of delayed type hypersensitivity reactions induced in chickens by infectious bronchitis virus. Avian Pathol 17:371–383.

28. Cook, J.K.A. 1984. The classification of new serotypes of infectious bronchitis virus isolated from poultry flocks in Britain between 1981 and 1983. Avian Pathol 13:733–741.

29. Cook, J.K.A., and M.B. Huggins. 1986. Newly isolated serotypes of infectious bronchitis virus: Their role in disease. Avian Pathol 15:129–138.

30. Cook, J.K.A., H.W. Smith, and M.B. Huggins. 1986. Infectious bronchitis immunity: Its study in chickens experimentally infected with mixtures of infectious bronchitis virus and Escherichia coli. J Gen Virol 67:1427–1434.

31. Cook, J.K.A., A.J. Brown, and C.D. Bracewell. 1987. Comparison of the hemagglutination inhibition test and the serum neutralization test in tracheal organ cultures for typing infectious bronchitis virus strains. Avian Pathol 16:505–511.

32. Cook, J.K.A., T.F. Davidson, M.B. Huggins, and P.I. McLaughlan. 1991. Effect of in ovo bursectomy on the course of an infectious bronchitis virus infection in line C White Leghorn chickens. Arch Virol 118:225–234.

33. Cook, J.K.A., K. Otsuki, N.R. Da Silva Martins, M.M. Ellis, and M. B. Huggins. 1992. The secretory antibody response of inbred lines of chickens to avian infectious bronchitis virus infection. Avian Pathol 21:681–692.

34. Coria, M.F. 1969. Intracellular avian infectious bronchitis virus: Detection by fluorescent antibody techniques in nonovarian kidney cell culture. Avian Dis 13:540–547.

35. Coria, M.F., and J.K. Peterson. 1971. Adaptation and propagation of avian infectious bronchitis virus in embryonic turkey kidney cell cultures. Avian Dis 15:22–27.

36. Coria, M.F., and A.E. Ritchie. 1973. Serial passage of 3 strains of avian infectious bronchitis virus in African Green monkey kidney cells (VERO). Avian Dis 17:697–704.

37. Cowen, B.S., and S.B. Hitchner. 1975. pH stability studies with avian infectious bronchitis virus (Coronavirus) strains. J Virol 15:430–432.

38. Cowen, B.S., R.F. Wideman, H. Rothenbacher, and M.O. Braune. 1987. An outbreak of avian urolithiasis on a large commercial egg farm. Avian Dis 31:392–397.

39. Cowen, B.S., R.F. Wideman, M.O. Braune, and R.L. Owen. 1987. An infectious bronchitis virus isolated from chickens experiencing a urolithiasis outbreak. I. In vitro characterization studies. Avian Dis 31:878–883.

40. Crinion, R.A.P. 1972. Egg quality and production following infectious bronchitis virus exposure at one day old. Poult Sci 51:582–585.

41. Crinion, R.A.P., and M.S. Hofstad. 1972. Pathogenicity of four serotypes of avian infectious bronchitis virus for the oviduct of young chickens of various ages. Avian Dis 16:351–363.

42. Crinion, R.A.P., R.A. Ball, and M.S. Hofstad. 1971. Abnormalities in laying chickens following exposure to infectious bronchitis virus at one day old. Avian Dis 15:42–48.

43. Csermelyi, M., R. Thijssen, F. Orthel, A.G. Burger, B. Kouwenhoven, and D. Lutticken. 1988. Serological classification of recent infectious bronchitis virus isolates by the neutralization of immunofluorescent foci. Avian Pathol 17:139–148.

44. Cumming, R.B. 1963. Infectious avian nephrosis (uraemia) in Australia. Aust Vet J 39:145–147.

45. Cumming, R.B. 1969. The control of avian infectious bronchitis/nephrosis in Australia. Aust Vet J 45:200–203.

46. Cumming, R.B. 1970. Studies on Australian infectious bronchitis virus IV. Apparent farm-to-farm airborne transmission of infectious bronchitis virus. Avian Dis 14:191–195.

47. Cunningham, C.H. 1970. Avian infectious bronchitis. Adv Vet Sci Comp Med 14:105–148.

48. Cunningham, C.H., M.P. Spring, and K. Nazerian. 1972. Replication of avian infectious bronchitis virus in African Green monkey kidney cell line VERO. J Gen Virol 16:423–427.

49. Darbyshire, J.H. 1978. Organ culture in avian virology: A review. Avian Pathol 7:321–335.

50. Darbyshire, J.H. 1980. Immunity to avian infectious bronchitis virus. In M.E. Rose, L.N. Payne, and B.M. Freeman (eds.). Avian Immunology. British Poultry Science, Edinburgh, Scotland, pp. 205–226.

51. Darbyshire, J.H. 1985. A clearance test to assess protection in chickens vaccinated against avian infectious bronchitis virus. Avian Pathol 14:497–508.

52. Darbyshire, J.H., and R.W. Peters. 1985. Humoral antibody response and assessment of protection following primary vaccination of chicks with maternally derived antibody against avian infectious bronchitis virus. Res Vet Sci 38:14–21.

53. Darbyshire, J.H., J.K.A. Cook, and R.W. Peters. 1975. Comparative growth kinetic studies on avian infectious bronchitis virus in different systems. J Comp Pathol 85:623–630.

54. Darbyshire, J.H., J.G. Rowell, J.K.A. Cook, and R.W. Peters. 1979. Taxonomic studies on strains of avian infectious bronchitis virus using neutralization tests in tracheal organ cultures. Arch Virol 61:227–238.

55. Davelaar, F.G., and B. Kouwenhoven. 1976. Changes in the Harderian gland of the chicken following conjunctival and intranasal infection with infectious bronchitis virus in one- and 20-day old chickens. Avian Pathol 5:39–50.

56. Davelaar, F.G., and B. Kouwenhoven. 1980. Vaccination of 1-day-old broilers against infectious bronchitis by eye drop application or coarse droplet spray and the effect of revaccination by spray. Avian Pathol 9:499–510.

57. Davelaar, F.G., B. Kouwenhoven, and A.G. Burger. 1984. Occurrence and significance of infectious bronchitis virus variant strains in egg and broiler production in the Netherlands. Vet Q 6:114–120.

58. Davies, H.A., and M.R. Macnaughton. 1979. Comparison of the morphology of three coronaviruses. Arch Virol 59:25–33.

59. Davies, H.A., R.R. Dourmashkin, and M.R. Macnaughton. 1981. Ribonucleoprotein of avian infectious bronchitis virus. J Gen Virol 53:67–74.

60. Drury, L.N., W.C. Patterson, and C.W. Beard. 1969. Ventilating poultry houses with filtered air under positive pressure to prevent airborne diseases. Poult Sci 48:1640–1646.

61. DuBose, R.T. 1967. Adaptation of the Massachusetts strain of infectious bronchitis virus to turkey embryos. Avian Dis 11:28–38.

62. Eck, J.H.H. van. 1983. Effects of experimental infection of fowl with EDS'76 virus, infectious bronchitis virus, and/or fowl adenovirus on laying performance. Vet Q 5:11–25.

63. Estola, T. 1966. Studies on the infectious bronchitis virus of chickens isolated in Finland with reference to the serological survey of its occurrence. Acta Vet Scand (Suppl) 18:1–111.

64. Estola, T. 1967. Sensitivity of suckling mice to various strains of infectious bronchitis virus. Acta Vet Scand 8:86–87.

65. Fulton, R.M., W.M. Reed, and H.L. Thacker. 1993. Cellular responses of the respiratory tract of chickens to infection with Massachusetts 41 and Australian T infectious bronchitis viruses. Avian Dis 37:951–960.

66. Geilhausen, H.E., F.B. Ligon, and P.D. Lukert. 1973. The pathogenesis of virulent and avirulent avian infectious bronchitis virus. Arch Gesamte Virusforsch 40:285–290.

67. Gelb, J., Jr. 1989. Infectious bronchitis. In H.G Purchase, L.H. Arp, C.H. Domermuth, and J E. Pearson (eds.). A Laboratory Manual for the Isolation and Identification of Avian Pathogens, 3rd ed. American Association of Avian Pathologists, Kennett Square, PA, pp. 124–127.

68. Gelb, J., Jr., and S.L. Killian. 1987. Serum antibody responses of chickens following sequential inoculations with different infectious bronchitis virus serotypes. Avian Dis 31:513–522.

69. Gelb, J., Jr., P.A. Fries, C.K. Crary, Jr., J.P. Donahoe, and D.E. Roessler. 1987. Sentinel bird approach to isolating infectious bronchitis virus. J Am Vet Med Assoc 190:1628.

70. Gentry, R.F., and M.O. Braune. 1972. Prevention of virus inactivation during drinking water vaccination of poultry. Poult Sci 51:1450–1456.

71. Gillette, K.G. 1973. Plaque formation by infectious bronchitis virus in chicken embryo kidney cell cultures. Avian Dis 17:369–378.

72. Glahn, R.P., R.F. Wideman, Jr., and B.S. Cowen. 1989. Order of exposure to high dietary calcium and Gray strain infectious bronchitis virus alters renal function and the incidence of urolithiasis. Poultry Sci 68:1193–1204.

73. Gough, R.E., and D.J. Alexander. 1978. Comparison of serological tests for the measurement of the primary immune response to avian infectious bronchitis virus vaccines. Vet Microbiol 2:289–301.

74. Gough, R.E., C.J. Randall, M. Dagless, D.J. Alexander, W.J. Cox, and D. Pearson. 1992. A "new" strain of infectious bronchitis virus infecting domestic fowl in Great Britain. Vet Rec 130:493–494.

75. Hanson, L.E., F.H. White, and J.O. Alberts. 1956. Interference between Newcastle disease and infectious bronchitis viruses. Am J Vet Res 17:294–298.

76. Hawkes, R.A., J.H. Darbyshire, R.W. Peters, A.P.A. Mockett, and D. Cavanagh. 1983. Presence of viral antigens and antibody in the trachea of chickens infected with avian infectious bronchitis virus. Avian Pathol 12:331–340.

77. Hitchner, S.B., and P.G. White. 1955. Growth curve studies of chick embryo propagated infectious bronchitis virus. Poult Sci 34:590–594.

78. Hofstad, M.S. 1981. Cross-immunity in chickens using seven isolates of avian infectious bronchitis virus. Avian Dis 25:650–654.

79. Hofstad, M.S. 1984. Avian infectious bronchitis. In M.S. Hofstad, H.J. Barnes, B.W. Calnek, W.M. Reid, and H.W. Yoder, Jr. (eds.). Diseases of Poultry, 8th ed. Iowa State University Press, Ames, IA, pp.429–443.

80. Hofstad, M.S., and H.W. Yoder, Jr. 1966. Avian infectious bronchitis—virus distribution in tissues of chicks. Avian Dis 10:230–239.

81. Holmes, H.C. 1973. Neutralizing antibody in nasal secretions of chickens following administration of avian infectious bronchitis virus. Arch Gesamte Virusforsch 43:235–241.

82. Hopkins, S.R. 1974. Serological comparisons of strains of infectious bronchitis virus using plaque purified isolants. Avian Dis 18:231–239.

83. Hopkins, S.R., and C.W. Beard. 1985. Studies on methods for determining the efficacy of oil emulsion vaccines against infectious bronchitis virus. J Am Vet Med Assoc 187:305.

84. Hopkins, S.R., and H.W. Yoder, Jr. 1986. Reversion to virulence of chicken passaged infectious bronchitis vaccine virus. Avian Dis 30:221–223.

85. Ignjatovic, J., and L. Galli. 1994. The S1 glycoprotein but not the N or M proteins of avian infectious bronchitis virus induces protection in vaccinated chickens. Arch Virol 138:117–134.

86. Ignjatovic, J., and P.G. Mcwaters. 1991. Monoclonal antibodies to three structural proteins of avian infectious bronchitis virus: Characerization of epitopes and antigenic differentiation of Australian strains. J Gen Virol 72:2915–2922.

87. Jackwood, M. W., H.M. Kwon, and D.A. Hilt. 1992. Infectious bronchitis virus detection in allantoic fluid using the polymerase chain reaction and a DNA probe. Avian Dis 36:403–409.

88. Janse, M.E., D. Van Rooselaar, and G. Koch. 1994. Leukocyte subpopulations in kidney and trachea of chickens infected with infectious bronchitis virus. Avian Pathol 23:513–523.

89. Jia, W., K. Karaca, C.R. Parrish, and S.A. Naqi. 1995. A novel variant of avian infectious bronchitis virus resulting from recombination among three different strains. Arch Virol 140:259–271.

90. Johnson, R.B., and W.W. Marquardt. 1975. The neutralizing characteristics of strains of infectious bronchitis virus as measured by the constant virus variable serum method in chicken tracheal cultures. Avian Dis 19:82–90.

91. Jones, R.C., and A.G. Ambali. 1987. Re-excretion of an enterotropic infectious bronchitis virus by hens at point of lay after experimental infection at day old. Vet Rec 120:617–620.

92. Jordan, F.T.W., and T.J. Nassar. 1973. The combined influence of age of embryo and temperature and duration of incubation on the replication and yield of avian infectious bronchitis (IB) virus in the developing chick embryo. Avian Pathol 2:279–294.

93. Jungherr, E.L., T.W. Chomiak, and R.E. Luginbuhl. 1956. Immunologic differences in strains of infectious bronchitis. Proc 60th Annu Meet US Livestock Sanit Assoc, pp. 203–209.

94. Kant, A., G. Koch, D.J. van Roozelaar, J.G. Kusters, J.G. Poelwijk, and B.A.M. van der Zeijst. 1992. Location of antigenic sites defined by neutralizing monoclonal antibodies on the S1 avian infectious bronchitis virus glycopolypeptide. J Gen Virol 73:591–596.

95. Karaca, K., and S. Naqi. 1993. A monoclonal antibody-based ELISA to detect serotype-specific infectious bronchitis virus antibodies. Vet Microbiol 34:249–257.

96. Karaca, K., S.A. Naqi, P. Palukatis, and B. Lucio. 1990. Serological and molecular characterization of three enteric isolates of infectious bronchitis virus of chickens. Avian Dis 34:899–904.

97. Karaca, K., S. Naqi, and J. Gelb. 1992. Production and characterization of monoclonal antibodies to three infectious bronchitis virus serotypes. Avian Dis 36:903–915.

98. King, D.J. 1984. Observations on the preparation and stability of infectious bronchitis virus hemagglutination antigen from virus propagated in chicken embryos and chicken kidney cell cultures. Avian Dis 28:504–513.

99. King, D.J. 1988. A comparison of infectious bronchitis virus hemagglutination-inhibition test procedures. Avian Dis 32:335–341.

100. King, D.J., and S.R. Hopkins. 1983. Evaluation of the hemagglutination inhibition test for measuring the response of chickens to avian infectious bronchitis virus vaccination. Avian Dis 27:100–112.

101. King, D.J., and S.R. Hopkins. 1984. Rapid serotyping of infectious bronchitis virus isolates with the hemagglutination inhibition test. Avian Dis 28:727–733.

102. Klieve, A.V., and R.B. Cumming. 1988. Immunity and cross-protection to nephritis produced by Australian infectious bronchitis viruses used as vaccines. Avian Pathol 17:829–839.

103. Klieve, A.V., and R.B. Cumming. 1988. Infectious bronchitis: Safety and protection in chickens with maternal antibody. Aust Vet J 65:396–397.

104. Koch, G., L. Hartog, A. Kant, and D.J. van Roozelaar. 1990. Antigenic domains on the peplomer protein of avian infectious bronchitis virus: Correlation with biological functions. J Gen Virol 71:1929–1935.

105. Kusters, J.G., H.G.M. Neisters, N.M.C. Bleumink–Pluym, F.G. Davelaar, M.C. Horzinek, and B.A.M. van der Zeigst. 1987. Molecular epidemiology of infectious bronchitis virus in the Netherlands. J Gen Virol 68:343–352.

106. Kusters, J.G., H.G.M. Niesters, J.A. Lenstra, M.C. Horzinek, and B.A.M. van der Zeijst. 1989. Phylogeny of antigenic variants of avian coronavirus IBV. Virology 169:217–221.

107. Kusters, J.G., E.J. Jager, H.G.M. Niesters, and B.A.M. van der Zeijst. 1990. Sequence evidence for RNA recombination in field isolates of avian coronavirus infectious bronchitis virus. Vaccine 8:605–608.

108. Kwon, H.M., M.W. Jackwood, and J. Gelb, Jr. 1993. Differentiation of infectious bronchitis virus serotypes using polymerase chain reaction and restriction fragment length polymorphism analysis. Avian Dis 37:194–202.

109. Kwon, H.M., M.W. Jackwood, T.P. Brown, and D.A.

Hilt. 1993. Polymerase chain reaction and a biotin-labelled DNA probe for detection of infectious bronchitis virus in chickens. Avian Dis 37:149–156.

110. Lai, M.M.C., C.-L. Liao, Y.-J. Lin, and X. Zhang. 1994. Coronavirus: How a large RNA viral genome is replicated and transcribed. Infect Agents Dis 3:98–105.

111. Lambrechts, C., M. Pensaert, and R. Ducatelle. 1993. Challenge experiments to evaluate cross-protection induced at the trachea and kidney level by vaccine strains and Belgian nephropathogenic isolates of avian infectious bronchitis virus. Avian Pathol 22:577–590.

112. Li, D., and D. Cavanagh. 1988. Coronavirus IBV-induced membrane fusion occurs at near-neutral pH. Arch Virol 122:307–316.

113. Lin, Z., A. Kato, Y. Kudou, and S. Ueda. 1991. A new typing method for the avian infectious bronchitis virus using polymerase chain reaction and restriction enzyme fragment length polymorphism. Virology 116:19–31.

114. Lin, Z., A. Kato, Y. Kudou, K. Umeda, and S. Ueda. 1991. Typing of recent infectious bronchitis virus isolates causing nephritis in chickens. Arch Virol 120:145–149.

115. Loomis, L.N., C.H. Cunningham, M.L. Gray, and F. Thorp, Jr. 1950. Pathology of the chicken embryo infected with infectious bronchitis virus. Am J Vet Res 11:245–251.

116. Lucio, B., and J. Fabricant. 1990. Tissue tropism of three cloacal isolates and Massachusetts strain of infectious bronchitis virus. Avian Dis 34:865–870.

117. Lukert, P.D. 1965. Comparative sensitivities of embryonating chicken's eggs and primary chicken embryo kidney and liver cell cultures to infectious bronchitis virus. Avian Dis 9:308–316.

118. Lukert, P.D. 1980. Infectious bronchitis. In S.B. Hitchner, C.H. Domermuth, H.G. Purchase, and J.E. Williams (eds.). Isolation and Identification of Avian Pathogens, 2nd ed. American Association of Avian Pathologists, Kennett Square, PA, pp. 70-72.

119. Macdonald, J.W., and D.A. McMartin. 1976. Observations on the effects of the H52 and H120 vaccine strains of the infectious bronchitis virus in the domestic fowl. Avian Pathol 5:157–173.

120. Macnaughton, M.R., H.J. Hasony, M.H. Madge, and S.E. Reed. 1981. Antibody to virus components in volunteers experimentally infected with human coronavirus 229E group viruses. Infect Immun 31:845–849.

121. Marquardt, W.W., D.B. Snyder, and B.A. Schlotthober. 1981. Detection and quantification of antibodies to infectious bronchitis virus by enzyme-linked immunosorbent assay. Avian Dis 25:713–722.

122. Meulemans, G., M.C. Carlier, M. Gonze, P. Petit, and M. Vandenbroeck. 1987. Incidence, characterization, and prophylaxis of nephropathogenic avian infectious bronchitis viruses. Vet Rec 120:205–206.

123. Miller, L., and V.J. Yates. 1968. Neutralization of infectious bronchitis virus by human sera. Am J Epidemiol 88:406–409.

124. Mockett, A.P.A., J.K.A. Cook, and M.B. Huggins. 1987. Maternally-derived antibody to infectious bronchitis virus: Its detection in chick trachea and serum and its role in protection. Avian Pathol 16:407–416.

125. Naqi, S. A. 1990. A monoclonal antibody-based immunoperoxidase procedure for rapid detection of infectious bronchitis virus in infected tissues. Avian Diseases 34:893–898.

126. Naqi, S. A., K. Karaca, and B. Bauman. 1993. A monoclonal antibody-based antigen capture enzyme-linked immunosorbent assay for identification of infectious bronchitis virus serotypes. Avian Pathol 22:555–564.

127. Otsuki, K., and M. Tsubokura. 1981. Plaque formation by avian infectious bronchitis virus in primary chick embryo fibroblast cells in the presence of trypsin. Arch Virol 70:315–320.

128. Otsuki, K., H. Yamamoto, and M. Tsubokura. 1979. Studies on avian infectious bronchitis virus (IBV) 1. Resistance of IBV to chemical and physical treatments. Arch Virol 60:25–32.

129. Otsuki, K., K. Noro, H. Yamamoto, and M. Tsubokura. 1979. Studies on avian infectious bronchitis virus (IBV) 2. Propagation of IBV in several cultured cells. Arch Virol 60:115–122.

130. Otsuki, K., T. Nakamura, Y. Kawaoka, and M. Tsubokura. 1988. Interferon induction by several strains of avian infectious bronchitis virus, a coronavirus, in chickens. Acta Virol 32:55–59.

131. Otsuki, K., M.B. Huggins, and J.K.A. Cook. 1990. Comparison of the susceptibility to infectious bronchitis virus infection of two inbred lines of White Leghorn chickens. Avian Pathol 19:467–475.

132. Parr, R.L., and E.W. Collisson. 1993. Epitopes on the spike protein of a nephropathogenic strain of infectious bronchitis virus. Arch Virol 133:369–383.

133. Pensaert, M., and C. Lambrechts. 1994. Vaccination of chickens against a Belgian nephropathogenic strain of infectious bronchitis virus B1648 using attenuated homologous and heterologous strains. Avian Pathol 23:631–41.

134. Powell, P.C. 1987. Immune mechanisms in infections of poultry. Vet Immunol Immunopathol 15:87–113.

135. Ratanasethakul, C., and R.B. Cumming. 1983. The effect of route of infection and strain of virus on the pathology of Australian infectious bronchitis. Aust Vet J 60:209–213.

136. Ratanasethakul, C., and R.B. Cumming. 1983. Immune response of chickens to various routes of administration of Australian infectious bronchitis vaccine. Aust Vet J 60:214–216.

137. Riddell, C. 1987. Avian Histopathology. American Association of Avian Patholology, Kennett Square, PA.

138. Rosenberger, J.K., and J. Gelb, Jr. 1987. Response of several avian respiratory viruses as affected by infectious bursal disease virus. Avian Dis 22:95–105.

139. Rosenberger, J.K., S.S. Cloud, M. Murphy, J. Gelb, Jr., E. Odor, M. Salem, and C. Pope. 1992. Characterization of several infectious bronchitis virus isolates obtained from Delmarva broilers. Proc 64th Northeastern Conf Avian Dis, The Pennsylvania State University, University Park, PA, p. 13.

140. Schalk, A.F., and M.C. Hawn. 1931. An apparently new respiratory disease of baby chicks. J Am Vet Med Assoc 78:413–422.

141. Schultze, B., D. Cavanagh, and G. Herrler. 1992. Neuraminidase treatment of avian infectious bronchitis coronavirus reveals a hemagglutinin activity that is dependent on sialic acid-containing receptors on erythrocytes. Virology 189:792–794.

142. Siddell, S.G. (ed) 1995. The Coronaviridae. Plenum Press, New York.

143. Siller, W.G. 1981. Renal pathology of the fowl: A review. Avian Pathol 10:187–262.

144. Smith, H.W, J.K.A. Cook, and Z.E. Parsell. 1985. The experimental infection of chickens with mixtures of infectious bronchitis virus and Escherichia coli. J Gen Virol 66:777–786.

145. Spackman, D., and I.R.D. Cameron. 1983. Isolation of infectious bronchitis virus from pheasants. Vet Rec 113:354–355.

146. Stern, D.F., and B.M. Sefton. 1982. Coronavirus proteins: Biogenesis of avian infectious bronchitis virus virion proteins. J Virol 44:794–803.

147. Stone, H.D., M. Brugh, S.R. Hopkins, H.W. Yoder, and C.W. Beard. 1978. Preparation of inactivated oil-emulsion vaccines with avian viral or mycoplasma antigens. Avian Dis 22:666–674.

148. Thompson, G., S.A. Naqi, and B. Bauman. 1993.

Respiratory immunity to IBV in immunocompetent and immunocompromised chickens. Proc Xth Int Congr World Vet Poultry Assoc, Sydney, Australia, p. 178.

149. Thornton, D.H., and J.C. Muskett. 1975. Effect of infectious bronchitis vaccination on the performance of live Newcastle disease vaccine. Vet Rec 96:467–468.

150. Timms, L.M., and C.D. Bracewell. 1981. Cell mediated and humoral immune response of chickens to live infectious bronchitis vaccines. Res Vet Sci 31:182–189.

151. Timms, L.M., and C.D. Bracewell. 1983. Cell mediated and humoral immune response of chickens to inactivated oil-emulsion infectious bronchitis vaccine. Res Vet Sci 34:224–230.

152. Tomley, F.M., A.P.A. Mockett, M.E.G. Boursnell, M.M. Binns, J.K.A. Cook, T.D.K. Brown, and G.L. Smith. 1987. Expression of the infectious bronchitis virus spike protein by recombinant vaccinia virus and induction of neutralizing antibodies in vaccinated mice. J Gen Virol 68:2291–2298.

153. Van Roekel, H., M.K. Clarke, K.L. Bullis, O.M. Olesiuk, and F.G. Sperling. 1951. Infectious bronchitis. Am J Vet Res 12:140–146.

154. Wadey, C.N., and J.T. Faragher. 1981. Australian infectious bronchitis viruses: Identification of nine subtypes by a neutralization test. Res Vet Sci 30:70–74.

155. Wainright, P.O., P. Villegas, M. Brugh, and P.D. Lukert. 1989. Characterization of infectious bronchitis virus using monoclonal antibodies. Avian Dis 33:482–490.

156. Wakenell, P.S., and J.M. Sharma. 1986. Chicken embryonal vaccination with avian infectious bronchitis virus. Am J Vet Res 47:933–938.

157. Wang, L., D. Junker, and E.W. Collisson. 1993. Evidence of natural recombination within the S1 gene of infectious bronchitis virus. Virology 192:710–716.

158. Wang, L., D. Junker, L. Hock, E. Ebiary, and E.W. Collisson. 1994. Evolutionary implications of genetic variations in the S1 gene of infectious bronchitis virus. Virus Res 34:327–338.

159. Wege, H., St. Siddell, and V. ter Meulen. 1982. The biology and pathogenesis of coronaviruses. Curr Top Microbiol Immunol 99:165–200.

160. Winterfield, R.W., and S.B. Hitchner. 1962. Etiology of an infectious nephritis-nephrosis syndrome of chickens. Am J Vet Res 23:1273–1279.

161. Winterfield, R.W., A.M. Fadly, and A.A. Bickford. 1972. The immune response to infectious bronchitis virus determined by respiratory signs, virus infection, and histopathological lesions. Avian Dis 16:260–269.

162. Yagyu, K., and Ohta, S. 1990. Detection of infectious bronchitis virus antigen from experimentally infected chickens by indirect immunofluorescent assay with monoclonal antibody. Avian Dis 34:246–252.

163. Zwaagstra, K.A., B.A.M. van der Zeijst, and J.G. Kusters. 1992. Rapid detection and identification of avian infectious bronchitis virus. J Clin Microbiol 30:79–84.

19 Laryngotracheitis

Trevor J. Bagust and James S. Guy

INTRODUCTION. Laryngotracheitis (LT) is a viral respiratory tract infection of chickens that may result in severe production losses due to mortality and/or decreased egg production. Severe epizootic forms of infection are characterized by signs of respiratory depression, gasping, expectoration of bloody mucus, and high mortality. Mild enzootic forms of infection increasingly are encountered in developed poultry industries and manifest variously as mucoid tracheitis, sinusitis, conjunctivitis, general unthriftiness, and low mortality. Laryngotracheitis virus (LTV) is a pathogen normally selected for exclusion from specific-pathogen–free chicken flocks.

HISTORY. The disease was first described in 1925 (98), but some reports indicate that it may have existed earlier (10, 56). It has been identified as laryngotracheitis, infectious laryngotracheitis, and avian diphtheria. Some early investigators also referred to the disease as infectious bronchitis. The term *laryngotracheitis* was used as early as 1930 (11, 47) and the name infectious laryngotracheitis was adopted in 1931 by the Special Committee on Poultry Diseases of the American Veterinary Medical Association. The cause of LT was first shown to be a filterable virus by Beaudette (13). Laryngotracheitis also was the first major avian viral disease for which an effective vaccine was developed (65).

INCIDENCE AND DISTRIBUTION. Laryngotracheitis virus has been identified in most countries and remains a serious disease where susceptible poultry populations occur, especially in large numbers (18). In areas of intensive production and large concentrations of poultry such as in the United States, Europe, China, Southeast Asia, and Australia, LT is usually well controlled in layer flocks by the use of modified live-virus vaccines. For intensive broiler production, the short growth cycle and high level of quarantine on sites can reduce the need for prophylactic vaccination. Within developed countries, LT viruses have tended to persist as endemic infections within backyard and fancier chicken flocks.

ETIOLOGY

Classification. Laryngotracheitis virus is classified as a member of the family *Herpesviridae* in the subfamily *Alphaherpesvirinae*. The virus is taxonomically identified as *Gallid herpesvirus 1* (122).

Morphology. Electron micrographs of LTV-infected chicken embryo cell cultures demonstrate the presence of icosahedral viral particles similar in morphology to herpes simplex virus. Watrach et al. (142) described the hexagonal nucleocapsids of LTV to be 80–100 nm in diameter. The nucleocapsids have icosahedral symmetry and are composed of 162 elongated hollow capsomeres (Fig. 19.1) (35, 142). The complete virus particle has a diameter of 195–250 nm and consists of an irregular envelope surrounding the nucleocapsid. The envelope contains fine projections representing viral glycoprotein spikes on its surface.

Chemical Composition. The nucleic acid of LTV is comprised of DNA having a buoyant density of 1.704 g/mL, a value consistent with those of other herpesviruses (109). The molecular weight of LTV DNA is approximately 100×10^6, with the genome having two isomeric forms (92, 94). Laryngotracheitis virus DNA has been reported to have a guanine plus cytosine ratio of 45% (109), which is lower than that for many other animal herpesviruses. The DNA genome consists of a linear 155-kb double-stranded molecule comprised of unique long and short segments flanked by inverted repeats (74, 95). Sequence data from the LTV thymidine kinase gene and upstream overlapping genes show DNA homology between LTV and various other alphaherpesviruses (48, 83). The glycoproteins of the virus, like other herpesviruses, are responsible for stimulating humoral and cell-mediated immune responses. Five major envelope glycoproteins with molecular weights of 205, 160, 115, 90, and 60 kD have been reported by York et al. (153, 155) to be the major immunogens of LT virus. Detailed characterization of LTV glycoproteins is under way in several laboratories; LTV gB, gC, gD, gX, gK, and the unique gp60 have been sequenced (see 7).

Virus Replication. Replication of LTV appears to be similar to that of other alphaherpesviruses such as pseudorabies virus and herpes simplex virus (110, 49, 123). The virus initiates infection by attachment to cell receptors followed by fusion of the envelope with the host cell plasma

527

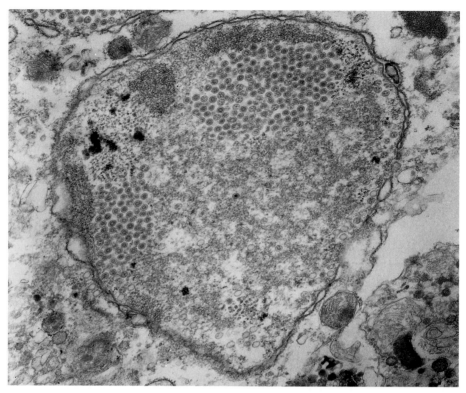

19.1.   Electron micrograph of laryngotracheitis virus. Aggregates of virus particles forming an inclusion body in nucleus of cultured chicken embryo kidney cell. Notice the peripheral accumulations of chromatin and centrally located amorphous material; the latter forms part of the inclusion body. ×18,500. (Watrach)

membrane. The nucleocapsid is released into the cytoplasm and transported to the nuclear membrane; viral DNA is released from the nucleocapsid and migrates into the nucleus through nuclear pores. Transcription and replication of viral DNA occur within the nucleus.

Transcription of LTV DNA occurs in a highly regulated, sequentially ordered cascade similar to that of other alphaherpesviruses (64, 110). Approximately 70 virus-coded proteins are produced; several are enzymes and DNA-binding proteins that regulate viral DNA replication, but most are viral structural proteins. Viral DNA replication occurs by a rolling circle mechanism with the formation of concatemers (15). DNA concatemers are cleaved into monomeric units and packaged into preformed nucleocapsids within the nucleus. DNA-filled nucleocapsids acquire an envelope by migration through the inner lamellae of the nuclear membrane (49). Enveloped particles then migrate through the endoplasmic reticulum and accumulate within vacuoles in the cytoplasm (49). Enveloped virions are released by cell lysis or by vacuolar membrane fusion and exocytosis.

Resistance to Chemical and Physical Agents.   Enveloped LTV infectivity is sensitive to the effects of lipolytic agents such as chloroform and ether (42, 101). Laryngotracheitis virus infectivity survives for several months when stored at 4 C in suitable diluents such as glycerol or nutrient broth. Thermostability of LTV infectivity has been reported to vary considerably. The infectivity of LTV has been reported to be rapidly inactivated by heat when exposed to 55 C for 15 minutes or 38 C for 48 hrs (see 78). Meulemans and Halen (101), however, found that 1% of the infectivity of a Belgian strain was retained after 1 hr at 56 C. Benton and Cover reported that LTV is destroyed in 44 hr at 37 C in tracheal tissues within chicken carcasses or in chorioallantoic membranes (CAMs) after 5 hr at 25 C (32). These results are, however, greatly at variance with several earlier reports (78) that indicate the capability of LTV infectivity to survive in tracheal exudates and chicken carcasses for periods of 10–100 days at ambient temperatures of 13–23 C. Additional studies are needed to resolve these discrepancies.

A solution of 3% cresol or 1% lye will inactivate

LTV in less than 1 minute; laboratory bench surfaces can be readily decontaminated with commercial iodophors or halogen-detergent mixtures. Some recent trials with microaerosolized hydrogen peroxide have indicated that the complete inactivation of LTV infectivity was achieved with a 5% hydrogen peroxide mist as a fumigant for poultry house equipment (104).

Strain Classification. Laryngotracheitis virus strains vary in virulence for chickens (32, 78, 111, 112), virulence for chicken embryos (71), plaque size and morphology in cell culture (125), and plaque size and morphology on CAMs of embryonated chicken eggs (112). Naturally occurring LTV strains vary in virulence from highly virulent strains that produce high morbidity and mortality in exposed chickens to strains of low virulence that produce mild-to-inapparent infection (32, 78, 111, 112). Laryngotracheitis virus strains appear to be antigenically homogenous based on virus-neutralization, immunofluorescence tests, and cross-protection studies (32, 133); however, minor antigenic variation among strains has been suggested by the finding that some strains are neutralized poorly by heterologous antisera (112, 125, 133).

Differentiation of LTV strains of varying virulence, particularly wild-type and modified live-vaccine viruses, is an important practical problem. Several methods for differentiating LTV viruses have been identified including analysis of virulence for chicken embryos (71), restriction endonuclease analyses of viral DNA (51, 92, 95), and DNA hybridization assays (93). Assessment of mortality patterns in embryonated chicken eggs was proposed as a biologic system for differentiating LTV strains (71) and mortality patterns correlated closely with virulence. Restriction endonuclease cleavage of viral DNA and electrophoretic separation of DNA fragments has been shown to distinguish different LTV strains (92, 95). Restriction endonuclease analysis of LTV DNA has been used extensively in epidemiologic studies of field outbreaks to differentiate wild-type and modified live-vaccine viruses (4, 51, 84, 86). Reciprocal DNA:DNA hybridization using cloned DNA fragments also has been shown to discriminate LTV strains (93), but additional testing of this method is needed.

Laboratory Host Systems. Laryngotracheitis virus may be propagated in embryonated chicken eggs and a variety of avian cell cultures. In embryonated chicken eggs the virus causes formation of opaque plaques on the CAM resulting from necrosis and proliferative tissue reactions (Fig. 19.2). Chorioallantoic membrane plaques generally have opaque edges and a central depressed area of necrosis. Plaques are observed as early as 2 days postinoculation (PI) and embryo deaths occur 2–12 days PI. Survival time of inoculated embryos decreases with additional egg passages (19, 21, 24).

Laryngotracheitis virus has been propagated in a variety of avian cell cultures including chicken embryo liver (CEL), chicken embryo lung, chicken

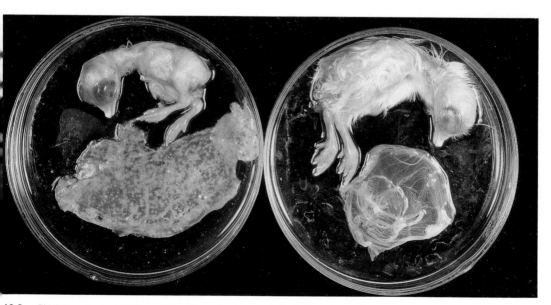

19.2. Chicken embryos at 14 days of age. Normal embryo and chorioallantoic membrane (CAM) (*right*). Laryngotracheitis virus–infected embryo is stunted, and CAM has numerous foci of proliferation (*left*).

embryo kidney (CEK), and chicken kidney (CK) cell cultures (27, 66, 100, 99). Hughes and Jones (66) compared several different laboratory host systems for efficiency of LTV isolation and propagation. The CEL and CK cells were found to be the preferred culture systems, with CEK cells, chicken embryo lung cells, and CAM inoculation of embryonated chicken eggs being less sensitive. Chicken embryo fibroblast cells, Vero cells, and quail-origin cells have been determined to be poor substrates for LTV propagation (66, 129).

Viral cytopathology may be observed in cell culture as early as 4–6 hr PI with a high multiplicity of infection. Cytopathology consists of increased refractiveness and swelling of cells, chromatin displacement, and rounding of the nucleoli. Cytoplasmic fusion results in formation of multinucleated giant cells. Intranuclear inclusion bodies can be detected as early as 12 hr PI, with the highest concentration occurring 30–36 hr PI (Fig. 19.3). Large cytoplasmic vesicles develop in the multinucleated cells and become more basophilic as cells degenerate (118).

Laryngotracheitis virus also may be propagated in avian leukocyte cultures. Initially, LTV was shown to replicate in avian leukocyte cultures derived from chicken buffy coat (28), and later the virus was shown to replicate in macrophage cultures obtained from bone marrow and spleen (23). Calnek et al. (26) determined that macrophage cul-

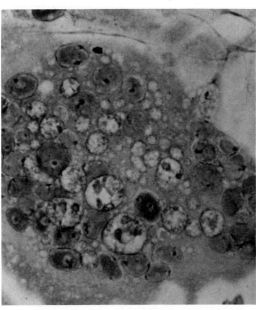

19.3. Chicken embryo kidney cell monolayer 72 hr after inoculation with laryngotracheitis virus. Large giant cell with numerous nuclei containing inclusion bodies. May-Grünwald-Giemsa, ×320.

tures were as susceptible to LTV infection as CK cells, but replication of most LTV strains examined was restricted. Both cell genotype and virus genotype influenced the extent of restriction of virus replication. Other cell types including lymphocytes, thymocytes, buffy-coat leukocytes, and activated T cells were either refractory or nearly refractory to LTV infection.

Laryngotracheitis virus recently has been shown to replicate in LMH cells, a continuous avian cell line derived from a chemically induced chicken liver tumor (129). Propagation of LTV in LMH cells requires adaptation; thus, they are unsuitable for diagnostic purposes involving primary isolation. They may, however, be useful for other purposes; for example, in research laboratories studying virus–host cell interactions.

PATHOGENESIS AND EPIZOOTIOLOGY

Natural and Experimental Hosts. The chicken is the primary natural host of LTV. Although the disease affects all ages, the most characteristic signs are observed in adult birds. Viral multiplication is limited to respiratory tissues, with little or no evidence of viremia (8, 63).

Several workers described a form of LT in pheasants and pheasant-chicken crosses (34, 65, 88). Winterfield and So (147) were able to induce lesions in the upper respiratory tract of young turkeys. They also reported the isolation of LTV from the trachea of a peafowl. Previous failures to infect turkeys (20, 131) indicated an age-dependent resistance in this species. Starlings, sparrows, crows, doves, ducks, pigeons, and guinea fowl appear to be refractory to LTV (12, 22, 131), although experimental infection of ducks producing subclinical disease and seroconversion has been reported (148). Embryonated eggs of turkeys and chickens are susceptible to LTV; duck eggs are susceptible to a lesser degree (78, 148), whereas eggs of guinea fowl and pigeons are not susceptible.

Transmission. Natural portals of entry for LTV are through the upper respiratory and ocular routes (13, 14). Ingestion can also be a mode of infection, although it may be that exposure of nasal epithelium following ingestion is required with this route (121). Transmission occurs more readily from acutely infected birds than through contact with clinically recovered carrier birds.

Laryngotracheitis virus infection of the upper respiratory tract of susceptible chickens is followed by intense viral replication. Several studies have independently confirmed that infectious virus usually is present in tracheal tissues and secretions for 6–8 days PI (8, 63, 114, 121); the virus may remain at very low levels up to 10 days PI (145). No clear evidence exists for a viremic phase of infection. Extratracheal spread of LTV to trigeminal ganglia 4–7 days after tracheal exposure was detected (8) in 40% of chickens exposed to a virulent Australian LTV strain. Reactivation of latent LTV from the trigeminal ganglia 15 months after vaccination of a flock has since been reported from Germany (81). Williams et al. (145), with the use of polymerase chain reaction (PCR) technology, have confirmed more recently that the trigeminal ganglion is the principal site of LTV latency. Hughes et al. (68) reported the reexcretion of LT virus from latently infected chicks following the stress of rehousing and the onset of reproduction.

Clinically inapparent LTV infection of the respiratory tract is a major feature of LT persistence. Pioneering observations by Komarov and Beaudette (91) and Gibbs (45), who collected laryngeal and tracheal swabs and inoculated susceptible chickens, indicated a "field" carrier rate of approximately 2% for periods up to 16 mo after a disease outbreak. In more recent studies with tracheal organ cultures explanted from chickens experimentally infected with Australian wild-type LTV and vaccine strains, latent tracheal infections were demonstrated for similar periods in 50% or more of infected chickens (5, 138). Repeated tracheal swabbing of small groups of chickens that had been experimentally infected with either a mildly pathogenic U.K. field strain or LT vaccine strains detected intermittent and apparently spontaneous shedding of LTV between 7 and 20 wk after infection (67, 69). Treatment with immunosuppressive drugs (e.g., cyclophosphamide, dexamethasone) has not yet proved successful in reactivation of latent LTV (5, 67, 68).

Mechanical transmission can occur by use of contaminated equipment and litter (14, 38, 46, 90). Egg transmission of virus contained in the interior or exterior of the egg has not been demonstrated.

Incubation, Morbidity, and Mortality.
Clinical signs generally appear 6–12 days following natural exposure (87, 130). Experimental inoculation via the intratracheal route results in a shorter incubation period of 2–4 days (16, 76, 130).

Severe epizootic forms of the disease cause high morbidity (90–100%) and variable mortality; mortality generally varies from 5% to 70% and averages 10–20% (10, 57, 130). Mild enzootic forms of the disease have been described in Great Britain, Australia, the United States, and New Zealand (32, 96, 112, 130, 143); these result in morbidity as low as 5% with very low mortality (0.1–2%) (117).

Signs.
Laryngotracheitis virus causes an acute respiratory disease in chickens. Characteristic clinical signs include nasal discharge and moist rales followed by coughing and gasping (Fig. 19.4) (10, 87). Marked dyspnea and expectoration of blood-stained mucus is characteristic of severe epizootic

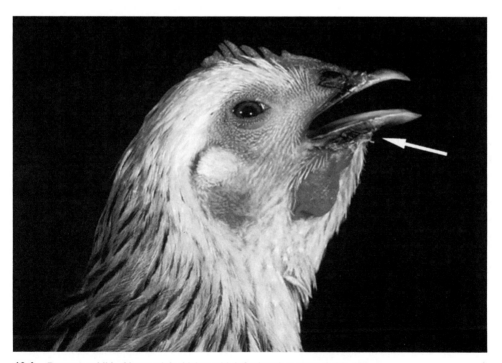

19.4. Dyspnea exhibited by an adult chicken with infectious laryngotracheitis. Note dried blood exudate around nostril and along the lower beak (*arrow*). (Munger)

forms of the disease (10, 56, 57, 75, 130).

Severe epizootic forms of LT were commonly described in earlier years; however, in recent years mild enzootic forms of LT have been more commonly observed in the intensive poultry producing areas of Europe, Australia, New Zealand and the United States (32, 96, 112, 130, 143). Clinical signs associated with mild enzootic forms include unthriftiness, reduction in egg production, watery eyes, conjunctivitis, swelling of infraorbital sinuses, persistent nasal discharge, and hemorrhagic conjunctivitis.

The course of the infection varies with the severity of lesions. Generally, most chickens recover in 10–14 days, but extremes of 1–4 wk have been reported (10, 57).

Gross Lesions.

Gross lesions may be found in the conjunctiva and throughout the respiratory tract of LTV-infected chickens, but they are most consistently observed in the larynx and trachea. Tissue changes in tracheal and laryngeal tissues may be mild, consisting only of excess mucus (96), or severe with hemorrhage and/or diphtheritic changes. In mild forms of LT, gross lesions may consist only of conjunctivitis, sinusitis, and mucoid tracheitis (37, 96). In severe forms, mucoid inflammation is observed early in infection with degeneration, necrosis, and hemorrhage occurring in later stages. Diphtheritic changes commonly are present and may be seen as mucoid casts that extend the entire length of the trachea. In other cases, severe hemorrhage into the tracheal lumen may result in blood casts (Fig. 19.5A), or blood may be mixed with mucus and necrotic tissue. Inflammation may extend down the bronchi into the lungs and air sacs.

Edema and congestion of the epithelium of the conjunctiva and infraorbital sinuses may be the only gross lesion observed in mild forms of LT.

Histopathology.

Microscopic changes vary with the stage of the disease (see Figs. 19.5B–F). Electron microscopic studies have shown that the first cellular change occurs in the nucleus of epithelial cells during formation of viral capsids (118). Viral capsids bud through the nuclear membrane, acquiring lipid envelopes, and aggregate into large masses within vacuoles in the cytoplasm. The cloudy swelling observed in light microscopic studies of early cellular changes has been associated with the presence of these large masses of viral particles in the cytoplasm (141).

Early microscopic changes in tracheal mucosa include the loss of goblet cells and infiltration of mucosa with inflammatory cells. As the viral infection progresses, cells enlarge, lose cilia, and become edematous. Multinucleated cells (syncytia) are formed and lymphocytes, histiocytes, and plasma cells migrate into the mucosa and submucosa after 2–3 days. Later, cell destruction and desquamation result in a mucosal surface either covered by a thin layer of basal cells or lacking any epithelial covering; blood vessels within the lamina propria may protrude into the tracheal lumen. Hemorrhage may occur in cases of severe epithelial destruction and desquamation with exposure and rupture of blood capillaries.

Intranuclear inclusion bodies are found in epithelial cells by 3 days PI (113). Inclusion bodies generally are present only in the early stages of infection (1–5 days) (54, 139); they disappear as infection progresses, a result of the necrosis and desquamation of epithelial cells.

Immunity.

A variety of immune responses are generated following LTV infection (79). Virus-neutralizing antibodies become detectable within 5–7 days PI, peak around 21 days, then wane over the next several months to low levels. Virus-neutralizing antibodies may be detectable for a year or more (62). Antibodies may be detected in tracheal secretions from approximately 7 days PI (5, 154) and plateau at days 10–28 PI. The numbers of IgA- and IgG-synthesizing cells in the trachea increased substantially in experimentally infected chickens between days 3 and 7 PI (154). Cell-mediated immunity (CMI) has not been extensively studied owing to the complexity of CMI studies; however, delayed-type hypersensitivity responses to LTV have been demonstrated (150). The duration of CMI responses to LTV following infection is not known.

Humoral immune responses to LTV, although associated with infection, are not the primary mechanism of protection, and a poor correlation generally has been found between serum antibody titers and immune status of flocks (79). In addition, Fahey and York (39), with the use of bursectomized chickens, have demonstrated that mucosal antibody is not essential in preventing replication of virus in vaccinated chickens. The principal mediator of LT resistance is the local cell-mediated immune response in the trachea (39). Bursectomized and cyclophosphamide-treated chickens fail to mount humoral immune responses following LT vaccination but develop full immunity (40, 119). Fahey et al. (41) demonstrated that LT resistance could be transferred using spleen cells and peripheral blood leukocytes from congenic immune donors.

Maternal antibody to LTV is transmitted to offspring via the egg (17), but this antibody does not confer protection to infection or interfere with vaccination (40, 135). Chickens less than 2 wk of age do not respond as well to vaccination as do older birds (2, 33, 44), although chickens can be successfully vaccinated as early as 1 day of age (136).

In chickens older than 2 wk of age, LT vaccina-

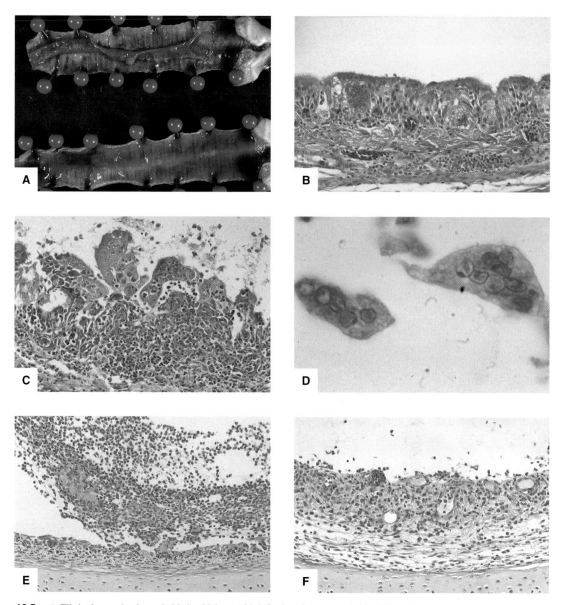

19.5. *A.* Fibrinohemorrhagic tracheitis in chickens with infectious laryngotracheitis. (Munger).
B–F. Microscopic tracheal lesions of infectious laryngotracheitis. *B.* Early infectious
laryngotracheitis lesions in the trachea. Mucosa is slightly thickened. There is a mild infiltration of lymphocytes in the mucosa and submucosa especially around vessels. A large
multinucleated syncytial cell has developed in the mucosa. *C.* Numerous syncytial cells
have separated from the mucosa, which is now heavily infiltrated by lymphocytes.
Presence of syncytial cells in the tracheal lumen is characteristic of infectious laryngotracheitis. *D.* High magnification of sloughed syncytial cells showing numerous intranuclear
inclusions. *E.* Later in the disease, epithelium, blood, and inflammatory exudate form a
membrane that separates and sloughs into the lumen. This may occlude the trachea and
cause death from asphyxiation or serve as a medium for bacterial proliferation. Expelling
the exudate by coughing is a classic clinical sign of infectious laryngotracheitis. *F.* The
amount of epithelium that survives depends on virulence of the strain. This bird was infected with the Illinois strain, which is highly virulent. As a result, there has been complete loss of epithelium, leaving lamina propria exposed.

tion or field exposure confers protection against challenge, which is partial by 3–4 days postvaccination and complete by 6–8 days (16, 43, 59). Waning of immunity has been detected as early as 8–15 wk postvaccination (61), but substantial flock immunity generally is observed for 15–20 wk after vaccination (2, 44, 107). Vaccine breaks in the field are most commonly observed after 15–20 wk postvaccination, but the value of revaccination is questionable (79).

Sinkovic (135) and Fahey et al. (40) determined that susceptibility of chickens to LTV declined with age; they found that meat-type males were more susceptible than meat-type females. They also reported that high environmental temperatures (35 C) cause higher mortality from LTV infection in heavy adult breeds than in light adult breeds.

DIAGNOSIS. In general, LT diagnosis requires laboratory assistance as other respiratory pathogens of poultry can cause similar clinical signs and lesions. Only in cases of severe acute disease with high mortality and expectoration of blood can LT be reliably diagnosed on the basis of clinical signs. Laboratory diagnosis may be achieved based on detection of intranuclear inclusion bodies, virus isolation, detection of LT virus antigens in tracheal tissues or respiratory mucus, detection of LT virus DNA, or serology (137).

Laryngotracheitis is characterized by the development of pathognomonic intranuclear inclusion bodies in respiratory and conjunctival epithelial cells (Fig. 19.5C,D). Intranuclear inclusion bodies may be detected in tissues stained with Giemsa or hematoxylin and eosin. Cover and Benton (32) reported that the choice of fixative was important for detection of inclusion bodies; they found that a fixative having a low pH was required. Diagnosis of LT based on demonstration of inclusion bodies in tissues has been shown to be considerably less sensitive than virus isolation. Keller and Hebel (85) showed that inclusion bodies could be detected in 57% of 60 specimens, while virus was isolated from 72% of the same specimens. Similarly, Guy et al. (54) found that histopathologic detection of inclusion bodies was a highly specific method for diagnosis of LT when compared with virus isolation, but sensitivity was poor.

Rapid methods for histopathologic identification of LTV inclusion bodies have been described by Pirozok et al. (108) and Sevoian (132); both techniques require as little as 3 hr for preparation of tissues as compared with 24–48 hr with the use of conventional histologic processing methods. Pirozok et al. (108) developed a method employing Carbowax, a water-soluble embedding medium that eliminates the need for dehydration steps, thus markedly decreasing processing time. Sevoian

(132) developed a procedure in which fixation and dehydration of tissues was done simultaneously.

Isolation of LTV may be accomplished by inoculation of suspensions of respiratory exudate, conjunctival exudate, or tissue onto the CAM of 9- to 12-day-old embryonated chicken eggs or onto susceptible cell cultures (see Laboratory Host Systems). Clinical samples may include trachea, larynx, lungs, conjunctiva, or exudate collected by swabbing these sites. Samples must be collected early in the course of infection, as experimental studies indicate that LTV is not detected or detected inconsistently after approximately 6 days of infection (8, 54, 149). Samples should be transported promptly to the laboratory, preferably on wet ice.

The CAM route of inoculation is utilized commonly for LTV isolation; it is the most sensitive of the embryonated egg inoculation routes and results in titers 2 $\log_{10}$ or greater than other routes (60, 77). Chicken embryo liver cells and CK cells are the cell cultures of choice for LTV isolation. In a comparison of the CAM inoculation route and a variety of cell cultures, Hughes and Jones (66) found CEL cells to be the most sensitive laboratory host system for LTV isolation, although CK cells were a satisfactory alternative. Both CEL and CK cells were superior to CAM inoculation of embryonated eggs. A maximum of two passages in CEL and CK cell cultures are required for LTV detection (5, 66).

A variety of different procedures have been described for rapid diagnosis of LT including fluorescent antibody (FA) procedures, an immunoperoxidase (IP) procedure, enzyme-linked immunosorbent assays (ELISA), electron microscopy, DNA hybridization techniques, and PCR techniques. Wilks and Kogan (144) reported the detection of LTV proteins in tracheal tissue from day 2 through day 14 PI using an FA procedure, but others (8, 63) have reported shorter periods (6–8 days PI) for successful detection using FA procedures. With the use of an IP procedure, Guy et al. (53) were able to detect LTV proteins in tracheal tissues from day 1 to day 9 PI (Fig. 19.6); the IP procedure was shown to be more sensitive than FA for detection of LTV in tissues. As well, ELISA procedures for detection of LTV proteins in tracheal exudate have been developed (105, 149). York and Fahey (149) described an antigen capture ELISA using monoclonal antibodies to LTV. This ELISA was shown to be as accurate as virus isolation, but faster, and more accurate than either FA or agar gel precipitation tests (80) for detecting LTV.

Rapid diagnosis of LT also has been accomplished using direct electron microscopic examination of tracheal scrapings (66, 140). Diagnosis is dependent upon visualization and morphologic identification of herpesviruses and, thus, is successful only when large numbers of virus particles are

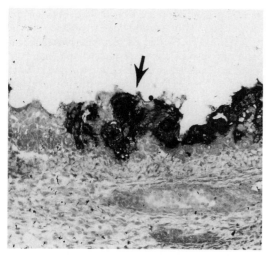

19.6. Immunoperoxidase staining of trachea of chicken killed on the 4th day following intratracheal inoculation. Staining is localized to large focal areas of the tracheal mucosa (*arrow*). ×150.

present in clinical samples. Hughes and Jones (66) found that virus particles were observed only when clinical samples contained a minimum titer of 3.5 $\log_{10}$ of infectious virus.

Recently, methods for detection of LTV DNA in clinical samples have been described (82, 89, 134, 146, 145). Keam et al. (82) and Key et al. (89) described procedures for detection of LTV DNA utilizing dot-blot hybridization assays and cloned LTV DNA fragments labeled with digoxigenin. These procedures were shown to be highly sensitive for detection of LTV in acutely infected chickens, as well as convalescent chickens when detection was no longer possible using virus isolation and ELISA. These procedures also were shown to provide rapid methods for detection of chickens latently infected with LTV. Polymerase chain reaction procedures for detection of LTV DNA were described by Shirley et al. (134) and Williams et al. (146). These procedures were shown to be more sensitive than virus isolation, and they could identify LTV in samples that were contaminated with other microorganisms, particularly adenoviruses, that prevented isolation of the virus (146).

Serology. A variety of techniques for demonstration of LTV antibodies in serum have been described, including agar-gel immunodiffusion (AGID), virus neutralization (VN), indirect fluorescent antibody (IFA) test, and ELISA. These procedures also may be utilized for identification of LTV in infected cell cultures and CAMs.

Burnet (25) first described a VN test to detect LT antibodies in chicken serum using embryonated chicken eggs inoculated by the CAM route with subsequent enumeration of CAM lesions. The use of cell cultures greatly simplified these procedures; VN antibodies may be measured by assay in cell cultures seeded in tubes, petri dishes, or microwell plates (30, 120, 124). Enzyme-linked immunosorbent assay systems recently have been developed for detection and quantitation of LTV antibodies (102, 105, 152). Direct comparison of the AGID, VN, IFA, and ELISA demonstrated that all were valid systems for detecting and quantifying LTV antibodies (1). Although ELISA was shown to possess slightly greater sensitivity than VN, it was comparable to IFA; AGID was the least sensitive. Both ELISA and IFA have the advantages of speed and sensitivity; however, ELISA lacks the subjectivity inherent to IFA and is more suitable for testing large numbers of sera.

TREATMENT. No drug has been shown to be effective in reducing the severity of lesions or relieving disease signs. If a diagnosis of LT is obtained early in an outbreak, vaccination of unaffected birds may induce adequate protection before they become exposed.

PREVENTION AND CONTROL

Management Procedures. Laryngotracheitis virus infections resulting from field exposure or vaccination will result in latently infected carrier birds; thus, it is extremely important to avoid mixing vaccinated or recovered birds with susceptible chickens. Special precautions should be taken to obtain a complete history when mixing breeding stock. Use of sound biosecurity measures will avoid exposing susceptible chickens via contaminated fomites.

The importance of site quarantine and hygiene in preventing the movement of potentially contaminated personnel, feed, equipment, and birds is central to successful prevention and control of LT. Rodent and dog control measures should also be in place (90). The persistent LT disease threat posed by backyard and exhibition poultry flocks (97, 99) should be recognized and guarded against.

Cooperative control of LT outbreaks by collaboration between government and industry is most desirable. Correctly implemented (97), this approach may obviate the need for widespread use of LT vaccine. Where outbreaks have been contained, recovered flocks should be moved for processing under quarantine as soon as possible. Experience with LT outbreaks in Pennsylvania (36) indicates that this interval can be as short as 2 wk after the last clinical signs of LT are observed on a site.

For control of an LT outbreak, the most effective approach is a coordinated effort to obtain a rapid diagnosis, institute a vaccination program, and prevent further virus spread (6). Vaccination in the face of an outbreak will both limit virus spread and shorten duration of the disease. Spread of LTV between sites can be prevented by appropriate biosecurity measures. Laryngotracheitis virus infectivity is readily inactivated outside the host chicken by disinfectants and warm temperatures, thus carryover between successive flocks in a house can be prevented by adequate cleanup.

Immunization. Vaccination has proven to be a satisfactory method for developing resistance in susceptible chicken populations (see Immunity). Since vaccination can result in latently infected carrier birds, it is recommended for use only in geographic areas where the disease is endemic. The appropriate regulatory agency should be contacted to determine approved vaccines and vaccine application procedures.

MODIFIED LIVE-VIRUS VACCINES. Successful immunization against LT initially was accomplished using virulent virus applied to the cloaca (22). Later, it was demonstrated that immunity could be provided by vaccination of chickens with attenuated (modified live) viruses via infraorbital sinuses (133), intranasal instillation (16), feather follicles (103), eye drop (136), and orally through drinking water (128). Field strains of LTV have been attenuated by sequential passage in cell cultures (43, 72, 73) and embryonated chicken eggs (127), and via feather follicle inoculation of chickens (70, 103).

Careful attention must be given to procedures of vaccine administration to ensure adequate immunization. Care must be taken to ensure that an adequate concentration of infectious virus is administered to provide effective vaccination of chickens. Raggi and Lee (116) found that LT vaccine must contain more than 10^2 plaque-forming units/mL to induce satisfactory immunity when administered by routes other than the oral route. A virus concentration of 10^5 embryo infective doses was necessary for satisfactory oral vaccination (58). Modified live-LT vaccines must be handled with care in order to ensure adequate concentrations of infective virus; manufacturers' instructions for storage, resuspension, dilution, and application should be followed.

Administration of modified live-LT vaccine in drinking water or by spray are desirable methods for rapid, mass application of these vaccines; however, several problems have been associated with these routes of inoculation. Robertson and Egerton (121) demonstrated that administration of LT vaccines by the drinking water route results in a high proportion of chickens that fail to develop protective immunity. Successful vaccination via the drinking water requires that vaccine virus contact susceptible nasal epithelial cells as a result of aspiration of virus through the external nares or choanae. The studies of Robertson and Egerton (121) showed that this occurred infrequently in chickens vaccinated by the drinking water route. Application of LT vaccines by spray may result in adverse reactions as a result of insufficient attenuation of vaccine virus, deep penetration of respiratory tract due to small droplet size of spray (115), or excessive dose (31).

Modified live-LT vaccines have been associated with a variety of adverse effects including spread of vaccine virus to nonvaccinates (3, 29, 55, 128), insufficient attenuation, production of latently infected carriers (5), and increased virulence as a result of in vivo passage (53). Laryngotracheitis vaccine viruses have been shown to spread readily from vaccinated to nonvaccinated chickens (3, 29, 55, 128). Such spread should be avoided, as spread to nonvaccinates results in in vivo passage and possible reversion of vaccine virus to virulence (53), or it may result in disease in unvaccinated chickens due to insufficient attenuation of vaccine virus. Spread of vaccine viruses may be prevented by biosecurity measures that prevent flock-to-flock spread and vaccination methods that ensure simultaneous infection with LT vaccine virus of all susceptible birds on a farm.

Guy et al. (51, 52, 53) have provided evidence indicating involvement of modified live-LT vaccine viruses in field outbreaks. They suggested that modified live-LT vaccine viruses increase in virulence as a result of vaccine virus spread and in vivo (bird-to-bird) passage. In studies comparing six modified live-LT vaccine viruses and field LTV isolates, vaccine viruses were shown to be indistinguishable from field isolates based on DNA-restriction endonuclease analyses (51), but the virulence of all vaccine viruses was low compared with field isolates (52). Two modified live-vaccine viruses, a chicken embryo–origin (CEO) virus and a tissue culture–origin (TCO) virus, were sequentially passaged in specific-pathogen-free chickens to determine whether virulence of vaccine viruses could increase after sequential in vivo passage (53). Sequential passage of modified live-LT vaccine viruses resulted in increased virulence of the CEO virus but not the TCO virus. After 10 sequential passages in chickens, the CEO virus possessed virulence comparable to that of a highly virulent reference strain (Illinois N71851 strain, ATCC VR-783). Guy et al. (53) suggested that increased virulence of modified live-LT vaccine viruses occurred in field situations as a result of drinking-water vaccination and poor biosecurity that potentiated spread of vaccine viruses to nonvaccinates and sequential in vivo passage of these viruses.

INACTIVATED AND GENETICALLY ENGINEERED VACCINES. Experimental vaccines have been prepared from inactivated whole LTV (9, 40) or affinity-purified preparations of LTV glycoproteins (151). These vaccines have been shown to stimulate immune responses in chickens and varying degrees of protection to LTV challenge. Practical field use of these types of vaccines, however, is unlikely due to high cost of preparation and delivery.

Genetically engineered LTV vaccines recently have been developed (50, 106, 126). Guo et al. (50) described the construction of a recombinant LTV expressing the ß-galactosidase marker gene through insertion into an open reading frame of the LTV DNA. Okamura et al. (106) successfully inserted the *Lac-Z* marker gene into the thymidine kinase region of LTV DNA and isolated a stable recombinant. Saif et al. (126) reported the use of a herpesvirus of turkeys (HVT) recombinant containing LTV genes for immunization of chickens. This recombinant vaccine produced protection against LTV challenge similar to that induced by modified live-virus vaccines. A variety of strategies for development of genetically engineered LT vaccines recently were reviewed by Bagust and Johnson (7). They suggested that this type of vaccine could be used in conjunction with quarantine and hygiene measures for regional LTV eradication programs.

Eradication. Eradication of LTV from intensive poultry production sites appears to be highly feasible owing to several biologic and ecologic properties of the virus (7). These properties include the high degree of host specificity of the virus, fragility of infectivity outside the chicken, and antigenic stability of the LTV genome (7). The chicken is the primary host species and reservoir host; wildlife reservoirs are believed either to be nonexistent or of minor importance in LTV ecology. Backyard and fancier chicken flocks are likely reservoirs of LTV; thus, any eradication effort would require identification and inclusion of these birds (97). Laryngotracheitis virus strains are antigenically homogeneous; thus, a single LTV vaccine produces cross-protective immunity for all LTV strains.

Eradication of LTV will be facilitated in the future by development of genetically engineered vaccines that induce protective immunity without development of latently infected carrier chickens (7). It is likely that such vaccines will be available around the year 2000.

REFERENCES

1. Adair, B.M., D. Todd, E.R. McKillop, and K. Burns. 1985. Comparison of serological tests for detection of antibodies to infectious laryngotracheitis virus. Avian Pathol 14:461–469.

2. Alls, A.A., J.R. Ipson, and W.D. Vaughan. 1969. Studies on an ocular infectious laryngotracheitis vaccine. Avian Dis 13:36–45.

3. Andreasen, J.R., Jr., J.R. Glisson, M.A. Goodwin, R.S. Resurreccion, P. Villegas, and J. Brown. 1989. Studies of in-fectious laryngotracheitis vaccines: Immunity in layers. Avian Dis 33:524–530.

4. Andreasen, J.R., J.R. Glisson, and P. Villegas. 1990. Differentiation of vaccine strains and Georgia field isolates of infectious laryngotracheitis virus by their restriction endonuclease fragment patterns. Avian Dis 34:646–656.

5. Bagust, T.J. 1986. Laryngotracheitis (Gallid-1) herpesvirus infection in the chicken. 4. Latency establishment by wild and vaccine strains of ILT virus. Avian Pathol 15:581–595.

6. Bagust, T.J. 1992. Laryngotracheitis. In Veterinary Diagnostic Virology: A Practitioner's Guide. Mosby Year Book, St. Louis, MO, pp. 40–43.

7. Bagust, T.J., and M.A. Johnson. 1995. Avian infectious laryngotracheitis: Virus-host interactions in relation to prospects for eradication. Avian Pathol 24:373–391.

8. Bagust, T.J., B.W. Calnek, and K.J. Fahey. 1986. Gallid-1 herpesvirus infection in the chicken. 3. Reinvestigation of the pathogenesis of infectious laryngotracheitis in acute and early post-acute respiratory disease. Avian Dis 30:179–190.

9. Barhoom, S.A., A. Forgacs, and F. Solyom. 1986. Development of an inactivated vaccine against laryngotracheitis (ILT)—serological and protection studies. Avian Pathol 15:213–221.

10. Beach, J.R. 1926. Infectious bronchitis of fowls. J Am Vet Med Assoc 68:570–580.

11. Beach, J.R. 1930. The virus of laryngotracheitis of fowls. Science 72:633–634.

12. Beach, J.R. 1931. A filterable virus, the cause of infectious laryngotracheitis of chickens. J Exp Med 54:809–816.

13. Beaudette, F.R. 1930. Infectious bronchitis. N J Agric Exp Stn Annu Rep 51:286.

14. Beaudette, F.R. 1937. Infectious laryngotracheitis. Poult Sci 16:103–105.

15. Ben-Porat, T., and S. Tokazewski. 1977. Replication of herpesvirus DNA. II. Sedimentation characteristics of newly synthesized DNA. Virol 79:292–301.

16. Benton, W.J., M.S. Cover, and L.M. Greene. 1958. The clinical and serological response of chickens to certain laryngotracheitis viruses. Avian Dis 2:383–396.

17. Benton, W.J., M.S. Cover, and W.C. Krauss. 1960. Studies on parental immunity to infectious laryngotracheitis of chickens. Avian Dis 4:491–499.

18. Biggs, P.M. 1982. The world of poultry disease. Avian Pathol 11:281–300.

19. Brandly, C.A. 1935. Some studies on infectious laryngotracheitis. The continued propagation of the virus upon the CAM of the hen's egg. J Infect Dis 57:201–206.

20. Brandly, C.A. 1936. Studies on the egg-propagated viruses of infectious laryngotracheitis and fowl pox. J Am Vet Med Assoc 88:587–599.

21. Brandly, C.A. 1937. Studies on certain filterable viruses. 1. Factors concerned with the egg propagation of fowl pox and infectious laryngotracheitis. J Am Vet Med Assoc 90:479–487.

22. Brandly, C.A., and L.D. Bushnell. 1934. A report of some investigations of infectious laryngotracheitis. Poult Sci 13:212–217.

23. Bülow, V., and A. Klasen. 1983. Effects of avian viruses on cultured chicken bone-marrow-derived macrophages. Avian Pathol 12:179–198.

24. Burnet, F. 1934. The propagation of the virus of infectious laryngotracheitis on the CAM of the developing egg. Br J Exp Pathol 15:52–55.

25. Burnet, F. 1936. Immunological studies with the virus of infectious laryngotracheitis of fowls using the developing egg technique. J Exp Med 63:685–701.

26. Calnek, B.W., K.J. Fahey, and T.J. Bagust. 1986. In vitro infection studies with infectious laryngotracheitis virus. Avian Dis 30:327–336.

27. Chang, P.W., V.J. Yates, A.H. Dardiri, and D.E. Fry.

1960. Some observations on the propagation of infectious laryngotracheitis virus in tissue culture. Avian Dis 4:384–390.

28. Chang, P.W., F. Sculo, and V.J. Yates. 1977. An in vivo and in vitro study of infectious laryngotracheitis virus in chicken leukocytes. Avian Dis 21:492–500.

29. Churchill, A.E. 1965. The development of a live attenuated infectious laryngotracheitis vaccine. Vet Rec 77:1227–1234.

30. Churchill, A.E. 1965. The use of chicken kidney tissue cultures in the study of the avian viruses of Newcastle disease, infectious laryngotracheitis, and infectious bronchitis. Res Vet Sci 6:162–169.

31. Clarke, J.K., G.M. Robertson, and D.A. Purcell. 1980. Spray vaccination of chickens using infectious laryngotracheitis virus. Aust Vet 56:424–428.

32. Cover, M.S., and W.J. Benton. 1958. The biological variation of infectious laryngotracheitis virus. Avian Dis 2:375–383.

33. Cover, M.S., W.J. Benton, and W.C. Krauss. 1960. The effect of parental immunity and age on the response to infectious laryngotracheitis vaccination. Avian Dis 4:467–473.

34. Crawshaw, G.J., and B.R. Boycott. 1982. Infectious laryngotracheitis in peafowl and pheasants. Avian Dis 26:397–401.

35. Cruickshank, J.G., D.M. Berry, and B. Hay. 1963. The fine structure of infectious laryngotracheitis virus. Virology 20:376–378.

36. Davidson, S., and K. Miller. 1988. Recent laryngotracheitis outbreaks in Pennsylvania. Proc 37th West Poult Conf. Sacramento, CA, pp. 135–136.

37. Davidson, S., R. Eckroade, and K. Miller. 1988. Laryngotracheitis—the Pennsylvania experience. Proc 23rd Natl Meet Poult Health Condemnations. Ocean City, MD, pp. 14–19.

38. Dobson, N. 1935. Infectious laryngotracheitis in poultry. Vet Rec 15:1467–1471.

39. Fahey, K.J., and J.J. York. 1990. The role of mucosal antibody in immunity to infectious laryngotracheitis virus in chickens. J Gen Virol 71:2401–2405.

40. Fahey, K.J., T.J. Bagust, and J.J. York. 1983. Laryngotracheitis herpesvirus infection in the chicken: The role of humoral antibody in immunity to a graded challenge infection. Avian Pathol 12:505–514.

41. Fahey, K.J., J.J. York, and T.J. Bagust. 1984. Laryngotracheitis herpesvirus infection in the chicken. 2. The adoptive transfer of resistance to a graded challenge infection. Avian Pathol 13:265–275.

42. Fitzgerald, J.E., and L.E. Hanson. 1963. A comparison of some properties of laryngotracheitis and herpes simplex viruses. Am J Vet Res 24:1297–1303.

43. Gelenczei, E.F., and E.W. Marty. 1964. Studies on a tissue-culture modified infectious laryngotracheitis virus. Avian Dis 8:105–122.

44. Gelenczei, E.F., and E.W. Marty. 1965. Strain stability and immunologic characteristics of a tissue-culture modified infectious laryngotracheitis virus. Avian Dis 9:44–56.

45. Gibbs, C.S. 1933. The Massachusetts plan for the eradication and control of infectious laryngotracheitis. J Am Vet Med Assoc 83:214–217.

46. Gibbs, C.S. 1934. Infectious laryngotracheitis field experiments: Vaccination. Mass Agric Exp Stn Bull 305:57–58.

47. Graham, R.F., F. Throp, Jr., and W.A. James. 1930. Subacute or chronic infectious avian laryngotracheitis. J Infect Dis 47:87–91.

48. Griffin, A.M., and M.E.G. Boursnell. 1990. Analysis of the nucleotide sequence of DNA from the region of the thymidine kinase gene of infectious laryngotracheitis virus: Potential evolutionary relationships between the herpesvirus subfamilies. J Gen Virol 71:841–850.

49. Guo, P., E. Scholz, J. Turek, R. Nordgreen, and B. Maloney. 1993. Assembly pathway of avian infectious laryngotracheitis virus. Am J Vet Res 54:2031–2039.

50. Guo, P., E. Scholz, B. Maloney, and E. Welniak. 1994. Construction of recombinant avian infectious laryngotracheitis virus expressing the ß-galactosidase gene and DNA sequencing of the insertion region. Virology 202:771–781.

51. Guy, J.S., H.J. Barnes, L.L. Munger, and L. Rose. 1989. Restriction endonuclease analysis of infectious laryngotracheitis viruses: Comparison of modified-live vaccine viruses and North Carolina field isolates. Avian Dis 33:316–323.

52. Guy, J.S., H.J. Barnes, and L.G. Smith. 1990. Virulence of infectious laryngotracheitis viruses: Comparison of modified-live vaccine viruses and North Carolina field isolates. Avian Dis 34:106–113.

53. Guy, J.S., H.J. Barnes, and L.G. Smith. 1991. Increased virulence of modified–live infectious laryngotracheitis vaccine virus following bird-to-bird passage. Avian Dis 35:348–355.

54. Guy, J.S., H.J. Barnes, and L.G. Smith. 1992. Rapid diagnosis of infectious laryngotracheitis using a monoclonal antibody-based immunoperoxidase procedure. Avian Pathol 21:77–86.

55. Hilbink, F.W., H.L. Oei, and D.J. van Roozelaar. 1987. Virulence of five live virus vaccines against infectious laryngotracheitis and their immunogenicity and spread after eyedrop or spray application. Vet Q 9:215–225.

56. Hinshaw, W.R. 1931. A survey of infectious laryngotracheitis of fowls. Calif Agric Exp Stn Bull 520:1–36.

57. Hinshaw, W.R., E.C. Jones, and H.W. Graybill. 1931. A study of mortality and egg production in flocks affected with laryngotracheitis. Poult Sci 10:375–382.

58. Hitchner, S.B. 1969. Virus concentration as a limiting factor in immunity response to laryngotracheitis vaccines [abst]. J Am Vet Med Assoc 154:1425.

59. Hitchner, S.B. 1975. Infectious laryngotracheitis: The virus and the immune response. Am J Vet Res 36:518–519.

60. Hitchner, S.B., and P.G. White. 1958. A comparison of embryo and bird infectivity using five strains of laryngotracheitis virus. Poult Sci 37:684–690.

61. Hitchner, S.B., and R.W. Winterfield. 1960. Revaccination procedures for infectious laryngotracheitis. Avian Dis 4:291–303.

62. Hitchner, S.B., C.A. Shea, and P.G. White. 1958. Studies on a serum neutralization test for diagnosis of laryngotracheitis in chickens. Avian Dis 2:258–269.

63. Hitchner, S.B., J. Fabricant, and T.J. Bagust. 1977. A fluorescent-antibody study of the pathogenesis of infectious laryngotracheitis. Avian Dis 21:185–194.

64. Honess, R.W., and B. Roizman. 1974. Regulation of herpesvirus macromolecular synthesis. I. Cascade regulation of the synthesis of three groups of viral proteins. J Virol 14:8–19.

65. Hudson, C.B., and F.R. Beaudette. 1932. The susceptibility of pheasants and a pheasant bantam cross to the virus of infectious bronchitis. Cornell Vet 22:70–74.

66. Hughes, C.S., and R.C. Jones. 1988. Comparison of cultural methods for primary isolation of infectious laryngotracheitis virus from field materials. Avian Pathol 17:295–303.

67. Hughes, C.S., R.C. Jones, R.M. Gaskell, F.T.W. Jordan, and J.M. Bradbury. 1987. Demonstration in live chickens of the carrier state in infectious laryngotracheitis. Res Vet Sci 42:407–410.

68. Hughes, C.S., R.M. Gaskell, R.C. Jones, J.M. Bradbury, and F.T.W. Jordan. 1989. Effects of certain stress factors on the re-excretion of infectious laryngotracheitis virus from latently infected carrier birds. Res Vet Sci 46:247–276.

69. Hughes, C.S., R.A. Williams, R.M. Gaskell, F.T.W. Jordan, J.M. Bradbury, M. Bennett, and R.C. Jones. 1991. Latency and reactivation of infectious laryngotracheitis vaccine virus. Arch Virol 121:213–218.

70. Hunt, S. 1959. The feather follicle method of vacci-

nating baby chicks with laryngotracheitis vaccine. Proc Poult Sci Conv, pp. 29–30. Sydney, Australia.

71. Izuchi, T., and A. Hasagawa. 1982. Pathogenicity of infectious laryngotracheitis virus as measured by chicken embryo inoculation. Avian Dis 26:18–25.

72. Izuchi, T., A. Hasegawa, and T. Miyamoto. 1983. Studies on a live virus vaccine against infectious laryngotracheitis of chickens. I. Biological properties of attenuated strain C7. Avian Dis 27:918–926.

73. Izuchi, T., A. Hasegawa, and T. Miyamoto. 1984. Studies on the live virus vaccine against infectious laryngotracheitis of chickens. II. Evaluation of the tissue-culture-modified strain C7 in laboratory and field trials. Avian Dis 28:323–330.

74. Johnson, M.A., C.T. Prideaux, K. Kongsuwan, M. Sheppard, and K.J. Fahey. 1991. Gallid herpesvirus 1 (infectious laryngotracheitis virus): Cloning and physical maps of the SA-2 strain. Arch Virol 119:181–198.

75. Jordan, F.T.W. 1958. Some observations of infectious laryngotracheitis. Vet Rec 70:605–610.

76. Jordan, F.T.W. 1963. Further observations of the epidemiology of infectious laryngotracheitis of poultry. J Comp Pathol 73:253–264.

77. Jordan, F.T.W. 1964. The control of infectious laryngotracheitis. Zentralbl Veterinaermed [B] 11:15–32.

78. Jordan, F.T.W. 1966. A review of the literature on infectious laryngotracheitis. Avian Dis 10:1–26.

79. Jordan, F.T.W. 1981. Immunity to infectious laryngotracheitis. In M. E. Ross, L. N. Payne, and B. M. Freeman (eds.). Avian Immunology. British Poultry Science Ltd., Edinburgh, Scotland, pp. 245–254.

80. Jordan, F.T.W., and R.C. Chubb. 1962. The agar gel diffusion technique in the diagnosis of infectious laryngotracheitis (I.L.T.) and its differentiation from fowl pox. Res Vet Sci 3:245–255.

81. Kaleta, E.F., T.H. Redman, U. Heffels-Redman, and K. Frese. 1986. Zum Nachweis der Latenz des attenuierten virus der infektiosen laryngotracheitis des Huhnes im trigeminus-ganglion. Dtsch Tieraerztl Wochenschr 93:40–42.

82. Keam, L.J.J. York, M. Sheppard, and K.J. Fahey. 1991. Detection of infectious laryngotracheitis virus in chickens using a non-radioactive DNA probe. Avian Dis 35:257–262.

83. Keeler, C.L., D.H. Kingsley, and C.R.A. Burton. 1991. Identification of the thymidine kinase gene of infectious laryngotracheitis virus. Avian Dis 35:920–929.

84. Keeler, C.L., J.W. Hazel, J.E. Hastings, and J.K. Rosenberger. 1993. Restriction endonuclease analysis of Delmarva field isolates of infectious laryngotracheitis virus. Avian Dis 37:418–426.

85. Keller, K., and P. Hebel. 1962. Diagnostico de las incusiones de laryngotraqueitis infecciosa en frotis y cortes histologicos. Zooiatria (Chile) 1:1.

86. Keller, L.H., C.E. Benson, S. Davison, and R.J. Eckroade. 1992. Differences among restriction endonuclease DNA fingerprints of Pennsylvania field isolates, vaccine strains and challenge strains of infectious laryngotracheitis virus. Avian Dis 36:575–581.

87. Kernohan, G. 1931. Infectious laryngotracheitis in fowls. J Am Vet Med Assoc 78:196–202.

88. Kernohan, G. 1931. Infectious laryngotracheitis in pheasants. J Am Vet Med Assoc 78:553–555.

89. Key, D.W., B.C. Gough, J.B. Derbyshire, and E. Nagy. 1994. Development and evaluation of a non-isotopically labeled DNA probe for the diagnosis of infectious laryngotracheitis. Avian Dis 38:467–474.

90. Kingsbury, F.W., and E.L. Jungherr. 1958. Indirect transmission of infectious laryngotracheitis in chickens. Avian Dis 2:54–63.

91. Komarov, A. and F.R. Beaudette. 1932. Carriers of infectious bronchitis. Poult Sci 11:335–338.

92. Kotiw, M., C.R. Wilks, and J.T. May. 1982. Differentiation of infectious laryngotracheitis virus strains using restriction endonucleases. Avian Dis 26:718–731.

93. Kotiw, M., M. Sheppard, J.T. May, and C.R. Wilks. 1986. Differentiation between virulent and avirulent strains of infectious laryngotracheitis virus by DNA:DNA hybridization using a cloned DNA marker. Vet Microbiol 11:319–330.

94. Lieb, D.A., J.M. Bradbury, R.M. Gaskell, C.S. Hughes, and R.C. Jones. 1986. Restriction endonuclease patterns of some European and American isolates of infectious laryngotracheitis virus. Avian Dis 30:835–837.

95. Lieb, D.A., J.M. Bradbury, C.A. Hart, and K. McCarthy. 1987. Genome isomerism in two alphaherpesviruses: Herpes saimiri-1 (herpesvirus tamaerinus) and avian infectious laryngotracheitis virus. Arch Virol 93:287–294.

96. Linares, J.A., A.A. Bickford, G.L. Cooper, B.R. Charlton, and P.R. Woolcock. 1994. An outbreak of infectious laryngotracheitis in California broilers. Avian Dis 38:188–192.

97. Mallinson, E.T., K.F. Miller, and C.D. Murphy. 1981. Cooperative control of infectious laryngotracheitis. Avian Dis 25:723–729.

98. May, H.G., and R.P. Tittsler. 1925. Tracheo-laryngotracheitis in poultry. J Am Vet Med Assoc 67:229–231.

99. McNulty, M.S., G.M. Allan, and R.M. McCracken. 1985. Infectious laryngotracheitis in Ireland. Irish Vet J 39:124–125.

100. Meulemans, G., and P. Halen. 1978. A comparison of three methods for diagnosis of infectious laryngotracheitis. Avian Pathol 7:433–436.

101. Meulemans, G., and P. Halen. 1978. Some physio-chemical and biological properties of a Belgian strain (U 76/1035) of infectious laryngotracheitis virus. Avian Pathol 7:311–315.

102. Meulemans, G., and P. Halen. 1982. Enzyme-linked immunosorbent assay (ELISA) for detecting infectious laryngotracheitis viral antibodies in chicken serum. Avian Pathol 11:361–368.

103. Molgard, P.C., and J.W. Cavett. 1947. The feather follicle method of vaccinating with fowl laryngotracheitis vaccine. Poult Sci 26:263–267.

104. Neighbour, N.K., L.A. Newberry, G.R. Bayyari, J.K. Skeeles, J.N. Beasley, and R.W. McNew. 1994. The effect of microaerosolized hydrogen peroxide on bacterial and viral pathogens. Poult Sci 73:1511–1516.

105. Ohkubo, Y., K. Shibata, T. Mimura, and I. Taskashima. 1988. Labeled avidin-biotin enzyme-linked immunosorbent assay for detecting antibody to infectious laryngotracheitis virus in chickens. Avian Dis 32:24–31.

106. Okamura, H., M. Sakaguchi, T. Honda, A. Taneno, K. Matsuo, and S. Yamada. 1994. Construction of recombinant laryngotracheitis virus expressing the lac-Z gene of E. coli with thymidine kinase gene. J Vet Med Sci 56:799–801.

107. Picault, J.P., M. Guittet, and G. Bennejean. 1982. Innocuite et activite de differents vaccins de la laryngotracheite infectieuse aviaire. Avian Pathol 11:39–48.

108. Pirozok, R.P., C.F. Helmbolt, and E.L. Jungherr. 1957. A rapid histological technique for the diagnosis of infectious avian laryngotracheitis. J Am Vet Med Assoc 130:406–407.

109. Plummer, G., C.R. Goodheart, D. Henson, and C.P. Bowling. 1969. A comparative study of the DNA density and behavior in tissue culture of fourteen different herpesviruses. Virology 39:134–137.

110. Prideaux, C.T., K. Kongsuwan, M.A. Johnson, M. Sheppard, and K.J. Fahey. 1992. Infectious laryngotracheitis virus growth, DNA replication, and protein synthesis. Arch Virol 123:181–192.

111. Pulsford, M.F. 1963. Infectious laryngotracheitis of poultry. Part I. Virus variation, immunology and vaccination. Vet Bull 33:415–420.

112. Pulsford, M.F., and J. Stokes. 1953. Infectious laryngotracheitis in South Australia. Aust Vet J 29:8–12.

113. Purcell, D.A. 1971. The ultrastructural changes pro-

duced by infectious laryngotracheitis virus in tracheal epithelium of the fowl. Res Vet Sci 12:455–458.

114. Purcell, D.A., and J.B. McFerran. 1969. Influence of method of infection on the pathogenesis of infectious laryngotracheitis. J Comp Path 79:285–291.

115. Purcell, D.A., and P.G. Surman. 1974. Aerosol administration of the SA-2 vaccine strain of infectious laryngotracheitis virus. Aust Vet J 50:419–420.

116. Raggi, L.G., and G.G. Lee. 1965. Infectious laryngotracheitis outbreaks following vaccination. Avian Dis 9:559–565.

117. Raggi, L.G., J.R. Brownell, and G.F. Stewart. 1961. Effect of infectious laryngotracheitis on egg production and quality. Poult Sci 40:134–140.

118. Reynolds, H.A., A.W. Watrach, and L.E. Hanson. 1968. Development of the nuclear inclusion bodies of infectious laryngotracheitis. Avian Dis 12:332–347.

119. Robertson, G.M. 1977. The role of bursa-dependent responses in immunity to infectious laryngotracheitis. Res Vet Sci 22:281–284.

120. Robertson, G.M., and J.R. Egerton. 1977. Micro-assay systems for infectious laryngotracheitis virus. Avian Dis 21:133–135.

121. Robertson, G.M., and J.R. Egerton. 1981. Replication of infectious laryngotracheitis virus in chickens following vaccination. Aust Vet J 57:119–123.

122. Roizman, B. 1982. The family Herpesviridae: General description, taxonomy and classification. In B. Roizman (ed.). The Herpesviruses, vol. 1. Plenum Press, New York, pp. 1–23.

123. Roizman, B. and A.E. Sears. 1990. Herpes Simplex Viruses and Their Replication. In B.N. Fields (ed.). Virology. Raven Press, New York, pp. 9–35.

124. Rossi, C.R., H.A. Reynolds, and A.M. Watrach. 1969. Studies of laryngotracheitis virus in avian tissue cultures. 1. Plaque assay in chicken embryo kidney tissue cultures. Arch Virol 28:219–228.

125. Russell, R.G., and A.J. Turner. 1983. Characterization of infectious laryngotracheitis viruses, antigenic comparison of neutralization and immunization studies. Can J Comp Med 47:163–171.

126. Saif, Y.M., J.K. Rosenberger, S.S. Cloud, M.A. Wild, J.K. McMillen, and R.D. Schwartz. 1994. Efficacy and safety of a recombinant herpesvirus of turkeys containing genes from infectious laryngotracheitis virus. Proc Am Vet Med Assoc, Minneapolis, MN, p. 154.

127. Samberg, Y., and I. Aronovici. 1969. The development of a vaccine against avian infectious laryngotracheitis. 1. Modification of a laryngotracheitis virus. Refu Vet 26:54–59.

128. Samberg, Y., E. Cuperstein, U. Bendheim, and I. Aronovici. 1971. The development of a vaccine against avian infectious laryngotracheitis. IV. Immunization of chickens with modified laryngotracheitis vaccine in the drinking water. Avian Dis 15:413–417.

129. Schnitzlein, W.M., J. Radzevicius, and D.N. Tripathy. 1994. Propagation of infectious laryngotracheitis virus in an avian liver cell line. Avian Dis 38:211–217.

130. Seddon, H.R., and L. Hart. 1935. The occurrence of infectious laryngotracheitis in fowls in New South Wales. Aust Vet J 11:212–222.

131. Seddon, H.R., and L. Hart. 1936. Infectivity experiments with the virus of laryngotracheitis of fowls. Aust Vet J 12:13–16.

132. Sevoian, M. 1960. A quick method for the diagnosis of avian pox and infectious laryngotracheitis. Avian Dis 4:474–477.

133. Shibley, G.P., R.E. Luginbuhl, and C.F. Helmboldt. 1962. A study of infectious laryngotracheitis virus. I. Comparison of serologic and immunogenic properties. Avian Dis 6:59–71.

134. Shirley, M.W., D.J. Kemp, M. Sheppard, and K.J. Fa-

hey. 1990. Detection of DNA from infectious laryngotracheitis virus by colourimetric analyses of polymerase chain reactions. J Virol Methods 30:251–260.

135. Sinkovic, B.S. 1974. Studies on the control of ILT in Australia. PhD dissertation. University of Sydney, Australia.

136. Sinkovic, B. and S. Hunt. 1968. Vaccination of day-old chickens against infectious laryngotracheitis by conjunctival instillation. Aust Vet J 44:55–57.

137. Tripathy, D.N., and L.E. Hanson. 1989. Laryngotracheitis. In H.G. Purchase, L.H. Arp, C.H. Domermuth, and J.E. Pearson, (eds.). A Laboratory Manual for the Isolation and Identification of Avian Pathogens, 3rd ed. American Association of Avian Pathologists, Kennett Square, PA, pp. 85–88.

138. Turner, A.J. 1972. Persistence of virus in respiratory infections of chickens. Aust Vet J 48:361–363.

139. VanderKop, M.A. 1993. Infectious laryngotracheitis in commercial broiler chickens. Can Vet J 34:185.

140. Van Kammen, A., and P.B. Spradbrow. 1976. Rapid diagnosis of some avian virus diseases. Avian Dis 20:748–751.

141. Watrach, A.M., A.E. Vatter, L.E. Hanson, M.A. Watrook, and H.E. Rhoades. 1959. Electron microscopic studies of the virus of infectious laryngotracheitis. Am J Vet Res 20:537–544.

142. Watrach, A.M., L.E. Hanson, and M.A. Watrach. 1963. The structure of infectious laryngotracheitis virus. Virology 21:601–608.

143. Webster, R.G. 1959. Studies on infectious laryngotracheitis in New Zealand. NZ Vet J 7:67–71.

144. Wilks, C.R., and V.G. Kogan. 1979. An immunofluorescence diagnostic test for avian infectious laryngotracheitis. Aust Vet J 55:385–388.

145. Williams, R.A., M. Bennett, J.M. Bradbury, R.M. Gaskell, R.C. Jones, and F.T.W. Jordan. 1992. Demonstration of sites of latency of infectious laryngotracheitis virus using the polymerase chain reaction. J Gen Virol 73:2415–2430.

146. Williams, R.A., C.E. Savage, and R.C. Jones. 1994. A comparison of direct electron microscopy, virus isolation, and a DNA amplification method for the detection of avian infectious laryngotracheitis virus in field material. Avian Pathol 23:709–720.

147. Winterfield, R.W., and I.G. So. 1968. Susceptibility of turkeys to infectious laryngotracheitis. Avian Dis 12:191–202.

148. Yamada, S., K. Matsuo, T. Fukuda, and Y. Uchinuno. 1980. Susceptibility of ducks to the virus of infectious laryngotracheitis. Avian Dis 24:930–938.

149. York, J.J., and K.J. Fahey. 1988. Diagnosis of infectious laryngotracheitis using a monoclonal antibody ELISA. Avian Pathol 17:173–182.

150. York, J.J., and K.J. Fahey. 1990. Humoral and cell-mediated immune responses to the glycoproteins of infectious laryngotracheitis herpesvirus. Arch Virol 115:289–297.

151. York, J.J., and K.J. Fahey. 1991. Vaccination with affinity-purified glycoproteins protects chickens against infectious laryngotracheitis herpesvirus. Avian Pathol 20:693–704.

152. York, J.J., K.J. Fahey, and T.J. Bagust. 1983. Development and evaluation of an ELISA for the detection of antibody to infectious laryngotracheitis virus in chickens. Avian Dis 27:409–421.

153. York, J.J., S. Sonza, and K.J. Fahey. 1987. Immunogenic glycoproteins of infectious laryngotracheitis herpesvirus. Virology 161:340–347.

154. York, J.J., J.G. Young, and K.J. Fahey. 1989. The appearance of viral antigen and antibody in the trachea of naive and vaccinated chickens infected with infectious laryngotracheitis virus. Avian Pathol 18:643–658.

155. York, J.J., S. Sonza, M.R. Brandon, and K.J. Fahey. 1990. Antigens of infectious laryngotracheitis herpesvirus defined by monoclonal antibodies. Arch Virol 115:147–162.

20 Newcastle Disease and Other Avian *Paramyxoviridae* Infections

Dennis J. Alexander

INTRODUCTION. The virus families *Paramyxoviridae* and *Rhabdoviridae* form the first virus order to be defined, the *Mononegavirales,* i.e., the single-stranded, nonsegmented, negative-sense RNA viruses. The taxonomy and nomenclature of the family *Paramyxoviridae* has been modified recently (228) and now has four genera forming two subfamilies. The subfamily *Paramyxovirinae* has three genera: *Rubulavirus,* which includes Newcastle disease virus and the other avian paramyxoviruses; *Paramyxovirus;* and *Morbillivirus.* The subfamily *Pneumovirinae* consists of a single genus, *Pneumovirus,* which includes avian pneumovirus. Nine serogroups of avian paramyxoviruses have been recognized: PMV-1 to PMV-9 (9). Of these, Newcastle disease virus (NDV) (PMV-1) remains the most important pathogen for poultry, but PMV-2 and PMV-3 can be responsible for serious disease. The prototype viruses and the recognized natural hosts for each serogroup are shown in Table 20.1. Detailed descriptions of serotypes not shown to affect poultry and serotypes usually infecting feral waterfowl have been reviewed by Alexander (6, 7, 9, 11).

Newcastle disease virus may vary widely in the type and severity of the disease it produces. This has often caused some problems with nomenclature, usually when the disease was first recognized in a country. As a result, Newcastle disease has been termed pseudo-fowl pest, pseudovogel-pest, atypische Geflugelpest, pseudo-poultry plague, avian pest, avian distemper, Ranikhet disease, Tetelo disease, Korean fowl plague, and avian pneumoencephalitis. There have been very few synonyms used for the other avian paramyxoviruses. The term *Yucaipa* viruses has been applied to PMV-2 viruses, as the first isolate was PMV-2/chicken/California/Yucaipa/56, the prototype of the serogroup. Isolates of the PMV-5 serotype have occasionally been referred to as "Kunitachi" viruses, again after the prototype virus.

Newcastle disease is complicated in that different isolates and strains of the virus may induce enormous variation in the severity of disease, even in a given host such as the chicken. To simplify matters, division into forms of disease based on clinical signs in chickens has been made as summarized by Beard and Hanson (45): 1) Doyle's form (95), an acute, lethal infection of all ages of chickens. Hemorrhagic lesions of the digestive tract are frequently present, and this form of disease has been termed viscerotropic velogenic Newcastle disease (VVND). 2) Beach's form (41), an acute, often lethal infection of chickens of all ages. Characteristically, respiratory and neurological signs are seen, hence the term *neurotropic velogenic* (NVND). 3) Beaudette's form (48). This appears to be a less pathogenic form of NVND in which deaths are usually seen only in young birds. Viruses causing this type of infection are of the mesogenic pathotype and may be used as secondary live vaccines. 4) Hitchner's form (146). This form is represented by mild or inapparent respiratory infections caused by viruses of the lentogenic pathotype, which are commonly used as live vaccines. 5) Asymptomatic-enteric form (184); chiefly gut infections with lentogenic viruses causing no obvious disease.

The clinical diseases that may result from avian pneumovirus infections of turkeys or chickens have been termed turkey rhinotracheitis (TRT) and swollen head syndrome (SHS), respectively. These disease signs are not specific for avian pneumovirus infections and can be confused with disease resulting from infections with other organisms such as *Bordetella avium* in turkeys, which is covered in Chapter 13. Nevertheless, it is now universally accepted that the conditions referred to as TRT or SHS can occur as a result of infection with the same avian pneumovirus. The more severe form of associated disease probably results from dual or secondary infection with other organisms, and for SHS, the characteristic "swollen head" appears as a result of infection with secondary adventitious bacteria, usually *Escherichia coli.*

HISTORY

NEWCASTLE DISEASE VIRUS (PMV-1). It is generally considered that the first outbreaks of Newcastle disease occurred in 1926, in Java, Indonesia (163), and in Newcastle-upon-Tyne, England (95). There are reports of disease outbreaks in Central Europe similar to what we now recognize as Newcastle disease, which predate 1926 (131), and Levine (173), citing Ochi and Hashimoto, indicated that the disease may have been present in Korea as early as 1924. The name Newcastle disease was coined by Doyle as a temporary measure because he wished to avoid a descriptive name that might be confused with other diseases (96).

It later became clear that other less severe diseases were caused by viruses indistinguishable from NDV. In the United States, a relatively mild respiratory disease, often with nervous signs, was first described in the 1930s and subsequently termed *pneumoencephalitis* (41). It was shown to be due to a virus indistinguishable from NDV in serologic tests (42). Within a few years, numerous NDV isolations that produced extremely mild or no disease in chickens were made around the world (33, 146, 185, 248).

AVIAN PARAMYXOVIRUS TYPE 2 (PMV-2). In 1956, Bankowski et al. (36) isolated a paramyxovirus (94) from a chicken suffering from infectious laryngotracheitis in Yucaipa, California. It was serologically distinct from NDV (Table 20.1) and caused only mild respiratory disease in chickens. Serologic surveys of poultry in the United States indicated that this virus was widespread, more frequently infecting turkeys than chickens (37, 62). Subsequent investigations suggested that viruses of the same serotype were common in poultry around the world (9).

Testing during quarantine of imported caged birds since the early 1970s has frequently resulted in the isolation of PMV-2 viruses, primarily from passerines but also from psittacines (9, 246). Surveillance of wild birds during the 1970s often resulted in the isolation of PMV-2 viruses, most frequently from passerine species (9).

AVIAN PARAMYXOVIRUS TYPE 3 (PMV-3). Paramyxoviruses representing a third serotype were isolated from turkeys in Ontario in 1967 and Wisconsin in 1968 and later detected serologically in turkeys in other states of the United States (267). Serologically related viruses have now been reported from turkeys in several countries in Europe.

PMV-3 viruses are also frequently isolated from captive caged birds in most countries where quarantine is imposed, most often from psittacine species, although passerines are also susceptible (9). There is evidence that these viruses differ antigenically from the turkey PMV-3 viruses (29).

AVIAN PNEUMOVIRUS. A clinical disease syndrome indistinguishable from conditions now known to be related to avian pneumovirus infections has been reported from a number of countries since the late 1960s (178). In some of these countries, most notably the United States, however, it has been established that the causative organism is *Bordetella avium* and this organism and disease are dealt with in Chapter 13. Because of the differing etiologies and the difficulty in isolating the causative virus, it is impossible to state categorically when the condition was first recognized. Early reports attributing a viral etiology to both TRT and SHS in chickens came from South Africa where both diseases had appeared during the 1970s (67, 204). But it was not until the isolation of the causative virus and the development of a serologic test in 1986 that some estimation of the true prevalence and distribution of the disease could be made.

DISTRIBUTION

NEWCASTLE DISEASE. Vaccination of poultry throughout the world makes assessment of the geographic distribution of Newcastle disease difficult. Nevertheless, international recording and reporting of Newcastle disease is carried out by the Food and Agriculture Organization of the United Nations (102), which formed the basis of several assessments of the geographic distribution of the disease (167, 168). Spradbrow (254) concluded that Newcastle disease is still widespread in many countries of Asia, Africa, and the Americas; only countries of Oceania appeared to have relative freedom from disease. In Europe during the 1980s, only rare sporadic outbreaks occurred (156). Since 1991, however, there has been an increase in incidence with a series of related outbreaks affecting poultry in Belgium, The Netherlands, Luxembourg, Germany, Spain, Malta, and France. Outbreaks in Portugal during this period and in Italy during 1994 appear to be unrelated (13).

The distribution of Newcastle disease is dependent on the attempts at eradication and control made in different countries. The success of such measures is, in turn, dependent on the nature of the poultry industry, i.e., countries with mostly village chicken flocks have far greater problems than those with mostly large commercial flocks. Similarly, in Germany the vast majority of the large number of outbreaks recorded during 1993–1994 were in backyard flocks for which control is difficult (276).

The nature of the spread of Newcastle disease also affects the distribution. Alexander (10) considered that three panzootics of Newcastle disease had occurred since the first recognition of the disease. The first represented the initial outbreaks of disease and appears to have arisen in Southeast Asia. Doyle (96) considered that the disease moved slowly through Asia to Europe and that isolated outbreaks such as in England in 1926 were chance introductions ahead of the mainstream. This theory of panzootic spread of Newcastle disease would mean that virus, which had apparently arisen in 1926, took over 30 years to spread worldwide and was still important in most countries in the early 1960s.

In marked contrast, the second panzootic appears to have begun in the Middle East in the late 1960s and to have reached most countries by 1973. The more rapid spread of the second panzootic could be because the poultry industry had undergone a major revolution in that it had developed into a major commercial industry with considerable international trade. In addition, the virus responsible for this panzootic appeared to be associated with imported caged psittacine species. The enormous trade in these birds, which involved rapid, airborne shipments, was considered to be a major factor in the spread of the disease (104, 273).

The serious effects of the second panzootic on the poultry industries of most countries led to the development of vaccines and regimens that provided significant protection to poultry. In addition, most countries imposed new control measures for the importation of exotic caged birds. Another group of domesticated birds that was generally ignored as a potential source of Newcastle disease, however, existed in large numbers in most countries. This group consisted of the pigeons and doves (*Columba livia*) that are kept for racing, show, or food purposes and in most European countries may represent several million birds. These were the birds primarily affected by the third panzootic of ND. The disease, which resembled the neurotropic form in chickens but without respiratory signs, apparently arose in the Middle East in the late 1970s (157). By 1981, it had reached Europe (52) and then spread rapidly to all parts of the world, largely as a result of contact between birds at races and shows and the large international trade in such birds. The variant nature of the virus enabled unequivocal demonstration of infection in 24 countries (22, 26, 218). Spread to chickens has occurred in several countries including Great Britain where 20 outbreaks in unvaccinated chickens occurred in 1984 as a result of feed that had been contaminated by infected pigeons (23).

Avian Paramyxovirus Type 2. PMV-2 viruses are found in feral birds, chiefly passerines, in European, Asian, African, and American countries (8, 117), probably accounting for their common isolation from imported caged birds (8). Isolations from domestic poultry have been rare, although problems associated with such viruses have been recorded in United States, Canada, the former Soviet Union, Japan, Italy, Israel, India, and France in chickens or turkeys (6, 8).

Avian Paramyxovirus Type 3. PMV-3 viruses have also been isolated from imported exotic birds but, unlike PMV-2 viruses, there have been no reports of PMV-3 viruses from feral birds (8). PMV-3 virus infections of domestic poultry have been restricted to turkeys in Canada and United States (267), Great Britain (180), France (30), and Germany (288). There have been no reports of naturally occurring infections of chickens with PMV-3 viruses although they are fully susceptible.

Avian Pneumovirus. Lister and Alexander (178) listed the countries reporting disease signs similar to TRT and the prevalence of the disease in those countries prior to the isolation and identification of avian pneumoviruses. Retrospective assessment of serology or isolation of viruses indicated that the disease seen in many of these countries was related to avian pneumovirus infections. The virus has been isolated from turkeys and/or chickens in France, Great Britain, Italy, Spain, Hungary, Germany, The Netherlands, South Africa, Taiwan, and Israel. Antibodies to the virus have been demonstrated in chickens and/or turkeys in Great Britain, France, Italy, South Africa, Israel, Germany, The Netherlands, Spain, Austria, and Greece. In South Africa, SHS, or "dikkop" as it is termed there, appears to have been prevalent for a number of years.

ETIOLOGY

Classification. Members of the *Paramyxoviridae* family are RNA viruses showing helical capsid symmetry with a nonsegmented, single-stranded genome of negative polarity. They are enveloped and this is formed from modified cell membrane as the virus is budded from the cell surface after capsid assembly in the cytoplasm (191).

The subfamily *Paramyxovirinae* consists of three genera. The genus *Morbillivirus* includes measles, rinderpest, and the distemper viruses; no members have been isolated from avian species. The genus *Paramyxovirus* is formed from Sendai virus and other mammalian parainfluenza viruses. The genus *Rubulavirus* is formed from mumps virus, human parainfluenza viruses 2 and 4, Newcastle disease virus (PMV-1), and the avian paramyxoviruses (PMV-2 to PMV-3).

The subfamily *Pneumovirinae* has only one genus, *Pneumovirus,* which consists of the respiratory syncytial viruses, mouse pneumovirus, and the avian pneumoviruses. Avian pneumovirus isolates fulfill the morphologic and structural criteria for inclusion in the genus and do not possess hemagglutination or neuraminidase activities (76, 113, 174). The mRNA produced in avian pneumovirus infections is similar in profile to that of respiratory syncytial virus (70). The gene order in avian pneumoviruses, however, appears to be different from that of respiratory syncytial viruses (287).

CLASSIFICATION OF AVIAN PARAMYXOVIRUSES. Tumova et al. (268) suggested grouping avian paramyxoviruses on the basis of their antigenic relatedness in hemagglutination inhibition (HI) tests. The prefixes PMV-1, PMV-2, etc. were adopted to signify serotype, and the nomenclature proposed for naming influenza isolates (277) was used for the avian paramyxovirus isolates (Table 20.1).

There has been no attempt to make more specific definition of a serotype, and further viruses have been grouped based on their relationships in HI tests. When neuraminidase inhibition (151, 159, 208, 267), serum neutralization (267) or agar gel diffusion (2, 20, 151, 160) tests have been used, however, similar groups have resulted.

Despite the consistency of the serologic groupings, there are some cross relationships between viruses of the different serotypes (see 9). Usually, these have been very minor, although Lipkind et al. (175, 177) considered them sufficient to suggest a phylogenic relationship between PMV-1, -3, -4, -7, -8, and -9 and between PMV-2 and -6. However, the relationship between PMV-1 and -3 viruses appears to be closer and more important than the others.

Smit and Rondhuis suggested there were low serologic reactions between NDV and PMV-3/parakeet/Netherlands/75 (249), which were later confirmed (15). In addition, prior infection of chickens with some PMV-3 viruses conferred protection against challenge with a virulent NDV strain (18). More recently, a monoclonal antibody against the pigeon variant PMV-1 inhibited PMV-3 viruses isolated from exotic birds in HI tests and bound to cells infected with these PMV-3 viruses (26, 77). Since turkey PMV-3 isolates also show relationships with PMV-1 viruses, however, and none could be demonstrated to react with this monoclonal antibody, other epitopes may be shared by the two serotypes.

Morphology. Negative contrast electron microscopy of members of the *Rubulavirus* genus reveals very pleomorphic virus particles. Generally, they are rounded and 100–500 nm in diameter, although filamentous forms of about 100 nm across and of variable length are often seen. The surface of the virus particle is covered with projections about 8 nm in length. In most electron micrographs of avian paramyxoviruses, the "herring bone" nucleocapsid, about 18 nm across, may be seen either free or emerging from disrupted virus particles (Fig. 20.1).

Negative contrast electron microscopy of avian pneumovirus reveals pleomorphic fringed particles, usually roughly spherical, of 80–200 nm in diameter, although occasionally round particles with diameters of 500 nm or more can be seen (Fig. 20.2). Fringed filamentous forms 80–100 nm in diameter and up to 1000-nm long may be present (Fig. 20.3), particularly in preparations from organ culture propagation. Collins and Gough (76) reported the surface projections to be 13–14 nm in length and the helical nucleocapsid to be 14 nm in diameter with an estimated pitch of 7 nm per turn.

Table 20.1. Representative strains of the avian *Paramyxovirus* serotypes

Prototype Virus	Primary Host	Other Hosts	Related Disease in Poultry
PMV-1/Newcastle disease virus	Numerous avian hosts	See text	Spectrum of disease
PMV-2/chicken/ Yucaipa/56	Passerines, turkeys	Chickens, psittacines, rails	Respiratory disease, egg production losses, serious if complicated
PMV-3/turkey/ Wisconsin/68[a]	Turkeys	None	Egg production losses, respiratory disease
PMV-3/parakeet/ Netherlands/75[a]	Psittacines	Passerines	No infections known
PMV-4/duck/ Hong Kong/D3/75	Ducks	Geese, rails	Inapparent infections in commercial ducks
PMV-5/budgerigar/ Japan/Kunitachi/75	Budgerigars	None	No infections known
PMV-6/duck/ Hong Kong/199/77	Ducks, geese	Turkeys	Inapparent in ducks and geese, respiratory disease and egg losses in turkeys
PMV-7/dove/ Tennessee/4/75	Pigeons, doves	None	No infections known
PMV-8/goose/ Delaware/1053/75	Ducks, geese	None	No infections known
PMV-9/duck/ New York/22/78	Ducks	None	Inapparent infections in commercial ducks

[a]Monoclonal antibodies allow host-related distinction between PMV-3 isolates.

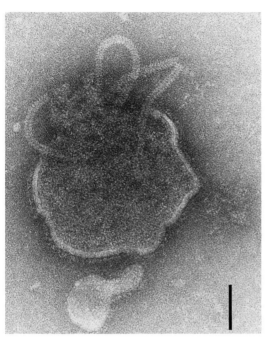

20.1. Negative contrast electron micrograph of Newcastle disease virus strain Ulster 2C showing a partially disrupted particle with nucleocapsid emerging. ×202,000, bar = 100 nm. (Collins)

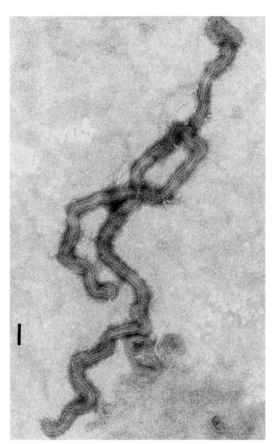

20.3. Negative contrast electron micrograph of avian pneumovirus filamentous particles. ×100,000, bar = 100 nm. (Collins)

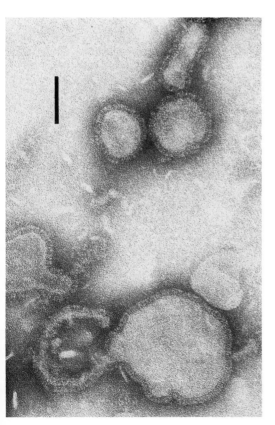

20.2. Negative contrast electron micrograph of avian pneumovirus particles. ×160,000, bar = 100 nm. (Collins)

Chemical Composition. Paramyxoviruses characteristically consist of a single molecule of single-stranded RNA of about 5×10^6 molecular weight (161), which makes up about 5% by weight of the virus particle. Nucleotide sequencing of the NDV genome has shown it to consist of 15,156 nucleotides (199).

Virus particles have about 20–25% w/w lipid derived from the host cell and about 6% w/w carbohydrate. The overall molecular weight for an average virus particle is about 500×10^6, with a density in sucrose of 1.18–1.20 g/mL.

VIRUS POLYPEPTIDES. Polyacrylamide gel electrophoresis (PAGE) of disrupted purified virus particles usually reveals a minimum of seven polypeptides for avian paramyxoviruses (16); however, one of these is the host protein actin, which is incorporated into the virus particle. The genome of NDV codes for six proteins (199), which have been described by Samson (241): L protein—this is the RNA-directed RNA polymerase associated with the nucleocapsid; HN—responsible for the hemagglutinin and neuraminidase activities, forming the larger of the two types of projections seen on the surface of paramyxovirus particles; F—fusion protein, forming the smaller of the surface projections; NP—nucleocapsid protein; P—phosphorylated, nucleocapsid-associated; M—matrix. Comparable polypeptides have been seen for the other avian paramyxoviruses, although minor variations in molecular weights has meant that PAGE profiles could be used to show similarities between isolates that coincide with the serogroups (16).

Characteristically, pneumoviruses have been reported to have about seven structural and three nonstructural virus-specified proteins of which two are glycosylated (224). Collins and Gough (76) described seven structural polypeptides for a TRT virus isolate of which two were glycosylated. In in vitro and in vivo polypeptide synthesis studies, Ling and Pringle (174) reported similar structural polypeptides and at least two nonstructural proteins.

Biologic Activities.

Several biologic activities are associated with paramyxoviruses, which characterize the group.

HEMAGGLUTINATION ACTIVITY. The ability of NDV and other avian paramyxoviruses to agglutinate red blood cells (RBCs) is due to the binding of the hemagglutinin-neuraminidase (HN) protein to receptors on the surface of the RBCs. This property and the specific inhibition of agglutination by antisera (66) have proven powerful tools in the diagnosis of the disease.

Chicken RBCs are usually used in hemagglutination (HA) tests, but NDV will cause agglutination of all amphibian, reptilian, and avian cells (166). Winslow et al. (283) showed that human, mouse, and guinea pig RBCs were agglutinated by all NDV strains tested, but the ability to agglutinate cattle, goat, sheep, swine, and horse cells varied with the strain of NDV. Other avian paramyxoviruses also appear to be able to agglutinate a wide range of RBCs, but the exact range may vary with isolate as well as serotype. Paramyxoviruses will agglutinate cells other than RBCs if they possess the correct receptors.

NEURAMINIDASE ACTIVITY. The enzyme neuraminidase (mucopolysaccharide N-acetyl neuraminyl hydrolase EC 3.2.1.18) is also part of the HN molecule and present in all members of the *Paramyxovirus* genus. An obvious consequence of the possession of this enzyme is the gradual elution of agglutinated RBCs (4). The exact function of the neuraminidase in virus replication is unknown, but it seems likely that it removes virus receptors from the host cell and this prevents the reattachment of released virus particles.

CELL FUSION AND HEMOLYSIS. Newcastle disease virus and other paramyxoviruses may bring about hemolysis of RBCs or fusion of other cells by essentially the same mechanism. Attachment at the receptor site during replication is followed by fusion of the virus membrane with the cell membrane and this may result in the fusion of two or more cells (similar to the syncytial formation that occurs when virus particles are budded from cells). The rigid membrane of the RBCs usually results in lysis from the virus membrane fusion.

Avian pneumoviruses do not possess HA or neuraminidase activity.

Virus Replication.

The strategy for replication employed by paramyxoviruses is that of the negative strand viruses in general, as detailed by Peeples (219).

The initial step is attachment of the virus to cell receptors, mediated by the HN polypeptide. Fusion of the viral and cell membranes is brought about by action of the fusion (F) protein, and, thus, the nucleocapsid complex enters the cell.

Intracellular virus replication takes place entirely within the cytoplasm. Because the virus RNA has negative sense, it is necessary for the viral RNA-directed RNA-polymerase (transcriptase) to produce complementary transcripts of positive sense that may act as messenger RNA and utilize the cell's mechanisms enabling translation into proteins and virus genomes. The F protein is synthesized as a nonfunctional precursor, F0, which requires cleavage to F1 and F2 by host proteases. The HN of some strains of NDV may also require posttranslational cleavage. The significance of this cleavage in the pathogenicity of NDV strains is discussed below.

The viral proteins synthesized in an infected cell are transported to the cell membrane, which becomes modified by their incorporation. Following alignment of the nucleocapsid close to modified regions of the cell membrane, virus particles are budded from the cell surface.

Resistance to Agents.

The infectivity of avian paramyxoviruses may be destroyed by physical and chemical treatments such as heat, irradiation (including light and ultraviolet rays), oxidation processes, pH effects, and various chemical compounds. The rate at which infectivity is destroyed depends on the strain of virus, the length of time of exposure, the quantity of virus, and the nature of the suspending medium and interactions between treatments. No single treatment can guarantee destruction of all virus but may result in a low probability of infective virus remaining. Lancaster (166) and Beard and Hanson (45) provided detailed reviews.

Strain Classification

NEWCASTLE DISEASE VIRUS (PMV-1).
The term *strain* is generally used to mean a well-characterized isolate of the virus. The important objective in characterizing viruses is to group similar viruses. For NDV isolates, this has inevitably meant the distinction between viruses of high and low pathogenicity for chickens or perhaps more pertinently between enzootic and epizootic virus.

Pathogenicity tests are useful markers and guides to the importance of the isolate. They give no further information, however, and do not indicate epizootiologic links between strains with the same virulence. Certain unrelated biologic properties of viruses have been shown to vary with different strains and isolates, and these have been used to characterize and group isolates showing similar properties.

PATHOGENICITY TESTS. The first attempt to distinguish between, or to group, isolates by a laboratory test was by assessment of virulence. Hanson and Brandly suggested that strains of NDV could be conveniently grouped as "velogenic," "mesogenic," and "lentogenic" based on chicken embryo mortality at <60 hr, 60–90 hr and >90 hr, respectively, after allantoic inoculation (136). The values obtained gave a guide to the disease produced in infected chickens. These terms have come to be applied to high-virulence, moderate-virulence, and low-virulence viruses regardless of the method of assessment.

Other tests devised to distinguish between strains give a direct assessment of the clinical signs or deaths in infected birds. This enables quantification by designating scores according to the degree of severity and calculating a pathogenicity index. The most widely used tests are the intracerebral pathogenicity index (ICPI) in day-old chicks and the intravenous pathogenicity index (IVPI) in 6-wk-old chickens.

PLAQUE FORMATION. Plaque formation, size, and morphology have been used to characterize viruses (133). Newcastle disease viruses of low virulence do not form plaques in cell cultures without the addition of diethylaminoethyl (DEAE) and magnesium (Mg^{2+}) ions (39) or trypsin (232) to the agar overlay. Plaques may be of two morphologic types, clear or red (244), and the size produced appears to be related to the virulence of the virus for chickens (226).

ELUTION. The rate of elution of chicken RBCs agglutinated by the virus has been used as a method of broadly grouping NDV isolates as rapid or slow eluters (253).

THERMOSTABILITY. The thermostability of the HA activity of NDV isolates varies (138) and has been used as a characterization test. This property has proven a useful tool in epizootiologic studies (137) and a rapid method for distinguishing between some avirulent and virulent viruses.

STRUCTURAL POLYPEPTIDES. Variations and similarities of structural polypeptides between different strains have been reported (16, 202). Nagy and Lomniczi (207) used structural polypeptide analysis by PAGE after enzyme treatment to show close relationships between viruses isolated during the same epizootic but differences from other strains.

OLIGONUCLEOTIDE FINGERPRINTING. McMillan and Hanson (187, 188) used oligonucleotide fingerprinting of the genomic RNA to compare different strains and isolates of NDV. This approach demonstrated identity of viruses from the same source and differences from other isolates, but it does not lend itself to routine diagnostic use.

LECTIN BINDING. McMillan et al. (189) demonstrated that different strains of NDV showed variation in lectin binding profiles, which could be useful for differentiation and grouping.

ANTIGENICITY. Virus neutralization (VN) or agar gel diffusion techniques have shown minor antigenic variation between different strains and isolates of NDV (116, 220, 245). For all practical purposes, however, isolates of NDV have been considered to represent a single antigenically homogeneous group.

Monoclonal antibody (MAB) technology provided a new approach to antigenic differentiation of NDV strains and isolates (3, 22, 26, 97, 149, 151, 165, 195, 210, 236, 256).

Monoclonal antibodies may detect slight variations in antigenicity, such as single amino acid changes at the epitope to which the antibody is directed. As a result, they are capable of detecting differences not only between strains but between subpopulations of virus (135). Some workers have used MABs to distinguish between specific viruses. For example, two groups have described MABs that distinguish between the common vaccine strains, Hitchner B1 and La Sota (97, 195), while other MABs can separate vaccine viruses from epizootic virus in a given area (256).

The most comprehensive use of MAB for strain characterization and classification has been by Russell and Alexander (236) and Alexander et al. (22, 25, 26). They used MABs to place strains and isolates of NDV into groups on the basis of their ability to react with the different MABs. Viruses in the same MAB group shared biologic and epizootiologic properties.

Monoclonal antibody typing was also used to establish the uniqueness of the variant NDV responsible for the pigeon panzootic and to confirm its presence in many countries (22, 26, 218). During the epizootic of NDV in Great Britain in 1984, rapid identification of the pigeon variant enabled early tracing of the source of disease to contaminated feed ingredients, and subsequent control of the disease.

NUCLEOTIDE SEQUENCING. Nucleotide sequencing, mainly of the HN or F genes has now been done on sufficient NDV strains to allow limited phylogenetic analyses (240, 266). These demonstrate genetic groupings that relate to biologic properties such as virulence and/or to the geographic origins of the strains examined. Russell et al. (239) pointed out the similarity between groups of viruses formed on a genetic basis and those formed on the basis of similarities in antigenicity detected using MABs.

AVIAN PARAMYXOVIRUS TYPE 2. No attempt has been made to classify strains of PMV-2 viruses. Considerable antigenic and structural diversity has been recorded among these viruses (6, 16) but these have not been related to any epizootiologic or biologic properties.

AVIAN PARAMYXOVIRUS TYPE 3. PMV-3 virus isolates also show considerable diversity. There appears to be antigenic differentiation between those isolated from exotic birds and those from turkeys. This has been confirmed by MABs to PMV-3/turkey/England/MPH/81. With the use of these, Anderson et al. (29) showed that while some antibodies reacted with isolates from either source, others bound specifically to turkey viruses. Turkey isolates from the United States and Germany were distinguishable from turkey isolates from Great Britain and France and possibly more closely related to exotic bird isolates. This division of PMV-3 isolates into two groups was supported by studies with a MAB to a PMV-1 pigeon variant isolate that was also able to react with PMV-3 isolates from exotic birds but not with those from turkeys (77).

AVIAN PNEUMOVIRUS. Early work, at a time when there were very few available isolates of avian pneumoviruses, suggested that there was little strain difference detectable by a variety of immunologic tests or polypeptide profiles (40, 120). More recently, field experience of serologic monitoring and vaccination problems has suggested there may be significant antigenic diversity amongst the viruses (171). Studies aimed at assessing antigenic variability have shown that viruses from different geographic locations may show marked variation in serologic tests (79, 86, 129, 171, 264). In three studies (79, 86, 171), MABs have been produced to an avian pneumovirus isolate and these have been used to further demonstrate considerable antigenic differences between strains. Cook et al. (86) reported some interesting relationships revealed by their panel of MABs. For example, virus obtained in South Africa in 1978 was closely related to isolates from Great Britain made in 1985 and 1990, whereas these viruses were quite different from an isolate made in France in 1986. Examination of isolates made in South Africa in 1978 and 1988 showed that little antigenic variation had taken place in the 10-yr period. Cook et al. (86) also reported high levels of relatedness between chicken and turkey isolates on the basis of pairs of viruses from South Africa and France.

Laboratory Host Systems for Avian Paramyxoviruses

ANIMALS. Newcastle disease virus can infect and multiply in a range of nonavian (166) as well as avian (155) species following laboratory infection. The chicken, however, remains the most readily available and frequently used laboratory animal, as well as the most important natural host of the disease.

CHICKEN EMBRYOS. All avian paramyxoviruses replicate in embryonated chicken eggs. Because of their availability (especially from specific-pathogen–free sources), their sensitivity for virus growth, and the high titers to which viruses grow in them, they are generally used for virus isolation and propagation.

Newcastle disease virus strains and isolates vary in their capacity and time taken to kill chick embryos. Virus titers are also influenced by strain, with the highest titers obtainable by those causing slow or no death (121). With some strains, embryo death and virus growth is affected by the presence of maternal antibodies in the yolk (105).

The route of inoculation is also important (45). Inoculation of NDV via the yolk sac, as compared with the allantoic cavity, produced more rapid embryo deaths and caused deaths by strains that do not consistently kill by the latter route (100). For other avian paramyxoviruses, yolk sac or amniotic inoculation may be the route of choice for isolation or replication (119, 209).

CELL CULTURES. Newcastle disease virus strains can replicate in an enormous range of cells. For example, Lancaster (166) listed 18 primary cell types and 11 cell lines as susceptible. Many more have been added to the list since his 1966 report. Cytopathic effects (CPE) are usually the formation of syncytia with subsequent cell death, with the CPE having some relationship to the strain's virulence for chickens (226). Plaque formation in chick embryo cells is restricted to velogenic and mesogenic viruses unless Mg^{2+} ions and DEAE (39) or trypsin (232) is added to the overlay.

Because of relatively poor growth of NDV and other paramyxoviruses in most cell culture systems, they are generally impracticable for virus propagation for most purposes.

Laboratory Host Systems for Avian Pneumovirus.

Initial problems in the laboratory diagnosis and determination of the etiology of TRT were due primarily to a lack of a suitable laboratory propagation system. The infectious nature of the disease could be demonstrated by typical clinical signs appearing in susceptible turkey poults placed in contact with infected birds or inoculated with filtered mucus from affected birds (24).

Inoculation of infective mucus into the yolk sac of turkey or chicken embryos resulted in embryo mortality after 4 or 5 passages, but virus was demonstrated to be at a very low titer (24). Similarly, inoculation of turkey or chicken tracheal organ cultures resulted in ciliostasis, but again, virus only replicated to low titers (112, 183). Isolates adapted to embryos or tracheal organ cultures, however, were capable of replication in cultures of chick embryo cells, turkey embryo cells, VERO cells, and BS-C-1 cells, with a characteristic cytopathic effect of syncytium formation and relatively high virus titers.

Pathogenicity

Newcastle Disease. The pathogenicity of NDV strains varies greatly with the host. Chickens are highly susceptible, but ducks and geese may be infected and show few or no clinical signs, even with strains lethal for chickens (142).

In chickens, the pathogenicity of NDV is determined chiefly by the strain of virus, although dose, route of administration, age of the chicken, and environmental conditions all have an effect. In general, the younger the chicken, the more acute the disease. With virulent viruses in the field, young chickens may experience sudden deaths without major clinical signs, while in older birds the disease may be more protracted and with characteristic clinical signs. Breed or genetic stock appears to have very little effect on the susceptibility of chickens to the disease (75). Natural routes of infection (nasal, oral, ocular) appear to emphasize the respiratory nature of the disease (44), while intramuscular, intravenous, and intracerebral routes appear to enhance the neurologic signs (45).

Avian Pneumovirus. Despite the high morbidity and often high mortality associated with TRT in the field, the pathogenicity of avian pneumovirus isolates has been difficult to assess in the laboratory. Experimentally infected birds often show recognizable signs of TRT, but these are milder than those seen in the field. Chickens show, at most, only mild respiratory disease in laboratory infections. An isolate of avian pneumovirus from chickens with SHS was able to produce TRT in infected turkey poults (221). Presumably, the difference in pathogenicity between laboratory and field infections is related to the conditions under which the birds are kept and the presence or absence of exacerbative organisms.

MOLECULAR BASIS FOR PATHOGENICITY. During the replication of NDV, it is necessary for the precursor glycoprotein F0 to be cleaved to F1 and F2 for the progeny virus particles to be infective (see 233). This posttranslation cleavage is mediated by host cell proteases (205). If cleavage fails to take place, noninfectious virus particles are produced. Trypsin is capable of cleaving F0 for all NDV strains and in vitro treatment of noninfectious virus will restore infectivity (206).

The importance of F0 cleavage was easily demonstrated, since viruses normally unable to replicate or produce plaques in cell culture systems were able to do both if trypsin was added to the agar overlay or culture fluid. While all viruses could replicate and produce infectious progeny in the allantoic cavity, the viruses pathogenic for chickens could replicate in a wide range of cell types in vitro with or without added trypsin, whereas strains of low virulence could replicate only when trypsin was added (231, 232). Thus, F0 molecules of virulent viruses can be cleaved by a host protease or proteases found in a wide range of cells and tissues, but F0 molecules in viruses of low virulence were restricted in their sensitivity and these viruses can grow only in certain host cell types.

The deduced amino acid sequences of the F0 precursor, obtained from nucleotide sequencing of the F gene for 17 NDV strains, were obtained by Collins et al. (78). These, with nine sequences published earlier (71, 114, 186, 199, 243, 265), enabled comparison of 11 viruses of low virulence and of 15 that were velogenic or mesogenic. For all viruses, the amino acid at residue 116, the C terminus of the F2 protein at the site of cleavage, was arginine. The viruses of low virulence all had leucine at residue 117, the N terminus of the F1 protein, and another basic amino acid at residue 113. In contrast, all velogenic or mesogenic viruses had phenylalanine at residue 117 and, with one exception, basic amino acids at residues 115 and 112 in addition to those at 113 and 116. The exception was the pigeon variant PMV-1 virus examined, which was identical to the virulent viruses but lacked a basic amino acid at position 112. Further studies have indicated that this variation was usual for pigeon variant PMV-1 viruses but had no significance in the variability of pathogenicity for chickens recorded with these viruses (80).

Thus, it would appear that the mechanism controlling the pathogenicity of NDV is very similar to that described for influenza viruses (274). The presence of additional basic amino acids in virulent strains means that cleavage can be effected by protease or proteases present in a wide range of host tissues and organs, but in lentogenic viruses, cleavage can occur only with proteases recognizing a single arginine, i.e., trypsinlike enzymes. Lentogenic viruses therefore only replicate in areas with trypsinlike enzymes, such as the respiratory and intestinal tracts, whereas virulent viruses can replicate in a range of tissues and organs, resulting in a fatal systemic infection (231).

Garten et al. (106) indicated that proteolytic activation of the HN glycoprotein also played a role in virulence. Although there are less data than for F, the sequences of the HN for several strains have been determined. It appears the HN0 precursor seen for the avirulent strains Ulster 2C (201) and D26 (242) is never produced in more virulent strains. The lentogenic Hitchner B1 (154); mesogenic Beaudette C (200); two velogenic strains, Australia Victoria (186) and Italien (275); and the pigeon variant virus (80), all have termination codons located before the end of the HN gene so the HN0 protein is not produced and posttranslational cleavage is not required.

PATHOGENESIS AND EPIZOOTIOLOGY

Natural and Experimental Hosts. From the available literature, Kaleta and Baldauf (155) concluded that in addition to the domestic avian species, natural or experimental infection with NDV has been demonstrated in at least 236 species from 27 of the 50 orders of birds. These authors stressed the variation in severity of clinical signs, even with different species of a genus. Nevertheless, they considered it possible to make tentative groupings based on susceptibility to the disease. The most resistant species appear to be aquatic birds, while the most susceptible are gregarious birds forming temporary or permanent flocks. There are far less data available with other avian paramyxoviruses. The general groups of birds reported to be infected with the different serotypes are shown in Table 20.1 and in more detailed reviews (6, 9). Isolations of avian paramyxoviruses from different species have been rarely associated with specific disease episodes. PMV-3 viruses have been related to disease in certain psittacine species such

as encephalitis with high mortality in parakeets of the *Neophema* and *Psephotus* genera (249), steatorrhea and pancreatic lesions in Neophema parakeets (271), and high mortality in lovebirds, *Agapornis roseicollis* (145). PMV-5 viruses appear to have a very limited host range being isolated only from budgerigars, *Melopsittacus undulatus,* in which infection resulted in high mortality (208).

Turkeys and chickens, apparently of any age, are known natural hosts of avian pneumovirus. Additionally, Picault et al. (221) found avian pneumovirus antibodies in flocks of guinea fowl (*Numida meleagris*) and were able to produce a rhinotracheitislike disease in this species with virus isolated from TRT-affected turkeys. In experimental infections with a TRT isolate, Gough et al. (124) demonstrated susceptibility with clinical signs in turkeys, chickens, and pheasants and an immune response to the virus in guinea fowl. Pigeons, geese, and ducks appeared to be refractory to the virus.

Transmission. In reviewing the modes of transmission of NDV between birds, Alexander (12) concluded that infection may take place by either inhalation or ingestion and that spread from one bird to another depends on the availability of the virus in an infectious form. It is tempting to assume that NDV is primarily transmitted by fine aerosols or large droplets that are inhaled by susceptible birds. Experimental evidence to prove this conclusively is, however, lacking. It is clear that infectious virus may be present in aerosols and that birds placed in an atmosphere containing such aerosols become infected. This is the basis for mass application of live vaccines by spray and aerosol generators (192). In naturally occurring infections, large and small droplets containing virus will be liberated from infected birds as a result of replication in the respiratory tract or as a result of dust and other particles, including feces. These virus-laden particles may be inhaled or impinge upon the mucous membranes, resulting in infection. The ability of such aerosols to form and to support infectious virus for a sufficient period for transmission, however, depends on many environmental factors.

During the course of infection of most birds with NDV, large amounts of virus are excreted in the feces. Ingestion of feces results in infection; this is likely to be the main method of bird-to-bird spread for avirulent enteric NDV and the pigeon variant virus (21), neither of which normally produces respiratory signs in infected birds.

Vertical transmission, i.e., passing of virus from parent to progeny via the embryo, is controversial. The true significance of such transmission in epizootics of Newcastle disease is not clear. Experimental assessment using virulent viruses is usually hampered by cessation of egg laying in infected birds. Infected embryos have been reported during naturally occurring infections of laying hens with virulent virus (45, 169), but this generally results in the death of the infected embryo during incubation. Cracked or broken infected eggs may serve as a source of virus for newly hatched chicks, as may virus-laden feces contaminating the outside of eggs. Virus may also penetrate the shell after laying (279), further complicating the assessment of true vertical or transovarian transmission. Infected chicks may be hatched from eggs infected with vaccinal or other lentogenic viruses that do not necessarily cause death of the embryo (81, 105). In naturally occurring infections, it is not clear how the embryos become infected, although La Sota vaccine has been shown to be present in most of the reproductive organs after vaccination (225).

Pospisil et al. (222) were able to demonstrate the presence of lentogenic virus in chick embryos and young progeny, including day-old chicks, of a vaccinated laying flock. Capua et al. (69), investigating the unexpected isolation of virulent virus from chick embryos, were able to isolate virulent NDV from cloacal swabs taken from the birds that had laid the eggs, despite high antibody titers to NDV, and from their hatched progeny.

The infectious nature of TRT was established by contact transmission from affected to susceptible turkey poults, or by inoculation with filtered or unfiltered mucus, nasal washings, or other materials from the respiratory tract of affected birds (178). Cook et al. (85) demonstrated that the virus was transmissible from infected to susceptible turkey poults placed in direct contact for a 9-day period after infection. These authors stressed the apparent importance of direct contact as, in their experiments, virus failed to spread to susceptible birds housed in the same room but in a different pen.

Spread. Lancaster and Alexander (12, 166, 169) reviewed the modes of spread of NDV. The following virus sources or methods have been implicated in various epizootics: 1) movement of live birds—feral birds, pet/exotic birds, game birds, racing pigeons, commercial poultry; 2) other animals; 3) movement of people and equipment; 4) movement of poultry products; 5) airborne spread; 6) contaminated poultry feed; 7) water; and 8) vaccines.

The importance of any of these factors will depend on the situation in which the epizootic occurs. In countries where poultry are kept exclusively in birdproof housing, the ability of feral birds to invade affected flocks and transfer the disease will be minimal, whereas birds kept on open range are more likely to be infected with strains carried by feral birds. In Canada and the northern United States, outbreaks of ND occurred in cormorants and pelicans in 1990 and 1992 (35, 269, 284). A virus,

indistinguishable from the cormorant viruses using MAB panels, was also isolated from turkeys showing signs of neurotropic velogenic ND that had been kept on range in the vicinity of diseased cormorants from which NDV had been isolated (269). Similarly, despite the huge international trade in exotic caged birds and the frequent isolation of virulent NDV from such birds (246), the threat of introduction and spread by this source (as in the California epizootic in 1971–72) (270) has been greatly reduced by strict importation quarantine procedures. Smuggled birds or those removed prematurely from quarantine may, however, still pose a threat (246), and since 1973, virulent NDV has been isolated from pet birds in the United States every year except 1978 and 1990 (214). There was particular concern in 1991 when outbreaks occurred in pet birds in six states (65, 214), but there was no spread to poultry. Airborne spread has been considered to be important in some epizootics such as the 1970–71 outbreaks in England (150) but unimportant in others such as the 1971–72 California outbreaks (270), even though the same virus appears to be involved.

In some cases, more than one factor combines in the spread of the disease. For example, the 1984 outbreaks of Newcastle disease in Great Britain were considered to be spread by feed that had been contaminated by infected feral pigeons (23).

Without doubt, the greatest potential for spread of NDV is by humans and their equipment. Humans may be infected in the conjunctival sac with NDV and this could pose a method of spread, but a more probable method is the mechanical transfer of infective material (most probably feces). Modern transportation enables personnel to travel rapidly to any country in the world, so spread by humans should not be treated as merely a local or national threat.

Vaccination crews moving from farm to farm have been implicated in the spread of NDV (270), as have incomplete inactivation (252) and contamination (47) of vaccines.

There is little information on the spread of other avian paramyxoviruses. For PMV-2 and PMV-3 serotypes, infection of poultry leads to shedding from the respiratory and intestinal tracts, so it is assumed that the methods of spread of NDV would also apply to these. PMV-2 viruses have been shown to infect feral passerines that may invade poultry houses, but in the absence of any wild bird host for PMV-3 viruses, it seems most likely that this subtype has been introduced into different countries by importation of infected poultry or by humans.

In most countries where TRT has appeared as a new disease, it has spread rapidly. For example, in the United Kingdom, the disease had been reported from most of the turkey-producing areas of England and Wales within 9 wk of the first outbreak of the disease (24). The methods by which such spread takes place are unclear, and even on a single site, spread is unpredictable. Contaminated water, movement of affected or recovered poults, movement of personnel and equipment, feed trucks, etc. have all been implicated in some outbreaks, while airborne spread or vertical transmission also have been put forward as possibilities. At present, only contact spread has been confirmed.

Incubation Period. The incubation period of ND after natural exposure has been reported to vary from 2 to 15 days (average 5–6). The speed with which signs appear, if at all, is variable depending on the infecting virus, the host species and its age and immune status, infection with other organisms, environmental conditions, the route of exposure, and the dose.

Clinical Signs, Morbidity, and Mortality

NEWCASTLE DISEASE. Newcastle disease virus isolates can be broadly grouped into pathotypes on the basis of clinical signs, which in turn are affected by the strain of virus. Other factors also important in establishing the severity of the disease are the host species, age, immune status, coinfection with other organisms, environmental stress, social stress, route of exposure, and the virus dose (184).

With extremely virulent viruses, the disease may appear suddenly, with high mortality occurring in the absence of other clinical signs. In outbreaks in chickens due to the VVND pathotype, clinical signs often begin with listlessness, increased respiration, and weakness, ending with prostration and death. During the panzootic caused by this type of virus in 1970–73, disease in some countries such as Great Britain (28) and Northern Ireland (184) was marked by severe respiratory signs, but in other countries these were absent. This type of ND may cause edema around the eyes and head. Green diarrhea is frequently seen in birds that do not die early in infection, and prior to death, muscular tremors, torticollis, paralysis of legs and wings, and opisthotonos may be apparent. Mortality frequently reaches 100% in flocks of fully susceptible chickens.

The neurotropic velogenic form of disease has been reported mainly from the United States. In chickens, it is marked by sudden onset of severe respiratory disease followed a day or 2 later by neurologic signs. Egg production falls dramatically, but diarrhea is usually absent. Morbidity may reach 100%. Mortality is generally considerably lower, although up to 50% in adult birds and 90% in young chickens have been recorded.

Mesogenic strains of NDV usually cause respiratory disease in field infections. In adult birds, there may be a marked drop in egg production that may last for several weeks. Nervous signs may occur but are not common. Mortality in fowl is usually low, except in very young susceptible birds, but may be considerably affected by exacerbating conditions.

Lentogenic viruses do not usually cause disease in adults. In young, fully susceptible birds, serious respiratory disease problems can be seen, often resulting in mortality, following infection with the more pathogenic La Sota strains with complicating infections. Vaccination or infection of broilers close to slaughter with these viruses can lead to colisepticemia or airsacculitis, with resulting condemnation.

The virus responsible for the panzootic in pigeons during the 1980s induced clinical signs in field infections of pigeons (272) and chickens (23) unlike those from other viruses. In both species, the predominant clinical features were diarrhea and nervous signs. In adult chickens, precipitous falls in egg production were seen while high mortality was recorded in younger birds. This virus did not induce respiratory signs in uncomplicated infections of pigeons or chickens.

The clinical signs produced by specific viruses in other hosts may differ widely from those seen in chickens. In general, turkeys are as susceptible as chickens to infection with NDV, but clinical signs are usually less severe (58, 184). Although readily infected, ducks and geese are usually regarded as resistant even to the strains of NDV most virulent for chickens. However, outbreaks of severe disease in ducks infected with NDV have been described (142). Outbreaks of virulent ND have been reported in most game bird species (166, 169) and the disease appears similar to that in chickens (50).

AVIAN PARAMYXOVIRUS TYPE 2. PMV-2 viruses have been associated with mild respiratory or inapparent diseases in chickens and turkeys (37, 62, 103). Unlike NDV, PMV-2 infections have been reported to be more severe in turkeys than chickens, and Lang et al. (170) reported severe respiratory disease, sinusitis, elevated mortality, and low egg production in turkey flocks infected with PMV-2 complicated by the presence of other organisms. PMV-2 viruses have been reported to be widespread in turkeys in Israel and associated with severe respiratory disease in complicated infections (176). In experiments conducted under field conditions, Bankowski et al. (38) demonstrated that PMV-2 infections of laying turkeys resulted in egg production losses with reduced hatchability and poult yield, but fertility was unaffected.

AVIAN PARAMYXOVIRUS TYPE 3. PMV-3 virus infections of domestic poultry appear to have been restricted to turkeys. Clinical signs are usually egg production problems, although these have been occasionally preceded by mild respiratory disease (19, 30, 34, 180, 267). Egg production usually declined rapidly with a large number of white-shelled eggs, although hatchability and fertility were rarely affected.

AVIAN PARAMYXOVIRUS TYPE 6. PMV-6 isolates have also been obtained from turkeys showing mild respiratory disease and egg production problems. Viruses of this serotype have been isolated frequently from domestic ducks in which the virus appears to be apathogenic (182, 247).

AVIAN PNEUMOVIRUS. Lister and Alexander (178) summarized the various clinical signs reported for TRT in general. Much of the variation reported may relate to the secondary adventitious organisms that frequently appear as a problem with TRT. Signs in young poults typically include snicking, rales, sneezing, nasal discharge (often frothy), foamy conjunctivitis, swelling of infraorbital sinuses, and submandibular edema. In laying birds, there may be a drop in egg production of up to 70% (259), along with slight respiratory distress. In some adult flocks of turkeys, serologic conversion to the virus has been recorded without any observation of clinical signs. When disease is seen, morbidity in birds of all ages is usually described as 100%, or very high. There is considerable variation in mortality, ranging from as low as 0.4% to as high as 90% of the flock. It is usually highest in young poults.

The clinical signs of SHS in broiler breeders were described by O'Brien (211) as swelling of the periorbital and infraorbital sinuses, torticollis, cerebral disorientation, and depression. Usually less than 4% of the flock were affected, although on occasions widespread respiratory signs were also present (286). Marked egg production losses have also been associated with SHS. Broiler chickens with confirmed avian pneumovirus infections have had more severe respiratory disease, and a greater proportion showing head swelling than has been seen in adult birds (204).

Gross Lesions. As with clinical signs, the gross lesions and the organs affected in birds infected with NDV are dependent on the strain and pathotype of the infecting virus, in addition to the host and all the other factors that may affect the severity of the disease. There are no pathognomonic lesions associated with any form of the disease. Gross lesions may also be absent.

Nevertheless, the presence of hemorrhagic lesions in the intestine of infected chickens has been used to distinguish VVND viruses from NVND viruses, a distinction of regulatory control importance in the diagnosis of ND in the United States (134, 139). These lesions are often particularly prominent in the proventriculus, ceca, and small intestine. They are markedly hemorrhagic and appear to result from necrosis of the intestinal wall or lymphoid foci such as cecal tonsils.

Generally, gross lesions are not observed in the central nervous system of birds infected with NDV, regardless of the pathotype (184).

Gross pathologic changes are not always present in the respiratory tract, but when observed they consist predominantly of hemorrhagic lesions and marked congestion of the trachea (14). Airsacculitis may be present even after infection with relatively mild strains, and thickening of the air sacs with catarrhal or caseous exudates is often observed (45).

Chickens and turkeys infected in lay with velogenic viruses usually reveal egg yolk in the abdominal cavity. The ovarian follicles are often flaccid and degenerative. Hemorrhage and discoloration of the other reproductive organs may occur.

Gross lesions of velogenic viscerotropic Newcastle disease in susceptible chickens inoculated by the eyedrop route are illustrated in Fig. 20.4.

Histopathology. The histopathology of NDV infections is as varied as the clinical signs and gross lesions, and can be greatly affected by the same parameters. In addition to the strain of virus and host, the method of infection may also be of paramount importance. For example, Beard and Easterday (44) were able to demonstrate similar histopathologic changes in the tracheas of chickens infected with either lentogenic or velogenic viruses by the aerosol route. Most published descriptions of the histologic changes following NDV infections are related to the virulent pathotypes and several descriptive reports or reviews of the literature have covered the histologic changes in the various organs during infection (44, 45, 184, 278). Briefly, the major changes are as follows.

NERVOUS SYSTEM. Lesions seen in the central nervous system are those of a nonpurulent encephalomyelitis with neuronal degeneration, foci of glial cells, perivascular infiltration of lymphocytes, and proliferation of endothelial cells. Lesions are usually seen in the cerebellum, medulla, mid brain, brain stem and spinal cord, but rarely in the cerebrum.

VASCULAR SYSTEM. Hyperemia, edema, and hemorrhage are found in the blood vessels of many organs. Other changes that may be seen consist of hydropic degeneration of the media, hyalinization of capillaries and arterioles, development of hyaline thrombosis in small vessels, and necrosis of endothelial cells of the vessels.

LYMPHOID SYSTEM. Regressive changes found in the lymphopoietic system consist of disappearance of lymphoid tissue. Hyperplasia of the reticulohisti-ocytic cells in various organs, especially the liver, may take place in subacute infections. Necrotic lesions are found throughout the spleen. Focal vacuolation and destruction of lymphocytes may be seen in the cortical areas and germinal centers of the spleen and thymus. Marked degeneration of the medullary region is seen in the bursa (257).

INTESTINAL TRACT. The hemorrhagic-necrotic lesions seen in the intestinal tract with infections of some virulent forms of ND appear to develop in lymphoid aggregates. Other lesions are related to changes in the vascular system.

RESPIRATORY TRACT. The effect of NDV infection on membranes of the upper respiratory tract may be severe and related to the degree of respiratory distress. Lesions may extend throughout the length of the trachea. Cilia may be lost within 2 days of infection. In the mucosa of the upper respiratory tract, congestion, edema, and dense cellular infiltration of lymphocytes and macrophages may be seen, particularly following aerosol exposure (44). The process appears to clear rapidly, and birds examined as early as 6 days after infection may be free from inflammation.

Cheville et al. (73) infected birds with two U.S. viscerotropic isolates, Texas 219 and Florida Largo. Marked lesions of the lung were seen with both viruses, the former producing hyperemia and edema of the parabronchi, the latter more extensive lesions consisting of hemorrhage and erythrophagocytosis in the alveolar areas of the parabronchi.

Edema, cell infiltration, and increased thickness and density of the air sacs may occur in chickens.

Avian Pneumovirus. Experimental avian pneumovirus infection of turkeys resulted in deciliation of the trachea beginning 48 hr after intranasal infection and resulting in complete removal of cilia by 96 hr after infection (153). Cytoplasmic eosinophilic inclusions were reported in the ciliated epithelial cells of the nasal cavities and trachea in experimentally infected turkey poults (112), and these lesions were seen in both turkeys and chickens 7 days after infection (221).

REPRODUCTIVE SYSTEM. Histopathologic changes in the reproductive tract are extremely variable. Biswal and Morrill (53) reported that the greatest functional damage was to the uterus or shell-forming portion of the oviduct. Changes in female reproductive organs included atresia of follicles with infiltration of inflammatory cells and formation of lymphoid aggregates. Similar aggregates were present in the oviduct.

20.4. Gross lesions of velogenic viscerotropic Newcastle disease in susceptible chickens inoculated by the eyedrop route. *A.* Facial edema. *B.* Hemorrhage, congestion, and conjunctivitis in reflected eyelid. *C-D.* Splenic necrosis on the capsular surface (*C*) and cut surface (*D*). *E-F.* Necrosis and hemorrhage in intestinal lymphoid aggregates evident from the serosal surface (*E*) and mucosal surface (*F*). *G.* Enlarged and necrotic cecal tonsils. *H.* Peritonitis with fibrin deposition. *I.* Ovarian follicles with hemorrhagic stigmata. *J.* Hemorrhage in the mucosa of the proventriculus. (*A-I*, King and Swayne; *J*, Beard)

OTHER ORGANS. Small focal areas of necrosis are seen in the liver and, sometimes with hemorrhage, in the gallbladder and heart. Lymphocyte infiltration has been reported in the pancreas. In infections with the viscerotropic velogenic viruses hemorrhage and ulceration of the skin may occur, and congestion and petechiae of the combs and wattle are common. Conjunctival lesions may be associated with hemorrhage.

Immunity. There have been few attempts to study the immune response in avian pneumovirus or other avian paramyxovirus infections; therefore, this section is restricted to NDV.

CELL-MEDIATED IMMUNITY. The initial immune response to infection with NDV is cell mediated and may be detectable as early as 2–3 days after infection with live vaccine strains (109, 263). This presumably explains the early protection against challenge that has been recorded in vaccinated birds before a measurable antibody response is seen (27, 118). The importance of cell-mediated immunity in protection conferred by vaccines is not clear, and a strong secondary response to challenge similar to the antibody response does not seem to occur (263).

HUMORAL IMMUNITY. Antibodies capable of protecting the host can be measured in VN tests. Since the VN response appears to parallel the HI response, however, the latter test is frequently used to assess protective response, especially after vaccination (28). Antibodies directed against either of the functional surface glycopolypeptides, the HN and the F polypeptides, can neutralize NDVs (234). In fact, MABs specific for epitopes on the F polypeptide have been shown to induce greater neutralization than those directed against HN in in vitro and in vivo tests (194, 196). Therefore, the successful reliance on the simple HI test to assess protection up to now may have been fortuitous.

When chickens survive NDV infection long enough, antibodies are usually detectable in the serum within 6–10 days. The levels largely depend

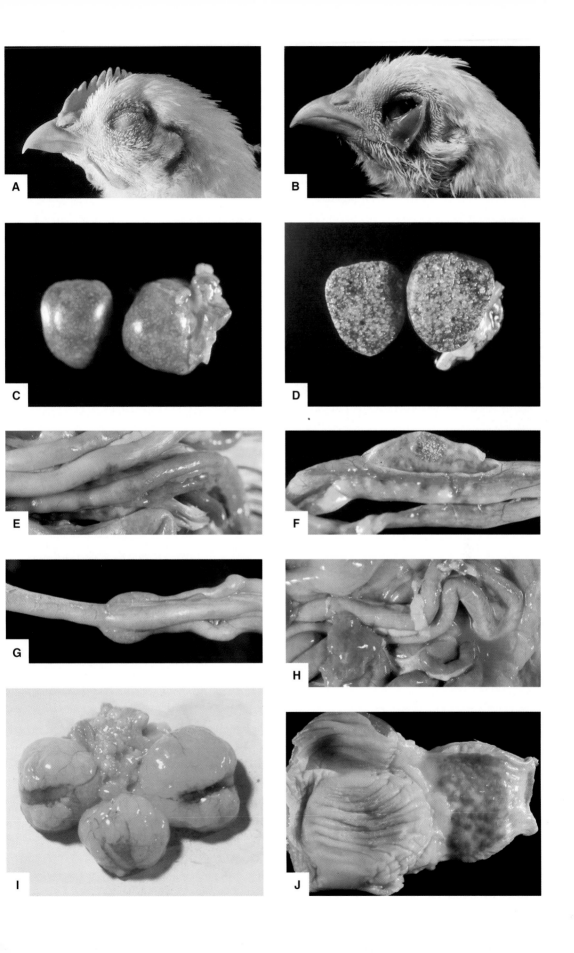

on the infecting strain, but generally, peak response is at about 3–4 wk. Decline in antibody titer varies with the titer achieved but is much slower than their development. Hemagglutination inhibition antibodies may remain detectable for up to 1 yr in birds recovered from infection with mesogenic viruses or after a series of immunizations. Reinfection or immunization some weeks after the titer begins to decline produces a secondary response (28).

LOCAL IMMUNITY. Antibodies appear in secretions of the upper respiratory tract and intestinal tract of chickens at about the time humoral antibodies can be first detected. In the upper respiratory tract, the immunoglobulins appear to be chiefly IgA with some IgG (216). Similar excretions occur in the Harderian gland following ocular, but not parenteral, infection (216, 223). Malkinson and Small (181) demonstrated effective local immunity when they found that birds may be susceptible to infection at one site but protected at another. The exact function of local immunity in protection is not clear, although a role in protection of the respiratory tract independent of humoral immunity has been proposed (148). Intraocular vaccination with Hitchner B1 resulted in replication of virus in the Harderian gland, which could be prevented by the presence of maternal IgG in lachrymal fluid (235). Replication of virus in the Harderian gland resulted in the production of lachrymal IgG, IgA, and IgM (235). In particular, the Harderian gland became the main site for IgA-antibody forming cells in the chicken (238). Russell and Ezeifeka (237) stressed that IgM may be the class of antibody most actively involved in the clearance of virus in intraocular infections.

PASSIVE IMMUNITY. Hens with antibodies to NDV will pass these on to their progeny via the egg yolk (141). Levels of antibody in day-old chicks will be directly related to titers in the parent. Allan et al. (28) estimated that each twofold decay in maternally derived HI titer takes about 4.5 days. Maternal immunity is protective and, thus, must be taken into account when timing primary vaccination of chicks.

IMMUNOSUPPRESSION. Suppression of the immune response has important effects on both the pathogenicity of infecting NDV strains and the protection levels achieved by vaccination. Under natural conditions immunosuppression may occur due to infection with other viruses such as infectious bursal disease virus. The subsequent immunodeficiency may result in a more severe disease caused by some NDV strains and a failure to respond adequately to vaccination (101, 111, 217, 230). Immunosuppression from chicken infectious anemia virus also has been implicated in the failure of

chickens to respond well to secondary inactivated NDV vaccine (61).

DIAGNOSIS.   The objective in the diagnosis of ND is to reach a decision on whether or not to impose control measures. None of the clinical signs or lesions of ND may be regarded as pathognomonic, and the wide variation in disease with virus strain, host species, and other factors means that at best, these can only serve as a suggestion of ND. Similarly, the presence of lentogenic NDV strains in birds in most countries and the almost universal use of live vaccines means that mere demonstration of infection, without definition of the infecting virus, is rarely adequate cause for control measures to be imposed. Additionally, ND may cause such devastating epizootics and can have such far-reaching effects on trade in poultry products that control measures are usually defined at a national or international level.

Serology.   The presence of specific antibodies to NDV in the serum of a bird gives little information on the infecting strain of NDV and, therefore, has limited diagnostic value.

Nevertheless, in certain circumstances the demonstration that infection has taken place is sufficient for the needs of the diagnostician. Postvaccinal serology can be used to confirm successful application of vaccine and an adequate immune response by the bird.

SEROLOGIC TESTS FOR NEWCASTLE DISEASE VIRUS ANTIBODIES. Antibodies to Newcastle disease virus may be detected in poultry sera by a variety of tests including single radial immunodiffusion (74), single radial hemolysis (140), agar gel precipitin (107), VN in chick embryos (43), and plaque neutralization (45). Enzyme-linked immunosorbent assays (ELISA), which lend themselves to semiautomated techniques, have become popular, especially as part of flock screening procedures (251), and a variety of such tests have been described (5, 193, 198, 229, 250, 282). Good correlation has been reported between ELISA and HI tests (5, 63, 92). Conventionally, antibodies to NDV and the other avian paramyxoviruses have been detected and quantitated by the HI test. Many methods for HA and HI tests have been described.

Sera from other species (including turkeys) may cause low-titer, nonspecific agglutination of chicken RBCs, complicating the test. Such agglutination may be removed by adsorption with chicken RBCs before testing.

The HA and HI tests are not greatly affected by minor changes in the methodology, although Brugh et al. (64) stressed the critical nature of the antigen/antiserum incubation period in test standardization. Surveys have not always reported good reproducibility in HI tests among different laboratories (46).

SEROLOGIC TESTS FOR OTHER AVIAN PARAMYX-OVIRUSES. The same serologic tests used for NDV (PMV-1) can be used for the other avian paramyxoviruses. PMV-5 viruses have been reported as not agglutinating RBCs (208). Gough et al. (125) reported, however, the isolation of virus clearly related to PMV-5 viruses that agglutinated guinea pig RBCs well and chick RBCs to a lesser extent. Hemagglutination inhibition antibodies to PMV-3 viruses may be detected in turkeys and chickens showing high vaccine-induced titers to NDV, and ND-vaccinated birds infected with PMV-3 viruses show a rise in HI titer to both viruses (19, 61).

SEROLOGIC TESTS FOR AVIAN PNEUMOVIRUS. Antibodies to avian pneumovirus may be detected in standard VN tests in organ cultures (40) or chicken embryo fibroblast (CEF) microcultures (120). Immunofluorescence assays (40), and immunodiffusion tests with *N*-lauroylsarcosine-disrupted virus (120), also can detect antibodies. The most frequently used method to assess antibodies to avian pneumovirus, however, has been the ELISA (40, 72, 112, 126, 285).

Direct Detection of Viral Antigens.
Immunohistologic techniques offer a rapid method for the specific demonstration of the presence of virus or viral antigens in organs or tissues. Immunofluorescence techniques for thin sections of trachea (144) or impression smears (190) and an immunoperoxidase technique for thin sections (132, 179) have been described and used in NDV infections.

Virus Isolation of Newcastle Disease Virus.
At present, the only unequivocal method of ND diagnosis, which also allows characterization of the infecting strain, is virus isolation.

CULTURE SYSTEM. Virulent ND viruses can be propagated in many cell culture systems, and viruses of low virulence can be induced to replicate in some of them. It is possible to use primary cell cultures or even cell lines for routine isolation of NDV. The embryonated chicken egg, however, represents an extremely sensitive and convenient vehicle for the propagation of NDV and is used almost universally in diagnosis.

Embryonated chicken eggs should be obtained from a specific-pathogen–free (SPF) flock and incubated for 9–10 days at 37 C before use. If SPF eggs cannot be obtained, eggs from a flock free of

NDV antibodies should be used. It is possible to propagate NDV strains in eggs containing yolk antibodies, but the virus titer is usually greatly reduced and such eggs should be avoided for diagnostic use.

SAMPLES. The two main sites of replication of NDV in infected poultry appear to be the respiratory and intestinal tracts, so specimens taken should always include either feces, intestinal contents or cloacal swabs, and tracheal swabs or trachea depending on the circumstances. Other specimens taken from carcasses should reflect the clinical signs prior to death and organs obviously affected.

Newcastle disease virus is relatively stable for long periods in nonputrefying tissues provided the ambient temperature is low (166). Gough et al. (123), however, considered the transport of samples in a frozen or chilled state as very important in virus isolation. Omojola and Hanson (212) suggested that bone marrow may be a useful sample in countries where transport is slow, temperatures high, and refrigeration not available, as they were able to isolate virus from this site after several days at 30 C.

ISOLATION METHOD. Ideally, each sample should be treated separately. It is common, however, to pool organ and tissue samples, although tracheal and fecal samples are best kept separate. Antibiotic media is used to make 20% w/v suspensions of feces or finely minced tissues and organs. Swabs are placed in sufficient antibiotic medium to ensure full immersion.

The suspensions are held at room temperature for 1–2 hr, then centrifuged at 1000 g for 10 min. Each of five embryonated eggs should then be inoculated with 0.2 mL of the supernatant fluid into the allantoic cavity. The eggs are placed at 37 C and examined regularly.

Eggs dead or dying, or after a minimum of 4 days and a maximum of 7 days, should be chilled to 4 C and the allantoic/amniotic fluid harvested. The presence of virus can be detected by an HA test; nonhemagglutinating fluids should be passaged at least one more time. Hemagglutination may be caused by bacteria, and possible contamination should be assessed by culture. If bacteria are present, the contaminated fluids can be passed through a 450-nm membrane filter before repassaging in eggs.

ISOLATION OF OTHER AVIAN PARAMYX-OVIRUSES. The samples taken and methods involved for the isolation of other avian paramyxoviruses are identical to those for NDV. Inoculation of 6- to 7-day-old embryonated eggs via the yolk sac should also be considered, as greater success has been reported for this route with some viruses. PMV-5 viruses do not grow after inoculation into the allantoic cavity and require amniotic inoculation of embryonating eggs or propagation in primary cultures of chick embryo cells (208).

ISOLATION AND IDENTIFICATION OF AVIAN PNEUMOVIRUS. Initially, virus isolation proved extremely difficult due to the fastidious nature of the virus, the frequency with which other organisms could be isolated, and the timing of the virus isolation attempts (178). Successful virus isolation was achieved in chicken or turkey embryos or chicken organ cultures and these have been used on a routine basis.

CHOICE AND TIMING OF SAMPLES FOR ISOLATION. Although virus has been isolated from trachea, lung, and viscera of affected turkey poults, by far the most fruitful source of virus has been nasal secretions or tissue scraped from the sinuses of affected birds. It is extremely important to obtain samples as early as possible after infection. Isolation of virus is rarely successful from birds showing severe signs; presumably the extreme signs are a result of secondary, adventitious bacterial infections in birds predisposed by earlier virus infection. This probably accounts for the lack of success in isolating virus from chickens with SHS, as the characteristic signs appear to be due to secondary *Escherichia coli* infection.

ISOLATION PROCEDURES. Twenty-percent (v/v) suspensions of nasal secretions/exudate and sinus material in phosphate-buffered saline containing antibiotics are held at room temperature for 1–2 hr, clarified by centrifugation at 1000 x g for 10 min, and then passed through a 450-nm porosity membrane filter. Six- to 7-day-old, specific-pathogen-free (SPF) embryonated chicken eggs should be inoculated via the yolk sac. Tracheal organ cultures from chick embryos or young chicks are susceptible to infection, but those from turkeys are generally more sensitive and should be used if they are from a SPF flock, or at least a flock free of specific antibodies. Blind passages should be made using allantoic-amniotic fluid harvested 10 days after inoculation, or supernatant fluids from tracheal organ cultures 7 days after inoculation. On passage in eggs, the virus first causes stunting of the embryo; after 4–5 passages, it consistently causes death. In organ cultures, the virus may cause ciliostasis within 2–3 passages.

Viruses adapted so that they are lethal to embryos or cause rapid ciliostasis generally grow to only very low titers. At this stage they are usually capable of growth in CEF cell cultures, although production of full cytopathic effects may require further passaging in CEF cells. Viruses adapted to CEF cultures grow to high titers, enabling electron microscopy and VN tests with specific antiserum to confirm the identity of the virus. As an alternative, VN tests for confirmatory diagnosis may be done in tracheal organ cultures, observing inhibition of ciliostasis by specific antiserum.

Differential Diagnosis. Viral HA activity may be due to any of the nine avian paramyxovirus serotypes or any of the 15 influenza type A hemagglutinin subtypes that are known to infect birds. Demonstration that the virus is of a specific serotype can usually be carried out by a simple HI test with specific polyclonal antisera.

Newcastle disease virus (PMV-1) shows some cross-reaction in HI tests with several of the other avian paramyxovirus serotypes, especially PMV-3 psittacine isolates, using polyclonal antisera (11). While the potential for misdiagnosis can largely be eliminated by the use of control sera and antigens in conventional tests, the use of MABs in routine diagnosis can give an unequivocal result.

Virus Characterization. For ND, the widespread presence of lentogenic strains in feral birds and the use of such viruses as live vaccines means that isolation of NDV is rarely sufficient to confirm a diagnosis of disease. For such confirmation and to meet statutory requirements that may be in force (51), further virus characterization such as pathogenicity testing is necessary.

PATHOGENICITY TESTS. The importance and impact of an NDV isolate will be directly related to the virulence of that isolate. Since field disease may be an unreliable measure of the true virulence of the virus, it is necessary to carry out laboratory assessment of the pathogenicity of the virus. At present, three in vivo tests are used for this purpose: 1) mean death time (MDT) in eggs, 2) ICPI, and 3) IVPI. Examples of the values obtained in these three methods are shown for some well-characterized NDV strains in Table 20.2.

Some modifications of these tests have been made for specific purposes. For example, Hanson (134) used a method similar to the IVPI test, which involved swabbing the cloaca and conjunctiva of 8-wk-old chickens with undiluted allantoic fluid to distinguish between VVND viruses and other velogenic viruses.

Although these pathogenicity tests have proved invaluable in distinguishing between vaccine, enzootic, and epizootic viruses during outbreaks, there are some drawbacks to the tests and difficulties in the interpretation of results. For example, Pearson et al. (218) reported 10 NDV isolates from pigeons to have ICPI values between 1.2 and 1.45 and a range of IVPI values of 0 to 1.3, suggesting the viruses to be at least mesogenic; however, the

Table 20.2.   Examples of pathogenicity indices obtained for strains of Newcastle disease virus

Virus Strain	Pathotype	ICPI[a]	IVPI[b]	MDT[c]
Ulster 2C	Lentogenic	0.0	0.0	>150
Queensland V4	Lentogenic	0.0	0.0	>150
Hitchner B1	Lentogenic	0.2	0.0	120
F	Lentogenic	0.25	0.0	119
La Sota	Lentogenic	0.4	0.0	103
H	Mesogenic	1.2	0.0	48
Mukteswar	Mesogenic	1.4	0.0	46
Roakin	Mesogenic	1.45	0.0	68
Beaudette C	Mesogenic	1.6	1.45	62
GB Texas	Velogenic	1.75	2.7	55
NY Parrot 70181 1972	Velogenic	1.8	2.6	51
Italien	Velogenic	1.85	2.8	50
Milano	Velogenic	1.9	2.8	50
Herts '33/56	Velogenic	2.0	2.7	48
Pigeon/England/561/83		1.5	0.0	120
Chicken/England/702/84		1.9	2.1	60

Note: Data from (10, 28).
[a] ICPI, intracerebral pathogenicity index in day-old chicks.
[b] IVPI, intravenous pathogenicity index in 6-week-old chickens.
[c] MDT, mean death time (hr) for chicken embryos infected with one minimum lethal dose of virus.

lowest MDT recorded was 98 hr, a characteristic of lentogenic viruses. In addition, work by Alexander and Parsons (17) on NDV (PMV-1) isolates from pigeons showed that both ICPI and IVPI values increased after passage through chickens or embryonated chicken eggs. This suggests that isolates from birds other than poultry may not show their potential virulence for chickens in conventional pathogenicity tests.

IN VITRO TESTS FOR PATHOGENICITY.   Only NDVs possessing additional basic amino acids at the cleavage site of the fusion protein are rendered infectious by nontrypsinlike proteases. Rott, therefore, suggested (232) that the ability of NDV isolates to form plaques in cell culture systems in the absence of trypsin represents a simple in vitro method for the detection of virulent viruses.

VIRUS PROPERTY PROFILES.   Newcastle disease virus isolates show a marked variation in biologic and biochemical properties (see Etiology), and some workers used these properties to develop distinct profiles enabling the grouping of viruses for the purposes of diagnosis (45, 134). Under specific circumstances, single properties of the virus may be sufficient to distinguish between avirulent and virulent isolates and be usefully employed in diagnosis.

MONOCLONAL ANTIBODIES.   In addition to their use in routine diagnosis, panels of MABs can be employed to characterize and group isolates by establishing profiles. Such typing on an antigenic basis represents a powerful tool for the diagnostician and epizootiologist, allowing rapid grouping and differentiation of NDV isolates (26, 234).

PREVENTION AND CONTROL.   Regardless of whether control is applied at the international, national, or farm levels, the objective is either to prevent susceptible birds from becoming infected or to reduce the number of susceptible birds by vaccination. For the former strategy, each method of disease spread must be considered in prevention policies.

International Control Policies.   The raising of poultry and trade in their products are now organized on an international basis, frequently under the management of multinational companies. There is a desire to trade both poultry products and genetic stock. The threat of ND, however, has proved to be a great restraint on such trade. Bennejean (51) considered that worldwide control of ND will be approached only if all countries report outbreaks within their borders to international agencies. International agreements on these and other points are not simple, owing to the enormous variation in the extent of disease surveillance in different countries.

A prerequisite to formulating control policies, particularly internationally, would be agreement on what constitutes disease and to what viruses control policies should apply. Some countries do not vaccinate and would not want any form of NDV introduced to their domestic poultry. Others allow only specific live vaccines and consider some vaccines to be unacceptably virulent. Yet other countries have the continued presence of circulating highly virulent virus, which is not seen as overt disease because of vaccination. Bennejean (51) suggested that any infection with virus having an ICPI greater than 0.7 should be reported as an outbreak of ND. Such a definition would probably be acceptable in countries where only lentogenic and inactivated vaccines are used, but completely unacceptable where mesogenic vaccines are used or where enzootic mesogenic viruses exist. Nevertheless, this definition has been adopted by countries of the European Union for the application of statutory control measures (89).

National Control Policies.   At the national level, control policies are directed at prevention of introduction of virus and prevention of spread within the country. To prevent the introduction of NDV, most countries have restrictions on trade in poultry products, eggs, and live poultry; these vary greatly.

Because of the link between exotic caged birds

and the spread of ND during the 1970–74 panzootic (104, 273), and the known ability of psittacine birds to excrete NDV for many weeks after infection (98), most importing countries have established quarantine procedures for importations.

The panzootic of ND (PMV-1) in racing pigeons in the 1980s (272) produced a unique situation, in view of the potential spread to poultry (281). Due to the large number of international pigeon races that take place each year, national policies were created in some countries including banning of races, restricting races, or enforcing vaccination of participating pigeons.

In many countries legislation exists to control ND outbreaks that may occur. Some countries have adopted eradication policies with compulsory slaughter of infected birds, their contacts and products. Such policies usually include restrictions of movement or marketing of birds within a defined quarantine area around the outbreak. Others require prophylactic vaccination of birds even in the absence of outbreaks, while some have a policy of "ring vaccination" around outbreaks to establish a buffer zone.

Higgins and Shortridge (143) stressed the importance of tailoring control policies to the country and warned against the dogmatic application of policies successful in one country to another that may differ socially, economically, and climatically.

Control and Prevention at the Farm Level.
Possibly the most important factors in preventing the introduction of NDV and its spread during outbreaks are the conditions under which the birds are reared and the degree of biosecurity practiced at the farm. Chapter 1 provides a comprehensive discussion of disease prevention through sanitation and security practices.

Control for Other Avian Paramyxoviruses.
Few, if any, countries have national control policies for the other avian paramyxoviruses, although, in some, vaccination is permitted for PMV-3 viruses. Thus, despite the frequent isolation of PMV-2 and PMV-3 viruses from passerine and psittacine birds in quarantine (9), little is usually done to restrict the introduction of such birds.

At the farm level, birdproofing of poultry houses should greatly reduce the possibility of introduction of paramyxoviruses such as PMV-2 by feral birds. Other preventive measures taken for NDV will equally apply to the other PMV types. Lang et al. (170) suggested depopulation for turkey flocks infected with PMV-2 virus if complicated by other organisms.

Control for Avian Pneumovirus.
Turkey rhinotracheitis is greatly exacerbated by poor management practices such as inadequate ventilation, overstocking, poor litter conditions, poor general hygiene, and mixed age groups (93, 259). Debeaking or vaccination with live NDV, if done at a critical time, might also increase the incidence and severity of clinical signs and mortality. Andral et al. (31) stressed the difficulty in eradicating TRT from multiage sites where complete cleaning and disinfection cannot take place.

Attempts to treat TRT and SHS with antibiotics have met with varied success. Some success in reducing the severity of the disease with an antibiotic regimen, presumably by controlling secondary adventitious bacteria, has been reported (93, 130). Similar attempts at treatment of the disease in Great Britain, however, met with little success (32, 260).

Newcastle Disease Vaccination.
Ideally, vaccination against ND would result in immunity against infection and replication of the virus. Realistically, ND vaccination usually protects the bird from the more serious consequences of disease, but virus replication and shedding may still occur, albeit at a reduced level (127, 215, 270).

Allan et al. (28) have produced a comprehensive description of all aspects of ND vaccination and vaccine production. More recently, detailed reviews have been published by Meulemans (192) on the use of vaccination in the control of ND, by Cross (91) on vaccine production, and by Thornton (262) on quality control of vaccines.

It should be emphasized that there are no circumstances in which vaccination can be regarded as an alternative to good management practice, biosecurity, or good hygiene in rearing domestic poultry.

HISTORICAL ASPECTS OF VACCINATION. Early studies demonstrated that inactivated infective material conferred protection on inoculated chickens, but problems in production and standardization discouraged its use on a large scale. Studies in the 1930s on the attenuation of virulent NDV strains by Iyer and Dobson led to the development of mesogenic vaccine strains that are still in use in some parts of the world (128, 152).

The identification of ND in the United States led, initially, to the use of inactivated vaccines (147). The later observation that some of the enzootic viruses produced only mild disease resulted in the development of the mesogenic live vaccine Roakin (49) and, subsequently, the milder Hitchner B1 (146) and La Sota (115) strains, which are now the most widely used vaccines.

Inactivated vaccines, usually with the virus adsorbed to aluminum hydroxide, were most widely used in Europe up to the 1970–74 panzootic, but their poor performance resulted in adoption of live vaccination with B1 and La Sota in most countries.

This panzootic also supplied the impetus for the development of modern inactivated vaccines based on oil-emulsions, which have proven highly effective.

VACCINATION POLICIES. Some governments have legislation affecting the use and quality control of vaccines. Policies vary enormously, in line with the enzootic status or perceived threat of ND. Some countries, such as Denmark, ban the use of any vaccine, while others, e.g., The Netherlands, enforce vaccination of all poultry. Countries of the European Union have legislated to define the pathogenicity of viruses that will be allowed for use as vaccines in Member States. The Master Seed of live vaccines must be tested, under specified dose conditions, and shown to have an ICPI value of less than 0.4, while the Master Seed of viruses used in inactivated vaccines must have an ICPI value less than 0.7 (90).

LIVE VACCINES

Virus Strains. It is convenient to divide live NDV vaccines into two groups, lentogenic and mesogenic, the mesogenic being suitable only for secondary vaccination of birds due to their greater virulence (Table 20.3). Even within the lentogenic group, however, there is a considerable range in virulence, as demonstrated by Borland and Allan (54) who developed a stress index test to assess the potential effects of vaccines on susceptible chickens. The immune response increases as the pathogenicity of the live vaccine increases(227). Therefore, to obtain the desired level of protection without serious reaction, vaccination programs are needed that involve sequential use of progressively more virulent viruses, or live virus followed by inactivated vaccine. Commonly used live vaccines and their pathogenicity indices for chickens are listed in Table 20.3.

Application of Live Vaccines. The objective of live vaccines is to establish an infection in the flock, preferably in each bird at the time of application. Individual bird treatments such as intranasal instillation, eyedrop, and beak-dipping are often used for lentogenic vaccines. Mesogenic vaccines usually require inoculation by wing-web stabbing or intramuscular injection.

The main appeal of live vaccines is that they may be administered by inexpensive mass application techniques. Probably the most common method of application used worldwide is via the drinking water. Generally, water is withheld from the birds for a number of hours and then vaccine is applied in fresh drinking water at concentrations carefully calculated to give each bird a sufficient dose. Addition of vaccine to header tanks has also been used successfully. Drinking water application must be carefully monitored as the virus may be inactivated by excessive ambient heat, impurities in the water, and even the type of pipes or vessels used to distribute the drinking water. To some extent, virus viability can be stabilized by the addition of dried skim milk powder to the drinking water (108).

Mass application of live vaccines by sprays and aerosols is also very popular due to the ease with which large numbers of birds can be vaccinated in a short time. It is important to achieve the correct size of particles by controlling the conditions under which the aerosol is generated (28, 192). Aerosol application is usually limited to secondary vaccination to avoid severe vaccine reactions. Coarse sprays of large particles do not penetrate deeply into the respiratory tract of birds and give less reaction, so these may be more suitable for the mass application of vaccine to young birds. Coarse spraying of chicks at day-old may result in the establishment of infection in the flock with the vaccinal virus despite maternally derived immunity. It is believed, however, that in these circumstances, infections are es-

Table 20.3. Newcastle disease viruses used as live vaccines

Virus	Pathotype	ICPI[a]	IVPI[b]	Derivation	Recommended use in chickens	Routes[c]
Strain H	Mesogenic	1.4	0.0	Laboratory attenuated by passage in eggs	Secondary	im,sc
Mukteswar	Mesogenic	1.4	0.0	Laboratory attenuated by passage in eggs	Secondary	im,sc
Komarov	Mesogenic	1.4	0.0	Laboratory attenuated by intra-cerebral passage in ducklings	Secondary	im,sc,io
Roakin	Mesogenic	1.45	0.0	Field isolate	Secondary	im,ww
La Sota	Lentogenic	0.4	0.0	Field isolate	Secondary	in,io,dw,sp,aer
F (Asplin)	Lentogenic	0.25	0.0	Field isolate	Primary	in,io,dw,sp,aer
Hitchner B1	Lentogenic	0.2	0.0	Field isolate	Primary	in,io,dw,sp,aer,bd
V4	Lentogenic	0.0	0.0	Field isolate	Primary	in,io,sp,aer,oral

[a] ICPI, intracerebral pathogenicity index in day-old chicks.
[b] IVPI, intravenous pathogenicity index in 6-wk-old chickens.
[c] aer = aerosol, bd = beak dipping, dw = drinking water, im = intramuscular, in = intranasal, io = intraocular, oral = in food, sc = subcutaneous, sp = coarse spray, ww = wing web.

tablished by the nasal or ocular route as a result of head rubbing on the backs of other birds and not necessarily directly by the spray (192). Aerosol and coarse-spray generators are available commercially (162); in the United States, a cabinet for coarse-spraying of day-old chicks is widely used (110).

A vaccine, based on the Australian V4 virus, has been developed specifically for use in village flocks in tropical countries. The recommended method of administration of the vaccine is in coated, pelleted feed that is fed to the chickens. Initial laboratory and field trials suggest that this method is efficacious (87), but later studies have recorded problems probably related to the type of feed used as a vehicle (255).

Advantages and Disadvantages of Live Virus Vaccination. Live vaccines are usually sold as freeze-dried allantoic fluid from infected embryonated eggs and are relatively inexpensive and easy to administer and lend themselves to mass application. Local immunity is stimulated by infection with live viruses, and protection occurs very soon after application. Vaccine viruses may spread from birds that have been successfully vaccinated to those that have not.

There are several disadvantages, the most important of which is that the vaccine may cause disease, depending upon environmental conditions and the presence of complicating infections. Because of this, it is important to use extremely mild virus for primary vaccination and, as a result, multiple applications of vaccine(s) are usually needed. Maternally derived immunity may prevent successful primary vaccination with live virus. Although the ability of vaccinal virus to spread may be an advantage within the flock, spread to susceptible flocks, especially on multiage sites can cause severe disease problems, particularly if dual infections with exacerbating organisms occur. Live vaccines may be easily killed by chemicals and heat and, if not carefully controlled during production, can contain contaminating viruses.

INACTIVATED VACCINES

Production Methods. Inactivated vaccines are usually produced from infective allantoic fluid treated with ß-propiolactone or formalin to kill the virus and then mixed with a carrier adjuvant. Early inactivated vaccines used aluminum hydroxide adjuvants but the development of oil emulsion–based vaccines proved a major advancement. Different oil-emulsion vaccines vary in their formulation of emulsifiers, antigen, and water-to-oil ratios; most now use mineral oil (91).

Various seed viruses used in the production of the oil-emulsion vaccines include Ulster 2C, B1, La Sota, Roakin, and several virulent viruses. The selection criterion should be the amount of antigen produced when the virus is grown in embryonated eggs. Apathogenic viruses grow to the highest titers (122); therefore, it would seem an unnecessary risk to use a virus virulent for chickens.

One or more other antigens may be incorporated into the emulsion with NDV, and bivalent or polyvalent vaccines may include infectious bronchitis virus, infectious bursal disease virus, egg drop syndrome virus, and reovirus (192).

Application of Inactivated Vaccines. Inactivated vaccines are administered by injection, either intramuscularly or subcutaneously.

Advantages and Disadvantages of Inactivated Vaccines. Inactivated vaccines are far easier to store than viable vaccines. They are expensive to produce and to apply because of the labor needed for their application. The labor expense can be partly offset by the use of polyvalent vaccines. Inactivated oil-emulsion vaccines are not as adversely affected by maternal immunity as live vaccines and can be used in day-old chicks (59). Quality control of inactivated vaccines is often difficult, and mineral oils may cause serious problems to the vaccinator if accidentally injected (258). The major advantages of inactivated vaccine are the very low level of adverse reactions in vaccinated birds, the ability to use them in situations unsuited for live vaccines, especially if complicating pathogens are present, and the extremely high levels of protective antibodies of long duration that can be achieved.

VACCINATION PROGRAMS. Vaccination programs and vaccines may be controlled by government policies. They should always be tailored to suit the prevailing disease situation and other factors, which include availability of vaccine, maternal immunity, use of other vaccines, presence of other organisms, size of flock, expected life of the flock, available labor, climatic conditions, past vaccination history, and cost.

Timing of vaccination of broiler chickens can be especially difficult due to the presence of maternal antibodies. Because of their short life, broiler chickens are sometimes not vaccinated in countries where there is a low risk of ND.

Vaccination of laying hens always requires more than one dose of vaccine to maintain immunity through their lives (28). Actual programs depend on local conditions. In many countries, local customs or circumstances result in too little vaccination, overvaccination, or mistiming of vaccination, all of which may have serious consequences. The problems and pressures that may face the poultry farmer in tropical developing countries can frequently result in what has been described as "vaccine abuse" (143).

INTERPRETATION OF VACCINE RESPONSE. For NDV, the immune response is usually estimated by the HI titers obtained. Single vaccination with live lentogenic virus will produce a response in susceptible birds of about 2^4 to 2^6, but HI titers as high as 2^{11} or more may be obtained following a vaccination program involving oil-emulsion vaccine. The actual titers obtained and their relationship to the degree and duration of immunity for any given flock and program are difficult to predict. Allan et al. (28) presented predictions of the outcome of challenge of vaccinated young chickens with highly virulent NDV.

VACCINATION OF OTHER POULTRY. Although vaccines developed primarily for chickens may be used effectively in other species, some differences in response may be apparent. For example, turkeys generally show a lower response and as a result, they are often vaccinated first with La Sota followed by oil-emulsion vaccine (60). There is, however, some evidence that La Sota may cause some reaction in the respiratory tract (192), and that aerosol vaccination with lentogenic viruses causes pathologic lesions of the trachea (1). There is still considerable investigation into vaccination programs involving live and inactivated vaccines for use in turkeys (158, 164).

Guinea fowl and partridges have been successfully vaccinated with La Sota and/or oil-emulsion vaccines. Considerable investigation into the most suitable vaccines and regimens for pigeons has taken place due to the panzootic occurring in these birds during the 1980s (272).

FUTURE DEVELOPMENTS. Recently developed molecular biology technology has enabled a much greater understanding of the pathogenicity (233) and antigenicity (234) of NDV and enabled cloning of the genes most closely involved (199). Groups working in this area have reported protective immunization with the HN gene expressed in recombinant fowl poxvirus (55) and recombinant avian cells (88) or the F gene expressed in recombinant fowl poxvirus (56, 261), vaccinia virus (197), pigeon poxvirus (172), and turkey herpesvirus (203).

The capacity of MABs to detect antigenic variation in NDV isolates may have an important application in assessing antigenic relationships between field and vaccine viruses and ensuring close similarity between the two.

VACCINATION FOR OTHER AVIAN PARAMYXOVIRUSES. The other avian paramyxoviruses do not cause overt disease with high mortality and,

thus, their economic impact is considerably less than NDV. Nevertheless, the egg production problems that have been associated with infections of turkeys by PMV-3 viruses can be sufficiently severe to warrant vaccination, and for several years, oil-emulsion vaccines to this serotype have been available in Europe and the United States (57, 99). They appear to be effective at preventing the serious egg production losses associated with PMV-3 infections in laying turkeys.

VACCINATION FOR AVIAN PNEUMOVIRUSES. Both inactivated and live attenuated vaccines are now available commercially. Problems in reproducing the diseases in the laboratory made work on attenuation difficult, but several groups have now reported the attenuation of TRT virus and the effective use of such viruses as vaccines (68, 82, 83, 84, 280).

Live and inactivated TRT virus–based vaccines have been used in both turkeys and chickens, but results in the field have been variable (171, 213). Currently, it is not clear whether apparent vaccine failures are due to antigenic variation reported in avian pneumoviruses (see above), interference by concurrent infections with other, possibly immunosuppressive, organisms, or some other cause.

REFERENCES

1. Abdul-Aziz, T.A., and L.H. Arp. 1983. Pathology of the trachea in turkeys exposed by aerosol to lentogenic strains of Newcastle disease virus. Avian Dis 27:1002–1011.

2. Abenes, G.B., H. Kida, and R. Yanagawa. 1983. Avian paramyxoviruses possessing antigenically related HN but distinct M proteins. Arch Virol 77:71–76.

3. Abenes, G.B., H. Kida, and R. Yanagawa. 1986. Biological activities of monoclonal antibodies to the hemagglutinin-neuraminidase (HN) protein of Newcastle disease virus. Jpn J vet Sci 48:353–362.

4. Ackerman, W.W. 1964. Cell surface phenomena of Newcastle disease virus. In R.P. Hanson (ed.). Newcastle disease virus an evolving pathogen. University of Wisconsin Press, Madison, WI, pp. 153–166.

5. Adair, B.M., M.S. McNulty, D. Todd, T.J. Connor, and K. Burns. 1989. Quantitative estimation of Newcastle disease virus antibody levels in chickens and turkeys by ELISA. Avian Pathol 18:175–192.

6. Alexander, D.J. 1980. Avian Paramyxoviruses. Vet Bull 50:737–752.

7. Alexander, D.J. 1982. Avian paramyxoviruses—other than Newcastle disease virus. World Poult Sci J 38:97–104.

8. Alexander, D.J. 1985. Avian Paramyxoviruses. Proc 34th West Poult Dis Conf, pp. 121–125.

9. Alexander, D.J. 1986. The classification, host range and distribution of avian paramyxoviruses. In J.B. McFerran and M.S. McNulty (eds.). Acute Virus Infections of Poultry. Martinus Nijhoff, Dordrecht, The Netherlands, pp. 52–66.

10. Alexander, D.J. 1988. Historical Aspects. In D.J. Alexander (ed.). Newcastle Disease. Kluwer Academic Publishers, Boston, MA, pp. 1–10.

11. Alexander, D.J. 1988. Newcastle Disease Virus—An Avian Paramyxovirus. In D.J. Alexander (ed.). Newcastle Disease. Kluwer Academic Publishers, Boston, MA, pp. 11–22.

12. Alexander, D.J. 1988. Newcastle Disease: Methods of

Spread. In D.J. Alexander (ed.). Newcastle Disease. Kluwer Academic Publishers, Boston, MA, pp. 256–272.

13. Alexander, D.J. 1995. Newcastle disease in countries of the European Union. Avian Pathol 24:545–551.

14. Alexander, D.J., and W.H. Allan. 1974. Newcastle disease virus pathotypes. Avian Pathol 3:269–278.

15. Alexander, D.J., and N.J. Chettle. 1978. Relationship of parakeet/Netherlands/449/75 virus to other avian paramyxoviruses. Res Vet Sci 25:105–106.

16. Alexander, D.J., and M.S. Collins. 1981. The structural polypeptides of avian paramyxoviruses. Arch Virol 67:309–323.

17. Alexander, D.J., and G. Parsons. 1986. Pathogenicity for chickens of avian paramyxovirus type 1 isolates obtained from pigeons in Great Britain during 1983–1985. Avian Pathol 15:487–493.

18. Alexander, D.J., N.J. Chettle, and G. Parsons. 1979. Resistance of chickens to challenge with the virulent Herts '33 strain of Newcastle disease virus induced by prior infection with serologically distinct avian paramyxoviruses. Res Vet Sci 26:198–201.

19. Alexander, D.J., M. Pattisson, and I. Macpherson. 1983. Avian paramyxoviruses of PMV-3 serotype in British turkeys. Avian Pathol 12:469–482.

20. Alexander, D.J., V.S. Hinshaw, M.S. Collins, and N. Yamane. 1983. Characterization of viruses which represent further distinct serotypes (PMV-8 and PMV-9) of avian paramyxoviruses. Arch Virol 78:29–36.

21. Alexander, D.J., G. Parsons, and R. Marshall. 1984. Infection of fowls with Newcastle disease virus by food contaminated with pigeon faeces. Vet Rec 115:601–602.

22. Alexander, D.J., P.H. Russell, G. Parsons, E.M.E. Abu Elzein, A. Ballough, K. Cernik, B. Engstrom, M. Fevereiro, H.J.A. Fleury, M. Guittet, E.F. Kaleta, U. Kihm, J. Kosters, B. Lomniczi, J. Meister, G. Meulemans, K. Nerome, M. Petek, S. Pokomunski, B. Polten, M. Prip, R. Richter, E. Saghy, Y. Samberg, L. Spanoghe, and B. Tumova. 1985. Antigenic and biological characterisation of avian paramyxovirus type 1 isolates from pigeons—an international collaborative study. Avian Pathol 14:365–376.

23. Alexander, D.J., G.W.C. Wilson, P.H. Russell, S.A. Lister, and G. Parsons. 1985. Newcastle disease outbreaks in fowl in Great Britain during 1984. Vet Rec 117:429–434.

24. Alexander, D.J, E.D. Borland, C.D. Bracewell, N.J. Chettle, R.E. Gough, S.A. Lister, and P.J. Wyeth. 1986. A preliminary report of investigations into turkey rhinotracheitis in Great Britain. State Vet J 40:161–169.

25. Alexander, D.J., J.S. Mackenzie, and P.H. Russell. 1986. Two types of Newcastle disease virus isolated from feral birds in Western Australia detected by monoclonal antibodies. Aust Vet J 63:365–367.

26. Alexander, D.J., R.J. Manvell, P.A. Kemp, G. Parsons, M.S. Collins, S. Brockman, P.H. Russell, and S.A. Lister 1987. Use of monoclonal antibodies in the characterisation of avian paramyxovirus type 1 (Newcastle disease virus) isolates submitted to an international reference laboratory. Avian Pathol 16:553–565.

27. Allan, W.H., and R.E. Gough. 1976. A comparison between the haemagglutination inhibition and complement fixation tests for Newcastle disease. Res Vet Sci 20:101–103.

28. Allan, W.H., J.E. Lancaster, and B. Toth. 1978. Newcastle disease vaccines—their production and use. FAO Animal Production and Health Series No. 10. FAO, Rome, Italy.

29. Anderson, C., R. Kearsley, D.J. Alexander, and P.H. Russell. 1987. Antigenic variation in avian paramyxovirus type 3 detected by mouse monoclonal antibodies. Avian Pathol 16:691–698.

30. Andral, B., and D. Toquin. 1984. Infectious a myxovirus: Chutes de ponte chez les dindes reproductrices I Infections par les paramyxovirus aviaires de type III. Recl Med Vet 160:43–48.

31. Andral, B., C. Louzis, D. Trap, J.A. Newman, D. Toquin, and G. Bennejean. 1985. Respiratory disease (rhinotracheitis) in turkeys in Brittany, France, 1981–1982. I. Field observation and serology. Avian Dis 29:35–42.

32. Anonymous. 1985. Turkey rhinotracheitis of unknown etiology in England and Wales. Vet Rec 117:653–654.

33. Asplin, F.D. 1952. Immunisation against Newcastle disease with a virus of low virulence (Strain F) and observations on subclinical infection in partially resistant fowls. Vet Rec 64:245–249.

34. Bahl, A.K., and M.L. Vickers. 1982. Egg drop syndrome in breeder turkeys associated with turkey para-influenza virus-3 (TPIV-3). Proc 31st West Poult Dis Conf, p. 113.

35. Banerjee, M., W.M. Reed, S.D. Fitzgerald, and B. Panigrahy. 1994. Neurotropic velogenic Newcastle disease in cormorants in Michigan: Pathology and virus characteristion. Avian Dis 38:873–878.

36. Bankowski, R.A., R.E. Corstvet, and G.T. Clark. 1960. Isolation of an unidentified agent from the respiratory tract of chickens. Science 132:292–293.

37. Bankowski, R.A., R.D. Conrad, and B. Reynolds. 1968. Avian influenza and paramyxoviruses complicating respiratory disease diagnosis in poultry. Avian Dis 12:259–278.

38. Bankowski, R.A., J. Almquist, and J. Dombrucki. 1981. Effect of paramyxovirus Yucaipa on fertility, hatchability and poult yield of turkeys. Avian Dis 25:517–520.

39. Barahona, H.H., and R.P. Hanson. 1968. Plaque enhancement of Newcastle disease virus (lentogenic strains) by magnesium and diethylaminoethyl dextran. Avian Dis 12:151–158.

40. Baxter-Jones, C., J.K.A. Cook, J.A. Frazier, M. Grant, R.C. Jones, A.P.A. Mockett, and G.P. Wilding. 1987. Close relationship between TRT virus isolates. Vet Rec 120:562.

41. Beach, J.R. 1942. Avian pneumoencephalitis. Proc Annu Meet US Livestock Sanit Assoc 46:203–223.

42. Beach, J.R. 1944. The neutralization in vitro of avian pneumoencephalitis virus by Newcastle disease immune serum. Science 100:361–362.

43. Beard, C.W. 1980. Serologic Procedures. In S.B. Hitchner, C.H. Domermuth, H.G. Purchase, and J.E. Williams (eds). Isolation and Identification of Avian Pathogens. American Association of Avian Pathologists, Kennett Square, PA, pp. 129–135.

44. Beard, C.W., and B.C. Easterday. 1967. The influence of route of administration of Newcastle disease virus on host response. J Infect Dis 117:55–70.

45. Beard, C.W., and R.P. Hanson. 1984. Newcastle Disease. In M.S. Hofstad, H.J. Barnes, B.W. Calnek, W.M. Reid, H.W. Yoder (eds.). Diseases of Poultry, 8th ed. Iowa State University Press, Ames, IA, pp. 452–470.

46. Beard, C.W., and W.J. Wilkes. 1985. A comparison of Newcastle disease hemagglutination-inhibition test results from diagnostic laboratories in the southeastern United States. Avian Dis 29:1048–1056.

47. Beard, P.D., J. Spalatin, and R.P. Hanson. 1970. Strain identification of NDV in tissue culture. Avian Dis 14:636–645.

48. Beaudette, F.R., and J.J. Black. 1946. Newcastle disease in New Jersey. Proc Annu Meet US Livestock Sanit Assoc 49:49–58.

49. Beaudette, F.R., J.A. Bivins, and B.R. Miller. 1949. Newcastle disease immunization with live virus. Cornell Vet 39:302–334.

50. Beer, J.V. 1976. Newcastle disease in the pheasant, Phasianus colchicus, in Britain. In L.A. Page (ed.). Wildlife Diseases. Plenum Press, New York, pp. 423–430.

51. Bennejean, G. 1988. Newcastle disease: Control policies. In D.J. Alexander (ed.). Newcastle Disease. Kluwer Academic Publishers, Boston, MA, pp. 303–317.

52. Biancifiori, F., and A. Fioroni. 1983. An occurrence of

Newcastle disease in pigeons: Virological and serological studies on the isolates. Comp Immunol Microbiol Infect Dis 6:247–252.

53. Biswal, G., and C.C. Morrill. 1954. The pathology of the reproductive tract of laying pullets affected with Newcastle disease. Poult Sci 33:880–897.

54. Borland, L.J., and W.H. Allan. 1980. Laboratory tests for comparing live lentogenic Newcastle disease vaccines. Avian Pathol 9:45–59.

55. Boursnell, M.E.G., P.F. Green, A.C.R. Samson, J.I. Campbell, A. Deuter, R.W. Peters, N.S. Millar, P.T. Emmerson, and M.M. Binns. 1990. A recombinant fowlpox virus expressing the hemagglutinin-neuraminidase gene of Newcastle disease virus (NDV) protects chickens against challenge by NDV. Virology 176:297–300.

56. Boursnell, M.E.G., P.F. Green, J.I. Campbell, A. Deuter, R.W. Peters, F.M. Tomley, A.C.R. Samson, P. Chambers, P.T. Emmerson, and M.M. Binns. 1990. Insertion of the fusion gene from Newcastle disease virus into a non-essential region in the terminal repeats of fowlpox virus and demonstration of protective immunity induced by the recombinant. J Gen Virol 71:621–628.

57. Box, P. 1987. PMV3 disease of turkeys. Int Hatch Prac 2:4–7.

58. Box, P.G., B.I. Helliwell, and P.H. Halliwell. 1970. Newcastle disease in turkeys. Vet Rec 86:524–527.

59. Box, P.G., I.G.S. Furminger, W.W. Robertson, and D. Warden. 1976. The effect of Marek's disease vaccination on the immunisation of day-old chicks against Newcastle disease, using B1 and oil emulsion vaccine. Avian Pathol 5:299–305.

60. Box, P.G., I.G.S. Furminger, W.W. Robertson, and D. Warden. 1976. Immunisation of maternally immune turkey poults against Newcastle disease. Avian Pathol 5:307–314.

61. Box, P.G., H.C. Holmes, A.C. Bushell, and P.M. Finney. 1988. Impaired response to killed Newcastle disease vaccine in chicken possessing circulating antibody to chicken anaemia agent. Avian Pathol 17:713–723.

62. Bradshaw, G.L., and M.M. Jensen. 1979. The epidemiology of Yucaipa virus in relationship to the acute respiratory disease syndrome in turkeys. Avian Dis 23:539–542.

63. Brown, J., R.S. Resurreccion, and T.G. Dickson. 1990. The relationship between the hemagglutination-inhibition test and the enzyme-linked immunosorbent assay for the detection of antibody to Newcastle disease. Avian Dis 34:585–587.

64. Brugh, M., C.W. Beard, and W.J. Wilkes. 1978. The influence of test conditions on Newcastle disease hemagglutination-inhibition titers. Avian Dis 22:320–328.

65. Bruning-Fann, C., J. Kaneene, and J. Heamon. 1992. Investigation of an outbreak of velogenic viscerotropic Newcastle disease in pet birds in Michigan, Indiana, Illinois and Texas. J Am Vet Med Assoc 2011:1709–1714.

66. Burnet, F.M. 1942. The affinity of Newcastle disease virus to the influenza virus group. Aust J Exp Biol Med Sci 20:81–88.

67. Buys, S.B., and J.H. Du Preez. 1980. A preliminary report on the isolation of a virus causing sinusitis in turkeys in South Africa and attempts to attenuate the virus. Turkeys (June):36,46.

68. Buys, S.B., J.H. Du Preez, and H.J. Els. 1989. The isolation and attenuation of a virus causing rhinotracheitis in turkeys in South Africa. Onderstepoort J Vet Res 56:87–98.

69. Capua, I., M. Scacchia, T. Toscani, and V. Caporale. 1993. Unexpected isolation of virulent Newcastle disease virus from commercial embryonated fowls' eggs. J Vet Med B 40:609–612.

70. Cavanagh, D., and T. Barrett. 1988. Pneumovirus-like characteristics of the mRNA and proteins of turkey rhinotracheitis virus. Virus Res 11:241–256.

71. Chambers, P., N.S. Millar, and P.T. Emmerson. 1986. Nucleotide sequence of the gene encoding the fusion glyco-

protein of Newcastle disease virus. J Gen Virol 67:2685–2694.

72. Chettle, N.J., and P.J. Wyeth. 1988. The use of an ELISA test to detect antibodies to turkey rhinotracheitis. Br Vet J 144:282–287.

73. Cheville, N.F., H. Stone, J. Riley, and A.E. Ritchie. 1972. Pathogenesis of virulent Newcastle disease in chickens. J Am Vet Med Assoc 161:169–179.

74. Chu, H.P., G. Snell, D.J. Alexander, and G.C. Schild. 1982. A single radial immunodiffusion test for antibodies to Newcastle disease virus. Avian Pathol 11:227–234.

75. Cole, R.K., and F.B. Hutt. 1961. Genetic differences in resistance to Newcastle disease. Avian Dis 5:205–214.

76. Collins, M.S., and R.E. Gough. 1988. Characterisation of a virus associated with turkey rhinotracheitis. J Gen Virol 69:909–916.

77. Collins, M.S., D.J. Alexander, S. Brockman, P.A. Kemp, and R.J. Manvell. 1989. Evaluation of mouse monoclonal antibodies raised against an isolate of the variant avian paramyxovirus type 1 responsible for the current panzootic in pigeons. Arch Virol 104:53–61.

78. Collins, M.S., J.B. Bashiruddin, and D.J. Alexander. 1993. Deduced amino acid sequences at the fusion protein cleavage site of Newcastle disease viruses showing variation in antigenicity and pathogenicity. Arch Virol 128:363–370.

79. Collins, M.S., R.E. Gough, and D.J. Alexander. 1993. Antigenic differentiation of avian pneumovirus isolates using polyclonal antisera and mouse monoclnal antibodies. Avian Pathol 22:469–479.

80. Collins, M.S., I. Strong, and D.J. Alexander. 1994. Evaluation of the molecular basis of pathogenicity of the variant Newcastle disease viruses termed `pigeon PMV-1 viruses.' Arch Virol 134:403–411.

81. Coman, I. 1963. Possibility of the elimination of strain F virus of Asplin (1949) in the eggs of inoculated hens. Lucr Inst Past Igiena Anim Buc 12:337–344.

82. Cook, J.K.A., and M.M. Ellis. 1990. Attenuation of turkey rhinotracheitis virus by alternative passage in embryonated chicken eggs and tracheal organ cultures. Avian Pathol 19:181–185.

83. Cook, J.K.A., M.M. Ellis, C.A. Dolby, H.C. Holmes, P.M. Finney, and M.B. Huggins. 1989. A live attenuated turkey rhinotracheitis vaccine. 1. Stability of the attenuated strain. Avian Pathol 18:511–522.

84. Cook, J.K.A., H.C. Holmes, P.M. Finney M.M. Ellis, M.B. Huggins, and C.A. Dolby. 1989. A live attenuated turkey rhinotracheitis virus vaccine. 2. The use of the attenuated strain as an experimental vaccine. Avian Pathol 18:523–534.

85. Cook, J.K.A., M.M. Ellis, and M.B. Huggins. 1991. The pathogenesis of turkey rhinotracheitis virus in turkey poults inoculated with the virus alone or together with two strains of bacteria. Avian Pathol 119:181–185.

86. Cook, J.K.A., B.V. Jones, M.M. Ellis, J. Li, and D. Cavanagh. 1993. Antigenic differentiation of strains of turkey rhinotracheitis virus using monoclonal antibodies. Avian Pathol 22:257–273.

87. Copland J.W. 1987. Newcastle disease in poultry. A new food pellet vaccine. Aust Centre for Int Agric Res Monogr No 5. ACIAR, Canberra.

88. Cosset, F-L., J-F. Bouquet, A. Drynda, Y. Chebloune, A. Rey-Senelonge, G. Kohen, V.M. Nigon, P. Desmettre, and G. Verdier. 1991. Newcastle disease virus (NDV) vaccine based on immunization with avian cells expressing the NDV hemagglutinin-neuraminidase glycoprotein. Virology 185:862–866.

89. Council of the European Communities 1992. Council Directive 92/66/EEC of 14 July 1992 introducing Community measures for the control of Newcastle disease. Off J Eur Commun L260:1–20.

90. Council of the European Communities. 1993. Com-

mission Decision of 8. February 1993 laying down the criteria to be used against Newcastle disease in the context of routine vaccination programmes. Off J Eu Commun L59:35.

91. Cross, G.M. 1988. Newcastle disease—vaccine production. In D.J. Alexander (ed.). Newcastle Disease. Kluwer Academic Publishers, Boston, MA, pp. 333–346.

92. Cvelic-Cabrilo, V., H. Mazija, Z. Bidin, and W.L. Ragland. 1992. Correlation of haemagglutination inhibition and enzyme-linked immunosorbent assays for antibodies to Newcastle disease virus. Avian Pathol 21:509–512.

93. Dayon, J.F., and F. Pecquerie. 1982. Rhinotracheite 81 de la dinde: le constat sur le terrain. L'Aviculteur 423:65–70.

94. Dinter, Z., S. Hermodsson, and L. Hermodsson. 1964. Studies on myxovirus Yucaipa: Its classification as a member of the paramyxovirus group. Virology 22:297–304.

95. Doyle, T.M. 1927. A hitherto unrecorded disease of fowls due to a filter-passing virus. J Comp Pathol Therap 40:144–169.

96. Doyle, T.M. 1935. Newcastle disease of fowls. J Comp Pathol Therap 48:1–20.

97. Erdei, J., J. Erdei, K. Bachir, E.F. Kaleta, K.F. Shortridge, and B. Lomniczi. 1987. Newcastle disease vaccine (La Sota) strain specific monoclonal antibody. Arch Virol 96:265–269.

98. Erickson, G.A. 1976. Viscerotropic velogenic Newcastle disease in six pet bird species: Clinical response and virus-host interactions. PhD Dissertation. Iowa State University, Ames, IA.

99. Eskelund, K.H. 1988. Vaccination of turkey breeder hens against paramyxovirus type 3 infection. Proc 37th West Poult Dis Conf, pp. 43–45.

100. Estupinan, J., J. Spalatin, and R.P. Hanson. 1968. Use of yolk sac route of inoculation for titration of lentogenic strains of NDV. Avian Dis 12:135–138.

101. Faragher, J.T., W.H. Allan, and P.J. Wyeth. 1974. Immunosuppressive effect of infectious bursal disease agent in vaccination against Newcastle disease. Vet Rec 95:385–388.

102. Food and Agriculture Organisation. 1985. In M. Bellver-Gallent (ed.). Animal Health Yearbook, FAO Animal Production and Health Series No. 25. FAO, Rome, Italy.

103. Franciosi, C., P.N. D'Aprile, and M. Petek. 1981. Isolamento di un paramixovirus Yucaipa dal tacchino. Boll Ist Sieroter Milan 60:225–228.

104. Francis, D.W. 1973. Newcastle and psittacines, 1970–71. Poult Dig 32:16–19.

105. French, E.L., T.D. St George, and J.J. Percy. 1967. Infection of chicks with recently isolated Newcastle disease viruses of low virulence. Aust Vet J 43:404–409.

106. Garten, W., W. Berk, Y. Nagai, R. Rott, and H-D. Klenk. 1980. Mutational changes of the protease susceptibility of glycoprotein F of Newcastle disease virus: Effects on pathogenicity. J Gen Virol 50:135–147.

107. Gelb, J., and C.G. Cianci. 1987. Detergent-treated Newcastle disease virus as an agar gel precipitin test antigen. Poult Sci 66:845–853.

108. Gentry, R.F., and M.O. Braune. 1972. Prevention of virus inactivation during drinking water vaccination of poultry. Poult Sci 51:1450–1456.

109. Ghumman, J.S., and R.A. Bankowski. 1975. In vitro DNA synthesis in lymphocytes from turkeys vaccinated with LaSota, TC and inactivated Newcastle disease vaccines. Avian Dis 20:18–31.

110. Giambrone J.J. 1985. Laboratory evaluation of Newcastle disease vaccination programs for broiler chickens. Avian Dis 29:479–487.

111. Giambrone, J.J., C.S. Eidson, R.K. Page, O.J. Fletcher, B.O. Barger, and S.H. Kleven. 1976. Effect of infectious bursal agent on the response of chickens to Newcastle disease and Marek's disease vaccination. Avian Dis 20:534–544.

112. Giraud, P., G. Bennejean, M. Guittet, and D. Toquin.
1986. Turkey rhinotracheitis in France: Preliminary investigations on a ciliostatic virus. Vet Rec 118:81.

113. Giraud, P., F.X. Le Gros, D. Toquin, J.F. Bouquet, and G. Bennejean. 1988. Turkey rhinotracheitis: Viral identification of the causal agent. Proc 37th West Poult Dis Conf, pp. 61–62.

114. Glickman, R.L., R.J. Syddall, R.M. Iorio, J.P. Sheehan, and M.A. Bratt. 1988. Quantitative basic residue requirements in the cleavage-activation site of the fusion glycoprotein as a determinant of virulence for Newcastle disease virus. J Virol 62:354–356.

115. Goldhaft, T.M. 1980. Historical note on the origin of the La Sota strain of Newcastle disease virus. Avian Dis 24:297–301.

116. Gomez-Lillo, M., R.A. Bankowski, and A.D. Wiggins. 1974. Antigenic relationships among viscerotropic velogenic and domestic strains of Newcastle disease virus. Am J Vet Res 35:471–475.

117. Goodman, B.B., and R.P. Hanson. 1988. Isolation of avian paramyxovirus-2 from domestic and wild birds in Costa Rica. Avian Dis 32:713–717.

118. Gough, R.E., and D.J. Alexander. 1973. The speed of resistance to challenge induced in chickens vaccinated by different routes with a B1 strain of live NDV. Vet Rec 92:563–564.

119. Gough, R.E., and D.J. Alexander. 1983. Isolation and preliminary characterisation of a paramyxovirus from collared doves (Streptopelia decaocto). Avian Pathol 12:125–134.

120. Gough, R.E., and M.S. Collins. 1989. Antigenic relationships of three turkey rhinotracheitis viruses. Avian Pathol 18:227–238.

121. Gough, R.E., W.H. Allan, D.J. Knight, and J.W.G. Leiper. 1974. The potentiating effect of an interferon inducer (BRL 5907) on oil-based inactivated Newcastle disease vaccine. Res Vet Sci 17:280–284.

122. Gough, R.E., W.H. Allan, and D. Nedelciu. 1977. Immune response to monovalent and bivalent Newcastle disease and infectious bronchitis inactivated vaccines. Avian Pathol 6:131–142.

123. Gough, R.E., D.J. Alexander, M.S. Collins, S.A. Lister, and W.J. Cox. 1988. Routine virus isolation or detection in the diagnosis of diseases of birds. Avian Pathol 17:893–907.

124. M.S. Collins, W.J. Cox, and N.J. Chettle. 1988. Experimental infection of turkeys, chickens, ducks, geese, Guinea fowl, pheasants and pigeons with turkey rhinotracheitis virus. Vet Rec 123:58–59.

125. Gough, R.E., R.J. Manvell, S.E.N. Drury, P.F. Naylor, D. Spackman, and S.W. Cooke. 1993. Deaths in budgerigars associated with a paramyxovirus-like agent. Vet Rec 133:123.

126. Grant, M., C. Baxter-Jones, and G.P. Wilding. 1987. An enzyme-linked immunosorbent assay for the serodiagnosis of turkey rhinotracheitis infection. Vet Rec 120:279–280.

127. Guittet, M., H. Le Coq, M. Morin, V. Jestin, and G. Bennejean. 1993. Proceedings of the Xth World Veterinary Poultry Association Congress, Sydney, 1993. p 179.

128. Haddow, J.R., and J.A. Idnani. 1946. Vaccination against Newcastle (Ranikhet) disease. Indian J Vet Sci 16:45–53.

129. Hafez, H.M. 1992. Comparative investigation on turkey rhinotracheitis (TRT) virus isolates from different countries. Dtsch Tierarztl Woshenschr 99:486–488.

130. Hafez, H.M., J. Emele, and H. Woernle. 1990. Rhinotracheitis der puten (TRT): Serologische Verfolgungsuntersuchung, wirtschaftliche parameter sowie Erfahrung mit dem Einsatz von Enrofloxacin zur Bekampfungder sekundarinfektionen. Tierarztl Umschau 45:111–114.

131. Halasz, F. 1912. Contributions to the knowledge of fowlpest. Vet Doctoral Dissertation. Commun Hungar Roy Vet Schl. Patria, Budapest, pp. 1–36.

132. Hamid, H., R.S.F. Campbell, C.M. Lamihhane, and R. Graydon. 1988. Indirect immunoperoxidase staining for Newcastle disease virus (NDV). Proc 2nd Asian/Pacific Poult Health Conf. Australitan Veterinary Poultry Association, Sydney, Australia, pp. 425–427.

133. Hanson, R.P. 1975. Newcastle disease. In S.B. Hitchner, C.H. Domermuth, H.G. Purchase, and J.E. Williams (eds.). Isolation and Identification of Avian Pathogens. American Association of Avian Pathologists, Kennett Square, PA, pp. 160–173.

134. Hanson, R.P. 1980. Newcastle disease. In S.B. Hitchner, C.H. Domermuth, H.G. Purchase, and J.E. Williams (eds.), Isolation and Identification of Avian Pathogens. American Association of Avian Pathologists, Kennett Square, PA, pp. 63–66a.

135. Hanson, R.P. 1988. Heterogeneity within strains of Newcastle disease virus: Key to survival. In D.J. Alexander (ed.). Newcastle Disease. Kluwer Academic Publishers, Boston, MA, pp. 113–130.

136. Hanson, R.P., and C.A. Brandly. 1955. Identification of vaccine strains of Newcastle disease virus. Science 122:156–157.

137. Hanson, R.P., and J. Spalatin. 1978. Thermostability of the hemagglutinin of Newcastle disease virus as a strain marker in epizootiological studies. Avian Dis 22:659–665.

138. Hanson, R.P., E. Upton, C.A. Brandly, and N.S. Wilson. 1949. Heat stability of hemagglutinin of various strains of Newcastle disease virus. Proc Soc Exp Biol Med 70:283–287.

139. Hanson, R.P., J. Spalatin, and G.S. Jacobson. 1973. The viscerotropic pathotype of Newcastle disease virus. Avian Dis 17:354–361.

140. Hari Babu, Y. 1986. The use of a single radial haemolysis technique for the measurement of antibodies to Newcastle disease virus. Indian Vet J 63:982–984.

141. Heller, E.D., D.B. Nathan, and M. Perek. 1977. The transfer of Newcastle serum antibody from the laying hen to the egg and chick. Res Vet Sci 22:376–379.

142. Higgins, D.A. 1971. Nine disease outbreaks associated with myxoviruses among ducks in Hong Kong. Trop Anim Health Prod 3:232–240.

143. Higgins, D.A., and K.F. Shortridge. 1988. Newcastle disease in tropical and developing countries. In D.J. Alexander (ed.). Newcastle disease. Kluwer Academic Publishers, Boston, MA, pp. 273–302.

144. Hilbink, F., M. Vertommen, and J.T.W. Van't Veer. 1982. The fluorescent antibody technique in the diagnosis of a number of poultry diseases: Manufacture of conjugates and use. Tijdschr Diergeneeskd 107:167–173.

145. Hitchner, S.B., and K. Hirai. 1979. Isolation and growth characteristics of psittacine viruses in chicken embryos. Avian Dis 23:139–147.

146. Hitchner, S.B., and E.P. Johnson. 1948. A virus of low virulence for immunizing fowls against Newcastle disease (avian pneumoencephalitis). Vet Med 43:525–530.

147. Hofstad, M.S. 1953. Immunization of chickens against Newcastle disease by formalin-inactivated vaccine. Am J Vet Res 14:586–589.

148. Holmes, H.C. 1979. Resistance of the respiratory tract of the chicken to Newcastle disease virus infection following vaccination: The effect of passively acquired antibody on its development. J Comp Pathol 89:11–20.

149. Hoshi, S., T. Mikami, K. Nagata, M. Onuma, and H. Izawa. 1983. Monoclonal antibodies against a paramyxovirus isolated from Japanese sparrow-hawks (Accipter virugatus gularis). Arch Virol 76:145–151.

150. Hugh-Jones, M., W.H. Allan, F.A. Dark, and G.J. Harper. 1973. The evidence for the airborne spread of Newcastle disease. J Hyg Camb 71:325–339.

151. Ishida, M., K. Nerome, M. Matsumoto, T. Mikami, and A. Oye. 1985. Characterization of reference strains of

Newcastle disease virus (NDV) and NDV-like isolates by monoclonal antibodies to HN subunits. Arch Virol 85:109–121.

152. Iyer, S.G., and N. Dobson. 1940. A successful method of immunization against Newcastle disease of fowls. Vet Rec 52:889–894.

153. Jones, R.C., C. Baxter-Jones, G.P. Wilding, and D.F. Kelly. 1986. Demonstration of a candidate virus for turkey rhinotracheitis in experimentally inoculated turkeys. Vet Rec 119:599–600.

154. Jorgensen, E.D., P.L. Collins, and P.T. Lomedico. 1987. Cloning and nucleotide sequence of Newcastle disease virus hemagglutinin-neuraminidase mRNA: Identification of a putative sialic acid binding site. Virology 156:12–24.

155. Kaleta, E.F., and C. Baldauf. 1988. Newcastle disease in free-living and pet birds. In D.J. Alexander (ed.). Newcastle Disease. Kluwer Academic Publishers, Boston, MA, pp. 197–246.

156. Kaleta, E.F., and U. Heffels-Redmann (eds.). 1992. Proceedings of the CEC Workshop on Avian Paramyxoviruses, Rauischholzhausen, Germany, 1992.

157. Kaleta, E.F., D.J. Alexander, and P.H. Russell. 1985. The first isolation of the PMV-1 virus responsible for the current panzootic in pigeons? Avian Pathol 14:553–557.

158. Kelleher, C.J., D.A. Halvorson, and J.A. Newman. 1988. Efficacy of viable and inactivated Newcastle disease virus vaccines in turkeys. Avian Dis 32:342–346.

159. Kessler, N., M. Aymard, and A. Calvet. 1979. Study of a new strain of paramyxoviruses isolated from wild ducks: Antigenic and biological properties. J Gen Virol 43:273–282.

160. Kida, H., and R. Yanagawa. 1981. Classification of avian paramyxoviruses by immunodiffusion on the basis of the antigenic specificity of their M protein antigens. J Gen Virol 52:103–111.

161. Kolakofsky, D., E. Boy de la Tour, and H. Delius. 1974. Molecular weight determination of Sendai and Newcastle disease virus RNA. J Virol 13:261–268.

162. Kouwenhoven, B. 1993. Newcastle disease. In J.B. McFerran and M.S. McNulty (eds.). Virus Infections of Vertebrates 4: Virus Infections of Birds. Elsevier, Amsterdam, pp. 341–361.

163. Kraneveld, F.C. 1926. A poultry disease in the Dutch East Indies. Ned Indisch Bl Diergeneeskd 38:448–450.

164. Kumar, M.C. 1988. New methods for immunizing turkeys against Newcastle disease. Turkey World (May–June):48–50.

165. Lana, D.P., D.B. Snyder, D.J. King, and W.W. Marquardt. 1988. Characterization of a battery of monoclonal antibodies for differentiation of Newcastle disease virus and pigeon paramyxovirus-1 strains. Avian Dis 32:273–281.

166. Lancaster, J.E. 1966. Newcastle disease—a review 1926–1964. Monograph No 3. Canadian Department of Agriculture, Ottawa.

167. Lancaster, J.E. 1977. Newcastle disease—A review of the geographical incidence and epizootiology. World Poult Sci J 33:155–165.

168. Lancaster, J.E. 1981. Newcastle disease. In E.P.J. Gibbs (ed.). Virus diseases of food animals, vol II. Disease Monographs. Academic Press, New York, pp. 433–465.

169. Lancaster, J.E., and D.J. Alexander. 1975. Newcastle disease: Virus and spread. Monograph No. 11, Canadian Department of Agriculture, Ottawa.

170. Lang, G., A. Gagnon, and J. Howell. 1975. Occurrence of paramyxovirus Yucaipa in Canadian poultry. Can Vet J 16:233–237.

171. Le Gros, F.X., P. Prevel, and D. Gaudry. 1994. Avian pneumovirus: Recent information resulting from vaccination difficulties. Proceedings of the Seminar: New and Evolving Virus Diseases of Poultry. European Commission, Brussels, pp. 135–155.

172. Letellier, C., A. Burny, and G. Meulemans. 1991.

Construction of a pigeonpox virus recombinant: Expression of the newcastle disease virus (NDV) fusion glycoprotein and protection of chickens against NDV challenge. Archiv Virol 118:43–56.

173. Levine, P.P. 1964. World dissemination of Newcastle disease. In R.P. Hanson (ed.). Newcastle Disease, An Evolving Pathogen. University of Wisconsin Press, Madison, WI, pp. 65–69.

174. Ling, R., and C.R. Pringle. 1988. Turkey rhinotracheitis virus: In vivo and in vitro polypeptide synthesis. J Gen Virol 69:917–923.

175. Lipkind, M., and E. Shihmanter. 1986. Antigenic relationships between avian paramyxoviruses. I. Quantitative characteristics based on hemagglutination and neuraminidase inhibition tests. Arch Virol 89:89–111.

176. Lipkind, M., E. Shihmanter, Y. Weisman, A. Aronovici, and D. Shoham. 1982. Characterization of Yucaipa-like avian paramyxoviruses isolated in Israel from domesticated and wild birds. Ann Virol 133E:157–161.

177. Lipkind, M., D. Shoham, and E. Shihmanter. 1986. Isolation of a paramyxovirus from pigs in Israel and its antigenic relationships with avian paramyxoviruses. J Gen Virol 67:427–439.

178. Lister, S.A., and D.J. Alexander. 1986. Turkey rhinotracheitis: A review. Vet Bull 56:637–663.

179. Lockaby, S.B., F.J. Hoerr, A.C. Ellis, and M.S. Yu. 1993. Immunohistochemical detection of Newcastle disease virus in chickens. Avian Dis 37:433–437.

180. Macpherson, I., R.G. Watt, and D.J. Alexander. 1983. Isolation of avian paramyxovirus, other than Newcastle disease virus, from commercial poultry in Great Britain. Vet Rec 112:479–480.

181. Malkinson, M., and P.A. Small. 1977. Local immunity against Newcastle disease virus in the newly hatched chicken's respiratory tract. Infect Immun 16:587–592.

182. Marius-Jestin, V., M. Cherbonnel, J.P. Picault, and G. Bennejean. 1987. Isolement chez des canards mulards d'une souche hypervirulente de virus de la peste du canard et d'un paramyxovirus aviaire de type 6. Comp Immunol Microbiol Infect Dis 10:173–186.

183. McDougall, J.S., and J.K.A. Cook. 1986. Turkey rhinotracheitis: Preliminary investigations. Vet Rec 118:206–207.

184. McFerran, J.B., and R.M. McCracken. 1988. Newcastle disease. In D.J. Alexander (ed.). Newcastle Disease. Kluwer Academic Publishers, Boston, MA, pp. 161–183.

185. McFerran, J.B., and R. Nelson. 1971. Some properties of an avirulent Newcastle disease virus. Arch Ges Virusforsch 34:64–74.

186. McGinnes, L.W., and T.G. Morrison. 1986. Nucleotide sequence of the gene encoding the Newcastle disease virus fusion protein and comparisons of paramyxovirus fusion protein sequences. Virus Res 5:343–356.

187. McMillan, B.C., and R.P. Hanson. 1980. RNA oligonucleotide fingerprinting: A proposed method of identifying strains of Newcastle disease virus. Avian Dis 24:1016–1020.

188. McMillan, B.C., and R.P. Hanson. 1982. Differentiation of exotic strains of Newcastle disease virus by oligonucleotide fingerprinting. Avian Dis 26:332–339.

189. McMillan, B.C., S.F. Rehmani, and R.P. Hanson. 1986. Lectin binding and the carbohydrate moieties present on Newcastle disease virus strains. Avian Dis 30:340–344.

190. McNulty, M.S., and G.M. Allan. 1986. Application of immunofluorescence in veterinary viral diagnosis. In M.S. McNulty and J.B. McFerran (eds.). Recent Advances in Virus Diagnosis. Martinus Nijhoff, Dordrecht, The Netherlands, pp. 15–26.

191. Melnick, J.L. 1982. Taxonomy and nomenclature of viruses, 1982. Prog Med Virol 28:208–221.

192. Meulemans, G. 1988. Control by vaccination. In D.J.

Alexander (ed.). Newcastle Disease. Kluwer Academic Publishers, Boston, MA, pp. 318–332.

193. Meulemans, G., M.C. Carlier, M. Gonze, P. Petit, and P. Halen. 1984. Diagnostic serologique de la maladie de Newcastle par les tests d'inhibition de l'hemagglutination et Elisa. Zetralbl Veterinaermed [B] 31:690–700.

194. Meulemans, G., M. Gonze, M.C. Carlier, P. Petit, A. Burny, and Le Long. 1986. Protective effects of HN and F glycoprotein-specific monoclonal antibodies on experimental Newcastle disease. Avian Pathol 15:761–768.

195. Meulemans, G., M. Gonze, M.C. Carlier, P. Petit, A. Burny, and Le Long. 1987. Evaluation of the use of monoclonal antibodies to hemagglutination and fusion glycoproteins of Newcastle disease virus for virus identification and strain differentiation purposes. Arch Virol 92:55–62.

196. Meulemans, G., C. Letellier, D. Espion, Le Long, and A. Burny. 1988. Importance de la proteine F dans l'immunite au virus de la maladie de Newcastle. Bull Acad Vet France 61:51–62.

197. Meulemans, G., C. Letellier, M. Gonze, M.C. Carlier, and A. Burny. 1988. Newcastle disease virus F glycoprotein expressed from a recombinant vaccinia virus vector protects chickens against live virus challenge. Avian Pathol 17:821–827,

198. Miers, L.A., R.A. Bankowski, and Y.C. Zee. 1983. Optimizing the enzyme-linked immunosorbent assay for evaluating immunity in chickens to Newcastle disease. Avian Dis 27:1112–1125.

199. Millar, N.S., and P.T. Emmerson. 1988. Molecular cloning and nucleotide sequencing of Newcastle disease virus. In D.J. Alexander (ed.). Newcastle Disease. Kluwer Academic Publishers, Boston, MA, pp. 79–97.

200. Millar, N.S., P. Chambers, and P.T. Emmerson. 1986. Nucleotide sequence analysis of the haemagglutinin-neuraminidase gene of Newcastle disease virus. J Gen Virol 67:1917–1927.

201. Millar, N.S., P. Chambers, and P.T. Emmerson. 1988. Nucleotide sequence of the fusion and haemagglutinin-neuraminidase glycoprotein genes of Newcastle disease virus, strain Ulster: Molecular basis for variations in pathogenicity between strains. J Gen Virol 69:613–620.

202. Moore, N.F., and D.C. Burke. 1974. Characterization of the structural proteins of different strains of Newcastle disease virus. J Gen Virol 25:275–289.

203. Morgan, R.W., J. Gelb, C.R. Pope, and P.J.A. Sondermeijer. 1993. Efficacy in chickens of a herpesvirus of turkeys recombinant vaccine containing the fusion gene of Newcastle disease virus: Onset of protection and effect of maternal antibodies. Avian Dis 37:1032–1040.

204. Morley, A.J., and D.K. Thomson. 1984. Swollen head syndrome in broiler chickens. Avian Dis 28:238–243.

205. Nagai, Y., H-D. Klenk, and R. Rott. 1976. Proteolytic cleavage of the viral glycoproteins and its significance for the virulence of Newcastle disease virus. Virology 72:494–508.

206. Nagai, Y., H. Ogura, and H-D. Klenk. 1976. Studies on the assembly of the envelope of Newcastle disease virus. Virology 69:523–538.

207. Nagy, E., and B. Lomniczi. 1984. Differentiation of Newcastle disease virus strains by one-dimensional peptide mapping. J Virol Methods 9:227–235.

208. Nerome, K., M. Nakayama, M. Ishida, H. Fukumi, and A. Morita. 1978. Isolation of a new avian paramyxovirus from a budgerigar. J Gen Virol 38:293–301.

209. Nerome, K., M. Ishida, A. Oya, and S. Bosshard. 1983. Genomic analysis of antigenically related avian paramyxoviruses. J Gen Virol 64:465–470.

210. Nishikawa, K., S. Isomura, S. Suzuki, E. Wanatabe, M. Hamaguchi, T. Yoshida, and Y. Nagai. 1983. Monoclonal antibodies to the HN glycoprotein of Newcastle disease virus. Biological characterization and use for strain comparisons. Virology 130:318–330.

211. O'Brien, J.D.P. 1985. Swollen head syndrome in broiler breeders. Vet Rec 117:619–620.

212. Omojola, E., and R.P. Hanson. 1986. Collection of diagnostic specimens from animals in remote areas. World Anim Rev 60:38–40.

213. Pages-Mante, A. 1994. Studies on swollen head syndrome in Spain. Proceedings of the Seminar: New and Evolving Virus Diseases of Poultry. European Commission, Brussels, pp. 89–109.

214. Panigrahy, B., D.A. Senne, J.E. Pearson, M.A. Mixson, and D.R. Cassidy. 1993. Occurrence of velogenic viscerotropic Newcastle disease in pet and exotic birds in 1991. Avian Dis 37:254–258.

215. Parede, L., and P.L. Young. 1990. The pathogenesis of velogenic Newcastle disease virus infection of chickens of different ages and different levels of immunity. Avian Dis 34:803–808.

216. Parry, S.H., and I.D. Aitken. 1977. Local immunity in the respiratory tract of the chicken. II The secretory immune response to Newcastle disease virus and the role of IgA. Vet Microbiol 2:143–165.

217. Pattison, M., and W.H. Allan. 1974. Infection of chicks with infectious bursal disease and its effect on the carrier with Newcastle disease virus. Vet Rec 95:65–66.

218. Pearson, J.E., D.A. Senne, D.J. Alexander, W.D. Taylor, L.A. Peterson, and P.H. Russell. 1987. Characterization of Newcastle disease virus (avian paramyxovirus-1) isolated from pigeons. Avian Dis 31:105–111.

219. Peeples, M.E. 1988. Newcastle disease virus replication. In D.J. Alexander (ed.). Newcastle Disease. Kluwer Academic Publishers, Boston, MA, pp. 45–78.

220. Pennington, T.H. 1978. Antigenic differences between strains of NDV. Arch Virol 56:345–351.

221. Picault, J.P., P. Giraud, P. Drouin, M. Guittet, G. Bennejean, I. Lamande, D. Toquin, and C. Gueguen. 1987. Isolation of a TRT-like virus from chickens with swollen head syndrome. Vet Rec 121:135.

222. Pospisil, Z., D. Zendulkova, and B. Smid. 1991. Unexpected emergence of Newcastle disease virus in very young chicks. Acta Vet Brno 60:263–270.

223. Powell, J.R., I.D. Aitken, and B.D. Survashe. 1979. The response of the Harderian gland of the fowl to antigen given by the ocular route. II Antibody production. Avian Pathol 8:363–373.

224. Pringle, C.R. 1985. Pneumoviruses. In B.W.J. Mahy (ed.). Virology—A Practical Approach, IRL Press, Oxford, United Kingdom, pp. 95–117.

225. Raszewska, H. 1964. Occurence of the La Sota strain NDV in the reproductive tract of laying hens. Bull Vet Inst Pulawy 8:130–136.

226. Reeve, P., and G. Poste. 1971. Studies on the cytopathogenicity of Newcastle disease virus: Relationship between virulence, polykaryocytosis and plaque size. J Gen Virol 11:17–24.

227. Reeve, P., D.J. Alexander, and W.H. Allan. 1974. Derivation of an isolate of low virulence from the Essex '70 strain of Newcastle disease virus. Vet Rec 94:38–41.

228. Rima, B., D.J. Alexander, M.A. Billeter, P.L. Collins, D.W. Kingsbury, M.A. Lipkind, Y. Nagai, C. Orvell, C.R. Pringle, and V. ter Meulen. 1995. Paramyxoviridae. In F.A. Murphy, C.M. Fauquet, D.H.L. Bishop, S.A. Ghabrial, A.W. Jarvis, G.P. Martelli, M.A. Mayo, and M.D. Summers (eds.). Virus Taxonomy. Sixth Report of the International Committee on Taxonomy of Viruses. Springer-Verlag, Vienna, pp. 268–274.

229. Rivetz, B., Y. Weisman, M. Ritterband, F. Fish, and M. Herzberg. 1985. Evaluation of a novel rapid kit for the visual detection of Newcastle disease virus antibodies. Avian Dis 29:929–942.

230. Rosenberger, J.K., and J. Gelb. 1978. Response to several avian respiratory viruses as affected by infectious bursal disease virus. Avian Dis 22:95–105.

231. Rott, R. 1979. Molecular basis of infectivity and pathogenicity of myxoviruses. Arch Virol 59:285–298.

232. Rott, R. 1985. In vitro Differenzierung von pathogenen und apathogenen aviaren Influenzaviren. Ber Munch Tieraerztl Wochenschr 98:37–39.

233. Rott, R., and H-D. Klenk. 1988. Molecular basis of infectivity and pathogenicity of Newcastle disease virus. In D.J. Alexander (ed.). Newcastle Disease. Kluwer Academic Publishers, Boston, MA, pp. 98–112.

234. Russell, P.H. 1988. Monoclonal antibodies in research, diagnosis and epizootiology of Newcastle disease. In D.J. Alexander (ed.). Newcastle Disease. Kluwer Academic Publishers, Boston, MA, pp. 131–146.

235. Russell, P.H. 1993. Newcastle disease virus: Virus replication in the Harderian gland stimulates lacrimal IgA; the yolk sac provides early lacrimal IgG. Vet. Immunol Immunopathol 37:151–163.

236. Russell, P.H., and D.J. Alexander. 1983. Antigenic variation of Newcastle disease virus strains detected by monoclonal antibodies. Arch Virol 75:243–253.

237. Russell, P.H., and G.O. Ezeifeka. 1995. The Hitchner B1 strain of Newcastle disease virus induces high levels of IgA, IgG and IgM in newly hatched chicks. Vaccine 113:61–66.

238. Russell, P.H., and G. Koch. 1993. Local antibody forming cell responses to the Hitchner B1 and Ulster strains of Newcastle disease virus. Vet Immunol Immunopathol 37:165–180.

239. Russell, P.H., A.C.R. Samson, and D.J. Alexander. 1990. Newcastle disease virus variations. In E. Kurstak, R.G. Marusyk, F.A. Murphy, and M.H.V. Regenmortel (eds.). Applied Virology Research, vol. II. Plenum, New York, pp. 177–195.

240. Sakaguchi, T., T. Toyoda, B, Gotoh, N.M. Inocencio, K. Kuma, T. Miyata, and Y. Nagai. 1989. Newcastle disease virus evolution 1. Multiple lineages defined by sequence variability of the hemagglutinin-neuraminidase gene. Virology 169:260–272.

241. Samson, A.C.R. 1988. Virus structure. In D.J. Alexander (ed.). Newcastle Disease. Kluwer Academic Publishers, Boston, MA, pp. 23–44.

242. Sato, H., M. Oh-Hira, N. Ishida, Y. Imamura, S. Hattori, and M. Kawakita. 1987. Molecular cloning and nucleotide sequence of P, M and F genes of Newcastle disease virus avirulent strain D26. Virus Res 7:241–255.

243. Schaper, U.M., F.J. Fuller, M.D.W. Ward, Y. Mehrotra, H.O. Stone, B.R. Stripp, and E.V. De Buysscher. 1988. Nucleotide sequence of the envelope protein genes of a highly virulent, neurotropic strain of Newcastle disease virus. Virology 165:291–295.

244. Schloer, G., and R.P. Hanson. 1968. Plaque morphology of Newcastle disease virus as influenced by cell type and environmental factors. Am J Vet Res 29:883–895.

245. Schloer, G., J. Spalatin, and R.P. Hanson. 1975. Newcastle disease virus antigens and strain variation. Am J Vet Res 36:505–508.

246. Senne, D.A., J.E. Pearson, L.D. Miller, and G.A. Gustafson. 1983. Virus isolations from pet birds submitted for importation into the United States. Avian Dis 27:731–744.

247. Shortridge, K.F., D.J. Alexander, and M.S. Collins. 1980. Isolation and properties of viruses from poultry in Hong Kong which represent a new (sixth) distinct group of avian paramyxoviruses. J Gen Virol 49:255–262.

248. Simmons, G.C. 1967. The isolation of Newcastle disease virus in Queensland. Aust Vet J 43:29–30.

249. Smit, T., and P.R. Rondhuis. 1976. Studies on a virus isolated from the brain of a parakeet (Neophema sp). Avian Pathol 5:21–30.

250. Snyder, D.B., W.W. Marquadt, E.T. Mallinson, and E. Russek. 1983. Rapid serological profiling by enzyme-linked immunosorbent assay. I Measurement of antibody activity titer against Newcastle disease virus in a single dilution.

Avian Dis 27:161–170.

251. Snyder, D.B., W.W. Marquadt, E.T. Mallinson, P.K. Savage, and D.C. Allen. 1984. Rapid serological profiling by enzyme-linked immunosorbent assay. III Simultaneous measurements of antibody titers to infectious bronchitis virus, infectious bursal disease and Newcastle disease virus in a single serum dilution. Avian Dis 28:12–24.

252. Spalatin, J.S., and R.P. Hanson. 1966. Recovery of a Newcastle disease virus strain indistinguishable from Texas GB. Avian Dis 10:372–374.

253. Spalatin, J., R.P. Hanson, and P.D. Beard. 1970. The hemagglutination-elution pattern as a marker in characterizing Newcastle disease virus. Avian Dis 14:542–549.

254. Spradbrow, P.B. 1988. Geographical distribution. In D.J. Alexander (ed.). Newcastle Disease. Kluwer Academic Publishers, Boston, MA, pp. 247–255.

255. Spradbrow, P.B. (ed.). 1992. Newcastle disease in village chickens. Control with thermostable oral vaccines. Proceedings of an International Workshop, Kuala Lumpur, Malaysia 1991. ACIAR, Canberra.

256. Srinivasappa, G.B., D.B. Snyder, W.W. Marquardt, and D.J. King. 1986. Isolation of a monoclonal antibody with specificity for commonly employed vaccine strains of Newcastle disease virus. Avian Dis 30:562–567.

257. Stevens, J.G., R.M. Nakamura, M.L. Cook, and S.P. Wilczynski. 1976. Newcastle disease as a model for paramyxovirus-induced neurological syndromes: Pathogenesis of the respiratory disease and preliminary characterization of the ensuing encephalitis. Infect Immun 13:590–599.

258. Stones, P.B. 1979. Self injection of veterinary oil-emulsion vaccines. BMJ 1:1627.

259. Stuart, J.C. 1986. Field experience in the UK with turkey rhinotracheitis. Turkeys 34:24–26.

260. Stuart, J.C. 1989. Rhinotracheitis: Turkey rhinotracheitis (TRT) in Great Britain. In C. Nixey, and T.C. Grey (eds.). Recent Advances in Turkey Science. Butterworths, London, pp. 217–224.

261. Taylor, J., C. Edbauer, A. Rey-Senelonge, J-F. Bouquet, E. Norton, S. Goebel, P. Desmettre, and E. Paoletti. 1990. Newcastle disease virus fusion protein expressed in a fowlpox virus recombinant confers protection in chickens. J Virol 64:1441–1450.

262. Thornton, D.H. 1988. Quality control of vaccines. In D.J. Alexander (ed.). Newcastle Disease. Kluwer Academic Publishers, Boston, MA, pp. 347–365.

263. Timms, L., and D.J. Alexander. 1977. Cell-mediated immune response of chickens to Newcastle disease vaccines. Avian Pathol 6:51–59.

264. Toquin, D., N. Eterradossi, M. Guittet, and G. Bennejean. 1994. Infectious rhinotracheitis in turkeys: Antigenic differences revealed by ELISA. Proceedings of the Seminar: New and Evolving Virus Diseases of Poultry. European Commission, Brussels, pp. 111–121.

265. Toyoda, T., T. Sakaguchi, K. Imai, N. Mendoza Inocencio, B. Gotoh, M. Hamaguchi, and Y. Nagai. 1987. Structural comparison of the cleavage-activation site of the fusion glycoprotein between virulent and avirulent strains of Newcastle disease virus. Virology 158:242–247.

266. Toyoda, T., T. Sakaguchi, H. Hirota, B. Gotoh, K. Kuma, T. Miyata, and Y. Nagai. 1989. Newcastle disease virus evolution II. Lack of gene recombination in generating virulent and avirulent strains. Virology 169:273–282.

267. Tumova, B., J.H. Robinson, and B.C. Easterday. 1979. A hitherto unreported paramyxovirus of turkeys. Res Vet Sci 27,135–140.

268. Tumova, B., A. Stumpa, V. Janout, M. Uvizl, and J. Chmela. 1979. A further member of the Yucaipa group isolated from the common wren (Troglodytes troglodytes). Acta Virol 23:504–507.

269. USAHA. 1993. Report of the committee on transmissible diseases of poultry and other avian species. Proc 96th Annu Meet US Anim Health Assoc, 1992. United States Animal Health Association, Richmond, VA, pp. 348–366.

270. Utterback, W.W., and J.H. Schwartz. 1973. Epizootiology of velogenic viscerotropic Newcastle disease in southern California, 1971–1973. J Am Vet Med Assoc 163:1080–1090.

271. Uyttebroek, E., R. Ducatelle, and D.J. Alexander. 1991. Steatorrhea and pancreatic lesions in Neophema parrots with paramyxovirus serotype 3 infection. Vlaams Diergeneeskd Tijdschr 60:55–58.

272. Vindevogel, H., and J.P. Duchatel. 1988. Panzootic Newcastle disease virus in pigeons. In D.J. Alexander (ed.). Newcastle Disease. Kluwer Academic Publishers, Boston, MA, pp. 184–196.

273. Walker, J.W., B.R. Heron, and M.A. Mixson. 1973. Exotic Newcastle disease eradication program in the United States of America. Avian Dis 17:486–503.

274. Webster, R.G., and R. Rott. 1987. Influenza virus A pathogenicity: The pivotal role of hemagglutinin. Cell 50:665–666.

275. Wemers, C.D., S. de Henau, C. Neyt, D. Espion, C. Letellier, G. Meulemans, and A. Burny. 1987. The hemagglutinin-neuraminidase (HN) gene of Newcastle disease virus strain Italien (ndv Italien): Comparison with HNs of other strains and expression by a vaccinia recombinant. Arch Virol 97:101–113.

276. Werner, O. 1994. Newcastle disease: Current situation in Germany. In D.J. Alexander (ed.). Proceedings of the Joint First Annual Meetings of the National Newcastle Disease and Avian Influenza Laboratories of the European Communities, 1993. CEC, Brussels, pp. 52–57.

277. WHO Expert Committee. 1980. A revision of the system of nomenclature for influenza viruses: A WHO memorandum. Bull WHO 58:585–591.

278. Wilczynski, S.P., M.L. Cook, and J.G. Stevens. 1977. Newcastle disease as a model for paramyxovirus-induced neurologic syndromes. Am J Pathol 89:649–666.

279. Williams, J.E., and L.H. Dillard. 1968. Penetration patterns of Mycoplasma gallisepticum and Newcastle disease virus through the outer structures of chicken eggs. Avian Dis 12:650–657.

280. Williams, R.A., C.E. Savage, and R.C. Jones. 1991. Development of a live attenuated vaccine against turkey rhinotracheitis. Avian Pathol 20:45–55.

281. Wilson, G.W.C. 1986. Newcastle disease and paramyxovirus 1 of pigeons in the European Community. World Poult Sci J 42:143–153,

282. Wilson, R.A., C. Perrotta, B. Frey, and R.J. Eckroade. 1984. An enzyme-linked immunosorbent assay that measures protective antibody levels to Newcastle disease virus in chickens. Avian Dis 28:1079–1085.

283. Winslow, N.S., R.P. Hanson, E. Upton, and C.A. Brandly. 1950. Agglutination of mammalian erythrocytes by Newcastle disease virus. Proc Soc Exp Biol 74:174–178.

284. Wobeser, G., F.A. Leighton, R. Norman, D.J. Myers, D. Onderka, M.J. Pybus, J.L. Neufeld, G.A. Fox, and D.J. Alexander. 1993. Newcastle disease in wild waterbirds in western Canada, 1990. Can Vet J 34:353–359.

285. Wyeth, P.J., R.E. Gough, N.J. Chettle, and R. Eddy. 1986. Preliminary observations on a virus associated with turkey rhinotracheitis. Vet Rec 119:139.

286. Wyeth, P.J., N.J. Chettle, R.E. Gough, and M.S. Collins. 1987. Antibodies to TRT in chickens with swollen head syndrome. Vet Rec 120:286–287.

287. Yu, Q., P.J. Davis, J. Li, and D. Cavanagh. 1992. Cloning and sequencing of the matrix protein (M) gene of turkey rhinotracheitis virus reveal a gene order different from that of respiratory syncytial virus. Virology 186:426–434.

288. Zeydanli, M.M., T. Redmann, E.F. Kaleta, and D.J. Alexander. 1988. Paramyxoviruses (PMV) isolated from turkeys with respiratory disease. Proc 37th West Poult Dis Conf, pp. 46–50.

21 Avian Encephalomyelitis

B. W. Calnek, R. E. Luginbuhl, and C. F. Helmboldt

INTRODUCTION. Avian encephalomyelitis (AE) is an infectious viral disease affecting young chickens, pheasants, quail, and turkeys. It is characterized by ataxia and rapid tremors, especially of the head and neck; because of the latter it was often called epidemic tremor.

No public health significance has been attached to this disease. The disease was of great economic importance to the poultry industry prior to the widespread use of vaccines in the early 1960s.

HISTORY. Jones (42, 43) first encountered AE in 1930 in 2-wk-old commercial Rhode Island Red chicks showing tremors. In 1931, two additional outbreaks were observed in 1- and 4-wk-old chicks raised on different farms but originating from the same breeding flock. During the next 2 yr, additional outbreaks were observed in Connecticut, Maine, Massachusetts, and New Hampshire, which led to AE being tagged "New England disease."

In 1934, Jones (43) reproduced the disease in susceptible chicks by intracerebral (IC) inoculation with filtrates of brain material from spontaneous cases. It was not until the mid-1950s, however, that Schaaf reported the first successful control of the disease by immunization (74). The epizootiology of AE was clarified by Calnek et al. in 1960 (19) and the development of an orally administered vaccine (20) soon followed. Additional historical details are provided by Tannock and Shafren (89) and van der Heide (92).

INCIDENCE AND DISTRIBUTION. Avian encephalomyelitis occurs virtually worldwide (see 89, 92). Nearly all flocks eventually become infected with the virus, but the incidence of clinical disease is very low unless a breeder flock is not vaccinated and becomes infected after the commencement of egg production.

ETIOLOGY

Characteristics of the Virus. Avian encephalomyelitis virus (AEV) was first shown to be filterable by Jones (43). The diameter of the virus, based on filtration studies, was found to range from 20 to 30 nm, or 16 to 25 nm, by Olitsky and Bauer (67) and Butterfield et al. (13), respectively. By electron microscopic (EM) examination of purified AEV, Gosting et al. (31) found the virions to have hexagonal profiles lacking envelopes and to be 24–32 nm in diameter; later EM studies by Tannock and Shafren (88) determined the mean diameter to be 26.1 ± 0.4 nm. Crystalline arrays observed in Purkinje cells from the brains of infected chickens had particles with diameters estimated to be 22 nm (21) or 25 nm (33). Gosting et al. (31) further detected a fivefold symmetry with 32 or 42 capsomeres, in contrast to an earlier report by Krauss and Ueberschaer (48), who proposed an icosahedral symmetry with only 12 capsomeres.

The virus has a buoyant density of 1.31–1.33 g/mL (13, 31, 88) and a sedimentation coefficient of 148 S (31). It is resistant to chloroform, acid, trypsin, pepsin, and DNase and is protected against effects of heat by divalent magnesium ions (8, 13). Based on these characteristics and resistance of AEV to DNase, Butterfield et al. (13) proposed that it be classified as an enterovirus belonging to the family *Picornaviridae*. Confirmatory evidence that AEV is an RNA virus came from studies showing that viral replication in vitro was unaffected by a DNA inhibitor, 5-bromo-2'-deoxyuridine (80). Tannock and Shafren (88) initially detected four virus-specific proteins (VP 1–4) with molecular weights of 43,000, 35,000, 33,000, and 14,000, respectively. They noted in a later report (79), however, that one of the proteins was actually contaminating ovalbumin and that the other three VPs (1–3) were similar in size to those of poliovirus. They also reported that there were no differences between a field isolate and the embryo-adapted Van Roekel (VR) strain of virus when they were compared using a radioimmunoprecipitation assay, in keeping with earlier comparisons of physical, chemical, and serologic properties of the two types of virus by Butterfield et al. (13).

Biologic Properties. Although all isolates of AEV are serologically similar, there are two distinct pathotypes of virus. One, represented by natural field strains, is enterotropic. These strains infect chickens readily via the oral route and are shed in the feces. They are relatively nonpathogenic except in susceptible chicks infected by vertical transmission or by early horizontal transmission, in which

571

case they cause neurologic signs. Neurologic disease also occurs following experimental infection by intracerebral inoculation of susceptible chickens.

Embryo-adapted strains constitute the other pathotype. These viruses are highly neurotropic and cause severe neurologic signs following intracerebral inoculation (invariable incidence) or parenteral routes such as intramuscular or subcutaneous inoculation (variable incidence). They not infect via the oral route except with very high doses and they do not spread horizontally (17, 40, 41, 59, 79, 98). Adaptation may occur after multiple passages in antibody-free chicken embryos (20, 58, 102), probably the result of selection of laboratory mutants (58). The most commonly used adapted strain is the VR strain, which had been passaged repeatedly by intracerebral inoculation of chickens (93). The VR strain already had the phenotype of adapted strains when first inoculated into embryos after 150 chicken passages (16, 85).

Both pathotypes can replicate in embryos derived from a susceptible flock, but natural strains do not cause obvious signs or gross lesions. On the other hand, adapted strains are pathogenic for embryos, causing muscular dystrophy (Fig. 21.1) and immobilization of skeletal muscles (16, 45). The virus was detected in brains of inoculated embryos 3–4 days postinoculation (PI), and peak titers were found 6–9 days PI (10, 16). Histopathologic changes in embryos infected with egg-adapted virus have been described as uniform in character but variable in intensity and location and consisting of encephalomalacia and muscular dystrophy (45). Muscular changes consisted primarily of

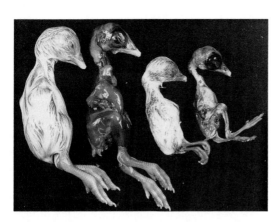

21.1. Chicken embryos on the *right* were inoculated via the yolk sac with the Van Roekel strain of avian encephalomyelitis virus on the 6th incubation day. Control embryos are on the *left*. The affected embryos, examined on the 18th incubation day, show extreme muscular dystrophy (most evident in the embryo with the skin removed) and rigidity of the legs.

eosinophilic swelling and necrosis, fragmentation, and loss of striations of affected fibers with rare sarcolemmal proliferation and heterophil infiltration. Neural lesions were characterized by severe local edema, gliosis, vascular proliferation, and pyknosis.

Laboratory Host Systems.   Virus may be propagated in the baby chick, chicken embryos from susceptible flocks and a variety cell culture systems. Chicks and embryos must be from a susceptible flock except in the case of intracerebral inoculation of chicks. Several routes of inoculation in embryos have been used (45, 85, 102), but the yolk sac is generally considered the route of choice. Gross lesions (see above section) are observed only with adapted strains. Tannock and Shafren (89) reviewed numerous reports on cell-culture propagation of AEV, beginning with the first successful replication of the VR strain of AEV in chicken embryo brain cultures in 1967 by Mancini and Yates (53). Subsequently, fibroblasts, kidney cells and neuroglial cells from chicken embryos, and pancreatic cells from young chicks, were used to cultivate both adapted and field strains of virus (3, 46, 47, 54, 55, 64, 73). Titers, particularly with natural strains, were generally low (rarely exceeding $10^{3.5}$ EID_{50}/mL) and cytopathic effects have not been described. Replication in cell cultures is detected by inoculation of embryos (adapted strains only) or by tests for antigen using immunofluorescence or enzyme-linked immunosorbent assays (ELISA). Nicholas et al. (64) suggested that chicken embryo neuroglial cells may provide an excellent substrate for production of AEV antigen suitable for serologic tests such as immunodiffusion and ELISA. Shafren and Tannock (79) compared the VR strain, a field isolate, and a vaccine strain for ability to grow in chicken embryo brain cultures; titers with the VR strain, after a 2-day eclipse, were 8 to 10 times higher than those with the other strains, and virus was largely cell associated. Abe (1) failed to demonstrate replication of AEV in a variety of established mammalian cell lines.

PATHOGENESIS AND EPIZOOTIOLOGY

Natural and Experimental Hosts.   Avian encephalomyelitis virus has a limited host range. Chickens, pheasants, coturnix quail, and turkeys have all succumbed to naturally occurring infection (see reviews 11, 92). Experimental infection of young quail chicks (32) caused clinical signs and the infection spread to breeding quail in the same room. Infection of the adults resulted in reduced egg production and hatchability, and clinical AE developed in chicks hatched from eggs laid during the outbreak. The naturally occurring disease in turkeys is essentially the same as that in chickens (35). Ducklings, poults, young pigeons, and guinea fowl also have been infected experimentally. Mice, guinea pigs, rabbits, and monkeys were refractory to virus introduced intracerebrally (56, 63, 68, 94, 95). Van Steenis (97) found naturally occurring AEV antibodies in serums from partridge, pheasant, and turkeys, but not in serums from finches, sparrows, starlings, pigeons, jackdaws, rooks, doves, or ducks. The latter four species also failed to develop antibodies after oral exposure to AEV. Bodin et al. (4) compared adult pheasants and red and gray partridges for sensitivity to intramuscular or oral–nasal inoculation with the VR strain of virus. All became infected, but the severity of disease based on signs and lesions was greatest in gray partridges and least in pheasants. Embryonated eggs from the three species were also susceptible to infection.

Transmission. The IC route of inoculation has given the most consistent results in reproducing AE in chickens. Other routes by which infection has been experimentally established are intraperitoneal, subcutaneous, intradermal, intravenous, intramuscular, intrasciatic, intraocular, oral, and intranasal inoculation (13, 19, 25, 44, 66, 76, 94).

Under natural conditions, AE is essentially an enteric infection (19). Ingestion is the usual portal of entry (19, 34); exposure via the respiratory tract may be unimportant other than through the coincident exposure of the alimentary tract (19). Virus is shed in the feces for a period of several days and, because it is quite resistant to environmental conditions, it remains infectious for long periods of time. The period during which virus is excreted in feces is dependent in part on the age of the bird when infected. Very young chicks may excrete virus for more than 2 wk, whereas those infected after 3 wk of age may shed virus for only about 5 days (101). Shafren and Tannock (78) found virus in feces from 4 to 10 days after exposure to a field strain of AEV. Infected litter is a source of virus that is easily transmitted horizontally by tracking or fomites. Infection spreads rapidly from bird to bird within a pen or house once introduced, and from pen to pen on farms where no special precautions are taken to prevent spread. Birds in isolated flocks of a single age group were found to be less likely to have encountered infection than chickens on farms with multiple-age groups. Virus spread was found to be less rapid among birds in cages than in those on the floor (19, 26, 77).

Vertical transmission is a very important means of virus dissemination, based on both field evidence and experimental results (19, 44, 76, 91, 96). Taylor and Schelling (90) reported that 57% of breeder flocks tested in North America had been exposed to the virus by 5 mo of age; however, 96% were serologically positive by 13 mo. Although the source of infection for susceptible flocks is unknown, it is likely that it is carried from infected farms by people or fomites. When susceptible flocks are exposed after sexual maturity, the hens infect a variable proportion of their eggs. Calnek et al. (19) showed that infected embryos and chicks came from eggs laid during the period 5–13 days after experimental infection of susceptible breeders. Jungherr and Minard (44) reported that hatchability of eggs from an infected flock was not affected. Conversely, Taylor et al. (91) observed a high embryo death pattern during the last 3 days of incubation. The percentage of embryos that hatched declined from a 78.6% preinfection level to 59.6% during the clinical stage, and increased to 75.4% postinfection. Eggs produced just prior to and during the period of depressed egg production showed decreased hatchability and increased embryo mortality during the last 3 days of incubation. Furthermore, only chicks from the group with depressed hatchability showed signs of AE; chicks hatched prior to and after the affected hatch appeared normal. Similar observations have been reported by other workers (19, 71).

Calnek et al. (19) demonstrated that virus transmission can occur in the incubator. Chicks hatched from eggs inoculated at 6 days' incubation manifested signs on the 1st day of age; by the 6th day, 49 of 52 showed clinical evidence of AE. Chicks from uninoculated eggs hatched with the infected birds first manifested signs on the 10th day, and 15 of 18 chicks developed clinical signs. An isolated control group of 19 chicks remained negative.

The possibility of a carrier status is unknown. Richey (71) incriminated a ready-to-lay pullet flock housed in the same building, but in a separate pen, as the source of infection for outbreaks that occurred in several susceptible breeding flocks at 45 wk of age. The pullet flock had experienced an acute outbreak of AE at 3 wk of age; it was suggested that a carrier existed in the flock. While certain aspects of transmission have been well established, other phases remain unknown.

Incubation Period. Studies conducted by Calnek et al. (19) demonstrated that the incubation period in chicks infected by embryo transmission was 1–7 days, whereas chicks infected by contact transmission or oral administration had a minimum incubation period of 11 days.

Signs. Avian encephalomyelitis presents an interesting syndrome. In naturally occurring outbreaks it usually makes its appearance when chicks are 1–2 wk of age, although affected chicks have been observed at the time of hatching. Affected chicks first show a slightly dull expression of the eyes, followed by a progressive ataxia from incoordination of the muscles, which may be detected readily by exercising the chicks. As the ataxia grows more pronounced, chicks show an inclination to sit on their hocks. When disturbed, they may move about, exhibiting little control over speed and gait; finally, they come to rest or fall on their sides. Some may refuse to move or may walk on their hocks and shanks. The dull expression becomes more pronounced and is accompanied by a weakened cry. Fine tremors of the head and neck may become evident, the frequency and magnitude of which may vary. Exciting or disturbing the chicks may bring on the tremor, which may continue for variable periods and recur at irregular intervals. Ataxic signs usually, but not always, appear before the tremor. In some cases, only tremor has been observed. Ataxia usually progresses until the chick is incapable of moving about, and this stage is followed by inanition, prostration, and finally death. Chicks with marked ataxia and prostration are frequently trampled by their penmates. Some chicks with definite signs of AE may survive and grow to maturity, and in some instances signs may disappear completely. Survivors may later develop blindness from an opacity giving a bluish discoloration to the lens (7, 69).

There is a marked age resistance to clinical signs in birds exposed after they are 2–3 wk of age (see Pathogenesis). Mature birds may experience a temporary drop in egg production (5–10%) but do not develop neurologic signs.

Morbidity and Mortality. Morbidity from the naturally occurring disease has been observed only in young stock. The usual morbidity rate is 40–60% if all the chicks come from the infected flock. Mortality averages 25% and may exceed 50%. These rates are considerably lower if many of the chicks composing the flock originate from breeder flocks of immune birds.

Pathogenesis. There are significant differences between embryo-adapted AEV and field strains of the virus in terms of pathogenesis. This is largely because the adapted strains generally lose the enterotropic properties that characterize the natural strains. Consequently, adapted strains are relatively noninfectious by the oral route of exposure, do not replicate in the intestine, and are not excreted in the feces following infection by parenteral inoculation (17, 19; see also 89).

Localization of viral antigen using virus isolation, immunodiffusion, immunofluorescence, and ELISA techniques has been reported by van der Heide (92), Braune and Gentry (6), Ikeda and coworkers (36, 38, 41), Miyamae and coworkers (57, 59, 60, 61, 62), and Shafren and Tannock (78, 79). In young chicks exposed orally to field strains of AEV, primary infection of the alimentary tract, especially in the duodenum, is rapidly followed by a viremia and subsequent infection of the pancreas and other visceral organs (liver, heart, kidney,

spleen) and skeletal muscle, and finally the central nervous system (CNS). Alimentary tract infections involve muscular layers, and pancreatic infections are found in both the acinar and islet cells, persisting more in the latter. Viral antigen is relatively abundant in the CNS where Purkinje cells and the molecular layer of the cerebellum are apparently favored sites of virus replication. Chicks with clinical signs at 10–30 days of age tend to have viral antigen mostly in the CNS and pancreas; lesser amounts of antigen have been seen in heart and kidney and only very small amounts in liver and spleen. Persistence of the virus infection is common in the CNS, alimentary tract, and pancreas. Interestingly, the CNS and the pancreas are the only sites uniformly infected by embryo-adapted strains of AEV, although small amounts of virus may be found transiently in other tissues including the liver, heart and spleen.

Van der Heide (92) was unable to find viral antigen when tissues from experimentally infected mature birds were examined. However, Miyamae (60) did detect viral antigen in viscera and intestinal tract of 2-yr-old hens infected orally with field strains of AEV. In the intestinal tract, viral antigen was found in the epithelial tunica mucosa, circular muscle layer and/or muscularis mucosa, and in the tunica propria mucosa, but the detection rate was lower than has been reported for young chicks. No viral antigen was found in the CNS; presumably this lack of infection correlates with the absence of clinical disease in infected adults. As in young chicks, infection of older birds with embryo-adapted AEV has a more limited tissue distribution and/or lower titers of AEV in tissues other than those of the CNS when compared with infection with field strains (38, 39).

Cheville (21) and Westbury and Sinkovic (98, 99, 100, 101) did much to clarify certain aspects of the pathogenesis of the naturally occurring or experimental disease. Age at exposure was especially important; Cheville noted that birds infected at 1 day of age generally died, whereas those infected at 8 days developed paresis but usually recovered, and infection at 28 days caused no clinical signs. Bursectomy but not thymectomy abrogated the age resistance. Westbury and Sinkovic also noted disease when infection was initiated at 14 or less days of age, but not when it occurred at 20 or more days. They confirmed Cheville's conclusion that humoral immunity was the basis of age resistance. In their studies, they correlated young age (thus immunologic incompetence) with extended viremia, persistence of virus in the brain, and development of clinical disease. Presumably, the immune response of an immunologically competent bird would stop the spread of infection before it reached the CNS. Age resistance was not expressed when experimental infection was induced by IC inoculation of virus. Interestingly, Calnek et al. (19) found clinical signs in contact-exposed young chicks to have a minimum incubation period of 10–11 days, the same time that virus-neutralizing (VN) antibodies can be detected in adult birds.

Gross Lesions. The only gross lesions associated with AE in chicks are whitish areas (due to masses of infiltrating lymphocytes) in the muscularis of the ventriculus. These are subtle changes and require favorable conditions to be discerned. No changes have been described for infected adult birds, other than the lens opacities described under Signs.

Histopathology. The principal changes are in the CNS and some viscera. The peripheral nervous system is not involved—a point of importance in differential diagnosis.

In the CNS, the lesions are those of a disseminated, nonpurulent encephalomyelitis and a ganglionitis of the dorsal root ganglia. The most frequently encountered addition is a striking perivascular infiltrate seeming to occur in all portions of the brain and spinal cord (Figs. 21.2, 21.3) except the cerebellum, where it is confined to the nucleus (n.) cerebellaris. Infiltrating small lymphocytes may pile up several layers to form an impressive cuff.

Microgliosis occurs as diffuse and nodular aggregates. The glial lesion is seen chiefly in the cerebel-

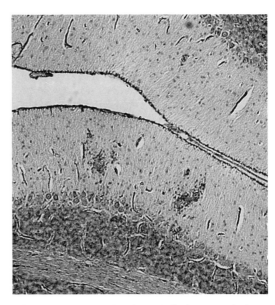

21.3. Perivascular infiltration and gliosis are seen in the nucleus cerebellaris. H & E, ×63 (Jakowski).

lar molecular layer, where it tends to be compact (Fig. 21.4). A loose gliosis is usually found in the n. cerebellaris, brain stem, midbrain, and optic lobes, and less often in the corpus straita. In the midbrain, two nuclei—n. rotundus and n. ovoidalis—are invariably affected with a loose microgliosis that can be considered pathognomonic. Another lesion of pathognomonic significance is central chromatolysis (axonal reaction) of the neurons in the nuclei of the brain stem, particularly those of the medulla ob-

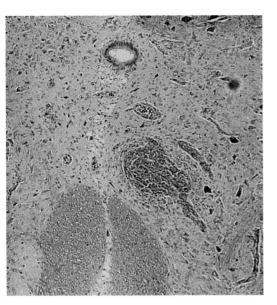

21.2. Spinal cord at lumbar level of chick. Large glial nodule and several perivascular infiltrates of lymphocytes are in gray matter. Central canal is at top.

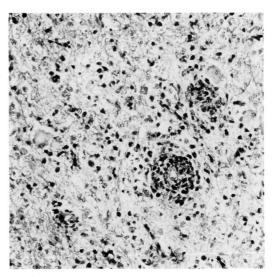

21.4. Cerebellum of chick. Glial foci common in avian encephalomyelitis are in the molecular layer. H & E, ×75.

longata (Fig. 21.5). If several sagittal sections are made, one can almost always find this alteration. The dying neuron is surrounded by satellite oligodendroglia and, later, microglia phagocytize the remains; the central chromatolysis is never seen without an attending cellular reaction.

Hishida et al. (33) examined brain and spinal cord lesions from experimentally infected chicks on a sequential basis using light- and electron-microscopy and immunofluorescence techniques. They considered the most characteristic changes to be degeneration of Purkinje cells in the cerebellum and motor neurons in the medulla oblongata and spinal cord. The central chromatolysis observed in the neurons was thought to be reversible, whereas affected Purkinje cells always became necrotic. Purkinje cells contained abundant viral antigen and cystalline arrays of virus particles in the cytoplasm, confirming the observations of Cheville (21). Degenerated neuronal cells showed dilatation of rough-surfaced endoplasmic reticulum, a reduction in ribosomes, and mitochondrial degeneration (21, 33, 103).

The dorsal root ganglia often contain rather tight aggregates of small lymphocytes amid the neurons. The lesion is always confined to the ganglion and never enters the nerves (Fig. 21.6).

In general, signs cannot be correlated with sever-

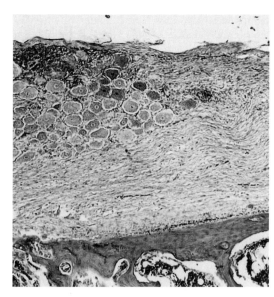

21.6. Dorsal root ganglion of lumbar level of chick. Dense infiltrate of lymphocytes is confined to ganglion. Sciatic nerve is unaffected. H & E, ×75.

ity of lesions or distribution in the CNS.

Visceral lesions appear to be hyperplasia of the lymphocytic aggregates scattered in a random fashion throughout the bird. In the proventriculus, there are normally a few small lymphocytes in the muscular wall; in AE, these are obvious dense aggregates that are certainly pathognomonic (Fig. 21.7). Similar lesions occur in the ventriculus muscle, but

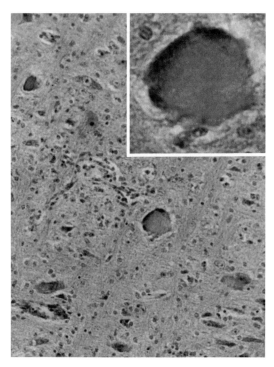

21.5. Medulla oblongata of chick. There is diffuse gliosis, and in the center a neuron is undergoing central chromatolysis. H & E, ×75. *Inset* shows tigrolysis and loss of nucleus, ×480.

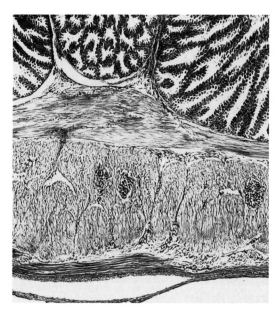

21.7. Proventriculus of chick. Dense lymphocytic foci are in muscular wall. This lesion is pathognomonic. H & E, ×30.

unfortunately they also occur in Marek's disease. In the pancreas, circumscribed lymphocytic follicles are normal (49), but in AE the number increases several times (Fig. 21.8). In the myocardium and particularly the atrium, there are aggregates of lymphocytes considered to be the result of AE (84). Lymphocytes in the myocardium of young chicks are not unusual, however; one may consider them a lesion only if they are widespread and accompanied by previously noted alterations.

There appears to be an excellent correlation between clinical signs and histologic lesions. In one study, 11% had signs but no lesions, while 8% had lesions but no signs (44). Later, Jungherr believed that all birds with clinical signs had histologic lesions. This was based on more intensive research that in turn was based on multiple sections of brain and viscera. Experimentally inoculated chicks killed in sequential fashion invariably yield lesions 1–2 days before clinical signs. Recovered birds free from signs have CNS lesions for at least 1 wk and probably much longer.

Immunity. Birds recovered from naturally occurring and experimental infection develop circulating antibodies capable of neutralizing the virus (see reviews 11, 14, 15, 89).

Cheville (21), and later Westbury and Sinkovic (99), clearly showed that humoral, but not cellular, immunity was important in curtailing infection. If the response is rapid, as is usual in birds over 21 days of age, the CNS infection apparently does not progress to the point where clinical signs may develop.

ACTIVE. When chickens are immunologically competent, the serologic response can be relatively rapid. Data from Calnek et al. (19) suggested that chicks from eggs laid as early as 11 days after exposure already carried passively acquired antibodies, since they were resistant to contact exposure after hatching. Also, positive VN tests, i.e., those with a neutralization index (NI) of 1.1 or greater (16), can be found after 11–14 days PI (20, 100), and positive immunodiffusion (ID) tests as early as 4–10 days PI (37).

Flocks of chickens with positive serology rarely if ever have recurrent outbreaks of AE.

PASSIVE. Antibodies are transferred to progeny from the dam via the embryo and can be demonstrated in egg yolk (86). Birds from immune dams were not fully susceptible to oral inoculation until 8–10 wk of age, and antibodies were demonstrated in the serum until 4–6 wk of age (20). Passively acquired antibodies can prevent development of clinical disease (101) and prevent or reduce the period of virus excretion in feces (19, 101). They also render embryonating eggs resistant to virus inoculated via the yolk sac, forming the basis for the embryo-susceptibility test (see Diagnosis).

DIAGNOSIS

Isolation and Identification of Causative Agent.
The brain is an excellent source of virus for isolation, although other tissues and organs induce the disease when injected into chicks (44, 93). Miyamae (61) found that in addition to the brain, the pancreas and duodenum were especially reliable sources of virus.

The need to titrate vaccine virus makes a sensitive method for virus detection very important. One system for assay of virus is to inoculate embryos (obtained from a susceptible flock) via the yolk sac when 5–7 days of age, allow these to hatch, and observe chicks for signs of disease during the first 10 days (9, 34). When clinical signs appear, brain, proventriculus, and pancreas should be examined for lesions as described under Histopathology. Additionally or alternatively, brain, pancreas, and duodenum from affected chicks can be examined for specific viral antigen by immunofluorescence (5, 6, 57, 61, 92) or ID (36) tests. A newly described monoclonal antibody (65), which recognizes a common epitope among AEV strains, may be a useful addition to the reagents available for virus detection in vaccine titrations, or for other assays.

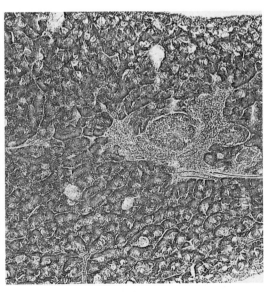

21.8. Pancreas of young chick. Several follicles of lymphocytes are present. This lesion is significant only when abnormal numbers of follicles are present. H & E, ×30.

Berger (3) infected chicken embryo brain cell cultures and then used indirect fluorescent antibody (FA) test to detect viral antigen. He found it to be more sensitive than the embryo inoculation method. Nicholas et al. (64) compared several methods for detection of AEV. Inoculation of brain cell cultures followed by indirect FA test was found to be convenient, but inoculation of 2-wk-old susceptible chicks followed by serologic tests such as ELISA or ID was slightly more sensitive. They considered the latter to be the method of choice for detection of AEV.

Serology. Chickens exposed to AEV develop antibodies that can be measured with the standard VN test (16, 86), indirect FA test (22), the ID test (29, 37, 50), ELISA (27, 82, see also 87), and passive hemagglutination test (2).

The VR embryo–adapted strain is recommended to determine the neutralizing capacity of the serum or plasma. Six-day-old embryos inoculated via the yolk sac with virus dilutions mixed with serum are examined for characteristic lesions 10–12 days PI. An NI of 1.1 or greater is considered as positive evidence of previous exposure to AEV. Among samples from a recently exposed flock, the NI may vary from 1.5 to 3.0. Antibodies may be detected as early as the 2nd wk after exposure and remain at significant levels for at least several months. Calnek and Jehnich (16) reported that in many instances birds having no detectable VN antibodies (NI less than 1.1) would resist IC challenge with as many as 10,000 EID_{50} of virus.

Another method to determine immunity of a flock is the embryo susceptibility (ES) test (86). Fertile eggs from the flock to be tested are incubated, along with control eggs from a known susceptible flock. After 6 days, each embryo is inoculated via the yolk sac with 100 EID_{50} of egg-adapted virus. Embryos are examined 10–12 days PI for characteristic lesions. If 100% of embryos are affected, the flock is considered susceptible; less than 50% affected indicates immunity. Intermediate figures should be considered nondefinitive and may indicate recent exposure.

Titers in the indirect FA test appear to parallel those of the VN test. Choi and Miura (22) and Dovadola et al. (24) found the indirect FA test to be as useful as the ES test for assessing immunity in turkey breeder flocks.

Standard procedures for ID tests were first reported by Ikeda (36, 37), who used concentrated tissue extracts from infected embryos as the antigen. Antibodies could be found as early as 4–10 days postexposure, and these persisted for at least 28 mo. Rare false-positives and false-negatives were reported when the ID test was compared with the VN test. Girshick and Crary (29), who used a similar

antigen, confirmed Ikeda's general results but did not find discrepancies between the ID and VN tests.

Ahmed et al. (2) described a passive hemagglutination test which they found to be more sensitive than the ID test and equal to the ES test in sensitivity.

An ELISA test using purified viral antigen compared well with the VN test and was found more suitable than the ID test for evaluation of immunity (27, 52, 72, 87). The use of a negative-antigen–subtraction step may enhance the ability to discriminate between positive and negative sera (78). Smart et al. (83) determined ELISA to correlate well with the ES test. They used ELISA to diagnose active infections with AEV by an increase in titer with sequential serum samples. Garrett et al. (28) were able to correlate ELISA titers in hens with the resistance of progeny embryos to challenge with AEV.

Differential Diagnosis. In spontaneous cases a tentative and frequently definite diagnosis of disease can be made when a complete history of the flock and typical specimens are provided for histopathology.

Histopathologic evidence of gliosis, lymphocytic perivascular infiltration, axonal type of neuronal degeneration in the CNS, and hyperplasia of the lymphoid follicles in certain visceral tissues usually can be considered as a basis for a positive diagnosis. Virus isolation or a rise in titer with serologic tests gives a more specific diagnosis.

Avian encephalomyelitis should not be confused with other avian diseases manifesting similar clinical signs, such as Newcastle disease, equine encephalomyelitis infection, nutritional disturbances (rickets, encephalomalacia, riboflavin deficiency), and Marek's disease.

Avian encephalomyelitis is predominantly a disease of 1- to 3-wk-old chicks. Since Newcastle disease may strike at this time, a problem of differential diagnosis can arise. Certain lesions are peculiar to AE: central chromatolysis as opposed to peripheral chromatolysis of Newcastle disease, gliosis in the n. rotundus and n. ovoidalis that is not observed in Newcastle disease, lymphocytic foci in the muscular wall of the proventriculus, and circumscribed lymphocytic follicles in the pancreas. Newcastle disease rarely causes an interstitial pancreatitis.

Encephalomalacia generally appears 2–3 wk later than AE, and from the standpoint of clinical history, the signs should be no problem. Histologically, it causes severe degenerative lesions in no way similar to AE.

Marek's disease, which occurs still later, presents little difficulty. The peripheral nerve involvement and state of lymphomatosis of the viscera are two criteria not seen in AE.

PREVENTION AND CONTROL. No satisfactory treatment is known for acute outbreaks in young chicks. Removal and segregation of affected chicks may be indicated under certain conditions, but they generally will not develop into profitable stock. Once a flock has experienced an outbreak of AE, no further evidence of it is likely to be observed (76).

Control of AE is achieved by vaccination of breeder flocks during the growing period to assure that they do not become infected after maturity, thereby preventing dissemination of the virus by the egg-borne route. Also, maternal antibodies protect progeny against contact to AEV during the critical first 2–3 wk. Vaccination may also be used with commercial egg-laying flocks to prevent a temporary drop in egg production associated with AE. Vaccines used to control AE in chickens have been shown to be efficacious in turkeys as well (23).

Inactivated vaccines have been developed (12, 18, 51, 75) and may be useful in flocks already in production or where the use of a live virus is contraindicated. Most flocks, however, are vaccinated with a live, embryo-propagated virus, such as strain-1143 (20), which can be administered by naturally occurring routes such as via drinking water or by spraying (9, 20, 26). Live virus vaccines, which can be stored frozen or after lyophilization (8, 70), are similar to field virus in that they spread readily within a flock. This allows for administration per os to a small percentage of the birds in a flock, which then spread infection to others, although this method is generally unsatisfactory for birds in wire cages (26, 77). Shafren et al. (81) found that serologic responses to vaccine administered ocularly to 10% (but not 5%) of a flock were as good as those following drinking-water administration of virus to the entire flock. Vaccination by wing-web inoculation of AEV is also practiced in many flocks, but, as noted below, this method may carry some risk of clinical signs (30). Generally, vaccination is done after 8 wk of age, and at least 4 wk before egg production.

It is very important that embryo adaptation of strains used for live virus vaccines does not occur because 1) adapted virus loses its ability to infect via the intestinal tract and is, therefore, no longer efficacious when administered by naturally occurring routes (20), and 2) adapted virus, like field strains, can cause clinical disease when administered by the wing-web route (17). Glisson and Fletcher (30) observed clinical encephalitis in broiler-breeder pullets given embryo-propagated AEV vaccine by the wing-web route and concluded that the most probable explanation was that the vaccine virus was inadvertently adapted during manufacture. Adaptation is detected by careful monitoring of inoculated embryos used in production of vaccine for characteristic signs (see Etiology), and any adapted virus can be eliminated from vaccine seed virus stocks by passage in susceptible chicks inoculated orally.

REFERENCES

1. Abe, T. 1968. A search for susceptible cells to avian encephalomyelitis (AE) virus. Jap J Vet Res 16:88–89.
2. Ahmed, A.A.S., I.M. Abou El-Azm, N.N.K. Ayoub, and B.I.M. E.-Toukhi. 1982. Studies on the serological detection of antibodies to avian encephalomyelitis virus. Avian Pathol 11:253–262.
3. Berger, R.G. 1982. An in vitro assay for quantifying the virus of avian encephalomyelitis. Avian Dis 26:534–541.
4. Bodin, G., J.L. Pellerin, A. Milon, M.F. Geral, X. Berthelot, and R. Lautie. 1981. Etude de la contamination experimentale du gibier a plumes (faisans, perdrix rouges, perdrix grises), par le virus de l'encephalomyelite infectieuse aviare. Revue Med Vet 132:805–816.
5. Braune, M.O., and R.F. Gentry. 1971. Avian encephalomyelitis virus. I. Pathogenesis in chicken embryos. Avian Dis 15:638–647.
6. Braune, M.O., and R.F. Gentry. 1971. Avian encephalomyelitis virus. II. Pathogenesis in chickens. Avian Dis 15:648–653.
7. Bridges, C.H., and A.I. Flowers. 1958. Iridocyclitis and cataracts associated with an encephalomyelitis in chickens. J Am Vet Med Assoc 132:79–84.
8. Bülow, V.v. 1964. Studies on the physico-chemical properties of the virus of avian encephalomyelitis (AE) with special reference to purification and preservation of virus suspensions. Zentralbl Veterinaermed [B] 11:674–686.
9. Bülow, V.v. 1965. Avian encephalomyelitis (AE). Cultivation, titration, and handling of the virus for live vaccines. Zentralbl Veterinaermed [B] 12:298–311.
10. Burke, C.N., H. Krauss, and R.E. Luginbuhl. 1965. The multiplication of avian encephalomyelitis virus in chicken embryo tissues. Avian Dis 9:104–108.
11. Butterfield, W.K. 1975. Avian encephalomyelitis: The virus and immune response. Am J Vet Res 36:557–559.
12. Butterfield, W.K., R.E. Luginbuhl, C.F. Helmboldt, and F.W. Sumner. 1961. Studies on avian encephalomyelitis. III. Immunization with an inactivated virus. Avian Dis 5:445–450.
13. Butterfield, W.K., C.M. Helmboldt, and R.E. Luginbuhl. 1969. Studies on avian encephalomyelitis. IV. Early incidence and longevity of histopathologic lesions in chickens. Avian Dis 13:53–57.
14. Calnek, B.W., and J. Fabricant. 1981. Immunity to infectious avian encephalomyelitis. In M.E. Rose, L.N. Payne and B.M. Freeman (eds.). Avian Immunology. British Poultry Science, Edinburgh, Scotland, pp. 235–244.
15. Calnek, B.W. 1993. Avian Encephalomyelitis. In J.B. McFerran and M.S. McNulty (eds.). Virus Infections of Vertebrates. 4. Virus Infections of Birds. Elsevier Science, Amsterdam, The Netherlands, pp. 469–478.
16. Calnek, B.W., and H. Jehnich. 1959. Studies on avian encephalomyelitis. I. The use of a serum-neutralization test in the detection of immunity levels. Avian Dis 3:95–104.
17. Calnek, B.W., and H. Jehnich. 1959. Studies on avian encephalomyelitis. II. Immune responses to vaccination procedures. Avian Dis 3:225–239.
18. Calnek, B.W., and P.J. Taylor. 1960. Studies on avian encephalomyelitis. III. Immune response to beta-propiolactone inactivated virus. Avian Dis 4:116–122.
19. Calnek, B.W., P.J. Taylor, and M. Sevoian. 1960. Studies on avian encephalomyelitis. IV. Epizootiology. Avian Dis 4:325–347.
20. Calnek, B.W., P.J. Taylor, and M. Sevoian. 1961. Studies on avian encephalomyelitis. V. Development and applica-

tion of an oral vaccine. Avian Dis 5:297–312.

21. Cheville, N.F. 1970. The influence of thymic and bursal lymphoid systems in the pathogenesis of avian encephalomyelitis. Am J Pathol 58:105–125.

22. Choi, W.P., and S. Miura. 1972. Research Note—Indirect fluorescent antibody technique for the detection of avian encephalomyelitis antibody in chickens. Avian Dis 16:949–951.

23. Deshmukh, D.R., C.T. Larsen, T.A. Rude, and B.S. Pomeroy. 1973. Evaluation of live-virus vaccine against avian encephalomyelitis in turkey breeder hens. Am J Vet Res 34:863–867.

24. Dovadola, E., M. Petek, P. D'Aprile, and F. Cancellotti. 1973. Detection of avian encephalomyelitis virus antibodies in turkey breeder flocks by the embryo-susceptibility and immunofluorescence tests. Proc 5th Int Congr World Vet Poult Assoc, pp. 1501–1506.

25. Feibel, F., C.F. Helmboldt, E.L. Jungherr, and J.R. Carson. 1952. Avian encephalomyelitis—Prevalence, pathogenicity of the virus, and breed susceptibility. Am J Vet Res 13:260–266.

26. Folkers, C., D. Jaspers, M.E.M. Stumpel, and E.A.E. Wittebrongel. 1976. Vaccination against avian encephalomyelitis with special reference to the spray method. Dev Biol Stand 33:364–369.

27. Garrett, J.K., R.B. Davis, and W.L. Ragland. 1984. Enzyme-linked immunosorbent assay for detection of antibody to avian encephalomyelitis virus in chickens. Avian Dis 28:117–130.

28. Garrett, J.K., R.B. Davis, and W.L. Ragland. 1985. Correlation of serum antibody titer for avian encephalomyelitis virus (AEV) in hens with the resistance of progeny embryos to AEV. Avian Dis 29:878–880.

29. Girshick, T., and C.K. Crary, Jr. 1982. Preparation of an agar-gel precipitating antigen for avian encephalomyelitis and its use in evaluating the antibody status of poultry. Avian Dis 26:798–804.

30. Glisson, J.R., and O.J. Fletcher. 1987. Clinical encephalitis following avian encephalomyelitis vaccination in broiler pullets. Avian Dis 31:383–385.

31. Gosting, L.H., B.W. Grinnell, and M. Matsumoto. 1980. Physico-chemical and morphological characteristics of avian encephalomyelitis virus. Vet Microbiol 5:87–100.

32. Hill, R.W., and R.G. Raymond. 1962. Apparent natural infection of Coturnix quail hens with the virus of avian encephalomyelitis. Case report. Avian Dis 6:226–227.

33. Hishida, N., Y. Odagiri, T. Kotani, and T. Horiuchi. 1986. Morphological changes of neurons in experimental avian encephalomyelitis. Jap J Vet Sci 48:169–172.

34. Hoekstra, J. 1964. Experiments with avian encephalomyelitis. Br Vet J 120:322–335.

35. Hohlstein, W.M., D.R. Deshmukh, C.T. Larsen, J.H. Sautter, B.S. Pomeroy, and J.R. MCDowell. 1970. An epiornithic of avian encephalomyelitis in turkeys in Minnesota. Am J Vet Res 31:2233–2242.

36. Ikeda, S. 1977. Immunodiffusion tests in avian encephalomyelitis. l. Standardization of procedure and detection of antigen in infected chickens and embryos. Natl Inst Anim Health Q (Tokyo) 17:81–87.

37. Ikeda, S. 1977. Immunodiffusion tests in avian encephalomyelitis. II. Detection of precipitating antibody in infected chickens in comparison with neutralizing antibody. Natl Inst Anim Health Q (Tokyo) 17:88–94.

38. Ikeda, S., and K. Matsuda. 1976. Susceptibility of chickens to avian encephalomyelitis virus. IV. Behavior of the virus in laying hens. Natl Inst Anim Health Q 16:83–89.

39. Ikeda, S., and K. Matsuda. 1976. Susceptibility of chickens to avian encephalomyelitis virus. V. Behavior of a field strain in laying hens. Natl Inst Anim Health Q 16:90–96.

40. Ikeda, I., K. Matsuda, and K. Yonaiyama. 1976. Susceptibility of chickens to avian encephalomyelitis virus. III.

Behavior of the virus in growing chicks. Natl Inst Anim Health Q 16:33–38.

41 Ikeda, S., K. Matsuda, and K. Yonaiyama. 1976. Susceptibility of chickens to avian encephalomyelitis virus. II. Behavior of the virus in day-old chicks. Natl Inst Health Q l6:1–7.

42. Jones, E.E. 1932. An encephalomyelitis in the chicken. Science 76:331–332.

43. Jones, E.E. 1934. Epidemic tremor, an encephalomyelitis affecting young chickens. J Exp Med 59:781–798.

44. Jungherr, E., and E.L. Minard. 1942. The present status of avian encephalomyelitis. J Am Vet Med Assoc 100:38–46.

45. Jungherr, E.L., F. Sumner, and R.E. Luginbuhl. 1956. Pathology of egg-adapted avian encephalomyelitis. Science 124:80–81.

46. Kamada, M., G. Sato, and S. Miura. 1974. Characterization of multiplication of embryo-adapted avian encephalomyelitis virus in chick embryo brain cell cultures. Jpn J Vet Res 22:32–42.

47. Kodama, H., G. Sato, and S. Miura. 1975. Avian encephalomyelitis virus in chicken pancreatic cell cultures. Avian Dis 19:556–565.

48. Krauss, H., and S. Ueberschär. 1966. Zur Ultrastruktur des Virus der aviaeren Enzephalitis. Berl Munch Tierarztl Wochenschr 79:480–482.

49. Lucas, A.M. 1951. Lymphoid tissue and its relationship to so-called normal lymphoid foci and to lymphomatosis. VI. A study of lymphoid areas in the pancreas of doves and chickens. Poult Sci 30:116–124.

50. Lukert, P.D., and R.B. Davis. 1971. New methods under investigation for the evaluation of the immune status of breeder hens to avian encephalomyelitis. II. Preliminary studies with an immunodiffusion test for avian encephalomyelitis antibodies. Avian Dis 15:935–938.

51. MacLeod, A.J. 1965. Vaccination against avian encephalomyelitis with a betapropialactone inactivated vaccine. Vet Rec 77:335–338.

52. Malkinson, M., Y. Weisman, A. Stavinski, I. Davidson, U. Orgad, and M.S. Dison. 1986. Application of ELISA to study avian encephalomyelitis in a flock of turkeys. Vet Rec 119:503–504.

53. Mancini, I.O., and V.J. Yates. 1967. Cultivation of avian encephalomyelitis virus in vitro. I. In chick embryo neuroglial cell culture. Avian Dis 11:672–679.

54. Mancini, I.O., and V.J. Yates. 1968. Cultivation of avian encephalomyelitis virus in vitro. II. In chick embryo fibroblastic cell culture. Avian Dis 12:278–284.

55. Mancini, I.O., and V.J. Yates. 1968. Cultivation of avian encephalomyelitis virus in chicken embryo kidney cell culture. Avian Dis 12:686–688.

56. Mathey, W.J., Jr. 1955. Avian encephalomyelitis in pheasants. Cornell Vet 45:89–93.

57. Miyamae, T. 1974. Ecological survey by the immunofluorescent method of virus in enzootics of avian encephalomyelitis. Avian Dis 18:369–377.

58. Miyamae, T. 1976. Emergence pattern of egg-adapted avian encephalomyelitis virus by alternating passage in chickens and embryos. Avian Dis 20:425–428.

59. Miyamae, T. 1977. Immunofluorescent study on egg-adapted avian encephalomyelitis virus infection in chickens. Am J Vet Res 38:2009–2012.

60. Miyamae, T. 1981. Localization of viral protein in avian-encephalomyelitis-virus-infected hens. Avian Dis 25:1065–1069.

61. Miyamae, T. 1983. Invasion of avian encephalomyelitis virus from the gastrointestinal tract to the central nervous system in young chickens. Am J Vet Res 44:508–510.

62. Miyamae, T. and S. Miura. 1971. Patterns of virus

multiplication in chickens infected orally with wild and egg adapted encephalomyelitis viruses. Jpn J Vet Sci 33:40–41.

63. Mohanty, G.C., and J.L. West. 1968. Some observations on experimental avian encephalomyelitis. Avian Dis 12:689–693.

64. Nicholas, R.A.J., A.J. Ream, and D.H. Thornton. 1987. Replication of avian encephalomyelitis virus in chick embryo neuroglial cell cultures. Arch Virol 96:283–287.

65. Ohishi, K., M. Senda, H. Yamamoto, H. Nagai, M. Norimatsu, and H. Sasaki. 1994. Detection of avian encephalomyelitis viral antigen with a monoclonal antibody. Avian Pathol 23:49–59.

66. Olitsky, P.K. 1939. Experimental studies on the virus of infectious avian encephalomyelitis. J Exp Med 70:565–582.

67. Olitsky, P.K., and J.H. Bauer. 1939. Ultrafiltration of the virus of infectious avian encephalomyelitis. Proc Soc Exp Biol Med 42:634–636.

68. Olitsky, P.K., and H. Van Roekel. 1952. Avian encephalomyelitis (epidemic tremor). In H.E. Biester and L.H. Schwarte (eds.). Diseases of Poultry, 3rd ed. Iowa State University Press, Ames, IA, pp. 619–628.

69. Peckham, M.C. 1957. Lens opacities in fowls possibly associated with epidemic tremors. Case report. Avian Dis 1:247–255.

70. Polewaczyk, D.E., Z. Zolli, Jr., and W.D. Vaughn. 1972. Efficacy studies for a freeze-dried avian encephalomyelitis vaccine. Poult Sci 51:1851.

71. Richey, D.J. 1962. Avian encephalomyelitis (epidemic tremor). Southeast Vet 13:55–57.

72. Richter, V.R., J. Kosters, and S. Kuhavanta-Kalkosol. 1985. Vergleichende untersuchungen zur anwendung eines enzyme-linked-immunosorbent-assay (ELISA) zum antikorpernachweis gegen den erreger der aviaren encephalomyelitis. Zentralbl Veterinarmed [B] 32:116–127.

73. Sato, G., M. Kamada, T. Miyamae, and S. Miura. 1971. Propagation of non-egg-adapted avian encephalomyelitis virus in chick embryo brain cell culture. Avian Dis 15:326–333.

74. Schaaf, K. 1958. Immunization for the control of avian encephalomyelitis. Avian Dis 2:279–289.

75. Schaaf, K. 1959. Avian encephalomyelitis immunization with inactivated virus. Avian Dis 3:245–256.

76. Schaaf, K., and W.F. Lamoreaux. 1955. Control of avian encephalomyelitis by vaccination. Am J Vet Res 16:627–633.

77. Schneider, T. 1967. Beobachtungen ueber die Durchseuchung von Zuchtthuehnerbestaenden nach Lebendvaccination mit dem Virus der aviaeren Encephalomyelitis (AE) der Huehner. Arch Gefluegelkd 31:342–348.

78. Shafren, D.R., and G.A. Tannock. 1988. An enzyme-linked immunosorbent assay for the detection of avian encephalomyelitis virus antigens. Avian Dis 32:209–214.

79. Shafren, D.R., and G.A. Tannock. 1991. Pathogenesis of avian encephalomyelitis viruses. J Gen Virol 72:2713–2719.

80. Shafren, D.R., and G.A. Tannock. 1992. Further evidence that the nucleic acid of avian encephalomyelitis virus consists of RNA. Avian Dis 36:1031–1033.

81. Shafren, D.R., G.A. Tannock, and P.J. Groves. 1992. Antibody responses to avian encephalomyelitis virus vaccines when administered by different routes. Aust Vet J 69:272–275.

82. Smart, I.J., and D.C. Grix. 1985. Measurement of antibodies to infectious avian encephalomyelitis virus by ELISA. Avian Pathol 14:341–352.

83. Smart, I.J., D.C. Grix, and D.A. Barr. 1986. The application of the ELISA to the diagnosis and control of avian encephalomyelitis. Aust Vet J 63:297–299.

84. Springer, W.T., and S.C. Schmittle. 1968. Avian encephalomyelitis. A chronological study of the histopathogenesis in selected tissues. Avian Dis 12:229–239.

85. Sumner, F.W., E.L. Jungherr, and R.E. Luginbuhl. 1957. Studies on avian encephalomyelitis. I. Egg adaption of the virus. Am J Vet Res 18:717–723.

86. Sumner, F.W., R.E. Luginbuhl, and E.L. Jungherr. 1957. Studies on avian encephalomyelitis. II. Flock survey for embryo susceptibility to the virus. Am J Vet Res 18:720–723.

87. Sytuo, B., and M. Matsumoto. 1981. Detection of chicken antibodies against avian encephalomyelitis virus by an enzyme-linked immunoassay. Poult Sci 60:1742.

88. Tannock, G.A., and D.R. Shafren. 1985. A rapid procedure for the purification of avian encephalomyelitis viruses. Avian Dis 29:312–321.

89. Tannock, G.A., and D.R. Shafren. 1994. Avian encephalomyelitis: A review. Avian Pathol 23:603–620.

90. Taylor, J.R.E., and E.P. Schelling. 1960. The distribution of avian encephalomyelitis in North America as indicated by an immunity test. Avian Dis 4:122–133.

91. Taylor, L.W., D.C. Lowry, and L.G. Raggi. 1955. Effects of an outbreak of avian encephalomyelitis (epidemic tremor) in a breeding flock. Poult Sci 34:1036–1045.

92. Van der Heide, L. 1970. The fluorescent antibody technique in the diagnosis of avian encephalomyelitis. Univ Maine Tech Bull 44:1–79.

93. Van Roekel, H., K.L. Bullis, and M.K. Clarke. 1938. Preliminary report on infectious avian encephalomyelitis. J Am Vet Med Assoc 93:372–375.

94. Van Roekel, H., K.L. Bullis, and M.K. Clarke. 1939. Infectious avian encephalomyelitis. Vet Med 34:754–755.

95. Van Roekel, H., K.L. Bullis, O.S. Flint, and M.K. Clarke. 1940. Avian encephalomyelitis. Mass Agric Exp Stn Annu Rep Bull 369:94.

96. Van Roekel, H., K.L. Bullis, and M.K. Clarke. 1941. Transmission of avian encephalomyelitis. J Am Vet Med Assoc 99:220.

97. Van Steenis, G. 1971. Survey of various avian species for neutralizing antibody and susceptibility to avian encephalomyelitis virus. Res Vet Sci 12:308–311.

98. Westbury, H.A., and B. Sinkovic. 1978. The pathogenesis of infectious avian encephalomyelitis. I. The effect of the age of the chicken and the route of administration of the virus. Aust Vet J 54:68–71.

99. Westbury, H.A., and B. Sinkovic. 1978. The pathogenesis of infectious avian encephalomyelitis. II. The effect of immunosuppression on the disease. Aust Vet J 54:72–75.

100. Westbury, H.A., and B. Sinkovic. 1978. The pathogenesis of infectious avian encephalomyelitis. III. The relationship between viraemia, invasion of the brain by the virus, and the development of specific serum neutralising antibody. Aust Vet J 54:76–80.

101. Westbury, H.A., and B. Sinkovic. 1978. The pathogenesis of infectious avian encephalomyelitis. IV. The effect of maternal antibody on the development of the disease. Aust Vet J 54:81–85.

102. Wills, F.K., and I.M. Moulthrop. 1956. Propagation of avian encephalomyelitis virus in the chick embryo. Southwest Vet 10:39–42.

103. Yamagiwa, S., T. Yamashita, and C. Itakura. 1969. Poliomyelitis of newborn chicks (epidemic tremor of chickens, avian encephalomyelitis). II. Electron microscopic observations of degenerated nerve cells. Jpn J Vet Sci 31:173–177.

22 Influenza

B. C. Easterday, Virginia S. Hinshaw, and David A. Halvorson

INTRODUCTION. Influenza is an infection and/or disease syndrome caused by any type A influenza virus, a member of the *Orthomyxoviridae* family. Influenza A viruses are responsible for major disease problems in birds, as well as in humans and lower mammals (46, 67, 98, 123). Literally thousands of viruses, belonging to many different antigenic subtypes based on hemagglutinin (HA) and neuraminidase (NA) surface antigens, have been recovered from domestic and wild avian species throughout the world. Infections among domestic or confined birds have been associated with a variety of disease syndromes ranging from subclinical to mild upper respiratory disease to loss of egg production to acute generalized fatal disease.

In domestic species, influenza viruses have caused considerable economic losses. The U.S. government expended over $60 million in 1983–84 to eradicate a highly pathogenic H5N2 virus in poultry in the Pennsylvania–Virginia–New Jersey outbreak. The potential cost of the disease without the eradication program was estimated to be many times higher (109). The $60 million included the cost of eradication (diagnosis, quarantine, flock disposal, cleanup, decontamination, epidemiologic investigation, and other regulatory procedures) and indemnity payments to flock owners. Consumers paid an estimated additional $349 million to cover the increased retail cost of table eggs as a result of lost egg production in the quarantine area (109). More limited outbreaks of avian influenza are also quite costly. For example, on one chicken farm in Australia in 1985, an outbreak involving a highly pathogenic virus cost over $2 million to eradicate (41).

The economic impact is not limited to chickens; losses have been suffered by turkey producers for many years in several countries in Europe, in the United States, and in Israel (10, 118, 139, 172, 185). An epidemic in Minnesota in 1978 cost turkey producers in excess of $5 million (140); the estimated cost of outbreaks in Minnesota since 1977 totaled more than $10 million (139).

In most cases, losses cannot be predicted when an influenza outbreak appears, because many factors influence the outcome of infection. These factors include the variation in the biologic characteristics of the virus, concurrent infection, environmental stresses, age and sex of the bird, etc., with the result being that the morbidity and mortality rates range from negligible to near 100%. Any calculation of economic impact must include all of those factors that impinge on the cost of production, e.g., medication, extra feed, extra care, quarantine measures, vaccines, decreased carcass quality, cleaning and sanitizing, and loss of local and international trade. Unfortunately, there are insufficient data to provide a reasonable estimate of avian influenza losses on a nationwide basis for any country.

In contrast to domestic or confined birds, free-flying birds typically do not experience significant disease problems due to influenza viruses; yet, these infections are widespread in many of these birds (67, 75). Influenza viruses are readily recovered from migratory waterfowl, particularly ducks, throughout the world. There is considerable speculation about the epidemiologic significance of this very large reservoir of viruses in wild birds: that this reservoir can serve as a source of viruses for other species, including humans, lower mammals, and birds, and that such a high rate of infection provides the opportunity for the maintenance and emergence of "new" and potentially highly pathogenic strains through the process of mutation and/or genetic reassortment. The genetic diversity of avian influenza viruses in the wildlife reservoirs may be important in the overall survival of these viruses in nature.

Because of the significant losses from avian influenza, international symposia were convened in 1981, 1986, and 1992 to exchange information on this virus; the first (142) focused on definition of highly pathogenic strains and identification of sources of the virus; the second (143), on the virus and on the problems and possible solutions in outbreaks involving highly pathogenic influenza viruses in chickens and turkeys; and the third (144), on the circulation of the virus and plans for dealing with localized outbreaks of mild disease and future outbreaks of highly pathogenic avian influenza. Influenza is an international problem, so solutions will require international efforts and cooperation.

HISTORY. Fowl plague, now known to be caused by highly pathogenic strains of avian influenza viruses, was described by Perroncito as a serious disease of chickens in Italy in 1878 and caused by a "filterable" agent (virus) by Centanni and Savunozzi in 1901 (169). It was not until 1955, however, that it was demonstrated that fowl plague viruses were actually type A influenza viruses (155). Viruses related to the original "fowl plague" isolates (surface antigens-H7N1 and H7N7) caused high mortality among chickens, turkeys, and other species. Disease outbreaks involving these particular strains have been reported in many areas of the world during this century, including North and South America, North Africa, the Middle and Far East, Europe, Great Britain, and the former Soviet Union. Highly pathogenic strains belonging to the H5 subtype were detected in chickens in Scotland, chick/Scot/59 (H5N1) and common terns, tern/S.A./61 (H5N3); both species suffered severe disease problems. These isolations led to the speculation that all H7 and H5 viruses were highly pathogenic, but this was not found true. As an example, a virus, avirulent for chickens, with an H7 HA was recovered from turkeys in Oregon in 1971 (21, 22). Since that time, many other viruses with the H5 and H7 HAs have been isolated from domestic and wild birds in various areas of the world, and many of these are avirulent for any species (5, 67). It should be mentioned, however, that historically, the most severe disease problems have been due to viruses of the H5 and H7 subtypes.

From 1950 to 1960, the discoveries that the fowl plaque virus was an influenza A virus and that influenza viruses could be recovered from many different domestic and wild avian species initiated increased efforts to understand avian influenza viruses. Since detailed histories of the isolation of influenza viruses in this century are available (5, 46, 67), only more recent events are described here.

Reports of severe disease outbreaks involving highly pathogenic influenza A viruses during the past 20 yr have, fortunately, been infrequent. Alexander (6) listed five substantiated outbreaks since 1975; these occurred in Australia (1975 and 1985), England (1979), the United States (1983–84), and Ireland (1983–84). In the United States, the only severe outbreaks were reported in 1929 (169) and 1983–84, indicating the infrequency of such events. Much information on the outbreak in Pennsylvania during 1983–84 is presented in the *Proceedings of the 2nd International Symposium on Avian Influenza* (143), but some specific aspects (47) are mentioned here. The first isolates were obtained in April, 1983, from chickens experiencing acute respiratory disease with 0–15% mortality and declining egg production. The viruses were identified as H5N2 and, based on chicken inoculation, were not classified as being highly pathogenic. This problem continued at a low level, with about six in-

fected flocks present at any given time until October 1983 when mortality increased to 50–89%, with the birds experiencing severe depression, tremors, and a complete cessation of egg production. Viruses isolated from these birds were also H5N2 but were designated as highly pathogenic based on chicken inoculation. This apparent change in the disease led the U.S. Department of Agriculture to declare an "extraordinary emergency" with the goal of eradication. The eradication effort included strict quarantine; total poultry population surveillance with destruction of all flocks with clinical, serologic, or virologic evidence of H5N2 influenza; environmental cleanup followed by decontamination; and intensive education on biosecurity (52). Over the next 2 yr, this effort had to include not only poultry farms, but also live-bird markets in metropolitan areas such as New York City because these markets were found to be involved in the maintenance of the virus and exposure of poultry flocks (58). The highly pathogenic strain was successfully eliminated; however, avirulent H5N2 viruses have since been recovered from farms and live-bird markets in several states.

The first observation of clinical signs compatible with avian influenza in Mexico is thought to have been in the fall of 1993. The virus was identified as avian influenza with H5N2 surface antigens in the spring of 1994, and it was classified at that time as being of low pathogenicity. Experience in the field was compatible with that determination. A nationwide serologic survey determined that poultry flocks in 11 states of central Mexico had been infected. Flocks in the north and southeast of Mexico were serologically negative at that time.

In December, 1994, and January, 1995, flocks in the states of Puebla (predominantly layer chickens) and Queretaro (predominantly broiler chickens) experienced greatly increased mortality and declines in egg production. Virus isolated from these flocks produced signs and lesions compatible with highly pathogenic avian influenza in laboratory tests. Numerous flocks representing millions of chickens in three states to the south and north of Mexico City were subsequently infected with the highly pathogenic virus. The state of Yucatan and some states bordering the United States have since been determined to have seropositive flocks. Vaccination with inactivated, oil-emulsion vaccine has apparently been effective in reducing mortality and egg-production losses, but nonvaccinated sentinels left in the vaccinated flocks have seroconverted at a high rate, indicating that the nonpathogenic virus is likely circulating in the flocks.

The events in Mexico over the past several years represent the most widespread and lengthy known occurrence of avian influenza virus in poultry. The change in the pathogenicity of the virus after many months of circulating in poultry flocks was not un-like the experience in Pennsylvania in 1983, al-though the molecular basis of those changes dif-fered (80).

A report from Pakistan (125) described a severe type H7 avian influenza outbreak that began in De-cember 1994 in broiler breeders. It eventually af-fected all classes of poultry from 7 to 66 wk of age, with an overall mortality of 63% in the area of the initial outbreak. There was also an outbreak of highly pathogenic avian influenza (H7N3) in chick-ens in 1994 in Queensland, Australia. The birds on the affected premises were slaughtered and nearby flocks were monitored by serology. The HA-cleav-age site contained a sequence that differed from the previous three highly pathogenic H7 avian in-fluenza (AI) viruses isolated from disease outbreaks in Australia (159).

Since the first influenza isolates from turkeys in North America in 1963 (104), these viruses have frequently caused disease problems. Viruses found in turkeys on open range are often thought to have been introduced by migratory waterfowl (62, 67). An interesting situation in turkeys has developed during the last decade in that H1N1 viruses typi-cally associated with pigs have been responsible for outbreaks in turkeys (72) characterized by respira-tory disease and diminished egg production (120). This swine–turkey connection was the first indica-tion that mammalian viruses could be responsible for infection and disease in birds. Studies on H1N1 isolates from pigs and birds throughout the world (12, 13, 73) suggest that swine viruses are being transmitted to turkeys and, in addition, that H1N1 viruses from ducks are being transmitted to pigs in some areas of the world.

Although evidence for the infection of wild birds existed prior to the 1970s, it was not until then that the high infection rate among migratory waterfowl was recognized. Surveillance studies revealed the widespread distribution of influenza viruses in these birds, particularly ducks (66, 69), and more recently in shorebirds (93). Such studies (67, 70) have shown that virtually all known antigenic subtypes of type A influenza viruses and combinations of HA and NA surface antigens exist in the avian wildlife reservoir; the viruses are typically avirulent for the hosts; the viruses possess broad host ranges, includ-ing other birds and mammals; genetic reassortment between their viruses occurs in the natural setting; and intestinal replication of the viruses in these birds may be an important factor in the efficient transmission of these viruses among waterfowl and potentially to other species. This reservoir in wildlife occupies an important role in the ecology of influenza.

During the last 10 yr, viruses typically found in avian species have been recovered from outbreaks of disease in mammals, such as seals (74, 108, 181) and mink (49, 101), and have been detected in whales (76). These findings suggest that the associ-ation between birds and mammals in the natural set-ting may lead to transmission of avian viruses, re-sulting in significant disease problems.

INCIDENCE AND DISTRIBUTION. Avian influenza viruses are distributed throughout the world in many domestic birds, including turkeys, chickens, guinea fowl, chukars, quail, pheasants, geese, and ducks, and in wild species, including ducks, geese, sandpipers, sanderlins, ruddy turn-stones, terns, swans, shearwaters, herons, guille-mots, puffins, and gulls (see 5, 7, 10, 46, 67, 123). Migratory waterfowl, particularly ducks, have yielded more viruses than any other group, while domestic turkeys and chickens have experienced the most substantial disease problems due to in-fluenza. Influenza viruses have also been isolated from caged birds, including mynahs, parakeets, par-rots, cockatoos, weaverbirds, finches, and hawks (4, 86, 160, 164, 165). These birds were often being held in quarantine and the significance of infection in these birds is not yet clear. Passerine birds have yielded relatively few influenza viruses, particu-larly in view of the size of this bird population. There have been some isolations from passerine birds in contact with sick domestic birds, e.g., star-lings in Israel (112) and Australia (41). Studies on the Australian isolate, A/starling/Victoria/5156/85 (H7N7) (131), led the authors to suggest that highly pathogenic viruses were transmitted between do-mestic poultry and passerine birds.

Precise distribution and prevalence of influenza viruses are difficult to determine because of the sampling anomalies. The World Health Organiza-tion has encouraged and supported surveillance programs to increase the available data on the prevalence and distribution. Even so, most surveil-lance efforts are conducted by investigators who have a specific interest in avian influenza and/or the ecology of influenza.

Distribution data on avian influenza are clearly influenced by the distribution of both domestic and wild species, the locality of poultry production, mi-gratory routes, season, and disease reporting sys-tems. Prevalence is also influenced by some of the same factors. Accurate prevalence rates are difficult to determine because of the variety of surveillance systems and procedures employed. For any one episode of avian influenza in a domestic species, a reasonable prevalence rate can be determined; how-ever, the prevalence and distribution are not pre-dictable. For example, in turkeys in Minnesota, the prevalence has been very high some years and nearly nonexistent during others (139). The absence is not due to residual immunity but, rather, to an unexplained absence of the viruses. Waterfowl have been viewed as a significant source of viruses for turkeys on open range and this may be important in areas such as Minnesota and Wisconsin, which are located along a major flyway. Investigators there (62, 63) have recovered many influenza viruses from free-flying and sentinel ducks during the fall migration and have established that the outbreaks in turkeys coincide with the presence of the migratory ducks. Even so, it is difficult to predict which virus will appear and cause problems in the turkeys at any given time.

Surveillance of migratory waterfowl in North America has indicated that up to 60% of juvenile birds may be infected as they congregate in marshalling areas prior to migration (69, 75). As the birds migrate, the rate of virus recovery drops precipitously. Since ducks have been shown to excrete virus for as long as 30 days (180), this means that few cycles of transmission would be required to maintain the viruses. It seems possible that the viruses are maintained in the wild duck population by passage to susceptible birds, even at a low level, throughout the year until the next breeding season results in a new group of susceptible juveniles. Transmission can readily occur due to the excretion of high quantities of the virus in the feces, resulting in heavily contaminated lake or pond water (68). Recent studies (93) on shorebirds (such as sanderlins, ruddy turnstones, and sandpipers) and gulls suggested that they constitute a significant reservoir of viruses. The involvement of wild birds, particularly waterfowl, with influenza viruses underlines the need for producers of domestic, commercial birds to provide separation between domestic and wild bird populations.

There have been only three incidents of influenza viruses in chickens in North America since the last fowl plague outbreak in 1929: Alabama in 1975 (83, 84), Minnesota in 1979 (61), and Pennsylvania during 1983–84 (48). There are reports of influenza infections in chickens in several other countries including Belgium, Scotland, Italy, the former Soviet Union, Australia, Hong Kong, Belgium, France, and Israel (5, 118). Influenza infections of domestic ducks have been detected in many areas of the world, including North America (154). Influenza in turkeys has also been reported in many countries, including Hungary, France, Holland, Italy, Ireland, England, Canada, the United States, and Israel (5, 6). Alexander (5), Hinshaw et al. (70) and the symposia proceedings (142, 143, 144) provide information and tabulations of the countries, years, and subtypes of viruses in wild waterfowl, chickens, domestic ducks, and turkeys.

In considering the prevalence and distribution of influenza viruses in avian species, it becomes clear that many viruses circulate in birds throughout the world. In view of that, it is puzzling that avian influenza viruses are not responsible for more extensive poultry disease problems.

ETIOLOGY

Classification. Avian influenza viruses, along with all other influenza viruses, constitute the virus family *Orthomyxoviridae* (98, 123). These are medium-sized, pleomorphic RNA viruses with helical symmetry and glycoprotein projections from the envelope that have hemagglutinating and NA activity. There are three antigenically distinct types of influenza viruses: A, B, and C. The type specificity is determined by the antigenic nature of the nucleoprotein (NP) and matrix (M) antigens, which are closely related among all influenza A viruses. Types B and C are typically found only in humans. Type A influenza viruses are found in humans; in swine; in horses; occasionally in other mammals such as mink, seals, and whales; and in many avian species.

CLASSIFICATION BASED ON THE HEMAGGLUTININ AND NEURAMINIDASE. Type A viruses are divided into subtypes according to the antigenic nature of the HA and NA. There are currently 15 distinct HAs and nine distinct NAs. A standard system of nomenclature for influenza viruses was proposed in 1971 (186) and revised in 1980 (187). The name of an influenza virus includes the type (A, B, or C), host of origin (except human), geographic origin, strain number (if any), and year of isolation followed by the antigenic description of the HA (H) and NA (N) in parentheses. For example, a type A influenza virus isolated from turkeys in Wisconsin in 1968 and classified as H8N4 is designated A/turkey/Wisconsin/1/68 (H8N4). The H and N subtype designations, which include the previous and current descriptions, are listed in Table 22.1.

Table 22.1. Type A influenza subtype nomenclature

Hemagglutinin		Neuraminidase	
1980–Present	Previous	1980–Present	Previous
H1	H0, H1, Hsw1	N1	N1
H2	H2	N2	N2
H3	H3, Heq2, Hav7	N3	Nav2, Nav3
H4	Hav4	N4	Nav4
H5	Hav5	N5	Nav5
H6	Hav6	N6	Nav1
H7	Hav1, Heq1	N7	Neq1
H8	Hav8	N8	Neq2
H9	Hav9	N9	Nav6
H10	Hav2		
H11	Hav3		
H12	Hav10		
H13	Hav11		
H14	—		
H15	—		

Sources: (94, 150, 187).

CLASSIFICATION BASED ON PATHOGENICITY.
The term *fowl plague* was often used to refer either
to the clinical disease or to the virus involved in
outbreaks with high mortality. It had become clear
that a definition of fowl plague based on antigenic
characteristics (presence of H7) was inadequate because antigenically similar, if not identical, viruses
were frequently isolated from avian species and
they were avirulent (21). Therefore, it was important to develop recommendations for a uniform terminology for the highly pathogenic avian influenza
viruses, especially fowl plague (16). Unfortunately,
most, if not all, disease regulations for the control of
fowl plague were based on the H7 surface antigen
requirement.

Participants at an international symposium recommended that the term *fowl plague* be discarded,
except for historical purposes, and they proposed
criteria for defining "highly pathogenic" influenza
viruses (142). One recommendation was that 75%
mortality in experimentally inoculated birds be considered as one criterion for highly pathogenic
strains (16). Unfortunately, the initial H5N2 isolates
from chickens in the Pennsylvania outbreak failed
to produce 75% mortality and did not qualify as a
"highly pathogenic" virus (135). In view of this, the
U.S. Animal Health Association Committee on
Transmissible Diseases of Poultry and Other Avian
Species (145) has revised the original recommendations for determining whether an avian influenza
isolate should be classified as highly pathogenic
and, therefore, must be considered for eradication.
These recommendations are:

1. Any influenza virus that is lethal for six, seven,
   or eight of eight 4- to 6-week-old susceptible
   chickens within 10 days following intravenous
   inoculation with 0.2 mL of a 1:10 dilution of a
   bacteria-free, infectious allantoic fluid.
2. Any H5 or H7 virus that does not meet the criteria in item 1, but has an amino acid sequence at
   the hemagglutinin cleavage site that is compatible with highly pathogenic avian influenza
   viruses.
3. Any influenza virus that is not an H5 or H7 subtype, which kills one to five chickens and grows
   in cell culture in the absence of trypsin.

Morphology. The morphology and arrangement of the components in the influenza virion have
been reviewed (98, 123). Virions (see Fig. 22.1) are
roughly spherical with a diameter of 80–120 nm;
however, there are often filamentous forms of the
same diameter with varying lengths. The surface of
the virion is covered with closely spaced spikes or
projections 10–12 nm in length. A helical nucleocapsid is enclosed within the viral envelope. The
surface spikes with two different shapes are the HA,
which is a rod-shaped trimer, and the NA, which is
a mushroom-shaped tetramer. The virion may be
disrupted with detergents, resulting in the release of
the spikes, which retain their respective activities.
The HA is responsible for the attachment of the
virion to cell surface receptors (sialyloligosaccha-
rides) and is responsible for the hemagglutinating
activity of the virus. Antibodies against the HA are
very important in neutralization of the virus and
protection against infection. Neuraminidase enzyme activity is responsible for the release of new
virus from the cell by its action on the neuraminic
acid in the receptors. Antibodies to NA are also important in protection, apparently by restricting the
spread of virus from infected cells. The three-dimensional structures of the H3 HA (188) and the N2
(39) and N9 NAs (15) have now been determined,
and important antigenic domains, or epitopes, have
been defined.

The HA and NA, in addition to a small protein
called M2, are embedded in a lipid envelope derived from the plasma membrane of the host cell.
Underneath the viral envelope is the major structural protein M1, which surrounds the RNA molecules in association with the nucleoprotein and
three large proteins (PB1, PB2, and PA) that are responsible for RNA replication and transcription.

The viral genome is composed of eight segments
of single-stranded RNA of a negative sense. Those
eight segments code for 10 viral proteins, eight of
which are constituents of the virions (HA, NA, NP,
M1, M2, PB1, PB2, and PA). The RNA segment
with the smallest molecular weight codes for two
nonstructural proteins, NS1 and NS2. These can be
detected in the infected cell and NS1 has been associated with inclusions in the cytoplasm; however,
the functions of NS1 and NS2 are not yet defined.

The eight RNA segments, all with different molecular weights, can be isolated from the virus particles; the coding function for each segment is
known. The RNA segments of a virus can be separated by polyacrylamide gel electrophoresis. Comparison of the migration patterns of the RNAs of
different viruses, particularly reassortants (see section on antigenic shift), has been used to examine
the source of viral genes. In addition, the RNAs of
closely related influenza viruses can be compared
by oligonucleotide mapping to determine the degree of differences between strains—a sensitive
method to detect mutations. This approach was
used initially for comparing isolates of high and
low pathogenicity from chickens in Pennsylvania
(17). There has been a dramatic increase in information on RNA sequences of influenza viral genes
during the last 10 yr. The genetic sequence information is significant and includes partial sequence
data and, in some cases, complete data on all of the
eight viral genes. Specific information on genes of

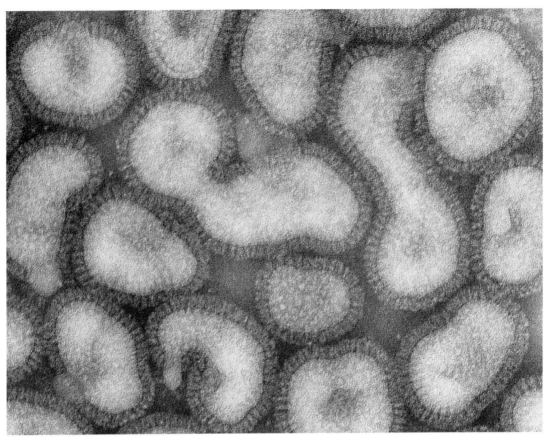

22.1.   Purified A/WSN/33 avian influenza virus. Negative stain with 2% phosphotungstic acid.
×282,100. (Gopal Murti)

avian viruses is also available; for example, the sequences of the HA genes of several avian subtypes, including H3 (50, 97), H5 (90, 92), and H7 (126, 138) are known in their entirety, and partial sequence data on 14 HAs are available (2). The available information is increasing at a rapid rate and should prove valuable in permitting determination of the genetic basis for important biologic properties such as pathogenicity, tissue tropism, and host range.

Chemical Composition.   The approximate composition of influenza virions is reported as 0.8–1.1% RNA, 70–75% protein, 20–24% lipid, and 5–8% carbohydrate (38). The lipids are located in the viral membrane; most are phospholipids with smaller amounts of cholesterol and glycolipid. Several carbohydrates (100) including ribose (in the RNA), galactose, mannose, fucose, and glucosamine are present in the virion mainly as glycoproteins or glycolipids. The virion proteins, as well as potential glycosylation sites, are all specified by

the viral genome, but the composition of the lipid and carbohydrate chains linked to glycoproteins or glycolipids of the viral membrane are determined by the host cell.

Virus Replication.   Replication of influenza viruses has been studied by many investigators and the process described in detail (99). Briefly, as described by Fenner et al. (51), the virus adsorbs to glycoprotein receptors containing sialic acid on the cell surface. The virus then enters the cell by receptor-mediated endocytosis. This includes exposure to a low pH in the endosome, resulting in a conformational change in the HA, which mediates membrane fusion. The nucleocapsid thus enters the cytoplasm and migrates to the nucleus. Influenza virus utilizes a unique mechanism to initiate transcription in that a viral endonuclease cleaves the 5′ cap from cellular mRNAs and uses this as a primer for transcription by the viral transcriptase. Six monocistronic mRNAs are produced and translated into the HA, NA, NP, and the three polymerases (PB1, PB2, and

PA). The mRNAs for NS and M genes undergo splicing and each yields two mRNAs, which are translated in different reading frames and thus produce the NS1, NS2, M1, and M2 proteins. The HA and NA are glycosylated in the rough endoplasmic reticulum, trimmed in the Golgi, and transported to the surface, where they remain embedded in the cell membrane. An important requirement for the HA is cleavage by host cell proteases into HA1 and HA2, which remain linked by disulfide bonds; cleavage is required for production of infectious virus. After production and assembly of viral proteins and RNA, the virus exits the cell by budding from the plasma membrane.

Although it is not yet clear how influenza virus actually kills host cells, recent studies (78) have shown that tissue culture cells infected with influenza virus undergo apoptosis (programmed cell death). The in vivo significance of apoptosis in influenza remains to be determined.

Antigenic Variation. The frequency of antigenic variation among influenza viruses is high and occurs in two ways, *drift* and *shift* (123). Antigenic drift involves minor antigenic changes in the HA and/or NA, whereas antigenic shift involves major antigenic changes in the HA and/or NA.

ANTIGENIC DRIFT. Antigenic drift is due to point mutations in the genes coding for the HA and/or NA proteins and is a reflection of selection of variants in an immune population. Antigenic drift has been most elegantly defined with influenza viruses from humans but is also known to occur with avian strains (12, 73, 82, 97). These studies have suggested that avian viruses show less antigenic drift than mammalian strains; the reason for this is not clear but could include lack of immunologic pressure in short-lived birds.

In defining the mechanisms of antigenic drift of human strains, four antigenic sites on the three-dimensional structure of the H3 HA of a human virus have been defined (188). This was based on sequence data from naturally occurring variants and variants selected with monoclonal antibodies. In essence, a single-point mutation can alter the structure of the surface protein (HA or NA) and, therefore, its antigenic and/or immunologic properties, resulting in an antigenic variant.

ANTIGENIC SHIFT. The segmented nature of the viral genome (8 segments of RNA) allows segments to reassort when a cell is infected with two different influenza viruses, potentially yielding 256 genetically different progeny viruses. That activity is called genetic reassortment. Genetic reassortment was initially demonstrated by antigenic analyses of the viruses produced during mixed infections (178).

Antigenic reassortant viruses, i.e., those with combinations of HA and NA of the parental viruses, were readily detected when a cell, embryo, or susceptible host was infected with two antigenically distinct viruses. Those exchanges that are detected by antigenic analysis involve only the segments that code for the HA and NA surface proteins (antigens); however, genetic exchanges can certainly involve genes other than those. In addition, viruses from different species also readily exchange genes.

It has been demonstrated "that mixed infections occur reasonably frequently in nature" (67). In such cases, two or more antigenically distinct influenza viruses have been recovered from cloacal samples of free-flying ducks. Experimentally, genetic reassortment takes place when ducks are infected with two antigenically distinct viruses. Thus, it is not surprising that viruses with almost every possible combination of antigenic subtypes have been recovered from ducks in nature.

Genetic reassortment between human and avian viruses is suggested as the mechanism by which "new" human pandemic strains arise (178). Thus, avian viruses may play a role in the influenza viruses in people by contributing genes to human strains.

Biologic Properties. The biologic property of pathogenicity of the avian influenza viruses is extremely variable and cannot be predicted based on the host of origin or antigenic subtype (HA) of the virus. Avian viruses of the H5 and H7 subtypes have been associated with severe disease in chickens, turkeys, ducks, and terns, e.g., chicken/Scotland/59 (H5N1), chicken/Penn/83 (H5N2), turkey/Ontario/7732/66 (H5N6), Tern/South Africa/61 (H5N3), and the fowl plague viruses (H7N1 and H7N7) (6). There are, however, many examples of H5 and H7 virus isolates that are not pathogenic, so antigenic configuration alone does not determine pathogenicity.

As with any virus, pathogenicity is a property of the interaction of the host and virus. An influenza virus that is pathogenic for one avian species will not necessarily be pathogenic for another avian species (9). For example, turkey/Ontario/7732/66 virus is highly pathogenic (100% mortality) for turkeys and chickens and at the same time nonpathogenic (no mortality) for other species, such as ducks (163). The tissue tropism of a virus may well be involved in its pathogenicity; for example, viruses restricted to the respiratory or intestinal tract will produce quite a different disease problem than a virus that becomes systemic and reaches vital organs. The basis for tissue tropism is not yet defined, but receptor specificities of human, equine, and avian viruses differ (148, 149). Studies (127) indicate that mutations in the receptor binding site of the viral HA can alter the ability of viruses to infect different hosts. It seems possible that receptor recognition is an important factor in both host range and tissue tropism, as well as pathogenicity. Since there is to date no cellular receptor identified for influenza viruses, the role of virus-receptor interactions in disease is unclear.

The molecular basis for pathogenicity is not totally defined. Rott and Scholtissek (151) suggested that pathogenicity is polygenic and can be disassociated from the HA and NA. On the other hand, there is substantial evidence (179) that the HA gene is extremely important in pathogenicity. The feature that is particularly relevant is the cleavability of the HA (29, 179).

As mentioned earlier, highly pathogenic viruses possess HAs that are readily cleaved in a variety of cells in vivo and in vitro. The ability of proteases in the host cell to accomplish this cleavage is considered important in determining the extent of replication. For example, the highly pathogenic viruses possess HAs that are cleaved in a number of different cells so infectious virus would be produced. The HAs of low to moderately influenza viruses, however, are typically not cleaved in many cells, so no infectious virus is produced. The highly pathogenic viruses have a series of basic amino acids at the carboxy-terminus of HA1, whereas avirulent viruses have a single basic amino acid at that site. It seems likely that the basic amino acids are involved in protease recognition and cleavage of the HA of highly pathogenic viruses.

Studies (89, 90, 91, 184) on both low and highly pathogenic H5N2 viruses from chickens in Pennsylvania suggested that this group of viruses all possessed the cleavage site sequence associated with highly pathogenic viruses; however, the HA of the early less pathogenic isolates had a glycosylation site in the cleavage region and the presence of this may have blocked efficient cleavage. A single mutation removing that glycosylation site resulted in a highly pathogenic strain. Thus, in this case, determination of the sequence around the cleavage site of the HAs would have indicated the dangerous nature of these particular viruses. Studies with another highly pathogenic H5 virus, turkey/Ontario/7732/66 (137) revealed that changes in neutralizing epitopes on the HA alter the virulence of the virus; thus, there may be different means by which changes on the HA alter the outcome of the viral infection.

In addition to assessing viruses for their in vivo pathogenicity, in vitro analyses provide useful information for evaluating virulence. Senne et al. (161) have compared in vitro and in vivo activities of H5N2 isolates from Pennsylvania and determined that chicken inoculations were inadequate to evaluate the virulence of these viruses. As mentioned above, cleavage of the HA is an important marker for highly pathogenic viruses and this can be measured in vitro. The ability of influenza viruses to produce plaques in tissue culture cells such as chick embryo fibroblasts (CEF) and Madin-Darby canine kidney (MDCK) cells in the absence of trypsin correlates with pathogenicity because it indicates that the HA of that strain is readily cleaved by cell proteases. In contrast, low to moderately pathogenic viruses cannot form plaques in the absence of trypsin because the HA remains uncleaved. The addition of trypsin to the cells will accomplish the cleavage and allow plaquing (29). Trypsin requirements correlate well with pathogenicity; however, there are exceptions. For example, mixed virus populations may be present and limit the usefulness of the procedure in predicting the pathogenicity of influenza isolates (30). In recent studies (136), highly pathogenic variants of turkey/Ont/7732/66 plaqued without trypsin in CEF but required trypsin to plaque in MDCK. This suggested that CEF may prove more reliable for evaluating this aspect. Another assay is analysis of HA cleavage by radioimmunoprecipitation of HA from tissue culture cells as described by Senne et al. (161).

The in vivo and in vitro analyses can identify a typical highly pathogenic strain. The presence of several basic amino acids at the carboxy-terminus of HA1, however, is probably the most reliable indicator that the virus has the potential to be highly pathogenic (179). Thus, this is the reason for the recommendation (145) that the sequence at the cleavage site in the HA be determined in evaluating pathogenicity of isolates.

Garcia et al. and Horimoto et al. reported that the change in the pathogenicity of the avian influenza viruses in Mexico was accompanied by substitution and insertion of six additional bases creating a two–amino-acid insert at the HA cleavage site (57, 80).

Resistance to Chemical and Physical Agents. Avian influenza A viruses are enveloped viruses and, thus, are relatively sensitive to inactivation by lipid solvents, such as detergents. Infectivity is also rapidly destroyed by formalin, ß-propiolactone, oxidizing agents, dilute acids, ether, sodium desoxycholate, hydroxylamine, sodium dodecylsulfate, and ammonium ions (55, 111). Avian influenza viruses are not endowed with unusual stability, so inactivation of the viruses themselves is not difficult. They are inactivated by heat, extremes of pH, nonisotonic conditions, and dryness.

LABORATORY SITUATION. Influenza viruses are generally grown in embryonated chicken eggs and are very stable in the allantoic fluid because the presence of protein protects the viruses. Infectivity, as well as hemagglutinating and NA activities of egg-grown virus, can be maintained for several weeks at 4 C. To maintain infectivity for the long-term, however, storage at -70 C or lyophilization is required. It should be mentioned that hemagglutinating and NA activities can be maintained even if the virus is no longer infectious. Formalin and ß-propiolactone have been used to eliminate infectivity, yet retain hemagglutinating and NA activities. Inactivation of these viruses in the laboratory situation can be accomplished with many common detergents and disinfectants (such as phenolic disinfectants or sodium hypochlorite).

FIELD SITUATION. In the field situation, influenza viruses are often released in nasal secretions and feces of infected birds so that the viruses are protected by the presence of organic material. This greatly increases their resistance to inactivation. An initial step is to heat the building to high temperatures for several days to inactivate the virus. The organic material, including manure, is then removed, followed by the cleaning of surfaces with detergent. The premises can then be decontaminated with sodium hypochorite solution, formalin or One-Stroke Environ[R] to decontaminate (54, 60).

Heavily contaminated manure represents a special problem in efforts to control influenza (52, 60). Litter and manure can be disposed of by burial, composting in a pile covered with plastic, or rototilling. It should be emphasized that influenza viruses can survive for long periods of time in the environment, particularly under cool and moist conditions. To exemplify this, infectious virus could be recovered from liquid manure for 105 days after depopulation during the wintertime influenza outbreak in chickens in Pennsylvania (52). Infectivity was retained in fecal material for as long as 30–35 days at 4 C and for 7 days at 20 C (23, 180). Influenza viruses have been recovered from lake and pond water where there were large concentrations of waterfowl, but not after the birds had left, suggesting that the viruses are not readily inactivated in the environment but may not survive for long periods (68). During disease outbreaks in domestic birds, recovery of virus from water troughs contaminated by secretions and feces is not unusual, but it is not known how long virus can survive in these areas.

Strain Classification. Strain classification of the avian influenza viruses is based on the HA and NA subtypes. There are currently 15 HAs and nine NAs and these have all been identified in various combinations in avian isolates. To identify the HA and NA of a virus, the isolate is tested in hemagglutination-inhibition (HI) and neuroaminidase-inhibition (NI) tests, using a panel of antisera specific for the different subtypes. These procedures have been described in detail in a manual entitled *Concepts and Procedures for Laboratory-Based Influenza Surveillance* (36) and by Kendal (95).

Comparison of viruses belonging to the same subtype is often accomplished by using postinfection sera from chickens and ferrets, and monoclonal antibodies. The use of monoclonal antibodies has enabled more detailed comparisons of related viruses appearing in the same or different species. For example, monoclonal antibodies to the H1 HA of H1N1 viruses present in turkeys and pigs have been used to establish the level of antigenic relatedness of their HAs (12, 73). Comparisons of viruses with these reagents are typically accomplished by HI, enzyme-linked immunosorbent assays (ELISA), and/or neutralization. Additional information on classification is given under "Virus Identification."

Laboratory Host Systems

CHICKEN EMBRYOS. All strains of avian influenza viruses grow readily in 9- to 11-day-old embryonated chicken eggs, making this is the most universally used method. The viruses grow to high levels in the egg and have a cleaved HA. Additional information is provided in the section on "Isolation and Identification of Causative Agent." Cultivation of influenza viruses in eggs is also used for vaccine production and for preparation of large quantities of virus for laboratory studies.

CELL CULTURE. Avian influenza viruses replicate in a limited number of cell cultures. Chicken embryo fibroblasts are the most commonly used primary cultures, whereas the most frequently used continuous cell line is the MDCK. Few influenza viruses will grow and produce plaques in cell cultures unless trypsin is added to the agar overlay to cleave the HA molecule for production of infectious virus. Using trypsin in the culture medium allows plaque assays with many strains in CEF or MDCK.

LABORATORY ANIMALS. Chickens, turkeys, and ducks have been the most commonly used species for laboratory studies because they have been the most commonly infected species under natural conditions. Generally, because of the considerable variation between species, it is advisable to use the natural avian host, preferably of the same age and species, for laboratory studies. Avian viruses also replicate in a number of experimentally inoculated mammals, such as ferrets, cats, hamsters, mice, monkeys, mink, and pigs (98).

Pathogenicity. There is a wide range of pathogenicity among the avian influenza viruses. Infections with these viruses may be inapparent or result in disease that ranges from mild transient syndromes to 100% morbidity and/or mortality. The signs of disease may be evident as respiratory, enteric or reproductive, and will vary with virus, species, age, concurrent infections, environment, and immune status of the host.

Given the very large number of influenza viruses that have been isolated from avian species, the number known to be highly pathogenic is extraordinarily small; however, there are a large number of viruses classified as low to moderately pathogenic. The method for detecting such viruses has been described under "Classification." Viruses isolated from free-flying waterfowl typically are nonpathogenic, especially for the species from which they were isolated.

There are many situations in which influenza viruses produce marked morbidity and mortality under field conditions, yet appear to produce no disease in experimentally inoculated birds. Studies by Toshiro et al. (170) have suggested that the concurrent bacterial infections play a major role in disease related to the low to moderately pathogenic influenza viruses. This could occur because the bacteria provide enzymes capable of cleaving the HA of these low or moderately virulent influenza viruses, enabling them to replicate and spread to a greater extent in that host. This is an interesting explanation for the ability of some strains to cause significant disease problems in the field but not in experimentally inoculated birds.

PATHOGENESIS AND EPIZOOTIOLOGY

Natural and Experimental Hosts. Many avian species, domestic or wild, can be infected with influenza viruses that may or may not cause disease. More influenza viruses have been isolated from ducks than any other species. Other avian species from which the viruses have been isolated include guinea fowl, domestic geese, quail (*Coturnix japonica*), pheasants, partridge, mynah birds, passerines, psittacines (parrots, parakeets and budgerigars), gulls, shorebirds, and seabirds.

Among the domestic avian species, turkeys have been the most frequently involved in disease outbreaks of influenza, whereas chickens have been less frequently involved.

Influenza A viruses, antigenically and genetically most closely related to avian viruses, have been isolated from two disease outbreaks in harbor seals (*Phoca vitulina*) in the United States (73). The infected seals experienced pneumonia and significant morbidity and mortality was produced. During studies on infected seals in the laboratory, an individual developed conjunctivitis due to the seal virus, A/Seal/Mass/1/80 (H7N7); several field

workers had experienced the same problem (182). The infection was limited to conjunctivitis and cleared with no sequelae. There have been two reports of influenza virus isolates most related to avian viruses from whales (76); whether these viruses are involved in a disease process in these animals is not yet known.

The H1N1 viruses typically found in pigs have also been detected in turkeys in the United States during the last decade. Antigenic and genetic comparisons of these viruses (12, 13, 73, 157) indicate that the turkey viruses are very closely related to those continually circulating in pigs and, thus, are of swine origin. It has been suggested that the viruses from pigs were introduced either by direct or indirect contact with pigs or by people infected with these viruses.

Scholtissek and Naylor (156) have raised an interesting suggestion that pigs represent a "mixing vessel" for viruses from avian and mammalian species. Thus, close contact between these groups, as in coculture of fish, ducks, and pigs, might facilitate the emergence of "new" strains.

Avian influenza viruses have also been responsible for disease outbreaks in mink (49, 101).

Experimentally, pigs, ferrets, cats, mink, monkeys, and humans (26, 71, 98) can be infected with influenza viruses originating from avian species.

Transmission and Carriers. Infected birds excrete virus from the respiratory tract, conjunctiva, and feces; thus, likely modes of transmission include both direct contact between infected and susceptible birds and indirect contact including aerosol (droplets) or exposure to virus-contaminated fomites. Since infected birds can excrete high levels of virus in their feces, spread is readily accomplished by virtually anything contaminated with fecal material, e.g., birds and mammals, feed, water, equipment, supplies, cages, clothes, delivery vehicles, and insects. Thereby, viruses are readily transported to other areas by people and equipment shared in production, live-haul, or live-bird marketing.

Alexander (5) categorized the sources of primary introduction of infection for domestic poultry as 1) other species of domestic poultry; 2) exotic captive birds; 3) wild birds; and 4) other animals. In category 1, there are examples of spread from one domestic species to another on the same or adjacent farms, e.g., ducks to chickens, and turkeys to chickens, guinea fowl, and pheasants. It is likely that most are due to mechanical transmission as described above. In category 2, while the potential for such spread appears to be real, there are no known introductions of influenza viruses into domestic poultry by infected exotic caged birds, as has been observed for Newcastle disease virus.

Category 3 is the commonly considered source for infection in domestic poultry, i.e., wild birds, particularly migratory waterfowl. There is substantial circumstantial evidence to incriminate wild birds for the introduction of influenza into domestic poultry flocks. For example, turkeys and migratory waterfowl are frequently spatially and temporally related. Studies in Minnesota (62, 87) have indicated that influenza viruses appear in the turkeys concurrently with the arrival of migratory birds. Given the high frequency of influenza viruses in duck feces, such sources should remain suspect. In addition, feces introduced into water supplies could serve as a source of virus for fecal–oral transmission to other birds.

In the Pennsylvania outbreak, surveillance studies (77, 132) demonstrated that many viruses, including a nonpathogenic H5N2 isolate, were present in wild birds in the area; however, there was no evidence that wild birds were disseminating the highly pathogenic virus. In addition, experimental studies (190) showed that ducks and gulls were poor hosts for this virus. The possibility that wild birds were involved in the initial introduction cannot be excluded. During the recent outbreak in turkeys in Ireland involving a highly pathogenic strain, turkey/Ireland/1378/83 (H5N8), a virus of the same subtype was isolated from healthy domestic ducks on an adjacent farm (121). Genetic studies (92) indicated that these viruses were closely related and replicated in ducks and chickens, but they only produced disease in chickens. Surveillance studies (121) suggested that the initial outbreak in domestic ducks may have occurred through contact with wild birds. Although much of the evidence implicating wild birds as a source is circumstantial, it is sufficient to view these birds as a real source. Wild birds have also been considered important in the influenza problems in seals, in that birds and seals frequently share habitats.

In category 4, there is evidence that turkeys may become infected with viruses from pigs; how frequently this might occur is difficult to estimate. As indicated previously, viruses of swine origin have been detected in turkeys and were presumably transmitted from pigs to turkeys, either mechanically or by people infected with the virus.

There is ample evidence for horizontal transmission of influenza viruses but no evidence to indicate that the viruses can be transmitted vertically. It should be noted, however, that virus can be present within or on the surface of eggs when the hen is infected, as demonstrated by the isolation of H5N2 viruses from chicken eggs during the Pennsylvania outbreak (35). After experimental infection of hens with the H5N2 virus from Pennsylvania, almost all eggs laid on postinfection days 3 and 4 contained virus (23).

Successful experimental routes of exposure include aerosol, intranasal, intrasinus, intratracheal, oral, conjunctival, intramuscular, intraperitoneal, intracaudal air sac, intravenous, cloacal, and intracranial administration of the various viruses.

Incubation Period. The incubation periods for the various diseases caused by these viruses range from as short as a few hours to 3 days in individual birds and up to 14 days in a flock. The incubation period is dependent on the dose of virus, the route of exposure, the species exposed, and the ability to detect clinical signs.

Signs. The signs of disease are extremely variable and depend on the species affected, age, sex, concurrent infections, virus, environmental factors, etc. Signs may reflect abnormalities of the respiratory, enteric, reproductive, or nervous systems. The signs most commonly reported include pronounced depression and decreased activity; decreased feed consumption and emaciation; increased broodiness of hens and decreased egg production; mild to severe respiratory signs including coughing, sneezing, rales, and excessive lacrimation; huddling; ruffled feathers; edema of head and face; cyanosis of unfeathered skin; nervous disorder; and diarrhea. Any of these signs may occur singly or in various combinations.

In some cases, the disease is rapidly fulminating and birds are found dead without previous signs. Some viruses cause severe disease in one species and inapparent infections in others under experimental conditions. Similarly, viruses that are identical antigenically may have quite different biologic characteristics, with one producing severe disease in a given species and the other being an inapparent infection (9, 163). In the recent situation of H5N8 viruses in turkeys and ducks in Ireland (121), there were significant disease problems in the turkeys and none in the ducks; thus, the species involved is quite significant. In all but the case of the mass mortality among common terns (27), influenza virus infections in wild birds have been inapparent with no obvious signs of disease.

In the outbreak in chickens in Pennsylvania (1, 47), initially there was an acute respiratory disease with increasing mortality and declining egg production. When the virus became highly pathogenic, however, there were other problems, including high mortality (50–89%) and significant declines in feed and water consumption and egg production. Respiratory signs were less prominent, but the birds were severely depressed and some had tremors or unusual attitudes of the head.

Morbidity and Mortality. Morbidity and mortality rates are as variable as the signs and are dependent on the species and virus, as well as age, environment, and concurrent infections. The more frequent observation is one of high morbidity and low mortality. Morbidity rates generally are poorly defined, largely because of the very large size of flocks involved and the ill-defined signs of disease in many of the outbreaks. On the other hand, in the case of highly pathogenic viruses, the morbidity and mortality can reach 100%.

Gross Lesions. The gross lesions observed in several avian species have been extremely varied with regard to their location and severity, depending greatly on the species and the pathogenicity of the infecting virus. The gross lesions that have been described generally are from observations in chickens and turkeys with naturally occurring or experimental infections (46). There are a few descriptions of lesions in terns, domestic ducks, and battery-reared quail, partridge, and pheasants.

In many cases, there are few striking lesions because the disease is mild. Mild lesions may be observed in the sinuses, characterized by catarrhal, fibrinous, serofibrinous, mucopurulent, or caseous inflammation. There may be edema of the tracheal mucosa with an exudate that varies from serous to caseous. Air sacs may be thickened and have a fibrinous or caseous exudate. Catarrhal to fibrinous peritonitis and "egg yolk peritonitis" may be observed. Catarrhal to fibrinous enteritis may be observed in the ceca and/or intestine, especially in turkeys. Exudates may be found in the oviducts of laying birds.

In the case of highly pathogenic viruses, there may be no prominent lesions because the birds die very quickly, before gross lesions can develop. However, a variety of congestive, hemorrhagic, transudative, and necrotic changes (see Fig. 22.2) have been described with highly pathogenic viruses such as fowl plague virus (H7N7), tern/S.A./61 (H5N3), chicken/Scotland/59 (H5N1), turkey/Ontario/7732/66 (H5N9), turkey/Ontario/6213/65 (H5N1), and chicken/Pennsylvania/83 (H5N2). With these viruses, initial changes may include edema of the head with swollen sinuses, and cyanotic, congested, and hemorrhagic wattles and combs. Congestion and hemorrhage may also be seen on the legs. As the disease progresses, internal lesions vary greatly. Necrotic foci were frequently observed in the liver, spleen, kidneys, and lungs in chickens experimentally infected with fowl plague virus (85), but similar lesions were not observed in terns experiencing infection with tern/S.A./61 (153). Congestive and hemorrhagic lesions were common in birds infected with the pathogenic strains, turkey/Ontario/7732/66 and turkey/Ontario/6213/65 (105, 106, 129, 130, 152). Descriptions of lesions observed in a number of individual

22.2. Gross lesions associated with experimental infection of white leghorn (WL) or White Rock (WR) chickens with highly pathogenic (HP) avian influenza viruses. A–D. Lesions in adult WL chickens, 47 to 59 wk of age, exposed to HP A/chicken/NJ/12508/86 (H5N2) derivative influenza virus by the intranasal/intratracheal routes. A. Multifocal necrosis and hemorrhage of comb and wattles 7 days postinfection (DPI). (Brugh) B. Severe edema, necrosis and hemorrhage of comb and wattles, 7 DPI. (Brugh) C. Bilateral ventral medial pneumonia with edema, 3 DPI. (Brugh) D. Petechial hemorrhages in epicardial fat, 4 DPI. (Brugh) E–H. Intranasal (IN) or intravenous (IV) exposure of immature chickens to HP A/chicken/Queretaro/14588-660/95 (H5N2) virus stock. E. Severe necrosis of comb and wattles, 12-wk-old WL, IN exposure, 4 DPI. (Swayne) F. Severe edema and necrosis of comb and wattles, 12-wk-old WL, IN exposure, 4 DPI. (Swayne) G. Severe subcutaneous hemorrhages of leg shanks, 4-wk-old WR, IV exposure, 4 DPI. (Swayne) H. Petechial hemorrhages around the ducts of the proventricular glandular region, 16-wk-old WL, IN exposure, 4 DPI. (Swayne)

outbreaks have been described in detail previously (46).

Gross lesions in chickens in the Pennsylvania outbreak, as described by Acland et al. (1), were characterized by severe swelling of the comb and wattles, with periorbital edema. Lesions of the comb were dramatic, ranging from vesicles to severe swelling and cyanosis, ecchymosis, and frank necrosis. Sometimes there was swelling of the feet, with ecchymotic discoloration. Visceral lesions included petechial hemorrhage of various serosal and mucosal surfaces, particularly the mucosal surface of the proventriculus near the junction with the ventriculus. The pancreas often had blotchy light yellow and dark red areas along its length. In some birds, gross lesions were limited to dehydration. The lesions were very similar to those described for fowl plague by Stubbs and Beaudette in the 1920s (169).

Not all the highly pathogenic strains produce the same gross lesions. Van Campen et al. (173) infected chickens with turkey/Ontario/7732/66 (H5N9) and showed that this virus causes severe destruction of lymphoid tissues as evidenced grossly by the mottled appearance of the spleen. However, naturally occurring and experimental infections of chickens with other virulent strains, such as tern/S.A./61 and Ck/Penn/83, did not cause lymphoid damage. The basis for the differences among these viruses is unknown.

When examining birds for gross lesions, an important consideration is that influenza virus infection may be accompanied by bacterial involvement,

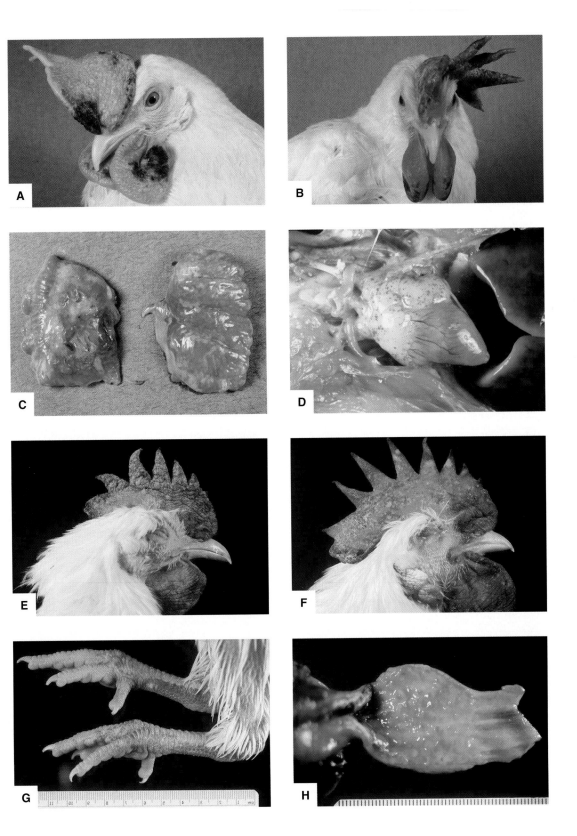

so lesions may reflect the effects of both virus and bacteria.

Histopathology. Histopathologic descriptions of avian influenza infection have been limited primarily to those conditions with severe overt disease and obvious gross changes, involving highly pathogenic viruses.

Classic "fowl plague," as described in 1926 (59), was characterized by edema, hyperemia, hemorrhages and foci of perivascular lymphoid cuffing, chiefly in the myocardium, spleen, lungs, brain, wattles, and to a lesser extent, liver and kidney. Parenchymal degeneration and necrosis were present in spleen, liver, and kidney. Brain lesions (53, 158) included foci of necrosis, perivascular lymphoid cuffing, glial foci, vascular proliferation, and neuronal changes. Chickens dying after intravenous inoculation of highly virulent fowl plaque virus have widespread edema, hyperemia, and hemorrhage, and also foci of necrosis in the spleen, liver, lung, kidney, intestine, and pancreas in decreasing order of frequency (85). Brain lesions were similar to those described earlier (53, 158).

The histologic changes caused by other highly pathogenic influenza viruses in various species, particularly chickens and turkeys, have some similarities, as well as differences, to the changes caused by fowl plague viruses.

In chickens inoculated with tern/S.A./61 (H5N3) (28), foci of necrosis and lymphoid infiltration were seen in spleen, myocardium, brain, eyes, ocular muscles, comb, and skeletal muscle. Splenic lesions were chiefly proliferation of reticular cells in the red pulp accompanied by heterophil accumulation. Severe myocarditis with focal areas of necrotic muscle was also evident. Despite high virus titers, there were no lesions in the lung (and no respiratory signs). After 5 or 6 days, a diffuse encephalitis developed in both the cerebrum and cerebellum, characterized by widespread perivascular cuffing with mononuclear cells, necrosis of neuronal cells, edema and a diffuse cellularity, and some hemorrhage. In contrast to the extensive lesions observed with tern/S.A./61, lesions in chickens infected with another highly pathogenic virus, chick/Scot/59 (H5N1), were much less severe. Distinguishing features between the lesions caused by these two viruses were degree of cardiac, brain, ocular, and cutaneous involvement, being less severe or absent with chick/Scot/59.

One of the most striking lesions observed in turkeys infected with turkey/Ont/6213/66 (H5N1) or turkey/Ont/7732/66 (H5N9) was pancreatitis with extensive necrosis of acinar cells (130, 152). Degenerative and necrotic changes were observed in other organs including the liver, brain and meninges, myocardium, and cutaneous tissues

(104, 130). Progressive myocardial necrosis and myocarditis accompanied by marked alterations in the myocardial ultrastructure have been described in detail (116). These changes coincided with high levels of virus in myocardial tissue, the maximum levels of serum glutamic-oxalacetic transaminase and lactic dehydrogenese, and cardiac arrhythmias. Resende (146) described necrotic depletion of lymphoid centers in turkeys infected with turkey/Ont/7732/66. Recent studies (173) indicate that turkey/Ontario/7732/66 also produces severe lymphoid necrosis in experimentally inoculated chickens; this necrosis was evident in lymphoid cells present in the spleen, thymus, bursa, intestinal tract, and lung. A prominent feature in these birds was necrosis of lymphoid nodules present in the lamina propria of the bronchioles, whereas the respiratory epithelium of the airways was relatively spared and no respiratory disease was evident.

Histopathologic examination of chickens naturally infected during the Pennsylvania outbreak have been very well described by Acland et al. (1). They defined the major microscopic lesions as mild to severe diffuse, nonsuppurative encephalitis; very mild to severe diffuse necrotizing pancreatitis; and very mild to severe subacute necrotizing myositis involving numerous skeletal muscles and most severe in the external ocular muscles and leg muscles. They also noted that the microscopic lesions were more severe in broilers than in layers; possible explanations include variable age or strain of bird, virus pathogenicity, or stage of disease.

There has been little examination of tissues from wild birds, such as ducks, which become infected with influenza viruses but typically do not develop disease. Cooley et al. (40) described pneumonic lesions in mallards experimentally infected with the highly pathogenic virus, turkey/Ont/7732/66. These lesions were characterized by rapid infiltration of lymphocytes and macrophages. There were no obvious clinical signs in these birds, suggesting that although healthy in appearance, ducks may experience damage to the respiratory tract during infection. Experimental studies (110) suggest reproductive and growth effects in ducks. There are currently no reports of characteristic disease or lesions in naturally infected waterfowl, so whether this occurs during naturally occurring infection is not known.

In summary, the lesions caused by at least six influenza viruses considered to be highly pathogenic share some similarities, but have some distinctive features. For example, multiple focal lymphoid necrosis was characteristic of infection with turkey/Ontario/7732/66 but not with turkey/Ontario/6213/66 or chick/Penn/83, whereas pancreatic necrosis was a noteworthy lesion with the latter two viruses. Myocarditis, as described with tern/S.A./61 infection, was not observed in the chicken/Scotland/59 infection but was found with the turkey/Ontario/7732/66 and chick/Penn/83 infections. Skeletal muscle lesions, along with brain and comb lesions, were observed in birds infected with chick/Penn/83 or tern/S.A./61, but infection with tern/S.A./61 did not produce pancreatic lesions. The basis for differences is not yet understood.

DIAGNOSIS. A diagnosis of influenza A virus infection is conclusively demonstrated by the isolation and identification of the virus, but detection of antibodies to the virus is a very useful indirect diagnostic tool. Since clinical symptoms can vary dramatically, clinical diagnosis is considered presumptive, except in an epizootic.

Isolation and Identification of Causative Agent. Viruses are recovered commonly from the trachea and/or cloaca of either live or dead birds, because the viruses typically replicate in the respiratory and/or intestinal tracts. Tissues, secretions, or excretions from these tracts are appropriate for virus isolation. In the case of systemic infections produced by highly pathogenic viruses, virtually every organ can yield virus because of the high levels of viremia.

Dry cotton, Dacron, or alginate swabs of various sizes may be used to swab the trachea and/or cloaca. A nasopharyngeal swab may be used for collecting materials from the trachea and cloaca of very small birds. The swabs should be placed in a sterile transport medium (1–2 mL) containing high levels of antibiotics to reduce bacterial growth. Organs can be collected and placed into sterile plastic tubes or bags. In the examination of organs for virus, efforts should be made to collect and store internal organs from the respiratory and intestinal tract tissues separately because isolation of virus from internal organs, generally an indication of systemic spread, is more often associated with the highly pathogenic viruses.

If the samples for virus isolation can be tested within 48 hr after collection, they may be kept at 4 C; however, if the samples must be held for additional time, storage at −70 C is recommended. Freezing at −20 C is not usually advisable, but storage in liquid nitrogen or with dry ice is satisfactory. Before processing, tissues can be ground as a 10% suspension in the transport medium and clarified by low-speed centrifugation.

Methods for the isolation and identification of influenza viruses have been described in detail (19, 36, 133). Embryonated chicken eggs are most commonly used for virus isolation because avian influenza viruses grow very well in them. Chicken embryos, 10–11 days old, are inoculated via the allantoic cavity with approximately 0.1–0.2 mL of sample. To increase the probability of growth of

virus, both the allantoic and amniotic routes may be used on the same egg.

The death of inoculated embryos within 24 hr after inoculation usually results from bacterial contamination and these eggs should be discarded. A few viruses may grow rapidly and kill the embryos by 48 hr; however, in most cases the embryos will not die. After 72 hr, or at death, the eggs should be removed from the incubator, chilled, and allantoic fluids collected. Viral replication is demonstrated by chicken erythrocyte hemagglutinating activity in the allantoic fluid.

Generally, if there is virus present in the samples, there will be sufficient growth in the first passage to result in hemagglutination. If no hemagglutinating activity is detected, a sample of the collected egg fluids may be injected into eggs (second passage) and the procedure repeated. Repeated passage of samples is, however, laborious and increases the risk of laboratory contamination; thus, these concerns must be considered when using multiple passage.

Long-term storage of viruses should be done at −70 C. Lyophilization of viruses is also appropriate for long-term storage; however, these stocks should be tested periodically to ensure infectivity.

Virus Identification. Standard methods for testing the egg fluids for the presence of hemagglutinating activity using chicken erythrocytes by macro- or micro-techniques are employed (19, 36, 133). Allantoic fluid positive for hemagglutination is used for virus identification.

It is important to determine whether the hemagglutinating activity detected in the allantoic fluid is due to influenza virus or other hemagglutinating viruses, such as paramyxoviruses like Newcastle disease virus (NDV). Thus, the isolate is tested in HI assays against Newcastle disease antiserum. If negative, the virus is then tested for the presence of the Type A NP (nucleoprotein) to establish that an influenza A virus is present. The type-specific NP or matrix protein may be detected by the double immunodiffusion test (18, 44) or the single-radial-hemolysis test (44). More recently, monoclonal antibodies that react with the nucleoprotein or matrix proteins have proved useful in identifying these antigens in ELISA (176).

The next step in the identification procedure is to determine the antigenic subtype of the surface antigens, HA and NA. The HA is identified in the HI test (36) using a panel of antisera prepared against the 14 distinct HAs. Typing is facilitated by using antisera against the isolated HA or against reassortant viruses with irrelevant NAs; this helps avoid steric inhibition due to antibodies against the NA (95). An influenza virus with a new HA would not be detected in tests utilizing antisera to the known

HA subtypes. Therefore, it is important that a procedure be used to determine that the unknown hemagglutinating agent is an influenza virus, usually by testing for the type-specific antigens (NP or MP) as described above.

The NA subtype is usually identified by NI assays with antisera prepared against the nine known NAs (36, 133). A micro-NI assay (175) has been developed to assist in the processing of large numbers of isolates and to economize on reagents and handling, so this NI assay is often the first assay done on an isolate.

If laboratories are unfamiliar with the techniques or do not have the necessary antisera, final identification can be accomplished by state, federal, or World Health Organization–designated influenza reference laboratories.

Serology.   Serologic tests are used to demonstrate the presence of antibodies, which may be detected as early as 7–10 days after infection. Several techniques are used for serologic surveillance and diagnosis. The most commonly used are the HI test to detect antibodies to the HA and double-immunodiffusion to detect antibodies to the NP. Other serologic tests (18, 19, 44, 98, 133) to detect antibodies include virus neutralization, complement fixation (generally unsatisfactory for avian serum), NI, and single radial hemolysis. More recently, ELISA assays have been developed to detect antibodies to avian influenza viruses (119, 166). In serologic surveillance programs, a test for the detection of anti-NP antibody is frequently used, since this detects antibodies to a cross-reactive antigen shared by all influenza A viruses.

In serologic assays, it is important to be aware that there is considerable variation in the immune response among the various avian species. For example, antibodies to the NP are generally prominent in turkeys and pheasants but may be undetectable in ducks known to have been infected (163). In addition, antibodies may be induced in ducks, as well as other species, but fail to be detected in conventional HI tests performed with intact virus (96, 114).

In the case of poultry, the detection of antibodies to the nucleoprotein, HA, or NA of influenza virus is considered indicative of recent infection. To prove that influenza virus is responsible for a current disease problem, it is important that acute and convalescent sera be collected. The acute serum sample is collected from affected birds as soon as possible after the onset of the disease. A convalescent phase serum should be collected 14–28 days after onset (79). Paired acute and convalescent serum samples are used to compare the levels of antibodies before and after infection. For example, the sera can be tested in HI assays for antibodies to a suspected virus; a fourfold rise in antibody titer in a convalescent serum would be indicative of very recent infection with that particular influenza virus. Serum should be kept frozen (−20 C) until tested. Sodium azide (0.01%) may be added to the serum as a preservative.

The sera of many species contain nonspecific inhibitors that may interfere with the specificity of the HI and other tests. Since these inhibitors are especially active against certain viruses, they present a very practical problem in serologic testing and the identification of viruses. Therefore, sera should be treated to reduce or destroy such activity, although it should be recognized that some treatments may lower specific antibody levels. The two most commonly used treatments for these inhibitors have been receptor-destroying enzyme (RDE) and potassium periodate (36, 44). In addition to the nonspecific inhibitors of hemagglutination, sera from other birds, such as turkey and goose, may cause agglutination of the chicken erythrocytes used in the HI test. This may mask low levels of HI activity. Such hemagglutinating activity can be removed by pretreatment of the serum with chicken erythrocytes (128). This problem may sometimes be avoided by using erythrocytes in the HI test of the same species as the serum being tested.

Direct Detection.   The direct demonstration of influenza viruses or viral proteins in samples from animals is not routinely used for diagnosis at this time. However, immunofluorescence techniques have been used for rapid diagnosis of influenza in humans (3, 65, 113, 117). Skeeles et al. (162) described the use of fluorescent antibody tests for rapid detection of avian influenza virus in tissue samples during the Pennsylvania disease outbreak, and Kodihalli et al. (102) described an antigen-capture ELISA to detect viral antigens in samples. At this time, monoclonal antibodies are proving quite useful for localizing viral antigen in tissues by immunoperoxidase staining (173), and radiolabeled gene probes for in situ hybridization can locate cells involved in viral replication in tissues of infected birds (174). These tools are not yet applicable to routine situations; however, their use in the future is a realistic consideration.

Differential Diagnosis.   Because of the broad spectrum of signs and lesions reported with infections of avian influenza viruses in several species, a definitive diagnosis must be made by virologic and serologic methods. Other infections that must be considered in the differential diagnosis include Newcastle disease virus and other paramyxoviruses, and chlamydia, mycoplasma, and other bacteria. Concurrent infections with influenza viruses and mycoplasma or other bacteria have been commonly observed (46).

TREATMENT. Presently, there is no practical specific treatment for avian influenza virus infections. Amantadine hydrochloride and rimantadine hydrochloride are effective in the prophylaxis of human influenza infections (43). Amantadine has also been shown to be effective against influenza A virus infection of quail (45), turkeys (107), and chickens (24, 183). The results of these studies are similar in several aspects. Rinaldi used amantadine for treatment of infection in a large flock of Japanese quail in Italy and the mortality rate was reduced by approximately 50%, but the rate of infection was unaffected. Similarly the severity of disease caused by the turkey/Ontario/7732/66, under experimental conditions, was markedly reduced when the turkeys were treated with amantadine hydrochloride. In recent studies in chickens (24, 183), amantadine and rimantadine administered in the drinking water reduced the mortality; however, the birds were still infected and shed virus. Additionally, there was a rapid emergence of amantadine-resistant viruses that killed hens receiving the drug. Amantadine was present in serum, muscle, and liver of treated birds. After withdrawal of the drug, the levels in serum and tissue fell to virtually zero within 24 hr; however, the level in the albumin and yolk of eggs was maintained at least 3 days. At this time, this drug is not approved for use in birds for consumption.

All other treatments used have been of a supportive nature to relieve respiratory distress. Antibiotic treatment has been employed to reduce the effects of concurrent mycoplasma and bacterial infections.

PREVENTION AND CONTROL. Methods for prevention and control of influenza virus infection center on preventing the initial introduction of the virus and controlling spread if it is introduced. One critical aspect in reaching the goal of prevention and control is the education of the poultry industry regarding how the viruses are introduced, how they spread, and how such events can be prevented.

Prevention. The most likely source of virus for birds is other infected birds, so the basic means for the prevention of infection of poultry with influenza viruses is the separation of susceptible birds from infected birds and their secretions and excretions. "Biosecurity," as it applies to any infectious disease, should be the first line of defense (see Chapter 1). Transmission can occur when susceptible and infected birds are in close contact or when infectious material from infected birds is introduced into the environment of susceptible birds. Such introductions take place by the contamination of equipment, footwear and clothing, vehicles, insemination equipment, feed, water, etc. The presence of virus in fecal material is a likely means for movement of the virus by equipment and people. Another considera-

tion is that there should be no contact with recovered birds because the length of time they shed virus is not clearly defined.

The reservoir of influenza viruses in wild birds should be considered as a potential source for domestic birds, particularly those on open range, so it is important to reduce the contact between these two groups. Swine may serve as a source of virus for turkeys, with the virus transmitted mechanically or by infected people or pigs (72).

Control. In the case of influenza outbreaks in birds involving viruses from low to high pathogenicity, efforts focus on containing the original disease problem. The outbreaks in Pennsylvania during 1983–84 and in Mexico during 1994–95 show that apparently "nonpathogenic" AI viruses have the potential for gaining virulence. In both instances, highly pathogenic influenza emerged after a nonpathogenic H5 virus circulated in poultry flocks for several months. This illustrates the need for prompt responses to mild influenza outbreaks. Prevention and control of mild influenza outbreaks are the most important steps to prevent many outbreaks of highly pathogenic influenza.

There is not a uniform control program for nonpathogenic AI in the United States, since each state takes a slightly different approach. Control programs in Minnesota (60, 141) and Pennsylvania (31) provide information on measures that have been used successfully by poultry producers to handle their influenza problems. Recommendations and responsibilities for containing influenza outbreaks have been described (52).

Poss et al. (141) have reported on an industry program for control of mild AI in Minnesota, which includes education, preventing exposure, monitoring, reporting, and a "responsible response." Once the disease is detected, there must be an appropriate response, and because the disease is unpredictable, the response must be prompt and complete. Prior to the isolation of the virus and determination of its pathogenicity, vigorous influenza control measures must already be in place. If a virus is determined to be highly pathogenic, it could take up to 4 wk from initial illness until a government emergency can be declared, so voluntary industry efforts to control the initial outbreak are critically important.

Each influenza outbreak must first be controlled before the disease can be eradicated. Because the economic penalties of influenza are severe, the control program should not additionally penalize the growers. The first step in the Minnesota response is voluntary isolation of the flock by the grower to prevent transmission to other flocks. The second part of the response is orderly marketing. Most of the influenza virus shed from an infected flock occurs during the first 2 wk of infection. Usually by 4 wk after the initiation of the infection, virus cannot be detected. Orderly and well-timed marketing of birds or eggs is appropriate.

The third part of the response is flock-scheduling changes. After the last flock on a farm becomes infected, it has been possible, with a 4-wk delay, to move birds back onto a farm, manage the flocks separately, and prevent the infection of the newly added flocks. This approach requires a certain amount of sophistication and a lot of dedication, but it is possible to eliminate influenza without a total depopulation of the premises. This is important for a producer, because the cost of depopulation of a multiage farm with mild influenza is approximately twice the direct cost of the disease losses.

Influenza virus is excreted from both the respiratory and the digestive tracts. Thus, within a poultry house, bird-to-bird transmission is probably by aerosol and droppings. Poultry manure appears to be the most likely source of transmission from flock to flock.

All methods for controlling the spread of influenza are based on preventing the contamination of, and controlling the movement of, people and equipment (60). Persons that have direct contact with birds or their manure have been the cause of most disease transmission between houses or premises. Equipment that comes in direct contact with birds or their manure should not be moved from farm to farm, and it is important to keep the traffic area near the poultry house from becoming contaminated with manure.

With a highly pathogenic influenza virus like chick/Penn/83, governmental eradication procedures (quarantine, slaughter, disposal, and cleanup) are employed. The decision to eradicate is based on successful control of the outbreak, the nature and extent of the problem, and the biologic properties of the virus. During the 1983–84 eradication effort in Pennsylvania, more than 17 million birds were destroyed. Area quarantines were essential to prevent spread and to accomplish eradication. Epidemiologic surveillance requiring field personnel and laboratory support (134, 135) was critical to detect new outbreaks and contain them. In Pennsylvania, surveillance efforts revealed that live-bird markets were a source of virus, and elimination of that source, as well as infected farms, had to be accomplished (58).

The legal authority to conduct an emergency disease eradication program is shared by the state and federal government, the state being responsible for intrastate quarantine regulation and the federal government being responsible for interstate and international regulations.

VACCINES. Inactivated influenza virus vaccines have been used in a variety of species and their effectiveness in alleviating clinical signs and mortality is well documented. Birds are susceptible to infection with influenza viruses belonging to any of the 15 HA subtypes and there is no way to predict their exposure to any particular one. It is not practical to practice preventive vaccination against all possible subtypes. On the other hand, once an outbreak occurs and the subtype of the virus is identified, vaccination may be a useful tool (64).

Considerations that influence decisions on influenza vaccination have been discussed by Beard (20). In the case of the many outbreaks caused by viruses of low to moderate pathogenicity, producers have been allowed to use inactivated vaccines. The limitation of vaccination in this situation is that serologic surveillance is impeded and viral infection can occur and persist in the absence of disease. To counter this, nonvaccinated sentinel birds should be placed in vaccinated flocks. Periodic testing of these for the presence of antibodies to influenza virus would determine if the flock has been exposed to the virus. Vaccinated flocks cannot be considered influenza virus–free, but vaccine use does typically reduce the amount of virus shed in experimentally vaccinated and challenged birds, thereby reducing the potential spread of the virus to other birds (64). Vaccinated flocks can then be identified and monitored for the presence of AI until sold. It has been suggested that carefully controlled use of vaccines in a mild AI outbreak may delay and reduce the chance of the emergence of a highly pathogenic virus (177); however, there is no evidence to support this possibility.

There are currently no fully licensed influenza vaccines for birds in the United States, although vaccines under limited licensure are used, particularly in turkeys (64, 115). Numerous experimental studies (8, 11, 14, 32, 33, 34, 88, 167, 168, 183, 189) have demonstrated that inactivated monovalent and polyvalent virus vaccines, with adjuvants, are capable of inducing antibody and providing protection against mortality, morbidity and egg-production declines. It should also be noted that upon challenge, these vaccinated birds often become infected and excrete virus although they exhibit no disease signs. Such vaccines could potentially reduce the severity of disease and the spread of virus in the field situation, but the virus would not be eliminated from the population. Because of this, and because eradication of highly pathogenic AI has been the goal, vaccination has been prohibited in the United States.

Approaches other than use of inactivated virus vaccines are currently being evaluated; several have been discussed by Murphy and Kendall (122). The use of genetic engineering has been applied to isolate the HA genes, particularly H5 and H7, and place them into viral vectors such as fowl poxvirus (25, 171), vaccinia virus (37, 42), baculovirus (103), and retrovirus (81). Another approach is to inoculate the DNA directly into chickens (56, 147).

These different approaches have been used successfully to immunize and protect birds. Thus, opportunities to develop a variety of effective vaccines clearly exists; the debate (20) centers on the role they should play in controlling influenza viruses of varying pathogenicity in different domestic bird populations in different geographic regions.

An interesting application of avian influenza viruses has been their use as gene donors for making live attenuated vaccines for potential use in humans (124). Whether these vaccines will be used is not yet known.

Based on the multitude of influenza A viruses in birds, it seems likely that the future, like the past, will include avian disease problems involving influenza viruses.

ROLE OF AVIAN SPECIES IN MAMMALIAN INFLUENZA.
Avian influenza viruses may play a role in the evolution of new human strains by contributing viral genes to human strains via genetic reassortment (178). Antigenic and genetic evidence supports the suggestion that the HA gene in the virus responsible for the 1968 pandemic in humans originated from a virus circulating in ducks. Direct transmission of viruses between birds and humans does not generally occur. The harbor seal isolate that resulted in conjunctivitis in a laboratory worker demonstrates, however, that a virus similar to avian viruses was infectious for mammals, including humans. Furthermore, there is evidence to suggest that the H1N1 viruses present in pigs, turkeys, and ducks may be involved in interspecies transmission (73), so a swine–avian–human connection could conceivably have public health significance. In experimental infections of humans, some avian influenza viruses have been shown to replicate to a limited extent (26). Therefore, the evidence suggests that avian influenza viruses have the potential to infect mammals, including humans. On the other hand, there are no reports of avian viruses producing disease outbreaks in human populations, so the potential public health concern is based primarily on circumstantial evidence and not actual events. Although the interspecies exchange of these viruses may well be an infrequent event, potential of interspecies transmission must not be excluded.

REFERENCES

1. Acland, H.M., L.A. Silverman-Bachin, and R.J. Eckroade. 1984. Lesions in broiler and layer chickens in an outbreak of highly pathogenic avian influenza virus infection. Vet Pathol 21:564–569.

2. Air, G.M. 1981. Sequence relationships among the hemagglutinin genes of 12 subtypes of influenza A virus. Proc Natl Acad Sci USA 78:7639–7643.

3. Al-Attar, M., K. Nielsen, and W.R. Mitchell. 1981. The application of the soluble antigen fluorescent antibody test for the diagnosis of avian influenza. Can J Comp Med 45:140–146.

4. Alexander, D.J. 1981. Isolation of influenza A viruses from exotic birds in Great Britain. In R.A. Bankowski (ed.). Proceedings of the First International Symposium on Avian Influenza. Carter Composition Corp., Richmond, VA, pp. 79–92.

5. Alexander, D.J. 1982. Avian Influenza: Recent developments. Vet Bull 52:341–359.

6. Alexander, D.J. 1987. Criteria for the definition of pathogenicity of avian influenza viruses. In Proceedings of the Second International Symposium on Avian Influenza. United States Animal Health Association, Athens, GA, pp. 228–245.

7. Alexander, D.J., and R.E. Gough. 1986. Isolations of avian influenza virus from birds in Great Britain. Vet Rec 118:537–538.

8. Alexander, D.J. and G. Parsons. 1980. Protection of chickens against challenge with virulent influenza A viruses of Hav5 subtype conferred by prior infection with influenza A viruses of Hsw1 subtype. Arch Virol 66:265–269.

9. Alexander, D.J., G. Parsons, and R.J. Manvell. 1986. Experimental assessment of the pathogenicity of eight avian influenza A viruses of H5 subtype for chickens, turkeys, ducks and quail. Avian Pathol 15:647–662.

10. Alexander, D.J., T.M. Murphy, and M.S. McNulty. 1987. Avian influenza in the British Isles during 1981 to 1985. In Proceedings of the Second International Symposium on Avian Influenza. United States Animal Health Association, Athens, GA, pp. 70–78.

11. Allan, W.H., C.R. Madeley, and A.P. Kendal. 1971. Studies with avian influenza A viruses: Cross protection experiments in chickens. J Gen Virol 12:79–84.

12. Austin, F.J. and R.G. Webster. 1986. Antigenic mapping of an avian H1 influenza virus hemagglutinin and interrelationships of H1 viruses from humans, pigs and birds. J Gen Virol 67:983–992.

13. Aymard, M., A.R. Douglas, J.M. Gourreau, C. Kaiser, J. Million and J.J. Skehel. 1985. Antigenic characterization of influenza A (H1N1) viruses recently isolated from pigs and turkeys in France. Bull WHO 63:537–542.

14. Bahl, A.K., and B.S. Pomeroy. 1977. Efficacy of avian influenza oil-emulsion vaccine in breeder turkeys. J Am Vet Med Assoc 171:1105.

15. Baker, A.T., J.N. Varghese, W.G. Laver, G.M. Air, and P.M. Colman. 1987. Three-dimensional structure of neuraminidase of subtype N9 from an avian influenza virus. Proteins 2:111–117.

16. Bankowski, R.A. 1981. Introduction and objectives of the symposium. In R.A. Bankowski (ed.). Proceedings of the First International Symposium on Avian Influenza. Carter Composition Corp., Richmond, VA, pp. vi–xiv.

17. Bean, W.J., Y. Kawaoka, J.M. Wood, J.E. Pearson, and R.G. Webster. 1985. Characterization of virulent and avirulent A/Chicken/Pennsylvania/83 influenza A viruses: Potential role of defective interfering RNAs in nature. J Virol 53:151–160.

18. Beard, C.W. 1970. Avian influenza antibody detection by immunodiffusion. Bull WHO 42:779–785.

19. Beard, C.W. 1980. Isolation and Identification of Avian Pathogens. In S.B. Hitchner, C.H. Domermuth, H.G. Purchase, and J.E. Williams (eds.). Am Assoc Avian Pathol, Kennett Square, PA, pp. 67–69.

20. Beard, C.W. 1987. To vaccinate or not to vaccinate. In Proceedings of the Second International Symposium on Avian Influenza. United States Animal Health Association, Athens, GA, 258–263.

21. Beard, C.W., and B.C. Easterday. 1973. A turkey/Oregon/71, an avirulent influenza isolate with

the hemagglutinin of fowl plague virus. Avian Dis 17:173–181.

22. Beard C.W., and D.H. Helfer. 1972. Isolation of two turkey influenza viruses in Oregon. Avian Dis 16:1133–1136.

23. Beard, C.W., M. Brugh, and D. C. Johnson. 1984. Laboratory studies with the Pennsylvania avian influenza viruses (H5N2). Proc 88th Meet US Anim Health Assoc, pp. 462–473.

24. Beard, C.W., M. Brugh, and R.G. Webster. 1987. Emergence of amantadine-resistant H5N2 avian influenza virus during a simulated layer flock treatment program. Avian Dis 31:533–537.

25. Beard, C.W., W.M. Schnitzlein, and D.N. Tripathy. 1991. Protection of chickens against highly pathogenic avian influenza virus (H5N2) by recombinant fowlpox viruses. Avian Dis 35:356–359.

26. Beare, A.S. 1982. Personal communication.

27. Becker, W.B. 1966. The isolation and classification of tern virus: Influenza virus A/tern/South Africa/1961. J Hyg 64:309–320.

28. Becker, W.B., and C.J. Uys. 1967. Experimental infection of chickens with influenza A/tern/South Africa/1961 and chicken/Scotland/1959 viruses. J Comp Pathol 77:159–165.

29. Bosch, F.X., W. Garten, H.-D. Klenk, and R. Rott. 1981. Proteolytic cleavage of influenza virus haemagglutinins: Primary structure of the connecting peptide between HA1 and HA2 determines proteolytic cleavability and pathogenicity of avian influenza viruses. Virology 113:725–735.

30. Brugh, M. 1987. Highly Pathogenic virus recovered from mildly or non-pathogenic H4N8 and H5N2 avian influenza virus isolates. In Proceedings of the Second International Symposium on Avian Influenza. United States Animal Health Association, Athens, GA, pp. 309–313.

31. Brugh, M. and D.C. Johnson. 1987. Epidemiology of Avian Influenza in Domestic Poultry. In Proceedings of the Second International Symposium on Avian Influenza. United States Animal Health Association, Athens, GA, pp. 177–186.

32. Brugh, M., and H.D. Stone. 1987. Immunization of chickens against influenza with hemagglutinin-specific (H5) oil emulsion vaccine. In Proceedings of the Second International Symposium on Avian Influenza. United States Animal Health Association, Athens, GA, pp. 283–292.

33. Brugh, M., C.W. Beard, and H.D. Stone. 1979. Immunization of chickens and turkeys against avian influenza with monovalent and polyvalent oil emulsion vaccines. Am J Vet Res 40:165–169.

34. Butterfield, W.K., and C.H. Campbell. 1979. Vaccination of chickens with influenza A/turkey/Oregon/71 virus and immunity challenge exposure to five strains of fowl plague virus. Vet Microbiol 4:101–107.

35. Cappucci, D.T., D.C. Johnson, M. Brugh, T.M. Smith, C.F. Jackson, J.E. Pearson, D.A. Senne. 1985. Isolation of avian influenza virus (subtype H5N2) from chicken eggs during a natural outbreak. Avian Dis 29:1195–1200.

36. Centers for Disease Control. 1982. Concepts and Procedures for Laboratory Based Influenza Surveillance. Centers for Disease Control, United States Department of Health and Human Services, Washington, DC.

37. Chambers, T., Y. Kawaoka, and R.G. Webster. 1988. Protection of chickens from lethal influenza infection by vaccinia expressed hemagglutinin. Virology 167:414–421.

38. Choppin, P.W., and R.W. Compans. 1975. The structure of influenza virus. In E.D. Kilbourne (ed.). The Influenza Viruses and Influenza. Academic

Press, New York, pp. 15–47.

39. Colman, P.M., J.N. Varghese, and W.G. Laver. 1983. Structure of the catalytic and antigenic sites in influenza virus neuraminidase. Nature 303:41–44.

40. Cooley, J., H. Van Campen, M.S. Philpott, B.C. Easterday and V.S. Hinshaw. 1989. Pathological lesions in the lungs of ducks infected with influenza A viruses. Vet Pathol 26:1–5.

41. Cross, G.M. 1987. The status of avian influenza in poultry in Australia. In Proceedings of the Second International Symposium on Avian Influenza. United States Animal Health Association, Athens, GA, pp. 96–103.

42. De, B.K., M.W. Shaw, P.A. Rota, M.W. Harmon, J.J. Esposito, R. Rott, N.J. Cox and A.P. Kendal. 1988. Protection against virulent H5 avian influenza virus infection in chickens by an inactivated vaccine produced with recombinant vaccinia virus. Vaccine 6:257–261.

43. Dolin, R., R.C. Reichman, H.P. Madore, R. Maynard, P.N. Linton and J. Webber-Jones. 1982. A controlled trial of amantadine and rimantadine in the prophylaxis of influenza A infection. N Engl J Med 307:580–584.

44. Dowdle, W.R., and G.C. Schild. 1975. Laboratory propagation of human influenza viruses, experimental host range, and isolation from clinical materials. In E.D. Kilbourne (ed.). The Influenza Viruses and Influenza. Academic Press, New York, pp. 243–268.

45. Easterday, B.C. 1975. Animal influenza. In E.D. Kilbourne (ed.). The Influenza Viruses and Influenza. Academic Press, New York, pp. 449–481.

46. Easterday, B.C. and C.W. Beard. 1984. Avian Influenza. In M.S. Hofstad, H.J. Barnes, B.W. Calnek, W.M. Reid, and H.W. Yoder (eds.). Diseases of Poultry, 8th ed. Iowa State University Press, Ames, IA, pp. 482–496.

47. Eckroade, R.J., and L.A. Silverman-Bachin. 1987. Avian influenza in Pennsylvania: The beginning. In Proceedings of the Second International Symposium on Avian Influenza. United States Animal Health Association, Athens, GA, pp. 22–32.

48. Eckroade, R.J., L.A. Silverman, and H.M. Acland. 1984. Avian influenza in Pennsylvania. Proc 33rd West Poult Dis Conf, pp. 1–2.

49. Englund, L. and B. Klingeborn. 1986. Avian influenza A virus causing an outbreak of contagious interstitial pneumonia in mink. Acta Vet Scand 27:497–504.

50. Fang, R., W. Min Jou, D. Huylebroeck, R. Devos and W. Fiers. 1981. Complete structure of A/Duck/Ukraine/63 influenza hemagglutinin gene: Animal virus as progenitor of human H3 Hong Kong 1968 influenza hemagglutinin. Cell 25:315–323.

51. Fenner, F., P.A. Bachmann, E.P.J. Gibbs, F.A. Murphy, M.J. Studdert, D.O. White (eds.). 1987. Veterinary Virology. Academic Press, Orlando, FL, pp. 473–484.

52. Fichtner, G.J. 1987. The Pennsylvania/Virginia experience in eradication of avian influenza (H5N2). In Proceedings of the Second International Symposium on Avian Influenza. United States Animal Health Association, Athens, GA, pp. 33–38.

53. Findlay, G.M., R.D. MacKenzie and R.O. Stern. 1937. The histopathology of fowl pest. J Pathol Bacteriol 45:589–596.

54. Foreign Animal Disease Report. 1987. Approved Disinfectants. United States Department of Agriculture, Washington, DC, p. 143.

55. Franklin, R.M., and E. Wecker. 1959. Inactivation of some animal viruses by hydroxylamine and the structure of ribonucleic acid. Nature 84:343–345.

56. Fynan, E.F., R.G. Webster, D.H. Fuller, J.R. Haynes, J.C. Santoro, and H.L. Robinson. 1993. DNA vaccines: Protective immunizations by parenteral, mucosal and gene-gun inoculations. Proc Natl Acad Sci USA 90:11,478–11,482.

57. Garcia, M. J.M. Crawford, J.W. Latimer, E. Rivera-Cruz, and M.L. Perdue. 1996. Heterogenicity in the hemagglutinin gene and emergence of the highly pathogenic phenotype among recent H5N2 avian influenza viruses from Mexico. J Gen Virol 77: (in press).

58. Garnett, W. H. 1987. Status of avian influenza in poultry: 1981–1986. In Proceedings of the Second International Symposium on Avian Influenza. United States Animal Health Association, Athens, GA, pp. 61–66.

59. Gerlach, F. and J. Michalka. 1926. Ueber die in Jahre 1925 in Oesterreich beobachtete Gefluegelpest. Dtsch Tieraerztl Wochenschr 34:897–902.

60. Halvorson, D.A. 1987. Avian influenza: A Minnesota cooperative control program. In Proceedings of the Second International Symposium on Avian Influenza. United States Animal Health Association, Athens, GA, pp. 327–336.

61. Halvorson, D.A., D. Karunakaran, and J.A. Newman. 1980. Avian influenza in caged laying chickens. Avian Dis 288–294.

62. Halvorson, D.A., D. Karunakaran, D. Senne, C. Zelleher, C. Bailey, A. Abraham, V. Hinshaw, and J. Newman. 1983. Epizootiology of avian influenza—simultaneous monitoring of sentinel ducks and turkeys in Minnesota. Avian Dis 27:77–85.

63. Halvorson, D.A., C.J. Kelleher, D.A. Senne. 1985. Epizootiology of avian influenza: Effect of season on incidence in sentinel ducks and domestic turkeys in Minnesota. Appl Environ Microbiol 49: 914–919.

64. Halvorson, D.A., D. Karunakaran, A.S. Abraham, J.A. Newman, V. Sivanandan, and P.E. Poss. 1987. Efficacy of vaccine in the control of avian influenza. In Proceedings of the Second International Symposium on Avian Influenza. United States Animal Health Association, Athens, GA, pp. 264–270.

65. Hers, J.F.P. 1962. Fluorescent antibody technique in respiratory viral disease. Am Rev Respir Dis 88:316–332.

66. Hinshaw, V.S. 1987. The nature of avian influenza in migratory waterfowl, including interspecies transmission. In Proceedings of the Second International Symposium on Avian Influenza. United States Animal Health Association, Athens, GA, pp. 133–141.

67. Hinshaw, V.S. and R.G. Webster. 1982. The natural history of influenza A viruses. In A.S. Beare (ed.). Basic and Applied Influenza Research. CRC Press, Inc., Boca Raton, FL, pp. 79–104.

68. Hinshaw, V.S., R.G. Webster, and B. Turner. 1979. Waterborne transmission of influenza A viruses. Intervirology 11:66–68.

69. Hinshaw, V.S., R.G. Webster and B. Turner. 1980. The perpetuation of orthomyxoviruses and paramyxoviruses in Canadian waterfowl. Can J Microbiol 26:622–629.

70. Hinshaw, V.S., R.G. Webster, R.G. Rodriquez. 1981. Influenza Viruses: Combinations of hemagglutinin and neuraminidase subtypes isolated from animals and other sources. Arch Virol 67:191–201.

71. Hinshaw, V.S., R.G. Webster, B.C. Easterday, and W.J. Bean. 1981. Replication of avian influenza A viruses in mammals. Infect Immun 34:354–361.

72. Hinshaw, V.S., R.G. Webster, W.J. Bean, J. Downie, and D.A. Senne. 1983. Swine influenza-like viruses in turkeys: A potential source of virus for humans? Science 220:206–208.

73. Hinshaw, V.S., D.J. Alexander, M. Aymard, P.A. Bachmann, B.C. Easterday, C. Hannoun, H. Kida, M. Lipkind, J.S. MacKenzie, K. Nerome, G.C. Schild, C. Scholtissek, D.A. Senne, K.F. Shortridge, J.J. Skehel, R.G. Webster. 1984. Antigenic comparisons of swine-influenza-like H1N1 isolates from pigs, birds and humans: an international collaborative study. Bull WHO 62:871–878.

74. Hinshaw, V.S., W.J. Bean, R.G. Webster, J.E. Rehg, P. Fiorelli, G. Early, J.R. Geraci and D.J. St. Aubin. 1984. Are seals frequently infected with avian influenza viruses? J Virol 51:863–865.

75. Hinshaw, V.S., J.M. Wood, R.G. Webster, R. Deibel and B. Turner. 1985. Circulation of influenza viruses and paramyxoviruses in waterfowl originating from two different areas of North America. Bull WHO 63:711–791.

76. Hinshaw, V.S., V.F. Nettles, L.F. Schorr, J.M. Wood, and R.G. Webster. 1986. Influenza virus surveillance in waterfowl in Pennsylvania after the H5N2 avian outbreak. Avian Dis 30:207–212.

77. Hinshaw, V.S., W.J. Bean, J. Geraci, P. Fiorelli, G. Early, and R.G. Webster. 1986. Characterization of two influenza A viruses from a pilot whale. J Virol 58:655–656.

78. Hinshaw, V.S., C.W. Olsen, N. Dybdahl-Sissoko, and D. Evans. 1994. Apoptosis: A mechanism of cell killing by influenza A and B viruses. J Virol 68:3667–3673.

79. Homme, P.J. and B.C. Easterday. 1970. Antibody response in turkeys to influenza A/turkey/Wisconsin/1966 virus. Avian Dis 14:277–284.

80. Horimoto, T., E. Rivera, J. Pearson, D. Senne, S. Krauss, Y. Kawaoka, and R.G. Webster. 1995. Origin and molecular changes associated with emergence of a highly pathogenic H5N2 influenza virus in Mexico. Virology 213:223-230.

81. Hunt, L.A., D.W. Brown, H.L. Robinson, C.W. Naeve, and R.G. Webster. 1988. Retrovirus-expressed hemagglutinin protects against lethal influenza virus infections. J Virol 62:3014–3019.

82. Ito, T., H. Kida, R. Yanagawa. 1985. Antigenic analysis of H4 influenza isolates using monoclonal antibodies to defined antigenic sites on the hemagglutinin of A/Budgerigar/Hokkaido/1/77 strain. Arch Virol 84:251–259.

83. Johnson, D.C. and B.G. Maxfield. 1976. An occurrence of avian influenza virus infection in laying chickens. Avian Dis 20:422–424.

84. Johnson, D.C., B.G. Maxfield, and J.I. Moulthrop. 1977. Epidemiologic studies of the 1975 avian influenza outbreak in chickens in Alabama. Avian Dis 21:167–177.

85. Jungherr, E.L., E.E. Tyzzer, C.A. Brandly, and H.E. Moses. 1946. The comparative pathology of fowl plague and Newcastle disease. Am J Vet Res 7:250–288.

86. Kaleta, E.F. 1987. The epidemiology of avian influenza in pet birds and free living birds other than migratory waterfowl. In Proceedings of the Second International Symposium on Avian Influenza. United States Animal Health Association, Athens, GA, pp. 142–149.

87. Karunakaran, D., V.S. Hinshaw, P. Poss, J. Newman and D. Halvorson. 1983. Influenza A outbreaks in Minnesota turkeys due to subtype H10N7 and possible transmission by waterfowl. Avian Dis 27:357–366.

88. Karunakaran., D., J.A. Newman, D.A. Halvorson, and A. Abraham. 1987. Evaluation of inactivated influenza vaccines in market turkeys. Avian Dis 31:498–503.

89. Kawaoka, Y., and R.G. Webster. 1985. Evolution of the A/Chicken/Pennsylvania/83 (H5N2) influenza virus. Virology 146:130–137.

90. Kawaoka, Y., C.W. Naeve, and R.G. Webster. 1984. Is virulence of H5N2 influenza viruses in chickens associated with loss of carbohydrate from the hemagglutinin? Virology 139:303–316.

91. Kawaoka, Y., W.J. Bean, and R.G. Webster. 1987. Molecular characterization of the A/Chicken/Pennsylvania/83 (H5N2) influenza viruses. In Proceedings of the Second International Symposium on Avian Influenza. United States Animal Health Association, Athens, GA, pp. 197–206.

92. Kawaoka, Y., A. Nestorowicz, D.J. Alexander, and R.G. Webster. 1987. Molecular analyses of the hemagglutinin genes of H5 influenza viruses: Origin of a virulent turkey strain. Virology 158:218–227.

93. Kawaoka, Y., T.M. Chambers, W.L. Sladen, and R.G. Webster. 1988. Is the gene pool of influenza viruses in shorebirds and gulls different from that in wild ducks? Virology 163:247–250.

94. Kawaoka, Y., S. Yamnikova, T.M. Chambers, D.K. Lvov, and R.G. Webster. 1990. Molecular characterization of a new hemagglutinin, subtype H14, of influenza A virus. Virology 179:759–767.

95. Kendal, A.P. 1982. Newer techniques in antigenic analysis with influenza viruses. In A.S. Beare (ed.). Basic and Applied Influenza Research. CRC Press, Inc. Boca Raton, FL, pp. 51–78.

96. Kida, H., R. Yanagawa, and Y. Matsuoka. 1980. Duck influenza lacking evidence of disease signs and immune response. Infect Immun 30:547–553.

97. Kida, H., Y. Kawaoka, C.W. Naeve, and R.G. Webster. 1987. Antigenic and genetic conservation of H3 influenza virus in wild ducks. Virology 159:109–119.

98. Kilbourne, E.D. 1987. Influenza. Plenum Press, New York.

99. Kingsbury, D. 1985. Orthomyxo- and paramyxoviruses and their replication. In B. Fields (ed.). Virology. Raven Press. New York, pp. 1157–1178.

100. Klenk, H.D., W. Keil, H. Niemann, R. Geyer, and R.T. Schwarz. 1983. The characterization of influenza A viruses by carbohydrate analysis. Curr Top Microbiol Immunol 104:247–257.

101. Klingeborn, B., L. Englund, R. Rott, N. Juntti, and G. Rockborn. 1985. An avian influenza A virus killing a mammalian species—the mink. Arch Virol 86:347–351.

102. Kodihalli, S., V. Sivanandan, K.V. Nagaraja, S.M. Goyal, D.A. Halvorson. 1993. Antigen capture enzyme immunoassay for detection of avian influenza virus in turkeys. Am J Vet Res 54:1385–1390.

103. Kuroda, K., C. Hauser, R. Rott, H.D. Klenk and W. Doerfler. 1986. Expression of the influenza virus hemagglutinin in insect cells by a baculovirus vector. EMBO 5:1359–1365.

104. Lang, G., A.E. Ferguson, M.C. Connell, and C.G. Wills. 1965. Isolation of an unidentified hemagglutinating virus from the respiratory tract of turkeys. Avian Dis 9:495–504.

105. Lang, G., B.T. Rouse, O. Narayan, A.E. Ferguson, and M.C. Connell. 1968. A new influenza virus infection in turkeys. I. Isolation and characterization of virus 6213. Can Vet J 9:22–29.

106. Lang, G., O. Narayan, B.T. Rouse, A.E. Ferguson, and M.C. Connell. 1968. A new influenza A virus infection in turkeys. II. A highly pathogenic variant, A/turkey/Ontario/7732/66. Can Vet J 9:151–160.

107. Lang. G., O. Narayan, and B.T. Rouse. 1970. Prevention of malignant avian influenza by 1-adamantanamine hydrochloride. Arch Gesamte Virusforsch 32:171–184.

108. Lang, G., A. Gagnon, J.R. Geraci. 1981. Isolation of influenza A virus from seals. Arch Virol 68:189–195.

109. Lasley, F.A. 1987. Economics of avian influenza: Control vs noncontrol. In Proceedings of the Second International Symposium on Avian Influenza. United States Animal Health Association, Athens, GA, pp. 390–399.

110. Laudert, E.A., V. Sivandandan, and D.A. Halvorson. 1993. Effect of intravenous inoculation of avian influenza virus on reproduction and growth in mallard ducks. J Wildl Dis 29:523–526.

111. Laver, W.G. 1963. The structure of influenza viruses. II. Disruption of the virus particle and separation of neuraminidase activity. Virology 20:251–262.

112. Lipkind, M., Y. Weisman, E. Shihmanter, D. Shoham. 1981. Studies on the ecology of avian influenza viruses in Israel. In R.A. Bankowski (ed.). Proceedings of the First International Symposium on Avian Influenza. Carter Composition Corp. Richmond, VA, p. 30.

113. Liu, C. 1961. Diagnosis of influenza infection by means of fluorescent antibody staining. Am Rev Respir Dis. 83:130–132.

114. Lu, B.L., R.G. Webster, and V.S. Hinshaw. 1982. Failure to detect hemagglutination-inhibiting antibodies with intact avian influenza virions. Infect Immun 38:530–535.

115. McCapes, R.H., and R.A. Bankowski. 1987. Use of avian influenza vaccines in California turkey breeders—Medical rationale. In Proceedings of the Second International Symposium on Avian Influenza. United States Animal Health Association, Athens, GA, pp. 271–278.

116. McKenzie, B.E., B.C. Easterday, and J.A. Will. 1972. Light and electron microscopic changes in the myocardium of influenza-infected turkeys. Am J Pathol 69:239–254.

117. McQuillin, J., C.R. Madeley, and A.P. Kendal. 1985. Monoclonal antibodies for the rapid diagnosis of influenza A and B virus infections by immunofluorescence. Lancet 2:911–914.

118. Meulemans, G. 1987. Status of Avian Influenza in Western Europe: 1981–1987. In Proceedings of the Second International Symposium on Avian Influenza. United States Animal Health Association, GA, pp. 77–83.

119. Meulemans, G., M.C. Carlier, M. Gonze, P. Petit. 1987. Comparison of hemagglutination-inhibition, agar gel precipitin and enzyme-linked immunosorbent assay for measuring antibodies against influenza viruses in chickens. Avian Dis 31:560–563.

120. Mohan, R., Y.M. Saif, G.A. Erickson, G.A. Gustafson, and B.C. Easterday. 1981. Serologic and epidemiologic evidence of infection in turkeys with an agent related to the swine influenza virus. Avian Dis 25:11–16.

121. Murphy, T. M. 1987. The control of avian influenza in Ireland. In Proceedings of the Second International Symposium on Avian Influenza. United States Animal Health Association, Athens, GA, pp. 39–50.

122. Murphy, F.A. and A.P. Kendall. 1987. Biotech-

nology and Modern Vaccine Development. In Proceedings of the Second International Symposium on Avian Influenza. United States Animal Health Association, Athens, GA, pp. 434–443.

123. Murphy, B.R. and R.G. Webster. 1985. Influenza Viruses. In B. Fields (ed.). Virology. Raven Press. New York, pp. 1179–1240.

124. Murphy, B.R., A.J. Buckler-White, W.T. London, J. Harper, E.L. Tierney, N.T. Miller, L.J. Reck, R.M. Chanock, and V.A Hinshaw. 1984. Avian-human reassortant influenza A viruses derived by mating avian and human influenza A viruses. J Infect Dis 150:841–50.

125. Naeem, K., and M. Hussain. 1995. An outbreak of avian influenza in poultry in Pakistan. Vet Rec 137:439.

126. Naeve, C.W., and R.G. Webster. 1983. Sequence of the hemagglutinin gene from influenza virus A/Seal/Mass/1/80. Virology 129:298–308.

127. Naeve, C.W., R.G. Webster and V.S. Hinshaw. 1984. Mutations in the hemagglutinin receptor-binding site can change the biological properties of an influenza virus. J Virol 51:567–569.

128. Nakamura, R.M., and B.C. Easterday. 1967. Serological studies of influenza in animals. Bull WHO 37:559–567.

129. Narayan, O., G. Lang, and B.T. Rouse. 1969. A new influenza A virus infection in turkeys. IV. Experimental susceptibility of domestic birds to virus strain Turkey/Ontario/7732/1966. Arch Gesamte Virusforsch 26:149–165.

130. Narayan, O., G. Lang, and B.T. Rouse. 1969. A new influenza A virus infection in turkeys. V. Pathology of the experimental disease by strain Turkey/Ontario/7732/1966. Arch Gesamte Virusforsch 26:166–182.

131. Nestorowicz, A., Y. Kawaoka, W.J. Bean, and R.G. Webster. 1987. Molecular analysis of the hemagglutinin genes of Australian H7N7 influenza viruses: Role of passerine birds in maintenance or transmission? Virology 160:411–418.

132. Nettles, V.F., J.M. Wood, and R.G. Webster. 1985. Wildlife surveillance associated with an outbreak of lethal H5N2 avian influenza in domestic poultry. Avian Dis 29:733–741.

133. Palmer, D.F., M.T. Coleman, W.R. Dowdle and G.C. Schild. 1975. Advanced Laboratory Techniques for Influenza Diagnosis. United States Department of Health, Education and Welfare Immunology Series No. 6, Procedure Guide. Center for Disease Control, Atlanta, GA.

134. Pearson, J.E., and D.A. Senne. 1987. Diagnostic procedures for avian influenza. In Proceedings of the Second International Symposium on Avian Influenza. United States Animal Health Association, Athens, GA, pp. 222–227.

135. Pearson, J.E., D.A. Senne, E.A. Carbrey, G.A. Gustafson, J.G. Landgraf, D.R. Cassidy, and G.A. Erickson. 1987. Laboratory support for the Pennsylvania/Virginia avian influenza outbreak. In Proceedings of the Second International Symposium on Avian Influenza. United States Animal Health Association, Athens, GA, pp. 39–50.

136. Philpott, M.S., B.C. Easterday and V.S. Hinshaw. 1989. Phenotypic and antigenic variants of a virulent influenza A virus selected by replication in ducks. J Wildl Dis 25:507–513.

137. Philpott, M.S., B.C. Easterday, and V.S. Hinshaw. 1989. Neutralizing epitopes of the H5 hemagglutinin of a virulent avian influenza virus and their relationship to pathogenicity. J Virol 63:3453–3458.

138. Porter, A.G., C. Barber, N.H. Carey, R.A. Hallewell, G. Threlfall and J.S. Emtage. 1979. Complete nucleotide sequence of an influenza virus hemagglutinin gene from cloned DNA. Nature 282:471–477.

139. Poss, P.E., and D.A. Halvorson. 1987. The nature of avian influenza in turkeys in Minnesota. In Proceedings of the Second International Symposium on Avian Influenza. United States Animal Health Association, Athens, GA, pp. 112–117.

140. Poss, P.E., D.A. Halvorson, D. Karunakaran. 1981. Economic impact of avian influenza in domestic fowl in the United States. In R.A. Bankowski (ed.). Proceedings of the First International Symposium on Avian Influenza. Carter Composition Corp. Richmond, VA, pp. 100–111.

141. Poss, P.E., K.A. Friendshuh, and L.T Ausherman. 1987. The control of avian influenza. In Proceedings of the Second International Symposium on Avian Influenza. United States Animal Health Association, Athens, GA, pp. 318–326.

142. Proceedings 1st International Symposium on Avian Influenza. 1981. Carter Composition Corp., Richmond, VA.

143. Proceedings 2nd International Symposium on Avian Influenza. 1987. United States Animal Health Association, Athens, GA.

144. Proceedings 3d International Symposium on Avian Influenza. 1992. United States Animal Health Association, Athens, GA.

145. Proceedings 98th Annual Meeting of the US Animal Health Association. 1994. Report of the committee on transmissible diseases of poultry and other avian species. Spectrum Press, Richmond, VA, p. 522.

146. Resende, M. 1980. Comparative pathogenesis of virulent and avirulent avian influenza viruses in turkeys. PhD Thesis. University of Wisconsin–Madison, Madison, WI.

147. Robinson, H.L., L.A. Hunt, and R.G. Webster. 1993. Protection against a lethal influenza virus challenge by immunization with a haemagglutinin-expressing plasmid DNA. Vaccine 11:957–960.

148. Rogers, G.N., and J.C. Paulson. 1983. Receptor determinants of human and animal influenza virus isolates: Differences in receptor specificity of the H3 hemagglutinin based on species of origin. Virology 127:361–373.

149. Rogers, G.N., T.J. Pritchett, J.L. Lane, and J.C. Paulson. 1983. Differential sensitivity of human, avian, and equine influenza A viruses to a glycoprotein inhibitor of infection: selection of receptor specific variants. Virology 131:394–408.

150. Rohm, C., N. Zhou, J. Suss, J. MacKenzie, and R.J. Webster. 1996. Characterization of a novel influenza hemagglutinin, H15: Criteria for determination of influenza A subtypes. Virology 217:508–516.

151. Rott, R., and C. Scholtissek, 1982. The molecular basis of biological properties of influenza viruses. In A.S. Beare (ed.). Basic and Applied Influenza Research. CRC Press, Inc., Boca Raton, FL, pp. 189–210.

152. Rouse, B.T., G. Lang, and O. Narayan. 1968. A new influenza A virus infection in turkeys. J Comp Pathol Ther 78:525–533.

153. Rowan, M.K. 1962. Mass mortality among European common terns in South Africa in April—May 1961. Br Birds 55:103–114.

154. Sandhu, T.S. and V.S. Hinshaw. 1981. Influenza A virus infection in domestic ducks. In R.A. Bankowski (ed.). Proceedings of the First International Symposium on Avian Influenza. Carter Com-

position Corp., Richmond, VA, pp. 93–99.

155. Schafer, W. 1955. Vergleichende sero-immunologische Untersuchungen uber die viren der influenza und klassichen Gefluegelpest Z Naturforsch 10b:81–91.

156. Scholtissek, C. and E. Naylor. 1988. Fish farming and influenza pandemics. Nature 331:215.

157. Scholtissek, C., H. Burger, P.A. Bachmann, and C. Hannoun. 1983. Genetic relatedness of hemagglutinins of the H1 subtype of influenza A viruses isolated from swine and birds. Virology 129:521–523.

158. Seifried, O. 1931. Gefluegelpest-Encephalitis. Pathologische Histologic. Lubarsch-Ostertag Ergebnisse der allgemeinen Pathologic und Pathologischen. Anat Menschen Tierernaehr 24:661–65.

159. Selleck, P. 1996. Personal communication.

160. Senne, D.A., J.E. Pearson, L.D. Miller, and G.A. Gustafson. 1983. Virus isolations from pet birds submitted for importation into the United States. Avian Dis 27:731–744.

161. Senne, D.A., J.E. Pearson, Y. Kawaoka, E.A. Carbrey, and R.G. Webster. 1987. Alternative methods for evaluation of pathogenicity of chicken Pennsylvania H5N2 viruses. In Proceedings of the Second International Symposium on Avian Influenza. United States Animal Health Association, Athens, GA, pp. 246–257.

162. Skeeles, J.K., R.L. Morrissey, A. Nagy, F. Helm, T.O. Bunn, M.J. Langford, R.E. Long, and R.O. Apple. 1984. The use of fluorescent antibody (FA) techniques for the rapid diagnosis of avian influenza (H5N2) associated with the Pennsylvania outbreak of 1983/1984. Proc 35th N Central Avian Dis Conf, p. 32.

163. Slemons, R.D., and B.C. Easterday. 1972. Host response differences among five avian species to an influenza virus A/turkey/Ontario/7732/66 (Hav5 N?). Bull WHO 47:521–525.

164. Slemons, R.D., R.S. Cooper, and J.S. Orsborn. 1973. Isolation of type A influenza viruses from imported exotic birds. Avian Dis 17:746–751.

165. Slemons, R.D., D.C. Johnson, and T. G. Malone. 1973. Influenza type A isolated from imported exotic birds. Avian Dis 17:458–459.

166. Snyder, D.B., W.W. Marquardt, F.S. Yancey, P.K. Savage. 1985. An enzyme-linked immunosorbent assay for the detection of antibody against avian influenza virus. Avian Dis 29:136–44.

167. Stone, H.A. 1987. Efficacy of avian influenza oil-emulsion vaccines in chickens of various ages. Avian Dis 31:483–490.

168. Stone, H.D. 1988. Optimization of hydrophilic-lipophil balance for improved efficacy of Newcastle disease and avian influenza oil-emulsion vaccine. Avian Dis 32:68–73.

169. Stubbs, E.L. 1965. Fowl Plague. In H.E. Biester, and L.H. Schwarte (eds.), Diseases of Poultry, 5th ed. Iowa State University Press, Ames, pp. 813–822.

170. Tashiro, P. Ciborowski, H.D. Klenk, G. Pulverer, R. Rott. 1987. Role of Staphylococcus protease in the development of influenza pneumonia. Nature 325:536–537.

171. Tripathy, D.N., and W.M. Schnitzlein. 1991. Expression of avian influenza virus hemagglutinin by recombinant fowlpox virus. Avian Dis 35:186–191.

172. Tumova, B. 1987. Avian influenza and paramyxoviruses in central and eastern Europe: A review. In Proceedings of the Second International Symposium on Avian Influenza. United States Animal Health Association, Athens, GA, pp. 84–89.

173. Van Campen, H., B.C. Easterday and V.S. Hinshaw. 1989. Virulent influenza A viruses: Their effect on avian lymphocytes and macrophages. J Gen Virol 70:2887–2895.

174. Van Campen, H., B.C. Easterday and V.S. Hinshaw. 1989. Pathogenesis of a virulent avian influenza A virus: Lymphoid infection and destruction. J Gen Virol 70:467–472.

175. Van Deusen, R.A., V.S. Hinshaw, D.A. Senne, D. Pellacani. 1983. Micro neuraminidase-inhibition assay for classification of influenza A virus neuraminidases. Avian Dis 27:745–750.

176. Walls, H.H., M.W. Harmon, J.J. Slagle, C. Stocksdale and A.P. Kendal. 1986. Characterization and evaluation of monoclonal antibodies developed for typing influenza A and influenza B viruses. J Clin Microbiol 23:240–245.

177. Webster, R.G. 1996. Personal communication.

178. Webster, R.G., and W.G. Laver. 1975. Antigenic variation of influenza viruses. In E.D. Kilbourne (ed.). The Influenza Viruses and Influenza. Academic Press, New York, pp 270–314.

179. Webster, R.G. and R. Rott. 1987. Influenza virus A pathogenicity: The pivotal role of hemagglutinin. Cell 50:665–666.

180. Webster, R.G., M. Yakhno, V.S. Hinshaw, W.J. Bean, and K.G. Murti. 1978. Intestinal influenza: Replication and characterization of influenza viruses in ducks. Virology 84:268–278.

181. Webster, R.G., V.S. Hinshaw, W.J. Bean, K.L. van Wyke, J.R. Geraci, D.J. St. Aubin and G. Petursson. 1981. Characterization of an influenza A virus from seals. Virology 113:712–724.

182. Webster, R.G., J.R. Petursson, K. Skirnisson. 1981. Conjunctivitis in human beings caused by influenza A virus of seals. N Engl J Med 304:911.

183. Webster, R.G., Y. Kawaoka., W.J. Bean, C.W. Beard, and M. Brugh. 1985. Chemotherapy and vaccination: A possible strategy for the control of highly virulent influenza virus. J Virol 55:173–176.

184. Webster, R.G., Y. Kawaoka, and W.J. Bean, Jr. 1986. Molecular changes in A/Chicken/Pennsylvania/83 (H5N2) influenza virus associated with acquisition of virulence. Virology 149:165–173.

185. Weisman, Y., M. Lipkind, E. Shihmanter, A. Aronovici. 1987. Current situation on avian influenza in Israel from 1981–1986. In Proceedings of the Second International Symposium on Avian Influenza. United States Animal Health Association, Athens, GA, pp. 90–95.

186. WHO Expert Committee. 1971. A revised system of nomenclature for influenza viruses. Bull WHO 45:119–124.

187. WHO Expert Committee. 1980. A revision of the system of nomenclature for influenza viruses: A WHO memorandum. Bull WHO 58:585–591.

188. Wiley, D.C., I.A. Wilson, J.J. Skehel. 1981. Structural identification of the antibody-binding sites of Hong Kong influenza hemagglutinin and their involvement in antigenic variation. Nature 289:373–378.

189. Wood, J.M., Y. Kawaoka, L.A. Newberry, E. Bordwell, and R.G. Webster. 1985. Standardization of inactivated H5N2 influenza vaccine and efficacy against lethal A/Chicken/Pennsylvania/1370/83 infection. Avian Dis 29:867–872.

190. Wood, J.M., R.G. Webster, V.F. Nettles. 1985. Host range of A/chicken/Pennsylvania/83 (H5N2) influenza virus. Avian Dis 29:198–207.

23 Adenovirus Infections

INTRODUCTION

J. B. McFerran

Infectious canine hepatitis (ICH) virus was the first adenovirus isolated (12), although Cowdry and Scott (2) had predicted that the intranuclear inclusions they saw in ICH cases would be found to be due to a filterable agent.

The first avian adenovirus was isolated when material from a case of lumpy skin disease in cattle was inoculated into embryonated hens' eggs (14). Other early unintentional isolates of fowl adenoviruses were the chicken embryo lethal orphan (CELO) isolates made in embryonated eggs (16) and the GAL viruses from chicken cell cultures (1). The first isolate of an avian adenovirus from diseased birds was from an outbreak of respiratory disease in bobwhite quail (*Colinus virginianus*) by Olson (10).

Human adenoviruses were isolated during investigations of respiratory disease (5) and were initially called adenoidal–pharyngeal–conjunctival viruses, but the name adenoviruses was subsequently adopted (4).

General properties required for classifying an isolate as an adenovirus have been defined by a number of international committees (9, 11, 15). They recognize the family *Adenoviridae* with two genera, *Mastadenovirus* and *Aviadenovirus*, with human adenovirus type 2 and CELO virus as the respective type species. One of the features distinguishing these two genera is that they do not share the same group antigen (13).

The second report on *Adenoviridae* (15) suggested substitution of species for type and defined a species on the basis of its quantitative neutralization with animal antisera. A species has either no cross-reaction with others or shows a homologous-to-heterologous titer ratio of >16 in both directions. If neutralization shows cross-reactivity in either or both directions (titer ratio, 8:16), distinctiveness of species is assumed if 1) hemagglutinins are unrelated or 2) substantial biophysical/biochemical differences of DNAs exist. It should be noted, however, that the majority of avian adenoviruses do not hemagglutinate.

It is possible to subdivide avian adenoviruses into three groups. Group I includes the conventional group I adenoviruses, or avian adenovirus group I isolates from chickens, turkeys, geese, and other avian species, which share a common group antigen (6, 7, 17). Group II includes the viruses of turkey hemorrhagic enteritis, marble spleen disease, and avian adenovirus group II splenomegaly virus of chickens. These viruses share a common group antigen that is distinct from the group I viruses (3). Group III are the viruses associated with egg drop syndrome 1976 and similar viruses from ducks, which only partially share the Group I common antigen (8).

REFERENCES

1. Burmester, B.R., G.R. Sharpless, and A.K. Fontes. 1960. Virus isolated from avian lymphomas unrelated to lymphomatosis virus. J Natl Cancer Inst 24:1443–1447.

2. Cowdry, E.V., and G.H. Scott. 1930. A comparison of certain intranuclear inclusions found in the livers of dogs without history of infection with intranuclear inclusions characteristic of the action of filterable viruses. Arch Pathol 9:1184–1196.

3. Domermuth, C.H., C.R. Weston, B.S. Cowen, W.M. Colwell, W.B. Gross, and R.T DuBose. 1980. Incidence and distribution of avian adenovirus group II splenomegaly of chickens. Avian Dis 24:591–594.

4. Enders, J.F., J.A. Bell, J.H. Dingle, T. Francis, H.R. Hilleman, R.J. Huebner, and A.M. Payne. 1956. Adenoviruses: Group name proposed for new respiratory-tract virus. Science 124:119–120.

5. Huebner, R.J, W.P. Rowe, T.G. Ward, R.J. Parrott, and J.A. Bell. 1954. Adenoidal-pharyngeal-conjunctival agents. New Engl J Med 257:1077–1086.

6. Kawamura, H., F. Shimizu, and H. Tsubahara. 1964. Avian adenovirus: Its properties and serological classification. Natl Inst Anim Health Q (Tokyo) 4:183–193.

7. McFerran, J.B., B. Adair, and T.J. Connor. 1975. Adenoviral antigens (CELO, QBV, GAL). Am J Vet Res 36:527–529.

8. McFerran, J.B., T.J. Connor, and B.M. Adair. 1978. Studies on the antigenic relationship between an isolate (127) from the egg drop syndrome 1976 and a fowl adenovirus. Avian Pathol 7:629–636.

9. Norrby, E., A. Bartha, P. Boulanger, R.S. Dreizin, H.S. Ginsberg, S.S. Kalter, H. Kawamura, W.P. Rowe, W.C. Russell, R.W. Schlesinger, and R. Wigand. 1976. Adenoviridae. Intervirology 7:117–125.

10. Olson, N.O. 1950. A respiratory disease (bronchitis) of quail caused by a virus. Proc 54th Annu Meet US Livestock Sanit Assoc, pp. 171–174.

11. Pereira, H.G., R.J. Huebner, H.S. Ginsberg and J. Van der Veen. 1963. A short description of the adenovirus group. Virology 20:613–620.

12. Rubarth, S. 1947. An acute virus disease with liver lesions in dogs (hepatitis contagiosa canis). A pathologico-anatomical and etiological investigation. Acta Pathol Microbiol Scand 24:(Suppl 69):1–222.

13. Sharpless, G.R. 1962. GAL virus. Ann NY Acad Sci 101:515–519.

14. Van den Ende, M.P., P.A. Don, and A. Kipps. 1949. The isolation in eggs of a new filterable agent which may be the cause of bovine lumpy skin disease. J Gen Microbiol 3:174–182.

15. Wigand, R., A. Bartha, R.S. Dreizin, H. Esche, H.S. Ginsberg, M. Green, J.C. Hierholzer, S.S. Kalter, J.B. McFerran, U. Pettersson, W.C. Russell and G. Waddell. 1982. Adenoviridae: Second Report. Intervirology 18:169–176.

16. Yates, V.J., and D.E. Fry. 1957. Observations on a chicken embryo lethal orphan (CELO) virus. Am J Vet Res 18:657–660.

17. Zsak, L., and J. Kisary. 1984. Characterisation of adenoviruses isolated from geese. Avian Pathol 13:253–264.

GROUP I ADENOVIRUS INFECTIONS

J. B. McFerran

INTRODUCTION. In contrast with the clear association of group II and group III (egg drop syndrome) adenoviruses with disease, the role of group I avian adenoviruses as pathogens is not well defined. While the majority of isolates appear to have a limited role, if any, as primary pathogens, there is growing evidence that some genotypes are primary pathogens. Adenoviruses do appear to have a role as secondary pathogens in association with chicken infectious anemia virus (CIAV) and infectious bursal disease virus (IBDV). It is not possible to assess their economic importance until their role is better delineated. They have no known public health importance. Several reviews are available (6, 75, 76, 84).

INCIDENCE AND DISTRIBUTION. Group I avian adenoviruses are widely distributed throughout the world. Domestic avian species of all ages are susceptible. Other avian species appear to be susceptible to infection with chicken serotypes as well as serotypes of their own, but this has not been fully investigated.

ETIOLOGY

Morphology and Physical Properties.
Details have been reviewed by McFerran (75). The adenovirus virion is a nonenveloped, icosahedral structure 70–90 nm in diameter, composed of 252 capsomeres, surrounding a core 60–65 nm in diameter. Capsomeres are arranged in triangular faces with six capsomeres along each edge. There are 240 nonvertex capsomeres (hexons) of 8–9.5 nm diameter and 12 vertex capsomeres (penton bases). Vertex capsomeres carry projections called fibers (111). Mammalian adenoviruses have one fiber on each penton base. The Phelps strain of fowl adenovirus serotype 1 (F1) was reported to have two fibers, one of 42.5 nm and the other of 8.5 nm, but other workers found only one fiber. In a study of 11 fowl serotypes (50), all had two fibers on the penton bases and there was a relationship between fiber length and antigenic properties; different serotypes, which showed some relationship in serum neutralization tests, had fibers of similar length.

In thin-section studies, particles of approximately 70-nm diameter with a central nucleoid of approximately 40 nm can be seen in the nucleus of infected cells (Fig. 23.1).

Densities between 1.32 and 1.37 g/mL in cesium chloride (CsCl) have been estimated for fowl adenoviruses. Similar differences in density, which have been attributed to differences in DNA content and base composition in different isolates, also have been found in human adenoviruses.

Chemical Composition.
The nucleic acid is double-stranded DNA, which accounts for 11.3 to 13.5% of the virion, with the remainder being protein. Others, however, have reported 17.3% DNA in F1 and estimated the guanine-cytosine (G-C) content of DNA at 54%, intermediate between the G-C contents of highly oncogenic (47–49%) and nononcogenic serotypes (57–59%) of human adenoviruses. Between 11 and 14 structural polypeptides have been described for F1.

Virus Replication.
Adenoviruses replicate in the nucleus, producing basophilic inclusions (Figs. 23.2 and 23.3). Human adenoviruses have been classified on their cytopathology into subgroups A and B. It also has been possible to subgroup avian adenoviruses into similar subgroups with F1, F2, F4, F5 (340), and F8 (H6 and TR 59) belonging to subgroup A and F3, F5 (TR 22), F6, F7, F8 (784), F9, and turkey adenovirus serotypes 1 (T1) and 2 (T2) belonging to subgroup B (1).

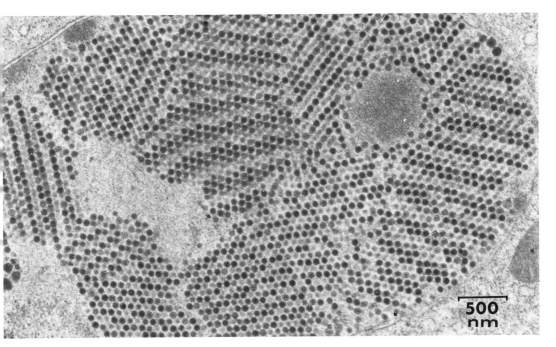

23.1. Adenovirus-infected chick liver cell (48 hr postinfection). Adenovirus particles almost fill the nucleus. (Adair)

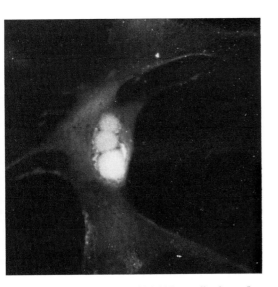

23.2. Growth of F8 (764) in chick kidney cell cultures. Intranuclear inclusions stained by fluorescein isothiocyanate-labelled antibody. (Adair)

Subgroup A viruses produce refractile, pearllike inclusions, which progress into a central basophilic inclusion surrounded by a clear halo. Immunofluorescence staining demonstrates peripheral accumulation of antigen in the area corresponding to the halo. In subgroup B, there is development of nonrefractile, irregular eosinophilic inclusions that in-

crease in size to fill the nucleus. Large circular bodies, probably corresponding to eosinophilic inclusions, are revealed by immunofluorescent staining (Fig. 23.2). In the cases of F5 and F8, different isolates fall into different subgroups. However, these are strains with broad antigenicity and their type of replication may aid classification (1).

These divisions appear to have wider implications. Subgroup A viruses tend to cause sporadic outbreaks of disease in humans and persist in the tonsils, whereas subgroup B viruses cause epidemics and do not normally persist in the tonsils. There also appear to be relationships between human adenoviral subgroups in cytopathology, G-C content, hemagglutinating characteristics, and oncogenicity (75).

Ultrastructurally, virus particles, some with electron-dense and some with electron-lucent cores, accumulate in the nucleus, often forming crystalline lattices (Fig. 23.1). Four types of inclusions comprised of viral protein and some with viral DNA, differing in density and morphology, have been identified, as well as large protein paracrystals with a well-defined morphology. These inclusions correspond to similar ones described for human adenoviruses (2).

Resistance to Physical and Chemical Agents. All avian adenoviruses tested so far have shown typical adenovirus properties (see reviews 6, 75, 76). They are resistant to lipid solvents

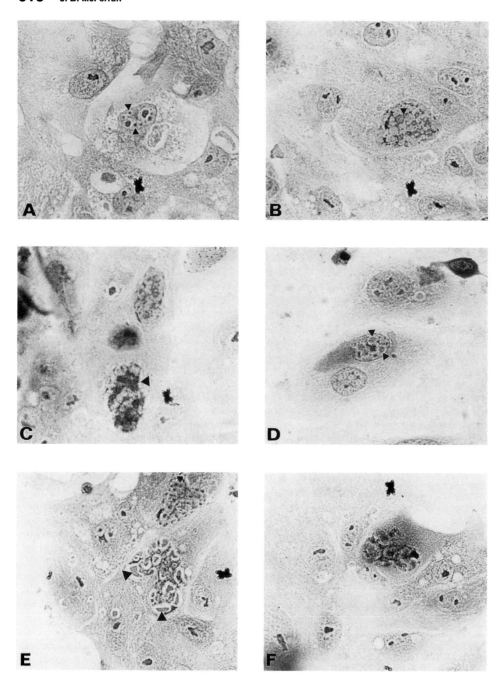

23.3. Cytopathic effects of avian adenoviral subgroups on chick kidney cell cultures. *A-C.* Effect of subgroup I. F1, F2, F4, F5 (340), F8 (H6 and TR59). *A.* Early stage—refractile inclusions in nucleus. *B.* Middle stage—formation of basophilic aggregation around refractile inclusions. *C.* Late stage—concentration of basophilic material in nucleus. *D-F.* Effect of group II. F3, F5 (TR22), F6, F7, F8 (784), F9, and T1 and T2. *D.* Early stage— irregular eosinophilic bodies in nucleus. *E.* Middle stage—formation of multiple eosinophilic inclusion bodies surrounded by granular, basophilic material. *F.* Late stage— condensation to form large intranuclear inclusions. (Adair)

such as ether and chloroform, sodium deoxycholate, trypsin, 2% phenol, and 50% alcohol. They are resistant to variations in pH between 3 and 9. They are inactivated by a 1:1000 concentration of formaldehyde. They are inhibited by DNA inhibitors, e.g., IuDR and BuDR.

Although it is accepted that adenoviruses in general are inactivated in aqueous solution after exposure to 56 C for 30 min, and that heat stability is reduced by divalent ions, the avian adenoviruses show more variability and are apparently more heat resistant. Some strains survive 60 C and even 70 C for 30 min. One F1 virus fell rapidly in titer after 180 min at 56 C, while another F1 strain apparently survived 18 hr at 56 C. Even strains tested in the same laboratory have shown differences in thermostability, suggesting these differences were not just a matter of technique. Although most workers found that divalent cations destabilize adenoviruses, some have found no effect. These divergent results may be due to technique, and it is important to standardize suspending media and pH carefully.

Hemagglutination. Hemagglutination has been reviewed by McFerran (75). F1 virus hemagglutinates rat cells. Optimal agglutination of erythrocytes occurs between pH 6 and 9 at temperatures between 20 and 45 C. The hemagglutinin is stable to treatment with trypsin, RNase, DNase, and neuraminidase. It is inactivated by 15 min at 56 C, and 0.2% formaldehyde reduces its titer eightfold. F1

has not agglutinated a wide range of other erythrocytes. Although a number of strains of F1 were found not to hemagglutinate sheep cells, the FAV1 (Indiana C) strain did, suggesting variation within serotypes. There is no evidence for hemagglutination by any of the other fowl serotypes, or turkey or duck isolates (14).

Strain Classification. Avian adenoviruses have been classified by their serologic relationships, growth in cell cultures (1, 2), and on nucleic acid characteristics (118).

A number of workers have compared the strains by neutralization tests (19, 53, 64, 65, 67, 77, 79). There is agreement over the number of serotypes (or species), but some disagreement over serotype designations (see Table 23.1). Twelve fowl serotypes have been recognized, but there are undoubtedly more that have been isolated but not yet classified.

A major problem has been the discovery of prime strains and strains with broad antigenicity (34, 80). As more strains are tested, two apparently unrelated serotypes can be shown to be related by isolates partly sharing antigens. If the need arises at any time for identification of field isolates, it is important that antiserums are chosen that give as clear-cut differentiation as possible. Monoclonal typing antibody may solve this problem and nucleic acid analysis should prove helpful (12, 118). However, whereas Zsak and Kisary (118) classified 7 and 8 as having restriction pattern E and 10 as restriction

Table 23.1. Serologic classification of Group I avian adenoviruses[a]

Serotype No.		Proposed Type Strain	Japan	Northern Ireland	United States	Hungary	Restriction Patterns
European	American						
Chicken							
1	1	Celo (Phelps)	OTE	112	QBV, Phelps	H1	A12
2	2	GAL1	SR48	685	P7	H3	D
3	3	SR49	SR49	75	-	H5	D
4	4	KR5	KR5	506	J2	H2	C
5	8	340	TR22	340	M2, Tipton	-	B
6	5	CR119	CR119	168	-	-	E
7	11	YR36/X11	YR36	122	X11	-	E
8	6	TR59	TR59	58	T8	H6	E
9	7	764	-	764	B3	-	E
10	9	A2	-	93	A2	-	D
11	10	C2B	-	-	C2B	-	C
12	12	380	-	380	-	-	D
Duck							
1		GR	-	-	-	-	NR[b]
Goose							
1		HA	-	-	-	-	NR
2		N1	-	-	-	-	NR
3		569	-	-	-	-	NR

Note: The group II avian adenoviruses and the egg drop syndrome virus are not included in this table.

[a]References: CELO (Phelps) (113); GAL1 (17); OTE, SR48, SR49, KR5, TR22, CR119, YR36, TR59 (64); 112, 685, 75, 506, 340, 168, 122, 58, 764, 93, 380 (77, 79); QBV (87); Tipton (46); P7, J2, M2, X11, T8, B3, A2, C2B (19); H1-H6 (67); GR (14); HA, N1, 569 (117).

[b]NR, not reported.

pattern D, Barr and Scott (12) classified their 7, 8, and 10 isolates as all having restriction pattern E.

Turkey isolates are not included in Table 23.1 because they have not been compared. Two serotypes of adenovirus in turkeys exist in Northern Ireland (80) and three serotypes have been described in the United States (44), but these have not been compared.

Laboratory Host Systems. Most chicken isolates have been made in chick kidney (CK) or chicken embryo liver (CEL) cells. Although it has been claimed that CEL cells are more sensitive, there appears to be little difference when examining clinical material. However, CEL cells are preferable for diagnostic work because of their greater sensitivity to other viruses. Fowl adenoviruses form plaques in CK. Chicken tracheal organ cultures and chicken embryo fibroblasts are not sensitive (see review 76).

Adenoviruses have been isolated from turkeys and a variety of other birds, including ducks (14), guinea fowl (88), pigeons, budgerigars, and mallard ducks (81), using chicken cell cultures. There are viruses in turkeys, however, that grow only in turkey cells and do not grow or grow poorly in chicken cells (104). It may be that if other avian species are examined using homologous cell systems, an extended range of viruses will be recognized.

Although it is probable that all avian adenoviruses multiply in the embryonated egg, not all chicken or turkey isolates cause recognizable lesions. The chorioallantoic membrane route of inoculation was found to be more sensitive for virus isolation than the allantoic cavity (64). High virus titers of all prototype strains except SR49 killed embryos, but when low titers were used, only Ote killed embryos. When material from naturally occurring infections was used (16), only three isolations were made in embryonated eggs compared with 45 in cell culture. Most adenovirus isolates made in eggs have been serotype 1 or 5, which are not the most prevalent viruses when either serologic surveys (55) or virus isolation studies (36, 114) have been done. However, inoculations into the yolk sac, and to a lesser degree onto the chorioallantoic membrane, supports growth of 11 recognized serotypes (32). Signs and lesions produced in the embryo are death, stunting, curling, hepatitis, splenomegaly, congestion and hemorrhage of body parts, and urate accumulations in the kidneys. Hepatocytes usually contain basophilic or eosinophilic, intranuclear inclusion bodies.

Pathogenicity. Because the role of group I adenoviruses as primary pathogens is not clearly established, factors determining pathogenicity are not clear. There are indications that different serotypes, and even strains of the same serotype, can vary in their ability to produce illness and death (15, 29), respiratory disease (41), or grow and persist in embryo tendon explants (51). A relationship has been found between genotype and virulence, but not between serotype and virulence, with some isolates (45). Although F1 produces a variety of tumors when inoculated into hamsters and will transform human and hamster cells (75), attempts to demonstrate oncogenicity with other avian serotypes have been unsuccessful (47).

In many studies, the route of inoculation has been extremely important; many isolates have failed to cause disease when given by natural routes or by direct spread, but were highly pathogenic when given by parenteral injection. This suggests that many adenoviruses are potential pathogens but require some other agent to allow them to cause disease. Age of the bird is also important. It has been possible to produce mortality (29) in day-old chicks by injection, but not in 10-day-old birds. Virulence could be associated with strain of virus, age of bird, and titer, with the minimum lethal dose ranging from 4 to >300,000 $TCID_{50}$ (12).

Infectious bursal disease virus enhances pathogenicity of avian adenoviruses (48, 98). Ability of avian adenoviruses to cause hepatitis and death also was considerably enhanced by the presence of CIAV (15). In contrast, presence of an adenovirus-associated parvovirus may reduce the growth of the adenovirus in cell cultures as well as pathogenicity and oncogenicity (75).

PATHOGENESIS AND EPIZOOTIOLOGY

Natural and Experimental Hosts. The chicken adenovirus is ubiquitous in fowl as demonstrated by many antibody surveys (55, 114) and from the high isolation rates of adenoviruses from specimens taken from normal and sick birds (36, 64, 67, 78). In addition to infecting chickens, fowl adenovirus serotypes have been recovered from turkeys, pigeons, budgerigars, and a mallard duck (23, 81), and probable fowl isolates have come from guinea fowl (88) and pheasants (18).

Particles that are probably adenoviruses have been seen in thin sections of tissue taken from kestrels (106); herring gulls (70); peach-faced lovebirds (110); a rose-ringed parakeet (39); budgerigars, rosella, and red-rumped parakeets (85); eclectus parrots (90); common murre (71); a cockatiel (105); and a tawny frogmouth (92).

In addition to being infected with chicken serotypes, turkeys are also infected with adenoviruses that grow in cells of turkey origin but either do not grow or only grow poorly in cells of fowl origin (104). Antibody to these viruses is widespread.

Adenoviruses have been isolated from geese and antibody is widespread. These viruses are unrelated to the recognized fowl serotypes but grow in cells of both goose and fowl origin (95, 117). A group I adenovirus has been isolated from a Muscovy duck (14). This virus is unrelated to recognized fowl or turkey serotypes but does grow in chicken as well as duck cells.

Attempts to grow avian adenoviruses in mammals have met with very limited success. F1 has produced fibrosarcomas, hepatomas, ependymomas, and adenocarcinomas when injected into hamsters (75), and another isolate has produced hepatitis in hamsters (47).

Transmission.   Vertical transmission is very important. Adenoviruses are transmitted through the embryonated egg and are often unmasked in cell cultures prepared from embryos and young chicks from infected flocks (76). This has been one of the strongest motivations for establishing SPF flocks. There is evidence that adenovirus infection can remain latent and undetected by the double immunodiffusion test for at least one generation in an SPF flock (49).

Although adenoviruses can be isolated from day 1 onward, viruses are normally excreted from wk 3 onward. In broilers, peak excretion occurred between 4 and 6 wk of age (75). In layer replacements, virus excretion was at maximum from 5 to 9 wk, but was still at 70% after 14 wk; six serotypes were isolated from four farms (114). In a study beginning with 8-wk-old birds (36), excretion continued at a high level until 14 wk and eight different serotypes were found on seven farms. It is not uncommon to isolate two or even three serotypes from one bird, suggesting that there is little cross protection. Certainly birds can excrete one serotype in spite of high levels of neutralizing antibody to other serotypes. There is a second period, around peak egg production, when adenoviruses are often present. Presumably, the stress of egg production or high levels of sex hormones cause reactivation of virus. This would ensure maximum egg transmission to the next generation.

Horizontal spread is also important. Virus is present in feces, the tracheal and nasal mucosa, and kidneys; therefore, virus could be transmitted in all excretions, but highest titers are found in the feces. There is a juvenile as well as an adult pattern of excretion. A 35-day-old bird showing the adult pattern has a lower peak titer of fecal virus with an earlier decline in virus titer, and it excretes for a shorter time than a newly hatched chick, which exhibits the juvenile pattern (26). Horizontal spread appears to be mainly by direct fecal contact but also by aerial contact over short distances, with a slow spread taking weeks (28). This pattern has also been seen in

experimentally infected and in adventitiously infected SPF flocks, and contrasts markedly with the normal pattern usually found in commercial flocks in which most birds in a flock are often excreting adenoviruses. In these circumstances, it is probable that there are many foci of infection due to reactivation of latent viruses. Commercial flocks are often derived from a number of parent flocks, each with their own range of serotypes, and there is considerable mixing of serotypes and birds may be infected concurrently with more than one virus. Aerial spread between farms does not appear to be important, but spread by fomites, personnel, and transport can be very important.

Incubation Period and Signs in Fowl.   Although adenoviruses have been associated with a number of clinical conditions, evidence for them being primary pathogens is conflicting. The incubation period for adenoviruses is short (24–48 hr) following infection by natural routes.

EFFECT ON EGG PRODUCTION.   Some workers have reported adenovirus infection caused a 10% fall in egg production (27) or affected eggshell quality (112). In another similar study, however, experimental infection of birds with four strains did not produce any effect on egg quality and only one strain had a minimal effect on egg numbers (35). Adenoviruses can be isolated from commercial flocks, even when there are exceptionally high levels of production and fertility, and adenovirus infections of SPF flocks in lay are often associated with little or no effect on either egg production or shell quality.

EFFECT ON FOOD CONVERSION AND GROWTH. There have been reports of adenovirus infection resulting in decreased food consumption (35). Although birds injected with adenovirus may have depressed body weights and even high mortality (29, 54), there is little evidence to suggest that naturally occurring infection causes either reduced food utilization or growth. However, growth retardation did occur in naturally infected birds kept under experimental conditions (101). Chickens inoculated with adenovirus had reduced weight gain accompanied by excess fat deposition and depressed cholesterol and triglyceride levels (42).

INCLUSION BODY HEPATITIS.   There have been many different serotypes associated with naturally occurring outbreaks of inclusion body hepatitis (IBH). Among those recorded are F1 (112); F2, F3, and F4 (53, 82); F5 (46, 81); F6, F7, and F8 (65); F7 and F10 (12); F8 (56, 72, 82); F9 (57); and F12 (101).

Some workers have been successful in reproducing liver lesions with basophilic intranuclear inclusions (56, 73, 97) (see Fig. 23.4A) or both liver and pancreatic lesions (96) following parenteral inoculation of very young chicks. When 12-mo-old birds were injected intravenously with an F1 virus (62), no clinical signs were seen but there was degeneration, necrosis, and a cellular response in livers and a mild response in the trachea and lungs. Occasionally, liver lesions have developed following natural routes of infection in older birds (46), but more typically, no disease results even when unnatural routes of exposure are used (72, 74).

Outbreaks of IBH in chickens under 3 wk of age with mortality up to 30% has occurred in Australia (12). Inclusion body hepatitis has been reproduced by inoculating day-old chicks by nasal and ocular routes with 24 isolates belonging to serogroups 6, 7, and 8. When these were analyzed using restriction enzymes, it was found they all had a high genomic relationship possessing a group E genotype (45).

Immunosuppression produced by infectious bursal disease (IBD) aids adenoviruses in producing IBH (48, 98). In both Northern Ireland and New Zealand, however, IBH occurred in chickens before IBD was present in the country (24), and IBH has occurred spontaneously in SPF birds without IBD (93). When birds are infected with both CIAV and adenovirus, there is increased incidence of hepatitis and death (15).

In New Zealand, mainly serotype 8 but also serotypes 1 and 12 were isolated from IBH outbreaks. All belonged to the E genotype (24), but differed from the Australian IBH group E genotype (101). These isolates produced focal hepatitis in 2-day-old birds infected orally. In contact, birds did not develop IBH but showed severe growth retardation (99).

Inclusion body hepatitis is characterized by sudden onset of mortality peaking after 3–4 days and usually stopping on day 5 but occasionally continuing for 2–3 wk. Morbidity is low; sick birds adopt a crouching position with ruffled feathers and die within 48 hr or recover (58, 72, 82). Mortality may reach 10% and occasionally as high as 30% (12). It is normally seen in meat-producing birds 3–7 wk of age, but it has been reported in birds as young as 7 days old (12) and as old as 20 wk (65). There is evidence that in an integrated broiler operation, disease occurs in chickens from certain breeder flocks (72).

INCLUSION BODY HEPATITIS IN OTHER BIRDS. A number of outbreaks of IBH have been recorded in pigeons. In addition to hepatitis, pancreatitis has also been found (30, 52, 66, 82, 108). Inclusion body hepatitis has been diagnosed in a group of eclectus parrots (90), kestrels (106), and a merlin (102).

HYDROPERICARDIUM SYNDROME. In 1987, a new condition—hydropericardium syndrome or Angara disease—was recognized in Pakistan and within a year it had devastated the national broiler industry. It caused between 20 and 60% mortality, with very low morbidity. Typically, mortality starts at 3 wk, peaks for 4–8 days in wk 4 and 5, and then declines (11).

Adenoviruses are associated with this condition, but there is evidence that another agent may also be involved (5, 11, 22). The agent spreads well laterally among birds, and people appear to be important vectors (8, 9). Liver suspension is infectious both orally and nasally. Higher mortalities follow subcutaneous inoculation and the possibility that the initial massive spread throughout Pakistan was the result of a contaminated vaccine has been raised (8).

There are similarities between the signs and pathology of this syndrome and IBH, but it is not clear if they are distinct. Recently, outbreaks of disease in both North and South America have been described with higher mortalities than usual for IBH and with some hydropericardium (33).

The disease has also been seen in pigeons (86). It was possible to reproduce the disease in broilers using livers from infected pigeons and the disease in pigeons was controlled using the poultry vaccine.

For more detailed information, see Hydropericardium-hepatitis Syndrome (Angara Disease), Chapter 37.

RESPIRATORY DISEASE. Adenoviruses have been frequently isolated from both the upper and lower respiratory tract of birds with respiratory disease (63, 78, 96). A survey of records of virus isolations, clinical, and necropsy findings over a 20-yr period, involving hundreds of adenovirus isolations, indicated no primary role for adenoviruses in fowl respiratory disease. Before infectious bronchitis was controlled and *Mycoplasma gallisepticum* and *Mycoplasma synoviae* were eradicated, however, respiratory disease outbreaks were considerably more severe when adenoviruses were isolated from the respiratory tract. Schmidt et al. (103) recorded similar findings when mixed infectious bronchitis–mycoplasma–adenovirus infections mimicked infectious laryngotracheitis. Catarrhal tracheitis and multifocal pneumonic lesions, similar to lesions resulting from experimental adenovirus infections, were found in 13 outbreaks leading to the conclusion that adenoviruses were a significant cause of respiratory disease (40).

Experimental infections have produced equivocal results. Using aerosol exposure, mild respiratory disease was produced (7). Following intratracheal inoculation, respiratory disease usually occurred (27, 74), but occasionally no signs were noted (37).

TENOSYNOVITIS. Adenoviruses have been isolated from chickens with tenosynovitis, but experimental work has not confirmed their involvement (61).

Signs in Turkeys.

Adenoviruses have been isolated from clinical outbreaks of respiratory disease, diarrhea, and depressed egg production, but attempts to reproduce disease have generally been unsuccessful (107).

Signs in Geese and Ducks.

Three serotypes isolated from geese did not reproduce disease in goslings (117). In outbreaks of high mortality associated with hepatitis, adenoviruslike particles were seen in the liver (94).

A diphtheroid, stenosing tracheitis, with occasional bronchitis and pneumonia were seen in up to 10% of 7- to 21-day-old Muscovy ducks. Tracheal epithelial cells contained numerous adenoviruses (13). A similar condition has recently been described in geese in Canada (95), where an isolated parent flock became infected and produced two hatches in which mortality reached 12% in 4- to 11-day-old goslings.

Signs in Guinea Fowl.

Two strains of adenovirus were isolated from naturally occurring outbreaks of pancreatitis in guinea fowl. One strain induced severe disease and death with respiratory and pancreatic lesions after oral and nasal infection of day-old guinea fowl (88). Foci of necrosis with large basophilic and smaller eosinophilic inclusion bodies were seen in guinea fowl suffering from necrotic pancreatitis (91). Recently, a serotype 1 isolate from guinea fowl with necrotizing pancreatitis reproduced the condition experimentally (69).

Signs in Ostriches.

Adenoviruses have been associated with illness, death, and poor hatchability on ostrich farms (89), and an isolate from an ostrich caused pancreatitis in guinea fowl (21).

Lesions

RESPIRATORY DISEASE. In naturally occurring outbreaks, mild to moderate catarrhal tracheitis with excess mucus were the only gross lesions noted (40). Hyperemia of the lungs, cloudy air sacs, and petechial hemorrhages in the pharynx and larynx were described after experimental infection (7).

Microscopically, the main lesions were loss of cilia, necrosis of some epithelial cells, intranuclear inclusion bodies, and infiltration of mononuclear cells into the lamina propria. Multifocal or occasionally diffuse interstitial pneumonia was found (7, 40, 41).

Following aerosol exposure, epithelial hyperplasia, edema, and infiltration by mononuclear cells were seen in air sacs (7).

INCLUSION BODY HEPATITIS. In the literature, there are several descriptions of a disease primarily affecting the liver and also one where the primary lesions appeared to be in the hemopoietic system. It is probable that the aplastic anemia described was due to infection with CIAV (116) (see Chapter 30).

The main lesions are pale, friable, swollen livers. Petechial or ecchymotic hemorrhages may be present in the liver and skeletal muscles (58, 72, 82).

There are inclusion bodies in the hepatocytes. These inclusions can be eosinophilic, large, round or irregularly shaped with clear pale halo (58, 59) or occasionally basophilic inclusions (60, 82) (Fig. 23.4A,B). In Australia, basophilic inclusions predominate (12, 65). Virus particles were detected only in cells with basophilic inclusions; eosinophilic inclusions were composed of fibrillar, granular material (60). In New Zealand, lesions included atrophy of bursa and thymus, aplastic bone marrow, and hepatitis. Inclusions were eosinophilic. Bursal and thymic atrophy in the absence of IBD is interesting (24).

HYDROPERICARDIUM SYNDROME. There is an accumulation of clear straw-colored fluid in the pericardial sac, pulmonary edema, swollen and discolored liver, and enlarged kidneys with distended tubules showing degenerative changes. There are multiple areas of focal necrosis with mononuclear infiltration in the heart and liver. Basophilic inclusions are present in the hepatocytes (11). For more detailed information, see Hydropericardium-Hepatitis Syndrome (Angara Disease), Chapter 37.

NECROTIZING PANCREATITIS AND GIZZARD EROSIONS. Focal pancreatitis and gizzard erosions have been described in chickens in the absence of IBH. Intranuclear inclusion bodies containing adenovirus antigen were demonstrated in necrotic pancreatic acinar cells and epithelial cells of the gizzard (109). Pancreatitis associated with adenoviral infection has been recorded in guinea fowl (91).

Immunity. Group I avian adenoviruses have a common group antigen that is distinct from that of human adenoviruses (64, 80). There are differences in the degree of sharing between these antigens. For example, F1 gave a strong reaction with its own antiserum but failed to detect antibody to F2 and F4 (64). A microtiter fluorescent test (3) confirmed these differences in titer.

Turkey group I adenoviruses have a common antigen detected in double immunodiffusion tests, and this distinguishes them from the group II (turkey hemorrhagic enteritis) adenoviruses (43,

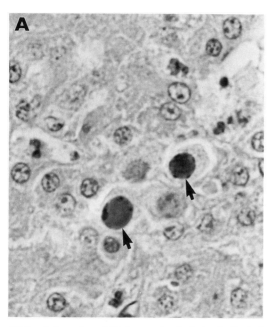
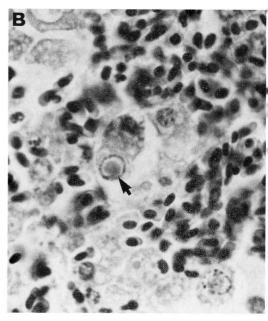

23.4. *A.* Large basophilic intranuclear inclusion bodies in liver of a chicken experimentally infected with F8. *B.* Eosinophilic intranuclear inclusion body in hepatocyte of a chicken with naturally occurring inclusion body hepatitis.

80). The isolate from a Muscovy duck also shares an antigen with F1 (14).

Following infection, birds rapidly develop neutralizing antibody detectable after 1 wk and reaching peak titers at 3 wk (115). They may develop transient precipitating antibody (27) or they may fail to do so (80, 115). This apparent failure is probably due to the insensitivity of the double immunodiffusion test because an antibody response is detectable using immunofluorescence (3).

Development of serum-neutralizing antibody coincides with cessation of virus excretion. Young chicks excrete virus longer because of slower development of neutralizing antibody (26).

It has been found that birds were resistant to reinfection with the same serotype 45 days after primary infection (25). In another study (115), however, birds were reinfected with the same strain after 8 wk, eliciting a secondary response of both neutralizing and precipitating antibodies; virus excretion also occurred despite humoral antibody. Peaks of virus excretion were found when birds were 2.5, 4.5, and 7.5 mo of age (68), consistent with the theory that local immunity lasts about 8 wk but then regresses allowing virus to replicate again on mucosal surfaces.

Serum-neutralizing antibody induced by an inactivated vaccine had no effect on virus excretion in feces but did reduce pharyngeal excretion, possibly by preventing hematogenous spread of virus from the intestine to the pharynx. It is, therefore, possible that resistance to challenge found after infection is due to short-lived local immunity while circulating antibodies protect mainly against invasion of internal organs. The apparent correlation between appearance of circulating antibody and cessation of virus excretion is more likely due to concurrent development of both local immunity, which is more transient, and humoral immunity, which is more persistent. Support for this hypothesis is provided by the finding that maternal antibody does not protect against natural routes of infection (25) but does protect against intraabdominal infection (46, 54). There is evidence that infection with some strains of adenovirus results in severe depletion of lymphocytes in the bursa, thymus, and spleen, causing an immunologic impairment (100).

DIAGNOSIS

Isolation and Identification of Virus.

Specimens of choice are feces, pharynx, kidney, and affected organs, e.g., livers, in cases of IBH. These should be made into a 10% suspension and, in the case of chickens, inoculated onto either chick embryo liver cells or chick kidney cells. Chick embryo fibroblasts and tracheal organ cultures are not sensitive. Although three passages have been used (16, 36), generally two blind passages of 7 days' duration each are sufficient. If attempting to isolate adenoviruses from other avian species, it is preferable to use cells from the avian species being investigated, although chicken cells can be used. However, there are turkey isolates that either grow poorly or not at all in chick cell cultures (104). Embryonated eggs are insensitive for primary isolation of most serotypes of adenoviruses, although Cowen (32) has showed that the yolk sac is a sensitive route for isolating laboratory strains representative of 11 serotypes. It remains to be shown whether this route is equally sensitive with field material, but it clearly should be tried in laboratories lacking cell culture technology.

Once an agent is isolated in cell cultures, the easiest method to confirm that it is an adenovirus is to stain the cells with an antiserum labeled with a fluorescent dye. Direct examination of cell lysate by electron microscopy also gives a quick and positive answer and has the added advantage that parvoviruses can also be detected if present. If these techniques are not available, then H&E staining of monolayers will demonstrate the presence of intranuclear basophilic inclusions. To identify a serotype, it is necessary to conduct virus neutralization tests with the isolate against standard reference antiserums to all known serotypes. This labor-intensive process can be reduced by using the "antiserum pool" modification (36).

Serology.   Antibody to the group antigen can be detected using the double immunodiffusion (DID) test, but its apparent sensitivity in naturally occurring outbreaks is often due to multiple infection with adenovirus serotypes, making it unreliable for detecting infection in SPF flocks (27, 49, 80). However, use of a trivalent antigen incorporating three adenovirus serotypes increases sensitivity of the DID test (31). The indirect immunofluorescent test is much more sensitive and rapid, and is inexpensive (3), but its interpretation requires skill. The enzyme-linked immunosorbent assay (ELISA) has been used to detect group antibodies and it is inexpensive and sensitive (20, 38, 83).

Type-specific antibody has normally been detected using the serum-neutralization test, but it can also be detected using ELISA (83).

The main problem with any serologic test for adenoviruses is interpreting the results; antibodies are common in both healthy and diseased birds and birds are frequently infected with a number of serotypes. Virus genotype may be of more interest than serotype for predicting disease-producing capability. Furthermore, presence of humoral antibody gives no indication of the state of local immunity at mucosal surfaces.

PREVENTION AND CONTROL.   As both IBDV and CIAV potentiate pathogenicity of adenoviruses, the first step must be to control or eliminate these two viruses.

Adenoviruses are resistant and, although it is possible to eliminate them from most environmentally controlled houses with impervious floors and walls that can be made airtight, the value of attempted eradication of adenovirus from commercial flocks is questionable. This is because the virus is so effectively spread vertically through the embryonated egg that viruses would almost certainly be introduced into the next flock, and, therefore, control would have to start at primary breeder level. Furthermore, experience with SPF flocks has indicated that horizontal spread would be a major problem and it would be exceedingly difficult to keep a commercial flock from becoming infected.

As evidence mounts that certain genotypes may be primary pathogens, the possibility of vaccination is more appealing. Maternal antibody titers of 64 or greater prevented IBH, but the birds did experience growth retardation (99). A vaccine prepared by inactivating homogenates of liver from infected birds has been used extensively with apparent success in Pakistan to control the hydropericardium syndrome (4, 10).

REFERENCES

1. Adair, B.M. 1978. Studies on the development of avian adenoviruses in cell cultures. Avian Pathol 7:541-550.

2. Adair, B.M., W.L. Curran, and J.B. McFerran. 1979. Ultrastructural studies of the replication of fowl adenoviruses in primary cell cultures. Avian Pathol 8:133-144.

3. Adair, B.M., J.B. McFerran, and V.M. Calvert. 1980. Development of a microtitre fluorescent antibody test for serological detection of adenovirus infection in birds. Avian Pathol 9:291-300.

4. Afzal, M., and I. Ahmad. 1990. Efficacy of an inactivated vaccine against hydropericardium syndrome in broilers. Vet Rec 126:59-60.

5. Afzal, M., R. Muneer, and G. Stein. 1991. Studies on the aetiology of hydropericardium syndrome (Angara disease) in broilers. Vet Rec 128:591-593.

6. Aghakhan, S.M. 1974. Avian adenoviruses. Vet Bull 44:531-552.

7. Aghakhan, S.M., and M. Pattison. 1974. Pathogenesis and pathology of infections with two strains of avian adenovirus. J Comp Pathol 84:495-503.

8. Ahmad, K., I. Ahmad, M.A. Akram-Muneer, and M. Ajmal. 1992. Experimental transmission of Angara disease in broiler fowls. Stud Res Vet Med 1:53-55.

9. Akhtar, S., S. Zahid, and M.I. Khan. 1992. Risk factors associated with hydropericardium syndrome in broiler flocks. Vet Rec 131:481-484.

10. Anjum, A.D. 1990. Experimental transmission of hydropericardium syndrome and protection against it in commercial broiler chickens. Avian Pathol 19:655-660.

11. Anjum, A.D., M.A. Sabri, and Z. Iqbal. 1989. Hydropericarditis syndrome in broiler chickens in Pakistan. Vet Rec 124:247-248.

12. Barr, D.A., and P. Scott. 1988. Adenoviruses and IBH. Proc 2nd Asian/Pacific Poult Health Conf [Proc 112]. Post Graduate Comm Vet Sci, University of Sydney, Australia, pp. 323-326.

13. Bergmann, Von. V., R. Heidrich, and E. Kinder. 1985. Pathomorphologische und Elektronenmikroskopische Fest-

stellung einer Adenovirus-tracheitis bei Moschusenten (Cairina moschata). Monatschefte fur Vet Med 40:313-315.

14. Bouquet, J.F., Y. Moreau, J.B. McFerran, and T.J. Connor. 1982. Isolation and characterisation of an adenovirus isolated from Muscovy ducks. Avian Pathol 11:301-307.

15. Bülow V.v., R. Rudolph, and B. Fuchs. 1986. Folgen der Doppelinfektion von Kuken mit adenovirus oder Reovirus und dem Erreger der aviaren infektiosen Anamie (CAA). J Vet Med [B] 33:717-726.

16. Burke, C.N., R.E. Luginbuhl, and E.L. Jungherr. 1959. Avian enteric cytopathogenic viruses. I. Isolation. Avian Dis 3:412-419.

17. Burmester, B.R., G.R. Sharpless, and A.K. Fontes. 1960. Virus isolated from avian lymphomas unrelated to lymphomatosis virus. J Nat Cancer Inst 24:1443-1447.

18. Cakala, A. 1966. Szczep wirusa CELO wyosobniony z bazantow. Med Wet 22:261-264.

19. Calnek, B.W., and B.S. Cowen. 1975. Adenoviruses of chickens: Serologic groups. Avian Dis 19:91-103.

20. Calnek, B.W., W.R. Shek, N.A. Menendez, and P. Stiube. 1982. Serological cross-reactivity of avian adenovirus serotypes in an enzyme-linked immunosorbent assay. Avian Dis 26:897-906.

21. Capua, I., R.E. Gough, P. Scaramozzino, R. Lelli, and A. Gatti. 1994. Isolation of an adenovirus from an ostrich (Struthio camelus) causing pancreatitis in an experimentally infected guinea fowl (Numida meleagris). Avian Dis 38:642-646.

22. Cheema, A.H., J. Ahmad, and M. Afzal. 1989. An adenovirus infection of poultry in Pakistan. Rev Sci Tech Int Epizootics 8:789-795.

23. Cho, B.R. 1976. An adenovirus from a turkey pathogenic to both chicks and turkey poults. Avian Dis 20:714-723.

24. Christensen, N.H., and Md. Saifuddin. 1989. A primary epidemic of inclusion body hepatitis in broilers. Avian Dis 33:622-630.

25. Clemmer, D.L. 1965. Experimental enteric infection of chickens with an avian adenovirus (strain 93). Proc Soc Exp Biol Med 118:943-948.

26. Clemmer, D.I. 1972. Age associated changes in fecal excretion patterns of strain 93 chick embryo lethal orphan virus in chicks. Infect Immun 5:60-64.

27. Cook, J.K.A. 1972. Avian adenovirus alone or followed by infectious bronchitis virus in laying hens. J Comp Pathol 82:119-128.

28. Cook, J.K.A. 1974. Spread of an avian adenovirus (CELO virus) to uninoculated fowls. Res Vet Sci 16:156-161.

29. Cook, J.K.A. 1974. Pathogenicity of avian adenoviruses for day-old chicks. J Comp Pathol 84:505-515.

30. Coussement, W.H., R. Ducatelle, P. Lemahieu, R. Froyman, L. Devriese, and J.H. Hoorens. 1984. Pathology of adenovirus infection in pigeons. Vlaam Diergeneeskd Tijdschr 53:277-283.

31. Cowen, B.S. 1987. A trivalent antigen for the detection of type 1 avian adenovirus precipitin. Avian Dis 31:351-354.

32. Cowen, B.S. 1988. Chicken embryo propagation of type I avian adenoviruses. Avian Dis 32:347-352.

33. Cowen, B.S. 1992. Inclusion body hepatitis—anaemia and hydropericardium syndromes: aetiology and control. World's Poult Sci J 48:247-254.

34. Cowen, B., B.W. Calnek, and S.B. Hitchner. 1977. Broad antigenicity exhibited by some isolates of avian adenovirus. Am J Vet Res 38:959-962.

35. Cowen, B., B.W. Calnek, N.A. Menendez, and R.F. Ball. 1978. Avian Adenoviruses—effect on egg production, shell quality and feed consumption. Avian Dis 22:459-470.

36. Cowen, B., G.B. Mitchell, and B.W. Calnek. 1978. An adenovirus survey of poultry flocks during the growing and laying periods. Avian Dis 22:115-121.

37. Cox, J.C. 1966. An avian adenovirus isolated in Australia. Aust Vet J 42:482.

38. Dawson, G.J., L.N. Orsi, V.J. Yates, P.W. Chang, and A.D. Pronovost. 1980. An enzyme-linked immunosorbent assay for detection of antibodies to avian adenovirus and avian adenovirus-associated virus in chickens. Avian Dis 24:393-402.

39. Desmidt, M., R. Ducatelle, E. Uyttebroek, G. Charlier, and J. Hoorens. 1991. Respiratory adenovirus-like infection in a rose-ringed parakeet (Psittacula krameri). Avian Dis 35:1001-1006.

40. Dhillon, A.S., and F.S.B. Kibenge. 1987. Adenovirus infection associated with respiratory disease in commercial chickens. Avian Dis 31:654-657.

41. Dhillon, A.S., and R.W. Winterfield. 1984. Pathogenicity of various adenovirus serotypes in the presence of Escherichia coli in chickens. Avian Dis 28:147-153.

42. Dhurandhar, N.V., P. Kulkarni, S.M. Ajinkya, and A. Sherikar. 1992. Effect of adenovirus infection on adiposity in chicken. Vet Microbiol 31:101-107.

43. Domermuth, C.H., J.R. Harris, W.B. Gross, and R.T. DuBose. 1979. A naturally occurring infection of chickens with a hemorrhagic enteritis/marble spleen disease. Avian Dis 23:479-484.

44. Easton, G.D., and D.G. Simmons. 1977. Antigenic analysis of several turkey respiratory adenoviruses by reciprocal-neutralization kinetics. Avian Dis 21:605-611.

45. Erny, K.M., D.A. Barr, and K.J. Fahey. 1991. Molecular characterisation of highly virulent fowl adenoviruses associated with outbreaks of inclusion body hepatitis. Avian Pathol 20:597-606.

46. Fadly, A.M., and R.W. Winterfield. 1973. Isolation and some characteristics of an agent associated with inclusion body hepatitis, hemorrhages and aplastic anaemia in chickens. Avian Dis 17:182-193.

47. Fadly, A.M., R.W. Winterfield, and H.J. Olander. 1976. The oncogenic potential of some avian adenoviruses causing diseases in chickens. Avian Dis 20:139-145.

48. Fadly, A.M., R.W. Winterfield, and H.J. Olander. 1976. Role of the bursa of Fabricius in the pathogenicity of inclusion body hepatitis and infectious bursal disease viruses. Avian Dis 20:467-472.

49. Fadly, A.M., B.J. Riegle, K. Nazerian, and E.A. Stephens. 1980. Some observations on an adenovirus isolated from specific pathogen-free chickens. Poult Sci 59:21-27.

50. Gelderblom, H., and I. Maichle-Laupper. 1982. The fibers of fowl adenoviruses. Arch Virol 72:289-298.

51. Georgiou, K., R.C. Jones, and J.R.M. Guneratne. 1983. Organ cultures studies on adenoviruses isolated from tenosynovitis in chickens. Avian Pathol 12:199-212.

52. Goodwin, M.A., and J.F. Davis. 1990. Inclusion body hepatitis in pigeons. Proc 39th West Poult Dis Conf, March 4-6 1990, Sacramento, CA, p. 35.

53. Grimes, T.M., and D.J. King. 1977. Serotyping avian adenoviruses by a microneutralization procedure. Am J Ves Res 38:317-321.

54. Grimes, T.M., and D.J. King. 1977. Effect of maternal antibody on experimental infections of chickens with a type 8 avian adenovirus. Avian Dis 21:97-112.

55. Grimes, T.M., D.H. Culver, and D.J. King. 1977. Virus-neutralizing antibody titers against 8 avian adenovirus serotypes in breeder hens in Georgia by a microneutralization procedure. Avian Dis 21:220-229.

56. Grimes, T.M., D.J. King, S.H. Kleven, and O.J. Fletcher. 1977. Involvement of a type-8 avian adenovirus in the etiology of inclusion body hepatitis. Avian Dis 21:26-38.

57. Grimes, T.M., D.J. King, O.J. Fletcher, and R.K. Page. 1978. Serologic and pathogenicity studies of avian adenovirus isolated from chickens with inclusion body hepatitis. Avian Dis 22:177-180.

58. Howell, J., D.W. McDonald, and R.G. Christian. 1970. Inclusion body hepatitis in chickens. Can Vet J 11:99-101.

59. Itakura, C., M. Yasuba, and M. Goto. 1974.

Histopathological studies on inclusion body hepatitis in broiler chickens. Jpn J Vet Sci 36:329-340.

60. Itakura, C., S. Matsushita, and M. Goto. 1977. Fine structure of inclusion bodies in hepatic cells of chickens naturally affected with inclusion body hepatitis. Avian Pathol 6:19-32.

61. Jones, R.C., and K. Georgiou. 1984. Experimental infection of chickens with adenoviruses isolated from tenosynovitis. Avian Pathol 13:13-23.

62. Kawamura, H., and T. Horiuchi. 1964. Pathological changes in chickens inoculated with CELO virus. Natl Inst Anim Health Q (Tokyo) 4:31-39.

63. Kawamura, H., T. Sato, H. Tsubahara, and S. Isogai. 1963. Isolation of CELO virus from chicken trachea. Natl Inst Anim Health Q (Tokyo) 3:1-10.

64. Kawamura, H., F. Shimizu, and H. Tsubahara. 1964. Avian adenovirus: its properties and serological classification. Natl Inst Anim Health Q (Tokyo) 4:183-193.

65. Kefford, B., R. Borland, J.F. Slattery, and D.C. Grix. 1980. Serological identification of avian adenoviruses isolated from cases of inclusion body hepatitis in Victoria, Australia. Avian Dis 24:998-1006.

66. Ketterer, P.J., B.J. Trimmins, H.C. Prior, and J.G. Dingle. 1992. Inclusion-body hepatitis associated with an adenovirus in racing pigeons in Australia. Aust Vet J 69:90-91.

67. Khanna, P.N. 1964. Studies on cytopathogenic avian enteroviruses. I. Their isolation and serological classification. Avian Dis 8:632-637.

68. Khanna, P.N. 1965. Studies on cytopathogenic avian enteroviruses. II. Influence of age on virus excretion and incidence of certain serotypes in a colony of chicks. Avian Dis 9:27-32.

69. Kles, V., M. Morin, G. Plassiart, M. Guittet, and G. Bennejean. 1991. Isolation of an adenovirus involved in a guinea fowl pancreatitis outbreak. J Vet Med [B] 38:610-620.

70. Leighton, F.A. 1984. Adenovirus-like agent in the bursa of Fabricius of herring gulls (Larus argentatus Pontoppidan) from Newfoundland, Canada. J Wildl Dis 20:226-230.

71. Lowenstine, L.J., and D.M. Fry. 1985. Adenovirus-like particles associated with intranuclear inclusion bodies in the kidney of a common murre (Uria aalge). Avian Dis 29:208-213.

72. Macpherson, I., J.S. McDougall, and A.P. Laursen-Jones. 1974. Inclusion body hepatitis in a broiler integration. Vet Rec 95:286-289.

73. McCracken, R.M., J.B. McFerran, R.T. Evans, and T.J. Connor. 1976. Experimental studies on the aetiology of inclusion body hepatitis. Avian Pathol 5:325-339.

74. McDougall, J.S., and R.W. Peters. 1974. Avian adenoviruses. A study of 8 field isolates. Res Vet Sci 16:12-18.

75. McFerran, J.B. 1981. Adenoviruses of vertebrate animals. In E. Kurstak and C. Kurstak (eds.). Comparative Diagnosis of Viral Diseases III. Academic Press, New York, pp. 102-165.

76. McFerran, J.B., and B.M. Adair. 1977. Avian adenoviruses—A review. Avian Pathol 6:189-217.

77. McFerran, J.B., and T.J. Connor. 1977. Further studies on the classification of fowl adenovirus. Avian Dis 21:585-595.

78. McFerran, J.B., W.A.M. Gordon, S.M. Taylor, and P.J. McParland. 1971. Isolation of viruses from 94 flocks of fowl with respiratory disease. Res Vet Sci 12:565-569.

79. McFerran, J.B., J.K. Clarke, and T.J. Connor. 1972. Serological classification of avian adenoviruses. Arch Virusforsch 39:132-139.

80. McFerran, J.B., B. Adair, and T.J. Connor. 1975. Adenoviral antigens (CELO, QBV, GAL). Am J Vet Res 36:527-529.

81. McFerran, J.B., T.J. Connor, and R.M. McCracken. 1976. Isolation of adenoviruses and reoviruses from avian species other than domestic fowl. Avian Dis 20:519-524.

82. McFerran, J.B., R.M. McCracken, T.J. Connor, and R.T. Evans. 1976. Isolation of viruses from clinical outbreaks of inclusion body hepatitis. Avian Pathol 5:315-324.

83. Mockett, A.P.A., and J.K.A. Cook. 1983. The use of an enzyme-linked immunosorbent assay to detect IgG antibodies to serotype-specific and group specific antigens of fowl adenovirus serotypes 2, 3 and 4. J Virol Methods 7:327-335.

84. Monreal, G., 1992. Adenoviruses and adeno-associated viruses of poultry. Poult Sci Rev 4:1-27.

85. Mori, F., A. Touchi, T. Suwa, C. Itakura, A. Hashimoto, and K. Hirai. 1989. Inclusion bodies containing adenovirus-like particles in the kidneys of psittacine birds. Avian Pathol 18:197-202.

86. Naeem, K., and H.S. Akram. 1995. Hydropericardium syndrome outbreak in a pigeon flock. Vet Rec 136:296-297.

87. Olson, N.O. 1950. A respiratory disease (bronchitis) of quail caused by a virus. Proc 54th Annu Meet US Livestock Sanit Assoc, pp. 171-174.

88. Pascucci, S., A. Rinaldi, and A. Prati. 1973. CELO virus in guinea-fowl: characterization of two isolates. Proc 5th Int Conf World Vet Poult Assoc, pp. 1524-1531.

89. Raines, A.M. 1993. Adenovirus infection in the ostrich (Struthio camelus). Proc Annu Conf Assoc Avian Vet, Nashville, TN, 31 August-4 September 1993, pp. 304-312.

90. Ramis, A., M.J. Marlasca, N. Majo, and L. Ferrer. 1992. Inclusion body hepatitis (IBH) in a group of eclectus parrots (Eclectus roratus). Avian Pathol 21:165-169.

91. Reece, R.L., and D.A. Pass. 1986. Inclusion body pancreatitis in guinea fowl (Numida meleagris). Aust Vet J 63:26-27.

92. Reece, R.L., D.A. Pass, and R. Butler. 1985. Inclusion body hepatitis in a tawny frogmouth (Podargus strigoides: Caprimulgiformes). Aust Vet J 62:426.

93. Reece, R.L., D.C. Grix, and D.A. Barr. 1986. An unusual case of inclusion body hepatitis in a cockerel. Avian Dis 30:224-227.

94. Riddell, C. 1984. Virus hepatitis in domestic geese in Saskatchewan. Avian Dis 28:774-782.

95. Riddell, C., J.V. Hurk, van-den, S. Copeland, G. Wobeser, and J.V. Van-den-Hurk. 1992. Virus tracheitis in goslings in Saskatchewan. Avian Dis 36: 158-163.

96. Rinaldi, A., G Mandelli, D. Cessi., A. Valeri, and G. Cervio. 1968. Proprieta di un ceppo di virus CELO isolato dal Pollo in Italia. Clin Vet (Milan) 91:382-404.

97. Rosenberger, J.K., R.J. Eckroade, S. Klopp, and W.C. Krauss. 1974. Characterization of several viruses isolated from chickens with inclusion body hepatitis and aplastic anaemia. Avian Dis 18:399-409.

98. Rosenberger, J.K., S. Klopp, R.J. Eckroade, and W.C. Krauss. 1975. The role of the infectious bursal agent and several avian adenoviruses in the hemorrhagic-aplastic-anaemia syndrome and gangrenous dermatitis. Avian Dis 19:717-729.

99. Saifuddin, Md., and C.R. Wilks. 1990. Reproduction of inclusion body hepatitis in conventionally reared chickens inoculated with a New Zealand isolate of avian adenovirus. NZ Vet J 38:62-65.

100. Saifuddin, Md., and C.R. Wilks. 1992. Effect of fowl adenovirus infection on the immune system of chickens. J Comp Pathol 107:285-294.

101. Saifuddin, Md., C.R. Wilks, and A. Murray. 1992. Characterisation of avian adenoviruses associated with inclusion body hepatitis. NZ Vet J 40:52-55.

102. Schelling, S.H., D.S. Garlick, and J. Alroy. 1989. Adenoviral hepatitis in a Merlin (Falco columbarius). Vet Pathol 26:529-530.

103. Schmidt, U., H. Hantschel, P. Schulze, and H. Linsert. 1970. Untersuchungen uber eine Mischinfektion von aviarem. Adenovirus und dem virus der infektiosen bronchitis. Arch Exp Vetmed 24:587-607.

104. Scott, M., and J.B. McFerran. 1972. Isolation of adenoviruses from turkeys. Avian Dis 16:413-420.

105. Scott, P.C., R.J. Condron, and R.L. Reece. 1986. Inclusion body hepatitis associated with adenovirus-like particles in a cockatiel (Psittaciformes:Nymphicus hollandicus). Aust Vet J 63:337-338.

106. Sileo, L., J.C. Franson, D.L. Graham, C.H. Domermuth., B.A. Rattner, and O.H. Patee. 1983. Hemorrhagic enteritis in captive American kestrels (Falco sparverius). J Wildl Dis 19:244-247.

107. Sutjipto, S., S.E. Miller, D.G. Simmons, and R.C. Dillman. 1977. Physicochemical characterization and pathogenicity studies of two turkey adenovirus isolants. Avian Dis 21:549-556.

108. Takase, K., N. Yoshinaga, T. Egashira, T. Uchimura, and M. Yamamoto. 1990. Avian adenovirus isolated from pigeons affected with inclusion body hepatitis. Jpn J Vet Sci 52:207-215.

109. Tanimura, N., K. Nakamura, K. Imai, M. Maeda, T. Gobo, S. Nitta, T. Ishihara, and H. Amano. 1993. Necrotizing pancreatitis and gizzard erosion associated with adenovirus infection in chickens. Avian Dis 37:606-611.

110. Wallner-Pendleton, E., D.H. Helfer, J.A. Schmitz, and L. Lowenstine. 1983. An inclusion body pancreatitis in Agapornis. Proc 32nd West Poult Dis Conf, p. 99.

111. Wigand, R., A. Bartha, R.S. Dreizin, H. Esche, H.S. Ginsberg, M. Green, J.C. Hierholzer, S.S. Kalter, J.B. Mc-Ferran, U. Pettersson, W.C. Russell, and G. Wadell. 1982. Adenoviridae: Second Report. Intervirology 18:169-176.

112. Winterfield, R.W., A.M. Fadly, and A.M. Gallina. 1973. Adenovirus infection and disease. I. Some characteristics of an isolate from chickens in Indiana. Avian Dis 17:334-342.

113. Yates, V.J., and D.E. Fry. 1957. Observations on a chicken embryo lethal orphan (CELO) virus. J Vet Res 18:657-660.

114. Yates, V.J., Y.O. Rhee, D.E. Fry, A.M. El Mishad, and K.J. McCormick. 1976. The presence of avian adenoviruses and adenovirus associated viruses in healthy chickens. Avian Dis 20:146-152.

115. Yates, V.J., Y.O. Rhee, and D.E. Fry. 1977. Serological response of chickens exposed to a type 1 avian adenovirus alone or in combination with the adeno-associated virus. Avian Dis 21:408-414.

116. Yuasa, N., T. Taniguchi, and I. Yoshida. 1979. Isolation and some characteristics of an agent inducing anaemia in chicks. Avian Dis 23:366-385.

117. Zsak, L., and J. Kisary. 1984. Characterisation of adenoviruses isolated from geese. Avian Pathol 13:253-264.

118. Zsak, L., and J. Kisary. 1984. Grouping of fowl adenoviruses based upon the restriction patterns of DNA generated by BAM HI and Hind III. Intervirology 22:110-114.

QUAIL BRONCHITIS

Willie M. Reed and Sherman W. Jack

INTRODUCTION. Quail bronchitis (QB) is a naturally occurring, acute, highly contagious, fatal respiratory disease of young bobwhite quail (*Colinus virginianus*). The disease is of major economic significance to gamebird breeders and has a worldwide distribution (1, 2). Quail bronchitis is characterized by rapid onset, high morbidity, and high mortality and mainly affects captive-reared birds. The etiologic agent is QB virus (QBV). Quail bronchitis and chicken embryo lethal orphan (CELO) viruses—both serotype I avian adenoviruses—are considered to be the same agent and are not distinguishable using conventional techniques (3, 19). Both viruses produce similar disease and lesions in bobwhite quail and chicken embryos.

Few type I avian adenoviruses, other than QBV and CELO, have been evaluated for pathogenicity in bobwhite quail with the exception of Indiana C adenovirus. Recent studies (10) have demonstrated that young bobwhite quail are susceptible to infection with Indiana C adenovirus, and the clinical disease and pathologic manifestations are indistinguishable from both naturally occurring and experimental infection with QBV.

While QBV is infectious for domestic poultry, including chickens and turkeys, as well as other avian species, resulting in seroconversion, the infection is generally asymptomatic. Although QB/CELO virus has induced neoplasms in laboratory animals, there is no known public health significance (14).

HISTORY, INCIDENCE, AND DISTRIBUTION. Quail bronchitis was first described by Olson (15) from a 1949 outbreak in West Virginia. A similar disease in quail had been reported as early as 1933 by Levine, however, and an agent similar to QBV was isolated by Beaudette in 1939. Following Olson's report, several outbreaks were reported in Texas in 1956–57 and in Virginia in 1959 (4, 5). Infection occurred in 3-wk-old to mature bobwhite quail with mortality in some pens reaching 80%. Chukar partridges on the gamebird farm did not develop the disease. Circumstantial evidence indicated transmission of QBV from inapparently infected chickens or captive gamebirds other than quail to the affected bobwhite quail.

Since the early descriptions, QB has been frequently diagnosed as the cause of mortality in captive-reared bobwhite quail. The true incidence and distribution of infection are unknown, but asymptomatic infection in older birds is believed to be widespread. Infection had not been identified in wild bobwhite quail until 1981 when King et al. (13) reported antibodies against serotype 1 avian adenovirus in 23% of mature, free-ranging bobwhite quail collected from a research station.

ETIOLOGY.

Quail bronchitis is caused by an avian adenovirus. It contains a DNA genome and is icosahedral, nonenveloped, and ranges in size from 69 to 75 nm in diameter (6). Based on virus neutralization, QBV is a group I/serotype 1 adenovirus indistinguishable from the Phelps strain of CELO virus (19, 14). QBV/CELO serves as the type strain for group I/serotype 1 avian adenoviruses. Other techniques have been used to classify avian adenoviruses (e.g., physicochemical properties, hemagglutination, and restriction endonuclease mapping), but they have failed to further clarify the taxonomy of these agents. As with other adenoviruses, avian adeno-associated virus (AAAV) may occur with QBV (22).

Laboratory Hosts and Pathogenicity.

Quail bronchitis virus is readily propagated in embryonating chicken eggs and in cultures of chicken kidney or liver cells. While QBV will grow in chicken fibroblasts, this system is less suitable for cultivation because virus multiplication is poor. Propagation may be interfered with by concurrent AAAV infection (14, 22) or by maternal antibodies in yolk of embryonating eggs (20, 21).

In most diagnostic laboratories, initial isolation is performed in embryonating chicken eggs, sometimes requiring several blind passages before typical lesions and mortality patterns develop. A common and proven route of inoculation is via the allantoic cavity. High yields of virus can be detected in allantoic fluid 48–96 hr postinfection (PI). Isolation and propagation of QBV using the yolk sac route in antibody-free embryonating eggs is also an effective method. Infection of the embryo by the yolk sac or allantoic cavity results in dwarfing, curling, and stunting of the embryo in 2–4 days. Examination of affected embryos reveals widespread congestion and hemorrhage and enlargement of the liver, with varying degrees of necrosis and hepatitis with intranuclear inclusion bodies.

Experimental inoculation of hamsters leads to various kinds of neoplasms, depending primarily on route of inoculation. Subcutaneous inoculation results in fibrosarcomas, hepatomas, or hepatic carcinomas, while intracranial inoculation leads to development of ependymomas (1, 14). Quail bronchitis virus/CELO has not been found to be oncogenic in mice or chickens (14).

PATHOGENESIS AND EPIZOOTIOLOGY

Natural and Experimental Hosts.

Bobwhite quail are the principal species that develop clinical signs and mortality due to infection with QBV. Clinical disease has been reported in Japanese quail. Chickens and turkeys may be experimentally infected but develop few or only mild clinical signs. Inapparent infections of chickens are suggested by serologic evidence (18, 19).

Transmission, Carriers, and Vectors.

Quail bronchitis is highly contagious, as demonstrated by explosive morbidity and mortality in susceptible flocks. Most signs are seen in quail < 6 wk of age. Although not experimentally documented, transmission is probably by aerosol. However, fecal–oral or mechanical transmission has been documented for other avian adenoviruses, and QBV has been isolated from cecal tonsil during experimental infections (12). Serologic evidence of infection of other gallinaceous birds may suggest that even though they fail to develop clinical signs, these species may serve as a vector for QBV.

Incubation Period, Signs, Morbidity, and Mortality.

Quail bronchitis is often a catastrophic disease of captive-reared bobwhite quail, which is manifested by respiratory distress that leads to death in young quail. Morbidity and mortality from field cases frequently exceeds 50% and may be much higher in flocks affected at <3 wk of age. In experimental infections of 1-wk-old quail, mortality began 2 days following intratracheal infection and subsided by day 9 (7). Mortality in quail inoculated at 3 wk of age occurred between 6 and 11 days PI. Death is uncommon in birds older than 6 wk of age.

Frequently, the first reported sign in the flock is a sudden increase in mortality. Closer inspection, however, frequently reveals "sick" birds that demonstrate decreased feed consumption, ruffled feathers, huddling under brooders, wing droop, open-mouthed breathing, "snicks," and nasal–ocular discharge. Following infection, signs may develop as early as 2 days, but generally develop in 3–7 days. Severity of infection varies depending on the age at which the bird is infected. Quail bronchitis is most severe in quail less than 3 wk of age. Older birds frequently are asymptomatic, but develop antibodies to group I/serotype 1 adenovirus. This suggests that survivors may be immune to subsequent virus exposure, but the persistence of these antibodies and the level of immunity have not been investigated. Antibodies against QBV have been identified in recently hatched quail that did not exhibit adverse signs of infection. These antibodies were lost at between 4 and 6 wk of age, suggesting that they were maternal antibodies.

Gross Lesions and Histopathology.

The principal lesions of QB are in the respiratory tract (8). Nasal–ocular discharge may also be noted. Opacity and filling of the trachea by pale, moist, necrotic, and sometimes hemorrhagic exudate is common (Fig. 23.5A). On cross section, the mucosa is markedly thickened (Fig. 23.5B). Similar exudate may be found in the anterior air sacs. Histologically, tracheal lesions may include epithelial deciliation, cell swelling, karyomegaly, necrosis, desquamation, and leukocyte infiltration (Fig. 23.5C). Basophilic, intranuclear viral inclusions are common in intact or desquamated tracheal epithelium. Electron microscopic changes are similar to those seen histologically but also demonstrate phagocytosed viral particles.

In the lungs, red, consolidated areas surround the bronchial hilus (Fig. 23.5D). On section, bronchi frequently contain exudate similar to that in the trachea, indicative of a necrotizing, proliferative bronchitis. Inflammatory exudates consisting of lymphocytes, heterophils, and fluid may extend into surrounding pulmonary parenchyma, but the intensity of the leukocyte response varies and may be confounded by secondary bacterial infections. Histologically, bronchial changes are similar to those in the trachea, except that bronchi may demonstrate more epithelial proliferation. Most lesions are associated with large basophilic intranuclear inclusions (Fig. 23.5E).

Lesions in the liver include multifocal pale pinpoint to 3 mm necrotic foci. Histologically, these foci are characterized by hepatocellular necrosis, infiltrated to varying degrees by lymphocytes and fewer heterophils. Inclusion bodies are occasionally seen in hepatocytes adjacent to necrotic foci and/or biliary epithelium.

Lesions occur in the spleen and bursa of Fabricius but can be difficult to identify in quail less than 3 wk of age. The spleen may be mottled and slightly enlarged. Histologically, affected spleens have multifocal, often extensive zones of necrosis characterized by lymphocytolysis with increased fibrillar eosinophilic intercellular material, with minimal leukocyte infiltration. Adenoviral inclusions are rare in the spleen. Histologic lesions of the bursa of Fabricius include necrosis of lymphocytes, frequently accompanied by generalized lymphoid depletion and follicular atrophy. Intranuclear viral inclusions are common in bursal epithelium. Experimentally, some quail also develop necrotizing pancreatitis associated with adenoviral inclusions.

Immunity. The duration of immunity in QB is not known, but survivors of both naturally occurring and experimental infections were refractory to challenge with QBV for at least 6 mo, and significant antibody levels developed in serum of quail following infection (2, 3, 15). Young chicks with maternal antibody are also refractory to challenge with QBV, but maternal antibody is not believed to prevent virus multiplication.

23.5. *A-E.* Quail bronchitis. *A.* Trachea from a young quail chick infected with quail bronchitis virus (QBV). There is opacity of the trachea due to the presence of necrotic exudate. *B.* Cross section of trachea from a young quail chick infected with QBV. The mucosa of the section on the *left* is extremely thickened, causing partial obstruction, while the section on the *right* is minimally affected. *C.* Microscopic section of trachea from a QBV-infected quail. There is epithelial deciliation, cell swelling, necrosis, desquamation, and leukocyte infiltration. *D.* Quail chick infected with QBV. The lungs are congested and contain red consolidated areas surrounding the bronchial hilus. *E.* Microscopic section of pulmonary bronchus from a quail infected with QBV. There is epithelial cell proliferation, leukocyte infiltration, and luminal exudate. Basophilic intranuclear inclusions are within epithelial cells. *F, G.* Hemorrhagic enteritis. *F.* Turkey, 7 wk old. Duodenal loop is dark purple due to bloody contents (one section opened to show contents). Note splenic enlargement and mottling. There is also inflammation of a thoracic air sac (*left*) typical of acute colisepticemia which often follows hemorrhagic enteritis virus (HEV) infection. (Barnes) *G.* Markedly enlarged and mottled spleen in turkey with HEV infection. (Barnes)

DIAGNOSIS. In quail chicks, sudden onset of rales, sneezing, or coughing that spreads rapidly through the flock and results in mortality suggests QB. Excess mucus in the trachea, bronchi, and air sacs is added evidence of the disease. Severity of signs, rapidity of spread, and presence of lesions are less marked in older quail. Isolation and identification of an agent indistinguishable from QBV (or CELO virus) would confirm the diagnosis. Inoculation of 9- to 11-day-embryonating chicken eggs via the chorioallantoic sac with suspensions of trachea, air sacs, or lungs has been used for isolation of the virus. Yates et al. (22) recommended suspensions of fecal samples or homogenates of the posterior small intestine (ileum) or colon. Jack et al. (11, 12) reported good success in isolating QBV from the liver of naturally infected birds and from the bursa of Fabricius and cecal tonsils of experimentally infected birds. Three to five blind passages are made with allantoamnionic fluid harvested from chilled eggs up to 6 days or more PI, or earlier from embryos that died 24 hr PI or later or that exhibit signs of stunting in daily candling. According to Yates et al. (22), a few strains seem to require inoculation via the yolk sac in 5- to 7-day embryos.

Embryo mortality (increasing with number of passages), stunting, thickening of the amnion, necrotic foci or mottling of the liver, and accumulation of urates in the mesonephros are typical changes caused by QBV or CELO virus. Neutralization of the isolated virus by specific QBV or

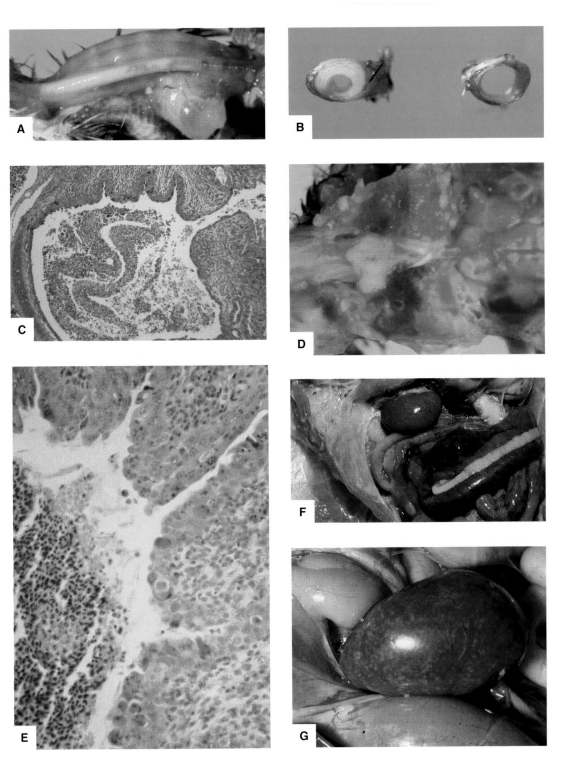

CELO virus antiserum would confirm identification of the virus and the diagnosis.

In general, information pertaining to isolation, propagation, and identification of CELO or any group I/serotype 1 avian adenovirus, would be applicable to QBV. Yates et al. (22) noted preference for chick embryo kidney or kidney cell cultures, and Jack and Reed (9, 10) have described propagation of QBV in chicken embryo liver tissue. The agar gel precipitation (AGP) test may be used to place an isolated virus in the avian adenovirus group, but it does not identify the serotype. Serotype classification is based on virus neutralization (9). In the absence of virus isolation or with failure to isolate a virus, the AGP test using stock antigen on paired sets of serum samples may be of value. A markedly higher percentage of positive precipitin tests among samples collected during convalescence (2.5 to 4 wk after initial signs) than among sera collected during the acute phase (1st few days of signs) should add weight to a presumptive diagnosis of QB based on clinical observations.

Pulmonary aspergillosis may be differentiated from pox by the presence of caseous plugs in lungs or deposits in air sacs with pockets of grayish or greenish spore accumulations. Although bacterial infections might complicate the disease, none is known to cause rapid development of signs, lesions, and mortality typical of QB. DuBose (2) suggested that Newcastle disease might present a clinical picture similar in part to QB, but clinical Newcastle disease has not been described in bobwhite quail. Histologic identification of intranuclear inclusion bodies morphologically characteristic of adenovirus in tracheal or bronchial epithelium is highly suggestive of infection with QBV (8).

TREATMENT, PREVENTION, AND CONTROL.

There is no specific treatment for QB. Increased warmth in the brooder house, adequate ventilation but no drafts, and avoidance of crowding are suggested supportive measures during an outbreak. Prevention is based on protecting susceptible quail from all possible sources of QBV or CELO virus. In addition to the usual sanitation procedures and measures to prevent entry of infectious agents onto the premises, care should be taken to keep adult quail, as well as other avian species, away from young quail. Control measures on a farm should be started immediately, when even a tentative diagnosis of QB has been made. In addition to general measures to prevent transmission from group to group, hatching operations may need to be deferred until 2 wk after signs have disappeared in order to prevent an outbreak in the presence of highly susceptible young quail.

Attempted eradication of QBV from bobwhite quail on a large gamebird farm was unsuccessful but may have been responsible for preventing losses and clinical QB over a 2½-yr period (3). In that effort, 80% of the 10,000 quail hatched during the previous year died from the disease. In addition to measures described above, older quail were marketed, and only survivors from hatches that had been affected <4 wk of age were kept for breeders. Virus-neutralization antibody at a high level was detected in 3½-mo-old quail hatched 2 yr later, but no signs of QB were detected in the intervening period up to the time the farm closed the following winter. Winterfield and Dhillon (16) used a type 1 adenovirus serotype in quail chicks as a vaccine against QB. The isolate, designated Indiana C virus, was isolated from chickens (17). It proved nonpathogenic for quail in a laboratory trial and was subsequently used on a farm where QB was endemic and losses were extensive. It was reported that the disease quickly subsided. In recent studies (10), however, experimental inoculation of quail at 1 or 3 wk of age resulted in mortality rates of 33–100%. In quail inoculated at 6 or 9 wk of age, mortality ranged from 0 to 10%. Gross and histologic lesions included necrotizing tracheitis and bronchitis with pneumonia, necrotizing hepatitis and splenitis, and lymphoid depletion of the bursa of Fabricius. Based on these findings, Indiana C appears to be highly pathogenic for bobwhite quail and is not recommended for use as a vaccine to prevent QB. More studies on potential use of vaccines to prevent QB are needed.

REFERENCES

1. Aghakhan, S.M. 1974. Avian adenoviruses. Vet Bull 44:531-552.
2. DuBose, R.T. 1967. Quail bronchitis. Bull Wildl Dis Assoc 3:10-13.
3. DuBose, R.T., and L.C. Grumbles. 1959. The relationship between quail bronchitis virus and chicken embryo lethal orphan virus. Avian Dis 3:321-344.
4. DuBose, R.T., L.C. Grumbles, and A.I. Flowers. 1958. The isolation of a nonbacterial agent from quail with a respiratory disease. Poult Sci 37:654-658.
5. DuBose, R.T., L.C. Grumbles, and A.I. Flowers. 1960. Differentiation of quail bronchitis virus and infectious bronchitis virus by heat stability. Am J Vet Res 21:740-743.
6. Dutta, S.K., and B.S. Pomeroy. 1967. Electron microscopic studies of quail bronchitis virus. Am J Vet Res 28:296-299.
7. Jack, S.W., and W.M. Reed. 1989. Experimentally-induced quail bronchitis. Avian Dis 34:433-437.
8. Jack, S.W., and W.M. Reed. 1990. Pathology of quail bronchitis. Avian Dis 34:44-51.
9. Jack, S.W., and W.M. Reed. 1990. Further characterization of an avian adenovirus associated with inclusion body hepatitis in bobwhite quail. Avian Dis 34:526-530.
10. Jack, S.W., and W.M. Reed. 1994. Experimental infection of bobwhite quail with Indiana C adenovirus. Avian Dis 38:325-328.
11. Jack, S.W., W.M. Reed, and T.A. Bryan. 1987. Inclusion body hepatitis in bobwhite quail (Colinus virginianus). Avian Dis 31:662-665.
12. Jack, S.W., W.M. Reed, and T. Burnstein. 1994. Pathogenesis of quail bronchitis. Avian Dis 38:548-556.

13. King, D.J., S.R. Pursglove, Jr., and W.R. Davidson. 1981. Adenovirus isolation and serology from wild bobwhite quail (Colinus virginianus). Avian Dis 25:678-682.

14. Monreal, G. 1992. Adenoviruses and adeno-associated viruses of poultry. Poult Sci Rev 4:1-27.

15. Olson, N.O. 1950. A respiratory disease (bronchitis) of quail caused by a virus. Proc 54th Annu Meet US Livest Sanit Assoc, pp. 171-174.

16. Winterfield, R.W., and A.S. Dhillon. 1980. Unpublished data.

17. Winterfield, R.W., A.M. Fadly, and A.M. Gallina. 1973. Adenovirus infection and disease. I. Some characteristics of an isolate from chickens in Indiana. Avian Dis 17:334-342.

18. Yates, V.J. 1960. Characterization of the chicken-em-bryo-lethal-orphan (CELO) virus. PhD dissertation, University of Wisconsin, Madison, WI.

19. Yates, V.J., and D.E. Fry. 1957. Observations on a chicken embryo lethal orphan (CELO) virus. Am J Vet Res 18:657-660.

20. Yates, V.J., P.W. Chang, A.H. Dardiri, and D.E. Fry. 1960. A study in the epizootiology of the CELO virus. Avian Dis 4:500-505.

21. Yates, V.J., D.V. Ablashi, P.W. Chang, and D.E. Fry. 1962. The chicken-embryo-lethal-orphan (CELO) virus as a tissue-culture contaminant. Avian Dis 6:406-411.

22. Yates, V.J., Y.-O. Rhee, and D.E. Fry. 1975. Comments on adenoviral antigens (CELO, QBV, GAL). Am J Vet Res 36:530-531.

HEMORRHAGIC ENTERITIS, MARBLE SPLEEN DISEASE, AND RELATED INFECTIONS

F. William Pierson and C. H. Domermuth

INTRODUCTION. Hemorrhagic enteritis (HE) is an acute viral disease of turkeys 4 wk of age and older. It is characterized by depression, bloody droppings, and death. Clinical disease usually persists in affected flocks for 7–10 days. Due, however, to the immunosuppressive nature of HE, secondary bacterial infections may extend the course of illness and mortality for an additional 2–3 wk (see Pathogenesis and Epizootiology).

Marble spleen disease (MSD) is a condition affecting confinement-reared pheasants 3–8 mo of age. The causative virus is serologically indistinguishable from that of HE virus. The clinical disease, however, is predominantly respiratory in nature, with death occurring as a result of asphyxia.

Avian adenovirus group II splenomegaly (AAS) of chickens and evidence of similar infections in other gallinaceous fowl are also described in this chapter.

HISTORY. Hemorrhagic enteritis was first observed by Pomeroy and Fenstermacher (69) in Minnesota and later by Gale and Wyne (33) in Ohio. The disease reached epidemic proportions in Texas in the early 1960s and in Virginia in the mid-1960s (35). It occurs in both confined and range flocks and exhibits a strong tendency to infect successive flocks on the same premises.

Complete records of losses from HE have not been kept; however, estimates within the United States exceeded $3 million per year prior to development of a vaccine. Losses due to immunosuppression and subsequent secondary bacterial infections may have actually been much higher.

Information developed on HE prior to 1984 has been reviewed (10, 68).

In 1966, the first reported outbreak of MSD in ring-necked pheasants was described by Mandelli et al. (48). This was the first evidence that group II avian adenoviruses were also present in Europe.

INCIDENCE AND DISTRIBUTION. Hemorrhagic enteritis has been a serious problem in at least 10 states and has been observed throughout the world where turkeys are raised. Various pathotypes of HE virus (HEV), which produce insignificant or no mortality, are known (15). Seroconversion studies performed by the authors suggest that infection with HEV is widespread among adult turkeys. Marble spleen disease virus (MSDV) has been documented in confinement pheasant operations throughout the United States, Canada, Europe, and Australia (4, 10, 47, 50, 70, 74, 76, 77, 78). Similarly, a high incidence of antibody in mature chickens suggests that most flocks have been infected with AAS virus (AASV).

ETIOLOGY. Hemorrhagic enteritis was first transmitted with both unfiltered and filtered intestinal contents obtained from turkeys that had died from the disease (35). It was later transmitted by intravenous (IV) inoculation of filtered serum (7) and the causative agent was found to be concentrated predominately in the spleen (11).

Classification. Morphologic, histologic, immunologic, and chloroform-resistance studies indicate that HEV, MSDV, and AASV are all members f the family *Adenoviridae* and the genus *Aviadenvirus* (10).

These viruses are believed to constitute an immunologically distinct group of avian adenoviruses, which has been designated as avian adenovirus roup (type) II (18) to distinguish it from the larger roup of adenoviruses [chicken embryo lethal orphan (CELO) and others], which share a different roup antigen and are classified as avian adenovirus roup (type) I. This classification is based on observations that convalescent HE turkey antiserum protects pheasants against MSD (13) and that MSD nd AAS viruses are indistinguishable from HEV in gar-gel immunodiffusion tests (10). As a group, hey have been shown to be serologically distinct rom CELO virus (18) and four other turkey adenovirus isolates (10).

Members of avian adenovirus group II can be differentiated from one another by restriction enonuclease fingerprinting (87) and monoclonal antibody affinity (82, 88).

Morphology. Hemorrhagic enteritis and MSD irions are nonenveloped, icosohedral, and reportedly vary in diameter between 70 and 80 nm and 70–90 nm, respectively (10). Differences in size, however, are probably within the limits of experimental error. Hemorrhagic enteritis virus readily passed filters with porosities of 220 and 100 nm but not 10 nm (10). Thin-section tissue preparations examined by electron microscopy revealed that HE nd MSD viral particles had a total capsomere count of 252, occurred in empty and dense forms, nd were arranged intranuclearly in loosely packed aggregates or crystalline arrays (10).

By using polyacrylamide gel electrophoresis and Western blotting techniques, a total of 11 distinct structural polypeptides have been identified with molecular weights ranging between 14 and 97 kD 58) and 9.5 and 96 kD (84). Six of these proteins ave been further characterized. They include a 96-kD polypeptide believed to be a monomer of the major outer capsid or hexon protein, 51/52-kD and 29-kD polypeptides believed to be the vertex penton base and fiber proteins, a 57-kD homologue of human adenovirus group 2 IIIa protein, and two core nucleoproteins of 12.5 kD and 9.5 kD each 84). On transmission electron microscopy, group II avian adenoviruses have been observed to possess only one penton fiber at each vertex (84). This distinguishes them from group I viruses, which possess two fibers at each vertex. Among group II avian adenoviruses, antigenic differences and variations in electrophoretic migration of penton base and fiber proteins have been noted (84, 88). Antigenic differences also appear to exist with regard to several other structural proteins (88).

Sucrose gradient studies reported for HEV reveal that it possesses a density of 1.34 g/mL. Marble spleen disease virus produces a band in cesium chloride gradients at a density of 1.32–1.33 g/mL.

Chemical Composition. Nucleic acid of density gradient-purified MSDV was obtained by phenol extraction, assayed for deoxyribose by direct colorimetric diphenylamine reaction, and determined to be DNA (41). The virus has an estimated genomic length of 25.5 kb which makes it relatively short in comparison with the viruses of avian adenovirus group I, and surprisingly suggests that HEV may be no more closely related to this group than to the mammalian adenoviruses (43).

Virus Replication. Early electron micrographic studies suggested that HEV and MSDV replication took place in nuclei of reticuloendothelial cells (10). Recent studies have revealed these cells to be more specifically mononuclear and primarily lymphoid, although some monocytes or macrophages do appear to contain viral antigen (71, 83). Enzyme-linked immunosorbent assays, as well as immunofluorescent and immunoperoxidase staining, have revealed the presence of infected cells in a variety of tissues including intestine, bursa of Fabricius, thymus, liver, kidney, peripheral blood leukocytes, lung, and spleen (25, 31, 39, 71, 72, 79). On the basis of immunodiffusion and immunoperoxidase studies, the spleen is the major site of viral replication (10, 71).

Resistance to Chemical and Physical Agents. Infectivity of HEV can be destroyed by heating at 70 C for 1 hr; drying at 37 or 25 C for 1 wk (7); or by treatment with 0.0086% sodium hypochlorite (8), 1.0% sodium lauryl sulfate, 0.4% Chlorocide, 0.4% Phenocide, 0.4% Wescodyne, or 1.0% Lysol (7). Infectivity is not destroyed by heating at 65 C for 1 hr; storage for 4 wk at 37 C, 6 mo at 4 C, 4 yr at -40 C; maintenance at pH 3 at 25 C for 30 min; or by treatment with 50% chloroform or 50% ethyl ether.

Strain Classification. Hemorrhagic enteritis virus, MSDV, and AASV have been classified only as to source (turkeys, chickens, pheasants), although it is common for isolates to be referred to as virulent or avirulent based on the degree of pathology they produce.

Laboratory Host Systems. Early attempts to propagate HEV in chicken and turkey embryos and in cell cultures were unsuccessful (10). More recent work indicates, however, that inoculation of specific-pathogen–free turkey eggs with MSDV on day 24 of embryonation does result in infection and viral replication with peak antigen levels being detected in spleen, intestine, and liver 6 days postinoculation (PI) (1). There have been several attempts to infect lymphocytes. Perrin et al. (64) inoculated spleen cells with HEV and were subsequently able to recover virus, but they did not show that it was other than the inoculum virus. Fasina and Fabricant (24) demonstrated in vitro infection of chicken, turkey, and pheasant spleen cells by immunofluorescence, but no demonstrable virus release occurred. Successful serial passage of HEV and MSDV in vitro was accomplished by Nazerian and Fadly (55) using a turkey lymphoblastoid B-cell line derived from a Marek's disease virus–induced tumor. This cell line, known as MDTC-RP19, has since become the standard system for in vitro viral isolation and HE and MSD vaccine production. A successful alternative in vitro system for vaccine production using normal turkey peripheral blood leukocytes has also been described by van den Hurk (80).

Pathogenicity.   Mortality in field outbreaks of HE has varied from over 60% (35) to less than 0.1%. In experiments in which spleen size and presence of precipitating antigen indicated 100% infection, mortality was reported to vary between 80% for the most pathogenic strain and 0% for the least. Present information suggests that the ability of a given strain to produce mortality is a fairly stable characteristic.

Mortality rates in pheasants naturally infected with MSDV have been reported to be 5–20% over a period of 10 days to several wk (50). As with HEV, variations in pathogenicity among MSDV isolates would be expected. Pheasants experimentally infected with cell-culture–propagated MSDV and avirulent and virulent HEV, however, showed typical gross and microscopic splenic lesions but no lung lesions or mortality (23). It has been suggested that other environmental factors may be involved in occurrence of lung lesions and mortality in field outbreaks (23).

PATHOGENESIS AND EPIZOOTIOLOGY

Natural and Experimental Hosts.   Until recently, turkeys, pheasants, and chickens were the only known natural hosts for group II avian adenoviruses. It is now suspected that guinea fowl (5, 49) and psittacines (34) may also be naturally infected. With regard to wild birds, a serologic survey of 42 species revealed no evidence of infection outside the order Galliformes (14). Even wild populations of galliforms, i.e., turkeys, appear to be at little risk of infection (37) due to their elusive nature. When infection does occur, host genetics appear to influence the severity of clinical disease and lesion

formation in both turkeys (46) and pheasants. Laboratory experiments indicate that pheasant MSDV isolates will infect turkeys (16) and turkey HEV isolates will infect pheasants. Similarly, chicken isolates will infect turkeys (17, 18, 19).

Lesions have been produced by experimental infection with HEV in a variety of other gallinaceous species including golden pheasants, peafowl, chickens, bobwhite quail, and chukars. Death, however, has not been reported in species other than the natural hosts.

AGE OF HOST MOST COMMONLY AFFECTED.   In the first reported outbreaks, HE occurred in turkeys 6–11 wk of age (33, 69). More recent field observations suggest that it has a tendency to affect birds 7–9 wk of age. Turkeys 13 days of age and younger have been reported to be refractory to HEV infection in the absence of maternal antibody (21), suggesting perhaps a need for some sort of target cell maturation. A recent report detailing successful in ovo infection of specific-pathogen–free turkeys at day 24 of embryonation (1) seems to confound this premise. Due to maternal antibody, poults younger than 3½–4 wk of age are considered to be refractory to HE. Fadly and Nazerian (21) reported that this effect may last up to 6 wk. In the absence of maternal antibody, poults are susceptible (20). This was presumably the situation in the single reported case of spontaneous infection in 2½-wk-old poults (36).

Marble spleen disease in pheasants occurs naturally in birds 3–8 mo of age (4, 50). It has also been reproduced experimentally in mature adult pheasants (13). As with turkeys, some evidence suggests that pheasants are refractory to infection up to about 4 wk of age, either as a result of undetectable, low maternal antibody levels or a developmental lack of target cells (29).

In chickens with AAS, field infection is observed as splenomegaly in young or market-age broilers (17, 36) or as splenomegaly with pulmonary congestion and edema in mature birds (19).

Transmission, Carriers, and Vectors.   Hemorrhagic enteritis virus can be transmitted orally or cloacally by inoculation of susceptible poults with infectious feces (35, 42). Virus can remain infectious for several weeks in carcasses protected from drying or in liquid suspensions of infectious feces. Hemorrhagic enteritis virus has been recovered from contaminated litter, and the disease is known to reoccur in houses where it has appeared before. Unlike group I adenoviruses, there is no epidemiologic evidence for egg transmission. Outside of mechanical vectors, other carriers and vectors have not been implicated in transmission of HEV. These observations strongly suggest that the usual route of HEV transmission is from infected to susceptible flocks via fomites contaminated with infectious feces or litter.

Incubation Period. Hemorrhagic enteritis mortality occurs about 5–6 days after oral or cloacal inoculation or 3–4 days after IV inoculation of dilute extracts of infectious spleen (11). In a naturally infected flock, all signs of disease usually subside within 6–10 days after first observing bloody droppings. Mortality in experimentally induced MSD occurred in pheasants 6 days after oral inoculation with pheasant-derived virus (13). Mortality has not been produced in chickens inoculated with AASV, but splenomegaly has been observed 5–7 days after oral inoculation (17) as well as pulmonary congestion and edema resembling field lesions (86).

Clinical Signs. Hemorrhagic enteritis is characterized by a rapid progression of clinical signs over a 24-hr period (10, 68). These include depression, bloody droppings, and death. Feces containing frank blood are frequently present on the skin and feathers surrounding vents of moribund and dead birds. The same may be forced from the vents of such birds if moderate pressure is applied to the abdominal area. Death of pheasants infected with MSDV and of chickens infected with AASV is considered to be peracute or acute due to respiratory compromise. Therefore, signs, if present, would consist of mild depression, weakness, dyspnea, and finally asphyxia. Occasionally, a premortem nasal discharge has been noted (26).

Morbidity and Mortality. In field outbreaks, all or nearly all birds are infected, as indicated by seroconversion (11) and resistance to experimental challenge. Depressed, clinically affected poults usually die within 24 hr or otherwise recover completely. Field mortality ranges from less than 1 to slightly over 60%, with the average being approximately 10–15%. Mortality of 80% often occurs in laboratory experiments in which 100% infection is achieved. Mortality in MSDV-infected, pen-reared pheasants has been reported to be 2–3%, but may reach as high as 5–20% over a course of 10 days to several weeks (10, 50). In mature chickens with AAS, 8.9% mortality has been reported (19).

Gross Lesions. Dead poults routinely appear pale due to blood loss, but are often in good flesh and have feed in their crops. Small intestines are usually distended, are dark red to black, and are filled with reddish-brown, bloody contents (Fig. 23.5F) [*Note*: Figure 23.5 can be found in the section entitled Quail Bronchitis in this chapter]. The

intestinal mucosa is congested and in some individuals covered with a yellow, fibrinonecrotic membrane. Lesions are usually more pronounced in the proximal small intestine but often extend distally in severe cases. Spleens of infected birds are characteristically enlarged, friable, and marbled or mottled in appearance (Fig. 23.5G); however, those of dead poults tend to be smaller and less marbled presumably due to blood loss and subsequent splenic contraction. Usually, lungs are congested, but other vascular organs are pale. Enlarged livers and petechial hemorrhages in various tissues of dead poults have been reported but are too inconsistent to be of diagnostic value (10).

Gross lesions in pheasants infected by MSDV consist of enlarged, characteristically mottled or marbled spleens and edematous, congested lungs (4, 50). No evidence of intestinal lesions is reported. In broiler and mature chickens infected by AASV, gross splenic lesions resemble those of MSDV in pheasants (17, 19).

Histopathology. Pathologic changes that characterize HE are most evident in lymphoreticular and gastrointestinal systems. Splenic lesions

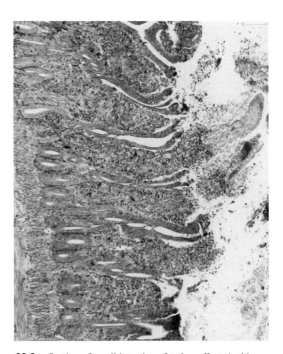

23.6. Section of small intestine of turkey affected with hemorrhagic enteritis. Lesions include severe congestion of the mucosa, degeneration of epithelial cells covering tips of villi, sloughing of epithelial cells and tip of villus, and hemorrhage into the lumen. H & E,×550.

present at death (Fig. 23.6) include hyperplasia of white pulp, lymphoid necrosis, and intranuclear inclusions in lymphoreticular cells (10, 71). Sequentially, proliferation of white pulp surrounding splenic ellipsoids is evident as early as 3 days PI with HEV. This leads to large, irregular, confluent islands of white pulp, which are grossly visible as mottling 4–5 days PI (71). H&E and immunoperoxidase staining have revealed numerous intranuclear inclusions in these zones between 3 and 5 days PI. Morphologic characteristics of infected cells are most consistent with lymphoid cells, primarily lymphoblasts (71), and are most probably B cells rather than reticular or endothelial cells as previously described. Presence of inclusions in splenic mononuclear phagocytes has also been noted (51). By 4–5 days PI, white pulp begins to undergo necrosis, and by 6–7 days PI, it has completely involuted with only occasional plasma cells appearing in red pulp (71). In addition to splenic changes, lymphoid depletion has also been noted in both cortical and medullary areas of thymus (39) and bursa of Fabricius (39, 71) between 3 and 9 days PI.

In general, lesions in the gastrointestinal tract include severe congestion of intestinal mucosa, degeneration and sloughing of villous epithelium, and hemorrhage in the villous tips. Hemorrhage is believed to result from endothelial disruption rather than destruction. Saunders et al. (71) noted that blood vessels in the lamina propria were intact but that red cells appeared to move out of vessels by diapedesis. This is consistent with the implication that histamine and eicosenoid compounds are involved in gastrointestinal lesion formation (61). Increased numbers of lymphoreticular cells positive for intranuclear inclusions have been observed in the lamina propria (39) in addition to mast cells (62), plasma cells, and heterophils (71). These histopathologic changes are most pronounced in the duodenum just posterior to the pancreatic ducts (Fig. 23.7), but similar, less severe lesions may also occur in proventriculus, gizzard, distal small intestine, ceca, cecal tonsils, and bursa of Fabricius (10).

Additionally, cells containing HEV intranuclear inclusions have been observed in liver, bone marrow, peripheral blood leukocytes, lung, pancreas, brain, and renal tubular epithelium (10, 39, 51, 79).

Marble spleen disease virus and AASV produce intranuclear inclusions and splenic lesions similar to those of HEV, but without significant gastrointestinal involvement. Instead, the site of vascular compromise in the pheasant and chicken appears to be the lung, with congestion and edema being the most consistent findings (4, 19, 31).

Multiple hypotheses regarding the mechanism of lesion formation in group II avian adenoviral infections have been proposed (20, 39, 62, 63, 71, 75); following is a synoptic composite. After oral inocu-

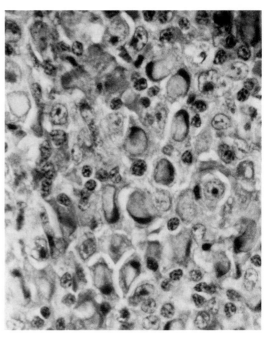

23.7.   Section of spleen of turkey affected with hemorrhagic enteritis. Nuclei of infected cells contain characteristic intranuclear inclusions. H & E, ×550.

lation, initial viral replication appears to occur in bursal-dependent, lymphoid target cells within the gastrointestinal tract. This is followed by a primary viremia that results in infection of large numbers of target cells, primarily in the spleen and peripheral blood. A massive, secondary release of viral particles and unassembled components into the circulation then occurs with cytotoxic viral proteins inducing a T-cell–dependent, chemically mediated inflammatory response at host-specific, predisposed tissue sites. This results in localized disruption of capillary endothelium and vascular leakage.

Immunosuppression.   Group II avian adenoviruses appear to be lymphotropic and lymphocytopathic (27, 39, 71, 75, 83). Both adherent mononuclear macrophages and nonadherent mononuclear cells (83) bearing IgM (75) have been reported to support viral replication. It has also been noted that B-cell depletion impairs viral replication and lesion formation (20, 27, 75) and that during the acute phase of HEV infection a marked depletion of IgM-bearing cells in the spleen and peripheral blood occurs (75). Thus, it is suggested that B cells and macrophages may serve as primary viral targets (75). This is further corroborated by the fact that HEV and MSDV produce a transient inhibition of antibody responses to sheep erythrocytes (30, 52) and Newcastle disease virus (54) and cause suppression of B- and T-cell mitogenic responses in vitro (30, 52, 53, 54).

Elevations in CD8 (CT8)-bearing cytotoxic/suppressor T lymphocytes have been reported 8–10 (65) and 16 days PI (75). This may be indicative of a protective response or it may reflect efforts to downregulate the immune system to slow viral replication.

Hemorrhagic enteritis virus alone (73) or in combination with other agents including *Bordetella avium,* Newcastle disease virus, and *Mycoplasma meleagridis* has been shown to predispose turkeys to secondary infection with *Escherichia coli* in the field (66). Similar findings have been reported under laboratory conditions (44, 45, 59, 67). Paramyxovirus type 2, chlamydial (2), and staphylococcal infections have also been reported secondary to HEV exposure. Surprisingly, improved weight gains and reduced oocyst shedding have been reported to occur in turkeys concomitantly infected with HEV or MSDV and *Eimeria meleagrimitis* (60). The mechanism for this beneficial interaction is not understood.

Immunosuppression appears to occur with virulent as well as avirulent strains of HEV and MSDV (45, 65). Therefore, although virulent strains may certainly be considered pathogenic, avirulent strains should not be considered apathogenic.

Immunity

ACTIVE. Poults recovering from either naturally occurring outbreaks of HE or experimental infections are refractory to challenge. Protection does not appear to be virus strain specific. Strains that cause less than 1% mortality induce immunity, which prevents infection with pathogenic strains normally producing much greater mortality (15). Antibodies against HEV may be detected as early as 3 days PI by enzyme-linked immunosorbent assay (ELISA) (81). Such immunity appears to be long lasting if not lifelong. One flock monitored by the authors over a 4-yr period demonstrated a seroconversion rate of 100% at 4 wk PI and was still found to be 83% positive 40 mo later.

Cell-mediated immunity undoubtedly plays a role in active protection against group II avian adenoviral infections and lesion formation; however, this role is not fully understood. Inoculation of turkeys with HEV causes an increase in splenic CD4 (CT4)-bearing T cells 4–6 days PI (75). CD8 (CT8)-bearing cytotoxic/suppressor T cells also appear to increase PI (65, 75), which may protect against further viral replication but could also increase susceptibility to secondary bacterial infections. Selective in vivo T-cell depletion with cyclosporin A enhances splenic lesion formation and viral replication in MSDV-infected pheasants (32)

and reduces intestinal lesion formation in HEV infected turkeys (75).

PASSIVE. When present, even at undetectable levels, maternal antibody provides protection from clinical HE for up to 6 wk posthatch and has been reported to interfere with vaccination for up to 5 wk posthatch (21). Passive immunity can be conferred by injection of birds with convalescent antiserum obtained from recovered flocks. In laboratory experiments, 0.5–1.0 mL of antiserum prevented gross lesions, and as little as 0.1–0.25 mL prevented intestinal lesions (9). Administered in this fashion, hyperimmune serum has been shown to afford some protection from lesion formation for up to 5 wk (21).

DIAGNOSIS

Isolation and Identification of Causative Agent.
Large concentrations of HEV can be found in sanguinous intestinal contents (35) or splenic tissue obtained from dead or moribund poults. Splenic material from MSDV-infected pheasants and AASV-infected chickens is also a suitable source of viral antigens. Hemorrhagic enteritis seronegative turkeys, preferably 5–10 wk of age, can be inoculated per os (PO) with intestinal contents or PO or IV with a crude saline extract of minced spleen. With virulent isolates, death often occurs about 3 days after IV and 5–6 days after PO inoculation. Poults that do not die usually have enlarged, marbled spleens that contain virus. Sera obtained at these times also contain virus (11). Alternatively, a lymphoblastoid B-cell line of turkey origin (MDTC-RP19) can be used to isolate and propagate HEV in vitro (55, 56).

Positive identification of group II avian adenoviruses in fresh or frozen tissue is commonly accomplished by testing saline tissue extracts using an agar gel precipitin (AGP) method (11, 12). Less common but more contemporary methods include antigen-capture ELISA (72, 40, 57, 81), restriction endonuclease fingerprinting (87), and polymerase chain reactions (PCR). Viral antigens can be identified in fixed tissues using immunofluorescent (25) or immunoperoxidase methods (31, 28, 38, 71).

Serology.
Hemorrhagic enteritis virus antibodies can be detected in plasma or serum of recovered birds by AGP (11, 12) as early as 2 wk, but practically are detected no sooner than 3 wk PI. It is advisable to test acute and convalescent sera if a diagnosis is to be made based on serology. Antibodies produced against HEV, MSDV, and AASV are indistinguishable. Maternal antibody may be detected using AGP, but this method generally lacks sufficient sensitivity beyond 1 wk of age (81). More sen-

sitive ELISA have been developed to detect and quantitate HEV maternal antibody and seroconversion postinfection (6, 40, 56, 57, 72, 81). These assays are capable of detecting maternal antibody in turkey sera until about 4–5 wk of age, although most birds are seronegative by 3 wk of age (21, 81). Seroconversion can be detected as early as 3 days PI (81).

Differential Diagnosis. In turkeys, an enlarged, marbled spleen without demonstrable HEV antigen on AGP, and the absence of intestinal bleeding, should evoke consideration of reticuloendotheliosis or lymphoproliferative disease as possible differential diagnoses. Enlarged, congested spleens in turkeys are often mistakenly attributed to HEV but most commonly result from bacterial septicemia, e.g., colibacillosis or erysipelas. Gastrointestinal bleeding and mucosal hyperemia may be associated with acute septicemia, viremia, or toxemia, e.g., colibacillosis, avian influenza. These are rarely observed, however, without other signs indicative of their respective infections. Parasitism such as coccidiosis and toxic substances, i.e., heavy metals and chemicals, should also be considered.

Pheasants and chickens that die acutely with signs of respiratory distress but without enlarged, marbled spleens should be tested for other respiratory pathogens including Newcastle disease, avian influenza, infectious laryngotracheitis, and infectious bronchitis. Atmospheric asphyxiants such as carbon monoxide, carbon dioxide, and natural gas should also be considered in confinement operations. Splenic enlargement and marbling without evidence of MSDV or AASV antigen on AGP should warrant histopathologic evaluation for neoplastic diseases such as Marek's disease, lymphoid leukosis, and reticuloendotheliosis.

TREATMENT, PREVENTION, AND CONTROL

Treatment. At the first sign of an outbreak, HE can be treated by subcutaneous or intramuscular injection of 0.5–1.0 mL of convalescent antiserum obtained from healthy flocks at slaughter (9). Treatment has not been described for MSD of pheasants or AAS of chickens, but it is presumed that a similar approach may be effective.

Due to the immunosuppressive nature of group II avian adenoviruses, treatment for secondary bacterial infections, primarily colibacillosis, must often be considered. Selection of an appropriate antibiotic based on culture and sensitivity is always advised.

Management Procedures. Prevention and control of HE, MSD, and AAS begin with good biosecurity, since transportation of infected litter or

feces from flock to flock is the most common mode of transmission. Contaminated facilities may be cleaned and disinfected with 0.0086% sodium hypochlorite solution or other viricidal agents including phenolic derivatives plus drying at 25 C for 1 wk (7, 8). In most commercial operations, however, especially those having multiple ages of birds, total elimination of the virus is considered impractical. In such cases, vaccination remains the most viable measure for control and prevention of clinical disease.

Immunization. Avirulent isolates of HEV and MSDV have been successfully used as live, water-administered vaccines (15). Two forms of vaccine are currently in widespread use. One is a crude homogenate prepared from spleens of 4- to 6-wk-old turkeys inoculated with MSDV or avirulent HEV (15); the other is one produced in vitro using the MDTC-RP19 cell line in suspension culture (22). Both vaccines appear to produce adequate seroconversion and protection (3) and both are used extensively in the United States; however, only the latter is available commercially. A third method of vaccine production involving propagation of avirulent virus in peripheral blood leukocytes has also been described (83) and is in use in Canada. Other vaccines, including a purified hexon subunit (85), and genetically engineered, recombinant products are under development (43).

Successful in ovo vaccination of specific-pathogen–free turkeys has recently been described (1), but standard vaccination of healthy turkeys is usually performed between 4 and 6 wk of age. Addition of a vaccine stabilizer, i.e., powdered milk, to the water, elimination of any in-line disinfectants, and temporary discontinuation of water chlorination is essential to the survival of vaccine virus and to successful vaccination. Flocks experiencing less than 100% protection from the initial vaccination are subsequently protected by lateral transmission within 2–3 wk. Despite this, double vaccination is occasionally employed.

Live, avirulent, water-administered vaccines are available and effective for controlling MSD of pheasants (16, 23). No vaccine for AAS of chickens currently exists nor does its development seem necessary.

REFERENCES

1. Ahmad, J., and J.M. Sharma. 1993. Protection against hemorrhagic enteritis and Newcastle Disease in turkeys by embryo vaccination with monovalent and bivalent vaccines. Avian Dis 37:485-491.

2. Andral, B., M. Metz, D. Toquin, J. LeCoz, and J. Newman. 1985. Respiratory disease (rhinotracheitis) of turkeys in Brittany, France. III. Interaction of multiple infecting agents. Avian Dis 29:233-243.

3. Barbour, E.K., P.E. Poss, M.K. Brinton, J.B. Johnson, and N.H. Nabbut. 1993. Evaluation of cell culture propagated

and in vivo propagated hemorrhagic enteritis vaccines in turkeys. Vet Immunol Immunopathol 35:375-383.

4. Bygrave, A.C., and M. Pattison. 1973. Marble spleen disease in pheasants (Phasianus colchicus). Vet Rec 92:534-535.

5. Cowen, B.S., H. Rothenbacher, L.D. Schwartz, M.O. Braune, and R.L. Owen. 1988. A case of acute pulmonary edema, splenomegaly, and ascites in guinea fowl. Avian Dis 32:151-156.

6. Davidson, I., A. Aronovici, Y. Weisman, and M. Malkinson. 1985. Enzyme immunoassay studies on the serological response of turkeys to hemorrhagic enteritis virus. Avian Dis 29:43-52.

7. Domermuth, C.H., and W.B. Gross. 1971. Effect of disinfectants and drying on the virus of hemorrhagic enteritis of turkeys. Avian Dis 15:94-97.

8. Domermuth, C.H., and W.B. Gross. 1972. Effect of chlorine on the virus of hemorrhagic enteritis of turkeys. Avian Dis 16:952-953.

9. Domermuth, C.H., and W.B. Gross. 1975. Hemorrhagic enteritis of turkeys. Antiserum — efficacy, preparation and use. Avian Dis 19:657-665.

10. Domermuth, C.H., and W.B. Gross. 1984. Hemorrhagic enteritis and related infections. In M.S. Hofstad, H.J. Barnes, B.W. Calnek, W.M. Reid, and H.W. Yoder, Jr. (eds.). Diseases of Poultry, 8th ed. Iowa State University Press, Ames, IA, pp. 511-516.

11. Domermuth, C.H., W.B. Gross, R.T. DuBose, C.S. Douglass, and C.B. Reubush, Jr. 1972. Agar gel diffusion precipitin test for hemorrhagic enteritis of turkeys. Avian Dis 16:852-857.

12. Domermuth, C.H., W.B. Gross, and R.T. DuBose. 1973. Microimmunodiffusion test for hemorrhagic enteritis of turkeys. Avian Dis 17:439-444.

13. Domermuth, C.H., W.B. Gross, R.T. DuBose, and E.T. Mallinson. 1975. Experimental reproduction and antibody inhibition of marble spleen disease of pheasants. J Wildl Dis 11:338-342.

14. Domermuth, C.H., D.J. Forrester, D.O. Trainer, and W.J. Bigler. 1977. Serologic examination of wild birds for hemorrhagic enteritis of turkey and marble spleen disease of pheasants. J Wildl Dis 13:405-408.

15. Domermuth, C.H., W.B. Gross, C.S. Douglass, R.T. DuBose, J.R. Harris, and R.B. Davis. 1977. Vaccination for hemorrhagic enteritis of turkeys. Avian Dis 21:557-565.

16. Domermuth, C.H., W.B. Gross, L.D. Schwartz, E.T. Mallinson, and R. Britt. 1979. Vaccination of ring-necked pheasant for marble-spleen disease. Avian Dis 23:30-38.

17. Domermuth, C.H., J.R. Harris, W.B. Gross, and R.T. DuBose. 1979. A naturally occurring infection of chickens with a hemorrhagic enteritis/marble spleen disease type of virus. Avian Dis 23:479-484.

18. Domermuth, C.H., C.R. Weston, B.S. Cowen, W.M. Colwell, W.B. Gross, and R.T. DuBose. 1980. Incidence and distribution of avian adenovirus group II splenomegaly of chickens. Avian Dis 24:591-594.

19. Domermuth, C.H., L. van der Heide, and G.P. Faddoul. 1982. Pulmonary congestion and edema (marble spleen disease) of chickens produced by group II avian adenovirus. Avian Dis 26:629-633.

20. Fadly, A.M., and K. Nazerian. 1982. Evidence for bursal involvement in the pathogenesis of hemorrhagic enteritis of turkeys. Avian Dis 26:525-533.

21. Fadly, A.M., and K. Nazerian. 1989. Hemorrhagic enteritis of turkeys: Influence of maternal antibody and age at exposure. Avian Dis 33:778-786.

22. Fadly, A.M., K. Nazerian, K. Nagaraja, and G. Below. 1985. Field vaccination against hemorrhagic enteritis of turkeys by a cell-culture live-virus vaccine. Avian Dis 29:768-777.

23. Fadly, A.M., B.S. Cowen, and K. Nazerian. 1988. Some observations on the response of ring-necked pheasants to inoculation with various strains of cell-culture-propagated type II avian adenovirus. Avian Dis 32:548-552.

24. Fasina, S.O., and J. Fabricant. 1982. In vitro studies of hemorrhagic enteritis virus with immunofluorescent antibody technique. Avian Dis 26:150-157.

25. Fasina, S.O., and J. Fabricant. 1982. Immunofluorescence studies on the early pathogenesis of hemorrhagic enteritis virus infection in turkeys and chickens. Avian Dis 26:158-163.

26. Fitzgerald, S.D., and W.M. Reed. 1989. A review of marble spleen disease of ring-necked pheasants. J Wildl Dis 25:455-461.

27. Fitzgerald, S.D., and W.M. Reed. 1991. Pathogenesis of marble spleen disease in bursectomized and non-bursectomized ring-necked pheasants following oral inoculation with cell-culture-propagated virus. Avian Dis 35:579-584.

28. Fitzgerald, S.D., and A. Richard. 1995. Comparison of four fixatives for routine splenic histology and immunohistochemical staining for group II avian adenovirus. Avian Dis 39:425-431.

29. Fitzgerald, S.D., W.M. Reed, and T. Burnstein. 1991. The influence of age on the response of ring-necked pheasants to infection with marble spleen disease virus. Avian Dis 35:960-964.

30. Fitzgerald, S.D., A.L. Fitzgerald, W.M. Reed, and T. Burnstein. 1992. Immune function in pheasants experimentally infected with marble spleen disease virus. Avian Dis 36:410-414.

31. Fitzgerald, S.D., W.M. Reed, and T. Burnstein. 1992. Detection of type II avian adenoviral antigen in tissue sections using immunohistochemical staining. Avian Dis 36:341-347.

32. Fitzgerald, S.D., W.M. Reed, A.M. Furukawa, E. Zimels, and L. Fung. 1995. Effect of T-lymphocyte depletion on the pathogenesis of marble spleen disease virus infection in ring-necked pheasants. Avian Dis 39:68-73.

33. Gale, C., and J.W. Wyne. 1957. Preliminary observations on hemorrhagic enteritis of turkeys. Poult Sci 36:1267-1270.

34. Gomez-Villamandos, J.C., J.M. Martin de las Mulas, J. Hervas, F. Chancon-M. de Lara, J. Perez, and E. Mozos. 1995. Spleno-enteritis caused by adenovirus in psittacine birds: A pathological study. Avian Pathol 24:553-563.

35. Gross, W.B., and W.E.C. Moore. 1967. Hemorrhagic enteritis of turkeys. Avian Dis 11:296-307.

36. Harris, J.R., and C.H. Domermuth. 1977. Hemorrhagic enteritis in two-and-one-half-week-old turkey poults. Avian Dis 21:120-122.

37. Hopkins, B.A., J.K. Skeeles, G.E. Houghten, D. Slagle, and K. Gardner. 1990. A survey of infectious diseases in wild turkeys (Meleagridis gallopavo silvestris) from Arkansas. J Wildl Dis 26:468-472.

38. Hussain, I., and K.V. Nagaraja. 1993. A monoclonal antibody-based immunoperoxidase method for rapid detection of haemorrhagic enteritis virus of turkeys. Res Vet Sci 55:98-103.

39. Hussain, I., C.U. Choi, B.S. Rings, D.P. Shaw, and K.V. Nagaraja. 1993. Pathogenesis of hemorrhagic enteritis virus infection in turkeys. J Vet Med 40:715-726.

40. Ianconescu, M., E.J. Smith, A.M. Fadly, and K. Nazerian. 1984. An enzyme-linked immunosorbent assay for detection of hemorrhagic enteritis virus and associated antibodies. Avian Dis 28:677-692.

41. Iltis, J.P. 1976. Experimental transmission of marble spleen disease in turkeys and pheasants with demonstration, characterization and classification of the causative virus. Diss Abstr 36:4890-B.

42. Itakura, C., H.C. Carlson, and G.N. Lang. 1974. Experimental transmission of hemorrhagic enteritis of turkeys. Avian Pathol 3:279-292.

43. Jucker, M.T., J.R. McQuiston, J.V. van den Hurk, S.M. Boyle, and F.W. Pierson. 1996. Characterization of the haem-

orrhagic enteritis virus genome and the sequence of the putative penton base and core protein genes. J Gen Virol 77:469-479.

44. Kwaga, J.K., B.J. Allen, J.V. van den Hurk, H. Seida, and A.A. Potter. 1994. A carAB mutant of avian pathogenic Escherichia coli serogroup O2 is attenuated and effective as a live oral vaccine against colibacillosis in turkeys. Infect Immun 62:3766-3772.

45. Larsen, C.T., C.H. Domermuth, D.P. Sponenberg, and W.B. Gross. 1985. Colibacillosis of turkeys exacerbated by hemorrhagic enteritis virus. Laboratory studies. Avian Dis 29:729-732.

46. Le Gros, F.X., D. Toquin, M. Guittet, G. Bennejean. 1989. Sensibilite comparee de quatre varietes genetiques de dinde a des souches virulentes ou attenuees du virue de l'enterite hemorragique. Avian Pathol 18:147-160.

47. Lucientes, J., J.F. Garcia-Marin, and J.J. Badiola. 1984. Outbreak of marble spleen disease in Spain. Med Vet 1:59-61.

48. Mandelli, G., A. Rinaldi, and G. Cervio. 1966. A disease involving the spleen and lungs in pheasants: Epidemiology, symptoms, and lesions. Clin Vet (Milano) 89:129-138.

49. Massi, P., D. Gelmett, G. Sironi, M. Dottori, A. Lavazza, and S. Pascucci. 1995. Adenovirus-associated haemorrhagic disease in guinea fowl. Avian Pathol 24:227-237.

50. Mayeda, B., G.B. West, A.A. Bickford, and B.R. Cho. 1982. Marble spleen disease in pen-raised pheasants in California. Proc Am Assoc Vet Lab Diag 25:261-270.

51. Meteyer, C.U., H.O. Mohammed, R.P. Chin, A.A. Bickford, D.W. Trampel, P.N. Klein. 1992. Relationship between age of flock seroconversion to hemorrhagic enteritis virus and appearance of adenoviral inclusions in the enteritis and renal tubule epithelia of turkeys. Avian Dis 36:88-96.

52. Nagaraja, K.V., D.J. Emery, B.L. Patel, B.S. Pomeroy, and J.A. Newman. 1982. In vitro evaluation of B-lymphocyte function in turkeys infected with hemorrhagic enteritis virus. Am J Vet Res 43:502-504.

53. Nagaraja, K.V., B.L. Patel, D.A. Emery, B.S. Pomeroy, and J.A. Newman. 1982. In vitro depression of the mitogenic response of lymphocytes from turkeys infected with hemorrhagic enteritis virus. Am J Vet Res 43:134-136.

54. Nagaraja, K.V., S.Y. Kang, and J.A. Newman. 1985. Immunosuppressive effects of virulent strain of hemorrhagic enteritis virus in turkeys vaccinated against Newcastle disease. Poult Sci 64:588-590.

55. Nazerian, K., and A. Fadly. 1982. Propagation of virulent and avirulent turkey hemorrhagic enteritis virus in cell culture. Avian Dis 26:816-827.

56. Nazerian, K., and A.M. Fadly. 1987. Further studies on in vitro and in vivo assays of hemorrhagic enteritis virus (HEV). Avian Dis 31:234-240.

57. Nazerian, K., L.F. Lee, and W.S. Payne. 1990. A double-antibody enzyme-linked immunosorbent assay for the detection of turkey hemorrhagic enteritis virus antibody and antigen. Avian Dis 34:425-432.

58. Nazerian, K., L.F. Lee, and W.S. Payne. 1991. Structural polypeptides of type II avian adenoviruses analyzed by monoclonal and polyclonal antibodies. Avian Dis 35:572-578.

59. Newberry, L.A., J.K. Skeeles, D.L. Kreider, J.N. Beasley, J.D. Story, R.W. McNew, and B.R. Berridge. 1993. Use of virulent hemorrhagic enteritis virus for the induction of colibacillosis in turkeys. Avian Dis 37:1-5.

60. Norton, R.A., J.K. Skeeles, and L.A. Newberry. 1993. Evaluation of the interaction of Eimeria meleagrimitis with hemorrhagic enteritis virus or marble spleen disease virus in turkeys. Avian Dis 37:290-294.

61. Opengart, K.N. 1991. Studies on the immunopathologic mechanisms of intestinal lesion formation in turkey poults infected with hemorrhagic enteritis virus. PhD dissertation. Virginia Polytechnic Institute and State University, Blacksburg, VA.

62. Opengart, K., P. Eyre, and C.H. Domermuth. 1992. Increased numbers of duodenal mucosal mast cells in turkeys inoculated with hemorrhagic enteritis virus. Am J Vet Res 53:814-819.

63. Ossa, I.E., J. Alexander, and G.G. Schurig. 1982. Role of splenectomy in prevention of hemorrhagic enteritis and death from hemorrhagic enteritis virus in turkeys. Avian Dis 27:1106-1111.

64. Perrin, G., C. Louzis, and D. Toquin. 1981. L'enterite hemorragique du dindon: Culture du virus in vitro. Bull Acad Vet Fr 54:231-235.

65. Pierson, F.W. 1993. The roles of multiple infectious agents in the predisposition of turkeys to colibacillosis. PhD dissertation. Virginia Polytechnic Institute and State University, Blacksburg, VA.

66. Pierson, F.W., V.D. Barta, D. Boyd, and W.S. Thompson. 1996. The association between exposure to multiple infectious agents and the development of colibacillosis in turkeys. J Appl Poult Res 5:347–357.

67. Pierson, F.W., C.T. Larsen, and C.H. Domermuth. 1996. The production of colibacillosis in turkeys following sequential exposure to Newcastle disease virus or Bordetella aviaum, avirulent hemorrhagic enteritis virus, and Escherichia coli. Avian Dis 40:837–840.

68. Pomeroy, B.S. 1972. Hemorrhagic enteritis. In M.S. Hofstad, B.W. Calnek, C.F. Helmboldt, W.M. Reid, and H.W. Yoder, Jr. (eds.). Diseases of Poultry, 6th ed. Iowa State University Press, Ames, IA, pp. 253-255.

69. Pomeroy, B.S., and R. Fenstermacher. 1937. Hemorrhagic enteritis in turkeys. Poult Sci 16:378-382.

70. Rachac, V., and K. Marjankova. 1983. Occurrence of marble spleen disease in pheasants in southern Bohemia. Veterinarstvi 33:359-361.

71. Saunders, G.K., F.W. Pierson, and J.V. van den Hurk. 1993. Haemorrhagic enteritis virus infection in turkeys: A comparison of virulent and avirulent virus infections, and a proposed pathogenesis. Avian Pathol 22:47-58.

72. Silim, A., and J. Thorsen. 1981. Hemorrhagic enteritis: Virus distribution and sequential development of antibody in turkeys. Avian Dis 25:444-453.

73. Sponenberg, D.P., C.H. Domermuth, and C.T. Larsen. 1985. Field outbreaks of colibacillosis of turkeys associated with hemorrhagic enteritis virus. Avian Dis 29:838-842.

74. Stoikov, V., and I. Nikiforov. 1983. Clinical features, epidemiology and pathology of marble spleen disease in pheasants. Veterinarnomed Nauk 20:89-97.

75. Suresh, M., and J.M. Sharma. 1995. Hemorrhagic enteritis virus induced changes in the lymphocyte subpopulations in turkeys and the effect of experimental immunodeficiency on viral pathogens. Vet Immunol Immunopathol 45:139-150.

76. Szankowska, Z., E. Kubissa, M. Piotrowska, H. Panufnik. 1982. Outbreak of marble spleen disease in pheasants in Poland. Med Wet 38:288-290.

77. Sztojkov, V., F. Ratz, and E. Saghy. 1978. Marble spleen disease of pheasants in Hungary. Magy Alltorvosok Lapja 33:223-226.

78. Tham, V.L., and N.F. Thies. 1988. Marble spleen disease of pheasants. Aust Vet J 65:130-131.

79. Trampel, D.W., C.U. Meteyer, A.A. Bickford. 1992. Hemorrhagic enteritis virus inclusions in turkey renal tubular epithelium. Avian Dis 36:1086-1091.

80. van den Hurk, J. 1985. Propagation of hemorrhagic enteritis virus in normal (nontumor derived) cell culture. J Am Vet Med Assoc 187:307.

81. van den Hurk, J.V. 1986. Quantitation of hemorrhagic enteritis virus antigen and antibody using enzyme-linked immunosorbent assay. Avian Dis 30:662-671.

82. van den Hurk, J. 1988. Characterization of group II avian adenoviruses using a panel of monoclonal antibodies. Can J Vet Res 52:458-467.

83. van den Hurk, J.V. 1990. Efficacy of avirulent hemorrhagic enteritis virus propagated in turkey leukocyte cultures

for vaccination against hemorrhagic enteritis in turkeys. Avian Dis 34:26-35.

84. van den Hurk, J.V. 1992. Characterization of the structural proteins of hemorrhagic enteritis virus. Arch Virol 126:195-213.

85. van den Hurk, J.V., and S. van Drunen Littel-van den Hurk. 1993. Protection of turkeys against hemorrhagic enteritis by monoclonal antibody and hexon immunization. Vaccine 11:329-335

86. Veit, H.P., C.H. Domermuth, and W.B. Gross. 1981. Histopathology of avian adenovirus group II splenomegaly of chickens. Avian Dis 25:866-873.

87. Zhang, C., and K.V. Nagaraja. 1989. Differentiation of avian adenovirus type II strains by restriction endonuclease fingerprinting. Am J Vet Res 50:1466-1470.

88. Zhang, C.L., K.V. Nagaraja, V. Sivanandan, and J.A. Newman. 1991. Identification and characterization of viral polypeptides from type-II avian adenoviruses. Am J Vet Res 52:1137-1141.

EGG DROP SYNDROME

J. B. McFerran

INTRODUCTION. Since its initial description (53), egg drop syndrome 1976 (EDS 76) has become a major cause of lost egg production throughout the world. It is caused by an adenovirus, probably introduced into chickens through a contaminated vaccine. Egg drop syndrome 76 is characterized by otherwise healthy birds producing thin-shelled or shell-less eggs. Once established in a breeding organization, the condition is more often seen as a failure to achieve production targets, and eggshell changes are less apparent, although still present. Since its initial recognition, it has become apparent that sporadic outbreaks of EDS 76 occur as a result of fowl becoming infected through direct or indirect contact with infected wild or domestic waterfowl.

The virus affects only avian species and, therefore, has no public health significance.

HISTORY. A condition of laying hens was described by Dutch workers in 1976 (53), and hemagglutinating adenoviruses were isolated (35). Using serologic studies with one of these isolates and flock records it was possible to establish the disease pattern (35, 37). It appeared that the virus was transmitted vertically and that horizontal transmission between flocks was not a feature; the virus often remained latent until birds were approaching peak egg production. Because of the absence of antibody to the virus in chickens prior to 1974 and the failure of the virus to grow in mammalian cells, as well as its poor growth in turkey cells and optimal growth in duck cells, it was suggested that this was probably a duck adenovirus. This suggestion was quickly confirmed by isolation of EDS 76 virus from normal ducks and demonstration of antibody in many duck flocks (9, 13).

INCIDENCE AND DISTRIBUTION. Egg drop syndrome 76 virus has been isolated from chickens in Australia (19), Belgium (38), China (61), France (41), Great Britain (9), Hungary (62), India (29), Israel (33), Italy (60), Japan (57), Northern Ireland (37), Singapore (44), South Africa (11), and Taiwan (31). Serologic evidence of infection has been found in chickens in Brazil (25), Denmark (5), Mexico (42), New Zealand (24), and Nigeria (39).

ETIOLOGY

Classification. Egg drop syndrome 76 virus is classified as an adenovirus on the basis of its morphology, replication, and chemical composition. While the avian adenovirus group antigen is not detected by immunodiffusion or immunofluorescence, if birds infected with another avian adenovirus are kept until antibody to this virus is no longer detectable and are then infected with EDS 76 virus, they develop antibody to both the adenovirus and EDS 76, indicating that there is a shared antigen (36). Egg drop syndrome 76 is not related to 11 fowl and two turkey prototype adenoviruses using serum neutralization (SN) or hemagglutination inhibition (HI) tests (3). Southern blotting detected homologous sequences in EDS DNA and bovine adenovirus DNA, but no homology was detected with FAV 1 DNA and bovine adenovirus DNA (59).

Morphology. The size of EDS 76 virus observed in negatively stained preparations has been reported to range from 76 nm (37) to 80 ± 5 nm (28). These sizes are within those acceptable for adenoviruses (56).

Using preparations made from a cesium chloride (CsCl) gradient, typical adenovirus morphology with triangular faces having six capsomeres on the edge and a single 25-nm fiber projecting from each vertex was demonstrated (28). In normal preparations, this structure is not obvious (37, 57). Although EDS 76 particles are clearly adenoviruses with well-defined capsomeres with hollow centers, it is possible to distinguish them from conventional adenoviruses (Fig. 23.8). In thin sections of infected chick embryo liver cells, virus particles of 70–75 nm are seen in the nucleus (3). Particles of 68–80 nm in diameter have been described in nuclei of epithelial cells of oviduct mucosa (50).

Density in Cesium Chloride.
Differences in the reported density of EDS 76 virus in CsCl have been reported. Todd and McNulty (51) found that infectious virus particles banded at densities of 1.32 and 1.30 g/mL. The heavier particles, however, did not agglutinate chicken erythrocytes and appeared by electron microscopy to be slightly damaged. Particles with a density of 1.30 g/mL hemagglutinated and appeared undamaged. A band of empty, disrupted, noninfectious hemagglutinating particles was present at a density of 1.28 g/mL. In contrast, Kraft et al. (28) reported presence of two bands of infectious, hemagglutinating particles at 1.32 g/mL, with noninfectious disrupted particles banding at 1.30 g/mL. Yamaguchi et al. (57) reported hemagglutinating particles banding at 1.30 g/mL and infectious particles with a density of 1.33 g/mL, while Takai et al. (49) found infectivity and hemagglutinin associated with a band at 1.33 g/mL and hemagglutinin also in a band at 1.29. This discrep-

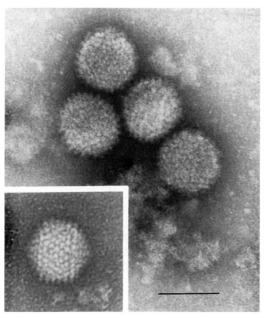

23.8. Four particles of egg drop syndrome (EDS) 76 virus. Although individual capsomeres are well resolved, typical adenovirus morphology is not apparent. *Inset:* type 8 fowl adenovirus particle showing well-defined, triangular faces. *Bar* = 80 nm.

ancy was explained, at least in part, by Zsak and Kisary (62), who reported that density and hemagglutinating ability of EDS 76 particles depended on the method used for virus purification and whether the virus was grown in cell cultures or embryonated eggs.

Chemical Composition.
Labeling with H^3-thymidine and inhibition with iododeoxyuridine showed that EDS 76 virus contained DNA (3, 28, 51, 57). The molecular weight of the DNA is estimated at 22.6×10^6 d compared with 28.9×10^6 d for fowl adenovirus type 1 (Phelps) and restriction endonuclease patterns indicate no relationship between these two viruses (62). The EDS 76 virus has 13 structural polypeptides; at least 7 of these correspond with polypeptides of fowl adenovirus type 1 (51).

Hemagglutination.
The EDS 76 virus agglutinates erythrocytes of chickens, ducks, turkeys, geese, pigeons, and peacocks but does not agglutinate rat, rabbit, horse, sheep, cattle, goat, or pig erythrocytes (3, 31).

The hemagglutinin (HA) is resistant. At 56 C, there is an initial fourfold fall in titer after 16 hr, but the titer remains stable for 4 days and is finally undetectable after 8 days. It survived 60 C but is destroyed by 70 C for 30 min. It retains its activity for long periods at 4 C (3, 38). It is resistant to trypsin, 2-mercaptoethanol, ethylenediaminetetraacetic acid (EDTA), papain, ficin, and 0.5% formaldehyde at 37 C for 1 hr, but the titer is greatly reduced by potassium periodate and 0.5% glutaraldehyde (49). However, purified soluble HA is destroyed by trypsin (51). Alpha-chymotrypsin destroyed the virus receptor on chicken erythrocytes, whereas trypsin and neuraminidase had no effect (49).

Virus Replication.
Egg drop syndrome 76 virus replicates in the nucleus in a similar fashion to avian adenoviruses belonging to group A (1, 2, 3). Intranuclear inclusions are seen in hematoxylin- and eosin-stained preparations of infected cell cultures (3), in epithelial cells of the infundibulum, tubular shell gland, pouch shell gland, isthmus, and nasal mucosa; and in spleen of experimentally infected chickens (47, 50). In ultrathin sections, virus particles and type I–IV inclusions similar to other avian adenoviruses are obvious in the nucleus (2, 3).

Resistance to Chemical and Physical Agents.
The EDS 76 virus is stable to treatment with chloroform and variations in pH between 3 and 10. It is inactivated by heating for 30 min at 60 C, survives for 3 hr at 56 C, and is stable in monovalent but not divalent cations (3, 57). Infectivity

was not demonstrated after treating with 0.5% formaldehyde or 0.5% glutaraldehyde (49).

Strain Classification. Only one serotype has been recognized (17, 57). With the use of restriction endonuclease analysis, however, it has been possible to divide a number of isolates into three genotypes (52). One includes isolates made over an 11-yr period from infected European chickens. A second group are viruses isolated from ducks in the United Kingdom. One virus isolated from chickens in Australia forms the third group.

Laboratory Host Systems. The EDS 76 virus grows to highest titers in duck kidney, duck embryo liver, and duck embryo fibroblast cells. It also grows well in chick embryo liver cells, less well in chick kidney cells, and rather poorly in chicken embryo fibroblasts. Growth in turkey cells is poor, and no replication could be detected in a range of mammalian cells (3). The virus grows to high titers in goose cell cultures (62). In chick liver cells, peak virus and intracellular hemagglutinin (HA) titers are reached after 48 hr and peak extracellular HA titers occur at 72 hr (57).

The virus grows very well when inoculated into the allantoic sac of embryonated duck or goose eggs producing titers of 1/16,000–1/32,000. No growth has been detected in embryonated chicken eggs (3, 63).

Pathogenicity. While all chicken isolates appear to be of similar virulence, isolates from ducks in the United States produced no effect on egg production (54) or only affected egg size (12) when chickens were infected. Isolates from ducks and chickens in Europe behaved identically in chickens (7).

PATHOGENESIS AND EPIZOOTIOLOGY

Natural and Experimental Hosts. Although disease outbreaks have been in laying hens, it is probable that the natural hosts are ducks and geese. Antibody is widespread in domesticated ducks (5, 8, 9, 13, 19, 32, 33) and domestic geese (8, 63). In a study of ducks in the Atlantic flyway in the United States, antibody was found in ruddy, ring-necked, wood, bufflehead, lesser scaup, mallard, northern shoveler, and gadwall ducks; and in mergansers, coots, and grebes (22, 43). Antibody has also been detected in Muscovy ducks and cattle egrets (33), Canada geese, (43), herring gulls (8), and in owls, a stork, and a swan (26).

Virus has been isolated from healthy domestic ducks (9, 54). Virus has also been recovered from diseased ducks (20), but the disease could not be reproduced using the isolate. A virus was isolated from ducks with a fall in egg production and severe diarrhea (6), and it has been suggested that EDS may cause rough, thin shells and decreased egg production in ducks (30).

Infection also is common in geese (26, 32, 63). Experimentally infected goslings and geese showed neither illness nor change in egg production (63).

Quail (*Coturnix coturnix japonica*) are susceptible to infection and develop classic signs (18). There has been no evidence of naturally occurring infection of turkeys or pheasants, but they can be experimentally infected (8, 40, 60). Guinea fowl may be infected naturally or experimentally (21) and soft-shelled eggs may be produced; however, guinea fowl became infected but remained clinically normal when exposed to a fowl isolate (55).

Because EDS 76 virus was initially primarily transmitted vertically there was often an apparent breed association in chickens. A wide range of breeds, however, are equally susceptible to experimental infection, although analysis of naturally occurring outbreaks suggests that broiler breeders and heavy breeds producing brown eggs are more severely affected than white-egg producers. When two brown and one white-egg layer strains were infected (23), egg production was depressed in the white layer strain. There was little depression in egg production of the brown layers, but they produced more eggs with shell defects; one brown egg–producing strain laid almost three times as many affected eggs as the white egg–laying strain.

Birds of all ages are susceptible to infection. If EDS 76 virus is introduced onto a site, effects on egg production can be seen in all ages of laying hens. However, when birds seemingly become infected around peak egg production (37), this may be due to reactivation of latent virus.

Pathogenesis. Following experimental oral infection of adult hens, there is limited virus replication in the nasal mucosa and a viremia (47). At 3–4 days postinfection (PI), virus replication occurs in lymphoid tissue throughout the body; especially spleen and thymus. In addition, the infundibulum of the oviduct is consistently affected. At 7–20 days PI, there is massive viral replication in the pouch shell gland (Fig. 23.9) and, to much lesser extents, in other parts of the oviduct. This replication is associated with a pronounced inflammatory response in the pouch shell gland and production of abnormally shelled eggs (45, 50, 58).

Unlike conventional adenoviruses, EDS does not replicate in the intestinal mucosa, and presence of virus in the feces is probably due to contamination with oviduct exudate (47).

Transmission. It is now possible to divide EDS outbreaks into three types. In the initially ob-

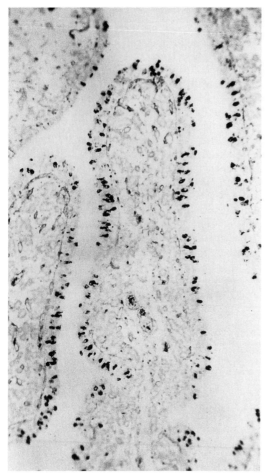

23.9. Pouch shell gland from hen experimentally infected with egg drop syndrome (EDS) virus. Note the viral nucleic acid in surface epithelial layer, demonstrated by a biotinylated purified virus genome probe. (Allan)

served classic form, primary breeders were infected and the main method of spread was vertically through the embryonated egg (37). Although the number of infected embryos is probably low with this type (10), spread is very efficient. In many cases, chicks infected in ovo do not excrete virus or develop HI antibody until the flock has achieved >50% egg production. At this stage, the virus is unmasked and excreted, resulting in rapid spread due to multiple foci of infection.

Probably arising from the classic form, virus has become established in some areas in commercial egg-laying flocks. In India, 32.6% of poultry flocks were found to be infected (29). This endemic form is often associated with a common egg-packing station. Both normal- and abnormal-shelled eggs laid during the period of virus growth in the pouch shell gland contain virus both on their exterior and inte-

rior (46). This leads to contamination of egg trays. Droppings also contain virus, but this excretion is intermittent and often of low titer (15), and in the adult bird may result from contamination of feces by oviduct exudate (47). Apart from direct spread between birds, there is evidence that spread can occur when birds are transported in inadequately cleaned trucks or when unused food has been taken from one site to another. There is also evidence that needles or blades used for vaccination or bleeding of viremic birds, if not properly sterilized, can transmit infection. Lateral spread is slow and intermittent, taking up to 11 wk to spread through a cage house; in one case, spread to an adjoining pen was prevented by a wire fence. Spread between birds on litter is usually faster (15, 53).

Spread from both domestic or wild ducks, geese, and possibly other wild birds to hens through drinking water contaminated by droppings appears to give rise to a third type of outbreak. This type is very important in some areas. These cases tend to be sporadic, but there is always the danger of an infected flock becoming the focus for an endemic infection.

Signs. Following experimental infection, most workers have found the first signs after 7–9 days (16, 34), but in some experiments they have not occurred until 17 days PI (38).

The first sign is loss of color in pigmented eggs. This is quickly followed by production of thin-shelled, soft-shelled, or shell-less eggs (Fig. 23.10). Thin-shelled eggs often have a rough, sandpaper-like texture, or a granular roughening of the shell at one end. If obviously affected eggs are discarded, there is no effect on fertility or hatchability and no long-term effect on egg quality. If birds are infected in late production, forced molting of the flock will restore egg production to normal. The fall in production can be very rapid or extend over weeks. Outbreaks usually last 4–10 wk, and egg production can be reduced by up to 40%; however, there is usually compensation later in lay, so that the total number lost is typically 10–16 eggs/bird. If the disease results from reactivation of latent virus, the fall usually occurs when production is between 50% and peak level. Small eggs have been described in naturally occurring outbreaks (37), but no effect on egg size was found in experimental infections (34). Watery albumen has been described (38, 53), although no effect on albumen has been seen by other workers (17, 34, 58). Age at time of infection may be important, however; birds infected at 1 day of age subsequently laid apparently normal eggs except for impaired albumen quality and smaller size (16).

If some birds have acquired antibody before latent virus is unmasked, an apparently different clin-

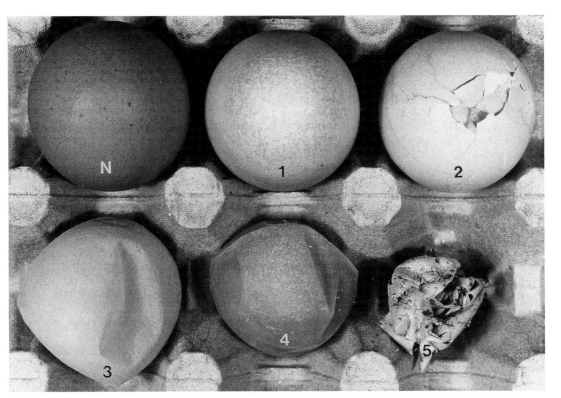

23.10.   Eggs from hens infected with egg drop syndrome (EDS) 76 virus. Changes range from
normal brown egg (N), to loss of shell pigment (1 and 2), thinning at the pole (1), thin-
shelled (2), soft-shelled (3), and shell-less eggs (4). Eggs may be eaten or broken, but
many membranes (5) may be found.

ical syndrome is seen. There is failure to achieve
predicted egg production and onset of lay may be
delayed. If a careful examination is made, it can
usually be established that there is a series of small
clinical episodes of classic EDS. Presumably, birds
with antibody slow down spread of virus. A similar
picture is often seen in birds in cage units, where
spread can be slow and EDS not suspected.

Affected birds remain otherwise healthy. Although inappetence and dullness have been described in some affected flocks, these are not consistent findings. Transient diarrhea described by
some authors is probably due to the exudate from
the oviduct (47). EDS 76 virus does not cause clinical disease in growing chickens in the field. Oral
infection of susceptible day-old chicks resulted in
increased mortality in the 1st wk of life (16), but
there was no increase in mortality in many flocks of
chickens produced by infected parent flocks.

Gross Lesions. In naturally occurring outbreaks, inactive ovaries and atrophied oviducts are
often the only recognized lesions and these are not

consistently present. In one outbreak, uterine edema
was (31). The absence of lesions may be a reflection
of the difficulty in selecting birds undergoing acute
disease.

Following experimental infection, edema of uterine folds and presence of exudate in the pouch shell
gland commonly occur within 9–14 days PI (45,
50). There is also mild splenomegaly, flaccid
ovules, and eggs in various stages of formation in
the abdominal cavity (45, 50).

Histopathology.   The   major   pathologic
changes occur in the pouch shell gland. Virus replicates in epithelial cell nuclei, producing intranuclear inclusion bodies from 7 days PI onward (45,
50). Many affected cells are sloughed into the lumen, and there is a rapid and severe inflammatory
response involving macrophages, plasma cells, and
lymphocytes, together with variable numbers of
heterophils in the lamina propria and epithelium
(Fig. 23.11). Inclusion bodies are not seen after the
3rd day of abnormal egg production, but viral antigen persists for up to 1 wk (45).

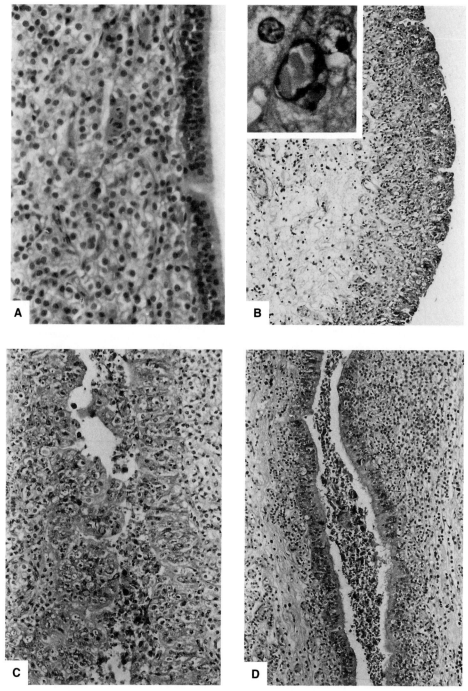

23.11. *A.* Normal uterine mucosa. Surface epithelium consists of a single layer of columnar cells, many of which are ciliated; underlying these are tubular glands. (Smyth) *B.* Pronounced edema of uterine submucosa, atrophy of tubular glands, and infiltration of entire mucosa by mononuclear cells are present at 8 days postinoculation (PI). *Inset:* intranuclear inclusion body in superficial epithelial cell. Note margination of nuclear chromatin and three eosinophilic inclusions in the nucleus. (Smyth) *C.* Uterine surface epithelium is markedly hyperplastic 11 days PI; there is complete loss of cilia. (Smyth) *D.* Exudate in uterine lumen consists of degenerating epithelial cells and heterophils mixed with mucus. Epithelium is devoid of cilia, tubular glands are almost absent, and uterine wall is infiltrated with lymphocytes and heterophils. (Smyth)

Immunity.   After experimental infection, antibody can be detected by indirect fluorescent antibody (IFA), enzyme-linked immunosorbent assay (ELISA), SN and HI tests in 5 days and double immunodiffusion (DID) tests in 7 days (4). They reach a peak in about 4–5 wk. Immunoprecipitating antibodies are more transient than others.

Birds still excrete virus even in the presence of high HI antibody, but some birds that excrete virus fail to develop antibody (16).

Antibody is transferred through the yolk sac, and chicks have high HI titers (geometric mean titers, 6–9 $\log_2$). This antibody has a half-life of 3 days (17). Active antibody production is not stimulated until chicks are 4–5 wk of age, and maternal antibody is nearly undetectable (17). When the disease was being eradicated it was found that some flocks, although 100% free from detectable antibody on two or three occasions, nevertheless suddenly developed EDS. It was assumed that some chicks infected in ovo failed to develop antibody until they came into egg production and then excreted virus. It is not known if all chicks developed antibody at this point, but it is possible they did not, because less than 100% of birds in infected flocks have antibody.

If a flock as a whole develops antibody to EDS 76 virus before coming into lay, egg production will not be affected (10).

DIAGNOSIS

Isolation and Identification of Causative Agent.   The most sensitive indicator system is either embryonated duck or goose eggs from a flock free of EDS 76 virus infection, or duck or goose cell cultures. If these are unavailable, chicken cells should be used. Chicken embryo liver cells are more sensitive than chicken kidney cells; chicken embryo fibroblasts are insensitive (3). Embryonating chicken eggs are not suitable. Not only are duck or goose cells or embryonated duck or goose eggs more sensitive, they also have the advantage that many chicken viruses do not grow in these systems.

It is not sufficient to rely on embryo death or cytopathic effects with EDS 76 viruses. Allantoic fluid from goose or duck eggs or cell culture supernatant should be checked after each passage for presence of hemagglutinins for avian erythrocytes (0.8% chick erythrocyte suspension is suitable). Alternatively, immunofluorescence using a labeled antiserum to EDS 76 virus can be used to detect growth in cells. Conjugated antiserum to conventional avian adenoviruses is unsuitable. If duck cells are used, a minimum of two passages are required, and with chick cells two to five passages are necessary before declaring a specimen negative. The need for extensive passage is partly due to poor growth of these viruses on primary isolation in chick cells and partly because it is difficult to select the bird at the correct phase in the disease process.

Serology.   The HI, ELISA, SN, FA, and DID tests are of equal sensitivity (4). When birds were infected with a number of adenovirus serotypes, however, and consequently had high levels of adenovirus group antibody, there were positive reactions in the ELISA, FA, or DID tests, but not in the HI or SN tests (4). The HI test is the one of choice for diagnosis. Antigen can be prepared in either embryonated duck eggs or cell culture. Higher HA titers are obtained if duck eggs are used, but HA titers in the thousands can be obtained using chick embryo liver cell cultures. A suitable HI test uses 4 HA units of antigen, an initial 1:4 serum dilution, and 0.8% chicken erythrocytes. The EDS 76 virus agglutinates erythrocytes from chickens, geese, turkeys, and ducks but not mammals. There is no hemolysin. If nonspecific hemagglutinins are present in serum, they can be removed by adsorption with a 10% erythrocyte suspension, or homologous erythrocytes can be used. The SN test, using 100 $TCID_{50}$, 1 hr at 37 C reaction time, and duck or chick cell cultures as the indicator system, is sensitive and specific. When using chick cell cultures, it often helps if the end-points are read by presence of hemagglutinins in the supernatant fluid rather than by cytopathology. The SN test is really only required to confirm an unusual HI test result, as in an eradication program or detection of HI antibody in a new species.

Many flocks containing birds infected in ovo do not show antibody during the growing period; it is only apparent immediately following clinical signs. Therefore, even a negative serologic test of all birds in a flock at, say, 20 wk of age gives no guarantee of freedom from infection.

Selection of Specimens.   Because of the absence of obvious clinical signs and the often slow spread of infection, it can be very difficult to select correct birds for either virus isolation or serology. The finding that abnormal eggs contain virus, however, and that these eggs are produced after the bird has antibody, has allowed a rational approach to diagnosis (46). To isolate virus, affected eggs can be fed to antibody-free adult laying hens. Once they produce abnormal eggs, they should be killed and virus isolations attempted using the pouch shell gland. For serologic diagnosis, all the birds in cages where abnormal eggs are being produced should be bled for serology. If the birds are on litter, then care must be taken to select samples throughout the house, as it is usually not possible to determine which birds are producing abnormal eggs.

Differential Diagnosis.   Egg drop syndrome 76 should be suspected whenever there is failure to achieve predicted egg production levels or if there are falls in production, especially if birds are healthy and eggshell changes precede or are concurrent with the decline. Shell-less eggs are usually a feature but are often missed because birds eat them. Therefore, an inspection should take place early in the morning before eggs can be eaten; if birds are on litter, a careful search will reveal egg membranes. While shell-less, soft-shelled, and thin-shelled eggs are characteristic, misshapen and ridged eggs are not a feature. In an infected flock in which vertical transmission has occurred, most if not all cases occur around peak egg production, but any age of flock can be infected by lateral spread.

While signs of EDS 76 are suggestive, diagnosis must not be made on them alone but should be confirmed by an HI test before embarking on a vaccination program.

TREATMENT.   There is no successful treatment. Various treatments have been tried (vitamins, increasing calcium or protein in the ration), but in controlled trials no effect could be demonstrated.

PREVENTION AND CONTROL

Management Procedures.   Since classic EDS 76 is primarily spread by vertical transmission through the egg, birds should be derived from uninfected flocks. Endemic EDS is often associated with a common egg-packing station where contaminated egg trays can be a major factor in spread. Virus is also present in droppings and lateral spread is possible because the virus is resistant. There is circumstantial evidence for spread by personnel and transport, and, therefore, sensible hygienic precautions are required.

Infected birds have a viremia; thus, it is important that bleeding needles, needles for inoculating vaccines, and other equipment should be sterilized between uses.

If there are infected and noninfected breeding flocks within the same organization, separate hatcheries, staff, and transport should be used. If this is not possible, separate setters and hatchers should be used, and hatches should be on different days of the week. The minimum possible procedure (and this is not recommended) is to use separate hatchers and to sex, vaccinate, and dispatch the clean stock before doing anything with potentially infected chicks. It is especially important to keep basic or grandparent breeding stock of an infected breed separate from noninfected birds of another breed, and these eggs should never be incubated in the same hatchery.

In certain areas of the world, especially where birds have water derived from dams, lakes or rivers, EDS infection has been common. These outbreaks have been controlled either by using water from wells or by chlorination of the water. In units where ducks or geese are kept, they should be carefully segregated from chickens. If possible, all housing should be made wild bird–proof. It is established that wild ducks and geese are often infected, but it is not known how widespread infection is in other avian species.

Eradication.   Egg drop syndrome 76 was successfully eradicated from a breeding organization in Northern Ireland. The method was based on a number of postulations: chickens produced from infected eggs may be latently infected and fail to develop antibody; the virus will become unmasked and be excreted around peak egg production, and antibody will develop, which will prevent or reduce further excretion; and lateral spread is poor.

The eradication program was based on the elite and grandparent flocks aged 40 wk or more. At this stage, these flocks had produced abnormal eggs and had HI antibody. Chicks hatched from these eggs were divided into small groups of about 100 (separated by netting wire). They were HI tested at a 10–25% level at about 6-wk intervals. If one or two reactors were found, they were removed; 100% of the pen and 100% of adjoining pens were then tested twice at weekly intervals. If reactors were found or reactors kept appearing in a pen, the whole pen was removed and the in-contact pens were tested. At 40 wk, a 100% test was carried out on all birds, and eggs were collected for the next generation. This program was successful; subsequently, the grandparent and parent flocks were found to be free of infection.

Immunization.   An oil-adjuvant inactivated vaccine is widely used and gives good protection against clinical disease. Birds are vaccinated between 14 and 16 wk of age. If uninfected birds are vaccinated, HI titers of 8–9 $\log_2$ can be expected; if the flock has been exposed previously to EDS 76 virus, titers of 12–14 $\log_2$ can be found. An antibody response can be detected by the 7th day, with peak titers between the 2nd and 5th wk. Immunity lasts at least 1 yr (10, 16, 27, 48). While properly vaccinated birds are protected against disease and do not appear to excrete virus, improperly vaccinated birds with low-HI titers excreted virus when challenged (14).

Where vertical or lateral transmission is a possibility, flocks in danger can be protected by vaccination in the growing period. If one or more houses on a multiage laying site becomes infected by lateral spread, careful evaluation must be undertaken before vaccinating the healthy birds in lay. Undoubtedly, the healthy birds can be protected by vaccination, but the cost of vaccinating them and the effects of the handling to administer the inactivated vaccine must be weighed against the economic returns achieved from the protection. It is possible to limit the spread of virus on a site by good hygiene. It is especially important to remember that the infected egg is the most dangerous source of virus.

REFERENCES

1. Adair, B.M. 1978. Studies on the development of avian adenoviruses in cell cultures. Avian Pathol 7:541–550.

2. Adair, B.M., W.L. Curran, and J.B. McFerran. 1979. Ultrastructural studies of the replication of fowl adenovirus in primary cell cultures. Avian Pathol 8:133–144.

3. Adair, B.M., J.B. McFerran, T.J. Connor, M.S. McNulty, and E.R. McKillop. 1979. Biological and physical properties of a virus (strain 127) associated with the egg drop syndrome 1976. Avian Pathol 8:249–264.

4. Adair, B.M., D. Todd, J.B. McFerran, and E.R. McKillop. 1986. Comparative serological studies with egg drop syndrome virus. Avian Pathol 15:677–685.

5. Badstue, P.B., and B. Smidt. 1978. Egg drop syndrome 76 in Danish poultry. Nord Vet Med 30:498–505.

6. Bartha, A. 1984. Dropped egg production in ducks associated with adenovirus infection. Avian Pathol 13:119–126.

7. Bartha, A., and J. Meszaros. 1985. Experimental infection of laying hens with an adenovirus isolated from ducks showing EDS symptoms. Acta Vet Hung 33:125–127.

8. Bartha, A., J. Meszaros, and J. Tanyi. 1982. Antibodies against EDS 76 avian adenovirus in bird species before 1975. Avian Pathol 11:511–513.

9. Baxendale, W. 1978. Egg drop syndrome 76. Vet Rec 102:285–286.

10. Baxendale, W., D. Lutticken, R. Hein, and I. McPherson. 1980. The results of field trials conducted with an inactivated vaccine against the egg drop syndrome 76 (EDS 76). Avian Pathol 9:77–91.

11. Bragg, R.R., D.M. Allwright, and L. Coetzee. 1991. Isolation and identification of adenovirus 127, the causative agent of egg drop syndrome (EDS), from commercial laying hens in South Africa. Onderstepoort J Vet Res 58:309–310.

12. Brugh, M., C.W. Beard, and P. Villegas. 1984. Experimental infection of laying chickens with adenovirus 127 and with a related virus isolated from ducks. Avian Dis 28:168–178.

13. Calnek, B.W. 1978. Hemagglutination-inhibition antibodies against an adenovirus (virus-127) in White Pekin ducks in the United States. Avian Dis 22:798–801.

14. Cook, J.K.A. 1983. Egg Drop Syndrome 1976 (EDS-76) virus infection in inadequately vaccinated chickens. Avian Pathol 12:9–16.

15. Cook, J.K.A., and J.H. Darbyshire. 1980. Epidemiological studies with egg drop syndrome 1976 (EDS-76) virus. Avian Pathol 9:437–443.

16. Cook, J.K.A., and J.H. Darbyshire. 1981. Longitudinal studies on the egg drop syndrome 1976 (EDS 76) in the fowl following experimental infection at 1-day old. Avian Pathol 10:449–459.

17. Darbyshire, J.H., and R.W. Peters. 1980. Studies on EDS 76 virus infection in laying chickens. Avian Pathol 9:277–290.

18. Das, B.B., and H.K. Pradhan. 1992. Outbreaks of egg drop syndrome due to EDS-76 virus in quail (Coturnix coturnix japonica). Vet Rec 131:264–265.

19. Firth, G.A., M.J. Hall, and J.B. McFerran. 1981. Isolation of a hemagglutinating adeno-like virus related to virus 127 from an Australian poultry flock with an egg drop syndrome. Aust Vet J 57:239–242.

20. Gough, R.E., M.S. Collins, and D. Spackman. 1982. Isolation of a haemagglutinating adenovirus from commercial ducks. Vet Rec 110:275–276.

21. Guittet, M., J.P. Picault, and G. Bennejean. 1981. Experimental soft-shelled eggs disease (EDS 76) in guinea fowl (Numida meleagridis). Proc VIIth Int Cong World Vet Poult Assoc, Oslo, Norway, p. 22.

22. Gulka, C.M., T.H. Piela, V.J. Yates, and C. Bagshaw. 1984. Evidence of exposure of waterfowl and other aquatic birds to the hemagglutinating duck adenovirus identical to EDS 76 virus. J Wildl Dis 20:1–5.

23. Higashihara, M., M. Hiruma, T. Houdatsu, S. Takai, and M. Matumoto. 1987. Experimental infection of laying chickens with egg drop syndrome 1976 virus. Avian Dis 31:193–196.

24. Howell, J. 1982. Egg drop syndrome in Ross Brown hens: An interim report. Surveillance 9:10–11.

25. Hwang, M.H., J.M. Lamas, O. Hipolito, and E.N. Silva. 1980. Egg drop syndrome 1976 a serological survey in Brazil. Proc 6th European Poultry Conf, Hamburg, Germany, pp. 371–378.

26. Kaleta, E.F., S.E.D. Khalaf, and O. Siegmann. 1980. Antibodies to egg drop syndrome 76 virus in wild birds in possible conjunction with egg-shell problem. Avian Pathol 9:587–590.

27. Khalaf, S.E.D., E.F. Kaleta, and O. Siegmann. 1982. Comparative studies on the kinetics of hemagglutination inhibition and virus neutralising antibodies following vaccination of chickens against egg drop syndrome 1976 (EDS 76). Dev Biol Stand 51:127–137.

28. Kraft, V., S. Grund, and G. Monreal. 1979. Ultrastructural characterisation of isolate 127 of egg drop syndrome 1976 virus as an adenovirus. Avian Pathol 8:353–361.

29. Kumar, R., G.C. Mohanty, K.C. Verma, and Ram-Kumar. 1992. Epizootiological studies on egg drop syndrome in poultry. Indian J Anim Sci 62:497–501.

30. Liu, M.R.S. 1986. Occurrence and pathology of rough and thin shelled eggs in ducks. J Chin Soc Vet Sci 12:65–76.

31. Lu, Y.S., D.F. Lin, H.J. Tsai, Y.L. Lee, S.Y. Chui, C. Lee, and S.T. Huang. 1985. Outbreaks of egg drop syndrome—1976 in Taiwan and isolation of the etiological agent. J Chin Soc Vet Sci 11:157–165.

32. Lu, Y.S., H.J. Tsai, D.F. Lin, S.Y. Chiu, Y.L. Lee, and C. Lee. 1985. Survey on antibody against egg drop syndrome 1976 virus among bird species in Taiwan. J Chin Soc Vet Sci 11:151–156.

33. Malkinson, M., and Y. Weisman. 1980. Serological survey for the prevalence of antibodies to egg drop syndrome 1976 virus in domesticated and wild birds in Israel. Avian Pathol 9:421–426.

34. McCracken, R.M., and J.B. McFerran. 1978. Experimental reproduction of the egg drop syndrome 1976 with a hemagglutinating adenovirus. Avian Pathol 7:483–490.

35. McFerran, J.B., H.M. Rowley, M.S. McNulty, and L.J. Montgomery. 1977. Serological studies on flocks showing depressed egg production. Avian Pathol 6:405–413.

36. McFerran, J.B., T.J. Connor, and B.M. Adair. 1978. Studies on the antigenic relationship between an isolate (127) from the egg drop syndrome 1976 and a fowl adenovirus. Avian Pathol 7:629–636.

37. McFerran, J.B., R.M. McCracken, E.R. McKillop, M.S. McNulty, and D.S. Collins. 1978. Studies on a depressed egg production syndrome in Northern Ireland. Avian Pathol 7:35–47.

38. Meulemans, G., D. Dekegel, J. Peeters, E. Van Meirhaeghe, and P. Halen. 1979. Isolation of an adeno-like virus from laying chickens affected by egg drop syndrome 1976. Vlaams Diergeneeskd Tijdschr 2:151–157.

39. Nawathe, D.R., and A. Abegunde. 1980. Egg drop syndrome 76 in Nigeria: Serological evidence in commercial farms. Vet Rec 107:466–467.

40. Parsons, D.G., C.D. Bracewell, and G. Parsons. 1980. Experimental infection of turkeys with egg drop syndrome 1976 virus and studies on the application of the haemagglutination inhibition test. Res Vet Sci 29:89–92.

41. Picault, J-P. 1978. Chutes de ponte associees a la production d'oeufs sans coquille ou a coquille fragile: Proprietes

de l'agent infectious isole au cours de la maladie. L'Aviculteur 379:57–60.

42. Rosales, G., A. Antillon, and C. Morales. 1980. Reporte en Mexico sobre la presencia de anticuerpos contra el adenovirus causante del sindrome de la baja en postura (CEPA BC-14) en parvadas de gallinas domesticas. Proc 29th West Poult Dis Conf, pp. 192–196.

43. Schloer, G.M. 1980. Frequency of antibody to adenovirus 127 in domestic ducks and wild waterfowl. Avian Dis 24:91–98.

44. Singh, K.Y., and M. Chew-Lim. 1981. Breeder farm egg drop syndrome 1976 (EDS 76) in Singapore. Singapore Vet J 5:8–13.

45. Smyth, J.A. 1988. A study of the pathology and pathogenesis of egg drop syndrome (EDS) virus infection in fowl. PhD Thesis. The Queen's University of Belfast, Belfast, Northern Ireland.

46. Smyth, J.A., and B.M. Adair. 1988. Lateral transmission of egg drop syndrome 76 virus by the egg. Avian Pathol 17:193–200.

47. Smyth, J.A., M.A. Platten, and J.B. McFerran. 1988. A study of the pathogenesis of egg drop syndrome in laying hens. Avian Pathol 17:653–666.

48. Solyom, F., M. Nemesi, A. Forgacs, E. Balla, and T. Perenyi. 1982. Studies on EDS vaccine. Dev Biol Stand 51:105–121.

49. Takai, S., M. Higashihara, and M. Matumoto. 1984. Purification and hemagglutinating properties of egg drop syndrome 1976 virus. Arch Virol 80:59–67.

50. Taniguchi, T., S. Yamaguchi, M. Maeda, H. Kawamura, and T. Horiuchi. 1981. Pathological changes in laying hens inoculated with the JPA-1 strain of egg drop syndrome 1976 virus. Natl Inst Anim Health Q (Tokyo) 21:83–93.

51. Todd, D., and M.S. McNulty. 1978. Biochemical studies on a virus associated with Egg Drop Syndrome 1976. J Gen Virol 40:63–75.

52. Todd, D., M.S. McNulty, and J.A. Smyth. 1988. Differentiation of egg drop syndrome virus isolates by restriction endonuclease analysis of virus DNA. Avian Pathol 17:909–919.

53. Van Eck, J.H.H. F.G. Davelaar, T.A.M. Van den Heuvel-Plesman, N. Van Kol, B. Kouwenhoven, and F.H.M. Guldie. 1976. Dropped egg production, soft shelled and shellless eggs associated with appearance of precipitins to adenovirus in flocks of laying fowl. Avian Pathol 5:261–272.

54. Villegas, P., S.H. Kleven, C.S. Eidson, and F. Arnold. 1979. Adenovirus 127 and egg drop syndrome 76: Studies in the USA. Proc 28th West Poultry Dis Conf, pp. 62–64.

55. Watanabe, T., and H. Ohmi. 1983. Susceptibility of guinea fowls to the virus of infectious laryngotracheitis and egg drop syndrome 1976. J Agric Sci (Japan) 28:193–200.

56. Wigand, R., A. Bartha, R.S. Dreizin, H. Esche, H.S. Ginsberg, M. Green, S.S. Hierholzer, S.S. Kalter, J.B. McFerran, U. Pettersson, W.C. Russell, and G. Wadell. 1982. Adenoviridae: Second report. Intervirology 18:169–176.

57. Yamaguchi, S., H. Imada, H. Kawamura, T. Taniguchi, H. Saio, and K. Shimamatsu. 1981. Outbreaks of egg drop syndrome—1976 in Japan and its etiological agent. Avian Dis 25:628–641.

58. Yamaguchi, S., T. Imada, H. Kawamura, T. Taniguchi, and M. Kawakami. 1981. Pathogenicity and distribution of egg drop syndrome 1976 virus (JPA-1) in inoculated laying hens. Avian Dis 25:642–649.

59. Zakharchuk, A.N., Kruglyak, V.A., Akopian, T.A., Naroditsky, B.S., and Tikchonenko, T.I. 1993. Physical mapping and homology studies of egg drop syndrome (EDS-76) adenovirus DNA. Arch Virol 128:171–176.

60. Zanella, A., A. Di Donato, A. Nigrelli, and G. Poli. 1980. Egg drop syndrome (EDS 76). Etiopathogenesis, epidemiology, immunology and control of the disease. Clin Vet 103:459–469.

61. Zhu, G.Q., and Wang, Y.K.. 1994. Study on egg drop syndrome 1976 (EDS-76) and its control. J Jiangsu Agric Coll 15:5–13.

62. Zsak, L., and J. Kisary. 1981. Some biological and physico-chemical properties of egg drop syndrome (EDS) avian adenovirus strain B8/78. Arch Virol 68:211–219.

63. Zsak, L., A. Szekely, and J. Kisary. 1982. Experimental infection of young and laying geese with egg drop syndrome 1976 adenovirus strain B8/78. Avian Pathol 11:555–562.

24 Pox

Deoki N. Tripathy and Willie M. Reed

INTRODUCTION. Pox is a common viral disease of domestic birds (chickens, turkeys, pigeons, and canaries) and has been reported in more than 60 species of wild birds representing 20 families. It is a slow-spreading disease characterized by the development of discrete nodular proliferative skin lesions on the nonfeathered parts of the body (cutaneous form) or fibrino-necrotic and proliferative lesions in the mucous membrane of the upper respiratory tract, mouth, and esophagus (diphtheritic form).

In the mild cutaneous form of the disease, flock mortality is usually low, but it may be high with generalized infection, when in diphtheritic form, or when the disease is complicated by other infections or poor environmental conditions.

Avian pox is not of public health significance. It does not generally affect mammals; however, a poxvirus isolated from a rhinoceros (71) was characterized as fowl poxvirus.

HISTORY. Pox has long been observed in several avian species. The term *fowl pox* initially included all pox infections of birds, but now it is often used to refer to the disease of commercial poultry, e.g., chickens and turkeys. Woodruff and Goodpasture (145, 146, 147) presented evidence that the virus particles (Borrel bodies) within the inclusion bodies (Bollinger bodies) were the etiologic agent of fowl poxvirus. Ledingham and Aberd (65) demonstrated that antisera produced against fowl poxvirus after immunization or following recovery agglutinated a suspension of elementary bodies of fowl poxvirus.

INCIDENCE AND DISTRIBUTION. Avian poxviruses infect birds of both sexes and all ages and breeds. Naturally occurring poxvirus infections have been reported in approximately 60 species of wild birds, representing about 20 families (57). The disease is worldwide in distribution (89).

ETIOLOGY. Avian poxviruses (fowl, turkey, pigeon, canary, junco, quail, sparrow, and starling) are members of the genus *Avipoxvirus* of the family *Poxviridae* (41, 134). Cross-protection studies indicate that psittacine poxvirus and mynah poxvirus are perhaps different members of the genus (16, 98, 100). Fowl poxvirus is the type species of the genus.

Morphology. Like other genera of the *Poxviridae* family, all avian poxviruses show identical morphology. The mature virus (elementary body) is brick shaped and measures about 250 x 354 nm. It consists of an electron-dense centrally located biconcave core or nucleoid and two lateral bodies in each concavity and envelope (Fig. 24.1). The outer coat is composed of random arrangements of surface tubules (26) (Fig. 24.2). In a recent study, Dubochet et al. (36) did not find a dumbbell-shaped core or lateral bodies when vaccinia virus was analyzed by cryoelectron microscopy. Instead, a brick-shaped homogenous core was detected, suggesting that the dumbbell shapes of the core and lateral bodies were preparation artifacts in negatively stained, conventionally embedded samples.

Chemical Composition. The main components of the virus are protein, DNA, and lipid. The virus has a particle weight of 2.04×10^{-14} g and contains 7.51×10^{-15} g protein, 4.03×10^{-16} g DNA, and 5.54×10^{-15} g lipid (96). Nearly one-third of fowl poxvirus is lipid. Squalene as a major lipid component, and elevation of cholesterol esters was detected in virus preparation from infected chick scalp epithelium (67, 139). The average weight of the inclusion body is about 6.1×10^{-7} mg, 50% of which is extractable lipids. The protein content per inclusion body is 7.69×10^{-8} mg, and the average weight of DNA per inclusion is 6.64×10^{-9} mg (95).

Hemagglutinin has been detected in some strains of pigeon poxvirus (47, 113) and in a strain of fowl poxvirus (137).

VIRAL GENOME. Electron microscopic studies of contour length measurements revealed that the fowl poxvirus genome was a single linear, double-stranded DNA molecule of approximately 200×10^6 daltons (54). However, sedimentation analyses in neutral and alkaline sucrose gradients (46) and summation of the molecular weights of the DNA

Contributions of Dr. Charles H. Cunningham to previous chapters are gratefully acknowledged.

643

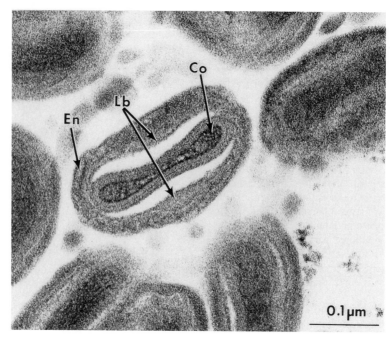

24.1. Ultrathin section of an avian poxvirus from cutaneous eyelid lesion in a dove. Co, core; Lb, lateral bodies; En, envelope. (Basgall)

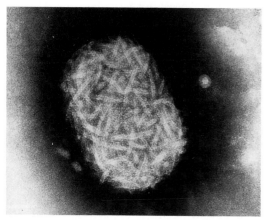

24.2. Negatively stained fowl poxvirus showing random distribution of surface tubules. (Carter and Cheville, Avian Dis)

fragments obtained after restriction endonuclease digestion indicated the molecular weight of fowl poxvirus genome to be approximately 160–185 x 10^6 d (84). The G+C content of fowl poxvirus DNA is about 35%. The fowl poxvirus genome size has been estimated to be from 254 to 300 kb (32, 77, 151).

The electrophoretic profiles of restriction enzyme-digested fowl poxvirus and vaccinia virus DNAs are distinct (84, 103). In spite of this apparent lack of genomic similarity, at least some con-servation has been maintained at the nucleotide and amino acid levels. A 3.1-kb fowl poxvirus DNA fragment, which hybridizes to vaccinia virus Hind III J fragment, contains six open reading frames similar in size, sequence, and relative positions to those contained in the corresponding DNA fragments in vaccinia virus (35). However, the fowl poxvirus counterpart to the internally located vaccinia virus thymidine kinase (TK) gene is located elsewhere. Similar observations have been made by Binns et al. (14). The TK gene of fowl poxvirus has been identified and sequenced (20, 22). It has an open reading frame of 183 codons, which is homologous at the nucleotide and deduced amino acid levels with the vaccinia virus TK gene. The DNA fragment containing quail poxvirus TK gene has been cloned and identified (104). It shows moderate homology to the fowl poxvirus TK gene. Even though fowl and quail poxviruses belong to the same genus, their genomic profiles are markedly different. It appears that fowl and quail poxvirus TK genes may be confined to different loci of their genomes.

The nucleotide sequence of the DNA polymerase gene of fowl poxvirus has been reported (13). When the DNA sequence of fowl poxvirus enzyme is compared with that of vaccinia virus DNA polymerase, only approximately 60% of the nucleotides are conserved. A strong homology is observed, however, when amino acid sequences of fowl poxvirus and vaccinia virus DNA polymerases are compared.

POLYPEPTIDES. Twenty-eight polypeptides were detected in purified fowl poxvirus by Obijeski et al. (88). Mockett et al. (76) observed about 30 structural polypeptides in fowl poxvirus, most of which were immunogenic. Twenty-one fowl poxvirus-coded polypeptides were resolved by ^{35}S methionine pulse labeling, and 57 major structural polypeptides were identified in purified fowl poxvirus preparations (93). Several major and minor immunogenic polypeptides of fowl poxvirus strains have been resolved by immunoblotting (86, 103).

Replication.   The cytoplasmic site of DNA synthesis and packaging within the infectious virus particle is characteristic of poxviruses. Noteworthy information on replication of poxviruses has been reviewed by Moss (23, 82). Replication of avian poxviruses appears to be similar in dermal or follicular epithelium of chicken, ectodermal cells of the chorioallantoic membrane (CAM), and embryo skin cells. Differences in the host cell and virus strain, however, may reflect in the time scale and virus output.

Biosynthesis of fowl poxvirus in dermal epithelium involves two distinct phases: a host response characterized by marked cellular hyperplasia during the first 72 hr and synthesis of infectious virus from 72 to 96 hr (27, 28).

The replication of viral DNA in dermal epithelium begins between 12 and 24 hr postinfection (PI) and is followed by the first appearance of infectious virus at 22–24 hr. Epithelial hyperplasia between 36–48 hr ends in a 2.5-fold increase in cell number at 72 hr. The rate of viral DNA synthesis is low during the first 60 hr of infection. Enhancement in the rate of viral DNA synthesis occurs between 60 and 72 hr concomitantly with a sharp decline of cellular DNA synthesis. Between 72 and 96 hr, the synthesis of viral DNA becomes progressively more

prominent, and no further hyperplasia is observed (27, 28). Swallen (110) demonstrated by autoradiography that chicken epidermis infected for 48 hr with fowl poxvirus shows a threefold higher percentage of labeled nuclei as compared with controls, indicating that infection is associated with an increased incidence of intranuclear DNA synthesis. Both viral RNA and DNA were detected by hybridization in the nucleus of infected cells 24–72 hr after infection (45).

Infection of chicken embryo skin cell culture involves an increase in virus titer at 16 hr after infection with evidence of cytopathic effects (CPE). Although the viral titer continues to increase for up to 36 hr, the rate of titer increase declines between 36 and 48 hr PI. A total increase in fowl poxvirus titer of 100-fold is observed over the growth period. Fowl poxvirus DNA replication occurs between 12 and 16 hr PI, which continues up to 48 hr PI (93).

Ultrastructural studies have been made on the morphogenesis of the virus in various developmental stages that lead to mature virions (4, 5, 29, 101). After adsorption to and penetration of the cell membrane by fowl poxvirus, 1 hr after infection of dermal epithelium (5) and 2 hr after infection of CAM (4), there is uncoating of the virus before synthesis of new virus from the precursor material. At 48 hr, areas of viroplasm with incomplete membranes around them are present in the cytoplasm. Inclusion bodies are present at 72 hr after infection of dermal epithelium (5) and at 96 hr after infection of the CAM (4). The type A inclusions may contain virions within or toward the periphery. Similar inclusions have been observed in fowl, canary, and pigeon poxviruses and perhaps occur in all avian poxviruses. Fowl poxvirus emerges from cells of the CAM by a budding process, with acquisition of an additional outer membrane obtained from the cell membrane (Fig. 24.3).

An avian poxvirus isolated from *Junco hyemalis*

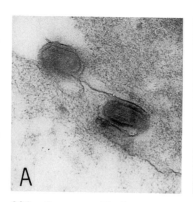 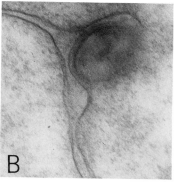 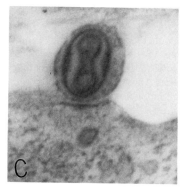

24.3.   Emergence of fowl poxvirus from cells of chorioallantoic membrane. *A, B.* Particles appear to be budding from surface, and cell membrane appears to surround virus. *C.* Virus is separated from cell and completely enclosed by outer layer obtained from cell membrane. *A.* ×43,000; *B, C.* ×62,000. (Arhelger and Randall, Virology)

produced nuclear inclusions in addition to cytoplasmic inclusions (12). However, the intranuclear inclusions are devoid of viral particles.

Although poxviruses are assembled exclusively in the cytoplasm of infected cells, Gafford and Randall (45) found that the nucleus participates in the complexities of fowl poxvirus replication, since viral RNA and DNA were detected in the nucleus of infected cells 24–72 hr PI.

Resistance to Chemical and Physical Agents. Resistance to ether treatment is listed as one of the taxonomic criterion for poxviruses (68). While some authors (96) stated that the virus was sensitive to both ether and chloroform, others (113) reported that a pigeon poxvirus and its two mutants were resistant to both chloroform and ether. A poxvirus isolate from a peacock was ether resistant but chloroform sensitive (2). Fowl poxvirus is known to withstand 1% phenol and 1:1000 formalin for 9 days but is inactivated by 1% caustic potash when freed from its matrix. Heating at 50 C for 30 min or 60 C for 8 min also inactivates the virus (3). Trypsin is without effect on the DNA or whole virus (97). When desiccated, the virus shows marked resistance. It can survive in dried scabs for months or even years.

Strain Classification. A nucleoprotein precipitinogen is common to all poxviruses (144). Avian poxviruses are antigenically and immunologically distinguishable from each other, but varying degrees of cross relationships do exist. Attempts have been made to differentiate strains by immunologic methods, e.g., complement-fixation, passive hemagglutination, agar gel precipitation, immunoperoxidase, virus neutralization, and immunofluorescence. Genomic characterization by restriction endonuclease analysis of DNA and antigenic characterization of immunogenic proteins by immunoblotting has been useful to some extent in detecting minor differences among the strains tested (86, 103). While fowl, pigeon, and junco poxvirus DNAs have similar genomic profiles, restriction endonuclease analysis of quail, canary, and mynah poxvirus DNA revealed marked differences from fowl poxvirus. Similarly, quail poxvirus shows distinct antigenic differences from fowl poxvirus by immunoblotting, although some common proteins are also detected (49).

Laboratory Host Systems

BIRDS. Avian poxviruses affect a wide range of birds of various families by naturally occurring or artificial infection. Chickens commonly used to determine the pathogenicity of new avian poxvirus isolates may not be suitable hosts because of their lack of susceptibility.

A substantial degree of host specificity exists among some avian poxviruses, especially those that infect wild birds. A poxvirus from a flicker (*Colaptes auratus*) (59) revealed strict host specificity when several species of wild and domestic birds were tested for susceptibility (60). Avian poxvirus strains isolated from various species of thrushes (*Turdidae*) did not protect chickens against fowl poxvirus (61). Differences in host susceptibility were also observed when a poxvirus isolated from parrots was inoculated into susceptible parrots and chickens. Although it was more pathogenic for parrots than chickens, it did not provide protection against fowl poxvirus. Further, vaccination of chickens with either fowl or pigeon poxvirus vaccine did not provide protection against the psittacine poxvirus (16). A poxvirus from a Canada goose (*Branta canadensis*) was transmissible to domestic geese but not to chickens or to domestic ducks (33). Sparrows and canaries were highly susceptible to a poxvirus isolated during an outbreak from sparrows, but produced mild, local cutaneous reaction in chickens, turkeys, and pigeons (50). Chickens and pigeons were found refractory to infection with an avian poxvirus isolated from a buzzard (*Accipiter nisus*) by Tantwai et al. (114). In an aviary housing over 100 birds of a variety of species, only Rothchild's mynahs (*Leucospar rothchildii*) were infected with an avian poxvirus. The virus, however, was pathogenic for starlings in the surroundings, but did not infect chickens. Mynahs and starlings are members of the family *Sturnidae* and starling pox has been reported specific for that family (64). Poxvirus strains from magpies (*Pica pica*) and great tits (*Parus major*) did not infect young chickens (53); however, an avian poxvirus isolated from a black-backed magpie produced lesions in chickens but was related more closely to pigeon than fowl poxvirus (31). Poxvirus strains from various species of grouse immunized chickens against fowl poxvirus challenge (60). High pathogenicity for chickens of a virus isolated from captive peacocks (*Pavo cristatus*) in a zoologic park indicated a close relationship of this virus to fowl poxvirus (2). The peacocks had been vaccinated with a fowl poxvirus vaccine but were the only birds affected among other wild and domestic birds in the aviary. An isolate of poxvirus from previously vaccinated turkeys was antigenically different from fowl poxvirus (143). Poxvirus isolated from cutaneous proliferative lesions of greater hill mynah (*Gracula religiosa*) imported from Malaysia produced severe necrotizing and proliferative lesions in chickens and bobwhite quail previously vaccinated with fowl, pigeon, or quail poxviruses (98, 100).

Studies on differentiation of fowl, canary, turkey, and pigeon poxviruses based on pathogenicity for chickens, turkeys, pigeons, ducks, and canaries (48,

69) have been summarized (125). Canaries are highly susceptible to canary poxvirus, but show resistance to turkey, fowl, and pigeon poxviruses. The pigeon poxvirus produces milder infection in chickens and turkeys, but is more pathogenic for pigeons. Susceptibility of ducks to turkey poxvirus and not to fowl poxvirus has been suggested for differentiation of these two closely related viruses.

AVIAN EMBRYOS. Developing chicken embryos are commonly employed for propagation of avian poxvirus on the CAM (34, 145). Duck and turkey embryos have been used, as well as other species of avian embryos. Typically, infection of chicken embryo CAM results in compact, proliferative pock lesions that may be focal or diffuse (Fig. 24.4).

Macroscopic lesions considered to be characteristic for some avian poxviruses have been described (69). Occasionally, isolates from wild birds fail to grow on the CAM of chicken embryos.

Quantitative assay of viral infectivity may be by the embryo infective dose-50% (EID_{50}) method or by the "pock counting enumerative dose" response (34).

CELL CULTURE. Avian poxviruses can be propagated in cell cultures of avian origin, e.g., chicken embryo fibroblasts, chicken embryo dermis and kidney cells, and duck embryo fibroblasts. A permanent cell line "QT 35" (81) of Japanese quail origin will support growth of some avian poxviruses after adaptation. Some isolates, especially from turkeys, however, fail to grow in this cell line even after repeated passages (122).

Cytopathic Effects. Characteristic CPE produced by the avian poxviruses in chicken embryo fibroblasts are an initial phase of rounding of the cells

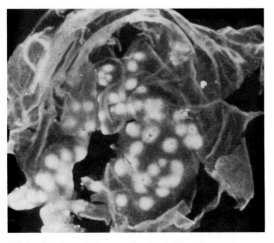

24.4. Fowl pox lesions on the chorioallantoic membrane.

followed by a second phase of degeneration and necrosis. The time sequence of these events and the variations observed with different viruses have been reported (69). Quantitative assay is by the cell culture dose-50% method based on CPE (34).

Plaque Formation. Differences in the plaque-forming ability of avian poxviruses have been observed. Adaptation of the virus in cell culture is necessary, since not all strains produce plaques (7, 79, 113). Plaque formation in monolayers of chicken embryo fibroblast cell cultures by some avian poxviruses has been shown sufficiently characteristic to be considered as an aid in differentiation (69). Plaques are evident by 3–4 days PI in quail cells with certain avian poxviruses after adaptation (103).

PATHOGENESIS AND EPIZOOTIOLOGY

Natural and Experimental Hosts. Fowl and turkey poxvirus infections are economically important diseases in domestic poultry. Among companion birds, avian poxvirus infections most often occur in blue-fronted Amazon parrots and in large aviaries of canaries where the disease is likely to be enzootic because of intimate contact. Canary and psittacine pox is, therefore, of special significance for aviculturists, as this infection can result in high losses in a short time. Severe outbreaks of quail pox in pen-raised quails have been reported. As naturally occurring infection has been reported in approximately 60 species of wild birds representing about 20 families, as well as in caged birds (57, 92), it seems that all avian species are susceptible to avian poxviruses. The infection can occur in susceptible birds of any age.

Pathogenesis of fowl poxvirus infection in chickens inoculated intradermally or intratracheally was similar, with only minor differences. In chickens infected intradermally, the virus was first detected in the skin at the inoculation site on day 2 and in lungs on day 4, followed by detectable viremia on day 5. In chickens infected intratracheally, the virus was first detected in the lungs on day 2, followed by viremia on day 4. The virus was recovered from liver, spleen, kidney, and brain of birds of both groups (109). In chickens inoculated intravenously, miliary nodules were observed in the kidneys 10–18 days PI in addition to cutaneous and diphtheritic lesions on the mucous membrane of the upper respiratory tract. Characteristic microscopic changes including inclusion bodies were observed in the epithelial cells of renal tubules 4–14 days PI, and in the epithelial reticular cells of the thymic medulla 4–10 days PI (112).

Transmission. Poxvirus infection occurs through mechanical transmission of the virus to the injured or lacerated skin. Individuals handling birds at the time of vaccination may carry the virus on their hands and clothing and may unknowingly deposit the virus in the eyes of susceptible birds. Insects also serve as mechanical vectors of the virus, resulting in ocular infection. The virus may reach the laryngeal region via the lacrimal duct to cause infection of the upper respiratory tract (39). In a contaminated environment, the aerosol generated by feathers and dried scabs containing poxvirus particles provides suitable condition for both cutaneous and respiratory infection. Cells of the mucosa of the upper respiratory tract and mouth appear to be highly susceptible to the virus as initiation of infection may occur in the absence of apparent trauma or injury.

Mosquitoes have been shown to be capable of infecting a number of different birds after a single feeding on a bird infected with avian poxvirus. Eleven species of Diptera have been reported as vectors of avian poxvirus (1). The mite, *Dermanyss gallinae,* has been implicated in the spread of fowl poxvirus (107). Mechanical transmission of fowl poxvirus from infected toms to turkey hens through artificial insemination has been reported (74).

In some flocks, the virus may exist as a latent infection (126). Duran Reynals and Bryan (37) showed that cutaneous treatment of chickens and pigeons with methylcholanthrene activated a latent fowl poxvirus infection. Kirmse (59) observed persistent cutaneous lesions of avian poxvirus infection in a yellow-shafted flicker over a period of 13 mo during which intracytoplasmic inclusions were demonstrable in the lesion.

Recently, poxviruses have been isolated in the Midwest, Southeast, and Northwest United States from previously vaccinated flocks experiencing high mortality due to the diphtheritic form and/or cutaneous form of pox. In cross-protection studies, some of these isolates had little or no immunologic relationship to strains of poxviruses used in commercial vaccines, while other isolates had some immunologic relationship to pigeon poxviruses (99). Currently available vaccines are not effective in providing protective immunity against challenge with these "variant" poxviruses (43, 99).

Incubation Period. Incubation period of the naturally occurring disease varies from about 4 to 10 days in chickens, turkeys, and pigeons and is about 4 days in canaries.

Signs. The disease may occur in one of the two forms, cutaneous or diphtheritic, or both. The signs vary depending upon the susceptibility of the host, virulence of the virus, distribution of the lesions, and other complicating factors. The cutaneous form of the disease is characterized by appearance of nodular lesions on the comb, wattle, eyelids, and other nonfeathered areas of the body. In the diphtheritic form (wet pox), cankers or diphtheritic yellowish lesions occur on the mucous membrane of mouth, esophagus, or trachea with accompanying Coryza-like mild or severe respiratory signs when lesions involve the trachea.

Morbidity and Mortality. Morbidity rate of pox in chickens and turkeys varies from a few birds being infected to involvement of the entire flock if a virulent virus is present and no control measures are taken. Birds affected with the cutaneous form of the disease are more likely to recover than those with the diphtheritic form involving the respiratory tract.

Effects of pox in chickens usually involve emaciation and poor weight gain; egg production is temporarily retarded if layers are infected. The course of the disease is about 3–4 wk, but if complications are present duration may be considerably longer.

In turkeys, retardation of growth development of market birds is of greater financial importance than mortality. Blindness due to cutaneous eye lesions and starvation cause most of the losses. If pox occurs in breeding birds, decreased egg production and impaired fertility may result. In uncomplicated mild infections, the course of the disease in a flock may be 2–3 wk. Severe outbreaks often last 6, 7, or even 8 wk.

Flock mortality in chickens and turkeys is usually low, but in severe cases it may be as high as 50%. In pigeons and psittacines, morbidity and mortality rates are similar to those in chickens. Pox in canaries can cause mortality as high as 80–100%. Significant mortality has been observed in quail infected with quail poxvirus.

Gross Lesions. The characteristic lesion of the cutaneous form of pox in chickens is a local epithelial hyperplasia involving epidermis and underlying feather follicles, with formation of nodules that first appear as small white foci and then rapidly increase in size and become yellow. In chickens infected intradermally, few primary lesions appear by the 4th day. Papules are formed by the 5th or 6th day. This is followed by the vesicular stage, with formation of extensive thick lesions (75). Adjoining lesions may coalesce and become rough and gray or dark brown (see Fig. 24.5). After about 2 wk, sometimes sooner, lesions have areas of inflammation at the base and become hemorrhagic. Formation of a scab, which may last for another 1–2 wk, ends with desquamation of the degenerated epithelial layer. If the scab is removed early in its development, there is a moist, seropurulent exudate underneath covering a hemorrhagic granulating surface. When the scab drops off naturally, a smooth scar may be

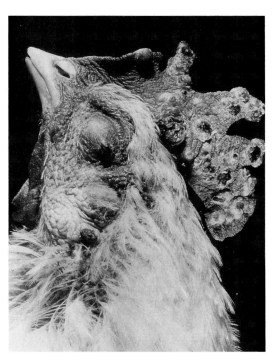

24.5. Fowl pox (cutaneous form). (Shivaprasad)

present; in mild cases, there may be no noticeable scar.

In the diphtheritic form, slightly elevated, white opaque nodules develop on the mucous membranes. Nodules rapidly increase in size and often coalesce to become a yellow, cheesy, necrotic, pseudodiphtheritic, or diphtheritic membrane (Fig. 24.6). If the membranes are removed they leave bleeding erosions. The inflammatory process may extend into sinuses, particularly the infraorbital sinus (resulting in swelling) and also into the pharynx and larynx (resulting in respiratory disturbances) and esophagus.

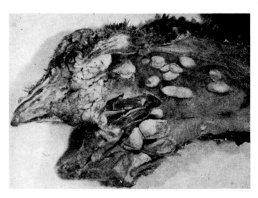

24.6. Fowl pox lesions in mouth and esophagus of turkey. (Hinshaw)

The first indication of pox in turkeys is seen as minute yellowish eruptions on the dewlap, snood, and other head parts. They are soft and easily removed in this pustular stage, leaving an inflamed area covered with a sticky serous exudate. The corners of the mouth, eyelids, and oral membranes are commonly affected. Lesions enlarge and become covered with a dry scab or a yellow-red or brown wartlike mass. In young poults, the head, legs, and feet may be completely covered with lesions. The disease may even spread to the feathered parts of the body. In an unusual outbreak of poxvirus in breeding turkeys, proliferative lesions occurred in the oviduct, cloaca, and skin surrounding the vent (74).

Histopathology. The most important feature of infection (whether the lesion is cutaneous, diphtheritic, or from the infected CAM) is hyperplasia of the epithelium and enlargement of cells, with associated inflammatory changes. Characteristic eosinophilic A-type cytoplasmic inclusion bodies (Bollinger bodies) are observable by light microscopy (Fig. 24.7).

Histopathologic changes of tracheal mucosa include initial hypertrophy and hyperplasia of mucus-producing cells, with subsequent enlargement of epithelial cells that contain eosinophilic cytoplasmic inclusion bodies. Often, clusters of epithelial

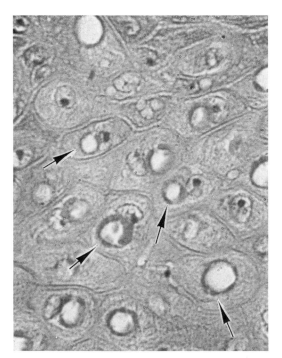

24.7. Cutaneous epithelium infected with fowl poxvirus. Infected cells are enlarged and contain cytoplasmic inclusion bodies (*arrows*).

cells resemble a papilloma (111). Inclusion bodies may be present in various stages of development, depending on the time after infection. The inclusion body may occupy almost the entire cytoplasm, with resulting cell necrosis.

Immunity. Actively acquired immunity against avian poxviruses results from recovery from naturally occurring infection or vaccination. Cell-mediated and humoral immunity following vaccination or naturally occurring infection provides protection (8, 78, 126). Cell-mediated immunity develops earlier than the humoral antibody response.

DIAGNOSIS. Methods for diagnosis, prevention, and control are also available in other publications (34, 123, 124).

Clinical Diagnosis. Cutaneous lesions typical of avian pox (see Fig. 24.5) must be confirmed by either histopathology (presence of cytoplasmic inclusions) or virus isolation. The diphtheritic form of the disease (see Fig. 24.6) in chickens with associated respiratory signs must be differentiated from infectious laryngotracheitis, an infection caused by a herpesvirus.

Lesions caused by pantothenic acid or biotin deficiency in young chicks (6) or by T-2 toxin (30, 149) could be mistaken for pox lesions. Diphtheritic pox lesions in doves and pigeons may be mistaken for lesions caused by *Trichomonas gallinae,* which are diagnosed by microscopic examination of smears or by culture.

Microscopy. Elementary bodies (Borrel bodies) of fowl poxvirus can be detected in smears prepared from lesions and stained with Wright's stain or by the Gimenez method (127). Tissue sections from cutaneous (see Fig. 24.7) or diphtheritic lesions may be processed by conventional methods (27) or by using a solution that fixes and dehydrates tissues simultaneously (105) for detection of cytoplasmic inclusions. Various histochemical and histopathologic techniques are described by Thompson and Hunt (121).

Electron microscopy can be employed for demonstration of virus particles in lesions and exudate by negative staining or in ultrathin sections of the infected tissues (73, 101, 138). Type A inclusions with virions around the periphery or virus-filled inclusions may be observed on electron microscopic examination.

Isolation and Identification of Virus

BIRD INOCULATION. Avian poxviruses can be transmitted to susceptible birds by applying a suspension of the lesion material from infected birds to scarified comb or denuded feather follicles of the thigh, or by the wing-web stick method. Fowl poxvirus can be transmitted readily from chicken to chicken, with typical cutaneous lesions developing in 5–7 days (see Fig. 24.5). In atypical cases, microscopy of lesion specimens may be advisable, as well as bird inoculation.

EMBRYO INOCULATION. A suspension of specimen from a dermal or diphtheritic lesion is inoculated on the CAM of 9- to 12-day-old developing chicken embryos from a specific-pathogen–free flock; 5–7 days after inoculation the CAM is examined for pock lesions (see Fig. 24.4). Occasionally, some isolates fail to grow on the CAM of chicken embryos (33, 59).

CELL CULTURE. Cell cultures are not generally employed for initial isolation of avian poxviruses. Adaptation of the virus to this host system is sometimes necessary, since not all strains produce CPE on initial inoculation.

IMMUNOLOGY AND SEROLOGY

Protection Tests. Protection tests are generally used to determine immunogenicity of fowl and pigeon pox vaccines. At least five susceptible birds are vaccinated according to directions of the manufacturer. An additional five nonvaccinated and isolated birds of the same source and age are kept as controls. At least 10 days after vaccination, vaccinated and control birds are challenged with a different strain of fowl poxvirus capable of causing clinical signs of pox in at least 80% of the control birds. The challenge virus may be applied to the skin of denuded feather follicles of the thigh, to scarified comb, or by the wing-web method at a site opposite that used for vaccination. The birds should be examined for takes (see Immunization). For satisfactory immunization, at least 80% of the controls should have lesions of fowl pox and at least 80% of the vaccinated birds should not.

Cross-protection tests for the antigenic relationship of the avian poxviruses are not generally practical for routine diagnosis but may be necessary for their antigenic characterization (98, 142).

Immunodiffusion. Immunodiffusion may be used for differential identification of fowl and pigeon poxviruses or antibody from those of other avian viral diseases (56, 136).

As precipitating antibodies are detectable for only a short duration after infection, serum must be collected at the appropriate time, usually 15–20 days after known infection.

Passive Hemagglutination. A passive hemagglutination test detects antibodies in serum of chickens earlier than the immunodiffusion test (31, 132).

Neutralization. Virus neutralization in cell culture (80) or chicken embryos (7) may be used; however, this procedure is not practical as a routine diagnostic test.

Fluorescent Antibody and Enzyme-Linked Immunosorbent Assay Tests. An indirect fluorescent antibody, immunoperoxidase, or enzyme-linked immunosorbent assay (ELISA) test can be used for detection of antibody (24, 76, 133).

Immunoblotting. Immunogenic proteins of vaccine and field strains of fowl poxvirus can be compared by immunoblotting. Common antigens are detected among strains (Fig. 24.8A). However, the strains can be differentiated by unique proteins of differing electrophoretic mobilities (86, 103).

Restriction Endonuclease Analysis of Avian Poxvirus DNA. Restriction endonuclease analysis is among the most sensitive methods for comparing closely related DNA genomes, since a single base change in recognition sequence may cause a change in restriction endonuclease profile. Müller et al. (84) reported differences of fowl poxvirus from vaccinia virus by the examination of the pattern of DNA fragments by their relative mobilities. Recently genomes of fowl, pigeon, and junco poxviruses were compared by restriction enzyme analysis using Bam HI and HindIII endonuclease digestion and subsequent agarose gel electrophoresis (103). The genetic profiles of these strains were similar, with a high proportion of comigrating fragments, although most strains could still be distinguished by presence or absence of one or two DNA fragments (Fig. 24.8B). The characteristic electrophoretic profile of restriction endonuclease digested DNA has facilitated comparison of other members of the *Avipoxvirus* genus. Genomic profiles of quail, canary, and mynah poxviruses are different from the profile of fowl poxvirus (122).

Genomic Fragments as Diagnostic Probes. Cloned genomic fragments of fowl poxvirus can be used effectively as nucleic acid probes for diagnosis of fowl poxvirus infection (128, 135). In this procedure, viral DNA isolated from lesions is hybridized with either ^{32}p-labeled or nonradioactive labeled genomic probes. This method is especially useful for differentiation of the diphtheritic form of fowl pox from infectious laryngotracheitis when tracheal lesions are present (44).

Polymerase Chain Reaction. Genomic DNA sequences of various sizes can be amplified by poly-merase chain reaction (PCR) using specific primers (130). This technique is useful when an extremely small amount of virus is present in the sample.

TREATMENT, PREVENTION, AND CONTROL.
There is no specific treatment for birds infected with avian poxviruses. Proper husbandry should be practiced to alleviate environmental stress.

Immunization. Two types of live virus vaccines are used for immunization of birds against pox: fowl pox and pigeon pox vaccines. These should contain a minimum concentration of 10^5 EID_{50}/mL (48, 141) to establish satisfactory takes for good immunity. Fowl pox and pigeon pox vaccines labeled "chick embryo origin" are prepared from the infected CAM. Fowl pox vaccine labeled "tissue culture origin" is prepared from chicken embryo fibroblast cultures. A fowl poxvirus vaccine strain adapted to chicken embryo dermis cell cultures was more economical with more uniformity than conventional vaccine prepared on the CAM of chicken embryos (40).

Success of a vaccination program depends on potency and purity of the vaccine and its application under conditions for which it is specifically intended. Vaccination essentially produces a mild form of the disease. Directions for use of vaccine as supplied by the producer should be followed explicitly. Vaccine should not be used in a flock affected with other diseases or in generally poor condition. All birds within a house should be vaccinated on the same day. Other susceptible birds on the premises should be isolated from those being vaccinated. If pox appears in a flock in an initial outbreak, with only a few birds affected, nonaffected birds should be vaccinated.

A vaccine vial should be opened immediately before use. Only one vial should be opened at a time, and the entire contents should be used within 2 hr. After vaccine is prepared, the vaccinator's hands should be washed thoroughly. Vaccine should contact the bird only at the site for vaccination. Extreme precautions should be taken not to contaminate other parts of the bird, the premises, or miscellaneous equipment.

All contaminated vaccine equipment, unused vaccine, empty vials, etc., should be decontaminated, preferably by incineration. No prepared vaccine should be saved for later use.

FOWL POX VACCINE. The "chick embryo origin" vaccine contains live, nonattenuated fowl poxvirus capable of producing serious disease in a flock if used improperly.

Fowl pox vaccine is applied by the wing-web method to 4-wk-old chickens and to pullets about

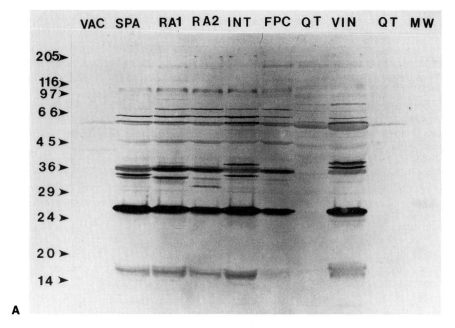

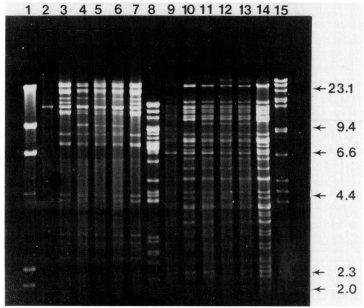

24.8. Strain variation in antigenic and DNA composition. *A.* Immunoblotting of soluble antigens of avian poxviruses. Antigens prepared from uninfected cells (QT) or cells infected
with vaccinia (VAC) or fowl poxvirus strains Spafas (SPA), Randall-1 (RA1), Randall-2
(RA2), Intervet (INT), C (FPC), and Vineland (VIN). Proteins were separated by sulfate–polyacrylamide gel electrophoresis (SDS–PAGE) and transferred to nitrocellulose.
Viral antigens were detected by reaction with chicken antifowl pox virus serum. (Schnitzlein, Virus Res) *B.* Agarose gel electrophoresis analysis of avian poxvirus DNA from
strains FPC (lanes 2 and 9), Vineland (lanes 3 and 10), UI (lanes 4 and 11), Sterwin
(lanes 5 and 12), Salsbury (lanes 6 and 13), CEVA (lanes 7 and 14), and vaccinia (lanes 8
and 15) after cleavage with BamHI (lanes 2 through 8) or HindIII (lanes 9 through 15).
Lane 1 is a HindIII digestion profile of lambda phage DNA, and the size of its fragments
(kb) are shown on the *right-hand side* of the gel. (Schnitzlein, Virus Res)

1–2 mo before egg production is expected to start. It is also used to revaccinate chickens held for the 2nd yr of egg production. The vaccine is not to be used on hens while they are laying.

Attenuated fowl poxvirus vaccines of cell culture origin can be used effectively on chicks as young as 1 day of age and have been used at times in combination with Marek's disease vaccine (38, 108).

Oral vaccination with an attenuated cell culture vaccine has been reported effective in Germany (70). Comparative immunity of fowl poxvirus vaccines by intramuscular, feather follicle, oral, and intranasal routes in chickens of different age groups was recently evaluated by Sharma and Sharma (106). They reported that oral vaccination did not provide protection over 50%, while other methods provided 80–100% protection. Nagy et al. (85) reported that 1-day-old chicks can be effectively vaccinated against fowl pox through drinking water when the vaccine contains a sufficiently high concentration of virus (10^6 cell culture infective dose-50%/mL).

Turkeys may be vaccinated by the wing-web method, but the virus may spread and infect the head region. The site of choice for vaccination is about midway on the thigh. Initially, turkeys are vaccinated when they are 2–3 mo old, but those to be used as breeders should be revaccinated before production. Revaccination at 3- to 4-mo intervals during the laying season might be of some advantage, depending on the level of risk.

Fowl pox vaccine is not to be used on pigeons.

PIGEON POX VACCINE. Pigeon pox vaccine contains live, nonattenuated, naturally occurring virus for pigeons. If used improperly, the vaccine can cause a severe reaction in these birds. The virus is less pathogenic for chickens and turkeys.

Pigeon pox vaccine may be applied by the wing-web method and can be used on chickens of any age. It is generally used, however, on 4-wk-old chickens and about 1 mo before egg production is expected to start. When birds younger than 4 wk are vaccinated, they should be revaccinated before start of production. Birds held for the 2nd yr of production should be revaccinated.

Turkeys can be vaccinated at any age by the wing-web or thigh stick methods. Day-old poults can be vaccinated if necessary, but it is better to wait until they are about 8 wk old for a better immune response. Revaccination may be necessary and advisable during the growing period. Turkeys retained as breeders should be revaccinated.

Pigeons can be vaccinated by the wing-web method. The vaccine can be applied by the feather follicle method, but this is not generally employed. Differences in the immunizing properties of pigeon pox vaccines have been observed (148).

Recently, an experimental bivalent pox vaccine composed of fowl and pigeon poxviruses has been demonstrated to provide protective immunity against fowl pox in chickens (42).

CANARY POX VACCINE. A live chicken embryo-attenuated canary poxvirus vaccine has been used effectively in canaries under experimental conditions (52, 72). A modified live-virus canary poxvirus vaccine is currently available commercially in the United States.

QUAIL POX VACCINE. A live vaccine of quail poxvirus origin is available commercially for use in quail, chickens, and turkeys. It does not provide protection against fowl poxvirus infection (142).

TURKEY POX VACCINE. A live nonattenuated vaccine is commercially available for use in turkeys. The vaccine does not provide adequate protection against fowl, pigeon, or quail poxviruses (143).

VACCINE TAKES. The flock should be examined about 7–10 days after vaccination for evidence of "takes." A "take" consists of swelling of the skin or a scab at the site where vaccine was applied and is evidence of successful vaccination. Immunity will normally develop in 10–14 days after vaccination. If the vaccine is properly applied to susceptible birds, the majority should have takes. In large flocks, at least 10% of the birds should be examined for takes.

The lack of a take could be the result of vaccine being applied to an immune bird, use of a vaccine of inadequate potency (after the expiration date or subjected to deleterious influences), or improper application.

PROPHYLACTIC VACCINATION. Immunization against pox consists of vaccinating susceptible birds prior to the time the disease is likely to occur. This is usually done during spring and summer in areas where the disease occurs in fall and winter. In tropical climates, where the disease may occur throughout the year, vaccination may be done at any time when warranted without regard to the season.

Vaccination is indicated under three conditions: 1) When a flock on the premises was infected the previous year. All young stock produced on the premises or introduced from other sources should receive fowl pox vaccine. 2) If pox was present the previous year and pigeon pox vaccine was used, birds should be revaccinated with fowl pox vaccine, because immunity from pigeon pox vaccine is not of long duration. 3) In areas where pox is prevalent, fowl pox vaccine should be used for protection against infection from neighboring flocks.

RECOMBINANT VACCINES

Recombinant Fowl Poxvirus Vaccines. The pox viruses have some unique features, e.g., cytoplasmic site of multiplication, large genome, and unique viral enzymes and transcription system, which allow the expression of a foreign gene in a faithful manner. Since the first demonstration in 1982 of the insertion and expression of the herpes simplex virus TK gene, a large variety of genes from specific pathogens, representing genetic elements responsible for specific immune responses, have been inserted into the genome of vaccinia virus. The early recombinant DNA studies on vaccinia virus (83) provided great impetus toward development of fowl poxvirus as an expression vector for genes from poultry pathogens. At approximately 300 kb (32, 151), the genome of fowl poxvirus is large enough to accommodate a significant amount of foreign DNA without a corresponding reduction in virus infectivity. The physical and biologic characteristics of fowl poxvirus endow it with several advantages for use as an expression vector. First, fowl poxvirus vaccines have been used in commercial poultry for over 70 years. The vaccine virus causes a mild, localized self-limiting infection. In addition, fowl poxvirus has a narrow host range affecting only avian species. The virus can be propagated in primary cultures of chicken embryo fibroblasts, chicken-embryo kidney cells, or skin cells, and also in permanent cell lines such as the Japanese quail cell line, QT35. Finally, because of its large size, genes from more than one pathogen probably can be inserted into its genome in order to create a polyvalent vaccine.

In order to develop a live recombinant fowl poxvirus, it is important to insert stably the foreign gene(s) of interest from a poultry pathogen into the fowl poxvirus genome, express the gene(s) optimally, and still maintain the infectivity of the virus. Thus, the generation of a fowl poxvirus expression vector requires 1) a suitable nonessential region in the fowl poxvirus genome for insertion of foreign genetic material so that virus replication is not disrupted, 2) a foreign gene that encodes for a protective antigen of a poultry pathogen, 3) a strong poxvirus promoter that will optimally regulate the expression of the inserted foreign gene(s), 4) a donor plasmid that incorporates these three features, and 5) a method for the selection and/or detection of recombinant progeny virus.

Nonessential Region. Several nonessential regions, including some in the terminal inverted repeats, have been identified in the fowl poxvirus genome (18, 21, 90, 116, 150). One commonly used insertion site for foreign sequences in the fowl poxvirus genome is the TK gene. This gene was first identified based on its ability to marker-rescue

TK⁻ vaccinia virus (20). Subsequently, the TK genes of fowl and quail poxviruses were identified by using a degenerate oligonucleotide probe representing a conserved region in the 3′ portion of several TK genes (103). The TK gene of pigeon poxvirus (66) was identified based upon the close genetic relationship between fowl and pigeon poxviruses. Since TK activity is not required for avian poxvirus multiplication, the encoding gene provides a convenient site for the insertion of a foreign gene(s). In addition, insertional inactivation of the TK gene reduces the virulence of the recombinant fowl poxvirus as compared to the unaltered parental virus (129).

Regulatory Sequences (Promoters). Since fowl poxvirus encodes its DNA-dependent RNA polymerase, which does not recognize promoters from other organisms, poxvirus promoters are necessary for expression of the inserted foreign genes. Poxvirus promoters are relatively conserved, and thus are recognized by heterologous poxviruses (20, 21, 102, 116, 131). Initially, therefore, vaccinia virus promoters were used in lieu of fowl poxvirus transcription regulatory elements in creating recombinant fowl poxviruses. Although homologous fowl poxvirus promoters have since been identified (15, 62, 63, 151) and a synthetic, early-late transcriptional regulatory element was recently utilized (25, 150), two vaccinia virus promoters, the early-late P7.5 and the late P11, are still predominately used for the construction of recombinant avian poxviruses.

Donor Plasmid. To create a recombinant virus, a donor plasmid that directs the insertion of foreign DNA into the fowl poxvirus genome must be constructed. In such a plasmid, contiguous fowl poxvirus DNA sequences are interrupted by a foreign gene(s) regulated by poxvirus promoter(s). Following introduction of this plasmid into virus-infected cells, in vivo recombination occurs in the cytoplasm between the homologous sequences of the replicating fowl poxvirus genome and those that flank the foreign genes in the plasmid DNA. This interaction results in the insertion of the foreign transcriptional unit into the fowl poxvirus genome.

Procedure for Selection of Recombinant Viruses. Since more than 99% of the progeny virus from a transfection is of parental type, a method for the selection and/or identification of recombinant virus is required. Although insertion of a foreign gene into the TK locus causes elimination of TK activity, in the absence of a TK⁻ avian cell line, recombinant virus progeny could not be selected based on this phenotype. Thus, recombinant viruses are usually identified and/or selected based on expression of a marker gene that is inserted adjacent to the other foreign gene. If the *Escherichia coli lacZ* gene is used for this purpose, recombinant viruses are screened for their ability to express ß-galactosidase (*lacZ* gene product) by the inclusion of the enzyme's histochemical substrates, X-gal or Bluo-gal, in agarose overlays of infected cells (91, 94, 102). Plaques arising from infection by recombinant viruses appear blue, due to hydrolysis of these compounds, against a background of colorless plaques generated by nonrecombinant viruses. Alternatively, recombinants carrying the *E. coli* xanthine phosphoribosyl transferase gene as a marker can be selected due to their resistance to mycophenolic acid (21). In addition, recombinant viruses have been identified by plaque hybridization using a DNA probe specific for the inserted foreign gene (18, 116) and by differences in plaque morphology (66).

Using molecular techniques described above, recombinant fowl or pigeon poxvirus vaccines capable of expressing genes from several poultry pathogens have been created. These include the hemagglutinin (HA) gene of avian influenza virus (10, 11, 21, 116, 129), the fusion (F) protein and the hemagglutinin-neuraminidase (HN) gene of Newcastle disease virus (17, 18, 19, 55, 66, 90, 118), the gB gene of Marek's disease virus (87, 150), the VP2 gene of infectious bursal disease virus (9, 51), the gB gene of infectious laryngotracheitis virus (58), and the envelope glycoprotein gene of reticuloendotheliosis virus (25). In most cases, foreign genes of avian pathogens inserted into the genome of avian poxvirus are expressed and also provide specific protection.

AVIAN POXVIRUSES AS EXPRESSION VECTORS FOR GENES FROM MAMMALIAN PATHOGENS.
The natural host range of avian poxviruses is limited to avian species. However, these viruses can initiate an abortive infection in vitro in cell lines of nonavian origin. Although infectious progeny virus is not produced, foreign antigens are synthesized authentically and processed and presented on the cell surface. In this regard, the rabies virus glycoprotein (117) and the measles virus fusion protein have been expressed in recombinant fowl poxvirus (140). Similarly, another avipoxvirus, canary poxvirus, has also been used to express the rabies virus glycoprotein gene (119), the measles virus fusion and hemagglutinin glycoproteins (120), and feline leukemia virus *env* and *gag* genes (115). These reports indicate that avian poxvirus vectors can be designed to function not only as poultry vaccines, but also as mammalian vaccines.

REFERENCES
1. Akey, B.L., J.K. Nayar, and D.J. Forrester. 1981. Avian pox in Florida wild turkeys: Culex nigripalpus and Wyeomyia vanduzeei as experimental vectors. J Wildl Dis 17:597–599.

2. Al Falluji, M.M., H.H. Tantawi, A. Albana, and S. Al Sheikhly. 1979. Pox infection among captive peacocks. J Wildl Dis 15:597–600.

3. Andrews, C., H.G. Pereira, and P. Wildy. 1978. Viruses of Vertebrates, 4th ed. Bailliere Tindall, London, United Kingdom, pp. 356–389.

4. Arhelger, R.B., and C.C. Randall. 1964. Electron microscopic observations on the development of fowlpox virus in chorioallantoic membrane. Virology 22:59–66.

5. Arhelger, R.B., R.W. Darlington, L.G. Gafford, and C.C. Randall. 1962. An electron microscopic study of fowlpox infection in chick scalps. Lab Invest 11:814–825.

6. Austic, R.E., and M.L. Scott. 1984. Nutritional deficiency diseases. In M.S. Hofstad, B.W. Calnek, W.M. Reid, and H.W. Yoder, Jr. (eds.). Diseases of Poultry, 8th ed. Iowa State University Press, Ames, IA, pp. 38–64.

7. Baxendale, W. 1971. Studies of three avian pox viruses and the development of an improved fowlpox vaccine. Vet Rec 88:5–10.

8. Baxendale, W. 1981. Immunity to fowlpox. In M.E. Rose, L.N. Payne, and B.M. Freeman (eds.). Avian Immunology. British Poultry Science, Edinburgh, Scotland, pp. 255–261

9. Bayliss, C.D., R.W. Peters, J.K.A. Cook, R.L. Reece, K. Howes, M.M. Binns, and M.E.G. Boursnell. 1991. A recombinant fowlpox virus that expresses the VP2 antigen of infectious bursal disease virus induces protection against mortality caused by the virus. Arch Virol 120:193–205.

10. Beard, C.W., W.M. Schnitzlein, and D.N. Tripathy. 1991. Protection of chickens against highly pathogenic avian influenza virus (H5N2) by recombinant fowlpox viruses. Avian Dis 35:356–359.

11. Beard, C.W., W.M. Schnitzlein, and D.N. Tripathy. 1992. Effect of route of administration on the efficacy of a recombinant fowlpox virus against H5N2 avian influenza. Avian Dis 36:1052–1055.

12. Beaver, D.L., and W.J. Cheatham. 1963. Electron microscopy of juncopox. Am J Pathol 42:23–40.

13. Binns, M.M., L. Stenzler, F.M. Tomley, J. Campbell, and M.E.G. Boursnell. 1987. Identification of a random sequencing strategy of fowlpoxvirus DNA polymerase gene, its nucleotide sequence and comparison with other viral DNA polymerases. Nucleic Acids Res 15:6563–6573.

14. Binns, M.M., F.M. Tomley, J. Campbell, and M.E.G. Boursnell. 1988. Comparison of a conserve region in fowlpox virus and vaccinia virus genomes and the translocation of the fowlpox virus thymidine kinase gene. J Gen Virol 69:1275–1283.

15. Binns, M.M., M.E.G. Boursnell, F.M. Tomley, and J. Campbell. 1989. Analysis of the fowlpox virus gene encoding the 4b core polypeptide and demonstration that it possesses efficient promoter sequences. Virology 170:288–291.

16. Boosinger, T.R., R.W. Winterfield, D.S. Feldman, and A.S. Dhillon. 1982. Psittacine poxvirus: Virus isolation and identification, transmission and cross-challenge studies in parrots and chickens. Avian Dis 26:437–444.

17. Boursnell, M.E.G., P.F. Green, J.I.A. Campbell, A. Deuter, R.W. Peters, F.M. Tomley, A.C.R. Samson, P. Chambers, P.T. Emmerson, and M.M. Binns. 1990. Insertion of the fusion gene of Newcastle disease virus into a non-essential region in the terminal repeats of fowlpox virus and demonstration of protective immunity induced by the recombinant. J Gen Virol 71:621–628.

18. Boursnell, M.E.G., P.F. Green, J.I.A. Campbell, A. Deuter, R.W. Peters, F.M. Tomley, A.C.R. Samson, P.T. Emmerson, and M.M. Binns. 1990. A fowlpox virus vaccine vector with insertion sites in the terminal repeats: Demonstration of its efficacy using the fusion gene of Newcastle disease virus. Vet Microbiol 23:305–316.

19. Boursnell, M.E.G., Green, P.F., Samson, A.C.R., Campbell, J.I.A., Deuter, A., Peters, R.W., Miller, N.S., Emmerson, P.T., and M.M. Binns. 1990. A recombinant fowlpox

virus expressing the hemagglutinin-neuraminidase gene of Newcastle disease virus (NDV) protects chickens against challenge by NDV. Virology 178:297–300.

20. Boyle, D.B., and B.E.H. Couper. 1986. Identification and cloning of the fowl pox virus thymidine kinase gene using vaccinia virus. J Gen Virol 67:1591–1600.

21. Boyle, D., and B.E.H. Couper. 1988. Construction of recombinant fowlpox viruses as vectors for poultry vaccines. Virus Res 10:343–356.

22. Boyle, D.B., B.E.H. Couper, A.J. Gibbs, L.J. Seigman, and G.W. Both. 1987. Fowlpox virus thymidine kinase: Nucleotide sequence and relationships to other thymidine kinases. Virology 156:355–365.

23. Buller, R.M.L., and G.J. Palumbo. 1991. Poxvirus pathogenesis. Microbiol Rev 55:80–122.

24. Buscaglia, C., R.A. Bankowski, and L. Miers. 1985. Cell-culture virus-neutralization test and enzyme-linked immunosorbent assay for evaluation of immunity in chickens against fowl pox. Avian Dis 29:672–680.

25. Calvert, J.G., K. Nazerian, W. Witter, and N. Yanagida. 1993. Fowlpox virus recombinants expressing the envelop glycoprotein of an avian reticuloendotheliosis retrovirus induce neutralizing antibodies and reduce viremia in chickens. J Virol 67:3069–3076.

26. Carter, J.K.Y., and N.F. Cheville. 1981. Isolation of surface tubules of fowlpox virus. Avian Dis 25:454–462.

27. Cheevers, W.P., and C.C. Randall. 1968. Viral and cellular growth and sequential increase of protein and DNA during fowlpox infection in vivo. Proc Soc Exp Biol Med 127:401–405.

28. Cheevers, W.P., D.J. O'Callaghan, and C.C. Randall. 1968. Biosynthesis of host and viral deoxyribonucleic acid during hyperplastic fowlpox infection in vivo. J Virol 2:421–429.

29. Cheville, N.F. 1966. Cytopathic changes in fowlpox (turkey origin) inclusion body formation. Am J Pathol 49:723–737.

30. Chi, M.S., and C.J. Mirocha. 1978. Necrotic oral lesions in chickens fed diacetoxyscirpenol, T-2 toxin, and crotocin. Poult Sci 57:807–808.

31. Chung, Y.S., and P.B. Spradbrow. 1977. Studies on poxvirus isolated from a magpie in Queensland. Aust Vet J 53:334–336.

32. Coupar, B.E.H., T. Teo, and D.B. Boyle. 1990. Restriction endonuclease mapping of the fowlpox virus genome. Virology 179:159–167.

33. Cox, W.R. 1980. Avian pox infection in a Canada goose (Branta canadensis). J Wildl Dis 16:623–626.

34. Cunningham, C.H. 1973. A Laboratory Guide in Virology. 7th ed. Burgess, Minneapolis, MN.

35. Drillien, R., D. Spehner, D. Villeval, and J.P. Lecocq. 1987. Similar genetic organization between a region of fowlpox virus DNA and the vaccinia virus HindIII J fragment despite divergent location of the thymidine kinase gene. Virology 160:203–209.

36. Dubochet, J., M. Adrian, K. Richter, J. Garces, and R. Wittek. 1994. Structure of intracellular mature vaccinia virus observed by cryoelectron microscopy. J Virol 68:1935–1941.

37. Duran-Reynals, F., and E. Bryan. 1952. Studies on the combined effects of fowl poxvirus and methylcholanthrene in chickens. Ann NY Acad Sci 54:977–991.

38. Eidson, C.S., P. Villegas, and S.H. Kleven. 1975. Efficacy of turkey herpesvirus vaccine when administered simultaneously with fowl pox vaccine. Poult Sci 54:1975–1981.

39. Eleazer, T.H., J.S. Harrel, and H.G. Blalock. 1983. Transmission studies involving a wet fowl pox isolate. Avian Dis 27:542–544.

40. El-Zein, A., S. Nehme, V. Ghoraib, S. Hasbani, and B. Toth. 1974. Preparation of fowlpox vaccine on chicken-embryo-dermis cell culture. Avian Dis 18:495–506.

41. Esposito, J.J., D. Baxby, D. Black, S. Dales, G. Darai, K. Dumbell, R. Granados, W.K. Joklik, G. McFadden, B.

Moss, R. Moyer, D. Pickup, A. Robinson, H. Rouhandeh, and D. Tripathy. 1991. Family Poxviridae. In R.I.B. Francki, C.M. Fauquet, D.L. Knudson, and F. Brown (eds.). Classification and Nomenclature of Viruses. Fifth Report of the International Committee on Taxonomy of Viruses. Springer-Verlag Wein, New York, NY, pp. 91–102.

42. Fatunmbi, O.O., and W.M. Reed. 1993. Use of a bivalent vaccine in the control of avian pox in chickens. Proc 44th North Cent Avian Dis Conf, pp. 94–95.

43. Fatunmbi, O.O., and W.M. Reed. 1994. The control of "variant" fowl pox virus infections using a commercial modified live virus fowl pox vaccine. Proc 45th North Cent Avian Dis Conf, pp. 83–84.

44. Fatunmbi, O.O., W.M. Reed, D.L. Schwartz, and D.N. Tripathy. 1995. Dual infection of chickens with pox and infectious laryngotracheitis (ILT) confirmed with specific pox and ILT DNA DOT-BLOT hybridization assays. Avian Dis 39:925-930.

45. Gafford, L.G., and C.C. Randall. 1976. Virus-specific RNA and DNA in nuclei of cells infected with fowlpox virus. Virology 69:1–14.

46. Gafford, L.G., B.E. Mitchell Jr., and C.C. Randall. 1978. Sedimentation characteristics and molecular weights of three poxvirus DNAs. Virology 89:229–239.

47. Garg, S.K., M.S. Sethi, and S.K. Negi. 1967. Hemagglutinating property of pigeon pox virus strains. Ind J Microbiol 7:101–102.

48. Gelenczei, E.F., and H.N. Lasher. 1968. Comparative studies of cell-culture-propagated avian poxviruses in chickens and turkeys. Avian Dis 12:142–150.

49. Ghildyal, N., W. Schnitzlein, and D.N. Tripathy. 1989. Genetic and antigenic differences between fowl pox and quailpox viruses. Arch Virol 106:85-92.

50. Giddens, W.E., L.J. Swago, J.D. Handerson Jr., R.A. Lewis, D.S. Farner, A. Carlos, and W.C. Dolowy. 1971. Canary pox in sparrows and canaries (Fringillidae) and in Weavers (Ploceidae). Vet Pathol 8:260–280.

51. Heine, H.G., and D.B. Boyle. 1993. Infectious bursal disease virus structural protein VP2 expressed by a fowlpox virus recombinant confers protection against disease in chickens. Arch Virol 131:277–292.

52. Hitchner, S.B. 1981. Canary pox vaccination with live embryo-attenuated virus. Avian Dis 25:874–881.

53. Holt, G., and J. Krogsrud. 1973. Pox in wild birds. Acta Vet Scand 14:201–203.

54. Hyde, J.M., L.G. Gafford, and C.C. Randall. 1967. Molecular weight determination of fowl poxvirus DNA by electron microscopy. Virology 33:112–120.

55. Iritani, Y., S. Aoyama, S. Takigami, Y. Hayashi, R. Ogawa, N. Yanagida, S. Saeki, and K. Kamogawa. 1991. Antibody response to Newcastle disease virus (NDV) of recombinant fowlpox virus (FPV) expressing a hemagglutinin-neuraminidase of NDV into chickens in the presence of antibody to NDV or FPV. Avian Dis 35:659–661.

56. Jordan, F.T.W., and R.C. Chubb. 1962. The agar gel diffusion technique in the diagnosis of infectious laryngotracheitis (ILT) and its differentiation from fowlpox. Res Vet Sci 3:245–255.

57. Karstad, L. 1971. Pox. In J.W. Davis, R.C. Anderson, L. Karstad, and D.O. Trainer (eds.). Infectious and Parasitic Diseases of Wild Birds. Iowa State University Press, Ames, IA, pp. 34–41.

58. Keeler, C.L., J.K Rosenbereger, S.S Cloud, D.J. Poulsen, K. Nazerian, and A. Yanagida. 1992. A recombinant fowlpox virus protects chickens against challenge by infectious laryngotracheitis virus (ILTV) [abst]. Proc 129th Annu Meet Am Vet Med Assoc, p. 137.

59. Kirmse, P. 1967. Host specificity and long persistence of pox infection in the flicker (Colaptes auratus). Bull Wildl Dis Assoc 3:14–20.

60. Kirmse, P. 1969. Host specificity and pathogenicity of pox viruses from wild birds. Bull Wildl Dis Assoc 5:376–386.

61. Kirmse, P., and H. Loftin. 1969. Avian pox in migrant and native birds in Panama. Bull Wildl Dis Assoc 5:103–107.

62. Kumar, S., and D.B. Boyle. 1990a. Mapping of early/late gene of fowlpox virus. Virus Res 15:175–186.

63. Kumar, S., and D.B. Boyle. 1990b. A poxvirus bidirectional promoter element with early/late and late functions. Virology 179:151–158.

64. Landolt, M., and R.M. Kocan. 1976. Transmission of avian pox from starlings to rothchild's mynahs. J Wildl Dis 12:353–356.

65. Ledingham, J.C.G., and M.B. Aberd. 1931. The aetiological importance of the elementary bodies in vaccinia and fowlpox. Lancet 221:525–526.

66. Letellier, C., Burny, A., and G. Meulemans. 1991. Construction of a pigeonpox virus recombinant: Expression of the Newcastle disease virus (NDV) fusion glycoprotein and protection of chickens against NDV challenge. Arch Virol 118:43–56.

67. Lyles, D.S., C.C. Randall, L.G. Gafford, and H.B. White, Jr. 1976. Cellular fatty acids during fowlpox virus infection of three different host systems. Virology 70:227–229.

68. Matthews, R.E.F. 1982. Classification and nomenclature of viruses. Intervirology 17:42–46.

69. Mayr, A. 1963. Neue Verfahren für die Differenzierung der Geflü gelpokenviren. Berl Munch Tierarztl Wochenschr 76:316–324.

70. Mayr, A., and K. Danner. 1976. Oral immunization against pox. Studies on fowlpox as a model. 14th Congr Int Assoc Biol Stand Dev Biol Stand 33:249–259.

71. Mayr, A., and H. Mahnel. 1970. Charakteisierung eines Vom Rhinozeros isolierten Hühnerpockenvirus. Arch Gesamte Virusforsch 31:51–60.

72. Mayr, A., F. Hartig, and I. Bayr. 1965. Entwicklung eines Impfstoffes gegen die Kanarienpocken auf der Basis eines attenierten Kanarienpocken-Kulturvirus. Zentralbl Vet Med Reihe [B] 12:41–49.

73. McFerran, J.B., J.K. Clarke, and W.L. Curran. 1971. The application of negative contrast electron microscopy to routine veterinary virus diagnosis. Res Vet Sci 12:253–257.

74. Metz, A.L., L. Hatcher, J.A. Newman, and D.A. Halvorson. 1985. Venereal pox in breeder turkeys in Minnesota. Avian Dis 29:850–853.

75. Minbay, A., and J.P. Kreier. 1973. An experimental study of the pathogenesis of fowlpox infection in chickens. Avian Dis 17:532–539.

76. Mockett, A.P.A., D.J. Southee, F.M. Tomley, and A. Deuter. 1987. Fowlpox virus: Its structural proteins and immunogens and the detection of viral-specific antibodies by ELISA. Avian Pathol 16:493–504.

77. Mockett, B., M. Binns, M. Boursnell, and M. Skinner. 1992. Comparison of the locations of homologous fowlpox and vaccinia virus genes reveals major genome reorganization. J Gen Virol 73:2661–2668.

78. Morita, C. 1973a. Role of humoral and cell-mediated immunity on the recovery of chickens from fowl poxvirus infection. J Immunol 111:1495–1501.

79. Morita, C. 1973b. Studies on fowlpox viruses. I. Plaque formation of fowlpox virus on chick embryo cell culture. Avian Dis 17:87–92.

80. Morita, C. 1973c. Studies on fowlpox viruses. II. Plaque-neutralization test. Avian Dis 17:93–98.

81. Moscovici, C., M.G. Moscovici, H. Jimenez, M.M.C. Lai, M.J. Hayman, and P.K. Vogt. 1977. Continuous tissue culture cell lines derived from chemically induced tumors of Japanese quail. Cell 11:95–103.

82. Moss, B. 1990. Poxviridae and their replication. In B.N. Fields, D.M. Knipe, R.M. Chanock, J.L. Melnick, B. Roizman, and R.E. Shope (eds.). Virology, 2nd Ed. Raven Press, New York, pp. 2079–2111.

83. Moss, B. 1991. Vaccinia virus: A tool for research and vaccine development. Science 252:1662–1667.

84. Müller, H.K., R. Wittek, W. Schaffner, D. Schümperli, A. Menna, and R. Wyler. 1977. Comparison of five poxvirus genomes by analysis with restriction endonucleases Hind III, Bam HI and Eco RI. J Gen Virol 38:135–147.

85. Nagy, E., A.D. Maeda-Machang'u, P.J. Krell, and J.B. Derbshire. 1990. Vaccination of 1-day-old chicks with fowlpox virus by the aerosol, drinking water, or cutaneous routes. Avian Dis 34:677–682.

86. Nazerian, K., S. Dhawale, and W.S. Payne. 1989. Structural Proteins of two different plaque-size phenotypes of fowlpox virus. Avian Dis 33:458–465.

87. Nazerian, K., L.F. Lee, N. Yanagida, and R. Ogawa. 1992. Protection against Marek's Disease by a fowlpox virus recombinant expressing the glycoprotein B of Marek's Disease virus. J Virol 66:1409–1413 .

88. Obijeski, J.F., E.L. Palmer, L.G. Gafford, and C.C. Randall. 1973. Polyacrylamide gel electrophoresis of fowlpox and vaccinia virus proteins. Virology 51:512–516.

89. Odend'hal, S. 1983. The Geographical Distribution of Animal Viral Diseases. Academic Press, New York, NY.

90. Ogawa, R., N. Yanagida, S. Saeki, S. Saito, S. Ohkawa, H. Gotoh, K. Kodama, K. Kamogawa, K. Sawaguchi, and Y. Iritani. 1990. Recombinant fowlpox viruses inducing protective immunity against Newcastle disease and fowlpox viruses. Vaccine 8:486–490.

91. Parks, R.J., P.J. Krell, J.B. Derbyshire, and E. Nagy. 1994. Studies of fowlpox virus recombination in the generation of recombinant vaccines. Virus Res 32:283–297.

92. Petrak, M.L. 1982. Diseases of Cage and Aviary Birds. Lea and Febiger, Philadelphia, PA.

93. Prideaux, C.T., and D.B. Boyle. 1987. Fowlpox virus polypeptides: Sequential appearance and virion associated polypeptides. Arch Virol 96:185–199.

94. Prideaux, C.T., S. Kumar, and D.B. Boyle. 1990. Comparative analysis of vaccinia virus promoter activity in fowlpox and vaccinia virus recombinants. Virus Res 16:43–58.

95. Randall, C.C., and L.G. Gafford. 1962. Histochemical and biochemical studies of isolated viral inclusions. Am J Pathol 40:51–62.

96. Randall, C.C., L.G. Gafford, R.W. Darlington, and J. Hyde. 1964. Composition of fowlpox virus and inclusion matrix. J Bacteriol 87:939–944.

97. Randall, C.C., L.G. Gafford, R.L. Soehner, and J.M. Hyde. 1966. Physiochemical properties of fowlpox virus deoxyribonucleic acid and its anomalous infectious behavior. J Bacteriol 91:95–100.

98. Reed, W.M., and O.O. Fatunmbi. 1993. Pathogenicity and immunological relationship of quail and Mynah poxviruses to fowl and pigeon poxviruses. Avian Pathol 22:395–400.

99. Reed, W.M., and O.O. Fatunmbi. 1994. Characterization and immunogenicity of "variant" strains of avian poxviruses. Proc 131st Annu Meet Am Vet Med Assoc, p. 124.

100. Reed, W.M., and D.L. Schrader. 1989. Immunogenicity and pathogenicity of Mynah pox virus. Poult Sci 68:631–638.

101. Sadasiv, E.C., P.W. Chang, and G. Gluka. 1985. Morphogenesis of canary poxvirus and its entrance into inclusion bodies. Am J Vet Res 46:529–535.

102. Schnitzlein, W.M., and D.N. Tripathy. 1990. Utilization of vaccinia virus promoters by fowlpox virus recombinants. Anim Biotech 1:161–174.

103. Schnitzlein, W.M., N. Ghildyal, and D.N. Tripathy. 1988. Genomic and antigenic characterization of avipoxviruses. Virus Res 10:65–76.

104. Schnitzlein, W.M., N. Ghildyal, and D.N. Tripathy. 1988. A rapid method for identifying the thymidine kinase genes of avipoxviruses. J Virol Methods 20:341–352.

105. Sevoian, M. 1960. A quick method for the diagnosis of avian pox and infectious laryngotracheitis. Avian Dis 4:474–477.

106. Sharma, D.K., and S.N. Sharma. 1988. Comparative immunity of fowl pox virus vaccines. J Vet Med B 35:19–23.

107. Shirinov, F.B., A.I. Ibragimova, and Z.G. Misirov. 1972. Spread of fowl poxvirus by the mite Dermanyssus gallinae. Veterinariya (Moscow) 4:48–49. [Abst Vet Bull 42:5206].

108. Siccardi, F.J. 1975. The addition of fowlpox and pigeonpox vaccine to Marek's vaccine in broilers. Avian Dis 19:362–365.

109. Singh, G.K., N.P. Singh, and S.K. Garg. 1987. Studies on pathogenesis of fowlpox: Virological study. Acta Virol 31:417–423.

110. Swallen, T.O. 1963. A radioautographic study of the lesions of fowlpox using thymidine-H^3. Am J Pathol 42:485–491.

111. Tanizaki, E., T. Kotani, and Y. Odagiri. 1986. Pathological changes of tracheal mucosa in chickens infected with fowlpox virus. Avian Dis 31:169–175.

112. Tanizaki, E., T. Kotani, Y. Odagiri, and T. Horiuchi. 1989. Pathologic changes in chickens caused by intravenous inoculation with fowlpox virus. Avian Dis 33:333–339.

113. Tantwai, H.H., M.M. Al Falluji, and M.O. Shony. 1979. Heat-selected mutants of pigeon poxvirus. Acta Virol 23:249–252.

114. Tantwai, H.H., S. Al Sheikhly, and F.K. Hussain. 1981. Avian pox in buzzard (Accipiter nisus) in Iraq. J Wildl Dis 17:145–146.

115. Tartaglia, J., O. Jarrett, J.C. Neil, P. Desmettre, and E. Paoletti. 1993. Protection of cats against feline leukemia virus by vaccination with a canarypox virus recombinants, ALVAC-FL. J Virol 67:2370–2375.

116. Taylor, J., R. Weinberg, Y. Kawaoka, R.G. Webster, and E. Paoletti. 1988. Protective immunity against avian influenza induced by a fowlpox virus recombinant. Vaccine 6:504–508.

117. Taylor, J., R. Weinberg, B. Languet, P. Desmettre, and E. Paoletti. 1988. Recombinant fowlpox virus inducing protective immunity in non-avian species. Vaccine 6:497–503.

118. Taylor, J., C. Edbauer, A. Rey-Senelonge, J.F. Bouquet, E. Norton, S. Goebel, P. Desmettre, and E. Paoletti. 1990. Newcastle disease virus fusion protein expressed in a fowlpox virus recombinant confers protection in chickens. J Virol 64:1441–1450.

119. Taylor, J., C. Trimarchi, R. Weinberg, B. Languet, F. Guillemin, P. Desmettre, and E. Paoletti. 1991. Efficacy studies on a canarypox-rabies recombinant virus. Vaccine 9:190–193.

120. Taylor, J., R. Weinberg, J. Tartaglia, C. Richardson, G. Alkhatib, D. Briedis, M. Appel, E. Norton, and E. Paoletti. 1992. Nonreplicating viral vectors as potential vaccines: Recombinant canarypox virus expressing measles virus fusion (F) and hemagglutinin (HA) glycoproteins. Virology 187:321–328.

121. Thompson, S.W., and R.D. Hunt. 1966. Selected Histochemical and Histopathological Methods. Charles C. Thomas, Springfield, IL, pp. 885–887.

122. Tripathy, D.N. 1988. Unpublished data.

123. Tripathy, D.N. 1989. Pox. In Purchase, H.G., L.H. Arp, C.H. Domermuth, and J.E. Pearson (eds.). A Laboratory Manual for the Isolation and Identification of Avian Pathogens, 3rd. ed. American Association of Avian Pathologists, Kennett Square, PA pp. 103–105.

124. Tripathy, D.N. 1993. Avipox Viruses. In J.B. McFerran, and M.S. McNulty (eds.). Virus Infections of Vertebrates, vol 4. Virus Infections of Birds. Elsevier Science, Amsterdam, The Netherlands, pp. 5–15.

125. Tripathy, D.N., and C.H. Cunningham. 1984. Avian pox. In M.S. Hofstad, H.J. Barnes, B.W. Calnek, W.M. Reid, and H.W. Yoder Jr. (eds.). Diseases of Poultry, 8th ed. Iowa State University Press, Ames, IA, pp. 524–534.

126. Tripathy, D.N., and L.E. Hanson. 1975. Immunity to fowlpox. Am J Vet Res 36:541–544.

127. Tripathy, D.N., and L.E. Hanson. 1976. A smear technique for staining elementary bodies of fowlpox. Avian Dis 20:609–610.

128. Tripathy, D.N., and J. Radzevicius. 1991. Evaluation of cloned DNA fragments of fowlpox virus as diagnostic probes [abst]. Proc 42nd North Cent Avian Dis Conf, p. 61.

129. Tripathy, D.N., and W.M. Schnitzlein. 1991. Expression of avian influenza virus hemagglutinin by recombinant fowlpox virus. Avian Dis 35:186–191.

130. Tripathy, D.N., and W.M. Schnitzlein. 1995. Polymerase chain reaction (PCR) for diagnosis of fowlpox [abstr]. Proc 132nd Annu Meet Am Vet Med Assoc, p. 152.

131. Tripathy, D.N., and R. Wittek. 1990. Regulation of foreign gene in fowlpox virus by a vaccinia virus promoter. Avian Dis 34:218–220.

132. Tripathy, D.N., L.E. Hanson, and W.L. Myers. 1970. Passive hemagglutination test with fowlpox virus. Avian Dis 14:29–38.

133. Tripathy, D.N., L.E. Hanson, and A.H. Killinger. 1973. Immunoperoxidase technique for detection of fowlpox antigen. Avian Dis 17:274–278.

134. Tripathy, D.N., L.E. Hanson, and R.A. Crandell. 1981. Poxviruses of veterinary importance; diagnosis of infections. Chapter 6. In E. Kurstak and C. Kurstak (eds.). Comparative Diagnosis of Viral Diseases, vol. III. Academic Press, New York, NY, pp. 267–346.

135. Tripathy, D.N., J. Radzevicius, and W.M. Schnitzlein. 1992. Specific genomic probes for differentiation of fowlpox and laryngotracheitis viruses [abstr]. Proc 129th Annu Meet Am Vet Med Assoc, p. 126.

136. Uppal, P.K., and P.R. Nilakantan. 1970. Studies on the serological relationships between avianpox, sheep pox, goat pox and vaccinia viruses. J Hyg Camb 68:349–358.

137. Uppal, P.K., and P.R. Nilakantan. 1974. Hemagglutination by fowlpox, sheep pox and vaccinia viruses. Indian Vet J 51:451–456.

138. Van Kammen, A., and P.B. Spradbrow. 1976. Rapid diagnosis of some avian virus diseases. Avian Dis 20:748–751.

139. White, H.B., S.S. Powell, L.G. Gafford, and C.C. Randall. 1968. The occurrence of squalene in lipid of fowlpox virus. J Biol Chem 243:4517–4525.

140. Wild, F., P. Giraudon, D. Spehner, R. Drillien, and J.P. Lecocq. 1990. Fowlpox virus recombinant encoding the measles virus fusion protein: Protection of mice against fatal measles encephalitis. Vaccine 8:441–442.

141. Winterfield, R.W., and S.B. Hitchner. 1965. The response of chickens to vaccination with different concentrations of pigeon pox and fowl pox viruses. Avian Dis 9:237–241.

142. Winterfield, R.W., and W. Reed. 1985. Avian pox: Infection and immunity with quail, psittacine, fowl, and pigeon pox viruses. Poult Sci 64:65–70.

143. Winterfield, R.W., W.M. Reed, and H.L. Thacker. 1985. Infection and immunity with a virus isolate from turkeys. Poult Sci 64:2076–2080.

144. Woodroofe, G.M., and F. Fenner. 1962. Serological relationship within the poxvirus group: An antigen common to all members of the group. Virology 16:334–341.

145. Woodruff, A.M., and E.W. Goodpasture. 1931. The susceptibility of the chorio-allantoic membrane of chick embryo to infection with the fowlpox virus. Am J Pathol 7:209–222.

146. Woodruff, C.E., and E.W. Goodpasture. 1929. The infectivity of isolated inclusion bodies of fowlpox. Am J Pathol 5:1–10.

147. Woodruff, C.E., and E.W. Goodpasture. 1930. The relation of the virus of fowl-pox to the specific cellular inclusions of the disease. Am J Pathol 6:713–720.

148. Woodward, H., and D.C. Tudor. 1973. The immunizing effect of commercial pigeon pox vaccines on pigeons. Poult Sci 52:1463–1468.

149. Wyatt, R.D., B.A. Weeks, P.B. Hamilton, and H.R. Brumeister. 1972. Severe oral lesions in chickens caused by ingestion of dietary fusariotoxin T-2. Appl Microbiol 24:251–257.

150. Yanagida, N., R. Ogawa, Y. Li, L.F. Lee, and K. Nazerian. 1992. Recombinant fowlpox viruses expressing the glycoprotein B homolog and the pp38 gene of Marek's Disease Virus. J Virol 66:1402–1408.

151. Zantinge, J.L. 1995. Characterization and transcriptional analysis of the fowlpox virus genome. PhD Thesis. The University of Guelph, Ontario, Canada.

25 Duck Hepatitis

P. R. Woolcock and J. Fabricant

INTRODUCTION. Duck hepatitis (DH) is a highly fatal, rapidly spreading viral infection of young ducklings characterized primarily by hepatitis. It can be caused by any of three different viruses, namely duck hepatitis virus (DHV) types 1, 2, and 3. DHV types 2 and 3 were first recognized as separate entities because they induced hepatitis in DHV type 1–immune ducklings. Duck hepatitis is of economic importance to all duck-growing farms because of the high potential mortality if not controlled. The three virus types are not known to have any public health significance.

In addition to the three viruses that are etiologically associated with liver disease in ducks, a member of the hepadnavirus group (hepatitis B viruses) is also found in wild and domestic ducks. Although the duck hepatitis B virus is not known to cause disease or lesions in ducks, it is briefly described in a separate section at the end of this chapter.

DUCK HEPATITIS TYPE 1

HISTORY AND DISTRIBUTION. An acute disease of ducklings, characterized by enlarged livers mottled with hemorrhages, was observed in 1945 by Levine and Hofstad (72). The disease affected ducklings during the 1st wk of age, and death was rapid after signs were observed. While the disease could be transmitted in ducklings, no agent was isolated. During the spring of 1949, Levine and Fabricant (71) studied a highly fatal disease, which is now known as DH type 1, in young White Pekin ducks on Long Island, New York. The disease spread rapidly; before the summer was over, practically all 70-odd duck farms in the area had suffered losses. At first, ducks 2–3 wk old were succumbing. On severely affected farms, mortalities up to 95% were not uncommon in some broods. Successive lots of ducks almost invariably became infected. Later, occasional broods would escape with little mortality. It is estimated that 15% of the total number of ducklings started for that year died from the disease—a total of 750,000 birds. In the United States, the disease has also been diagnosed in other duck-raising areas. Duck hepatitis type 1 is worldwide in distribution (106); the most recent reports of new isolations include China (48) and Korea (89).

ETIOLOGY. Duck hepatitis virus type 1 was first isolated in chicken embryos by Levine and Fabricant (71). No serologic relationship was demonstrated between this virus and that causing duck plague (duck virus enteritis); likewise, no neutralization of DHV type 1 occurred when tested with convalescent serum from cases of human and canine virus hepatitis (26). Duck hepatitis virus type 1 contains RNA and has been classified as a picornavirus (105). It bears no relationship to the hepadna virus infection caused by duck hepatitis B virus (DHBV) as described by Mason et al. (81). Duck hepatitis B virus has been found in domestic ducks in China and the United States.

Morphology. Duck hepatitis virus type 1 has been estimated to be 20–40 nm in size (95). Richter et al. (97) observed 30-nm particles in thin liver sections by electron microscopy (EM). Tauraso et al. (105) confirmed the size to be less than 50 nm by filtration studies.

Biologic Properties. Fitzgerald and Hanson (30) were unable to demonstrate hemagglutination of chicken, duck, sheep, horse, guinea pig, mouse, snake, swine, and rabbit red blood cells (RBCs) by cell culture–grown DHV type 1.

Cell cultures infected with DHV type 1 failed to hemadsorb green and rhesus monkey, hamster, mouse, rat, rabbit, guinea pig, human O, goose, duck, and day-old chicken RBCs. High-titered virus

661

suspensions would not hemagglutinate RBCs of the same species when tested at a pH range of 6.8–7.4 and at temperatures of 4, 24, and 37 C (105).

Resistance to Chemical and Physical Agents.

Duck hepatitis virus type 1 is resistant to ether and chloroform, relatively heat stable, and capable of survival for long periods under usual environmental conditions.

Duck hepatitis virus type 1 resisted treatment with ether or fluorocarbon (90), chloroform, pH 3 and trypsin (105), and 30% methanol or ammonium sulfate (53). Using cell culture–grown virus, Davis (18) reported that DHV type 1 resisted pH 3 for 9 hr, but longer exposure (48 hr) reduced virus titer. The virus was not inactivated by 2% lysol or 0.1% formalin (6); 15% creolin, naphthalysol, or xylonaphtha; or 20% anhydrous sodium carbonate (91). Complete inactivation was reported with 1% formaldehyde or 2% caustic soda within 2 hr at 15–20 C, 2% calcium hypochlorite within 3 hr at 15–20 C (91), and 3% chloramine in 5 hr or 0.2% formalin in 2 hr (25). Haider (49) reported complete virus inactivation with 5% phenol, undiluted Wescodyne (an inorganic iodine solution), and undiluted Clorox (sodium hypochlorite solution).

Heating the virus at 50 C for 1 hr had no effect on virus titer (105). Most of the virus was inactivated at 56 C after 30 min (53). Asplin (6) reported, however, that it would survive at 56 C for 60 min but not at 62 C for 30 min. Dvorakova and Kozusnik (25) reported that 23 hr were required for complete inactivation at 56 C. Duck hepatitis virus type 1 survived for 21 days at 37 C (90). Heat stability was unaffected by 1 M divalent cation (Mg^{2+}) (109). Davis (18), using cell culture–grown type 1 virus, showed that it had a half-life of 48 min at 50 C, but that the presence of molar NaCl, Na_2SO_4, $MgCl_2$, or $MgSO_4$ protected the virus from inactivation at that temperature.

Under more natural environmental conditions, the virus survived at least 10 wk in uncleaned infected brooders and for longer than 37 days in moist feces stored in a cool shed (6). At 4 C, the virus survived over 2 yr (6, 25) and at -20 C for as long as 9 yr (53).

Variability.

Viruses differing, or serologically distinct, from DHV type 1 have been recognized as causes of hepatitis in ducklings and have been reported from India (94) and Egypt (103). The Indian isolate is known to be distinct from DHV type 1, but its relationship to the other DHV types is unknown.

A variant strain of DHV type 1, named DHV type 1a, has been described by Sandhu et al. (101). The origin of the virus is unknown, but all known isolates can be traced back to a single location. With the use of cross-neutralization tests in embryonating chicken eggs, they showed, with somewhat variable results, a partial cross-reaction between types 1 and 1a. They also showed partial cross-protection in passively immunized ducklings challenged with each of the viruses. Woolcock (see 120) had also reported differences between these two viruses in plaque-reduction assays in duck embryo kidney cells. Both DHV type 1 and DHV type 1a are serologically distinct from DHV type 3.

Laboratory Host Systems

EMBRYOS. Levine and Fabricant (71) were the first to propagate the virus in the allantoic sac of 9-day-old chicken embryos. From 10 to 60% of the embryos died by the 5th or 6th day and were stunted or edematous (Fig. 25.1A). Hwang and Dougherty (62) passaged a DHV type 1 strain as two lines in 10-day-old chicken embryos. The serially passaged lines became nonpathogenic for newly hatched ducklings at the 20th and 26th transfers. The virus titer in chicken embryos was 1–3 $\log_{10}$ lower than when grown in ducklings.

Hwang (54) developed a chicken embryo lethal strain of DHV type 1 by serial embryo passages. Using a homogenate of dead embryos and chorioallantoic membrane (CAM) in embryonic fluid, mortality reached 100% at the 63rd passage. More consistent results were obtained when 5- to 7-day-old embryos were inoculated via the yolk sac.

Toth (107) found titers of 80th passage–adapted virus to be highest at about 53 hr postinoculation (PI): embryo, $10^{7.50}$; CAM $10^{5.79}$; and amnioallantoic fluid $10^{3.62}$. A high-titer live vaccine could be harvested from all these parts 53–69 hr PI. Essentially similar results were reported by Pan (86).

Mason et al. (80) noted a somewhat higher titer of attenuated DHV type 1 in chicken embryos that reached a peak (10^8) in 48 hr. The latent period was between 6 and 24 hr.

Goose embryos were found to be susceptible to the virus, and embryo deaths occurred 2–3 days after allantoic inoculation (4).

CELL CULTURES. Various attempts to grow and assay DHV type 1 in cell cultures of duck and chicken embryo origin have been described (30, 31, 56, 64, 80, 90). Maiboroda (75) followed development of DHV type 1 in monolayers of duck kidney cells with a direct fluorescent antibody (FA) technique. Fluorescence was observed after 8 hr, reached a maximum after 2–4 days, and was confined to the cytoplasm. Cytopathic effects (CPE) (rounding of cells) and maximum virus titers occurred after 2 days. Maiboroda and Kontrimavichus (76) produced growth and CPE in goose embryo kidney cells. Kurilenko and Strelnikov (70) reported similar results in piglet kidney cell culture.

Davis and Woolcock (21) showed that attenuated DHV type 1 grew in embryo cell cultures of goose, turkey, quail, pheasant, guinea fowl, and chicken origin, while virulent virus strains grew to varying degrees in only guinea fowl, quail, and turkey embryo cells. Golubnichi et al. (40) reported successful growth and a high level of cytopathogenicity in duck embryo fibroblasts inoculated with chick embryo–adapted DHV type 1. They recommended this procedure for vaccine production and virus neutralization (VN) tests.

Woolcock et al. (121) described a plaque assay for attenuated DHV type 1 in primary monolayers of duck embryo kidney (DEK) cells. The concentration of fetal calf serum in the overlay medium affected plaque size. Subsequently, Chalmers and Woolcock (15) demonstrated that several mammalian sera had an inhibitory effect on the virus, which was nonspecific and only occurred when the serum was in direct contact with the virus. The virus-inhibitory substance in fetal calf serum appeared to be present in the albumin fraction. There was no or minimal inhibitory effect in sera from ducks or chickens. Woolcock (115) reported plaque assays for both virulent and attenuated DHV type 1 in primary duck embryo liver (DEL) cells and compared the results of in vitro assays with those obtained in ovo and in vivo. Kaleta (65) described a microneutralization assay using attenuated DHV type 1 in primary DEK cells; Woolcock (116) modified this assay to monitor immune responses to vaccines.

Pathogenicity.

Asplin (5) and Reuss (96) reported loss of pathogenicity of DHV type 1 for ducklings after chicken embryo passages. Hwang (54) found one virus strain to have lost its pathogenicity for ducklings after 20 or more passages in chicken embryos. He also found that the same strain had lost its pathogenicity for ducklings after the sixth passage in duck embryo fibroblasts, but the virus retained its pathogenicity for chicken embryos (55).

Hwang and Dougherty (62) reported that chicken embryo–passaged strains, while nonpathogenic for ducklings, did multiply in the tissues but at a lower titer than field strains. Field strains were found in fairly high concentrations in duckling brain; chicken embryo–passaged strains could not be detected or were present in low concentrations in the brain.

A similar attenuation of pathogenicity has been reported when DHV type 1 was passaged in duck embryos (11). Embryo passage–attenuated DHV type 1 strains are still capable of causing very mild and transitory histologic changes after inoculation (100, 104), and reversion to virulence occurs after back-passage in young ducklings (118, 119).

When Kapp et al. (66) encountered heavy losses from DH type 1 in several flocks of ducklings 3–4 wk old, they suspected inadequate rations as contributory causes. This was borne out experimentally when eight of nine 3-wk-old ducks that had been fed the farm ration died after virus exposure. No mortality occurred in controls on normal feed. It was concluded that faulty diet had impaired liver function, which predisposed ducklings to hepatitis at an unusually advanced age.

Friend and Trainer (33, 35, 36) fed low levels of polychlorinated biphenyl, DDT, and dieldrin to mallard ducklings for 10 days; 5 days later, birds were infected with DHV type 1. Birds receiving toxic substances had significantly higher mortality than controls not previously fed the chemicals. It appears that inadequate diet or ingestion of toxic substances exacerbates pathogenic effects of the virus.

Lu et al. (73) reported an outbreak of infectious-bill-atrophy syndrome in ducklings in Taiwan, which they believe was caused by a parvovirus infection in association with DHV. The exact role of DHV in this syndrome was not clearly defined.

Sandhu et al. (101) reported that the pathologic responses to DHV types 1 and 1a were similar.

PATHOGENESIS AND EPIZOOTIOLOGY

Natural and Experimental Hosts.

In naturally occurring outbreaks, DH type 1 occurred only in young ducklings. Adult breeders on infected premises did not become clinically ill and continued in full production. Field observations indicated that chickens and turkeys were resistant. Rahn (93), however, found that day-old and wk-old poults exposed to DHV type 1 developed signs, lesions, and neutralizing antibody. Poults, after either oral or intraperitoneal exposure, had mottled livers and enlarged gallbladders and spleens. Duck hepatitis virus type 1 was isolated from livers up to 17 days after oral exposure of day-old poults. Schoop et al. (102) and Reuss (95) failed to infect chickens experimentally. Reuss could not transmit the disease to rabbits, guinea pigs, white mice, or dogs. Asplin (6) reported that young chickens can contract an inapparent infection and pass it on through contact with other chicks. Experimental infections in goslings (4) and mallard ducklings (34) have been reported. In experimentally exposed birds, no mortality occurred in chicks, muscovy ducklings, or pigeon squabs; low mortality occurred in young turkeys and quail, while high mortality occurred in young pheasants, geese, and guinea fowl. All exposed birds became infected with DHV type 1 (60).

Transmission, Carriers, and Vectors.

Under field conditions, DH type 1 spreads rapidly

to all susceptible ducklings in the flock. Although high mortality and rapid spread of the disease on farms indicate extreme contagiousness, occasional exceptions have been observed. In one pen, 65% of the ducks died, while in an adjoining pen separated only by a 14-in. curb, mortality was negligible.

The first efforts to transmit the disease to small groups of three or four caged ducklings by injection and feeding of egg-propagated virus were not successful. In another experiment, with tissues from a naturally occurring outbreak, some ducklings became infected. Transmission was most easily accomplished by intramuscular (IM) injection and feeding egg-propagated virus and infected organs to larger groups of ducklings (10–20) kept on litter under a hover. The incubation period was 24 hr in most experiments, and nearly all deaths took place by the 4th day. Uninoculated ducklings placed in the same pens with inoculated birds contracted the disease and died somewhat later than injected ducks.

Egg transmission presumably does not take place. Newly hatched ducklings produced by breeders on infected premises remained well when taken where no ducks were being kept. Asplin (5) confirmed this finding.

Priz (92) found that aerosol infection of ducklings with Yagotinski strain of DHV type 1 was lethal.

Hanson and Tripathy (52) reported successful infection with attenuated DHV type 1 by the oral route, although Toth and Norcross (110) suggested that in this case, the portal of entry was really the pharynx or upper respiratory tract, since the virus administered in a capsule failed to produce infection.

Recovered ducks may excrete virus in feces for up to 8 wk PI (95). Asplin (6) reported that there is strong field evidence to incriminate wild birds as mechanical carriers of the virus over short distances. He also suggested the possibility that an unknown host acting as a healthy carrier might be responsible for new outbreaks at great distances. However, Asplin (8) found no serologic evidence of DHV type 1 in VN tests of sera from 520 wild aquatic fowl of six species. These negative results were fortified by failure of Ulbrich (112) to find VN antibodies in 36 wild ducks (four species) taken from ponds where DH type 1 had occurred in domestic ducks. In addition, all of 153 wild duck embryonated eggs from an infected area were susceptible to experimental infection.

Of possible significance in the epizootiology of the disease is the report of Demakov et al. (22) indicating that brown rats (*Rattus norvegicus*) could act as a reservoir host of DHV type 1. Ingested virus remained alive in the body up to 35 days and the virus was excreted 18–22 days PI. Serum antibodies were also present 12–24 days PI.

Vectors are not known to be a factor in transmission of DH type 1.

Signs. Onset and spread of DH type 1 are very rapid, with practically all mortality occurring within 3–4 days. Affected ducklings at first fail to keep up with the brood. Within a short time, they stop moving and squat down with eyes partially closed. Birds fall on their sides, kick spasmodically with both legs, and die with heads drawn back (Fig. 25.1B). Death occurs within an hour or so after signs are noted. During the height of severe outbreaks, the rapidity with which ducklings die is astonishing.

Farmer et al. (27, 28) described duck fatty kidney syndrome and focal pancreatic necrosis, which were considered to be aspects of DH type 1. Between 1978 and 1983, losses up to 30% were recorded on certain duck-rearing farms in the United Kingdom. Two age groups, 1–2 wk and 4–6 wk old, were affected despite routine vaccination with type 1 vaccine. Gross lesions were characterized by pale swollen livers and kidneys, and swollen mottled spleens. Histologic evidence was indicative of DH type 1. Despite vaccination with attenuated DHV type 1, and the age of the older group of birds, the authors suggested that this syndrome was a manifestation of DH type 1. They acknowledged, however, that DHV type 2, which was subsequently diagnosed in East Anglia (46, 47), may have played a role in this syndrome.

Morbidity and Mortality. Morbidity is 100% and mortality is variable in young ducklings infected with DHV type 1. In some broods less than 1 wk old, mortality may reach 95%. In ducklings 1–3 wk of age, mortality may be 50% or less. In ducklings 4–5 wk of age, morbidity and mortality are low or negligible.

Gross Lesions. Principal lesions due to DHV type 1 are found in the liver, which is enlarged and contains punctate or ecchymotic hemorrhages (Fig. 25.1C). Frequent reddish discoloration or mottling of the liver surface is seen. The spleen is sometimes enlarged and mottled. In numerous cases, the kidneys are swollen and renal blood vessels congested.

Histopathology. Microscopic changes in uncomplicated, experimentally induced DHV type 1 infections have been studied (26). Primary changes in the acute disease consisted of necrosis of hepatic cells (Fig. 25.1D); survivors with more chronic lesions showed widespread bile duct hyperplasia (Fig. 25.1E). Varying degrees of inflammatory cell response and hemorrhage occurred. Regeneration of liver parenchyma was observed in ducklings that did not die. Ten-day-old chicken embryos inoculated with DHV type 1 were killed and examined histologically at 12-hr intervals for periods up to 10

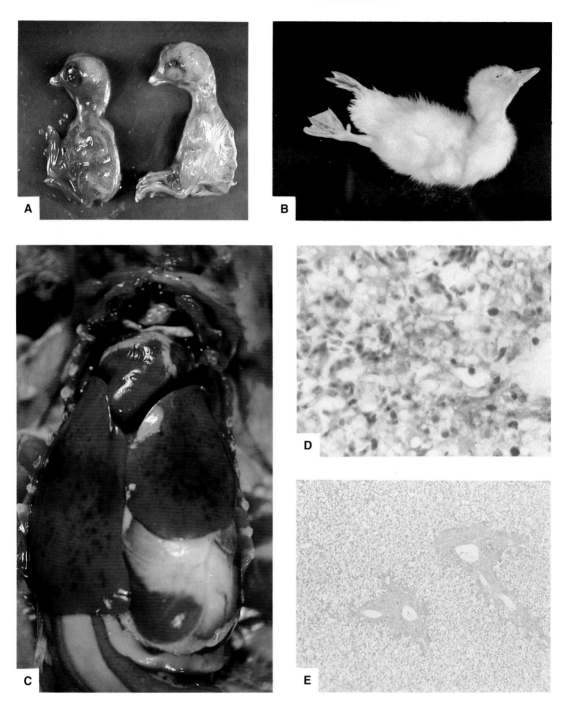

25.1. *A.* Normal 15-day-old chick embryo (*right*). Fifteen-day-old chicken embryo inoculated 6 days previously with duck hepatitis virus (DHV) type 1 (*left*). Note small size, hemorrhage, and edema. *B.* Duckling dead from infection with DHV type 1. Note typical opisthotonos. *C.* Liver with hemorrhagic lesions caused by DHV type 1 infection. *D.* Microscopic lesions in liver of duckling 24 hr after infection. Note massive liver cell necrosis and hemorrhage. H & E, ×1000. *E.* Microscopic lesions in liver of duckling 7 days after infection. Note extensive bile duct proliferation. H & E, ×250.

days PI (32). Histologic changes included proliferation of granulocytes in various organs, focal necrosis of the liver, bile duct hyperplasia, and subcutaneous edema. Inclusion bodies were not found. Six-day-old ducklings were infected intranasally and intramuscularly with DHV type 1 and killed 14–24 hr later. Their livers were examined by EM. One hr after infection, there was an occasional breakup of glycogen within the liver cells. Spherical particles 100–300 nm in diameter and of unknown origin were visible. Changes seen in peracute cases were degenerative, and there was extensive cell necrosis after 24 hr. Viruslike particles were detected at 1 hr and 18–20 hr PI (1).

Adamiker (2) examined spleen and muscle of ducks infected with DHV type 1 by EM. The spleen showed regressive changes from the 6th hr PI and became necrotic by the 24th hr. There were degenerative changes in the nuclei of plasma cells that may have been caused by the virus. Virus particles were not identified. Only slight changes were seen in muscles.

Biochemical Effects. Ahmed et al. (3) reported that in clinical cases of DH type 1, there were lower serum levels of total protein and albumen and elevated levels of alkaline phosphatase, glutamic pyruvic transaminase (GPT), bilirubin, and creatinine. Mennella and Mandelli (82) noted that serum levels of GPT and glutamic oxaloacetic transaminase were increased in relation to severity of infection. Buynitzky et al. (12, 13) indicated that even in clinically inapparent DHV type 1 infection in mallards, liver enzyme patterns were altered, with a consequent alteration in metabolism of DDT. This may partially explain the interrelationship between chlorinated hydrocarbons and DH type 1 (33, 35, 36).

Immunity. Recovery from DH type 1 results in solid immunity and VN antibodies in the serum. Active immunity can be induced in adult ducks by injection of certain strains of virus (6). Some strains require repeated injections to obtain high levels of antibody (96). Passive immunity can be conferred to ducklings by injection of serum from recovered or immunized birds. Passive antibodies may also be transferred through yolk to hatched ducklings to protect them. Malinovskaya (78), investigating the antibody response to DHV type 1 vaccine in breeder ducks and 7-day-old ducklings, showed by a passive hemagglutination (HA) test that duck serum contained more 7S antibodies (cysteine sensitive) than 19S antibodies (cysteine resistant). Decline of the 7S antibodies halved the hemagglutination-inhibition titers in 43% of serum samples taken 3–7 days PI. In ducklings experimentally infected between 3 and 21 days of age, the main type of antibody response was 19S during the ensuing 20 days; but in ducklings infected at 30 days of age, 19S antibody was formed first, but 7S antibody began to appear after 15 days. Davis and Hannant (20) reported that VN antibody was present 4 days postvaccination of 2-day-old ducklings. The antibodies were shown to be in the macroglobulin and 7S fractions by Sephadex G200 chromatography and had τ or β_2 mobility by immunoelectrophoresis.

DIAGNOSIS

Virus Isolation and Identification. Duck hepatitis virus type 1 may be isolated by inoculating infective liver suspensions or blood into the allantoic sac of 8- to 10-day-old chicken embryos. In embryos that die 5–8 days PI, gross lesions consist of cutaneous hemorrhage and edema, dwarfing, and enlarged greenish livers with necrotic foci. On subsequent passages, the proportion of embryos that die with specific lesions tends to increase.

If available, 10- to 14-day-old duck embryos from susceptible breeder ducks are preferable to chicken embryos, since embryo mortality and lesions occur sooner after inoculation and at earlier embryo passages (49, 109). A still more sensitive and reliable method of virus diagnosis is reproduction of typical signs and lesions of DHV type 1 by inoculation of virus-susceptible 1- to 7-day-old ducklings.

A rapid and accurate diagnosis of DH type 1 can be made using the direct FA technique on livers of naturally occurring cases or inoculated duck embryos (75, 113).

Primary DEL cells were shown to be particularly sensitive to the virulent field strain Quodling (Q) of DHV type 1; CPE was best detected as plaques in cultures overlaid with agarose (115).

Serology. Serologic tests have not been useful in diagnosing acute outbreaks of DHV type 1. However, from the time the virus was first recognized (71), the VN test has been used for other purposes: virus identification, titration of serologic response to vaccination, and epidemiologic surveys.

Hwang (57) described an accurate, reproducible DHV type 1 neutralization test in chicken embryos. Modifications of this procedure were described (44, 110). Haider (49) described several modified VN tests in duck embryos or ducklings, and Golubnichi et al. (40) described a VN test with virus adapted to tissue culture. Malinovskaya (77) reported that a passive HA test was more sensitive than the VN test. Ivashhenko (63) examined the use of an indirect HA test for the diagnosis of DHV type 1 and showed a 90% correspondence between indirect HA and VN results.

Murty and Hanson (83) described the use of an agar gel diffusion precipitin (AGDP) test for identification of DHV type 1. Later studies by Wachendorfer (114) and Toth and Norcross (110) claimed that reactions seen by Murty and Hanson were not specific or related to DHV type 1 or antibodies. Zhao et al. (122) compared enzyme-linked immunosorbent assay (ELISA), VN, and AGDP for the detection of DHV type 1 antibodies in duck sera. In a report containing several errors, they claimed ELISA and VN to be comparable in sensitivity, but they did not quantitate their VN test results; AGDP was reported to be considerably less sensitive, but exactly what was being measured must be questioned in the light of other reports (110, 114).

Woolcock et al. (121) first described a plaque-reduction test for VN antibody. This assay was considerably more sensitive than VN assays in eggs. Chalmers and Woolcock (15) showed that sera collected from 16 uninfected ducks had 50% plaque reduction titers (VN_{50}) ranging between 1:12 and 1:250 with an average of 1:59. They suggested that the maximum VN_{50} titer for negative control serum should be taken as 1:250. Woolcock (115) reported a plaque reduction assay in DEL cells and showed that type 1 virus was only neutralized by type 1 antiserum and not by antisera to type 2 or type 3. He also reported that a VN_{50} of 1:64 in embryonated chicken eggs was equivalent to a VN_{50} in excess of 1:3200 in DEK cells. Kaleta (65) described a microneutralization assay for DHV type 1 in DEK cells. He claimed the assay to be more practical, rapid, and economical than alternative tests but considered the plaque reduction assay more sensitive. Woolcock (116) adapted this microneutralization assay to monitor the VN antibody responses of ducks to vaccines in field and laboratory trials.

Differential Diagnosis. The sudden onset, rapid spread, and acute course of the disease caused by DHV type 1 are characteristic. Hemorrhagic lesions in livers of ducklings up to 3 wk of age are practically pathognomonic. Occurrence of similar disease outbreaks, caused by serologic variants of type 1 virus or by DHV type 2 and DHV type 3, offers the main problem in differential diagnosis.

Chalmers et al. (16) reported an outbreak of DHV type 1 associated with *Chlamydia psittaci* in 4- to 6-wk-old birds and suggested a possible synergistic effect as the cause of the persistent 15% mortalities recorded. Gough and Wallis (45) reported DHV type 1 associated with influenza virus in 2- to 5-wk-old mallard ducks reared on a game farm. The DHV type 1 isolated was of low virulence, and it is suggested that the influenza virus may have exacerbated the hepatitis infection.

Other potential causes of acute mortality in ducklings include salmonellosis and aflatoxicosis. The latter disease may cause ataxia, convulsions, and opisthotonos as well as microscopic lesions of bile duct hyperplasia suggestive of DH but does not cause the same characteristic liver hemorrhages. None of the other common lethal diseases of ducks occur frequently in this young age group.

TREATMENT. As soon as the cause and nature of DH type 1 were recognized by Levine and Fabricant (71), it became apparent that ducklings might be protected by administration of serum from immune ducks. This procedure proved to be highly successful in laboratory experiments and in the field. For many years, the Duck Research Laboratory at Eastport, Long Island, kept a bank of antiserum processed from blood collected at the time of slaughter from recovered birds. Intramuscular injection of 0.5 mL DHV type 1 antiserum into each duckling of a brood at the time of the first deaths in an outbreak was an effective control method.

Rispens (99) suggested passive immunization by injection of yolk from eggs produced by hyperimmune breeder ducks. This procedure was modified (50) by substituting yolk from eggs produced by specific-pathogen–free chickens hyperimmunized with DHV type 1.

PREVENTION AND CONTROL

Management Procedures. Duck hepatitis type 1 can be prevented by strict isolation, particularly during the first 4–5 wk. In areas where the disease is prevalent, however, it is very difficult to obtain the necessary degree of isolation.

Panikar (87) and Kaszanyitzky and Tanyi (67) demonstrated the feasibility of eradicating DH type 1 in selected areas where isolation can be achieved. In both studies, vaccination of breeder ducks was used as part of the program.

Immunization. Resistance against DH type 1 may be conferred to ducklings by three methods: injection of immune serum or yolk as described under Treatment; immunization of breeding stock to ensure high levels of passively transferred antibody in the hatched ducklings; and direct active immunization of ducklings with live avirulent strains of DHV type 1.

Attenuated DHV type 1 strains suitable for vaccine use have been produced by passage in chicken embryos (5, 37, 38, 40, 61, 102) or duck embryos (99). Up to this time, various strains of chicken embryo–passaged DHV type 1 have been used most frequently as vaccines.

Davis (19) reported that triple plaque-purified strains of DHV type 1 vaccines could revert to virulence as readily as noncloned virus. This finding has been confirmed with various egg-passage levels of DHV type 1 (117). Davis suggested rapid passage as a method to increase genetic stability.

BREEDERS. Asplin (5) developed a chicken embryo–attenuated strain of virus for immunizing breeders. The method was to inoculate 0.5 mL undiluted egg-propagated virus IM 2–4 wk before collecting hatching eggs. Reuss (96) found it necessary, with the strain of virus he used, to make repeated injections in breeders to obtain sufficient antibody levels to protect hatched ducklings against challenge with virulent virus. The optimum age, dosage, route of inoculation, strain of virus, and interval between initial and subsequent vaccinations are not known (6).

Rispens (99) recommended two doses of attenuated virus vaccine administered to breeders at least 6 wk apart; passive immunity was transmitted to progeny for about 9 mo after the second vaccination.

Hwang (58), Rinaldi et al. (98), Nikitin and Panikar (84), and Doroshko and Bezrukavaya (24) all confirmed that two or three doses of attenuated virus vaccine were necessary to secure satisfactory levels of protection of progeny. Bezrukavaya (11) secured effective protection by vaccination of breeders with duck embryo–attenuated vaccine. Demakov et al. (23) reported that effectiveness of the chicken embryo–attenuated strain was improved by aluminum hydroxide adsorption and a saponin adjuvant. Malinovskaya (79) looked at the effect of chemical stimulators on postvaccinal immunity against DHV type 1 by assaying for passive HA and VN antibodies. Dibazol had no effect, but saponin, methyluracil, and ascorbic acid promoted an accelerated antibody response, which was particularly pronounced 15 days postvaccination.

Golubnichi and Malinovskaya (39) monitored the immune response, following up to three immunizations over a 3-mo period, by assaying HA and VN antibody. The antibody titers in sera of laying ducks necessary to protect their offspring was 1:64 for HA and 1:32 for VN antibodies.

The application of inactivated vaccines also has been investigated. Gough and Spackman (44) reported that effective levels of duckling protection can be secured by administering three doses of inactivated DHV type 1 oil-emulsion vaccine. These workers also reported that live DHV type 1 vaccine at 2–3 days of age, followed by inactivated vaccine at 22 wk, produced significantly higher VN antibody levels than did three doses of inactivated vaccine. Finally, they reported that inactivated vaccine prepared from virus grown in duck eggs gave a better antibody response than virus grown in chicken eggs. Woolcock (116), investigating the use of inactivated DHV type I vaccines in breeder ducks, showed that in order to ensure an adequate immune response to the inactivated virus, it was necessary to prime the ducks with DH type 1–modified live virus (MLV). He showed that ducks primed with MLV at

12 wk of age, and boosted with inactivated DHV type 1 vaccine at 18 wk, developed VN antibody titers 16-fold higher than those in ducks that received only the MLV priming. This level of immunity was sufficient to protect ducklings hatched through a complete laying cycle (8 mo), as demonstrated by challenging progeny with virulent DHV type 1. Inactivated vaccines prepared from MLV grown in embryos or from virulent type 1 virus grown in ducklings were both equally effective. Woolcock (116) also investigated various immunization schedules, using inactivated virus alone, and monitored the VN antibody response of individual ducks in a microtiter assay using primary DEL cells. Only 7 (11%) of 63 ducks developed titers of 6 $\log_2$ or greater, which was considered the minimum protective level, and these responses were only in birds given multiple inoculations of inactivated vaccine.

DUCKLINGS. Asplin (5) used his chicken embryo–attenuated strain of DHV type 1 to vaccinate ducklings by the foot web–stab method. Reuss (96) also reported successful immunization experiments with an attenuated strain.

Newly hatched ducklings injected IM with an attenuated DHV type 1 developed resistance in 3 days (59). Oral exposure required up to 6 days for protection to occur. There was evidence that vaccination would be of benefit even at the start of an outbreak.

Lyophilized, attenuated strains of DHV type 1 induced a considerable degree of protection in day-old ducklings inoculated by the IM, intranasal, or foot-web route (123). Crighton and Woolcock (17) and Gazdzinski (38) also reported successful immunization of ducklings by the (subcutaneous) SC and IM routes, respectively, with chicken embryo–passaged DHV type 1. Golubnichi et al. (40) used tissue culture–passaged DHV type 1 for duckling immunization. Effective mass vaccination of ducklings by the aerosol and drinking water routes have been reported (52, 68, 69, 85, 88, 111). Ducklings vaccinated orally at 2–3 days of age did not show an increased immune response when revaccinated at 17 days (9). Balla et al. (10) examined administration in the field of DHV type 1 vaccine by SC and drinking water routes. They reported that two doses given in the drinking water at 2–3 days of age were as effective as one dose given orally at 2 days of age.

Balla and Veress (9) examined the antibody response of ducklings of different immune status to SC and oral vaccination with live attenuated DHV type 1. They found that susceptible ducklings and those hatched with maternally derived immunity both responded to vaccination with 1600–9600 EID_{50} given during the first 3 wk of life. The maternally immune birds responded only marginally less. They also showed that a dose of 300–600 EID_{50}/duckling between 2 and 21 days and of 100 EID_{50} at 35 days was sufficient for seroconversion to occur irrespective of the ducklings' immune status. Exposure to an aerosol vaccine for 5–6 min at 2–5 days of age produced a good response in susceptible birds but not in maternally immune ducklings; 30-min exposure to aerosol vaccine gave a good response, which was not boosted by reexposure at 16 days. They did not report any results covering challenge of any of these ducklings with virulent virus. Luff and Hopkins (74) also looked at the effect of maternally derived immunity on vaccination of ducklings with live attenuated DHV type 1. Ducklings were vaccinated when about 12 hr old and were challenged with virulent DHV type 1 at 24

hr, and 3 and 6 days. Their results suggested that partially protective levels of maternally derived antibody did not adversely affect either the speed of onset or the extent of protection afforded by the currently available live vaccine. Unfortunately, findings were limited to the first 6 days of life.

In contrast to the results reported by Luff and Hopkins, field experience has indicated that successful practical duckling vaccination is dependent on the absence of maternal antibodies and is influenced by time and severity of exposure to virulent virus. Vaccination is also less effective when ducklings are exposed to virulent virus early in life, especially in endemic areas and on heavily infected premises. Judicious application of proper hygiene and sanitation methods could do much to solve this problem.

DUCK HEPATITIS TYPE 2

Duck hepatitis type 2, although similar to DH type 1 as a pathologic entity, is caused by an entirely different agent. The first report of an outbreak of DH type 2 in ducklings was from Norfolk, England, in 1965 (7). The affected flock had been vaccinated with attenuated DHV type 1. An agent was isolated which was shown, by cross-protection studies in ducklings, to be different from DHV type 1 and was named DHV type 2 (7). The disease disappeared from commercial flocks by 1969 but reappeared in 1983/84 on three farms, again in Norfolk, England (47). Losses in that outbreak varied between 10 and 25% in 3- to 6-wk-old birds, and up to 50% in 6- to 14-day-old birds. Outbreaks on affected farms were often sporadic, affecting some batches of ducks and not others. There are no reports of the disease occurring outside of East Anglia, England, and since the outbreaks in the mid-1980s, there have been no more outbreaks of the disease in that area (43).

Duck hepatitis virus type 2 particles have an astroviruslike morphology and a diameter between 28 and 30 nm as seen by EM (46). Aggregates containing more than 1000 virus particles have been observed in liver suspensions. On this basis, DHV type 2 has been classified as an astrovirus, and it has been suggested that it should be renamed duck astrovirus (41). It has been compared with astrovirus isolates from chickens and turkeys by cross-protection and transmission studies, and found to be antigenically distinct (42). The virus is resistant to chloroform, pH 3.0, trypsin treatment, and heating at 50 C for 60 min. Formaldehyde fumigation and stan-

dard disinfection procedures have eliminated the infection from contaminated premises (42).

Duck hepatitis virus type 2 replicated in embryonated chicken eggs following several blind passages in the amniotic sac (47). Few embryos died in less than 7 days, but infected embryos appeared stunted and had greenish necrotic livers in which astroviruslike particles could be demonstrated by EM. Attenuation of pathogenicity occurred after serial passage in chicken embryos (47). Various duck and chicken cell cultures appear to be refractory to infection (47, 115).

Ducks appear to be the only species affected by DHV type 2, and no wildlife reservoirs nor vectors have been detected. All recorded outbreaks have initially involved ducks kept on open fields; therefore, wildfowl, gulls, and other wild birds have been suspected as being vectors (41).

Infection occurs through oral, cloacal, and subcutaneous routes. Deaths occur within 1–4 days, usually within 1–2 hr after the appearance of clinical signs, which include polydypsia with loose droppings, excessive urate excretion, and sometimes convulsions and acute opisthotonos (42). Affected ducks usually die in good condition and both the time of death and the mortality rate (10–50%) depend on the age of the ducks (47). Survivors excrete virus for at least 1 wk after infection (42) and rear normally, with little evidence of retarded growth (47). Mature ducks are refractory to the disease (47).

The target organs for DHV type 2 appear to be

liver and kidneys (47). Significantly more virus is present in the liver, which is usually pale pink with multiple, small punctate hemorrhages, often forming confluent bands. The spleen is invariably enlarged and "sago-like" in appearance due to scattered pale foci. Kidneys are often swollen with blood vessels injected and standing out from the pale kidney substance. The alimentary tract is usually devoid of food. Occasionally, small hemorrhages are seen in the intestinal wall and on the heart fat. Microscopic changes in the acute disease are characterized by extensive necrosis of the hepatocyte cytoplasm and bile duct hyperplasia is usually present and widespread.

Gough (42) found that survivors of DH type 2 were immune to further infection. Detectable antibody levels following infection were shown to be low, using a varying virus-constant serum neutral-ization test in embryonated chicken eggs (41).

The most reliable diagnostic method for DHV type 2 is EM examination of liver homogenates for the detection of astroviruslike particles. The virus can only be isolated, with difficulty, following repeated passage in the amniotic sac of embryonated chicken or duck eggs. Inoculation of susceptible ducklings with virus gives a variable response; mortality up to 20% may occur within 2–4 days PI (47).

Inoculation of susceptible ducklings with convalescent serum obtained from DHV type 2–infected ducks has been used successfully to control the disease in the field (42). An experimental live attenuated virus vaccine also protected ducklings from challenge with virulent virus, but this vaccine has never been produced commercially (43).

DUCK HEPATITIS TYPE 3

Duck hepatitis type 3 was first reported by Toth (108) who observed hepatitis causing mortality and morbidity in ducklings immune to DHV type 1, on Long Island in the United States. The disease was less severe than DH type 1 and mortality rarely exceeded 30%. Based on differences from both DHV type 1 and DHV type 2, the agent was named DHV type 3 (51). The disease is only known to have occurred in the United States.

Haider and Calnek (51) reported that DHV type 3 contained RNA, based on insensitivity to IUdR, and was resistant to chloroform and pH 3.0 but sensitive to 50 C irrespective of the presence of 1 M $MgCl_2$. Electron microscopy of cultured duck kidney (DK) cells infected with the virus revealed crystalline arrays containing particles about 30 nm in diameter in the cytoplasm. Based on these observations, they suggested that DHV type 3 be classified as a picornavirus, but that it was unrelated to DHV type 1, since no common antigens could be demonstrated in VN and FA tests.

Nine- to 10-day-old duck embryos inoculated onto the CAM were susceptible to DHV type 3 (51). During the first passages embryo deaths were erratic and did not occur until the 8th or 9th day PI, but this was reduced with higher passages. In severely affected embryos, the CAMs were discolored and the surface of the affected areas had a dry, crusty or cheesy appearance. Underneath, the CAM was edematous and thickened up to 10 times normal. Embryo lesions included stunting, edema, skin hemorrhages, flaccid appearance, gelatinous fluid accumulations and enlargement of liver, kidneys, and spleen. Attenuation of pathogenicity for ducklings, accompanied by increased pathogenicity for duck embryos, occurred following serial passage in embryonated duck eggs inoculated by the CAM route. Chicken embryos were not susceptible to inoculation with DHV type 3.

Liver and kidney cell cultures of duck embryo or duckling origin were shown to support replication of the virus. This was demonstrated by a direct FA test to show foci of positively infected cells (51). Woolcock (115) reported that the type 3 virus failed to produce plaques in primary DEK and DEL cell monolayers.

Duck hepatitis virus type 3 has a low pathogenicity for ducklings experimentally infected, and only ducklings appear to be affected by the virus. Subcutaneous or IM inoculation of liver homogenate from infected ducklings into susceptible day-old ducklings is unreliable. Intravenous inoculation may increase the effectiveness. Mortality and virus yields from liver could be increased if ducklings received two or three doses of cyclophosphamide (2 mg/dose) on days 1–3 and were challenged with virus on the 6th day of age (14).

Ducklings dying from DHV type 3 infection show the typical appearance of type 1 infection, i.e., outstretched legs and opisthotonos (108). Mortality rarely exceeds 30%, but gross pathologic changes are similar to those caused by DHV type 1.

An active immune response to DHV type 3 can be stimulated in adult ducks by inoculation of attenuated virus. This immunity may be passively transferred, via the yolk, to progeny.

Duck hepatitis virus type 3 infection may be tentatively identified by inoculation of liver suspension onto the CAM of 10-day-old embryonated duck eggs if embryo lesions and mortality pattern develop as described above. Alternatively, virus may be isolated and identified in DK or DEK cultures examined by immunofluorescence 48–72 hr PI, using DHV type 3–specific antiserum. A direct FA test in duckling livers and DEK or DK cells has been described for DHV type 3 (51). A serum neutralization test in embryonated duck eggs is possible. Differential diagnosis is similar to that described for type 1 virus.

Convalescent sera obtained from DHV type 3–infected ducks has been used effectively in the field to control outbreaks. A live attenuated vaccine has been used experimentally in breeder ducks to confer passive immunity to ducklings, but this vaccine has not been available commercially.

DUCK HEPATITIS B VIRUS INFECTION

Duck hepatitis B virus (DHBV) infection is widely distributed in domestic ducks and several species of migratory wild ducks. It is commonly found in the liver and serum. The virus is a small (40 nm diameter) DNA virus belonging to the hepadnavirus group which includes human and woodchuck hepatitis B viruses. In contrast to these mammalian hepadna viruses, DHBV has not been associated with significant lesions or clinical disease in either chronic congenitally acquired infection or acute experimentally induced infection.

A recent detailed review of the characteristics of this virus can be found in (29).

REFERENCES

1. Adamiker, D. 1969. Elektronenmikroskopische Untersuchungen zur Virushepatitis der EntenkÜken. Zentralbl Veterinaermed (B) 16:620–636.
2. Adamiker, D. 1970. Die Virushepatitis der EntenkÜken im elektronenmikroskopischen Bild. Teil II: Befunde an der Milz und am Muskel. Zentralbl Veterinaermed (B) 17:880–889.
3. Ahmed, A.A.S., Y.Z. El-Abdin, S. Hamza, and F.E. Saad. 1975. Effect of experimental duck virus hepatitis infection on some biochemical constituents and enzymes in the serum of white Pekin ducklings. Avian Dis 19:305–310.
4. Akulov, A.V., L.M. Kontrimavichus, and A.D. Maiboroda. 1972. Susceptibility of geese to duck hepatitis virus. Veterinariya 3:47; Abstr Vet Bull 42:4629.
5. Asplin, F.D. 1958. An attenuated strain of duck hepatitis virus. Vet Rec 70:1226–1230.
6. Asplin, F.D. 1961. Notes on epidemiology and vaccination for virus hepatitis of ducks. Off Int Epizoot Bull 56:793–800.
7. Asplin, F.D. 1965. Duck hepatitis: Vaccination against two serological types. Vet Rec 77:1529–1530.
8. Asplin, F.D. 1970. Examination of sera from wildfowl for antibodies against the viruses of duck plague, duck hepatitis and duck influenza. Vet Rec 87:182–183.
9. Balla, L., and T. Veress. 1984. Immunization experiments with a duck virus hepatitis vaccine. I. Antibody response of ducklings of different immune status after subcutaneous, oral and aerosol vaccination. Magy Allatorv Lapja 39:395–400; Abstr Vet Bull 1985:100.

10. Balla, L., T. Veress, E. Horvath, and G. Hegedus. 1984. Immunization experiments with a duck virus hepatitis vaccine. II. Efficacy of vaccination by drinking water in large duckling flocks. Magy Allatorv Lapja 39:401–404; Abstr Vet Bull 1985:100.
11. Bezrukavaya, I.J. 1978. Vaccine against duck virus hepatitis from strain ZM. Sborn Rab Puti Ob Vet Blago Prom Zivot (Kiev), pp. 90–95; Abstr Landwirtsch Zentralbl Abt IV 1981:1061.
12. Buynitzky, S.J., G.J. Tritz, and W.L. Ragland. 1977. Correlation of induced drug metabolism with titer of duck hepatitis virus in chickens. Res Commun Chem Pathol Pharmacol 17:275–282.
13. Buynitzky, S.J., G.O. Ware, and W.L. Ragland. 1978. Effect of viral infection on drug metabolism and pesticide disposition in ducks. Toxicol Appl Pharmacol 46:267–278.
14. Calnek, B.W. 1988. Personal communication.
15. Chalmers, W.S.K., and P.R. Woolcock. 1984. The effect of animal sera on duck hepatitis virus. Avian Pathol 13:727–732.
16. Chalmers, W.S.K., H. Farmer, and P.R. Woolcock. 1985. Duck hepatitis virus and Chlamydia psittaci outbreak. Vet Rec 116:223.
17. Crighton, G.W., and P.R. Woolcock. 1978. Active immunisation of ducklings against duck virus hepatitis. Vet Rec 102:358–361.
18. Davis, D. 1987. Temperature and pH stability of duck hepatitis virus. Avian Pathol 16:21–30.
19. Davis, D. 1987. Triple plaque purified strains of duck hepatitis virus and their potential as vaccines. Res Vet Sci 43:44–48.
20. Davis, D., and D. Hannant. 1987. Fractionation of neutralising antibodies in serum of ducklings vaccinated with live duck hepatitis virus vaccine. Res Vet Sci 43:276–277.
21. Davis, D., and P.R. Woolcock. 1986. Passage of duck hepatitis virus in cell cultures derived from avian embryos of different species. Res Vet Sci 41:133–134.
22. Demakov, G.P., S.N. Ostashev, V.N. Ogorodnikova, and M.A. Shilov. 1975. Infection of brown rats with duck hepatitis virus. Veterinariya 3:57–58; Abstr Vet Bull 45:4375.
23. Demakov, G.P., V.N. Ogorodnikova, A.P. Semenovykh, and F.A. Nabatov. 1979. Improvement of prophylaxis of duck viral hepatitis. Vestn Skh Nauki 10:85–87.
24. Doroshko, I.N., and I. Yu. Bezrukavaya. 1975. Field trials of duck viral hepatitis vaccine. Veterinariya 1:52–53; Abstr Vet Bull 45:2458.
25. Dvorakova, D., and Z. Kozusnik. 1970. The influence

of temperature and some disinfectants on duck hepatitis virus. Acta Vet Brno 39:151–156.

26. Fabricant, J., C.G. Rickard, and P.P. Levine. 1957. The pathology of duck virus hepatitis. Avian Dis 1:256–275.

27. Farmer, H., W.S.K. Chalmers, and P.R. Woolcock. 1986. Recent advances in duck viral hepatitis. In J.B. McFerran and M.S. McNulty (eds.). Acute Virus Infections of Poultry. Martinus Nijhoff Publishers, Dordrecht, pp. 213–222.

28. Farmer, F., W.S.K. Chalmers, and P.R. Woolcock. 1987. The duck fatty kidney syndrome-an aspect of duck viral hepatitis. Avian Pathol 16:227–236.

29. Fernholz, D., H. Wetz, and H. Will. 1993. Hepatitis B viruses in birds. In J.B. McFerran, and M.S. McNulty (eds.). Virus Infections of Birds. Elsevier, Amsterdam, pp. 111–119.

30. Fitzgerald, J.E., and L.E. Hanson. 1966. Certain properties of a cell-culture-modified duck hepatitis virus. Avian Dis 10:157–161.

31. Fitzgerald, J.E., L.E. Hanson, and M. Wingard. 1963. Cytopathic effects of duck hepatitis virus in duck embryo kidney cell cultures. Proc Soc Exp Biol Med 114:814–816.

32. Fitzgerald, J.E., L.E. Hanson, and J. Simon. 1969. Histopathologic changes induced with duck hepatitis virus in the developing chicken embryo. Avian Dis 13:147–157.

33. Friend, M., and D.O. Trainer. 1970. Polychlorinated biphenyl: Interaction with duck hepatitis virus. Science 170:1314–1316.

34. Friend, M., and D.O. Trainer. 1972. Experimental duck virus hepatitis in the mallard. Avian Dis 16:692–699.

35. Friend, M., and D.O. Trainer. 1974. Experimental DDT-duck hepatitis virus interaction studies in mallards. J Wildl Manage 38:887–895.

36. Friend, M., and D.O. Trainer. 1974. Experimental dieldrin-duck hepatitis virus interaction studies in mallards. J Wildl Manage 38:896–902.

37. Gazdzinski, P. 1979. Attenuation of duck hepatitis virus and evaluation of its usefulness for duckling immunisation. I. Studies on attenuation of the virus. Bull Vet Inst Pulawy 23:80–89.

38. Gazdzinski, P. 1979. Attenuation of duck hepatitis virus and evaluation of its usefulness for duckling immunisation. II. Studies on application of the attenuated strain of DVH for vaccination of ducklings. Bull Vet Inst Pulawy 23:89–98.

39. Golubnichi, V.P., and G.V. Malinovskaya. 1984. Dynamics of postvaccinal antibodies in blood serum against duck hepatitis virus. Vet Nauk Proiz (Minsk) 22:72–75; Abstr Agro Selekt 1985:1973.

40. Golubnichi, V.P., G.P. Tishchenko, and V.I. Korolkov. 1976. Preparation of tissue culture antigens of duck hepatitis virus. Vet Nauk Proiz Tr (Minsk) 14:88–90; Abstr Landwirtsch Zentralbl Abt IV 1977:2251.

41. Gough, R.E. 1986. Duck hepatitis type 2 associated with an astrovirus. In J.B. McFerran and M.S. McNulty (eds.). Acute Virus Infections of Poultry. Martinus Nijhoff, Dordrecht, pp. 223–230.

42. Gough, R.E. 1988. Personal communication.

43. Gough, R.E. 1995. Personal communication.

44. Gough, R.E., and D. Spackman. 1981. Studies with inactivated duck virus hepatitis vaccines in breeder ducks. Avian Pathol 10:471–479.

45. Gough, R.E., and A.S. Wallis. 1986. Duck hepatitis type I and influenza in mallard ducks (Anas platyrhynchos). Vet Rec 119:602.

46. Gough, R.E., M.S. Collins, E. Borland, and L.F. Keymer. 1984. Astrovirus-like particles associated with hepatitis in ducklings. Vet Rec 114:279.

47. Gough, R.E., E.D. Borland, I.F. Keymer, and J.C. Stuart. 1985. An outbreak of duck hepatitis type II in commercial ducks. Avian Pathol 14:227–236.

48. Guo, Y.P., and W.S. Pan. 1984. Preliminary identifications of the duck hepatitis virus serotypes isolated in Beijing, China. Chin J Vet Med 10:2–3; Abstr Vet Bull 1986:378.

49. Haider, S.A. 1980. Duck virus hepatitis. In S.B. Hitchner, C.H. Domermuth, H.G. Purchase, and J.E. Williams (eds.). Isolation and Identification of Avian Pathogens, 2nd ed. American Association of Avian Pathologists, Kennett Square, PA, pp. 75–76.

50. Haider, S.A. 1982. Personal communication.

51. Haider, S.A., and B.W. Calnek. 1979. In vitro isolation, propagation, and characterization of duck hepatitis virus type III. Avian Dis 23:715–729.

52. Hanson, L.E., and D.N. Tripathy. 1976. Oral immunization of ducklings with attenuated duck hepatitis virus. Dev Biol Stand 33:357–363.

53. Hanson, L.E., H.E. Rhoades, and R.L. Schricker. 1964. Properties of duck hepatitis virus. Avian Dis 8:196–202.

54. Hwang, J. 1965. A chicken-embryo-lethal strain of duck hepatitis virus. Avian Dis 9:417–422.

55. Hwang, J. 1965. Duck hepatitis virus in duck embryo fibroblast cultures. Avian Dis 9:285–290.

56. Hwang, J. 1966. Duck hepatitis virus in duck embryo liver cell cultures. Avian Dis 10:508–512.

57. Hwang, J. 1969. Duck hepatitis virus-neutralization test in chicken embryos. Am J Vet Res 30:861–864.

58. Hwang, J. 1970. Immunizing breeder ducks with chicken embryo-propagated duck hepatitis virus for production of parental immunity in their progenies. Am J Vet Res 31:805–807.

59. Hwang, J. 1972. Active immunization against duck hepatitis virus. Am J Vet Res 33:2539–2544.

60. Hwang, J. 1974. Susceptibility of poultry to duck hepatitis viral infection. Am J Vet Res 35:477–479.

61. Hwang, J., and E. Dougherty III. 1962. Serial passage of duck hepatitis virus in chicken embryos. Avian Dis 6:435–440.

62. Hwang, J., and E. Dougherty III. 1964. Distribution and concentration of duck hepatitis virus in inoculated ducklings and chicken embryos. Avian Dis 8:264–268.

63. Ivashhenko, V. 1982. The use of indirect hemagglutination reaction for the diagnosis of virus hepatitis of ducklings. Eksp Inf Inst Ptits 109:32–34; Abstr Landwirtsch Zentralbl Abt IV 1983:174.

64. Kaeberle, M.L., J.W. Drake, and L.E. Hanson. 1961. Cultivation of duck hepatitis virus in tissue culture. Proc Soc Exp Biol Med 106:755–757.

65. Kaleta, E. F. 1988. Duck viral hepatitis type I vaccination: monitoring of the immune response with a microneutralization test in Pekin duck embryo kidney cell culture. Avian Pathol 17:325–332.

66. Kapp, P., F. Karsai, and I. Weiner. 1969. On the pathogenesis of virus hepatitis of ducks. Magy Allatorv Lapja 24:289–294; Abstr Vet Bull 40:112.

67. Kaszanyitzky, E.J., and J. Tanyi. 1980. Studies on the laboratory diagnosis and epizootiology of duck virus hepatitis. Magy Allatorv Lapja 35:808–814.

68. Korolkov, V.I., and G.P. Tishchenko. 1975. Laboratory trials of a duck hepatitis vaccine. Tr Beloruss NI Vet Inst 13:79–83.

69. Korolkov, V.I., and V.P. Golubnichi, P.S. Khandogin, and M.A. Karvus. 1979. Aerosol vaccination method for virus hepatitis of ducklings. Vet Nauk Proiz Tr (Minsk) 17:82–83; Abstr Landwirtsch Zentralbl Abt IV 1980:2235.

70. Kurilenko, A.N., and A.P. Strelnikov. 1976. Cytopathic effect of duck hepatitis virus in transplantable piglet kidney cell culture. Sb Nauk Trud Moscow Vet Akad 85:122–124; Abstr Vet Bull 1978:317.

71. Levine, P.P., and J. Fabricant. 1950. A hitherto-undescribed virus disease of ducks in North America. Cornell Vet 40:71–86.

72. Levine, P.P., and M.S. Hofstad. 1945. Duck disease investigation. Annu Rep New York State Vet Coll, Ithaca, pp. 55–56.

73. Lu, Y.S., D.F. Lin, Y.L. Lee, Y.K. Liao, and H.J. Tsai.

1993. Infectious bill atrophy syndrome caused by parvovirus in a co-outbreak with duck viral hepatitis in ducklings in Taiwan. Avian Dis 37:591–596.

74. Luff, P.R., and I.G. Hopkins. 1986. Live duck virus hepatitis vaccination of maternally immune ducklings. Vet Rec 119:502–503.

75. Maiboroda, A.D. 1972. Formation of duck hepatitis virus in culture cells. Veterinariya (8):50–52; Abstr Vet Bull 42:6905.

76. Maiboroda, A.D., and L.M. Kontrimavichus. 1968. Propagation of duck hepatitis virus in goose-embryo cells. Byull Vses Inst Eksp Vet (4):5–7.

77. Malinovskaya, G.V. 1980. Use of passive hemagglutination reaction to determine antibodies in hyperimmune serum against virus hepatitis of ducklings. Tr Beloruss Inst Eksp Vet Minsk 18:54–56; Abstr Landwirtsch Zentralbl Abt IV 1981:1796.

78. Malinovskaya, G.V. 1982. Formation of 19S and 7S antibodies during immunogenesis and pathogenesis of duck viral hepatitis. Vet Nauk Proiz (Minsk) 19:68–70; Abstr Vet Bull 53:3209.

79. Malinovskaya, G.V. 1984. Influence of chemical stimulators on postvaccinal immunity against duck viral hepatitis. Vet Nauk Proiz (Minsk) 22:75–78; Abstr Agro Selekt 1985:1973.

80. Mason, R.A., N.M. Tauraso, and R.K. Ginn. 1972. Growth of duck hepatitis virus in chicken embryos and in cell cultures derived from infected embryos. Avian Dis 16:973–979.

81. Mason, W.S., G. Seal, and J. Summers. 1980. Virus of Pekin ducks with structural and biological relatedness to human hepatitis B virus. J Virol 36:829–836.

82. Mennella, G.R., and G. Mandelli. 1977. Glutamic-oxaloacetic (GOT) and glutamic-pyruvic (GPT) transaminases in the blood serum in experimental viral hepatitis of ducklings. Arch Veterinar Ital 28:187–190.

83. Murty, D.K., and L.E. Hanson. 1961. A modified microgel diffusion method and its application in the study of the virus of duck hepatitis. Am J Vet Res 22:274–278.

84. Nikitin, M.G., and I.I. Panikar. 1974. Specific prophylaxis of duck virus hepatitis. Veterinariya (8):51–53; Abstr Vet Bull 45:692.

85. Nikitin, M.G., I.I. Panikar, and V.V. Garkavaya. 1976. Aerosol immunization against duck virus hepatitis. Vestn Skh Nauki (1):124–26.

86. Pan, W.S. 1981. Growth curve and distribution of chick-embryo-adapted duck hepatitis virus in embryonated chicken eggs. Acta Vet Zootech Sin 12:259–262; Abstr Vet Bull 1982:494.

87. Panikar, I.I. 1979. Eradicating duck hepatitis virus from flocks. Veterinariya 4:35–36.

88. Panikar, I., and V. Gostrik. 1981. Aerosol vaccination of ducklings against duck virus hepatitis. Ptitsevodstvo (11):35; Abstr Landwirtsch Zentralbl Abt IV 1982:1475.

89. Park, N.Y. 1985. Occurrence of duck virus hepatitis in Korea. Korean J Vet Res 25:171–174.

90. Pollard, M., and T.J. Starr. 1959. Propagation of duck hepatitis virus in tissue culture. Proc Soc Exp Biol Med 101:521–524.

91. Polyakov, A.A., and G.D. Volkovskii. 1969. Survival of duckling hepatitis virus outside the host and methods of disinfection. Vses Inst Vet Sanit 34:278–290; Abstr Vet Bull 40:4843.

92. Priz, N.N. 1973. Comparative study of virus hepatitis in animals (dogs and ducks) using different routes of influence. Vopr Virusol (6):696–700; Abstr Vet Bull 44:2746.

93. Rahn, D.P. 1962. Susceptibility of turkeys to duck hepatitis virus and turkey hepatitis virus. MS Thesis, University of Illinois.

94. Rao, S.B.V., and B.R. Gupta. 1967. Studies on a filterable agent causing hepatitis in ducklings, and biliary cirrho-

sis and blood dyscrasia in adults. Indian J Poult Sci 2:18–30.

95. Reuss, U. 1959. Virusbiologische Untersuchungen bei der Entenhepatitis. Zentralbl Veterinaermed 6:209–248.

96. Reuss, U. 1959. Versuche zur aktiven und passiven Immunisierung bei der Virushepatitis der Entenküken. Zentralbl Veterinaermed 6:808–815.

97. Richter, W.R., E.J. Rozok, and S.M. Moize. 1964. Electron microscopy of virus like particles associated with duck viral hepatitis. Virology 24:114–116.

98. Rinaldi, A., G. Mandelli, G. Cervio, and A. Valeri. 1970. Immunization of the duck against viral hepatitis. Atti Soc Ital Sci Vet 24:663–665.

99. Rispens, B.H. 1969. Some aspects of control of infectious hepatitis in ducklings. Avian Dis 13:417–426.

100. Roszkowski, J., W. Kozaczynski, and P. Gazdzinski. 1980. Effect of attenuation on the pathogenicity of duck hepatitis virus, histopathological study. Bull Vet Inst Pulawy 24:41–48.

101. Sandhu, T.S., B.W. Calnek, and L. Zeman. 1992. Pathologic and serologic characterization of a variant of duck hepatitis type I virus. Avian Dis 36:932–936.

102. Schoop, G., H. Staub, and K. Erguney. 1959. Virus hepatitis of ducks. V. Attempted adaptation of the virus to chicken embryos. Monatsh Tierheilkd 11:99–106.

103. Shalaby, M.A., M.N.K. Ayoub, and I.M. Reda. 1978. A study on a new isolate of duck hepatitis virus and its relationship to other duck hepatitis virus strains. Vet Med J Cairo Univ 26:215–221.

104. Syurin, V.N., I.I. Panikar, and I.M. Shchetinskii. 1977. Immunogenesis and pathogenesis of viral hepatitis of ducks. Veterinariya 8:53–55.

105. Tauraso, N.M., G.E. Coghill, and M.J. Klutch. 1969. Properties of the attenuated vaccine strain of duck hepatitis virus. Avian Dis 13:321–329.

106. Tempel, E., and J. Beer. 1968. Die virushepatitis der enten. In H. Rohrer (ed.). Handbuch der Virusinfektionen bei Tieren, vol. 3. Gustav Fischer, Jena, Germany, pp. 1019–1032.

107. Toth, T.E. 1969. Chicken-embryo-adapted duck hepatitis virus growth curve in embryonated chicken eggs. Avian Dis 13:535–539.

108. Toth, T.E. 1969. Studies of an agent causing mortality among ducklings immune to duck virus hepatitis. Avian Dis 13:834–846.

109. Toth, T.E. 1975. Duck virus hepatitis. In S.B. Hitchner, C.H. Domermuth, H.G. Purchase, and J.E. Williams (eds.). Isolation and Identification of Avian Pathogens. American Association of Avian Pathologists, College Station, Texas, pp. 192–196.

110. Toth, T.E., and N.L. Norcross. 1981. Humoral immune response of the duck to duck hepatitis virus: Virus-neutralizing vs. virus-precipitating antibodies. Avian Dis 25:17–28.

111. Tripathy, D.N., and L.E. Hanson. 1986. Impact of oral immunisation against duck viral hepatitis in passively immune ducklings. Prevent Vet Med 4:355–360.

112. Ulbrich, F. 1971. Significance of wild ducks in the transmission of duck viral hepatitis. Monatsh Veterinaermed 26:629–631.

113. Vertinskii, K.I., B.F. Bessarabov, A.N. Kurilenko, A.P. Strelnikov, and P.M. Makhno. 1968. Pathogenesis and diagnosis of duck viral hepatitis. Veterinariya 7:27–30; Abstr Vet Bull 39:2074.

114. Wachendörfer, G. 1965. Das Agar-präzipitationsverfahren bei der Entenhepatitis, der Newcastle-Krankheit und besonders der klassischen Schweinepest-Seine Leistungsfähigkeit und Grenzen in der Virusdiagnostik. Zentralbl Veterinaermed 12:55–66.

115. Woolcock, P.R. 1986. An assay for duck hepatitis virus type I in duck embryo liver cells and a comparison with other assays. Avian Pathol 15:75–82.

116. Woolcock, P.R. 1991. Duck hepatitis virus type I: studies with inactivated vaccines in breeder ducks. Avian Pathol 20:509–522.

117. Woolcock, P.R. 1995. Unpublished data.

118. Woolcock, P.R., and G.W. Crighton. 1979. Duck virus hepatitis: Serial passage of attenuated virus in ducklings. Vet Rec 105:30–32.

119. Woolcock, P.R., and G.W. Crighton. 1981. Duck virus hepatitis: The effect of attenuation on virus stability in ducklings. Avian Pathol 10:113–119.

120. Woolcock, P.R., and J. Fabricant. 1991. Duck virus hepatitis. In B.W. Calnek, H.J. Barnes, C.W. Beard, W.M. Reid, and H.W. Yoder, Jr., eds. Diseases of Poultry, 9th ed. Iowa State University Press, Ames, Iowa, pp. 597–608.

121. Woolcock, P.R., W.S.K. Chalmers, and D. Davis. 1982. A plaque assay for duck hepatitis virus. Avian Pathol 11:607–610.

122. Zhao, X., R.M. Phillips, G. Li, and A. Zhong. 1991. Studies on the detection of antibody to duck hepatitis virus by enzyme-linked immunosorbent assay. Avian Dis 35:778–782.

123. Zubtsova, R.A. Laboratory trial of live vaccine against duck hepatitis containing GNKI attenuated strains. 1971. Tr Gos Nauchn-Kontrol Inst Vet Prep 17:127–132; Abstr Vet Bull 42:1870.

26 Duck Virus Enteritis (Duck Plague)

T. S. Sandhu and Louis Leibovitz

INTRODUCTION. Duck virus enteritis (DVE) is an acute, contagious herpesvirus infection of ducks, geese, and swans, characterized by vascular damage, tissue hemorrhages, digestive mucosal eruptions, lesions of lymphoid organs, and degenerative changes in parenchymatous organs.

Synonyms for the disease are *duck plague, eendenpest* (Dutch), *peste du canard* (French), *entenpest* (German), and *duck virus enteritis* (72). Although Bos (4) first used the term *duck plague*, it was proposed as the official name by Jansen and Kunst in 1949 (34). Subsequently, *DVE*, based on principal features of the disease and to distinguish it from fowl plague, has become the preferred term.

In duck-producing areas of the world where the disease has been reported, DVE has produced significant economic losses in market ducklings and laying breeder ducks due to mortality, condemnations, and decreased egg production. The first outbreak in the United States in 1967 caused losses in excess of $1 million during a 1-yr period for the small, but concentrated, duck industry of Long Island, New York (47).

Since the first reports of DVE in free-flying anseriforms (ducks, geese, and swans) (42, 48), serious outbreaks in migratory waterfowl with high mortality have occurred (20). Outbreaks in zoos and game farm flocks have also been reported (28, 46, 54).

Prior to the 1973 massive outbreak in migratory waterfowl in the Mississippi flyway, the United States Department of Agriculture considered the disease exotic; however, DVE is now considered enzootic because of its wide geographic distribution in North America. For a review of the disease in North American waterfowl, see Brand (5).

HISTORY. In 1923 Baudet (2) reported an outbreak of an acute, hemorrhagic disease of domestic ducks in the Netherlands. Bacterial cultures were negative, and the disease was experimentally reproduced in domestic ducks by injection of sterile filtered liver suspensions. Although presented as a previously unknown viral infection of ducks not infecting chickens, it was concluded the disease was due to a specific duck-adapted strain of fowl plague

(influenza) virus. Subsequently, more outbreaks were reported in the Netherlands. DeZeeuw (18) substantiated Baudet's findings and again indicated specificity of the virus for ducks. Although chickens, pigeons, and rabbits were refractory to experimental infection, he also believed the agent to be a specific duck-adapted strain of fowl plague virus. DeZeeuw suspected that wild waterfowl were carriers of the disease, as they were found within outbreak areas.

Bos (4) reexamined findings of the earlier workers and observed new outbreaks. He further characterized lesions, clinical course, and immune response of ducks by experimental study and was unable to infect chickens, pigeons, rabbits, guinea pigs, rats or mice experimentally. He concluded that the disease was not due to fowl plague virus but was a new distinct viral disease of ducks, which he termed "duck plague." This conclusion was based on the high degree of specificity of the agent for ducks, both in experimental and naturally occurring infections, persistence of the disease as a uniform entity in the Netherlands, and the longer incubation period. He differentiated it from Newcastle disease. These observations have been further supported by more detailed studies on virus propagation, incidence and distribution, pathology, and immunity (29, 30, 31, 32, 33, 34, 35, 36).

INCIDENCE AND DISTRIBUTION. In addition to the Netherlands, DVE has been suspected in China (35) and confirmed in France (21, 52), Belgium (17), India (56, 57), Thailand (59), England (1, 24), Canada (25, 77), Hungary (74), Denmark (60), Austria (58), and Vietnam (75).

In 1967, the first reported outbreak in North America was observed in White Pekin ducks in the concentrated duck-producing area of Long Island (47). In addition, outbreaks in wild, free-flying waterfowl on Long Island have occurred at seven different locations (42, 48). The disease has been reported in 21 states, with repeated outbreaks in New York, Pennsylvania (27), Maryland (55), California (66), Virginia, and Wisconsin. An extensive survey for duck enteritis virus (DEV) in North American wild waterfowl failed to detect the virus, indicating that the disease is not enzootic in them (6).

Concentrated large numbers of susceptible domestic ducks and geese enhance the probability of disease detection. In contrast, lack of information on DVE in wild waterfowl, small domestic flocks, ornamental bird collections, and zoos results from limited surveillance and inadequate sampling. Accordingly, the reported incidence of DVE in domestic ducks may be misleading when compared with its natural occurrence in other anseriforms.

In the Netherlands, a higher incidence of DVE was noted in the spring (30); however, on Long Island, no seasonal increase was noted. In contrast, a higher incidence of DVE in wild, free-flying anseriforms on Long Island was observed in the fall of 1967 (42).

ETIOLOGY. The causative agent of DVE is a herpesvirus.

Morphology. Electron microscopy of virus-infected cells revealed virus particles in both nucleus and cytoplasm (Fig. 26.1) (7). Bergmann and Kinder (3) and Tantaswasdi et al. (68) studied structure and maturation of DEV in the cells of infected ducklings. They recorded spherical nucleocapsids

about 91–93 nm in diameter with nucleoids (cores) approximately 61 nm in diameter in the nuclei of the host cells. Virus particles about 126–129 nm in diameter, probably the result of envelopment of nucleocapsids by the nuclear membrane, were seen in the cytoplasm and perinuclear spaces. Larger mature particles varying in size from 156 to 384 nm in diameter were observed in the tubular system of the endoplasmic reticulum in the cytoplasm. These consisted of enveloped nucleocapsids encased in an osmiophilic matrix and surrounded by an additional membrane. These morphological structures differentiate DEV from other animal herpesviruses (3).

Biologic Properties. DEV is nonhemagglutinating (29) and nonhemadsorbing (15). It produces intranuclear inclusions in infected chicken and duck embryo cell cultures (26) (Fig. 26.2). The virus has the ability to form plaques in cell cultures (15). In the presence of complement, antibodies to DEV are capable of lysing infected duck embryo fibroblasts (40).

Chemical Composition. The virion contains DNA (7). RNase had no effect on ultrastructural morphology of the virus, while exposure to DNase led to removal of the central core without affecting the envelope. Fluorescence of intranuclear inclusion bodies in cell cultures stained with acridine orange was also consistent with presence of DNA (26). Inactivation by pancreatic lipase indicates virions contain an essential lipid (26).

Replication. Development of the virus in cell cultures was studied by electron microscopy and growth curves of intracellular and extracellular virus (3, 7, 68). Examination of thin sections revealed development forms only in the nucleus 12 hr postinoculation. By 24 hr, in addition to viral forms

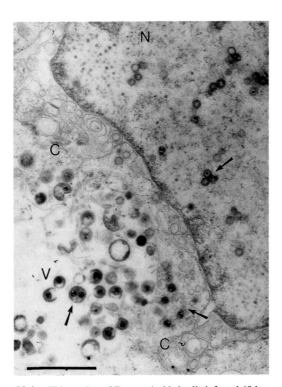

26.1. Thin section of Epon-embedded cells infected 48 hr with Long Island isolate of duck enteritis virus. Virus particles (*arrows*) appear in several forms in the nucleus (N), cytoplasm (C), and a cytoplasmic vacuole (V). Bar = 1 μm. (Breese and Dardiri).

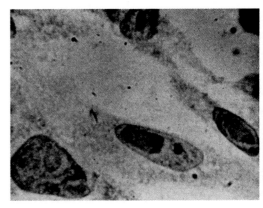

26.2. Inclusion bodies in duck embryo fibroblasts infected with duck virus enteritis. ×10,000. (Plum Island Animal Disease Laboratory).

in the nucleus, larger particles with an envelope were observed in the cytoplasm. Virus titrations of similar cell cultures demonstrated new cell-associated virus 4 hr postinoculation, with maximum titer at 48 hr. Extracellular virus was first detected 6–8 hr postinoculation and reached maximum titer at 60 hr (7). Increased incubation temperatures of tissue cultures (39.5–41.5 C) favored viral replication, especially less virulent strains (8).

Resistance to Chemical and Physical Agents.

The virus was found to be sensitive to ether and chloroform (26). Exposing virus for 18 hr at 37 C to trypsin, chymotrypsin, and pancreatic lipase markedly reduced or inactivated it, while papain, lysozyme, cellulase, DNase, and RNase had no effect. Cells treated with DNase showed intranuclear inclusions, but there was marked reduction in fluorescence when stained with acridine orange (26).

Thermal inactivation studies (26) revealed that infectivity was destroyed after heating for 10 min at 56 C or 90–120 min at 50 C. At room temperature (22 C), infectivity was lost after 30 days. Drying over calcium chloride at 22 C resulted in inactivation after 9 days.

Exposure of the virus for 6 hr at pH levels of 7, 8, and 9 resulted in no loss of titer, but a measurable titer reduction was noted at pH 5, 6, and 10. At pH 3 and 11, the virus was rapidly inactivated. A marked difference in inactivation rates was noted between pH 10 and 10.5 (26).

Strain Classification.

While differences in virulence among DEV strains have been noted, all appear immunologically identical (26, 33, 67). The virus is immunologically distinct from other avian viruses, including fowl plague, Newcastle disease, and duck hepatitis viruses (4, 15, 34, 49), and herpesviruses (63).

Laboratory Host Systems.

Duck enteritis virus can be propagated in duck embryo fibroblast tissue culture (79) incubated at 39.5–41.5 C (8), or on the chorioallantoic membrane (CAM) of 9- to 14-day-old embryonating duck eggs (29). Virus can also be grown in duck embryo liver or kidney cells (23). Duck enteritis virus can be adapted to grow in embryonating chicken eggs (29); however, they are unsatisfactory for primary isolation. It has been propagated in chicken embryo cell cultures (15) and muscovy duck fibroblasts (38).

A cytopathic effect occurs in cell cultures (39); a cell culture plaque assay method for titrating DEV concentrations and plaque inhibition by neutralizing antisera have been developed (15).

PATHOGENESIS AND EPIZOOTIOLOGY

Natural and Experimental Hosts.

Natural susceptibility to DVE has been limited to members of the family *Anatidae* (ducks, geese, swans) of the order Anseriformes, although the virus can be adapted by serial passage to grow in embryonating chicken eggs and chickens up to 2 wk of age (32, 33). Infection has not been reported in other avian species or mammals. Naturally occurring outbreaks have occurred in a variety of domestic ducks (*Anas platyrhynchos*), including White Pekin, khaki campbell, Indian runner, hybrids, and native ducks of mixed breeding. Outbreaks are quite common in muscovy ducks (*Cairina moschata*) (29, 48). Naturally occurring infections have also been reported in domestic geese (*Anser anser*) (36) and mute swans (37). Gray call ducks have been found resistant to lethal infection (73). Outbreaks of DVE in domestic ducks are frequently associated with aquatic environments cohabited by wild waterfowl (18, 48).

Susceptibility of various species of anseriforms to experimental DVE has been studied (73). In addition to domesticated species, they found mallards (*A. platyrhynchos*), Garganey teal (*A. querquedula*), gadwall (*A. strepera*), European widgeon (*A. penelope*), wood ducks (*Aix sponsa*), shovelers (*Spatula clypeata*), common pochards (*Aythya ferina*), common eiders (*Somateria mollissima*), white-fronted geese (*Anser albifrons*), bean geese (*A. fabalis*), and mute swans (*Cygnus olor*) susceptible to lethal infection. European teal (*A. crecca*) and pintails (*A. acuta*) were resistant to lethal effects but produced antibodies against DVE as a result of experimental exposure. Mallards were more resistant to lethal effects and were considered a possible natural reservoir of infection. A recent experimental study (76) showed blue-winged teal (*A. discors*) and Canada geese were extremely susceptible to DVE and experienced high mortalities. Blue-winged teal had few gross lesions at necropsy.

Of the order Charadriiformes, herring gulls (*Larus argentatus*) and black-headed gulls (*L. ridibundus*) were not susceptible to experimental infection and failed to produce antibodies against DVE (73).

The first reported outbreaks of spontaneous DVE in wild waterfowl were diagnosed on Long Island, New York (42, 47). It was detected in mallards, black ducks (*A. rubripes*), a Canada goose (*Branta canadensis*), a bufflehead (*Bucephala albeola*), a greater scaup (*Aythya marila*), and a mute swan.

A major epornitic of DVE occurred at Lake Andes, South Dakota, in 1973, with an estimated loss of 43,000 ducks and geese out of a total population of 100,000 (20). Duck virus enteritis was diagnosed in black ducks, mallards, pintail-mallard hybrids, redheads (*Aythya americana*), common mergansers, common goldeneyes (*Bucephala clangula*), canvasbacks (*Aythya valisineria*), American widgeon (*Mareca americana*), wood ducks, and Canada geese.

Transmission. Duck virus enteritis can be transmitted by direct contact between infected and susceptible birds, or indirectly by contact with a contaminated environment. Since waterfowl are dependent on an aquatic medium to provide a common vehicle for feeding, drinking, and body support, water appears to be the natural means of virus transmission from infected to susceptible individuals. Support for this concept is found in the history of new outbreaks in domestic ducks, which have been limited to birds having access to open bodies of water cohabited by free-flying waterfowl. Once infection is established, it can be maintained in the absence of open water or infected birds if susceptible populations are moved onto recently contaminated premises.

New foci of infection may be established by movement of infected waterfowl into susceptible flocks or onto bodies of water previously free of virus contamination. Course and direction of the infection are defined by population densities and rate of transmission between infected and susceptible waterfowl. Population densities in concentrated duck-producing areas encourage rapid spread of DVE, with high mortality. Breeder ducks are usually selected and placed in a defined area and maintained in the same location for the balance of their productive life. Once a breeder population is exposed, DVE is self-limiting. In contrast, market ducks are progressively moved as they mature and relocated in areas formerly occupied by the next oldest age group. Infection in market ducklings tends to be a continuous recycling as susceptible birds are sequentially moved to contaminated environments.

Experimentally, DVE can be transmitted via oral, intranasal, intravenous, intraperitoneal, intramuscular, and cloacal routes. Potential transmission by bloodsucking arthropods may be possible during viremia. While virus has been recovered from an egg removed from the cloaca of an infected domestic duck (32), it has not been recovered from eggs laid during a naturally occurring outbreak. Experimental vertical transmission has been reported in persistently infected waterfowl (9).

A carrier state has been suspected in wild ducks (12, 18, 73). Contact between domestic and wild anseriforms is common and frequently mediated by use of open bodies of water for duck production. Experimentally stressed carrier mallards shed more virus (11).

Incubation Period and Age. In domestic ducks, the incubation period ranges from 3 to 7 days. Once overt signs appear, death usually follows within 1 to 5 days. Naturally occurring infection has been observed in ages ranging from 7-day-old ducklings to mature breeder ducks.

Signs. In domestic breeder ducks, sudden, high, persistent flock mortality is often the first observation. Mature ducks die in good flesh. Prolapse of the penis may be evident in dead mature male breeders. In laying flocks, a marked drop in egg production may be noted during the period of highest mortality.

As DVE progresses within a flock, more signs are observed. Photophobia, associated with half-closed, pasted eyelids, inappetence, extreme thirst, droopiness, ataxia, ruffled feathers, nasal discharge, soiled vents, and watery diarrhea appear. Affected ducks are unable to stand; they maintain a posture with drooping outstretched wings and head down, suggesting weakness and depression. Sick ducks forced to move may have tremors of head, neck, and body.

Young market ducklings 2–7 wk of age show dehydration, loss of weight, blue beaks, and often a blood-stained vent.

Mortality. Total mortality in domestic ducks may range from 5 to 100%. Morbidity, based on the observation that sick birds usually die, closely approaches mortality. Adult breeder ducks tend to experience greater mortality than young ducks. No differences in mortality rates were found in mallard and White Pekin ducks infected with DVE and *Riemerella anatipestifer*, indicating that these organisms do not act synergistically (53). However, mallards immunosuppressed with cyclophosphamide and challenged with a sublethal dose of DEV had higher mortality (22).

Gross Lesions. The specific pathologic response to DEV is dependent on species affected (42); age, sex, and susceptibility of the affected host; stage of infection; and virulence and intensity of virus exposure (47, 48).

Lesions of DVE are those of vascular damage, eruptions at specific locations on the mucosal surface of the gastrointestinal tract, lesions of lymphoid organs, and degenerative sequelae in parenchymatous organs. These collective lesions, when present, are diagnostic of DVE.

Petechial, ecchymotic, or larger extravasations of blood may be found on or in the myocardium and other visceral organs and their supporting structures, including the mesentery and serous membranes. On the epicardium, especially within coronary grooves, closely packed petechiae give the surface a red "paintbrush" appearance (Fig. 26.3A). The latter lesion is observed more frequently in mature breeder ducks than in young market ducklings. When heart chambers are exposed, endocardial mural and valvular hemorrhages may also be observed.

Surfaces of liver, pancreas, intestine, lungs, and kidney may be covered with petechiae. In mature laying females, hemorrhages may be observed in deformed, discolored, ovarian follicles and massive hemorrhage from the ovary may fill the abdominal cavity. Lumina of intestines and gizzard are often filled with blood. The esophageal–proventricular sphincter appears as a hemorrhagic ring.

Specific digestive mucosal lesions are found in the oral cavity (12), esophagus, ceca, rectum, and cloaca. Each of these lesions undergoes progressive alterations during the course of the disease. Initially, macular surface hemorrhages appear, which are later covered by elevated, yellow white crusty plaques. Subsequently, the lesion becomes organized into a green superficial scab devoid of its former hemorrhagic base. Lesions range in size from approximately 1 to 10 mm in length. In the esophagus and cloaca, lesions may become confluent; however, close inspection will often reveal their composite structure. In the esophagus, macules occur parallel to longitudinal folds. When macular concentrations are numerous, small lesions may merge to form larger ones, suggesting a patchy diphtheritic membrane (Fig. 26.3B). In young ducklings, individual lesions in the esophagus are less frequent; sloughing of the entire mucosa is more common, and the lumen becomes lined with a thick yellow-white membrane. Oral erosions can be found at openings of sublingual salivary gland ducts in chronically infected waterfowl (12). Meckel's diverticulum may be hemorrhagic and contain a fibrinous core (61).

In ceca, macular lesions are singular, separated, and well defined between mucosal folds. The external surface of affected ceca often presents a barred, congested appearance.

Rectal lesions are usually few in number with greatest concentration at the posterior portion of the rectum, adjacent to the cloaca.

In the cloaca, macular lesions are densely packed; initially, the entire mucosa appears reddened. Later, individual plaquelike elevations become green and form a continuous scalelike band lining the lumen of the organ.

All lymphoid organs are affected. The spleen tends to be normal or smaller in size, dark, and mottled. The thymus has multiple petechiae and yellow focal areas on the surface and cut section, and is surrounded by clear yellow fluid that infiltrates and discolors subcutaneous tissues of the adjacent cervical region from the thoracic inlet to the upper third of the neck. The latter lesion is of importance in meat inspection and is easily detected when the opened neck of the carcass is observed on the processing line. The bursa of Fabricius is intensely reddened during early infection. The exterior becomes surrounded by clear yellow fluid that discolors adjacent tissue of the pelvic cavity. When the lumen of the bursa is opened, pinpoint yellow areas are found in an intensely reddened surface. Later, walls of the bursa become thin and dark, and the bursal lumen is filled with white coagulated exudate. Intestinal annular bands appear as intensely reddened rings visible from external and internal surfaces. Yellow pinpoint areas can be observed on the mucosal surface. Later, the entire band becomes dark brown and tends to separate at its margins from the mucosal surface. The multifocal necrosis of gut-associated lymphoid tissue causes ulceration covered by fibrinous pseudomembranes (Fig. 26.3C).

During early stages of infection, the entire liver surface is a pale copper color with an admixture of irregularly distributed pinpoint hemorrhages and white foci (Fig. 26.3D), giving it a heterogeneous, speckled appearance. Late stages of infection are characterized by dark bronze or bile-stained livers without hemorrhages; the white foci are larger and appear more distinct on the darker background.

Although the above lesions are representative, each age group responds distinctively. In ducklings, tissue hemorrhages are less pronounced and lymphoid lesions are more prominent. In mature domestic ducks with naturally regressed bursa of Fabricius and thymus, tissue hemorrhages and reproductive tract lesions predominate.

In geese, intestinal lymphoid disks (44) are analogous to annular bands in ducks. In a single Canada goose, lesions of the intestinal lymphoid disks resembled "button-like ulcers" (43). Similar intestinal lesions have been observed in an outbreak of DVE in Canada and Egyptian geese. In swans, diphtheritic esophagitis is a consistent lesion (37).

Histopathology. The initial lesion occurs in the walls of blood vessels. Smaller blood vessels, venules, and capillaries, instead of larger blood vessels, are more markedly involved. The endothelial lining is disrupted, and connective tissue of the wall becomes less compact, with visible separations at points where extravasations of blood pass from the lumen through the thin ruptured wall into surrounding tissues.

Hemorrhages are especially pronounced in certain locations: interlobular venules of the proventriculus, hepatic and portal venules at the margins of liver lobules, venules in the spaces between lung parabronchi, capillaries within intestinal villi, and star-shaped intralobular renal hemorrhages.

As a result of vascular damage, affected tissues undergo progressive degenerative changes. Microscopic changes can be found in any visceral organs including those without gross lesions.

Digestive lesions appear initially as hemorrhages of capillary arcades of submucosal papillae or folds. Hemorrhages become larger and confluent, elevating and separating the overlying mucosa. The affected epithelium above the hemorrhage becomes edematous, necrotic and raised into the lumen above normal adjacent mucosal surfaces (Fig. 26.3E). Later, margins of necrotic epithelium separate to define the borders of elevated plaques. Eosinophilic intranuclear and cytoplasmic inclusions have been seen in epithelial cells (68).

Hemorrhage from venules and capillaries fills lymphoid tissue within intestinal annular bands or lymphoid disks and lymphoid tissue of the esophageal–proventricular sphincter and spleen. Lymphocytes undergo karyorrhexis and pyknosis. Fragments of lymphocytes appear everywhere and are engulfed by phagocytes. In addition to cellular debris and hemorrhage within lymphoid follicles, there is marked swelling of reticulum cells, and their cytoplasm becomes subdivided and condensed into spherical and oval pale-staining bodies. Reticulum cells rupture and discharge their cytoplasmic contents into tissue spaces. An intranuclear inclusion body and delicate nuclear membrane and cell wall are remaining vestiges of reticulum cells.

Intestinal lymphoid lesions become large hemorrhagic infarcts. A layer of free blood separates lymphoid tissue from the mucosa, which undergoes coagulation necrosis. The necrotic mucosa forms a pseudomembrane higher than adjacent normal intestinal mucosa.

In the small intestines, sheets of epithelial cells are displaced from the surface of villi, many of which are broken and cast into the lumen. Abundant blood and cellular debris fill the lumen.

Within the bursa of Fabricius, submucosal and interfollicular capillary hemorrhages are found. There is a severe depletion of lymphocytes in the follicles, many of which have empty hollow cavities in the medulla. Corticomedullary epithelial cells, capillary networks, and large phagocytic cells containing fragmented lymphocytes form the circumference around these cavities.

In the thymus, free blood fills interfollicular spaces. Coagulation necrosis of central medullary reticulum cells and destruction of cortical lymphocytes are pronounced.

In mature female breeder ducks, congestive, hemorrhagic, and necrotic alterations occur in the oviduct. Follicles may be misshapen and blood stained. In the ovary of immature female breeder ducks, focal intestinal hemorrhages from capillaries and venules may be found.

In mature breeder drakes, focal capillary hemorrhages occur in interstitial tissues between seminiferous tubules. In parenchymatous organs such as liver, pancreas, and kidneys, hemorrhages and focal necrosis are found surrounding blood vessels.

Within necrotic foci in the liver, hepatic cords show a variety of changes including detachment and disassociation of hepatocytes from each other and their surrounding structure. A few necrotic liver cells become swollen or subdivided and discharge their cytoplasmic contents through a ruptured cell surface and are represented only by intranuclear inclusion bodies. Focal areas of necrosis may be filled with fibrin (Fig. 26.3F). Similar, but more limited, changes occur in pancreas and kidney (45).

Immunity. Field observations suggest that recovered birds are immune to reinfection by DEV. In an experimental study (10), superinfection of persistently infected mallard ducks resulted in death, indicating that protection against mortality was dependent on route of exposure, strain of the initial virus, and strain of superinfecting virus. It is assumed that both humoral and cell-mediated immunity are involved in protection (41, 71). Active immunity has been demonstrated following use of a modified live-virus vaccine (32). Maternal immunity has been reported in ducklings, but it declines rapidly. Progeny of breeder ducks vaccinated with a live-virus vaccine were fully susceptible. On the other hand, ducklings from breeders that had been vaccinated and challenged with a virulent virus were fully protected at 4 days of age, although less than 40% were protected at 13 days of age (70).

DIAGNOSIS. A presumptive diagnosis can be made on the basis of gross and histopathologic lesions. Isolation and identification of DEV confirms the diagnosis even in the absence of typical lesions. Primary virus isolation should be made by inoculation of susceptible 1-day-old White Pekin ducklings or the CAM of 9- to 14-day-old embryonated duck eggs. Characteristic lesions and mortality in susceptible ducklings are highly suggestive of DVE. Virus can also be isolated and propagated in White Pekin or muscovy duck embryo fibroblasts, liver, or kidney cells. Immunofluorescence tests can be used to detect viral antigens in cell cultures or tissue sections (19). Neutralization of such an isolate by known antiserum will confirm identification. Increase in virus neutralization (VN) titers following convalescence from DVE will demonstrate progress of the disease within a flock. A VN index of 1.75 or more indicates infection with DEV (14). A VN index of 0–1.5 has been found in sera of domestic and wild waterfowl not exposed to the disease. Use of chicken embryo–adapted virus in chicken eggs for VN studies is safer and more convenient than use of field-strain viruses inoculated onto the CAM of duck eggs (14). Other serologic procedures for detecting antibodies include a microtiter isolation and neutralization test using duck embryo fibroblasts (78), a reverse passive hemagglutination test (16), and enzyme-linked immunosorbent assay (ELISA) (65).

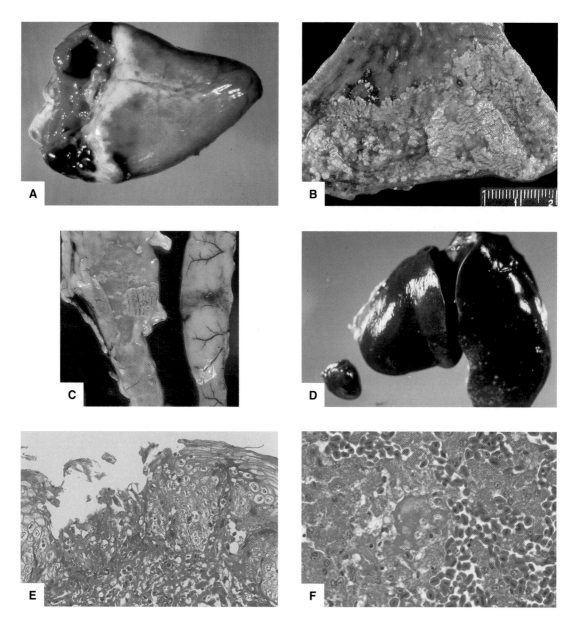

26.3. Duck virus enteritis (DVE) lesions in a muscovy duck. *A.* Petechial hemorrhages in the epicardium. (Munger). *B.* Extensive ulceration of esophageal mucosa. (Munger) *C.* Multifocal necrosis of gut-associated lymphoid tissue resulting in ulceration covered by fibrinous pseudomembranes. Note also the reddened ring visible on the external surface of the intestine. (Munger). *D.* Multiple pale foci in liver, and slightly smaller dark-colored spleen. *E.* Microscopic appearance of esophageal ulceration. Note lack of inflammatory response and presence of intranuclear inclusion bodies. ×225. (Munger, Barnes). *F.* Microscopically, liver shows focal areas of necrosis filled with fibrin. Intranuclear inclusion bodies can be seen in hepatacytes near areas of necrosis. ×360. (Munger, Barnes).

Differential diagnosis requires consideration of other diseases producing hemorrhagic and necrotic lesions in anseriforms. In domestic ducks, common diseases producing such changes are duck virus hepatitis, pasteurellosis, necrotic enteritis, coccidiosis, and specific intoxications. While Newcastle disease, fowl pox, and fowl plague are reported to produce similar changes in anseriforms, these diseases have been infrequently reported.

PREVENTION AND CONTROL.

There is no specific treatment for infection with DEV. Prevention is achieved by maintaining susceptible birds in environments free from exposure to the virus. These measures include addition of stock known to be free from infection and avoiding direct and indirect contact with possibly contaminated material. Introduction of the disease by free-flying anseriforms and contaminated aquatic environments must be prevented. Once DVE has been introduced, control can be effected by depopulation, removal of birds from the contaminated environments, sanitation, and disinfection. All possible measures should be taken to prevent dissemination of virus by free-flowing water. If authorized by government agencies, all susceptible ducklings should be vaccinated with a chicken embryo–adapted DVE vaccine. The vaccine can also be used in the face of an outbreak, as it provides protection immediately after vaccination due to an interference phenomenon (62). It should be noted, however, that birds in the period of incubation may not be protected.

In countries where the disease is not enzootic and is truly exotic, measures should be taken to further prevent entry and dissemination into geographic areas known to be free from DVE. This would include specific examination to prevent importation of infected anseriforms. Accordingly, there would be surveillance of ornamental bird collectors, zoos, and domestic growers of anseriforms. Efforts should be made to provide efficient detection of DEV by laboratory workers and waterfowl specialists so that its presence, status, and importance can be better defined.

Immunization.

Immunization has been used as a preventive measure and also for controlling disease outbreaks.

Inactivated vaccines have been tried but have not been as efficacious as modified live-virus vaccines (13).

A chicken embryo–adapted DEV strain, avirulent for domestic ducks, has been developed and used extensively with good success in the Netherlands (32). This vaccine strain has also been used to prevent and control DVE outbreaks on commercial duck farms in the United States and Canada. Vaccinated birds acquired resistance to infection as early as 1 day after vaccination due to interference phenomenon (31). The vaccine has been used successfully in outbreaks in commercial and captive waterfowl (54, 64). An apathogenic, immunogenic strain of DEV has recently been isolated and reported to be successful for active and passive immunization of ducks (50, 51).

The vaccine is administered in 0.5-mL doses by subcutaneous or intramuscular routes in domestic ducklings over 2 wk of age. Normally, the breeding flocks are vaccinated. Flocks maintained for more than a year are revaccinated annually. The vaccine strain does not spread among contacts. Apparently, vaccinated ducklings do not excrete inoculated virus to a degree that would be sufficient to bring about contact immunization (33, 69).

REFERENCES

1. Asplin, F. 1970. Examination of sera from wildfowl for antibodies against the viruses of duck plague, duck hepatitis and duck influenza. Vet Rec 87:182–183.
2. Baudet, A.E.R.F. 1923. Mortality in ducks in the Netherlands caused by a filtrable virus; fowl plague. Tijdschr Diergeneeskd 50:455–459.
3. Bergmann, V., and E. Kinder. 1982. Zu morphologie, reifung und wirkung des entenpestvirus im wirtsgewebe—Eine elektronenmikroskopische studie. Arch Exp Vet Med 36:455–463.
4. Bos, A. 1942. Some new cases of duck plague. Tijdschr Diergeneeskd 69:372–381.
5. Brand, C.J. 1987. Chapter 11: Duck plague. In M. Friend (ed.). Field Guide to Wildlife Diseases (General Field Procedures and Disease of Migratory Birds). United States Department of Interior Fish and Wildlife Services Resource Publication No. 167, Washington, DC.
6. Brand, C.J., and D.E. Docherty. 1984. A survey of North American migratory waterfowl for duck plague (duck virus enteritis) virus. J Wildl Dis 20:261–266.
7. Breese, S.S., Jr., and A.H. Dardiri. 1968. Electron microscopic characterization of duck plague virus. Virology 34:160–169.
8. Burgess, E.C., and T.M. Yuill. 1981. Increased cell culture incubation temperatures for duck plague virus isolation. Avian Dis 25:222–224.
9. Burgess, E.C., and T.M. Yuill. 1981. Vertical transmission of duck plague virus (DPV) by apparently healthy DPV carrier waterfowl. Avian Dis 25:795–800.
10. Burgess, E.C., and T.M. Yuill. 1982. Superinfection in ducks persistently infected with duck plague virus. Avian Dis 26:40–46.
11. Burgess, E.C., and T.M. Yuill. 1983. The influence of seven environmental and physiological factors on duck plague virus shedding by carrier mallards. J Wildl Dis 19:77–81.
12. Burgess, E.C., J.Ossa, and T.M. Yuill. 1979. Duck plague: A carrier state in waterfowl. Avian Dis 23:940–949.
13. Butterfield, W.K., and A.H. Dardiri. 1969. Serologic and immunologic response of ducks to inactivated and attenuated duck plague virus. Avian Dis 13:876–887.
14. Dardiri, A.H., and W.R. Hess. 1967. The incidence of neutralizing antibodies to duck plague virus in serums from domestic ducks and wild waterfowl in the United States of America. Proc 71st Annu Meet US Livest Sanit Assoc, pp. 225–237.
15. Dardiri, A.H., and W.R. Hess. 1968. A plaque assay for duck plague virus. Can J Comp Med Vet Sci 32:505–510.
16. Deng, M.Y., E.C. Burgess, and T.M. Yuill. 1984. De-

tection of duck plague virus by reverse passive hemagglutination test. Avian Dis 28:616–628.

17. Devos, A., N. Viaene, and H. Staelens. 1964. Duck plague in Belgium. Vlaams Diergeneeskd Tijdschr 33:260–266.

18. DeZeeuw, F.A. 1930. Nieuwe gevallen van eendenpest en de specificiteit van het virus. Tijdschr Diergeneeskd 57:1095–1098.

19. Erickson, G. A., J. S. Proctor, J. E. Pearson, and G. A. Gustafson. 1974. Diagnosis of duck virus enteritis (duck plague). Am Assoc Vet Lab Diag Proc 17:85–89.

20. Friend, M., and G.L. Pearson. 1973. Duck plague (duck virus enteritis) in wild waterfowl. US Dept Int Bur Sport Fish Wildl Bull, Washington, DC.

21. Gaudry, D., P. Precausta, G. de Saint-Aubert, J. Fontaine, J. Janson, R. Wemmenhove, and H. Kunst. 1970. Mise en evidence d'agents infectieux dans un elevage de Canards de Barbarie. Rev Med Vet 121:317–331.

22. Goldberg, D. R., T. M. Yuill, and E. C. Burgess. 1990. Mortality from duck plague virus in immunosuppressed adult mallard ducks. J Wildl Dis 26:299–306.

23. Gough, R. E., and D. J. Alexander. 1990. Duck virus enteritis in Great Britain, 1980 to 1989. Vet Record 126:595–597.

24. Hall, S.A., and J.R. Simmons. 1972. Duck plague (duck virus enteritis) in Britain. Vet Rec 90:691.

25. Hanson, J.A., and N.G. Willis. 1976. An outbreak of duck virus enteritis (duck plague) in Alberta. J Wildl Dis 12:258–262.

26. Hess, W.R., and A.H. Dardiri. 1968. Some properties of the virus of duck plague. Arch Gesamte Virusforsch 24:148–153.

27. Hwang, J., E.T. Mallinson, and R.E. Yoxheimer. 1975. Occurrence of duck virus enteritis (duck plague) in Pennsylvania, 1968–74. Avian Dis 19:382–384.

28. Jacobsen, G.S., J.E. Pearson, and T.M. Yuill. 1976. An epornitic of duck plague on a Wisconsin game farm. J Wildl Dis 12:20–26.

29. Jansen, J. 1961. Duck plague. Br Vet J 117:349–356.

30. Jansen, J. 1963. The incidence of duck plague. Tijdschr Diergeneeskd 88:1341–1343.

31. Jansen, J. 1964. The interference phenomenon in the development of resistance against duck plague. J Comp Pathol Ther 74:3–7.

32. Jansen, J. 1964. Duck plague (a concise survey). Indian Vet J 41:309–316.

33. Jansen, J. 1968. Duck plague. J Am Vet Med Assoc 152:1009–1016.

34. Jansen, J., and H. Kunst. 1949. Is duck plague related to Newcastle disease or to fowl plague? Proc 14th Int Vet Congr 2:363–365.

35. Jansen, J., and H. Kunst. 1964. The reported incidence of duck plague in Europe and Asia. Tijdschr Diergeneeskd 89:765–769.

36. Jansen, J., and R. Wemmenhove. 1965. Duck plague in domesticated geese (Anser anser). Tijdschr Diergeneeskd 90:811–815.

37. Keymer, I. F., and R. E. Gough. 1986. Duck virus enteritis (Anatid herpesvirus infection) in mute swans (Cygnus olor). Avian Pathol 15:161–170.

38. Kocan, R.M. 1976. Duck plague virus replication in Muscovy duck fibroblast cells. Avian Dis 20:574–580.

39. Kunst, H. 1967. Isolation of duck plague virus in tissue cultures. Tijdschr Diergeneeskd 92:713–714.

40. Lam, K.M. 1984. Antibody-and complement-mediated cytolysis against duck-enteritis-virus-infected cells. Avian Dis 28:1125–1129.

41. Lam, K. M., and W. Lin. 1986. Antibody-mediated resistance against duck enteritis virus infection. Can J Vet Res 50:380–383.

42. Leibovitz, L. 1968. Progress report: Duck plague surveillance of American Anseriformes. Bull Wildl Dis Assoc 4:87–90.

43. Leibovitz, L. 1969. The comparative pathology of duck plague in wild Anseriformes. J Wildl Manage 33:294–303.

44. Leibovitz, L. 1969. Duck plague. In J.W. Davis, R.C. Anderson, L. Karstad, and D.O. Trainer (eds.). Infectious and Parasitic Diseases of Wild Birds. Iowa State University Press, Ames, IA, pp. 22–33.

45. Leibovitz, L. 1971. Gross and histopathologic changes of duck plague (duck virus enteritis). Am J Vet Res 32:275–290.

46. Leibovitz, L. 1973. Necrotic enteritis of breeder ducks. Am J Vet Res 34:1053–1061.

47. Leibovitz, L., and J. Hwang. 1968. Duck plague on the American continent. Avian Dis 12:361–378.

48. Leibovitz, L., and J. Hwang. 1968. Duck plague in American Anseriformes. Bull Wildl Dis Assoc 4:13–14.

49. Levine, P.P., and J. Fabricant. 1950. A hitherto-undescribed virus disease of ducks in North America. Cornell Vet 40:71–86.

50. Lin, W., K.M. Lam, and W.E. Clark. 1984. Active and passive immunization of ducks against duck viral enteritis. Avian Dis 28:968–977.

51. Lin, W., K.M.Lam, and W.E. Clark. 1984. Isolation of an apathogenic immunogenic strain of duck enteritis virus from waterfowl in California. Avian Dis 28:641–650.

52. Lucam, F. 1949. La peste aviare en France. Proc 14th Int Vet Congr 2:380–382.

53. Mo, C.L. and E.C. Burgess. 1987. Infection of duck plague carriers with Pasteurella multocida and P. anatipestifer. Avian Dis 31:197–201.

54. Montali, R.J., M. Bush, and G.A. Greenwell. 1976. An epornitic of duck viral enteritis in a zoological park. J Am Vet Med Assoc 169:954–958.

55. Montgomery, R.D., G. Stein, Jr., M.N. Novilla, S.S. Hurley, and R.J. Fink. 1981. An outbreak of duck virus enteritis (duck plague) in a captive flock of mixed waterfowl. Avian Dis 25:207–213.

56. Mukerji, A., M.S. Das, B.B. Ghosh, and J.L. Ganguly. 1963. Duck plague in West Bengal. I and II. Indian Vet J 40:457–462.

57. Mukerji, A., M.S. Das, B.B. Ghosh, and J.L. Ganguly. 1965. Duck plague in West Bengal. III. Indian Vet J 42:811–815.

58. Pechan, V. P., H. Schweighardt, and E. Lauermann. 1985. Zum auftreten der entenpest in Oberosterreich. Wien Tierarztl Monatsschr 72:358–360.

59. Poomvises, P. 1976. Personal communication.

60. Prip, M., B. Jylling, J. Flensburg, and B. Bloch. 1983. An outbreak of duck virus enteritis among ducks and geese in Denmark. Nord Vet Med 35:385–396.

61. Proctor, S.J., G.L. Pearson, and L. Leibovitz. 1975. A color atlas of wildlife pathology. 2. Duck plague in free-flying water-fowl. Wildl Dis Color Fiche 67.

62. Richter, J.H.M., and M.C. Horzinek. 1993. Duck plague. In J.B. McFerran, and M.S. McNulty (eds.). Virus Infections of Birds. Elsevier Science Publishing Company, New York, pp. 77–90.

63. Roizman, B., L.E. Carmicheal, F. Deinhardt, G. de-Thé, A.J. Nahmias, et al. 1981. Herpesviridae: Definition, provisional nomenclature, and taxonomy. Intervirology 16:201–217.

64. Sandhu, T. 1992. Unpublished data.

65. Shawky, S. S. 1994. Unpublished data.

66. Snyder, S.B., J.G. Fox, L.H. Campbell, K.F. Tam, and A.O. Soave. 1973. An epornitic of duck virus enteritis (duck plague) in California. J Am Vet Med Assoc 163:647–652.

67. Spieker, J.O. 1977. Virulence assay and other studies of six North American strains of duck plague virus tested in wild and domestic waterfowl. PhD Dissertation. University of Wisconsin, Madison, WI.

68. Tantaswasdi, U., W. Wattanavijarn, S. Methiyapun, T. Kumagai, and M. Tajima. 1988. Light, immunofluorescent and electron microscopy of duck virus enteritis (duck

plague). Jpn J Vet Sci 50:1150–1160.

69. Toth, T.E. 1971. Active immunization of white pekin ducks against duck virus enteritis (duck plague) with modified-live virus vaccine: serologic and immunologic response of breeder ducks. Am J Vet Res 32:75–81.

70. Toth, T. E. 1971. Two aspects of duck virus enteritis: parental immunity, and persistence/excretion of virulent virus. Proc 74th Annu Meet US Anim Health Assoc 1970–1971, pp. 304–314.

71. Umamaheswararao, S., and B. V. Rao. 1993. Assay of cell mediated immune responses of ducks vaccinated against duck plague. Indian J Poult Sci 28:256–258.

72. USDA. 1967. Duck virus enteritis. Fed Reg 32:7012–7013.

73. Van Dorssen, C.A., and H. Kunst. 1955. Susceptibility of ducks and various other waterfowl to duck plague virus. Tijdschr Diergeneeskd 80:1286–1295.

74. Vetesi, F., V. Palya, S. Levay, and P. Kapp. 1982. A kacsapestis (duck plague) elofordulasa kacsaallomanyokban. Magy Allatorv Lapja 37:171–182.

75. Welling, R. 1993. Personal communication.

76. Wobeser, G. 1987. Experimental duck plague in blue-winged teal and Canada geese. J Wildl Dis 23:368–375.

77. Wobeser, G., and D.E. Docherty. 1987. A solitary case of duck plague in a wild mallard. J Wildl Dis 23:479–482.

78. Wolf, K., C.N. Burke, and M.C. Quimby. 1974. Duck viral enteritis: Microtiter plate isolation and neutralization test using the duck embryo fibroblast cell line. Avian Dis 18:427–434.

79. Wolf, K., C.N. Burke, and M.C. Quimby. 1976. Duck viral enteritis: A comparison of replication by CCL-141 and primary cultures of duck embryo fibroblasts. Avian Dis 20:447–454.

27 Viral Enteric Infections

INTRODUCTION
H. John Barnes

Collectively, infectious diseases affecting the digestive tract of commercial poultry likely result in more economic loss than those affecting any other system. Mortality can be considerable, but more typically, digestive tract diseases affect the value of the flock by depressing growth rate (decreased average daily gains), impairing efficient feed utilization (increased feed conversion ratios), decreasing flock uniformity, increasing susceptibility to and occurrence of other diseases, and increasing medication costs.

The effects of digestive tract disease continue long after clinical recovery of the flock. While compensatory growth may be possible following a brief period of feed deprivation, this does not happen when infectious diseases damage the intestinal mucosa; that growth potential has been effectively lost. When growth is depressed, supply organs (primarily viscera) preferentially receive nutrients at the expense of demand organs (primarily muscle). The result is decreased meat yield, especially high-value white meat, per carcass. Decreased average daily gains also result in decreased production efficiency. To obtain a projected quantity of product in the face of a 10% decreased growth, all production inputs must also be increased by a similar amount including number of breeders, hatchery capacity, number of farms, number of flocks produced, amount of feed prepared and delivered, and number of birds produced, handled, and processed. Yet all of these additional required inputs cannot be amortized across increased output—that remains unchanged because of the impact of digestive tract disease. The additional time required by flocks to reach market weights further erodes production efficiency by decreasing the number of birds raised on a given farm annually.

Feed constitutes the greatest single investment in a flock. Even slight differences in efficiency of feed utilization significantly impact flock value. Severe digestive diseases usually are accompanied by a virtual cessation of feed intake so, even though the birds are not growing, the net effect on feed utilization may be minimal. The more frequently occurring, less-severe digestive diseases affect growth while the birds maintain at least some feed consumption. Nutrients in the diet are often lost because of maldigestion and/or malabsorption. Nutrients that are absorbed are first utilized to combat the disease ("immunologic stress," see Chapter 2, Nutritional Diseases, Interactions Between Nutrition and Disease); remaining nutrients are utilized by the supply and demand organs in that order. The net result is that feed is used but much of it does not result in saleable product, which is reflected in an increased feed conversion ratio (quantity of feed:quantity of product) and decreased flock value.

Variations in the degree to which individual birds in a flock are affected by a digestive tract disease result in decreased uniformity, which persists and may even get worse as the flock matures. Lack of flock uniformity makes it difficult to make product forecasts or meet contracts for certain types of products. Processing efficiency is also directly influenced by flock uniformity. Procedures and equipment used for the "average" bird often do not work as well for over- or under-sized birds.

Digestive tract diseases influence the occurrence of other diseases. Direct mucosal damage can provide a portal of entry for other potential pathogens in the digestive system. Because birds lack mesenteric lymph nodes, foreign materials, including microorganisms, that cross the intestinal mucosal barrier enter the bloodstream and are processed in the liver. This can lead to hyperplasia of hepatic phagocytic (Kupffer) cells and focal to diffuse damage and inflammation (hepatitis). Failure to limit a pathogen to the liver may result in septicemia and localization at distant sites. Enteric-origin colisepticemia is a classic example of a disease that occurs this way.

Nutritional deficiencies, especially those related to fat-soluble vitamins and minerals, can occur as a result of maldigestion/malabsorption. It is common to see rickets in young, meat-type birds with digestive disease when they are still trying to grow; when growth has essentially stopped, thin, brittle bones (osteoporosis) are more common. Flocks that have experienced a digestive tract disease when they were young often have increased skeletal abnormalities as they become older.

Nutrient deficiencies, either directly or indirectly via immunologic stress, can affect the immune organs. During the first several weeks, the bursa of Fabricius and thymus develop at a rate much faster than the body as a whole. When the growth rate is slowed during this period because of digestive tract disease, these organs are highly labile to damage, which can lead to subsequent immunologic deficiency and increased susceptibility to other infectious diseases.

A variety of infectious agents can affect the digestive tract, but viruses cause the majority of primary infections that have the greatest impact on flock health and performance. Unfortunately, our knowledge of viral digestive tract diseases is rather limited compared with their importance as production constraints. Some, such as diseases caused by viruses discussed in this chapter and the chapter on adenoviruses (Chapter 23), are fairly well defined, although much about them still remains to be learned. The causes of the vast majority of infectious digestive tract disease occurrences remain largely unknown; often the disease may be so common and subtle that it even goes unrecognized. Information on these complex diseases of uncertain etiology can be found in Chapter 37.

While there are a number of problems inherent in the study of digestive tract diseases, the need is so great that a concerted effort to understand them better and to develop efficient prevention and control strategies must be undertaken.

CORONAVIRAL ENTERITIS OF TURKEYS (BLUECOMB DISEASE)

K. V. Nagaraja and B. S. Pomeroy

INTRODUCTION. Coronaviral enteritis (CE) is an acute, highly infectious disease affecting turkeys of all ages, characterized by loss of appetite, constant chirping, weight loss, depression, and wet droppings. Synonyms are *mud fever*, *bluecomb disease*, *transmissible enteritis*, and *infectious enteritis*.

In Minnesota between 1951 and 1971, CE was the most costly disease of turkeys. In 1966, CE accounted for 23% of all turkey mortality and over a half million dollars in lost income in that state. After 1971, there was a dramatic drop in incidence; less than 1% of total mortality in turkeys was caused by CE. The last focus of infection was eliminated in 1976 by controlled depopulation and decontamination with a rest period before restocking. There have been no reported outbreaks in Minnesota since 1977 (37). In other geographic areas, CE continues to be a cause of death. Once CE is introduced into areas with high concentrations of turkeys on a year-round basis, it is not easily eliminated and is encountered frequently in young birds.

HISTORY. Peterson and Hymas (38) described an unfamiliar disease of turkeys, known locally as "mud fever," with general characteristics of pullet disease in chickens, that had been observed in Washington state for the previous 7 yr. An extensive outbreak of CE caused severe losses in young turkeys in Minnesota in 1951 (41). A similar condition had been recognized sporadically in turkey flocks on range for several years previously. Subsequently, CE, similar to the disease in Minnesota, was recognized in other turkey-producing areas of the United States and Canada (19, 50) where it occurred as a serious problem in young turkeys.

Studies on the etiology of CE extended over a 20-yr period, and various agents were found associated with field outbreaks, including vibrio, reovirus, enterovirus, and papovavirus, but none was capable of reproducing CE experimentally (12, 21, 48, 52, 55, 57). Adams and Hofstad (1) first reproduced CE with an embryo-propagated virus.

INCIDENCE AND DISTRIBUTION. Coronaviral enteritis has been reported in several states in the United States, Canada, and Australia, but not in turkey-raising areas of Europe. Enteric diseases of undetermined cause, which may include CE, accounted for over 50% of enteritis cases reported in the United States and Canada (see also Chapter 37). More severe outbreaks occur in areas practicing multiple brooding and year-round turkey production.

ETIOLOGY

Classification. The causative agent is a coronavirus (33, 45). Characterization by electron microscopy (EM) of sucrose density gradient concentrates of buoyant density 1.16–1.24 g/mL revealed a particle of 135 nm (range 50–150 nm) diameter with an envelope manifesting a corona of petal-shaped projections (Fig. 27.1). Turkey coronavirus (TCV) reacted specifically with antibodies in hyperimmune serum, but not with normal serum or antibodies against four different coronaviruses. Transmission EM of intestine from infected poults and turkey embryos revealed small enveloped particles budding into membrane-lined cisternae within the cytoplasm of epithelial cells (3).

Physicochemical properties of TCV grown in embryonating turkey eggs indicate that it contains RNA (11). Chloroform treatment at 4 C for 10 min inactivates the virus. There is no reduction in infectivity at pH 3 at 22 C for 30 min. The virus is resistant to 50 C for 1 hr, even in the presence of 1 M magnesium sulfate.

Both Minnesota and Quebec TCV isolates agglutinate rabbit and guinea pig erythrocytes (RBCs), but not cattle, horse, sheep, mouse, goose, monkey, rooster, or chicken RBCs. By immuno-EM, hemag-glutination-inhibition, and Western immunoblotting assays, Quebec TCV isolates were found to be closely related to the Minnesota strain of TCV and the Mebus strain of bovine coronavirus (9).

Studies with TCV isolates from several states indicated a close immunologic relationship among them (42), but no relationship to a reovirus isolate causing severe enteritis in Georgia poultry (56).

Laboratory Host Systems

TURKEY AND CHICKEN EMBRYOS. Turkey coronavirus can be cultivated in embryonating turkey eggs >15 days of age and chicken eggs >16 days of age when inoculated via the amniotic cavity (1, 32, 33, 34). When turkey embryos at 23–24 days of age were infected, the agent was recovered from intestines, yolk, and bursa of Fabricius. Poults hatched from inoculated embryos developed CE and died (13). One hundred passages of the Minnesota TCV isolate were made in turkey eggs without loss of pathogenicity for young turkeys.

CELL CULTURES. Attempts have been made to cultivate TCV in a wide variety of cell cultures (26, 34). Turkey coronavirus has been serially propagated in HRT-18 cells, an established cell line derived from a human rectal adenocarcinoma (8). Ostrich embryo fibroblasts have developed cytopathic effects when inoculated with TCV (46). Survival of TCV in organ (4) and cell (13) cultures for up to 120 hr was observed, although virus multiplication apparently did not occur. There is in vitro interference against Newcastle disease virus in coronavirus-infected turkey embryo intestine cell cultures, a test with potential value for rapid identification of TCV (10).

PATHOGENESIS AND EPIZOOTIOLOGY

Hosts. Coronaviral enteritis affects turkeys of all ages. Chickens (26, 41, 50), pheasants (26), sea gulls (26), coturnix quail (24), and hamsters (24) are refractory to infection. Recently, enteritis suspected to be caused by coronavirus has been identified in ratites (20, 25), but it is unknown if this has any relationship to CE.

Transmission. Coronaviral enteritis is readily transmitted using unfiltered and filtered intestinal material administered by oral or rectal routes. Filtrates given intraperitoneally reproduce the disease, but intramuscular and subcutaneous inoculation fail to infect poults. Suspensions of heart, liver, spleen, kidney, and pancreas from infected turkeys did not cause CE when administered orally to 1-day-old poults. Cell-free filtrates of the bursa of Fabricius from infected birds were pathogenic for adult turkeys (31).

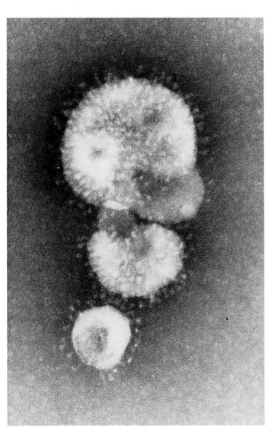

27.1. Turkey coronaviral enteritis (CE) virus. Three typical particles from infected turkey embryo intestine illustrating petal-shaped surface projections characteristic of coronaviruses. Particles have variable diameters, 50–150 nm; many appear hollow. ×200,000. (Ritchie)

Under natural conditions, CE spreads rapidly through a flock and from flock to flock on the same farm. Circumstantial evidence indicates that CE is spread from farm to farm by personnel, equipment, and vehicles. Free-flying birds may serve as mechanical vectors.

There is no evidence that CE is egg transmitted, but infection may be introduced into poults in a hatchery from contamination.

Turkey coronavirus is excreted in droppings of turkeys recovered from CE for several months, and remains viable in intestinal tracts stored at -20 C or lower for over 5 yr. Turkey coronavirus is readily destroyed by cleaning and sanitizing. In the field, it can only be eliminated in buildings that can be thoroughly cleaned and disinfected and allowed to remain empty for at least 3–4 wk before reintroducing birds. Turkey coronavirus may survive in pole barns, yards, and ranges from year to year even though depopulated of turkeys (41).

Incubation Period.

The typical incubation period is 2–3 days, but may vary from 1–5 days; clinical signs usually develop within 48 hr.

Signs.

In young poults and growing turkeys, CE appears suddenly; there is depression, subnormal body temperature, a drop in feed and water consumption, loss of body weight, and frothy or watery droppings. Poults constantly chirp, huddle together, and seek additional heat. In growing turkeys, the flock is depressed and sick birds show darkening of the head and skin accompanied by drooping wings, arched back, and retracted head. Droppings may be green to brown and contain mucus threads and casts. As the disease progresses, droppings contain mostly urates. When breeder hens in production are affected, a pattern of disease similar to that seen in growing turkeys occurs along with a rapid drop in egg production and chalky eggshells (41).

During experimental CE in 8- to 10-wk-old medium-sized white turkeys, reductions in body weight, ingestion and excretion of dry matter and water, and rectal temperature were comparable to those seen in control-fasted turkeys (17). The clinical course of CE often extends over a period of 10–14 days. Birds may require several weeks to regain lost weight. In mature birds, particularly males, some never regain satisfactory weight, and there is general unevenness in the flock.

Morbidity and Mortality.

Morbidity approaching 100% with weight loss depending on the degree birds go off feed and water is typical of CE. Morbidity loss may be high because of weight loss, stunted birds, and inability of the flock to grow at a normal rate. Experimentally, losses in young poults range from 50 to 100%. In older birds (6–8 wk old) mortality may approach 50%. In naturally occurring CE, losses range from 5 to 50% or occasionally even higher. In young turkeys (4–8 wk old), mortality can be kept minimal if supplemental heat is provided. In range turkeys 8 wk or older, losses may be low, but this is dependent on environmental conditions. In adverse weather, losses may be as high as 25–50%.

Infected poults have increased numbers of coliforms, clostridia, and non–lactose-fermenting bacteria (30). Gnotobiotic poults suffered only mild weight retardation, while conventional poults inoculated with intestinal filtrates from the infected gnotobiotes suffered severe disease. Gnotobiotes inoculated with intestinal filtrates and common enteric bacteria also suffered heavier losses than those inoculated with filtrate alone (26).

Gross Lesions.

Gross lesions are seen primarily in the intestinal tract. Contents of the duodenum, jejunum, and ceca are watery and gaseous. The duodenum may be swollen, pale and flaccid (Fig. 27.2). There may be gelatinous mucus and occasionally casts. Ceca are distended and filled with watery, yellow-brown contents having a fetid odor. Small petechial hemorrhages may be seen on the intestinal mucosa.

Breast muscle is usually dark and dehydrated, and the carcass is generally emaciated. Usually, internal organs are normal, but abnormalities are occasionally noted. The pancreas may have a chalky appearance with numerous white foci. Urate deposits are occasionally present in kidneys and ureters. Spleen is frequently smaller than normal (41).

Histopathology.

Intraluminal mononuclear cell exudate is present in the duodeno–jejunal area

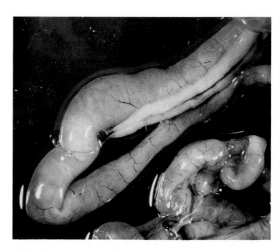

27.2. Turkey poult orally inoculated with turkey coronaviral enteritis (CE) virus at 7 days of age and necropsied at 4 days postinfection. Note swollen, pale, flaccid duodenum.

of experimentally and spontaneously infected turkeys (23). Histopathologic studies of 18-day-old poults experimentally infected with more purified virus preparations showed the following: at 2 days postinfection (PI), prominent concentrations of goblet cells on villi tips, cuboidal epithelial cells without microvilli, infiltration of lamina propria with mononuclear cells, and separation of epithelium from lamina propria; at 3 days PI, nearly all goblet cells had disappeared, and epithelial cells were "washed out" (2). A diminished cross-sectional intestinal diameter occurred along with a significantly decreased villus to crypt ratio (22). Lesions were most distinct in the jejunum but also seen in duodenum, ileum, and cecum. Over the following 2 wk, goblet cells reappeared, epithelial cells regained their microvilli and normal density, and infiltration of lamina propria gradually subsided. Argentaffin cell numbers decreased gradually until day 7, returning to normal by day 21.

Fasting produced similar signs and gross lesions in the intestinal tract (17), but not histopathologic changes (2, 14).

Transmission EM from infected poults corroborated histopathologic findings, but also showed damaged mitochondria, disrupted mucin production, and virus replication (3). Ultrastructural alterations include marked shortening of villi, loss of microvilli, epithelial desquamation, and hemorrhage in the jejunum, ileum, and cecum (3, 43).

Changes in the intestines of infected young turkeys, detected with scanning EM, began 1 day PI, progressed through day 3, and regressed on days 4 and 5. By 10 days PI, tissues were similar to those in controls. Diapedesis and catarrhal enteritis presented a striking picture with scanning EM compared with the equivocal lesions seen with light microscopy (22).

In combined fluorescent antibody (FA) tests and transmission EM studies of sequential intestinal samples from turkey embryos and poults infected with TCV (43), coronavirus antigens were first detected at 12 hr in a few cells at the base of villi. By 24 hr, villi were markedly shortened and immunofluorescent cells were observed over the entire villi. By 120 hr, villi had returned to normal, but specific fluorescence persisted in small groups of cells randomly located on villi and in crypts until 336 hr PI. Virus particles were detected only from 24 to 96 hr postinoculation.

Hematology. Hematologic changes in CE have been described, but are not consistent except for heterophilia (23, 47). Both lymphopenia and lymphocytosis, with and without monocytosis, were found by different investigators. Other changes in hematologic parameters (hypoproteinemia, hypoalbuminemia, hemoconcentration) apparently result from fasting rather than infection. In recovered turkeys, levels of alpha and gamma globulins are increased (42).

Immunity

ACTIVE. Turkeys that had recovered from experimental CE, challenged 3–4 wk later, or longer, resisted challenge (49). Turkeys surviving experimental infection at 4 days of age and challenged at 11 and 22 wk showed no clinical signs. Gross lesions were observed and FA tests on intestinal sections collected at 3 and 7 days PI were positive in control groups, but negative in immune groups (42). Field observations indicated flocks that had recovered from CE previously were resistant to subsequent attacks (41). IgM and IgG were present in the acute phase and IgA fraction at 14 days PI, but at 21 days PI, only IgG was present (5).

Intestinal secretions and bile from affected birds contained secretory IgA immunoglobulins against coronaviral antigen for at least 6 mo (27). Tissue localization of secretory antibodies in intestines of recovered birds was demonstrated by immunofluorescence (29).

Cell-mediated immune responses in turkeys infected with TCV may be important in determining immunity against infection (28).

PASSIVE. Poults given serum from recovered birds subcutaneously and subsequently exposed to experimental infection were not protected (41). When poults from recovered and susceptible breeding flocks were challenged with filtrates or infective intestinal material, they had little or no protection (53).

DIAGNOSIS. In turkeys of any age, typical signs with characteristic gross and microscopic lesions are suggestive of CE, but not diagnostic. Intestinal material from the small intestine, ceca, and bursa of Fabricius may be passed through a membrane filter of 220- or 300-nm porosity and injected into embryonating turkey eggs (>15 days) or 1- to 4-day-old poults for infectivity tests. The former has been used for routine cultivation of field isolates (34). Sections of intestinal tract from field cases and inoculated poults or embryos may be used for the direct FA test. A double-antibody enzyme-linked immunosorbent assay (ELISA) is more sensitive than EM for detecting coronaviruses in intestinal contents from turkey poults with diarrhea (6).

Immunology and Serology

FLUORESCENT ANTIBODY PROCEDURE. The direct FA test is highly useful for detecting TCV in intestinal epithelium from 1 to 28 days PI from field cases, infected turkey embryos, and poults. The indirect FA test detects antibodies in serum from 9 to at least 160 days PI. These tests permit detection of clinically affected, recovered, and carrier flocks (34, 35, 36, 37).

VIRUS NEUTRALIZATION. Tests may be done using turkey embryo intestinal homogenate as a source of virus, 1- to 4-day-old poults, and the suspected serum sample. The virus usually has a titer of 5 $\log_{10}$ poult-infectivity doses (PID)/mL. Pooled serum samples from recovered turkeys usually have a neutralizing index (NI) of 2–3 $\log_{10}$ PID. Pooled serum samples from susceptible turkeys usually have an NI of 0–1 $\log_{10}$ (42, 44).

Electron Microscopy. Examination of intestinal contents by negative-staining direct EM may provide a preliminary diagnosis of CE or identification of other enteric viruses. Particles resembling coronaviruses, presumably cell debris, are often seen, especially when whole intestine is prepared for examination. This, along with the pleomorphic nature of the virus, can make definitive morphologic recognition of TCV difficult. Coronavirus was more easily recognized by direct EM following precipitation with polyethylene glycol than by ultracentrifugation (7). Failure to identify coronaviruses on EM does not rule out the possibility of CE. A final diagnosis of CE must be made by FA or VN procedures.

Differential Diagnosis. In young poults, CE must be differentiated from inanition (starve-outs), water deprivation, and intestinal viral, bacterial, and protozoal infections. Medicated flocks may have secondary candidiasis. In growing and mature birds, increased numbers of trichomonads are found in contents of the ceca and rectum; their role in naturally occurring outbreaks is unknown. The possibility of known specific infections (e.g., erysipelas, fowl cholera, and histomoniasis) must be eliminated by appropriate diagnostic methods.

TREATMENT. No treatment regimen has been found completely effective in preventing CE. Antibiotics and other drugs help reduce mortality, most likely by controlling secondary infections. Individual oral treatment of turkeys with penicillin, chlortetracycline, and oxytetracycline (38), and penicillin, chlortetracycline, oxytetracycline, and streptomycin in feed or drinking water (39, 40, 41, 51) were effective in reducing death loss, but had little effect on morbidity. Three nitrofurans had prophylactic value in experimental infections, reducing mortality but having no effect on morbidity (54). These products are no longer approved for use in poultry flocks in the United States.

Force-feeding birds under laboratory conditions produced no beneficial effect (15, 16), nor did use of milk replacer, electrolytes, or glucose (18).

Treatment commonly used in outbreaks includes:

1. In the brooder house, provide additional heat until birds are comfortable, then decrease gradually as flock improves. Birds on range need protection from adverse weather.
2. Calf milk replacer, 25 lb/100 gal drinking water, is commonly used and mixed fresh each day.
3. Potassium chloride (KCl), 450 g/100 gal drinking water, is added to milk suspension.
4. An antibiotic is added to drinking water at the highest recommended level. Neomycin, oxytetracycline, chlortetracycline, streptomycin, penicillin, or bacitracin may be used.
5. Because secondary intestinal mycosis usually follows high levels of antibiotics, copper sulfate can be provided in the water. If approved for use, mycostatin may be used in feed.
6. Medicated drinking water is used 4–5 days, then untreated water is given 1 day and medication repeated an additional 4–5 days. It is usually about 10 days before the flock improves feed and water consumption.

PREVENTION AND CONTROL

Management Procedures. Prevention is the only means to achieve control of CE. The Minnesota turkey industry eliminated CE by controlled depopulation and decontamination of turkey buildings and surrounding areas with a rest period before restocking (37).

Farms that have had flocks with CE need to be completely depopulated of all turkeys and other fowl, followed by cleanup and disinfection of houses, equipment, and areas around permanent buildings. A period of depopulation for 3–4 weeks is highly desirable before repopulation, since feces from carrier birds remain the primary source of infection. Die-off of virus in feces and litter probably occurs faster in summer than winter.

Coronaviral enteritis may be introduced onto a turkey farm from outside sources. Observations point to processing trucks, loaders, equipment, and personnel that move from one farm to another without proper precautions. Other vectors may also be involved in transmission from active infections to new flocks in the area.

Immunization. Turkeys that recover from CE are immune to challenge but remain carriers for life. No licensed vaccine is available.

An exposure program is recommended only after all other methods of control have failed, and only on farms and in areas where CE is a continual problem.

REFERENCES

1. Adams, N.R., and M.S. Hofstad. 1971. Isolation of transmissible enteritis agent of turkeys in avian embryos. Avian Dis 15:426–433.

2. Adams, N.R., R.A. Ball, and M.S. Hofstad. 1970. Intestinal lesions in transmissible enteritis of turkeys. Avian Dis 14:392–399.

3. Adams, N.R., R.A. Ball, C.L. Annis, and M.S. Hofstad. 1972. Ultrastructural changes in the intestines of turkey poults and embryos affected with transmissible enteritis. J Comp Pathol 82:187–192.

4. Adams, N.R., M.S. Hofstad, and M.L. Frey. 1972. Growth of transmissible enteritis virus of turkeys in intestinal organ cultures. Arch Gesamte Virusforsch 38:97–99.

5. Carson, C.A., S.A. Naqi, an D.F. Hall. 1972. Serologic response of turkeys to an agent associated with infectious enteritis (bluecomb). Appl Microbiol 23:903–907.

6. Dea, S., and P. Tijssen. 1989. Detection of turkey enteric coronavirus by enzyme-linked immunosorbent assay and differentiation from other coronaviruses. Am J Vet Res 50:226–231.

7. Dea, S., G. Marsolais J., Beaubien, and R. Ruppanner. 1986. Coronaviruses associated with outbreaks of transmissible enteritis of turkeys in Quebec: Hemagglutination properties and cell cultivation. Avian Dis 30:319–326.

8. Dea, S., S. Garzon, and P. Tijssen. 1989. Isolation and trypsin-enhanced propagation of turkey enteric (bluecomb) coronaviruses in a continuous human rectal adenocarcinoma cell line. Am J Vet Res 50:1310–1318.

9. Dea, S., A. Verbeck, and P. Tijssen. 1991. Transmissible enteritis of turkeys: Experimental inoculation studies with tissue culture adapted turkey and bovine coronaviruses. Avian Dis 35:767–777.

10. Deshmukh, D.R., and B.S. Pomeroy. 1974. In vitro test for the detection of turkey bluecomb coronavirus interference against Newcastle disease virus. Am J Vet Res 35:1553–1556.

11. Deshmukh, D.R., and B.S. Pomeroy. 1974. Physicochemical characterization of a bluecomb coronavirus of turkeys. Am J Vet Res 35:1549–1552.

12. Deshmukh, D.R., C.T. Larsen, S.K. Dutta, and B.S. Pomeroy. 1969. Characterization of pathogenic filtrate and viruses isolated from turkeys with bluecomb. Am J Vet Res 30:1019–1025.

13. Deshmukh, D.R., C.T. Larsen, and B.S. Pomeroy. 1973. Survival of bluecomb agent in embryonating turkey eggs and cell cultures. Am J Vet Res 34:673–675.

14. Deshmukh, D.R., J.H. Sautter, B.L. Patel, and B.S. Pomeroy. 1976. Histopathology of fasting and bluecomb disease in turkey poults and embryos experimentally infected with bluecomb disease coronavirus. Avian Dis 20:631–640.

15. Duke, G.E., H.E. Dziuk, O.A. Evanson, and D.E. Nelson. 1970. Food metabolizability in normal and bluecomb diseased turkeys. Poult Sci 49:1037–1042.

16. Dziuk, H.E., G. E. Duke, O .A. Evanson, D. E. Nelson, and P. N. Schultz. 1969. Force-feeding turkeys during bluecomb disease. Poult Sci 48:843–846.

17. Dziuk, H.E., O.A. Evanson, and C.T. Larsen. 1969. Physiologic effects of fasting and bluecomb in turkeys. Am J Vet Res 30:1045–1056.

18. Dziuk, H.E., G.E. Duke, and O.A. Evanson. 1970. Milk replacer, electrolytes, and glucose for treating bluecomb in turkeys. Poult Sci 49:226–229.

19. Ferguson, A.E. 1961. Bluecomb-transmissible enteritis in turkeys. Can Poult Rev 85:74–76.

20. Frank, R.K., and J.W. Carpenter. 1992. Coronaviral enteritis in an ostrich (Struthio camelus) chick. J Zoo Wildl Med 23:103–107.

21. Fujisaki, Y., H. Kawamura, and D.P. Anderson. 1969. Reoviruses isolated from turkeys with bluecomb. Am J Vet Res 30:1035–1043.

22. Gonder, E., B.L. Patel, and B.S. Pomeroy. 1976. Scanning electron, light, and immunofluorescent microscopy of coronaviral enteritis of turkeys (bluecomb). Am J Vet Res 37:1435–1439.

23. Hilton, F.E. 1954. The pathology of bluecomb of turkeys. MS thesis. University of Minnesota, Minneapolis-St. Paul.

24. Hofstad, M.S., N. Adams, and M. L. Frey. 1969. Studies of filterable agent associated with infectious enteritis (bluecomb) of turkeys. Avian Dis 13:386–393.

25. Kennedy, M.A., and K.A. Brenneman. 1995. Enteritis associated with a coronavirus-like agent in a rhea (Rhea americana) chick. J Avian Med Surg 9:138–140.

26. Larsen, C.T. 1979. The etiology of bluecomb disease of turkeys. PhD thesis. University of Minnesota, Minneapolis-St. Paul.

27. Nagaraja, K.V., and B.S. Pomeroy. 1978. Secretory antibodies against turkey coronaviral enteritis. Am J Vet Res 39:1463–1465.

28. Nagaraja, K.V., and B.S. Pomeroy. 1980. Cell-mediated immunity against turkey coronaviral enteritis (bluecomb). Am J Vet Res 41:915–917.

29. Nagaraja, K.V., and B.S. Pomeroy. 1980. Immunofluorescent studies on localization of secretory immunoglobulins in the intestines of turkeys recovered from turkey coronaviral enteritis. Am J Vet Res 41:1283–1284.

30. Naqi, S.A., C.F. Hall, and D.H. Lewis. 1971. The intestinal microflora of turkeys: Comparison of apparently healthy and bluecomb-infected turkey poults. Avian Dis 15:14–21.

31. Naqi, S.A., B. Panigrahy, and C.F. Hall. 1972. Bursa of Fabricius, a source of bluecomb infectious agent. Avian Dis 16:937–939.

32. Naqi, S.A., B. Panigrahy, and C.F. Hall. 1975. Purification and concentration of viruses associated with transmissible (coronaviral) enteritis of turkeys (bluecomb). Am J Vet Res 36:548–552.

33. Panigrahy, B., S.A. Naqi, and C.F. Hall. 1973. Isolation and characterization of viruses associated with transmissible enteritis (bluecomb) of turkeys. Avian Dis 17:430–438.

34. Patel, B.L. 1975. Studies on immunofluorescent techniques for the diagnosis of turkey bluecomb disease (coronaviral enteritis). MS thesis. University of Minnesota, Minneapolis-St. Paul.

35. Patel, B.L., D.R. Deshmukh, and B.S. Pomeroy. 1975. Fluorescent antibody test for rapid diagnosis of coronaviral enteritis of turkeys (bluecomb). Am J Vet Res 36:1265–1267.

36. Patel, B.L., B.S. Pomeroy, E. Gonder, and C.E. Cronkite. 1976. Indirect fluorescent antibody test for the diagnosis of coronaviral enteritis of turkeys (bluecomb). Am J Vet Res 37:1111–1112.

37. Patel, B.L., E. Gonder, and B.S. Pomeroy. 1977. Detection of turkey coronaviral enteritis (bluecomb) in field epiornithics, using the direct and indirect fluorescent antibody tests. Am J Vet Res 38:1407–1411.

38. Peterson, E.H., and T.A. Hymas. 1951. Antibiotics in the treatment of unfamiliar turkey disease. Poult Sci 30:466–468.

39. Pomeroy, B.S. 1956. High level use of antibiotics. Proc 1st Int Conf Antibiot Agric. Natl Acad Sci Res Counc Pub 397, pp. 56–57.

40. Pomeroy, B.S. 1956. Use of furazolidone and antibiotics in bluecomb disease of turkeys. Proc 1st Natl Symp Nitrofurans Agric, Michigan State University, East Lansing, MI, pp. 75–78.

41. Pomeroy, B.S., and J.M. Sieburth. 1953. Bluecomb disease of turkeys. Proc 90th Annu Meet Am Vet Med Assoc, pp. 321–328.

42. Pomeroy, B.S. C.T. Larsen, D.R. Deshmukh, and B.L. Patel. 1975. Immunity to transmissible (coronaviral) enteritis of turkeys (bluecomb). Am J Vet Res 36:553–555.

43. Pomeroy, K.A., B.L. Patel, C.T. Larsen, and B.S. Pomeroy. 1978. Combined immunofluorescence and trans-

mission electron microscopic studies of sequential intestinal samples from turkey embryos and poults infected with turkey enteritis coronavirus. Am J Vet Res 39:1348–1354.

44. Reynolds, D., and Pomeroy, B.S. 1989. Enteritic viruses. In H.G. Purchase, L.H. Arp, C.H. Domermuth, and J.E. Pearson (eds.). Isolation and Identification of Avian Pathogens. American Association of Avian Pathologists, Kennett Square, PA, pp. 128–134.

45. Ritchie, A.E., D.R. Deshmukh, C.T. Larsen, and B.S. Pomeroy. 1973. Electron microscopy of coronavirus-like particles characteristic of turkey bluecomb disease. Avian Dis 17:546–558.

46. Rodgers, S.J., S.L. Vanhooser, R. D. Welsh, and T. G. Silkwood. 1994. Preliminary studies of primary ostrich fibroblasts for the isolation of ratite viruses. Avian Dis 38:866–872.

47. Schultz, P.N., D.E. Nelson, H.E. Dziuk, G.E. Duke, and C.T. Larsen. 1970. Hemic studies in normal and bluecomb diseased turkeys. Poult Sci 49:136–145.

48. Sharma, T.S. 1968. Characterization and comparative studies of vibrios associated with bluecomb disease (transmissible enteritis) of turkeys. PhD thesis. University of Minnesota, Minneapolis-St. Paul.

49. Sieburth, J.M. 1954. Bluecomb disease of turkeys. Antibiotic prophylactic and etiology. PhD thesis. University of Minnesota, Minneapolis-St. Paul.

50. Sieburth, J.M., and E.P. Johnson. 1957. Transmissible enteritis of turkeys (bluecomb disease). I. Preliminary studies. Poult Sci 36:256–261.

51. Sieburth, J.M., and B.S. Pomeroy. 1956. Bluecomb disease of turkeys. II. Antibiotic treatment of poults. J Am Vet Med Assoc 128:509–513.

52. Truscott, R.B. 1968. Transmissible enteritis of turkeys—disease reproduction. Avian Dis 12:239–245.

53. Tumlin, J.T., and B.S. Pomeroy. 1958. Bluecomb disease of turkeys. V. Preliminary studies on parental immunity and serum neutralization. Am J Vet Res 19:725–728.

54. Tumlin, J.T., and B.S. Pomeroy. 1958. The prophylactic effect of nitrofurans in feed on bluecomb disease, mortality, and weight gains in day-old poults. Proc 2nd Nat Symp Nitrofurans Agric, The University of Georgia, Athens, GA, p. 144.

55. Tumlin, J.T., B.S. Pomeroy, and R.K. Lindorfer. 1957. Bluecomb disease of turkeys. IV. Demonstration of a filterable agent. J Am Vet Med Assoc 130:360–365.

56. Wooley, R.E. 1973. Serological comparison of the Georgia and Minnesota strains of infectious enteritis in turkeys. Avian Dis 17:150–154.

57. Wooley, R.E., T.A. Dees, A.S. Cromack, and J.B. Gratzek. 1972. Infectious enteritis of turkeys: Characterization of two reoviruses isolated by sucrose density gradient centrifugation from turkeys with infectious enteritis. Am J Vet Res 33:157–164.

ROTAVIRUS INFECTIONS

M. S. McNulty

INTRODUCTION. Rotaviruses are now established as a major cause of enteritis and diarrhea in a wide range of mammalian species, including humans (70). Rotavirus infection in avian species was first reported in 1977 by Bergeland et al.(5), who found particles morphologically indistinguishable from rotaviruses in intestinal contents of poults with watery droppings and increased mortality. Since then, it has become apparent that rotaviruses infect many species of domesticated birds.

As in mammals, rotavirus infection in avian species is frequently associated with outbreaks of diarrhea. The economic significance of rotaviral enteritis to the poultry industry has not yet been defined, but by analogy with the situation in mammals, it is likely to be significant. Some mammalian rotaviruses have limited ability to infect other mammalian species, and rotaviruses from turkeys and pheasants can infect chickens (74). There is a report of the isolation of an avianlike group A rotavirus from a calf with diarrhea (9); however interspecies transmission of rotaviruses between birds and to mammals and vice versa is probably rare.

In this section, the term *rotavirus* includes those viruses described as atypical rotaviruses and rotaviruslike viruses.

INCIDENCE AND DISTRIBUTION. Rotaviral enteritis has been described in poults in the United Kingdom (22, 33, 34), United States (5, 11, 56, 73), and France (2). Rotavirus isolation from, or detection in, chicken feces has been documented in Argentina (4), Belgium (41), Brazil (1), the United Kingdom (34, 36, 37), United States (73), and the former Soviet Union (3). Rotaviral antibody has been reported in chickens in Japan (57), ducks in the United Kingdom (34), and pigeons in Belgium (72). Rotavirus was detected in feces of guinea fowl with transmissible enteritis in Italy, but their etiologic role is uncertain (50). Rotaviruses have been found in feces of diseased pheasant chicks in Italy (14), the United Kingdom (16, 17), and United States (53, 73), and were isolated from, or detected in, feces of ducks (61, 71) and pigeons (19, 43) in Japan and the United Kingdom. A chicken embryo lethal rotavirus was isolated from the liver and small intestine of a lovebird in England (18). This evidence suggests rotaviruses have a worldwide distribution in a wide variety of avian species.

ETIOLOGY

Classification. Rotaviruses are classified as a genus in the family *Reoviridae*.

Morphology.   Intact rotavirus particles have a double-shelled capsid and are approximately 70 nm in diameter. They have been described as reovirus-like but can be distinguished from reoviruses by their more clearly defined smooth outer edge (Fig. 27.3). The outer capsid shell may be lost, producing noninfectious or poorly infectious single-shelled particles (7) that resemble orbiviruses and are about 10 nm smaller than intact virions (Fig. 27.3). Double- and single-shelled particles of turkey rotavirus have densities in cesium chloride of 1.34 and 1.36 g/mL respectively (29). Double- and single-shelled group D rotavirus particles from a pheasant were reported to be larger, at 80 nm and 70 nm, respectively, than those of an avian group A rotavirus with densities of 1.347 and 1.365 g/mL, respectively

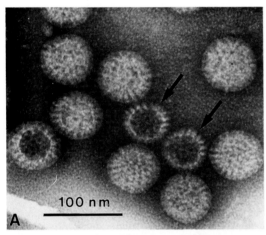

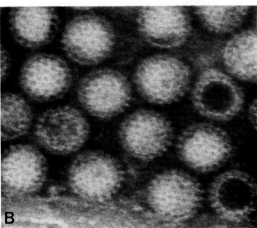

27.3.   *A.* Rotavirus particles in chicken feces showing intact particles with smooth outer edge and particles with serrated edges (*arrows*), lacking outer capsid shell. *B.* Reovirus isolated from guinea fowl feces. Intact rotavirus and reovirus particles can be differentiated by the more distinct, smooth outer margin of rotavirus. Methylamine tungstate stain.

(12). There is disagreement about the precise arrangement of capsomeres in rotaviruses. Models involving icosahedral arrangement of 32 (49), 180 (60), 320 (13), and 132 (55) capsomeres in the inner capsid shell have been proposed.

Chemical Composition.   Like their mammalian counterparts, avian rotaviruses possess a double-stranded RNA genome consisting of 11 segments ranging from about 0.2×10^6 to 2.1×10^6 in molecular weight (1, 4, 11, 16, 17, 18, 19, 31, 37, 39, 43, 56, 68, 69, 73).

Ten major virus polypeptides were detected in MA104 cells infected with a turkey rotavirus. Three polypeptides, designated VP1, VP2, and VP6, with approximate molecular weights of 125 kD, 100 kD, and 45 kD, were associated with the inner capsid. Polypeptides VP3, VP4, VP5s, and VP7, with molecular weights of 90 kD, 88 kD, 54–55 kD, and 37 kD, formed part of the outer capsid shell. The 37-kD polypeptide was glycosylated, and two nonstructural polypeptides (30 kD and 28 kD) were also identified as glycoproteins (28).

Virus Replication.   The morphogenesis of turkey and chicken rotaviruses has been investigated by thin-section electron microscopy (31, 37). Virus replication occurs in the cytoplasm. Both in cell cultures and in vivo, virus cores are formed within granular matrices of viral precursor material (viroplasm) that lies free in the cytoplasm. Developing virus particles are liberated into dilated cisternae of rough endoplasmic reticulum. Some particles appear to bud through ribosome-free areas of endoplasmic reticulum, acquiring an envelope in the process (Fig. 27.4). Virus is released by cell lysis.

Resistance to Chemical and Physical Agents.   There is little published information about resistance of avian rotaviruses to chemical and physical inactivation. Two isolates of turkey rotavirus were stable to treatment with chloroform for 30 min and to pH 3 for 2 hr. Heating at 56 C for 30 min decreased infectivity of both viruses 100-fold, both in the presence and absence of magnesium ions (29). Similarly, a pigeon rotavirus was stable to ether, chloroform, and sodium deoxycholate treatment (43).

Strain Classification.   The vast majority of mammalian rotaviruses share a group antigen. These have been termed group A or conventional rotaviruses to distinguish them from so-called atypical rotaviruses, which do not have this antigen. Atypical rotaviruses have been further divided into groups B, C, D, and E, based on possession of different group antigens and by terminal fingerprinting analysis of viral RNA (51, 52).

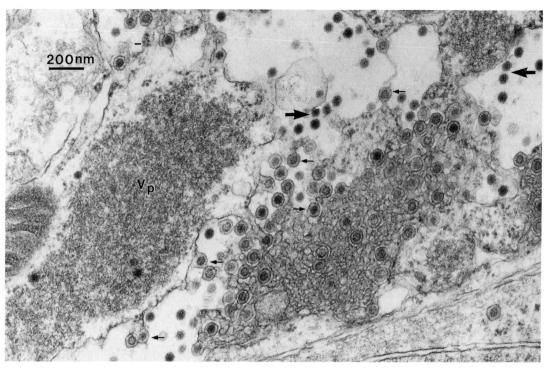

27.4. Electron micrograph of chicken embryo liver cell culture 48 hr postinfection with turkey rotavirus. Part of the cytoplasm of an infected cell is shown, with viroplasm (Vp) containing virus cores and virus particles gaining envelopes by budding (*small arrows*) from rough endoplasmic reticulum and from type 2 inclusion material. Nonenveloped virus particles (*large arrows*) are also present.

Some avian rotaviruses show antigenic relationship with mammalian group A rotaviruses by cross-immunofluorescence using hyperimmune or convalescent antisera (34, 36, 65, 73). Those avian rotaviruses antigenically related to mammalian group A rotaviruses are referred to as avian group A rotaviruses. This relationship was originally assumed to occur through sharing of the mammalian rotavirus group A antigen, but more recent work, using monoclonal antibodies, suggests a more complex relationship. Some monoclonal antibodies, specific for group A avian rotavirus VP6, the major inner capsid protein of the virus, react with all mammalian and avian group A rotaviruses, while others recognize only avian group A rotaviruses (25, 44). Conversely, other monoclonal antibodies that recognize mammalian group A rotaviruses do not recognize avian group A rotaviruses (15, 23). Thus, it appears that there are epitopes on VP6 of group A avian and mammalian rotaviruses that are distinct from the antigenic determinant common to all group A mammalian rotaviruses. Group A mammalian rotaviruses can be further classified into subgroups. Initial evidence suggested that group A avian rotaviruses belonged to neither mammalian

rotavirus subgroup (15, 23, 25, 63), but more recent work has shown that avian rotaviruses from pigeons, turkeys, and chickens react with subgroup 1–specific group A monoclonal antibodies, which detect a similar mammalian rotavirus antigen (44).

In addition to group A avian rotaviruses, three other antigenically distinct serogroups of rotavirus have been identified in chickens (40). The prototype virus of one of these groups, the 132 chicken isolate, has been classified as a group D rotavirus (52). So far, group D rotaviruses have been identified only in avian species. Rotaviruslike viruses of turkeys (56, 65, 66) are antigenically related by cross-immunofluorescence to the 132 chicken rotavirus isolate (32) and should also be regarded as group D rotaviruses. Similarly a rotaviruslike virus of pheasants has also been classified as a group D rotavirus (12). The antigenic relationship of the other two chicken serogroups to mammalian rotavirus groups B, C, and E has not yet been investigated. It is possible they represent two new groups. An avian serogroup antigenically distinct from groups A and D, designated atypical rotavirus, has been identified in turkeys in the United States (66).

Limited information exists about avian rotavirus

type antigens. Using a fluorescent focus-neutralization test, three serotypes were identified in a collection of six turkey and two chicken isolates of group A avian rotavirus (36). With the use of a more sensitive plaque-reduction test, however, two of the viruses classified as different serotypes had a prime strain relationship (23). Given the serotypic diversity of group A mammalian rotaviruses (8, 23), it is anticipated that similar diversity of serotypes will be identified among avian rotaviruses.

Analysis of the pattern of migration of genome segments, especially segment 5, the triplet consisting of segments 7, 8, and 9; and the doublet of segments 10 and 11, following polyacrylamide gel electrophoresis, has been extremely useful, both in preliminary characterization of avian rotaviruses and in investigating their epidemiology. An important advantage of this technique is that it does not require isolation and propagation of virus in cell cultures, but can be carried out on virus in intestinal contents or feces. Five major types of RNA profiles, termed *electropherogroups,* were recognized when turkey and chicken rotavirus RNAs were electrophoresed (68) (Fig. 27.5). Rotaviruses belonging

to electropherogroups 1, 2, 3, and 4 were detected in chickens, while electropherogroups 1, 2, 3, and 5 were found in turkeys.

Interestingly, four representative isolates, each belonging to different chicken electropherogroups, were also found to belong to different serogroups (40). Furthermore, turkey and pheasant group D rotaviruses from the United States have a similar pattern of migration of RNA segments to group D chicken rotavirus (12, 37, 40, 66, 68). This suggests electropherogrouping may be a useful indicator of group antigenic differences. It will be interesting to see if turkey viruses from the United States with genome profiles similar to those of electropherogroup 3 (26, 66), i.e., so-called atypical rotaviruses, are antigenically related to chicken rotaviruses with similar profiles from the United Kingdom.

Within each electropherogroup, minor variations, termed *electropherotypes,* were described in turkey and chicken rotaviruses from the United Kingdom (68). Similar variations have also been described in turkey rotaviruses in the United States (26, 67). These variations may be useful for classifying rotavirus strains, although minor electrophoretic differences do not necessarily imply serotypic differences (29).

Some group A and group D avian rotaviruses agglutinate a range of avian and mammalian erythrocytes (12, 20, 29, 43). Hemagglutination and hemagglutination-inhibition tests may also provide a means of strain classification.

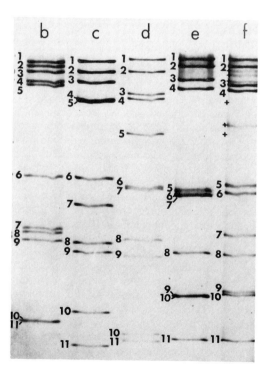

27.5. Genome profiles following electrophoresis of rotavirus RNAs in 5% polyacrylamide gel, showing profiles typical of avian electropherogroups 1 (lane b), 2 (lane c), 3 (lane d), 4 (lane f), and 5 (lane e). Genome segments are numbered 1–11; + indicates unidentified, contaminating bands. (Avian Pathol)

Laboratory Host Systems. Isolations of turkey and chicken rotaviruses were first made in primary chick kidney or chick embryo liver cell cultures (34, 36, 37). Since then, rotaviruses from chickens, turkeys, pheasants (73), and ducks (61) have been isolated in chick kidney cells. Although a chicken rotavirus grew better in chick kidney cells than in a continuous line of fetal rhesus monkey kidney cells (MA104) (45), primary isolation of turkey (27, 65), pheasant (14), and pigeon (43) rotaviruses has also been achieved in MA104 cells. The pigeon isolate also replicated to higher titer in MDBK cells than in chick embryo kidney cell cultures (43). Some group A rotaviruses are capable of infecting both nonstimulated avian splenic lymphocytes and transformed avian lymphoblastoid cell lines (58).

Serial propagation of rotaviruses in cell culture usually requires trypsin treatment of virus inoculum. Most isolates are noncytopathic on primary isolation; several passages in cell cultures are required before a cytopathic effect is seen. With the exception of the 132 chicken rotavirus isolate (37), rotaviruses isolated to date in cell cultures have all been group A avian rotaviruses.

A rotavirus from lovebirds was lethal for chick embryos following yolk sac inoculation. Passage of the virus in 6- to 8-day-old embryos resulted in death 4–6 days after inoculation (18). Similarly, group A rotaviruses from turkey poults were isolated in chick embryos following yolk sac inoculation. Dead embryos were hemorrhagic and stunted with no other visible lesions (11). So far, there is no information concerning replication of other avian rotaviruses in embryos.

Accounts of experimental propagation of avian rotaviruses in their natural hosts are numerous (42, 38, 50, 74, 75, 76, 77). Some group A avian rotaviruses are also capable of infecting avian species other than their natural hosts (73, 74, 75, 77).

PATHOGENESIS AND EPIZOOTIOLOGY

Natural and Experimental Hosts. As discussed above, turkeys, chickens, pheasants, ducks, guinea fowl, pigeons, and lovebirds are naturally infected with rotaviruses, and some have been experimentally infected. Most naturally occurring infections in turkeys, chickens, pheasants, and ducks involve birds <6 wk old. Paradoxically, older chickens (56–119 days) and turkeys (112 days) were more susceptible to experimental infection than birds in the first few weeks of life (74, 76). This observation is interesting; however, its relevance to the field situation is questionable because available evidence indicates that most turkeys and chickens will have been infected, and presumably have developed immunity, well before this age. Lack of age resistance to infection, however, is illustrated by an outbreak of diarrhea associated with rotavirus infection in commercial laying hens between 32 and 92 wk of age (24).

Longitudinal surveys have shown that flocks of broilers and turkeys frequently experience simultaneous or sequential infections with different rotavirus electropherogroups (40, 54, 64, 68).

Transmission, Carriers, and Vectors. Rotaviruses are excreted in feces in very large numbers (76). No information is available concerning survival of avian rotaviruses in feces, but, by extrapolation from mammals, environmental contamination is likely to be persistent. Horizontal transmission occurs readily between birds in direct and indirect contact. Egg transmission of rotaviruses has not been demonstrated, but rotavirus detection in 3-day-old turkey poults prompted speculation that transmission occurs either in or on the egg (64). There is no evidence for a carrier state in birds or biologic vectors.

Incubation Period, Signs, Morbidity, and Mortality. The incubation period is short. In experimentally infected turkeys, watery droppings were passed 2–5 days postinfection. Gross lesions at this time consisted of intestinal tract pallor and ceca distended with liquid contents. Rotavirus infection caused significant impairment of D-xylose absorption from the intestinal tract at 2 and 4 days postinfection (75). Mild (38) or no clinical signs (42, 74) were observed following experimental infection of chickens. When signs occurred, their onset coincided with peak virus excretion about 3 days postinfection. Birds passed increased quantities of cecal droppings, and, at necropsy, ceca were abnormally distended with fluid and gas (38). No mortality occurred in experimentally infected turkeys or chickens. Laying hens experimentally infected with rotavirus showed a drop in egg production 4–9 days postinfection (76). Rotavirus was detected in feces of experimentally infected chickens and turkeys from 24 hr postinfection, and in some birds, excretion continued for more than 16 days (38, 74, 75, 76).

Under field conditions, clinical signs associated with rotavirus infection in broilers have varied from subclinical infections to outbreaks of diarrhea severe enough to warrant attention to the litter, with associated dehydration, poor weight gains, and increased mortality (1, 4, 34, 36). In poults, variations in severity of clinical signs have also been observed including a very mild scour in the 1st wk of life, which caused mortality only if vent pecking occurred (22); a more severe disease in 12- to 21-day-old poults characterized by restlessness, litter eating, and watery droppings with mortality between about 4 and 7% (5); and (33) profuse scouring in 2- to 5-wk-old poults, with affected birds huddling together, mortalities from suffocation, and stunting of survivors. In other outbreaks, predominant signs have been diarrhea and wet litter.

Pheasant chicks 2- to 3-wk-old in the United States had diarrhea and increased mortality associated with rotavirus infection (53). In the United Kingdom, rotavirus infection was associated with stunting and increased mortality in pheasant chicks in the 1st wk of life (16, 17). Six of twenty 2-day-old pheasants inoculated with intestinal contents containing rotaviruses from naturally occurring cases died 5–6 days postinfection. At necropsy, ceca were distended with frothy, ocher-colored material. Hemorrhages were present in cecal walls of several chicks, and intestinal contents were fluid (17). In Italy, pheasants between 6 and 40 days of age showed depression, drooping wings, yellowish watery diarrhea, and dehydration; mortality was 20–30% (14). Diarrhea, lethargy, and loss of appetite were associated with rotavirus infection in 3- to 4-month-old racing pigeons in the United Kingdom (19).

Variations in severity of clinical signs associated

with rotavirus infections could be due to genuine differences in virulence of avian rotavirus strains, as has been shown for bovine rotavirus (6, 10), and/or interaction of rotavirus with additional factors such as other infectious agents (21) or environmental stress.

Morbidity is high. Most fecal specimens taken randomly from birds in affected flocks will contain rotaviruses.

Gross Lesions. The most common finding at necropsy is presence of abnormal amounts of fluid and gas in the intestinal tract and ceca. Secondary findings include dehydration, inflamed vents, anemia due to vent pecking, litter in the gizzard, and inflammation and encrustation with droppings of plantar surfaces of the feet (5, 22, 36, 38).

Histopathology. Immunofluorescence (IF) studies using chickens and turkeys experimentally infected with rotavirus have demonstrated the principal site of virus replication to be cytoplasm of mature villous absorptive epithelial cells in the small intestine. Infected cells were more numerous in the distal third of villi (Fig. 27.6). Small numbers of infected cells were also detected in colon epithelium, ceca, and lamina propria of some villi. No IF was observed in proventriculus, gizzard, spleen, liver, or kidney (38, 42, 74, 75, 76). Within the small intestine, different rotavirus strains may show preference for specific areas. A group A rotavirus grew

best in the duodenum, while a group D rotavirus favored the jejunum and ileum (38). In general, experimental infections using chickens and turkeys of differing ages showed that increasing amounts of viral antigen were synthesized in birds of increasing age (76).

Histopathologic lesions in experimentally infected turkeys consisted of basal vacuolation of enterocytes, separation of enterocytes from the lamina propria with subsequent desquamation, villous atrophy, enlargement of the lamina propria, scalloping of the villous surface, fusion of villi, and leukocytic infiltration of the lamina propria. In general, mean villous lengths were decreased and crypt depths increased following experimental infection, resulting in significantly decreased villus to crypt ratios (21, 59, 77). In experimentally infected chickens, only minimal leukocytic infiltration of the lamina propria was found in one study (77). Moderate villous atrophy, mainly in the ileum, however, has also been described in experimentally infected chickens (42). Changes observed in experimentally infected SPF turkeys are shown in Fig. 27.7.

No histopathologic changes were observed in poults with naturally acquired rotavirus infection (22). Degeneration and inflammation of villi of the duodenum and jejunum have also been reported, however, in poults with rotaviral enteritis (5). Lesions were not found in ileum, cecum, colon, cloaca, or other organs.

Neither gross nor microscopic lesions are pathognomonic for rotavirus infection.

Immunity. Chickens and turkeys inoculated orally with rotaviruses showed serum antibody responses as early as 4–6 days postinfection measured by indirect IF. In general, older birds developed higher antibody titers and responded faster than younger birds (74, 75, 76). Little is known about development or duration of immunity to rotaviruses following infection of birds. Using immunoglobulin class–specific enzyme-linked immunosorbent assay (ELISAs) (48) to follow antibody responses in chickens experimentally infected with a group A rotavirus, rotavirus-specific IgM, IgG, and IgA were detected in serum, whereas the intestinal antibody response consisted almost entirely of IgA. Embryonic bursectomized chicks recovered from infection and developed resistance to a subsequent homotypic challenge more slowly than intact chicks (46), indicating that the intestinal IgA response is not the sole mediator of recovery from infection and development of resistance to reinfection, but that it plays a part. Natural killer cell–like activity has been demonstrated in chick intraepithelial leukocytes against rotavirus-infected target cells, and it has been suggested that this may be an important in vivo immune response (47). Ma-

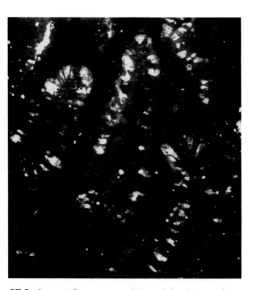

27.6. Immunofluorescent staining of duodenum of specific-pathogen–free chicken infected with rotavirus at 14 days of age and killed 3 days postinfection; rotavirus antigen is seen in villous epithelial cells. ×96. (Avian Pathol)

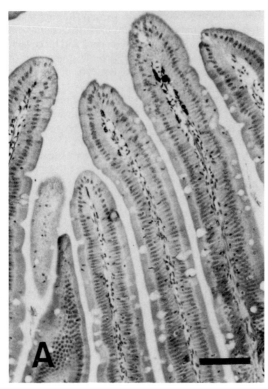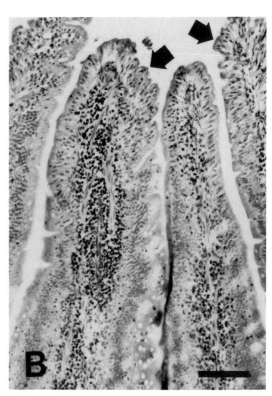

27.7. Duodenum of SPF turkey poults. *A.* Normal villi of an uninfected control poult at 10 days of age. *B.* Villi of a 10-day-old poult infected with Tu-2 at 7 days of age. Note the remarkable hypercellularity in the lamina propria, scalloping of the villous surface, and basal vacuolation of the epithelial cells at the tips (*arrows*). H&E stain, Bar = 0.1 mm. (Yason and Schat) (Avian Pathol)

ternally derived antibodies to rotavirus are passively transferred to the avian embryo through the egg yolk. They progressively decline in titer and are undetectable at 3–4 wk of age (32, 75). Presence of maternal antibody had no apparent effect on susceptibility of chickens and turkeys to experimental rotavirus infection (42, 75). Progeny of hyperimmunized turkey hens, however, were more resistant to experimental infection with rotavirus at 2 or 5 days of age, but not at 12 days of age, compared with poults without maternal antibodies to rotavirus (59).

DIAGNOSIS

Isolation and Identification of Causative Agent.
The classic way to diagnose rotavirus infections in the laboratory is to identify the virus in feces or intestinal contents by direct electron microscopy. This technique is relatively sensitive and detects rotaviruses of all serogroups. Material can be prepared in a variety of ways (35). The standard method is to extract an approximately 15% suspension of feces made in phosphate-buffered saline

with an equal volume of fluorocarbon. Following centrifugation at $3000 \times g$ for 15–30 min to separate aqueous and fluorocarbon phases, the aqueous phase is removed and centrifuged at approximately $12,000 \times g$ for 15 min using an Eppendorf 5414 bench centrifuge. This pelleting procedure gives similar results to those obtained by ultracentrifugation, but is quicker and simpler. The pellet is resuspended in a few drops of water and examined. Some workers use immune electron microscopy. While this technique requires availability of specific antisera, it allows rotaviruses of different serogroups to be distinguished (56, 66). The morphology of rotavirus is sufficiently distinct that experienced electron microscopists should have little difficulty identifying the virus with certainty. Rotaviruses can be confused with reoviruses, however, which are also frequently found in avian feces. The main distinguishing feature is the more clearly defined outer capsid shell of rotavirus (see Fig. 27.3).

Detection of rotavirus RNA in intestinal contents or feces provides an alternate means of diagnosis. Following extraction of RNA, electrophoresis on polyacrylamide gels, and silver staining, rotavirus

RNA can be identified by the pattern of migration of the 11 genome segments. This technique is almost as sensitive as electron microscopic techniques (30, 40, 62, 66), and provides a convenient means of distinguishing between different isolates. At present, this technique is used mostly by those interested in rotavirus epidemiology and classification.

Diagnosis of rotavirus infection by virus isolation in cell cultures is useful only for group A avian rotaviruses. It has proved extremely difficult to isolate other rotavirus serogroups in cell cultures (27, 40, 65). As infections with other serogroups constitute the majority of rotavirus infections in chickens (40, 68) and turkeys (54, 64), virus isolation in cell cultures cannot be recommended as a diagnostic technique. Even with group A avian rotaviruses, in most cases, serial passage can be achieved only by activation of virus infectivity with proteolytic enzymes such as trypsin. Furthermore, not all group A avian rotaviruses detected by electron microscopy grow in cell cultures. Those that do are often non-cytopathic on primary isolation, requiring immunofluorescence to detect virus growth. For isolation of group A avian rotaviruses, the MA104 cell line or primary cultures of chick embryo liver or chick kidney cells, trypsin treatment, and centrifugation of inoculum onto the cell monolayer are recommended (27, 34, 41, 43, 45, 61, 65, 73).

Serology. Serologic diagnosis of rotavirus infections is difficult and not recommended. The high prevalence of antibody (39, 43) makes results difficult to interpret. Few laboratories offer serologic tests for avian rotaviruses on a routine basis. Furthermore, the inability to adapt some avian serogroups to cell culture has resulted in gaps in the available battery of antigens.

Differential Diagnosis. Rotavirus infection must be differentiated from other conditions causing diarrhea. Since the clinical signs and pathology of rotavirus infection are not pathognomonic, laboratory diagnosis is necessary. It is important to remember, however, that rotavirus infection does not necessarily result in disease.

TREATMENT, PREVENTION, AND CONTROL.

The ubiquity of rotavirus infections in turkeys and chickens indicates that it is not practical to keep commercial flocks free from infection. At present, there is no specific treatment or means of control. The effect of diarrhea on the litter can be minimized by increasing ventilation rate and temperature and adding fresh litter. In those countries where litter is reused several times, infection will build up and problems are likely to be more severe than in situations in which houses are cleaned and fumigated, and fresh litter is used for each batch of birds. If severe problems arise, it is recommended that litter be removed and the house and equipment be thoroughly cleaned and fumigated with formaldehyde before restocking with a new flock.

Vaccines have not yet been developed. Given the number of serogroups and the difficulty in growing some rotaviruses in cell culture, there are obvious problems in vaccine development. Available knowledge of immunity to avian rotavirus suggests that live attenuated vaccines given orally might be more effective than parenterally administered inactivated vaccines.

REFERENCES

1. Alfieri, A.F., Resende, M., Resende, J.S., and A.A. Alfieri. 1989. Atypical rotavirus infections among broiler chickens in Brazil. Arq Bras Med Vet Zoot 41:81–82.
2. Andral, B., and D. Toquin. 1984. Observations au microscope electronique a partir de prelevements de dindes presentant des troubles pathologiques. Avian Pathol 13:389–417.
3. Bakulin, V., Aliev, A.S., Dzhavadov, E.D., Tul'skaya, I.I., Vashukova, S.S., Gorbachev, E.N., and S.N. Verbor. 1991. Morphology of avian rotavirus and the lesions it produces in chicks. Veterinariya (Moskva) 1:36–37.
4. Bellinzoni, R., Mattion, N., Vallejos, L., La Torre, J.L., and E.A. Scodeller. 1987. Atypical rotavirus in chickens in Argentina. Res Vet Sci 43:130–131.
5. Bergeland, M.E., J.P. McAdaragh, and I. Stotz. 1977. Rotaviral enteritis in turkey poults. Proc 26th West Poult Dis Conf, pp. 129–130.
6. Bridger, J.C. and D.H. Pocock. 1986. Variation in virulence of bovine rotaviruses. J Hyg (Camb) 96:257–264.
7. Bridger, J.C., and G.N. Woode. 1976. Characterization of two particle types of calf rotavirus. J Gen Virol 31:245–250.
8. Browning, G.F., Fitzgerald, T.A., Chalmers, R.M., and D.R. Snodgrass. 1991. A novel group A rotavirus G serotype: Serological and genomic characterization of equine isolate F123. J Clin Microbiol 29:2043–2046.
9. Brüssow, H., Nakagomi, O., Gerna, G., and W. Eichhorn. 1992. Isolation of an avian like group A rotavirus from a calf with diarrhea. J Clin Microbiol 30:67–73.
10. Carpio, M., J.E.C. Bellamy, and L.A. Babiuk. 1981. Comparative virulence of different bovine rotavirus isolates. Can J Comp Med 45:38–42.
11. Castro, A.E., Moore, J., Hammami, S., Manalac, R.B., and R.P. Chin. 1992. Direct isolation of rotaviruses from turkeys in embryonating chicken eggs. Vet Rec 130:379–380.
12. Devitt, C.M., and D.L. Reynolds. 1993. Characterization of a group D rotavirus. Avian Dis 37:749–755.
13. Esparza, J., and F. Gil. 1978. A study on the ultrastructure of human rotavirus. Virology 91:141–150.
14. Foni, E., Gelmetti, D., Nigrelli, A.D., Gatti, R., and V. Carra. 1989. Transmissible enteritis syndrome in pheasants for restocking: Experimental reproduction of the disease. Isolation of rotavirus. Sel Vet 30:879–888.
15. Gary, G.W., Jr., R. Black, and E. Palmer. 1982. Monoclonal IgG to the inner capsid of human rotavirus. Arch Virol 72:223–227.
16. Gough, R.E., G.W. Wood, M.S. Collins, D. Spackman, J. Kemp, and L.A.C. Gibson. 1985. Rotavirus infection in pheasant poults. Vet Rec 116:295.
17. Gough, R.E., G.W. Wood, and D. Spackman. 1986. Studies with an atypical avian rotavirus from pheasants. Vet Rec 118:611–612.
18. Gough, R.E., M.S. Collins, G.W. Wood, and S.A. Lister. 1988. Isolation of a chicken embryo-lethal rotavirus from a lovebird (Agapornis species). Vet Rec 122:363–364.

19. Gough, R.E., Cox, W.J., and J. Devoy. 1992. Isolation and identification of rotavirus from racing pigeons. Vet Rec 130:273.

20. Hancock, K., G.W. Gary, Jr., and E.L. Palmer. 1983. Adaptation of two avian rotaviruses to mammalian cells and characterization by haemagglutination and RNA electrophoresis. J Gen Virol 64:853–861.

21. Hayhow, C.S., and Y.M. Saif. 1993. Experimental infection of specific-pathogen-free turkey poults with single and combined enterovirus and group A rotavirus. Avian Dis 37:546–557.

22. Horrox, N.E. 1980. Some observations and comments on rotaviruses in turkey poults. Proc 29th West Poult Dis Conf, pp. 162–164.

23. Hoshino, Y., R.G. Wyatt, H.B. Greenberg, J. Flores, and A.Z. Kapikian. 1984. Serotypic similarity and diversity of rotaviruses of mammalian and avian origin as studied by plaque-reduction neutralization. J Infect Dis 149:694–702.

24. Jones, R.C., C.S. Hughes, and R.R. Henry. 1979. Rotavirus infection in commercial laying hens. Vet Rec 104:22.

25. Kang, S.Y., and L.J. Saif. 1991. Production and characterization of monoclonal antibodies against an avian group A rotavirus. Avian Diseases 35:563–571.

26. Kang, S.Y., K.V. Nagaraja, and J.A. Newman. 1986. Electropherotypic analysis of rotaviruses isolated from turkeys. Avian Dis 30:794–801.

27. Kang, S.Y., K.V. Nagaraja, and J.A. Newman. 1986. Primary isolation and identification of avian rotaviruses from turkeys exhibiting signs of clinical enteritis in a continuous MA104 cell line. Avian Dis 30:494–499.

28. Kang, S.Y., K.V. Nagaraja, and J.A. Newman. 1987. Characterization of viral polypeptides from avian rotavirus. Avian Dis 31:607–621.

29. Kang, S.Y., K.V. Nagaraja, and J.A. Newman. 1988. Physical, chemical, and serological characterization of avian rotaviruses. Avian Dis 32:195–203.

30. Lozano, L-F., Hammami, S., Castro, A.E., and B. Osburn. 1992. Comparison of electron microscopy and polyacrylamide gel electrophoresis in the diagnosis of avian reovirus and rotavirus infections. Avian Dis 36:183–188.

31. McNulty, M.S. 1980. Morphology and chemical composition of rotaviruses. In F. Bricout and R. Scherrer (eds.). Viral Enteritis in Humans and Animals. INSERM, Paris, France, pp. 111–140.

32. McNulty, M.S. 1988. Unpublished data.

33. McNulty, M.S., G.M. Allan, and J.C. Stuart. 1978. Rotavirus infection in avian species. Vet Rec 103:319–320.

34. McNulty, M.S., G.M. Allan, D. Todd, and J.B. McFerran. 1979. Isolation and cell culture propagation of rotaviruses from turkeys and chickens. Arch Virol 61:13–21.

35. McNulty, M.S., W.L. Curran, D. Todd, and J.B. McFerran. 1979. Detection of viruses in avian faeces by direct electron microscopy. Avian Pathol 8:239–247.

36. McNulty, M.S., G.M. Allan, D. Todd, J.B. McFerran, E.R. McKillop, D.S. Collins, and R.M. McCracken. 1980. Isolation of rotaviruses from turkeys and chickens: Demonstration of distinct serotypes and RNA electropherotypes. Avian Pathol 9:363–375.

37. McNulty, M.S., G.M. Allan, D. Todd, J.B. McFerran, and R.M. McCracken. 1981. Isolation from chickens of a rotavirus lacking the rotavirus group antigen. J Gen Virol 55:405–413.

38. McNulty, M.S., G.M. Allan, and R.M. McCracken. 1983. Experimental infection of chickens with rotaviruses: Clinical and virological findings. Avian Pathol 12:45–54.

39. McNulty, M.S., G.M. Allan, and J.B. McFerran. 1984. Prevalence of antibody to conventional and atypical rotaviruses in chickens. Vet Rec 114:219.

40. McNulty, M.S., D. Todd, G.M. Allan, J.B. McFerran, and J.A. Greene. 1984. Epidemiology of rotavirus infection in broiler chickens: Recognition of four serogroups. Arch Virol 81:113–121.

41. Meulemans, G., G. Charlier, and P. Halen. 1985. Detection de rotavirus aviaire et adaptation a la culture cellulaire. Ann Med Vet 127:43–48.

42. Meulemans, G., J.E. Peeters, and P. Halen. 1985. Experimental infection of broiler chickens with rotavirus. Br Vet J 141:69–73.

43. Minamoto, N., K. Oki, M. Tomita, T. Kinjo, and Y. Suzuki. 1988. Isolation and characterization of rotavirus from feral pigeon in mammalian cell cultures. Epidemiol Infect 100:481–492.

44. Minamoto, N., Sugimoto, O., Yokota, M., Tomita, M., Goto, H., Sugiyama, M., and T. Kinjo. 1993. Antigenic analysis of avian rotavirus VP6 using monoclonal antibodies. Arch Virol 131:293–305.

45. Myers, T.J., and K.A. Schat. 1989. Propagation of avian rotavirus in primary chick kidney cell and MA 104 cell cultures. Avian Dis 33:578–581.

46. Myers, T.J., and K.A. Schat. 1990. Intestinal IgA response and immunity to rotavirus infection in normal and antibody-deficient chickens. Avian Pathol 19:697–712.

47. Myers, T.J., and K.A. Schat. 1990. Natural killer cell activity of chicken intraepithelial leukocytes against rotavirus-infected target cells. Vet Immunol Immunopathol 26:157–170.

48. Myers, T.J., Schat, K.A., and A.P.A. Mockett. 1989. Development of immunoglobulin class-specific enzyme-linked immunosorbent assays for measuring antibodies against avian rotavirus. Avian Dis 33:53–59.

49. Palmer, E.L., M.L. Martin, and F.A. Murphy. 1977. Morphology and stability of infantile gastroenteritis virus: Comparison with reovirus and bluetongue virus. J Gen Virol 35:403–414.

50. Pascucci, S., M.E. Misciattelli, and L. Giovanetti. 1981. Transmissible enteritis of guinea fowl; electron microscopic studies and isolation of a rotavirus strain [abst]. Proc 8th Int Congr World Vet Poult Assoc, pp. 57.

51. Pedley, S., J.C. Bridger, J.F. Brown, and M.A. McCrae. 1983. Molecular characterization of rotaviruses with distinct group antigens. J Gen Virol 64:2093–2101.

52. Pedley, S., J.C. Bridger, D. Chasey, and M.A. McCrae. 1986. Definition of two new groups of atypical rotaviruses. J Gen Virol 67:131–137.

53. Reynolds, D.L., K.W. Theil, and Y.M. Saif. 1987. Demonstration of rotavirus and rotavirus-like virus in the intestinal contents of diarrheic pheasant chicks. Avian Dis 31:376–379.

54. Reynolds, D.L., Y.M. Saif, and K.W. Theil. 1987. A survey of enteric viruses of turkey poults. Avian Dis 31:89–98.

55. Roseto, A., J. Escaig, E. Delain, J. Cohen, and R. Scherrer. 1979. Structure of rotaviruses as studied by the freeze-drying technique. Virology 98:471–475.

56. Saif, L.J., Y.M. Saif, and K.W. Theil. 1985. Enteric viruses in diarrheic turkey poults. Avian Dis 29:798–811.

57. Sato, K., Y. Inaba, T. Shinozaki, and M. Matumoto. 1981. Neutralizing antibody to bovine rotavirus in various animal species. Vet Microbiol 6:259–261.

58. Schat, K.A., and T.J. Myers. 1987. Cultivation of avian rotaviruses in chicken lymphocytes and lymphoblastoid cell lines. Arch Virol 94:205–213.

59. Shawky, S.A., Saif, Y.M., and D.E. Swayne. 1993. Role of circulating maternal anti-rotavirus IgG in protection of intestinal mucosal surface in turkey poults. Avian Dis 37:1041–1050.

60. Stannard, L.M., and B.D. Schoub. 1977. Observations on the morphology of two rotaviruses. J Gen Virol 37:435–439.

61. Takase, K., F. Nonaka, M. Sakaguchi, and S. Yamada. 1986. Cytopathic avian rotavirus isolated from duck faeces in chicken kidney cell cultures. Avian Pathol 15:719–730.

62. Theil, K.W. 1987. A modified genome electropherotyping procedure for detecting turkey rotaviruses in

small volumes of intestinal contents. Avian Dis 31:899–903.

63. Theil, K.W., and C.M. McCloskey. 1989. Nonreactivity of American avian group A rotaviruses with subgroup-specific monoclonal antibodies. J Clin Microbiol 27:2846–2848.

64. Theil, K.W., and Y.M. Saif. 1987. Age-related infections with rotavirus, rotavirus-like virus, and atypical rotavirus in turkey flocks. J Clin Microbiol 25:333–337.

65. Theil, K.W., D.L. Reynolds, and Y.M. Saif. 1986. Isolation and serial propagation of turkey rotaviruses in a fetal rhesus monkey kidney (MA104) cell line. Avian Dis 30:93–104.

66. Theil, K.W., D.L. Reynolds, and Y.M. Saif. 1986. Comparison of immune electron microscopy and genome electropherotyping techniques for detection of turkey rotaviruses and rotavirus-like viruses in intestinal contents. J Clin Microbiol 23:695–699.

67. Theil, K.W., D.L. Reynolds, and Y.M. Saif. 1986. Genomic variation among avian rotavirus-like viruses detected by polyacrylamide gel electrophoresis. Avian Dis 30:829–834.

68. Todd, D., and M.S. McNulty. 1986. Electrophoretic variation of avian rotavirus RNA in polyacrylamide gels. Avian Pathol 15:149–159.

69. Todd, D., M.S. McNulty, and G.M. Allan. 1980. Poly-acrylamide gel electrophoresis of avian rotavirus RNA. Arch Virol 63:87–97.

70. Tzipori, S. 1985. The relative importance of enteric pathogens affecting neonates of domestic animals. Adv Vet Sci Comp Med 29:103–206.

71. Varley, J., Jones, R.C., Bradbury, J.M., and F.T.W. Jordan. 1993. A survey of the viral flora of two commercial Pekin duck flocks. Avian Pathol 22:703–714.

72. Vindevogel, H., L. Dagenais, B. Lansival, and P.P. Pastoret. 1981. Incidence of rotavirus, adenovirus and herpesvirus in pigeons. Vet Rec 109:285–286.

73. Yason, C.V., and K.A. Schat. 1985. Isolation and characterization of avian rotaviruses. Avian Dis 29:499–508.

74. Yason, C.V., and K.A. Schat. 1986. Experimental infection of specific-pathogen-free chickens with avian rotaviruses. Avian Dis 30:551–556.

75. Yason, C.V., and K.A. Schat. 1986. Pathogenesis of rotavirus infection in turkey poults. Avian Pathol 15:421–435.

76. Yason, C.V., and K.A. Schat. 1987. Pathogenesis of rotavirus infection in various age groups of chickens and turkeys: Clinical signs and virology. Am J Vet Res 48:977–983.

77. Yason, C.V., B.A. Summers, and K.A. Schat. 1987. Pathogenesis of rotavirus infection in various age groups of chickens and turkeys: Pathology. Am J Vet Res 48:927–938.

ASTROVIRUS INFECTIONS

D. L. Reynolds

INTRODUCTION. Astroviruses have been identified in cases of diarrhea and gastroenteritis in human infants (3), calves (12), lambs (9), and piglets (1). More recently, they have been detected in birds with enteric disease. The economic impact of astrovirus infections on the poultry industry has yet to be determined. Whether or not avian astroviruses can infect other animal species, including humans, constituting a public health concern, is also unknown.

HISTORY. Astroviruses were first identified in 1980 by McNulty et al. (4) from intestinal contents of 11-day-old turkey poults with diarrhea and increased mortality. Subsequently, astroviruses in flocks of young turkeys were reported in the United States in 1985 (8) and 1986 (5).

Avian astroviruses have not been propagated in vitro. Perhaps because of this, their presence in feces and intestinal contents of birds has eluded investigators until recently. Astroviruses have only been detected by direct electron microscopy (EM) or immune electron microscopy (IEM).

INCIDENCE AND DISTRIBUTION. Astrovirus infections are geographically widespread and usually the most prevalent virus infection, other than rotavirus infection, in poults 1–5 wk of age with enteric disease (5, 6, 8). In one study, astrovirus infections occurred in nearly 80% of affected flocks and was the most prevalent virus detected (6). Astroviruses have also been detected in normal healthy flocks, but far less frequently (< 30%). Astroviruses are seldom the only virus detected in flocks with enteric disease. Generally, they occur in combination with other enteric viruses, especially rotaviruslike virus (group D rotaviruses) (6).

Astrovirus infections usually occur within the first 4 wk of life and are rare in older turkeys (7). Although they have been detected as early as 3 days of age, astrovirus infections are more common after 7 days (7). When flocks were continuously monitored for enteric viral infections from 1 day of age until market, the first samples positive for viruses always contained astroviruses, either alone or with other viruses (7).

ETIOLOGY. Avian astroviruses have been classified and named solely on the basis of size and morphology determined by EM. Initially, they were reported to be 28–31 nm (mean, 30.1 nm) in diameter, with about 10% of virus particles displaying a 5- or 6-pointed star shape (4). Later, astroviruses were described as having an average diameter of 31 nm, with a few particles having a 5-pointed star shape (8). Subsequently, in the United States, only a small percentage of astroviruses had 5- or 6-pointed star-shaped morphology, with an average diameter of 29.6 nm (5) (Fig. 27.8). Avian astroviruses have not yet been classified into a viral taxon.

PATHOGENESIS AND EPIZOOTIOLOGY.
Turkeys appear to be the only avian species naturally infected by astroviruses, except possibly for astroviruslike particles identified from ducklings with hepatitis (2) (see Chapter 25). Astroviruses have been observed from turkey poults experiencing viral enteritis (see Chapter 31). Clinical signs of disease usually develop between 1 and 3 wk of age, and generally last 10–14 days. They vary somewhat, but typically include diarrhea, listlessness, litter eating, and nervousness. Severity ranges from mild to moderate with only slight mortality. Morbidity, occurring as decreased growth (stunting), is of greatest concern.

Experimental studies have shown that astroviruses can cause enteric disease in turkey poults (5, 10). When SPF poults were given an inoculum containing only astrovirus, they gained significantly less weight and absorbed significantly less D-xylose compared with uninoculated control poults. Commercial poults inoculated with astrovirus had decreased intestinal maltase by 3 days postinfection. The decrease in specific maltase activity in astrovirus-infected poults was transient, returning to normal by 10 days postinfection (11). Astrovirus-inoculated poults had watery to frothy, yellow-brown droppings. Onset of clinical signs in experimentally infected poults appeared as early as 2 days postinfection and persisted for 7 to 9 days.

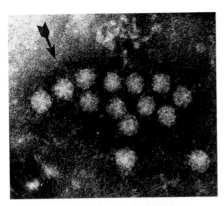

27.8. A star-shaped astrovirus particle (*arrow*) among an aggregate of astroviruses from intestinal samples of experimentally infected diarrheic poults, detected by immune electron microscopy. Average particle size is 29.6 nm. (Avian Diseases)

At necropsy, characteristic pathologic changes were dilated ceca containing yellow, frothy contents; and gaseous fluid, loss of tone (gut thinness), and hyperemia of the intestinal tract. The pathogenesis of diarrhea associated with astrovirus infections has been attributed to the osmotic effect of undigested, unabsorbed disaccharides (and other nutrients) attracting water to the intestinal lumen.

Astroviruses were detected in intestinal contents of poults prior to the onset of clinical disease and gross pathologic changes. This observation may explain why astroviruses are sometimes detected from normal-appearing, healthy poults, which are likely in an early stage of the disease. In addition, it was shown that shedding of astroviruses wanes before clinical signs and pathologic changes abate. Poults in the later stages of astrovirus infection may, therefore, display clinical signs and gross pathologic changes but not have detectable astrovirus present in their intestinal tract.

Astrovirus infections of poults induce histopathologic lesions of the small intestine characterized by mild crypt hyperplasia, resulting in increased crypt depth and area (10) (Fig. 27.9). Histopathologic changes were noted in the proximal jejunum as early as 1 day postinfection, with all portions of the small intestines affected by 5 days postinfection. Intestinal lesions persisted until 7 days postinfection and could not be detected after 10 days postinfection. Unlike some other intestinal viral infections, astrovirus infections do not induce villous atrophy. Astrovirus has been identified in the cytoplasm of enterocytes located along the sides and near the base of the intestinal villi. Crystalline arrays of viral particles, as well as free virus particles, have been observed within enterocytes as early as 2 days postinfection (Fig. 27.10A,B). Release of astrovirus into the intestinal lumen occurs as a consequence of enterocyte degeneration (Fig. 27.10C).

Astrovirus and group D rotavirus frequently occur together in naturally infected turkey poults (7). SPF poults, experimentally inoculated with this combination, shed astrovirus into their intestinal tract (detected by IEM) prior to shedding detectable levels of group D rotavirus. Also, they developed more pronounced clinical disease than that produced by astrovirus alone. Interactions between astroviruses and other viruses have not been reported.

The mode of transmission for astroviruses is assumed to be fecal–oral. Experimentally, poults inoculated orally with astrovirus developed infection (5, 10). Studies on naturally occurring transmission of astroviruses have not been reported.

No reports specifically address astrovirus immunity in poultry; however, SPF poults infected with astroviruses ceased intestinal shedding by 14 days postinfection, and convalescent sera aggregated astrovirus particles when used for IEM, indicating as-

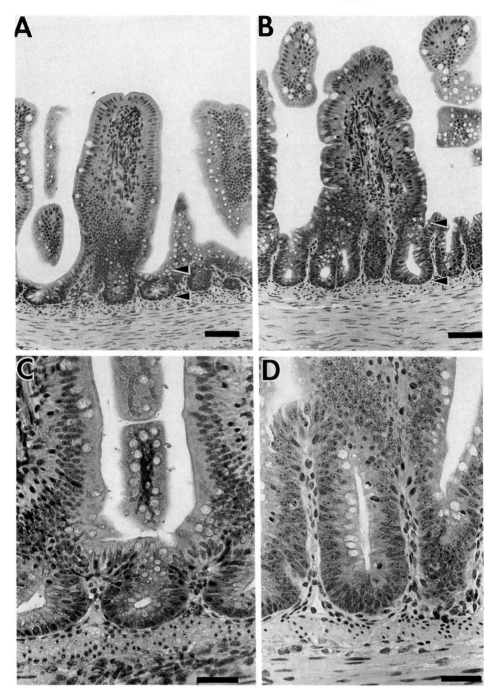

27.9. *A.* Jejunum from control poult with normal crypt depth (*between arrows*). *B.* Jejunum from an inoculated poult 3 days postinfection with significantly increased crypt depth (*between arrows*). Bar = 50 µm. *C.* Intestine from a normal control poult; compare with intestine from an infected poult shown in (*D*). *D.* Intestine from infected poult 7 days postinfection with crypt epithelial hyperplasia, resulting in significantly increased crypt depth. Most crypt epithelial cells contain multiple, prominent nucleoli. Bar = 30 µm. (Avian Diseases)

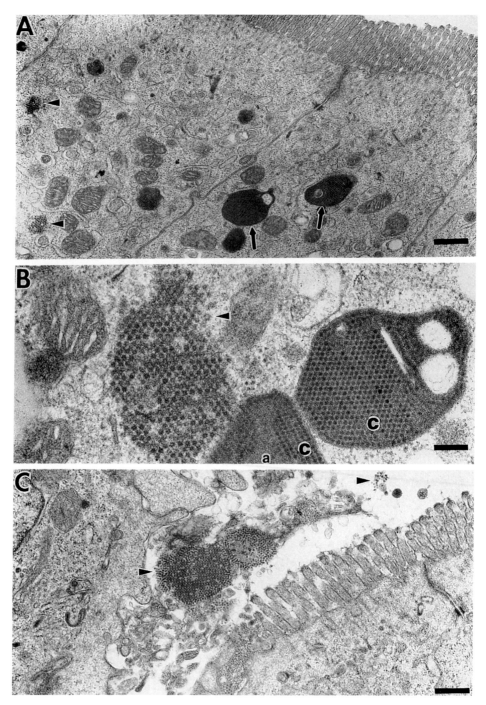

27.10. Ileal enterocytes from an astrovirus infected poult 2 days postinfection. *A*. Intracytoplasmic aggregates of astrovirus (*arrowheads*) and electron dense crystalline arrays of astrovirus particles (*arrows*). Bar = 606 nm. *B*. Intracytoplasmic aggregates of astrovirus and
free virions. Virions are approximately 30 nm in diameter and have an electron-lucent
center (*arrowhead*). Astrovirus virions are also organized into membrane-bound, crystalline arrays (c), which contain virions embedded within an electron-dense matrix (a).
Bar = 174 nm. *C*. Intestinal jejunal enterocytes (3 days postinfection). Luminal aggregates of astrovirus (*arrowheads*) within debris adjacent to enterocytes. Bar = 441 nm.
(Avian Diseases)

trovirus-specific antibodies (5). Whether convalescent birds are protected from further astrovirus infection has not been determined. This appears likely, however, for naturally infected turkeys, as astroviruses were rarely detected beyond 5 wk of age when commercial turkey flocks were monitored until market age (7). The effect of maternal antibodies on astrovirus infections is unknown.

DIAGNOSIS. Immune electron microscopy is the preferred method for identifying astroviruses from fecal and/or intestinal samples. This procedure is done by diluting the fecal/intestinal sample with sterile diluent such as phosphate-buffered saline (pH 7.2) to make a working solution. The diluted sample is thoroughly mixed by using a homogenizer or vortex mixer, and sonicated. Particulate matter and bacteria are removed by centrifugation at $500 \times g$ for 20 min and filtering the resulting supernatant fluid through a 450-nm porosity membrane filter. The filtrate is incubated with an appropriate dilution of antiserum containing astrovirus antibodies. Following incubation, the sample is pelleted by ultracentrifugation, negatively stained with phosphotungstic acid, and observed by EM. Aggregates of astrovirus can be easily observed at ×30,000 to 50,000 magnification. Although astroviruses have star-shaped morphology, only a small percentage of particles display this characteristic. It is quite difficult to diagnose astrovirus infections accurately without IEM. A definitive diagnosis of astrovirus infection is made by recognizing aggregates of typical astrovirus particles in the IEM preparation. In the author's experience, turkey astroviruses only occasionally display nonspecific agglutination; therefore, one must rely on IEM for aggregation of particles (see Fig. 27.8).

Differential diagnosis of astrovirus infections in turkey poults needs to include infectious, parasitic, and noninfectious agents that can cause enteric disease. Cultures for enteropathogenic bacteria such as *Salmonella* spp. and *Campylobacter* spp. should be done. Smears or tissue sections will demonstrate protozoa. Other enteric viruses need to be excluded including coronavirus and rotavirus. The latter needs to be highly considered and a method to detect rotavirus infections should be employed, as

there is evidence that astroviruses and rotaviruses often occur together and may be involved in the same disease entity (6).

TREATMENT, PREVENTION, AND CONTROL. There are no vaccines, chemotherapeutics, or other measures reported to be efficacious for control and/or prevention of astrovirus infections. Generally, good management practices emphasizing cleaning, disinfecting, litter management, and resting of facilities between flocks are recommended. Astrovirus infections have, however, continued to be problems for some producers with modern facilities employing high standards of management, suggesting that contemporary management practices may not have been entirely effective.

REFERENCES
1. Bridger, J.C. 1980. Detection by electron microscopy of caliciviruses, astroviruses and rotavirus-like particles in the faeces of piglets with diarrhoea. Vet Rec 107:532–533.
2. Gough, R.E., M.S. Collins, E. Borland, and L.F. Keymer. 1984. Astrovirus-like particles associated with hepatitis in ducklings. Vet Rec 114:279.
3. Kurtz, J.B., T.W. Lee, and D. Pickering. 1977. Astrovirus associated gastroenteritis in a children's ward. J Clin Pathol 30:948–952.
4. McNulty, M.S., W.L. Curran, and J.B. McFerran. 1980. Detection of astroviruses in turkey faeces by direct electron microscopy. Vet Rec 106:561.
5. Reynolds, D.L., and Y.M. Saif. 1986. Astrovirus: A cause of an enteric disease in turkey poults. Avian Dis 30:728–735.
6. Reynolds, D.L., Y.M. Saif, and K.W. Theil. 1987. A survey of enteric viruses of turkey poults. Avian Dis 31:89–98.
7. Reynolds, D.L., Y.M. Saif, and K.W. Theil. 1987. Enteric viral infections of turkey poults: Incidence of infection. Avian Dis 31:272–276.
8. Saif, L.J., Y.M. Saif, and K.W. Theil. 1985. Enteric viruses in diarrheic turkey poults. Avian Dis 29:798–811.
9. Snodgrass, D.R., and E.W. Gray. 1977. Detection and transmission of 30 nm virus particles (astroviruses) in faeces of lambs with diarrhoea. Arch Virol 55:287–291.
10. Thouvenelle, M.L., J.S. Haynes, and D.L. Reynolds. 1995. Astrovirus infection in hatchling turkeys: Histologic, morphometric and ultrastructural findings. Avian Dis 39:328–336.
11. Thouvenelle, M.L., J.S. Haynes, J.L. Sell, and D.L. Reynolds. 1995. Astrovirus infection in hatchling turkeys: Alterations in intestinal maltase activity. Avian Dis 39:343–348.
12. Woode, G.N., and J.C. Bridger. 1978. Isolation of small viruses resembling astroviruses and caliciviruses from acute enteritis of calves. J Med Microbiol 11:441–452.

AVIAN ENTEROVIRUSLIKE VIRUSES

M. S. McNulty and James S. Guy

INTRODUCTION. A number of enteroviruslike viruses (ELVs) have been identified in avian species in recent years. The term *enteroviruslike* is applied to these viruses, as they have not been fully characterized; definitive classification awaits further biologic, physicochemical, and molecular characterization. This section addresses those ELVs identified in domestic poultry, other than avian encephalomyelitis virus (see Chapter 21), avian nephritis virus (see Chapter 31), duck hepatitis virus types 1 and 3 (see Chapter 25), and turkey hepatitis virus (see Chapter 31).

The economic significance of avian ELVs is not yet known. There is no evidence that they are transmissible from avian species to humans or other mammals.

HISTORY, INCIDENCE, AND DISTRIBUTION.

Examination of feces from avian species using negative contrast electron microscopy (EM) has led to the discovery of several ELVs. The presence of ELVs in intestinal contents of young turkeys and chickens was described in the United Kingdom in 1979 (18). Subsequently, ELVs were identified in the feces of turkey poults in the United States (11, 24, 25, 26) and France (1), in chickens in Belgium (5), United States (8), and Malaysia (3), in guinea fowl with transmissible enteritis in Italy (15) and France (2), and in partridges (10) and pheasants in the United Kingdom (9). In Japan, ELVs were isolated from chicks affected by baby chick nephropathy (28) and from broilers with a stunting syndrome (31). Similar viruses were isolated from broilers with stunting syndrome or baby chick nephropathy in the United Kingdom (7). In addition, ELVs have been found in feces and enterocytes of cockatoos and galahs with enteric disease in Australia (22, 33). Based on these findings, it is likely that avian ELVs have a worldwide distribution.

ETIOLOGY

Classification. Enteroviruses comprise one of four genera within the family *Picornaviridae*. Genera within the family *Picornaviridae* are distinguished by their sensitivity to acid, buoyant density of the virion in CsCl, and clinical manifestations in the affected host (16). Enteroviruses are stable at acid pH, have a density of 1.33 g/mL in CsCl, and replicate preferentially in the intestinal tract. Most avian ELVs have been classified on the basis of size, morphology, cytoplasmic replication in ente-

rocytes, and resistance to acid pH. Information on genome structure of ELVs is available only for U.S. isolates from turkeys. United States turkey isolates possessed a single-stranded RNA genome of approximately 7.5 kb; in addition, these viruses were determined to have a buoyant density of 1.33 g/mL in CsCl (11, 13).

Morphology. *Picornaviridae* possess roughly spherical naked nucleocapsids 22–30 nm in diameter (icosahedral, with T=1). The virion lacks obvious surface structure and there are no surface projections (Fig. 27.11). The sizes described for most avian ELVs fall within a 22–30 nm range, although a range of 18–24 nm was described for U.S. turkey ELVs (11, 30).

Virus Replication. Replication of turkey ELVs has been investigated by both immunohistochemistry and thin-section EM (11, 14). Virus replication was shown to occur in the cytoplasm of intestinal enterocytes. Crystalline arrays composed of small, round viruslike particles approximately

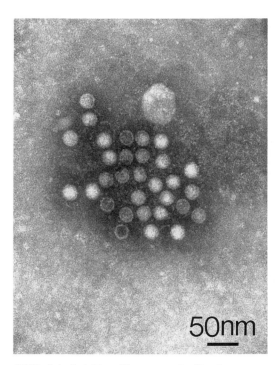

27.11. Spherical, 18- to 27-nm enteroviruslike viruses (ELVs) detected in feces of young turkeys with enteric disease, sodium phosphotungstate.

23 nm in diameter (Fig. 27.12) were observed (11, 14); an earlier study (30) described particles of 17.1 nm. Similar findings to the former were reported for a chicken ELV (6, 19).

A U.S. turkey ELV was shown by immunofluorescence and immunoperoxidase staining procedures to replicate primarily in the jejunum and ileum of experimentally infected poults (14). The virus replicated preferentially in those enterocytes located halfway between the tip and base of the villus. Viral antigen was found most abundantly in enterocytes situated immediately above crypt openings.

Resistance to Chemical and Physical Agents. Avian ELVs that have been tested have been found to be stable at pH 3 and unaffected by solvents such as chloroform and ether (17, 19, 20, 29, 31). There is no information about their sensitivity to disinfectants.

Strain Classification. Because of the difficulties with growing avian ELVs in cell culture and other laboratory host systems, very little information is available concerning their antigenic relationships. Using cross immunofluorescence, three

ELVs isolated from chickens, designated EF84/700 (20), FP3 (29), and 612 (17), were found to be antigenically distinct from each other and also from avian nephritis virus, avian encephalomyelitis virus, duck hepatitis type 1, and duck hepatitis virus type 3, which also belong to antigenically distinct serogroups (17, 21). Several ELVs isolated in Japan from chicks with baby chick nephropathy (28) and from broilers with a stunting syndrome (31) had biologic and physical properties similar to the G-4260 strain of avian nephritis virus, but were antigenically distinct from avian nephritis virus (27, 28).

Several ELVs isolated from broiler chickens with runting and stunting syndrome in the United Kingdom and Belgium were antigenically related to avian nephritis virus by cross-immunofluorescence and cross-neutralization tests (4, 21). Interestingly, these viruses differed in their pathogenicity, as determined by their ability to depress growth of orally inoculated broiler chicks (5, 19, 21). Variations in pathogenicity using different criteria were also observed among Japanese isolates of avian nephritis virus (27, 32). Thus, it is possible that other avian ELVs that belong to the same serogroup may differ in pathogenicity.

A U.S. turkey ELV was shown to be antigenically

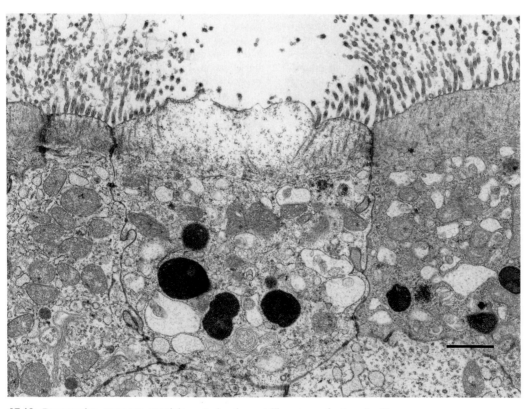

27.12. Degenerating enterocyte containing cytoplasmic crystalline arrays of enteroviruslike viruses (ELVs).

distinct from avian encephalomyelitis virus by cross immunofluorescence (11). Turkey ELVs were isolated in France by yolk sac inoculation of embryonated eggs; two strains were identified using cross-neutralization tests (1).

Laboratory Host Systems. Enteroviruslike viruses can be propagated in the laboratory by oral inoculation of neonatal birds of the same species from which they originally were isolated. Depending on the virus, inoculated birds may develop enteric disease and depressed growth rates. Intestinal contents examined by negative contrast EM 1–3 days postinfection (PI) will normally contain the inoculated virus. Caution must be exercised, however, in propagating ELVs in this manner as even specific-pathogen–free birds may be infected with ELVs.

Most chicken ELVs will grow in 6-day-old embryonated chicken eggs, with approximately 50% of embryos dying within 3–7 days PI. Some of these viruses also can be propagated in the chorioallantoic membrane of embryonated eggs. Immunofluorescent staining of impression smears of yolk sac membranes or cryostat sections of chorioallantoic membrane can be used to confirm virus growth. In addition, some ELVs, for example FP3 and 612, show limited growth in primary cultures of chicken embryo liver or chicken kidney cells. Growth of virus in cell culture is best detected by immunofluorescent staining (Fig. 27.13), as many of these viruses cause little, if any, cytopathology (17, 21).

A U.S. turkey ELV was propagated in embryonated turkey eggs (11). Inoculation of embryonated turkey eggs at 18 days of incubation resulted

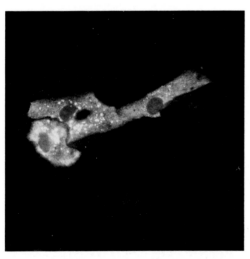

27.13. Immunofluorescent staining of chicken embryo liver cell culture infected with enteroviruslike

in replication of the virus in embryo intestines. At 6 days PI, turkey embryos were normal with the exception of intestinal tissues; duodenum, jejunum, and ileum were pale and dilated. The turkey ELV was detected in embryo intestines by thin-section EM, direct examination of intestinal contents by EM, and immunofluorescence.

An ELV from guinea fowl with transmissible enteritis was successfully propagated following inoculation of 7-day-old guinea fowl embryos via the yolk sac; however, embryo mortality and lesions were inconsistent (23).

Pathogenicity. The role of these other avian ELVs as pathogens requires clarification. While there is evidence that they may cause enteric disease in young turkeys, chickens, and guinea fowl, and baby chick nephropathy, further work is needed to define their importance.

PATHOGENESIS AND EPIZOOTIOLOGY

Natural and Experimental Hosts. Infections with ELVs have been described in turkeys, chickens, guinea fowl, partridges, pheasants, and psittacine species. The majority of infections in domestic poultry have been identified in young birds during the first few weeks of life. A chicken ELV was isolated from meconium of a dead-in-shell chicken embryo (29), however, indicating that infection with these viruses may occur in adulthood. These findings indicate that the epizootiology of these viruses may be similar to that of avian encephalomyelitis.

The principal site of replication of ELVs is the small intestinal epithelium (Fig. 27.14); some chicken ELVs also replicate in the kidney (7, 28). Thus, infection is spread horizontally through ingestion of infected feces, but other routes of spread cannot be ruled out. Isolation of a chicken ELV from meconium of a dead-in-shell chicken embryo indicates that this virus is vertically transmitted (29); it is likely that others are transmitted in this manner.

Incubation Period, Signs, Morbidity, and Mortality. In experimentally infected turkeys, a U.S. turkey ELV produced watery droppings by 4 days PI and significant reduction of body weight gain on days 4 and 8 PI, as compared with controls (30). The virus was shown in a subsequent study (14) to produce depression, watery droppings, and pasted vents in inoculated turkeys. Virus was detected in droppings of inoculated turkeys from days 2–14 PI.

Transient stunting of growth of variable severity was observed in broiler chickens dosed orally with ELVs (17, 21). Specific-pathogen–free chicks inoc-

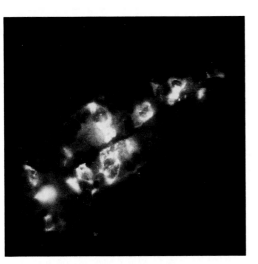

27.14. Specific immunofluorescence in epithelium of jejunal villus of chicken infected with enteroviruslike virus (ELV) (612 isolate). ×450.

ulated orally with Japanese ELVs showed diarrhea and variable mortality (up to 53.3%), dying between 2 and 6 days PI (28).

An ELV isolated from guinea fowl with transmissible enteritis in Italy suppressed weight gains of commercial guinea fowl when they were inoculated orally at 1 day of age (23).

Pathology.   Gross lesions in turkeys experimentally infected with a U.S. turkey enterovirus consisted of thin-walled, dilated ceca filled with yellow, foamy fluid; catarrhal secretions were detected in the small intestines (14, 30). Morphometric studies indicated shortening of the duodenal villi and elongation of crypts in the duodenum and ileum. In naturally occurring infections in turkeys, ELVs usually occur as a component of mixed infections. Interestingly, poults experimentally infected with a combined ELV/group A rotavirus inoculum were more severely affected in terms of clinical signs, body weight gain and lesion severity than poults that received either inoculum alone (12).

Chicks experimentally infected with Japanese ELVs and which died 2–6 days after inoculation showed nephrosis and visceral urate deposition. Survivors examined 14 days PI had interstitial nephrosis (28).

DIAGNOSIS.   Diagnosis of ELV infections in avian species most commonly is accomplished by EM examination of droppings or intestinal samples. Turkey ELVs have been identified in droppings and intestinal contents using both direct and immune EM procedures (11, 18, 30). For direct EM, turkey droppings or intestinal contents are prepared as sus-

pensions (10–29%) in phosphate-buffered saline and centrifuged at $800 \times g$ for 20 min to remove large particulate material. The supernatant fluid is centrifuged at $15,000 \times g$ for 20 min in a benchtop centrifuge, and the resultant pellet is resuspended in approximately 500 µL distilled water and 100 µL 2% phosphotungstic acid. After mixing, the material either is sprayed onto formvar-filmed copper grids or a drop of the material is placed on the grid for 1–3 min and removed by blotting on bibulous paper. Turkey ELVs also may be detected in droppings or intestinal contents using immune EM (25); however, this procedure requires availability of specific antisera.

An antigen-capture enzyme-linked immunosorbent assay (ELISA) was described for detection of turkey ELV in turkey intestinal contents (12). The procedure was shown to be a rapid, highly sensitive, and specific method for diagnosis of the virus. Confirmation that the particles observed by EM are animal viruses is achieved by isolation of the viruses in turkey or chicken embryos, or in cell cultures as described above. Antigenic characterization of the isolate is dependent on the availability of serogroup-specific antisera; immunofluorescent staining of impression smears or cryostat sections of yolk sac membranes or chorioallantoic membranes from inoculated embryos or of inoculated cell cultures will distinguish between isolates of known serogroups and aid in the identification of new serogroups.

Antibodies to ELVs have been detected by serum-neutralization and indirect immunofluorescence tests; however, because virus isolates and reference antisera are not widely distributed, serologic diagnosis is not recommended.

TREATMENT, CONTROL, AND PREVENTION.   The role of ELVs as avian pathogens has not yet been fully defined; consequently, no specific therapeutic or prophylactic measures are available.

REFERENCES
1. Andral, B., and D. Toquin. 1984. Observations and isolation of pseudopicornavirus from sick turkeys. Avian Pathol 13:377–388.
2. Andral, B., M. Lagadic, C. Louzis, J.P. Guillou, and J.M. Gourreau. 1987. Fulminating disease of guinea fowl: Aetiological studies. Point Veterinaire 19:515–520.
3. Chooi, K.F., and U. Chulan. 1985. Broiler runting/stunting syndrome in Malaysia. Vet Rec 116:354.
4. Decaesstecker, M., G. Charlier, and G. Meulemans. 1986. Significance of parvoviruses, entero-like viruses and reoviruses in the aetiology of the chicken malabsorption syndrome. Avian Pathol 15:769–782.
5. Decaesstecker, M., and G. Meulemans. 1989. Antigenic relationships between fowl enteroviruses. Avian Pathol 18:715–723.
6. Frazier, J.A., and R.L. Reece. 1990. Infectious stunting syndrome of chickens in Great Britain: Intestinal ultrastructural pathology. Avian Pathol 19:759–777.
7. Frazier, J.A., K. Howes, R.L. Reece, A.W. Kidd, and

D. Cavanagh. 1990. Isolation of non-cytopathic viruses implicated in the aetiology of nephritis and baby chick nephropathy and serologically related to avian nephritis virus. Avian Pathol 19:139–160.

8. Goodwin, M.A., J.F. Davis, M.S. McNulty, J. Brown and E.C. Player. 1993. Enteritis (so-called runting stunting syndrome) in Georgia broiler chicks. Avian Dis 37:451–458.

9. Gough, R.E., D.J. Alexander, M.S. Collins, S.A. Lister, and W.J. Cox. 1988. Routine virus isolation or detection in the diagnosis of diseases in birds. Avian Pathol 17:893–907.

10. Gough, R.E., M.S. Collins, D.J. Alexander, and W.J. Cox. 1990. Viruses and virus-like particles detected in samples from diseased game birds in Great Britain during 1988. Avian Pathol 19:331–343.

11. Guy, J.S., and H.J. Barnes. 1991. Partial characterization of a turkey enterovirus-like virus. Avian Dis 35:197–203.

12. Hayhow, C.S., and Y.M. Saif. 1993. Development of an antigen-capture enzyme-linked immunosorbent assay for detection of enterovirus in commercial turkeys. Avian Dis 37:375–379.

13. Hayhow, C.S., and Y.M. Saif. 1993. Experimental infection of specific-pathogen-free turkey poults with single and combined enterovirus and group A rotavirus. Avian Dis 37:546–557.

14. Hayhow, C.S., A.V. Parwani, and Y.M. Saif, 1993. Single-stranded genomic RNA from turkey enterovirus-like virus. Avian Dis 37:558–560.

15. Hayhow, C.S., Y.M. Saif, K.M. Kerr, and R.E. Whitmoyer. 1993. Further observations on enterovirus infection in specific-pathogen-free turkey poults. Avian Dis 37:124–134.

16. Lavazza, A., S. Pascucci, and D. Gelmetti. 1990. Rod-shaped virus-like particles in intestinal contents of three avian species. Vet Rec 126:581.

17. Matthews, R.E.F. 1982. Classification and nomenclature of viruses. Intervirology 17:1–199.

18. McNeilly, F., T.J. Connor, V.M. Calvert, J.A. Smyth, W.L. Curran, A.J. Morley, D. Thompson, S. Singh, J.B. McFerran, B.M. Adair, and M.S. McNulty. 1994. Studies on a new enterovirus-like virus isolated from chickens. Avian Pathol 23:313–327.

19. McNulty, M.S., W.L. Curran, D. Todd, and J.B. McFerran. 1979. Detection of viruses in avian faeces by direct electron microscopy. Avian Pathol 8:239–247.

20. McNulty, M.S., G.M. Allan, T.J. Connor, J.B. McFerran, and R.M. McCracken, 1984. An entero-like virus associated with the runting syndrome in broiler chickens. Avian Pathol 13:429–439.

21. McNulty, M.S., G.M. Allan, and J.B. McFerran. 1987. Isolation of a novel avian entero-like virus. Avian Pathol 16:331–337.

22. McNulty, M.S., T.J. Connor, F. McNeilly, and J.B. McFerran. 1990. Biological characterisation of avian enteroviruses and enterovirus-like viruses. Avian Pathol 19:75–87.

23. McOrist, S., D Madill, M. Adamson, and C. Philip. 1991. Viral enteritis in cockatoos (Cacatua spp.). Avian Pathol 20:531–539.

24. Pascucci, S., and A. Lavazza. 1994. A survey of enteric viruses in commercial avian species: Experimental studies of transmissible enteritis of guinea fowl. In M.S. McNulty and J. B. McFerran (eds.). New and Evolving Virus Diseases of Poultry. Commission of the European Communities, Brussels, Belgium, pp. 225–241.

25. Reynolds, D.L., Y.M. Saif, and K.W. Theil. 1987. A survey of enteric viruses of turkey poults. Avian Dis 31:89–98.

26. Saif, L.J., Y.M. Saif, and K.W. Theil. 1985. Enteric viruses in diarrheic turkey poults. Avian Dis 29:798–811.

27. Saif, Y.M., L.J. Saif, C.L. Hofacre, C. Hayhow, D.E. Swayne, and R.N. Dearth. 1990. A small round virus associated with enteritis in turkey poults. Avian Dis 34:762–764.

28. Shirai, J., K. Nakamura, K. Shinohara, and H. Kawamura. 1991. Pathogenicity and antigenicity of avian nephritis isolates. Avian Dis 35:49–54.

29. Shirai, J., N. Tanimura, K. Uramoto, M. Narita, K. Nakamura, and H. Kawamura. 1992. Pathologically and serologically different avian nephritis virus isolates implicated in etiology of baby chick nephropathy. Avian Dis 36:369–377.

30. Spackman, D., R.E. Gough, M.S. Collins, and D. Lanning. 1984. Isolation of an enterovirus-like agent from the meconium of dead-in-shell chicken embryos. Vet Rec 114:216–218.

31. Swayne, D.E., M.J. Radin, and Y.M. Saif. 1990. Enteric disease in specific-pathogen-free turkey poults inoculated with a small round turkey-origin enteric virus. Avian Dis 34:683–692.

32. Takase, K., K. Shinohara, M. Tsuneyoshi, M. Yamamoto, and S. Yamada, 1989. Isolation and characterisation of cytopathic avian enteroviruses from broiler chicks. Avian Pathol 18:631–642.

33. Takase, K., T. Uchimura, and M. Yamamoto. 1990. Comparative studies on the pathogenicity of the cytopathic avian enteroviruses (avian nephritis virus) isolated from broiler chicks. Avian Pathol 19:635–642.

34. Wylie, S.L., and D.A. Pass. 1989. Investigations of an enteric infection of cockatoos caused by an enterovirus-like agent. Aust Vet J 66:321–324.

28 Viral Arthritis

John K. Rosenberger and N. O. Olson

INTRODUCTION. Viruses that are members of the genus *Reovirus* can be separated into two subdivisions based on their mammalian or avian origins (37, 45). These two subdivisions are further differentiated by antigenic configuration, growth in cell culture, host specificity, and ability to induce hemagglutination in vitro.

Reoviruses have been isolated from a variety of tissues in chickens affected by assorted disease conditions including viral arthritis/tenosynovitis, stunting syndrome, respiratory disease, enteric disease, and malabsorption syndrome. They have frequently been found in chickens that were clinically normal (65). The nature of the disease that occurs following reovirus infection is very much dependent upon host age, virus pathotype, and route of exposure.

Economic losses caused by reovirus infections are frequently the result of crippling (viral arthritis/tenosynovitis) and a general lack of performance including diminished weight gains, poor feed conversion, and a reduced marketability of affected birds.

HISTORY. In 1954, Fahey and Crawley (13) made what was later confirmed by Petek et al. (59) to be the initial isolation of avian reovirus from the respiratory tract of chickens with chronic respiratory disease. The Fahey-Crawley virus, when inoculated into susceptible chickens, produced a moderate respiratory disease, liver necrosis, and an inflammation of the tendons and synovial membranes.

Olson et al. in 1957 (57) described a naturally occurring synovitis in chickens from which they were able to isolate an agent insensitive to chlortetracycline and furazolidone and serologically unrelated to either *Mycoplasma gallisepticum* or *M. synoviae*. This agent, later named the "viral arthritis agent" by Olson and Kerr (53), was eventually identified as a reovirus by Walker et al. in 1972 (89). Dalton and Henry (6) used the term *tenosynovitis* to define the changes in the tendons and tendon sheaths associated with a condition they considered different from that caused by *M. synoviae*. This difference was substantiated by Olson and Solomon (55) when they reported tenosynovitis in commercially produced chickens that had been derived from *M. synoviae*–free broiler chickens. An isolate obtained

from these birds had characteristics identical to those described for the "viral arthritis agent" and was shown to be antigenically similar to the Fahey-Crawley virus (56). Since the first reports of tenosynovitis in the United States and England, the disease has been described in many other countries. Several reviews document the incidence of reovirus-induced tenosynovitis (41, 64, 82).

Reoviruses have been associated with other disease conditions including ruptured gastrocnemius tendons, osteoporosis, pericarditis, myocarditis, hydropericardium, cloacal pasting, early mortality in poults, and most recently, malabsorption syndrome. In the case of the latter condition, the etiologic picture is not clear-cut. In addition to reoviruses, several other viruses as well as bacteria and noninfectious agents have been implicated (see Chapter 37, Emerging Diseases and Diseases of Complex or Unknown Etiology).

INCIDENCE AND DISTRIBUTION. Reovirus infections are prevalent worldwide in chickens, turkeys and other avian species. Viral arthritis/tenosynovitis is found primarily in meat-type chickens but has been diagnosed in egg-type birds (75) and turkeys (58). Reovirus-associated malabsorption syndrome has been reported in the United States, Europe, and Australia, but many of these associations are tenuous and need confirmation. Reoviruses are commonly found in the digestive and respiratory tracts of clinically normal chickens and turkeys (38, 59, 77, 94) and have been identified as contaminants in Marek's disease vaccine (91).

ETIOLOGY. As a group, reoviruses are nonenveloped with an icosahedral symmetry and a double-capsid structure. Intact virus particles have a diameter of approximately 75 nm and a density in cesium chloride of 1.36–1.37 g/mL (18, 73, 74, 79). The viral genome consists of dsRNA, which is segmented and can be further segregated into at least three size classes that contain a total of 10 discrete molecular species (19, 20, 79).

Reoviruses are heat resistant, being able to withstand 60 C for 8–10 hr, 56 C for 22–24 hr, 37 C for 15–16 wk, 22 C for 48–51 wk, 4 C for over 3 yr, −20 C for over 4 yr, and −63 C for over 10 yr (52). The titer of semipurified virus at 60 C is reduced, but not completely inactivated, in 5 hr. Heat treatment in the presence of magnesium chloride results in increased titers.

Reoviruses are not sensitive to ether but are slightly sensitive to chloroform. They are resistant to pH 3; hydrogen peroxide when incubated for 1 hr at room temperature; 2% Lysol; 3% formalin; and the DNA metabolic inhibitors actinomycin D, cytosine arabinoside, and 5-fluoro-2-deoxyuridine. They are inactivated by 70% ethanol, 0.5% organic iodine (28), and a 5% solution of hydrogen peroxide (50).

Attempts to demonstrate hemagglutination by avian reovirus have been generally unsuccessful (64) with two exceptions (9, 15).

Strain Classification. Reoviruses can be classified using serologic procedures or grouped according to their relative pathogenicity for chickens. Kawamura and Tsubahara and Kawamura et al. (37, 38) identified five serotypes of reovirus from 77 isolates originally obtained from feces, cloacal swabs, and tracheas. Sahu and Olson (72) found four serotypes from intestines, respiratory tract, and synovial isolates. Wood et al. (92) calculated the relatedness of reoviruses originating from the United States, the United Kingdom, Germany, and Japan and found at least 11 serotypes, although there was considerable cross neutralization among heterologous types. Hieronymus et al. (23) grouped five reovirus isolates into three serotypes, and Robertson and Wilcox (63) assigned 10 Australian isolates into three groups with considerable cross-reactivity. It is apparent that reoviruses frequently exist as antigenic subtypes, rather than distinct serotypes.

Rosenberger (68) inoculated specific-pathogen–free chickens by various routes with plaque-purified, antigenically similar viruses and demonstrated clear strain differences based on relative pathogenicity and virus persistence.

Laboratory Host Systems. Reoviruses grow readily in the embryonating chicken egg following inoculation via yolk sac or chorioallantoic membrane (CAM). The yolk sac is preferred for original isolation and generally results in embryo mortality 3 to 5 days after inoculation, with affected embryos exhibiting a purplish discoloration due to massive subcutaneous hemorrhage. Mortality in CAM-inoculated embryos usually occurs on the 7th to 8th day postinoculation; embryos are slightly dwarfed with occasional enlargement of the liver and spleen. Necrotic foci may occur in both the liver and spleen, particularly in embryos that survive longer than 7 days postinoculation. Small, discrete, slightly raised white lesions may be found on the CAM. Histologically, areas of necrosis of the ectoderm with only moderate stimulation of the epithelial cells are seen. Mesoderm adjacent to the lesion is edematous and contains numerous inflammatory cells. Edema alone may be found. Embryo mortality is less consistent following inoculation via the chorioallantoic sac.

The virus grows in primary chicken cell cultures of embryo, lung, kidney, liver, macrophages, and testicle. Primary chicken kidney cells from 2- to 6-wk-old chickens are satisfactory, but for plaques and isolation, primary embryo liver cells are preferred (2, 22). Chicken embryo fibroblasts are suitable for reovirus growth, but the virus often requires adaptation (2). Chicken-origin cell cultures infected with reoviruses are characterized by the formation of syncytia, which may occur as early as 24–48 hr, followed by degeneration, leaving holes in the monolayer and giant cells floating in the medium. Infected cells exhibit intracytoplasmic inclusions that may appear either eosinophilic or basophilic (64). Of many established cell lines tested, virus has been grown on Vero (72), BHK 21/13, 1TT, feline kidney (CRFK), Georgia bovine kidney (GBK), rabbit kidney (RK), porcine kidney (PK) cells (2), a Japanese quail cell line (QT35) derived from an induced fibrosarcoma (5), and chicken lymphoblastoid cells (76).

Pathogenicity. Although normally associated with arthritis/tenosynovitis, reoviruses have been identified as the etiology of other disease conditions as well, including growth retardation, pericarditis, myocarditis, hydropericardium, enteritis, hepatitis, bursal and thymic atrophy, osteoporosis, and acute and chronic respiratory syndromes (64). The pathogenicity of selected reovirus isolates was enhanced by coinfection with *Eimeria tenella* or *E. maxima* (70, 71). Exposure to infectious bursal disease virus or particular dietary regimes increased the severity of tenosynovitis resulting from infections with the WVU-2937 isolate (3, 4, 80). Reoviruses may also exacerbate disease conditions caused by other pathogens including chicken anemia agent (12), *Escherichia coli,* and Newcastle disease virus (69). The increased susceptibility to other infectious agents following or concomitant with reovirus exposure may result from immune system compromise (62).

PATHOGENESIS AND EPIZOOTIOLOGY

Natural and Experimental Hosts. Although reoviruses have been found in many avian species, chickens and turkeys are the only recognized natural or experimental hosts for reovirus-induced arthritis/tenosynovitis. Reoviruses have been isolated from turkeys with arthritis (58), and Van der Heide et al. (87) found a turkey isolate to be pathogenic for chickens. The turkey isolate was neutralized by chicken reovirus S1133 antiserum. High mortality in turkey poults has also been associated with reovirus (77), although turkeys were shown to be more resistant than chickens to reovirus-induced tenosynovitis (1). McFerran et al. (46) identified a reovirus in turkey feces that shared the group-specific antigen with chicken isolates but was not neutralized by available reference antiserum.

Reoviruses were found in clinically affected ducks, pigeons, geese, American woodcock, and Psittacine species, but a firm etiologic relationship was not always established (8, 64). A disease in Muscovy ducks characterized by a general malaise, diarrhea, and stunted growth has been reported in several countries (14, 36, 43) and reproduced experimentally with isolated reoviruses (14, 43). Attempts to establish active infection in the canary, pigeon, guinea pig, rat, mouse, hamster, and rabbit failed; however, Phillips et al. (60) reported liver lesions in neonatal mice after oral and nasal infection, and Nersessian et al. (51) produced stunted growth and incoordination in suckling mice inoculated intracerebrally with several turkey isolates.

Age-Associated Resistance. Kerr and Olson (39) were the first to report on age-related resistance to reovirus-induced arthritis/tenosynovitis. The disease can be readily reproduced in 1-day-old chickens free of maternal antibody (30, 86), whereas older chickens are infected, but the disease is generally less severe and the incubation period longer. Similar results were reported by Rosenberger (68) with reoviruses isolated from birds with an apparent stunting and tenosynovitis. Jones and Georgiou (30) suggested the age-associated susceptibility may be related to the inability of young birds to develop an effective immune response.

Transmission. Horizontal transmission of reovirus has been extensively documented (64, 82). There is considerable variation, however, among strains of virus in their ability to spread laterally. Although reovirus may be excreted from both the intestinal and respiratory tracts for at least 10 days postinoculation, virus generally appears to be shed from the intestine for longer periods, suggesting fecal contamination as a primary source of contact infection (33, 42). Roessler (66) demonstrated that 1-day-old chickens are more susceptible to reovirus introduced via the respiratory route than orally. Virus may persist for long periods in the cecal tonsils and hock joints, particularly in birds infected at a young age (31, 44), implicating carrier birds as potential sources of infection for penmates.

Menendez et al. (48) and Van der Heide and Kalbac (83) have clearly demonstrated avian reoviruses can be vertically transmitted. Menendez et al. showed that following oral, tracheal, and nasal inoculation of 15-mo-old breeders, virus was present in chicks from eggs laid 17, 18, and 19 days postinfection. Egg transmission rate was low (1.7%). Reoviruses were also isolated from chicken embryo fibroblast cell cultures prepared from embryonated eggs derived from experimentally infected hens (83).

Incubation Period. The incubation period differs depending upon virus pathotype, age of host, and route of exposure (64, 82). For inoculated 2-wk-old chickens, the incubation period varied from 1 day (foot pad inoculation) to 11 days (intramuscular, intravenous, intrasinus inoculation). The incubation period following intratracheal inoculation and contact exposure was 9 and 13 days, respectively (55).

Often, infections are inapparent and demonstrable only by serology or virus isolations. Mature birds inoculated by oral and respiratory routes with the FDO isolate had virus in all organs tested at 4 days postinfection. The number of virus isolations was greatly reduced by 2 wk, and no virus was present 20 days postinfection. There was frequent localization of virus in the flexor and extensor tendons of the pelvic limb, although gross lesions were not evident (49). Foot pad inoculation of 1-day-old chickens with an arthrotropic reovirus (R2) produced a more rapid progression of disease than either the oral, subcutaneous, or articular routes (27). When infected by the oral route, which appears to be a likely mode of naturally transmitted virus, the initial site of viral replication, which occurred within 2 to 12 hr postexposure, was the epithelium of the intestine and the bursa of Fabricius. This was followed by virus distribution in a wide range of tissues, including the hock joint, within 24–48 hr (35). Many reoviruses cause microscopic inflammatory changes in the digital flexor and metatarsal extensor tendons without development of gross lesions (54).

When disease (viral arthritis/tenosynovitis) does occur from naturally occurring infection, it is usually seen in young birds 4–7 wk old, but may be seen in much older chickens as well (82). Morbidity can be as high as 100%, while mortality is generally less than 6%.

Signs. In acute infections, lameness is present and some chickens are stunted. With chronic infection, lameness is more pronounced, and in a small percentage of infected chickens, the hock joint is immobilized. In a flock of 36,000 broilers, the infection, first diagnosed as infectious synovitis, appeared in 8 of 16 pens when the chicks were 3–4 wk old. Approximately 550 birds died or were removed because of lameness by 7–8 wk. Another 4,500 birds were stunted.

In another flock of approximately 15,000 broilers, no clinical signs of viral arthritis/tenosynovitis were observed, but approximately 5% of the birds had enlargement in the area of the gastrocnemius or digital flexor tendons when observed at slaughter. At 9 wk, birds from this flock had an average weight of only 3.66 lb, feed conversion was 2.45, mortality totaled 5%, and the condemnation rate was 2.6%. Virus was isolated from two birds condemned for toxemia; of 80 serum samples obtained from this flock, 89% had reovirus antibodies detected in a precipitin test. This inapparent infection probably caused the poor performance of these broilers.

Similar observations have been made by other workers (18, 29). Rupture of the gastrocnemius tendon, especially in male roaster birds 12- to 16-wk-old, is often associated with reovirus infection (29, 34). A similar lesion has been seen in 5- to 8-wk-old turkeys (58). The typical uneven gait in bilateral rupture of the tendon results from inability of the bird to immobilize the metatarsus. The latter is often accompanied by ruptured blood vessels.

Gross Lesions. Gross lesions in naturally infected chickens are observed as swellings of digital flexor and metatarsal extensor tendons. The latter lesion is evident by palpation just above the hock and may be readily observed when feathers are removed (Fig. 28.1).

Swellings of the foot pad and hock joint are less frequent. The hock usually contains a small amount of straw-colored or blood-tinted exudate; in a few cases there is a considerable amount of purulent exudate resembling that seen with infectious synovitis. Early in the infection, there is marked edema of the tarsal and metatarsal tendon sheaths (Fig. 28.2). Petechial hemorrhages are frequent in the synovial membranes above the hock (Fig. 28.3B).

Inflammation of tendon areas progresses to a chronic-type lesion characterized by hardening and fusion of tendon sheaths. Small pitted erosions develop in the articular cartilage of the distal tibiotarsus. These erosions enlarge, coalesce, and extend into underlying bone (Fig. 28.3 B,C). An overgrowth of fibrocartilaginous pannus develops on the articular surface. Condyles and epicondyles are frequently involved (40). In inoculated chickens, the diaphysis of the proximal metatarsal of the affected limb is enlarged.

Histopathology. Histologic changes have been described by Kerr and Olson (40). In general, they are the same for naturally occurring and experimental infections. During the acute phase (7–15 days following foot pad inoculation), edema, coagulation necrosis, heterophil accumulation, and perivascular infiltration are seen. There also are hypertrophy and hyperplasia of synovial cells, infiltration of lymphocytes and macrophages, and a proliferation of reticular cells. These latter lesions cause parietal and visceral layers of the tendon sheaths to become markedly thickened. The synovial cavity is

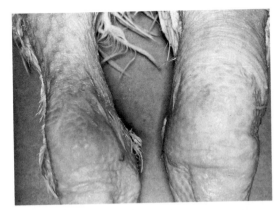

28.1. An 8-wk-old broiler showing marked swelling of digital flexor and metatarsal extensor tendons. Diagnosis can frequently be made on the basis of the bilateral swelling of these tendons.

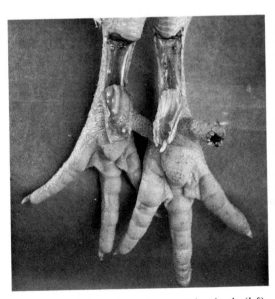

28.2. Marked edema of digital flexor tendon sheaths (*left*); normal (*right*).

filled with heterophils, macrophages, and sloughed synovial cells. Periostitis characterized by increased osteoclasts develops. During the chronic phase (starting by 15 days postinfection), the synovial membrane develops villous processes, and lymphoid nodules are seen. After 30 days, inflammatory changes become more chronic. There is an increase in the amount of fibrous connective tissue and a pronounced infiltration or proliferation of reticular cells, lymphocytes, macrophages, and plasma cells.

The same general inflammatory changes develop in the tarsometatarsal and hock joint areas. Development of sesamoid bones in the tendon of the af-

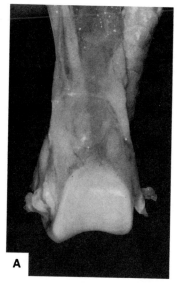
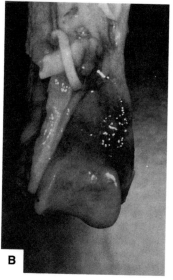
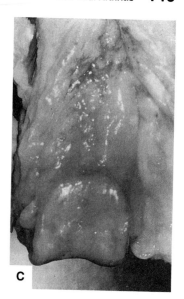

28.3. Viral arthritis lesions in distal posterior tibia of inoculated chickens. *A.* Normal. *B.* Cartilage erosions and hemorrhages of synovial membrane 35 days postinoculation. *C.* Erosions of cartilage and marked thickening of synovial membrane 212 days postinoculation.

fected limb is inhibited. Some tendons are completely replaced by irregular granulation tissue, and large villi form on the synovial membrane.

At 54 days postinfection, orally infected birds showed chronic fibrosis of tendon sheaths, with fibrous tissues invading tendons and resulting in ankylosis and immobility (85).

Linear growth of cartilage cells in the proximal tarsometatarsal bone becomes narrow and irregular. Erosions on the hock joint cartilage are accompanied by a granulation pannus. Osteoblasts become active and lay down a thickened layer of bone beneath the erosion. Osteoblastic activity is present on the condyles, epicondyles, and accessory tibia, producing osteoneogenesis and subsequent exostosis. (40). Ultrastructurally, the gastrocnemius tendon and sheath in broilers infected with reovirus at 1 day of age by the oral route were characterized by degenerative changes in fibroblasts including cytoplasmic vacuolization, membrane disruption, loss of ribosomes from the endoplasmic reticulum and generalized mitochondrial and cellular disruption (25).

Lesions found in the heart have been described in detail (40, 55). An infiltration of heterophils between myocardial fibers is a constant finding. In some cases, it is accompanied by proliferating mononuclear cells, probably reticular cells. The pathogenicity of avian reoviruses for day-old chicks revealed the arthrogenic potential for all strains and marked hepatic necrosis (21).

Erythrocyte, hematocrit, and total leukocyte determinations are generally within the normal range, although there may be a rise in the heterophil percentage and a decrease in the lymphocyte percentage.

Immunity. Avian reoviruses possess a group-specific antigen discernable with gel diffusion techniques and a serotype-specific antigen demonstrable with neutralizing antibody in plaque-reduction or chicken embryo assays (64, 82). Neutralizing antibodies can be detected 7–10 days following infection, and precipitating antibodies at approximately 2 wk. Neutralizing antibody appears to persist longer than precipitating antibody, but this may simply be a reflection of assay sensitivity. The importance of antibody in establishing protection is not well understood, since birds may become persistently infected in the presence of high levels of circulating antibody (32). It is apparent, however, that maternal antibody can afford a degree of protection to 1-day-old chickens against naturally occurring and experimental challenges (84, 86). Relative protection afforded by antibody appears to be as much related to serotype homogeneity, virus virulence, and host age as to antibody titer (61, 68, 86).

Interferon production by avian reoviruses has been demonstrated in vitro and in vivo. The S1133 attenuated strain induced interferon in chick embryo cell cultures, while in vivo interferon was detected in the lungs but not in other tissues (10, 11, 90). A more pathogenic reovirus elicited the production of interferon detectable in serum samples (10, 11). Hill et al. (24) reported that suppression of T-cell–mediated immunity by cyclosporin A resulted in increased mortality in reovirus-infected birds, but the relative severity of tendon lesions was unaffected.

DIAGNOSIS. A presumptive diagnosis of viral arthritis may be made on the basis of signs and lesions. Involvement of primarily the metatarsal extensor and digital flexor tendons (see Fig. 28.2), and heterophil infiltration in the heart, assist in differentiating the infection from bacterial and mycoplasmal synovitis. Demonstration of reoviruses in the tendon sheaths by fluorescent antibody techniques (64) or virus isolation in chickens embryos or chicken embryo liver cells provides further evidence (64, 82). The relative pathogenicity of a reovirus obtained from an affected joint can be confirmed by inoculation into the foot pad of susceptible 1-day-old chickens. If pathogenic, the virus will induce a pronounced inflammation of the foot pad within 72 hr postinoculation.

Reoviruses can be readily differentiated from other viruses by their typical physicochemical characteristics and the presence of a group-specific antigen demonstrable with the agar gel precipitin test. For preparation of the antigen, 9- to 11-day-old embryonating chicken eggs are inoculated by the CAM route and CAMs are harvested from dead or affected embryos within 7 days postinoculation. The CAMs are then homogenized and used as antigen (56). The precipitin test can be utilized to identify isolates as reovirus if known positive antiserum is available, or it can be used as an indication of antibody status in affected flocks.

Serology. Reovirus group-specific antibody can be readily detected with the agar gel precipitin test (37, 56) or indirect fluorescent antibody (IFA) assay (26). The IFA test is more sensitive and, therefore, better suited for quantitative evaluations. Virus neutralization, based on plaque reduction in chicken kidney or chicken embryo liver cell cultures, has been routinely utilized for determining serotype differences with rabbit or chicken antiserum (64, 82). Although several serotypes have been described, there is considerable homogeneity among reovirus isolates, with many being classified as antigenic subtypes rather than distinct serotypes. In vitro measurements of reovirus antibody specificity may not always correlate with protection against homologous and heterologous challenge of birds with maternally derived antibody (93), and the type specificity of neutralizing antibody is less for chickens immunized with inactivated reovirus than for chickens immune following infection (47).

Slaght et al. (78) were the first to describe an enzyme-linked immunosorbent assay (ELISA) for detecting avian reovirus antibody. The S1133 strain was used as antigen and found to react with antibodies to the Reo-25 and WVU-2937 isolates; ho-mologous antibody gave the highest titer. The ELISA systems now available from commercial sources are apparently suitable for assessing reovirus antibody levels on a flock basis (81).

PREVENTION AND CONTROL. The ubiquitous nature of the avian reoviruses and their inherent stability, coupled with modern, high-density confinement rearing practices, suggests that elimination of virus exposure may be difficult. The virus can be transmitted both vertically and horizontally and, because of its resistance to inactivation, may in addition be frequently carried by mechanical means. Thorough cleaning of a poultry house appears to prevent infection with pathogenic virus in subsequent groups following removal of an infected flock from the premises. Common disinfectants have not been adequately tested, but lye and 0.5% organic iodine solutions are thought to be effective inactivating agents.

Chickens are most susceptible to pathogenic reoviruses at 1 day of age and then develop an age-associated resistance beginning as early as 2 wk. Because of this enhanced period of susceptibility, vaccines and vaccination programs have evolved that are directed at providing protection at 1 day of age. Active immunization can be achieved by vaccination with viable attenuated reovirus that is normally applied by the subcutaneous route (88), although immunization by coarse-spray application of vaccine has also been utilized (17). Protection from subsequent challenge can be demonstrated, but the S1133-derived reovirus vaccines may interfere with Marek's disease vaccination if administered simultaneously (67). Reovirus vaccination of breeding stock can be done with viable or inactivated vaccines or combinations of both. If a live vaccine is used, it should be administered prior to the onset of egg production to prevent transovarian transmission of the vaccine virus (16). The advantages of this type of immunization program include immediate protection of 1-day-old progeny provided by maternal antibody, and a limitation of the potential for vertical transmission that has been shown to be economically significant (7). Vaccination of breeders is an efficacious method of controlling viral arthritis/tenosynovitis and other pathogenic reoviruses, but it should be recognized that protection is assured against homologous serotypes only (61).

REFERENCES

1. Al Afaleq, A,. and R.C. Jones. 1989. Pathogenicity of three turkey and three chicken reoviruses for poults and chicks with particular reference to arthritis/tenosynovitis. Avian Pathol 18:433–440.

2. Barta, V., W.T. Springer, and D.L. Miller. 1984. A comparison of avian and mammalian cell cultures for the propagation of avian reovirus WVU 2937. Avian Dis 28:216–223.

3. Cook, M.E., W.T. Springer, K.M. Kerr, and J.A. Herbert. 1984. Severity of tenosynovitis in reovirus-infected

chickens fed various dietary levels of choline, folic acid, manganese, biotin, or niacin. Avian Dis 28:562–573.

4. Cook, M.E., W.T. Springer, and J.A. Herbert. 1984. Enhanced incidence of leg abnormalities in reovirus WVU 2937-infected chickens fed various dietary levels of selected vitamins. Avian Dis 28:548–561.

5. Cowen, B.S. and M.O. Braune. 1988. The propagation of avian viruses in a continuous cell line (QT35) of Japanese quail origin. Avian Dis 32:282–297.

6. Dalton, P.J., and R. Henry. 1967. Tenosynovitis in poultry. Vet Rec 80:638.

7. Dobson, K.N. and J.R. Glisson. 1992. Economic impact of a documented case of reovirus infection in broiler breeders. Avian Dis 36:788–791.

8. Docherty, D.E., K.A. Converse, W.R. Hansen, and G.W. Norman. 1994. American woodcock (Scolopox minor) mortality associated with a reovirus. Avian Dis 38:899–904.

9. Dutta, S.K., and B.S. Pomeroy. 1967. Isolation and characterization of an enterovirus from baby chicks having an enteric infection. I. Isolation and pathogenicity. Avian Dis 11:1–9.

10. Ellis, M.N., C.S. Eidson, J. Brown, and S.H. Kleven. 1983. Studies on interferon induction and interferon sensitivity of avian reoviruses. Avian Dis 27:927–936.

11. Ellis, M.N., C.S. Eidson, O.J. Fletcher, and S.H. Kleven. 1983. Viral tissue tropisms and interferon production in White Leghorn chickens infected with two reovirus strains. Avian Dis 27:644–651.

12. Engstrom, B.E., O. Fossum and Margaretha Luthman. 1988. Blue wing disease of chickens: Experimental infection with Swedish isolate of chicken anemia agent and an avian reovirus. Avian Pathol 17:33–50.

13. Fahey, J.E. and J.F. Crawley. 1954. Studies on chronic respiratory disease of chickens. II. Isolation of a virus. Can J Comp Med 18:13–21.

14. Gaudry, D., J. Tektoff, and J.M. Charles. 1972. A propos d'un nouveau virus isole chez le canard de Barbarie. Bull Soc Sci Vet Med Comp Lyon 74:137–143.

15. Gershowitz, A. and R.E. Wooley. 1973. Characterization of two reoviruses isolated from turkeys with infectious enteritis. Avian Dis 17:406–414.

16. Giambrone, J.J., T.L. Hathcock, and S.B. Lockaby. 1991. Effect of a live reovirus vaccine on reproductive performance of broiler breeder hens and development of viral tenosynovitis in progeny. Avian Dis 35:380–383.

17. Giambrone, J.J., T. Dormitorio, and S.B. Lockaby. 1992. Coarse-spray immunization of one-day-old broilers against enteric reovirus infections. Avian Dis 36:364–368.

18. Glass, S.E., S.A. Naqi, C.F. Hall, and K.M. Kerr. 1973. Isolation and characterization of a virus associated with arthritis of chickens. Avian Dis 17:415–424.

19. Gouvea, V.S., and T.J. Schnitzer. 1982. Polymorphism of the genomic RNAs among the avian reoviruses. J Gen Virol 61:87–91.

20. Gouvea, V.S., and T.J. Schnitzer. 1982. Polymorphism of the migration of double-stranded RNA genome segments of avian reoviruses. J Virol 43:465–471.

21. Gouvea, V., and T.J. Schnitzer. 1982. Pathogenicity of avian reoviruses: examination of six isolates and a vaccine strain. Infect Immun 38:731–738.

22. Guneratne, J.R.M., R.C. Jones, and K. Georgiou. 1982. Some observations on the isolation and cultivation of avian reoviruses. Avian Pathol 11:453–462.

23. Hieronymus, D.R.K., P. Villegas, and S.H. Kleven. 1983. Identification and serological differentiation of several reovirus strains isolated from chickens with suspected malabsorption syndrome. Avian Dis 27:246–254.

24. Hill, J.E., G.N. Rowland, K.S. Latimer, and J. Brown. 1989. Effects of cyclosporin A on reovirus-infected broilers. Avian Dis 33:86–92.

25. Hill, J.E., G.N. Rowland, W.L. Steffens, and M.B. Ard. 1989. Ultrastructure of the gastrocnemius tendon and

sheath from broilers infected with reovirus. Avian Dis 33:79–85.

26. Ide, P.R. 1982. Avian reovirus antibody assay by indirect immunofluorescence using plastic microculture plates. Can J Comp Med 46:39–42.

27. Islam, M.R., R.C. Jones and D.F. Kelly. 1988. Pathogenesis of experimental reovirus tenosynovitis in chickens: influence of the route of infection. J Comp Pathol 98:325–336.

28. Jackson, G.G., and R.L. Mulloon. 1973. Viruses causing common respiratory infection in man. IV. Reoviruses and adenoviruses. J Infect Dis 128:811–866.

29. Johnson, D.C., and L. Van der Heide. 1971. Incidence of tenosynovitis in Maine broilers. Avian Dis 15:829–834.

30. Jones R.C., and K. Georgiou. 1984. Reovirus-induced tenosynovitis in chickens: The influence of age at infection. Avian Pathol 13:441–457.

31. Jones, R.C., and F.S.B. Kibenge. 1984. Reovirus-induced tenosynovitis in chickens: The effect of breed. Avian Pathol 13:511–528.

32. Jones, R.C. and B.N.C. Nwajei. 1985. Reovirus-induced tenosynovitis: persistence of homologous challenge virus in broiler chicks after vaccination of parents. Res Vet Sci 39:39–41.

33. Jones, R.C., and O. Onunkwo. 1978. Studies on experimental tenosynovitis in light hybrid chickens. Avian Pathol 7:171–181.

34. Jones, R.C., F.T.W. Jordan, and S. Lioupis. 1975. Characteristics of reovirus isolated from ruptured gastrocnemius tendons of chickens. Vet Rec 96:153–154.

35. Jones, R.C., M.R. Islam and D.F. Kelly. 1989. Early pathogenesis of experimental reovirus infection in chickens. Avian Pathol 18:239–253.

36. Kaschula, V.R. 1950. A new virus disease of the Muscovy duck (Cairina moschata) present in Natal. J S Afr Vet Med Assoc 21:18–26.

37. Kawamura, H., and H. Tsubahara. 1966. Common antigenicity of avian reoviruses. Natl Inst Anim Health Q (Tokyo) 6:187–193.

38. Kawamura, H., F. Shimizu, M. Maeda and H. Tsubahara. 1965. Avian reovirus: its properties and serological classification. Natl Inst Anim Health Q (Tokyo) 5:115–124.

39. Kerr, K.M., and N.O. Olson. 1964. Control of infectious synovitis. The effect of age of chickens on the susceptibility to three agents. Avian Dis 8:256–263.

40. Kerr, K.M. and N.O. Olson. 1969. Pathology of chickens experimentally inoculated or contact-infected with an arthritis producing virus. Avian Dis 13:729–745.

41. Kibenge, F.S.B. and G.E. Wilcox. 1983. Tenosynovitis in chickens. Vet Bull 53:431–444.

42. Macdonald, J.W., C.J. Randall, M.D. Dagless, and D.A. McMartin. 1978. Observations on viral tenosynovitis (viral arthritis) in Scotland. Avian Pathol 7:471–482.

43. Malkinson, M., K. Perk, and Y. Weisman. 1981. Reovirus infection of young Muscovy ducks (Cairina moschata). Avian Pathol 10:433–440.

44. Marquardt, J., W. Herrmanns, L.C. Schulz and W. Leibold. 1983. A persistent reovirus infection of chickens as a possible model of human rheumatoid arthritis (RA). Zentralbl Veterinaermed 30B:274–282.

45. Mathews, R.E.F. 1982. Classification and nomenclature of viruses. Intervirology 17:1–200.

46. McFerran, J.B., T.J. Connor and R.M. McCracken. 1976. Isolation of adenoviruses and reoviruses from avian species other than domestic fowl. Avian Dis 20:519–524.

47. Meanger, J., R. Wickramasinghe, C.E. Enriquez, M.D. Robertson and G.E. Wilcox. 1995. Type-specific antigenicity of avian reoviruses. Avian Pathol 24:121–124.

48. Menendez, N.A., B.W. Calnek, and B.S. Cowen. 1975. Experimental egg-transmission of avian reovirus. Avian Dis 19:104–111.

49. Menendez, N.A., B.W. Calnek, and B.S. Cowen. 1975.

Localization of avian reovirus (FDO isolate) in tissues of mature chickens. Avian Dis 19:112–117.

50. Neighbor, N.K., L.A. Newberry, G.R. Baygori, J.K. Skeeles, J.N. Beasly, and R.W. McNew. 1994. The effect of microaerosolized hydrogen peroxide on bacterial and viral poultry pathogens. Poult Sci 73:1511–1516.

51. Nersessian, B.N., M.A. Goodwin, R.K. Rage, S.H. Kleven, and J. Brown. 1986. Studies on orthoreoviruses isolated from young turkeys. III. Pathogenic effects in chicken embryos, chicks, poults, and suckling mice. Avian Dis 30:585–592.

52. Olson, N.O., and K.M. Kerr. 1966. Some characteristics of an avian arthritis viral agent. Avian Dis 10:470–476.

53. Olson, N.O., and K.M. Kerr. 1967. The duration and distribution of synovitis-producing agents in chickens. Avian Dis 11:578–585.

54. Olson, N.O., and M.A. Khan. 1972. The effect of intranasal exposure of chickens to the Fahey-Crawley virus on the development of synovial lesions. Avian Dis 16:1073–1078.

55. Olson, N.O., and D.P. Solomon. 1968. A natural outbreak of synovitis caused by the viral arthritis agent. Avian Dis 12:311–316.

56. Olson, N.O., and R. Weiss. 1972. Similarity between arthritis virus and Fahey-Crawley virus. Avian Dis 16:535–540.

57. Olson, N.O., D.C. Shelton, and D.A. Munro. 1957. Infectious synovitis control by medication-effect of strain differences and pleuropneumonia-like organisms. Am J Vet Res 18:735–739.

58. Page, R.K., O.J. Fletcher, and P. Villegas. 1982. Infectious tenosynovitis in young turkeys. Avian Dis 26:924–927.

59. Petek, M., B. Felluga, G. Borghi, and A. Baroni. 1967. The Crawley agent: An avian reovirus. Arch Gesamte Virusforsch 21:413–424.

60. Phillips, P.A., N.F. Stanley, and M. Walters. 1970. Murine disease induced by avian reovirus. Aust J Exp Biol Med Sci 48:277–284.

61. Rau, W.E., L. Van der Heide, M. Kalbac, and T. Girshick. 1980. Onset of progeny immunity against viral arthritis/tenosynovitis after experimental vaccination of parent breeder chickens and cross immunity against six reovirus isolates. Avian Dis 24:648–657.

62. Rinehart, C.L., and J.K. Rosenberger. 1983. Effects of avian reoviruses on the immune responses of chickens. Poult Sci 62:1488–1489.

63. Robertson, M.D., and G.E. Wilcox. 1984. Serological characteristics of avian reoviruses of Australian origin. Avian Pathol 13:585–594.

64. Robertson, M.D., and G.E. Wilcox. 1986. Avian reovirus. Vet Bull 56:155–174.

65. Robertson, M.D., G.E. Wilcox and F.S.B. Kibenge. 1984. Prevalence of reoviruses in commercial chickens. Aust Vet J 61:319–322.

66. Roessler, D.E. 1986. Studies on the pathogenicity and persistence of avian reovirus pathotypes in relation to age resistance and immunosuppression. PhD Thesis. University of Delaware, Newark.

67. Rosenberger, J.K. 1983. Reovirus interference with Marek's disease vaccination. Proc 32nd West Poult Dis Conf, pp. 50–51.

68. Rosenberger, J.K. 1983. Characterization of reoviruses associated with runting syndrome in chickens. Proc No 66. International Union of the Immunological Society, Sydney, Australia, pp. 141–152.

69. Rosenberger, J.K., P.A. Fries, S.S. Cloud and R.A. Wilson. 1986. In vitro and in vivo characterization of Escherichia coli. II. Factors associated with pathogenicity. Avian Dis 29:1094–1107.

70. Ruff, M.D. and J.K. Rosenberger, 1985. Concurrent infections with reoviruses and coccidia in broilers. Avian Dis 29:465–478.

71. Ruff, M.D. and J.K. Rosenberger, 1985. Interaction of

low-pathogenicity reoviruses and low levels of infection with several coccidia species. Avian Dis 29:1057–1065.

72. Sahu, S.P. and N.O. Olson. 1975. Comparison of the characteristics of avian reoviruses isolated from the digestive and respiratory tract, with viruses isolated form the synovia. Am J Vet Res 36:847–850.

73. Schnitzer, T.J., T. Ramos, and V. Gouvea. 1982. Avian reovirus polypeptides: analysis of intracellular virus-specified products, virions, top component and cores. J Virol 43:1006–1014.

74. Schnitzer, T.J., J. Rosenberger, D.D. Huang, V. Gouvea, T. Ramos, and K. Hassett. 1983. Molecular biology and pathogenicity of avian reoviruses. In R.W. Compons and D.H. Bishop (eds.). Double-stranded RNA Viruses. Elsevier, New York, pp. 383–390.

75. Schwartz, L.D., R.F. Gentry, H. Rothenbacher and L. Van der Heide. 1976. Infectious tenosynovitis in commercial white leghorn chickens. Avian Dis 20:769–773.

76. Shapouri, M.R.S., S.K. Reddy, and A. Silim. 1994. Interaction of avian reovirus with chicken lymphoblastoid cell lines. Avian Pathol 23:287–296.

77. Simmons, D.G., W.M. Colwell, K.E. Muse, and C.E. Brewer. 1972. Isolation and characterization of an enteric reovirus causing high mortality in turkey poults. Avian Dis 16:1094–1102.

78. Slaght, S.S., T.J. Yang, L. Van der Heide and T.N. Fredrickson. 1978. An enzyme-linked immunosorbent assay (ELISA) for detecting chicken anti-reovirus antibody at high sensitivity. Avian Dis 22:802–805.

79. Spandidos, D.A., and A.F. Graham. 1976. Physical and chemical characterization of an avian reovirus. J Virol 19:968–976.

80. Springer, W.T., N.O. Olson, K.M. Kerr, and C.J. Fabacher. 1983. Responses of specific-pathogen-free chicks to concomitant infections of reovirus (WVU-2937) and infectious bursal disease virus. Avian Dis 27:911–917.

81. Thayer, S.G., P. Villegas, and O.J. Fletcher. 1987. Comparison of two commercial enzyme-linked immunosorbent assays and conventional methods for avian serology. Avian Dis 31:120–124.

82. Van der Heide, L. 1977. Viral arthritis/tenosynovitis: A review. Avian Pathol 6:271–284.

83. Van der Heide, L., and M. Kalbac. 1975. Infectious tenosynovitis (viral arthritis): characterization of a Connecticut viral isolant as a reovirus and evidence of viral egg transmission by reovirus-infected broiler breeders. Avian Dis 19:683–688.

84. Van der Heide, L., and R.K. Page. 1980. Field experiments with viral arthritis/tenosynovitis vaccination of breeder chickens. Avian Dis 24:493–497.

85. Van der Heide, L., J. Geissler, and E.S. Bryant. 1974. Infectious tenosynovitis: serologic and histopathologic response after experimental infection with a Connecticut isolate. Avian Dis 18:289–296.

86. Van der Heide, L., M. Kalbac, and W.C. Hall. 1976. Infectious tenosynovitis (viral arthritis): Influence of maternal antibodies on the development of tenosynovitis lesions after experimental infection by day-old chickens with tenosynovitis virus. Avian Dis 20:641–648.

87. Van der Heide, L., M. Kalbac, M. Brustolon, and M.G. Lawson. 1980. Pathogenicity for chickens of a reovirus isolated from turkeys. Avian Dis 24:989–997.

88. Van der Heide, L., M. Kalbac, and M. Brustolon. 1983. Development of an attenuated apathogenic reovirus vaccine against viral arthritis/tenosynovitis. Avian Dis 27:698–706.

89. Walker, E.R., M.H. Friedman, and N.O. Olson. 1972. Electron microscopic study of an avian reovirus that causes arthritis. J Ultrastruct Res 41:67–79.

90. Winship, T.R., and P.I. Marcus. 1980. Interferon induction by viruses. VI. Reovirus: Virion genome dsRNA as the interferon inducer in aged chick embryo cells. J Interferon Res 1:155–167.

91. Woernle, H., A. Brunner, and K.F. Kussaul. 1974.

Nachweis aviären Reo-Viren im Agar-Gel-Präzipitationstest. Tieraerztl Umsch 29:307–312.

92. Wood, G.W., R.A.J. Nicholas, C.N. Hebert and D.H. Thornton. 1980. Serological comparisons of avian reoviruses. J Comp Pathol 90:29–38.

93. Wood, G.W., J.C. Muskett, and D.H. Thorton. 1986. Observations on the ability of avian reovirus vaccination of hens to protect their progeny against the effects of challenge with homologous and heterologous strains. J Comp Pathol 96:125–129.

94. Wooley, R.E., T.A. Dees, A.S. Cromack, and J.B. Gratzek. 1972. Infectious enteritis of turkeys: characterization of two reoviruses isolated by sucrose density gradient centrifugation from turkeys with infectious enteritis. Am J Vet Res 33:157–164.

29 Infectious Bursal Disease

Phil D. Lukert and Y. M. Saif

INTRODUCTION. Infectious bursal disease (IBD) is an acute, highly contagious viral infection of young chickens. Lymphoid cells, especially B cells, are the primary target cell and the lymphoid tissue of the cloacal bursa is most severely affected. It was described as a specific new disease by Cosgrove (22) in 1962, and was referred to as "avian nephrosis" because of the extreme kidney damage found in birds that succumbed to infection. The economic importance of this disease is manifested in two ways. The first is due to the clinical disease and mortality in chickens 3 wk of age and older. The second, and more important, manifestation is a severe prolonged immunosuppression of chickens infected at an early age. Sequelae of the immunosuppression include gangrenous dermatitis, inclusion body hepatitis–anemia syndrome, *Escherichia coli* infections, and vaccination failures. The IBD virus does not affect humans and has no public health significance.

HISTORY. Early studies to identify the etiologic agent of IBD (avian nephrosis) were clouded by the presence of infectious bronchitis virus (IBV) in the kidneys of field cases of the disease. Winterfield and Hitchner (171) described an IBV isolate (Gray) that came from a field case of nephrosis not unlike the newly reported IBD syndrome. Because of the similarity between kidney lesions induced by Gray virus and those seen in avian nephrosis as described by Cosgrove (22), it was believed that Gray virus was the causative agent. Later studies, however, revealed that birds immune to Gray virus could still be infected with the IBD agent and would develop pathologic changes in the cloacal bursa specific for the disease. In subsequent studies with IBD, Winterfield et al. (172) succeeded in isolating an agent in embryonating eggs. The mortality pattern was irregular and the agent was difficult to maintain in serial passage. The isolate was referred to as "infectious bursal agent" and was identified as the true cause of IBD; Gray virus was identified as an isolate of IBV with nephrotropic tendencies. Hitchner (53) subsequently proposed the term *infectious bursal disease* as the name of the disease causing specific pathognomonic lesions of the cloacal bursa.

In 1972, Allan et al. (1) reported that IBD virus (IBDV) infections at an early age were immunosuppressive. The recognition of the immunosuppressive capability of IBDV infections greatly increased the interest in the control of these infections. The existence of a second serotype was reported in 1980 (97). Control of IBD viral infections has been complicated by the recognition of "variant" strains of serotype 1 IBDV that were found in the Delmarva poultry-producing area (127, 133). These strains caused disease in the presence of maternal immunity against "standard" strains (131, 133). These variants were either already present in nature and were selected by immune pressure, or they were mutants that occurred and flourished, again due to immune pressure.

INCIDENCE AND DISTRIBUTION. Infections with serotype 1 IBDV are of worldwide distribution and occur in all major poultry-producing areas. The incidence of infection in these areas is high; essentially all flocks are exposed to the virus during the early stages of life. Because of vaccination programs carried out by most producers, all chickens eventually become seropositive to IBDV. Clinical cases are rare in the United States, however, because infections are either modified by maternal antibody or are due to variant strains that do not cause disease but can induce severe immunosuppression. Highly virulent strains originally isolated in the Netherlands and characterized by Chettle et al. in 1989 (15) are the cause of severe outbreaks with high mortality in many parts of the world.

Serotype 2 IBDV infections are also widespread and occur in chickens (66, 133), turkeys (5, 17, 68), and ducks (97). No serotype 2 isolates have been demonstrated to be either pathogenic or immunosuppressive.

ETIOLOGY

Classification. Infectious bursal disease virus is a member of the *Birnaviridae* family (13, 29, 104). The family has one genus, *Birnavirus,* and the prototype is infectious pancreatic necrosis virus of fish. Other viruses in the *Birnaviridae* family include Tellina virus of bivalve mollusks and Drosophila X virus of the fruit fly (29). Viruses in that family have genomes consisting of two segments of double-stranded (ds)RNA (90, 104, 156), hence the name *birnaviruses.* Before the recognition of the *Birnaviridae* family and before there was adequate information on its morphology and physicochemical characteristics, IBDV was placed at times in the *Picornaviridae* (19, 89) or *Reoviridae* families (42, 79, 85, 120).

Morphology. The virus is a single-shelled, nonenveloped virion with icosahedral symmetry and a diameter varying from 55 to 65 nm (50, 112, 116) (see Fig. 29.1). The capsid symmetry is askew, with a triangulation number of T = 13 and a dextro-handedness (116).

Buoyant density of complete particles in cesium chloride gradients has been reported to range from 1.31 to 1.34 g/mL (8, 34, 68, 103, 112, 120, 161). Lower density values were reported for incomplete virus particles.

Chemical Composition. The dsRNA of the IBDV genome has two segments (8, 29, 69, 104) as shown by polyacrylamide gel electrophoresis. Jackwood et al. (69) reported that the two segments of five serotype 1 viruses migrated similarly when coelectrophoresed. The RNA segments from serotype 2 viruses migrated similarly, but differed from serotype 1 viruses when coelectrophoresed, suggesting that RNA migration patterns could be used to differentiate IBDV isolates that differ serotypically. Becht (9) reported similar results when comparing isolates of each serotype.

Four viral proteins designated VP1, VP2, VP3, and VP4 were recognized early (8, 28, 29, 112, 161). The approximate molecular weights of the

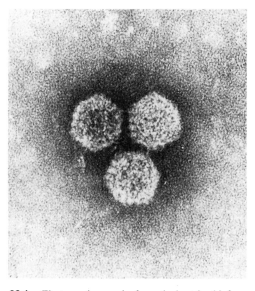

29.1. Electron micrograph of negatively stained infectious bursal disease (IBD) viral particles. ×200,000. (Reed)

four proteins are 90 kD, 41 kD, 32 kD, and 28 kD, respectively. Additional proteins, such as VPX, have been observed and are thought to have a precursor–product relationship (28). A novel viral protein (VP5) having a molecular weight of 21 kD was described (107). Becht et al. (9) compared isolates of serotypes 1 and 2 and reported viral proteins with molecular weights in the same range as those observed by Jackwood et al. and Kibenge et al. (69, 78). It was not possible to differentiate between strains of serotype 1 viruses based on differences in structural proteins (164). VP2 and VP3 are the major proteins of IBDV. In serotype 1 viruses, they constitute 51 and 40% of the virus proteins, respectively (29), whereas VP1 (3%) and VP4 (6%) are minor proteins. VP1 is the viral RNA polymerase and VP4 is a viral protease (57, 109, 155). The function of the newly described VP5 is currently not known (107). The small segment of the IBDV genome (B) codes for VP1, whereas the large segment (A) encodes the rest of the viral proteins (3, 57, 101).

A conformational dependent (discontinuous) neutralizing epitope was detected on VP2, and a conformational independent (continuous) epitope was found on VP3. Antibodies to these epitopes passively protected chickens (4). It was reported earlier (35) that VP3 had the antigenic determinants for serotype specificity, but later studies indicated that these determinants were on VP2 (4, 9). According to Becht (9), monoclonal antibodies to VP2 differentiated between the two serotypes of the virus, whereas monoclonal antibodies to VP3 recognized a group-specific antigen from both serotypes. A panel of monoclonal antibodies against VP3 of serotypes 1 and 2 was mapped to four segments of the VP3 gene, and two of these sites were specific for one serotype only (92). Snyder et al. (151) developed a monoclonal antibody to VP2 that neutralized both serotypes of the virus, indicating the existence of multiple epitopes on VP2. The molecular basis for pathogenicity of the virus has not been determined.

The chemistry of the virus has been reviewed in detail by Kibenge et al. (76).

Virus Replication. Kibenge et al. (76) has reviewed this subject. In general, little is known about the biochemical events associated with replication of birnaviruses. Several laboratory hosts for IBDV are described later in this chapter. The virus was shown to attach to chicken embryo kidney cells maximally 75 min after inoculation (85). The multiplication cycle in chicken embryo cells is 10–36 hr and the latent period is 4–6 hr (8, 69, 85, 112). In Vero and BGM-70 cells, a longer (48-hr) multiplication cycle was described (72, 77, 88). Viral polypeptides were detected in chicken bursal lymphoid cells grown in vitro and in their culture media at 90 min and 6 hr postinfection, respectively (103). The cell receptor recognition site on the virus is not known.

The mechanism of viral RNA synthesis has not been clearly determined. A dsRNA-dependent RNA polymerase, VP1, was described (155). Genome-linked proteins have been demonstrated, indicating that the virus replicates its nucleic acid by a strand displacement mechanism. RNA polymerase activity could be demonstrated without pretreatment of the virus, indicating that transcription and replication occur following cell penetration without uncoating of the virus (155).

Becht (8) reported that synthesis of host proteins is not shut off in chicken embryo fibroblasts (CEFs) infected with IBDV.

Resistance to Chemical and Physical Agents. Infectious bursal disease virus is very stable. Benton et al. (10) found that IBDV resisted treatment with ether and chloroform, was inactivated at pH 12 but unaffected by pH 2, and was still viable after 5 hr at 56 C. The virus was unaffected by exposure for 1 hr at 30 C to 0.5% phenol and 0.125% thimerosal. There was a marked reduction in virus infectivity when exposed to 0.5% formalin for 6 hr. The virus was also treated with various concentrations of three disinfectants (an iodine complex, a phenolic derivative, and a quaternary ammonium compound) for a period of 2 min at 23 C. Only the iodine complex had any deleterious effects. Landgraf et al. (80) found that the virus survived 60 C but not 70 C for 30 min, and 0.5% chloramine killed the virus after 10 min. Invert soaps with 0.05% sodium hydroxide either inactivated or had a strong inhibitory effect on the virus (139).

Certainly, the hardy nature of this virus is one reason for its persistent survival in poultry houses even when thorough cleaning and disinfection procedures are followed.

Strain Classification. McFerran et al. (97), in Northern Ireland, were the first to report antigenic variations among IBDV isolates of European origin. They presented evidence for the existence of two serotypes, designated 1 and 2, and showed only 30% relatedness between several strains of serotype 1 and the designated prototype of that serotype. Similar findings were reported in the United States (68, 84), and the American serotypes were designated I and II. Later studies (98) indicated the relatedness of the European and American isolates of the second serotype, and use of the Arabic numerals 1 and 2 to describe the two serotypes of IBDV was proposed. Antigenic relatedness of only 33% between two strains of serotype 2 was reported (98), indicating an antigenic diversity similar to that of serotype 1 viruses.

The two serotypes are differentiated by virus-neutralization (VN) tests, but they are not distinguishable by fluorescent antibody tests or enzyme-linked immunosorbent assay (ELISA). Immunization against serotype 2 does not protect against serotype 1. The reverse situation cannot be tested because there are no virulent serotype 2 viruses for challenge (60, 71). The first isolates of serotype 2 (68) originated from turkeys and it was thought that this serotype was host specific. Later studies showed, however, that viruses of serotype 2 could be isolated from chickens (61), and antibodies to serotype 2 IBDVs are common in both chickens and turkeys (66, 133).

Variant viruses of serotype 1 were described (128, 133). Vaccine strains available at the time they were isolated did not elicit full protection against the variants, which are antigenically different from the standard serotype 1 isolates.

Jackwood and Saif (67) conducted a cross-neutralization study of eight serotype 1 commercial vaccine strains, five serotype 1 field strains, and two serotype 2 field strains. Six subtypes were distinguished among the 13 serotype 1 strains studied. One of the subtypes included all of the variant isolates. Snyder et al. (152), using monoclonal antibodies, suggested that a major antigenic shift in serotype 1 viruses had occurred in the field. The highly virulent strains that were first described in Europe (15) are thought to be antigenically similar to the classic serotype 1 viruses.

Laboratory Host Systems

CHICKEN EMBRYOS. Initially, most workers had difficulty in isolating virus or, if successful, in serially transferring virus using chicken embryos. Landgraf et al. (80) reported a typical experience using the allantoic sac route of inoculation. On the first passage, all inoculated embryos died; on the second, 30% died; and on the third, there was no embryo mortality.

Continued studies (53) uncovered three factors that could explain these difficulties: 1) Embryonating eggs that originated from flocks recovered from the disease were highly resistant to growth of the virus. 2) In early virus passage, the allantoamnionic fluid (AAF) had a very low virus content while the chorioallantoic membrane (CAM) and embryo each had a much higher and nearly equal virus content. 3) Comparison of the allantoic sac, yolk sac, and CAM as routes of inoculation showed the allantoic sac to be the least desirable, yielding embryo-infective dose-50% (EID_{50}) virus titers of 1.5–2.0 $\log_{10}$ lower than those obtained after inoculation by the CAM route. The yolk sac route gave titers that were intermediate.

Winterfield (170) increased virus concentration in the AAF by serial passage in embryonating eggs. Hitchner (53) used isolate 2512, obtained from

Winterfield in the 46th embryo passage, to perform a multistep growth curve study. He found that virus concentration reached a peak 72 hr postinoculation.

Injection of the virus into 10-day-old embryonating eggs resulted in embryo mortality from the 3rd to 5th day postinoculation. Gross lesions observed in the embryo were edematous distention of the abdominal region; cutaneous congestion and petechial hemorrhages, particularly along feather tracts; occasional hemorrhages on toe joints and in the cerebral region; mottled-appearing necrosis and ecchymotic hemorrhages in the liver (latter stages); pale "parboiled" appearance of the heart; congestion and some mottled necrosis of kidneys; extreme congestion of lungs; and pale spleen, occasionally with small necrotic foci. The CAM had no plaques, but small hemorrhagic areas were observed at times. Lesions induced in embryos by IBDV variants differ from those induced by standard isolates. Splenomegaly and liver necrosis are characteristic of the lesions induced by the variants, but there is little mortality (131).

CELL CULTURE. Many strains of IBDV have been adapted to cell cultures of chicken embryo origin, and cytopathic effects have been observed. Cell culture–adapted virus may be quantified by plaque assay or microtiter techniques. Rinaldi et al. (126) and Petek et al. (123) were able to culture egg-adapted strains of IBDV in CEFs, which proved more sensitive to the virus than either embryonating eggs or suckling mice.

Lukert and Davis (85) successfully adapted wild-type virus from infected bursas to growth in cells derived from the chicken embryo bursa. After four serial passages in chicken embryo bursa cells, the virus grew in chicken embryo kidney cells and produced plaques under agar. This virus was subsequently propagated in CEFs and used as an attenuated live virus vaccine (144). In addition to cells of chicken origin, the virus has been grown in turkey and duck embryo cells (99), mammalian cell lines derived from rabbit kidneys (RK-13) (126), monkey kidneys (Vero) (77, 88), and baby grivet monkey kidney cells (BGM-70) (72).

Jackwood et al. (72) compared three mammalian cell lines (MA-104, Vero, and BGM-70) for their ability to support several strains of IBDV serotypes 1 and 2, including serotype 1 variants. The viruses replicated in the three cell lines, but cytopathic effects were most pronounced in the BGM-70 cells. The growth curve of one strain tested in BGM-70 cells was similar to that in CEFs, and VN titers in BGM-70 cultures compared well with those in CEFs. BGM-70 cells are used routinely for serology by one of the authors (135).

A continuous fibroblast cell line of Japanese quail origin was found to support the replication of IBDV and several other viral pathogens of poultry (23). These viruses, already adapted to tissue culture, produced a cytopathic effect in the quail cells.

Hirai and Calnek (49) propagated virulent IBDV in normal chicken lymphocytes and in a lymphoblastoid B-cell line derived from an avian leukosis virus–induced tumor. The virus would not replicate in six T-cell lymphoblastoid cell lines initiated from Marek's disease tumors. Their work showed that IgM-bearing B lymphocytes were the probable target cells of IBDV. This was subsequently verified in a study on normal lymphocytes of chickens (110). Lymphocytes from the cloacal bursa and thymus were purified and separated into T cells, B cells, and null cells. The B cells bearing surface IgM were susceptible to IBDV, but the T cells and null cells were not.

Müller (102) enriched Ig-bearing cells by rosetting and cell sorting, and observed that IBDV replicated preferentially in a population of proliferating cells and that susceptibility did not correlate with expression of immunoglobulins on their surface. A B-lymphoblastoid cell line from a chicken with lymphoid lesions (48) was found to be superior to CEF, chicken kidney cells, and BGM-70 cells in propagating several attenuated and pathogenic viruses (163).

Isolation of IBDV from field cases of the disease may be difficult. McFerran et al. (97) found it very difficult to isolate and serially propagate the virus in cell cultures of chicken embryo origin. Lee and Lukert (81) attempted isolations of IBDV from turkeys and chickens as well as from samples of challenge strains received from other laboratories. Turkey strains (five of five) were readily adapted to CEF cells after three to 10 blind passages. Only two of nine chicken strains could be adapted to CEF cells; the other seven strains could be grown only in chicken embryo bursa cells, even after 20 bursal cell passages.

BGM-70 cells were used successfully for isolation of IBDV from the bursas of naturally infected chickens (134). Usually, a cytopathic effect was detected after two or three blind passages.

One aspect that should be considered concerning in vitro replication of the virus is the possibility of development of defective particles. Müller et al. (106) reported that serial passages of undiluted virus in chicken embryo cells resulted in fluctuations in infectivity and the development of a stable small-plaque–forming virus that interfered with the replication of the standard virus and favored the generation of defective particles. The defective particles had lost the large segment of dsRNA. Passage of the virus six times in BGM-70 cells or CEF resulted in loss of pathogenicity, but similar passages in chicken embryos did not affect the pathogenicity of the virus (43).

Pathogenicity. Chickens are the only animals

known to develop clinical disease and distinct lesions when exposed to IBDV. Field viruses exhibit different degrees of pathogenicity in chickens. Vaccine viruses also have varying pathogenic potential in chickens, as discussed later in this chapter.

There has been considerable interest in studying the potential pathogenicity of viruses belonging to serotype 2 in chickens and turkeys. Jackwood et al. (71) reported a lack of clinical signs and either gross or microscopic lesions in chickens inoculated with a serotype 2 isolate. Sivanandan et al. (143), however, observed typical IBDV lesions in chickens inoculated with the same isolate. In later studies (60), five isolates of serotype 2, three of chicken origin and two of turkey origin (including the isolate studied by Jackwood et al. and Sivanandan et al.), were found nonpathogenic in chickens.

In turkey poults inoculated at 1–8 days of age, an isolate of serotype 2 from turkeys failed to cause disease, or gross or microscopic lesions in the cloacal bursa, thymus, or spleen (70); however, the virus was infectious and the poults responded serologically to the infection. Nusbaum et al. (113) studied experimental infection in 1-day-old poults with isolates representing serotypes 1 and 2 that originated from turkeys. Virus-infected cells were detected by immunofluorescence in the bursa, thymus, spleen, and the harderian gland of infected birds, but no clinical disease resulted. Only slight gross changes were observed, and no histologic differences were seen between infected and noninfected birds. In general, the distribution of fluorescing (infected) cells from these tissues seemed to indicate that the majority were not lymphocytes. The number of plasma cells in the harderian gland was reduced at 28 days of age. As indicated earlier, the effect of the host system on pathogenicity of the virus may be profound (43, 162).

PATHOGENESIS AND EPIZOOTIOLOGY

Pathogenesis. In sequential studies of tissues from orally infected chickens using immunofluorescence, viral antigen was detected in macrophages and lymphoid cells in the cecum at 4 hr after inoculation; and an hour later, virus was detected in lymphoid cells in the duodenum and jejunum (105). The virus first reaches the liver, where it is detected 5 hr postinoculation. It then enters the bloodstream, where it is distributed to other tissues including the bursa; the bursal infection is followed by a second massive viremia.

Natural and Experimental Hosts. For many years, the chicken was considered the only species in which natural infections occurred. All breeds were affected and it was observed by many investigators that white leghorns exhibited the most severe reactions and had the highest mortality rate.

Meroz (100), however, found no difference in mortality between heavy and light breeds in a survey of 700 outbreaks of the disease.

The period of greatest susceptibility to clinical disease is between 3 and 6 wk of age. Susceptible chickens younger than 3 wk do not exhibit clinical signs but have subclinical infections that are economically important as a result of severe immunosuppression of the chicken. This immunosuppressive effect of IBDV was first recognized by Allan et al. (1) and Faragher et al. (37) and is discussed later in this chapter.

The reason for the apparent age susceptibility of chickens to IBD has been the subject of several research publications regarding the pathogenesis of IBDV infections. Fadly et al. (33) treated 3-day-old chicks with cyclophosphamide and found they were refractory to clinical signs and lesions when challenged at 4 wk of age. Kaufer and Weiss (75) found similar results with birds surgically bursectomized at 4 wk of age. When they were challenged immediately, or 1 wk later, there was no clinical disease, whereas 100% of control nonbursectomized chickens died. Bursectomized chickens challenged with virulent virus produced 1000 times less virus than control birds, produced VN antibodies by the 5th day, and had only very discrete and transient necrosis of lymphatic tissues.

Several studies on the pathogenesis of IBDV infections have been conducted. Skeeles et al. (145) attempted to demonstrate that the hemorrhagic lesions were a result of formation of immune complexes, as proposed by Ivanyi and Morris (63). Histologic lesions in the cloacal bursa resemble an Arthus reaction (necrosis, hemorrhage, and large numbers of polymorphonuclear leukocytes). This reaction is a type of localized immunologic injury caused by antigen–antibody-complement complexes that induce chemotactic factors, which cause hemorrhage and leukocyte infiltration. They found that 2-wk-old and 8-wk-old chicks produced rapid and high levels of antibody by 72 hr postinfection, but that 2-wk-old chickens had very little complement compared with 8-wk-old chickens. They postulated that the reason 2-wk-old chickens did not develop Arthus-type lesions was a lack of sufficient complement. They also showed that complement was depleted in 8-wk-old chickens at 3, 5, and 7 days postinfection compared with uninfected controls. A later study by Skeeles et al. (148) with another IBDV isolate failed to substantiate the depletion of complement at 3 days postinfection.

Kosters et al. (79) and Skeeles et al. (145, 148) found increased clotting times in IBDV-infected chickens and suggested that such coagulopathies would contribute to the hemorrhagic lesions observed with this disease. Skeeles et al. (148) found that 17-day-old chickens did not exhibit clotting defects, but at 42 days they had greatly increased clotting times and became clinically ill; 4 of 11 died. The key to the pathogenesis of IBDV in birds of different ages may lie with the factors involved in the clotting of blood and/or an immunologic injury. The pathogenesis is certainly not straightforward and simple.

Naturally occurring infections of turkeys and ducks have been recorded (74, 97, 99, 117). Serologic evidence and isolation of IBDV from these species indicate that natural infections do occur. McNulty et al. (99) examined turkey serums from several flocks and could not detect IBDV antibodies prior to 1978, suggesting that IBDV infections of turkeys were a relatively new occurrence.

Giambrone et al. (39) found that experimental IBDV infections of turkeys were subclinical in 3- to 6-wk-old poults, producing microscopic lesions in the bursa. Virus-infected cells in the bursa were detected by immunofluorescence. Neutralizing antibody was detected 12 days postinfection, and the virus could be reisolated after five serial passages in chicken embryos. Weisman and Hitchner (169) could not reisolate virus from their 6- to 8-wk-old IBDV-infected poults, but they observed an increase in VN antibody. Infection was subclinical and no damage to the bursa was evident. These authors were not able to infect Coturnix quail with a chicken strain of IBDV. Experimentally infected guinea fowl did not develop lesions or antibodies (114). A serotype 1 virus was isolated from two 8-wk-old ostrich chicks that had lymphocyte depletion in the bursa of Fabricius, spleen, and/or thymus (173).

Transmission, Carriers, and Vectors. Infectious bursal disease is highly contagious and the virus is persistent in the environment of a poultry house. Benton et al. (11) found that houses from which infected birds were removed were still infective for other birds 54 and 122 days later. They also demonstrated that water, feed, and droppings taken from infected pens were infectious after 52 days.

There is no evidence that IBDV is transmitted through the egg or that a true carrier state exists in recovered birds. Resistance of the virus to heat and disinfectants is sufficient to account for virus survival in the environment between outbreaks. Snedeker et al. (149) demonstrated that the lesser mealworm (Alphitobius diaperinus), taken from a house 8 wk after an outbreak, was infectious for susceptible chickens when fed as a ground suspension. In another study (96), the virus was isolated from several tissues of surface-sterilized lesser mealworm adults and larvae that were fed the virus earlier.

Howie and Thorsen (55) isolated IBDV from mosquitoes (Aedes vexans) that were trapped in an area where chickens were being raised in southern Ontario. The isolate was nonpathogenic for chick-

ens. Okoye and Uche (115) detected IBDV antibodies by the agar-gel precipitin (AGP) test in six of 23 tissue samples from rats found dead on four poultry farms that had histories of IBDV infection. There has been no further evidence to support a conclusion that either mosquitoes or rats act as vectors or reservoirs of the virus.

Incubation Period and Signs. The incubation period is very short, and clinical signs of the disease are seen within 2–3 days after exposure. Helmboldt and Garner (47) detected histologic evidence of infection in the cloacal bursa within 24 hr. Müller et al. (105), using immunofluorescence techniques, observed infected gut-associated macrophages and lymphoid cells within 4–5 hr after oral exposure to IBDV. Virus-infected cells were present in the cloacal bursa by 11 hr after oral exposure and 6 hr after direct application of virus to the bursa.

One of the earliest signs of infection in a flock is the tendency for some birds to pick at their own vents. Cosgrove (22), in his original report, described soiled vent feathers, whitish or watery diarrhea, anorexia, depression, ruffled feathers, trembling, severe prostration, and finally, death. Affected birds became dehydrated, and in terminal stages of the disease, had a subnormal temperature.

Morbidity and Mortality. In fully susceptible flocks, the disease appears suddenly and there is a high morbidity rate, usually approaching 100%. Mortality may be nil but can be as high as 20–30%, usually beginning on the 3rd day postinfection and peaking and receding in a period of 5–7 days. In the late 1980s, strains of very virulent IBDV (vvIBDV) became a problem in Europe. Several of these isolates caused mortality rates of 90% (15) to 100% (168) in 4-wk-old susceptible Leghorn chickens. A 1970 isolate (52/70) (14) was compared with two vvIBDV isolates in one study; it caused 50% mortality compared with 90% for the vvIBDV strains (15).

Initial outbreaks on a farm are usually the most acute. Recurrent outbreaks in succeeding broods are less severe and frequently go undetected. Many infections are silent, owing to age of birds (less than 3 wk old), infection with avirulent field strains, or infection in the presence of maternal antibody.

Gross Lesions. Birds that succumb to the infection are dehydrated, with darkened discoloration of pectoral muscles. Frequently, hemorrhages are present in the thigh and pectoral muscles (Fig. 29.2). There is increased mucus in the intestine, and renal changes (22) may be prominent in birds that die or are in advanced stages of the disease. Such lesions are most probably a consequence of severe dehydration. In birds killed and examined during the course of infection, kidneys appear normal.

The cloacal bursa appears to be the primary target organ of the virus. Cheville (16) made a detailed study of bursal weights for 12 days postinfection. It is important that the sequence of changes be understood when examining birds for diagnosis. On the 3rd day postinfection, the bursa begins to increase in size and weight because of edema and hyperemia (Fig. 29.3). By the 4th day, it usually is double its normal weight and the size then begins to recede. By the 5th day, the bursa returns to normal weight, but it continues to atrophy, and from the 8th day

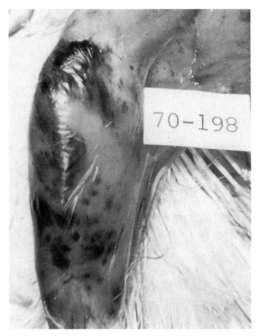

29.2. Hemorrhages of leg muscle typical in infectious bursal disease (IBD).

forward, it is approximately one-third its original weight.

By the 2nd or 3rd day postinfection, the bursa has a gelatinous yellowish transudate covering the serosal surface. Longitudinal striations on the surface become prominent, and the normal white color turns to cream color. The transudate disappears as the bursa returns to its normal size, and the organ becomes gray during and following the period of atrophy.

Isolates of variant IBDV were reported not to induce an inflammatory response (128, 138), although one variant strain (IN) did so (44).

The infected bursa often shows necrotic foci and at times petechial or ecchymotic hemorrhages on the mucosal surface. Occasionally, extensive hemorrhage throughout the entire bursa has been observed (see Fig. 29.3); in these cases, birds may void blood in their droppings.

The spleen may be slightly enlarged and very often has small gray foci uniformly dispersed on the surface (125). Occasionally, hemorrhages are observed in the mucosa at the juncture of the proventriculus and gizzard.

Compared with a moderately pathogenic strain of the virus, the vvIBDV strains caused a greater decrease in thymic weight index and more severe lesions in the cecal tonsils, thymus, spleen, and bone marrow, but bursal lesions were similar. It was also shown that pathogenicity correlated with lesion production in nonbursal lymphoid organs, suggesting that pathogenicity may be associated with antigen distribution in nonbursal lymphoid organs (158).

Histopathology. Histologic lesions of IBD occur primarily in the lymphoid structures, i.e., cloacal bursa, spleen, thymus, harderian gland, and cecal tonsil. Histopathology at the level of light microscopy has been studied by Helmboldt and

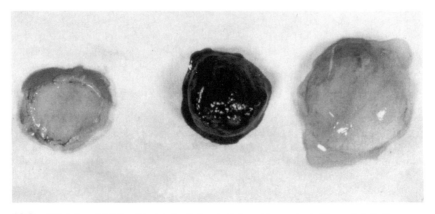

29.3. Edematous (*right*) and hemorrhagic (*center*) cloacal bursas typical in acute infectious bursal disease (IBD) at 72–96 hr postinfection. The bursa on the *left* is normal.

Garner (47), Cheville (16), Mandelli et al. (94), and Peters (124). Changes were most severe in the cloacal bursa. As early as 1 day postinfection, there was degeneration and necrosis of lymphocytes in the medullary area of bursal follicles. Lymphocytes were soon replaced by heterophils, pyknotic debris, and hyperplastic reticuloendothelial cells. Hemorrhages often appeared but were not a consistent lesion. All lymphoid follicles were affected by 3 or 4 days postinfection. The increase in bursal weight seen at this time was caused by severe edema, hyperemia, and marked accumulation of heterophils. As the inflammatory reaction declined, cystic cavities developed in medullary areas of follicles, necrosis and phagocytosis of heterophils and plasma cells occurred, and there was a fibroplasia in interfollicular connective tissue (16). Proliferation of the bursal epithelial layer produced a glandular structure of columnar epithelial cells containing globules of mucin. During the suppurative stage, scattered foci of lymphocytes appeared but did not form healthy follicles during the observation period of 18 days postinoculation (47). Some of the histologic changes observed in the cloacal bursa are shown in Fig. 29.4. A recent isolate (variant A) of IBDV was reported to cause extensive lesions in the cloacal bursa, but an inflammatory response was lacking (138).

The spleen had hyperplasia of reticuloendothelial cells around the adenoid sheath arteries in early stages of infection. By the 3rd day, there was lymphoid necrosis in the germinal follicles and periarteriolar lymphoid sheath. The spleen recovered from the infection rather rapidly, with no sustained damage to the germinal follicles.

The thymus and cecal tonsils exhibited some cellular reaction in the lymphoid tissues in early stages of infection, but, as in the spleen, the damage was less extensive than in the bursa, and recovery was more rapid. A variant virus (A) was reported to cause milder lesions in the thymus than a standard isolate (IM) (138).

Survashe et al. (157) and Dohms et al. (31) found that the harderian gland was severely affected following infection of 1-day-old chicks with IBDV. Normally, the gland is infiltrated and populated with plasma cells as the chicken ages. Infection with IBDV prevented this infiltration. From 1 to 7 wk of age, glands of infected chickens had populations of plasma cells five- to 10-fold fewer than those of uninfected controls (31). In contrast, broilers inoculated with IBDV at 3 wk of age had plasma cell necrosis in the harderian gland 5–14 days postinoculation, and the plasma cells were reduced by 51% at 7 days after inoculation (32). Reduction in plasma cells, however, was transient and the numbers were normal after 14 days. Follicular necrosis was noticed in the cloacal bursa of infected birds from 1 to 7 days postinoculation.

Histologic lesions of the kidney are nonspecific (124) and probably occur because of severe dehydration of affected chickens. Helmboldt and Garner (47) found kidney lesions in less than 5% of birds examined. Lesions observed were large casts of homogeneous material infiltrated with heterophils.

The liver may have slight perivascular infiltration of monocytes (124).

Naqi and Millar (111) followed the sequential changes in the surface epithelium of the cloacal bursa of IBDV-infected chicks by scanning electron microscopy. They observed a reduction in number and size of microvilli on epithelial cells at 48 hr postinoculation. There was gradual loss of the button follicles normally seen at the surface, and by 72 hr, most had involuted. By 96 hr, there were numerous erosions of the epithelial surface. The surface was intact by the 9th day postinoculation, but follicles were involuted, leaving deep pits.

Immunity. Viruses of both serotypes of IBDV share common group antigen(s) that can be detected by the fluorescent antibody test and ELISA (58, 68). Hence, it is not possible to distinguish serotypes or their antibodies by these tests. The common (group) antigens for both serotypes are on VP2 (40 kD) and VP3 (32 kD). VP2 also has serotype-specific group antigens that induce VN antibodies (4, 9). Becht et al. (9) reported that antibodies against VP3 do not have any protective effect. In vivo studies (59, 71) corroborated this observation, since chickens having antibodies to serotype 2 viruses were not protected against serotype 1 viruses. The current thought is that VP2 has the major antigens that induce protection (4, 9).

Traditionally, serotype 1 viruses have been used for studies of the immune response to IBDV. All known isolates of serotype 2 were reported to be nonpathogenic in chickens and turkeys (70, 71, 60) or of very low pathogenicity (20, 113, 122). The discovery of variant strains of serotype 1 has heightened interest in furthering the knowledge of the immune response to IBDV. It was interesting that variants were originally isolated from chickens that had VN antibodies to serotype 1 (128, 133). Inactivated vaccines and a live vaccine made from variant strains protected chickens from disease caused by either variant or standard strains, whereas inactivated vaccines made from standard strains did not protect, or only partially protected, against challenge with variant strains (59, 132).

In recent studies (59), five different subtypes of serotype 1 IBDV were tested as inactivated vaccines against a variant strain of a different subtype. Vaccines made with 10^8 but not 10^5 tissue-culture-infective doses–50% were protective against a challenge dose of 10^2 EID_{50}. Even the higher vaccine dose did not protect against challenge with $10^{3.5}$ EID_{50}. Based on these results, it was suggested that

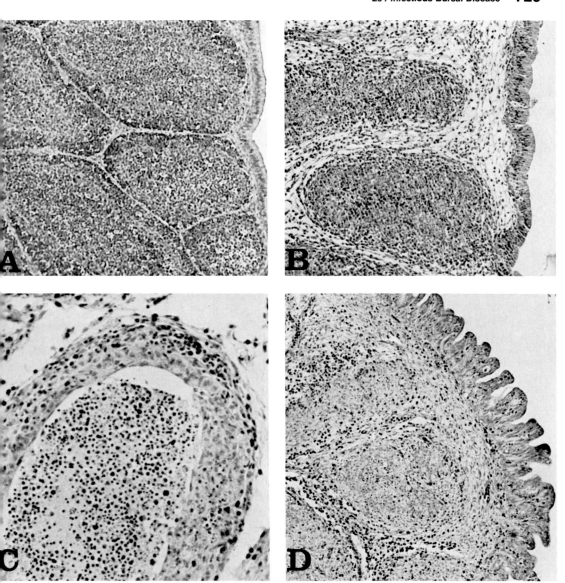

.4. Photomicrographs of 6-wk-old birds affected with infectious bursal disease virus (IBDV). Tissues are cloacal bursa fixed in 10% buffered saline and stained with H & E. *A.* Normal tissue. Large active follicles consist of lymphoid cells that form discrete follicles with little interfollicular tissue. Covering epithelium is simple columnar. ×40. *B.* Bursa approximately 24 hr postinfection. Note interfollicular edema mixed with phagocytic cells, many of which are heterophils. Follicles are already beginning to degenerate. ×40. *C.* Single follicle approximately 60 hr postinfection. Medullary portion is now a mass of cellular debris surrounded by cortical remnants. Only reticular cells exist in any number, but scattered among them are a few lymphocytes that will later regenerate. ×250. *D.* Terminal phase of severe infection. Only ghosts of follicles remain, while heterophils (scattered dark cells) are actively engaged in phagocytosis. ×40. (Helmboldt).

all the subtypes of serotype 1 share a minor antigen(s) that elicits protective antibodies.

ACTIVE IMMUNITY. Field exposure to the virus, or vaccination with either live or killed vaccines, stim-

ulates active immunity. Antibody response may be measured by several methods—VN, AGP, or ELISA tests. Antibody levels are normally very high after field exposure or vaccination, and VN titers greater than 1:1000 are common. Adult birds are resistant to oral exposure to the virus, but produce antibody after intramuscular or subcutaneous inoculation of IBDV (54).

PASSIVE IMMUNITY. Antibody transmitted from the dam via the yolk of the egg can protect chicks against early infections with IBDV, with resultant protection against the immunosuppressive effect of the virus. The half-life of maternal antibodies to IBDV is between 3 and 5 days (147). Therefore, if the antibody titer of the progeny is known, the time that chicks will become susceptible can be predicted. Lucio and Hitchner (82) demonstrated that after antibody titers fell below 1:100, chicks were 100% susceptible to infection, and titers from 1:100 to 1:600 gave approximately 40% protection against challenge. Skeeles et al. (147) reported that titers must fall below 1:64 before chickens can be vaccinated effectively with an attenuated strain of IBDV. Use of killed vaccines in oil emulsions (including variant strains) to stimulate high levels of maternal immunity is extensive in the field. Studies by Lucio and Hitchner (82) and Baxendale and Lutticken (6) indicated that oil emulsion IBD vaccines can stimulate adequate maternal immunity to protect chicks for 4–5 wk, while progeny from breeders vaccinated with live vaccines are protected for only 1–3 wk. As with many diseases, passively acquired immunity to IBDV can interfere with stimulation of an active immune response.

Immunosuppression.

Allan et al. (1) and Faragher et al. (37) first reported immunosuppressive effects of IBDV infections. Suppression of the antibody response to Newcastle disease virus was greatest in chicks infected at 1 day of age. There was moderate suppression when chicks were infected at 7 days, and negligible effects when infection was at 14 or 21 days (37). Hirai et al. (51) demonstrated decreased humoral antibody response to other vaccines as well. Not only was response to vaccines suppressed, but chicks infected early with IBDV were more susceptible to inclusion body hepatitis (33), coccidiosis (2), Marek's disease (18, 136), hemorrhagic-aplastic anemia and gangrenous dermatitis (130), infectious laryngotracheitis, (129), infectious bronchitis (121), chicken anemia agent (178), and salmonellosis and colibacillosis (174).

A paradox associated with IBDV infections of chickens is that while there is immunosuppression against many antigens, the response against IBDV itself is normal, even in 1-day-old susceptible chickens (146). There appears to be a stimulation of the proliferation of B cells committed to anti-IBDV antibody production.

The effect of IBD on cell-mediated immune (CMI) responses is transient and less obvious than that on humoral responses. Panigraphy et al. (118) reported that IBDV infections at a young age

caused a delayed skin graft rejection; however, other workers (38, 56) found no effect from early IBDV infections on skin graft rejection or tuberculin-delayed hypersensitivity reaction. Sivanandan and Maheswaran (142) observed suppression of CMI responsiveness, using the lymphoblast transformation assay. They found that maximal depression of cellular immunity occurred 6 wk postinfection. Nusbaum et al. (113) detected a significant suppression of T-cell response to the mitogen concanavalin A in poults from 3 days to 4 wk postinfection. There was no reduction, however, in tuberculin reactions in IBDV-infected poults. In a sequential study of peripheral blood lymphocytes from chickens inoculated with IBDV, a transient depression of mitogenic stimulation was reported (21). Sharma and Lee (137) reported an inconsistent effect of IBDV infection on natural killer cell toxicity and a transient early depression of the blastogenic response of spleen cells to phytohemagglutinin. Craft et al. (24) demonstrated that a variant IBD virus strain (A) had a significantly more severe effect on the CMI response than a standard strain (Edgar) when given to 1-day-old chicks, and the CMI was suppressed for 5 wk. A similar transient suppression of the CMI was observed in chickens infected at 3 wk of age.

Another component of the immune system is the harderian gland, which is associated with the local immune system of the respiratory tract. Pejkovski et al. (121) and Dohms et al. (31) reported that IBDV infection of 1- to 5-day-old chicks produced a drastic reduction in plasma cell content of the harderian gland that persisted for up to 7 wk. There have been similar observations with IBDV infections of poults (113). In other studies on broilers infected with IBDV at 3 wk of age, extracts from the harderian gland and serum had reduced antibody titers to *Brucella abortus* (a T-cell–independent antigen) and sheep red blood cells (SRBC, a T-cell–dependent antigen). Compared with SRBC antibody response, diminished antibody responses to *B. abortus* were evident at a later time period. A variant virus of serotype 1 produced a similar effect in chickens (30).

Chickens infected with IBDV at 1 day of age were completely deficient in serum immunoglobulin G and produced only a monomeric immunoglobulin M (IgM) (62, 63). The number of B cells in peripheral blood was decreased following infection with IBDV, but T cells were not appreciably affected (52, 140). The virus appears to replicate primarily in B lymphocytes of chickens (49, 62, 177). Apparently, IBDV has a predilection for actively proliferating cells (102), and it was suggested that the virus affected "immature," or precursor, B lymphocytes to a greater extent than mature B lymphocytes (141).

DIAGNOSIS. Acute clinical outbreaks of IBD in fully susceptible flocks are easily recognized and a presumptive diagnosis can be readily made. The rapid onset, high morbidity, spiking mortality curve, and rapid recovery (5–7 days) from clinical signs are characteristic of this disease. Confirmation of the diagnosis can be made at necropsy by examination for characteristic grossly visible changes in the cloacal bursa. It should be remembered that there are distinctive changes in size and color of the bursa during the course of infection, i.e., enlargement due to inflammatory changes followed by atrophy (see Gross Lesions).

Infections of very young chicks, or chicks with maternal antibody, are usually subclinical and are diagnosed retrospectively at necropsy with observations of macroscopic and histologic bursal atrophy. Infections of chickens of any age with variant strains of IBDV will only be detected by histopathology of the cloacal bursa or by virus isolation.

Isolation and Identification of the Causative Agent.
The cloacal bursa and spleen are the tissues of choice for the isolation of IBDV, but the bursa is the most commonly used. Other organs contain the virus, but at a lower concentration and probably only because of the viremia. Tissues should be macerated in an antibiotic-treated broth or saline and centrifuged to remove the larger tissue particles. The supernatant fluid is then used to inoculate embryonating eggs or cell cultures.

Hitchner (53) demonstrated that the chorioallantoic membrane (CAM) of 9- to 11-day-old embryos was the most sensitive route for isolation of the virus. The virus could subsequently be adapted to the allantoic sac and yolk sac routes of inoculation. Death of infected embryos usually occurs in 3 to 5 days. Variant strains of IBD differ from standard viruses in that they induce splenomegaly and liver necrosis of embryos and produce little mortality (131). The embryonating egg may be the most sensitive substrate for isolation of IBDV. McFerran et al. (97) reported that three of seven chicken isolates of IBDV failed to grow in CEF cells; however, they could be propagated in embryonating eggs.

Isolation and propagation of IBDV in cell culture was discussed previously in this chapter (see Laboratory Host Systems). Since the virus has been shown to replicate in B lymphocytes, either primary cells derived from the cloacal bursa or continuous cell lines of B-cell origin would be the cells of choice for the isolation of the virus. It appears that some strains of virus are very fastidious, and, although they may replicate in embryonating eggs or B lymphocytes, they cannot readily be adapted to CEF cells or cells from other organs such as the kidney and liver (81, 97). The use of immunofluorescence tests and electron microscopy of infected embryos and cell cultures is valuable for the early detection and identification of IBDV. Cell cultures containing 50% bursal lymphocytes and 50% CEF have been used to isolate and serotype IBD viruses successfully (83). The fibroblasts serve as a matrix for the lymphocytes, and the infected lymphocytes are detected by immunofluorescence tests. BGM-70 cells may also be used for isolation of IBDV.

Identification of the virus by direct immunofluorescent staining of affected organs or direct examination by electron microscopy have proven to be an adjunct to the isolation and identification of IBDV (97). If antigen or virus is detected by these methods from field cases of disease, then every effort should be made to isolate the virus using both embryonating eggs and cell-culture techniques. The broad antigenic diversity of IBDV makes continued isolation and antigenic analysis of field viruses imperative. New variants will likely continue to appear and they should be recognized as soon as possible. Immunoperoxidase and immunofluorescence techniques were used to detect virus antigens in formalin-fixed, paraffin-embedded sections of the bursa of Fabricius (25).

Nucleic acid probes (64) and antigen-capture ELISA using monoclonal antibodies (151) to detect IBDV directly in tissues is beneficial for rapid diagnosis of field viruses. In detecting the virus, however, polyclonal antibodies were found more sensitive than monoclonal antibodies, and embryo inoculation was more sensitive than antigen-capture ELISA (45). The polymerase chain reaction (PCR) is also useful for detection of the virus. Reverse transcription with PCR followed by restriction endonuclease analysis was described (40, 65, 159) and used to differentiate between classic and variant strains of serotype 1. Latex agglutination and reverse passive hemagglutination tests were described to detect virus antigens in chicken organs (108). A Western blot assay was not useful for distinguishing viruses of different subtypes or serotypes (165).

Differential Diagnosis.
The sudden onset, morbidity, ruffled feathers, and droopy appearance of the birds in initial disease outbreaks are suggestive of an acute outbreak of coccidiosis. In some cases, there is blood in the droppings, which would further lead one to suspect coccidiosis. The muscular hemorrhages and enlarged edematous or hemorrhagic cloacal bursae would, however, suggest IBD.

Birds that die from IBD may show an acute nephrosis. Because of many other conditions that may cause nephrosis, and the inconsistency of kidney lesions, such lesions should not be sufficient cause for a diagnosis of IBD. Again, involvement of the cloacal bursa will usually distinguish IBD from other nephrosis-causing conditions. Water deprivation will cause kidney changes and possibly gray, atrophied bursae that closely resemble those associated with IBD infection. Unless this occurs as a flock condition, however, such changes would be seen in relatively few birds. A history of the flock would be essential in aiding in the differential diagnosis of these cases.

Certain nephrotrophic strains of infectious bronchitis virus cause nephrosis (171). These cases can be differentiated from infectious bursal disease by the lack of changes in the cloacal bursa and the respiratory signs that usually precede death. The possibility that the two diseases may occur simultaneously in a flock should not be overlooked.

The muscular hemorrhages and mucosal hemorrhages seen at the juncture of the proventriculus and gizzard are similar to those reported for so-called hemorrhagic syndrome (probably infectious anemia) and could be differentiated on the basis of bursal changes that accompany IBDV infections. It is not unlikely that before IBD was recognized, some cases were diagnosed as hemorrhagic syndrome.

Jakowski et al. (73) reported bursal atrophy in experimentally induced infection with four isolates of Marek's disease. The atrophy was observed 12 days postinoculation, but the histologic response was distinctly different from that found in IBD.

Grimes and King (41) reported that experimental infections of 1-day-old, specific-pathogen-free (SPF) chickens with a type-8 avian adenovirus produced small bursae and atrophy of bursal follicles at 2 wk postinfection. Several other organs such as the liver, spleen, pancreas, and kidneys were grossly affected, and intranuclear inclusion bodies were observed in the liver and pancreas.

Serology. The ELISA procedure is presently the most commonly used serologic test for the evaluation of IBDV antibodies in poultry flocks. Marquardt et al. (95) first described an indirect ELISA for measuring antibodies, and since that time, several workers (12, 93, 150, 154, 160) have reported on the use of ELISA and its comparison to VN test results. The ELISA procedure has the advantage of being a rapid test with the results easily entered into computer software programs. With these programs, one can establish an antibody profile on breeder flocks that will indicate the flock immunity level and provide information for developing proper immunization programs for both breeder flocks and their progeny. To perform an antibody profile on a flock for the evaluation of the efficacy of vaccination programs, no less than 30 serum samples should be tested; many producers submit as many as 50-100 samples. The antibody profiles may be performed with serum collected either from the breeders or from 1-day-old progeny. If progeny serums are used, titers will normally be 60–80% lower than those in the breeders. It should be rec-

ognized that the standard ELISA, using whole virus for antigen, does not differentiate between antibodies to serotypes 1 and 2 (58, 165).

Prior to the use of the ELISA, the most common procedure for antibody detection was the constant virus-diluting serum VN test performed in a microtiter system (145). The VN test is the only serologic test that will distinguish between the different serotypes of IBDV, and it is still the method of choice to discern antigenic variations between isolates of this virus. The indicator virus used for VN can make a significant difference in test results due to the fact that within a given serotype there are several antigenic subtypes (67). Most chicken serums from the field have high levels of neutralizing antibody to a broad spectrum of antigenically diverse viruses owing to a combination of field exposure, vaccine exposure, and cross-reactivity from high levels of antibody.

The other method used for the detection of IBDV antibodies is the AGP test. In the United Kingdom, a quantitative AGP test is routinely used (26); however, as used in the United States, the test is not quantitative. This test does not detect serotypic differences; it measures primarily group-specific soluble antigens.

TREATMENT. No therapeutic or supportive treatment has been found to change the course of IBDV infection (22, 119). Because of the rapid recovery of the affected flock, treatments might appear highly effective if nontreated controls are not maintained for comparison. There are no reports in the literature concerning the use of some of the newer antiviral compounds and interferon inducers for the treatment of IBD.

PREVENTION AND CONTROL. The epizootiology of this infection has not been studied extensively, but it is known that contact with infected birds and contaminated fomites readily causes spread of the infection. The relative stability of this virus to many physical and chemical agents increases the likelihood that it will be carried over from one flock to a succeeding flock. The sanitary precautions that are applied to prevent the spread of most poultry infections must be rigorously used in the case of IBD. The possible involvement of other vectors, e.g., the lesser mealworm, mosquitoes, and rats, has already been discussed; they could certainly pose extra problems for the control of this infection.

Management Procedures. Before the development of attenuated vaccine strains, intentional exposure of chicks to infection at an early age was used for controlling IBD. This was advised on farms that had a history of the disease, in which case the chicks would normally have maternal antibodies for protection. Also, young chicks less than 2 wk of age did not normally exhibit clinical signs of IBD. When the severe immunosuppressive effect of early IBD infections was discovered, the practice of "controlled exposure" with virulent strains became less appealing. On many farms, the cleanup between broods is not thorough and, due to the stable nature of the virus, it easily persists and provides an early exposure by natural means.

Immunization. Immunization of chickens is the principal method used for the control of IBD in chickens. Especially important is the immunization of breeder flocks in order to confer parental immunity to their progeny. Such maternal antibodies protect the chick from early immunosuppressive infections. Maternal antibody will normally protect chicks for 1 to 3 wk, but by boosting the immunity in breeder flocks with oil-adjuvated vaccines, passive immunity may be extended to 4 or 5 wk (6, 82).

The major problem with active immunization of young maternally immune chicks is determining the proper time of vaccination. This varies with the level of maternal antibody, route of vaccination, and virulence of the vaccine virus. Environmental stresses and management may be factors to consider when developing a vaccination program that will be effective. Monitoring of antibody levels in a breeder flock or its progeny (antibody profiling) can aid in determining the proper time to vaccinate.

There are many choices of live vaccines available, based on virulence and antigenic diversity. The most virulent vaccine is no longer commercially available. Presently available in the United States are strains of intermediate virulence and highly attenuated strains. Also available are some cell culture–adapted variant strains. Highly virulent, intermediate, and avirulent strains overcome maternal VN antibody titers of 1:500, 1:250, and less than 1:100, respectively (82, 147). Intermediate strains vary in their virulence and can induce bursal atrophy and immunosuppression in 1-day-old and 3-wk-old SPF chickens (86). If maternal VN antibody titers are less than 1:1000, chicks may be vaccinated by injection with avirulent strains of virus. The vaccine virus replicates in the thymus, spleen, and cloacal bursa, where it persists for 2 wk (87). Once the maternal antibody is catabolized, there is a primary antibody response to the persisting vaccine virus.

Oil-adjuvant, killed-virus vaccines are used to boost and prolong immunity in breeder flocks, but they are not practical or desirable for inducing a primary response in young chickens. Oil-adjuvant vaccines are most effective in chickens that have been "primed" with live virus either in the form of vaccine (175) or field exposure to the virus. Oil-adju-

vant vaccines presently may contain both standard and variant strains of IBDV. Antibody profiling of breeder flocks is advised to assess effectiveness of vaccination and persistence of antibody. Virus from bursal tissue of infected SPF chickens has been shown to yield a killed vaccine more potent than those prepared from virus grown in either embryos or cell culture (176). It was shown recently, however, that inactivated vaccine preparations derived from tissue culture or bursal homogenates, and containing similar antigen masses, elicited virus neutralizing antibodies that did not differ significantly in titer (43).

A universal vaccination program cannot be offered because of the variability in maternal immunity, management, and operational conditions that exist. If very high levels of maternal antibody are achieved and the field challenge is reduced, then vaccination of broilers may not be needed. Vaccination timing with attenuated and intermediate vaccines varies from as early as 7 days to 2 or 3 wk. If broilers are vaccinated at 1 day of age, the IBDV vaccine can be given by injection along with Marek's disease vaccine. Priming of breeder replacement chickens may be necessary, and many poultry producers vaccinate with live vaccine at 10–14 wk of age. Killed oil-adjuvant vaccines are commonly administered at 16–18 wk. Revaccination of breeders may be required if antibody profiling should indicate the need. Recombinant vaccines have been described, but none is currently available commercially (7, 27, 36, 46, 91, 153, 166, 167).

REFERENCES

1. Allan, W.H., J.T. Faragher, and G.A. Cullen. 1972. Immunosuppression by the infectious bursal agent in chickens immunized against Newcastle disease. Vet Rec 90:511–512.

2. Anderson, W.I., W.M. Reid, P.D. Lukert, and O.J. Fletcher. 1977. Influence of infectious bursal disease on the development of immunity to Eimeria tenella. Avian Dis 21:637–641.

3. Azad, A.A., S.A. Barrett, and K.J. Fahey. 1985. The characterization and molecular cloning of the double-stranded RNA genome of an Australian strain of infectious bursal disease virus. Virology 143:35–44.

4. Azad, A.A., M.N. Jagadish, M.A. Brown, and P.J. Hudson. 1987. Deletion mapping and expression in Escherichia coli of the large genomic segment of a birnavirus. Virology 161:145–152.

5. Barnes, H.J., J. Wheeler, and D. Reed. 1982. Serological evidence of infectious bursal disease virus infection in Iowa turkeys. Avian Dis 26:560–565.

6. Baxendale, W., and D. Lutticken. 1981. The results of field trials with an inactivated Gumboro vaccine. Dev Biol Stand 51:211–219.

7. Bayliss, C.D., R.W. Peters, J.K.A. Cook, R.L. Reece, K. Howes, M.M. Binns and M.E.G. Boursnell. 1991. A recombinant fowlpox virus that expresses the VP2 antigen of infectious bursal disease virus induces protection against mortality caused by the virus. Arch Virol 120:193–205.

8. Becht, H. 1980. Infectious bursal disease virus.

Curr Top Microbiol Immunol 90:107–121.

9. Becht, H., H. Müller, and H.K. Müller. 1988. Comparative studies on structural and antigenic properties of two serotypes of infectious bursal disease virus. J Gen Virol 69:631–640.

10. Benton, W.J., M.S. Cover, and J.K. Rosenberger. 1967. Studies on the transmission of the infectious bursal agent (IBA) of chickens. Avian Dis 11:430–438.

11. Benton, W.J., M.S. Cover, J.K. Rosenberger, and R. S. Lake, 1967. Physicochemical properties of the infectious bursal agent (IBA). Avian Dis 11:438–445.

12. Briggs, D.J., C.E. Whitfill, J.K. Skeeles, J.D. Story, and K.D. Reed. 1986. Application of the positive/negative ratio method of analysis to quantitate antibody responses to infectious bursal disease virus using a commercially available ELISA. Avian Dis 30:216–218.

13. Brown, F. 1986. The classification and nomenclature of viruses: Summary of results of meetings of the International Committee on Taxonomy of Viruses in Sendai. Intervirology 25:141–143.

14. Bygrave, A.C. and J.T. Faragher. 1970. Mortality associated and Gumboro disease. Vet Rec 86:758–759.

15. Chettle, N., J.C. Stuart, and P.J. Wyeth. 1989. Outbreak of virulent infectious bursal disease in East Anglia. Vet Rec 125:271–272.

16. Cheville, N.F. 1967. Studies on the pathogenesis of Gumboro disease in the bursa of Fabricius, spleen and thymus of the chicken. Am J Pathol 51:527–551.

17. Chin, R.P., R. Yamamoto, W. Lin, K.M. Lam and T.B. Farver. 1984. Serological survey of infectious bursal disease virus: Serotypes 1 and 2 in California turkeys. Avian Dis 28:1026–1036.

18. Cho, B.R. 1970. Experimental dual infections of chickens with infectious bursal and Marek's disease agents. I. Preliminary observation on the effect of infectious bursal agent on Marek's disease. Avian Dis 14:665–675.

19. Cho, Y., and S.A. Edgar. 1969. Characterization of the infectious bursal agent. Poult Sci 48:2102–2109.

20. Chui, C.H., and J.J. Thorsen. 1984. Experimental infection of turkeys with infectious bursal disease virus and the effect on the immunocompetence of infected turkeys. Avian Dis 28:197–207.

21. Confer, A.W., W.T. Springer, S.M. Shane, and J.F. Conovan. 1981. Sequential mitogen stimulation of peripheral blood lymphocytes from chickens inoculated with infectious bursal disease virus. Am J Vet Res 42:2109–2113.

22. Cosgrove, A.S. 1962. An apparently new disease of chickens—avian nephrosis. Avian Dis 6:385–389.

23. Cowen, B.S., and M.O. Braune. 1988. The propagation of avian viruses in a continuous cell line (QT35) of Japanese quail origin. Avian Dis 32:282–297.

24. Craft, D.W., J. Brown, and P.D. Lukert. 1990. Effects of standard and variant strains of infectious bursal disease virus on infections of chickens. Am J Vet Res 51:1192–1197.

25. Cruz-Coy, J.S., J.J. Giambrone, and F.J. Hoerr. 1993. Immunohistochemical detection of IBDV in formalin-fixed, paraffin-embedded chicken tissues using monoclonal antibody. Avian Dis 37:577–581.

26. Cullen, G.A., and P.J. Wyeth. 1975. Quantitation of antibodies to infectious bursal disease. Vet Rec 97:315.

27. Darteil, R., M. Bublot, E. Laplace, J-F. Bouquet, J-C. Audonnet, and M. Riviere. 1995. Herpesvirus of turkey recombinant viruses expressing infectious bursal disease virus (IBDV) VP2 immunogen induce protection against an IBDV virulent challenge in chickens. Virology 211:481–490.

28. Dobos, P. 1979. Peptide map comparison of the proteins of infectious bursal disease virus. J Virol 32:1046–1050.

29. Dobos, P., B. J. Hill, R. Hallett, D.T. Kells, H. Becht, and D. Teninges. 1979. Biophysical and biochemical characterization of five animal viruses with bisegmented double-stranded RNA genomes. J Virol 32:593–605.

30. Dohms, J.E. and J.S. Jaeger. 1988. The effect of infectious bursal disease virus infection on local and systemic antibody responses following infection of 3-week-old broiler chickens. Avian Dis 32:632–640.

31. Dohms, J.E., K.P. Lee, and J.K. Rosenberger. 1981. Plasma cell changes in the gland of harder following infectious bursal disease virus infection of the chicken. Avian Dis 25:683–695.

32. Dohms, J.E., K.P. Lee, J.K. Rosenberger, and A.L. Metz. 1988. Plasma cell quantitation in the gland of Harder during infectious bursal disease virus infection of 3-week-old broiler chickens. Avian Dis 32:624–631.

33. Fadly, A.M., R.W. Winterfield, and H.J. Olander. 1976. Role of the bursa of Fabricius in the pathogenicity of inclusion body hepatitis and infectious bursal disease virus. Avian Dis 20:467–477.

34. Fahey, K.J., I.J. O'Donnell, and A.A. Azad. 1985. Characterization by western blotting of the immunogens of infectious bursal disease virus. J Gen Virol 66:1479–1488.

35. Fahey, K.J., I.J. O'Donnell, and T.J. Bagust. 1985. Antibody to the 32K structural protein of infectious bursal disease virus neutralizes viral infectivity in vitro and confers protection on young chickens. J Gen Virol 66:2693–2702.

36. Fahey, K.J., K.M. Erny, and J. Crooks. 1989. A conformational immunogen on VP2 of infectious bursal disease virus that passively protects chickens. J Gen Virol 70:1473–1481.

37. Faragher, J.T., W.H. Allan, and C.J. Wyeth. 1974. Immunosuppressive effect of infectious bursal agent on vaccination against Newcastle disease. Vet Rec 95:385–388.

38. Giambrone, J.J., J.P. Donahoe, D.L. Dawe, and C.S. Eidson. 1977. Specific suppression of the bursa-dependent immune system of chicks with infectious bursal disease virus. Am J Vet Res 38:581–583.

39. Giambrone, J.J., O.J. Fletcher, P.D. Lukert, R.K. Page, and C.E. Eidson. 1978. Experimental infection of turkeys with infectious bursal disease virus. Avian Dis 22:451–458.

40. Giambrone, J.J., H.J. Liu, and T. Dormitorio. 1994. Genetic variation in infectious bursal disease virus using restriction fragment length polymorphism and sequence comparisons of polymerase chain reaction generated cDNA. Intl Symp on Infectious Bursal Disease, Germany, pp. 71–82.

41. Grimes, T.M., and D.J. King. 1977. Effect of maternal antibody on experimental infections of chickens with a type-8 avian adenovirus. Avian Dis 21:97–112.

42. Harkness, J.W., D.J. Alexander, M. Pattison, and A.C. Scott. 1975. Infectious bursal disease agent: Morphology by negative stain electron microscopy. Arch Virol 48:63–73.

43. Hassan, M.K., and Y.M. Saif. 1996. Influence of the host system on the pathogenicity, immunogenicity, and antigenicity of infectious bursal disease viruses. Avian Dis 40:553–561.

44. Hassan, M.K., M.Q. Al-Natour, L.A. Ward, and Y.M. Saif. 1996. Pathogenicity, attenuation and immunogenicity of infectious bursal disease virus. Avian Dis 40:567–571.

45. Hassan, M.K., Y.M. Saif, and S. Shawky. 1996. Comparison between antigen-capture ELISA and conventional methods used for titration of infectious bursal disease virus. Avian Dis 40:562–566.

46. Heine, H.-G. and D.B. Boyle. 1993. Infectious bursal disease virus structural protein VP2 expressed by a fowlpox virus recombinant confers protection against disease in chickens. Arch Virol 131:277–292.

47. Helmboldt, C.F., and E. Garner. 1964. Experimentally induced Gumboro disease (IBA). Avian Dis 8:561–575.

48. Hihara, H., H. Yamamoto, K. Arqi, W. Okazaki and T. Shimizu. 1980. Conditions for successful cultivation of tumor cells from chickens with lymphoid leucosis. Avian Dis 24:971–979.

49. Hirai, K., and B.W. Calnek. 1979. In vitro replication of infectious bursal disease virus in established lymphoid cell lines and chicken B lymphocytes. Infect Immun 25:964–970.

50. Hirai, K., and S. Shimakura. 1974. Structure of infectious bursal disease virus. J Virol 14:957–964.

51. Hirai, K., S. Shimakura, E. Kawamoto, F. Taguchi, S.T. Kim, C.N. Chang, and Y. Iritani. 1974. The immunodepressive effect of infectious bursal disease virus in chickens. Avian Dis 18:50–57.

52. Hirai, K., K. Kunihiro and S. Shimakura. 1979. Characterization of immunosuppression in chickens by infectious bursal disease virus. Avian Dis 23:950–965.

53. Hitchner, S.B. 1970. Infectivity of infectious bursal disease virus for embryonating eggs. Poult Sci 49:511–516.

54. Hitchner, S.B. 1976. Immunization of adult hens against infectious bursal disease virus. Avian Dis 20:611–613.

55. Howie, R.I., and J. Thorsen. 1981. Identification of a strain of infectious bursal disease virus isolated from mosquitoes. Can J Comp Med 45:315–320.

56. Hudson, L., H. Pattison, and N. Thantrey. 1975. Specific B lymphocyte suppression by infectious bursal agent (Gumboro disease virus) in chickens. Eur J Immunol 5:675–679.

57. Hudson, P.J., N.M. McKern, B.E. Power, and A.A. Azad. 1986. Genomic structure of the large RNA segment of infectious bursal disease virus. Nucleic Acids Res 14:5001–5012.

58. Ismail, N. and Y.M. Saif. 1990. Differentiation between antibodies to serotypes 1 and 2 infectious bursal disease viruses in chicken sera. Avian Dis 34:1002–1004.

59. Ismail, N., and Y.M. Saif. 1991. Immunogenicity of infectious bursal disease viruses in chickens. Avian Dis 35:460–469.

60. Ismail, N., Y.M. Saif, and P.D. Moorhead. 1988. Lack of pathogenicity of five serotype 2 infectious bursal disease viruses in chickens. Avian Dis 32:757–759.

61. Ismail, N., Y.M. Saif, W.L. Wigle, G.B. Havenstein, and C. Jackson. 1990. Infectious bursal disease virus variant from commercial leghorn pullets. Avian Dis 34:141–145.

62. Ivanyi, J. 1975. Immunodeficiency in the chicken. II. Production of monomeric IgM following testosterone treatment of infection with Gumboro disease. Immunology 28:1015–1021.

63. Ivanyi, J., and R. Morris. 1976. Immunodeficiency in the chicken. IV. An immunological study of infectious bursal disease. Clin Exp Immunol 23:154–165.

64. Jackwood, D.J. 1988. Detection of infectious bursal disease virus using nucleic acid probes [abst]. J Am Vet Med Assoc 192:1779.

65. Jackwood, D.J. and R.J. Jackwood. 1994. Infectious bursal disease viruses: Molecular differentiation of antigenic subtypes among serotype 1 virus. Avian Dis 38:531–537.

66. Jackwood, D.J., and Y.M. Saif. 1983. Prevalence of antibodies to infectious bursal disease virus serotypes I and II in 75 Ohio chicken flocks. Avian Dis 27:850–854.

67. Jackwood, D.H., and Y.M. Saif. 1987. Antigenic diversity of infectious bursal disease viruses. Avian Dis 31:766–770.

68. Jackwood, D.J., Y.M. Saif, and J.H. Hughes. 1982. Characteristics and serologic studies of two serotypes of infectious bursal disease virus in turkeys. Avian Dis 26:871–882.

69. Jackwood, D.J., Y.M. Saif, and J.H. Hughes. 1984. Nucleic acid and structural proteins of infectious bursal disease virus isolates belonging to serotypes I and II. Avian Dis 28:990–1006.

70. Jackwood, D.J., Y.M. Saif, P.D. Moorhead, and G. Bishop. 1984. Failure of two serotype II infectious bursal disease viruses to affect the humoral immune response of turkeys. Avian Dis 28:100–116.

71. Jackwood, D.J., Y.M. Saif, and P.D. Moorhead. 1985. Immunogenicity and antigenicity of infectious bursal disease virus serotypes I and II in chickens. Avian Dis 29:1184–1194.

72. Jackwood, D.H., Y.M. Saif, and J.H. Hughes. 1987. Replication of infectious bursal disease virus in continuous cell lines. Avian Dis 31:370–375.

73. Jakowski, R.M., T.N. Fredrickson, R.E. Luginbuhl and C.F. Helmboldt. 1969. Early changes in bursa of Fabricius from Marek's disease. Avian Dis 13:215–222.

74. Johnson, D.C., P.D. Lukert, and R.K. Page. 1980. Field studies with convalescent serum and infectious bursal disease vaccine to control turkey coryza. Avian Dis 24:386–392.

75. Kaufer, I., and E. Weiss. 1980. Significance of bursa of Fabricius as target organ in infectious bursal disease of chickens. Infect Immun 27:364–367.

76. Kibenge, F.S.B., A.S. Dhillon, and R.G. Russell. 1988. Biochemistry and immunology of infectious bursal disease virus. J Gen Virol 69:1757–1775.

77. Kibenge, F.S.B., A.S. Dhillon, and R.G. Russell. 1988. Growth of serotypes I and II and variant strains of infectious bursal disease virus in vero cells. Avian Dis 17:298–303.

78. Kibenge, F.S.B., A.S. Dhillon, and R.G. Russell. 1988. Identification of serotype II infectious bursal disease virus proteins. Avian Pathol 17:679–687.

79. Kosters, J., H. Becht, and R. Rudolph. 1972. Properties of the infectious bursal agent of chicken (IBA). Med Microbiol Immunol 157:291–298.

80. Landgraf, H., E. Vielitz, and R. Kirsch. 1967. Occurrence of an infectious disease affecting the bursa of Fabricius (Gumboro disease). Dtsch Tieraerztl Wochenschr 74:6–10.

81. Lee, L.H., and P.D. Lukert. 1986. Adaptation and antigenic variation of infectious bursal disease virus. J Chin Soc Vet Sci 12:297–304.

82. Lucio, B., and S.B. Hitchner. 1979. Infectious bursal disease emulsified vaccine: Effect upon neutralizing-antibody levels in the dam and subsequent protection of the progeny. Avian Dis 23:466–478.

83. Lukert, P.D. 1986. Serotyping recent isolates of infectious bursal disease virus. Proc 21st Natl Meet Poult Health Condemn, Ocean City, MD, pp. 71–75.

84. Lukert, P.D. 1988. Unpublished data.

85. Lukert, P.D., and R.B. Davis. 1974. Infectious bursal disease virus: Growth and characterization in cell cultures. Avian Dis 18:243–250.

86. Lukert, P.D., and L.A. Mazariegos. 1985. Virulence and immunosuppressive potential of intermediate vaccine strains of infectious bursal disease virus [abst]. J Am Vet Med Assoc 187:306.

87. Lukert P.D., and D. Rifuliadi. 1982. Replication of virulent and attenuated infectious bursal disease virus in maternally immune day-old chickens [abst]. J Am Vet Med Assoc 181:284.

88. Lukert, P.D., J. Leonard, and R.B. Davis. 1975. Infectious bursal disease virus: Antigen production and immunity. Am J Vet Res 36:539–540.

89. Lunger, P.D., and T.C. Maddux. 1972. Fine-structure studies of the avian infectious bursal agent. I. In vivo viral morphogenesis. Avian Dis 16:874–893.

90. MacDonald, R.D. 1980. Immunofluorescent detection of double-stranded RNA in cells infected with reovirus, infectious pancreatic necrosis virus, and infectious bursal disease virus. Can J Microbiol 26:256–261.

91. Macreadie, I.G., P.R. Vaughan, A.J. Chapman, N.M. McKern, M.N. Jagadish, H.G. Heine, C.W. Ward, K.J. Fahey, and A.A. Azad. 1990. Passive protection against infectious bursal disease virus by viral VP2 expressed in yeast. Vaccine 8:549–552.

92. Mahardika, G.N.K., and H. Becht. 1995. Mapping of cross-reacting and serotype-specific epitopes on the VP3 structural protein of infectious bursal disease virus. Arch Virol 140:765–774.

93. Mallinson, E.T., D.B. Snyder, W.W. Marquardt, E. Russek-Cohen, P. K. Savage, D.C. Allen, and F.S. Yancey. 1985. Presumptive diagnosis of subclinical infections utilizing computer-assisted analysis of sequential enzyme-linked immunosorbent assays against multiple antigens. Poult Sci 64:1661–1669.

94. Mandelli, G., A. Rinaldi, A. Cerioli, and G. Cervio. 1967. Aspetti ultrastrutturali della borsa di Fabrizio nella malattia di Gumboro de pollo. Atti Soc Ital Sci Vet 21:615–619.

95. Marquardt, W., R.B. Johnson, W.F. Odenwald, and B.A. Schlotthober. 1980. An indirect enzyme-linked immunosorbent assay (ELISA) for measuring antibodies in chickens infected with infectious bursal disease virus. Avian Dis 24:375–385.

96. McAllister, J.C., C.D. Steelman, L.A. Newberry, and J.K. Skeeles. 1995. Isolation of infectious bursal disease virus from the lesser mealworm, Alphitobius diaperinus (Panzer). Poult Sci 74(1):45–49.

97. McFerran, J.B., M.S. McNulty, E.R. McKillop, T.J. Conner, R.M. McCracken, D.S. Collins, and G.M. Allan. 1980. Isolation and serological studies with infectious bursal disease viruses from fowl, turkey and duck: Demonstration of a second serotype. Avian Pathol 9:395–404.

98. McNulty, M.S., and Y.M. Saif. 1988. Antigenic relationship of non-serotype 1 turkey infectious bursal disease viruses. Avian Dis 32:374–375.

99. McNulty, M.S., G.M. Allan, and J.B. McFerran. 1979. Isolation of infectious bursal disease virus from turkeys. Avian Pathol 8:205–212.

100. Meroz, M. 1966. An epidemiological survey of Gumboro disease. Refu Vet 23:235–37.

101. Morgan, M.M., I.G. Macreadie, V.R. Harley, P.J. Hudson, and A.A. Azad. 1988. Sequence of the small double-stranded RNA genomic segment of infectious bursal disease virus and its deduced 90-K Da product. Virology 163:240–242.

102. Müller, H. 1986. Replication of infectious bursal disease virus in lymphoid cell. Arch Virol 87:191–203.

103. Müller, H., and H. Becht. 1982. Biosynthesis of virus-specific proteins in cells infected with infectious bursal disease virus and their significance as structural elements for infectious virus and incomplete particles. J Virol 44:384–392.

104. Müller, H., C. Scholtissek, and H. Becht. 1979. Genome of infectious bursal disease virus consists of two segments of double-stranded RNA. J Virol 31:584–589.

105. Müller, R., I. K. Weiss, M. Reinacher and E. Weiss. 1979. Immunofluorescent studies of early virus propagation after oral infection with infectious bursal disease virus (IBDV). Zentralbl Veterinaermed Med [B] 26:345–352.

106. Müller, H., H. Lange, and H. Becht. 1986. Formation, characterization and interfering capacity of a small plaque mutant and of incomplete virus particles of infectious bursal disease virus. Virus Res 4:297–309.

107. Mundt, E., J. Beyer, and H. Müller. 1995. Identification of a novel viral protein in infectious bursal disease virus-infected cells. J Gen Virol 76:437–443.

108. Nachimuthu, K., G.D. Raj, A. Thangavelu and R.A. Venkatesan. 1995. Reverse passive hemagglutination test in the diagnosis of infectious bursal disease. Trop Anim Health Prod 27:43–46.

109. Nagy, E., R. Duncan, P. Krell, and P. Dobos. 1987. Mapping of the large RNA genome segment of infectious pancreatic necrosis virus by hybrid arrested translation. Virology 158:211–217.

110. Nakai, T., and K. Hirai. 1981. In vitro infection of fractionated chicken lymphocytes by infectious bursal disease virus. Avian Dis 25:831–838.

111. Naqi, S.A., and D.L. Millar. 1979. Morphologic changes in the bursa of Fabricius of chickens after inoculation with infectious bursal disease virus. Am J Vet Res 40:1134–1139.

112. Nick, H., D. Cursiefen, and H. Becht. 1976. Structural and growth characteristics of infectious bursal disease virus. J Virol 18:227–234.

113. Nusbaum, K.E., P.D. Lukert, and O.J. Fletcher. 1988. Experimental infection of one-day-old poults with turkey isolates of infectious bursal disease virus. Avian Pathol 17:51–62

114. Okoye, J.O.A., and G.C. Okpe. 1989. The pathogenicity of an isolate of infectious bursal disease virus in guinea fowls. Acta Vet Brno 58:91–96.

115. Okoye, J.O.A., and U.E. Uche. 1986. Serological evidence of infectious bursal disease virus infection in wild rats. Acta Vet Brno 55:207–209.

116. Ozel, M., and H. Gelderblom. 1985. Capsid symmetry of viruses of the proposed birnavirus group. Arch Virol 84:149–161.

117. Page, R.K., O.J. Fletcher, P.D. Lukert, and R. Rimler. 1978. Rhinotracheitis in turkey poults. Avian Dis 22:529–534.

118. Panigrahy, B., L.K. Misra, S.A. Naqi, and C.F. Hall. 1977. Prolongation of skin allograft survival in chickens with infectious bursal disease. Poult Sci 56:1745.

119. Parkhurst, R.T. 1964. On-the-farm studies of Gumboro disease in broilers. Avian Dis 8:584–596.

120. Pattison, M., D.J. Alexander, and J.W. Harkness. 1975. Purification and preliminary characterization of a pathogenic strain of infectious bursal disease virus. Avian Pathol 4:175–187.

121. Pejkovski, C., F.G. Davelaar, and B. Kouwenhoven. 1979. Immunosuppressive effect of infectious bursal disease virus on vaccination against infectious bronchitis. Avian Pathol 8:95–106.

122. Perelman, B., and E.D. Heller. 1983. The ef-

fect of infectious bursal disease virus on the immune system of turkeys. Avian Dis 27:66–76.

123. Petek, M., P.N. D'Aprile, and F. Cancellotti. 1973. Biological and physicochemical properties of the infectious bursal disease virus (IBDV). Avian Pathol 2:135–152.

124. Peters, G. 1967. Histology of Gumboro disease. Berl Munch Tierarztl Wochenschr 80:394–396.

125. Rinaldi, A., G. Cervio, and G. Mandelli. 1965. Aspetti epidemiologici, anatomo-clinici ed istologici di una nuova forma morbosa dei polli verosimilmente identificabile con la considdetta Malattia di Gumboro. Atti Conv Patol Aviare. Societa Italiana de Patologia Aviare, pp. 77–83.

126. Rinaldi, A., E. Lodetti, D. Cessi, E. Lodrini, G. Cervio, and L. Nardelli. 1972. Coltura del virus de Gumboro (IBA) su fibroblast de embrioni di pollo. Nuova Vet 48:195–201.

127. Rosenberger, J.K., and S.S. Cloud. 1985. Isolation and characterization of variant infectious bursal disease viruses [abst]. J Am Vet Med Assoc 189:357.

128. Rosenberger, J.K., and S.S. Cloud. 1986. Isolation and characterization of variant infectious bursal disease viruses [abst]. J Am Vet Med Assoc 189:357.

129. Rosenberger, J.K., and J. Gelb, Jr. 1978. Response to several avian respiratory viruses as affected by infectious bursal disease virus. Avian Dis 22:95–105.

130. Rosenberger, J.K., S. Klopp, R.J. Eckroade, and W.C. Krauss. 1975. The role of the infectious bursal agent and several avian adenoviruses in the hemorrhagic-aplastic-anemia syndrome and gangrenous dermatitis. Avian Dis 19:717–729.

131. Rosenberger, J.K., S.S. Cloud, J. Gelb, Jr., E. Odor, and J.E. Dohms. 1985. Sentinel bird survey of Delmarva broiler flocks. Proc 20th Natl Meet Poult Health Condemn, Ocean City, MD, pp. 94–101.

132. Rosenberger, J.K., S.S. Cloud, and A. Metz. 1987. Use of infectious bursal disease virus variant vaccines in broilers and broiler breeders. Proc 36th West Poult Dis Conf, pp. 105–109.

133. Saif, Y.M. 1984. Infectious bursal disease virus types. Proc 19th Natl Meet Poult Health Condemn, Ocean City, MD, pp. 105–107.

134. Saif, Y.M. 1988. Unpublished data.

135. Saif, Y.M. 1995. Unpublished data.

136. Sharma, J.M. 1984. Effect of infectious bursal disease virus on protection against Marek's disease by turkey herpes virus vaccine. Avian Dis 28:629–640.

137. Sharma, J.M. and L.F. Lee. 1983. Effect of infectious bursal disease virus on natural killer cell activity and mitogenic response of chicken lymphoid cells: Role of adherent cells in cellular immune suppression. Infect Immun 42:747–754.

138. Sharma, J.M., J.E. Dohms, and A.L. Metz. 1989. Comparative pathogenesis of serotype 1 and variant serotype 1 isolates of infectious bursal disease virus and the effect of those viruses on humoral and cellular immune competence of specific pathogen free on chickens. Avian Dis 33:112–124.

139. Shirai, J., R. Seki, R. Kamimura, and S. Mitsubayashi. 1994. Effects of invert soap with 0.05% sodium hydroxide on infectious bursal disease virus. Avian Dis 38:240–243.

140. Sivanandan, V., and S.K. Maheswaran. 1980. Immune profile of infectious bursal disease. I. Effect of infectious bursal disease virus on peripheral blood T and B lymphocytes in chickens. Avian Dis 24:715–725.

141. Sivanandan, V., and S.K. Maheswaran. 1980. Immune profile of infectious bursal disease (IBD). II. Effect of IBD virus on pokeweed-mitogen-stimulated peripheral blood lymphocytes of chickens. Avian Dis 24:734–742.

142. Sivanandan, V., and S.K. Maheswaran. 1981. Immune profile of infectious bursal disease. III. Effect of infectious bursal disease virus on the lymphocyte responses to phytomitogens and on mixed lymphocyte reaction of chickens. Avian Dis 25:112–120.

143. Sivanandan, V., J. Sasipreeyajan, D.A. Halvorson, and J.A. Newman. 1986. Histopathologic changes induced by serotype II infectious bursal disease virus in specific-pathogen-free chickens. Avian Dis 30:709–715.

144. Skeeles, J.K., and P.D. Lukert. 1980. Studies with an attenuated cell-culture-adapted infectious bursal disease virus: Replication sites and persistence of the virus in specific-pathogen-free chickens. Avian Dis 24:43–47.

145. Skeeles, J.K., P.D. Lukert, E.V. De Buysscher, O.J. Fletcher, and J. Brown. 1979. Infectious bursal disease virus infections. I. Complement and virus-neutralizing antibody response following infection of susceptible chickens. Avian Dis 23:95–106.

146. Skeeles, J.K., P.D. Lukert, E.V. De Buysscher, O.J. Fletcher, and J. Brown. 1979. Infectious bursal disease virus infections. II. The relationship of age, complement levels, virus-neutralizing antibody, clotting and lesions. Avian Dis 23:107–117.

147. Skeeles, J.K., P.D. Lukert, O.J. Fletcher, and J.D. Leonard. 1979. Immunization studies with a cell-culture-adapted infectious bursal disease virus. Avian Dis 23:456–465.

148. Skeeles, J.K., M.F. Slavik, J.N. Beasley, A.H. Brown, C.F. Meinecke, S. Maruca, and S. Welch. 1980. An age-related coagulation disorder associated with experimental infection with infectious bursal disease virus. Am J Vet Res 41:1458–1461.

149. Snedeker, C., F.K. Wills, and I.M. Moulthrop. 1967. Some studies on the infectious bursal agent. Avian Dis 11:519–528.

150. Snyder, D.B., W.W. Marquardt, E.T. Mallinson, E. Russek-Cohen, P. K. Savage, and D.C. Allen. 1986. Rapid serological profiling by enzyme-linked immunosorbent assay. IV. Association of infectious bursal disease serology with broiler flock performance. Avian Dis 30:139–148.

151. Snyder, D.B., D.P. Lana, B.R. Cho, and W.W. Marquardt. 1988. Group and strain-specific neutralization sites of infectious bursal disease virus defined with monoclonal antibodies. Avian Dis 32:527–534.

152. Snyder, D.B., D.P. Lana, P.K. Savage, F.S. Yancey, S.A. Mengel, and W.W. Marquardt. 1988. Differentiation of infectious bursal disease viruses directly from infected tissues with neutralizing monoclonal antibodies: Evidence of a major antigenic shift in recent field isolates. Avian Dis 32:535–539.

153. Snyder, D.B., V.N. Vakharia, S.A. Mengel-Whereat, G.H. Edwards, P.K. Savage, D. Lutticken, and M.A. Goodwin. 1994. Active cross-protection induced by a recombinant baculovirus expressing chimeric infectious bursal disease virus structural proteins. Avian Dis 38:701–707.

154. Solano, W., J.J. Giambrone, and V.S. Panangala. 1985. Comparison of a kinetic-based enzyme-linked immunosorbent assay (KELISA) and virus-neutralization test for infectious bursal disease virus. I. Quantitation of antibody in white leghorn hens. Avian Dis 29:662–671.

155. Spies, U., H. Müller, and H. Becht. 1987. Properties of RNA polymerase activity associated

with infectious bursal disease virus and characterization of its reaction products. Virus Res 8:127–140.

156. Steger, D., H. Müller, and D. Riesner. 1980. Helix-core transitions in double-stranded viral RNA: Fine resolution melting and ionic strength dependence. Biochem Biophys Acta 606:274–285.

157. Survashe, B.D., I.D. Aitken, and J.R. Powell. 1979. The response of the harderian gland of the fowl to antigen given by the ocular route. I. Histological changes. Avian Pathol 8:77–93.

158. Tanimura, N., K. Tsukamoto, K. Nakamura, M. Narita and M. Maeda. 1995. Association between pathogenicity of infectious bursal disease virus and viral antigen distribution detected by immunochemistry. Avian Dis 39:9–20.

159. Tham, K.M., L.W. Young, and C.D. Moon. 1995. Detection of infectious bursal disease virus by reverse transcription-polymerase chain reaction amplification of the virus segment A gene. J Virol Methods 53:201–212.

160. Thayer, S.G., P. Villegas, and O.J. Fletcher. 1987. Comparison of two commercial enzyme-linked immunosorbent assays and conventional methods for avian serology. Avian Dis 31:120–124.

161. Todd, D., and M.S. McNulty. 1979. Biochemical studies with infectious bursal disease virus: Comparison of some of its properties with infectious pancreatic necrosis virus. Arch Virol 60:265–277.

162. Tsai, H.J. and Y.M. Saif 1992. Effect of cell-culture passage on the pathogenicity and immunogenicity of infectious bursal disease virus. Avian Dis 36:415–422.

163. Tsukamoto, K., T. Matsumura, M. Mase, and K. Imai. 1995. A highly sensitive, broad-spectrum infectivity assay for infectious bursal disease virus. Avian Dis 39:575–586.

164. Ture, O. and Y.M. Saif. 1992. Structural proteins of classic and variant strains of infectious bursal disease viruses. Avian Dis 36:829–836.

165. Ture, O., H.J. Tsai and Y.M. Saif. 1993. Studies on antigenic relatedness of classic and variant strains of infectious bursal disease virus. Avian Dis 37:647–654.

166. Vakharia, V.N., D.B. Snyder, J. He, G.H. Edwards, P.K. Savage, and S.A. Mengel-Whereat. 1993. Infectious bursal disease virus structural proteins expressed in a baculovirus recombinant confer protection in chickens. J Gen Virol 74:1201–1206.

167. Vakharia, V.N., D.B. Snyder, D. Lutticken, S. A. Mengel-Whereat, P.K. Savage, G.H. Edwards, and M.A. Goodwin. 1994. Active and passive protection against variant and classic infectious bursal disease virus strains induced by baculovirus expressed structural proteins. Vaccine 12:452–456.

168. Van den Berg, T.P., M. Gonze and G. Meulemans. 1991. Acute infectious bursal disease in poultry: Isolation and characterization of a highly virulent strain. Avian Pathol 20:133–143.

169. Weisman, J., and S.B. Hitchner. 1978. Infectious bursal disease virus infection attempts in turkeys and coturnix quail. Avian Dis 22:604–609.

170. Winterfield, R.W. 1969. Immunity response to the infectious bursal agent. Avian Dis 13:548–557.

171. Winterfield, R.W., and S.B. Hitchner. 1962. Etiology of an infectious nephritis-nephrosis syndrome of chickens. Am J Vet Res 23:1273–1279.

172. Winterfield, R.W., S.B. Hitchner, G.S. Appleton, and A.S. Cosgrove. 1962. Avian nephrosis, nephritis and Gumboro disease. L & M News Views 3:103.

173. Woolcock, P.R., R.P. Chin, and Y.M. Saif. 1995. Personal communication.

174. Wyeth, P.J. 1975. Effect of infectious bursal disease on the response of chickens to S. typhimurium and E. coli infections. Vet Rec 96:238–243.

175. Wyeth, P.J., and G.A. Cullen. 1978. Transmission of immunity from inactivated infectious bursal disease oil-emulsion vaccinated parent chickens to their chicks. Vet Rec 102:362–363.

176. Wyeth, P.J., and G.A. Cullen. 1979. The use of an inactivated infectious bursal disease oil emulsion vaccine in commercial broiler parent chickens. Vet Rec 104:188–193.

177. Yamaguchi, S., I. Imada, and H. Kawamura. 1981. Growth and infectivity titration of virulent infectious bursal disease virus in established cell lines from lymphoid leucosis. Avian Dis 25:927–935.

178. Yuasa, N., T. Taniguchi, T. Noguchi, and I. Yoshida. 1980. Effect of infectious bursal disease virus infection on incidence of anemia by chicken anemia agent. Avian Dis 24:202–209.

30 Chicken Infectious Anemia

V. von Bülow and Karel A. Schat

INTRODUCTION. Chicken infectious anemia (CIA), a disease of young chickens, is caused by a unique small virus (46, 60, 76, 109, 157, 183). The disease is characterized by aplastic anemia and generalized lymphoid atrophy with a concomitant immunosuppression. Consequently, CIA is frequently complicated by secondary viral, bacterial, or fungal infections. The virus appears to play a major role in the etiology of a number of multifactorial diseases associated with hemorrhagic syndrome and/or aplastic anemia. CIA and closely associated syndromes have commonly been termed *hemorrhagic syndrome* (189), *anemia-dermatitis* (168), or *blue wing disease* (5, 39).

Terminology for the disease and the causative agent has varied. The agent was originally designated chicken anemia agent (CAA) (183), but after morphologic and biochemical characterization (46, 109, 157), it was renamed chicken anemia virus (CAV) (46, 118). Because the disease is commonly referred to as chicken infectious anemia, however, the causative virus is more logically referred to as chicken infectious anemia virus (CIAV). This terminology has been chosen for use in this chapter.

Chicken infectious anemia virus infection has been confirmed as the cause of disease in several cases in which syndromes suggestive of infectious anemia occurred in chicken flocks at 2–4 wk of age (17, 21, 32, 38, 59, 72, 91, 105, 135, 141, 148, 168, 173, 189). Growth was retarded and mortality was generally between 10 and 20%, but occasionally it reached 60%.

Therefore, CIAV-induced disease constitutes a serious economic threat, especially to the broiler industry (99). In chickens 6 or more wk of age, the etiologic significance of CIAV infection associated with aplastic anemia-hemorrhagic syndromes (58, 125, 186) has not definitely been established.

Chicken infectious anemia virus infection has only been recognized in chickens. Results of serologic tests (16) suggest that the virus has no public health significance.

HISTORY. Chicken infectious anemia virus (Gifu-1 strain) was first isolated in 1979 in Japan by Yuasa et al. (183). A major breakthrough was achieved in 1983 by Yuasa (175), who showed that CIAV, which does not replicate in any of the con- ventional monolayer cell cultures, is cytopathogenic for cultures of certain lymphoblastoid chicken cell lines, e.g., MDCC-MSB1 (MSB1). This enabled virus-neutralization (VN) tests to be performed in vitro (187) rather than in vivo (183), and it facilitated more extensive virologic studies. Moreover, the availability of CIAV-infected MSB1 cells made it feasible to detect anti-CIAV antibody in chicken serum or egg yolk by indirect immunofluorescence tests (19, 188), and to purify the virus from supernatant fluids of CIAV-infected cell cultures (46, 60, 76, 109, 157).

Virus identification was followed by studies that unraveled much of the pathogenesis and epizootiology of the infection. In the early 1990s, remarkable progress was made in research on the molecular biology of CIAV, as recently reviewed by Noteborn and Koch (117). This resulted in the development of refined diagnostic methods and new types of vaccines (89).

Aplastic anemia syndromes, including inclusion-body hepatitis, were described many years before CIAV was detected. Their possible etiologic association with CIAV infection has been reviewed and discussed in several papers dealing with CIA (14, 61, 102, 136, 189).

INCIDENCE AND DISTRIBUTION. Chicken infectious anemia virus appears to be ubiquitous in all major chicken-producing countries of the world. It has been isolated from chickens in Japan (58, 59, 125, 180, 183, 186, 189), European countries (18, 21, 27, 37, 38, 43, 72, 106, 118, 135), the United States (47, 91, 94, 105, 141), South America (9, 25, 164), China (93), Australia (32, 44), New Zealand (148), and South Africa (174). Furthermore, serologic evidence of widespread infection has been found with chicken sera from many countries all over the world (48, 82, 84, 94, 103, 104, 115, 165, 177, 188).

ETIOLOGY

Classification. Chicken infectious anemia virus has not yet been assigned to a specific virus family. Because it shares the characteristic of having circular, single-stranded DNA (see Virus DNA) with two other small animal viruses, porcine circovirus (PCV) (156) and psittacine beak and feather disease virus (PBFDV) (139), Lukert et al. (96) proposed placing these three viruses in a new virus family tentatively named *Circoviridae*. Noteborn and Koch (117) suggested, however, that CIAV belongs in its own novel virus family based on differences from PCV and PBFDV in terms of size, morphology, buoyant density, and sedimentation coefficient; the lack of DNA sequence similarities and the absence of shared antigenic determinants; and differences in transcriptional regulation (4, 119, 134, 159).

Morphology and Physical Properties.

Chicken infectious anemia virus virions consist of nonenveloped, icosahedral particles with an average diameter of 25 to 26.5 nm, as observed in preparations negatively stained with 1% uranyl acetate (46, 109). Based on threefold and fivefold rotational symmetry of the viral capsids, two types of virus particles are commonly detected. Type I particles show a pattern of one central hollow surrounded by six neighboring hollows with a center-to-center distance of 7.5 nm, forming a regular surface network (Fig. 30.1A). This arrangement suggests a regular T = 3 icosahedron with 32 morphologic subunits. Type II particles are characterized by 10 evenly spaced surface protrusions giving the impression of a cog-wheel structure (Fig 30.1B) (46, 109).

Thin sections of CIAV-infected MSB-1 cells, reacted with CIAV-specific monoclonal antibodies (mAb) and gold-labeled goat anti-mouse IgG, demonstrated the presence of intranuclear inclusions, often with a typical doughnut shape. In a mi-

nority of cells, virus particles were detected in the cytoplasm in association with microtubules (109).

Virions have a buoyant density in cesium chloride gradients variously reported as 1.33–1.34 g/mL (4, 157) or between 1.35 and 1.37 g/mL (46, 60). The sedimentation coefficient of CIAV has an estimated value of 91S in isokinetic sucrose gradients (4).

Virus DNA. The genome of CIAV consists of single-stranded, circular, covalently linked DNA (46, 157). The sequences of the Cux-1 and other isolates have been determined (29, 86, 111, 118, 138). The replicative form of the viral genome consists of 2298 or 2319 bp depending on the presence or absence of four or five 21-bp repeats. Most CIAV strains have four repeats, with a 12-bp insert in the middle. Todd et al. (163) reported that the fifth repeat was obtained after about 30 passages of the Cux-1 strain in MSB1 cells. In infected cells, both single-stranded and double-stranded DNA are present, but the virion contains only the circular minus-strand DNA (118, 134). In general, most strains analyzed thus far have been very similar, but some sequence differences between strains have been described. Todd et al. (161) assigned CIAV isolates to seven groups based on restriction-enzyme analysis of a polymerase chain reaction (PCR)-amplified 675-bp fragment coding for the N-terminal half of ORF3. It is not clear whether these groups differ biologically. In some instances, however, nucleotide differences result in changes in amino acid composition that would alter the predicted protein structure (138, 147).

Thus far, all sequenced strains have three par-

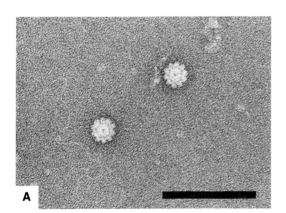
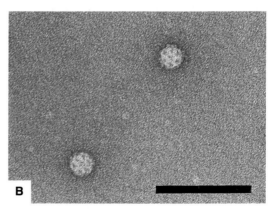

30.1. Electron micrographs of chicken infectious anemia virus (CIAV). Different structural aspects of the CIAV capsids become apparent in negative-stained preparations. Two types of particle projections are obvious. *A.* Particle projection type II characterized by 10 peripheral protrusions. ×250,000. Bar = 100 nm. (Gelderblom) *B.* Projection type I showing CIAV capsids that exhibit six stain-filled morphologic units that surround one central hole.

tially overlapping open reading frames (ORFs) coding for putative proteins of 52 (ORF1), 24 (ORF2) and 13 kDa (ORF3), one promoter region, and one polyadenylation signal. The Japanese strain CAA82-2 contains a fourth open reading frame (ORF4) (86), but its function has not been established. ORF3 is located within ORF2, while ORF2 partly overlaps ORF1. The promoter-enhancer region containing the 21-bp direct repeats is located upstream of ORF2. The repeat units and the 12-bp insert bind to different transcription factors of chicken T cells. Optimal transcription requires the binding of the transcription factors to both the direct repeats and the 12-bp insert (122). Deletion of the first two direct repeats reduces transcriptional activity by 40 to 50% (134). Only one unspliced, polycistronic mRNA of 2100 bases is produced, coding for the three ORFs. The use of internal AUG start codons for the synthesis of the 52-kDa and 13-kDa proteins is unique for DNA viruses (119, 134).

Viral Proteins and Antigens.   A 50-kDa viral protein (VP1) is commonly found in highly purified virus particles (157). This protein is probably the major capsid protein. The N-terminal 40 amino acids show a limited similarity to histone proteins, suggesting a DNA binding role perhaps with the virus capsid (29, 111). In addition, a 30-kDa protein (VP2) also has been associated with virions (11). The function of this protein has not yet been established. The third viral protein, VP3 (16 kDa), is associated with infected cells (26) but not with highly purified virus particles (11). VP3, also named apoptin, is a strong inducer of apoptosis in chicken thymocytes and chicken lymphoblastoid cell lines (121) as well as several malignant human lymphoblastoid cell lines (191) and human osteosarcoma cells (192). Truncated apoptin lacking the last 11 amino acids is unable to induce apoptosis. Intact VP3 is essential for the virus replication cycle (121).

Studies using neutralizing mAbs in Western blots suggest that the neutralizing epitope(s) is conformational in nature and may consist of VP1 and VP2 components (11). Support for this hypothesis was provided by Koch et al. (88, 89) in studies using recombinant baculovirus products. Neutralizing antibodies were induced after inoculation of chickens with insect cells containing both VP1 and VP2, but not cells containing only VP1 or VP2.

Virus Replication.   Virions probably enter the cell by conventional absorption and penetration. Low levels of the 2.0-kb polycistronic viral RNA transcript can be demonstrated at 8 hr postinfection of MSB-1 cells, with maximum levels attained at 48 hr (119, 134). In addition, a minor 4.0 kb transcript has been detected (134). VP3 can be detected at 6 hr, while VP2 is present at 12 hr postinfection. The capsid protein VP1 was not detectable until 30 hr postinfection (162). DNA replication probably occurs by the rolling-circle model (111).

In chickens, CIAV appears to replicate primarily in hematopoietic precursor cells in the bone marrow and in thymic precursor cells in the thymus cortex, where it has been shown to cause cell death by apoptosis (80).

Strain Classification.   No antigenic differences have been recognized among various Japanese, European, and American isolates of CAA using polyclonal chicken antibodies (13, 19, 38, 180). As a consequence, it is generally accepted that all strains belong to one serotype (102, 117); however, based on differences in reaction patterns with mAbs (108) and DNA sequence differences resulting in changes in the predicted protein folding patterns (138), it is expected that strains may differ in their pathogenicity.

Resistance to Chemical and Physical Agents.   Chicken infectious anemia virus is resistant to ethyl ether and chloroform and is stable at pH 3 for 3 hr. It is also resistant to treatment with 90% acetone for 24 hr (152). As a consequence, acetone-fixed slides of CIAV material may remain infectious and need to be sterilized prior to final disposal. In liver suspensions, CIAV is inactivated after treatment with 50% phenol for 5 min (183), but not after treatment with 5% phenol for 2 hr at 37 C. Treatment of liver suspensions with 0.1 N NaOH for 2 hr at 37 C or 24 hr at 15 C does not inactivate CIAV completely, but treatment with 1% glutaraldehyde for 10 min at room temperature (RT), 0.4% ß-propiolactone 24 hr at 4 C, or 5% formaldehyde 24 hr at RT inactivates the virus completely (178). Commercial disinfectants based on invert soap, amphoteric soap, or orthodichlorobenzene are not effective against CIAV. Treatments with iodine or hypochlorite are effective but require 2 hr at 37 C with final concentrations of 10% rather than the generally recommended concentrations of 2%. Formaldehyde or ethylene oxide fumigation for 24 hr does not inactivate CIAV completely (178).

Although CIAV is resistant to heating at 56 C or 70 C for 1 hr and at 80 C for 15 min (38, 58, 183), it is only partially resistant to heating at 80 C for 30 min, and it is completely inactivated within 15 min at 100 C (58). Inactivation of CIAV in infected chicken byproducts requires a core temperature of 95 C for 35 min or 100 C for 10 min (166).

Laboratory Host Systems.   Chicken infectious anemia virus can be propagated and assayed in 1-day-old chicks, in cell cultures, or in chicken embryos.

CHICKENS. One-day-old chicks inoculated with CIAV develop anemia and gross lesions in lymphoid tissues and bone marrow. These are most pronounced after 12–16 days (183). Mortality occurs between 12 and 28 days postinoculation and usually remains low, rarely exceeding 30%. Response to CIAV infection is enhanced by simultaneous inoculation of Marek's disease virus (MDV) or by treatment with betamethasone (20, 21, 23, 126), or by the use of embryonally bursectomized chicks (94). Chicks with maternal anti-CIAV antibody are resistant to CIAV infection (184).

CHICKEN EMBRYOS. Propagation of CIAV in chicken embryos following yolk sac inoculation has been reported by Bülow and Witt (17). Moderate virus yields were obtained after 14 days from all parts of the embryo, but not from yolk or chorioallantoic membrane. Lesions were not observed after inoculation with the Gifu-1 and Cux-1 strains of CIAV. Some strains, however, may cause significant embryo mortality between the 16th and 20th days of incubation. The GL-1 strain caused up to 50% mortality with embryos being small, hemorrhagic, and edematous (91).

CELL CULTURES. Yuasa (175) found cultures of the T-cell lymphoblastoid cell lines MDCC-MSB1 and MDCC-JP2 and the B-cell lymphoblastoid cell line LSCC-1104B1 to be suitable for propagation and assay of CIAV. Many other T-cell and B-cell lymphoblastoid cell lines, whether producers or nonproducers of the respective transforming viruses, turned out to be resistant to CIAV (21, 175). Also, cell cultures derived from a large variety of tissues of chickens and chicken embryos proved to be resistant to CIAV infection (175).

MSB1 cell cultures are presently preferred for in vitro cultivation, although sublines of MSB1 differ in their susceptibility to infection. Certain strains of CIAV, e.g., CIA-1 (94), may not replicate at all in one subline of MSB1 and poorly in another subline of MSB1, while both sublines are susceptible to infection with Cux-1 (138, 140, 147). Cell-associated infectivity peaks between about 36 and 42 hr after inoculation, coinciding with the maximum amount of intranuclear antigens detected by immunofluorescence. Cell-free titers peak at 48–72 hr after inoculation, and the rate of multiplication has been reported to range between 10- and 100-fold (19, 175). Virus titrations require subculturing of inoculated cells every 2–4 days until cells inoculated with the endpoint dilution of CIAV are destroyed.

Pathogenicity. Virulence of CIAV isolates may vary slightly based on the degree of age-resistance of the chicks being infected (180). Attenuation of CIAV by serial passage in cell culture has been reported; however, it is possible that a decrease in infectivity and immunogenicity in vivo was correlated with the attenuation (15). Todd et al. (163) found that Cux-1 became substantially less pathogenic after 173 passages in MSB1 cells. Attenuation resulted in genetically diverse virus populations. Molecularly cloned isolates from attenuated virus were, indeed, less pathogenic than the original isolate, but the attenuation may not be stable. One isolate reverted back to pathogenicity after 10 passages in young chicks.

PATHOGENESIS AND EPIZOOTIOLOGY

Natural and Experimental Hosts. The chicken is the only known host for CIAV. All ages are susceptible to infection, but susceptibility to disease rapidly decreases in immunologically intact chicks during the first 1–3 wk of life (58, 142, 180, 183, 185).

Antibodies to CIAV have not been detected in turkey or duck sera (103). Turkey poults inoculated at 1 day of age with high doses of the virus were resistant to infection and did not develop antibodies to CIAV (102).

Transmission. Chicken infectious anemia virus spreads both horizontally and vertically. Vertical transmission through the hatching egg is considered to be the most important means of dissemination (27, 69). Embryo infection also can be caused by semen of infected cocks (70).

Egg transmission only occurred from 8–14 days after experimental infection of hens (182), but field observations indicated that vertical transmission could occur during a period of 3–9 wk after exposure, with a peak at 1–3 wk, obviously depending on the rate of spread of infection and development of immunity to CIAV (5, 27, 39, 168).

The virus is present at high concentrations in the feces of chickens for 5–7 wk after infection (69, 187). Horizontal infection by direct or indirect contact most likely occurs via the oral route, but infection via the respiratory route as shown in experimentally infected chicks (142) may also be possible in the field. Chicken infectious anemia virus spreads easily among chickens in a group (185). In field flocks naturally exposed to CIAV, it commonly takes 2–4 wk until most birds have seroconverted (13, 103).

Incubation Period. In experimental infections, anemia and distinct histologic lesions can first be detected at 8 days after parenteral inoculation of virus. Clinical signs generally develop after 10–14 days, and mortality occurs beginning at 12–14 days after inoculation (61, 151, 183). It may, however, be more than 14–21 days before anemia develops, presumably depending on the genetic strain of experimental chicks and the properties of the inoculated virus strain (142).

Under field conditions, congenitally infected chicks show clinical signs and increased mortality beginning at 10–12 days of age, with a peak at 17–24 days (27, 39, 59, 83, 168). In heavily infected flocks, there can be a second peak of mortality at 30–34 days (39, 83), probably due to horizontal infection.

Clinical Signs.   The only specific sign of CIAV infection is anemia, with a peak at 14–16 days postinoculation. Anemia is characterized by hematocrit values ranging from 6 to 27%. Affected birds are depressed and more or less pale. Weight gain is depressed between 10 and 20 days after experimental infection. Affected birds may die between 12 and 28 days postinoculation. If mortality does occur, it does not exceed 30%. Surviving chicks completely recover from depression and anemia by 20–28 days after infection (21, 58, 142, 150, 183), although retarded recovery and increased mortality may be associated with secondary bacterial or viral infections. Secondary infections causing more severe clinical signs are frequently seen in field cases, but they may also occur inadvertently in experimental chicks (21, 40, 59, 168).

Morbidity and Mortality.   The outcome of CIAV infection is influenced by a number of viral, host, and environmental factors. Uncomplicated infectious anemia, especially if caused by horizontal infection, may result in nothing more than slightly increased mortality and transient poor performance of affected flocks, and, therefore, it could even go unobserved in commercial settings.

Maternal antibodies to CIAV (see Immunity) confer virtually complete protection against the disease (142, 184). Resistance due to passive immunity, however, can be at least partly overcome if chicks are immunosuppressed, e.g., by other viral infections (20, 23, 142).

Morbidity and mortality may be influenced by the virulence of the CIAV strain. The TK-5803 strain described by Goryo et al. (58) appears to be more virulent than either of the isolates studied by Yuasa and Imai (180). Dosage may have an effect on the severity of anemia or the proportion of affected chicks (107, 142, 183). The route of infection also plays a role in experimental infection, since infection by contact usually does not cause anemia in immunologically intact chicks, in contrast to the situation in immunologically compromised birds (142, 185). Oral, nasal, or ocular infection routes are much less effective than parenteral inoculation in inducing disease (142, 176).

In immunologically competent chicks, age resistance develops rapidly during the 1st wk of life and becomes complete by 3 wk or even earlier, depending on the virulence of the infecting CIAV strain (58, 142, 180, 185). Development of age resistance appears to be closely associated with the ability of the chicken to produce antibodies against the virus (180, 185). It is considerably delayed by immunosuppression, e.g., by simultaneous infection with infectious bursal disease virus (IBDV) (142, 185) or by bursectomy (73, 190). Circumstantial evidence indicates that commercial broiler chickens may become infected by horizontal transmission by 2–3 wk of age, after disappearance of maternal antibodies, resulting in poor performance due to subclinical effects of CIAV infection (110). This, however, could not be confirmed by others (56, 85).

Morbidity and mortality are considerably enhanced if chicks are dually infected with CIAV and MDV, reticuloendotheliosis virus (REV), or IBDV, probably due to virus-induced immunosuppression (18, 20, 21, 30, 129, 142, 185). Certain strains of reovirus also can be immunosuppressive in chickens (112, 113, 144), which may explain the enhanced pathogenicity of CIAV in the presence of reovirus as reported by Engström et al. (40). Chemical immunosuppression by betamethasone or cyclosporin A also aggravates signs and lesions (23). In field infections, various environmental and other factors causing a decrease of immunocompetence have, therefore, been suspected to enhance CIAV pathogenicity.

Nothing is known about genetic factors that might affect the outcome of CIAV infection. The disease occurs most frequently in broiler chickens, which could well be due to a variety of other factors.

Gross Lesions.   Thymic atrophy is the most consistent lesion (Fig. 30.2A), but bone marrow atrophy is the most characteristic lesion seen in affected chickens (Fig. 30.2B). Femoral bone marrow is fatty and yellowish or pink. In some instances, its color appears dark red, although distinct lesions can be detected by histologic examination. Thymic atrophy may result in an almost complete regression of the organ, which then has a dark reddish brown color. As infected chicks develop age resistance, thymic atrophy may become a much more consistent lesion than grossly visible bone marrow lesions (58, 81). Bursal atrophy is less obvious. In a small proportion of birds, the size of the bursa of Fabricius may be reduced. In many cases, the outer bursal wall appears translucent, so plicae become visible. Hemorrhages in the proventricular mucosa, and subcutaneous and muscular hemorrhages are sometimes associated with severe anemia (21, 58, 141, 150, 151). More pronounced hemorrhages or bursal atrophy, and lesions in other tissues, e.g., swollen and mottled livers, have also been reported but are likely to be associated with secondary infections with other agents.

HEMORRHAGIC-APLASTIC ANEMIA SYNDROME. Outbreaks of infectious anemia in field flocks are mostly associated with so-called hemorrhagic syndrome, with or without concurrent (gangrenous) dermatitis (Fig. 30.2C) (5, 8, 27, 35, 37, 39, 45, 67, 68, 137, 143, 148, 168, 189). Circumstantial evidence suggests that CIAV is also involved in the etiology of aplastic anemia associated with inclusion body hepatitis (see Chapter 23), with or without concurrent hemorrhagic syndrome and gangrenous dermatitis (33, 41, 64, 65, 66, 90, 114, 133). Infectious bursal disease virus is considered to be of particular importance among the factors that can enhance the severity of these syndromes (143). Hemorrhages seen in chickens with infectious bursal disease (see Chapter 29) may, in most instances, be a sequel of CIAV rather than IBDV infection.

Characteristic lesions of so-called hemorrhagic syndrome are intracutaneous, subcutaneous, and intramuscular hemorrhages (Figs. 30.2D,E). Punctuate hemorrhages may be present even more frequently in the mucosa of the distal part of the proventriculus (Fig. 30.2F). Intracutaneous or subcutaneous hemorrhages of the wings are often complicated by severe edema and subsequent dermatitis, which may become gangrenous due to bacterial infection (see Chapter 12). Subcutaneous hemorrhage of shanks and feet may result in formation of ulcers. Affected chicks also sometimes appear to be predisposed to develop pododermatitis (see Chapter 35).

Hemorrhages are not consistently seen in anemic chicks, although their occurrence is mostly correlated with the severity of anemia. Increased clotting time associated with thrombocytopenia, therefore, does not completely explain hemorrhages. Endothelial lesions and impaired liver functions, partly caused by viral infection and enhanced by secondary bacterial infection are likely to be more important in the pathogenesis of hemorrhagic diathesis.

Histopathology. Histopathologic changes in anemic chicks have been characterized as panmyelophthisis and generalized lymphoid atrophy (20, 21, 61, 136, 150, 151).

In the bone marrow, atrophy and aplasia involve all compartments and hematopoietic lineages (Fig. 30.3). Necrosis of residual small cell foci may occasionally be seen. Hematopoietic cells are replaced by adipose tissue or proliferating stroma cells. Regenerative areas consisting of proerythroblasts appear 16–18 days after experimental infection, and there is a hyperplasia of bone marrow between 24

and 32 days postinoculation in birds that recover.

Severe lymphoid depletion is seen in the thymus, bursa of Fabricius, and spleen and cecal tonsils, as well as in a wide range of other tissues. The thymus cortex and medulla become equally atrophic, with hydropic degeneration of residual cells and occasional necrotic foci (Fig. 30.4). In chicks that recover, repopulation of the thymus with lymphocytes becomes distinct at 20–24 days, and the morphology returns to normal by 32–36 days after infection.

Lesions in the bursa of Fabricius consist of atrophy of the lymphoid follicles with occasional small necrotic foci, infolded epithelium, hydropic epithelial degeneration, and proliferation of reticular cells (Fig. 30.5). Repopulation of lymphocytes until complete recovery is similar to that in the thymus.

In the spleen, atrophy of lymphoid tissue with hyperplasia of reticular cells is seen in the lymphoid follicles as well as in the Schweigger-Seidl sheaths. Necrotic foci in follicles or sheaths have rarely been observed.

In the liver, kidneys, lungs, proventriculus, duodenum, and cecal tonsils, lymphoid foci are depleted of cells, making them smaller and less dense than those in unaffected birds. Liver cells are swollen, and hepatic sinusoids may be dilated.

Small eosinophilic nuclear inclusions have been detected in altered, enlarged cells of affected tissues, predominantly in the thymus and bone marrow, where they are most frequent at 5–7 days after experimental infection (61, 145).

Hematology. Blood of severely affected chicks is more or less watery, the clotting time is increased, and the blood plasma is paler than normal. Hematocrit values begin to drop below 27% at 8–10 days after inoculation, are mostly in the range of 10–20% at 14–20 days, and may even drop to 6% in moribund birds. In convalescent chicks, hematocrit values increase after 16–21 days and return to normal (29–35%) by 28–32 days postinfection (61, 141, 151, 183). Anemia is commonly defined as a hematocrit value of less than or equal to 27%, but a limit of 25% also may be appropriate (141, 142). The definition of anemia may vary with the age and genetic constitution of chickens (49, 52, 54, 55).

Low hematocrit values in CIAV-infected chickens are due to a pancytopenia (150, 151, 183) with markedly decreased numbers of erythrocytes, white blood cells, and thrombocytes. Anisocytosis has been noticed as early as 8 days postinfection. Juvenile forms of erythrocytes, granulocytes, and thrombocytes begin to appear in the peripheral blood by 16 days after inoculation, and the incidence of immature erythrocytes may exceed 30% several days later. The blood picture in convalescent chicks returns to normal by 40 days (151).

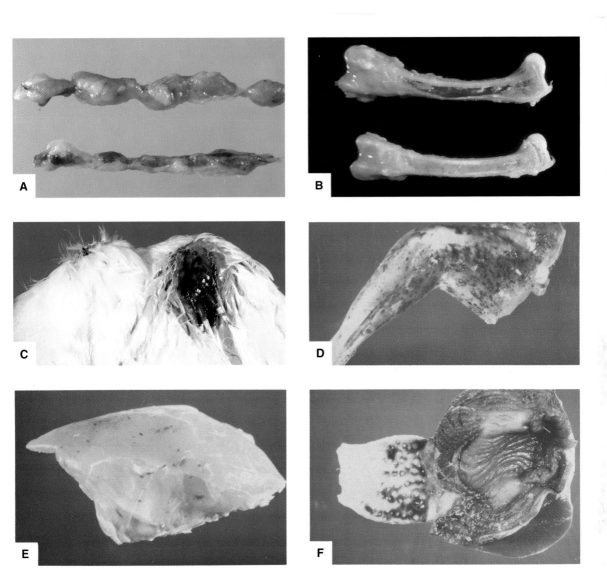

30.2. Lesions in chickens associated with chicken infectious anemia and hemorrhagic anemia disease. *A.* Control thymus (*top*) and thymus with chicken infectious anemia virus (CIAV)–induced atrophy (*bottom*), 14 days postinoculation with the CIA-1 strain of CIAV. (Lucio and Shivaprasad). *B.* Femur with normal dark red bone marrow (*top*) and femur with pale aplastic bone marrow (*bottom*), 14 days postinoculation with the CIA-1 strain of CIAV. (Lucio and Shivaprasad). *C.* Gangrenous dermatitis (blue wing disease). (Shivaprasad). *D.* Hemorrhages in thigh and leg muscles. (Peckham). *E.* Hemorrhages in breast muscle. (Peckham). *F.* Hemorrhages in proventriculus. (Peckham)

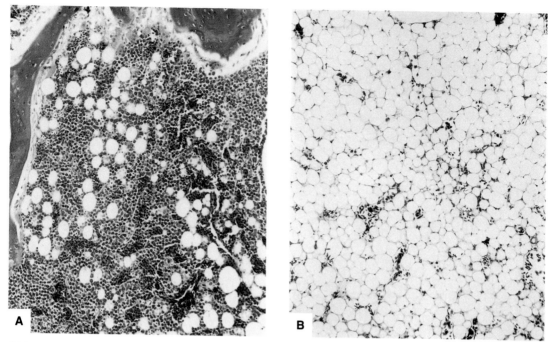

30.3. Femoral bone marrow from 14-day-old chickens. *A.* Uninfected control. *B.* Chicken infectious anemia virus–infected, 14 days postinoculation. Note atrophy of hematopoietic tissue and presence of fat cells. H & E, ×160. (Lucio and Shivaprasad)

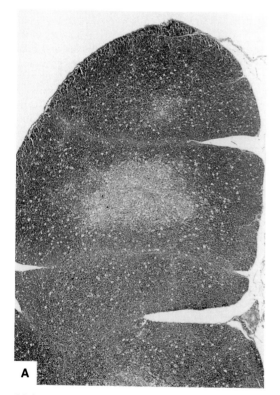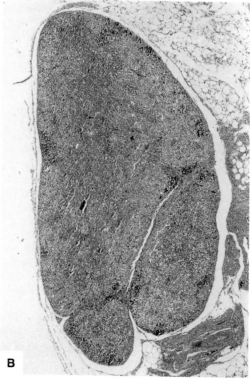

30.4. Thymus from 14-day-old chickens. *A.* Uninfected control. *B.* Chicken infectious anemia virus–infected, 14 days postinoculation. Note the absence of demarcation between medulla and cortex. H & E, ×63. (Lucio and Shivaprasad)

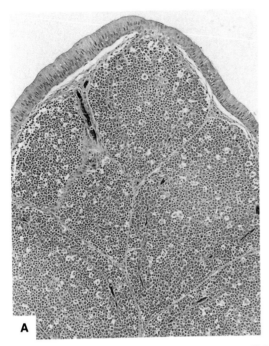 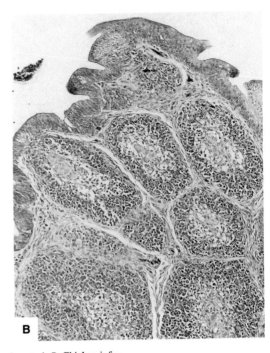

30.5. Bursa of Fabricius from 14-day-old chickens. *A.* Uninfected control. *B.* Chicken infectious anemia virus–infected, 14 days postinoculation. Note lymphoid depletion and atrophy of follicles. H & E, ×63. (Lucio and Shivaprasad)

Pathogenesis. The pathogenesis of CIAV infection has been elucidated by sequential histopathologic (61, 145, 151), ultrastructural (62, 63) and immunocytochemical studies (12, 71, 145). It was concluded from the morphologic findings that hemocytoblasts in the bone marrow and lymphoblasts in the thymus cortex are primarily involved in early cytolytic infection at 6–8 days postinoculation. Death of cortical thymocytes has been shown to be caused by apoptosis (80). Besides enlarged proerythroblasts and degenerating hematopoietic cells, macrophages with ingested degenerated hematopoietic cells have been observed in the bone marrow. In contrast to the thymus, depletion of lymphoid cells and occasional necrosis in the bursa of Fabricius, spleen, and lymphoid foci of other tissues have not been detected before 10–12 days postinoculation (21, 61, 145, 151). Repopulation of the thymus with lymphocytes, and of the bone marrow with proerythroblasts and promyelocytes, and recovery of hematopoietic activity from 16 days after inoculation all appear to coincide with the beginning of antibody formation (see Immunity). These events result in complete recovery by 32–36 days.

Immunocytochemical studies (2, 71, 145) showed that CIAV replicates in cortical thymic lymphoblasts, intrasinoidal and extrasinoidal hemocytoblasts, and reticular cells. As well, CIAV antigens

have been detected in mature T lymphocytes in the spleen (2). Infected cells in the thymus and bone marrow are most abundant at 6–7 days postinfection and can be detected until 10–12 days or even later. Viral antigen has also been demonstrated in lymphoid tissues of many other organs (145). Infection of proventriculus, ascending part of the duodenum, kidney, and lung could provide an explanation for virus shedding. Infected cells in these tissues usually cannot be detected for more than 22 days after infection at 1 day of age (145), although virus may persist in tissues until 28 days and in rectal contents until 49 days or later (187). Viral persistence is considerably enhanced in chickens immunosuppressed by bursectomy (190).

Susceptibility of chicks to CIAV infection has been reported to be dependent on properties of thymic precursor cells during prehatching and posthatching development (81). Age resistance to infectious anemia, however, is not due to disappearance or increased resistance of a specific target cell (101). Although CIAV has a tropism for lymphoid tissue, particularly for the thymus cortex (79), susceptibility of thymocytes or spleen cells to infection is not dependent on the expression of particular cell markers such as CD4 or CD8 (2, 79). On the other hand, transient severe depletion of CD4[+] and CD8[+] lymphocytes, or a selective decrease in cytotoxic T cells, may play an important role in the mechanism of CIAV-induced immunosuppression (2, 6, 30, 74, 79).

Immunity

ACTIVE. There is only a poor antibody response in susceptible chickens inoculated with CIAV at 1 day of age. Neutralizing antibody cannot be detected until 3 wk after inoculation. Even then, titers are low (1:80) and show little increase (1:320) until 4 wk. The antibody response is considerably enhanced in chickens inoculated intramuscularly at 2–6 wk of age, with neutralizing antibody detectable as early as 4–7 days and with maximum titers (1:1280–1:5120) at 12–14 days postinoculation (187, 188). Humoral antibody formation is delayed by about 1 wk if chickens are infected orally rather than intramuscularly. Yuasa et al. (187) reported that increasing antibody production coincides with decreasing virus concentrations in chicken tissues.

Seroconversion in horizontally infected breeder flocks may be detected as early as 8–9 wk of age, and most flocks have antibody to CIAV at 18–24 wk (77, 103). High titers of neutralizing antibody persist in all birds of a flock for at least 52 wk. The prevalence of immunofluorescent antibodies, however, may decrease with increasing age (77) and is frequently less than 100% in a flock (48, 103).

PASSIVE. Maternal antibodies provide complete protection of young chicks against CIAV-induced anemia (184), provided that the chicks are not immunologically compromised by other factors (20, 21). Maternally derived immunity, including protection against experimental challenge, persists for about 3 wk (103, 131). Furthermore, vertical transmission of the virus is unlikely to occur from actively immune hens. Outbreaks of infectious anemia in the field have, in fact, been found to be correlated with the absence of anti-CIAV antibody in the respective parent flocks (27, 167, 168, 189).

IMMUNOSUPPRESSION. There is strong circumstantial evidence that CIAV infection is immunosuppressive, at least in susceptible young chicks during clinical stages of the disease. Immunosuppression in anemic birds is indicated by an increased susceptibility to bacterial and fungal infections (21, 59, 137, 150, 173) and by enhanced pathogenicity of adenovirus (22), reovirus (40), and live attenuated Newcastle disease (ND) virus (34) in dually infected chicks. In experimental dual infection of 1-day-old specific-pathogen–free (SPF) chicks with CIAV and MDV, lymphoproliferative MD lesions were unexpectedly enhanced or reduced with low or high doses of MDV, respectively (78).

Under experimental conditions in which chicks are vaccinated against MD at 1 day of age and challenged with MDV within the first 8 days, CIAV infection up to 14 days of age can depress the MDV vaccinal immunity (126, 127, 128, 181). Conditions similar to these may occur rarely in the field. Impaired humoral immune response to inactivated ND vaccine may also occur (7, 31) but is not a usual phenomenon in commercial flocks (51).

Impairment of the immune response by CIAV infection may result directly from damage to hematopoietic and lymphopoietic tissues and subsequent generalized lymphoid depletion (see Histopathology, and Pathogenesis). In laboratory experiments, mitogenic stimulation (by concanavalin A or phytohemagglutinin) of splenocytes from chicks intramuscularly inoculated with the virus at 1–7 days of age was depressed at 7–15 days, but not at 18–21 days after infection (1, 6, 126, 127). This depression of cell functions also occurred in chickens orally infected at 3 wk of age but was delayed by 1 wk (98). Transient decreases in macrophage functions and cytokine production (97, 98) also are involved in the mechanism of CIAV-induced immunosuppression.

Minor lesions and some infected cells in the thymus may also be detected in SPF chickens experimentally infected at 5–6 wk of age, but there is insufficient damage to cause immunosuppression at that age (117, 170). Therefore, CIAV-induced immunosuppression appears closely associated with the presence of distinct gross and histologic signs of generalized lymphoid atrophy.

DIAGNOSIS

Isolation and Identification of CIAV.

Chicken infectious anemia virus can be isolated from virtually all tissues of infected chickens (187), with maximum virus titers detected at 7 days after infection. In chickens inoculated at 1 day of age, the virus content of tissues and rectal contents remains almost constant until 21 days and rapidly declines thereafter. Serum, however, loses its infectivity after 14 days (187). Whole blood and buffy coat were found to be infectious for at least 14 days even in birds with neutralizing antibody (18, 179). In chickens inoculated at 4–6 wk of age, maximum virus titers occurred in a variety of tissues and in rectal contents at 7 days after infection, rapidly decreasing to rather low levels by 14–21 days; however, CIAV has never been detected in the brain or serum of such birds (187).

Liver is a preferred source of CIAV because it most consistently contains high concentrations of the virus. Clarified liver homogenate can be heated for 5 min at 70 C (58) or treated with chloroform to eliminate or inactivate possible contaminants before use as an inoculum for cell cultures.

Bioassay by intramuscular or intraperitoneal inoculation of susceptible 1-day-old chicks is the most specific method available for primary isolation of CIAV. The infectivity of most strains is as much as 100-fold lower in chicks than in cell culture but can be increased by immunosuppression of experimental chicks (15). At either 14–16 days or at both 14 and 21 days after inoculation (141), chicks are examined for anemia, as indicated by hematocrit values below 27%, and for bone marrow atrophy that may also be present at a given time in some affected, but nonanemic, birds. Suspected tissues may be examined histologically, but this is usually not necessary to confirm the diagnosis.

MDCC-MSB1 cell cultures can be used for in vitro isolation attempts and virus titrations (19, 59, 75, 175, 186), although some CIAV strains don't readily replicate in these cells (24, 147). Freshly prepared cultures containing 2×10^5 cells/mL and seeded at 10^5 cells/cm² should be used. Appropriately prepared tissue homogenate, at a 1:20 or greater dilution (or serial 10-fold dilutions) should be inoculated at a rate of 0.1 mL/1 mL of culture. Subcultures of the MSB1 cells must be made every 2–4 days. Cell damage occurring after 1–6 (but sometimes up to 10) subcultures is suggestive of CIAV infection. Microscopic examination of cultures after 36 hr and not later than 48 hr after a subculture is recommended to distinguish between virus-induced cytopathic effects (Fig. 30.6) and

nonspecific cell degeneration. Isolation of CIAV should be verified by serologic procedures.

Viral Markers in Tissues

DETECTION BY ANTIBODIES. Viral infection can be demonstrated in chicken tissues by immunofluorescence or immunoperoxidase staining. Thymus, collected at 7–12 days after infection, is usually preferred for diagnostic tests (see Pathogenesis).

Tissue impression smears and cryostat sections, fixed with acetone, are used for either indirect or direct immunofluorescence staining employing polyclonal chicken or rabbit hyperimmune serum or monoclonal antibodies to CIAV (71, 73, 100, 108).

Immunoperoxidase assays are performed with formalin-fixed, paraffin-embedded sections (73, 100, 145). Optimization of the technique has been described in great detail by Smyth et al. (145). The most satisfactory results are obtained with monoclonal antibodies, since polyclonal antibodies may produce quite a high level of nonspecific background staining.

DNA PROBES. Detection of CIAV in formalin-fixed, paraffin-embedded thymus sections by in situ hybridization using a biotinylated DNA probe prepared by PCR has been described (3, 116).

Dot-blot hybridization assays using cloned ³²P-labeled DNA probes can detect viral DNA extracted from chicken tissues from 5 through 42 days after

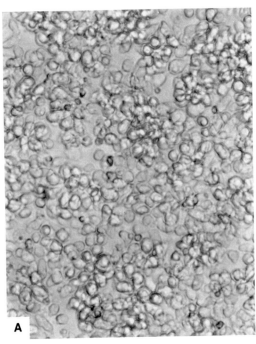
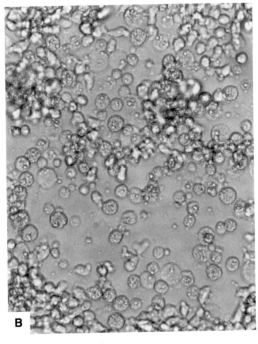

A   B

30.6. Lesions in cultured MSB1 cells 2 days after infection with chicken infectious anemia virus. *A.* Uninfected cells. *B.* Cells infected with a high dose of virus. Unstained. ×230.

infection (160) or from MSB1 cells infected with field isolates of CIAV (120).

POLYMERASE CHAIN REACTION. Polymerase chain reaction for detection of CIAV DNA in infected MSB1 cells, chicken tissues, or vaccines has been developed in several laboratories (36, 57, 120, 140, 146, 153, 154, 155, 161). The test proved to be specific and definitely more sensitive than cell-culture isolation of the virus. Very high sensitivity is achieved with a nested PCR, which, however, is also most sensitive to cross-contamination (146). A recently developed hot-start PCR for CIAV is also highly sensitive; furthermore, the use of a spike DNA as an internal control enables the validation of CIAV-negative samples and an estimation of the number of CIAV genomes present in the tested samples (36).

Polymerase chain reaction is most useful for research purposes and is expected to become the preferred method of detecting CIAV contamination of poultry vaccines.

ELECTRON MICROSCOPY. Chicken infectious anemia virus particles may be found in highly purified preparations of infected cell cultures. They are difficult to detect, however, and are not clearly identifiable in ultrathin sections of infected cultured cells or chicken tissues (62, 63, 80, 109), even though typical intranuclear inclusions, which are often ring-shaped, have been shown by immunologic techniques to be virus specific (109). No satisfactory results can be expected from electron microscopy (EM) examination of partially purified supernatant fluids of tissue homogenates (9). There is only one report of detection of CIAV in blood plasma of anemic chicks by direct EM (50).

Serology

VIRUS-NEUTRALIZATION TESTS. In the VN test (19, 187), serial twofold dilutions of serum or egg yolk are mixed with equal parts of a CIAV suspension containing 200–500 tissue-culture-infective-doses-50% (TCID$_{50}$)/0.1 mL, and the mixtures are incubated at 37 C for 60 min or at 4 C overnight before assay in MSB1 cell culture. Microtest plates are recommended if large numbers of sera have to be examined (75, 82). It may take up to 5 wk, requiring eight to nine subcultures, before the assay is completed; however, results can be obtained much earlier, and subcultures can be omitted, if the virus concentration in the mixture is increased to $10^{5.0}$ to $10^{5.5}$ TCID$_{50}$/0.1 mL (13, 19, 130). In this instance, inoculated cultures should be examined microscopically for CIAV-specific CPE after both 2 and 3 days. One subculture may be required if complete destruction of virus-control cultures is desired to establish the endpoint.

Qualitative VN tests for flock screening can be made with a constant serum dilution of 1:80–1:100 and a high dose of test virus as described above. Lower serum dilutions are not recommended because they can occasionally be cytotoxic or cause nonspecific inhibition of the virus. This type of test can be rendered semiquantitative by making a series of subcultures; the relative antibody level is indicated by the number of subcultures in which the inoculated cells stay alive (13, 19).

FLUORESCENT ANTIBODY TESTS. In the indirect fluorescent antibody (FA) test (19, 103, 188), CIAV-infected MSB1 cells collected just before the beginning of cell lysis, usually 36–42 hr after inoculation, are smeared on glass slides and acetone fixed for use as antigens. Cells are reacted first with appropriately diluted test serum and then with a fluorescein-labeled mammalian antiserum against chicken IgG. Fluorescent staining of rather small, irregularly shaped granules in the nucleus of enlarged cells (Fig. 30.7) is considered evidence for antibody in the test serum. The concurrent appearance of fluorescent, somewhat irregular circular structures is also specific, but less frequent. This pattern of immunofluorescence is considered typical of tests with neutralizing CIAV antibody (11, 108, 158). Positive reference serum should always

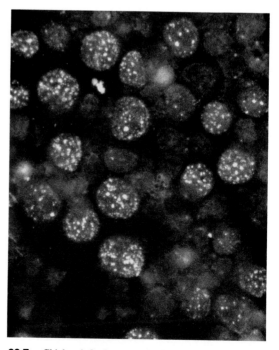

30.7. Chicken infectious anemia virus antigens detected by immunofluorescent staining in cytospin preparations of MSB1 cells harvested at 40 hr postinoculation. Antigens are seen in enlarged cells with characteristic intranuclear granular fluorescence. ×400.

be included in FA tests. Negative control sera are of little or no use because they usually have already been selected for nonreactivity in the indirect FA test. Noninfected cells as internal or external controls enable only the evaluation of several obvious types of nonspecific fluorescence and the degree of background staining that might mask specific reactions.

Most problems are encountered with nonspecific fluorescence primarily characterized by large spherical inclusions scattered in the nucleus of enlarged cells, predominantly at late stages after infection. Nonspecific staining and background staining masking specific reactions ("prozone phenomenon") can be largely reduced by using sufficiently diluted test sera, i.e., 1:40 to 1:100 or even more (103). Nonspecific staining due to direct binding of anti-IgG conjugates (95) may be controlled by selection of pretested conjugates.

The indirect FA test is less sensitive than the VN test in detecting low concentrations of CIAV antibody in chicken sera (13, 19, 28, 130).

ENZYME IMMUNOASSAYS. Various enzyme-linked immunosorbant assay (ELISA) techniques for the detection and measurement of CIAV antibodies in chicken sera have been developed. Todd et al. (158) described a highly specific and sensitive ELISA using a monoclonal antibody to capture CIAV partially purified from infected MSB1 cell cultures as the target antigen. The ELISA plates directly coated with partially purified virus appear to be equally suitable (10). Both techniques have been used in the production of commercially available ELISA kits. Highly purified CIAV also has been shown to be a suitable ELISA antigen (53, 92); however, it may not be easy to produce it at sufficient concentrations and quantities. Clarified lysates of infected MSB1 cells have been used as ELISA antigens (87, 130) but appear less suitable than purified or semipurified virions for routine testing. A very promising development is an ELISA based on a recombinant CIAV antigen, VP1 (132). ELISA generally is more sensitive than VN and indirect FA tests and is at least as specific as the indirect FA test. False-positive reactions that may occur in up to 18% of sera from SPF chickens were found to be associated with the transient presence of a particular protein fraction (124).

An indirect immunoperoxidase test using multispot slides or microtest plates coated with CIAV-infected MSB1 cells was found to be at least as sensitive as the indirect FA test, but less sensitive than the ELISA (28, 92, 164).

Differential Diagnosis. Infection criteria have only limited value in diagnosis of CIAV-induced disease because CIAV is virtually ubiquitous among chickens. Demonstration of the virus, viral antigens, or viral DNA may be considered etiologically significant if detected at sufficiently high levels in a high proportion of affected birds. In chickens under 6 wk of age, a typical combination of signs, hematologic changes, gross and microscopic lesions, and flock history (see Pathogenesis and Epizootiology) are suggestive of CIA. There are no particular lesions per se, however, that can be considered pathognomonic.

Aplastic anemia, but not a pancytopenia, with a concurrent atrophy of thymus and bursa of Fabricius, and depressed immune response also can be caused by osteopetrosis virus. Anemia induced by erythroblastosis virus can be distinguished from CIAV-induced anemia by microscopic examination of blood smears. Both MDV and IBDV induce atrophy of lymphoid tissues with typical histologic lesions but do not cause anemia in naturally infected chickens. Aplastic anemia that may be associated with acute IBDV occurs and disappears much earlier than CIAV-induced anemia (123). Adenovirus is a major cause of an inclusion body hepatitis–aplastic anemia syndrome that occurs most frequently between 5 and 10 wk of age (33). It does not, however, induce aplastic anemia in single infection of experimental chickens.

Intoxication with high doses of sulfonamides, or mycotoxins such as aflatoxin, can result in aplastic anemia and "hemorrhagic syndrome" (see Chapter 36). Aflatoxin also may impair the immune system. In the field, however, chickens are rarely exposed to doses of aflatoxin or sulfonamides that are sufficient to cause acute disease. On the other hand, subclinical intoxication of chickens might add to the pathogenicity of CIAV or vice versa.

TREATMENT. There is no specific treatment for chickens affected by CIAV infection. Treatment with broad-spectrum antibiotics to control bacterial infections usually associated with CIA might be indicated.

PREVENTION AND CONTROL. Immunization of parent flocks several wk before egg production efficiently prevents outbreaks of CIA in their progeny. Artificial exposure by transfer of litter from CIAV-infected flocks to young breeder flocks has been shown to be effective but is a dubious and risky procedure with regard to hygiene (168). Chicken infectious anemia virus infection of breeders via the drinking water with tissue homogenates from naturally affected chicks has also been effective (167, 168). This method, however, cannot be recommended as a standard procedure, because it is almost impossible to be sure of a sufficient CIAV concentration or the absence of other pathogens in the tissue preparations.

Two types of commercial live vaccines are presently available in several countries. Firstly,

Bülow and Witt (17) had suggested that virulent CIAV production in embryos could provide a live vaccine for application via the drinking water. Indeed, efficacious and safe vaccines free from extraneous agents have been produced in that manner (169, 170, 171, 172). Cell culture–propagated CIAV may also be suitable as a drinking water vaccine provided that the titer is adequate. Vaccination should be performed at about 13–15 wk of age, but never later than 3–4 wk before the first collection of hatching eggs to avoid the hazard of vaccine virus spread through the egg. Chicken infectious anemia virus does not cause immunosuppression in birds of that age (see Immunity). The second, more recent, vaccine consists of attenuated CIAV that has to be administered via parenteral routes (intramuscular, subcutaneous, or wingweb) to be fully effective (149). Vaccination can be omitted if humoral CIAV antibodies have been detected in the growing breeder chickens.

Attention should be paid to management and hygiene procedures to prevent immunosuppression by environmental factors or other infectious diseases and to prevent early exposure to CIAV. Eradication, however, is virtually impossible even from infected SPF premises (42), because of the high resistance of the virus to disinfection. Monitoring of breeder flocks for the presence of CIAV antibody should be done to avoid vertically transmitted CIAV infections or to test the efficacy of vaccinations.

REFERENCES

1. Adair, B.M., F. McNeilly, C.D.G. McConnell, D. Todd, R.T. Nelson, and M.S. McNulty. 1991. Effects of chicken anemia agent on lymphokine production and lymphocyte transformation in experimentally infected chickens. Avian Dis 35:783–792.

2. Adair, B.M., F. McNeilly, C.D.G. McConnell, and M.S. McNulty. 1993. Characterization of surface markers present on cells infected by chicken anemia virus in experimentally infected chickens. Avian Dis 37:943–950.

3. Allan, G.M., J.A. Smyth, D. Todd, and M.S. McNulty. 1993. In situ hybridization for the detection of chicken anaemia virus in formalin-fixed, paraffin-embedded sections. Avian Dis 37:177–182.

4. Allan, G.M., K.V. Phenix, D. Todd, and M.S. McNulty. 1994. Some biological and physico-chemical properties of porcine circovirus. J Vet Med B 41:17–26.

5. Bisgaard, M. 1983. An age related and breeder flock associated hemorrhagic disorder in Danish broilers. Nord Vet Med 35:397–407.

6. Bounous, D.I., M.A. Goodwin, R.L. Brooks, C.M. Lamichhane, R.P. Campagnoli, J. Brown, and D.B. Snyder. 1995. Immunosuppression and intracellular calcium signaling in splenocytes from chicks infected with chicken anemia virus, CL-1 isolate. Avian Dis 39:135–140.

7. Box, P.G., H.C. Holmes, A.C. Bushell, and P.M. Finney. 1988. Impaired response to killed Newcastle disease vaccine in chicken possessing circulating antibody to chicken anaemia agent. Avian Pathol 17:713–723.

8. Braunius, W.V. 1988. Blauwe vleugeltjes ziekte en chicken anemia agent bij slachtkuikens. Tijdschr Diergeneeskd 113:431–434.

9. Brentano, L., N. Mores, I. Wentz, D. Chandratilleke, and K.A. Schat. 1991. Isolation and identification of chicken

10. Brewer, J., J.M. Saunders, and N.J. Chettle. 1994. The development of an enzyme linked immunosorbent assay to detect antibodies to chicken anaemia virus, and its comparison with the indirect fluorescent antibody test. Proc Int Symp Infect Bursal Dis Chick Infect Anaemia, Rauischholzhausen, Germany, pp. 408–412.

11. Buchholz, U. and V. von Bülow. 1994. Characterization of chicken anaemia virus (CAV) proteins. Proc Int Symp Infect Bursal Dis Chick Infect Anaemia, Rauischholzhausen, Germany, pp. 366–375.

12. Buchholz, U., F. Taugner, R. Rudolph, und V.v.Bülow. 1993. Vergleichende immunhistologische Untersuchungen bei Küken nach experimenteller Infektion mit zwei verschiedenen Stämmen des Hühneranämievirus. In G. Monreal (ed.). Internationale Fachtagung über Geflügelkrankheiten. Deutsche Veterinärmedizinische Gesellschaft, Gießen, pp. 151–153.

13. Bülow, V.v. 1988. Unsatisfactory sensitivity and specificity of indirect immunofluorescence tests for the presence or absence of antibodies to chicken anaemia agent (CAA) in sera of SPF and broiler breeder chickens. J Vet Med B 35:594–600.

14. Bülow, V.v. 1991. Avian infectious anemia and related syndromes caused by chicken anaemia virus. Crit Rev Poult Biol 3:1–17.

15. Bülow V.v. and B. Fuchs. 1986. Attenuierung des Erregers der aviären infektiosen Anämie (CAA) durch Serienpassagen in Zellkulturen. J Vet Med B 33:568–573.

16. Bülow, V.v. and D. Lutticken. 1993. Unpublished data.

17. Bülow, V.v. and M. Witt. 1986. Vermehrung des Erregers der aviären infektiosen Anämie (CAA) in embryonierten Hühnereiern. J Vet Med B 33:664–669.

18. Bülow, V.v., B. Fuchs, E. Vielitz, and H. Landgraf. 1983. Frühsterblichkeitssyndrom bei Küken nach Doppelinfektion mit dem Virus der Marekschen Krankheit (MDV) und einem Anämie-Erreger (CAA). Zentralbl Veterinärmed [B] 30:742–750.

19. Bülow, V.v., B. Fuchs, and M. Bertram. 1985. Untersuchungen über den Erreger der infektiosen Anämie bei Hühnerküken (CAA) in vitro: Vermehrung, Titration, Serumneutralisationstest und indirekter Immunfluoreszenztest. Zentralbl Veterinärmed [B] 32:679–693.

20. Bülow, V.v., B. Fuchs, and R. Rudolph. 1986. Avian infectious anaemia caused by chicken anaemia agent (CAA). In J.B. McFerran and M.S. McNulty (eds.). Acute Virus Infections of Poultry. Martinus Nijhoff Publishers, Dordrecht, pp. 203–212.

21. Bülow, V.v., R. Rudolph, and B. Fuchs. 1986. Erhöhte Pathogenität des Erregers der aviären infektiosen Anämie bei Hühnerküken (CAA) bei simultaner Infektion mit dem Virus der Mareksschen Krankheit (MDV), Bursitisvirus (IBDV) oder Reticuloendotheliosevirus (REV). J Vet Med B 33:93–116.

22. Bülow, V.v., R. Rudolph, and B. Fuchs. 1986. Folgen der Doppelinfektion von Küken mit Adenovirus oder Reovirus und dem Erreger der aviären infektiosen Anämie (CAA). J Vet Med B 33:717–726.

23. Bülow, V.v., M. Witt, and R. Rudolph. 1987. Auswirkungen immunologischer Defekte bei Hühnerküken im Zusammenhang mit der aviären infektiosen Anämie. In Bericht des 17. Kongresses der Deutschen Veterinärmedizinischen Gesellschaft, pp. 384–390. Deutsche Veterinärmedizinische Gesellschaft, Gießen.

24. Bülow, V.v., S. Kling, and R. Rudolph. 1991. Recent results of research on chicken anemia virus in vivo and in vitro. Proc 128th Meet Am Vet Med Assoc, pp. 129–130.

25. Buscaglia, C., C.F. Crosetti, and P. Nervi. 1994. Identification of chicken infectious anaemia, isolation of the virus and reproduction of the disease in Argentina. Avian Pathol 23:297–304.

26. Chandratilleke, D., P. O'Connell, and K.A. Schat.

infectious anemia virus in Brazil. Avian Dis 35:793–800.

1991. Characterization of proteins of chicken infectious anemia virus with monoclonal antibodies. Avian Dis 35:854–862.

27. Chettle, N.J., R.K. Eddy, P.J. Wyeth, and S.A. Lister. 1989. An outbreak of disease due to chicken anaemia agent in broiler chickens in England. Vet Rec 124:211–215.

28. Chettle, N.J., R.K. Eddy, J. Saunders, and P.J. Wyeth. 1991. A comparison of serum neutralisation, immunofluorescence and immunoperoxidase tests for the detection of antibodies to chicken anaemia agent. Vet Rec 128:304–306.

29. Claessens, J.A.J., C.C. Schrier, A.P.A. Mockett, E.H.J.M. Jagt, and P.J.A. Sondermeijer. 1991. Molecular cloning and sequence analysis of the genome of chicken anaemia agent. J Gen Virol 72:2003–2006.

30. Cloud, S.S., H.S. Lillehoj, and J.K. Rosenberger. 1992. Immune dysfunction following infection with chicken anemia agent and infectious bursal disease virus. 1. Kinetic alterations of avian lymphocyte subpopulations. Vet Immunol Immunopathol 34:337–352.

31. Cloud, S.S., J.K. Rosenberger, and H.S. Lillehoj. 1992. Immune dysfunction following infection with chicken anemia agent and infectious bursal disease virus. 2. Alterations of in vitro lymphoproliferation and in vivo immune responses. Vet Immunol Immunopathol 34:353–366.

32. Connor, T.J., F. McNeilly, G.A. Firth, and M.S. McNulty. 1991. Biological characterisation of Australian isolates of chicken anaemia agent. Aust Vet J 68:199–201.

33. Cowen, B.S. 1992. Inclusion body hepatitis-anaemia and hydropericardium syndromes: Aetiology and control. World's Poulty Sci J 48:247–254.

34. de Boer, G.F., D.J. van Roozelaar, R.J. Moorman, S.H.M. Jeurissen, J.C. van den Wijngaard, F. Hilbink, and G. Koch. 1994. Interaction between chicken anaemia virus and live Newcastle disease vaccine. Avian Pathol 23:263–275.

35. Dorn, P., J. Weikel and E. Wessling. 1981. Anämie, Ruckbildung der lymphatischen Organe und Dermatitis— Beobachtungen zu einem neuen Krankheitsbild in der Geflügelmast. Dtsch Tierärztl Wochenschr 88:313–315.

36. Dren, Cs.N., G. Koch, A. Kant, C.A.J. Verschueren, A.J. van der Eb, and M.H.M. Noteborn. 1994. A hot start PCR for the laboratory diagnosis of CAV. Proc Int Symp Infect Bursal Dis Chick Infect Anaemia, Rauischholzhausen, Germany, pp. 413–420.

37. Drouin, P., J.P. Picault, G. Plassiart, Y. Cherel, D. Toquin, J.Y. Toux, M. Guittet, G. Bennejean, and M. Wyers. 1992. La maladie des ailes bleues chez le poulet—premières observations en France. Rec Med Vet 168:331–339.

38. Engström, B.E. 1988. Blue wing disease of chickens. Isolation of avian reovirus and chicken anaemia agent. Avian Pathol 17:23–32.

39. Engström, B.E. and M. Luthman. 1984. Blue wing disease of chickens: Signs, pathology and natural transmission. Avian Pathol 13:1–12.

40. Engström, B.E., O. Fossum, and M. Luthman. 1988. Blue wing disease of chickens: Experimental infection with a Swedish isolate of chicken anaemia agent and an avian reovirus. Avian Pathol 17:33–50.

41. Fadly, A.M. and R.W. Winterfield. 1973. Isolation and some characteristics of an agent associated with inclusion body hepatitis, hemorrhages, and aplastic anemia in chickens. Avian Dis 17:182–193.

42. Fadly, A.M., J.V. Motta, R.L. Witter, and R.M. Nordgren. 1994. Epidemiology of chicken anemia virus in specific-pathogen-free chicken breeder flocks. Proc Int Symp Infect Bursal Dis Chick Infect Anaemia, Rauischholzhausen, Germany, pp. 447–455.

43. Farkas, T., Cs. Dren, I. Nemeth, M. Dobos-Kovács, J. Povazsán, and E. Sághy. 1992. Isolation of chicken anaemia virus from broiler chickens. Acta Vet Hung 40:207–223.

44. Firth, G.A. and K. Imai. 1990. Isolation of chicken anemia agent from Australian poultry. Aust Vet J 67:301–302.

45. Froyman, R., J. Derijcke, and R. Vandermeersch.

1986. Een haemorrhagisch-anaemisch syndroom met dermatitis bij slachtkuikens. Tijdschr Diergeneeskd 111:639–642.

46. Gelderblom, H., S. Kling, R. Lurz, I. Tischer, and V. v. Bülow. 1989. Morphological characterization of chicken anaemia agent (CAA). Arch Virol 109:115–120.

47. Goodwin, M.A., J. Brown, S.L. Miller, M.A. Smeltzer, W.L. Steffens, and W.D. Waltman. 1989. Infectious anemia caused by a parvovirus-like virus in Georgia broilers. Avian Dis 33:438–445.

48. Goodwin, M.A., J. Brown, M.A. Smeltzer, C.K. Crary, T. Girshick, S.L. Miller, and T.G. Dickson. 1990. A survey for parvovirus-like virus (so-called chick anemia agent) antibodies in broiler breeders. Avian Dis 34:704–708.

49. Goodwin, M.A., J. Brown, K.S. Latimer, and S.L. Miller. 1991. Packed cell volume reference intervals to aid in the diagnosis of anemia and polycythemia in young leghorn chickens. Avian Dis 35:820–823.

50. Goodwin, M.A., W.L. Steffens, J. F. Davis, J. Brown, K.S. Latimer, and T.G. Dickson. 1991. Diagnoses of infections by the so-called chick anemia agent: Anemia and direct transmission electron microscopic detection of virus. Avian Dis 35:869–871.

51. Goodwin, M.A., J. Brown, M.A. Smeltzer, T. Girshick, S.L. Miller, and T.G. Dickson. 1992. Relationship of common avian pathogen antibody titers in so-called chicken anemia agent (CAA)-antibody-positive chicks to titers in CAA-antibody-negative chicks. Avian Dis 36:356–358.

52. Goodwin, M.A., J.F. Davis, and J. Brown. 1992. Packed cell volume reference intervals to aid in the diagnosis of anemia and polycythemia in young broiler chickens. Avian Dis 36:440–443.

53. Goodwin, M.A., C.M. Lamichhane, J. Brown, M.A. Smeltzer, S.L. Miller, T. Girshick, D.B. Snyder, and T.G. Dickson. 1992. Relationship of the enzyme-linked immunosorbent assay to indirect immunofluorescent antibody test for the detection of so-called chicken anemia agent antibodies in serum from broiler breeders. Avian Dis 36:512–514.

54. Goodwin, M.A., J.F. Davis, J. Brown , and T.G. Dickson. 1992. Incidence of anemia and polycythemia in clinically ill Georgia broilers. Avian Dis 36:685–687.

55. Goodwin, M.A., J. Brown, J.F. Davis, T. Girshick, S.L. Miller, R.M. Nordgren, and J. Rodenberg. 1992. Comparisons of packed cell volumes (PCVs) from so-called chicken anemia agent (CAA; a virus)-free broilers to PCVs from CAA-free specific-pathogen-free leghorns. Avian Dis 36:1063–1066.

56. Goodwin, M.A., M.A Smeltzer, J. Brown, T. Girshick, B.L. McMurray, and S. McCarter. 1993. Effect of so-called chicken anemia agent maternal antibody on chick serologic conversion to viruses in the field. Avian Dis 37:542–545.

57. Goodwin, M.A., J. Rodenberg, D.I. Bounous, R.M. Nordgren, C.M. Lamichhane, and J. Brown. 1994. Polymerase chain reaction for detection of the chicken anemia agent in formalin-fixed paraffin-embedded thymus sections. Proc Int Symp Infect Bursal Dis Chick Infect Anaemia, Rauischholzhausen, Germany, pp. 425–427.

58. Goryo, M., H. Sugimura, S. Matsumoto, T. Umemura, and C. Itakura. 1985. Isolation of an agent inducing chicken anaemia. Avian Pathol 14:483–496.

59. Goryo, M., Y. Shibata, T. Suwa, T. Umemura, and C. Itakura. 1987. Outbreak of anemia associated with chicken anemia agent in young chicks. Jpn J Vet Sci 49:867–873.

60. Goryo, M., T. Suwa, S. Matsumoto, T. Umemura, and C. Itakura. 1987. Serial propagation and purification of chicken anaemia agent in MDCC-MSB1 cell line. Avian Pathol 16:149–163.

61. Goryo, M., T. Suwa, T. Umemura, C. Itakura, and S. Yamashiro. 1989. Histopathology of chicks inoculated with chicken anaemia agent (MSB1-TK5803 strain). Avian Pathol 18:73–89.

62. Goryo, M., T. Suwa, T. Umemura, C. Itakura, and S.

Yamashiro. 1989. Ultrastructure of bone marrow in chicks inoculated with chicken anaemia agent (MSB1-TK5803 strain). Avian Pathol 18:329–343.

63. Goryo, M., S. Hayashi, K. Yoshizawa, T. Umemura, C. Itakura, and S. Yamashiro. 1989. Ultrastructure of the thymus in chicks inoculated with chicken anaemia agent (MSB1-TK5803 strain). Avian Pathol 18:605–617.

64. Grimes, T.M., D.J. King, S.H. Kleven, and O.J. Fletcher. 1977. Involvement of type-8 avian adenovirus in the etiology of inclusion body hepatitis. Avian Dis 21:26–38.

65. Hanley, J.E. 1962. Observations on avian aplastic anemia in Florida. Avian Dis 6:251–257.

66. Helmboldt, C.F. and M.N. Frazier. 1963. Avian hepatic inclusion bodies of unknown significance. Avian Dis 7:446–450.

67. Hoffmann, R., P. Dorn and H. Dangschat. 1973. Ein neues durch Panmyelopathie, Anämie und hämorrhagische Diathese gekennzeichnetes Syndrom beim Huhn. Zentralbl Veterinärmed [B] 20:741–746.

68. Hoffmann, R., E. Wessling, P. Dorn and H. Dangschat. 1975. Lesions in chickens with spontaneous or experimental infectious hepato-myelopoietic disease (inclusion body hepatitis) in Germany. Avian Dis 19:224–236.

69. Hoop, R.K. 1992. Persistence and vertical transmission of chicken anaemia agent in experimentally infected laying hens. Avian Pathol 21:493–501.

70. Hoop, R.K. 1993. Transmission of chicken anaemia virus with semen. Vet Rec 133:551–552.

71. Hoop, R.K. and R.L. Reece. 1991. The use of immunofluorescence and immunoperoxidase staining in studying the pathogenesis of chicken anaemia virus in experimentally infected chickens. Avian Pathol 20:349–355.

72. Hoop, R.K., F. Guscetti, and B. Keller. 1992. Ein Ausbruch von infektiöser Kükenanämie bei Mastküken in der Schweiz. Schweiz Arch Tierheilk 134:485–489.

73. Hu, L.-b., B. Lucio, and K.A. Schat. 1993. Abrogation of age-related resistance to chicken infectious anemia by embryonal bursectomy. Avian Dis 37:157–169.

74. Hu, L.-b., B. Lucio, and K.A. Schat. 1993. Depletion of CD4+ and CD8+ T lymphocyte subpopulations by CIA-1, a chicken infectious anemia virus. Avian Dis 37:492–500.

75. Imai, K. and N. Yuasa. 1990. Development of a microtest method for serological and virological examinations of chicken anaemia agent. Jpn J Vet Sci 52:873–875.

76. Imai, K., M. Maeda, and N. Yuasa. 1991. Immunoelectron microscopy of chicken anaemia agent. J Vet Med Sci 53:1065–1067.

77. Imai, K., S. Mase, K. Tsukamoto, H. Hihara, T. Matsumura, and N. Yuasa. 1993. A long term observation of antibody status to chicken anaemia virus in individual chickens of breeder flocks. Res Vet Sci 54:392–396.

78. Jeurissen, S.H.M. and G.F. de Boer. 1993. Chicken anaemia virus influences the pathogenesis of Marek's disease in experimental infections, depending on the dose of Marek's disease virus. Vet Q 15:81–84.

79. Jeurissen, S.H.M., J.M.A. Pol and G.F. de Boer. 1989. Transient depletion of cortical thymocytes induced by chicken anaemia agent. Thymus 14:115–123.

80. Jeurissen, S.H.M., F. Wagenaar, J.M.A. Pol, A.J. van der Eb, and M.H.M. Noteborn. 1992. Chicken anaemia virus causes apoptosis of thymocytes after in vivo infection and of cell lines after in vitro infection. J Virol 66:7383–7388.

81. Jeurissen, S.H.M., M.E. Janse, D.J. van Roozelaar, G. Koch, and G.F. de Boer. 1992. Susceptibility of thymocytes for infection by chicken anemia virus is related to pre- and posthatching development. Dev Immunol 2:123–129.

82. Jørgensen, P.H. 1990. A micro-scale serum neutralisation test for the detection and titration of antibodies to chicken anaemia agent—Prevalence of antibodies in Danish chickens. Avian Pathol 19:583–593.

83. Jørgensen, P.H. 1991. Mortality during an outbreak of blue wing disease in broilers. Vet Rec 129:490–491.

84. Jørgensen, P.H., L. Otte, O.L. Nielsen, and M. Bis-

gaard. 1994. Investigations on the epidemiology and economical impact of chicken anaemia virus infection in Danish broilers and broiler breeders. Proc Int Symp Infect Bursal Dis Chick Infect Anaemia, Rauischholzhausen, Germany, pp. 438–446.

85. Jørgensen, P.H., L. Otte, O.L. Nielsen and M. Bisgaard. 1995. Influence of subclinical virus infections and other factors on broiler flock performance. Br Poult Sci 36:455–463.

86. Kato, A., M. Fujino, T. Nakamura, A. Ishihama, and Y. Otaki. 1995. Gene organization of chicken anemia virus. Virology 209:480–488.

87. Kling, S. 1991. Versuche zum Antikörper- und Antigennachweis beim Hühner-Anämievirus nach Optimierung und Standardisierung des Western Blot und eines Nitrocellulose-ELISA am Modell von Geflügel-Herpesviren. Vet.-med. Dissertation, Freie Universität, Berlin, Germany.

88. Koch, G., D.J. van Roozelaar, C.A.J. Verschueren, A.J. van der Eb, and M.H.M. Noteborn. 1994. The formation of neutralising epitopes of chicken anaemia virus requires the synthesis of its proteins VP1 and VP2 in the same cell. Proc Int Symp Infect Bursal Dis Chick Infect Anaemia, Rauischholzhausen, Germany, pp. 498–506.

89. Koch, G., D.J. van Roozelaar, C.A.J. Verschueren, A.J. van der Eb, and M.H.M. Noteborn. 1995. Immunogenic and protective properties of chicken anaemia virus proteins expressed by baculovirus. Vaccine 13:763–770.

90. Kohler, H. and L. Hromatka Vasicek. 1974. Einschlußkorper-Hepatitis bei Broilern in Österreich. Wien Tierärztl Monatsschr 61:90–95.

91. Lamichhane, C.M., D.B. Snyder, M.A. Goodwin, S.A. Mengel, J. Brown, and T.G. Dickson. 1991. Pathogenicity of CL-1 chicken anemia agent. Avian Dis 35:515–522.

92. Lamichhane, C.M., D.B. Snyder, T. Girschick, M.A. Goodwin, and S.L. Miller. 1992. Development and comparison of serologic methods for diagnosing chicken anemia virus infection. Avian Dis 36:725–729.

93. Li, X.X., W.Y. Xu, and G.Y. Tang. 1994. Isolation and identification of the chicken anemia virus and serological survey in China. Proc Int Symp Infect Bursal Dis Chick Infect Anaemia, Rauischholzhausen, Germany, pp. 429–433.

94. Lucio, B., K.A. Schat, and H.L. Shivaprasad. 1990. Identification of the chicken anemia agent, reproduction of the disease, and serological survey in the United States. Avian Dis 34:146–153.

95. Lucio, B., K.A. Schat, and S. Taylor. 1991. Direct binding of protein A, protein G, and anti-IgG conjugates to chicken infectious anemia virus. Avian Dis 35:180–185.

96. Lukert, P., G.F. de Boer, J.L. Dale, P. Keese, M.S. McNulty, J.W. Randles, and I. Tischer. 1995. Family Circoviridae. In F.A. Murphy, C.M. Fauquet, D.H.L. Bishop, S.A. Ghabrial, A.W. Jarvis, G.P. Martelli, M.A. Mayo, and M.D. Summers (eds.). Virus Taxonomy—Classification and nomenclature of viruses, 6th Report of the International Committee on Taxonomy of Viruses. Springer-Verlag, Vienna, pp. 166–168.

97. McConnell, C.D.G., B.M. Adair, and M.S. McNulty. 1993. Effects of chicken anemia virus on macrophage function in chickens. Avian Dis 37:358–365.

98. McConnell, C.D.G., B.M. Adair, and M.S. McNulty. 1993. Effects of chicken anemia virus on cell-mediated immune function in chickens exposed to the virus by a natural route. Avian Dis 37:366–374.

99. McIlroy, S.G., M.S. McNulty, D.W. Bruce, J.A. Smyth, E.A. Goodall, and M.J. Alcorn. 1992. Economic effects of clinical chicken anemia agent infection on profitable broiler production. Avian Dis 36:566–574.

100. McNeilly, F., G.M. Allan, D.A. Moffett, and M.S. McNulty. 1991. Detection of chicken anaemia agent in chickens by immunofluorescence and immunoperoxidase staining. Avian Pathol 20:125–132.

101. McNeilly, F., B.M. Adair, and M.S. McNulty. 1994. In vitro infection of mononuclear cells derived from various

chicken lymphoid tissues by chicken anaemia virus. Avian Pathol 23:547–556.

102. McNulty, M.S. 1991. Chicken anaemia agent: A review. Avian Pathol 20:187–203.

103. McNulty, M.S., T.J. Connor, F. McNeilly, K.S. Kirkpatrick, and J.B. McFerran. 1988. A serological survey of domestic poultry in the United Kingdom for antibody to chicken anaemia agent. Avian Pathol 17:315–324.

104. McNulty, M.S., T.J. Connor, and F. McNeilly. 1989. A survey of specific pathogen-free chicken flocks for antibodies to chicken anaemia agent, avian nephritis virus and group A rotavirus. Avian Pathol 18:215–220.

105. McNulty, M.S., T.J. Connor, F. McNeilly, and D. Spackman. 1989. Chicken anemia agent in the United States: Isolation of the virus and detection of antibody in broiler breeder flocks. Avian Dis 33:691–694.

106. McNulty, M.S., T.J. Connor, F. McNeilly, M.F. McLoughlin, and K.S. Kirkpatrick. 1990. Preliminary characterisation of isolates of chicken anemia agent from the United Kingdom. Avian Pathol 19:67–73.

107. McNulty, M.S., T.J. Connor, and F. McNeilly. 1990. Influence of virus dose on experimental anaemia due to chicken anemia agent. Avian Pathol 19:167–171.

108. McNulty, M.S., D.P. Mackie, D.A. Pollock, J. McNair, D. Todd, K.A. Mawhinney, T.J. Connor, and F. McNeilly. 1990. Production and preliminary characterization of monoclonal antibodies to chicken anemia agent. Avian Dis 34:352–358.

109. McNulty, M.S., W.L. Curran, D. Todd, and D.P. Mackie. 1990. Chicken anemia agent: An electron microscopic study. Avian Dis 34:736–743.

110. McNulty, M.S., S.G. McIlroy, D.W. Bruce, and D. Todd. 1991. Economic effects of subclinical chicken anemia agent infection in broiler chickens. Avian Dis 35:263–268.

111. Meehan, B.M., D. Todd, J.L. Creelan, J.A.P. Earle, E.M. Hoey, and M.S. McNulty. 1992. Characterization of viral DNAs from cells infected with chicken anemia agent: Sequence analysis of the cloned replicative form and transfection capabilities of cloned genome fragments. Arch Virol 124:301–319.

112. Montgomery, R.D., P. Villegas, D.L. Dawe and J. Brown. 1985. Effect of avian reoviruses on lymphoid organ weights and antibody response in chickens. Avian Dis 29:552–560.

113. Montgomery, R.D., P. Villegas, D.L. Dawe and J. Brown. 1986. A comparison between the effect of an avian reovirus and infectious bursal disease virus on selected aspects of the immune system of the chicken. Avian Dis 30:298–308.

114. Naqi, S.A., L.G. Adams, B. Panigrahy, and A.R. Vivek. 1978. Experimental induction of hemorrhagic-aplastic anemia in chickens. I. Etiology. Avian Dis. 22:675–682.

115. Nicholas, R.A.J., B. Westbury, R.D. Goddard, and P.R. Luff. 1989. Survey of vaccines and SPF flocks for contamination with chick anaemia agent. Vet Rec 124:170–171.

116. Nielsen, O.L., P.H. Jørgensen, M. Bisgaard, and S. Alexandersen. 1995. In situ hybridization for the detection of chicken anaemia virus in experimentally-induced infection and field outbreaks. Avian Pathol 24:149–155.

117. Noteborn, M.H.M. and G. Koch. 1995. Chicken anaemia virus infection: Molecular basis of pathogenicity. Avian Pathol 24:11–31.

118. Noteborn, M.H.M., G.F. de Boer, D.J. van Roozelaar, C. Karreman, O. Kranenburg, J.G. Vos, S.H.M. Jeurissen, R.C. Hoeben, A. Zantema, G. Koch, H. van Ormondt, and A.J. van der Eb. 1991. Characterization of cloned chicken anemia virus DNA that contains all elements for the infectious replication cycle. J Virol 65:3131–3139.

119. Noteborn, M.H.M., O. Kranenburg, A. Zantema, G. Koch, G.F. de Boer, and A.J. van der Eb. 1992. Transcription of the chicken anemia virus (CAV) genome and synthesis of its 52-kDa protein. Gene 118:267–271.

120. Noteborn, M.H.M., C.A.J. Verschueren, D.J. van Roozelaar, S. Veldkamp, A.J. van der Eb, and G.F. de Boer. 1992. Detection of chicken anemia virus by DNA hybridisation and polymerase chain reaction. Avian Pathol 21:107–118.

121. Noteborn, M.H.M., D. Todd, C.A.J. Verschueren, H.W.F.M. de Gauw, W.L. Curran, S. Veldkamp, A.J. Douglas, M.S. McNulty, A.J. van der Eb, and G. Koch. 1994. A single chicken anemia virus protein induces apoptosis. J Virol 68:346–351.

122. Noteborn, M.H.M., C.A.J. Verschueren, A. Zantema, G. Koch, and A.J. van der Eb. 1994. Identification of the promoter region of chicken anemia virus (CAV) containing a novel enhancer-like element. Gene 150:313–318.

123. Nunoya, T., Y. Otaki, M. Tajima, M. Hiraga, and T. Saito. 1992. Occurrence of acute infectious bursal disease with high mortality in Japan and pathogenicity of field isolates in specific-pathogen-free chickens. Avian Dis 36:597–609.

124. O'Rourke, D., W.P. Michalski, and T.J. Bagust. 1994. Chicken anaemia virus antibody ELISA reactions: Practical experiences and problems in high-security SPF poultry flocks. Proc Int Symp Infect Bursal Dis Chick Infect Anaemia, Rauischholzhausen, Germany, pp. 456–464.

125. Otaki, Y., T. Nunoya, M. Tajima, H. Tamada, and Y. Nomura. 1987. Isolation of chicken anemia agent and Marek's disease virus from chickens vaccinated with turkey herpesvirus and lesions induced in chicks by inoculating both agents. Avian Pathol 16:291–306.

126. Otaki, Y., T. Nunoya, M. Tajima, A. Kato, and Y. Nomura. 1988. Depression of vaccinal immunity to Marek's disease by infection with chicken anemia agent. Avian Pathol 17:333–347.

127. Otaki, Y., M. Tajima, K. Saito, and Y. Nomura. 1988. Immune response of chicks inoculated with chicken anemia agent alone or in combination with Marek's disease virus or turkey herpesvirus. Jpn J Vet Sci 50:1040–1047.

128. Otaki, Y., T. Nunoya, M. Tajima, A. Kato, K. Saito and Y. Nomura. 1988. Chicken anemia agent infection as a possible cause of Marek's disease vaccination failures. In S. Kato, T. Horiuchi, T. Mikami, and K. Hirai (eds.). Advances in Marek's Disease Research. Japanese Association on Marek's Disease. Osaka, Japan, pp 364–366.

129. Otaki, Y., T. Nunoya, M. Tajima, K. Saito, and Y. Nomura. 1989. Enhanced pathogenicity of chicken anemia agent by infectious bursal disease virus relating to the occurrence of Marek's disease vaccination breaks. Jpn J Vet Sci 51:849–852.

130. Otaki, Y, K. Saito, M. Tajima, and Y. Nomura. 1991. Detection of antibody to chicken anemia agent: A comparison of three serological tests. Avian Pathol 20:315–324.

131. Otaki, Y., K. Saito, M. Tajima, and Y. Nomura. 1992. Persistence of maternal antibody to chicken anemia agent and its effect on the susceptibility of young chickens. Avian Pathol 21:147–151.

132. Pallister, J., K.J. Fahey, and M. Sheppard. 1994. Cloning and sequencing of the chicken anaemia virus (CAV) ORF-3 gene, and the development of an ELISA for the detection of serum antibody to CAV. Vet Microbiol 39:167–178.

133. Pettit, J.R. and H.C. Carlson. 1972. Inclusion-body hepatitis in broiler chickens. Avian Dis 16:858–863.

134. Phenix, K.V., B.M. Meehan, D. Todd, and M.S. McNulty. 1994. Transcriptional analysis and genome expression of chicken anaemia virus. J Gen Virol 75:905–909.

135. Picault, J.-P., D. Toquin, G. Plassiart, P. Drouin, J.-Y. Toux, M. Wyers, M. Guittet, and G. Bennejean. 1992. Reproduction experimentale de l'anemie infectieuse aviaire et mise en evidence du virus en France à partir de prelèvements de poulets presentant la "maladie des ailes bleues." Rec Med Vet 168:815–822.

136. Pope, C.R. 1991. Chicken anemia agent. Vet Immunol Immunopathol 30:51–65.

137. Randall, C.J., W.G. Siller, A.S. Wallis, and K.S. Kirk-

patrick. 1984. Multiple infections in young broilers. Vet Rec 114:270–271.

138. Renshaw, R.W., C. Soine, T. Weinkle, P.H. O'Connell, K. Ohashi, S. Watson, B. Lucio, S. Harrington, and K.A. Schat. 1996. A hypervariable region in VP1 of chicken anemia virus mediates rate of spread and cell tropism in tissue culture. J Virol (in press).

139. Ritchie, B.W., F.D. Niagro, P.D. Lukert, W.L. Steffens III, and K.S. Latimer. 1989. Characterization of a new virus isolated from cockatoos with psittacine beak and feather disease. Virology 171:83–88.

140. Rodenberg, J., C. de Wannemaeker, J. Heeren, D. Colau, G. Thiry, and R. Nordgren. 1994. Comparison of MSB1 isolation and polymerase chain reaction to determine the presence of CAV in avian biological products. Proc Int Symp Infect Bursal Dis Chick Infect Anaemia, Rauischholzhausen, Germany, pp. 421–424.

141. Rosenberger, J.K., and S.S. Cloud. 1989. The isolation and characterization of chicken anemia agent (CAA) from broilers in the United States. Avian Dis 33:707–713.

142. Rosenberger, J.K. and S.S. Cloud. 1989. The effects of age, route of exposure, and coinfection with infectious bursal disease virus on the pathogenicity and transmissibility of chicken anemia agent (CAA). Avian Dis 33:753–759.

143. Rosenberger, J.K., S. Klopp, R.J. Eckroade, and W.C. Krauss. 1975. The role of infectious bursal agent and several avian adenoviruses in the hemorrhagic-aplastic-anemia syndrome and gangrenous dermatitis. Avian Dis 19:717–729.

144. Sharma, J.M. and J.K. Rosenberger. 1987. Infectious bursal disease and reovirus infection of chickens: Immune responses and vaccine control. In Toivanen, A. and Toivanen P. (eds.). Avian Immunology: Basis and Practice, vol. 2. CRC Press, Boca Roton, FL, pp. 143–157.

145. Smyth, J.A., D.A. Moffett, M.S. McNulty, D. Todd, and D.P. Mackie. 1993. A sequential histopathologic and immunocytochemical study of chicken anemia virus infection at one day of age. Avian Dis 37:324–338.

146. Soine, C., S.K. Watson, E. Rybicki, B. Lucio, R.M. Nordgren, C.R. Parrish, and K.A. Schat. 1993. Determination of the detection limit of the polymerase chain reaction for chicken infectious anemia virus. Avian Dis 37:467–476.

147. Soine, C., R.H. Renshaw, P.H. O'Connell, S.K. Watson, B. Lucio, and K.A. Schat. 1994. Sequence analysis of cell culture- and non-cell culture-adapted strains of chicken infectious anemia virus. Proc Int Symp Infect Bursal Dis Chick Infect Anaemia, Rauischholzhausen, Germany, pp. 364–365.

148. Stanislawek, W.L. and J. Howell. 1994. Isolation of chicken anaemia virus from broiler chickens in New Zealand. N Z Vet J 42:58–62.

149. Steenhuisen, W., H.J.M. Jagt, and C.C. Schrier. 1994. The use of a live attenuated CAV vaccine in breeder flocks in the Netherlands. Proc Int Symp Infect Bursal Dis Chick Infect Anaemia, Rauischholzhausen, Germany, pp. 482–497.

150. Taniguchi, T., N. Yuasa, M. Maeda, and T. Horiuchi. 1982. Hematopathological changes in dead and moribund chicks induced by chicken anemia agent. Natl Inst Anim Health Q (Jpn) 22:61–69.

151. Taniguchi, T., N. Yuasa, M. Maeda, and T. Horiuchi. 1983. Chronological observations on hemato-pathological changes in chicks inoculated with chicken anemia agent. Natl Inst Anim Health Q (Jpn) 23:1–12.

152. Taylor, S.P. 1992. The effect of acetone on the viability of chicken anemia agent. Avian Dis 36:753–754.

153. Taylor, S.P. and A.J. Ryncarz. 1993. Rapid detection of low amounts of chicken anemia virus DNA using the polymerase chain reaction assay [abst]. Vet Microbiol 37:418.

154. Tham, K.M. and W.L. Stanislawek. 1992. Detection of chicken anaemia agent DNA sequences by the polymerase chain reaction. Arch Virol 127:245–255.

155. Tham, K.M. and W.L. Stanislawek. 1992. Polymerase chain reaction amplification for direct detection of chicken anemia virus DNA in tissues and sera. Avian Dis 36:1000–1006.

156. Tischer, I., H. Gelderblom, W. Vettermann, and M.A. Koch. 1982. A very small porcine virus with circular single-stranded DNA. Nature 295:64–65.

157. Todd, D., J.L. Creelan, D.P. Mackie, F. Rixon, and M.S. McNulty. 1990. Purification and biochemical characterization of chicken anaemia agent. J Gen Virol 71:819–823.

158. Todd, D., D.P. Mackie, K.A. Mawhinney, T.J. Connor, F. McNeilly, and M.S. McNulty. 1990. Development of an enzyme-linked immunosorbent assay to detect serum antibody to chicken anaemia agent. Avian Dis 34:359–363.

159. Todd, D., F.D. Niagro, B.W. Ritchie, W. Curran, G.M. Allan, P.D. Lukert, K.S. Latimer, W.L. Steffens III, and M.S. McNulty. 1991. Comparison of three animal viruses with circular single-stranded DNA genomes. Arch Virol 117:129–135.

160. Todd, D., J.L. Creelan, and M.S. McNulty. 1991. Dot blot hybridization assay for chicken anemia agent using a cloned DNA probe. J Clin Microbiol 29:933–939.

161. Todd, D., K.A. Mawhinney, and M.S. McNulty. 1992. Detection and differentiation of chicken anaemia virus isolates by using the polymerase chain reaction. J Clin Microbiol 30:1661–1666.

162. Todd, D., A.J. Douglas, K.V. Phenix, W.L. Curran, D.P. Mackie, and M.S. McNulty. 1994. Characterisation of chicken anaemia virus. Proc Int Symp Infect Bursal Dis Chick Infect Anaemia, Rauischholzhausen, Germany, pp. 349–363.

163. Todd, D., T.J. Connor, V.M. Calvert, J.L. Creelan, B.M. Meehan, and M.S. McNulty. 1995. Molecular cloning of an attenuated chicken anaemia virus isolate following repeated cell culture passage. Avian Pathol 24:171–187.

164. Toro, H., M.S. McNulty, and C. Gonzalez. 1994. Chicken anemia in Chile: Viral detection by immunohistochemistry. Proc Int Symp Infect Bursal Dis Chick Infect Anaemia, Rauischholzhausen, Germany, pp. 434–437.

165. Toro, H., M.S. McNulty, H. Hidalgo, S. Rosende, and T.J. Connor. 1994. Detection of chicken anemia virus antibodies in four poultry operations in Chile. Prev Vet Med 21:103–106.

166. Urlings, H.A.P., G.F. de Boer, D.J. van Roozelaar, and G. Koch. 1993. Inactivation of chicken anaemia virus in chickens by heating and fermentation. Vet Q 15:85–88.

167. Vielitz, E. and H. Landgraf. 1986. Zur Epidemiologie und Prophylaxe der infektiösen Anämie (CAA)-Dermatitis des Huhnes. In M. Larbier (ed.). Proc 7th Eur Poult Conf, vol. 2. World's Poult Sci Assoc, French Branch, Tours, pp. 1124–1129.

168. Vielitz, E. and H. Landgraf. 1988. Anaemia-dermatitis of broilers: Field observations on its occurrence, transmission and prevention. Avian Pathol 17:113–120.

169. Vielitz, E. and M. Voß. 1994. Experiences with a commercial CAV vaccine. Proc Int Symp Infect Bursal Dis Chick Infect Anaemia, Rauischholzhausen, Germany, pp. 465–481.

170. Vielitz, E., V. v. Bülow, H. Landgraf, and C. Conrad. 1987. Anämie des Mastgeflügels—Entwicklung eines Impfstoffes für Elterntiere. J Vet Med B 34:553–557.

171. Vielitz, E., V. v. Bülow, and C. Conrad. 1989. CAA: Experiences with an experimental vaccine. Proc 38th West Poult Dis Conf, March 6–9, 1989, Tempe, AZ, pp. 29–34.

172. Vielitz, E., V. v. Conrad, M. Voss, V. v. Bülow, P. Dorn, J. Bachmeier und U. Lohren. 1991. Impfungen gegen die infektiöse Anämie des Geflügels (CAA)—Ergebnisse von Feldversuchen. Dtsch Tierärztl Wochenschr 98:144–147.

173. Weikel, J., P. Dorn, H. Spiess, and E. Wessling. 1986. Ein Beitrag zur Diagnostik und Epidemiologie der infektiösen Anämie (CAA) beim Broiler. Berl Münch Tierärztl Wochenschr 99:119–121.

174. Wicht, J.V. and S.B. Maharaj. 1993. Chicken anaemia agent in South Africa. Vet Rec 133:147–148.

175. Yuasa, N. 1983. Propagation and infectivity titration of the Gifu-1 strain of chicken anemia agent in a cell line (MDCC-MSB1) derived from Marek's disease lymphoma. Natl Inst Anim Health Q (Jpn) 23:13–20.

176. Yuasa, N. 1989. CAA: Review and recent problems. Proc 38th West Poult Dis Conf, March 6–9, 1989, Tempe, AZ, pp. 14–20.

177. Yuasa, N. 1990. Survey of antibody to chicken anemia agent in sera from foreign countries. Bull Natl Inst Anim Health (Jpn) 95:9–10.

178. Yuasa, N. 1992. Effect of chemicals on the infectivity of chicken anaemia virus. Avian Pathol 21:315–319.

179. Yuasa, N. 1994. Pathology and pathogenesis of chicken anemia virus infection. Proc Int Symp Infect Bursal Dis Chick Infect Anaemia, Rauischholzhausen, Germany, pp. 385–389.

180. Yuasa, N. and K. Imai. 1986. Pathogenicity and antigenicity of eleven isolates of chicken anaemia agent (CAA). Avian Pathol 15:639–645.

181. Yuasa, N. and K. Imai. 1988. Efficacy of Marek's disease vaccine, herpesvirus of turkeys, in chickens infected with chicken anemia agent. In S. Kato, T. Horiuchi, T. Mikami, and K. Hirai (eds.). Advances in Marek's Disease Research. Japanese Association on Marek's Disease, Osaka, Japan, pp. 358–363.

182. Yuasa, N. and I. Yoshida. 1983. Experimental egg transmission of chicken anemia agent. Natl Inst Anim Health Q (Jpn) 23:99–100.

183. Yuasa, N., T. Taniguchi, and I. Yoshida. 1979. Isolation and some characteristics of an agent inducing anemia in chicks. Avian Dis 23:366–385.

184. Yuasa, N., T. Noguchi, K. Furuta, and I. Yoshida. 1980. Maternal antibody and its effect on the susceptibility of chicks to chicken anemia agent. Avian Dis 24:197–201.

185. Yuasa, N., T. Taniguchi, T. Noguchi, and I. Yoshida. 1980. Effect of infectious bursal disease virus infection on incidence of anemia by chicken anemia agent. Avian Dis 24:202–209.

186. Yuasa, N., T. Taniguchi, M. Goda, M. Shibatani, T. Imada, and H. Hihara. 1983. Isolation of chicken anemia agent with MDCC-MSB1 cells from chickens in the field. Natl Inst Anim Health Q (Jpn) 23:75–77.

187. Yuasa, N., T. Taniguchi, T. Imada, and H. Hihara. 1983. Distribution of chicken anemia agent (CAA) and detection of neutralizing antibody in chicks experimentally inoculated with CAA. Natl Inst Anim Health Q (Jpn) 23:78–81.

188. Yuasa, N., K. Imai, and H. Tezuka. 1985. Survey of antibody against chicken anaemia agent (CAA) by an indirect immunofluorescent antibody technique in breeder flocks in Japan. Avian Pathol 14:521–530.

189. Yuasa, N., K. Imai, K. Watanabe, F. Saito, M. Abe, and K. Komi. 1987. Aetiological examination of an outbreak of haemorrhagic syndrome in a broiler flock in Japan. Avian Pathol 16:521–526.

190. Yuasa, N., K. Imai, and K. Nakamura. 1988. Pathogenicity of chicken anaemia agent in bursectomised chickens. Avian Pathol 17:363–369.

191. Zhuang, S.-M., J.E. Landegent, C.A.J. Verschueren, J.H.F. Falkenburg, H. van Ormondt, A.J. van der Eb, and M.H.M. Noteborn. 1995. Apoptin, a protein encoded by chicken anemia virus, induces cell death in various human hematologic malignant cells in vitro. Leukemia 9:S118–S120.

192. Zhuang, S.-M., A. Shvarts, H. van Ormondt, A.G. Jochemsen, A.J. van der Eb, and M.H.M. Noteborn. 1995. Apoptin, a protein encoded by chicken anemia virus, induces p53-independent apoptosis in human osteosarcoma cells. Cancer Res 55:486–489.

31 Other Viral Infections

INTRODUCTION
B. W. Calnek

This chapter includes material on infections that require only a brief description. Two conditions previously included in this chapter have been moved to other sections in this book. It is believed that pneumovirus infections are more appropriately incorporated in Chapter 20 along with Newcastle disease virus and other paramyxoviruses. Chicken infectious anemia, because of its importance, is now afforded a separate chapter (Chapter 30). The former subchapter on chicken parvovirus has been eliminated because it now appears that the so-called parvovirus is very likely identical to the chicken infectious anemia virus. The section on goose parvovirus infection, however, remains, since the etiology of that disease is well documented. Descriptions of that disease, along with infectious nephritis, ar-

bovirus infections, miscellaneous herpesvirus infections, and turkey viral hepatitis, remain in this chapter.

Arbovirus infections can be significant in domestic poultry, as illustrated by those causing meningoencephalitis in turkeys or equine encephalitis in pheasants, but they are additionally important as human pathogens originating from avian reservoirs.

Of the miscellaneous herpesviruses, the pigeon herpesvirus is the most significant. Pseudorabies (Aujeszky's disease) is briefly mentioned only because chickens and pigeons are susceptible to infection with that virus. Herpesviruses that infect wild and exotic birds are not included, in keeping with the scope of this book.

MISCELLANEOUS HERPESVIRUS INFECTIONS
H. Vindevogel and J. P. Duchatel

INTRODUCTION. Herpesvirus infections have been described in several species of domestic and wild birds including pigeons (9, 34), psittacine birds (29), falcons (22), owls (4), cormorants (11), cranes (5), storks (17), and bobwhite quail (16).

All herpesvirus strains isolated from pigeons in Belgium, France, Australia, and Czechoslovakia have been found to be antigenically similar and to possess the same cultural characteristics (3, 15, 19, 34, 35). Therefore, only one pigeon herpesvirus type, pigeon herpesvirus 1 (PHV1) appears to exist. But following Kaleta (15), various breeds of racing and show pigeons may harbor two serologically different herpesviruses and some isolates may contain small- and large-plaque variants.

Pigeon herpesvirus 1 is antigenically different from turkey herpesvirus, Marek's disease virus, infectious laryngotracheitis virus, and duck virus en-

teritis herpesvirus (23, 34). It can also be clearly distinguished from the psittacine herpesvirus (Pacheco's disease virus) based on antigenic composition and plaque size in cell cultures (45).

Conversely, PHV1 cannot be serologically distinguished from the falcon (FHV) and the owl (OHV) herpesviruses, and it remains to be established whether these three herpesviruses are different isolates of the same virus (22, 23). All other herpesviruses isolated from wild birds differ antigenically from each other and from other avian herpesviruses except for the bobwhite quail herpesvirus and the crane herpesvirus, which are serologically related (16).

This subchapter will cover PHV1 infections in pigeons and will briefly mention pseudorabies virus infections that can be experimentally induced in pigeons and young chickens.

757

PIGEON HERPESVIRUS INFECTION

HISTORY.   The first observation of intranuclear inclusion bodies in the liver of pigeons, probably associated with PHV1 infection, was reported in 1945 (30). Since 1967, PHV1 has been isolated from diseased pigeons in numerous countries (9, 34).

INCIDENCE AND DISTRIBUTION.   The suspected geographic distribution of PHV1 is worldwide. The virus has been isolated in the United Kingdom (8), Czechoslovakia (19), Australia (3), Belgium (39), Hungary (33), Germany (12), France (20), and Italy (52). Infection has also been observed in the United States (24). In Europe, the vast majority of pigeons are infected, since more than 50% of them possess specific antibodies (14, 20, 34, 46). In Belgium, the presence of PHV1 was demonstrated in 60% of dove-cotes where pigeons were permanently affected with respiratory disease, and PHV1 could be isolated from the pharynx of 82% of pigeons affected with acute coryza (34, 47).

ETIOLOGY.   Belonging to the family of *Herpesviridae* (most probably alpha), PHV1 is called *Columbid herpesvirus 1* in the new nomenclature. It possesses the morphology and has the physicochemical properties of a typical herpesvirus (54).

All avian cell cultures tested to date were susceptible to PHV1, but the cytopathic effects varied (7, 40, 41). In chicken embryo fibroblast (CEF) cultures, the most consistent change is an increase in the size of cells with syncytia containing two to four nuclei. Initial alterations consist of margination of chromatin and the appearance of Cowdry type A intranuclear inclusion bodies 10 hr after inoculation. Viral antigen is first detected in the nucleus and later throughout the cytoplasm. Virus can be detected by 12 hr, and peak titers are reached by 36 hr after inoculation (40). The baby hamster kidney cell line (BHK) is also susceptible to infection with PHV1, but all the other mammalian cell lines tested so far have been refractory to the virus (41).

Plaques develop in cultures overlaid with carboxymethylcellulose, agarose, or specific antiserum (38, 39). Virus multiplication in cell cultures is inhibited by trisodium phosphonoformate (25, 26, 34) and acycloguanosine (31). Extracellular virus can be protected by the addition of 5% dimethylsulfoxide to the medium before freezing (39).

PATHOGENESIS AND EPIZOOTIOLOGY

Natural and Experimental Hosts.   The pigeon seems to be the natural host of PHV1 with virus infection remaining latent (34).

Pigeon herpesvirus 1 has been isolated from budgerigars (*Nymphicus hollandicus*) accidently infected after close contact with pigeons (42). Pigeons are susceptible to experimental infection by pharyngeal painting, which causes a mainly localized disease (38, 44), or by the intraperitoneal route, causing a systemic infection (10). Systemic infections can also be produced in budgerigars (*Melopsittacus undulatus*) by intranasal inoculation of the virus (35). Chickens, ducks, canaries, and hamsters are resistant to infection (10, 34, 36).

Transmission.   Susceptible pigeons can be infected through direct contact with infected birds. Egg transmission of PHV1 seems unlikely (37). Mature pigeons in infected flocks are asymptomatic carriers of the virus, and some of them may shed virus from time to time (44).

The vast majority of latently infected mature pigeons re-excrete virus in their throat during the breeding season and during squab gorging (56). They are, therefore, able to transmit directly the infection to the squabs soon after hatching. Although the squabs become infected, they are protected from the disease by maternal antibodies acquired through the egg yolk. Therefore, most of the squabs themselves become asymptomatic carriers after this initial infection (37).

Incubation Period, Shedding, and Latency.   Virus excretion begins 24 hr after inoculation and persists at a high titer for a minimum of 7-10 days in inoculated squabs. Typical lesions appear 1-3 days after infection when viral excretion reaches its peak. Mild episodes of recurrence, without clinical signs, occur spontaneously. High titers of specific antibodies do not prevent these recurrences, and, conversely, recurrent episodes are not more frequent when the animals are nearly devoid of specific antibodies. Pigeon herpesvirus 1 re-excretion can also be provoked by cyclophosphamide (Cy)-treatment of pigeons and this period of re-excretion may be accompanied by lesions (44).

Distribution of Pigeon Herpesvirus 1 in the Host.   In classic PHV1 infection, virus generally remains localized in the upper respiratory and digestive tracts. Naturally occurring or experimental pharyngeal infection, however, may be followed by viral dissemination throughout the body, with viral localization and development of lesions in organs such as trachea, spleen, liver, kidney, and brain (6, 8, 38, 39). Indeed, during the primary infection and during episodes of re-excretion following Cy-treatment, a transient viremia may occur (38). Moreover, PHV1 can be transmitted from cell to cell in the presence of high titers of specific antibodies (38). Thus, PHV1 can be spread either by tissue contiguity or by viremia, especially when pigeons are immunodepressed (34).

Signs. In the acute form of the disease, pigeons sneeze frequently and show conjunctivitis, and nostrils become obstructed with nasal mucus and moisture. Caruncles, which are normally white, turn yellow-gray.

In the chronic form, sinusitis and intense dyspnea may be observed if the primary viral infection is complicated by *Trichomonas columbae* or secondary mycoplasmal or bacterial invaders (*Mycoplasma columbinum, Mycoplasma columborale, Pasteurella multocida, Pasteurella hemolytica, Escherichia coli, Staphylococcus β-hemolysin, Streptococcus β-hemolytic*) (27, 34).

Morbidity and Mortality. Clinical disease is observed principally following primary infection of young pigeons not protected by maternal antibodies and in virus carriers in which the infection is complicated by virtue of debilitating factors (37).

Gross Lesions. The mucous membranes of the mouth, pharynx, and larynx are congested and, in severe cases, covered with foci of necrosis and small ulcers. The mucous membrane of the pharynx may be coated with diphtheritic membranes. When the viral infection is generalized (viremia), foci of necrosis can be observed in the liver. If the initial infection becomes complicated by bacterial infections, the trachea may be obstructed by caseous material and some birds may show airsacculitis and pericarditis (pigeon chronic respiratory disease) (34).

Histopathology. Multiple foci of necrosis are observed in the pharyngeal stratified squamous epithelium and in the salivary glands. Foci contain cells at different stages of degeneration and necrosis, and intranuclear inclusions are present in adjacent epithelial cells. Large foci may extend and form ulcers. Similar foci of necrosis can also be observed in the laryngeal and tracheal epithelium (38).

In generalized infections, pigeons present hepatitis; intranuclear inclusion bodies are found in many hepatic cells widely spread throughout the organ (8, 38, 39).

Lesions have also been described in the pancreas and the brain (6, 8, 10).

Immunity. Neutralizing antibodies appear in squabs at the end of the first week following infec-tion. Importance of these antibodies is difficult to evaluate with regard to re-emergence of active infection (44), but when acquired passively in the form of maternally derived antibodies, they are protective for squabs (37). As a herpesvirus infection, it might be presumed that cell-mediated immunity is important in PHV1 infections.

DIAGNOSIS

Isolation and Identification of Causative Agent.
Pigeon herpesvirus 1 can be easily isolated in CEF cultures from pharyngeal swabs of infected pigeons; also, but with more difficulty, from internal organs such as trachea, lungs, or liver. Isolates should be characterized by immunologic means such as immunofluorescence (34, 43).

Serology. Specific antibodies can be titrated by virus-neutralization tests or by indirect immunofluorescence and can be detected by counterimmunoelectroosmophoresis (34, 43).

Differential Diagnosis. Clinically acute PHV1 infection disease may be confused with Newcastle disease virus infection (lentogenic pneumotropic paramyxovirus 1 strains), and chronic PHV1 infection disease complicated by secondary bacterial invaders must be distinguished from the diphtheroid form of pox virus infection (53, 55). A diagnosis of PHV1 infection requires virus isolation or serologic evidence; however, both techniques may fail to demonstrate PHV1 infection in individual pigeons, the first because the animal may not be actively excreting virus and the second because of an absence of seroconversion in a latent carrier. For these reasons, several animals from the same dovecote must be simultaneously examined (34, 43).

TREATMENT PREVENTION AND CONTROL.
After primary infection, pigeons become asymptomatic carriers and may re-excrete virus. Chemotherapy trials with trisodium phosphonoformate and acycloguanosine failed to prevent infection (25, 26, 31, 48). Vindevogel et al. (49, 50, 51), therefore, compared the ability of inactivated (in oil adjuvant), or attenuated, vaccines to prevent clinical disease, the carrier state, and virus re-excretion. Both types of vaccine were able to reduce primary viral excretion and clinical signs after challenge. Nevertheless, neither attenuated nor inactivated vaccines were able to prevent appearance of carriers since most of the pigeons re-excreted virus after Cy-treatment. Vaccination did, however, help to prevent spontaneous viral re-excretion, thereby helping to control viral dissemination.

PSEUDORABIES (AUJESZKY'S DISEASE)

Pseudorabies virus [*Sus herpesvirus 1* (SHV1)] produces a generally mild disease in swine, its natural host, but a fatal disease in cattle. Other animals found infected in nature are dogs, cats, sheep, and rats (18, 21). The virus multiplies very well in chicken embryo fibroblast cultures (2).

Experimentally, SHV1 can infect chickens, chicken embryos, and pigeons (13, 18, 32). Chicken embryos succumb with encephalitis after inoculation on the chorioallantoic membrane, as do 2-day-old chicks after being inoculated subcutaneously (1). Adult chickens, however, are resistant to subcutaneous inoculation (28).

Toneva (32) attenuated a strain of SHV1 by serial passages in pigeons combining intramuscular and subcutaneous routes of inoculation (pigeon strain 80). Inoculated pigeons developed classic symptoms of encephalitis, i.e., torticollis, and disordered balance. The SHV1 pigeon strain 80 is avirulent for rabbits, mice, guinea pigs, and piglets after subcutaneous injection but remains lethal after intracerebral inoculation.

REFERENCES

1. Bang, F.B. 1942. Experimental infection of the chick embryo with the virus of pseudorabies. J Exp Med 76:263–270.
2. Beladi, I. 1962. Study on the plaque formation and some properties of the Aujeszky disease virus on chicken embryo cells. Acta Vet Acad Sci Hung 12:417–422.
3. Boyle, D.B., and J.A. Binnington. 1973. Isolation of a herpesvirus from a pigeon. Aust Vet J 49:54.
4. Burtscher, H. 1965. Die virusbedingte Hepatosplenitis infectiosa strigum. 1. Mitteilung: Morphologische Untersuchungen. Pathol Vet 2:227–255.
5. Burtscher, H., and W. Grünberg. 1979. Herpesvirus-Hepatitis bei Kranichen (Aves Gruidae). I. Pathomorphologische Befunde. Zentralbl Veterinaermed [B] 26:561–569.
6. Callinan, R.B., B. Kefford, R. Borland, and R. Garrett. 1979. An outbreak of disease in pigeons associated with a herpesvirus. Aust Vet J 55:339–341.
7. Cornwell, H.J.C., and A.R. Weir. 1970. Herpesvirus infection of pigeons. IV. Growth of the virus in tissue-culture and comparison of its cytopathogenicity with that of the viruses of laryngotracheitis and pigeon pox. J Comp Pathol 80:517–523.
8. Cornwell, H.J.C., and N.G. Wright. 1970. Herpesvirus infection of pigeons. I. Pathology and virus isolation. J Comp Pathol 80:221–227.
9. Cornwell, H.J.C., A.R. Weir, and E.A.C. Follett. 1967. A herpes infection of pigeons. Vet Rec 81:267–268.
10. Cornwell, H.J.C., N.G. Wright, and H.B. McCusker. 1970. Herpesvirus infection of pigeons. II. Experimental infection of pigeons and chicks. J Comp Pathol 80:229–232.
11. French, E.L., H.G. Purchase, and K. Nazerian. 1973. A new herpesvirus isolated from a nestling cormorant (Phalacrocorax melanoleucos). Avian Pathol 2:3–15.
12. Fritzche, K., U. Heffels, and E.F Kaleta. 1981. Ubersichtreferat: Virusbedingte Infektionen der Taube. Dtsch Tieraerztl Wochenschr 88:72–76.
13. Glover, R.E. 1939. Cultivation of the virus of Au-

jeszky's disease on the chorioallantoic membrane of the developing egg. Br J Exp Pathol 20:150–158.
14. Heffels, U., K. Fritzche, E.F. Kaleta, and U. Neumann. 1981. Serologische Untersuchungen zum Nachweis virusbedingter infektionen bei der Taube in der Bundesrepublik Deutschland. Dtsch Tieraerztl Wochenschr 88:97–102.
15. Kaleta, E.F. 1990. Herpesviruses of birds. A review. Avian Pathol 19:193–211.
16. Kaleta, E.F., H. J. Marschall, G. Glünder, and B. Stiburek. 1980. Isolation and serological differentiation of a herpesvirus from Bobwhite Quail (Colinus virginianus, L. 1758). Arch Virol 66:359–364.
17. Kaleta, E.F., T. Mikami, H.J. Marschall, U. Heffels, M. Heidenreich and B. Stiburek. 1980. A new herpesvirus isolated from black storks (Ciconia nigra). Avian Pathol 9:301–310.
18. Kaplan, A.S. 1969. Herpes simplex and pseudorabies viruses. In S. Gard, C. Hallauer, K.F. Meyer, (eds.). Virology monographs. Springer-Verlag, Vienna/New York, pp. 66–68, 80–82.
19. Krupicka, V., B. Smid, L. Valicek, and V. Pleva. 1970. Isolation of an herpesvirus from pigeons on the chorio-allantoic membrane of embryonated eggs. Vet Med (Praha) 15:609–612.
20. Landré, F., H. Vindevogel, P.P. Pastoret, A. Schwers, E. Thiry, and J. Espinasse. 1982. Fréquence de l'infection du pigeon par le Pigeon herpesvirus 1 et le virus de la maladie de Newcastle dans le Nord de la France. Rec Med Vet 158:523–528.
21. Lautié, R. 1969. Les maladies animales à virus. La maladie d'Aujeszky. In P. Lépine, P. Goret (eds.). Collection de monographies, direction scientifique. L'expansion scientifique Française éditeur.
22. Mare, C.J., and D.L. Graham. 1973. Falcon herpesvirus, the etiologic agent of inclusion body disease of falcons. Infect Immun 8:118–126.
23. Purchase, H.G., C.J. Mare, and B.R. Burmester. 1972. Antigenic comparison of avian and mammalian herpesviruses and protection tests against Marek's disease. Proc 76th Annu Meet US Anim Health Assoc, pp. 484–492.
24. Saik, J.E., E.R. Weintraub, R.W. Diters, and M.A.E. Egy. 1986. Pigeon herpesvirus: Inclusion body hepatitis in a free-ranging pigeon. Avian Dis 30:426–429.
25. Schwers, A., P.P. Pastoret, H. Vindevogel, P. Leroy, A. Aguilar-Setien, and M. Godart. 1980. Comparison of the effect of trisodium phosphonoformate on the mean plaque size of pseudorabies virus, infectious bovine rhinotracheitis virus and pigeon herpesvirus. J Comp Pathol 90:625–633.
26. Schwers, A., H. Vindevogel, P. Leroy, and P.P. Pastoret. 1981. Susceptibility of different strains of pigeon herpesvirus to trisodium phosphonoformate. Avian Pathol 10:23–29.
27. Shimizu, T., H. Erno, and H. Nagatomo. 1978. Isolation and characterization of Mycoplasma columbinum and Mycoplasma columborale, two new species from pigeons. Int J Syst Bact 28:538–546.
28. Shope, R.E. 1931. An experimental study of mad itch with special reference to its relationship to pseudorabies. J Exp Med 45:233–248.
29. Simpsons, C.F., J.E. Hanley, and J.M. Gaskin. 1975. Psittacine herpesvirus resembling Pacheco's parrot disease. J Infect Dis 131:390–396.
30. Smadel, J.E., E.B. Jackson, and J.W. Harman. 1945. A new virus of pigeons. I. Recovery of the virus. J Exp Med 81:385–398.
31. Thiry, E., H. Vindevogel, P. Leroy, P.P. Pastoret, A. Schwers, B. Brochier, Y. Anciaux, and P. Hoyois. 1983. In

vivo and in vitro effect of acyclovir on pseudorabies virus, infectious bovine rhinotracheitis virus and pigeon herpesvirus. Ann Rech Vét 14:239–245.

32. Toneva, V. 1961. Obtention d'une souche non-virulente du virus de la maladie d'Aujeszky au moyen de passages et de l'adaptation des pigeons. C R Acad Bulgare Sci 14:187–190.

33. Vetesy, F., and J. Tanyi. 1975. Occurrence of a pigeon disease in Hungary caused by a herpesvirus. Magyar Allatorv Lapja, pp. 193–197.

34. Vindevogel, H. 1981. Le coryza infectieux du pigeon. Thesis of "Agrégation de l'Enseignement Supérieur." University of Liège, Fac Vet Med.

35. Vindevogel, H., and J.P. Duchatel. 1977. Réceptivité de la perruche au virus herpès du pigeon. Ann Méd Vét 121:193–195.

36. Vindevogel, H., and J.P. Duchatel. 1979. 1. Etude de la récéptivité de différentes espèces animales au virus herpès du pigeon. 2. Résistance du pigeon au virus de la laryngotrachéite infectieuse aviaire. Ann Méd Vét 123:63–65.

37. Vindevogel, H., and P.P. Pastoret. 1980 . Pigeon herpes infection: Natural transmission of the disease. J Comp Pathol 90:409–413.

38. Vindevogel, H., and P.P. Pastoret. 1981. Pathogenesis of pigeon herpes infection. J Comp Pathol 91:415–426.

39. Vindevogel, H., P.P. Pastoret, G. Burtonboy, M. Gouffaux, and J.P. Duchatel. 1975. Isolement d'un virus herpès dans un elevage de pigeons de chair. Ann Rech Vét 6:431–436.

40. Vindevogel, H., J.P. Duchatel, and M. Gouffaux. 1977. Pigeon herpesvirus. I. Pathogenesis of pigeon herpesvirus in chicken embryo fibroblasts. J Comp Pathol 87:597–603.

41. Vindevogel, H., J.P. Duchatel, M. Gouffaux, and P.P. Pastoret. 1977. Pigeon herpesvirus. II. Susceptibility of avian and mammalian cell cultures to infection with pigeon herpesvirus. J Comp Pathol 87:605–610.

42. Vindevogel, H., J.P. Duchatel, and G. Burtonboy. 1978. Infection herpétique de psittacidés. Ann Méd Vét 122:167–169.

43. Vindevogel, H., A. Aguilar-Setien, L. Dagenais, and P.P. Pastoret. 1980. Diagnostic de l'infection herpétique du pigeon. Ann Méd Vét 124:407–418.

44. Vindevogel, H., P.P. Pastoret, and G. Burtonboy. 1980. Pigeon herpes infection: Excretion and re-excretion of virus after experimental infection. J Comp Pathol 90:401–408.

45. Vindevogel, H., P.P. Pastoret, P. Leroy, and F. Coignoul. 1980. Comparaison de trois souches de virus herpétique isolées de psittacidés avec le virus herpès du pigeon. Avian Pathol 9:385–394.

46. Vindevogel, H., L. Dagenais, B. Lansival, and P.P. Pastoret. 1981. Incidence of rotavirus, adenovirus and herpesvirus infection in pigeons. Vet Rec 109:285–286.

47. Vindevogel, H., A. Kaeckenbeeck, and P.P. Pastoret. 1981. Fréquence de l'ornithose-psittacose et de l'infection herpétique chez le pigeon voyageur et les psittacidés en Belgique. Rev Méd de Liège 36:693–696.

48. Vindevogel, H., P. P. Pastoret, and A. Aguilar-Setien. 1982. Assays of phosphonoformate-treatment of pigeon herpesvirus infection in pigeons and budgerigars, and Aujeszky's disease in rabbits. J Comp Pathol 92:177–180.

49. Vindevogel, H., P.P. Pastoret, and P. Leroy. 1982. Vaccination trials against pigeon herpesvirus infection (Pigeon herpesvirus 1). J Comp Pathol 92:484–494.

50. Vindevogel, H., P.P. Pastoret, and P. Leroy. 1982. Essais de vaccination contre l'infection herpétique du pigeon (Pigeon herpesvirus 1). 17th Int Congr Herpesvirus Man Anim: Standard Immunol Proc Dev Biol Stand 52:429–436.

51. Vindevogel, H., P.P. Pastoret, and P. Leroy. 1982. Comportement d'une souche atténuée de Pigeon herpesvirus 1 et de souches pathogènes lors d'infections successives chez le pigeon. Ann Rech Vét 13:143–148.

52. Vindevogel, H., P.P. Pastoret, E. Thiry and N. Peeters. 1982. Réapparition de formes graves de la maladie de Newcastle chez le pigeon. Ann Méd Vét 126:5–7.

53. Vindevogel, H., E. Thiry, P.P. Pastoret, and G. Meulemans. 1982. Lentogenic strains of Newcastle disease virus in pigeons. Vet Rec 110:497–499.

54. Vindevogel, H., P.P. Pastoret, and E. Thiry. 1983. Pigeon herpesvirus 1. WHO Collaborating Centre for Collection and Evaluation of Data on Comparative Virology. Munich, W. Germany.

55. Vindevogel, H., J.P. Duchatel, and P.P. Pastoret. 1984. Les dominantes pathologiques respiratoires chez le pigeon. Rec Med Vet 160:1031–1036.

56. Vindevogel, H., H. Debruyne, and P.P. Pastoret. 1985. Observation of Pigeon herpesvirus 1 re-excretion during the reproduction period in conventionally reared homing pigeons. J Comp Pathol 95:105–112.

AVIAN NEPHRITIS

Tadao Imada and Hitoshi Kawamura

INTRODUCTION. Avian nephritis, caused by a picornavirus (enterovirus), is an acute, highly contagious, typically subclinical disease of young chickens that produces lesions in the kidneys.

The causative agent, avian nephritis virus (ANV), was first isolated in chicken kidney cell (CKC) cultures from the rectal contents of apparently normal, 1-wk-old broiler chickens in Japan in 1976 (36). It has been shown to be a picornavirus, which is distinct from avian encephalomyelitis virus and duck hepatitis viruses, based on pathologic (7, 12) and immunologic (1, 13, 14, 18, 33) criteria. The pathogenicity of this virus was established by experimental infections of chickens and chicken embryos. As there have been a few reports on the disease associated with this virus infection in the field (27, 33), the economic importance is not well known, and public health significance is not known.

INCIDENCE AND DISTRIBUTION. The true incidence and distribution of the disease are not well known owing to the transient, usually subclinical nature of the infection and the difficulties with virus isolation. Runting and diarrhea in young chickens associated with an enteroviruslike particle serologically identical or related to ANV, but different biologically, have been reported in some countries (2, 4, 5, 6, 13, 15, 16, 24, 31). Avian nephritis virus has been shown to be widely distributed in chicken flocks in Japan (8, 34), some European countries (1, 3, 23), and several specific-pathogen–free (SPF) flocks (1, 17, 23). Antibody to ANV has been also detected in turkeys in Northern Ireland and England (1, 23).

ETIOLOGY

Classification and Morphology. Avian nephritis virus has been tentatively classified as a picornavirus based on the following properties: 1) the presence of RNA; 2) replication in the cytoplasm; 3) diameter of 28 nm; 4) resistance to ethyl ether, chloroform, trypsin, and acid (pH 3.0); 5) relative heat lability; and 6) partial stabilization at 50 C by molar magnesium chloride (36). The density in cesium chloride (CsCl) of the intact particles was not estimated because the virus is very unstable in a strong solution of CsCl. When the density is defined, the virus will probably be classified as an enterovirus belonging to the family *Picornaviridae*. It has been reported that serotypes of ANV exist (6, 29, 31, 33).

Laboratory Host Systems

CHICKEN EMBRYOS. When inoculated with ANV, 6-day-old embryos died 3–14 days postinoculation (PI). They manifested hemorrhage and edema of the whole body at 3–6 days PI and stunting at 7–14 days PI. When inoculated by the chorioallantoic membrane (CAM) route, high virus doses killed all embryos, but low virus doses allowed some infected embryos to hatch normally. In these eggs, the CAM showed edematous thickening or pocks at the inoculation site, and the embryos were stunted. Embryos inoculated by the allantoic cavity route sometimes became infected, but no virus was detected in allantoic fluids (6, 10).

CELL CULTURE. The representative strain (G-4260) of ANV grew in CKC with round cell–type cytopathic effect (CPE) and maximum virus titers at 24 hr PI (36). It did not grow in duck embryo fibroblasts, duck embryo kidney cells, or some established mammalian cell lines (HeLa, Vero, MDBK, PK-15, and MDCK). But the ability of ANV to replicate in vitro may be influenced by the conditions of the cell cultures and the strains of ANV (1, 4, 6, 18, 33).

Pathogenicity. Young chickens are the only animals known to develop clinical disease and distinct kidney lesions when exposed to ANV. Field viruses exhibit different degrees of pathogenicity in chickens. There are indications that different serotypes, and even strains with the same serotype, can vary in their ability to produce illness and death (4, 6, 7, 25, 29, 30, 31, 33). Avian nephritis virus had no apparent effect on egg production or egg quality in laying hens (11). Narita et al. (21, 22) showed that infectious bursal disease virus infection and cyclophosphamide treatment enhance the pathogenicity of ANV.

PATHOGENESIS AND EPIZOOTIOLOGY

Natural and Experimental Hosts. Infection has been recognized in chickens, and the antibody to ANV is recognized in turkey flocks. Attempts to establish active infection in other animals have not yet been carried out. Chickens of all ages may be infected, but it has been observed that 1-day-old chicks are the most susceptible (6, 9, 20). Transmission readily occurs by direct or indirect contact (9). Egg transmission has been suggested on the basis of field observations (1, 33), and virus can be isolated from chicks hatched from artificially infected embryonating eggs (10). In experimentally infected chicks, the virus was first detected in feces 2 days PI, with maximum virus shedding at 4–5 days PI. The virus is widely distributed, with maximum titers in the kidney and jejunum and lower titers in the bursa of Fabricius, spleen, and liver. The virus was consistently isolated from kidney, jejunum, and rectum, but not from brain and trachea during the first 10 days PI (7).

The clinical signs of ANV infection in 1-day-old chicks is only transient diarrhea, but not all chicks show the signs. Weight gain is depressed between 7 and 14 days PI. At necropsy at 4–21 days PI, mild to severe discoloration and swelling in the kidneys are observed, and in dead chicks within 2 weeks PI, visceral urate deposits (Fig. 31.1) are observed (6, 7, 12, 19, 20, 25, 26, 28). It has been reported that the concentration of serum uric acid or plasma urate value of ANV-infected 1-day-old chicks is transiently higher than that of uninfected chicks (19, 20, 21, 22, 28, 30).

Mortality may be influenced by the virulence of the ANV strain, strain of birds, and experimental conditions (6, 25, 30, 35).

Under field conditions, clinical signs associated with this virus infection in broiler chickens have varied from none (subclinical) to outbreaks of the so-called runting syndrome and baby chick nephropathy (6, 8, 13, 15, 27, 31, 33, 36). Nothing is known about clinical signs in turkeys.

Histopathology. Histopathologic lesions in the kidneys of experimentally infected chickens have been studied (6, 9, 10, 11, 12, 19, 20, 21, 22, 25, 26, 28, 29, 31). The primary changes consisted of necrosis and degeneration of epithelial cells of

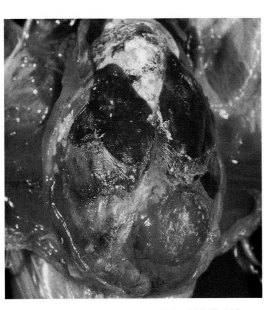

31.1. Visceral urate deposits in a chick which died 10 days postinfection. Chalklike urate crystals were deposited on the surface of the peritoneum and liver, although those on the surface of the liver were mostly removed during necropsy. The heart is white due to heavy urate deposits on the epicardium.

PI. There may be difficulties associated with isolation of enteric viruses in cell cultures (see Chapter 27, Rotavirus Infection, Diagnosis).

In embryonating eggs, infected embryos display hemorrhage and edema or stunting. Virus isolates may be further characterized by filtration through 50-nm–porosity membrane filters, or by inoculation of 1-day-old chicks with a 50% suspension of tissues harvested from embryos, followed by examination for lesions in the kidneys 3–7 days PI.

The IF technique is a useful diagnostic procedure. Viral antigens can be detected in the early acute phase of the disease by staining infected kidneys with specific anti-ANV fluorescent antibodies. This technique can also be used to detect viral antigens in cell cultures and embryos. In CKC infected with ANV, lumpy and granular antigens are seen in the cytoplasm as early as 12 hr PI.

Serology.   Chickens recovered from naturally occurring and experimental infections manifest an immunologic response that can be measured with a conventional virus-neutralization test, the indirect IF test, and enzyme-linked immunosorbent assay (ELISA) (3).

the proximal convoluted tubules with infiltration of granulocytes. The degenerating epithelial cells had acidophilic granules of various sizes in the cytoplasm (Fig. 31.2). Also, there was interstitial lymphocyte infiltration and moderate fibrosis. In later stages, at 14–28 days PI, lymphoid follicles developed. Avian nephritis virus particles and viral antigens were demonstrated by electron microscopy in the degenerating epithelium (Fig. 31.3) and immunofluorescence (IF), respectively. Specific viral antigens were recognized by IF also in the jejunum, but distinct microscopic lesions were not observed in the small intestine. The chicks that died revealed many urate tophi in the serosa and parenchyma throughout the body, including the kidneys.

DIAGNOSIS

Isolation and Identification of Causative Agent.   For isolation of the virus from infected chickens, suspensions of either the kidneys or the rectal contents made in cell culture medium can be used as inoculum. After freezing and thawing three times, and centrifuging to remove the large tissue particles, the supernatant fluid is inoculated onto monolayers of CKCs or injected by the yolk sac route into 6-day-old embryonating eggs that originated from an SPF flock with no antibody to ANV (35, 36). In infected CKC cultures, round cell–type CPE, without hemagglutinin, develops within 72 hr

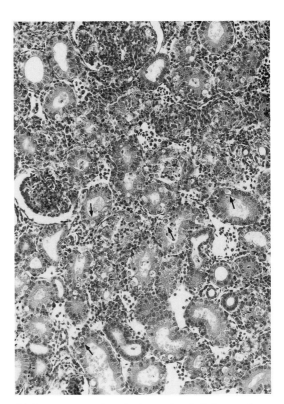

31.2.   Degenerated proximal convoluted tubules containing acidophilic granules (*arrows*) in epithelial cell cytoplasm, and lymphocytic infiltration in interstitium, 5 days postinfection. H & E, ×300.

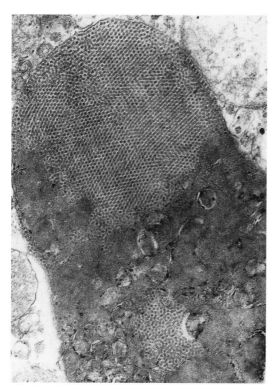

31.3. Crystalline array of virus particles in the cytoplasm of a kidney epithelial cell, 3 days postinfection. ×30,000.

Differential Diagnosis.   Certain nephrotoxic strains of infectious bronchitis virus (IBV) cause interstitial nephritis. It would be difficult to separate the two conditions on the basis of the histologic lesions (32). These cases may be differentiated from ANV infections by the fact that with infectious bronchitis there are some changes in the trachea, and infections in kidneys are usually preceded by respiratory signs. When a nephritis is noticed in especially young chickens, it is necessary to isolate the causative agent or conduct serologic tests. The possibility that the two diseases may occur simultaneously in a flock should not be overlooked.

TREATMENT, PREVENTION, AND CONTROL.   There is no specific treatment. Additional knowledge is needed to formulate measures for prophylaxis and control. It is important to know that the flocks are infected or not in view of the possible economic implications for the poultry industry.

REFERENCES

1. Connor, T.J., F. McNeilly, J.B. McFerran, and M.S. McNulty. 1987. A survey of avian sera from Northern Ireland for antibody to avian nephritis virus. Avian Pathol 16:15–20.

2. Decaesstecker, M., and G. Meulemans. 1989. Antigenic relationships between fowl enteroviruses. Avian Pathol 18:715–723.

3. Decaesstecker, M., and G. Meulemans. 1991. An ELISA for the detection of antibodies to avian nephritis virus and related entero-like viruses. Avian Pathol 20:523–530.

4. Decaesstecker, M., G. Charlier, J. Peeters, and G. Meulemans. 1989. Pathogenicity of fowl enteroviruses. Avian Pathol 18:697–713.

5. Frazier, J.A., and R.L. Reece. 1990. Infectious stunting syndrome of chickens in Great Britain: Intestinal ultrastructural pathology. Avian Pathol 19:759–777.

6. Frazier, J.A., K. Howes, R.L. Reece, A.W. Kidd, and D. Cavanagh. 1990. Isolation of non-cytopathic viruses implicated in the aetiology of nephritis and baby chick nephropathy and serologically related to avian nephritis virus. Avian Pathol 19:139–160.

7. Imada, T., S. Yamaguchi, and H. Kawamura. 1979. Pathogenicity for baby chicks of the G-4260 strain of the picornavirus "Avian nephritis virus." Avian Dis 23:582–588.

8. Imada, T., S. Yamaguchi, and H. Kawamura. 1980. Antibody survey against avian nephritis virus among chickens in Japan. Natl Inst Anim Health Q (Jpn) 20:79–80.

9. Imada, T., T. Taniguchi, S. Yamaguchi, T. Minetoma, M. Maeda, and H. Kawamura. 1981. Susceptibility of chickens to avian nephritis virus at various inoculation routes and ages. Avian Dis 25:294–302.

10. Imada, T., T. Taniguchi, S. Sato, S. Yamaguchi, and H. Kawamura. 1982. Pathogenicity of avian nephritis virus for embryonating hen's eggs. Natl Inst Anim Health Q (Jpn) 22:8–15.

11. Imada, T., M. Maeda, K. Furuta, S. Yamaguchi, and H. Kawamura. 1983. Pathogenicity and distribution of avian nephritis virus (G-4260 stain) in inoculated laying hens. Natl Inst Anim Health Q (Jpn) 23:43–48.

12. Maeda, M., T. Imada, T. Taniguchi, and T. Horiuchi. 1979. Pathological changes in chicks inoculated with the picornavirus "Avian nephritis virus." Avian Dis 23:589–596.

13. McFerran, J.B., and M.S. McNulty. 1986. Recent advances in enterovirus infections of birds. In J.B. McFerran and M.S. McNulty (eds.). Acute Virus Infections of Poultry. Martinus Nijhoff, Dordrecht, Netherlands, pp. 195–202.

14. McNeilly, F., T.J. Connor, V.M. Calvert, J.A. Smyth, W.L. Curran, A.J. Morley, D. Thompson, S. Singh, J.B. McFerran, B.M. Adair, and M.S. McNulty. 1994. Studies on a new enterovirus-like virus isolated from chickens. Avian Pathol 23:313–327.

15. McNulty, M.S., G.M. Allan, T.J. Connor, J.B. McFerran, and R.M. McCracken. 1984. An entero-like virus associated with the runting syndrome in broiler chickens. Avian Pathol 13:429–439.

16. McNulty, M.S., G.M. Allan, and J.B. McFerran. 1987. Isolation of a novel avian entero-like virus. Avian Pathol 16:331–337.

17. McNulty, M.S., T.J. Connor, and F. McNeilly. 1989. A survey of specific pathogen-free chicken flocks for antibodies to chicken anaemia agent, avian nephritis virus and group a rotavirus. Avian Pathol 18:215–220.

18. McNulty, M.S., T.J. Connor, F. McNeilly, and J.B. McFerran. 1990. Biological characterisation of avian enteroviruses and enterovirus-like viruses. Avian Pathol 19:75–87.

19. Narita, M., H. Kawamura, K. Nakamura, J. Shirai, K. Furuta, and F. Abe. 1990. An immunohistological study on the nephritis in chicks experimentally produced with avian nephritis virus. Avian Pathol 19:497–509.

20. Narita, M., K. Ohta, H. Kawamura, J. Shirai, K. Nakamura, and F. Abe. 1990. Pathogenesis of renal dysfunction in chicks experimentally induced by avian nephritis virus. Avian Pathol 19:571–582.

21. Narita, M., H. Kawamura, K. Furuta, J. Shirai, and K. Nakamura. 1990. Effects of cyclophosphamide in newly hatched chickens after inoculation with avian nephritis virus. Am J Vet Res 51:1623–1628.

22. Narita, M., S. Umiji, K. Furuta, J. Shirai, and K. Nakamura. 1991. Pathogenicity of avian nephritis virus in chicks

previously infected with infectious bursal disease virus. Avian Pathol 20:101–111.

23. Nicholas, R.A.J., R.D. Goddard, and P.R. Luff. 1988. Prevalence of avian nephritis virus in England. Vet Rec 123:398.

24. Reece, R.L., and J.A. Frazier. 1990. Infectious stunting syndrome of chickens in Great Britain: Field and experimental studies. Avian Pathol 19:723–758.

25. Reece, R.L., K. Howes, and J.A. Frazier. 1992. Experimental factors affecting mortality following inoculation of chickens with avian nephritis virus (G-4260). Avian Dis 36:619–624.

26. Shirai, J., K. Nakamura, M. Narita, K. Furuta, H. Hihara, and H. Kawamura. 1989. Visceral urate deposits in chicks inoculated with avian nephritis virus. Vet Rec 124:658–661.

27. Shirai, J., H. Obata, K. Nakamura, K. Furuta, H. Hihara, and H. Kawamura. 1990. Experimental infection in SPF chicks with avian reo and avian nephritis viruses isolated from broiler chicks showing runting syndrome. Avian Dis 34:295–303.

28. Shirai, J., K. Nakamura, M. Narita, K. Furuta, and H. Kawamura. 1990. Avian nephritis virus infection of chicks: Virology, pathology, and serology. Avian Dis 34:558–565.

29. Shirai, J., K. Nakamura, K. Shinohara, and H. Kawamura. 1991. Pathogenicity and antigenicity of avian nephritis isolates. Avian Dis 35:49–54.

30. Shirai, J., K. Nakamura, H. Nozaki, and H. Kawamura. 1991. Differences in the induction of urate deposition of specific-pathogen-free chicks inoculated with avian nephritis virus passaged by five different methods. Avian Dis 35:269–275.

31. Shirai, J., N. Tanimura, K. Uramoto, M. Narita, K. Nakamura, and H. Kawamura. 1992. Pathologically and serologically different avian nephritis virus isolates implicated in etiology of baby chick nephropathy. Avian Dis 36:369–377.

32. Siller, W.G. 1981. Renal pathology of the fowl-a review. Avian Pathol 10:187–262.

33. Takase, K., K. Shinohara, M. Tsuneyoshi, M. Yamamoto, and S. Yamada. 1989. Isolation and characterisation of cytopathic avian enteroviruses from broiler chicks. Avian Pathol 18:631–642.

34. Takase, K., K. Matsuo, and M. Yamamoto. 1990. A survey of avian sera for avian nephritis virus, strain AAF in Japan. J Jpn Vet Med Assoc 43:199–201.

35. Takase, K., T. Uchimura, M. Yamamoto, and S. Yamada. 1994. Susceptibility of embryos and chicks, derived from immunized breeding hens, to avian nephritis virus. Avian Pathol 23:117–125.

36. Yamaguchi, S., T. Imada, and H. Kawamura. 1979. Characterization of a picornavirus isolated from broiler chicks. Avian Dis 23:571–581.

ARBOVIRUS INFECTIONS

James S. Guy

INTRODUCTION. The term *arbovirus*, an abbreviation of *arthropod-borne-virus*, is used to describe a virus that replicates in a hematophagous (bloodsucking) arthropod and is transmitted by bite to a vertebrate host. Taxonomically, the term has been used to group those viruses that share the property of transmission by arthropod vectors. The most recent edition of the *International Catalog of Arboviruses* (38), published in 1985, lists 504 known arboviruses; since that time, an additional 31 arboviruses have been recognized (39). Over 100 have been isolated from avian species or ornithophilic arthropod vectors, but only four—eastern equine encephalitis (EEE) virus, western equine encephalitis (WEE) virus, Highlands J (HJ) virus, and Israel turkey meningoencephalitis (IT) virus—have been identified as causes of disease in domestic poultry and farm-reared gamebirds.

ETIOLOGY

Virus Classification. The arboviruses comprise a large, diverse group of viruses, with members in 12 different virus families. Six of those, the *Togaviridae, Flaviviridae, Bunyaviridae, Arenaviridae, Reoviridae* and *Rhabdoviridae* have arbovirus members that have been isolated from birds and ornithophilic arthropod vectors. The main characteristics of each of these virus families are presented below (45, 47, 68). The two families of arboviruses identified as causes of disease in poultry and game birds, i.e., *Togaviridae* and *Flaviviridae,* are emphasized.

TOGAVIRIDAE. Togaviruses are spherical enveloped viruses approximately 50–70 nm in diameter (Fig. 31.4). The genome consists of a single molecule of positive-sense, single-stranded RNA of approximately 12 kb, enclosed within a 28- to 35-nm diameter icosahedral core. Virions are composed of two or three envelope proteins (E1, E2, and sometimes E3) that are usually glycosylated, and a fourth core protein (C). The molecular weights (mw) of alphavirus E1 and E2 structural proteins are $50–59 \times 10^3$; that of E3, when present, is 10×10^3, and C has a mw of $30–34 \times 10^3$ (17). Togaviruses replicate in the cytoplasm, and assembly involves budding of nucleocapsids through host-cell plasma membranes. Some togaviruses exhibit pH-dependent hemagglutinating activity.

Four genera comprise the family *Togaviridae,* but only the *Alphavirus* genus contains arboviruses. The alphaviruses formerly were known as the arbovirus A group; the genus includes 27 viruses, the best known being EEE virus, WEE virus, Venezuelan equine encephalitis (VEE) virus, and HJ virus. Based on neutralization tests (37), the alphaviruses have been subdivided into six antigenic groups

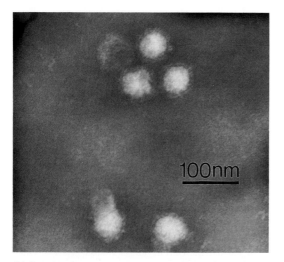

31.4. Negative-contrast electron micrograph of eastern equine encephalitis virus. ×150,000.

named for prototype viruses: EEE virus, WEE virus, VEE virus, Semliki Forest virus, Ndumu virus, and Middleburg virus. Individual viruses are placed within these antigenic groups based on demonstration of antigenic relatedness to a prototype virus.

FLAVIVIRIDAE. Flaviviruses formerly were known as Group B arboviruses and until recently were classified in the family *Togaviridae.* They now are recognized as a distinct virus family based on differences in virion structure, gene sequence, morphogenesis and replication strategy (68). Flaviviruses resemble togaviruses, with the exception that they are somewhat smaller: 40–50 nm in diameter. They replicate in the cytoplasm and acquire a lipid envelope by budding into cytoplasmic vesicles. The genome consists of a single molecule of positive-sense, single-stranded RNA of approximately 10 kb. Virions are composed of three structural proteins: an envelope glycoprotein with a mw of 51 to 59 × 10³, a core protein of 13 to 16 × 10³ mw, and a membranelike protein of 7 to 9 × 10³ mw. Flaviviruses exhibit pH-dependent hemagglutinating activity.

The family contains a single genus, *Flavivirus*, and about 70 virus members. Members of the *Fla-*

viviridae include IT virus and St. Louis encephalitis virus.

BUNYAVIRIDAE. Bunyaviruses are spherical, enveloped viruses 90–120 nm in diameter. The genome consists of three molecules of circular, negative-sense RNA with a total size of 13–21 kb. Virus replication occurs in the cytoplasm with budding through Golgi membranes.

ARENAVIRIDAE. Arenaviruses are enveloped, pleomorphic viruses, 50–300 nm (mean, 110–130 nm) in diameter. The genome consists of two molecules of circular, negative-sense RNA with a total size of 10–14 kb. Replication occurs in the cytoplasm with assembly and budding from the host cell plasma membrane.

REOVIRIDAE. Members of the *Reoviridae* family are nonenveloped, spherical viruses with a diameter of 60–80 nm. Ten linear segments of double-stranded RNA with a total size of approximately 18 kb comprise the genome. Replication and assembly occur in the cytoplasm. The family has four genera, but only the *Orbivirus* genus contains arboviruses isolated from birds.

RHABDOVIRIDAE. Rhabdoviruses are bullet-shaped, enveloped viruses, approximately 70–85 nm in diameter and 130–380 nm in length. The genome consists of a single molecule of negative-sense, single-stranded RNA with a total size of approximately 13–16 kb.

Laboratory Host Systems. Newborn and baby mice are highly susceptible to arboviruses when inoculated by the intracerebral (IC) route and some are susceptible following inoculation by peripheral routes (49, 57). Intracerebral inoculation of newborn mice, 1 to 4 days of age, is the preferred method for isolation of these viruses. Arboviruses also may be propagated in embryonated chicken eggs and in a variety of vertebrate and arthropod cell cultures. Vero cells, BHK-21 cells, and primary cultures of chicken and duck cells are frequently used for virus propagation. Cytopathic effects are readily produced by arboviruses in vertebrate cell cultures; they are not always produced in arthropod cell cultures.

ARBOVIRUS DISEASES OF BIRDS

The four arboviruses identified as causes of disease in domestic poultry and farm-reared game birds are Eastern equine encephalitis (EEE) virus, Western

equine encephalites (WEE) virus, Highlands J (HJ) virus, and Israel turkey meningeoencephalitis (IT) virus.

EASTERN EQUINE ENCEPHALITIS

HISTORY. Eastern equine encephalitis virus was first isolated in the eastern United States in 1933 from the brain of a horse with encephalitis (60). In 1938, the virus was identified by Tyzzer et al. (63) as the cause of an epornitic disease of penned pheasants. It was subsequently identified as a cause of disease in pigeons in 1938 (16), chukar partridges (46) and Pekin ducks (11) in 1960, and turkeys in 1961 (58).

INCIDENCE AND DISTRIBUTION. Eastern equine encephalitis is most commonly seen as a disease of horses. Many outbreaks of EEE in farm-raised ring-neck pheasants and chukar partridges have been identified, but it occurs only sporadically in other species of poultry and game birds. The disease occurs primarily in the eastern parts of North America, throughout Central America and the Caribbean, and in eastern parts of South America. In the United States, EEE has been identified in most states east of the Mississippi River, as well as Louisiana and Texas; it occurs most often in Atlantic seaboard states and Gulf Coast states. Reported isolations of EEE virus in Europe and Asia have not been confirmed.

Outbreaks generally occur in late summer and fall as a consequence of increasing numbers of mosquito vectors. Wallis et al. (67) demonstrated that increased population densities of mosquitoes coincided with the appearance of outbreaks. Hayes and Hess (23) studied weather patterns associated with EEE outbreaks in Massachusetts and New Jersey and noted that excessive rainfall during the preceding autumn months influenced the occurrence of the disease.

PATHOGENESIS AND EPIZOOTIOLOGY

Natural and Experimental Hosts. Outbreaks of EEE in avian species have been reported primarily in pheasants (36, 63); however, outbreaks in pigeons (16), chukar partridges (46, 52), turkeys (15, 58, 64), and ducks (11) also have been reported. Episodes of clinical disease in chickens and quail have not been reported, but both species are highly susceptible to experimental infection (62, 63).

Transmission. *Culiseta melanura,* an ornithophilic mosquito, has been determined to be the principal enzootic vector of EEE virus in North America (8, 29). The virus also has been identified in a variety of other mosquitoes including *Aedes sollicitans, Coquilletia perturbans, Culex pancossa, Cx. dunni,* and *Cx. sacchettae,* as well as

mites, lice, simuliid flies, and culicoides (10, 65, 66). *C. melanura* is the likely vector responsible for transmission to poultry and game birds; transmission to mammalian species most likely occurs by other mosquitoes such as *Aedes* spp. and *Coquillettia* spp., which feed on birds but also have a propensity to bite mammals (45).

Wild birds, primarily the smaller species of Passeriformes, are the principal vertebrate hosts of EEE virus (43, 45, 69). These birds rarely become ill but serve as maintenance and amplifying hosts for the virus in the transmission cycle. In experimental studies, a variety of wild birds were shown to develop viremias lasting up to 4 days; small passeriform birds were shown to develop viremias with maximal lethal-dose-50% (LD_{50}) titers greater than 10^6/mL (43).

Although EEE virus is transmitted principally by mosquitoes, direct transmission has been shown to occur among pheasants as a result of feather picking and cannibalism (28). In addition, pheasants have been experimentally infected by oral inoculation of the virus (54). Epornitics of EEE virus infection in pheasants are believed to be initiated by mosquito-borne infection of one or more birds in a flock, with subsequent spread within the flock occurring as a result of feather picking and cannibalism.

Transmission of EEE virus by semen also has been demonstrated (21); virus was shed in the semen of experimentally infected tom turkeys on days 1 to 5 postinfection (PI). Semen collected from infected tom turkeys at 1–2 days PI resulted in transmission to breeder hens after artificial insemination.

Clinical Signs and Pathology. Clinical disease produced by EEE virus in poultry and game birds usually is attributed to central nervous system (CNS) infection with or without involvement of viscera. However, EEE also may produce visceral infections with little or no involvement of CNS tissues.

PHEASANTS. Naturally infected pheasants develop signs of neurologic dysfunction consisting of depression, leg paralysis, torticollis, and tremors (3, 63). Clinical signs occurred in 40–100% of experimentally infected pheasants with mortality of 25–100% (22, 42, 54). Mortality rates up to 80% have been described for naturally occurring outbreaks.

Tyzzer et al. (63) and Jungherr et al. (36) described the pathology of EEE in pheasants. Gross lesions were not observed; however, histopathologic changes in the CNS consisted of vasculitis, patchy necrosis, neuronal degeneration, and meningeal inflammation.

TURKEYS. Outbreaks of EEE in turkeys in Wisconsin were characterized by drowsiness, incoordination, progressive weakness, and paralysis of legs and wings (58). Mortality in affected flocks was low, generally less than 5%. Infected turkeys had neurologic lesions consisting of calcification of blood vessel walls and cell processes, primarily in the cerebral cortex, the cerebellar folia, and the basal part of the medulla. Central nervous system lesions in intracerebrally inoculated birds included lymphocytic perivascular infiltration, neuronal degeneration, and endothelial cell swelling. Calcification of blood vessel walls was not observed in intracerebrally inoculated birds that died before 6 days PI.

Ficken et al. (15) serologically identified EEE virus as the cause of high mortality in young (1- to 4-wk-old) turkeys. Subsequent experimental studies demonstrated susceptibility of young turkeys to experimental infection (18). Two-week-old turkeys experimentally infected with EEE virus exhibited depression, somnolence, and high mortality. Viremia was detected in infected turkeys on days 1 and 2 PI, with peak viremia of $10^{5.5}$ detected on day 1 PI. Pathologic changes consisted of multifocal necrosis in the heart (Fig. 31.5A), kidney, and pancreas, and lymphoid necrosis and depletion in the thymus (Fig. 31.5B), spleen and bursa of Fabricius (Fig. 31.5C). No lesions were detected in brains.

Acute drops in egg production in turkey breeder hens due to EEE virus infection were reported by Wages et al. in 1993 (64). Decreased egg production in affected flocks was characterized by sudden onset and production of white, thin-shelled and shell-less eggs. No increase in mortality was observed, and acute ovarian regression was the only gross lesion observed. Experimental infection of turkey hens with EEE virus reproduced the disease observed in naturally affected flocks (20). Eastern equine encephalitis virus–infected turkey hens exhibited mild depression and inappetence, but only on day 1 PI. A precipitous decline in egg production began on day 2 PI, and production remained depressed for 15 days; no mortality was observed. Viremia of short duration (1–2 days), peaking at $10^{5.8}$ on day 1 PI, was detected in EEE-virus–infected hens.

CHUKAR PARTRIDGES. Chukar partridges infected with EEE virus exhibited clinical signs of depression, somnolence, and high mortality (30–80%)(52). Pale, focal areas were present on hearts of affected birds, and spleens were mottled and enlarged. Microscopic lesions consisted of gliosis, satellitosis, and perivascular lymphocytic infil-

tration in brains and myocardial necrosis with lymphocytic infiltration was observed in hearts.

DUCKS. White Pekin ducklings infected with EEE virus developed a paralytic disease characterized by sudden onset, posterior paresis, and paralysis; mortality rates in affected flocks were 2–60% (11). Histopathologic lesions consisted of edema of spinal cord white matter, lymphocytic meningitis, and microgliosis.

CHICKENS. Newly hatched chickens are highly susceptible to EEE virus and succumb rapidly to the infection, often without showing signs of CNS involvement. Byrne and Robbins (5) demonstrated that susceptibility of chickens to lethal EEE virus infection declined rapidly with age; they became refractory to lethal infection by 14 days of age. In contrast to their findings, susceptibility to lethal infection was demonstrated by Tyzzer and Sellards (62) in 3- to 13-day-old chickens and by Guy et al. (19) in 14-day-old chickens. These differences with respect to age-dependent susceptibility of chickens to EEE virus infection are unexplained, but may be due to differences in host genetics and/or differences in virulence of the EEE viruses used in the various studies.

Experimental infection of young chickens, 1–14 days of age, caused depression, somnolence, and high mortality; paralysis was infrequently observed (19, 62). The principal lesion, and the presumed cause of death, was myocarditis. Microscopic heart lesions consisted of multifocal necrosis with fragmentation of myocardial fibers, and infiltration with lymphocytes, plasma cells, and macrophages (Fig. 31.5E). Central nervous system lesions in infected chickens were inconsistently observed (19, 62). In brains, microscopic lesions consisted of occasional small foci of necrosis and mild perivascular cuffing (Fig. 31.5D). Multifocal necrosis of the liver (Fig. 31.5F) and lymphoid depletion and necrosis in the thymus, spleen, and bursa of Fabricius also were observed in EEE-virus–infected chickens (19). Ascites and right ventricular dilatation of the heart were observed in chickens that survived the acute effects of EEE virus infection, most likely as sequelae of myocardial damage (19).

DIAGNOSIS. Eastern equine encephalitis may be diagnosed by isolation and identification of the virus, detection of viral antigens using enzyme-linked immunosorbent assays (ELISAs) or serologic testing (57). The virus can be isolated by inoculation of blood or tissue homogenates (brain, spleen, liver, heart) into newborn mice by the intracerebral route, day-old chickens by subcutaneous or intramuscular routes, and 5- to 7-day-old embryonated chicken eggs by the yolk sac route (49, 57). In addition, a variety of cell cultures may be utilized

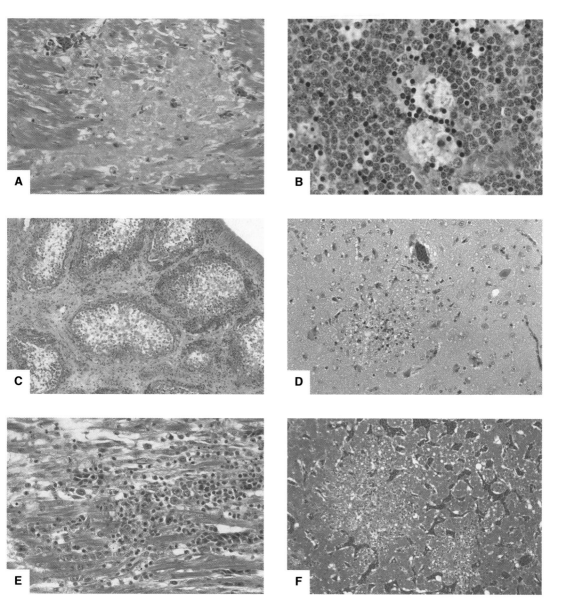

31.5. Microscopic lesions in turkeys and chickens experimentally infected with eastern equine encephalitis virus. *A*. Heart of turkey, 3 days postexposure. A large focal area of myocardial necrosis is present, with no inflammatory reaction. *B*. Thymus of turkey, 3 days postexposure. Aggregates of pyknotic nuclei within clear spaces indicate acute lymphocyte necrosis. *C*. Bursa of Fabricius of turkey, 3 days postexposure. Atrophy of bursal follicles with marked lymphoid depletion is present. *D*. Brain of chicken, 2 days postexposure. A focal area of necrosis is present with mild perivascular cuffing. Note emigration of mononuclear cells from an adjacent venule distended with erythrocytes. *E*. Heart of chicken, 5 days postexposure. Myocardial degeneration and necrosis with a mononuclear cell infiltrate. *F*. Liver of chicken, 5 days postexposure. Focal necrosis is present with minimal inflammatory cell response.

for isolation of the virus; Vero, BHK-21, and chicken or duck embryo cells are highly susceptible. Newborn mice and 1-day-old chickens generally die of encephalitis in 2–5 days. Chicken embryos generally die within 18–72 hr and have a hemorrhagic appearance. Cell cultures develop cytopathic effects (CPE) within 24–48 hr, and plaques develop under agar within 36–48 hr. Identification of EEE virus in inoculated animals, embryonated eggs, or cell cultures generally is accomplished by virus-neutralization (VN) tests or complement fixation (CF) tests.

The ELISA procedures for detection of EEE virus antigens have been described (26, 27, 55, 56). These procedures have been shown to be highly sensitive, detecting EEE virus in experimentally infected birds as early as 12 hr PI and in pools of insects in which only 1% of the insects were infected (26, 27, 55, 56).

Serologic tests useful for serologic diagnosis include VN, hemagglutination-inhibition (HI), ELISA, and CF. Of these, VN and HI tests are most commonly utilized. The HI test is rapid and relatively simple; it requires either goose or 1-day-old chicken erythrocytes, and antigen prepared from infected suckling mouse brains by the sucrose–acetone extraction method (9, 57). Avian serum contains nonspecific inhibitors of hemagglutination and these must be removed by kaolin adsorption before use in HI tests. A presumptive serologic diagnosis may be obtained by detection of EEE virus antibodies in serum collected from recovered birds. A definitive diagnosis is achieved by demonstrating a rising antibody titer in serum samples collected soon after onset of clinical signs and 1–2 wk later.

Guy et al. (20) recently demonstrated the value of serology for diagnosis of EEE virus–induced episodes of decreased egg production in turkey breeder hens. Serology was shown to be particularly important because the virus was found to be present in tissues of experimentally infected turkey breeder hens for only a very brief period (on days 1–2 PI) following experimental inoculation, yet marked drops in egg production became apparent only after day 2 PI. Virus isolation attempts may be profitable using ovary and eggs, as the virus was detectable for somewhat longer periods (days 1–5 PI) in these samples.

Differential Diagnosis. Eastern equine encephalitis must be distinguished from other causes of neurologic disease in poultry and game birds such as Newcastle disease virus, avian encephalomyelitis virus, botulism, and listeriosis. In cases of egg-production drops in turkeys, EEE virus, HJ virus, Newcastle disease virus, avian influenza virus, avian encephalomyelitis virus, paramyxovirus type 3, and turkey rhinotracheitis virus must be considered. These diseases generally are distinguished based on isolation and identification of the causative agent or by serologic analyses.

CONTROL. Eastern equine encephalitis is best prevented and controlled by measures aimed at reducing vector populations. Such measures include reduction of vector habitats by modifications of the environment or by chemical spraying. If feasible, farms that raise susceptible avian species should be located away from swamps and other areas that provide habitat for vectors.

Formalin-inactivated EEE vaccines, prepared for use in horses, have been used to protect pheasants against EEE epornitics (59), although their efficacy has been questioned (12).

WESTERN EQUINE ENCEPHALITIS

Western equine encephalitis virus has many characteristics in common with EEE virus. Although it is rarely associated with disease in avian species, a few cases have been reported. The WEE virus was attributed by Woodring in 1957 (70) as the cause of encephalitis and high mortality in turkeys in Wisconsin based on serologic studies; affected turkeys exhibited somnolence, tremors, and leg paralysis. Faddoul and Fellows (14) reported the isolation of WEE virus from the brain of a pheasant in Massachusetts, and Ranck et al. (52) identified the virus as the cause of high mortality in chukar partridges in Florida. The association of WEE virus with disease in these species, however, is tenuous because it is now generally accepted that WEE virus does not occur in the eastern United States, and that all WEE-related alphaviruses isolated in the eastern United States are actually strains of HJ virus (see below) (6, 61).

Western equine encephalitis is identified mainly in western parts of the United States and Canada, in Central America, and in South America. It is transmitted principally by *Culiseta tarsalis,* a mosquito vector that is relatively common in the United States west of the Mississippi River (8). Laboratory diagnosis of WEE is accomplished using the same procedures that are used for EEE.

HIGHLANDS J VIRUS INFECTION

Highlands J virus initially was isolated in 1960 from bluejays in Florida (25). Since that time, the virus has been identified as a cause of disease in chukar partridges (13, 52) and turkeys (15, 18, 20, 64). Ranck et al. reported that WEE virus was the cause of mortality in chukar partridges in Florida in 1964; however, this virus most likely was HJ virus. Antigenically, HJ virus is closely related to WEE virus and for many years was considered to be a variant of that virus (24, 25, 40). Recent serologic and oligonucleotide mapping studies, however, clearly differentiate these viruses and have identified HJ virus as a distinct virus in the WEE antigenic group of alphaviruses (6, 7, 37, 61). All viruses belonging to the WEE antigenic group isolated in the eastern United States have been determined to be HJ virus (6).

Ranck et al. (52) identified HJ virus infection as the cause of encephalitis in chukar partridges, and experimentally reproduced the disease by subcutaneous inoculation of young chukars. Experimentally infected chukars exhibited somnolence, ruffled feathers, and recumbency prior to death; lesions primarily consisted of encephalitis and myocardial necrosis. Eleazer and Hill (13) described a more recent outbreak in chukar partridges in South Carolina that resulted in similar clinical signs and high mortality (35%); myocarditis was consistently observed in affected birds, but lesions in the brain were uncommon.

Wages et al. (64) found HJ virus to be the cause of acute drops in egg production in turkey breeder hens. In addition, these viruses were serologically associated with mortality in young turkeys (15). Highlands J virus infection produced precipitous egg-production drops in experimentally infected turkey hens (20) and was mildly pathogenic for young turkeys (18). The clinical and pathologic characteristics of HJ virus infection in turkeys closely resemble those of EEE virus infection (see above).

Laboratory diagnosis of HJ virus infection is accomplished using the same procedures used for EEE virus and WEE virus. Highlands J virus is readily distinguished from WEE virus isolates by a variety of serologic procedures using polyclonal and monoclonal antibodies (41).

ISRAEL TURKEY MENINGOENCEPHALITIS

HISTORY. Israel turkey meningoencephalitis was first described in Israel by Komarov and Kalmar in 1960 (44). In 1961, Porterfield (51) identified the etiologic agent as a new virus belonging to the *Flaviviridae*. The disease also was identified in South Africa in 1978 (2).

INCIDENCE AND DISTRIBUTION. Israel turkey meningoencephalitis has been reported only in Israel and South Africa. Outbreaks of the disease occur seasonally in Israel, corresponding with the activity of arthropod vectors; generally they begin in late summer, peak in October, and disappear in early winter (30).

PATHOGENESIS AND EPIZOOTIOLOGY

Natural and Experimental Hosts. Israel turkey meningoencephalitis has been reported only in turkeys. The disease generally occurs only in birds older than 10 wk of age (53), but younger birds are equally susceptible. Experimental infection of turkeys less than 10 wk of age results in disease with an incubation period of 5 to 8 days (30). A viremia is detectable within 24 hr PI in experimentally infected turkeys and persists for 5–8 days (33). Field cases of IT are not observed in turkeys less than 10 wk of age, probably because they are raised in closed brooder houses until this time and lack exposure to arthropod vectors.

Newly hatched poults (35), Japanese quail (*Coturnix coturnix japonica*) (34) and suckling mice (31) are highly susceptible to IT virus inoculated by the intracerebral and intramuscular routes. Chickens, ducks, geese, and pigeons are refractory to infection (44).

Transmission. The seasonal incidence and sporadic occurrence in flocks on the same farms strongly suggest that IT is transmitted by insect vectors. The virus has been isolated from unsorted pools of mosquitoes (*Aedes* spp. and *Culex pipiens*) and culicoides trapped near affected turkey flocks (4). Experimentally, IT virus has been shown to infect *Aedes aegypti* and *Culex molestus* mosquitoes (48). Field observations and experimental studies indicated that virus transmission does not occur by direct contact between infected and uninfected birds (33, 35).

Clinical Signs and Pathology.
In field outbreaks, IT occurs with greatest incidence in turkeys 10–12 wk old. Affected turkeys exhibit neurologic dysfunction characterized by progressive paresis and paralysis, with variable mortality. Morbidity and mortality rates generally average 15–30% but may be as high as 80% (30). Affected birds initially exhibit an uncoordinated gait and walk with one or both wings drooping. As the disease progresses, birds become reluctant or unable to walk, and rest on their breasts with legs extended forward and wings spread laterally. Turkey breeder hens exhibit a severe drop in egg production, but egg quality, fertility, and hatchability are unaffected. Egg production returns to normal levels after recovery from infection.

Gross lesions include splenomegaly or atrophy of the spleen, catarrhal enteritis, and myocarditis (2, 32, 44). Ovarian regression, ruptured ovarian follicles, and peritonitis are observed in affected breeder hens (2). The principal microscopic lesions are nonpurulent meningoencephalitis characterized by submeningeal and perivascular lymphocytic infiltration, and focal myocardial necrosis (32, 44).

DIAGNOSIS.
Brain, spleen, liver, serum, and ovary are the preferred materials for virus isolation (31, 33). Homogenates of tissue or undiluted serum are inoculated into 6- to 8-day-old embryonated chicken eggs by the yolk sac route, or onto monolayers of chicken embryo fibroblasts (CEF). One or more passages in embryonated chicken eggs may be required before embryo mortality is observed; embryos die 3 to 6 days PI and show a distinct cherry-red discoloration. Suckling mice inoculated by the intracerebral or intramuscular routes also may be used for virus isolation (31).

A readily recognizable CPE is produced in infected CEF by 3 days PI (32, 33), although CEF cells are less sensitive than embryonated chicken eggs or suckling mice for isolation of IT virus. Identification of isolates usually is accomplished by VN tests.

Serologic diagnosis can be accomplished using HI or VN tests in CEF or BHK-21 cells (2, 32, 33, 50). The HI test requires either goose or day-old chicken erythrocytes and antigen prepared from infected suckling mouse brains by the sucrose–acetone extraction method (31, 48).

Differential Diagnosis.
Israel turkey meningoencephalitis must be differentiated from other causes of neurologic disease in turkeys, particularly Newcastle disease, EEE, WEE, and HJ virus infection. The known geographic distribution of these viruses and the greater severity of paralysis that is observed with IT as compared with EEE, WEE, and HJ are helpful in distinguishing these agents. Nervous signs may be observed with Newcastle disease, but paralysis generally does not occur.

CONTROL.
Israel turkey meningoencephalitis can be controlled by vaccination. Live attenuated vaccines have been prepared by serial passage of IT virus in embryonated chicken eggs (32), Japanese quail kidney cells (35), and BHK-21 cells (1). The Japanese quail kidney cell–attenuated virus has been shown to be highly efficacious and is commercially available. Reduction of insect vector populations in the vicinity of turkey farms also may be useful in controlling the disease.

REFERENCES
1. Barnard, B.J.H., and H.J. Geyer. 1981. Attenuation of turkey meningo-encephalitis virus in BHK21 cells. Onderstepoort J Vet Res 48:105-108.
2. Barnard, B.J.H., S.B. Buys, J.H. Du Preez, S.P. Greyling, and H.J. Venter. 1980. Turkey meningo-encephalitis in South Africa. Onderstepoort J Vet Res 47:89-94.
3. Beaudette, F.R., J.J. Black, C.B. Hudson, and J.A. Bivens. 1952. Equine encephalomyelitis in pheasants from 1947 to 1951. J Am Vet Med Assoc 121:478-483.
4. Braverman, Y., M. Rubina, and K. Frish. 1981. Pathogens of veterinary importance isolated from mosquitoes and biting midges in Israel. Insect Sci Appl 2:157-161.
5. Byrne, R.J., and M.L. Robbins. 1961. Mortality patterns and antibody response in chickens inoculated with eastern equine encephalitis virus. J Immunol 86:13-16.
6. Calisher, C.H., T.P. Monath, D.J. Muth, J.S. Lazuick, D. W. Trent, D.B. Francy, G.E. Kemp, and F.W. Chandler. 1980. Characterization of Fort Morgan virus, an alphavirus of the western equine encephalitis virus complex in an unusual ecosystem. Am J Trop Med Hyg 29:1428-1440.
7. Calisher, C.H., N. Karabotsos, J.S. Lazuick, T.P. Monath, and K.L. Wolff. 1988. Reevaluation of the western equine encephalitis antigenic complex of alphaviruses (family Togaviridae) as determined by neutralization tests. Am J Trop Med Hyg 38:447-452.
8. Chamberlain, R.W. 1958. Vector relationships of the arthropod-borne encephalitides in North America. Ann N Y Acad Sci 70:312-319.
9. Clarke, D.H., and J. Casals. 1958. Techniques for hemagglutination and hemagglutination-inhibition with arthropod-borne viruses. Am J Trop Med Hyg 7:561-573.
10. Crans, W.J., J. McNelly, T.L. Sulze, and A. Main. 1986. Isolation of eastern equine encephalitis virus from Aedes sollicitans during an epizootic in southern New Jersey. J Am Mosq Control Assoc 2:68-72.
11. Dougherty, E., 3rd, and J. I. Price. 1960. Eastern encephalitis in White Pekin ducklings on Long Island. Avian Dis 4:247-258.

12. Eisner, R.J., and S.R. Nusbaum. 1983. Encephalitis vaccination of pheasants: A question of efficacy. J Am Vet Med Assoc 183:280-281.

13. Eleazer, T.H., and J.E. Hill. 1994. Highlands J virus-associated mortality in chukar partridges. J Vet Diagn Invest 6:98-99.

14. Faddoul, G.P., and G.W. Fellows. 1965. Clinical manifestations of eastern equine encephalomyelitis in pheasants. Avian Dis 9:530-535.

15. Ficken, M.D., D.P. Wages, J.S. Guy, J.A. Quinn, and W.H. Emory. 1993. High mortality of domestic turkeys associated with Highlands J virus and eastern equine encephalitis virus infections. Avian Dis 37:585-590.

16. Fothergill, G.P., and J.H. Dingle. 1938. A fatal disease of pigeons caused by the virus of the eastern variety of equine encephalomyelitis. Science 88:549-50.

17. Garoff, H., C. Konder-Koch, and H. Riedel. 1982. Structure and assembly of alphaviruses. Curr Top Microbiol Immunol 99:1-50.

18. Guy, J.S., M.D. Ficken, H.J. Barnes, D.P. Wages, and L.G. Smith. 1993. Experimental infection of young turkeys with eastern equine encephalitis virus and Highlands J virus. Avian Dis 37:389-395.

19. Guy, J.S., H.J. Barnes, and L.G. Smith. 1994. Experimental infection of young broiler chickens with eastern equine encephalitis virus and Highlands J virus. Avian Dis 38:572-582.

20. Guy, J.S., H.J. Barnes, M.D. Ficken, L.G. Smith, W.H. Emory, and D.P. Wages. 1994. Decreased egg production in turkeys experimentally infected with eastern equine encephalitis virus or Highlands J virus. Avian Dis 38:563-571.

21. Guy, J.S., T.P. Siopes, H.J. Barnes, L.G. Smith, and W.H. Emory. 1995. Experimental transmission of eastern equine encephalitis virus and Highlands J virus via semen collected from infected tom turkeys. Avian Dis 39:337-342.

22. Hanson, R.P., S. Vadlamudi, D.O. Trainer, and R. Anslow. 1968. Comparison of the resistance of different aged pheasants to eastern encephalitis virus from different sources. Am J Vet Res 29:723-727.

23. Hayes, R.O., and A.D. Hess. 1964. Climatological conditions associated with outbreaks of eastern encephalitis. Am J Trop Med Hyg 13:851-858.

24. Hayes, C.G., and R.C. Wallis. 1977. Ecology of western equine encephalitis virus in the eastern United States. Adv Virus Res 21:37-83.

25. Henderson, J.R., N. Karabotsos, A.T.C. Bourke, R.C. Wallis, and R.M. Taylor. 1962. A survey of arthropod-borne viruses in south-central Florida. Am J Trop Med Hyg 11:800-810.

26. Hildreth, S.W., and B.J. Beaty. 1984. Detection of eastern equine encephalitis virus and Highlands J virus antigens within mosquito pools by enzyme-linked immunoassay (EIA) 1. A laboratory study. Am J Trop Med Hyg 33:965-972.

27. Hildreth, S.W., B.J. Beaty, H.K. Maxfield, R.F. Gilfillan, and B.J. Rosenau. 1984. Detection of eastern equine encephalitis virus and Highlands J virus antigens within mosquito pools by enzyme-linked immunoassay (EIA) 2. Retrospective field test of the EIA. Am J Trop Med Hyg 33:973-980.

28. Holden, P. 1955. Transmission of eastern equine encephalitis virus in ring-neck pheasants. Proc Soc Exp Biol Med 88:607-610.

29. Howard, J.S., and R.C. Wallis. 1974. Infection and transmission of eastern equine encephalitis virus with colonized Culiseta melanura (Coquillett). Am J Trop Med Hyg 23:522-525.

30. Ianconescu, M. 1976. Turkey meningo-encephalitis: A general review. Avian Dis 20:135-138.

31. Ianconescu, M. 1989. Turkey meningo-encephalitis. In H. G. Purchase, L.H. Arp, C.H. Domermuth, and J.E. Pearson (eds.), A Laboratory Manual for the Isolation and Identification of Avian Pathogens, 3rd ed. American Association of Avian Pathologists, Kennett Square, PA, pp. 163-164.

32. Ianconescu, M., A. Aharonovici, Y. Samberg, M. Merdinger, and K. Hornstein. 1972. An aetiological and immunological study of the 1971 outbreak of turkey meningo-encephalitis. Refu Vet 29:110-117.

33. Ianconescu, M., A. Aharonovici, Y. Samberg, K. Hornstein, and M. Merdinger. 1973. Turkey meningo-encephalitis: Pathologic and immunological aspects of the infection. Avian Pathol 2:251-262.

34. Ianconescu, M., A. Aharonovici, and Y. Samberg. 1974. The Japanese quail as an experimental host for turkey meningo-encephalitis virus. Refu Vet 31:100-108.

35. Ianconescu, M., K. Hornstein, Y. Samberg, A. Aharonovici, and M. Merdinger. 1975. Development of a new vaccine against turkey meningo-encephalitis using a virus passaged through Japanese quail (Coturnix coturnix japonica). Avian Pathol 4:119-131.

36. Jungherr, E.L., C.F. Helmboldt, S.F. Satriano, and R.E. Luginbuhl. 1958. Investigation of eastern equine encephalomyelitis. III. Pathology in pheasants and incidental observations in feral animals. Am J Hyg 67:10-20.

37. Karabotsos, N. 1975. Antigenic relationships of group A arboviruses by plaque-reduction neutralization testing. Am J Trop Med Hyg 24:527-532.

38. Karabotsos, N. 1985. International Catalog of Arboviruses, 3rd ed. American Society of Tropical Medicine and Hygiene. San Antonio, TX.

39. Karabotsos, N. 1995. Personal communication.

40. Karabotsos, N., A.T.C. Burke, and J.R. Henderson. 1963. Antigenic variation among strains of western equine encephalomyelitis virus. Am J Trop Med Hyg 12:408-412.

41. Karabotsos, N., A.L. Lewis, C.H. Calisher, A.R. Hunt, and J.T. Roehrig. 1988. Identification of Highlands J virus from a Florida horse. Am J Trop Med Hyg 39:603-606.

42. Kissling, R.E. 1958. Eastern equine encephalomyelitis in pheasants. J Am Vet Med Assoc 132:466-468.

43. Kissling, R.E. 1958. Host relationship of the arthropod-borne encephalitides. Ann N Y Acad Sci 70:320-327.

44. Komarov, A., and E. Kalmar. 1960. A hitherto undescribed disease-turkey meningoencephalitis. Vet Rec 72:257-261.

45. Monath, T.P., and D.W. Trent. 1981. Togaviral diseases of domestic animals. In E. Kurstak and C. Kurstak (eds.). Comparative Diagnosis of Viral Diseases, vol. 4. Academic Press, New York, pp. 331-440.

46. Moulthrop, I.M., and B.A. Gordy. 1960. Eastern viral encephalomyelitis in chukar (Alectoris graeca). Avian Dis 4:380-83.

47. Murphy, F.A., and D.W. Kingsbury. 1990. Virus Taxonomy. In B. N. Fields (ed.). Virology. Raven Press, New York, pp. 9-35.

48. Nir, Y. 1972. Some characteristics of Israel turkey virus. Arch ges Virusforsch 36:105-114.

49. Pearson, J.E. 1989. Arbovirus infections. In H.G. Purchase, L.H. Arp, C.H. Domermuth, and J.E. Pearson (eds.). A Laboratory Manual for the Isolation and Identification of Avian Pathogens, 3rd ed.. American Association of Avian Pathologists, Kennett Square, PA, pp. 161-162.

50. Peleg, B.A. 1963. A small-scale serological survey of Israel turkey meningo-encephalitis. Refu Vet 20:253-250.

51. Porterfield, J.S. 1961. Israel turkey meningoencephalitis virus. Vet Rec 73:392-393.

52. Ranck, F.M., Jr., J.H. Gainer, J.E. Hanley, and S.L. Nelson. 1965. Natural outbreak of eastern and western encephalitis in pen-raised chukars in Florida. Avian Dis 9:8-20.

53. Samberg, Y., M. Ianconescu, and K. Hornstein. 1972. Epizootiological aspects of turkey meningoencephalitis. Refu Vet 29:103-110.

54. Satriano, S.F., R.E. Luginbuhl, R.C. Wallis, E.L.

Jungherr, and L.H. Williamson. 1958. Investigation of eastern equine encephalomyelitis. Susceptibility and transmission studies with virus of pheasant origin. Am J Hyg 67:21–34.

55. Scott, T.W., and J.G. Olsen. 1986. Detection of eastern equine encephalitis viral antigen in avian blood by enzyme immunoassay: A laboratory study. Am J Trop Med Hyg 35:611–618.

56. Scott, T.W., J.G. Olsen, T.E. Lewis, J.W. Carpenter, L. H. Lorenz, L.A. Lembeck, S.R. Joseph, and B.B. Pagac. 1987. A prospective field evaluation of an enzyme immunoassay: Detection of eastern equine encephalitis virus in pools of Culiseta melanura. J Am Mosq Control Assoc 3:412–417.

57. Shope, R.E., and G.E. Sather. 1979. Arboviruses. In E.H. Lennette and N.J. Schmidt (eds.). Diagnostic Procedures for Viral, Rickettsial, and Chlamydial infections, 5th ed. American Public Health Service, Washington, DC, pp. 767–814

58. Spalatin, J., L. Karstad, J.R. Anderson, L. Lauerman, and R.P. Hanson. 1961. Natural and experimental infections in Wisconsin turkeys with the virus of eastern encephalitis. Zoonoses Res 1:29–48.

59. Sussman, O., D. Cohen, J.E. Gerende, and R.E. Kissling. 1958. Equine encephalitis vaccine studies in pheasants under epizootic and preepizootic conditions. Ann N Y Acad Sci 70:328–340.

60. TenBroeck, C., and M.H. Merrill. 1933. A serological difference between eastern and western equine encephalomyelitis virus. Proc Soc Exp Med 31:217–220.

61. Trent, D.W., and J.A. Grant. 1980. A comparison of New World alphaviruses in the western equine encephalomyelitis complex by immunochemical and oligonu-cleotide fingerprint techniques. J Gen Virol 47:261–282.

62. Tyzzer, E.E., and A.W. Sellards. 1941. The pathology of equine encephalomyelitis in young chickens. Am J Hyg 33:69–81.

63. Tyzzer, E.E., A.W. Sellards, and B.L. Bennett. 1938. The occurrence in nature of equine encephalomyelitis in the ring-necked pheasant. Science 88:505–506.

64. Wages, D.P., M.D. Ficken, J.S. Guy, T.S. Cummings, and S.R. Jennings. 1993. Egg-production drop in turkeys associated with alphaviruses: Eastern equine encephalitis virus and Highlands J Virus. Avian Dis 37:1163–1166.

65. Walder, R., O.M. Suarez, and C.H. Calisher. 1984. Arbovirus studies in the Guajira region of Venezuela: Activities of eastern equine encephalitis and Venezuelan equine encephalitis viruses during an interepizootic period. Am J Trop Med Hyg 33:699–707.

66. Wallis, R.C., and A.J. Main. 1974. Eastern equine encephalitis in Connecticut, progress and problems. Mem Conn Entomol Soc, pp. 117–144.

67. Wallis, R.C., J.J. Howard, A.J. Main, Jr., C. Frazier, and C. Hayes. 1974. With an epizootic of eastern equine encephalomyelitis in Connecticut. Mosq News 34:63–65.

68. Westaway, E.G., M.A. Brinton, S.Y. Gaidamovich, M.C. Horzinek, A. Igarashi, L. Kaarainen, D.K. Lvov, J.S. Porterfield, P.K. Russell, and D.W. Trent. 1985. Togaviridae. Intervirology 24:125–139.

69. Williams, J. E., O. P. Young, D. M. Watts, and T. J. Reed. 1971. Wild birds as eastern equine encephalitis and western equine encephalitis sentinels. J Wildl Dis 7:188–194.

70. Woodring, F.R. 1957. Naturally occurring infection with equine encephalomyelitis virus in turkeys. J Am Vet Med Assoc 130:511–512.

TURKEY VIRAL HEPATITIS

James S. Guy

INTRODUCTION. Turkey viral hepatitis (TVH) is a highly contagious, generally subclinical disease of turkeys characterized by multifocal hepatic necrosis with or without accompanying pancreatic necrosis. Turkey viral hepatitis was described simultaneously in North America in 1959 by Mongeau et al. (5) in Ontario and by Snoeyenbos et al. (8) in Massachusetts. The disease also has been reported in Italy (3) and the United Kingdom (4). The disease is believed to be widely distributed in North America, but the true incidence and distribution is not known because of the frequent subclinical nature of the disease and the absence of serologic diagnostic tests.

ETIOLOGY. The etiologic agent of TVH has not been characterized, although a viral etiology was suggested based on filtration experiments in which it passed a 100-nm filter (5, 8, 10). Agar-gel precipitin tests indicated a one-way antigenic relationship between the TVH agent and duck hepatitis virus, a picornavirus (11). Rabbit antiserum against TVH produced confluent precipitin bands with both TVH and duck hepatitis virus antigen; however, rabbit antiserum prepared against duck hepatitis virus did not react with TVH antigen. More recent studies have provided additional evidence indicating involvement of a picornavirus in this disease. In 1982, McDonald et al. (4) identified aggregates of 24 nm, picornaviruslike particles in the cytoplasm of degenerating hepatocytes in livers from turkeys with hepatitis and pancreatitis. In 1991, Klein et al. (2) isolated a picornaviruslike virus, 26–28 nm in diameter, with icosahedral morphology from liver and pancreas tissues collected from TVH-affected turkeys. Turkey viral hepatitis was experimentally reproduced by inoculation of young turkeys with this agent. While these studies suggest a picornavirus etiology for TVH, additional studies are needed in order to classify the virus definitively.

Resistance to Chemical and Physical Agents.

The virus is resistant to ether, chloroform, phenol, and creoline, but not formalin. In yolk, it survives 6 hr at 60 C, 14 hr at 56 C, and 4 wk at 37 C. It survived for 1 hr at pH 2 but not at pH 12 (10).

Laboratory Host Systems. The TVH virus can be propagated and assayed in embryonated chicken eggs, embryonated turkey eggs, and turkey poults (11). The virus has not been propagated in cell culture.

Virus propagation may be accomplished by yolk sac inoculation of 5- to 7-day-old embryonated chicken eggs (5, 7, 8). Attempts to grow the virus in embryonated chicken eggs using older embryos or different routes of inoculation generally have been unsuccessful. Virus was demonstrated in inoculated embryonated chicken eggs at 66 hr postinoculation (PI) and peak embryo-infective dose-50% (EID_{50}) virus titers of approximately $10^{3.5}$/mL were detected at 90 hr (9). The virus also may be propagated by yolk sac inoculation of embryonated turkey eggs up to 10 days of incubation; however, embryonated chicken eggs have been shown to be a superior host system, possibly due to the presence of maternal antibody in turkey eggs (3).

Turkey poults are susceptible to infection by intraperitoneal, intravenous, and intramuscular routes of exposure. Clinical signs seldom develop in experimentally infected poults, but infection may be demonstrated 5–10 days PI by necropsy and detection of characteristic lesions (6).

PATHOGENESIS AND EPIZOOTIOLOGY.
Turkey viral hepatitis has been recognized only in turkeys. Chickens, pheasants, ducks, quail, mice, and rabbits were refractory to infection (11). Transmission of infection readily occurs by both direct and indirect contact. Feces from infected turkeys is believed to be the principal source for virus transmission. The virus could be isolated consistently from liver and feces, and less frequently from bile, blood, and kidney, of experimentally infected birds during the first 28 days PI, but not thereafter. The virus could not be detected in tissues and feces after 28 days PI (8, 11). Vertical transmission via the egg has been suggested by field observations and by the isolation of virus from an ovarian follicle of an experimentally infected hen (7).

The incubation period in poults, as determined by the appearance of lesions, varied between 2 and 7 days in both intraperitoneally inoculated and contact-exposed poults (7, 8).

Signs, Morbidity, and Mortality. Turkey viral hepatitis is usually a subclinical infection. It is believed that the disease becomes apparent as a result of undefined factors such as concurrent infection with other agents and/or environmental stresses. Clinical signs are not well defined. Variable degrees of depression may be observed in affected flocks, but field cases are more commonly characterized by sudden death of apparently normal birds. Turkey viral hepatitis has been suggested as a cause of decreased egg production and decreased fertility and hatchability in eggs from turkey breeders, but an etiologic role for TVH virus in these conditions has not been conclusively determined (6).

Morbidity and mortality vary considerably among affected flocks. Usually morbidity and mortality are very low, with mortality occurring during a 7- to 10-day period (6). Morbidity rates of up to 100%, however, have occurred in some flocks, and a 25% mortality was reported in one flock (6). Levels of morbidity and mortality are believed to be influenced by other factors such as concurrent infection. Mortality in turkeys over 6 wk of age has not been reported.

Pathology. Gross lesions attributable to TVH have been detected only in the liver and pancreas. Livers generally are enlarged. Hepatic lesions consist of focal, gray, sometimes depressed areas up to several millimeters in diameter (Fig. 31.6). Lesion distribution is variable; birds that die usually exhibit very extensive lesions, which often coalesce and may be parItially masked by vascular congestion and focal hemorrhage. Pancreatic lesions are less consistently observed than hepatic lesions. Lesions in the pancreas generally are roughly circular,

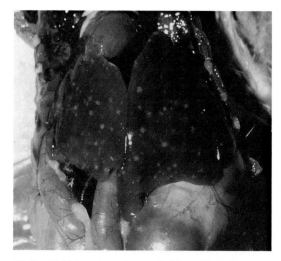

31.6. Multiple, pale tan to gray foci in the liver of a poult with turkey viral hepatitis. Lesions vary from 1 to several mm, are randomly scattered throughout the liver, are roughly circular, oval, or elliptical, often have an irregular, "frayed" border, and some have a darker, slightly depressed central area. (Barnes)

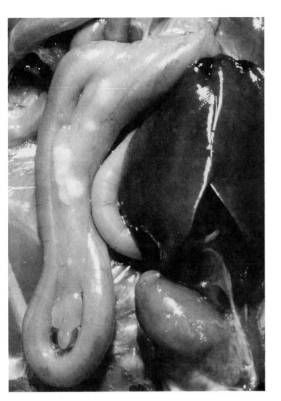

31.7. Poult with turkey viral hepatitis showing prominent pancreatic foci. (Barnes)

gray-pink, and may extend across a lobe (Fig. 31.7).

Vacuolation of hepatocytes occurs early in the course of infection, with dense infiltration by mononuclear leukocytes and proliferation of bile ductules. Lesions progress to overt focal necrosis with pooling of blood around the focus; necrotic cells are scattered among infiltrating lymphocytes. Late in the course of infection, lesions are comprised of proliferating reticuloendothelial cells that frequently form giant cells. Figure 31.8 A-D (see p. 776) illustrates the progressive changes in the liver.

Pancreatic lesions exhibit the same general histopathologic changes as those observed in livers. Acinar cell degeneration and necrosis are observed, along with infiltration of macrophages and lymphocytes.

Immunity. Immunologic aspects of TVH have received little attention. Tzianabos and Snoeyenbos were unable to detect neutralizing antibodies in sera from recovered turkeys, or hyperimmunized chickens, turkeys, and rabbits (11). Immunity to reinfection was observed, however, in previously infected turkeys; reexposure of recovered birds after an interval of 21 days resulted in less frequent and less extensive lesions than in infected controls (8). Recovery from TVH results in resistance to reinfection, but the duration of immunity has not been determined.

DIAGNOSIS. Presence of lesions in both the liver and pancreas of turkeys is highly suggestive of TVH. Similar lesions may, however, be produced in the liver by bacterial infections, particularly *Salmonella* spp. and *Pasteurella multocida,* and infections caused by group I and group II avian adenoviruses (1, 13), reovirus (12), and *Histomonas meleagridis* (7).

Virus isolation may be accomplished using a variety of tissues including liver, pancreas, spleen, kidney, or feces, but liver is the preferred sample. Homogenates of tissue or fecal suspensions are inoculated into 5- to 7-day-old embryonated chicken eggs by the yolk sac route; in positive cases, embryos generally die 4–11 days PI (8). Embryo mortality is delayed if virus titers are low, and, in some cases, a second passage may be required. Embryos exhibit cutaneous congestion and edema; embryos in which mortality is delayed may be dwarfed and have less congestion (8). Liver lesions containing necrotic foci are sometimes observed in embryos that survive to 11 days PI. Embryonic fluids do not hemagglutinate erythrocytes. Further characterization of isolates may be accomplished by yolk sac or intraperitoneal inoculation of poults with yolk harvested from infected embryonated eggs. Poults should be examined for lesions 5–10 days PI.

TREATMENT. There is no effective treatment. Prevention of stress and other infections may be helpful in preventing normally subclinical disease from developing into TVH.

REFERENCES

1. Cho, B.R. 1976. An adenovirus from a turkey pathogenic for both chicks and turkey poults. Avian Dis 20:714–723.
2. Klein, P.N., A.E. Castro, C.U. Meteyer, B. Reynolds, J. A. Swartzmann-Andert, G. Cooper, R.P. Chin, and H.L. Shivaprasad. 1991. Experimental transmission of turkey viral hepatitis to day-old poults and identification of associated viral particles resembling picornaviruses. Avian Dis 35:115–125.
3. Mandelli, G.A., A. Rinaldi, and G. Cervio. 1966. Gross and ultramicroscopic lesions in hepatopancreatitis in turkeys. Atti Soc Ital Sci Vet 20:541–545.
4. McDonald, J.W., C.J. Randall, and M.D. Dagless. 1982. Picorna-like virus causing hepatitis and pancreatitis in turkeys. Vet Rec 111:323.
5. Mongeau, J.D., R.B. Truscott, A.E. Ferguson, and M.C. Connell. 1959. Virus hepatitis in turkeys. Avian Dis 3:388–396.
6. Snoeyenbos, G.H. 1991. Turkey viral hepatitis. In B.W. Calnek, H.J. Barnes, C.W. Beard, W.M. Reid, and H.W. Yoder, Jr. (eds.). Disease of Poultry, 9th ed. Iowa State University Press, Ames, IA, pp. 699–701.
7. Snoeyenbos, G.H., and H.I. Basch. 1960. Further studies of virus hepatitis in turkeys. Avian Dis 4:477–485.

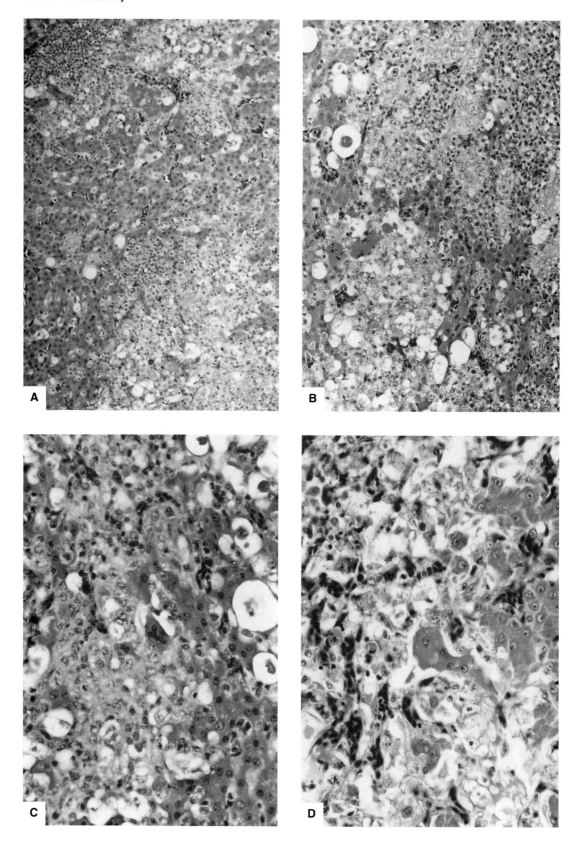

8. Snoeyenbos, G.H., H.I. Basch, and M. Sevoian. 1959. An infectious agent producing hepatitis in turkeys. Avian Dis 3:377–388.

9. Tzianabos, T. 1965. Turkey viral hepatitis. Some clinical, immunological, and physiochemical properties. PhD dissertation. University of Massachusetts, Amherst, MA.

10. Tzianabos, T., and G.H. Snoeyenbos. 1965. Some physiochemical properties of turkey hepatitis virus. Avian Dis 9:152–156.

11. Tzianabos, T., and G.H. Snoeyenbos. 1965. Clinical, immunological and serological observations on turkey virus hepatitis. Avian Dis 9:578–591.

12. Van der Heide, L. Kalbac, M. Brustolon and M.G. Lawson. 1980. Pathogenicity for chickens of a reovirus isolated from turkeys. Avian Dis 24:989–997.

13. Wilcock, B.P., and H.L. Thacker. 1976. Focal hepatic necrosis in turkeys with hemorrhagic enteritis. Avian Dis 20:205–208.

GOOSE PARVOVIRUS INFECTION

R. E. Gough

INTRODUCTION. Goose parvovirus infection, variously known as Derzsy's disease, so-called goose influenza, goose or gosling plague, goose hepatitis, goose enteritis, infectious myocarditis, or ascitic-hepato-nephritis, is a highly contagious disease affecting young geese and Muscovy ducks (*Cairina moschata*). The diverse names given to the condition reflect the multiple pathologic features of the disease. Depending on the age of affected goslings, the disease may present in either acute, subacute, or chronic forms (6, 51, 56). The acute form of the disease can result in 100% mortality in goslings under 10 days of age. Apart from geese and Muscovy ducks, the disease has not been reported in other avian species or mammals, including humans.

HISTORY. The first detailed description of a serious disease of goslings, which occurred in China in 1956 and was later shown to be caused by a parvovirus, was reported by Fang and Wang in 1981 (16) and later confirmed by Zheng et al. (67). During the 1960s, a similar disease was reported from many European countries, including Poland (62), Germany (40), Hungary (37), Bulgaria (1), Holland (61), France, the former Soviet Union, and Czechoslovakia (10). Initially, many authors referred to the disease as "goose influenza," which caused some confusion, as this name had originally been used for a disease of geese thought to be caused by a hemophilic bacterium (10). To distinguish the two diseases, it was suggested that the "new" disease be known as "so-called goose influenza" (12). During the following years, the disease was reported from all the major goose- and Muscovy duck–farming countries of Europe, and a variety of names were given to the condition.

Although several viruses had been implicated, it was not until 1971 that Schettler (58) confirmed that the disease was caused by a parvovirus. In 1978, it was recommended that the disease be called goose parvovirus (11).

INCIDENCE AND DISTRIBUTION. Goose parvovirus has been reported from all the major goose farming countries of Europe, including the former Soviet Union and Israel. The disease has also been reported from the People's Republic of China, several of its autonomous regions, Taiwan, Vietnam, and Japan. A disease with similar clinical and postmortem features has also been reported from Canada (53), although parvoviruses were not isolated. In countries such as France and Germany, where Muscovy ducks are farmed intensively, the disease is a serious problem.

ETIOLOGY. During the past 20 years, several etiologic agents have been proposed for the disease. Some early reports attributed the disease to reoviruses (8, 13, 40). It was suggested that adenoviruses were the etiologic agents, as they were fre-

31.8. Microscopic lesions of turkey viral hepatitis. (Barnes). *A.* Early lesions consist of multiple foci of vacuolar degeneration and coagulative necrosis. Cellular response primarily consists of lymphocytes and macrophages; heterophils are occasionally present but are not numerous. Pancreatic lesions are similar. In the liver, biliary hyperplasia is generally present, but the degree is highly variable among infected birds. *B.* As lesions mature, they advance along sinusoids, often investing islands of liver cells, creating an irregular margin. *C.* Frequently, liver cells within or adjacent to the lesions fuse together to form syncytial cells. *D.* Nuclear changes as seen here in hepatocytes adjacent to a lesion develop an appearance suggestive of inclusion bodies. Their nature is currently uncertain, but they are not believed to be of viral origin.

quently isolated or detected from outbreaks of disease in goslings (7, 27, 52). In subsequent, more detailed studies, however, it has been confirmed that the etiologic agent is a parvovirus (6, 9, 21, 35, 38, 58).

Classification. The virus is a member of the family *Parvoviridae*. No antigenic relationships with chicken or mammalian parvoviruses have been demonstrated (33, 48).

Morphology. Intact virions are unenveloped and hexagonal in shape (Fig. 31.9) with an estimated 32 capsomeres and a diameter of 20–22 nm (9, 21, 35, 58). The density of the virus in cesium chloride is approximately 1.38 g/mL (30).

Chemical Composition. Goose parvovirus, like its mammalian counterparts, has a single-stranded DNA genome (35, 58) of about 5600 bases (42). Using a Muscovy duck isolate, Le Gall-Recule and Jestin (42) identified three major proteins of 91, 78, and 58 kD and a fourth, lighter protein of 51 kD. Unlike several mammalian parvoviruses, hemagglutination activity, using a variety of red blood cells under different conditions, has not been demonstrated with goose parvovirus (58).

Virus Replication. The replication of goose parvovirus has not been investigated in detail, although in vitro studies by Kisary and Derzsy (35) have shown that viral replication takes place in the nucleus, and electron microscopy studies by Bergmann (2) have demonstrated the presence of large aggregates of parvovirus in the nuclei of cells from the hearts and bursae of infected goslings. Like other parvoviruses that are able to replicate without the presence of a helper virus, goose parvovirus is dependent on cells actively synthesizing DNA for its replication cycle (32).

Resistance to Chemical and Physical Agents. Goose parvovirus is very resistant to chemical and physical inactivation. Gough et al. reported no loss of titer occurred when the virus was heated at 65 C for 30 min (21). These authors also found that the virus was stable at pH 3.0 for 1 hr at 37 C. Schettler (58) tested an isolate against a variety of chemicals under different conditions and detected no significant loss of activity.

Strain Classification. The results of early studies using cross-neutralization and gosling-protection tests suggested that several serologically distinct strains of the virus existed (14). At the time of these studies, however, the etiology of the dis-

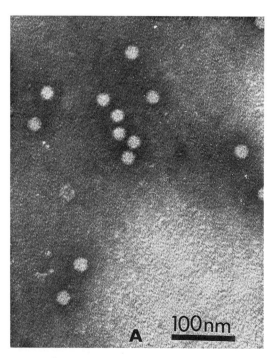
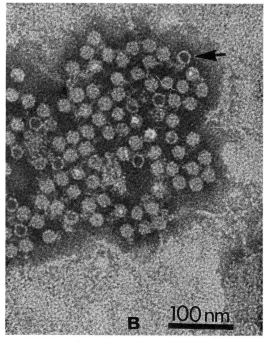

31.9. Electron micrographs of purified goose parvovirus. *A.* Purified virions. *B.* Virions in the feces of a naturally infected 10-day-old gosling, showing intact and hollow (*arrow*) particles.

ease had not been confirmed, and later work showed that several of the virus strains used were contaminated with reoviruses (15). Subsequent studies showed that all the goose parvoviruses tested were antigenically closely related (18, 22, 29). Recent studies with Muscovy duck isolates using cross-neutralization and restriction-endonuclease analysis have identified significant differences between Muscovy duck and goose isolates of parvovirus (26, 66).

Laboratory Host Systems. Goose parvovirus has only been isolated in embryonated goose or Muscovy duck eggs or primary cell cultures prepared from the embryos.

PATHOGENESIS AND EPIZOOTIOLOGY

Natural and Experimental Hosts. Geese and Muscovy ducks are the only species in which naturally occurring clinical disease has been observed. All breeds of domestic geese are susceptible and the disease has also been reported to occur in Canada geese (*Branta canadensis*) and snow geese (*Chen hypoborea atlantica*) following accidental infection (57). Other breeds of domestic poultry and ducks appear refractory to experimental infection (21, 25).

AGE OF HOST COMMONLY AFFECTED. The disease is strictly age dependent; thus, 100% mortality may occur in goslings under 1 wk of age, with negligible losses occurring in 4- to 5-wk-old birds. Although older geese do not show clinical signs of infection, they respond immunologically (12, 18, 31). Similar findings apply to the clinical disease in Muscovy ducks (25, 39, 69).

Transmission, Carriers, and Vectors. Infected birds excrete large amounts of virus in their feces resulting in a rapid spread of infection by direct and indirect contact. The most serious outbreaks occur in susceptible goslings following vertical transmission of the virus. In older geese that become subclinically infected, a latent infection may become established. These birds may then act as carriers of the disease and transmit the virus through their eggs to susceptible goslings in the hatchery (10, 34). No biologic vectors have been identified.

Incubation Period, Signs, Mortality, and Morbidity. In susceptible goslings the incubation period is age dependent. Experimental infection of day-old goslings results in the appearance of clinical signs 3–5 days later. In 2- to 3-wk-old birds, the incubation period may vary between 5 and 10 days (34, 56).

The clinical signs, morbidity, and mortality in susceptible goslings also vary according to the age of the birds. In goslings under 1 wk of age, the course of the disease may be very rapid with anorexia, prostration, and death occurring within 2–5 days. In older birds, or those with variable levels of maternally derived antibody, the disease follows a more protracted course with the appearance of characteristic clinical signs. Initially, affected birds exhibit anorexia, polydipsia, and weakness with a reluctance to move. There is a nasal and ocular discharge in many birds with associated head shaking. The uropygial glands and eyelids are often red and swollen, and a profuse white diarrhea is evident in many of the birds. Examination of the birds at this stage may reveal a fibrinous pseudomembrane covering the tongue and oral cavity. Goslings that survive the acute phase may develop a more prolonged disease characterized by profound growth retardation, loss of down around the back and neck, and marked reddening of the exposed skin. There may be an accumulation of ascitic fluid in the abdomen, which causes the goslings to stand in a "penguinlike" posture.

Mortality sometimes reaches 100% in goslings infected in the hatchers. In 2- to 3-wk-old goslings mortality levels may be below 10%, although morbidity levels may be high. Complicating factors such as poor management and secondary bacterial, fungal, or viral infections may influence the final mortality levels (34, 39). Goslings over 4 wk of age rarely show clinical signs although a "late-form" of the disease has been described in goslings 1–3 mo of age (6). Geese of all ages respond immunologically to goose parvovirus infection without necessarily showing clinical signs (31).

Gross Lesions. In acute cases with a short clinical course, lesions are commonly found in the heart, which has a pale myocardium characteristically rounded at its apex (Fig. 31.10). The liver, spleen, and pancreas may be swollen and congested (10). A variety of other gross lesions may also be present in cases with a more prolonged clinical course. Typically, a serofibrinous perihepatitis and pericarditis is present with large volumes of straw-colored fluid in the abdominal cavity. Pulmonary edema, liver dystrophy, and catarrhal enteritis may also be present. Less frequently, hemorrhages in the thigh and pectoral muscles may be seen. Diptheritic and ulcerative lesions may be observed in the mouth, pharynx, and esophagus, depending on the presence of secondary invaders.

Histopathology. Detailed histopathology studies of goose parvovirus infection by a number of workers have produced similar findings (5, 47, 49, 50). The main lesions reported were pronounced

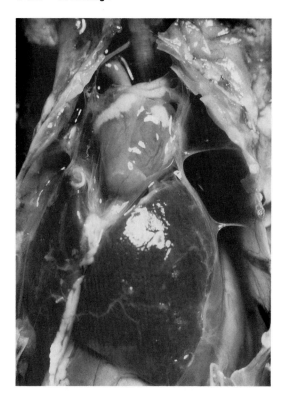

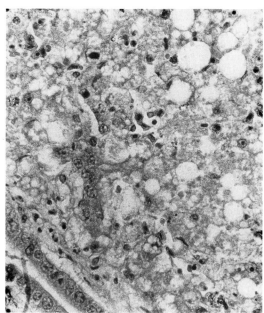

31.11. Liver section from a 10-day-old gosling infected with goose parvovirus showing widespread vacuolation and degeneration of hepatocytes.

31.10. Postmortem appearance of a 12-day-old gosling infected with goose parvovirus showing hydropericardium and ascites. The liver is coated with a fibrinous membrane.

degenerative changes in myocardial cells with associated loss of striation, fatty infiltration, and the presence of scattered Cowdry type A intranuclear inclusions. Similar histologic changes were also found in intestinal and smooth muscle cells. In the liver, the predominant lesions were degeneration of hepatocytes with vacuolation and fatty infiltration (Fig. 31.11). Small, eosinophilic inclusion–like bodies were sometimes seen in the cytoplasm of the vacuolated hepatocytes. Changes in the pancreas consisted of shrunken, necrotic acinar cells with fatty infiltration. Some lymphoblastic processes were occasionally observed in the spleen, bursa of Fabricius, and thymus, together with marked vacuolation of the kidneys .

Immunity. Adult breeding geese that have been naturally infected with parvovirus, either as goslings or adults, transfer maternal antibody via the egg yolk to their progeny (13, 19, 25). This passively acquired antibody may persist at a relatively high level until about 2 wk of age (31). The primary humoral response of geese to parvovirus infection is characterized by the initial production of IgM- and then IgG-type immunoglobulins (31). Using virus-neutralization (VN) and agar gel precipitin tests to measure parvovirus antibodies in the sera of geese that had survived the disease, high and persistent levels of antibody were detected for up to 80 mo after infection. The progeny of these geese were also found to be fully resistant to experimental challenge up to 4 wk of age (19). The results of studies by Kisary (31) suggested that goslings are not fully immunocompetent until 20 days of age.

DIAGNOSIS

Isolation and Identification of the Causative Agent. Goose parvovirus can be isolated from a variety of suitable postmortem specimens following inoculation of 10- to 15-day-old embryonated goose or Muscovy duck eggs via the allantoic cavity. Embryo mortality occurs 5–10 days postinoculation with hemorrhages and ocher-colored livers. The virus can also be isolated in primary cell cultures of goose or Muscovy duck embryos. Isolation of the virus is facilitated by inoculating cultures before they reach confluency (35). The virus produces a well-defined cytopathic effect 3–5 days postinfection. In hemotoxylin- and eosin-stained preparations, Cowdry type A intranuclear inclusions and syncytium formation are often present (35, 59). The presence of the virus can be confirmed by electron microscopic examination of infected cell cultures or neutralization with specific goose parvovirus antiserum. Immunofluorescence has also been used to detect the presence of antigen in both goose embryos (63) and infected cell cultures (58). Other methods of detecting goose parvovirus have been developed, including the immunoperoxidase technique (54) and reverse indirect hemagglutination test (64).

An agar gel diffusion technique has been described using hyperimmune rabbit antigoose parvovirus serum to precipitate parvovirus in allantoic fluid from infected goose embryos (3). Aggregates of goose parvovirus virions have also been detected by electron microscopy examination of ultrathin sections of heart and bursa of Fabricius from infected goslings (2) and in concentrated extracts of feces from goslings showing clinical signs of goose parvovirus (17). A digoxigenin-labeled DNA probe for the detection of Muscovy duck parvovirus has recently been described (43).

Serology. Confirmation of goose parvovirus infection can be obtained by serologic means. The most commonly used method is the VN test in embryonated goose or Muscovy duck eggs or primary cell cultures to detect the presence of goose parvovirus neutralizing antibodies. A VN test has also been developed for use in Khaki Campbell or Pekin duck eggs using a duck embryo–adapted goose parvovirus (20). Though less sensitive than the VN test, the agar gel diffusion test is a useful method of rapidly testing large numbers of sera for the presence of goose parvovirus antibodies (18, 45). Other serologic techniques developed include the spermagglutination-inhibition test (46), enzyme-linked immunosorbent assay tests (24, 26, 41), and plaque assay (60).

Differential Diagnosis. Apart from duck herpesvirus enteritis, there are no other known viral infections that cause high mortality in young geese or Muscovy ducklings. Equivocal results can arise, however, when viruses other than parvovirus are isolated, particularly reoviruses and adenoviruses. In such cases, it may be necessary to carry out serologic tests in order to confirm the diagnosis.

TREATMENT, PREVENTION, AND CONTROL.
There is no specific treatment for goose parvovirus infection. Antibiotic therapy has been used to reduce losses from secondary bacterial or fungal infections (12).

Because many outbreaks of goose parvovirus are directly attributed to transmission of the disease by congenitally infected goslings during hatching, the practice of incubating and hatching eggs that have originated from different breeding flocks should be discouraged. Only eggs from known parvovirus-free flocks should be incubated together, and good hatchery hygiene should be maintained.

On farms where outbreaks of the disease have occurred, the practice of breeding from geese that have survived the disease as goslings should also be discouraged, as these birds are potential carriers of the virus. All contact geese, whether goslings or adults, should be serologically tested in order to identify which birds have been infected horizontally. Positive reactors should be removed from the flock, as these birds may also become carriers of the virus.

Because the disease is confined to young geese or Muscovy ducklings, control measures have been developed to provide adequate immunity during the first 4–5 wk of life. Some of the early outbreaks of goose parvovirus occurring in China in 1962 were controlled by the use of hyperimmune serum in newly hatched goslings (16). Serum therapy was widely used when the disease subsequently appeared in Europe, using serum produced in hyperimmunized geese (10, 23, 25, 55). Passive immunization, however, was found to be expensive and time consuming, particularly because two doses of serum were often required to produce adequate immunity (36). Active immunization of adult breeding geese and Muscovy ducks with virulent virus has also been reported (25). The results showed that good protection against goose parvovirus was transferred to the progeny via the egg yolk.

One of the first vaccines against the disease was developed in China, and during the period 1962–79 about four million female geese were vaccinated (16). The virus was attenuated following multiple passage in embryonated goose eggs, and good protection to challenge was recorded in the progeny goslings. Other vaccines have been developed by attenuation of the virus in goose or Muscovy duck embryo cell cultures, for use in breeding geese and goslings (28, 36, 44, 65, 68). Duck embryo–adapted goose parvovirus vaccines have also been shown to induce a good immune response in goslings and breeder geese (4, 20).

In flocks of geese in which parvovirus has not been diagnosed, inactivated vaccines have been used (34, 51).

REFERENCES
1. Angelacev, A. 1966. Exudative septicaemia of goose influenza. Vet Sb Sofia 63:912.
2. Bergmann, V. 1987. Pathology and electron microscopical detection of virus in the tissues of goslings with Derzsy's disease (parvovirus infection). Arch Exp Vet Med 41:212–221.
3. Bondarenko, A.F. 1982. Improved diagnosis of parvoviral enteritis in geese. (Immunodiffusion test). Vet Moscow 11:68–69.
4. Chen, B.L., B.H. Ye, and J.H. Li. 1985. Duck embryo adapted vaccine for gosling plague. Acta Vet Zootech Sin 16:269–275.

5. Coudert, M., M. Fedida, G. Dannacher, M. Peillon, R. Labatut, and P. Ferlin. 1972. Viral disease of gosling. Recl Med Vet 148:455–472.

6. Coudert, M., M. Fedida, G. Dannacher, and M. Peillon. 1974. Parvovirus disease of goslings. Late form. Recl Med Vet 150:899–906.

7. Csontos, L. 1967. Isolation of an adenovirus from geese. Acta Vet Hung 17:217–219.

8. Dannacher, G., M. Coudert, M. Fedida, M. Peillon, and X. Fouillet. 1972. Etiology of the virus disease of geese. Recl Med Vet 148:1333–1349.

9. Dannacher, G., X. Fouillet, M. Coudert, M. Fedida, and M. Peillon. 1974. Etiology of the virus disease of geese: The beta virus. Recl Med Vet 150:49–58.

10. Derzsy, D. 1967. A viral disease of goslings. Acta Vet Hung 17:443–448.

11. Derzsy, D. 1978. A viral disease of goslings. In H. Rohrer (ed.). Handbuch der Virusinfektionen bei Tieren VI/2. VEB Gustav Fischer Verlag, pp. 919–949.

12. Derzsy, D., and J. Meszaros. 1969. Epidemiological problems of the so-called goose influenza and the possibilities of protection. Magy Allatorv Lapja 10:1–11.

13. Derzsy, D., I. Szep, and F. Szoke. 1966. Investigation on the etiology of the so-called goose influenza. Magy Allatorv Lapja 21:388–389.

14. Derzsy, D., C. Dren, M. Szedo, J. Surjan, B. Toth, and E. Iro. 1970. A viral disease of goslings. III. Isolation, properties and antigenic patterns of the virus strains. Acta Vet Hung 20:419–428.

15. Derzsy, D., J. Kisary, L.M. Kontrimavichus, and G.A. Nadtochey. 1975. Presence of reoviruses in certain goose embryo isolates from outbreaks of viral gosling disease and in chicken embryos. Acta Vet Hung 25:383–391.

16. Fang, D.Y., and Y.K. Wang. 1981. Studies on the etiology and specific control of goose parvovirus infection. Sci Agric Sin 4:1–8.

17. Gough, R.E. 1982. Unpublished data.

18. Gough, R.E. 1984. Application of the agar gel precipitin and virus neutralisation tests to the serological study of goose parvovirus. Avian Pathol 13:501–509.

19. Gough, R.E. 1987. Persistence of parvovirus antibody in geese that have survived Derzsy's disease. Avian Pathol 16:327–330.

20. Gough, R.E., and D. Spackman. 1982. Studies with a duck embryo adapted goose parvovirus. Avian Pathol 11:503–510.

21. Gough, R.E., D. Spackman, and M.S. Collins. 1981. Isolation and characterisation of a parvovirus from goslings. Vet Rec 108:399–400.

22. Hanh, N.V. 1974. A disease of goslings in Vietnam. Magy Allatorv Lapja 29:262–265.

23. Hansen, H.C. 1980. Derzsy's disease (parvovirus infection) in geese. Dansk Vet 63:191–194.

24. Have, P., and H.C. Hansen. 1981. Detection of goose parvovirus antibodies by microneutralisation and enzyme-linked immunosorbent assay. Proc 7th World Vet Poult Assoc, Oslo, Norway, p. 60.

25. Hoekstra, J., T. Smit, and C. van Brakel. 1973. Observations on the host range and control of goose virus hepatitis. Avian Pathol 2:169–178.

26. Jestin, V., M. Le Bras, M. Cherbonnel, G. Le Gall-Recule, and G. Bennejean. 1991. Demonstration of very pathogenic parvoviruses (Derzsy disease virus) in Muscovy duck farms. Recl Med Vet 167:849–857.

27. Kaleta, E.F. 1969. Celo-virus from goslings. Dtsch Tierarztl Wochenschr 76:427–428.

28. Kaleta, E.F. 1985. Immunisation of geese and Muscovy ducks against parvovirus hepatitis (Derzsy's disease). Report of a field trial with the attenuated live vaccine "Palmivax." Dtsch Tierarztl Wochenschr 92:303–305.

29. Kisary, J. 1974. Cross-neutralisation tests on parvoviruses isolated from goslings. Avian Pathol 3:293–296.

30. Kisary, J. 1976. Buoyant density of goose parvovirus strain B. Acta Microbiol Hung 23:205–207.

31. Kisary, J. 1977. Immunological aspects of Derzsy's disease in goslings. Avian Pathol 6:327–334.

32. Kisary, J. 1979. Interaction in replication between the goose parvovirus strain B and duck plague herpesvirus. Arch Virol 59:81–88.

33. Kisary, J. 1985. Indirect immunofluorescence as a diagnostic tool for parvovirus infection of broiler chickens. Avian Pathol 14:269–273.

34. Kisary, J. 1986. Diagnosis and control of parvovirus infection of geese (Derzsy's disease). In J.B. McFerran and M.S. McNulty (eds.). Acute Virus Infections of Poultry. Martinus Nijhoff, Dordrecht, Netherlands, pp. 239–242.

35. Kisary, J., and D. Derzsy. 1974. A viral disease of goslings. IV. Characterization of the causal agent in tissue culture systems. Acta Vet Hung 24:287–292.

36. Kisary, J., D. Derzsy, and J. Meszaros. 1978. Attenuation of the goose parvovirus strain B. Laboratory and field trials of the attenuated mutant for vaccination against Derzsy's disease. Avian Pathol 7:397–406.

37. Kis-Csatari, M. 1965. An outbreak of exudative septicaemia (goose influenza) in goslings. Magy Allatorv Lapja 20:148–151.

38. Kontrimavichus, L.M. 1975. Comparison of strains of virus isolated from goslings with enteritis. Tr Vses Inst Eksp Vet 43:212–224.

39. Kontrimavichus, L.M., V.F. Makogon, and V.V. Navrotskii. 1980. Epidemiological, clinical and pathological features of goose viral enteritis. Vet Moscow 7:34–35.

40. Krauss, H. 1965. Eine Verlustreiche aufzuchtkrankheit bei gansekuken. Berl Munch Tieraerztl Wochenschr 78:372–375.

41. Kwang, M.J., H.J. Tsai, Y.S. Lu, A.C.Y. Fei, Y.L. Lee, D.F. Lin, and C. Lee. 1987. Detection of antibodies against goose parvovirus by an enzyme-linked immunosorbent assay (ELISA). J Chin Soc Vet Sci 13:17–23.

42. Le Gall-Recule, G., and V. Jestin. 1994. Biochemical and genomic characterisation of Muscovy duck parvovirus. Arch Virology 139:121–131.

43. Le Gall-Recule, G., and V. Jestin. 1994. A digoxigenin-labelled DNA probe for the detection of Muscovy duck parvovirus. In M.S. McNulty and J.B. McFerran (eds.). New and Evolving Virus Diseases of Poultry. Commission of European Communities, Brussels, Belgium, pp. 157–166.

44. Lu, Y.S., Y.L. Lee, D.F. Lin, H.J. Tsai, C. Lee, and T.H. Fuh. 1985. Control of parvoviral enteritis in goslings in Taiwan: The development and field application of immune serum and an attenuated vaccine. Taiwan J Vet Med 46:43–50.

45. Malkinson, M. 1974. Application of the gel diffusion test to the study of the serological response to gosling hepatitis virus. Proc Goose Dis Symp, Doorn, Netherlands, pp. 47–51.

46. Malkinson, M., B.A. Peleg, R. Nily, and E. Kalmar. 1974. The assay of gosling hepatitis virus and antibody by spermagglutination and spermagglutination-inhibition. II. Spermagglutination-inhibition. Avian Pathol 3:201–209.

47. Mandelli, G., A. Valire, A. Rinaldi, and E. Lodetti. 1971. Histological and ultramicroscopical findings in a viral disease of goslings. Folia Vet Lat 1:121–170.

48. Mengeling, W.L., P.S. Paul, T.O. Bunn, and J.F. Ridpath. 1986. Antigenic relationships among autonomous parvoviruses. J Gen Virol 67:2839–2844.

49. Nadtochei, G.A., and E.V. Petelina. 1985. Ultrastructural changes in the liver and small intestine of geese infected with parvovirus. Tr Vses Inst Eksp Vet 62:103–112.

50. Nagy, Z., and D. Derzsy. 1968. A viral disease of goslings. II Microscopic lesions. Acta Vet Hung 18:3–18.

51. Nougayrede, P. 1980. Virus diseases of Palmipeds or domestic Anatidae. Recl Med Vet 156:471–477.

52. Peter, W. 1985. Parvovirus infection in geese. Mh Vet

Med 40:636–639.

53. Riddell, C. 1984. Viral hepatitis in domestic geese in Saskatchewan. Avian Dis 28:774–782.

54. Roszkowski, J., P. Gazdzinski, W. Kozaczynski, and M. Bartoszcze. 1982. Application of the immunoperoxidase technique for the detection of Derzsy's disease virus antigen in cell cultures and goslings. Avian Pathol 11:571–578.

55. Samberg, Y. R. Bock, and Z. Perlstein. 1972. A new infectious disease of goslings in Israel. Refu Vet 29:29–33.

56. Schettler, C.H. 1971. Virus hepatitis of geese. II. Host range of goose hepatitis virus. Avian Dis 15:809–823.

57. Schettler, C.H. 1971. Goose virus hepatitis in the Canada goose and Snow goose. J Wildl Dis 7:147–148.

58. Schettler, C.H. 1973. Virus hepatitis of geese. III. Properties of the causal agent. Avian Pathol 2:179–193.

59. Suvorov, A.V. 1982. Cytopathic changes produced in goose fibroblast cultures by goose parvovirus. Bull Vses Inst Eksp Vet 48:16–18.

60. Takehara, K., K. Hyakutake, T. Imamura, K. Mutoh, and M. Yoshimura. 1994. Isolation, identification and plaque titration of parvovirus from Muscovy ducks in Japan. Avian Dis 38:810–815.

61. van Cleef, S.A.M., and J.T. Miltenburg. 1966. A serious virus disease with an acute course and high mortality in goslings. Tijdschr Diergeneeskd 91:372–382.

62. Wachnik, Z., and J. Novaki 1962. Wirosowe zapaleine watroby u gesiat. Med Weter 18:344–347.

63. Winteroll, G. 1974. Fluorescent antibody studies on goose hepatitis. Proc Goose Dis Symp, Doorn Netherlands, pp. 65–67.

64. Xu, W.Y., and Y.S. Chou. 1981. Preliminary report on the reverse indirect hemagglutination test for goose hepatitis virus. Acta Vet Zootech Sin 12:23–26.

65. Yadin, H., D.J. Roozelaar, and J. Hoekstra. 1977. Vaccines against viral hepatitis in geese. Tijdschr Diergeneeskd 102:318–325.

66. Zadori, A., J. Erdei, J. Nagy, and J. Kisary. 1994. Characteristics of the genome of goose parvovirus. Avian Pathol 23:359–364.

67. Zheng, Y.M., J.B. Li, and Y.S. Zhou. 1985. Determination of the nucleic acid type of goose plague virus. J Jiangsu Agric Coll 6:7–10.

68. Zhou, Y.S., H.F. Tian, J.Y. Guo, and D.Y. Fang. 1984. Safety and potency tests of gosling plague vaccine in newly hatched goslings. Chin J Vet Med 10:2–4.

69. Ziedler, von K., W. Peter, and E. Sobanski. 1984. Studies into the pathogen of entero-hepatitis of Muscovy ducks. Mh Vet Med 39:374–377.

32 External Parasites and Poultry Pests

James J. Arends

INTRODUCTION. External parasites of poultry are arthropods that live on or in the skin and feathers. A few parasites of internal organs are included. Also important are insects that develop in poultry manure, dead carcasses, and moist organic debris, thereby causing sanitation and public relations problems. There are many parasite species of bird hosts and other arthropods related to poultry production; this chapter emphasizes those of the domesticated chicken, turkey, fowl, duck, goose, and pigeon of North America. Reference texts on these parasites are those by Georgi (24), Soulsby (43), Williams et al. (49), Lancaster and Meisch (35), and Kettle (32).

The external parasite problem has changed completely with evolution of the poultry industry to high-density confinement production units. Pests that were once common in poultry flocks are less frequently seen in modern poultry production facilities, and some of the previously minor pests have become major pest problems. Pests such as lice depend upon bird-to-bird transmission. Lice problems are less common in modern poultry practice than formerly, since fewer ages of birds are maintained on a single farm. With the increase in integrated poultry production, however, the chance of human management practices spreading a pest is increased. For example, the northern fowl mite, which can live off the host for long periods of time, may be transported on egg flats, other equipment, and clothing of company service personnel as well as on wild birds and rodents. Thus, mites remain major problems. Type of housing can be a deciding factor mitigating against some species of mites and flies. The chicken mite seldom infests caged-layer houses, since there are fewer hiding places, such as manure-coated roosts, in which to complete its life cycle. Instead, the crowding of birds favors the northern fowl mite, which completes its life cycle on the birds and moves freely among them. The housefly can be a problem in all types of poultry housing. If a breeding area is present and the temperature requirements are met, flies can increase to large numbers. While the housefly does not generally cause problems to birds, it is a possible nuisance to the surrounding human dwellings, and the frequency of complaints against poultry producers about fly numbers is increasing. Modern broiler facilities seldom have ectoparasite problems; chicks arrive with few or no parasites, and there is not enough time for parasites to increase to damaging numbers before birds are slaughtered.

Poultry management should stress an integrated approach to the control of pests that includes management measures that capitalize on the advantages of modern poultry systems. External parasite problems will be minimized by thorough cleaning of houses between flocks of birds, whole flock replacement rather than partial culling and replacement, smooth-house construction and mesh to keep out wild birds, a sound rodent management program, and maintenance of manure in a dry condition to discourage fly breeding.

Certain ectoparasites of birds (lice) actually eat the dead cells of the skin and its appendages. For many, however, skin merely serves as a medium through which they draw blood or lymph, and from which they obtain warmth and shelter. Ectoparasites may be closely confined to their hosts during the entire life cycle (lice), with transmission taking place by host contact. Others wander freely from bird to bird. Some are highly host specific, contradicting the viewpoint that chicken lice, e.g., can live on horses or other animals. Also, some species may maintain a rather loose relationship and do not always limit their activities to one particular host species or even to birds (gnats, mosquitoes, bedbugs, fleas). Fowl ticks and chicken mites attack birds only at night, hiding in cracks and nests during the day.

These variations in habit and pest biology are important when control measures are considered. Mites cannot be successfully controlled by any single method of attack because of habit variations among species. This indicates the prime necessity for accurate parasite identification to ensure that the proper integrated control approach is chosen. In case of doubt, various state and national diagnostic services may be called on for assistance.

Grateful acknowledgment is given for background materials, figures, references, and copyright permissions taken from earlier editions of this chapter written by E.A. Benbrook and E.C. Loomis.

CLASSIFICATION. Poultry ectoparasites are members of the animal phylum Arthropoda, characterized by possession of externally segmented bodies, jointed appendages, and chitinous exoskeletons. Adaptation to the parasitic mode of life, however, frequently involves modification in form and reduction in characters, so recognition is difficult.

Lice, flies, bugs, and fleas are members of the class Insecta, characterized by possession of a body divided into three regions (head, thorax, and abdomen), one pair of antennae attached to the head, three pairs of legs attached to the thorax, and trachea (air tubes) for breathing. Some adult insects have wings.

Insects undergo metamorphosis whereby immature stages may appear totally different from adults and do not show the characteristics given for the class Insecta. Examples are some fly maggots, which possess no legs, antennae, or obvious body divisions. Lice, on the other hand, are easily recognized as insects regardless of stage. For classification of insects, see Borror and DeLong (8).

Mites are members of the class Arachnida, order Acarina, characterized by fused body divisions, no antennae, and four pairs of legs (the first motile stage, larva, has three pairs). Ticks are very large mites, contrasting sharply with most mites, which are much smaller than most insects. Acarina never possess wings. For classification of mites, see Krantz (34).

Common names and scientific binomials used are those accepted by the Entomological Society of America (47).

DETECTION. Poultry seriously infested with the common parasites exhibit irritation and react by scratching and preening. Incipient infestations may be less obvious. Any unexplained production drop or increase in feed conversion is cause to look for external parasites. Lice and northern fowl mites can be found by examining the skin after parting the feathers. Good light and good eyes are needed to see these small parasites. An adequate light is a battery-pack lamp held on the head by its elastic band, leaving the hands free to ruffle the feathers. To monitor birds in a production facility, 20–50 birds should be checked a minimum of two times a month. Birds should be checked at random and should be chosen from all parts of the house. The vent, head, and legs should be closely examined. If parasites are found and cannot be identified at first glance, some of the parasites should be sent to a laboratory or to an entomologist to have the specific identity determined.

Bloodsucking parasites (bedbugs and chicken mites) that come to the birds only to feed are more difficult to detect. It is necessary to examine bedding, roosts, walls, cracks and crevices, and beneath manure clods. A sharp-pointed probe may be useful in prying under splintered wood to reveal ectoparasites. Nest material, dust, and other material collected in the house can be spread out on a white pan and examined. The arthropods can be seen crawling on the pan. This material can also be placed in a Berleze funnel, which is a funnel with a light over it, and the arthropods collected in a container placed below the funnel. The collection container should have alcohol in it to preserve arthropods that emerge from the funnel. Nighttime examination of birds may detect parasites that feed on them at night. A necropsy examination in the laboratory is required to locate parasites in internal organs.

GENERAL PESTICIDE CONTROL PROCEDURES. Control techniques and strategies will be discussed under sections describing each parasite, with a full description in *Integrated Pest Management Manual* for North Carolina (2). General recommendations of specific chemicals is difficult due to their ever changing availability. Prior to choosing a particular chemical for use, a specialist should be consulted on the best choice and use of the chemical. General information on insecticides, tolerances and residues, and methods of application are presented here to avoid repetition.

The synthetic pyrethroids, organophosphorus, carbamate, and pyrethroid insecticides are the main ectoparasite and fly control chemicals used for direct application to poultry, litter, or buildings. In general, chemical insecticides and disinfectants should not be mixed for application together (22). There is little reason to use the relatively ineffective older inorganic insecticides such as sulfur and lime. Application methods for many older insecticides require too much labor to be pertinent to modern poultry production. Among the botanical insecticides, pyrethrum remains very effective against flies and is a main ingredient of mist and aerosol fly sprays, particularly with synergists.

In the United States, insecticides for use on poultry must be accepted by the Environmental Protection Agency (EPA) as causing no hazardous residues in eggs, meat, or other edible poultry products. The EPA has set tolerances for use of a few insecticides on poultry or poultry premises. A few others have been declared safe after absence of food residues hazardous to consumers has been demonstrated. The Pesticides Regulation Division of the EPA issues label approvals after all regulations have been met. The list of approved insecticides is constantly changing. Each label should be checked to be sure that poultry or poultry housing is listed on the label.

The chlorinated hydrocarbon insecticides are banned from use on poultry or in poultry houses because of residues in eggs and meat. Under no circumstances should DDT, benzene hexachloride, toxaphene, chlordane, aldrin, dieldrin, endrin, or heptachlor be used on poultry houses, or on poultry feeds or feed ingredients.

Biologic control agents: parasites, entomopathic nematodes, predators (beetles), bacteria, and fungi are invaluable parts of any integrated pest management (IPM) program. In production facilities that utilize stored manure or built-up litter, i.e., caged-layer and breeder facilities, biocontrol agents are one of the most important tools in a fly management program. Currently, managing manure to foster the natural populations of these organisms is recommended, but work continues on the mass production of these organisms and it may soon be possible to obtain and release the proper organism in the facility and, thereby, reduce or eliminate pesticide use.

Insecticides are available as wettable powders (WP), emulsifiable concentrates (EC), and water-dispersible liquids (WDL), all of which are intended to be applied as a spray or mist. Insecticides are also available as dusts and as baits. These low-assay products are prepared, premixed, and ready to use. Care should be taken to be sure that feed and water are not contaminated when using a pesticide and that all label directions are strictly adhered to so that tolerances are not exceeded.

Tolerances and Residues. Listed in Table 32.1 are residue tolerances for common pesticides used for control of poultry pests, and time that must elapse between application and slaughter or sale of eggs to meet legal requirements. This time is often spoken of as "withdrawal time," in days prior to slaughter.

All other insecticides (except sulfur and lime sulfur, which require no tolerances) must be accepted as having no tolerance, thus no allowable residue. Fly-spray ingredients (pyrethrin and piperonyl butoxide) may be used on poultry or in poultry houses with no interval required between treatment and slaughter or gathering of eggs.

Insecticides should not be used on poultry or in poultry houses without carefully reading all precautions on the label. Illegal insecticide residues in eggs and meat will result if the wrong insecticides are used, the wrong concentration or volume is used, or the wrong application method is employed. In all treatment of poultry, contamination of feed and water must be avoided. All eggs should be gathered before starting to treat with insecticides. Off-flavors in eggs can be caused by direct contamination of eggshells. Ventilation should be supplied during dusting, spraying, or misting.

Pesticide residues may occur in eggs or meat from contaminants in feed, water, litter, or soil. Persistent chlorinated hydrocarbons (particularly DDT and dieldrin) have occasionally been found in poultry feeds, causing illegal residues. In some cases, contaminated carcasses have been seized and destroyed after processing. Residue levels in eggs approximate levels in feed, and contaminated eggs continue to be produced long after pesticide ingestion ceases. Because the EPA and Food and Drug Administration (FDA) are concerned with contamination of foods by pesticides, industrial chemicals (PCB), and toxins (aflatoxin), regular collections are made of poultry, meat, and eggs from market shelves for laboratory analysis of residues. Thus feed manufacturers should buy only pesticide-free ingredients, and poultry producers should not use

Table 32.1. Generic or common and trade names of insecticides with specific regulations regarding use with poultry

Generic or Common name	Trade Name	Primary U.S. Manufacturer	Tolerance, if Established (ppm)	Required Withdrawal Days Before Slaughter
Cyromazine	Larvadex	Ciba-Geigy	0.05, MBY[a]	ND[b]
Carbaryl	Sevin	Union Carbide	5, MF, 0, E	7
Chlorpyrifos	Dursban	Dow Chemical	0.05, FMBY; 1, E	ND
Coumaphos	Co-Ral	Bayvet	1, MBY	0
Dichlorvos	Vapona	Fermenta Animal Health	0.05, FMEBY	ND
Dimethoate	Cygon	American Cyanamid	0.02, MFEBY	0
Fenthion	Baytex	Bayvet	0.1, MFBY	ND
Fenvalerate (a pyrethroid)	Ectrin	Fermenta Animal Health	Pending	ND
Malathion	Malathion	American Cyanamid	4, MBY, 0.1, E	0
Methomyl	Malrin	E.I. DuPont de Nemours	0[c]	ND
Naled	Dibrom	Chevron Chemical	0.05, FMBYE	0
Permethrin (a pyrethroid)	Ectiban, Atroban	Coopers Animal Health	0.05, FMEBY	ND
Propoxyr	Baygon	Bayvet	0[c]	ND
Stirofos	Rabon	Fermenta Animal Health	0.75, F; 0.1, E	ND

[a]BY, by-products; E, eggs; F, fat; M, meat.

[b]ND, no documentation for drug withdrawal listed.

[c]Pesticides are listed as having a zero degree tolerance unless special documentation is approved.

contaminated local ingredients or keep birds in a known contaminated environment. Grain fumigants can be hazardous to chickens. Fumigated grain should be thoroughly aerated before feeding to poultry.

Application. Laborious individual bird application methods such as dusting or dipping are inappropriate to modern poultry production. The key to any successful application of an insecticide, and resulting control that meets expectations, is to make sure that the insecticide is applied directly to the site where the pest is located. If birds are being sprayed, the treatment must thoroughly cover the entire bird and the bird should be wet to the skin. If buildings are being treated, the sites where the pests are located must be treated if control is to be good. Methods of choice for caged layers include high pressure sprays (125 psi) from outside the cages. Other types of equipment can be used, but if the birds are not treated to ensure the application of the insecticide/ascaricide to the skin and feathers, control will not be acceptable.

DUSTING.   For conventional houses, dust can be applied to litter. Dust boxes may be used for birds kept on conventional litter or in cages. Dilute insecticides should be placed in a shallow (3-in.) dusting box, about 1×1.5 ft; use one box for every 30 birds, or put one box in each colony cage. Because of the large number of boxes required, this method is seldom used in modern poultry facilities. The use of electrostatic dusters and other dust application equipment has not been used in commercial poultry production. While these methods work well in small-scale tests, they have not worked well in large commercial houses where the dusts do not penetrate the feathers of the birds and control is poor due to the lack of penetration to the skin.

SPRAYING.   The usual cylindric compressed air sprayers are satisfactory, although slow, for treating roosts and walls, as are knapsack sprayers (continuously pumped during spraying) that give a continuous spray. Sprayers that are powered by an electric or gasoline motor that deliver pressures of 125 psi, and the use of a spray gun with a solid stream nozzle, are much more rapid and efficient. When spraying houses, high-pressure and large-volume output are most desirable to drive spray into all cracks and crevices. Be sure the sprayer is equipped with an agitator or pump bypass to ensure constant agitation, particularly if wettable powders are used. Dunning et al. (15) and Arends (2) describe portable spray units that are highly adaptable and versatile for use on poultry farms.

MISTING.   Electric mist machines (foggers) are ef-

ficient, rapid, and often labor-saving. Mist machines can be used efficiently to dispense fly spray. Mist machines are concentrate applicators and do not use the same mixtures as ordinary sprayers. Generally they use five to 10 times the concentration and one-third to one-tenth the volume. In all fog work, the container should be shaken frequently during spraying to keep insecticide from settling.

Recommended Treatments. Annual recommendations and guides for use of insecticides listed in Table 32.1, plus information on limitations of use and new EPA label information, can be obtained from state departments of agriculture, cooperative extension offices, or entomology departments at state universities in major poultry-producing regions of the United States.

INSECTS

LICE. Lice are common external parasites of birds. They belong in the order Mallophaga, the chewing lice, and are characterized by possession of chewing-type mandibles located ventrally on the head, incomplete metamorphosis, no wings, dorsoventrally flattened body, and short antennae with three to five segments. More than 40 species have been reported from domesticated fowl. Fortunately, as far as the poultry producer is concerned, all the various species of bird lice are controlled by the same methods. Birds frequently harbor several species at the same time.

The list of lice of North American poultry is from Emerson (18, 19), who also includes keys and illustrations of lice on chickens and turkeys. There are many species of bird lice, but only a few are commonly seen. Bird lice can be found on hosts that are not commonly produced commercially; that is, you may see lice from guinea fowl on chickens and turkeys if these birds can have physical contact. Pigeon lice are frequently found on domestic fowl if the pigeons nest above the fowl. The species of louse on infested birds should be determined if cross contamination from another bird species is suspected. If the lice are not controlled on both birds at the same time, the control program will fail. The more common louse species are listed below.

Chicken lice:
Cuclotogaster heterographa, chicken head louse (Fig. 32.1)
Goniocotes gallinae, fluff louse (Fig. 32.2)
Goniodes dissimilis, brown chicken louse
Lipeurus caponis, wing louse

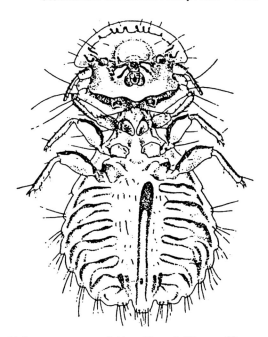

32.2. *Goniocotes,* probably *gallinae,* fluff louse. ×20. (Reis and Nobrega)

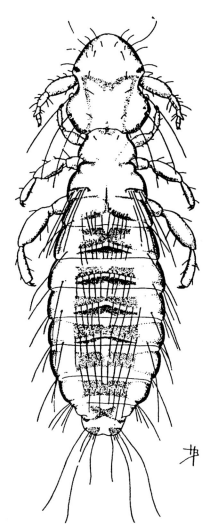

32.1. *Cuclotogaster heterographa,* chicken head louse. (USDA)

Menacanthus stramineus, chicken body louse (also turkey, guinea fowl)
Menopon gallinae, shaft louse (also on guinea fowl) (Fig. 32.3)

Turkey lice:
Chelopistes meleagridis, large turkey louse
Oxylipeurus polytrapezius, slender turkey louse
O. corpelentus, (common on wild turkeys)

Guinea fowl lice:
Goniodes numidae, guinea feather louse
Lipeurus numidae, slender guinea louse

Duck and goose lice:
Anaticola anseris, slender goose louse
A. crassicormis, slender duck louse

Trinoton anserinum, goose body louse
T. querquedulae, large duck louse

Pigeon lice:
Campanulotes bidentatus compar, small pigeon louse
Columbicola columbae, slender pigeon louse (Figs. 32.4, 32.5)

Lice will transfer from one bird species to another if these hosts are in close contact. The slender pigeon louse, however, is known to transfer between hosts by transmission with the hippoboscid pigeon fly (*Pseudolynchia canariensis*) (33). Only lice included in the host-parasite list for any one species of bird are likely to become established. Some species of lice occur wherever domestic birds are raised, but they are less frequently found on modern intensive poultry-production facilities. Lousiness (pediculosis) of birds is diagnosed by finding the straw-colored lice on skin or feathers of birds. Lice of domestic birds vary in size from less than 1 mm to over 6 mm in length. Mallophaga up to 10-mm long occur on wild birds. Lice spend the entire life cycle on the host. Eggs are attached to the feathers, often in clusters, and require 4–7 days to hatch (see Fig. 32.5). The entire life cycle takes about 3 wk for completion, including 4–5 days for incubation and three nymphal instars of 3 days each. One pair of lice may produce 120,000 descendants within a few months. Their normal life

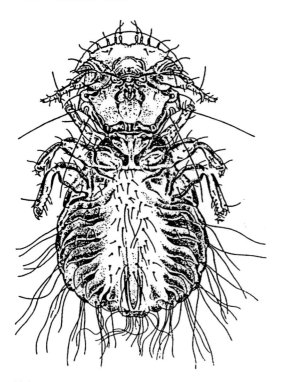

32.3.   *Menopon gallinae,* shaft louse. (Kriner)

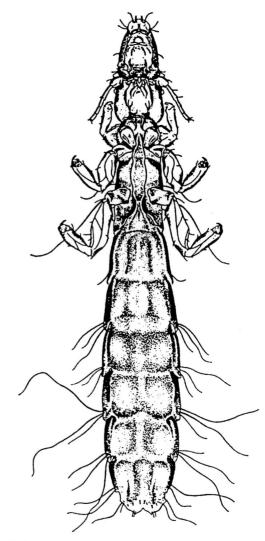

32.4.   *Columbicola columbae,* slender pigeon louse. ×42.
(Reis and Nobrega)

span is several months; but away from the birds, they can remain alive only 5 or 6 days. Although bird lice ordinarily eat feather products, *Menacanthus stramineus* may consume blood by puncturing soft quills near the bases and gnawing through the covering layers of the skin itself.

Severe lousiness in poultry originally was thought to follow malnutrition and lead to weight loss as well as low production. There is conflicting evidence on these hypotheses. Warren et al. (46) and Stockdale and Raun (44) found no effect on laying hens, even following rather heavy body louse infestation. Edgar and King (16) concluded that louse-free hens averaged about 11% greater egg production than did those moderately infested. Gless and Raun (25) revealed that an average of 23,000 chicken body lice per hen reduced egg production by 15%. DeVaney (11, 12) showed that decreases in egg production, hen weight, clutch size, and feed consumption correlated with populations of lice when lice-infested birds were compared with noninfested birds. Further research is needed to quantify economic effect and determine differences in effect according to the louse species involved. Breeding lines of chickens also may vary in louse susceptibility. Factors of grooming (related to birds without trimmed beaks) and relative humidity may also be important in determining variations in densities of chicken body lice on birds.

Lice are not highly pathogenic to mature birds,

but louse-infected chicks may die. Clinical evidence indicates that lice may irritate nerve endings, thus, interfering with the rest and sleep so necessary to immature animals. Lousiness frequently accompanies manifestations of poor health such as internal parasitism, infectious disease, and malnutrition, as well as poor sanitation.

The virus of equine encephalomyelitis has been isolated from *M. stramineus,* as has chlamydia of ornithosis from *Menopon gallinae* and from mites on chickens and turkeys. There are little data, however, to support the fact that these lice are actually important in transmission of these agents in the field.

Turkeys may be infested with the common chicken body louse (*M. stramieneus*), large turkey louse (*Chelopistes meleagridis*), and slender turkey

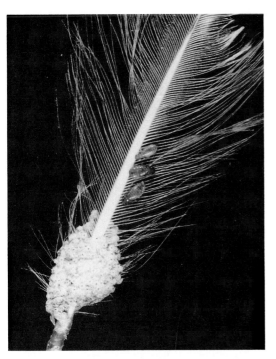

32.5. Eggs of *Columbicola columbae*, slender pigeon louse, at base of feather. ×48. (Reis and Nobrega)

louse (*Oxylipeurus polytrapezius*), which is occasionally found on wild turkeys. Rearing turkeys in close confinement and unsanitary quarters favors lice more than does range management. It is important that breeding males and females be examined frequently, since parasites may contribute to infertility. A common method of introducing lice to a noninfested facility is by the use of infested shipping crates, egg flats, or cartons that have been brought on the facility. All equipment used to transfer birds should be cleaned and disinfected before being used on another farm.

Control. Galliform wild or domestic birds should never be allowed to contact poultry flocks. Lice tend to increase during autumn and winter, so flocks should be examined for lice on a regular basis (a minimum of two times per month) and treated, if needed. If treatment is required, the birds should be treated two times on a 7- to 10-day interval. Only the mature and immature forms will be controlled, as none of the available chemicals are ovicidal (eggs are not killed). Retreatment (the second spraying) is necessary to control the lice that will hatch after the initial treatment. In all poultry houses, the egg-laden feathers will continue to be a source of reinfestation, and, when the house is depopulated, a through cleanup should be completed. In many cases, spraying of birds is the best choice for most poultry operations. When properly done,

spraying ensures that all birds in a house are treated, and with large numbers of birds, it is the most practical means currently available. Care should be taken when spraying the birds to ensure that the whole bird is treated, as it is common for lice to move to the neck of birds from the vent when populations are large. In caged-layer flocks it is important that the birds be checked on a regular basis. Monitoring is done by randomly checking birds two times a month throughout the house. By following this procedure, infestations can be seen prior to the time that the whole house is infested, and control can be implemented on 100 to 200 birds instead of 60,000. Lice on pigeons can be controlled by using the same methods and materials that are used on commercial poultry.

BUGS. The family Cimicidae in the order Hemiptera includes several bloodsucking parasites of birds. These insects are flattened dorsoventrally, and adults are 2- to 5-mm long × 1.5 to 3-mm wide with small pad-like wing remnants. Thus, they are able to creep into crevices and hide in the daytime. Color varies according to species from brown to yellow or red. The piercing-sucking mouthpart or "beak" is attached far forward on the head and is jointed, folding under the head and part of the thorax when not in use. Stink glands provide the common bedbug and its surroundings with an unpleasant odor. If attacked by large numbers of bugs, young birds may become anemic. Bites are usually followed by swelling and itching caused by injection of saliva into the wound.

Bedbug. The most widespread of these bugs is the common bedbug (*Cimex lectularius*) (Fig. 32.6), which attacks humans, most other mammals, and poultry. It is most prevalent in temperate and subtropical climates. Poultry houses and pigeon lofts may become heavily invaded.

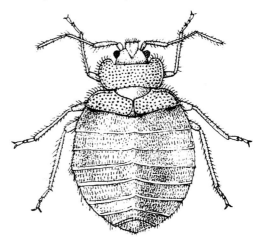

32.6. *Cimex lectularius,* common bedbug. (USDA)

The female bedbug lays several eggs per day in crevices until about 200 have been deposited. Depending on the temperature, the eggs hatch in 4–20 days, followed by five nymphal stages. The nymphs feed at each stage and hide in crevices to digest the blood meal and molt their skins. From egg hatching to adulthood requires 1–3 mo. Nymphs may withstand starvation for about 70 days, while adults live without food for 1–12 mo, depending on temperature. Feeding usually occurs at night; the bugs becoming engorged within 10 min. Large numbers of bedbugs can have a severe impact on production of poultry. Infested breeder houses have shown decreased egg production, increased feed consumption, and lower peak production.

In the tropics and subtropics, the closely related bedbugs, *C. hemipterus* and *C. boueti*, will also attack poultry. *C. columbarius* attacks pigeons in Europe.

Bird Bug.   The most important bird bug is the poultry bug (*Haemotosiphon modoru*), also known as the Mexican chicken bug, adobe bug, or *curuco*. It occurs in the southern and western United States and in Central America and has been found in nests of the California condor, and on the great horned owl in Oklahoma, and turkey in New Mexico and Arizona. It also attacks humans.

The swallow bug (*Oeciacus vicarius*) is commonly found in nests of swallows (particularly barn swallows) and may spread to poultry and humans.

Other cimicid bugs may be found occasionally on poultry in various countries outside the United States. *Ornithocoris toledoi* is a South American poultry pest known as the Brazilian chicken bug. *O. pallidus,* another South American species, has been found on chicks in Florida and Georgia.

Assassin Bug.   The family Reduviidae in the order Hemiptera includes many predacious bugs, but a few known as cone-nose bugs are minor bloodsucking pests of poultry (Fig. 32.7).

The body is cylindrical in shape, and the narrow head bears a stout beak that is curved back into a groove in the prosternum. They are larger than true bedbugs (up to 25 mm in length) and have well-developed wings; otherwise their morphology, life cycles, and behavior are somewhat similar. Species of reduviid bugs reported as attacking poultry in the United States include the bloodsucking cone-nose (*Triatoma sanguisuga*) (Maryland, Florida, California, Texas) and the western bloodsucking cone-nose (*T. protracta*) (Utah, California) (Fig. 32.7). *T. sanguisuga* was found to harbor the virus of equine encephalomyelitis in Kansas, with naturally occurring viral infections found in pigeons and pheasants.

Control.   Treatment should be directed against daytime hiding places of the bugs—in cracks and crevices of walls and floors and under roosts, nest boxes, and feeders. Spraying the birds will also be helpful if an infestation is large. In a house infested with bedbugs, it will be necessary to treat the house and all contents at cleanout. A residual chemical in combination with a fumigant is needed to flush the bugs from their hiding places and give control.

FLEAS.   Fleas (order Siphonaptera) are parasites in the adult stage but free-living as larvae. Adults vary in size from 1.5 mm, possess a tough laterally compressed body, piercing-sucking mouthparts, short antennae in grooves, and long legs adapted for leaping. They undergo complete metaphormosis, with larvae that are legless and wormlike, and pupae in tiny cocoons.

Fleas are brown to black and suck blood from various host species. They are cosmopolitan in distribution, although more abundant in temperate and warm climates. Female fleas deposit several white spherical eggs per day, which roll off the host into surrounding litter, where they incubate. Dampness and warmth are essential for further development. Within 1–2 wk, eggs hatch, liberating tiny maggot-like larvae that feed chiefly on flea "feces" and specialized blood released by female fleas to ensure food for the developing larvae. Fully grown larvae proceed to spin silken cocoons, entangling the threads with various particles of dust and dirt. The inactive pupal stage varies from 1 wk to several months, depending on the temperature. Emerging from the pupal cocoons, young fleas seek a host, suck blood, and are ready to reproduce within a few days. Immature fleas may live for weeks or months

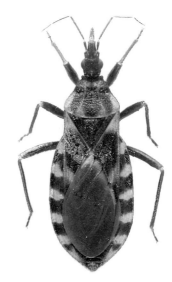

32.7.   *Triatoma,* probably *lectularia,* cone-nose assassin bug. (USDA)

without food. Adult fleas may also live for weeks without feeding, but live many months to a year when hosts are available. Their life cycle varies greatly, depending on such factors as temperature, humidity, exposure, and host availability. Birds returning to old haunts can become infested with fleas that have remained quiescent for long periods. Many species of fleas have been found on birds, but only three of six species reported from poultry in North America are important for review. To identify fleas and for distributional data, see Fox (20) and Hubbard (31).

Sticktight Flea.   The sticktight flea (*Echidnophaga gallinacea*) (Fig. 32.8) occurs more often in the southern United States, although occasionally it is found as far north as New York. Adults usually attach to skin of the head, often in clusters of 100 or more. Mouthparts are deeply embedded in the skin, so they are difficult to dislodge. The sticktight is unique among poultry fleas in that adults become sessile parasites and usually remain attached for days or weeks. Adult females forcibly eject their eggs so that they reach surrounding litter (Fig. 32.8). *E. gallinacea* has been reported from bird hosts (chicken, turkey, pigeon, blackbird, bluejay, hawk, owl, pheasant, quail, sparrow) as well as mammals (human, horse, cattle, swine, dog, fox, cat, badger, coyote, deer, ground squirrel, lynx, mouse, opossum, rabbit, raccoon, rat, ring-tailed cat, skunk).

This flea does not transmit infectious disease agents to chickens. Irritation and blood loss may damage poultry seriously, especially young birds in which death may occur. Production is lowered in older birds. The rickettsia that causes human endemic (murine) typhus has been experimentally transmitted from infected rats to guinea pigs through sticktight fleas, thus indicating a possible public health importance of this parasite.

European Chicken Flea.   The European chicken flea (*Ceratophyllus gallinae*) (Fig. 32.9) has been reported from Maine, Massachusetts, Connecticut, New York, Delaware, Michigan, and Iowa. Undoubtedly, it has a much wider distribution. Hosts include chickens, pigeons, bluebirds, sparrows, and tree swallows, as well as humans, dogs, chipmunks, rats, and squirrels. This flea stays on birds only long enough to feed, while its immature stages occur in nests and other surroundings.

Western Chicken Flea.   The western chicken flea (*Ceratophyllus niger*) is reported mainly from the Pacific coast and north to Alberta. It may attack various birds and mammals, including chickens, turkeys, cormorants, gulls, magpies, sparrows, and woodpeckers as well as humans, mice, and rats. It resembles *C. gallinae* in appearance and biology.

Others.   The cat flea (*Ctenocephalides felis*) has been found in poultry houses at pest levels. Most of these houses are using cats as a rodent control program, and it appears as if the cats start the flea population in the house and then the fleas move to the birds. Other pests are accidental, such as *Orchopeas howardii,* ordinarily found on squirrels. Similarly, the human flea (*Pulex irritans*) occasionally attacks poultry.

Control.   The most important control measures are removal of infested litter and thorough house spraying to kill immature fleas. Fresh litter should be put in the house and treated to kill adult fleas on birds and those that drop into litter. In Scotland, tests have shown control of *C. gallinae* by using the pyrethroid permethrin as a 0.125–0.25% spray to nest boxes and litter (45).

Poultry, dogs, cats, and rats should be screened from access under buildings, since they may serve

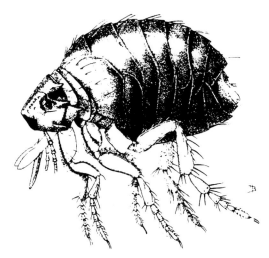

32.8. *Echidnophaga gallinacea*, sticktight flea. (USDA)

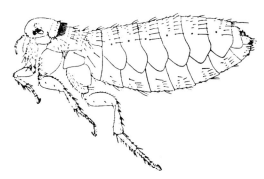

32.9. *Ceratophyllus gallinae*, European chicken flea. (Reis and Nobrega)

to perpetuate flea invasions. Sunlight, hot dry weather, excessive moisture, and freezing hinder development of fleas.

BEETLES. Beetles (order Coleoptera) possess chewing mouthparts and two pairs of wings, the first pair modified to horny wing covers and the second pair folded under the wing covers except during flight; they experience complete metamorphosis, with a wormlike grub stage followed by the resting pupal stage. No beetles are true parasites of birds, but a few may occasionally feed on living skin. Poultry will feed on beetles found in litter or on the range, thus providing an opportunity for ingestion of parasites or debris associated with the beetles. The following tapeworms can be transmitted by beetles: *Raillietina cesticillus, R. magninumida, Choanotaenia infundibulum, Hymenolepis carioca, H. diminuta,* and *H. cantaniana* (see Chapter 33 for specific host–parasite relationships). Darkling beetles have been shown to be reservoirs, or mechanical carriers, for a number of pathogens including *Aspergillus, Escherichia, Salmonella, Streptococcus,* and viruses causing Marek's disease and infectious bursal disease (7). These beetles also serve as an alternative source of food for small chicks and poults, increasing the possibility of disease in the birds as well as decreasing bird performance. Internal parasite problems in both broiler and turkey production have increased, and the intermediate host/vector of these parasites is the darkling beetle. Styrofoam insulation used in enclosed poultry houses may be invaded by various beetle species (lesser or yellow mealworms and dermestids), and severe damage, particularly to ceiling areas, requires expensive repair (21).

Darkling Beetle or Lesser Mealworm. Darkling beetles are cosmopolitan insects infesting poultry housed around the world. The beetles live in the litter, where they feed on spilled poultry feed, manure, and dead or moribund birds. The life cycle of darkling beetles (Fig. 32.10) requires from 1 to 3 mo for the development of the larvae and the adults can live for 1 yr (21). Darkling beetles are small (0.5 cm) and can be most easily seen under feeders or along the wall of the poultry house. The larvae are wormlike and will avoid light. It should be noted that there will be other species of beetles found in the litter as well darkling beetles. The other species of beetles are beneficial insects such as Histerids and Staphylinids and should not be confused with the litter beetle.

Beetles within a poultry house can number up to 1000 per square meter. They are important to the poultry industry as possible disease vectors by damage to insulation, and as pests. Geden and Axtell (21) reported that only adults and late instar larvae

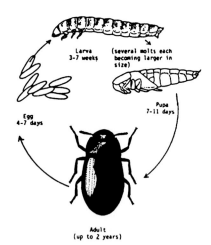

32.10. Life cycle of the darkling beetle.

seeking pupation sites were tunneling in the insulation and that the climbing activity was taking place at night. Beetles can be found throughout the poultry house; eggs, larvae, pupae, and adults are in litter and soil. Due to the beetles' ability to utilize many niches in the poultry house, control is difficult to achieve with any single approach.

Others. The yellow mealworm (*Tenebrio molitor*) is ordinarily found consuming grain products stored in mills, warehouses, bakeries, and groceries. Adult beetles are shiny brown to black and about 15-mm long. The yellow larvae or grubs (flour, meal, or branworms) are smooth, cylindrical wormlike creatures up to 30-mm long. They may infest setting hens, mainly attacking the feet, where loss of skin may be followed by severe hemorrhage. These grubs have been found to erode skin of young pigeons; other related mealworm beetle larvae may produce similar damage.

The larder beetle (*Dermestes lardarius*) and related species (*Dermestes maculatus*) ordinarily destroy stored grain products and meats (especially ham and bacon) and feed on hides, skins, furs, museum specimens, or decaying animal matter (notably accumulated droppings in pigeon lofts). The adult is black and about 7-mm long; the basal half of each wing cover is brownish yellow crossed by a band of three black spots. The larvae are up to 12-mm long, dark brown above, gray below, and covered with brown hairs. The larvae may attack skin of nestling pigeons. *Dermestes maculatus* has emerged as a problem in high-rise layer housing where deep-pit manure is used. The beetles feed on dead birds, feathers, and feed in the pits. This beetle will also tunnel insulation when seeking pupation sites; moreover, in addition to insulation, they tunnel into the structure itself. In some instances, the beetles have tunneled support beams so extensively that the building collapsed.

Silpha thoracica, S. opaca, Necrophorus ivestigator, and possibly other species of the beetle family Silphidae (carrion beetles) may also develop in pigeon droppings. Larvae, which are black and up to 15-mm long, are reported to invade the skin of squabs; wounds produced may be secondarily infested by fly maggots.

Control. Generally there is little point in attempting to control beetles on poultry ranges, but control in confined large-scale poultry housing is necessary. Stored grains and feeds should not be allowed to become infested with insects; infested material should be fumigated.

Control of lesser mealworms and hide beetles should be part of an integrated approach that utilizes all possible approaches to manage the population. Any control strategy that is chosen must take into account that there will be a number of eggs, larvae, pupae, and adults in the soil and walls of a building. These life stages will not come into contact with an insecticide immediately, and if the insecticide chosen does not have a long residual life, control of the beetles will be shortened. The best control approach is to clean out each house after each flock; however, due to the cost of bedding and labor, this practice is rarely followed. Another approach is to utilize carefully timed insecticide treatments. Houses should be treated with an insecticide immediately after the flock is removed. If treatment is delayed, a number of the beetles will move to inaccessible areas in the house, and the insecticide will not come into contact with the beetles. Posts and support poles and braces can be treated as a barrier to the beetles. At the present time, there is no one insecticide that would be a best choice for treatment at the time a flock is removed; any of the currently registered products is acceptable. To monitor the population of beetles in the house, a tube trap can be used (2). By examining the traps weekly, the population trend can be determined.

The darkling beetle is not tolerant of temperatures below 40 F. If the air temperature is less than 40 F, the house should be opened up at clean-out to allow the temperature of the litter to drop as low as possible. By using cultural controls, low temperature, clean-out schedules, and chemicals, beetle populations can be managed and maintained below damaging levels.

FLIES AND MOSQUITOES.

The order Diptera includes several families whose members annoy or suck blood from birds as well as mammals. All dipterans have two wings in the adult stage (except degenerate wingless forms) and pass through a complete metamorphosis, including a maggotlike larva and a puparium resting stage. Adult mouthparts are of the piercing-sucking or sponging types. The intermittent nature of their feeding and extensive flight-range render adult flies ideal vectors of disease. Certain species develop in poultry manure and may become so numerous as to create a health and public relations problem. For identification and information on flies associated with manure, see Axtell (6).

Mosquitoes. Although mosquitoes are not as important to poultry as to humans and other mammals, many species feed on poultry and transmit disease. Some 140 species have been described from North America; a number of these are known to suck avian blood.

Most mosquito species are about 5 mm in length, and wings are characteristically veined and scaled. Legs and abdomen are long and slender, and the female is provided with elongated mouthparts for piercing the skin. The male does not suck blood but feeds on plant juices, nectar, and other fluids. Mosquitoes deposit eggs on pools of water, moist soil, or surfaces subject to flooding. Larval and pupal stages develop in water, with adults emerging from pupal cases to mate and then seek a host. In warm weather, the life cycle is completed in about 7–14 days. Adults are most active on dull, quiet days, especially toward evening and at night.

Poultry production facilities that utilize lagoons can have problems with mosquitoes breeding in the lagoon if it is not properly maintained. Lagoons should have steep banks that are free of vegetation along the shoreline and should be relatively deep in order to provide the proper environment for anaerobic decomposition of the waste. If mosquito breeding is a problem and the lagoon requires chemical treatment, Dursban would be the chemical of choice.

Mosquitoes may attack poultry in dense numbers. *Psorophora confinnis* was responsible for the deaths of numerous chickens in Florida. The southern house mosquito (*Culex quinquefasciatus*) was found in dense numbers in chicken houses in Alabama, and their attacks on birds appeared to reduce egg production. The encephalitis mosquito in the western United States (*Culex tarsalis*) shows a host preference for birds, including chickens. Other mosquito species have been found to carry and transmit viral agents of eastern equine encephalomyelitis (EEE), St. Louis encephalitis (SLE), and western equine encephalomyelitis (WEE). Reeves (41) reviewed avian virus reservoirs and mosquito vectors and their relation to human disease. Fowl pox virus is transmitted by *Aedes stimulans, A. aegypti, A. vexans,* and many species of culicodies biting midges. *A. stimulans* may harbor the virus for 2 days, whereas *A. vexans* may infect birds up to 39 days after contacting the virus of fowl pox and pigeon pox. Vaccination programs for fowl pox are often instituted during seasons when dense mosquito populations are expected.

CONTROL. The best attack is prevention of mosquito development. The farm should be surveyed for all water areas that may produce mosquitoes, including swamps, ponds, stagnant pools, and water-filled containers of all types. Mosquito production can be stopped by removal of such containers, covering cisterns and water barrels, clearing pool and pond edges of emergent vegetation, employing drainage operations, and filling low areas that collect water.

For housed poultry, mosquitoes landing on surfaces inside or outside the house may be killed by residual insecticide deposits of the type recommended for fly control. Poultry in open houses or on range are most difficult to protect from mosquitoes. Pyrethrum fly sprays can be fogged in houses or on ranges to obtain quick kill of mosquitoes in an outbreak, but control will not last more than a few hours. Residual sprays can be applied to exterior surfaces of buildings or outdoors to vegetation from which poultry are excluded. If needed, breeding areas can be treated with larvicides using registered chemicals; biologic control agents also have been shown to be effective.

Area treatment with insecticides is fraught with danger of water contamination, wildlife, and fish kill. In many states, a permit must be obtained to treat stream and pond drainage basins. Mosquito control and local public health authorities should be consulted for current information prior to outdoor use of pesticides. Promotion of community-wide mosquito control is usually necessary, since water sources may be far from the poultry farm.

Biting Midges. *Culicoides* spp. (family Ceratopoginidae) are biting midges, "punkies," or "no-see-ums"; some 35 species have been reported from North America, and many attack birds and mammals. These are extremely small although easily seen as small blackish specks moving on the skin. In Virginia, some 20 species have been taken in chicken coops or found to feed on chickens and turkeys; *C. obsoletus, C. furens, C. sanguisuga,* and *C. crepuscularis* were most abundant. The agent of avian infectious synovitis remains alive in *C. variipennis* for at least 24 hr, but transmission by bites has not been proved for any *Culicoides* species. Some species may serve as intermediate hosts for *Haemoproteus nettionis,* a blood protozoan of domesticated ducks in Canada. Culicodies midges have been incriminated in the transmission of fowl pox in turkeys.

CONTROL. Controlling biting midges is very difficult. They will pass through ordinary screen mesh, but screens treated with 6% malathion solution have killed midges for more than 3 wk. Fogging with mosquito or fly sprays may alleviate the problem. Residual deposits applied for fly control will also help. Since habitats where these species develop are so variable, it is difficult and often impractical to use measures for source reduction. One area, however, that has become a breeding area near poultry housing is improperly managed lagoons. In many cases, the midges can be controlled by maintaining the lagoon properly on these facilities.

Blackflies. Blackflies (family Simuliidae) (Fig. 32.11) are also known as turkey or buffalo gnats. They are similar in size to mosquitoes but are dark, short, chunky, and humpbacked, with short legs: their wing venation is distinctive. More than 20 species have been reported to attack domestic poultry in North America. Blackflies usually suck blood during the day and may cause serious damage to humans and livestock; in dense numbers on poultry they may cause a severe anemia. They also transmit certain blood protozoa belonging to the genus *Leucocytozoon.*

Blackfly production sources are restricted to running water such as creeks, streams, or irrigation supply and drainage systems. Eggs are laid on rocks, sticks, or floating vegetation, or are dropped into streams. They may hatch in a few days, but some remain through summer or even until the following spring. Larvae attach to stones or other objects and reach the pupal stage after 3–10 wk. The pupal stage also occurs under water, lasting from a few days to 1 wk or more. Adults of some species emerge in spring, others during summer or early fall; some species may travel several miles to seek a blood meal. Overwintering occurs in the egg or larval stage. Most temperate zone species have one generation a year.

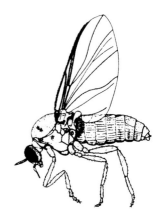

32.11.   Blackfly, family Simuliidae. (Travis)

Simuliids are most troublesome in the northern part of the temperate zone and the subarctic, but some important species are found in the tropics. Reports in the United States date back to the last century, when buffalo gnats were noted to swarm on poultry, forcing setting chickens and turkeys to leave their nests. It is reported that *Simulium bracteatum* fatally attacked goslings and that other *Simulium* species caused losses to chickens and turkeys in Canada. *S. jenningsi* and *S. slossonae* were found to attack turkeys in Virginia as far as 15 miles from their breeding places. In Kansas, egg losses of 50% in 8 days were recorded from chickens attacked by the turkey gnat (*S. meridionae*).

Disease transmission by gnats to poultry was initially proved in Nebraska, where *S. occidentale* transmitted *Leucocytozoon smithi*, a blood protozoon of turkeys. Many other blackfly species have been found to transmit *Leucocytozoon* spp. to poultry. *S. venustum* transmits *L. simondi* to tame and wild ducks in Michigan, while in Canada this organism is transmitted to ducks by *S. croxtoni, S. euryadminiculum*, and *S. rugglesi*. *S. slossonae* and *S. congareenarum* are vectors of *Leucocytozoon* spp. to turkeys in South Carolina. Noblet et al. (40) showed differences in seasonal incidence, levels of transmission, and blackfly vector habits related to *L. smithi* in turkeys in the coastal plains and sandhill areas of South Carolina. This information was overlooked, however, in selecting the location of a new turkey industry, and disease outbreaks resulted in great financial losses to a major poultry-producing company. Anderson (1) found that six species of blackflies in Canada transmitted the blood microfilariae of the nematode *Ornithofilaria fallinsensis* to domesticated and wild ducks. Ducks are no longer produced commercially in these localities.

CONTROL. Control is difficult because these pests develop in streams, often some distance from the poultry farm, where insecticide treatment may be harmful to fish. Successful reduction of larval and subsequent adult blackfly populations (and no fish kill) were obtained in infested streams treated monthly by helicopters using 2% temephos granules. Area-wide control programs have been developed using biologic control agents, *Bacillus thuringiensis* var. *israelenis* (Bti). These programs involve treatment of all breeding areas in a defined geographic area, with treatment taking place weekly. Measures recommended for mosquito control as well as cautions on watershed contamination by pesticides are also pertinent to blackfly control.

Housefly and Its Relatives. Nonbiting flies produced on poultry farms are a health and sanitation problem to the poultry producer and neighbors. Public pressure against poultry enterprises can force producers to move or go out of business if flies, odors, or blowing feathers are not controlled. Intensive modern poultry farms produce a tremendous amount of manure, which must be properly managed to ensure that it is not attractive to flies for breeding and that it does not cause an odor problem.

Location of poultry houses and manure disposal areas needs to be carefully planned to prevent filth fly problems from developing. The entire poultry industry has an important role in community responsibility to control flies in suburban and urban areas. Many poultry producers have met financial disaster as new residential developments have invaded formerly suburban locations where they had built their facilities. In many regions, state and county legislative action has strengthened public health codes, and local ordinances have resulted whereby poultry farms can be closed because of unabated fly sources found on their property. Poultry associations have assisted in drafting legislation and policing the few careless producers who have permitted public health problems to develop.

The common nonbiting flies on poultry farms in the United States include the housefly (*Musca domestica*) (Fig. 32.12); *Fannia* spp. (Fig. 32.13) including the little housefly (*Fannia canicularis*), coastal fly (*F. femoralis*), and latrine fly (*F. scalaris*); false stable fly (*Muscina stabulans*); several species of blowflies (Calliphoridae); and flesh flies (Sarcophagidae). So-called filth flies are a worldwide problem on poultry farms, with many other species of *Musca,* other genera, and indigenous Calliphoridae and Sarcophagidae involved. Identification of biting and nonbiting flies and notes

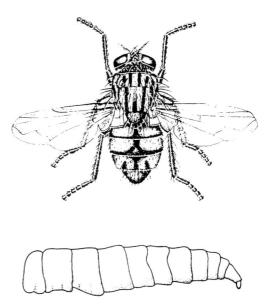

32.12. *Musca domestica,* housefly adult and smooth-tapered larva. (Coop Ext, Univ Calif)

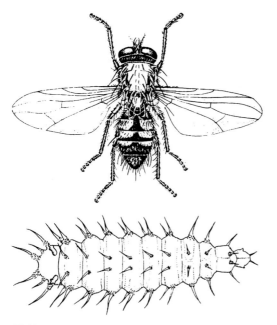

32.13. *Fannia* spp. adult and spinose larva. (Coop Ext Univ Calif)

on their biology were reported by Loomis et al. (38), and there is a monograph on fly biology and control by Axtell (6).

Filth flies lay eggs in manure (some sarcophagids deposit living larvae), in moist spilled feed, or on dead-bird carcasses. In hot weather, the housefly can complete its life cycle in 8 days, but in colder weather it may require over 6 wk. Larvae (maggots) develop in moist manure and then move to drier areas for pupation. The housefly does not diapause and survives northern winters by slow development in warm indoor locations such as enclosed poultry houses and dairy barns and in towns and cities. Other filth flies survive northern winters by hibernation as diapausing adults or in immature stages.

Flies have been incriminated as vectors of many mammalian, as well as avian, gastrointestinal diseases, largely through their habit of feeding on inoculum in excrement and regurgitating onto food or feeds (48). Newcastle disease virus was isolated from adult *F. canicularis, F. femoralis,* and *M. domestica* larvae during an outbreak of this disease in California. Houseflies and maggots are readily eaten by birds, affording transmission of helminths. They are intermediate hosts for the tapeworm *Choanotaenia infundibulum* of chickens and turkeys. Common housefly and blowfly species (Calliphoridae) are capable of carrying eggs of the cecal worm *Heterakis gallinae,* which may contain the protozoan agent of histomoniasis of turkeys.

Certain fly larvae feed on decomposing cadavers

and may ingest toxins of the bacterium *Clostridium botulinum.* If poultry eat such maggots, botulism ("limberneck") may occur. Larvae of the following species of flies have been incriminated as transmitters of botulinus toxins types A and C: *Lucilia illustris* and *Phaenicia sericata* (Calliphoridae); sarcophagid larvae; larvae of *Cochliomyia macellaria* (Calliphoridae), the secondary screwworm fly. Prompt burial, burning, or use of disposal pits for animal cadavers will do much to prevent botulism from these sources. To ensure safety, dead-bird disposal should be located at some distance from the poultry house.

It is known that common houseflies feeding on infected fowl cholera blood can transmit this disease when fed to turkeys. Larvae of fly species that often develop in tuberculous chicken cadavers can also transmit *Mycobacterium tuberculosis* when fed to nontuberculous chickens.

Invasion of birds by fly larvae (maggots) is not as common as in mammals. The black blowfly (*Phormia regina*) can deposit eggs in wounds on chickens, turkeys, and geese, and the ensuing maggots may destroy living tissue. Nests of wild birds may become infested by maggots of other species of flesh flies and blowflies, with disastrous effects on nestlings.

CONTROL. Fly control on poultry farms should be based on IPM principles that include cultural, biologic, and chemical control strategies. By utilizing an IPM approach that includes the judicious use of cultural (manure management), biologic (parasites and predators), and chemical (insecticides) control practices, flies can be maintained below threshold levels (5). Manure should be maintained in a moisture range of less than 60%. Manure moisture of 60 to 90% is ideal for fly development. Sufficient airflow should be provided over the manure to aid in its drying. Airflow over manure is critical to maintaining manure that is dry and will not support fly breeding. Airflow for the building should be checked to ensure that proper amounts are available for ventilation. If airflow is insufficient for the birds, it should be corrected. If, owing to the building design or other factors, airflow over manure is not correct, stirring fans should be added in the pits of layer houses. Also, if insulation levels in the house are insufficient, and airflow is therefore reduced in cold weather, moisture will build in the manure, and fly breeding will increase. All tall vegetation that might reduce the flow of air into the house should be cut. All watering devices should be maintained and water leaks repaired. The water supply should be tested and the salt levels determined so that diets can be adjusted to maintain proper salt content. High salt levels in water and feed increase water consumption and, in turn, increase the amount of water in the manure. Because wettness makes the manure more suitable for fly breeding, buildings in which birds have high salt consumption usually have more severe fly problems.

The selection of building site is also very important. The site should be well drained and constructed properly. Roofs should be in good condition in order to keep manure cones dry and the roof overhang should be large enough to ensure that rain will be carried away from the building and not pool next to the foundation, where it is often found leaking back into the manure. Clean-out should be completed on a schedule, remembering that in hot weather, the housefly maggot can develop in less than 1 wk, and other pest species in 2–3 wk. On-farm storage can be done by proper composting of manure in short windrows, or by covering with a black polyethylene tarpaulin to prevent fly production. If manure is stored in a shallow or deep pit under the birds, clean-out should be completed in the winter. This will allow time for a new dry pad of manure to develop prior to fly season. That will act as an absorbent pad as well as a reservoir for parasites and predators.

After all possible physical methods of maintaining dry manure have been completed, attention should be directed to the use and fostering of the natural and introduced biologic control organisms that are comprised of mites, beetles, and parasitic wasps. Biologic methods include the retention of indigenous as well as introduced predators and parasites of eggs, larvae, and pupae of filth flies such as predator mites (*Macrocheles muscaedomesticae, Fuscuropoda vegetans*); predator beetles (*Carcinops pumilo*) and other Histeridae; and parasitic hymenopterous wasps (*Muscidifurax, Spalangia* spp.) and other parasites of the eggs, larvae, and pupae of filth flies (5).

The success of releasing parasites into a poultry house to control a fly population has been mixed (5). In general, due to strain differences and rearing problems, the most successful approach with parasites has been to ensure that the environment of the poultry house is conducive to natural reproduction of the parasites.

Predators of filth flies include histerid beetles, macrochelid mites, and the muscid fly *Ophyra aenescens*. Geden et al. (23) reported that the daily destruction of fly larvae and eggs would range from 5 to 30 per predator. By maintaining the manure in the poultry house in a dry condition, the effectiveness of predators can be enhanced and in many cases chemicals will not be needed to maintain the fly population below threshold.

It is useful to have a method of evaluating a fly population within the poultry house. Monitoring methods should be simple and give an accurate assessment of the population so that the effectiveness of a control program can be measured. By using a monitoring system, treatment can be timed to give the maximum level of control before the population reaches problem levels. Methods for monitoring flies are grid counts, sticky fly ribbons, baited jug traps, and spot cards. The two simplest methods of monitoring are the baited jug trap and the spot cards. Jug traps consist of a plastic 1-gal milk jug with four 3-in. holes cut in the upper one-third of the jug. One ounce of fly bait that contains muscalure is placed in the bottom (39). Flies enter to feed in the jugs and die, with the number of flies being counted weekly in each trap to determine the level of flies in the house. A minimum of six traps should be used in each house; a threshold of an average of 350 flies per trap per week would indicate a need for treatment. This threshold will vary depending upon the location of the poultry house and the nearness of neighbors. A second method of fly monitoring is the use of spot cards. Index cards (3 × 5 in.) should be placed on fly resting sites, rafters, etc. A minimum of 10 cards should be used, with a threshold of 50 specs per card indicating a need for treatment (39). Visual monitoring should be done for fly larvae. Areas where manure is wet should be checked, and if larvae are seen, these areas should be treated.

The use of insecticides for fly control is an important component in an integrated fly control program. Insecticides that are registered for use in poultry buildings for fly control are the only insecticides that should be used to avoid residues in eggs or meat. Insecticides that are efficacious against flies will also kill predators and parasites, and care must be taken when using insecticides to ensure that the predator and parasite population is not decreased due to improper application of an insecticide.

Insecticides can be applied in four basic ways: space sprays/fogs, surface sprays/residuals, baits, and larvicides. Each method has merit and can be an aid in reducing the fly population in the poultry facility but must be used properly for the maximum benefit and lowest cost.

Space Sprays, Fogs, and Mists. The use of space sprays gives temporary control of adult flies. There is no residual or long-term effect of these applications with all the flies being killed at the time of application. Space sprays and mists should be applied early in the morning or late in the evening when most of the flies will be resting within the building. They can be applied with hand-held or tractor-mounted units. The equipment should break the insecticide into fine droplets and, in general, formulations that have an oil or petroleum product base will be more effective, although the oil may irritate animals. Piped-in systems that are designed to deliver a small amount of insecticide on a regular basis (hourly or six times daily) can also be installed in the facility. One key point that should be remembered when using a mist for fly control is that the mist must hang in the air as long as possible for full effectiveness. If a house is well ventilated and air is being rapidly moved at the time of application, control will be decreased due to the short time that the product and flies can come into contact. It may be necessary to close the curtains or stop the fans until after the treatment is completed.

Surface   Sprays/Residuals.   Residual surface sprays should be applied as a coarse spray to areas on which adult flies rest. These surfaces include posts, overhead beams/rafters, and vertical surfaces. Surface sprays may be applied with any type of sprayer at low pressure (40 psi), with the resting surfaces treated until thoroughly wet but without runoff. Insecticide formulations used are WDL, WP, and EC. In general, the WP formulations will give a longer-lasting residue than the other formulations. Dust, type of surface, and amount of sunlight on the surface will all have an effect on how long the product remains active.

Baits.   Commercial baits are generally formulated as granules and should be placed into pans or placed in protected areas. Bait can also be placed into fly traps. To increase effectiveness of dry baits, 1 part field-grade molasses may be diluted with 4 parts water in a 5-gal can and covered with a removable window screen lid on which the dry bait is placed. Some commercial baits have a fly attractant added such as muscamone, which greatly increases their effectiveness.

Larvicides.   Control of fly larvae in the manure is done with a larvicide. Larvicides can be applied as a liquid, dry, or in the feed of the birds. Penetration of the manure with a liquid is difficult, and it is adding water to manure that will make it more difficult to dry the manure to reduce breeding. Treating manure with a larvicide is also devastating to the predators and parasites living in the manure, causing a further imbalance of the fly larvae and predators and parasites. Using a larvicide should only be done on a spot-treatment basis where large numbers of larvae are seen. One exception to this is the larvicide cyromazine, which is toxic to fly larvae but not to the predators and parasites.

Stable Fly.   The stable fly (*Stomoxys calcitrans*) attacks most mammals and birds. This fly is similar in size and appearance to the common housefly but possesses a piercing beak. Stable flies develop in manure with high fiber content or in wet crop refuse

such as straw left in the field after grain harvest. Near the seacoast, they can be very annoying, since they develop in windrows of wet seaweed.

CONTROL.   Stable flies can be controlled by the same measures used against houseflies. Prevention requires cleanup of crop and other plant refuse, and proper manure management to prevent production of moist manure mixed with spilled feed. For control in poultry houses, measures recommended against houseflies are used.

Pigeon Fly.   The pigeon fly (*Pseudolynchia canariensis*) is a rather important parasite of domesticated pigeons in warm or tropical areas. It has been known since 1896 in the southern half of the United States and also occurs in many other countries. The pigeon fly is a member of the parasitic fly family Hippoboscidae, or louse flies. The body is dorsoventrally flattened, and the head is provided with a short stout beak. The life cycle is unusual in that the larva matures inside the female and pupates immediately upon being ejected. The pupal stage requires about 30 days; adults live about 45 days and deposit four or five young.

The adult pigeon fly is dark brown and about 6 mm in length, with two transparent wings somewhat longer than the body. These flies move rapidly through the feathers and suck blood, particularly from nestling pigeons 2–3 wk of age. They may also bite humans, inflicting a painful skin wound that persists for several days. Infested pigeons suffer from blood loss and irritation. The pigeon fly may also transmit a protozoan blood-cell parasite (*Haemoproteus columbae*), the cause of a malaria-like disease of pigeons.

CONTROL.   See control of mites.

MITES.   The common free-living ectoparasitic mites of poultry belong to the family Dermanyssidae and include the chicken mite, northern fowl mite, and tropical fowl mite. These mites possess relatively well-sclerotized free dorsal and ventral plates, claws and caruncles on the tarsi, one lateroventral stigma near each third coxa, and small chelicerae on long-sheathed bases. They are bloodsuckers and can run rapidly on skin and feathers. Of lesser importance are members of many other mite families that bore into the skin or infect various internal passages and organs.

Chicken Mite.   The chicken mite (*Dermanyssus gallinae*), also called red mite, roost mite, or poultry mite, is found worldwide and is particularly serious in warmer parts of the temperate zone in older poultry houses with roosts. The mite is rare in modern large commercial caged-layer operations, but is seen frequently in modern broiler breeder farms. It can be identified by the shape of the dorsal plate and by the long whiplike chelicerae that appear to be stylets (Fig. 32.14). The adult female measures about 0.7×0.4 mm, varying in color from gray to deep red, depending on its blood content. The life cycle may be completed in as little as 7 days. Adult females lay eggs in surroundings of the hosts 12–24 hr after their first blood meal. Eggs hatch in 48–72 hr when warm. The 6-legged larvae molt in 24–48 hr without feeding, becoming first-stage bloodsucking nymphs; they then molt to second-stage nymphs in another 24–48 hr and soon afterward molt to the adult stage. Chicken mites have lived up to 34 wk without food. Chickens are the commonest hosts, but these mites may occur on turkeys, pigeons, canaries, and several species of wild birds. Humans may also be attacked, and invasions of human dwellings (apartments, hospitals, doctors' offices) by mites from outdoor pigeon nests are frequently seen. English sparrows may transmit this parasite because of the habit of lining their nests with chicken feathers. These mites may not only produce anemia, thereby seriously lowering production and increasing feed consumption, but actually kill birds, particularly chicks and setting or laying hens. Birds in production may refuse to lay in infested nests. An increase in feed consumption accompanied by lower production are signs that poultry houses should be examined for mites. These mites often can be found by looking under loose clods of manure, under slats in a breeder house, in nests or in cracks and crevices of posts and roof bracing. They are evident as tiny red to blackish dots, often clustered together. Inspection during the night is usually necessary to find mites on birds. Occasionally these mites may be found on the shanks of both hens and roosters, but care must be taken to differentiate them from northern fowl mites that also appear on the legs.

Northern Fowl Mite. The northern fowl mite (NFM) (*Ornithonyssus sylviarum*) is the commonest and most important permanent parasite of poultry in all major poultry production areas of the United States. It is also recognized as a serious pest throughout the temperate zone of other countries. It is extremely common in almost all types of production facilities. It has been reported from many species of birds, including domesticated poultry, English sparrows, and numerous wild birds, as well as from rats and humans.

This mite is often confused with the chicken mite but can be distinguished by its possession of easily visible chelicerae and the shape of dorsal and anal plates (Fig. 32.15). Unlike the chicken mite, the northern fowl mite can easily be found on birds in the day as well as night, since it breeds continuously. In heavy infestations, feathers are blackened (Fig. 32.16) and skin is scabbed and cracked around the vent; when birds are handled, mites quickly crawl over the examiner's hands and arms. Parting the feathers reveals mites, their eggs, cast-off skins, and excrement on the body surface and feathers. Poultry producers often diagnose NFM infestation by seeing mites crawling on eggs. The proper way to monitor for NFM, however, is to check a sample of 20 to 60 birds in the house. In layer houses, birds should be removed from cages at random throughout the house and the vents examined for NFM.

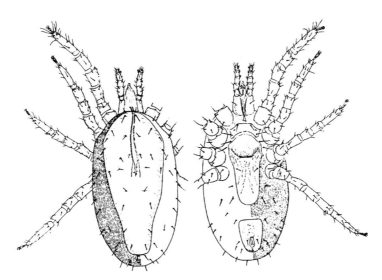

32.14 *Dermanyssus gallinae*, chicken mite. (Baker)

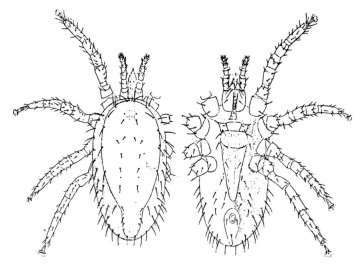

32.15.   *Ornithonyssus sylviarum,* northern fowl mite. (Baker)

Turkeys and broiler breeders should be caught and checked, with more males being checked than females. Birds from all sections of a house need to be examined, as it is common for NFM to start in one section and then slowly spread throughout the house. If the birds are monitored twice monthly, an NFM infestation can be caught before it causes economic damage, and a smaller number of birds will require treatment.

The life cycle of the NFM is completed in less than 1 wk on the birds. Eggs are laid on the feathers and hatch in 1 day. The larval instar and two nymphal instars develop in less than 4 days. In the north, mite densities increase in winter and usually drop to low numbers by summer. Occasionally, however, infestations are found in summer. This contrasts with the chicken mite, which is a pest during warm weather in northern areas but inactive in cold houses during winter. Mites may survive 3–4 wk in the absence of avian hosts.

The northern fowl mite is introduced into laying hen flocks from four main sources: infested hatcheries and contract–started pullet farms; trucks and crates used to carry old birds or infested pullets; personnel, equipment, or egg flats and crates; and wild birds. Sparrows, pigeons, etc. that nest in or near poultry houses are suspected, although tests to infest chicks with NFMs taken from sparrows have not proved successful.

These mites suck blood, and the resulting scabs may injure the appearance of dressed poultry. Of greater concern is the economic importance of this mite to egg production from infested caged layers. Recent investigations indicate the following factors

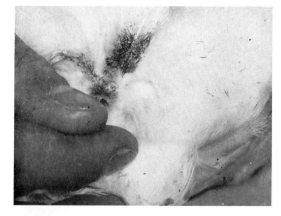

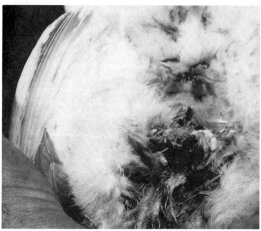

32.16.   Two levels of feather blackening and soiling by northern fowl mite. (Matthysse)

relating to mite densities on hens showing normal or reduced egg production: breed or strain differences (37;12), plasma corticosterone levels and cage stress (27), estrogen levels (28), and immune responses and genetic heritability (13, 17). Arends et al. (3) showed that in broiler breeder laying hens, NFM-infested birds produced 7.7 eggs per hen housed less than NFM-free birds, and that feed costs were increased from $0.01 to $0.06 per dozen eggs produced. These and other investigators agree that the NFM is deleterious to male birds, with extremely dense infestations causing lowered semen production, anemia, and even death.

Although WEE and SLE viruses have been recovered from the NFM obtained from wild birds, it is doubtful that this mite plays any important role in the epidemiology of encephalitides. The NFM may harbor the viruses of fowl pox and Newcastle disease of poultry after feeding on infected chickens, but proof of transmission is lacking. Chlamydia have been isolated from fowl mites (*Ornithonyssus* spp.) and from nonparasitic mites found in nests of turkeys 2½ mo after their abandonment because of ornithosis in the flock (9).

Tropical Fowl Mite.   The tropical fowl mite (*Ornithonyssus bursa*) (Fig. 32.17) is distributed throughout the warmer regions of the world and possibly replaces the NFM in these regions. It is a much less important pest in the United States. Hosts include poultry, pigeons, sparrows, myna birds, and humans. The tropical fowl mite closely resembles the NFM but can be distinguished by the shape of the dorsal plate and pattern of setae. This mite can pass its entire life cycle on chickens. Its biology and habits are similar to those of the NFM, although a greater proportion of its eggs are laid in the nests.

Control.   The chicken mite, NFM, and tropical fowl mite may be controlled by the same insecticides applied to birds, litter, nests, and the walls and roosts of the facility.

Initial control strategy should be focused on monitoring all birds and the facilities. Proper monitoring will reduce the spread of ectoparasites from farm to farm on service personnel, flats, repair personnel, replacement birds, and live haul equipment. By following an active monitoring system, infestations can be identified, and movement on and off these facilities restricted. By reducing the number of houses that are infested, the cost of control can be drastically reduced. This is especially true for most modern vertically integrated companies that may have large numbers of houses that are linked by feed trucks, egg trucks, and service personnel.

All egg flats and cases should be checked if they are coming off an infested farm. Operations that use plastic flats on racks should include procedures to ensure that they are washed with hot water and detergent prior to being redelivered to another farm. Operations that use fiber flats and cardboard cases should include inspection of them prior to sending them back to a farm. Data from field trials showed that as many as 19 adult NFM/egg case may be transported from an infested farm through the hatchery and on to another farm.

Birds can be treated with any of the registered insecticides. All flocks should be treated twice on a 5-

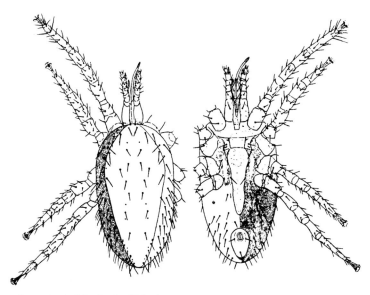

32.17.   *Ornithonyssus bursa,* tropical fowl mite. (Baker)

to 7-day interval for NFM and longer with other parasites. With lice and NFM, the birds should be treated to ensure that the skin is wet, since this is where the pests reside. The most efficient method to use in most poultry facilities is a solid stream spray at 40–125 psi. Care should be taken to ensure that the birds are wet to the skin, or control will be less than desired. Arthur and Axtell (4) found permethrin EC spray to be the most effective chemical registered lasting up to 9 wk after treatment when applied at 0.05%. Red mites can be controlled by treating both the birds and the facility. If the red mites persist in a house, the house should be retreated at cleanout.

Laelaptidae.   Occasionally, mites of the family Laelaptidae will infest chickens, e.g., *Haemolaelaps casalis,* which has also been found on pigeons.

Uropodidae.   Heavy infestations of scavenger mites found in the litter have frequently alarmed broiler producers as they prepare for a new batch of chicks. These mites, which are fungus feeders, often multiply in old litter and then climb through to the surface of new pine shavings used as top dressing. If examined with some magnification (×10) and identified as a member of the Uropodidae family, the producer may rest assured that the mite is harmless and that treatment or a last minute clean-out is unnecessary.

Chigger.   Chigger infestations are sporadic and localized; a heavily infested site may adjoin a habitat that appears similar to it in all respects but is free of these mites. Chiggers affect poultry mainly in the southern states and only birds that are housed outside on the ground. Larval mites of the family Trombiculidae are called chiggers. Nymphs and adults are free-living, usually in or on soil. Although over 700 species are known, only a few attack poultry. The larval chigger is six-legged and possesses a single dorsal plate bearing a pair of sensillae and four to six setae. The legs are seven-segmented and bear two claws and an empodial bristle. Unfed chigger larvae are 0.1–0.45 mm in diameter, hence, hardly visible unless engorged, when they appear as minute red dots. Adults occur on the ground, especially along fence rows or in undisturbed wooded or bushy areas. Larvae attach to the skin, often in groups, and inject a highly irritating substance into the wound, thereafter feeding on liquefied host tissue but not blood. Itching vesicles or even abscesses surrounded by a zone of hyperemia and edema may form at the points of attachments. Apparently, a toxemia may occur, as indicated by the mortality that follows infestation of chicks, especially quail.

The most important poultry chigger in the United States is *Neoschongastia americana* (Fig. 32.18), which is a serious pest of turkeys and wild birds and a minor pest of chickens all across the South (particularly Georgia, the Carolinas, Texas, Alabama, Arkansas, Missouri, and Kentucky) as well as Nebraska. This chigger also occurs in Central America and the West Indies. *N. americana* was not important in past years when turkeys were marketed almost exclusively for the Thanksgiving and Christmas holidays in contrast to current marketing throughout the year, including the summer period of chigger activity.

Feather Mites.   Most mites in the families Analgesidae, Pterolichidae, and Proctorphyllodidae and a few in Cheyletidae live on the feathers of birds or in the quills. These feather mites are rather host specific, and over 25 species are found on poultry throughout the world. Feather mites are rarely found on modern chicken farms because the cycle is broken by separation of the hatchery from producing flocks. Although reports from Germany cite no pathogenicity caused by feather mites on ducks, Indian workers claim pathogenicity with loss of vigor, poor laying performance, and clinical signs similar to those of depluming mite.

Feather mites (except *Syringophilus*) belong to the superfamily Analgesoidae of the suborder Sarcoptiformes.

The quill mite (*Syringophilus hipectinatus*) occurs inside quills of poultry, and wild birds harbor related species: *S. coluumbae* in pigeons and *S. mi-*

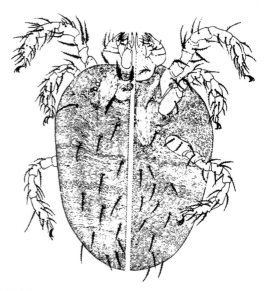

32.18. *Neoschongastia americana* larva, chigger of chickens. (Baker)

nor in house sparrows. These mites are elongate, with long setae on the body. Females measure up to 0.9 mm in length and 0.15 mm in width. The cycle of development from eggs to sexually mature adults takes from 38 to 41 days, and only males develop from eggs deposited by unfertilized females (parthenogenesis).

This species has been found on the chicken, turkey, and golden pheasant in Ohio and on chickens in New Jersey, Maryland, and Pennsylvania. These mites appear to cause partial or complete loss of feathers. The remaining quill stumps contain a powdery material in which mites may be detected under low-power magnification. No specific method for control has yet been described. It would appear advisable to dispose of affected birds, then disinfect and clean their quarters.

Other feather damaging mites (family Pterolichidae) include: *Falculifer rostratus* (Europe, United States) and *F. cornutus,* occurring chiefly between the barbs of the large wing feathers of pigeons; *Freyana chanayi* (United States), in the grooves on the underside of shafts on wing feathers of turkeys; *Dermoglyphus minor* and *D. elongatus* (United States), from inside chicken and turkey quills; and *Pterolichus obtusus* (United States), on flight and tail feathers of chickens. *Megninia cubitalis* (family Analgesidae) occurs on chickens and less so on turkeys in the United States, with *M. gallineulae* (Canada) on the legs and head region of chickens, *M. ginglymura* (depluming mite in India) on chickens and turkeys, and *M. columbae* (United States) on the neck and body areas of pigeons.

Records of economic damage by these mites are rare, although a few reports cite possible reduced egg production in relation to malnutrition, feather loss, and dermatitis in mite-infested body regions where crustlike lesions appear on the lower legs and the skin of combs and wattles. Other skin lesions of poultry can be caused by ectoparasite mites of the families Sarcoptidae and Epidermoptidae, but these parasites are rarely encountered on large poultry production farms.

Scaly-Leg Mites.

Knemidocoptes mutans (Sarcoptidae) (Fig. 32.19) is one of a dozen related species of scaly-leg mites occurring on various birds. They are most commonly found on older birds that should ordinarily be culled from flocks. The mites are almost spherical in shape and short-legged, with strongly striated epidermis, and the dorsal striations are not interrupted. Adult females are about 0.5 mm in diameter. The mites pass through their entire life cycle in the skin, with transmission to noninfested birds by contact with infested birds and their surroundings. Lesions are produced on nonfeathered portions of the host's legs and occasionally on skin of the comb and wattles.

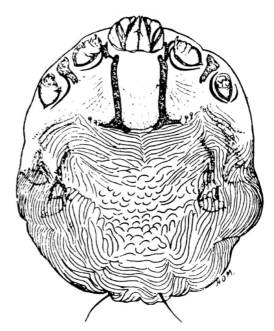

32.19. *Knemidocoptes mutans,* scaly-leg mite. (Soulsby)

Tunnels are bored into the epithelium, causing proliferation and formation of scales and crusts. Affected birds may be crippled if the infestation is severe.

CONTROL. Control of scaly-leg mites should begin by culling or isolating affected birds. Additions to the flock should be covered with an application of warm vegetable oil to loosen scabs, which can then be scraped from the leg, placed in a vial, and sent to a diagnostic laboratory for microscopic examination. If scaly-leg mites are found, it is best to dip the legs in a warm acaricidal solution recommended by a veterinarian. Houses should be cleaned frequently, especially the roosts, which should be sprayed as recommended for the chicken mite.

Depluming Mite. The depluming mite (*Knemidocoptes gallineae*) resembles the scaly-leg mite in general structure although it is smaller, the adult female being about 0.3 mm in diameter. Striations are interrupted on the dorsal surface to form raised sculpturing. The mites are more prevalent in spring and summer, at which time infestation may spread rapidly by contact. Mites burrow into basal shafts of feathers on the epidermis of chickens, pigeons, and pheasant. Intense irritation induces the host to pull out body feathers. These mites injure the bird by interfering with control of body heat. Some affected birds will lose weight and show lowered production.

CONTROL. Control of depluming mites is not easily accomplished. Prompt isolation of affected birds and disinfection of houses as recommended for chicken mites should come first.

Skin Mites. *Epidermoptes bilobatus* (Epidermoptidae) (Fig. 32.20) is a skin mite frequently reported from Europe and more rarely from South and North America. The adult female is about 0.17–0.22 mm in length. It occurs on chickens and apparently may or may not produce lesions but has been described as a cause of pityriasis. When lesions are produced, they consist first of a fine scaly dermatitis, followed by formation of thick, brownish, sharply edged scabs. The more severe lesions may be due partly to a concomitant fungus infection by *Lophophyton gallinae*; also, birds affected with epidermoptid mites often have depluming mites at the same time. Epidermoptic scabies may at times result in emaciation and even death. Pruritis is a common sign.

CONTROL. Treatment of infested birds is recommended as for depluming mites.

Internal Parasitic Mites. Internal passages of the respiratory system, air sacs, and subcutaneous tissue can be infested with sarcoptiform mites of the families Cytoditidae and Laminosioptidae, the mesostigmatid family Rhinonyssidae, and the prostigmatid family Speleogmatidae. These mites are an odd occurrence on modern poultry farms but may be commoner than reports would indicate, since diagnostic procedures seldom include a search for them.

Cyst Mite. The fowl cyst mite (*Laminosioptes cysticola*, family Laminosioptidae) (Fig. 32.21) has been reported mainly from chickens and also from turkeys, pheasant, geese, and pigeons in many parts of the world. The female mite measures about 0.25 × 0.11 mm. The gnathosoma is reduced and not visible from above, and the body bears a few long setae. The life cycle is unknown except that the female lays embryonated eggs and mites pass through all stages of their development under the skin or even in the deeper tissues of the host.

Initial infestation is on the skin, with more frequent findings in the loose subcutaneous connective tissue, occurring in the muscles, abdominal viscera, and lungs (pigeons), and on the peritoneum. These mites do not appear to influence the health of infested birds, although lesions may make carcasses unpalatable as food for humans. If lesions or mites are detected by the inspection service, the carcass is condemned.

Subcutaneous mites occur inside yellowish nodules up to several millimeters in diameter in the subcutis. These areas are often mistaken for tuberculous lesions. The nodules appear to be caseocal-

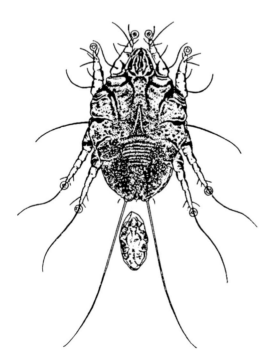

32.20. *Epidermoptes bilobatus*, epidermoptic scabies mite. ×200. (Reis and Nobrega)

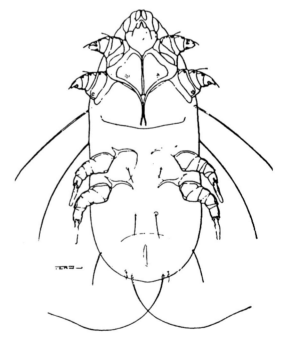

32.21. *Laminosioptes cysticola*, fowl cyst mite. ×376. (Hirst)

careous deposits formed by the bird to enclose mites after they die in the tissues. Large numbers of nodules are most often found in aged emaciated birds. *L. cysticola* has been reported in pigeons in which mites were surrounded by nodules in the lungs, causing death.

Careful examination of skin and subcutis of birds under a dissecting microscope might reveal presence of this parasite more frequently. Otherwise, diagnosis will depend on finding characteristic nodular lesions and by seeing mites or their remains in nodules that have been crushed under a coverglass in a drop of acidulated water.

CONTROL. No attempt has been made to control subcutaneous mites except by destruction of affected birds.

Air Sac Mite. Respiratory system mites of poultry include the air sac mite (*Cytodites nudus,* family Cytoditidae) (Fig. 32.22), which is found in bronchi, lungs, air sacs, and bone cavities. Air sac mites have been found in chickens, turkeys, pheasant, pigeons, canaries, and ruffled grouse from many parts of the world. Although not of common occurrence, these mites are often overlooked because of their small size and peculiar habitat.

The adult female mites are whitish specks, measuring about 0.6×0.4 mm. The mites appear nude because they bear but a few short setae. The gnathosoma is reduced, with minute chelicerae in a tube formed by coalescence of the palpi and gnathosoma. No details are known of the life cycle; speculation is that the mites lay eggs in the lower air passages and these are coughed up and probably swallowed, reaching the ground in droppings. The mode of infection is not known.

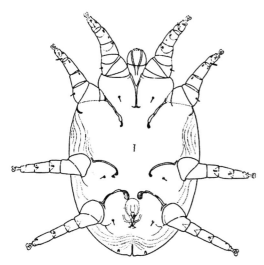

32.22. *Cytodites nudus,* air sac mite. (Baker)

There is considerable conflict as to the damage done by air sac mites. Some observers claim they are practically harmless because their presence has been noted in apparently healthy birds. Others state that the mites are responsible for emaciation, peritonitis, pneumonia, and obstruction of air passages and are predisposing factors for tuberculosis. Dense infestations have definitely been associated with weakness and grave loss in weight so that affected birds resemble clinical cases of tuberculosis. Lindt and Kutzer (36) found *C. nudus* to cause granulomatous pneumonia, which can be fatal.

Close inspection of the opened cadaver of an affected bird soon after death will show whitish dots moving slowly over the transparent air sac surfaces. Identification requires examination under $\times 100$ magnification.

CONTROL. Limited publications on control suggest destruction of the cadavers of affected birds, followed by disinfection and cleaning of the poultry house.

Other Respiratory System Mites. Other respiratory system mites of poultry and pigeons include a few members of the genera *Neonyssus, Rhinonyssus,* and *Sternostoma* of the family Rhinonyssidae and *Speleognathus* of the family Speleognathidae. None is an important pest of commercial poultry. *N. columbae, N. melloi,* and *S. striatus* are nasal mites from pigeons and *R. rhinolethrum* is from ducks and geese. These mites are about 0.5-mm long, oval, bear no setae, possess two dorsal plates, and have stigmata without peritremes.

CONTROL. *S. tracheacolum* has been controlled in Gouldian finches with 0.04 carbaryl on 50 g millet and 1 mL cod liver oil fed three times within 18–24 hr at weekly intervals.

TICKS. Ticks are large mites belonging to the superfamily Ixodoidea of the Acarina, characterized by possession of a pair of oval or kidney-shaped stigmata posterior or lateral to the coxae; the hypostome is modified as a piercing organ provided with recurved teeth, and there is a pitlike sensory organ on the tarsi of the first pair of legs (Haller's organ). Nonengorged adults of most common ticks are 2- to 4-mm long, but fully engorged females may reach more than 10 mm. Nonengorged tick larvae, however, are similar in size to adult mites. Ticks inhabiting poultry houses belong to the family Argasidae. They have no scutum (dorsal shield), and except for larvae, feed intermittently in all stages. The integument is leathery, wrinkled, and granulated in appearance. The capitulum (head) is ventrally placed near the anterior margin of the body (Fig. 32.23). Many hard-bodied ticks in the

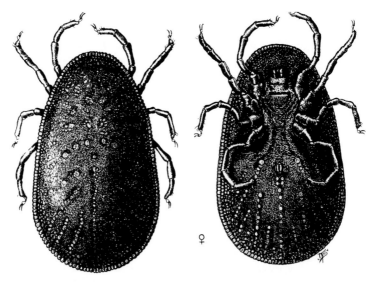

32.23. *Argas persicus* group, fowl tick. Dorsal view on *left*, ventral on *right*. (USDA)

family Ixodoidae will feed on range poultry. These ticks possess a scutum in all stages and feed only once in each stage, remaining on the host for several days. The scutum usually appears shiny, and the capitulum is terminal at the anterior of the tick (Fig. 32.24). Diagnostic keys by Cooley and Kohls (10) and Diamant and Strickland (14) are most useful to determine North American tick species.

Losses caused by ticks are threefold: loss of host blood, which may cause death; reduced production associated with anemia but also possibly due to tick-produced toxic substances; and transmission of disease such as avian spirochetosis, tularemia, piro-

plasmosis, anaplasmosis, dirofilariasis, and certain rickettsial diseases (notably Rocky Mountain spotted fever) and many viruses, including encephalitis.

Fowl Ticks. Soft-bodied ticks (Argasidae) are the most important ticks of poultry. The genus *Argas* (*persicus* group) consists of three species found on poultry, other fowl, and pigeons in the United States: *Argas persicus, A. sanchezi* and *A. radiatus.* Other species include *A. miniatus* in Central and South America, *A. robertsi* along with *A. persicus* in Australia, and *A. aboreus* on wild birds and chickens in South Africa.

Life cycles are about equal in time for *A. radiatus* and *A. sanchezi,* but temperature sensitivity limits *A. sanchezi* to two or three generations per year in southern Texas. These fowl ticks (chicken ticks, blue bugs, tampans, and adobe ticks) are distributed mainly in states along the Gulf of Mexico and the Mexican border. They are also established in many other tropical and temperate areas of the world. Although primarily parasites of birds, they may be found on mammals. In North America, they have been reported from the following hosts: chicken, turkey, duck, goose, guinea fowl, pigeon, canary, dove, hawk, magpie, owl, quail, sparrow, thrush, vulture, ostrich, and wild turkey; also, rarely, from cattle, dogs, and humans.

Mature blood-engorged females measure about 10×6 mm. Unfed ticks are relatively easily recognized by their flattened ovoid shape and tan to reddish brown color. Females may lay a total of 500–875 eggs in four or five separate batches but require a blood meal before laying each batch of eggs. Eggs are laid in sheltered crevices, including

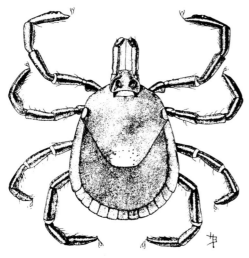

32.24. *Amblyomma americanum,* lone star tick. (USDA)

bark of trees. They hatch in from 6–10 days in warm weather to 3 mo during cool periods. Larvae (seed ticks) become hungry in 4–5 days and seek a host, although they may live for several months without feeding. They blood-feed for 4–5 days and then leave the host for a hiding place nearby and molt (shed skins) in 3–9 days to the first nymphal stage. Nymphs are active and feed only at night, but can do without food for as long as 15 mo. The first-stage nymphs feed in 10–45 min, leave the host and hide for 5–8 days, and molt to a second nymphal stage that is ready to feed in 5–15 days. Similarly, these second-stage nymphs feed and hide; adult ticks emerge from the nymphal skins ready to engorge with blood and mate about 1 wk later. Oviposition commences 3–5 days after mating. This complete life cycle takes about 7–8 wk during warm weather and longer during cold seasons. Fowl ticks remain inactive in cracks and crevices during cold weather, and adults may live without a blood meal for more than 4 yr.

Birds suffer chiefly from attacks of these ticks during the warm dry season. Loss of blood may reach proportions of a fatal anemia; at the least, there may be emaciation, weakness, slow growth, and lowered production. Ruffled feathers, poor appetite, and diarrhea are signs suggesting tick infestation.

The fowl tick is the most important poultry ectoparasite in many tropical countries, being a limiting factor in successful rearing of standard breeds of poultry (42). Turkeys usually suffer even more than chickens; recently hatched poults and chicks show the highest mortality. These ticks cause skin blemishes on turkeys, reducing market price.

The fowl tick is capable of transmitting the highly pathogenic spirochete *Borrelia anserina* in many parts of the world. Tick-borne avian spirochetosis has been reported in chickens and turkeys in the United States, with epizootics of avian spirochetosis in Arizona associated with infestations by the fowl tick. Fowl ticks have been reported to transmit *Aegyptianella pullorum* and fowl cholera (*Pasteurella multocida*) in some regions of the world. All postembryonal stages of the common fowl tick have been found infected with *A. pullorum* in some areas. In other areas, however, transmission of fowl cholera was not shown even though fowl ticks harbored *P. multocida* for 25 days. Aegyptianellosis has not been reported from the Americas.

Tick paralysis in chickens—a flaccid, afebrile motor paralysis—may result from attacks by *A. persicus* as well as by *A. walkerae* in Africa (26). Etiology of this sporadic disease is not understood, but most probably a specific paralytic toxin is contained and transmitted in the tick salivary secretions. Clinical signs may be confused with botulism or neural

signs of Marek's disease and also with transient paralysis, Newcastle disease, and possibly conditions caused by other bacterial or chemical toxins.

The pigeon tick (*A. reflexus*) is not in the persicus group. The subspecies *A. reflexus* attacks pigeons in Europe and Asia; *A. reflexus hermanni* is the pigeon tick of Africa (29, 30). In most areas, these ticks are not pests of chickens, but *A. reflexus hermanni* and *A. persicus* are found together on chickens in West Africa. *A. neghmei* is a pest of both chickens and pigeons in Chile. These argasid ticks (except *A. refexus hermanni*) have been reported as pests of humans, and *A. neghmei* is known to bite children in homes adjacent to adobe wall poultry houses in Chile. Probably both subspecies of *A. reflexus* are important vectors of fowl spirochetosis. *A. reflexus hermanni* in Egypt is suspected of transmitting West Nile and Chenuda virus and the Quaranfil virus group among pigeons and is implicated in transmission of Q fever rickettsia.

CONTROL. Control requires treatment of premises, because adult and nymphal ticks are on their hosts only a short time and then hide in the surroundings. The litter, walls, floors, and ceilings must be sprayed thoroughly, forcing spray into cracks and behind nest boxes. Outdoor runs and feed troughs, woodpiles, and tree trunks may be treated using approved insecticides. Other methods for fowl tick control include use of metal construction, elimination of tree roosting, using roosts suspended from ceilings, and converting to cage operation. Frequent inspection is necessary to combat ticks before their number has increased to a harmful extent. Fowl ticks are rarely found in modern, large commercial cage-layer operations.

Hard Ticks. Hard ticks (Ixodidae) of many species will feed on poultry as well as wild ground birds. Birds are preferred hosts of larvae and nymphs of some species of Hyalomma (Old World only) and Amblyomma ticks that are common in the adult stage on mammals. Ixodid ticks attach to hosts, mate, feed to repletion, and then drop off. Females oviposit several thousand eggs in a single batch on the ground and then die. The eggs hatch in 1–2 mo, and the six-legged larvae climb up on the vegetation to await a new vertebrate host. There is only one larval and one nymphal stage, and each feeds from 5 to 7 days on the host. Hard ticks are likely to be found only on birds that are on range or have access to range.

In the temperate zone, many ixodid ticks have but one generation a year, spending the winter in diapause as eggs or immature or mature ticks. Even in the tropics, some ticks require a year to complete their life cycle; others may complete the cycle in 2–4 mo. Ticks that do not find a host will live for a long period (over 2 yr has been recorded), so the cycle may be very prolonged. Premises and ranges will remain infested for long periods even when unoccupied.

RODENTS

Rodents are very common pests in and around poultry facilities, and a facility that does not have at least a few rodents is unusual. Rodents do a tremendous amount of damage if an effective control program is not implemented and maintained. Rodents' burrowing and gnawing activity can undermine foundations and destroy curtains and insulation. Rodents can eat or contaminate feed, which increases feed costs and affects feed conversions. Additional problems can be produced by the presence of these pests, since they are capable of carrying a variety of diseases and ectoparasites. Rats are commonly seen in layer and breeder facilities, while mice are problems in all types of production facilities. Rodents will increase the chance that disease agents will spread due to their feeding and defecation where birds feed. If present in large numbers, they may attack birds.

RATS.   The Norway Rat (*Rattus norvegicus*) is the most common rat found around poultry houses. Rats have three basic requirements: food, water, and harborage. If one of these items is missing from an area, there will not be a rat problem. Unfortunately, all of these items are usually present in and around poultry production facilities. Rats eat almost any type of food, including eggs and poultry feed; however, rats prefer fresh food. When fresh food is available, rodents will totally ignore spoiled food. An adult rat will eat and drink approximately 0.5–2 oz of food and water each day with 200 adult rats consuming 25 lb of feed daily.

Rat harborage around a poultry house is seen in the form of burrows in the ground and under the foundation, litter under the slats, and in wood piles, old nests, and other debris near the poultry houses. This type of harborage must be removed from the poultry house for any control program to be successful. Most rat activity, including feeding, occurs at night. Rats observed outside their harborage during the day indicate a large population. Rats are very territorial and when crowded, they become increasingly aggressive. The stronger and more aggressive rats drive the weaker rats away from the food, forcing them to feed during the day.

Rats have high reproductive rates, which can lead to large numbers of rodents in a fairly short period of time. A single pair of rats and their offspring could produce as many as 1500 rats in 1 yr if all the offspring survived. Rats will breed at an age of 3–5 mo and give birth approximately 3 wk after mating. Four to seven litters are produced in 1 yr with each litter having 6–12 young, and the female rat will breed again 1–2 days after giving birth. Although breeding will occur all year, increased breeding frequently occurs during the spring and fall. Generally speaking, rodent populations decrease during the winter; however, in a poultry house, the opposite is frequently true. This occurs because of immigration of rats into the building when the weather cools, not because of increased reproduction.

MICE.   The house mouse (*Mus musculus*) is the most common mouse found in and around poultry facilities. Mice require food, water, and harborage, and will eat almost any kind of food with about 1% of 1 oz of food consumed by an adult mouse each day. Mice are frequently active throughout the day, often feeding every hour. Peak activity, however, usually occurs at dusk and dawn. Mice require much less water than rats and are capable of utilizing water from the food they eat. Mice will burrow in the ground, burrow in insulation, or live in rolled-up curtains. Mice are able to reproduce at an age of 6–8 wk. They will give birth to five or six young approximately 3 wk after mating. Two to 4 days after giving birth, the female mouse can breed again. Generally, five to eight litters are produced in a year. Mice breed regularly throughout the year with no seasonal peak.

CONTROL.   There are three general aspects to rodent control. They are rodentproofing, sanitation, and rodent killing. Rodentproofing can be an effective long-term control measure. It is, however, impractical, if not impossible, to rodentproof a poultry facility. Access to the poultry building can be restricted by patching holes in the foundation or screening. Rodents will be forced to burrow into the house, which makes them easier to detect.

Sanitation is a form of cultural control and simply involves cleaning up around the poultry facility. Rodents are secretive creatures; they do not like to move about in open areas; therefore, mowing the grass and weeds on a regular basis creates a less favorable habitat. Removing piles of old wood, nests, or any other debris helps to make the area less attractive to rodents, and aids in making early detection possible. When debris or tall grass is present, rodents can burrow into a facility and go unnoticed. Rolling the house curtains up and down a couple of times a week during summer months will disturb any rodents that are in the curtains and discourage them from living and/or nesting in them.

After the cultural control measures have been completed, a rodent-killing program should be implemented. Rodent killing can take the form of baiting, fumigating, trapping, or even shooting. Under most circumstances, a properly conducted baiting program is the easiest and most effective means for killing rodents.

There are many products on the market that will kill rodents. The first group of safe and commonly used baits are the multiple dose anticoagulants (Table 32.2). Products that contain warfarin, fumarin, chlorophacinone, or diphacinone as an active ingredient are examples of this type of bait. Multiple-dose anticoagulants must be consumed for several consecutive days to be lethal. The effects are cumulative: if a rodent feeds on this type of bait for a day or so, then feeds on something else before returning to the bait for another few feedings, the rodent will not be controlled. It is, therefore, imperative that enough bait be available for the rodents to eat for several days. The specific number of days that a rat or mouse must feed on a multiple-dose anticoagulant poison depends on the bait being used and the amount consumed. These chemicals are relatively safe for humans and nontarget animals, because a single dose will not cause death.

The second type of rodenticide includes the single-dose anticoagulants. Products that contain bromadialone or brodifacoum are examples of this category of baits. A single feeding is sufficient to kill a rodent. They are safe; however, care should be taken to keep them out of reach of pets, livestock, and children, as they are potentially lethal if a large dose is consumed.

Currently, there are two other types of single-dose baits that are not anticoagulants. The first contains the active ingredient bromethalin, which affects the central nervous system, and cholecalciferol, which causes a calcium imbalance in the blood.

The last category of baits includes acute single-dose rodenticides such as zinc phosphide. These chemicals are very effective and useful for a quick knockdown of a large rodent population. These chemicals are highly toxic, however, and most of them are restricted to use by licensed pest control operators. Except under extreme circumstances, the other types of bait are equally effective and they are much safer.

For any baiting program to be effective, rodents must consume the bait and they need to consume a lethal amount. In order to accomplish this, care must be taken in the placement of bait. Random placement of bait around a poultry facility is rarely effective. Always remember that rodents will not go out of their way to eat poison bait if they have food readily available. Therefore, placing the bait in or closer to their harborage than their regular food source is important. One of the best and safest places to put the bait is down in the active rodent burrow. A great deal of bait, time, and money can be saved by determining which burrows are active before the baiting begins. This can be done by filling in all the burrows around the facility with soil or newspaper. These burrows should be rechecked the next day and all burrows that have been reopened should be baited. Bait stations are effective and a complete discussion of the use of stations can be found in Arends (2).

When using a multiple-dose rodenticide, be sure to put bait in all active burrows daily until the bait is no longer consumed. When bait is no longer taken, remove the uneaten bait and fill in the burrow. If a single-dose anticoagulant is used, the active burrows should be baited for 2 consecutive days, and 4 or 5 days later, all of the burrows should be filled and any that are active baited for 2 more days. When baiting for mice at ground level, this procedure should be used; however, mice frequently inhabit the upper areas of a poultry house. When this occurs, baiting at ground level will be ineffective. The bait must be placed within the mouse's territory. To accomplish this, put out a small amount of bait in many places rather than putting out a large quantity of bait in a few places. The bait can be placed on the sill, in the feed rooms, or scattered in the attic area if the facility has a drop ceiling. There are also baits that are sold in a block form that can be nailed or wired to the rafters, or a bait station can be used.

Acute rodenticides should only be used in extreme cases. The best time to use these compounds is when a very high rodent population is present and after the birds have been removed. The bait can then be placed in the poultry houses so that no animals other than rodents could be accidentally poisoned. Since the rodents' normal food source is absent during this period, the bait placement is not that crucial. The location of all bait placements should be recorded on paper and checked off when they are removed to make sure that no bait station is missed. Always remove and carefully dispose of any uneaten bait before the building is cleaned out.

Table 32.2. Rodenticides for use in poultry facilities

Active Ingredient	Type of Bait
Warfarin	Multiple-dose anticoagulant
Pival	Multiple-dose anticoagulant
Diphacinone	Multiple-dose anticoagulant
Chlorophacinone	Multiple-dose anticoagulant
Zinc phosphide[a]	Acute single dose
Bromethalin	Affects central nervous system
Brodifacoum	Single-dose anticoagulant
Bromadiolon	Single-dose anticoagulant
Cholecalciferol	Single feeding/multiple feeding

[a]Restricted to use by licensed pest-control operators.

Tracking powders and fumigants can also be used to kill rodents. Tracking powders are mixtures of rodent poisons and nontoxic powders, which are spread on the floor in active rodent runways. Rats and mice pick up the poisoned powder on their fur, tail, and feet as they run across it, and then ingest the poison when grooming.

Until recently, fumigants were frequently used to gas rodents trapped in their burrows or enclosed areas. Methyl bromide gas, chloropicrin fumigant, and other control measures are now being used as fumigants. Fumigants are extremely hazardous to humans and nontarget animals. All people, pests, and livestock must be removed from the area until the gas is totally dissipated. When using any pesticide, always read and follow label instructions carefully.

Claims that rodents can be driven away or negatively affected by ultrasonic sound or electromagnetic radiation remain unproven. In fact, several studies have indicated that ultrasonic sound and electromagnetic radiation do not drive rodents away or affect them adversely. The devices involved are very expensive and should be viewed skeptically until further research proves them worthwhile.

A rodent control program must be a continual effort if it is to be effective and efficient. Too often, control programs are implemented only after a severe problem exists. At that point, control requires a great deal of effort and expense and, when most of the rodents are killed, the control effort stops until the rodents become a serious problem again. This type of control program is a waste of time and money. It is much easier and less expensive to control and/or totally eliminate a small rodent population. This can be accomplished by checking the facility for rodent activity on a regular basis even after the control program has killed most of the rodents. Look for rodent signs both inside and outside at least every 2 wk, and start baiting as soon as any activity is observed. It is especially important to check inside partially slatted broiler breeder facilities. Frequently, in a facility of this type, the rodents will enter through a small number of burrows from outside and then live and reproduce in the litter under the slats. If rodents are under slats, the severity of the infestation can be underestimated if only the outside of the building is checked and the area under the slats are left uninspected.

REFERENCES

1. Anderson, R.C. 1956. The life cycle and seasonal transmission of Ornithofilaria fallisensis Anderson, a parasite of domestic and wild ducks. Can J Zool 34:485.

2. Arends, J.J. 1982. Integrated Pest Management Manual. North Carolina State University Extension Publishing, Raleigh, NC.

3. Arends, J.J., S.H. Robertson, and C.S. Payne. 1984. Impact of northern fowl mite on broiler breeder flocks in North Carolina. Poult Sci 63:1457–1461.

4. Arthur, F.H., and R.C. Axtell. 1982. Comparisons of permethrin formulations and application methods for northern fowl mite control on caged laying hens. Poult Sci 61:879–884.

5. Axtell, R.C. 1986. Fly management in poultry production cultural, biological, and chemical. Poult Sci 65:657–667.

6. Axtell, R.C. 1987. Fly control in confined livestock and poultry production. Ciba-Geigy Corporation, Greensboro, NC.

7. Axtell, R.C., and J.J. Arends. 1990. Ecology and management of arthropod pests of poultry. Ann Rev Entomol 35:101–126.

8. Borror, D.J., and D.M. DeLong. 1976. An Introduction to the Study of Insects. Holt/Rinehart/Winston, New York.

9. Chamberlain, R.W. 1968. In K. Maramorosch (ed.), Springer-Verlag, Berlin. Curr Top Microbiol Immunol 42:38–58

10. Cooley, R.A., and G.M. Kohls. 1944. The Argasidae of North America, Central America, and Cuba. Notre Dame University Press, South Bend, IN.

11. DeVaney, J.A. 1976. Effects of the chicken body louse, Menacanthus stramineus, on caged layers. Poult Sci 55:430–435.

12. DeVaney, J.A. 1979. The effects of the northern fowl mite, Ornithonyssus sylviarum, on egg production and body weight of caged white leghorn hens. Poult Sci 191–194.

13. DeVaney, J.A., and R.L. Ziprin. 1980. Acquired immune response of white leghorn hens to populations of northern fowl mite, Ornithonyssus sylviarum. Poult Sci 59:1742–1744.

14. Diamant, G., and R.K. Strickland. 1965. Manual on Livestock Ticks. United States Department of Agriculture, ARS, Washington, DC, pp. 91–94.

15. Dunning, L.L., E.C. Loomis, and V.E. Burton. 1971. Portable spray unit serves many farm and ranch purposes. Calif Agric 25:8–10.

16. Edgar, S.A., and D.F. King. 1950. Effect of the body louse, Eomenacanthus stramineus, on mature chickens. Poult Sci 29:214–219.

17. Eklund, J., E. Loomis, and H. Abplanalp. 1980. Genetic resistance of white leghorn chickens to infestation by the northern fowl mite, Ornithonyssus sylviarum. Arch Gefluegelkd 44:195–199.

18. Emerson, K.C. 1956. Mallophaga (chewing lice) occurring on the domestic chicken. J Kans Entomol Soc 29:63–79.

19. Emerson, K.C. 1962. Mallophaga (chewing lice) occurring on the turkey. J Kans Entomol Soc 35:196–201.

20. Fox, I. 1940. Fleas of Eastern United States. Iowa State College Press, Ames, IA.

21. Geden, C.J., and R.C. Axtell. 1987. Factors affecting climbing and tunneling behavior of the lesser mealworm (Coleoptoia: Tenebrionidae). J Econ Entomol 80:1197–1204.

22. Geden, C.J., T.D. Edwards, J.J. Arends, and R.C. Axtell. 1987. Efficacies of mixtures of disinfectants and insecticides. Poult Sci 66:659–665.

23. Geden, C.J., R.E. Stinner, and R.C. Axtell. 1988. Predation by predators of the house fly in poultry manure: Effects of predator density, feeding history, interspecific interference, and field conditions. Environ Entomol 17:320–329.

24. Georgi, J.R. 1980. Parasitology for Veterinarians, 3rd ed. Saunders, Philadelphia.

25. Gless, E.E., and E.S. Raun. 1959. Effects of chicken body louse infestation on egg production. J Econ Entomol 52:358–359.

26. Goethe, R., and K. Kunze. 1973. Parasitic Zoonosis Clinical and Experimental Studies. Academic Press, New York, pp. 369–382.

27. Hall, R.D., and W.B. Gross. 1975. Effect of social stress and inherited plasma corticosterone levels in chickens on populations of the northern fowl mite, Ornithonyssus sylviarum. J Parasitol 61:1096–1100.

28. Hall, R.D., W.B. Gross, and E.C. Turner, Jr. 1978. Preliminary observations on northern fowl mite infestations on estrogenized roosters and in relation to initial egg production in hens. Poult Sci 57:1088–1090.

29. Hoogstraal, H., and G.M. Kohls. 1960. Observations on the subgenus Argas (Ixodoidea, Argasidae, Argas). 1. Study of A. reflexus reflexus (Fabricius, 1794), the European bird argasid. Ann Entomol Soc Am 53:611–618.

30. Hoogstraal, H., and G.M. Khols. 1960. Observations on the subgenus Argas (Ixodoidea, Argasidae, Argas). 3. A biological and systematic study of A. reflexus hermanni Audouin, 1827 (revalidated), the African bird argasid. Ann Entomol Soc Am 53:743–755.

31. Hubbard, C.A. 1947. Fleas of Western North America. Iowa State College Press, Ames.

32. Kettle, D.S. 1985. Medical and Veterinary Entomology. John Wiley & Sons, New York.

33. Kiernans, J.E. 1975. A review of the phoretic relationship between Mallophaga (Phthiraptera: Insecta) and Hippoboscidae (Diptera: Insecta). J Med Entomol 12:71–76.

34. Krantz, G.W. 1970. A Manual of Acarology. Oregon State University Press, Corvallis, OR.

35. Lancaster, J.L., Jr., and M.V. Meisch. 1986. Arthropods in Livestock and Poultry Production. Halsted Press, New York.

36. Lindt, S., and E. Kutzer. 1965. Luftsackmilben (Cytodites nudus) als Ursache einer granulomatosen Pneumonie beim Huhn. Pathol Vet 2:264–276.

37. Loomis, E.C., E.L. Bramhall, J.A. Allen, R.A. Ernst, and L.L. Dunning. 1970. Effects of the northern fowl mite on white leghorn chickens. J Econ Entomol 63:1885–1889.

38. Loomis, E.C., J.P. Anderson, and A.S. Peal. 1980. Coop Ext Univ Calif Leafl 2506.

39. Lysyk, T.J., and R.C. Axtell. 1986. Field evaluation of three methods for monitoring populations of house flies (Musca domestica) (Diptera:Muscidae) and other filth flies in three types of poultry housing systems. J Econ Entomol 79:144–151.

40. Noblet, R., J.B. Kissam, and T.R. Atkins, Jr. 1975. Leucocytozoon smithi: Incidence of transmission by black flies in South Carolina (Diptera: Simuliidae). J Med Entomol 12:111–114.

41. Reeves, W.C. 1965. Ecology of mosquitoes in relation to arboviruses. Annu Rev Entomol 10:25–46.

42. Reid, W.M. 1956. Incidence and economic importance of poultry parasites under different ecological and geographical situations in Egypt. Poult Sci 35:926–933.

43. Soulsby, E.J.L. 1982. Helminths, Arthropods, and Protozoa of Domesticated Animals, 7th ed. Williams & Wilkins, Baltimore, MD.

44. Stockdale, H.J., and E.S. Raun. 1960. Economic importance of the chicken louse. J Econ Entomol 53:421–422.

45. Titchener, R.N. 1983. The use of permethrin to control an outbreak of hen fleas (Ceratophyllus gallinae). Poult Sci 62:608–611.

46. Warren, D.C., R. Eaton, and H. Smith. 1948. Influence of infestations of body lice on egg production in the hen. Poult Sci 27:641–642.

47. Werner, F.G. 1982. Common names of insects and related organisms. Entomology Society of American College Park, MD.

48. West, L.S. 1951. The Housefly: Its Natural History, Medical Importance and Control. Comstock, Ithaca, NY.

49. Williams, R.E., R.D. Hall, A.B. Broce, and P.J. Scholl. 1985. Livestock Entomology. John Wiley & Sons, New York.

33 Internal Parasites

NEMATODES AND ACANTHOCEPHALANS

M. D. Ruff and R. A. Norton

INTRODUCTION. Nematodes constitute the most important group of helminth parasites of poultry. In both the number of species and the amount of damage done, they far exceed the trematodes and cestodes.

This chapter is designed to aid the diagnostician in identifying predominant nematodes of poultry throughout the world. Those reported in chickens are listed in Table 33.1; those from other domestic poultry and/or commercially raised game birds are listed in Table 33.2. Nematodes from areas other than North America are mentioned in the text, but are not listed in the tables. Avian nematodes often have a broad host range. Accordingly, nematodes found in wild birds (see Table 33.3) may constitute a hazard for commercially raised birds. Only species commonly found are described in any detail in this chapter. For a more detailed description of individual species, early works, and additional information, the reader should refer to the original references listed in the previous editions of this book (80, 101) or to other reviews (1, 16, 18, 20, 60). A checklist and descriptions are available for parasites reported from the bobwhite quail and waterfowl (55, 66).

The genus and species names used in this chapter are those of Yamaguti (104), except where usage by recognized authorities supersedes his classification. Yamaguti described 25 families of nematodes from nine orders in avian species; 13 of these families (Strongyloididae, Trichuridae, Syngamidae, Trichostrongylidae, Subuluridae, Heterakidae, Ascarididae, Spiruridae, Thelaziidae, Gnathostomatidae, Physalopteridea, Acuariidae, Dipetalonematidae) contain species that infect poultry. Levine (60) used a similar classification but substituted Onchocercidae for Dipetalonematidae. The classification used for families in this chapter is that given in the CIH keys in a series on the nematode parasite of vertebrates edited by Anderson, Chabaud, and Willmott (3), which elevates many of the families (60, 104) to superfamily rank; thus, the number of families

containing parasites of poultry is increased to 21. Yorke and Maplestone (107) provided yet another key to orders and families.

GENERAL MORPHOLOGY. Nematodes, or roundworms, are usually spindle shaped with the anterior and posterior ends attenuated. The body covering, or cuticle, is often marked by transverse grooves. Longitudinal folds, or alae, may be present at the anterior (cervical alae) or posterior (caudal alae, Fig. 33.14) part of the body. The latter are found on the tail of the male worm, and in the case of certain groups, are modified to form a bursa (see Fig. 33.18B). Cuticular ornamentations are occasionally found on the anterior extremities and may take the form of spines, cordons, or shields (see Fig. 33.6A).

The mouth opening, located at the anterior end of the body, is usually surrounded by lips bearing sensory organs (Fig. 33.5A). In more generalized types of nematodes, the mouth leads directly into a cavity immediately anterior to the esophagus (Fig. 33.24A). The mouth cavity may be considerably reduced or absent in more specialized groups of nematodes. The esophagus may be simple (consisting of one undivided part) or more complex (consisting of a short anterior muscular part and a long posterior glandular part). A bulb may or may not be present at the posterior end (Fig. 33.20). The intestine follows the esophagus and is connected with the anal or cloacal opening in the posterior end of the body by a short rectum.

The nematodes are, with very few exceptions, sexually distinct. Sexual dimorphism is remarkably demonstrated by some species of nematodes such as *Tetrameres americana* (Fig. 33.7), in which the elongate male worm is much smaller than the globule-shaped female. The male can usually be distinguished from the female by the presence of two (rarely one) chitinous structures known as spicules, located in the posterior end of the body. The spicules (Fig. 33.20) have been considered as intro-

815

Table 33.1. Nematodes reported from chickens in the United States

Nematode	Location	Intermediate Host	Other Definitive Host
Baylisascaris procyonis	Brain		Raccoons (accidental parasite in chicken, turkey, partridge, quail)
Oxyspirura mansoni	Eye	Cockroach	Turkey, duck, grouse, guinea fowl, peafowl, pigeon, quail
Syngamus trachea	Trachea	None	Turkey, goose, guinea fowl, pheasant, peafowl, quail
Capillaria contorta	Mouth, esophagus, crop	None or earthworm	Turkey, duck, guinea fowl, partridge, pheasant, quail
C. annulata	Esophagus, crop	Earthworm	Turkey, goose, grouse, guinea fowl, partridge, pheasant, quail
Gongylonema ingluvicola	Crop, esophagus proventriculus	Beetle, cockroach	Turkey, partridge, pheasant, quail
Dispharynx nasuta	Proventriculus	Sowbug	Turkey, grouse, guinea fowl, partridge, pheasant, pigeon, quail
Tetrameres americana	Proventriculus	Grasshopper, cockroach	Turkey, duck, grouse, pigeon, quail
T. fissispina	Proventriculus	Amphipod, grasshopper, cockroach, earthworm	Turkey, duck, goose, guinea fowl, pigeon, quail
Cheilospirua hamulosa	Gizzard	Grasshopper, beetle	Turkey, grouse, guinea fowl, pheasant, quail
Ascaridia galli	Small intestine	None	Turkey, duck, goose, quail
Capillaria anatis	Small intestine, cecum, cloaca	None	Turkey, duck, goose, partridge, pheasant
C. bursata	Small intestine	Earthworm	Turkey, goose, pheasant
C. caudinflata	Small intestine	Earthworm	Turkey, duck, goose, grouse, guinea fowl, partridge, pheasant, pigeon, quail
Capillaria obsignata	Small intestine, cecum	None	Turkey, goose, guinea fowl, pigeon, quail
Heterakis gallinarum	Cecum	None	Turkey, duck, goose, grouse, guinea fowl, partridge, pheasant, quail
Subulura brumpti	Cecum	Earwig, grasshopper, beetle, cockroach	Turkey, dove, duck, grouse, guinea fowl, partridge, pheasant, quail
S. strongylina	Cecum	Beetle, cockroach, grasshopper	Guinea fowl, quail
Strongyloides avium	Cecum	None	Turkey, goose, grouse, quail
Trichostrongylus tenuis	Cecum	None	Turkey, duck, goose, guinea fowl, pigeon, quail

Table 33.2. Nematodes reported from poultry or commercially raised game birds other than chickens

Nematode	Location	Intermediate Host	Other Definitive Host
Cyathostoma bronchialis	Trachea	None or earthworm	Turkey, duck, goose, (chicken)
Cyrnea colini	Proventriculus	Cockroach	Turkey, grouse, prairie chicken, quail, (chicken)[a]
Tetrameres crami	Proventriculus	Amphipod	Duck
Microtetrameres helix	Proventriculus	Grasshopper	Pigeon
Amidostomum anseris	Gizzard	None	Duck, goose, pigeon
A. skrjabini	Gizzard	None	Duck, pigeon, (chicken)[a]
Ascaridia columbae	Small intestine	None	Pigeon, dove
A. dissimilis	Small intestine	None	Turkey
A. numidae	Small intestine	None	Guinea fowl
Ornithostrongylus quadriradiatus	Small intestine	None	Pigeon, dove
Heterakis dispar	Cecum	None	Duck, goose
H. isolonche	Cecum	None	Duck, grouse, pheasant, prairie chicken, quail
Capillaria columbae	Large intestine	None	Pigeon, dove

[a]Experimental

Table 33.3. Nematodes reported from wild birds in the United States that pose a potential problem for poultry or commercially raised game birds

Nematode	Location	Intermediate Host	Definitive Host
Oxyspirura petrowi	Eye	Unknown	Grouse, quail, pheasant, prairie chicken
Splendidofilaria californiensis	Heart	Unknown	Quail
Singhfilaria hayesi	Subcutaneous	Unknown	Turkey, quail
Splendidofilaria pectoralis	Subcutaneous	Unknown	Grouse
Chandlerella chitwoodae	Connective tissues	Unknown	Grouse
Aproctella stoddardi	Body cavity	Unknown	Turkey, dove, quail
Cardiofilaria nilesi	Body cavity	Mosquito	Chicken
Echinura uncinata	Esophagus, gizzard, proventriculus, small intestine	Water flea	Duck, goose
E. parva	Proventriculus, gizzard	Unknown	Duck, goose
Tetrameres pattersoni	Proventriculus	Grasshopper, cockroach	Quail
T. ryjikovi	Proventriculus	Unknown	Duck
Cyrnea neeli	Proventriculus, gizzard	Unknown	Turkey
C. pileata	Proventriculus	Unknown	Quail
Physaloptera acuticauda	Proventriculus	Unknown	Chicken, pheasant
Amidostomum acutum	Gizzard	None	Duck
A. raillieti	Gizzard	None	Duck, dove
Cheilospirura spinosa	Gizzard	Grasshopper	Grouse, partridge, pheasant, quail, turkey
Cyrnea eurycerea	Gizzard	Unknown	Pheasant, quail, turkey
Epomidiostomum uncinatum	Gizzard	None	Chicken, duck, goose, pigeon
Streptocara crassicauda	Gizzard	Amphipod	Chicken, duck
Ascaridia bonasae	Small intestine	None	Grouse
A. compar	Small intestine	None	Grouse, partridge, pheasant, quail
Porrocaecum ensicaudatum	Small intestine	Earthworm	Chicken, duck
Capillaria phasianina	Small intestine, cecum	Unknown	Partridge, pheasant, guinea fowl
C. tridens	Small intestine	Unknown	Turkey
Aulonocephalus lindquisti	Cecum, large intestine	Unknown	Quail
A. pennula	cecum	Unknown	Turkey
A. quaricensis	Cecum	Unknown	Quail

Note: Some of these have been reported from domestic poultry outside of the United States.

mittent organs for use during copulation, keeping the vulva and vagina open and, to some extent, guiding the sperm into the female. Eggs or larvae are discharged through the vulva, the position of which varies considerably in different groups of nematodes.

DEVELOPMENT. Nematodes of poultry have either a direct or an indirect type of development; about one-half require no invertebrate intermediate hosts, whereas the others depend on such intermediate hosts as insects, snails, and slugs for the early stage of development.

Nematodes normally pass through four developmental stages before reaching the fifth or final stage. Successive stages are preceded by shedding of the skin (molting). In some nematodes, the loosened skin or cuticle is retained for a short time as a protective covering; in others, it is shed at once.

Eggs deposited ultimately reach the outside in the droppings. Excorporeal existence is necessary for eggs to become infective for avian or arthropod hosts. The conditions existing within the definitive host are usually inimical to the development of the eggs. Outside the host in the required optimum moisture and temperature, these undergo development. Eggs of some nematodes require only a few days to complete embryonation; others require several weeks. For nematodes with direct life cycles, the final host becomes infected by eating embryonated eggs containing the second-stage larvae or free larvae. For those with indirect life cycles, the intermediate host ingests the embryonated eggs or free larvae and retains the larvae within the body tissues. The final host becomes infected either by eating the infected intermediate host or by injection of the larvae by a blood-feeding arthropod.

NEMATODES

NEMATODES OF THE DIGESTIVE TRACT

CAPILLARIA ANNULATA MOLIN 1858, CAPILLARI-IDAE

Synonyms. *C. oblata* Graham, Thorpe and Hectorne 1929; *Trichosoma delicatissum* Godoelst 1903; (64, 65).

Hosts. *C. annulata* has been reported in chicken, turkey, goose, grouse, guinea fowl, partridge, pheasant, and quail.

Location. *C. annulata* may be found in the mucosa of the esophagus and the crop.

Morphology. *C. annulata* are long, slender worms, similar in appearance to *C. contorta* but easily differentiated by a cuticular swelling just back of the head (Fig. 33.1A). The male is usually 1–26 mm in length and 52–74 µm in width; the tail ends in two inconspicuous round lateral flaps, united dorsally by a cuticular flap; the spicule sheath is beset with fine spines (Fig. 33.1B); and the spicule is 1.12–11.63 mm in length. The female is usually 25–60 mm in length and 77–120 µm in width; the posterior portion of the body (posterior to vulva) is about seven times as long as anterior portion; the vulva circular is located about opposite the termination of the esophagus; and the eggs are operculated (Fig. 33.1C), and are 55–66 × 26–28 µm.

Life Cycle. Eggs pass out in the droppings of infected birds. They develop to active embryos very slowly (from 24 days to over 1 mo). Wehr (99) demonstrated that two species of earthworms, *Eisenia foetidus* and *Allolobophora caliginosus,* served as intermediate hosts of this crop worm.

Pathogenicity. This worm has been associated with deaths of turkeys in Maryland. Burrowing into the crop mucosa causes a thickening of the crop wall and enlargement of the glands. Usually, there is inflammation of the crop and esophageal walls. In heavy infections, the inner surface of the crop becomes thickened, roughened, and badly macerated, with masses of worms concentrated primarily in the sloughing tissue.

In pheasants, quail, and other gallinaceous game birds, infections often prove fatal. Signs are principally malnutrition and emaciation, associated with severe anemia.

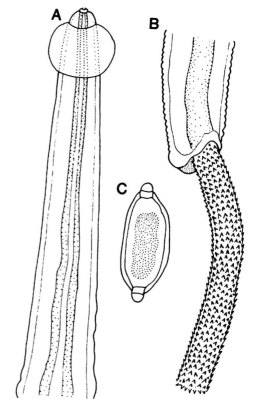

33.1.   *Capillaria annulata. A.* Head end. *B.* Male tail. (After Ciurea) *C.* Egg.

CAPILLARIA CONTORTA CREPLIN 1839, CAPILLARIIDAE

Synonyms.   *C. vanelli* Yamaguti 1935.

Hosts.   *C. contorta* has been reported in chicken, turkey, duck, guinea fowl, partridge, pheasant, and quail.

Location.   *C. contorta* may be found in mucosa of the esophagus, the crop, and sometimes the mouth.

Morphology.   *C. contorta* had a threadlike body, attenuated anteriorly and posteriorly; its head is without a cuticular swelling. The male is 8–17 mm in length and 60–70 µm in width; there are two terminal laterodorsal prominences on the tail end; the spicule very slender and transparent, about 800-µm long; and the spicule sheath is covered with fine hairlike processes (Fig. 33.2B). The female is 15–60 mm in length and 120–150 µm in width; and the vulva is prominent and circular, 140–180 µm posterior to beginning of intestine (Fig. 33.2A).

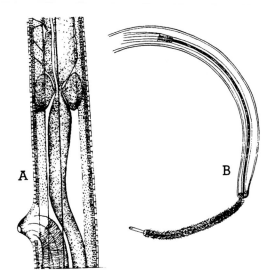

33.2. *Capillaria contorta. A.* Region of vulva. (After Eberth) *B.* Male tail. (After Travassos)

Life Cycle. Eggs are apparently deposited in tunnels in the crop mucosa and escape into the lumen of crop and esophagus with the sloughed mucosa. They are abundant in droppings from infected birds. Approximately 1 mo or slightly longer is required for embryos to develop. Worms mature in susceptible avian hosts 1–2 mo after embryonated eggs are ingested.

Pathogenicity. When present in large numbers, these worms are extremely pathogenic. In light infections, the wall of the crop and esophagus becomes slightly thickened and inflamed. In heavy infections, there is a marked thickening and inflammation with a flocculent exudate covering the mucosa, with more or less sloughing of the mucosa. The crop may become nonfunctional. In extremely heavy infections, the worms may invade the mouth and upper esophagus.

Infected birds become droopy, weak, and emaciated. Deaths have been observed among infected wild turkeys, Hungarian partridges, and quail in the United States. The birds are not inclined to move unless forced to; occasionally, they assume a penguinlike posture, with the head drawn close to the body.

ECHINURA UNCINATA (RUDOLPHI 1819) SOLOVIEV 1912, ACUARIIDAE

Hosts. *E. uncinata* has been reported in wild and domestic duck and goose, and in wild and domestic birds in Canada.

Location. *E. uncinata* may be found in the mucosa of the esophagus, proventriculus, gizzard, and small intestine. There is one report of this parasite in air sacs.

Morphology. *E. uncinata* is similar to *Cheilospirura* and *Dispharynx,* however, the cordons are not recurrent, and anastomose posteriorly (Fig. 33.3A). The male is 8–10 mm in length and 300–500 μm in width; the left spicule is 700–900 μm in length and the right spicule is 350 μm in length (Fig. 33.3B). The female is 12–18.5 mm in length and 515 μm in width; the tail is 250-μm long; the vulva is 1.0–1.4 mm from end of tail; and the eggs are 28–37 × 17–23 μm and embryonated when laid.

Life Cycle. Eggs are ingested by water fleas of the genus *Daphnia.* Larvae become infective after 12–14 days. Adults mature 51 days after ingestion.

Pathogenicity. Death is sometimes quite rapid and can occur without any previous signs. Nodules may form in the proventriculus; however, in chronic infections these may contain only inspissated pus, the worms having disappeared. Emaciation and listlessness can occur.

GONGYLONEMA INGLUVICOLA RANSOM 1904, GONGYLONEMATIDAE

Hosts. *G. ingluvicola* has been reported in chicken, turkey, partridge, pheasant, and quail.

Location. *G. ingluvicola* may be found in the mucosa of the crop, and sometimes in the esophagus and the proventriculus.

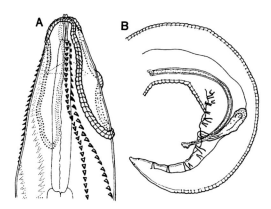

33.3. *Echinura uncinata. A.* Head. *B.* Male tail. (After Romanova)

Morphology. *G. ingluvicola* has an anterior end of body with a zone of shieldlike markings, few and scattered near the head, numerous and arranged in longitudinal rows farther back (Fig. 33.4A). The male is 17–20 mm in length and 224–250 µm in width; the cervical papillae are about 100 µm from head end; the tail has two narrow bursal asymmetrical membranes; the genital papillae are variable in number and asymmetrical; the preanal papillae number up to seven on the left side and up to five on the right side (Fig. 33.4B); the left spicule is as long or nearly as long (17–19 mm) as the body, and 7–9 µm in width with a barbed point; the right spicule is 100–120 µm in length and 15–20 µm in width. The female is 32–55 mm in length and 320–490 µm in width; and the vulva is 2.5–3.5 mm from the tip of the tail.

Life Cycle. Larval roundworms collected from the beetle *Copris minutus* and fed to a chicken permitted recovery of a single male specimen of species *Gongylonema*, tentatively identified as *G. ingluvicola* (20). Subsequently, cockroaches were infected by feeding embryonated eggs of *G. ingluvicola* derived from a mountain quail (19). Some of the larvae recovered from the cockroaches were fed to a chicken, but no worms were found on necropsy 79 days later.

Pathogenicity. The only damage associated with those worms is local lesions in the form of bur-

rows in the crop mucosa. The worms and burrows appear as white convoluted tracks in the crop wall and can be confused with *Capillaria* unless examined microscopically.

CYRNEA COLINI CRAM 1927, HABRONEMATIDAE

Synonym. *Seurocyrena colini* Strand 1929.

Hosts. *C. colini* has been reported in turkey, grouse, prairie chicken, and quail (and in chicken, experimentally). It is common in bobwhite quail of southeastern states and occasionally in bobwhite quail or closely related birds in some northeastern states. *C. colini* has also been reported from the turkey in Georgia, and from the prairie chicken in Wisconsin and Montana.

Location. *C. colini* may be found in the wall of the proventriculus, preferentially at its junction with the gizzard.

Morphology. *C. colini* are slender yellowish white worms, similar in appearance to *Cheilospirura hamulosa* but smaller and lacking the so-called cordons or cuticular ornamentations on the anterior part of the body; the tail of the male has winglike expansions or alae (Fig. 33.5B); the head structures are complicated with four lips; dorsal and ventral lips are prominent and bear four conspicuous projecting papillae and a prominent thumblike projection (Fig. 33.5A); the lateral lips are very large, each bearing two digitiform processes on inner surface and two winglike expansions on lateral surface. The male is 6-mm long and 250-µm wide; the buccal cavity is 58-µm deep; the esophagus is 2-mm long; the caudal alae is nearly circular, with 10 pairs of pedunculated papillae, the anterior ones larger than posterior; and the spicules are very unequal, with the left 2-mm long and the right, 365–400 µm. The female is 14–18 mm in length and 315-µm wide; the buccal cavity is 75-µm deep; the esophagus is about 2.8-mm long; the vulva is 915-µm anterior to anus; and the eggs are 40.5 × 22.5 µm.

Life Cycle. The cockroach *Blattella germanica* was infected with *C. colini* by feeding eggs (18). Larvae entered the body cavity, developed into the third stage in the tissues without encysting, and appeared fully developed by 18 days. Larvae were fed to quail 27 days later; mature worms were recovered 41 days subsequently.

Pathogenicity. Little or no pathologic change has been observed.

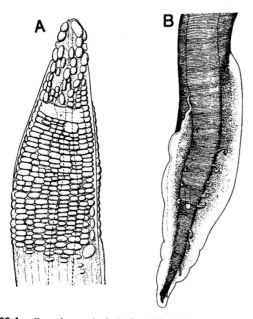

33.4. *Gongylonema ingluvicola.* A. Head. B. Male tail. (After Ransom)

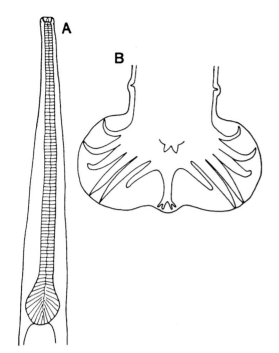

33.10. *A.* Head, *Amidostomum raillieti. B.* Male bursa, *Amidostomum skrjabini.* (After Boulenger)

CHEILOSPIRURA HAMULOSA (DIESING 1851) DIESING 1861, ACUARIIDAE.

Synonym. *Acuaria hamulosa* Diesing 1851.

Hosts. *C. hamulosa* has been reported in chicken, turkey, grouse, guinea fowl, pheasant, and quail.

Location. *C. hamulosa* may be found under the horny lining of the gizzard, usually in the cardiac and/or pyloric regions, where the lining is soft and pliable.

Morphology. *C. hamulosa* has two large triangular lateral lips. The four cuticular cordons double, irregularly wavy (Fig. 33.11A), and extending at least two-thirds the length of the body and sometimes almost to posterior extremity, not anastomosing or recurring anteriorly, are characteristic of this species. The male is 9–19 mm in length; spicules are unequal and dissimilar, the left long and slender, 1.6–1.8 mm × 12 μm, the right short and curved, 180–200 μm × 64 μm; the tail is tightly coiled; two very wide caudal alae are present; and there are 10 pairs of caudal papillae (Fig. 33.11B). The female is 16–25 mm in length; the vulva is slightly posterior to middle of body; the tail is pointed; and eggs are embryonated when deposited and are 40 × 27 μm.

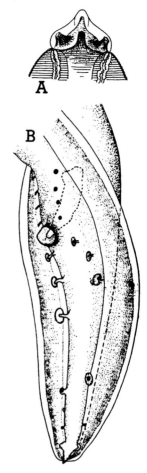

33.11. *Cheilospirura hamulosa. A.* Head. (After Drasche) *B.* Male tail. (After Cram)

Life Cycle. Grasshoppers, beetles, weevils, and sandhoppers serve as intermediate hosts. When eggs are fed to grasshoppers (*Melanoplus femurrubrum* and *M. differentialis*), the *C. hamulosa* larvae hatch and migrate into the body cavity (18). They develop, chiefly in the muscles, to the third stage, which is infective for the bird. This larva is easily recognized by the two prominent liplike structures at the anterior end of the body, the dorsal curvature of the posterior portion of the body, and the four digitiform processes at the tip of the tail.

Larvae were infective for chickens as early as 22 days and as late as 67 days after ingestion of eggs by the grasshoppers. At 11 days after feeding to chicks, larvae were on the underside of the corneous lining of the gizzard; 16 days after feeding, larvae showed characteristics of immature adults. By 25 days, worms began penetrating the muscular wall. Maturity was reached at about 76 days.

Pathogenicity. When present in small numbers, these worms are relatively nonpathogenic, although the lining of the gizzard may show small local lesions that may also involve the muscular tissue. Soft nodules enclosing parasites may be found in the muscular portion of the gizzard. In heavy infections, the wall of the gizzard may be seriously damaged. This parasite may weaken the wall, causing a rupture, with ultimate formation of a sac or pouch. There has been a single human infection reported (in the Philippines), a tumor in the conjunctiva.

CHEILOSPIRURA SPINOSA CRAM 1927, ACUARIIDAE

Hosts. *C. spinosa* have been reported in grouse, partridge, pheasant, quail, and wild turkey.

Location. *C. spinosa* may be found in the gizzard underneath the corneous lining.

Morphology. *C. spinosa* have four spiny cordons originating in pairs between the lips (Fig. 33.12A), not extending beyond the anterior third of the anterior esophagus. The male is 14–20 mm in length and 183–232 μm in width; spicules are unequal and very dissimilar, one being 660–720 μm in length and the other, 192-μm long; and the caudal alae are broad, similar in appearance to *C. hamulosa* (Fig. 33.12B). The female is 34–40 mm in length and 315–348 μm in width; the vulva is anterior to the middle of body; the anus is 250–300 μm from the posterior end; and eggs are 39–42 × 25–27 μm.

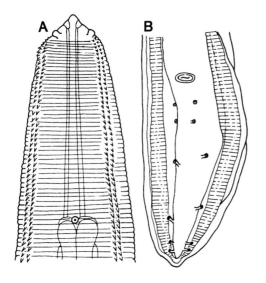

33.12. *Cheilospirura spinosa.* A. Head. B. Male tail. (After Cram)

Life Cycle. This worm, originally a parasite of grouse, was then probably spread to quail (18). Grasshoppers serve as the intermediate host, where development is similar to that seen with *C. hamulosa*. The tail structures on the third-stage larvae are similar in *C. spinosa*, rather than as in *C. hamulosa*. In the bobwhite quail, fourth-stage larvae were found underneath the gizzard lining 14 days after feeding (18). Worms with fully developed sexual characteristics were seen at 32 days.

Pathogenicity. Light infections seem to produce few problems in quail, although tortuous paths are found between the lining and muscular wall of the gizzard. In cases of heavy infection, the gizzard lining may become hemorrhagic and necrotic. Marked proliferative changes in the gizzard wall can occur with prolonged heavy infection.

EPOMIDIOSTOMUM UNCINATUM (LUNDAHL 1841) SEURAT 1918, AMIDOSTOMATIDAE

Synonym. *E. anatinum* Skrjabin 1915.

Hosts. *E. uncinatum* has been reported in duck, goose, and pigeon (and chicken, experimentally).

Location. *E. uncinatum* may be found under the horny lining of gizzard.

Morphology. *E. uncinatum* differs from *Amidostomum* in that the buccal capsule contains no teeth and the head has a pair of nodules (Fig. 33.13A). The male is 6.5–7.3 mm in length and 150-μm wide; spicules are 120–130 μm in length (Fig. 33.13B), dividing to form three terminations. The female is 10–11.5 mm in length and 230–240 μm in width; the tail is 140–170 μm in length (Fig. 33.13C); the vulva is 2.2–3.2 mm from the posterior end; and eggs are 74–90 × 45–50 μm.

Life Cycle. In larval development the ensheathed, third-stage larvae are infective 4 days after hatching (58).

ASCARIDIA BONASAE WEHR 1940, ASCARIDIIDAE

Host. *A. bonasae* has been reported in grouse.

Location. *A. bonasae* may be found in the lumen of the small intestine.

Morphology. Several authors have apparently reported *A. bonasae* as *A. galli,* although *A. bonasae* is small and does not infect the chicken. The male is 10–35 mm in length; and spicules are 1.8–2.7 mm in length and are equal. The female is 30–50 mm in length.

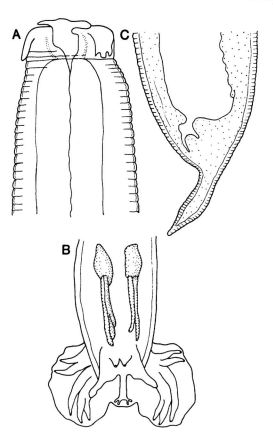

33.13. *Epomidiostomum uncinatum,* A. Head. B. Male tail. C. Female tail. (After Skrjabin)

Life Cycle. The life cycle of *A. bonasae* is similar to that of *A. galli.*

ASCARIDIA COLUMBAE (GMELIN 1790) TRAVASSOS 1913, ASCARIDIIDAE

Hosts. *A. columbae* has been reported in pigeon and dove.

Location. *A. columbae* is usually found in the lumen of the small intestine, but sometimes may be found in the esophagus, proventriculus, gizzard, liver, or body cavity.

Morphology. The *A. columbae* male is 50–70 mm in length; spicules are 1.2–1.9 mm in length and are equal. *A. columbae* has a fourth pair of ventral papillae located adjacent to the anus (Fig. 33.14A). The female is 20–95 mm in length.

Life Cycle. The life cycle of *A. columbae* is similar to that of *A. galli,* but *A. columbae* is more invasive. Second-stage larvae frequently penetrate the intestinal mucosa and reach the liver and lungs

(102) but do not develop further. Worms mature in about 37 days after embryonated eggs are consumed.

Pathogenicity. The invasion of the liver produces little effect until the larvae die; then, granulomatous lesions form with leucocyte infiltration.

ASCARIDIA COMPAR SCHRANK 1790, ASCARIDIIDAE

Hosts. *A. compar* has been reported in grouse, partridge, pheasant, and quail.

Morphology. *A. compar* is smaller than *A. galli,* but similar in appearance. The male is 36–48 mm in length; spicules are 1.8-mm long; and there are four pairs of preanal papillae, two near the preanal sucker, two just anterior to the anus (Fig. 33.14B). The female is 84–96 mm in length.

Life Cycle. The life cycle of *A. compar* is similar to that of *A. galli.*

ASCARIDIA DISSIMILIS PEREZ VIGUERAS 1931, ASCARIDIIDAE

Host. *A. dissimilis* has been reported in turkey.

Location. *A. dissimilis* may be found in the lumen of the small intestine.

Morphology. Although the literature contains numerous reports of both *A. galli* and *A. dissimilus* in turkeys, probably only *A. dissimilis* is the parasite found in the turkey (51). Only males can be accurately identified based on caudal papillae and spicule tips. The male is 35–65 mm in length; spicules are 1.3–2.2 mm in length, and the distal ends of the spicules are rounded; the first pair of preanal papillae are opposite the preanal sucker, the ventral pair of postanal papillae are only slightly separated and just behind the anus (Fig. 33.14C). The female is 50–105 mm in length.

Life Cycle. The life cycle of *A. dissimilus* is similar to that of *A. galli.* Eggs embryonate in 9–10 days. Larvae enter the intestinal mucosa, then mature in the lumen in about 30 days.

Pathogenicity. Significant levels of mortality in turkeys associated with high levels of *A. dissimilis* have been reported (42, 70). Surveys of commercial flocks in the south-central states in the United States have indicated that a high percentage of the flocks are parasitized with high levels of *A. dissimilis* (71). Aberrant migration of *A. dissimilis* larvae has also been associated with hepatic foci.

ASCARIDIA GALLI SCHRANK 1788, ASCARIDIIDAE

Synonyms. *A. lineata* Schneider 1866; *H. granulosa* Linstow 1906.

Hosts. *A. galli* has been reported in chicken, turkey, dove, duck, and goose.

Location. *A. galli* may be found in the lumen of the intestine, occasionally in the esophagus, crop, gizzard, oviduct, and body cavity.

Morphology. *A. galli* are large worms, thick yellowish white; their head has three large lips. The male is 50–76 mm in length and 490 μm–1.21 mm in width; the preanal sucker is oval or circular, with a strong chitinous wall with a papilliform interruption on its posterior rim; the tail has narrow caudal alae or membranes and 10 pairs of papillae; the first pair of ventral caudal papillae is anterior to the preanal sucker, the fourth pair is widely separated (Fig. 33.14D; compare with *A. dissimilis*); and spicules are nearly equal and narrow, end blunt with a slight

indentation. The female is 60–116 mm in length and 900 μm–1.8 mm in width; the vulva is in the anterior part of body; and the eggs are elliptical, thick shelled, and not embryonated at time of deposition (Fig. 33.15).

Life Cycle. The life history of *A. galli* is simple and direct. Infective eggs hatch in either the proventriculus or the duodenum of the susceptible host. The young larvae, after hatching, live free in the lumen of the posterior portion of the duodenum for the first 9 days, then penetrate the mucosa and cause hemorrhages. The young worms enter the lumen of the duodenum by the 17th or 18th day and remain there until maturity, at approximately 28–30 days after ingestion of embryonated eggs. Larvae may enter the tissues as early as the 1st day and remain there as late as the 26th day after infection. The large majority spend from the 8th to the 17th day in the intestinal mucosa. A few of the larvae penetrate deep into the tissue, while the majority undergo only a brief and shallow association with the intestinal mucosa during the "tissue phase." *A. galli* eggs are ingested by grasshoppers or earthworms, hatch, and are infective to chickens, although no development of the larvae occurs.

Under optimum conditions of temperature and moisture, eggs in the droppings become infective in 10–12 days; under less favorable conditions, a longer time is necessary. Eggs are quite resistant to low temperatures. Larvae were recovered from experimental birds fed embryonated eggs of this worm that had been exposed continuously to outdoor conditions at Beltsville, Maryland, for 66 wk (34). A 12-hr exposure to 43 C proved lethal for eggs in all stages of development.

Pathogenicity. *A. galli* infection causes weight depression in the host, which correlates with increasing worm burden (77). The nutritional state of the host is also important, since weight depression

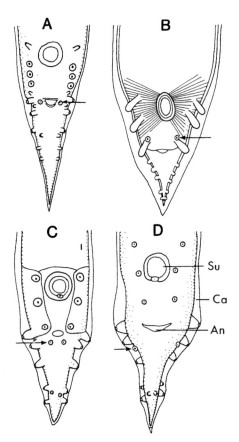

A B C D

33.14. Male tails. *A. Ascaridia columbae.* (After Wehr and Hwang). *B. Ascaridia compar.* (After Linstow) *C. Ascaridia dissimilis. D. Ascaridia galli.* (After Wehr)

Su
Ca
An

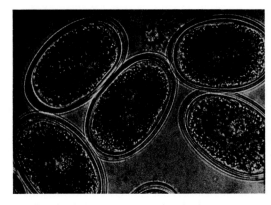

33.15. *Ascaridia galli* eggs freshly voided from a chicken.

is greater with high dietary levels of protein (15%) than with low levels (12.5%) (49). In severe infections, intestinal blockage can occur. Chickens infected with a large number of ascarids suffer from loss of blood, reduced blood sugar content, increased urates, shrunken thymus glands, retarded growth, and greatly increased mortality. However, no effects of infection on blood protein level, packed cell volume, or hemoglobin levels were found (47). *A. galli* can also have detrimental effects through interaction (synergism) with other disease conditions such as coccidiosis and infectious bronchitis. *A. galli* have also been shown to contain and transmit avian reoviruses.

One of the most striking effects of infection, at least from an aesthetic standpoint, is the occasional finding of this parasite in the hen's egg. Numerous reports of this phenomenon have been made in the literature (78). Presumably the worms migrate up the oviduct via the cloaca, with subsequent inclusion in the egg. Infected eggs can be detected by candling, thus, eliminating a potential consumer complaint. Some embarrassing law suits against the poultry industries could be avoided if egg candlers were encouraged to remove such eggs in packing plants.

Immunity. Age of the host and severity of exposure play roles in *A. galli* infections. Chickens 3 mo or older manifest considerable resistance to infection with *A. galli*. In older fowl, larvae are recovered that have undergone little or no development since emerging from the egg (93). Larval development is arrested in the third stage at high dose rates as a result of resistance, rather than a density-dependent phenomenon (48). Heavier breeds such as Rhode Island Reds and White and Barred Plymouth Rocks are more resistant to ascarid infections than are the lighter White Leghorns and White Minorcas.

The nutritional state of the bird also influences the development of immunity. Diets consisting chiefly of animal proteins with little or no plant protein aid the chicken in building resistance to infection with ascarids. Birds given a diet consisting principally of animal protein developed fewer worms than those given a diet low in animal protein. Diets high in vitamins A and B (complex) increase the fowl's resistance to *A. galli,* and diets low in these vitamins definitely favor parasitism. Increasing levels of dietary calcium and lysine decreased the length and number of worms recovered (21).

ASCARIDIA NUMIDAE LEIPER 1908, ASCARIDIIDAE

Synonym. *Heterakis numidae* Leiper 1908.

Host. *A. numidae* has been reported in guinea fowl.

Location. *A. numidae* may be found in the lumen of the small intestine, sometimes the cecum.

Morphology. *A. numidae* is much smaller than *A. galli*. The male is 19–35 mm in length; it has 10 pairs of caudal papillae, 2 of them preanal and 2 adanal; and spicules are equal, 3-mm long. The female is 30–50 mm in length.

Life Cycle. The larvae remain in the lumen for 4–14 days before penetrating the intestinal mucosa.

TAXONOMY OF *CAPILLARIA* FROM THE INTESTINE OF BIRDS.
Most species of *Capillaria* from birds have been described under a variety of names. Likewise, many species names have been used for several different capillaria. As a result, descriptions, host specificity, location in the intestine, geographic distribution, and even the validity of some species are confused (60, 62, 64, 76). This chapter uses essentially the species accepted by Levine (60) except for *C. dujardini,* which is considered a synonym for *C. obsignata*. The species *C. retusa, C. collaris,* and *C. longicallis,* commonly used in the literature, have been synonymized. The species *C. columbae* Rudolphi 1819 is retained for the capillaria in the large intestine of pigeons that possess a vulva with a projecting appendage (Table 33.4 and Fig. 33.16).

CAPILLARIA ANATIS (SCHRANK 1790) TRAVASSOS 1915, CAPILLARIIDAE

Synonym. *Capillaria brevicollis* Walton 1935.

Hosts. *C. anatis* has been reported in chicken, turkey, duck, goose, partridge, and pheasant.

Table 33.4. Characteristics of *Capillaria* from chickens in the United States

Characteristic	*C. anatis*	*C. bursata*	*C. caudinflata*	*C. obsignata*
Male				
Lateral caudalae	−	+	+	−
Spicule Sheath	Spines	No spines	Minute spines	No spine
Female				
Vulvar appendage	None	Semicircular	Pronounced	None

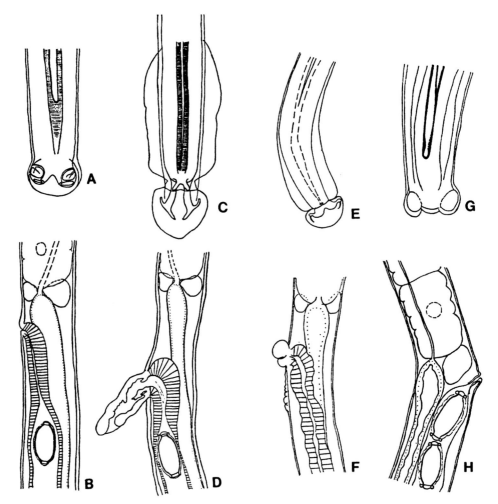

33.16. Male bursa (*A, C, E, G*) and female vulva (*B, D, F, H*) of *Capillaria obsignata* (*A, B*), *Capillaria caudinflata* (*C, D*), *Capillaria bursata* (*E, F*), and *Capillaria anatis* (*G, H*). (After Wakelin)

Location. *C. anatis* is usually found in the cecum, sometimes the small intestine.

Morphology. *C. anatis* are threadlike worms. The male is 8–15 mm in length; the spicule is 0.7–1.9 mm in length with a spiny sheath; and the tail has two lobes but no lateral caudal alae (Fig. 33.16G). The female is 11–28 mm in length; the vulva is without appendage (Fig. 33.16H); and eggs are 46–67 × 22–29 μm with a thick rugous outer shell.

Life Cycle. The life cycle of *C. anatis* is unknown.

CAPILLARIA BURSATA FREITAS AND ALMEIDA 1934, CAPILLARIIDAE

Hosts. *C. bursata* has been reported in chicken, turkey, goose, and pheasant.

Location. *C. bursata* may be found in the mucosa of the small intestine.

Morphology. Although some authors consider *C. bursa* to be a synonym of *C. caudinflata,* others give reasons for their each being recognized as a separate species (76, 97). The male is 11–20 mm in length and 44–51 μm in width; spicules are 1.1–1.6 mm in length; the sheath is without spines; and the bursa is round, supported by two dorsal and two-ventral projections (Fig. 33.16E). The female is 16–35 mm in length and 53–64 μm in width; the vulva has two semicircular valves (Fig. 33.16F); and eggs are 51–62 × 22–24 μm, with a shell with fine longitudinal ridges.

Life Cycle. Eggs are passed in the feces; larval development is complete in 8–15 days, depending on temperature. Eggs hatch after ingestion by earthworm. Larvae are infective after 22–25 days. Worms mature in final host 20–26 days after ingestion.

Capillaria caudinflata (Molin 1858) Wawilowa 1926, Capillariidae

Synonym. *C. longicollis* (Mehlis 1931) of Madsen 1945.

Hosts. *C. caudinflata* has been reported in chicken, turkey, duck, goose, guinea fowl, grouse, partridge, pheasant, pigeon, and quail.

Location. *C. caudinflata* may be found in the mucosa of the small intestine.

Morphology. The male *C. caudinflata* is 9–18 mm in length and 33–51 μm in width; the spicule is 0.7–1.2 mm, tapering to a fine point distally; the spicule sheath has fine thornlike spines on the proximal portion; and there are bursa present, supported dorsally by two T-shaped processes (Fig. 33.16C). The female is 12–25 mm in length and 38–62 μm in width; the vulva has characteristic appendage (Fig. 33.16D); and eggs are 47–58 × 20–24 μm, with a thick and finely sculptured shell.

Life Cycle. Turkeys were experimentally infected by feeding earthworms of the species *Allolobophora caliginosa* from infected poultry yards (2). This earthworm is an essential intermediate host or the successful transmission of *C. caudinflata* from turkey to turkey. Attempts to transmit this threadworm by using *Lumbricus terrestris* were unsuccessful. When earthworms (*Eisenia foetida*) were fed embryonated eggs of *C. caudinflata*, adults were recovered at necropsy from turkeys to which these earthworms had been fed.

Capillaria obsignata Madsen 1945, Capillariidae

Synonym. *C. collaris* Linstow 1873.

Hosts. *C. obsignata* has been reported in chicken, turkey, goose, guinea fowl, pigeon, and quail.

Location. *C. obsignata* may be found in the small intestine and the cecum.

Morphology. *C. obsignata* are hairlike worms (Fig. 33.17). The male is 7–13 mm in length and 49–53 μm in width, with the cloacal aperture almost terminal, and a small bursal lobe on either side, the two lobes connected dorsally by a delicate bursal membrane (Fig. 33.16A); the spicule is 1.1–1.5 mm in length; and the sheath has transverse folds without spines. The female is 10–18 mm in length and approximately 80 μm wide; the vulva is on slight prominence slightly posterior to the union of esophagus and intestine (Fig. 33.16B); and eggs are 44–46 × 22–29 μm, their shell with a reticulate pattern.

Life Cycle. *C. obsignata* has a direct development as detailed by Wakelin (97). Embryonation of the eggs was dependent on environmental conditions. No development occurred at 4 C. Development was complete in 13 days at 20 C and in 65–72 hours at 35 C. Temperatures above 37 C were detrimental to embryonation. Storage of embryonated eggs at low (-3.5 C) or high (50 C) temperatures reduced infectivity. No molting was observed in the egg; the larva, which hatched only after ingestion by the host, was considered first stage. Worms reached maturity in about 18 days. The prepatent period was 20–21 days after infection. Pigeons experimentally infected with *C. obsignata* and held under conditions designed to preclude reinfection will remain infected for about 9 mo.

Pathogenicity. Birds heavily infected with *C. obsignata* spend much of their time apart from the rest of the flock huddled on the ground, underneath the roosts, or in some corner of the room. Signs include emaciation, diarrhea, hemorrhagic enteritis,

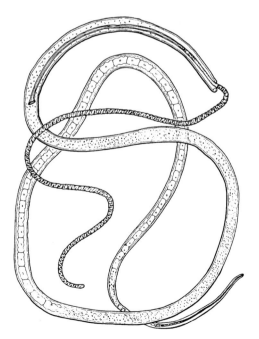

33.17. *Capillaria obsignata.* (After Gagarin)

and death. A catarrhal exudate in the upper intestine and some thickening of the wall are the most severe gross pathologic changes seen in heavy experimental infections (97). Changes, however, are variable and are not an inevitable consequence of massive infection. Effects on weight gain are also variable, with some weight depression with as few as 14 worms (59); in other cases, infections of 100–1000 worms cause no weight change (97). Perhaps the most significant effect of infection from a practical standpoint is the less efficient utilization of feed.

No significant differences in total white blood cells or packed cell volume between infected and uninfected birds were found (97). A significant increase in B and V globulin, total globulin, and total protein in infected chickens compared with uninfected controls was demonstrated (8). Conversely, in the pigeon, there was a marked decrease in total protein and albumen. A significant reduction in levels of plasma carotenoids and liver vitamin A with heavy infection was shown, although plasma vitamin A levels were only slightly reduced (11).

ORNITHOSTRONGYLUS QUADRIRADIATUS (STEVENSON 1904) TRAVASSOS 1914, HELIGMOSOMIDAE

Hosts.   *O. quadriradiatus* have been reported in pigeon and dove.

Location.   *O. quadriradiatus* may be found in the lumen of the small intestine.

Morphology.   *O. quadriradiatus* worms are delicate, slender, and red when freshly collected, apparently from ingested blood in intestine, and they have a cuticle about their head inflated to form vesicular enlargement (Fig. 33.18A). The male is 9 mm–12 mm in length; the bursa is bilobed, with no distinct dorsal lobe; the dorsal ray is much shorter than other rays, not extending halfway to bursal margin, bifurcating near its tip to form two short tips; there is a stumpy process present on each side

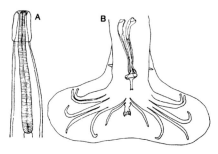

33.18.   *Ornithostrongylus quadriradiatus.* A. Head. B. Bursa of male. (After Stevenson)

near base of ray; spicules are equal, 150–160 μm in length, somewhat curved, each terminating in three pointed processes (Fig. 33.18B); and the telamon is 57–70 μm in length, with two longitudinal processes extending backward and forward along the dorsal wall of cloaca, and two lateral processes forming a partial ring through which the spicules protrude. The female is 18–24 mm in length; the vulva is near the end of tail; the vagina is short, followed by two powerful muscular ovejectors; the tail tapers to a narrow blunt end, bearing a short spine; and eggs segment when deposited.

Life Cycle.   This bloodsucking nematode occurs in the small intestine of pigeons and mourning doves in the United States. The oval thin-shelled eggs are voided in the droppings and hatch in approximately 19–25 hr under favorable conditions of moisture and temperature. After hatching, the larva molts twice within the next 3 or 4 days to reach the infective stage. The infective larva is swallowed by a pigeon or other susceptible host and grows to maturity in the small intestine. The female worm deposits eggs 5–6 days following ingestion of the larva.

Pathogenicity.   This roundworm can cause serious losses in pigeons due to catarrhal enteritis and blood loss during hemorrhage. Birds heavily infected become droopy, remain squatted on the ground or floor, and if disturbed, try to move but usually tip forward on the breast and head. Food is eaten sparingly and is frequently regurgitated, along with bile-stained fluid. There is a pronounced greenish diarrhea, and the bird gradually wastes away. Signs of difficult and rapid breathing usually precede death. Intestines of fatally infected birds are markedly hemorrhagic and have a greenish mucoid content with masses of sloughed epithelium.

HETERAKIS DISPAR (SCHRANK 1790) DUJARDIN 1845, HETERAKIDAE

Hosts.   *H. dispar* has been reported in duck and goose.

Location.   *H. dispar* may be found in the lumen of the cecum.

Morphology.   *H. dispar* is somewhat larger than *H. gallinarum*, but similar in appearance except for spicules. The male is 7–18 mm in length; has a preanal sucker 109–256 μm in diameter; and its spicules are short and essentially equal, 390–730 μm in length (Fig. 33.19A). The female is 16–23 mm in length; and eggs are 59–62 × 39–41 μm.

Life Cycle.   Similar to *H. gallinarum.*

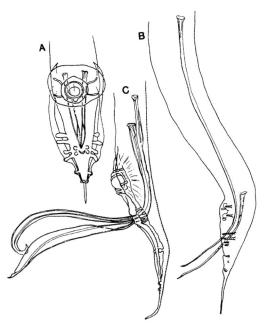

33.19. Male tails. *A. Heterakis dispar.* (After Madsen) *B. Heterakis gallinarum.* (After Lane) *C. Heterakis isolonche.* (After Cram et al.)

Pathogenicity. *H. dispar* is considered to be relatively nonpathogenic.

HETERAKIS GALLINARUM (SCHRANK 1788) MADSEN 1950, HETERAKIDAE

Synonyms. See Madsen (63).

Hosts. *H. gallinarum* has been reported in chicken, turkey, duck, goose, grouse, guinea fowl, partridge, pheasant, and quail.

Location. *H. gallinarum* may be found in the lumen of the cecum.

Morphology. The *H. gallinarum* worm is small and white; its head end is bent dorsally; the mouth is surrounded by three small equally sized lips; two narrow lateral membranes extend almost the entire length of body; and the esophagus ends in a well-developed bulb containing a valvular apparatus (Fig. 33.20A). The male is 7–13 mm in length; the tail is straight, ending in a subulate point; there are two large lateral bursal wings; the preanal sucker is well developed, with strongly chitinized walls and a small semicircular incision in posterior margin of the sucker wall; there are 12 pairs of caudal papillae, the two most posterior pairs being stout and superimposed; and spicules are dissimilar, the right one 0.85–2.8 (generally 2) mm in length, and the left one 0.37–1.1 mm in length with a curved tip (Fig. 33.19B). The female is 10–15 mm in length; the tail is long, narrow, and pointed; the vulva is not prominent and is slightly posterior to the middle of body; and eggs are thick shelled, ellipsoidal, unsegmented when deposited, similar in appearance to those of *A. galli,* and are 63–75 × 36–50 μm.

Life Cycle. Lund and Chute (61) found the greatest production of eggs for each egg ingested was with the ring-necked pheasant, followed by the guinea fowl and chicken. Eggs pass out in the feces in an unsegmented state. Oogenesis and eggshell formation have been described by Lee and Lestan (57). In approximately 2 wk or less, under favorable conditions of temperature and moisture, eggs reach the infective stage. When these are swallowed by a susceptible host, the embryos hatch in the upper part of the intestine; at the end of 24 hr, most of the young worms have reached the ceca. The larvae are closely associated with or occasionally embedded in the cecal tissue until 12 days postexposure, with peak association at 3 days. Tissue association increases with age of birds; nevertheless, a true tissue phase rarely occurs with *H. gallinarum.* At necropsy, most of the adult worms are found in the tips or blind ends of the ceca. Earthworms may also ingest the eggs of the cecal worms and may be the means of causing infection in poultry.

Pathogenicity. The ceca of experimentally infected birds show marked inflammation and thickening of the walls. In heavy infections, nodules form in the mucosa and submucosa, as the response of already sensitized ceca to subsequent infection (53). Hepatic granulomas containing the worms

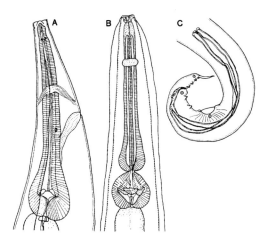

33.20. *A. Heterakis gallinarum,* head. *B. Subulura suctoria,* head. (After Skrjabin and Shikhobalova) *C. Subulura strongylina,* male tail. (After Barreto)

have also been reported in chickens (79).

The chief economic importance of the cecal worm lies in its role as a carrier of the blackhead organism *Histomonas meleagridis*. Blackhead may be produced in susceptible birds by feeding embryonated eggs of *H. gallinarum* taken from blackhead-infected birds. The protozoan parasite was found incorporated in the worm egg (95), and its presence was identified in the gut wall and in the reproductive systems of the male and female and in the developing eggs of this cecal worm (39). Direct transmission of *Histomonas meleagridis* was accomplished using larvae (81) and male worms (86).

HETERAKIS ISOLONCHE LINSTOW 1906, HETERAKIDAE

Synonym.   *Heterakis bonasae* Cram 1927.

Hosts.   *H. isolonche* has been reported in duck, grouse, pheasant, prairie chicken, and quail.

Location.   Adult *H. isolonche* may be found in the lumen of the cecum or mucosa; larvae, in the mucosa.

Morphology.   *H. isolonche* is similar to *H. gallinarum* but easily differentiated based on the spicules. The male is 5.9–15 mm in length; it has a preanal sucker, 70–15 µm in diameter; and spicules are long and essentially equal, 0.72–2.33 (generally 1.4–1.9) µm in length (Fig. 33.19C). The female is 9–12 mm in length; and eggs are 65–75 × 37–46 µm.

Life Cycle.   The life cycle of *H. isolonche* is similar to that of *H. gallinarum* but with a more extensive tissue phase. The second-stage larvae mature in the cecal mucosa and sometimes the adults are still found there.

Pathogenicity.   *H. isolonche* can be quite pathogenic, and mortality in pen-reared pheasants can exceed 50%. Diarrhea and weight depression are common. The invasion of the mucosa causes lymphocyte infiltration and granulation that leads to the formation of nodules in the cecal wall. These nodules may coalesce to form a thickened wall. In quail and grouse, these nodules do not seem to form and there is little pathology, even when worms are present in the large numbers.

SUBULURA BRUMPTI (LOPEZ-NEYRA 1922) CRAM 1926, SUBULURIDAE

Synonyms.   Some authors consider *S. brumpti* a synonym of *S. suctoria,* others consider it a separate species.

Hosts.   *S. brumpti* has been reported in chicken, turkey, dove, duck, grouse, guinea fowl, partridge, pheasant, and quail.

Location.   *S. brumpti* may be found in the lumen of the cecum.

Morphology.   *S. brumpti* are small nematodes with anterior end curved dorsally; the mouth is hexagonal, surrounded by six weakly developed lips, each with median papillae; there are two pairs of larger papillae located dorsally and ventrally, well-developed amphids laterally, and anterior portions of esophageal wall cuticularized, forming three teethlike structures; the esophagus is dilated posteriorly, followed by a bulb (Fig. 33.20B); and there are cephalic alae extending to anterior portion of intestine. The male is 6.9–10 mm in length and 340–420 µm in width; the esophagus is 0.98–1.1 mm in length; there are lateral alae extending to the middle of the esophagus; the tail is curved ventrally and ends in prolongation; there are caudal papillae (10 pairs) consisting of 3 pairs preanal, 2 pairs adanal, and 5 pairs postanal; caudal alae are narrow and not well developed; the preanal sucker is 170–220 µm long; spicules are similar and equal, 1.22–1.5 mm in length; and the gubernaculum is 150–210 µm in length. The female is 9–13.7 mm in length and 460–560 µm in width; the esophagus is 1–1.3 mm in length; the tail is straight and conical, ending in a sharp point; the vulva is anterior to the middle of the body; eggs are almost spherical, thin-shelled, 82–86 × 66–76 µm, and fully embryonated when deposited.

Life Cycle.   Eggs pass from definitive hosts in cecal droppings. At this time, they contain embryos infective to beetles and cockroaches, the reported intermediate hosts (5, 22). Larvae hatch in 4–5 hr, penetrate the intestinal wall, and enter the body cavity, where further development occurs (4, 22). The first larval molt occurs on the 4th or 5th day after infection; by the 7th or 8th day, the larva encapsulates on the intestinal wall. The molt to the second stage occurs between the 13th and 15th day after ingestion; shortly thereafter, the larva contracts in length and coils up within the capsule, becoming the third, or infective, stage. When the definitive host swallows an infected intermediate host, the larva migrates to the ceca and develops to the fourth stage within about 2 wk. The final molt takes place on about the 18th day after infection. The young adults continue to grow and develop, and eggs appear in the feces in about 6 wk after infection. Experimental infections of the beetle *Alphitobius diaperinus* when fed the parasitic ova may yield second-stage larvae 8 days postingestion; the encysted infective third-stage larvae can occur 12-16 days postingestion (50).

Pathogenicity. The cecum showed no evidence of larval penetration or any extensive inflammatory reactions, even though infection could persist as long as 8 mo (22). No noticeable lesions were produced by this worm in the ceca of the quail (20).

SUBULURA STRONGYLINA (RUDOLPHI 1819) RAILLIET AND HENRY 1912, SUBULURIDAE

Hosts. *S. strongylina* has been reported in chicken, guinea fowl, and quail. This parasite has been reported in chickens in South America and Puerto Rico but not in the United States. It has, however, been found in quail in southeastern United States.

Location. *S. strongylina* may be found in the lumen of cecum.

Morphology. The lateral cephalic alae are well developed and extend from head to the median part of the esophageal bulb. The male is 4.4–12 mm in length; there are lateral alae extending to the median part of bulb; the tail is curved into a V or an O shape; the preanal sucker is long and slender, 169-μm long; there are 11 pairs of caudal papillae; and spicules are equal, 890 μm–1.2 mm in length (Fig. 33.20C). The female is 5.6–18 mm in length; the vulva is slightly anterior to middle of body; and eggs are 84 × 67 μm, and embryonated when deposited.

Life Cycle. The exact life cycle of *S. strongylina* is unknown.

Pathogenicity. No noticeable lesions are produced in the ceca of quail.

SUBULURA SUCTORIA (MOLIN 1860) RAILLIET AND HENRY 1912, SUBULURIDAE

Synonym. *Heterakis suctoria* Molin 1860.

Hosts. *S. suctoria* has been reported in chicken, turkey, guinea fowl, partridge, pheasant, and quail.

Location. *S. suctoria* may be found in the lumen or the mucosa of the cecum, although sometimes in the small intestine.

Morphology. This worm is larger than *S. brumpti.* Apparently it has not been reported from the United States but has been found in the chicken in Mexico, Africa, South America, the Middle East, and Asia. The lateral cephalic alae are small and extend to the middle of the esophagus. The male is 11.8–13.8 mm in length and 359-μm wide; spicules

are equal and curved, 1–1.5 mm in length. The female is 20–33 mm in length; and eggs are 51–70 × 45–64 μm.

Life Cycle. The life cycle of *S. suctoria* is similar to that of *S. brumpti.* Beetles serve as intermediate hosts.

Pathogenicity. Barus and Blazek (7) reported little pathology.

STRONGYLOIDES AVIUM CRAM 1929, STRONGYLOIDIDAE

HOSTS. *S. avium* has been reported in chicken, turkey, goose, grouse, and quail. This extremely small roundworm has been reported from chickens in Puerto Rico (17). The junco (*Junco hyemalis*) in Virginia, and the coot (*Fulica americana*) in North Carolina, harbor naturally occurring infections.

Location. *S. avium* may be found in the cecum, sometimes in the small intestine.

Morphology. *S. avium* are characterized by parasitic generation consisting of only parthenogenic females in the intestine of the avian host; free-living generation consisting of both males (Fig. 33.21A) and females in soil. The parasitic adult is 2.2-mm long and 40–45 μm in width; the vulva has projecting lips, and is located 1.4 mm from head end (Fig. 33.21B and C); the uteri are divergent from vulva; ovaries are recurrent with simple "hairpin bends," their course not sinuous; and eggs have very thin shells, segmenting when deposited, and are 52–56 × 36–40 μm.

Life Cycle. Unlike most species of nematodes, the parasitic cycle of *S. avium* consists of females only. Eggs hatch soon after being passed in the droppings, sometimes as soon as 18 hr. Young worms develop in the soil to adult males and females. Shortly thereafter, the females give rise to young which feed, molt, and develop into other adult free-living males and females; or they transform into another type of larvae known as the infective larvae, that develop into parthenogenic females after being swallowed by a susceptible host.

Pathogenicity. During the early or acute stage of infection, the walls of the ceca are greatly thickened; typical pasty cecal contents almost disappear, the discharge being thin and bloody. If the fowl survives this acute stage, the ceca gradually become functional again and the thickening of the walls decreases. Young birds suffer most from infections. If infection is light or the birds are adults, little if any clinical effect is noted.

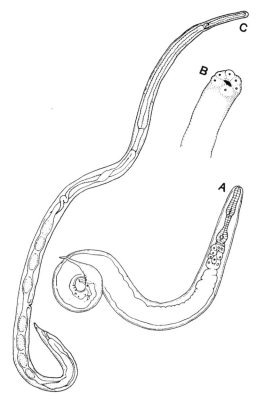

33.21. *Strongyloides avium. A.* Free-living male. (After Cram) *B.* Head, parasitic female. *C.* Parasitic (parthenogenic) female. (*B* and *C* after Sakamoto and Sarashina)

TRICHOSTRONGYLUS TENUIS MEHLIS 1846, TRICHOSTRONGYLIDAE

Hosts. *T. tenuis* has been reported in chicken, turkey, duck, goose, guinea fowl, pigeon, and quail.

Location. *T. tenuis* may be found in the cecum, sometimes in the small intestine.

Morphology. *T. tenuis* worms are small and slender; the body is gradually attenuated in front of the genital opening; the mouth is surrounded by three small, inconspicuous lips; the cuticle anterior end of body is lacking in conspicuous striations for a distance of about 200–250 μm from the extremity, then with a distinct serrated appearance for a distance of about 1–2 mm more. The male is 5.5–9 mm in length and 48-μm wide near the center of body; the cuticle is inflated on the ventral surface just anterior to the bursa; the bursa has one dorsal and two lateral lobes, the dorsal one not distinctly marked off from the lateral; each lateral lobe is supported by six rays (Fig. 33.22); the dorsal ray bifurcates at

its distal third, and each of these divisions again bifurcates and is very finely pointed; spicules are dark brown and slightly unequal in length, the longer being 120–164 μm and the shorter, 104–150 μm; both are much twisted, especially at distal ends, and provided with an earlike structure on proximal end; and both spicules are apparently surrounded in distal two-thirds by a thin membrane extending for a short distance beyond distal ends. The female is 6.5–11 mm in length and 77–100 μm in width at the level of the vulva; the vulva is in the posterior end of body, with crenelated edges; uteri are divergent; and eggs are thin shelled.

Life Cycle. This worm has a direct life cycle. *T. tenuis* from pheasants has been successfully transmitted to domestic turkey and guinea fowl. Experimental infections have also been induced in chickens (98). Eggs hatch within 36–48 hr after being passed in the droppings, and the larvae become infective within approximately 2 wk. Within this time, the larvae have molted twice. When picked up by a susceptible host, the infective larvae molt twice more within the ceca of the bird before finally becoming adults.

Pathogenicity. *T. tenuis* was associated with the disease that decimated the red grouse population in Scotland. A fatal dose can be as low as 500 infective larvae. Ceca become extended, and blood vessels show congestion. The mucosa of the ceca is inflamed, and the ridges are greatly thickened. Severe infection causes loss of weight and anemia. *T. tenuis* can also be fatal to young goslings under certain conditions.

Heavy mortality occurs usually in the fall, mainly in the young birds in that year's hatching, and again in the spring. These two seasons are not isolated epidemics, but rather are the peaks of a disease that continues in a chronic form the entire year.

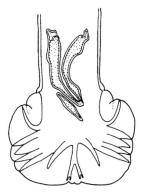

33.22. *Trichostrongylus tenuis.* Bursa of male. (After Railliet)

AULONOCEPHALUS LINDQUISTI CHANDLER 1934, SUBULURIDAE

Hosts. *A. lindquisti* have been reported in bobwhite quail and blue or scaled quail. The distribution seems somewhat restricted, being found mainly in western Texas.

Location. *A. lindquisti* is most commonly found in the cecum, although sometimes in the large intestine.

Morphology. *A. lindquisti* are bright pink worms; the cuticle is finely striated; cervical alae are present, 45–65 μm in breadth in the female but only 20–25 μm in breadth in the male; the head has six troughlike grooves about 65–70 μm in length radiating from the mouth (Fig. 33.23A); the esophagus is club shaped, 1.3–1.8 mm in length, with the bulb slightly longer than it is broad. The male is 8–10.6 mm in length and 420–490 μm in width; the gubernaculum is 170–190 μm in length; spicules are approximately equal, 1.16–1.3 mm in length (Fig. 33.23B). The female is 10–14.8 mm in length and 530–590 μm in width; the vulva is inconspicuous, ranging from slightly anterior to slightly posterior to the middle of the body; the tail terminates in

a thin spike; and eggs are broadly oval, 58 × 42–45 μm.

Life Cycle. The life cycle of *A. lindquisti* has not been described.

Pathogenicity. The pathologic effects of this species is unknown, but as many as 300 worms have been recovered from a single host.

OTHER NEMATODES OF THE DIGESTIVE TRACT. Numerous species of nematodes have been found in domestic poultry in other parts of the world but have not yet been reported from North America. The diagnostician should, however, be aware of their existence because the potential always remains for their appearance. Following are some of these species.

Esophagus and Crop. These include *Gongylonema crami* Smit 1927 from the chicken in Java, *G. congolense* Fain 1944 from the chicken and duck in Africa, and *G. sumani* Bhalerao 1933 from the chicken in India. *Capillaria cairinae* Freitas and Almeida 1935 is found in the esophagus of ducks in Brazil and *C. combologiodes* Erlich and Mikacie 1940, in the crop of turkeys in Europe. Larvae of *Spirocerca lupi* have been found encysted in the crop of chickens in the southern United States.

Proventriculus. *Parhadjelia neglecta* Lent and Freitas 1939 is a Habronematide resembling *Cyrnea* that has been reported in the submucosa of the proventriculus of the domestic duck in Brazil. *Echinuria jugadornata* Soloviev 1912 causes nodules at the junction of the proventriculus and gizzard of domestic ducks in the former Soviet Union. *Physaloptera acuticauda* Molin 1860 has been reported from chickens and pheasants in Brazil and falconiform birds in the United States. *Tetrameres* include *T. confusa* Travassos 1919 from the chicken, turkey, and pigeon in South America and Asia; *T. gigas* Travassos 1919 from the domestic duck in South America; *T. mohtedae* Bhalerao and Rao 1944 from the chicken in India; and *T. spinosa* Maplestone 1913 from the chicken and domestic duck in India.

Gizzard. Several other nematodes are found under the gizzard lining of domestic poultry. *Histiocephalus laticaudatus* (Rudolphi 1819) Diesing 1851 has been recovered from chickens and ducks, and *Streptocara pectinifera* (Neumann 1900) Skrjabin 1916, from chickens and guinea fowl in Europe. *Epomidiostomum orispinum* (Molin 1861) Seurat 1981 is in the domestic duck and goose in Europe and Africa, and *E. skrjabini* Petrov 1926, in the domestic goose in Asia.

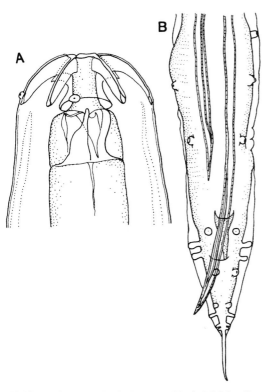

33.23. *Aulonocephalus lindquisti*. A. Head. B. Male tail. (After Chandler)

Small Intestine. *Abbreviata gemina* Linstow 1899, a *Physaloptera*-like worm, occurs in the chicken in Egypt. The anisakid *Contracaecum microcephalum* (Rudolphi 1809) Railliet and Henry 1912 infects domestic ducks in Europe, Asia, and Africa, and *Porrocaecum crassum* (Deslongchamps 1824) Railliet and Henry 1912 is in domestic ducks and guinea fowl in Europe. *Capillaria anseris* occurs in the domestic goose in Europe. *Hartertia gallinarum* (Theiler 1919) Cram 1927, which uses termites as an intermediate host, causes diarrhea and decreased growth and egg production in chickens in Africa.

Cecum. Numerous other species of *Heterakis* are found in the chicken throughout the world. These include *H. beramporia* Lane 1914, Asia; *H. bervispiculum* Gendre 1911, South America and Africa; *H. caudabrevis* Popova 1929, former Soviet Union; *H. indica* Maplestone 1931, India; and *H. linganensis* Li 1933, China. Turkeys in China are infected with *H. meleagris* Hsu 1957. *Subulura differens* Sonsino 1890 is widespread in chickens, guinea fowl, and quail in South America, Europe, Africa, and Asia, and sometimes is also found in the small intestine. Several *Capillaria* have been described including *C. monteividensis* Calzada 1937 and *C. uruguayensis* Calzada 1937 from chickens in Uruguay, and *C. spinulosa* (Linstow 1890) Travassos 1915 from ducks in Europe.

NEMATODES OF THE RESPIRATORY TRACT

CYATHOSTOMA BRONCHIALIS (MUEHLIG 1884) CHAPIN 1925, SYNGAMIIDAE

Hosts. *C. bronchialis* have been reported in duck, goose, and turkey (and chicken, experimentally).

Location. *C. bronchialis* may be found in the larynx, trachea, bronchi, and sometimes in the abdominal air sacs.

Morphology. *C. bronchialis* is very similar to *Syngamus,* but larger and less firmly united in copula; the buccal capsule is somewhat wider than deep, with usually six, but occasionally seven. triangular buccal teeth (Fig. 33.24A). The male is 8–12 mm in length and 200–600 μm in width; spicules are long and slender, 540–870 μm, with tips slightly incurved (Fig. 33.24B). The female is 16–30 mm in length, 750 μm–1.5 mm in width; the vulva has fairly prominent lips, situated in the posterior part of the anterior third of body; the tail is acute; and eggs are 68–90 × 43–60 μm, with slight operculum in mature ones.

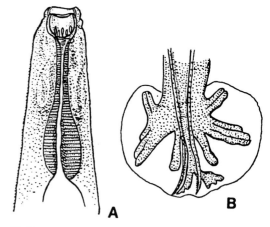

33.24. *Cyathostoma bronchialis.* A. Head. B. Male tail.

Life Cycle. The life cycle of this species of gapeworm can involve direct infections with third-stage larvae, but infections using infected earthworms are more successful. The third-stage larvae migrate to the lungs through the peritoneal cavity and air sacs (36), rather than through the bloodstream as does *S. trachea.* The larvae molt twice in the lung at 1 and 4 days postinfection. They migrate into the trachea at 6 days, copulate at 7 days, and reach maturity by 13 days postinfection. Eggs are first found in the tracheal mucus 13 days postinfection.

Pathogenicity. Morbidity of 80% with a mortality of 20% has been reported in a flock of domestic geese near Duluth, Minnesota (41). The course of the disease extended over a period of 5 mo, during which time the birds showed signs of respiratory distress by throwing back their heads and gaping for air. Severely affected birds died soon after the appearance of respiratory disturbances. The signs were similar to those of laryngotracheitis. Recovered birds showed growth retardation.

Experimentally infected domestic geese developed bronchitis of the primary, secondary, and tertiary bronchi (37). During prepatency, hyperplasia of the epithelium of the primary bronchi was the predominant lesion. During patency, generalized pneumonitis was most prominent in response to the aspirated nematode eggs. Feeding worms infected with the parasite caused dyspnea and mortality in 6-wk-old mandarin ducks (108). Similar worms from the same source were found to harbor 4–5 nematode larvae each.

SYNGAMUS TRACHEA (MONTAGU 1811) CHAPIN 1925, SYNGAMIDAE

Synonyms. *S. gracilis* Chapin 1925; *S. parvis* Chapin 1925.

Hosts. *S. trachea* has been reported in chicken, turkey, goose, guinea fowl, pheasant, peafowl, and quail.

Location. *S. trachea* may be found in the trachea, bronchi, and bronchioles.

Morphology. *S. trachea* is sometimes designated as "redworm" because of its color, or "forked worm" because the male and female are in permanent copulation so that they appear like the letter Y (Fig. 33.25A). *S. trachea* has an orbicular mouth, with a hemispheric chitinous capsule, usually with eight sharp teeth at the base; the mouth is surrounded by a chitinous plate, the outer margin of which is incised to form six festoons opposite each other. The male is 2–6 mm in length and 200-μm wide; the bursa is obliquely truncated, and is provided with rays, sometimes with strikingly asymmetrical dorsal rays; spicules are equal, slender, short, and 57–64 μm in length. The female is 5–20 mm in length (longer in the turkey) and 350-μm wide; the tail end is conical, bearing a pointed process; the vulva is prominent, about one-fourth of the body length from anterior end, but the position varies with age; and eggs are 90 × 49 μm, ellipsoidal, and operculated (Fig. 33.25B).

Life Cycle. The life history of this cosmopolitan is peculiar in that transmission from bird to bird may be successfully accomplished either directly (by the feeding of embryonated eggs or infective larvae) or indirectly (by ingestion of earthworms containing free or encysted gapeworm larvae they had obtained by feeding on contaminated soil). The female gapeworm deposits eggs through the vulvar opening underneath the bursa of the attached male onto the lumen of the trachea. The eggs reach the mouth cavity, are swallowed, and pass to the outside in the droppings. Following a period of incubation of approximately 8–14 days under optimum conditions of moisture and temperature, eggs embryonate, and soon after some may hatch, with the larvae living free in the soil. The earthworms *Eisenia foetidus* and *Allolobophora caliginosus* become infected with gapeworm larvae. Within the earthworm, the larvae penetrate the intestinal wall, enter the body cavity, and finally invade the body musculature in which they may encyst for an indefinite period. Gapeworm larvae in the earthworm remain infective to young chickens for as long as 4⅓ years. Slugs and snails may also serve as transfer or auxiliary hosts of larvae, and live larvae have been recovered from snails over a year after infection. Snails are not true intermediate hosts in the strict sense, since they are not necessary for the transfer of gapeworms to other bird hosts. *S. trachea* taken from various wild and domestic birds were more readily transferred to young chickens and with a greater degree of success if the earthworm was employed as an intermediary.

Some infective larvae penetrate the wall of the crop and esophagus and then penetrate the lungs directly. The majority, however, penetrate the duodenum and are carried to the lungs by the portal bloodstream via the liver and heart (6, 35). Larvae are found in the liver as early as 2 hr postinoculation and in the lungs as early as 4 hr. Larvae probably break out of the capillaries in the lung into the interlobular connective tissue and migrate into the parabronchia and atria via air capillaries. Molting and development to the adult stage can occur as early as 4 days postinfection, with copulation by 5 days in pheasants. Copulation of the worms in the chicken is seen 1 day later. Larvae can be recovered in the lungs up to 7 days. Worms are also found in the parabronchi and secondary bronchi up to 9 days. Adults enter the trachea as early as 7 days, and males are firmly attached to the tracheal wall by 11 days postinfection. Approximately 2 wk are required for the infective larvae to reach sexual maturity and for eggs to appear in the droppings. Although the role played by wild birds in the spread of gapeworm disease is still undecided, wild birds probably do not spread gapeworm disease in this country.

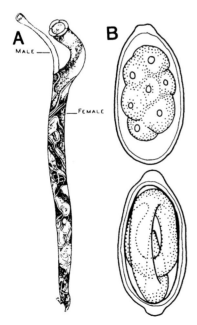

33.25. *Syngamus trachea.* A. Male and female worms. (After Wehr) B. Egg.

Pathogenicity. In the United States, *S. trachea* is the causative agent of "gapes" (labored breathing due to parasites) in chickens, turkeys, peacocks, and pheasants (Fig. 33.26); *Cyathostoma bronchialis* is the causative agent of this disease in geese.

In artificial rearing of pheasants, gapes is a serious menace in the United States. Confinement rearing of young birds has reduced the problem in chickens compared to a few years ago. However, this parasite continues to present an occasional problem with turkeys raised on range.

Young birds are most seriously affected with gapeworms. The rapidly growing worms soon obstruct the lumen of the trachea and cause the birds to suffocate. Turkey poults, baby chicks, and pheasant chicks are most susceptible to infection. Turkey poults usually develop gapeworm signs earlier and begin to die sooner after gapeworm infection than young chickens. Experimentally infected guinea fowls, pigeons, and ducks do not exhibit characteristic signs of gapeworm infections. Full-grown birds rarely show characteristic signs unless heavily infected.

Birds infected with gapeworms show signs of weakness and emaciation and usually spend much of their time with eyes closed and head drawn back against the body. From time to time, they throw their heads forward and upward and open the mouth wide to draw in air. An infected bird may give its head a convulsive shake in an attempt to remove the obstruction from the trachea so that normal breathing may be resumed. Little or no food is taken by

birds in the advanced stages of infection, and death usually ensues.

Examination of the trachea of infected birds shows that the mucous membrane is extensively irritated and inflamed; coughing is apparently the result of this irritation to the mucous lining. Lesions are usually found in the trachea of turkeys and pheasants, but seldom if ever in the trachea of young chickens and guinea fowl. These lesions or nodules are produced as a result of an inflammatory reaction at the site of attachment of the male worm, which remains permanently attached to the tracheal wall throughout the duration of its life. The female worms apparently detach and reattach from time to time in order to obtain a more abundant supply of food. Studies with radioactive isotopes have shown that the net blood loss with *S. trachea* is minimal. A marked heterophilia, monocytosis, eosinophilia, lymphocytopenia, and a decreased pack cell volume in infected turkey poults has been reported (46).

NEMATODES OF THE EYE

OXYSPIRURA MANSONI COBBOLD 1879, THELAZIIDAE

Hosts. *O. mansoni* has been reported in chicken, turkey, duck, grouse, guinea fowl, peafowl, pigeon, and quail.

Location. *O. mansoni* may be found beneath the nictitating membrane, conjunctival sacs, and nasolacrimal ducts.

Morphology. The body of *O. mansoni* is attenuated at both ends, anterior rounded, posterior pointed; the cuticle is smooth; there are no membranous appendages; the mouth is circular, surrounded by a six-lobed chitinous ring with two lateral and four submedian papillae in relation to the clefts of this ring; there are two pairs of subdorsal and one pair of subventral teeth in the mouth cavity; the buccal cavity has a short wide anterior portion and a long narrow posterior portion (Fig. 33.27A). The male is 8.2–16 mm in length and 350-μm wide; the tail is curved ventrally, without alae; there are four pairs of preanal and two pairs of postanal papillae; spicules are unequal (Fig. 33.27B), one 3–4.55 mm in length, and the other, 180–240 μm. The female is 12–20 mm in length and 270–430 μm in width; the vulva is 0.78–1.55 mm; the anus is 400–530 μm from the tip of the tail (Fig. 33.27C); and eggs are embryonated when deposited, 50–65 × 45 μm (Fig. 33.27D).

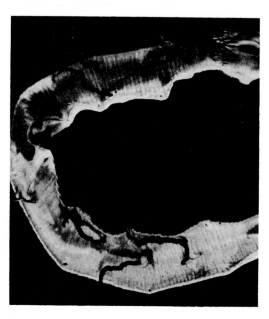

33.26. *Syngamus trachea.* Trachea showing attached gapeworms. (After Wehr)

Life Cycle. Eggs of the mature female worm are deposited in the eyes of the bird host, washed

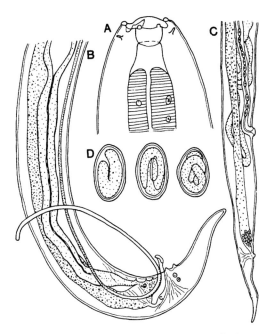

33.27. *Oxyspirura mansoni. A.* Head. *B.* Male tail. *C.* Female tail. *D.* Eggs. (*B-D* after Ransom)

down the tear ducts, swallowed, and passed in the droppings. The cockroach *Pycnoscelus (Leucophaea) surinamensis,* which is an omnivorous feeder, ingests the nematode eggs in the feces. Within approximately 50 days, the body cavity of the cockroach contains mature larvae, which are capable of infecting a susceptible host. Mature larvae are often contained within cysts deep in the adipose tissue or along the course of the alimentary tract of the insect host. Some larvae release themselves from the capsules and are found free in the body cavity and legs of the cockroach. When an infected cockroach is swallowed by a chicken or other susceptible host, the infective larva is freed in the crop, passes up the esophagus to the mouth and through the nasolacrimal duct to the eye.

Various wild birds become infected with the eyeworm of poultry and may serve as sources of infection for domestic birds. Such birds as the blackbird (*Agelaius phoeniceus*), bobolink (*Dolichonyx oryzivorus*), wild pigeon (*Columbia livia*), loggerhead shrike (*Lanius ludovicianus*), and blue jay (*Aphelocoma cyanea*) have been experimentally infected with the eyeworm of poultry. The eyeworm occurs naturally in the English sparrow, mynah, Chinese dove, Japanese quail, and pheasant (*Phasianus torquatus torquatus* and *P. versicolor versicolor*) in Hawaii. In Hawaii, the local wild birds appear to be of little importance in the dissemination of this poultry parasite (83).

Pathogenicity. Infected birds show a peculiar ophthalmia. They appear uneasy and continuously scratch at the eyes, which are usually watery and show severe inflammation. The nictitating membrane becomes swollen, projects slightly beyond the eyelids at the corners of the eyes, and is usually kept in continual motion, as if trying to remove some foreign object from the eye. The eyelids sometimes become stuck together, and a white cheesy material collects beneath them. If left untreated, severe ophthalmia may develop; as a result the eyeball may be destroyed. The worms are seldom, if ever, found in the eyes when severe signs are manifested, presumably due to unfavorable conditions existing there.

Oxyspirura petrowi Skryjabin 1929, Thelaziidae

Synonym. *O. lumsdeni* Addison and Anderson 1969.

Hosts. *O. petrowi* has been reported in grouse, pheasant, and prairie chicken.

Location. *O. petrowi* may be found beneath the nictitating membrane of eye.

Morphology. The body of *O. petrowi* is slender, yellow to cream color, bluntly rounded anteriorly, and attenuated posteriorly; cervical alae are present, with the cuticle transversely striated; the mouth has four submedian pairs and three circumoral pairs of cephalic papillae; there is an undivided cuticularized bursal capsule. The male is 6.3–8.6 mm in length and 185–330 μm in width; the right spicule is 121–320 μm in length and slender with a sharp tip. The female is 7.7–12.3 μm in length and 200–455 μm in width; the vulva is 500–700 μm from tip of tail; the anus is 242–400 μm from the posterior extremity; and eggs are embryonated and 35–44 μm × 15–31 μm.

Life Cycle. Over 70 species of *Oxyspirura* have been described as parasites in the eyes of birds. Of these species, only three, *O. mansoni. O. petrowi,* and *O. pusillae,* have been reported from North America north of Mexico. *O. petrowi* is a species of wide geographic range. It shows little host specificity (74) and has been found in 14 species of wild birds in Louisiana and five species in Michigan. Although this species has not been reported from the chicken, it is found in grouse and prairie chickens.

Pathogenicity. Infection with *O. petrowi* produces a condition similar to that seen with *O. mansoni.*

TISSUE-DWELLING NEMATODES OUTSIDE OF THE ENTERIC TRACT

APROCTELLA STODDARDI CRAM 1931, DIPETALONEMATIDAE

Synonym.   *Microfilaria fallisi* Brinkmann 1950.

Hosts.   *A. stoddardi* has been reported in turkey, dove, and quail. This species has been recovered from the bobwhite quail in the southern United States and from grouse in New England.

Location.   *A. stoddardi* may be found in the body cavity.

Morphology.   The body of *A. stoddardi* is slender; the cuticle divided into four fields, two medians longitudinally striated, two laterals smooth; the mouth is simple without definite lips (Fig. 33.28A). The male is 6–7.6 mm in length and 60–140 μm in width; the spicules are stout and curved, the right is 50–60 μm, and the left, 73–90 μm (Fig. 33.28B); and caudal papillae are absent. The female is 13–16.5 mm in length and 71–260 μm in width; the vulva is 1.3–1.6 mm from the anterior end, not opening on protuberance; the anus is 140–180 μm from the caudal extremity; and there are no eggs,

and unsheathed larvae are in uteri.

Life Cycle.   The life cycle is unknown, but a biting arthropod is hypothesized as intermediate host.

Pathogenicity.   Small numbers of *A. stoddardi* are not pathogenic; however, heavy infection may result in mortality in doves. A granulomatous pericarditis has also been reported.

SINGHFILARIA HAYESI ANDERSON AND PRESTWOOD 1969, ONCHOCERCIDAE

Hosts.   *S. hayesi* have been reported in turkey and quail, and have been recovered from the wild turkey in the southern United States, thus representing a potential problem in the domestic turkey.

Location.   *S. hayesi* may be found in subcutaneous tissues in the region of the esophagus, crop, and trachea.

Morphology.   *S. hayesi* have no structures on head (Fig. 33.29A); the cuticle have innumerable tiny, transverse thickenings. The male is 13.6-mm long and 250-μm wide; spicules are markedly dissimilar, the right is tooth shaped, 81-μm long, and the left, 125-μm long, divided into broad shaft and blade and short filament (Fig. 33.29B); the anus is subterminal, 28 μm from caudal extremity; the caudal papillae consist of one large pair postanal papillae and one large medial papilla anterior to anus. The female is 35–40 mm in length and 420–500 μm wide; the vulva is 390–400 μm from the cephalic extremity; and there are microfilariae in uteri.

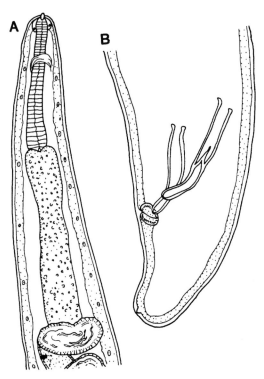

33.28.   *Aproctella stoddardi*. *A*. Head. *B*. Male tail. (After Anderson)

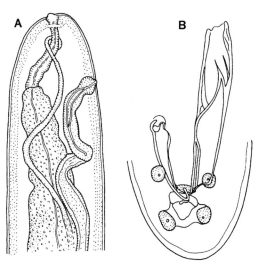

33.29.   *Singhfilaria hayesi*. *A*. Head. *B*. Mail tail. (After Anderson and Prestwood)

Life Cycle. The life cycle of *S. hayesi* is unknown.

Pathogenicity. Few pathologic lesions are found.

OTHER TISSUE-DWELLING NEMATODES.
The guinea worm *Avioserpens taiwana* (Sugimoto 1919) Chabaud, Campana, and Truong-Tan-Ngoc 1950 causes fibrous tumors in the subcutaneous tissue under the mandible and on the thigh of domestic ducks in Asia.

Fifteen genera of filaroids that infect birds have been recognized (3). Many species are not host specific. *Cardiofilaria pavlovsky*; and *Aproctella stoddardi* have been reported from at least seven families of birds. In general, filaroids cause little problems in domestic poultry. Those species shown in Table 33.1 are from game birds in North America. Other species that infect chickens but have not been reported in North America include the following: from India, *Aprocta babamii* Bhalerae and Rao 1944 from the heart, *Cardiofilaria mhowensis* (Jain, Alwar, Adwadhiya, and Pandit 1965) from the body cavity, and experimentally *Chandlerella quiscali* (Linstow 1904) Robinson 1971 (3).

Baylisascaris procynois and *Baylisascaris columnaris* from raccoons and skunks, respectively, are reported to cause avian cerebrospinal nematodiasis in a variety of birds including the chicken, bush turkey, partridge, and quail. This disease has been experimentally produced in chickens (54).

PREVENTION AND CONTROL.
Modern poultry practices, especially confinement rearing of broilers and pullets and caging of laying hens, have significantly influenced the quantity and variety of nematode infections in poultry. Many that caused extensive problems in "backyard" or "farmyard" flocks are seldom seen in commercial operations. Others such as *Ascaridia* are still found in older birds. In addition, increased pen-rearing of game birds has led to increasing nematode problems in these species.

For most nematodes, control measures consist of sanitation and breaking the life cycle, rather than chemotherapy. Confinement rearing on litter largely prevents infections with nematodes using outdoor intermediate hosts such as earthworms or grasshoppers. Conversely, nematodes with direct life cycles or those that utilize indoor intermediate hosts such as beetles may prosper. Treatment of the soil or litter to kill intermediate hosts may be beneficial (67). Insecticides suitable for litter treatment include carbaryl, tetrachlorvinphos (stirofos), or ronnel; however, treatment is usually made only between growouts. Extreme care should be taken to ensure that feed and water are not contaminated. Treatment

of soil on ranges to kill ova is only partially successful. Changing of litter can reduce infections, but oil treatment of floors is not very effective. After the old litter has been removed, spraying with permethrin or Ravap[R] (a mixture of Rabon and Vapona) has proven effective for beetle control. Edgar (24) feels that changing litter is unnecessary if medication is given on a regular basis.

Raising different species or different ages of birds together or in close proximity is a dangerous procedure as regards parasitism. Adult turkeys that are carriers of gapeworms can transmit the disease to young chicks or pheasants, although older chickens are almost entirely resistant to infection.

Chemotherapy. Because of economics, investigations into the efficacy of chemotherapy have been limited to parasites widespread enough to suggest a potential drug market. The increasing cost of testing to obtain Food and Drug Administration (FDA) approval for new compounds or new uses for approved compounds also makes unlikely future studies on chemical control of rare or infrequently occurring nematodes. Investigations may continue on the ascarids, capillarids, heterakids, and *Syngamus*. The reported types of drugs, effective levels, and means of administering compounds for control of these parasites vary considerably. Only certain compounds have been approved by the FDA. Poultry producers should be aware that the use of unapproved drugs is not legal in birds that will produce eggs or meat for market, and that approvals for drugs and levels are continually changing. Recent regulatory changes concerning the extra-label use of drugs not specifically approved in food animals have been made in the United States. These regulatory changes may affect the poultry industry. Commercial poultry operations should contact the attending veterinarian concerning the use of any extra-label durgs. Extreme care should be taken to obtain current information from appropriate sources before any medication is used. Label directions and dosages should be followed explicitly.

ASCARIDIA

APPROVED COMPOUNDS. Drugs currently approved for use in chickens are Hygromycin B or coumaphos in feed, or piperazine in feed or water. Only piperazine is approved for turkeys. Hygromycin B is fed at a level of 0.00088 0.00132%. Coumaphos is only approved for use in replacements (0.004%) or layers (0.003%). It is more commonly used for control of capillarids (see below) than for ascarids.

Piperazine compounds have been widely adopted as a method of treatment for ascaridiasis, since they are practically nontoxic. Piperazine may be administered to chickens in the feed (0.2–0.4%), water (0.1–0.2%) or as a single treatment (50–100 mg/bird). The rate for feed or water medication in turkeys is the same, however the single treatment dose is 100 mg/bird (under 12 wk) and 100–400 mg/bird (over 12 wk). A high concentration of piperazine in contact with worms at a given time is very important for maximum elimination. Therefore, to be most effective, piperazine should be consumed by birds in a period of a few hr. Piperazine in drinking water is the most practical method of application for commercial flocks. Since piperazine is available as a wide variety of salts, the level should be calculated on the basis of milligrams of active piperazine (25). Piperazine compounds exert a narcotizing effect, thus enabling worms to be removed by means of naturally occurring peristalsis. The worms are expelled alive. A combination of piperazine (0.11%) and phenothiazine (0.50–0.56%) as a 1-day treatment only is used for removal of both heterakids and ascarids.

EXPERIMENTAL DATA. Piperazine citrate administered at the rate of 8, 10, and 16 g/gal of drinking water for 1–4 days effectively removed all ascarids but not heterakids (9, 84). Piperazine carbon bisulfide, piperazine adipate, and piperazine citrate, tested against *A. galli* in chickens, completely eliminated all adult worms (45). The compounds were administered as single doses of 100–500 mg/kg body weight. Fenbendazole at 8–10 mg/kg for 3 or 4 days was also effective (87). Fenbendazole administered in the feed at the level of 30 ppm for 4 days or 60 ppm for 3 days was reported to have 100% efficacy against *A. galli* in chickens (75, 105). The same drug was as effective in eliminating *A. dissimilis* from experimentally infected turkeys when administered at 30 ppm for 3 or 6 days (69, 106).

Poultry producers sometimes utilize knowledge of the *Ascaridia* life cycle to plan a routine medication program at fixed time periods, rather than waiting until worms are present. This is most beneficial when large numbers of *A. galli* eggs are present in built-up litter.

EXPERIMENTAL COMPOUNDS. The three common nematodes of the chicken, *Ascaridia galli, Heterakis gallinarum,* and *Capillaria obsignata,* were effectively removed with 40 mg/kg of body weight of dl-tetramisole (10, 91). Levotetramizole (levamisole) given to turkeys naturally infected with *A. dissimilis, H. gallinarum,* and *C. obsignata* at the rate of 30 mg/kg of body weight was also effective (52). Levels of 0.06% or 0.03% levamisole in the drinking water removed 99% of adult *A. dissimilis,* 94–98% of larval *A. dissimilis,* and 99–100% of *H. gallinarum* and *C. obsignata* (73). Twenty-five milligrams per kilogram were found to

be effective (13). Levamisole hydrochloride eliminated 92% of the fourth-stage larvae and 96% of the adult *A. galli* in experimentally infected chickens, while pyrantel pamoate had a much lower level of efficacy for both larvae and adults (96). Levamisole, when given orally two times weekly at a rate of 40 mL/kg of body weight, was effective against mixed infection of *A. galli* and *T. tenuis* (56).

Pyrantel tartrate has a high efficacy against *A. galli* and some against *C. obsignata.* A single dose of 15–25 mg/kg body weight gave 99.6–100% removal of all adult *A. galli* from chicks, but was relatively ineffective against the larval stages (72).

CAPILLARIA

APPROVED COMPOUNDS. Coumaphos and Hygromycin B are both approved but only for use in chickens. Coumaphos is given to replacement pullets in the feed (0.004%) for 10–14 days prior to the onset of egg production. This treatment is repeated a minimum of 3 wk after the previous treatment if the birds are maintained on contaminated litter or exposed to infected birds. It is given to layers (0.003%) for 14 days as needed, but no sooner than 3 wk after the end of the preceding treatment. Hygromycin B may be administered in the feed at the rate of 8–12 g/ton (0.000882–0.00132%) but should be withdrawn 3 days prior to slaughter. Coumaphos (Meldane) was reported (26) to have activity against *A. galli, H. gallinarum, C. obsignata.*

EXPERIMENTAL COMPOUNDS. Capillariasis due to *C. obsignata* could be controlled in pigeons and chickens by administration of 1 cc of 10% methyridine solution subcutaneously in the pectoral region or into the leg (pigeon) and dorsal regions between the wings (chickens) (90). These authors stated that this drug must be administered with great care: 1) spilling of the drug on the skin may produce a small lesion; 2) nausea, slight ataxia, and incoordination were observed to some degree even with subeffective doses; and 3) death may sometimes result. The drug has no marked effect on coccidiosis and trichomoniasis and was only slightly effective against *Ascaridia.* Methyridine is an excellent drug for the removal of adults and larvae of *C. obsignata* from chickens (43, 44, 68).

Fenbendazole was reported to be over 97% effective in removing experimental infections of *C. obsignata* when administered to turkeys at 45 ppm for 6 days (69). A more significant efficacy (>99%) was reported by Pote and Yazwinski (75) with the same parasite in chickens. Other research has indicated slightly lower efficacies when chickens were fed Fenbendazole at 80 ppm for 3 days or 48 ppm for 5 days (105).

Methyridine injected subcutaneously beneath the

wing as a 5% aqueous solution was an effective anthelmintic for the removal of *C. obsignata* from the pigeon (103). Injections of 25–45 mg methyridine per bird were 99–100% effective against *C. obsignata* in naturally infected birds, but doses of 23 mg per bird removed only 62% of the worms. The anthelmintic action of the drug was relatively rapid, as indicated by elimination of the majority of the worms within 24 hr after treatment. Maretin (*N*-hydroxynaphthalimide diethy phosphate) was more effective than Coumaphos against *C. obsignata* in quail (23).

Individual doses of 25 and 50 mg/kg body weight of haloxon against *Capillaria* infections in chickens eliminated practically all the worms (12). Doses of 50–60 mg/kg haloxon were effective against adult worms, but larvae and immature stages were less sensitive (68). Piperazine citrate, phenothiazine, thiabendazole, and bephenium were inactive against *C. obsignata*.

Haloxon was apparently 46–100% effective against *C. contorta* in quail when administered at levels of 0.05–0.5% of the feed for 5–7 days (15). Results were best at the 0.075–0.5% levels. However, the highest concentration was toxic, and one-fourth of the birds died. Single oral doses of the drug were not uniformly effective and produced undesirable side effects, primarily ataxia.

Fenbendazole administered in the feed at the rate of 80 ppm for 3 consecutive days was found to have >99% efficacy in eliminating *C. obsignata* in broiler breeder hens (89). Efficacy greater than 99% was also achieved at 30 ppm for 6 days (75). An efficacy level in excess of 97% was obtained when experimentally infected turkeys were fed 45 ppm for 6 days (69).

HETERAKIS

APPROVED COMPOUNDS. Hygromycin B and Coumaphos (see above) are also approved for use in chickens but not in turkeys.

EXPERIMENTAL DATA. Phenothiazine is highly effective in the control of cecal worms in chickens (0.5 g/bird) and turkeys (1 g/bird) when given for 1 day only. Hygromycin B is approved for use in chickens when administered in the feed at 8–12 g/ton (0.00082–0.00132%). This product is not approved for turkeys. The drug must be withdrawn from the feed 3 days prior to slaughter.

Coumaphos is approved only for chickens and is administered at either 0.003% for layers or 0.004% for replacement chickens. The treatment regimen consists of continuous administration for 10–14 days prior to the onset of egg production. If the birds are exposed to contaminated litter, an additional treatment period of 10–14 days is repeated 3 wk after the first period. The same regimen is used for laying birds, but the drug is used at the lower level (0.003%).

Phenothiazine in 1-g doses removed 94% of the heterakids, but only 24% of the ascarids (14). Piperazine citrate, given by capsule in single doses containing 200 mg of piperazine, removed 66% of the heterakids and was completely effective against the ascarids. Single 1-g doses of a 7:1 mixture or a 12:1 mixture of phenothiazine and piperazine, however, removed 94% of the heterakids and 91% of the ascarids. It seems, therefore, that the combination of the two drugs is more effective against these roundworms than is either alone.

Hygromycin B has been used extensively in controlling combinations of ascaridiasis, heterakidiasis, and capillariasis. It shows greatest efficacy against *H. gallinarum* and may completely eliminate this nematode when fed at the rate of 0.0018–0.0026% for a period of 2 mo or longer. Reductions in worm numbers of *A. galli* and *C. obsignata* are less dramatic, but continuous use in successive flocks grown in the same house may drastically reduce worm numbers and can improve egg production. Economic benefits (including drug costs) have not been fully demonstrated, but the product has been found useful in cases in which few other drugs are cleared for use. Hygromycin B has found some acceptance on pen-raised game bird farms where losses due to intestinal nematodes have been severe. Fenbendazole had 100% efficacy in turkeys experimentally infected with *H. gallinarum* and given 120 ppm for 3 days or 45 ppm for 6 days (69). The compound had the same efficacy at 30 ppm for 6 days or 60 ppm for 3 days in experimentally infected chickens (75). A separate study indicated 100% efficacy could be achieved when experimentally infected birds were given 30 ppm Fenbendazole for 5 days (105).

SYNGAMUS

APPROVED COMPOUNDS. Thiabendazole is currently approved for use in pheasants only at a level of 0.05% for 2 wk.

EXPERIMENTAL COMPOUNDS. Thiabendazole is effective when administered to turkeys in the feed. Mash containing 0.5% thiabendazole fed to 4-wk-old turkey poults for 9–20 days removed 98% of the gapeworms from 117 birds (100). The drug appeared effective, whether treatment was initiated on postinfection day 30 or started on the day of infection. Continuous medication of pen-reared birds at levels of 0.1–4% has been recommended, but is not economical.

Several other compounds have been shown effective against *Syngamus*. Mebendazole (methyl *N*-[5-(6)-benzoyl-2-benzimidazolyl] carbonate) was 100% efficacious when fed prophylactically at 0.0064% and curatively at 0.0125% to turkey poults

(92). A level of 0.044% for 14 days has also been effective.

Cambendazole [5-(isopropoxycarbonyl-amino-2) (4-thizolyl)-benzimidazole] was found to be more efficacious than thiabendazole or disophenol (2,6-diiodo-4-nitrophenol) (29). The level of control with three treatments of cambendazole on days 3–4, 6–7, and 16–17 postinfection was 94.9% in chickens (2 × 50 mg/kg) and 99.1% in turkeys (2 × 20 mg/kg).

Levamisole at a1 level of 0.04% fed for 2 days or 2 g/gal drinking water for 1 day each mo has proven effective in game birds. Fenbendazole at 20 mg/kg for 3 to 4 days is also effective (87).

OTHER NEMATODES. *Amidostomum anseris* in geese can be treated with a variety of compounds. Cambendazole (60 mg/kg) was the most effective against both adults and larvae (30). Pyrantel (100 mg/kg) was effective against adults. Some success was also obtained with citarin (40 mg/kg). Mebendazole at 10 mg/kg given for 3 consecutive days completely eliminated *A. anseris* (32). Fenbendazole is also effective.

Tetramisole is not effective against *Dispharynx nasuta*, although mebendazole has some efficacy. *Subulura brumpti* can be partially controlled with several different tin compounds or tetramisole. Tetramisole also has some effect against *Strongyloides avium*. Piperazine has been used against *Tetrameres fissispina*.

Trichostrongylus tenuis can be controlled by cambendazole (30 mg/kg), pyrantel tartrate (50 mg/kg), thiabendazole (75 mg/kg), and citarin (40 mg/kg) (31). Mebendazole was completely effective at 10 mg/kg given for 3 consecutive days (32).

ACANTHOCEPHALANS

The Acanthocephala, or thorny-headed worms, are parasites occurring as adults in the intestinal tract of vertebrates.

They are elongate, roughly cylindrical, or spindle shaped. Several distinct body regions are recognizable; retractile proboscis, neck, and body proper. The retractile proboscis always bears a considerable number of recurved hooks arranged in rows. The number, form, and arrangement of the hooks are valuable diagnostic characteristics. The body proper forms the major portion of the worm. It is usually unarmed but may bear small spines of definite form and arrangement on some portion of the external surface. This group of worms is deprived of a digestive tract. Nutrition is provided for entirely by absorption through the body wall. The sexes are separate in all cases. The male is smaller and more slender than the female and often distinguished externally by a bell-shaped bursa that surrounds the genital pore.

So far as is known, all species of Acanthocephala require one or more intermediate hosts before reaching a stage of development at which they are infective for the final host. Various arthropods, snakes, lizards, and amphibians serve as hosts of the larval stages. Seasonal fluctuations in acanthocephalan populations have been seen in both wild and domestic ducks. It was speculated that these flucuations were due to the accessibility of water (85).

Only four species of thorny-headed worms have been reported as parasites of domestic poultry in North America, three of these as immature forms.

ONCICOLA CANIS KAUPP 1909. *Oncicola canis* (Kaupp 1909) was found in about 10% of the young turkeys around San Angelo, Texas (Fig. 33.30). The worms were encysted under the epithelial lining of the esophagus in numbers varying from a few to 100 or more. They were reported as the possible cause of death.

Adults occur in the dog and coyote. The presence of larval forms in young turkeys suggests that such occurrences are accidental, the young worms encysting when taken into an unsuitable host.

Larvae of *Oncicola oncicola*, a parasite of South American jungle cats have been recovered from chickens in Costa Rica.

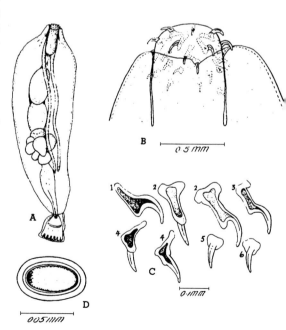

33.30. *Oncicola canis. A.* Male showing reproductive organs. *B.* Proboscis. *C.* Hooks from proboscis (numerals indicate row). *D.* Egg. (Price)

***PROSTHORHYNCHUS FORMOSUS* (VAN CLEAVE 1918) TRAVASSOS 1926.** A synonym for this species is *Plagiorhynchus formosus*. An immature male and two female specimens of *P. formosus* Van-Cleave 1918 were reported from the small intestine of a chicken collected at Vineland, New Jersey. Other bird hosts from which this species has been reported are the flicker (Bowie, Maryland), crow (Washington, D.C.), and robin (New Jersey) (Fig. 33.31). Several authors have suggested that this species is a potential hazard to domestic poultry; however, the level of experimental infections in chickens and turkeys is low (82).

***POLYMORPHUS BOSCHADIS* (SCHRANK 1788).** This worm (Fig. 33.32) has been reported from the duck in Canada. It causes serious injury and death in domesticated waterfowl, especially in young birds. It causes an inflammation of the intestine with subsequent anemia and cachexia. The birds are sick only a short time, the gait is staggering, and the head and wings droop.

OTHER ACANTHOCEPHALANS FROM POULTRY.
Other species infecting chickens, but not found in North America, include *Leipera-*

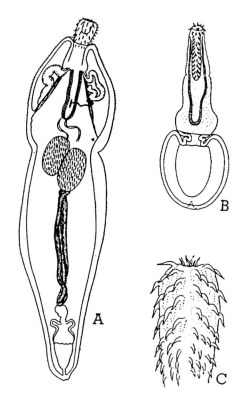

33.32. *Polymorphus boschadis. A.* Male. *B.* Larva from *Gamarus pulex. C.* Proboscis of larva. (Luhe)

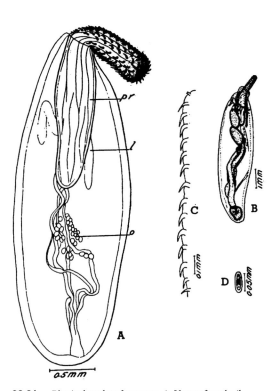

33.31. *Plagiorhynchus formosus. A.* Young female (l, lemniscus; o, ovary; pr, proboscis receptacle). (Jones) *B.* Male. *C.* Hooks from proboscis. *D.* Egg. (VanCleave)

canthus gallinarum, Mediorhynchus gallinarum, and *Neoschongastia gallinarum* in Asia; subcutaneous larvae of *Macracanthorhynchus hirudinaceus* in chickens in Brazil; *Prosthorhynchus transversus* in many passerine birds as well as the partridge and pheasant in Europe. The latter is experimentally infective for chickens.

REFERENCES
1. Addison, E.M., and R.C. Anderson. 1969. A review of the eye worms of the genus Oxyspirura (Nematode: Spiruroidea). J Wildl Dis 55:1–58.
2. Allen, R.W., and E.E. Wehr. 1942. Earthworm as possible intermediate host of Capillaria caudinflata of the chicken and turkey. Proc Helminthol Soc Wash 9:72–73.
3. Anderson, R.C., and O. Bain. 1976. CIH Keys to the Nematode Parasites of Vertebrates. No. 3. Keys to genera of the order Spirurida. Part 3. Diplotriaenoiden, Aprocloidea and Filarioidea. Commonwealth Agri Bureau, Farnham Royal, Bucks England.
4. Barus, V. 1970. Studies of the nematode Subulura sactoria II. Development in the intermediate host. Folia Parasitol (Prague) 17:49–59.
5. Barus, V. 1970. Studies on the Nematode Subulura sactoria. Folia Parasitol (Prague) 17:191–199.
6. Barus, V. and K. Blazek. 1965. Revision Der Exogenen Und Endogenen Phase Des Entwicklungszyklus Und Der Pathogenitat Von Syngamus (Syngamus) trachea (Montagu, 1811) Chapin, 1925 IM Organismus Des Endwirtes. Cesk Parasitol 12:47–70.

7. Barus, V. and K. Blazek. 1970. Studies on the nematode Subulura sactoria III. Development in the definitive host. Folia Parasitol (Prague) 17:141–151.

8. Berghen, P. 1966 Serum protein changes in Capillaria obsignata infections. Exp Parasitol 19:34–41.

9. Bradley, R.E. 1955. Observations on the anthelmintic effect of piperazine citrate in chickens. Vet Med 50:444–446.

10. Bruynooghe, D., D. Thienpont, and O.F.J. van Parijs. 1968. Use of tetramisole as an anthelmintic in poultry. Vet Rec 82:701–706.

11. Chubb, L.G., B.M. Freeman, and D. Wakelin. 1964. The effect of Capillaria obsignata, Madsen, 1945, on the vitamin A and ascorbic acid metabolism in the domestic fowl. Res Vet Sci 5:154–160.

12. Clarke, M.L. 1962. A mixture of diaveridine and sulphaquin-oxaline as a coccidiostat for poultry. I. Preliminary studies on efficiency against Eimeria tenella and E. necatrix infections and on toxicity in poultry. Vet Rec 74:845–848.

13. Clarkson, M.J. and M.K. Beg. 1970. The anthelmintic activity of L-tetramisole against Ascaridia galli and Capillaria obsignata in the fowl. Vet Rec 86:652–654.

14. Colglazier, M.L., A.O. Foster, F.D. Enzie, and D.E. Thompson. 1960. The anthelmintic action of phenothiazine and piperazine against Heterakis gallinae and Ascaridia galli in chickens. J Parasitol 46:267–270.

15. Colglazier, M.L., E.E. Wehr, R.H. Burtner, and L.M. Wiest, Jr. 1967. Haloxon as an anthelmintic against the cropworm Capillaria contorta in quail. Avian Dis 11:257–260.

16. Cram, E.B. 1927. Bird parasites of the nematode suborders Strongylata, Ascaridata and Spirurata. US Nat Mus Bull 140.

17. Cram, E.B. 1929. A new roundworm parasite, Strongyloides avium of the chicken with observations of its life history and pathogenicity. North Am Vet 10:27–30.

18. Cram, E.B. 1931. Developmental stages of some nematodes of the Spiruroidea parasite in poultry and game birds. US Dept Agric Tech Bull No. 227:1–27

19. Cram, E.B. 1933. Observations on the life history of Tetrameres patterson. J Parasitol 10:97–98.

20. Cram, E.B., M.F. Jones, and E.A. Allen. 1931. In H.L. Stoddard (ed.). The Bobwhite Quail: Its Habits, Preservation, and Increase. Charles Scribner's Sons, New York, pp. 240–296.

21. Cuca, M., A.C. Todd, and M.L. Sunde. 1968. Effect of levels of calcium and lysine upon the growth of Ascaridia galli in chicks. J Nutr 94:83–88.

22. Cuckler, Ashton C. and J.E. Alicata. 1944. The life history of Subulura brumpti, a cecal nematode of poultry in Hawaii. Trans Am Microbiol Soc 63:345–357.

23. Dawe, D.L., J. Brown, R., B. Davis, and F.E. Kellogg. 1969. Effectiveness of maretin and meldane as treatments for capillariasis in Bob Whites. Avian Dis 13:662–667.

24. Edgar, S.A. 1976. Personal communication.

25. Edgar, S.A., D.C. Davis, and J.A. Frazier. 1957. The efficacy of some piperazine compounds in the elimination of helminths from experimentally- and naturally-infected poultry. Poult Sci 36:495–510.

26. Eleazer, T.H. 1969. Case Report Coumaphus, a new anthelmintic for control of Capillaria obsignata, Heterakis gallinarum and Ascaridia galli in chickens. Avian Dis 13:228–230.

27. Enigk, K., and A. Dey-Hazra. 1968. Die perkutane infektion bei Amidostomum anseris (Strongyloidea, Nematoda). Z Parasitenk 31:155–165.

28. Enigk, K., and A. Dey-Hazra. 1968. Zur wirtsspezifitat von Amidostomum anseris (Strongyloidea, Nematoda). Z Parasitenk 31:266–275.

29. Enigk, K., and A. Dey-Hazra. 1970. Zur Behandlung der Syngamose der Hühnervögel. Dtsch Tieraerztl Wochenschr 77:609–613.

30. Enigk, K., and A. Dey-Hazra. 1971. Zur Behandlung der häufigsten nematodeninfektionen des hausgeflügels. Dtsch Tieraerztl Wochenschr 78:178–181.

31. Enigk, K., and A. Dey-Hazra. 1971. Zur verbreitung und behandlung des Trichostrongylus tenuis Befalles. Berl Munch Tierarztl Wchnschr 84:11–14.

32. Enigk, K., A. Dey-Hazra, and J. Batke. 1973. Zur Wirksamkeit Von Mebendazol Bei Helminthosen Von Huhn und Gans. Avian Pathol 2:67–74.

33. Ewing, S.A., J.L. West, and A.L. Malle. 1967. Tetrameres sp. (Nematoda: Spiruridae) found in pigeons (Columba livia) in Kansas and Oklahoma. Avian Dis 11:407–412.

34. Farr, M.M. 1956. Survival of the protozoan parasite Histomonas meleagridis in feces of infected birds. Cornell Vet 46:178–187.

35. Fernando, M.A., P.H.G. Stockdale, and C. Remmler. 1971. The route of migration development and pathogenesis of Syngamus trachea (Montagu, 1811) Chapin, 1925, in pheasants. J Parasitol 57:107–116.

36. Fernando, M.A., I.J. Hoover, and S.G. Ogungbade. 1973. The migration and development of Cyatostoma bronchialis in geese. J Parasitol 59:759–764.

37. Fernando, M.A., P.H.G. Stockdale, and S.G. Ogungbade. 1973. Pathogenesis of the lesions caused by Cyathostoma bronchialis in the respiratory tract of geese. J Parasitol 59:980–986.

38. Flatt, R.E., and L.R. Nelson. 1969. Tetrameres americana in laboratory pigeons (Columba livia). Lab Anim Care 19:853–856.

39. Gibbs, B.J. 1962. The occurrence of the protozoan parasite Histomonas meleagridis in the adults and eggs of the cecel worm Heterakis gallinae. J Protozool 9:288–293.

40. Goble, F.C. and H.L. Kutz. 1945. Notes on the gapeworms (Nematoda: Syngamidae) of galliform and passeriform birds in New York State. J Parasitol 31:323–331.

41. Griffiths, H.J., R.M. Leary, and R. Fenstermacher. 1954. A new record for gapeworm (Cyathostoma bronchialis) infections of domestic geese in North America. Am J Vet Res 15:298–299.

42. Hemsley, R.V. 1971. Fourth stage Ascaridia spp. larvae associated with high mortality in turkeys. Can Vet J 12:147–149.

43. Hendriks, J. 1962. The use of promintic as anthelmintic against experimental infections of Capillaria obsignata Madsen, 1945, in chickens. Tijdschr Diergeneeskd 87:314–322.

44. Hendriks, J. 1963. Methyridine in the drinking water against Capillaria obsignata, Madsen, 1945, in experimentally infected chickens. Tijdschr Diergeneeskd 88:418–424.

45. Horton-Smith, C. and P.L. Long. 1956. The anthelmintic effect of three piperazine derivatives on Ascaridia galli (Schrank 1788). Poult Sci 35:606–614.

46. Hwang, J.C. 1964. Hemogram of turkey poults experimentally infected with Syngamus trachea. Avian Dis 8:380–390.

47. Ikeme, M.M. 1971. Observations on the pathogenicity and pathology of Ascaridia galli. Parasitology 63:169–179.

48. Ikeme, M.M. 1971. Effects of different levels of nutrition and continuing dosing of poultry with Ascaridia galli eggs on the subsequent development of parasite populations. Parasitology 63:233–250.

49. Ikeme, M.M. 1971. Weight changes in chickens placed on different levels of nutrition and varying degrees of repeated dosage with Ascaridia galli eggs. Parasitology 63:251–260.

50. Karunamoorthy, G., D.J. Chellappa, and R. Anandan. 1994. The life history of Subulura brumpti in the beetle Aliphitobius diaperinus. Indian Vet J 71:12–15.

51. Kates, K.C., and M.L. Colglazier. 1970. Differential morphology of adult Ascaridia galli (Schrank 1788) and Ascaridia dissimilis Perez Vigueras, 1931. Proc Helminthol Soc Wash 37:80–84.

52. Kates, K.C., M.L. Colglazier, and F.D. Enzie. 1969. Comparative efficacy of levo-tetramisole, parbendazole, and piperazine citrate against some common helminths of

turkeys. Trans Am Microsc Soc 88:142–148.

53. Kaushik, R.K., and V.P.S. Deorani. 1969. Studies on tissue responses in primary and subsequent infections with Heterakis gallinae in chickens and on the process of formation of caecal nodules. J Helminthol 43:69–78.

54. Kazacos, K.R., and W.L. Wirtz. 1983. Experimental cerebrospinal nematodiasis due to Baylisascaris procyonis in chickens. Avian Dis 27:55–65.

55. Kellogg, F.E., and J.P. Calpin. 1971. A checklist of parasites and diseases reported from the Bobwhite Quail. Avian Dis 15:704–715.

56. Kuczynska, E., I. Ziomko, and T. Cencek. 1994. Intestinal roundworm infections in broilers and hens. Medycyna-Weterynaryjna 50:30–31.

57. Lee, D.L., and P. Lestan. 1971. Oogenesis and egg shell formation in Heterakis gallinarum (Nematoda). Proc Zool Soc London 164:189–196.

58. Leiby, P.D., and O.W. Olsen. 1965. Life history studies on Nematodes of the genera Amidostomum (Strongloidea) and Epomidiostomum (Trichostrongyloidea) occurring in the gizzards of waterfowl. Proc Helminthol Soc Wash 32:32–49.

59. Levine, P.P. 1938. Infection of the chicken with Capillaria Columbae (RUD). J Parasitol 24:45–52.

60. Levine, N.D. 1980. Nematode Parasites of Domestic Animals and of Man, 2nd ed. Burgess Publishing Co., Minneapolis, MN.

61. Lund, E.E., and A.M. Chute. 1972. Reciprocal responses of eight species of galliform birds and three parasites: Heterakis gallinarum, Histomonas meleagridis and Parahistomonas wenrichi. J Parasitol 58:940–945.

62. Madsen, H. 1945. The species of (nematodes, Trichinelloidea) parasite in the digestive tract of Danish gallinaceous and anatine game birds, with a revised list of species of Capillaria in birds. Dan Rev Game Biol 1:1–112.

63. Madsen, H. 1950. Studies on species of Heterakis (nematodes) in birds. Dan Rev Game Biol 1:1–42.

64. Madsen, H. 1951. Notes on the species of capillaria zeder, 1800 known from gallinaceous birds. J Parasitol 37:257–265.

65. Madsen, H. 1952. A study on the nematodes of Danish gallinaceous gamebirds. Dan Rev Game Biol 2:1–126.

66. McDonald, M.E. 1969. Catalogue of helminths of waterfowl (anatidae): Special Sci Rep Wildl (126). Fish Wildl Ser, 692 pp.

67. McGregor, J.K., A.A. Kingscote, and F.W. Remmler. 1961. Field trials in the control of gapeworm infections in pheasants. Avian Dis 5:11–18.

68. Norton, C.C., and L.P. Joyner. 1965. Experimental chemotherapy of infection with Capillaria obsignata. J Comp Pathol 75:137–145.

69. Norton, R.A., T.A. Yazwinski, and Z. Johnson. 1991. Research note: Use of fenbendazole for the treatment of turkeys with experimentally induced nematode infections. Poult Sci 70:1835–1837.

70. Norton, R.A., B.A. Hopkins, J.K. Skeeles, J.N. Beasley, and J.M. Kreeger. 1992. High mortality of domestic turkeys associated with Ascaridia dissimilis. Avian Dis 36:469–473.

71. Norton, R.A., B.A. Bayyari, J.K. Skeeles, W.E. Huff, and J.N. Beasley. 1994. A survey of two commercial turkey farms experiencing high levels of liver foci. Avian Dis 38:887–894.

72. Okon, E.D. 1975. Anthelmintic activity of pyrantel tartrate against Ascaridia galli in fowls. Res Vet Sci 18:331–332.

73. Pankavich, J.A., G.P. Poeschel, A.L. Shor, and A. Gallo. 1973. Evaluation of Levamisole against experimental infections of Ascaridia, Heterakis and Capillaria spp. in chickens. Am J Vet Res 34:501–505.

74. Pence, D.B. 1972. The genus oxyspirura (Nematoda: Thelaziidae) from birds in Louisiana. Proc Helminthol Soc Wash 39:23–28.

75. Pote, L.M., and T.A. Yazwinski. 1985. Efficacy of fenbendazole in chickens. Arkansas Farm Res 34:2.

76. Read, C.P. 1949. Studies on North American helminths of the genus Capillaria Zedor, 1800 (Nematoda) III. Capillarids from the lower digestive tract of North American birds. J Parasitol 35:240–249.

77. Reid, W.M., and J.L. Carmon. 1958. Effects of numbers of Ascarida galli in depressing weight gains in chicks. J Parasitol 44:183–186.

78. Reid, W.M., J.L. Mabon, and W.C. Harshbarger. 1973. Detection of worm parasites in chicken eggs by candling. Poult Sci 52:2316–2324.

79. Riddell, C., and A. Gajadhar. 1988. Cecal and hepatic granulomas in chickens associated with Heterakis gallinarum infection. Avian Dis 32:836–838.

80. Ruff, M.D. 1984. Nematodes and acanthocephalens. In M.S. Hofstad, H.J. Barnes, B.W. Calnek, W.M. Reid and H.W. Yoder, Jr. (eds.). Diseases of Poultry, 8th ed. Iowa State University Press, Ames, IA, pp. 614–648.

81. Ruff, M.D., L.R. McDougald, and M.F. Hansen. 1970. Isolation of Histomonas meleagridis from embryonated eggs of Heterakis gallinarum. J Protozool 17:10–11.

82. Schmidt, G.D., and O.W. Olsen. 1964. Life cycle and development of Prosthynohus formosus (Van Cleave, 1918) Travassos, 1926, an Acanthocephalan parasite of birds. J Parasitol 50:721–730.

83. Schwabe, C.W. 1951. Studies on Oxyspirura manson: The tropical eyeworm of poultry II life history. Pac Sci 5:18–35.

84. Shumard, R.F., and D.F. Eveleth. 1955. A preliminary report on the anthelmintic action of piperazine citrate on Ascaridia galli and Heterakis gallinae in hens. Vet Med 50:203–205.

85. Spakulova, M., V. Birova, and J.K. Macko. 1991. Seasonal changes in the species composition of nematodes and acanthocephalans of ducks in East Slovakia. Biologia 46:119–128.

86. Springer, W.T., J. Johnson, and W.M. Reid. 1969. Transmission of histomoniasis with male Heterakis gallinarum (Nematoda). Parasitology 59:401–405.

87. Ssenyonga, G.S.Z. 1982. Efficacy of fenbendazole against helminth parasites of poultry in Uganda. Trop Anim Health Prod 14:163–166.

88. Swales, W.E. 1933. Tetrameres crami Sp. Nov., a nematode parasitizing the proventriculus of a domestic duck in Canada. Can J Res 8:334–336.

89. Taylor, S.M., J. Kenny, A. Houston, and S.A. Hewitt. 1993. Efficacy, pharmacokinetics and effects on egg-laying and hatchability of two dose rates of in-feed fenbendazole for the treatment of Capillaria species infections in chickens. Vet Rec 133:519–521.

90. Thienpont, D., and J. Mortelmans. 1962. Methyridine in the control of intestinal capillariasis in birds. Vet Rec 74:850–852.

91. Thienpont, D., O.F.J. Vanparijs, A.H.M. Raeymaekers, J. Vanderberk, P.J.A. Demoen, R.P.H. Marsboom, C.J.E. Niemegeers, K. H.L. Schellekens, and P.A.J. Janssen. 1966. Tetramisole (R-8299), a new potent broad spectrum anthelmintic. Nature 209:1084–1086.

92. Thienpont, D.C., O.F.J. Vanparijs, and L.C. Hermans. 1973. Mebendazole, a new potent drug against Syngamus trachea in turkeys. Poult Sci 52:1712–1714.

93. Tongson, M.S., and B.M. McCraw. 1967. Experimental ascaridiasis: Influence of chicken age and infective egg dose on structure of Ascaridia galli populations. Exp Parasitol 21:160–172.

94. Tsvetaeva, N.P. 1960. Pathomorphological changes in the proventriculus of the ducks by experimental tetrameriasis. Helminthologia 2:143–150.

95. Tyzzer, E.E. 1926. Heterakis vesicularis Froelich 1791: A vector of an infectious disease. Proc Soc Exp Med 23:708–709.

96. Verma, N., P.K. Bhatnager, and D.P. Banerjee. 1991.

Comparative efficacy of three broad spectrum anthelmintics against Ascaridia galli in poultry. Indian J Anim Sci 61:834–835.

97. Wakelin, D. 1965. Experimental studies on the biology of Capillaria obsignata, Madson, 1945, a nematode parasite of the domestic fowl. J Helminthol 39:399–412.

98. Watson, H., D.L. Lee, and P.J. Hudson. 1988. Primary and secondary infection of the domestic chicken with Trichostrongylus tenuis (Nematoda), a parasite of red grouse, with observations on the effect on the cecal mucosa. Parasitol 97:89–99.

99. Wehr, E.E. 1936. Earthworms as transmitters of Capillaria annulata, the crop-worm of chickens. North Am Vet 17:18–20.

100. Wehr, E.E. 1967. Anthelmintic activity of thiabendazole against the gapeworm (Syngamus trachea) in turkeys. Avian Dis 11:44–48.

101. Wehr, E.E. 1972. In M.S. Hofstad, B.W. Calnek, C.F. Helmboldt, W.M. Reid, and H.W. Yoder, Jr. (eds.). Diseases of Poultry, 6th ed. Iowa State University Press, Ames, IA, pp. 844–883.

102. Wehr, E.E., and J.C. Hwang. 1964. The life cycle and morphology of Ascaridia columbae (Gmelin, 1790)

Travassps. 1913. (Nematoda: Ascarididae) in the domestic pigeon (Columba livia domestica). J Parasitol 50:131–137.

103. Wehr, E.E., M.I. Colglazier, R.H. Burtner, and L.M. Wiest, Jr. 1967. Methyridine, an effective anthelmintic for intestinal threadworm, capillaria obsignata in pigeons. Avian Dis 11:322–326.

104. Yamaguti, S. 1961. The nematodes of vertebrates. Parts I and II. Systema Helminthum. Vol. 3. Nematodes. Interscience, New York, pp. 1–679; 681–1261.

105. Yazwinski, T.A., P. Andrews, H. Holtzen, B. Presson, N. Wood, and Z. Johnson. 1986. Dose-titration of fenbendazole in the treatment of poultry nematodiasis. Avian Dis 30:716–718.

106. Yazwinski, T.A., M. Rosenstein, R.D. Schwartz, K. Wilson, and Z. Johnson. 1993. The use of fenbendazole in the treatment of commercial turkeys infected with Ascaridia dissimilis. Avian Pathol 22:177–181.

107. Yorke, W., and P.A. Maplestone, 1962. The Nematode Parasites of Vertebrates. Hafner, New York.

108. Zieris, H., and P. Betke. 1991. Cyathostoma bronchialis (Muhling 1884), Ordnung Strongylida, Familie Syngamidae bei Mandarinenten (Aix galericulata) als Todesursache. Monatschefte fur Vet 46:146–149.

CESTODES AND TREMATODES

W. Malcolm Reid and Larry R. McDougald

INTRODUCTION.   Many species of worm parasites appear during necropsy examination of the digestive tract or other internal organs of poultry. Some of these are large enough to cause concern for the damage they may be inflicting on the host. Others are so small that a hand lens may be required to distinguish them from intestinal contents. If flattened in shape, they are probably "flatworms" belonging to the phylum Platyhelminthes. Tapeworms are in the class Cestoda, and flukes are in the class Trematoda. Accurate identification is essential for effective control. Species identification may give direction to control measures aimed at eliminating the intermediate host, thus breaking the life cycle. Others may require treatment with anthelmintics.

CESTODES

INTRODUCTION.   A high percentage of chickens or turkeys may be infected with tapeworms if they are reared on range or in backyard flocks. These parasites are found more frequently in warmer seasons, when intermediate hosts are abun-

dant. Many species of tapeworms are now considered rare in intensive poultry-rearing regions because the birds do not come in contact with intermediate hosts. Beetles and houseflies inhabiting poultry houses still act as intermediate hosts for the two large chicken tapeworms known only by the scientific names *Raillietina cesticillus* and *Choanotaenia infundibulum*.

Some of the larger tapeworms may appear to block completely the intestine of an infected bird, thus producing concern on the part of the poultry producer. Different species vary considerably in pathogenicity, so identification to species is to be desired.

Unfortunately, diagnosticians have often been satisfied with a diagnosis of "cestodiasis" or "taeniasis" without making further attempts at identification. Prevention, flock prognosis, and treatment suggestions may vary with each species of tapeworm. Only after the species has been determined, can an assessment of flock damage and possible control measures be considered (Table 33.5). For identification of the less common species, specialized textbooks (8, 11, 15, 16) may be needed to supplement the keys and illustrations included in this text.

Tapeworms or cestodes are flattened, ribbon shaped, usually segmented worms. The term *proglottid* is used to describe these individual "segments," since the latter term is defined otherwise by

E. E. Wehr authored the chapter on cestodes in earlier editions of this text. W. W. Price, E. E. Byrd, and Newton Kingston authored a chapter on trematodes. Their contributions to materials included in this edition are gratefully acknowledged.

Table 33.5. Tapeworms and hosts from poultry in the United States

Tapeworm	Definitive hosts (occasional hosts)	Intermediate hosts	Degree of pathogenicity
Amoebotaenia cuneata	Chicken (turkey)	Earthworm	Mild
Choanotaenia infundibulum	Chicken (turkey)	Housefly, beetle	Moderate
Davainea proglottina	Chicken	Slug, snail	Severe
Hymenolepis carioca	Chicken (turkey, bobwhite quail)	Stable fly, dung beetle	Unknown
H. cantaniana	Chicken (turkey, peafowl, bobwhite quail)	Beetle	Mild or harmless
Raillietina cesticillus	Chicken (turkey, guinea fowl, bobwhite quail)	Beetle	Mild or harmless
R. tetragona	Chicken (guinea fowl, peafowl, bobwhite quail, turkey?)	Ant	Moderate to severe
R. echinobothrida	Chicken (turkey?)	Ant	Moderate to severe
R. magninumida	Guinea fowl (chicken, turkey)	Beetle	Unknown
Davainea meleagridis	Turkey	Unknown	Unknown
Drepanidotaenia watsoni	Wild turkey	Unknown	Unknown
Imparmargo baileyi	Wild turkey	Unknown	Unknown
Raillietina georgiensis	Wild turkey (domestic turkey)	Ant	Unknown
R. ransomi	Wild turkey	Unknown	Unknown
R. williamsi	Wild turkey	Unknown	Unknown
Metroliasthes lucida	Turkey (guinea fowl, chicken)	Grasshopper	Unknown
Diorchis nyrocae	Wild and domestic duck	Copepod crustacean	Unknown
Fimbriaria fasciolaris	Duck (chicken)	Copepod crustacean	Unknown
Hymenolepis anatina	Wild and domestic duck	Freshwater crustacean	Severe
H. compressa	Duck, goose	Unknown	Unknown
H. collaris	Wild and domestic duck (chicken)	Freshwater crustacean (snail=auxiliary)	Unknown
H. coronula	Duck	Crustacean, snail	Unknown
H. lanceolata	Goose, duck	Crustacean	Severe
H. megalops	Duck	Unknown	Unknown
H. parvula	Wild and domestic duck	Leech	Unknown

classic zoologists (see Fig. 33.33). One to several gravid proglottids are shed daily from the posterior end of the worm. Each proglottid contains one or more sets of reproductive organs, which may become crowded with a mass of eggs as the maturing proglottid becomes a gravid proglottid.

Tapeworms are characterized by complete absence of a digestive tract and obtain their nourishment by absorption from the gut contents of the host. Although the duodenum, jejunum, or ileum is the usual site for attachment, one species (*Hymenolepis megalops*) from ducks is found in the cloaca or bursa of Fabricius. Birds become infected by eating an intermediate host, thus allowing the larval stage of the tapeworm access to the intestine. This larval tapeworm is known as a cysticercoid (see Fig. 33.34C). The intermediate host may be an insect, crustacean, earthworm, slug, snail, or leech depending upon the species of tapeworm.

Most cestodes are host specific for a single or a few closely related birds. Identification of the genus and species may provide a clue to the probable in-

termediate host. The diagnostician may then be able to suggest practical control measures. Completion of a two-host life cycle depends upon a unique set of ecologic conditions. Thus, minor changes in flock management may cause a break in the life cycle and, thus, effect a useful control measure.

HISTORY, INCIDENCE, AND DISTRIBUTION.

Over 4000 species of tapeworms have been described from animals (14), with many of the earlier species bearing the genus name *Taenia*. Since no poultry tapeworms are currently listed in this genus, the term *taeniasis* is no longer appropriate and the term *cestodiasis* would be a better substitute for infection with poultry tapeworms. Slender threadlike forms (*Hymenolepis carioca*) may require some magnification to distinguish individual proglottids, thus indicating that they are tapeworms. Some short forms, e.g., *Davainea proglottina*, are almost microscopic. To differentiate them from villi, which they superficially resemble, may require examining the mucosal surface with low magnification. These tapeworms, however, are still large enough to be recognized unmagnified after they have been removed from the intestine.

CLASSIFICATION. Over 1400 species of tapeworms have been described from wild and domestic birds. Since most of them have no common name, they are best recognized by their genus and species names.

Three families (Davainidae, Dilepididae, Hymenolepidae) and 10 genera (*Amoebotaenia, Choanotaenia, Davainea, Diorchis, Drepanidotaenia, Imparmargo, Metroliasthes, Raillietina, Hymenolepis, Fimbriaria*) are recognized here, as they may appear in birds brought to diagnostic laboratories in the United States.

MORPHOLOGY AND LIFE CYCLES

ADULTS. The anatomic features needed to identify poultry tapeworms are illustrated by describing *Davainea proglottina* (Fig. 33.33). This species differs from most other tapeworms in possessing only one or two each of immature, mature, and gravid proglottids compared with dozens or hundreds in other species. The entire connected chain of proglottids is called a strobila. Besides the strobila,

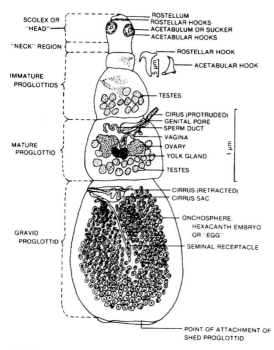

33.33. Adult tapeworm (*Davainea proglottina*). Although readily seen with the naked eye, this species has been called a "microscopic tapeworm," since it is often overlooked among villi in gross examination of the intestine.

two other regions, the scolex and the neck, are recognized. Anchorage is accomplished by the scolex with the assistance of four pairs of suckers or acetabula, which may possess one or two rows of acetabular hooks. If hooks are present, the species is described as armed; if absent, it is unarmed. A plunger-shaped organ known as the rostellum is frequently present at the anterior end. The rostellum may assist in anchorage by means of one or two rows of rostellar hooks and by the suction created by partial withdrawal of the rostellum into the scolex. The neck is an undifferentiated area between the scolex and the strobila from which new proglottids proliferate.

A set of both male and female reproductive organs are found in each proglottid. Morphologic differences in size and location of these organs are used in taxonomic descriptions of different species. Older gravid proglottids containing numerous eggs are shed individually or in short chains late in the day after the worm has absorbed and stored nutrients from the gut contents of the host. *D. proglottina* generally sheds one gravid proglottid per day, while *Raillietina cesticillus* may produce as many as 10–12.

ONCHOSPHERE. Within the uterus, the fertilized egg develops into a multicellular embryo called an oncosphere or hexacanth embryo. The onchosphere is a multicellular larva containing penetration glands and numerous muscular attachments to activate the hooks. Each gravid proglottid may contain several hundred of these multicellular embryos or "eggs." Distinctive membranes (Fig 33.34A) surrounding the eggs may be useful in identifying the species.

CYSTICERCOID. Intermediate hosts such as beetles, houseflies, slugs, or snails become infected by swallowing individual eggs from the feces, or they devour the entire proglottid after being attracted by odor or movement. The six-hooked embryo hatches from the egg in the gut of the intermediate host and penetrates the gut wall. The larva reorganizes and changes in polarity to become a cysticercoid (Fig. 33.34C,D). This development requires a minimum of 2 wk depending upon temperature. The cysticercoid remains within the body cavity of the intermediate host until the latter is eaten by the bird host. The cysticercoid is activated by the bile in the definitive host and attaches to the intestine to begin the formation of a strobila. The first gravid proglottids appear in the feces 2–3 wk after the cysticercoid is swallowed by the definitive host.

DIAGNOSIS AND IDENTIFICATION. Distinctive characteristics of different species of chicken tapeworms may best be demonstrated by

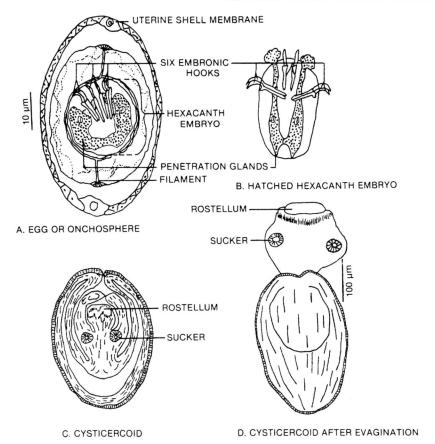

UTERINE SHELL MEMBRANE

SIX EMBRONIC HOOKS

HEXACANTH EMBRYO

PENETRATION GLANDS

FILAMENT

10 μm

A. EGG OR ONCHOSPHERE

B. HATCHED HEXACANTH EMBRYO

ROSTELLUM

SUCKER

100 μm

ROSTELLUM

SUCKER

C. CYSTICERCOID

D. CYSTICERCOID AFTER EVAGINATION

33.34. Larval stages of the chicken tapeworm (*Raillietina cesticillus*). *A.* The egg is encapsulated by a membrane derived from the uterus wall. Eggs are occasionally found free in feces, but more often, several hundred are enclosed in a single gravid proglottid. *B.* Hexacanth embryos escape from shell membranes. Active hooks and enzymes from secretory glands assist in penetration of gut wall of the beetle intermediate host. *C.* Cysticercoid that has developed from the hexacanth embryo in the hemocoele of a beetle. *D.* Scolex in the cysticercoid has evaginated after exposure to bile and enzymes in gut of the fowl.

examining 1) the scolex (Figs. 33.33, 33.35), 2) the eggs (Figs. 33.34A, 33.37,) or 3) individual proglottids of recently shed, live specimens (Figs. 33.33, 33.36) (11). Although differential staining can be used to show internal organs of mature proglottids, this procedure is too slow for most diagnostic laboratories. Preservation in alcohol or formalin, although required before staining, often obscures useful characteristics needed for rapid identification. The intestine is best opened with scissors under water, thus permitting the strobila to float free, revealing the area to which the scolex is attached. Recovery of the scolex is worth considerable effort, as its characteristics alone may indicate the species. Freeing the scolex may be accomplished by 1) teasing apart the mucosa with two dissecting needles, 2)

cutting a deep gouge into the mucosa under the attachment point with a sharp scalpel, or 3) leaving the intestine submerged in saline for a few hours in the refrigerator. Wet-mount preparations of the scolex examined under a cover glass with ×100 or higher magnification may reveal sufficient characteristics to make a species identification. Hook characteristics may require measurement with an ocular micrometer under higher magnification. Semipermanent cleared preparations of scolices may be made by using a drop of Hoyer's solution (prepared by adding to 50 mL of distilled water the following ingredients in this order: gum arabic flakes, 30 g; chloral hydrate, 200 g; and glycerin, 20 g). Distinctive egg characteristics may be demonstrated by teasing apart a gravid proglottid under a coverglass (Fig. 33.37). Wet preparations of mature or gravid proglottids under low magnification may reveal diagnostic characteristics such as the location, size, and shape of the cirrus pouch and the location of the genital pore and the gonads. If further details of the internal structure of the proglottid are required for identification, it may be necessary to kill, fix, stain, destain, dehydrate, and permanently mount the specimen (1).

TAPEWORMS OF CHICKENS. A dichotomous key is given to the eight species of tapeworms commonly found in chickens from the continental United States. In such keys, successive selections must be made between 1a and 1b, 2a and 2b, etc., until a species name is designated. After viewing a portion of the worm under the microscope, make a comparison of the appropriate figures organized under scolices (Fig. 33.35), eggs (Fig 33.37), or proglottids (Fig. 33.36). With rare species, additional descriptions from other texts may be required (16).

Key to Species

1a. Minute forms, less than 1 cm in length. A very limited number of proglottids with the terminal proglottid being gravid with eggs.........2
1b. Longer than 1 cm..........3
2a. Wedge-shaped worm. Contains about 20 proglottids. Posterior proglottids wide, short (Figs. 33.35C,33.36E, 33.37)........*Amoebotaenia cuneata*
2b. Contains only 2–5 proglottids, rarely 9. Posterior proglottids as long as wide (Fig. 33.33)........*Davainea proglottina*
3a. Threadlike, never more than 1.5-mm wide; fragile scolex is usually lost; often more than 100 worms in a single bird; proglottids short and wide, genus *Hymneolepis*........4
3b. Robust worms, gravid proglottids wider than 2 mm........5
4a. Mature worms with gravid proglottids present less than 12 mm in length (Fig 33.35A)........*H. cantaniana*
4b. Mature specimens with a total length including gravid proglottids of more than 12 mm (Figs 33.35B, 33.36D)........*H. carioca*
5a. 5–12 embryos enclosed in single capsule; verify by opening terminal proglottid; view under a coverglass (Fig. 33.37F)........6
5b. Embryos in single egg capsules enclosed in distinct membranes (Examine under high power)........7
6a. Cirrus sac small (75–100 μm in length). Suckers markedly oval in shape (Figs. 33.35E, 33.36A)........*R. tetragona*
6b. Cirrus sac large (130–180 μm). Suckers round

(Figs. 33.35F, 33.36B)........*R. echinobothrida*
7a. Outer membrane prolonged in 2 elongated filaments (Fig 33.37B)........*Choanotaenia infundibulum*
7b. Outer membrane smooth and round, 2 elongated filaments (Fig. 33.34A, 33.37D)........ *R. cesticillus*

Species descriptions are given for these eight chicken tapeworms to assist in verifying tentative identifications.

AMOEBOTAENIA CUNEATA (LINSTOW 1872)

Diagnostic Characteristics. This short (<4 mm, 25–30 proglottids) tapeworm may be recognized as whitish projections among the villi of the duodenum (Fig. 33.35C); a triangular anterior end with a pointed scolex gives the entire worm a wedge-shaped anterior. Suckers unarmed, rostellum armed with a single row of 12–14 distinctive hooks 25–32 μm in length, 12–15 testes located transversely in a single row across the posterior end of the proglottid (33.36E), genital pores usually alternate regularly, located at extreme anterior point of proglottid margin; six-hooked embryos single, surrounded by a distinctive granular layer (Fig. 33.37A); embryonal hooks, 6 μm.

Life History. Several species of earthworms belonging to the genera *Allotophora, Pheritima, Ocnerodrilus,* and *Lumbricus* act as intermediate hosts for this tapeworm. Literature descriptions of pathogenicity range from "comparatively slight" to "cause of death." No controlled experiments have been reported.

CHOANOTAENIA INFUNDIBULUM (BLOCH 1779)

Diagnostic Characteristics. This large robust tapeworm is extremely white and is readily seen attached to the upper half of the intestine. Mature worms up to 23 cm in length; large rostellum armed with a single row of 16–22 large (25–30 μm) hooks, suckers unarmed (Fig. 33.35G); genital pores irregularly alternate; 25–60 testes are grouped in posterior portion of proglottid (Fig. 33.36C); eggs are with distinctive elongated filaments (Fig. 33.37B); and embryonal hooks are 18-μm long.

Life History and Pathogenicity. Houseflies and several species of beetles are proven natural hosts. Other insects including nine families of beetles, grasshoppers, and termites are proven experimental hosts. Gravid proglottids are released 13 days after swallowing an infected fly. No controlled experiments testing pathogenicity have been reported.

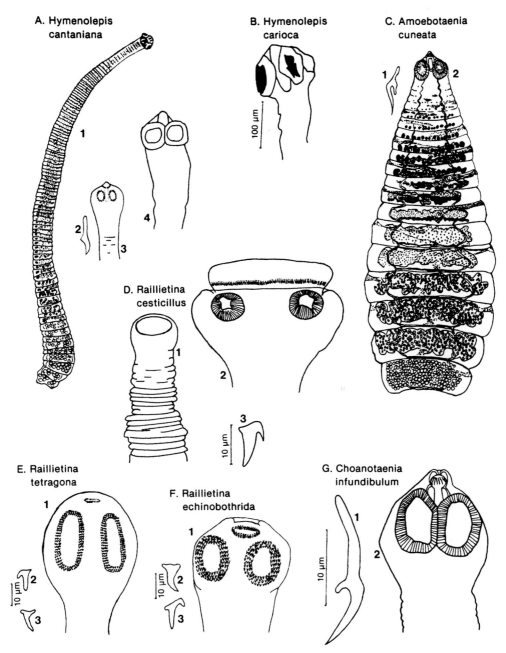

A. Hymenolepis cantaniana

B. Hymenolepis carioca

C. Amoebotaenia cuneata

D. Raillietina cesticillus

E. Raillietina tetragona

F. Raillietina echinobothrida

G. Choanotaenia infundibulum

33.35. Tapeworms of chickens. Scolex characteristics: *A. Hymenolepis cantaniana. 1.* Scolex and strobilia (Ransom); *2.* Hook (Yamaguti); *3.* Scolex (Neveu-Lemaire); *4.* Scolex (Wehr). *B. H. carioca* scolex. *C. Amoebotaenia cuneata* (Monnig). *1.* Rostellar hook; *2.* Entire worm. *D. Raillietina cesticillus. 1.* Scolex (Ackert); *2.* Scolex (Monnig); *3.* Rostellar hook (Ransom). *E. R. tetragona. 1.* Scolex (Monnig); *2.–3.* Rostellar and acetabular hooks (Ransom). *F. R. echinobothrida. 1.* Scolex (Monnig); *2.–3.* Rostellar and acetabular hooks (Ransom). *G. Choanotaenia infundibulum. 1.* Hook (Ransom); *2.* Scolex (Monnig)

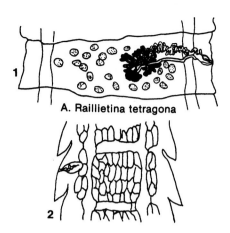

A. Raillietina tetragona

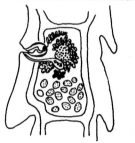

B. Raillietina echinobothrida

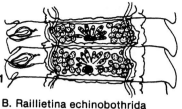

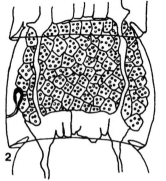

C. Choanotaenia infundibulum

D. Hymenolepis carioca

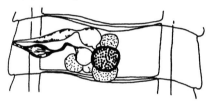

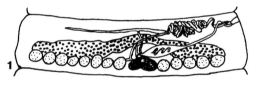

F. Raillietina cesticillus

E. Amoebotaenia cuneata

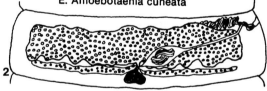

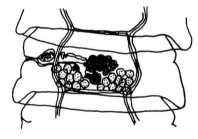

33.36. Mature and gravid proglottids of chicken tapeworms. *A. Raillietina tetragona. 1.* Mature proglottid (Ransom); *2.* Gravid proglottid showing egg capsules (Neveu-Lemaire). *B. R. echinobothrida. 1.* Mature proglottid (Fuhrmann); *2.* Gravid proglottid (Lang). *C. Choanotaenia infundibulum* (Fuhrmann). *D. Hymenolepis carioca* (Sawada). *E. Amoebotaenia cuneata. 1.* Mature proglottid; *2.* Gravid proglottid filled with eggs (Fuhrmann). *F. Raillietina cesticillus*: mature proglottid (Monnig).

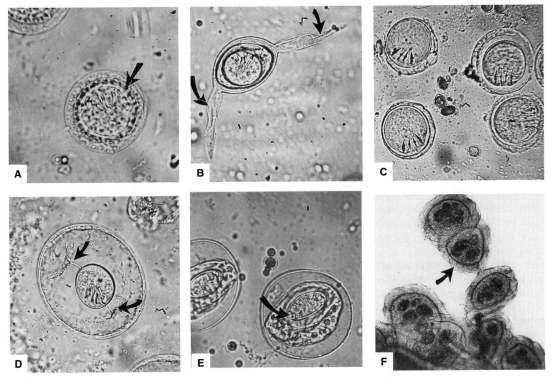

33.37. Eggs of chicken tapeworms (high power). *A. Amoebotaenia sphenoides* showing distinctive granular layer. *B. Choanotaenia infundibulum* with elongated filaments. *C. Davainea proglottina*. *D. Raillietina cesticillus* showing distinctive funnel-shaped structures between membranes found only in fully developed gravid proglottids. *E. Hymenolepis carioca* or *H. cantaniana* showing football-shaped embryophore with granular accumulations at the poles. *F.* Capsules containing 6–12 eggs. Found in the chicken (*Raillietina tetragona, R. echinobothrida*) and two turkey tapeworms (*R. georgiensis, R. williamsi*).

Davainea proglottina (Davaine 1860)

Diagnostic Characteristics. This microscopic tapeworm may be recognized in the duodenal mucosa by protrusion of the gravid proglottids above the villi if the open intestine is floated in water. Eggs are without distinctive membranes, but embryonal hooks are distinctive, 10–11 μm long (Fig. 33.37C). Mature worms measure up to 4 mm in length; never with more than nine proglottids; suckers are armed with 3–6 rows of hooks (Fig. 33.33); the rostellum is armed; genital pores regularly alternate and are located near the anterior margin; and the cirrus is disproportionately large.

Life History. Several species of slugs and snails host larval stages of this tapeworm. More than 1500 cysticercoids have developed along the digestive tract of susceptible slugs, where they have remained infective for more than 11 mo. Tapeworms may live as long as 3 yr; over 3000 worms have been recovered from a single bird.

Pathogenicity. This parasite is one of the more harmful species in young birds. In controlled experiments, a 12% reduction in growth rate has been reported (5). Uncontrolled reports include emaciation, dull plumage, slow movements, breathing difficulties, thickened mucosal membranes that produce hemorrhage and fetid mucus, leg weakness, paralysis, and death.

Hymenolepis cantaniana (Polonio 1860)

Diagnostic Characteristics. This short hymenolepid tapeworm (maximum length 2 cm) superficially resembles the longer *H. carioca*. It is usually listed as unarmed, but rostellar hooks have been described by European investigators (Fig. 33.35A); the fragile rostellum is frequently lost;

genital pores are unilateral, anterior to middle of proglottid; eggs are similar to those of *H. carioca*; embryonal hooks measure 13–14 μm.

Life History.   Dung beetles (Scarabeidae) are intermediate hosts; each beetle may carry 100 or more cysticercoids. A unique larval development involves budding, which produces many cysticercoids from a single onchosphere. This tapeworm is considered relatively nonpathogenic, although no controlled experiments have been reported.

HYMENOLEPIS CARIOCA (MAGALHAES 1898)

Diagnostic Characteristics.   Several thousand specimens of this extremely slender species have been found in the duodenum of a single chicken or turkey. The worm is so slender (about 1 mm in diameter) that the hundreds of inconspicuous proglottids look more like a thread than a worm. Suckers are unarmed; rostellar sacs are present; rostellum is rudimentary (Fig. 33.35B); there are three testes, usually in a straight row; genital pores are unilateral, located anterior to middle of proglottid margin (Fig. 33.36D); an inner membrane enveloping the onchosphere is elongated into a football shape with granular deposits at poles (Fig. 33.37E); embryonal hooks measure 10–12 μm.

Life History.   Twenty-six species belonging to nine families of beetles and one species of termite are experimental or natural intermediate hosts; dung and ground beetles are the most common source of infection. Reports incriminating the housefly are probably erroneous.

Pathogenicity.   Experimental infections establishing several hundred worms per bird had no effect on weight gains. These results indicate that this species is relatively nonpathogenic.

RAILLIETINA CESTICILLUS (MOLIN 1858)

Diagnostic Characteristics.   Scolex of this large robust tapeworm (up to 15-cm long) embeds deeply in the mucosa of the duodenum or jejunum. The distinctive, wide, flat, rostellum bears a double row of 300–500 hammer-shaped hooks. The flattened rostellum acts as a retractable piston drawing into an outer sleeve of the scolex, thus, providing a firm grip on the mucosa (Fig. 33.35D1,D2); there are four unarmed weak suckers; genital pores alternate irregularly (Fig. 33.36F); there are 20–30 testes posteriad in proglottid; single eggs are encapsulated in uterine membranes; and mature eggs have two distinctive funnel-shaped filaments between the middle and inner membranes (Fig. 33.37D).

Life History.   Over 100 species of beetles belonging to 10 families are proven natural or experimental intermediate hosts. A minute histerid beetle (*Carcinops pumilio*) is the natural intermediate host in broiler houses. The darkling beetle (*Alphitobius diaperinus*), houseflies, grasshoppers, ants, and lepidopterous larvae have proved negative as experimental hosts. As many as 930 cysticercoids have been found in a single ground beetle.

Pathogenicity.   Early reports attribute this parasite with causing emaciation, degeneration and inflammation of villi, reduction of blood sugar and hemoglobin, and reduced growth rate. None of these early reports could be confirmed in extensive controlled experiments with broilers and layers maintained on optimum nutritional diets (2). Experimental infections (135 worms/bird) produced by feeding 300 cysticercoids caused no reduction in weight gain in broilers or reduced egg production in layers when compared with uninfected controls.

RAILLIETINA TETRAGONA (MOLIN 1858)

Diagnostic Characteristics.   These are moderately large tapeworms measuring up to 25 cm long × 3 mm wide. Scolex (Fig. 33.35E1) anchors in the posterior half of the intestine; the rostellum is armed with 90–100 hooks, 6–8 μm in length, arranged in a single or double row (Fig. 33.35E2); suckers are oval shaped, armed with 8–12 rows of minute hooks, 3–8 μm in length (Fig. 33.35E); genital pores are usually unilateral (Fig. 33.36A); the uterus breaks up into capsules containing 6–12 eggs (Figs. 33.36A2, 33.37F), similar to *R. echinobothrida* from chickens, and *R. williamsi* and *R. georgensis* from turkeys; and the cirrus sac is small (75–100 μm in length), more anterior in proglottid margin than with *R. echinobothrida*.

Life History.   Several species of small ants that nest under rocks or boards act as intermediate hosts. The minimum prepatent period after feeding cysticercoids to chickens is 13 days.

Pathogenicity.   Weight loss was demonstrated in controlled experiments (9) with white leghorns and hybrids infected with an average of 12–16 worms/bird. Decreases in egg production in four breeds of hens occurred after administering 50 cysticercoids/bird, causing reduced glycogen levels in livers and the intestinal mucosa of infected chickens.

RAILLIETINA ECHINOBOTHRIDA (MEGNIN 1881)

Diagnostic Characteristics.   This species resembles *R. tetragona* but differs in the following characteristics: the strobila is larger (34 cm long × 4 mm wide); the scolex has rounded suckers containing 200–250 hooks, 10–13 μm in length (Fig. 33.35F) with 8–15 rows of hooks 5–15 μm in length (Fig. 33.35F2,3); genital pores are in the posterior half of the proglottid (Fig. 33.36B2); the cirrus sac is large (130–180 μm in length); and gravid proglottids frequently loosen from each other in the center, making a windowlike arrangement not found in *R. tetragona.*

Life History. As with *R. tetragona,* numerous species of ants have been found naturally infected with cysticercoids. Concurrent infections with both *R. echinobothrida* and *R. tetragona* cysticercoids have been found in ants.

Pathogenicity. *R. echinobothrida* is usually listed as one of the most pathogenic tapeworms, since its presence has often been associated with nodular disease of chickens. Nadakal et al. (10) reported parasitic granulomas approximately 1–6 mm in diameter at the sites of worm attachment 6 mo after experimental infection with 200 cysticercoids. The condition was associated with catarrhal hyperplastic enteritis as well as lymphocytic, polymorphonuclear, and eosinophilic infiltration.

TAPEWORMS OF TURKEYS. Six species of tapeworms from domestic and/or wild turkeys have been reported from the United States (12). Since these tapeworms are readily transferred between wild and domestic turkeys, wild turkeys provide a reservoir for these parasites of domestic birds. No controlled experiments on pathogenicity have been reported for any species. Descriptions included here are limited to the two species with known life cycles. Scolex (Fig. 33.38) and proglottid characteristics (Fig. 33.39) of different species are organized in separate figures to facilitate comparisons if complete specimens are unavailable.

Raillietina georgiensis (Reid and Nugara 1961)

Description and Diagnostic Characteristics. This species is a large (15–38 cm long × 3.5-mm wide) robust tapeworm from domestic and wild turkeys. Scolex (Fig. 33.38A) is armed with a double row of 230 moderate length (12–23 μm) rostellar hooks, and 8–10 circles of acetabular hooks, 8–13 μm long (Fig. 33.38A2,A3); genital pores are unilateral, located in middle of the proglottid (Fig. 33.39A); eggs are in uterine capsules, similar to *R. tetragona* and *R. echinobothrida.*

Life History. A small brownish ant (*Pheidole vinelandica*) that frequents turkey ranges has been

found naturally infected; gravid proglottids appear in droppings within 3 wk after turkeys have fed on infected ants. This tapeworm was introduced to a domestic farm by wild turkeys.

Pathogenicity. Enteritis is present if parasites are found in large numbers. Some host damage is assumed on the basis of a close relationship to *R. echinobothrida* from chickens.

Metroliasthes lucida (Ransom 1900)

Description and Diagnostic Characteristics. This species is a long tapeworm (20 cm) from turkeys and guinea fowl, rarely in chickens. There are unarmed scolex and suckers, 200–250 μm in diameter (Fig. 33.38C); genital pores irregularly alternate, near middle of margin in mature proglottids but posterior in gravid proglottids; uterus consists of two sacs side by side, visible to the naked eye in gravid proglottids, and is known as the parauterine organ (Fig. 33.39C2,C3); eggs have three membranes, 75 × 50 μm.

Life History. Several species of grasshoppers serve as intermediate hosts; cysticercoid development requires 15–42 days depending on temperature. Pathogenicity is unknown.

TAPEWORMS OF DUCKS AND GEESE. Domestic ducks and geese frequently become infected with numerous species of tapeworms introduced by wild ducks and geese. Some of these species have occasionally been reported in chickens. Two of the more common species are described below. Life cycles usually involve crustaceans or other aquatic invertebrates. No controlled pathogenicity studies have been made on any of these species.

Fimbriaria fasciolaris (Pallas 1781)

Description and Diagnostic Characteristics. This large (5–43 cm in length × 1–5 mm in width) twisted tapeworm of ducks also occurs in chickens and 31 species of wild birds. This distinctive flaring anterior neck region is known as the pseudoscolex; strobila is unsegmented, but crossstriations give the impression of segmentation (Fig. 33.40A1); there are minute scolex (Fig. 33.40A3,A4) attached to pseudoscolex, 100–130 μm wide; suckers are unarmed; the retractile rostellum has 10–12 hooks 17–22 μm in length (Fig. 33.40A2); genital pores are unilateral and closely crowded together; onchospheres are 35–45 μm in diameter, hooks are 16-μm in length.

Life History. Cysticercoids develop in copepod

A. Raillietina georgiensis

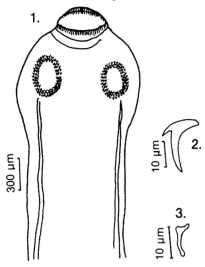

B. Raillietina williamsi

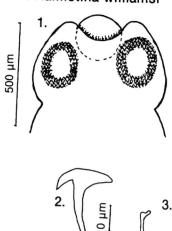

C. Metroliasthes lucida

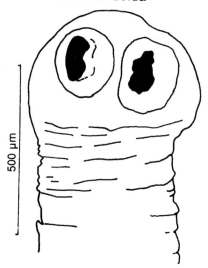

D. Raillietina ransomi

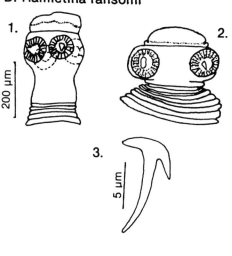

33.38.   Scolices of turkey tapeworms. *A. Raillietina georgiensis. 1.* Scolex; *2.* Rostellar hook; *3.* Acetabular hook (Reid and Nugara). *B. R. williamsi. 1.* Scolex; *2.* Rostellar hook; *3.* Acetabular hook (Williams). *C. Metroliasthes lucida* scolex (Ransom). *D. R. ransomi. 1.–2.* Scolex; *3.* Rostellar hook (Williams).

crustaceans (*Diaptomus* sp., *Cyclops* sp.); intermediate hosts are ingested with drinking water to infect the definitive host. Pathogenicity is unknown.

HYMENOLEPIS MEGALOPS (NITZSCH, IN CREPLIN 1829)

Description and Diagnostic Characteristics.   This cosmopolitan tapeworm of waterfowl

(Fig. 33.40B) is 3–6 mm in length and readily recognized by the large scolex (1–2 mm in width) attached to the cloaca or the bursa of Fabricius. Suckers and rostellum are unarmed, the latter containing a rudimentary central pit; eggs are not in capsules.

Life History.   Onchospheres develop into cysticercoids after 18 days in ostracod crustacea. The definitive host is infected by eating ostracods.

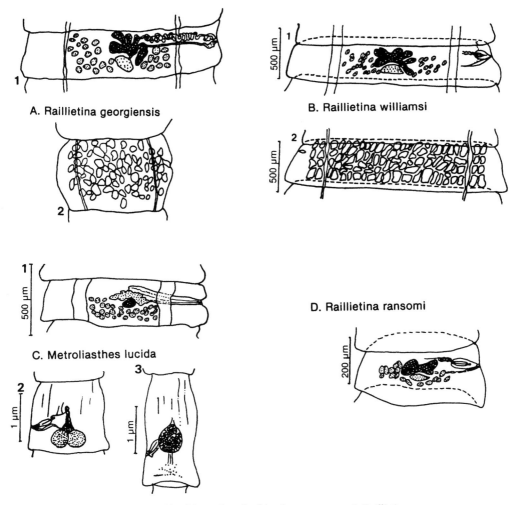

33.39. Mature and gravid proglottids of domestic and wild turkey tapeworms. *A. Raillietina georgiensis* (Reid and Nugara). *B. R. williamsi. 1.* Mature proglottid; *2.* Gravid proglottid showing position of egg capsules, each containing several eggs (Williams). *C. Metroliasthes lucida. 1.*Mature proglottid; *2.* Proglottid showing two-part uterus and developing parauterine organ; *3.* Gravid proglottid (Ransom). *D. R. ransomi* mature proglottid (Williams).

Pathogenicity. Reports range from "severe damage" to "mortality if other cestodes (*H. coronula, H. furcigera*) are also present."

PREVENTION AND CONTROL. During the past 40 yr, changes from backyard or range management to confinement rearing in large houses has brought on marked reductions in tapeworm infections in chickens and turkeys. Many flocks no longer have easy access to the required insect or other invertebrate hosts. *Davainea proglottina*, one of the most pathogenic species, was reported from 23% of the chickens submitted to the diagnostic laboratory in New York state in 1932. No cases have been found in recent years, probably because poultry no longer has easy access to garden slugs.

Prevention of contact with the intermediate host is the first step to consider in tapeworm control. Elimination of intermediate hosts may provide additional benefits besides tapeworm control. If *Choanotaenia infundibulum* appears in a cage layer facility, housefly control will benefit the producer by preventing nuisance and public health complaints (see Chapter 32). If *Raillietina cesticillus* tapeworms appear in broiler houses, beetle control measures for the darkling beetle (*Alphitobius diaperinus*) may also eliminate the true intermediate host *Carcinops pumilio*, which is a minute histerid

A. Fimbriaria fasciolaris

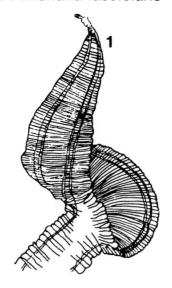

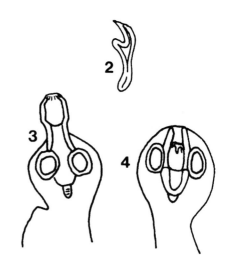

B. Hymenolepis megalops

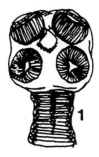

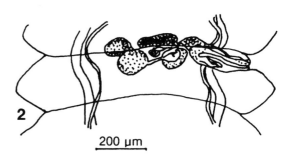

200 μm

33.40.   Tapeworms of ducks and geese. *A. Fimbriaria fasciolaris. 1.* Pseudoscolex showing irregular distension of the anterior end and the minute scolex (Todd); *2.* Rostellar hook (Fuhrmann); *3.* Scolex with rostellum extended; *4.* Scolex with rostellum withdrawn (Neveu-Lemaire). *B. H. megalops. 1.* Scolex; *2.* Mature proglottid (Yamaguti).

beetle. After species identification has given an indication of the intermediate host, some specific control measures may be recommended.

TREATMENT.   If a tapeworm infection appears during a necropsy examination in a diagnostic laboratory, the client usually asks first for a drug to remove the worms. The diagnostician should warn the client that expulsion of the parasite will be a very short-term remedy if the intermediate host as a source of infection is still present.

In the United States, only a single drug is approved for use in poultry. Butynorate (dibutyltin dilaurate) is approved for treatment of six species of chicken tapeworms (*Raillietina cesticillus, R. tetragona, Choanotaenia infundibulum, D. proglottina, Hymenolepis carioca,* and *Amoebotaenia*

sphenoides) (3). Although butynorate is available in a feed additive used for prevention of turkey coccidiosis, it is not registered for use against tapeworms.

TREMATODES

INTRODUCTION.   Trematodes (flukes) are flat, leaflike, parasitic organisms belonging to the phylum Platyhelminthes, class Trematoda. They differ from the cestodes (class Cestoda) in having a digestive system, and they do not form proglottids. The life cycle of all trematodes parasitizing birds requires a molluscan as an intermediate host; some species also use a second intermediate host. Since adult trematodes and larval metacercariae invade almost every cavity and tissue of birds, they may show up unexpectedly at necropsy.

Over 500 species belonging to some 125 genera and 27 families are known to occur in the four orders of birds most likely to be submitted to diagnostic laboratories as domestic or pet birds (4). Twenty of these flukes are considered potentially dangerous to poultry in the Western Hemisphere. These flukes belong to four orders: Anseriformes (ducks and geese), Galliformes (chickens and turkeys), Columbiformes (pigeons and allies), and Passeriformes (perching birds). Flukes are less host specific than tapeworms, so wild birds often introduce infection in areas where domestic poultry is reared. Since many snails live in ponds and streams, ducks and geese are the most frequently parasitized. The oviduct fluke (*Prosthogonimus* sp.), which is a frequent parasite of many species of wild birds, sometimes causes problems with ducks and chickens (6). This species will be used to illustrate fluke morphology and life history. *P. macrorchis* is the species name recognized in United States, while this fluke is known as *P. ovatus* or by other specific names in other countries.

MORPHOLOGY AND LIFE HISTORY.
The body of the adult fluke (Fig. 33.41) is a flattened oval, and it bears two suckers. The digestive system consists of the mouth (within the oral sucker), the pharynx, a short esophagus, and two intestinal ceca. An anus is lacking in the trematodes. Two testes and one ovary are present in the same individual. After fertilization, the zygote is enclosed along with yolk cells from the vitellaria by an egg shell. Large numbers of eggs are stored in a prominent convoluted

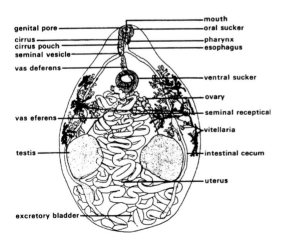

33.41. Morphology of an adult trematode (*Prosthogonimus macrorchis*) (Macy).

uterus. The excretory system, which originates in a series of flame cells bearing a tuft of cilia, drains with a series of collecting tubules that empty through an excretory pore near the posterior end of the parasite. The arrangement pattern of these collecting tubules is used as a family characteristic in classification of flukes.

LIFE CYCLE. Adult flukes continually shed eggs, which pass out with the feces of the host. These eggs contain an embryo that develops into a larval stage known as a miracidium. In this group of trematodes, the miracidium hatches after the egg is swallowed by a susceptible snail. Larval development continues within the snail through a succession of stages known as sporocysts and cercariae. The cercariae emerge from the snail and swim about in a lake or pond. Some are drawn into the brachial basket of a dragonfly naiad. The cercaria encysts (metacercaria) and remains in the insect until either the naiad or an infected adult dragonfly is eaten by a bird (Fig 33.42).

IDENTIFICATION. Twenty-four trematodes that occasionally appear in diagnostic laboratories have been described with keys by Kingston (4). More extensive listings of species are provided by Yamaguti (17), McDonald (7), and Schell (13). The latter text also describes methods of identifying, collecting, preserving, and staining trematodes with emphasis on North American families and genera.

PATHOGENICITY. *Prosthogonimus* sp., popularly known as the oviduct fluke, has caused economic losses to poultry producers by 1) drastically reducing egg production after a recent infection, and 2) occasionally being enveloped within a hen's egg and later discovered by a complaining customer. Other organs of the bird invaded by flukes include 1) metacercarial cysts in the skin of chickens and turkeys (*Collyriclum faba*), 2) small adult flukes in the conjunctival sac of the eye (*Philophthalmus gralli*), 3) adults in the liver, pancreas, and bile duct of ducks and turkeys (*Amphimerus elongatus*), 4) adults in the collecting tubules of the excretory system of chickens, turkeys, and pigeons (*Tanaisia bragai*), 5) adults and eggs in the circulatory system of ducks by three species of blood fluke, and 6) 14 species of flukes that invade various areas of the digestive tract.

CONTROL. If the life cycle is known and evidence of pathogenicity or economic loss is clear, changes in poultry management may prevent the problem. For example, oviduct flukes are easily controlled by fencing in chicken flocks, thus preventing access to lakes or streams where dragonfly naiads live (6).

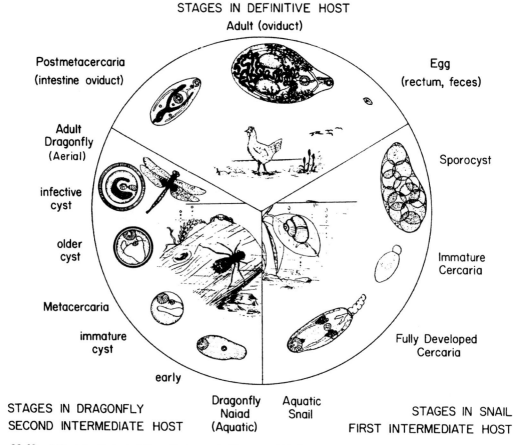

33.42. Life cycle of a typical digenetic trematode (*P. macrorchis*) (Macy).

Chemotherapy for control or prevention of trematode infections is not available for use in poultry.

REFERENCES

1. Ash, L R. and T.C. Orihel. 1987. Parasites: A Guide to Laboratory Procedures and Identification. American Society of Clinical Pathologists, Chicago, IL.

2. Botero, H. and W.M. Reid. 1969. The effects of the tapeworm Raillietina cesticillus upon body weight gains of broilers, poults and on egg production. Poult Sci 48:536–542.

3. Kerr, K.B. 1952. Butynorate, an effective and safe substance for the removal of R. cesticillus from chickens. Poult Sci 31:328–336.

4. Kingston, N. 1984. Trematodes. In M.S. Hofstad, H.J. Barnes, B.W. Calnek, W.M. Reid and H.W. Yoder, Jr. (eds.). Diseases of Poultry, 8th ed. Iowa State University Press, Ames, IA, pp. 668–690.

5. Levine, P.P. 1938. The effect of infection with Davainea proglottina on the weights of growing chickens. J Parasitol 24:550–551.

6. Macy, R.W. 1934. Studies on the taxonomy, morphology and biology of Prosthogonimus macorchis Macy, a common oviduct fluke of domestic fowls in North America. Minn Agric Exp Tech Bull 98:1–64.

7. McDonald, M.E. 1981. Key to trematodes reported in waterfowl. US Dept Int Fish Wildl Serv Resource Pub 142, Washington, DC.

8. Monnig, H.O. 1934. Veterinary Helminthology and Entomology. Baillerie, Tindall and Cox, London, England.

9. Nadakal, A.M., and K.V. Nair. 1979. Studies on the metabolic disturbances caused by Raillietina tetragona (Cestoda) infection in domestic fowl. Indian J Exp Biol 17:310–311.

10. Nadakal, A.M., K. Mohandas, K.O. John, and K. Muraleedharan. 1973. Contribution to the biology of the fowl cestode Raillietina echinobothrida with a note on its pathogenicity. Trans Am Microsc Soc 92:273–276.

11. Reid, W.M. 1962. Chicken and turkey tapeworms. Handbook. University of Georgia Poultry Department, Athens, GA.

12. Reid, W.M. 1984. Cestodes. In M.S. Hofstad, H.J., Barnes, B.W. Calnek, W.M. Reid, and H.W. Yoder, Jr. (eds.). Diseases of Poultry 8th ed. Iowa State University Press, Ames, IA, pp. 649–667.

13. Schell, S.C., 1985. Handbook of Trematodes of North America North of Mexico. University Press, Moscow, ID.

14. Schmidt, G.D. 1986. Handbook of Tapeworm Identification. CRC Press, Boca Raton, FL.

15. Wardle, R.A. and J.A. McLeod. 1952. The Zoology of Tapeworms. University of Minnesota Press, Minneapolis, MN.

16. Yamaguti, S. 1959. Systema Helminthum, vol. 2: The Cestodes of Vertebrates. Interstate, New York.

17. Yamaguti, S. 1971. Synopsis of Digenetic Trematodes of Vertebrates, vols. 1 and 2. Keigaku, Tokyo, Japan.

34 Protozoa

INTRODUCTION

Larry R. McDougald

Protozoa are common in poultry and other birds, and some cause moderate or severe disease. Parasitic diseases differ from viral and bacterial diseases by 1) the presence of a complicated life cycle, 2) the methods of transmission, 3) the lack of useful serologic methods for diagnosis, and 4) the means of control. Disinfection and quarantine have been of little use in control of the diseases, and control programs emphasize chemotherapy or chemoprevention rather than immunization. Prevention of coccidiosis with anticoccidial drugs administered through the feed allowed better uniformity of treatment and centralized decisions on the use of drugs. This system has proved more reliable than on-farm control and is practiced universally.

Emphasis of confinement rearing and high-density flocks have increased the infection pressure from diseases that have short, direct life cycles. In contrast, parasitic diseases that depend on an intermediate host for transmission have been practically eliminated.

Rational and effective control of all parasitic diseases depends upon accurate diagnosis of the parasite and also on the extent of the infection. Diagnosis usually depends on gross and microscopic examination of birds taken from a flock for necropsy, or on microscopic examination of feces of live birds.

Protozoa were historically placed in a single phylum, containing all one-celled animals. The complex organization and vastly different structure of protozoa led to the separation of various classes into seven different phyla (1). Two of these phyla contain species that are important parasites of poultry. The phylum Apicomplexa is characterized by the presence of an apical complex in sporozoites, and all are essentially intracellular parasites. Parasitic genera in this phylum include *Eimeria, Isospora, Haemoproteus, Leucocytozoon, Plasmodium, Toxoplasma, Sarcocystis, Wenyonella, Tyzzeria*, and *Cryptosporidium*.

The second phylum, Sarcomastigophora, includes the flagellates and amebas. Generally, they possess pseudopodia or flagella or both as locomotor organelles. Genera in this phylum that are important to poultry include *Histomonas, Trypanosoma, Chilomastix, Entamoeba, Endolimax*, and *Hexamita*.

Encephalitozoon cuniculi, a protozoan in a third phylum, Microspora, recently has been discovered infecting chickens. The protozoan is egg-transmitted and infection can be associated with embryo mortality but is usually inapparent. Affected birds may show inactivity, lameness, mild diarrhea, and weight loss. Parasites have been identified in the digestive tract, urogenital organs, and muscle. In embryos, brain and heart also were found to be infected (2, 3).

REFERENCES

1. Levine, N.D. 1985. Veterinary Protozoology. Iowa State Univ Press, Ames, IA. 414 pp.
2. Reetz, J. 1993. Naturlich Mikrosporidien (Encephalitozoon cuniculi) Infecktionen bei Hühnern. Tierärztlich Praxis 21:429–435.
3. Reetz, J. 1994. Naturlich Übertragung von Mikrosporidien (Encephalitozoon cuniculi) über das Nühnerei. Tierärztlich Praxis 22:147–150.

COCCIDIOSIS

Larry R. McDougald and W. Malcolm Reid

INTRODUCTION. Coccidiosis is a disease of almost universal importance in poultry production. The protozoan parasites of the genus *Eimeria* mul-tiply in the intestinal tract and cause tissue damage, with resulting interruption of feeding and digestive processes or nutrient absorption; dehydration;

blood loss; and increased susceptibility to other disease agents. Historically, the spectacular onset of coccidiosis with bloody diarrhea and high mortality inspired awe and dread on the part of poultry growers and fanciers. Like many parasitic diseases, coccidiosis is largely a disease of young animals because immunity quickly develops after exposure and gives protection against later disease outbreaks. Unfortunately, there is no cross-immunity between species of *Eimeria* in birds, and later outbreaks may be the result of different species. The short, direct life cycle and high reproductive potential of coccidia in poultry intensifies the potential for severe outbreaks of disease in the modern poultry house, where 15–30,000 chickens may be reared in total confinement.

Coccidiosis may strike any type of poultry in any type of facility. The disease may be mild, resulting from ingestion of a few oocysts, and may escape notice, or may be severe as a result of ingestion of millions of oocysts. Most infections are relatively mild, but because of the potential for the disastrous outbreak and the resulting financial loss, almost all young poultry are given continuous medication with low levels of anticoccidial drugs, which prevent the infection or reduce infections to a low, immunizing level. Immunity is not as important in broiler chickens, which may be kept only for 6–8 wk before market, as in layers, turkeys, and breeder birds, which may be kept much longer. Vaccines against coccidiosis have met with limited success, and have been used mostly in breeder pullets and in turkeys. Vaccination of broilers has rarely been practiced because even light infections with some species of coccidia can affect weight gain, feed conversion, and pigmentation of the skin.

CLASSIFICATION AND TAXONOMIC RELATIONSHIPS.

The biology and taxonomy of coccidia were reviewed by Long (18) and Pellerdy (25). Although several genera of coccidia are known to infect some types of birds, those most often encountered in poultry belong to the genus *Eimeria* described in this section or the genus *Cryptosporidium* discussed in another section of this chapter. Species of *Eimeria* are frequently described from the morphology of the oocyst, a thick-walled zygote shed in fecal matter by the infected host. Oocysts are enclosed in a thick outer shell and consist of a single cell that begins the process of sporulation to yield the infective stage in about 48 hr. Infective oocysts contain four sporocysts, which in turn contain two sporozoites (Fig. 34.1).

The closely related parasites *Sarcocystis* and *Toxaplasma,* as well as avian malaria, are discussed in the subchapter Other Blood and Tissue Protozoa.

When oocysts are ingested, the oocyst wall is crushed in the gizzard, and the sporozoites are released from sporocysts by the action of chymotrypsin and bile salts in the small intestine. Sporozoites enter epithelial cells or are taken into intraepithelial lymphocytes, where development may begin. Species of coccidia are identified on the basis of: 1) oocyst morphology, 2) host specificity, 3) immune specificity, 4) appearance and location of gross lesions within the natural host, and 5) length of the prepatent period. The host specificity of *Eimeria* in birds and mammals is very strict, so that parasites from different species of birds or animals can be considered different species even though they may have similar-appearing oocysts.

Life Cycle. Coccidiosis differs from bacterial and viral diseases in the self-limiting nature of its development. The life cycle of *E. tenella* (Fig. 34.2) is typical of all *Eimeria,* although some species vary in the number of asexual generations and the time required for each developmental stage. After the oocyst wall is crushed in the gizzard and the sporozoites are released, the sporozoites enter cells in the mucosa of the intestine and begin the cell cycle leading to reproduction. At least two generations of asexual development, called schizogony or merogony, lead to a sexual phase, where small, motile microgametes seek out and unite with macrogametes. The resulting zygote matures into an oocyst, which is released from the intestinal mucosa and is shed in the feces. With each species, the reproductive potential from a single ingested oocyst is fairly constant. The entire process takes 4-6 days, depending on species, although oocysts may be shed for several days after patency is reached. In some species (*E. tenella, E. necatrix*), the maximum tissue damage may occur when second-generation schizonts rupture to release merozoites. Other species may have small schizonts, which cause lit-

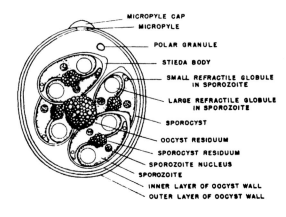

34.1. Diagram of sporulated oocyst of genus *Eimeria.*

tle damage, but the gametocytes may elicit a strong reaction with cellular infiltration and thickened, inflamed tissues.

Relationship between Coccidiosis and Other Poultry Diseases.

The tissue damage and changes in intestinal tract function may allow colonization by various harmful bacteria, such as *Clostridium perfringens,* leading to necrotic enteritis (12, 19), or *Salmonella typhimurium* (2, 3).

Immunosuppressive diseases may act in concert with coccidiosis to produce a more severe disease. Marek's disease may interfere with development of immunity to coccidiosis (4), and infectious bursal disease (IBD) may exacerbate coccidiosis, placing a heavier burden on anticoccidial drugs (21).

COCCIDIOSIS IN CHICKENS.

Coccidiosis remains one of the most expensive and common diseases of poultry production in spite of advances in chemotherapy, management, nutrition and genetics. The disease is often diagnosed in birds brought to diagnostic laboratories (1), but the vast majority of cases are diagnosed in the field, and handled by poultry service personnel. The current expense for preventive medication exceeds $90 million in the USA and over $300 million worldwide.

Incidence and Distribution.

Coccidia are almost universally found wherever chickens are raised. Their strict host specificity eliminates wild birds as sources of infection. The most common means of spread of coccidia is mechanical, by personnel who move between pens, houses, or farms. Coccidial infections are self-limiting and depend largely on the number of oocysts ingested and on the immune status of the bird. Surveys in North and South America revealed coccidia present in almost all broiler farms (22, 23). Very high percentages of positive flocks were also reported from Europe (5, 17). Oocysts in the litter or droppings of broiler chickens are usually most numerous at 4–5 wk of age, and generally decline thereafter. Few oocysts are found after birds are removed from a farm, be-

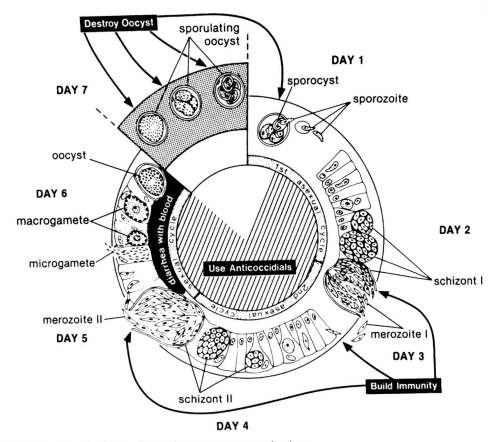

34.2. The 7-day life cycle of *E. tenella* includes two or more asexual and one sexual cycle during the 6 days after an oocyst has been swallowed by the host. The new generation of oocysts must sporulate (day 7) after being passed by the host before becoming infective.

cause poultry litter or droppings are poor environments for their survival. The ubiquitous nature of poultry coccidia precludes the possibility of elimination or prevention of coccidia by quarantine, disinfection, and sanitation.

Etiology. Nine species of *Eimeria* have been described from chickens (Table 34.1), but some are questionable. Similarly, several species of *Cryptosporidium* were described, but possibly only one or two names are valid owing to the lack of species specificity. *Cryptosporidium* spp. are often diagnosed, but clinical disease is not often seen (9). Concurrent infection with two or more species of coccidia is common.

Characteristics useful in identification of species are as follows: 1) location of the lesions in the intestine, 2) appearance of the gross lesion, 3) oocyst size, shape, and color, 4) size of schizonts and merozoites, 5) location of parasites in tissues (type of cell parasitized), 6) minimum prepatent period in experimental infections, 7) minimum time for sporulation, 8) immunogenicity against pure strains. In recent years, more emphasis has been placed on biochemical and physiologic identification of coccidia. A promising new tool for species identification is electrophoresis of metabolic enzymes (28). For diagnostic purposes, the traditional characteristics are adequate, and a satisfactory diagnosis can be made from Table 34.2. Cross-immunity and biochemical studies require pure species isolates propagated from single oocysts. Monoclonal antibodies are useful in serologic diagnosis, but have not been suitably specific to distinguish species, probably because of common antigens. The severity of infection is often graded on a scale of 0–4 as described by Johnson and Reid (16), where 0 = normal and 4 = maximum lesion.

EIMERIA ACERVULINA TYZZER **1929.** This species is the most frequently encountered in commercial poultry in North and South America. Oocysts are ovoid and often show thinning of the shell at the small end. The average size of oocysts is 18.3 × 14.6 µm, but the range is 17.7–20.2 × 13.7–16.3 µm.

PATHOGENICITY. Severity of infection may vary with the isolate, the number of oocysts ingested and the immune state of the bird. Ingestion of 1000, 30,000, 100,000 or 1,000,000 oocysts by young White Rock chicks resulted in mild to severe coccidiosis, with lesion scores ranging from 1+ (1000 oocysts) to 4+ (1,000,000 oocysts) (26). Reduction in rate of weight gain was also proportional to the infective dose. Heavy infections often cause lesions to coalesce, and sometimes mortality may result. Light to moderate infections may produce little effect on weight gain and feed conversion, but may cause loss of carotenoid and xanthophyll pigments from the blood and skin because of reduced absorption in the small intestine. The intestinal mucosa may be thickened, resulting in poor feed conversion. Egg production may be reduced in laying birds.

GROSS LESIONS AND HISTOPATHOLOGY. Lesions can often be seen from the serosal surface of the small intestine. The intestinal mucosa may at first be thin and covered with white plaques, which tend to arrange in transverse fashion and cause a ladderlike appearance because of the striations. The intestine may be pale and contain watery fluid. The gross lesion in light infections is limited to the duodenal loop, with only a few plaques/cm, but in heavy infections lesions may extend some distance through the small intestine, and plaques may overlap or coalesce; they are generally smaller in heavy infections due to crowding. The lesions are comprised of schizonts, gametocytes, and developing oocysts. Microscopy of smears from intestinal lesions usually reveals numerous oocysts.

Histopathology of the small intestine reveals the ovoid gametocytes lining the mucosal cells on the villi. In moderate to heavy infections, the tips of villi are broken off, leading to truncation and fusion of villi and thickening of the mucosa. Some cells may contain more than one parasite. Schiff's reagent will stain the macrogametes and developing oocysts a brilliant red, because of the polysaccharide used in oocyst wall formation.

EIMERIA BRUNETTI LEVINE **1942.** About 10–20% of field isolates in recent surveys in the United States and South America contained *E. brunetti* (22). The oocysts of *E. brunetti* average 24.6 × 18.8 µm, and are easily confused with *E. tenella*. This species is found in the lower small intestine, usually from the yolk sac diverticulum to near the cecal juncture. In severe cases, the lesion may extend from the gizzard to the cloaca and extend into the ceca (Fig. 34.3 E–H). Most field infections are difficult to recognize based on gross lesions and can be confirmed only with the aid of microscopy.

PATHOGENICITY. Although less serious than *E. tenella* or *E. necatrix*, *E. brunetti* is capable of producing moderate mortality, loss of weight gain, poor feed conversion and other complications. Inoculation with 100,000–200,000 oocysts will frequently cause 10–30% mortality and reduced gain in survivors. Light infections of *E. brunetti* are easily overlooked unless careful attention is paid to the lower small intestine. Such infections can cause reduced weight gain and poor feed conversion even though gross lesions are not clearly apparent.

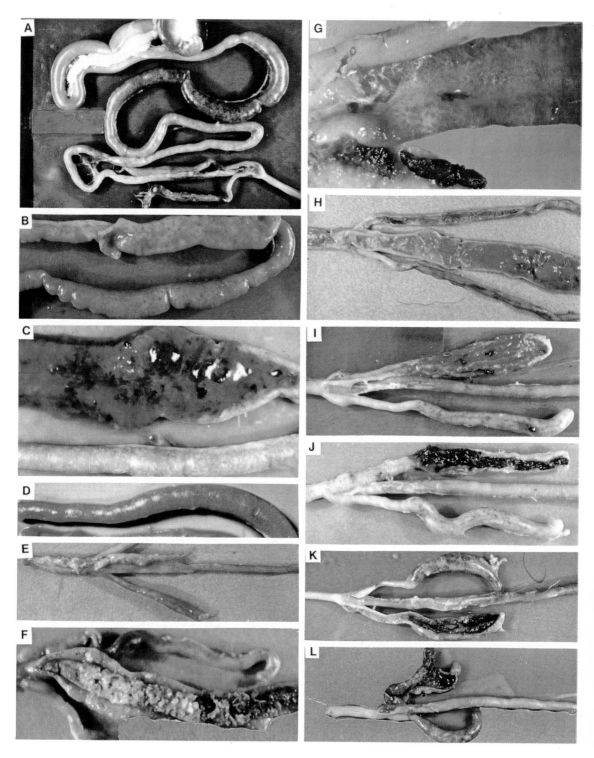

34.4. *A. Eimeria necatrix* showing ballooning in midgut. *B. E. necatrix* (+2). *C. E. necatrix D. E. necatrix* (+4). (Long et al., [British] Crown copyright 1976). *E. E. brunetti* from bacteria-free chick. *F. E. brunetti* (+4). *G. E. brunetti* (+3). *H. E. brunetti* (+4) (Long et al. [British] Crown copyright 1976). *I. E. tenella* (+2). *J. E. tenella* (+3). *K. E. tenella* (+4). *L. E. tenella* (+4) with cecal core.

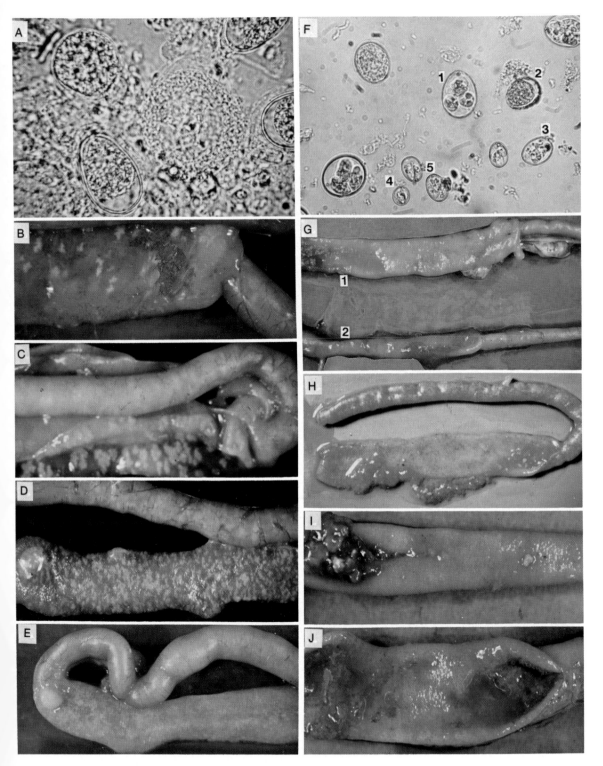

34.3. *A.* Oocysts and a microgametocyte (*center*) of *Eimeria maxima* (Long et al., [British] Crown copyright 1976). *B. E. acervulina* (+2). *C. E. acervulina* (+2). *D. E. acervulina* (+3). *E. E. acervulina* (+4). *F. 1.* Sporulated *E. maxima* with distinctive brownish walls; *2.* Unsporulated *E. maxima* showing roughened outer wall; *3.* Probably *E. tenella*; *4.* End view, probably *E. mitis*; *5.* Side view, probably two *E. mitis. G. 1.* normal midgut; *2. E. maxima* midgut (+1). *H. E. maxima* midgut (+2 or +3) (Long et al., [British] Crown copyright 1976). *I. E. maxima* (+3). *J. E. maxima* close-up view (+4).

Table 34.2.   Anticoccidial drugs for treatment of coccidiosis in chickens

Trade or Empirical Name (Manufacturer)	Feed or Water	Active Ingredient: Treatment, Duration	First Approval by FDA	Drug Withdrawal (Days before Slaughter)
Sulfamethazine (American Cyanamid)	Water	0.1%: 2 days; 0.05%: 4 days	1947	10
SQ,[a] sulfaquinoxaline (Merck): Sulquin[a] (Salsbury)	Feed	0.1%: 2-3 days on, 3 off followed by 0.05%: 2 on, 3 off, 2 on	1948	10
Amprol,[a] amprolium (Merck)	Water	0.012-0.024%: 3-5 days; 0.006%: 1-2 weeks	1960	0
Esb3,[a] sodium sulfachloropyrazine monohydrate (Squibb)	Water	0.03%: 3 days	1967	4
Agribon,[a] Albon,[a] sulfadimethoxine (Hoffmann-La Roche)	Water	0.05%: 6 days	1968	5

FDA, Food and Drug Administration.
[a] Registered trade name.

GROSS LESIONS AND HISTOPATHOLOGY. At early stages of infection, the mucosa of the lower small intestine may be covered with tiny petechiae and have some thickening and loss of color. In heavy infections, the mucosa is badly damaged, with coagulation necrosis appearing on days 5–7 post infection (PI) and with a caseous eroded surface over the entire mucosa. The coagulated blood and mucosa will be apparent in the droppings. Thickening of the mucosa and edematous swelling occurs in severe infections, especially on the 6th day PI.

The asexual stages of first- and second-generation schizogony generally occur in the upper small intestine. Histopathology on the 4th day of infection reveals schizonts, cellular infiltration, and some damage to the mucosa. By the 5th day, many of the tips of villi are broken off. Merozoites invade the epithelium and develop into sexual stages in the lower small intestine and ceca. In severe cases, the villi may be completely denuded, and in some instances only the basement membranes remain.

Eimeria hagani Levine **1938.**   The taxonomic status of *E. hagani* is in doubt because the original description was incomplete. This species reportedly produced hemorrhagic spots, catarrhal inflammation, and watery intestinal contents and was moderately pathogenic. Unless research is forthcoming to establish the characteristics of this species and existence in field infections, it will likely be declared invalid.

Eimeria maxima Tyzzer **1929.**   The mid–small intestine is often parasitized with *E. maxima*, from below the duodenal loop past the yolk sac di-

verticulum, but in heavy infections the lesions may extend throughout the small intestine. *E. maxima* is an easy species to recognize because of the characteristic large oocysts, 30.5 × 20.7 µm (21.5–42.5 × 16.5–29.8), which usually have a distinctive yellowish color (Fig. 34.4A,F,G,H,I,J). There is often an abundance of yellow-orange mucus and fluid in the midgut. This species can be differentiated from *E. necatrix* by the lack of large schizonts associated with the lesions, and from *E. brunetti* by the larger oocysts and the appearance of the lesions.

PATHOGENICITY.   This species is moderately pathogenic. Infection with 200,000 oocysts is usually sufficient to cause poor weight gain, morbidity, diarrhea, and sometimes mortality. There is often extreme emaciation, pallor, roughening of feathers, and inappetence. Producers interested in maintaining good skin color in chickens must be concerned with subclinical infections because of the effect of this species on absorption of the xanthophyll and carotenoid pigments in the small intestine.

GROSS LESIONS AND HISTOPATHOLOGY.   Minimal tissue damage occurs with the first two asexual cycles, which develop superficially in the epithelial cells of the mucosa. When the sexual stages develop in deeper tissues on the 5th to 8th days PI, lesions develop because of congestion and edema, cellular infiltration, and thickening of the mucosa. Infected host cells become enlarged, pushing into the subepithelial zone. Microscopic hemorrhages occur near the tips of the villi, and foci of infection can be seen from the serosal surface. The intestine may be flaccid and filled with fluid, and the lumen

Table 34.1. DIFFERENTIAL CHARACTERISTICS FOR 9 SPECIES OF CHICKEN COCCIDIA ◉

DIAGNOSTIC CHARACTERISTICS IN RED

	CHARACTERISTICS	E. acervulina	E. brunetti	E. maxima	E. mitis †	E. mivati ‡	E. necatrix	E. praecox	E. tenella	SPECIES OF DOUBTFUL VALIDITY — E. hagani
MACROSCOPIC LESIONS	ZONE PARASITIZED									
	MACROSCOPIC LESIONS	light infection whitish round lesions sometimes in ladder-like streaks heavy infection plaques coalescing, thickened intestinal wall	coagulation necrosis mucoid, bloody enteritis in lower intestine	thickened walls, mucoid, blood-tinged exudate, petechiae	no discrete lesions in intestine, mucoid exudate	light infection rounded plaques of oocysts heavy infection thickened walls coalescing plaques	ballooning, white spots (schizonts), petechiae mucoid blood-filled exudate	no lesions, mucoid exudate	onset hemorrhage into lumen later thickening, whitish mucosa, cores clotted blood	pinhead hemorrhages petechiae — non available
MICROSCOPIC CHARACTERISTICS	OOCYSTS REDRAWN FROM ORIGINALS (millimicrons)									
	LENGTH × WIDTH / µ LENGTH = / WIDTH =	AV = 18.3 × 14.6 / 17.7 - 20.2 / 13.7 - 16.3	24.6 × 18.8 / 20.7 - 30.3 / 18.1 - 24.2	30.5 × 20.7 / 21.5 - 42.5 / 16.5 - 29.8	15.6 × 14.2 / 11.7 - 18.7 / 11.0 - 18.0	15.6 × 13.4 / 11.1 - 19.9 / 10.5 - 16.2	20.4 × 17.2 / 13.2 - 22.7 / 11.3 - 18.3	21.3 × 17.1 / 19.8 - 24.7 / 15.7 - 19.8	22.0 × 19.0 / 19.5 - 26.0 / 16.5 - 22.8	19.1 × 17.6 / 15.8 - 20.9 / 14.3 - 19.5
	OOCYST SHAPE AND INDEX / LENGTH/WIDTH	ovoid / 1.25	ovoid / 1.31	ovoid / 1.47	subspherical / 1.09	ellipsoid to broadly ovoid / 1.16	oblong ovoid / 1.19	ovoidal / 1.24	ovoid / 1.16	broadly ovoid / 1.08
	SCHIZONT MAX IN MICRONS	10.3	30.0	9.4	15.1	17.3	65.9	20	54.0	
LIFE HISTORY CHARACTERISTICS	PARASITE LOCATION IN TISSUE SECTIONS	epithelial	2nd generation schizonts subepithelial	gametocytes subepithelial	epithelial	epithelial	2nd generation schizonts subepithelial	epithelial	2nd generation schizonts subepithelial	epithelial
	MINIMUM PREPATENT PERIOD-HR	97	120	121	93	93	138	83	115	99
	SPORULATION TIME MINIMUM (HR)	17	18	30	15	12	18	12	18	18

† = From Norton and Joyner (1980)
‡ = As described by Edgar and Siebold (1964)
◉ = Compiled from various sources (1982)

Peter L. Long and W. Malcolm Reid
Department of Poultry Science
The University of Georgia, Athens

often contains yellow or orange mucus and blood. This condition has been described as "ballooning." Microscopic pathology is characterized by edema and cellular infiltration, developing schizonts through day 4, and sexual stages (macrogametes and microgametes) in deeper tissues on days 5–8. In severe infections, there is considerable disruption of the mucosa.

***EIMERIA MITIS* TYZZER 1929.**   The lower small intestine is the normal site of this parasite, from the yolk sac diverticulum to the cecal necks. The lesions are normally indistinct with this species, but the potential for pathogenic effects on weight gain and morbidity was recently demonstrated.

PATHOGENICITY.   Infection with 1–1.5 million oocysts will reduce weight gain and cause morbidity and loss of pigmentation. The lack of distinct gross lesions causes this species to be overlooked or misdiagnosed in subclinical infections.

GROSS LESIONS AND HISTOPATHOLOGY.   Clinically, the gross lesion is very slight and can be easily overlooked. The lower small intestine appears pale and flaccid, and microscopic examination of smears from the mucosal surface may reveal numerous tiny oocysts (15.6×14.2 µm). The infection is easily distinguished from *E. brunetti* by the smaller, round oocysts. In light infections, the appearance of the gross lesion may be similar to *E. brunetti*. The gross lesion of this species is unremarkable because the developing parasites do not tend to localize in colonies as do other species, and the schizonts and gametocytes are superficial in the mucosa.

***EIMERIA MIVATI* EDGAR AND SIEBOLD 1964.**   This parasite was first identified as a small strain of *E. acervulina* (7). The parasitized zone reportedly extends from the duodenal loop to the ceca and cloaca. Early lesions appear in the duodenum and later in the midgut and lower small intestine. In light infections, isolated lesions resemble those of *E. acervulina,* but are more circular in shape. These lesions, representing colonies of gametocytes and developing oocysts, may be seen from the serosal surface of the gut. Infection with 1,000,000 oocysts of *E. mivati* causes reduced weight gain and morbidity. Occasional mortality occurs in experimental infections.

Recent work with isoenzymes has caused some workers to question the validity of *E. mivati*. Examination of laboratory cultures has failed to produce a bona fide culture of *E. mivati,* but there have been no extensive field studies aimed at settling this controversy. While there is no convincing evidence for the existence of this species, not all field obser-

vations can be easily explained within the taxonomic limits of other described species. Further work will be needed to settle the taxonomic status of this species.

***EIMERIA NECATRIX* JOHNSON 1930.**   Because of the spectacular lesions in the small intestine, this species was one of the best known by early poultry producers. The lesion is found in the small intestine in approximately the same location as *E. maxima* (Fig. 34.3 A-D). Probably because of the low reproductive capability of *E. necatrix,* it is not able to compete with other coccidia and is diagnosed mostly in older birds such as brooder pullets or layer pullets 9–14 wk old. The intestine is often dilated to twice its normal size (ballooning) and the lumen may be filled with blood. The oocysts are near in size to those of *E. tenella* and are found only in the ceca. The sexual stages do not develop in the intestine where the lesions are found, but in the ceca where they compete for space with *E. tenella*. The developing gametocytes are scattered and not found in colonies.

PATHOGENICITY, GROSS LESIONS, AND HISTOPATHOLOGY.   Some gross lesions may be associated with first-generation schizogony at 2–3 days PI. By the 4th day PI, the intestine may be ballooned, the mucosa thickened, and the lumen filled with fluid, blood, and tissue debris. From the serosal surface, the foci of infection can be seen as small white plaques or red petechiae. Smears examined microscopically on the 4–5th days may contain numerous clusters of large (66 µm) schizonts, often containing hundreds of merozoites. The clusters of schizonts deep in the mucosa often penetrate the submucosa and damage the layers of smooth muscle and destroy blood vessels. In these instances, the foci are large enough to be seen from the serosal surface. Later, scar tissue may be seen where epithelial regeneration is incomplete. Few pathogenic effects are seen with the invasion of the cecal mucosa by the third-generation schizonts and gametocytes because of the scattered, noncolonizing nature of these stages. The third-generation schizonts produce only 6–16 merozoites, compared with the hundreds of merozoites produced by the second-generation schizonts in the small intestine.

Lesions may extend throughout the small intestine in severe infections, causing dilation (ballooning) and thickening of the mucosa. The lumen may be filled with blood and pieces of mucosal tissue. From the serosal surface, the infection may be seen as white or red foci, or in dead birds the foci will be white and black, giving the appearance of "salt and pepper." Microscopic examination of smears from the mucosal surface reveals numerous clusters of large schizonts, which are characteristic for this species and distinguishes it from others that overlap in habitat. Also, oocysts are never associated with lesions of this species.

Infection with 75,000–100,000 oocysts is sufficient to cause severe weight loss, morbidity, and mortality. Survivors may be emaciated, suffer secondary infections, and lose pigmentation. Droppings of infected birds often contain blood, fluid, and mucus. This species and *E. tenella* are the most pathogenic of the chicken coccidia. Naturally occurring infections have caused mortality in excess of 25% in commercial flocks, and in experimental infections 100% mortality is possible.

***EIMERIA PRAECOX* JOHNSON 1930.** This species is named from the short prepatent period (about 83 hrs); hence a "precocious" parasite. Even though *E. praecox* is often overlooked because there are no prominent lesions, there may be reduced weight gain, loss of pigmentation, extreme loss of fluids, and poor feed conversion.

PATHOGENICITY, GROSS LESIONS, AND HISTO-PATHOLOGY. The gross lesion consists of watery intestinal contents and sometimes mucus and mucoid casts. Most of the infection is confined to the duodenal loop. Small pinpoint hemorrhages may be seen on the mucosal surface on the 4th and 5th days of infection. Recent studies suggest that this species may cause morbidity and reduced weight gain (10). Dehydration may result from the extreme fluid loss caused by severe infections. The epithelial cells of the sides of the villi (but not the tips) are most often infected. There may be several parasites in each cell. Three to four asexual generations are followed by the sexual stages. The oocysts are generally larger than those of other species found in the duodenum. At 21.3×17.1 μm, they are larger than *E. acervulina*, *E. mivati*, and *E. mitis* and smaller than *E. maxima*. Little tissue reaction has been described.

***EIMERIA TENELLA* (RAILLIET AND LUCET 1891) FANTHAM 1909.** Coccidiosis caused by *E. tenella* is the best known of the avian types, partly because of the spectacular disease it causes, and partly because of its widespread importance in commercial broilers. This species inhabits the ceca and adjacent intestinal tissues, causing a severe disease characterized by bleeding, high morbidity and mortality, lost weight gain, emaciation, and other signs attributed to coccidiosis. Diagnosis is dependent upon finding cecal lesions with accompanying clusters of large schizonts or (later) oocysts (Fig. 34.3 I–L).

PATHOGENICITY, PATHOGENESIS, AND EPIZOOTIOLOGY. Experimental inoculation with 100,000

sporulated oocysts can cause morbidity, mortality, and greatly reduced weight gain, making this one of the most pathogenic species in chickens. Inoculation with 1000–3000 oocysts is sufficient to cause bloody droppings and other signs of infection. The most pathogenic stage is the second-generation schizont, which matures at 4 days PI. Like *E. necatrix,* this species produces colonies of large schizonts, which may contain hundreds of merozoites. The schizonts develop deep in the lamina propria, so that the mucosa is badly disrupted when the schizonts mature and merozoites are released. Onset of mortality in a flock is rapid. Most of the mortality occurs between 5 and 6 days PI, and in acute infections it may follow the first signs of infection by only a few hours. Blood loss may reduce the erythrocyte count and hematocrit value as much as 50%. The maximum effect on weight gain is seen at 7 days PI. Some of the weight lost from dehydration may be regained quickly, but growth will always lag behind that of uninfected birds. The exact cause of death is not known, but toxic factors are suspected. Blood loss alone does not account for mortality. In a few cases, death may result from gangrenous or ruptured cecal pouches. Extracts of infected cecal pouches produce acute blood coagulation and death when injected intravenously into other chicks. The possible role of bacterial products in mortality from coccidiosis is suggested by the lack of mortality from *E. tenella* in germ-free chicks.

GROSS LESIONS AND HISTOPATHOLOGY. Even during maturation of the first generation of schizonts, small foci of denuded epithelium may be seen. By the 4th day PI, the second-generation schizonts are maturing and hemorrhages are apparent. The cecal pouch may become greatly enlarged and distended with clotted blood and pieces of cecal mucosa in the lumen. On the 6th and 7th days, the cecal core becomes hardened and drier; eventually it is passed in the feces. Regeneration of the epithelium is rapid and may be complete by the 10th day. The infection can usually be seen from the serosal surface of the ceca as dark petechiae and foci, which become coalesced in more severe infections. The cecal wall is often greatly thickened because of edema and infiltration, and later scar tissue.

Microscopically, the first-generation schizonts are widely scattered and mature at 2–3 days PI. Small focal areas of hemorrhage and necrosis may appear near blood vessels of the inner circular muscles of the muscularis layer. Heterophil infiltration of the submucosa proceeds rapidly as the large second-generation schizonts develop in the lamina propria. These are found in clusters or colonies that generally are progeny of a single first-generation schizont. Maturation of the second-generation parasites is accompanied by excessive tissue damage, bleeding, disruption of the cecal glands, and often complete destruction of the mucosa and muscularis layer. Oocysts are seen on microscopic examination on the 6th and 7th days, when macrogametes and motile microgametes can often be seen. Regeneration of the epithelium and glands may be complete by the 10th day in light infections, but the epithelium may never completely recover in severe infections. Lost muscularis mucosa is not replaced and the submucosa becomes densely fibrosed.

Epizootiology

NATURAL AND EXPERIMENTAL HOSTS. The chicken is the only natural host of the species described above. Reports of these species of *Eimeria* infecting other birds can be considered spurious. Cross-transmission of *Eimeria* spp. from chickens to other host species has been unsuccessful except for a few instances where immunocompromised birds were used.

Chickens of all ages and breeds are susceptible to infection. Immunity develops quickly, limiting further infection. Newly hatched birds are sometimes not fully susceptible to infection because of insufficient chymotrypsin and bile salts in the intestines to cause excystation. Outbreaks are common at 3–6 wk of age and are rarely seen in poultry flocks at less than 3 wk. Surveys of coccidia in broiler houses in Georgia demonstrated the manner in which oocysts of coccidia build up during growth of a flock, then decline as the birds become immune to further infection (27). This "self-limiting" nature of coccidial infections is widely known in chickens and other poultry. There is no stimulation of cross-immunity between species of coccidia. Thus, several outbreaks of coccidiosis are possible in the same flock, with different species involved in each. Breeder pullets and layer pullets are at greatest risk because they are kept on litter for 20 wk or more. Normally the infections with *E. acervulina, E. tenella,* and *E. maxima* are seen at 3–6 wk of age, then *E. necatrix* at 8–18 wk of age.

Coccidiosis rarely occurs in layers and breeders because of prior exposure to coccidia and resulting immunity. In a few instances, a flock may not be exposed to a particular species, or the immunity may lapse because of other diseases. Outbreaks of any species in layers can reduce or eliminate egg production for several wk.

TRANSMISSION AND VECTORS. Ingestion of viable sporulated oocysts is the only natural method of transmission. Infected chickens may shed oocysts in the feces for several days or wk. The oocysts in feces become infective through the process of sporulation within 2 days. Susceptible birds in the same flock may ingest the oocysts through the litter-pecking activities common to chickens.

Although there are no natural intermediate hosts for the *Eimeria* spp., oocysts can be spread mechanically by many different animals, insects, contaminated equipment, wild birds, and dust. Oocysts are generally considered resistant to environmental extremes and to disinfectants, although survival time varies with conditions. Oocysts may survive for many wk in soil, but survival in poultry litter is limited to a few days because of the ammonia released by composting and the action of molds and bacteria. Viable oocysts have been reported from the dust inside and outside broiler houses, as well as from insects in poultry litter (27). The darkling beetle, common in broiler litter, is a mechanical carrier of oocysts. Transmission from one farm to another is facilitated by movement of personnel and equipment between farms and by the migration of wild birds, which may mechanically spread the oocysts. New farms may remain free of coccidia for most of the first growout of chickens until the introduction of coccidia to a completely susceptible flock. Such outbreaks, which are usually more severe than those experienced on older farms, are often called "the new-house coccidiosis syndrome."

Oocysts may survive for many wk under optimal conditions but will be quickly killed by exposure to high or low temperatures or drying. Exposure to 55 C or freezing kills oocysts very quickly. Even 37 C is fatal when continued for 2–3 days. Sporozoites and sporocysts can be frozen in liquid nitrogen with appropriate cryopreservation technique, but oocysts cannot be adequately infiltrated with cryoprotectants to effect survival. Threat of coccidiosis is less during hot dry weather and greater in cooler wetter weather.

Diagnosis. Coccidiosis can best be diagnosed from birds killed for immediate necropsy. Attempts to identify characteristic lesions in birds that have been dead for 1 hr or longer are frustrated by the postmortem changes that begin quickly in the intestine. The entire intestinal tract should be examined. A microscope should be available for use in looking for special diagnostic characteristics such as the large schizonts of *E. necatrix* or the small round oocysts of *E. mitis.* The finding of a few oocysts by microscopic examination of smears from the intestine indicates the presence of infection, but not a diagnosis of clinical coccidiosis. Coccidia are often present in the intestines of birds 3–6 wk old in most flocks. Coccidiosis should be diagnosed if the gross lesions are serious, or if other economic parameters are threatened. Diagnosis should be based on finding of lesions and confirmatory microscopic stages on necropsy of typical birds from the flock, rather than from culls.

Microscopic Examination. Many stages of coccidia can be seen in smears taken from the suspected lesion. A small amount of mucosal scraping should be diluted with saline on a slide, then covered with a coverslip. Oocysts or macrogametes are most easily seen, but in many cases the lesion is caused by maturing schizonts. Presence of clusters of large schizonts in the midgut area is pathognomonic for *E. necatrix,* while a similar finding in the ceca indicates *E. tenella.*

Oocyst size and shape are less useful as diagnostic characteristics in chickens than once thought, because of the extensive overlapping in size of the species. Measurement of 30–50 oocysts of the predominant type of oocyst usually gives a good indication of the size of the unknown species. This information is useful in conjunction with other observations in the identification of species in field cases.

Lesion Scoring. The severity of lesions is generally proportionate to the number of oocysts ingested by the bird and correlates with other parameters such as weight loss and droppings scores. The most commonly used system was devised by Johnson and Reid (16). By this system a score of 0 to 4 is assigned to a bird where 0 = normal and 4 = most severe case. This technique is most useful in experimental infections, where the dose of oocysts and medicaments are controlled, and the species are known. In the field, lesion scoring is generally useful in gauging the severity of infections. Even though there are several species of coccidia that may be present at some time, only four separate sections of the intestine are usually scored. These are 1) the duodenum (upper), 2) the midgut from the duodenum past the yolk sac diverticulum, 3) the lower small intestine from the yolk sac diverticulum to the cecal junctures, and 4) the ceca.

Droppings Score. In laboratory infections, the droppings score may be used in the same manner as lesion score for a rapid and fairly reliable rating of the infection (24). The extent of abnormal droppings is rated on a scale of 0–4, where 4 = maximum diarrhea, with mucus, fluid, and/or blood.

Histopathology Methods. Ordinary methods in histopathology are satisfactory for routine examination of tissues infected with coccidia. Staining of sections with H & E or other common histologic stains will demonstrate developing stages. There are specialized techniques that will identify specific stages: Staining with Schiff's reagent gives a brilliant red color with the polysaccharide associated with the refractile body and with wall-forming bodies in the macrogamete. Monoclonal antibodies conjugated with fluorescent markers such as fluorescein are highly useful in research because specific stages of parts of cells can be readily identified.

Procedures Used in Species Identification. One of the oldest techniques takes advantage of the lack of cross-immunity when birds are infected with one species of coccidia. If pure cultures of coccidia are used to infect groups of birds repeatedly, they will become immune to that species. If a test culture produces patent infections in immunized birds, it must be of a different species. In this way, by process of elimination, the species can be determined. This technique is time consuming and requires extensive laboratory isolation facilities and access to pure cultures of known species of coccidia, but has proved extremely useful as a research tool. Pure species cultures of coccidia are difficult to maintain because they must be propagated in strict isolation to prevent contamination.

Preservation of Coccidia for Experimental Work. Droppings or litter collected in the field, or intestinal contents in the diagnostic lab, can be saved for isolation of coccidia in a solution of 2–4% potassium dichromate. Aeration of oocyst suspensions is necessary to allow sporulation. A good-quality aquarium pump is highly effective and can be regulated with valves and tubes to service several bottles at one time. For short-term storage, suspensions of oocysts may be refrigerated.

Prevention and Control

CONTROL OF COCCIDIOSIS BY CHEMOTHERAPY. Early emphasis in chemotherapy was centered on the treatment of outbreaks with sulfonamides or other compounds after signs of infection were apparent. Soon, the concept of preventive medication emerged with the realization that most of the damage is done once signs of coccidiosis are widespread in a flock. Today almost all broiler flocks receive preventive medication, and treatment is used as a last resort (Table 34.3). The historical aspects of chemotherapy have been reviewed extensively by McDougald (20).

CHARACTERISTICS OF ANTICOCCIDIAL DRUGS. All types of drugs used for coccidiosis control are unique in the mode of action, the way in which parasites are killed or arrested, and the effects of the drug on the growth and performance of the bird. Following are the most important characteristics.

Spectrum of Activity. There are several important

Table 34.3. Preventive anticoccidials approved by FDA for use in feed formulation

Trade or Empirical Name, Approved Level (Manufacturer)	Trade Name	First Approval by FDA	Drug Withdrawal (Days before (Slaughter)
Sulfaquinoxaline, 0.015-0.025% (Merck)	SQ, Sulquin	1948	10
Nitrofurazone, 0.0055% (Hess & Clark; Smith-Kline)	nfz, Amifur	1948	5
Arsanilic acid or sodium arsanilate, 0.04% for 8 days (Abbott)	Pro-Gen	1949	5
Butynorate, 0.0375% for turkeys (Solvay)	Tinostat	1954	28
Nicarbazin, 0.0125% (Merck)	Nicarb	1955	4
Furazolidone, 0.0055-0.011% (Hess & Clark)	nf-180	1957	5
Nitromide, 0.025% + sulfanitran, 0.03% + roxarasone, 0.005% (Solvay)	Unistat-3	1958	5
Oxytetracycline, 0.022% (Pfizer)	Terramycin	1959	3
Amprolium, 0.0125-0.025% (MSD-AGVET)	Amprol	1960	0
Chlortetracycline, 0.022% (American Cyanamid)	Aureomycin	1960	(see feeding restrictions)
Zoalene, 0.004-0.0125% (Solvay)	Zoamix	1960	(higher levels, 5 days)
Amprolium, 0.0125% + ethopabate, 0.0004/0.004% (Merck)	Amprol Plus, Amprol Hi-E	1963	0
Buquinolate, 0.00825% (Norwich-Eaton)	Bonaid	1967	0
Clopidol or meticlorpindol, 0.0125-0.025% (A. L. Laboratories)	Coyden	1968	0 days at 0.0125%; 5 days at 0.025%
Decoquinate 0.003% (Rhone-Poulenc)	Deccox	1970	0
Sulfadimethoxine, 0.0125% + ormetoprin, 0.0075% (Hoffmann-La Roche)	Rofenaid	1970	5
Monensin, 0.01-0.0121% (Elanco)	Coban	1971	0
Robenidine, 0.0033% (American Cyanamid)	Robenz, Cycostat	1972	5
Lasalocid, 0.0075-0.0125% (Hoffmann-La Roche)	Avatec	1976	3
Salinomycin, 0.004-0.0066% (Agri-Bio)	Bio-Cox	1983	0
Halofuginone, 3 ppm (Hoechst-Roussell Agri-Vet)	Stenorol	1987	5
Narasin, 54-72g/T (Elanco)	Monteban	1988	0
Madurimicin, 5-6 ppm (American Cyanamid)	Cygro	1989	5
Narasin + nicarbazin,54-90 g/T (Elanco)	Maxiban	1989	5
Semduramycin, 25 ppm (Pfizer)	Aviax	1995	0

Source: (8)
FDA, Food and Drug Administration.

species of coccidia in chickens, several more in turkeys, and many others in other hosts. A drug may be efficacious against one or several of these parasites; very few drugs are equally efficacious against all.

Mode of Action. Each class of chemical compound is unique in the type of action exerted on the parasite, and even in the developmental stage of the parasite most affected. The chemical mode of action of some drugs is known to be a highly detailed event, while the action of other drugs remains a mystery. The sulfonamides and related drugs compete for the incorporation of PABA and metabolism of folic acid. Amprolium competes for absorption of thiamine by the parasite. The quinoline coccidiostats and clopidol inhibit energy metabolism in

the cytochrome system of the coccidia. The polyether ionophores upset the osmotic balance of the protozoan cell by altering the permeability of cell membranes for alkaline metal cations.

The coccidia are prone to attack by drugs at various stages in development in the host. Totally unrelated drugs may attack the same stage of parasite. The quinolones and ionophores arrest or kill the sporozoite or early trophozoite. Nicarbazin, robenidine, and zoalene destroy the first- or second-generation schizont, and the sulfonamides act on the developing schizonts and also on the sexual stages. Diclazuril acts in early schizogony with *E. tenella*, but is delayed to later schizogony with *E. acervulina* and to the maturing macrogamete with *E. maxima*. The time of action in the life cycle has been construed as having significance in the use of drugs in certain types of programs in which immunity is desired, but there is no good evidence that this is true under practical conditions.

Coccidiocidal vs. Coccidiostatic. Some drugs kill the parasite, but others only arrest development. When coccidiostatic medication is withdrawn, arrested parasites may continue to develop and contaminate the environment with oocysts. In such cases, a relapse of coccidiosis is possible. In general, the coccidiocidal drugs have been more successful than those that are coccidiostatic.

Effects of Drugs on the Chicken. Most compounds used in animal feeds have good "selective toxicity," providing toxicity for the parasite but being nontoxic to vertebrates. Unfortunately, toxicity and side effects of drugs on the host are possible where formulation errors lead to overdose. Sometimes a drug may exhibit side effects at the recommended use level. Some of the toxicity may be the result of management, genetics, nutrition, or other interaction, and in other cases the margin of safety is just too narrow. Environmental interaction is possible with nicarbazin, which interacts with high temperatures to produce excess mortality. Also nicarbazin is highly toxic to layers, first causing a bleaching of brown-shelled eggs, mottling of yolks, reduced hatchability, and reduced production. The ionophores are highly toxic at elevated doses, causing a transient paralysis in mild overdoses, or a permanent paralysis and mortality in more severe cases. Monensin was once thought to interact with methionine to reduce feather growth, but this relationship is not clear. Under some conditions, lasalocid will stimulate water consumption and excretion, resulting in a wet litter. With slight overdoses, most of the ionophores depress weight gain under laboratory conditions. A withdrawal period of 5–7 days is often practiced to allow "compensatory growth" to make up for the lost gain. The ionophores are known for their toxicity to other animals. Thus, monensin and salinomycin are highly toxic to horses. The lethal dose-50% (LD_{50}) for monensin in horses is about 2 mg/kg body weight. Salinomycin is highly toxic to turkeys at levels above 15 g/ton and causes excessive mortality at the level recommended for use in chickens (60 g/ton), while monensin and lasalocid are well tolerated in turkeys at the level used for chickens.

PROGRAMS FOR USE OF ANTICOCCIDIAL DRUGS IN BROILERS. In broilers, the objective is usually to produce the maximum growth and feed efficiency with minimum of disease, while in layers or breeders the objective may be immunization (Fig. 34.5).

Continuous Use of a Single Drug. Often, a single product will be used from day 1 to slaughter, or with a withdrawal period of 3–7 days. Most products are approved for use until slaughter, but producers withdraw medication for economic or other reasons.

Shuttle or Dual Programs. The use of one product in the starter and another in the grower feed is called a "shuttle" program in the United States and a "dual" program in other countries. The shuttle program is usually intended to improve coccidiosis control. Intensive use of the polyether ionophore drugs for many years produced strains of coccidia in the field that have "reduced sensitivity" to the ionophores. It is a common practice to use another drug such as nicarbazin or halofuginone in either the starter or grower feed to bolster the anticoccidial control and take some pressure off of the ionophore. The use of shuttle programs is thought to reduce buildup of drug resistance. In 1988, approximately 80% of the producers used some type of shuttle program.

Rotation of Products. It is considered sound management to make changes in anticoccidial drug use. Most producers consider changes in the spring and in the fall. Rotation of drugs may improve productivity because of the buildup of isolates or species of coccidia that have reduced sensitivity after products have been used for a long time. Producers often notice a boost in productivity for a few months after a change of anticoccidial drugs.

DRUG RESISTANCE. The development of tolerance of drugs by coccidia after exposure to medication is the most serious limitation to the effectiveness of products. Surveys reveal widespread drug resistance in coccidia in the United States, South America, and Europe (11, 14, 15, 17, 20, 23). Even though coccidia develop less resistance to some drugs than to others, long-term exposure to any drug will produce a loss in sensitivity and, eventually, resistance. Drug resistance is a genetic phenomenon, and once established in a line of coccidia, will remain for many years or until selection pressure and genetic drift forces return to sensitivity in the population. Drugs such as the quinolones and clopidol have a well-defined mode of action, and resistance develops quickly as coccidia are selected with cytochromes, which do not bind as readily to the drug. The polyether ionophores, in contrast, have a more complicated mode of action involving the mechanisms of active transport of alkaline metal cations across cell membranes, and it has taken many years for coccidia to become tolerant, and in some cases, completely resistant. Many other drugs appear to be intermediate in selecting resis-

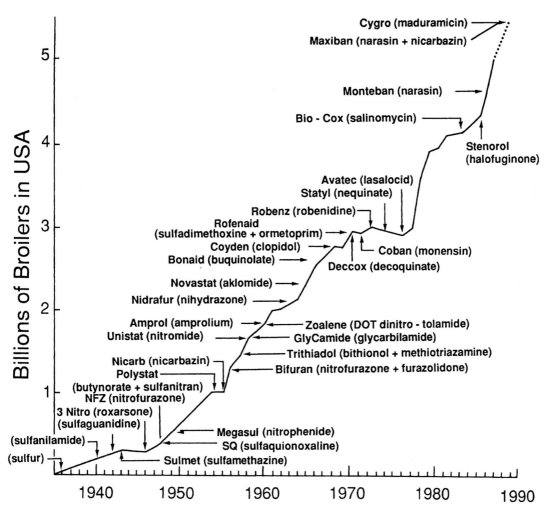

34.5. Broiler production (USDA figures) and year of introduction of new anticoccidial drugs. Generic names begin with lower case letters and trade names begin with capital letters. (Avian Dis)

tance in coccidia. The primary defense against drug resistance is the use of less intensive programs, shuttle programs, and frequent rotation of drugs. Rotation of programs, used alone, will not prevent the development of resistance because the periods of use of drugs between changes is often adequate for resistance development.

ANTICOCCIDIAL DRUGS USED FOR BROILERS IN THE UNITED STATES. The products currently approved for use in chickens in the United States are listed in Table 34.3. Not all are still available commercially, but the approvals remain. Those used at present include monensin, salinomycin, and lasalocid (polyether ionophores), nicarbazin, amprolium + ethopabate, decoquinate, clopidol, sul

fadimethoxine + ormetoprim and sulfaquinoxaline. Other products listed with approvals but lacking in significant activity include chlortetracycline, oxytetracycline, and nitrofurans. These products may prevent mortality from coccidiosis when given at high levels because of antibacterial activity, but are not of much value in general use. The polyether ionophores became the drugs of choice for prevention of coccidiosis in 1972, and remain the most extensively used today. Other drugs, such as nicarbazin and halofuginone, are used mostly in shuttle programs as an adjunct to the ionophores.

New drugs pending approval in the United States, which are used in Europe, South America, or Asia, include diclazuril and toltazuril (synthetic triazines).

DRUGS AND PROGRAMS USED IN BREEDERS AND LAYERS. Pullets started on the floor and later reared as caged layers do not need immunity to coccidiosis. They are often protected against coccidiosis with preventive medication, as with broilers until they are moved to cages. Breeder pullets that will be kept on the floor during lay should have an immunity to coccidiosis. Natural immunity after mild infection is usually achieved by one of two approaches. Controlled exposure can be given by means of commercial products (Coccivac, Immucox, or Paracox). The program calls for a light, harmless initial exposure, which must be reinforced by two to three repeated natural life cycles. Careful supervision of management is required to provide adequate immunity. The second approach relies upon a natural exposure assuming the presence of oocysts of important species. A broad-spectrum anticoccidial drug is fed to provide protection for 6–12 wk. Some producers reduce the level of the drug during the final 4 wk in a "step-down" program. Occasionally, oocyst numbers may be insufficient to provide adequate exposure to all species. Outbreaks of *E. necatrix* have sometimes occurred at 8–16 wk after all medication has been stopped. Climatic and seasonal conditions may add to the inherent uncertainties of this method. Neither program is foolproof, and damaging outbreaks may occur.

NEW VACCINES TO PREVENT COCCIDIOSIS. The considerable research on coccidiosis vaccines in recent years has produced interesting results and may eventually lead to a commercial product. Along conventional lines, Coccivac-style vaccines have been prepared from live but attenuated lines of oocysts. The success of these vaccines may depend more on a novel approach to administration rather than attenuation. One product is encapsulated in alginate beads, then mixed into the starter feed for "trickle administration." Another is be given by spraying the oocysts directly into feed or water in the poultry house.

Monoclonal antibody technology has led to identification of coccidial proteins protective against infection when inoculated into young chicks. These proteins can be made in quantity if the gene that encodes the protein is cloned into a bacterial cell. Research is in progress identifying broad-spectrum antigens and appropriate routes of administration.

DISINFECTION AND SANITATION. Older recommendations for coccidiosis control often suggest directions for sanitation and disinfection to prevent outbreaks. Most of these are no longer considered valid since: 1) there have been too many failures in such programs; 2) oocysts are extremely resistant to common disinfectants; 3) complete house sterilization is never complete; and 4) an oocyst-sterile environment for floor-maintained birds could prevent early establishment of immunity.

If birds are kept in self-cleaning cages, immunity is not essential, and outbreaks of coccidiosis occur only rarely, usually in single rows of cages in which there has been accidental fecal contamination of feed or water.

COCCIDIOSIS IN TURKEYS. Coccidiosis in turkeys is common, but is often unrecognized because the lesions in turkeys are less spectacular than those in chickens. Several species infect turkeys, but only about four are economically important. Typical signs of coccidiosis in turkeys are watery or mucoid diarrhea, ruffled feathers, anorexia, and general signs of illness. Recovery is quick, so lesions could go undetected at necropsy. Several species have been found in commercial turkey farms throughout the United States (6). Coccidia infecting domestic turkeys also infect wild turkeys. Range-rearing of turkeys can add significantly to the exposure of wildlife to coccidiosis and other diseases.

Turkeys of all ages are susceptible to primary infection, but birds older than 6–8 wk are considered more resistant to the disease; they can suffer weight loss and morbidity, but are not killed as easily as are younger birds. Reductions in rate of weight gain are often unrecognized until adequate coccidiosis control measures have been instituted.

Etiology. Seven species of *Eimeria* have been described in turkeys in the United States. Identifying characteristics of each species are listed in Table 34.4. *E. innocua* and *E. subrotunda* have been so rarely recovered that the validity of these species should be listed as doubtful.

Species described from the turkey include *Isospora* and *Cryptosporidium* (see next section) as well as *Eimeria*. The strictly intestinal *Eimeria* spp. contrast with *Cryptosporidium*, which may cause both respiratory and intestinal infection (13). The pathogenic species of *Eimeria* are *E. adenoeides*, *E. meleagrimitis*, *E. gallopavonis*, and *E. dispersa*. Differentiation of oocysts of the pathogenic species from those of milder species is difficult because some of the species are poorly described.

***EIMERIA ADENOEIDES* MOORE AND BROWN 1951.** Gross lesions appear primarily in the ceca, but extend to the lower small intestine and cloaca. Cecal contents are often hardened into a core consisting of mucosal debris. The cecal and/or intestinal wall is often swollen and edematous. Oocysts are ellipsoidal and have a high shape index (length/width = 1.54). The oocysts average 25.6×16.6 µm.

Table 34.4. Diagnostic characteristics of Eimeria in turkeys

SPECIES → CHARACTERISTICS ↓	E. adenoeides	E. dispersa	E. gallopavonis	E. innocua	E. meleagridis	E. meleagrimitis	E. subrotunda
Lesions (■ Lesions; ▦ Occasional lesions; ▒ Parasites no lesion; □ Species distinctive)							
Macroscopic lesions	liquid feces with mucus and flecks of blood, loose whitish cecal cores	cream-colored serosal surface, dilation of intestine, yellowish mucoid feces	edema, ulceration of mucosal ileum, yellow exudate, flecks of blood in feces	none	cream-colored ceca, formation of caseous plug, a few petechial hemorrhages	spotty congestion and petechiae from duodenum to ileum, dilation of jejunum, casts	none
Length × Width (in um)	Av = 25.6 × 16.6	Av = 26.1 × 21.0	Av = 27.1 × 17.2	Av = 22.4 × 20.9	Av = 24.4 × 18.1	Av = 19.2 × 16.3	Av = 21.8 × 19.8
Length =	18.9 – 31.3	21.8 – 31.1	22.7 – 32.7	18.57 – 25.86	20.3 – 30.8	15.8 – 26.9	16.48 – 26.42
Width =	12.6 – 20.9	17.7 – 23.9	15.2 – 19.4	17.34 – 24.54	15.4 – 20.6	13.1 – 21.9	14.21 – 24.44
Oocyst shape and index length/width	ellipsoidal	broadly oval	ellipsoidal	subspherical	ellipsoidal	ovoid	subspherical
	1.54	1.24	1.52	1.07	1.34	1.17	1.10
Minimum sporulation	24 hr	35 hr	15 hr	under 45 hr	24 hr	18 hr	48 hr
Prepatent period (minimum)	103 hr	120 hr	105 hr	114 hr	110 hr	103 hr	95 hr
Refractile body	yes	no	yes	no	yes	yes	no
Pathogenicity	++++	+	++++	none	none	++++	none

NOTE: *Characteristics compiled from original descriptions.*

PATHOGENICITY. *E. adenoeides* is one of the most pathogenic of the turkey coccidia. Experimental infections of 25,000–100,000 oocysts in young poults may produce mortality up to 100% on the 5th or 6th day PI. Turkeys several months old may lose considerable weight after infection. Outward signs of infection are apparent after 4 days PI. Feces are frequently fluid, may be blood-tinged, and may contain mucous casts. White or gray caseous cores may be produced in the ceca. The lesions heal quickly, so no evidence of infection may be seen soon after the acute phase unless the cecal core remains.

GROSS LESIONS AND HISTOPATHOLOGY. By the 4th day PI, the intestine may suffer congestion, edema, petechial hemorrhage, and mucus secretion. Five days PI, the ceca contain white caseous material, which condenses into a core. The serosal surface of the intestine appears pale and may be edematous and dilated.

Invasion of the submucosa by heterophils occurs throughout the intestine, especially in the lower small intestine and ceca. Epithelial cells at the tips of villi are most often invaded, but deep glands may also be parasitized. Edema is common deep in the muscular layers as the infection progresses. After the 5th day, regeneration of lost mucosa is rapid.

***EIMERIA DISPERSA* TYZZER 1929.** The small intestine, principally the midgut region, is commonly parasitized, but some infection may occur in the cecal necks. Oocysts are large (average, 26.1 × 21.0 µm) and broadly ovoid (index = 1.24). Sporozoites lack a refractile body, and the oocyst wall is distinctively contoured and lacks the double wall common to other species. The prepatent period is 120 hr, longer than for other species.

PATHOGENICITY. Compared with some of the other species, the pathogenicity is low, but infection with 1,000,000–2,000,000 oocysts can cause reduction in rate of weight gain and diarrhea in young poults.

NATURAL AND EXPERIMENTAL HOSTS. The natural host of this species is apparently the bobwhite quail, in which the parasite is more pathogenic than in turkeys. This is the only *Eimeria* in chickens or turkeys known to infect more than one species. Experimental inoculation has produced patent infections in domestic and wild turkeys, Hungarian partridge (Perdix perdix), ruffed grouse (*Bonasa umbellus*), sharp-tailed grouse (*Pediocetes phasianellus campestris*), Japanese and bobwhite quail, and other pheasants. Infection in chickens often requires immunosuppression.

GROSS LESIONS AND HISTOPATHOLOGY. Three

days PI, the duodenum appears cream colored on the serosal surface. Later, the entire intestine may become dilated with thickening of the wall. Dilation continues on the 5th and 6th days, along with secretion of a cream-colored mucoid material containing denuded epithelium from the duodenum. Individual villi may become so dilated as to be visible to the naked eye.

The duodenum shows edema and progressively increasing congestion of capillaries. Separation of the epithelium and basement membranes may result in the lamina propria being exposed to a fibrin network or an open fluid-filled space. Necrosis is common on distal tips of villi. Parasites do not invade the glands.

***EIMERIA GALLOPAVONIS* HAWKINS 1952.** Lesions are restricted to the area posterior to the yolk sac diverticulum and tend to be most severe in the lower small intestine and large intestine. Some foci of infection may be seen in the ceca. Oocysts are elongate, averaging 17.1 × 17.2 µm (index = 1.52).

PATHOGENICITY. Experimental infection with 50,000–100,000 oocysts causes mortality of 10–100% in 2- to 6-wk-old poults. Mortality occurs 5–6 days PI.

GROSS LESIONS AND HISTOPATHOLOGY. Marked inflammatory and edematous changes on the 5th to 6th day are followed by sloughing of soft white caseous necrotic material containing numerous oocysts and flecks of blood on the 7th and 8th days.

***EIMERIA MELEAGRIDIS* TYZZER 1929.** Visible lesions may be seen in the ceca with yellow-white caseous cores, but this species is considered virtually nonpathogenic. Oocysts resemble those of other pathogenic species in the ceca, and differentiation is difficult.

PATHOGENICITY. Most studies have characterized this species as almost nonpathogenic. Two to five million oocysts produce little effect on growth of 4- to 8-wk-old poults. Earlier reports indicating greater pathogenicity may have come from mixed infections with *E. adenoeides*.

GROSS LESIONS AND HISTOPATHOLOGY. Nonadherent cream-colored caseous cecal cores are characteristics of infection in young poults. The core may be passed intact. The mucosa is somewhat thickened and may contain petechial hemorrhages in dilated portions of the ceca. The plugs disappear 5.5–6 days PI, and many oocysts may be found in cecal contents.

Edema and lymphocytic infiltration may be seen

histologically, but less extensively than with *E. adenoeides* and *E. gallopavonis*. First-generation schizonts develop in surface epithelium of the small intestine, but later stages occur in the cecal epithelium.

EIMERIA MELEAGRIMITIS TYZZER 1929.

Infection with E. meleagrimitis is primarily upper intestinal, but may spread throughout the small intestine in heavy infections. This is the most pathogenic of the upper-intestinal coccidia in turkeys. The oocysts are small (average, 19.2×16.3 µm) and ovoid.

PATHOGENICITY. Experimental infection of young poults produces morbidity and mortality, lost weight gain, dehydration, and general unthriftiness. Inoculation of 200,000 oocysts produces some mortality and morbidity, but this species is not as pathogenic as *E. adenoeides*.

GROSS LESIONS AND HISTOPATHOLOGY. Infected birds show signs of dehydration. In the duodenum, enlargement and congestion are marked on the 5th and 6th days of infection. Large amounts of mucus and fluid may be found in the lumen. Feces may contain occasional flecks of blood and mucous casts 5–7 days PI.

The tips of villi are most commonly parasitized, and the epithelium may be completely denuded, although hemorrhage is rare. Eosinophilic infiltration may begin as early as 2 hr PI and is extensive at the height of the infection.

UNDESCRIBED SPECIES. Several species of coccidia that do not fit descriptions of established species have been isolated from wild or domestic turkeys, but have not been adequately described or named. Thus, some difficulty may be expected in speciating coccidia found in field cases unless the pathology and appearance are distinctive.

Prevention and Control of Turkey Coccidiosis.

Drugs effective in chickens are generally effective in turkeys, but the optimal level of application may vary and the toxicity of some drugs is significantly higher in turkeys than in chickens.

TREATMENT. As in chickens, treatment of outbreaks in turkeys is less desirable than prevention by chemotherapy or immunization. When treatment is necessary, application of amprolium (0.012–0.025% in water) or a sulfonamide (dosage depending on drug, often given 2 days on drug, 3 days off, and 2 days on, sometimes repeated a 2nd wk). The toxicity of sulfonamides limits their usefulness for turkeys.

CONTROL BY CHEMOTHERAPY. Most producers use anticoccidial drugs continuously in the feed at least 8 wk. Generally, poults are confined to a brooding facility at that time. Later, the birds may be moved to range or to other facilities. Drugs approved for use in feed include amprolium (0.0125–0.25%), butynorate (0.0275%), sulfaquinoxaline (0.0175%), sulfadimethoxine (0.006–0.25%) + ormetoprim (0.00375%), or monensin (54–90 g/ton), halofuginone (1.5–3.0 ppm), and lasalocid (75–125 ppm).

PREVENTION WITH PLANNED IMMUNIZATION. The principle of immunization by exposure to a small number of pathogenic oocysts of the important species of *Eimeria* was developed with chickens and is represented by a single product for turkeys in the United States (Coccivac-T, Sterwin, Millsboro, Delaware) and in Canada (Immucox, Vetech, Guelph, Ontario). The inoculum is sprayed on the feed during the first 1–7 days and causes a mild infection. There are risks inherent in use of virulent strains of coccidia, and occasional treatment at 3–4 wk of age is necessary if one of the species multiplies too rapidly, but the program has been used with success in most instances.

COCCIDIOSIS IN GEESE.

Numerous species of coccidia have been described from domestic and wild geese. The most prevalent and damaging in commercial flocks are *E. truncata,* which causes renal coccidiosis, and *E. anseris* which causes intestinal coccidiosis. Renal coccidiosis may produce high mortality from blockage of kidney function in young goslings. Coccidia may be introduced into domestic flocks by migrating and resident wild geese.

EIMERIA TRUNCATA RAILLET AND LUCET 1891.

Flock losses due to renal coccidiosis have been reported as high as 87% in Iowa. Geese aged 3–12 wk are affected, although the disease is most acute in goslings. Signs of infection include depression, weakness, diarrhea with whitish feces, and anorexia. Eyes become dull and sunken and wings are drooped. Survivors may show vertigo and torticollis. Birds quickly develop immunity to reinfection.

Oocysts and endogenous stages of *E. truncata* are found only in the kidneys or cloaca near the junction of the ureters. Diagnosis of *E. truncata* is assured by finding the distinctive oocysts in the kidneys and ureters. Oocysts average 21.3×16.7 µm and have truncated ends.

NATURAL AND EXPERIMENTAL HOSTS. Although thorough cross-infection experiments have not been done in most cases, *E. truncata* has been reported from domestic and wild geese, ducks, and swans.

GROSS LESIONS AND HISTOPATHOLOGY. The kidneys may be enlarged and protrude from the sacral bed. The normal reddish brown is altered to light grayish yellow or grayish red. Pinhead-sized grayish white foci or hemorrhagic petechiae may be seen; they contain numerous oocysts and accumulations of urates. Invading and growing parasites may distort the kidney tubules to many times the normal size. Eosinophils and signs of necrosis are present in focal areas.

EIMERIA ANSERIS KOTLAN 1933. The oocysts average 19.2 × 16.6 µm. Differentiation from the 14 species listed by Pellerdy (25) may be difficult.

PATHOGENICITY. *E. anseris* may produce anorexia, tottering gait, debility, diarrhea and morbidity, and sometimes mortality. The small intestine becomes enlarged and filled with thin reddish brown fluid. Catarrhal inflammatory lesions are most intense in middle and lower portions of the small intestine. There may be large whitish nodules or a fibrinous diphtheroid necrotic enteritis. Under dry pseudomembranous flakes, the oocysts and endogenous stages of the parasite are found in large numbers. Parasite stages invade epithelial cells of the posterior half of the intestine in closely packed rows. Developing gametocytes penetrate deeply into subepithelial tissues of the villi.

TREATMENT. Various sulfonamide drugs have been used in treatment of renal and intestinal coccidiosis of geese. Some studies indicated a favorable response, but, unfortunately, there have been no controlled experiments.

COCCIDIOSIS IN DUCKS. Coccidiosis in ducks is sporadic but is of sufficient frequency to warrant more attention from researchers. Cases involving moderate to heavy mortality have been reported on domestic duck farms in New York, New Jersey, Hungary, and Japan. Coccidia were recovered from every farm sampled on Long Island, New York. Clinical and subclinical coccidiosis appears to be quite common, and can produce morbidity and mortality as well as poor performance.

SPECIES OF COCCIDIA AND DESCRIPTIONS. Although 13 species of coccidia have been reported from domestic and wild ducks, the descriptions are often insufficient to use in diagnosis (25). Many species will remain in doubt until further work is completed. Coccidia in ducks may be of Eimeria, Wenyonella, or Tyzzeria. The genus can readily be determined from the sporulated oocyst. The oocysts of Eimeria have four sporocysts, each containing two sporozoites; Wenyonella have four sporozoites, each with four sporozoites; and Tyzzeria have eight naked sporozoites not contained within sporocysts.

Tyzzeria perniciosa Allen 1936, from domestic ducks in the United States, have thin-walled oocysts measuring 10–12.3 × 9–10.8 µm and sporulate to produce eight free sporozoites.

Wenyonella philiplevinei Leibovitz 1968 is the best described of the coccidia from ducks. It is found in the lower intestine from the posterior jejunal annular band to the cloaca. The prepatent period is 93 hr. The oocysts have three-layered walls, measure 15.5–21 × 12.5–16 µm (average, 18.7 × 14.4), have a micropyle at one end, 1–2 polar granules, and no oocyst residuum. Sporulation results in four sporocysts/oocyst, each containing four sporozoites.

PATHOGENICITY OF DUCK COCCIDIOSIS. Signs of infection with *T. perniciosa* usually include anorexia, weight loss, weakness, distress, morbidity, and up to 70% mortality. Hemorrhagic areas are common in the anterior portion of the intestine but may be found throughout. Bloody or cheesy exudate is common. The epithelial lining may be sloughed in long sheets. Parasite invasion may extend through the mucosal and submucosal layers as deep as the muscular layers. Acute hemorrhage as early as the 4th day may be followed by death on the 5th to 6th day.

With *W. philiplevinei,* the effects are limited to 72–96 hrs PI. Occasional petechial hemorrhages appear in the posterior ileal mucosa. Diffuse congestion is found in lower intestinal mucosa. In severe infections, mortality may occur on the 4th day.

COCCIDIOSIS IN PIGEONS. Coccidiosis in pigeons is similar to, but less severe than, that caused in chickens by *E. necatrix.* Young pigeons suffer the greatest losses, but mortality may occur in birds as old as 3–4 mo.

The most frequently occurring species of coccidia in pigeons is *E. labbeana* (Labbe 1896) Pinto 1928. Oocysts are spherical or subspherical, averaging 19.1 × 17.4 µm.

PATHOGENICITY. Mortality of 15–70% has been reported in young pigeons in various parts of the world. Subclinical infections may persist in older birds for long periods. Immunity does not appear to be as "self-limiting" as reported for other species. Common signs of infection are anorexia, greenish diarrhea, marked dehydration, and emaciation. Droppings may be blood tinged, and the entire digestive tract may be inflamed. The common condition of "going light" is frequently attributed to coccidiosis.

TREATMENT. Favorable response has been reported after use of sulfonamides in drinking water at the same or half the level recommended for chickens. A product was introduced in 1987 in France and Belgium for specific use in pigeons. The active ingredient is Clazuril, a close relative of the Diclazuril under development for use in chickens. This product is highly effective in treating coccidiosis in pigeons.

REFERENCES

1. AAAP Committee on Disease Reporting. 1987. Summary of commercial poultry disease reports. Avian Dis 31:926–982.
2. Arakawa, A., E. Baba and T. Fukata. 1981. Eimeria tenella infection enhances Salmonella typhimurium infections in chickens. Poult Sci 60:2203–2209.
3. Baba, E., T. Fukata and A. Arakawa. 1982. Establishment and persistence of Salmonella typhimurium infection stimulated by Eimeria tenella in chickens. Poult Sci 61:1410.
4. Biggs, P.M., P.L. Long, S.G. Kenzy and D.G. Rootes. 1969. Investigations into the association between Marek's disease and coccidiosis. Acta Vet 38:65–75.
5. Braunius, W.W. 1986. Incidence of Eimeria species in broilers in relation to the use of anticoccidial drugs. Proc Georgia Coccidiosis Conference, University of Georgia, Athens, pp. 409–414.
6. Edgar, S.A. 1986. Coccidiosis in turkeys: Biology and incidence. Proc Georgia Coccidiosis Conference, University of Georgia, Athens, pp. 116–123.
7. Edgar, S.A., and C.T. Siebold. 1964. A new coccidium of chickens, Eimeria mivati sp. n. (Protozoa: Eimeriidae), with details of its life history. J Parasitol 50:193–204.
8. Feed Additive Compendium. 1989. Miller Publishing Co., Minneapolis, MN.
9. Fletcher, O.J., J.F. Munnell and P.K. Page. 1975. Cryptosporidiosis of the bursa of Fabricius in chickens. Avian Dis 19:630–639.
10. Gore, T.C., and P.L. Long. 1982. The biology and pathogenicity of a recent field isolate of Eimeria praecox, Johnson 1930. J Protozool 29:82–85.
11. Hamet, N. 1986. Resistance to anticoccidial drugs in poultry farms in France from 1975 to 1984. Proc Georgia Coccidiosis Conference, University of Georgia, Athens, pp. 415–421.
12. Helmbolt, C.F., and E.S. Bryant. 1971. The pathology of necrotic enteritis in domestic fowl. Avian Dis 15:775–780.

13. Hoerr, J.F., F.M. Ranck and T.F. Hastings. 1978. Respiratory cryptosporidiosis in turkeys. J Am Vet Med Assoc 173:1591–1593.
14. Jeffers, T.K. 1974. Eimeria tenella: Incidence, distribution and anticoccidial drug resistance of isolants in major broiler producing areas. Avian Dis 18:74–84.
15. Jeffers, T.K. 1974. Eimeria acervulina and Eimeria maxima: Incidence and anticoccidial drug resistance of isolants in major broiler producing areas. Avian Dis 18:331–342.
16. Johnson, J., and W.M. Reid. 1970. Anticoccidial drugs: Lesion scoring techniques in battery and floor-pen experiments with chickens. Exp Parasitol 28:30–36.
17. Litjens, J.B. 1986. The relationship between coccidiosis and the use of anticoccidials in broilers in the southern part of the Netherlands. Proc Georgia Coccidiosis Conference, University of Georgia, Athens, pp. 442–448.
18. Long, P.L. 1982. The Biology of the Coccidia. University Park Press, Baltimore.
19. Maxey, B.W., and R.K. Page. 1977. Efficacy of lincomycin feed medication for the control of necrotic enteritis in broiler-type chickens. Poult Sci 56:1909–1913.
20. McDougald, L.R. 1986. Current drugs and programs. Proc Georgia Coccidiosis Conference, University of Georgia, Athens, pp. 237–238.
21. McDougald, L.R., T. Karlsson and W.M. Reid. 1979. Interaction of infectious bursal disease and coccidiosis in layer replacement chickens. Avian Dis 23:999–1005.
22. McDougald, L.R., A.L. Fuller and J. Solis. 1986. Drug sensitivity of 99 isolates of coccidia from broiler farms. Avian Dis 30:690–694.
23. McDougald, L.R., J.M.L. DaSilva, J. Solis and M. Braga. 1987. A survey of sensitivity to anticoccidial drugs in 60 isolates of coccidia from broiler chickens in Brazil and Argentina. Avian Dis 31:287–292.
24. Morehouse, N.F., and R.R. Barron. 1970. Coccidiosis: Evaluation of coccidiostats by mortality, weight gains, and fecal scores. Exp Parasitol 28:25–29.
25. Pellerdy, L.P. 1974. Coccidia and Coccidiosis, 2nd ed. Akademine Kiado, Budapest.
26. Reid, W.M., and J. Johnson. 1970. Pathogenicity of Eimeria acervulina in light and heavy coccidial infections. Avian Dis 14:166–177.
27. Reyna, P.S., G.F. Mathis and L.R. McDougald. 1982. A survey of sensitizing anticoccidial drugs to 60 isolates from broiler chickens in Brazil and Argentina. Avian Dis 31:287–292.
28. Shirley, M.W. 1986. Studies on the immunogenicity of the seven attenuated lines of Eimeria given as a mixture to chickens. Avian Pathol 15:629–638.

CRYPTOSPORIDIOSIS

William L. Current

INTRODUCTION. Cryptosporidiosis is caused by small coccidian parasites of the genus *Cryptosporidium* that live within the microvillous region of epithelial cells of the respiratory and gastrointestinal tracts of vertebrates. Naturally occurring infections have been reported from at least nine different avian hosts. In chickens, turkeys, and quail, these parasites are primary pathogens that can produce respiratory and/or intestinal disease, resulting in morbidity and mortality. Reviews of the biology of *Cryptosporidium* spp. are now available (5, 11, 12, 30).

HISTORY AND TAXONOMY. Clarke (2) in 1895, observed what may have been a species of *Cryptosporidium* in mice. The type species *C. muris* was described 12 yr later from laboratory mice by Tyzzer (40), who later also described many of the life cycle stages and a second species, *C. parvum* (41, 42). Only a few of the 19 additional named species of *Cryptosporidium* from a variety of vertebrate hosts are now considered valid. At the time of this writing, there appear to be two species (*C. baileyi* and *C. meleagridis*) infecting both chickens and turkeys, and perhaps a third, unnamed, species infecting quail. *Cryptosporidium baileyi* is believed to be responsible for both intestinal (cloaca and bursa of Fabricius) and respiratory infections in chickens and turkeys. The species believed to be responsible for intestinal (small intestine) infections associated with diarrheal disease in turkeys is *C. meleagridis*. A species believed to be distinct from *C. baileyi* and *C. meleagridis* is responsible for intestinal (small intestine) cryptosporidiosis associated with high mortality in quail.

LIFE CYCLE AND MORPHOLOGY. Taxonomic distinctions among the genera of coccidia are based mainly on the differences in oocyst structure. In contrast to other coccidia found in poultry, *Cryptosporidium* spp. oocysts do not have sporocysts surrounding the sporozoites, four of which lie naked within the oocyst wall (Fig. 34.6).

The life cycle of *Cryptosporidium,* like other true coccidia belonging to the suborder Eimeriorina, can be divided into 6 major developmental events (Fig. 34.7): excystation (release of infective sporozoites), merogony (asexual multiplication within epithelial cells), gametogony (formation of male and female gametes), fertilization (union of gametes), oocyst wall formation (to produce an environmentally resistant form), and sporogony (the formation of infective sporozoites within the oocyst wall).

The life cycle (8) differs in several respects from that of *Eimeria* spp. infecting poultry. The intracellular stages of *Cryptosporidium* spp. are confined to the microvillous region of the host cell, and the oocysts, which sporulate within the host cell, are infective when released in the feces. Some oocysts do not form environmentally resistant walls; their sporozoites are surrounded by only a single unit membrane. When released from the parasitophorous vacuole of the host cell, the unit membrane ruptures and these invasive forms penetrate adjacent host cells and reinitiate the developmental cycle. The majority of oocysts, however, develop a multilayered, environmentally resistant, thick wall and are passed in the feces. It is this thick-walled form that transmits the infection to other susceptible hosts. The thin-walled, autoinfective oocysts and the type I meronts (asexual stages) can recycle allowing a small number of ingested oocysts to produce a severe infection. In the absence of new exposures, the immune-deficient host may develop a

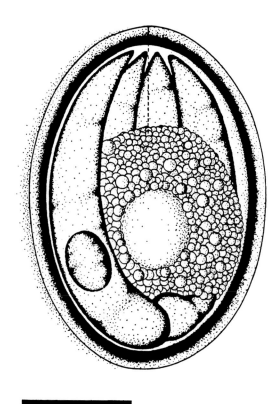

2 μM

34.6. Composite line drawing of an oocyst of *Cryptosporidium baileyi*. Note the four sporozoites surrounding the oocyst residuum, and the suture in the two-layered oocyst wall. (J Protozool)

persistent, life-threatening disease. Another feature of *Cryptosporidium* spp., which differs from *Eimeria* spp. in mammalian and avian hosts, is frequent establishment of infections in the mucosal epithelium of a wide variety of organs. For example, *C. baileyi* can infect the cloaca, the bursa of Fabricius, the upper and lower respiratory tracts, and the eyelids.

Oocyst morphology may be useful for species identification (Table 34.5). Only *C. baileyi* can be identified on the basis of morphology alone since it is larger and more ovoid than *C. meleagridis* and the other species infecting quail. *Cryptosporidium* isolated from quail will not infect chickens or turkeys. Thus, the species infecting quail can be distinguished from *C. meleagridis* on the basis of the host in which they are found. Oocysts of all three species are fully sporulated when passed in the feces and contain four crescent-shaped sporozoites that surround a centrally located oocyst residuum. Oocyst walls of all three species are about 0.5-μm thick, colorless, and have no micropyle (Fig. 34.6).

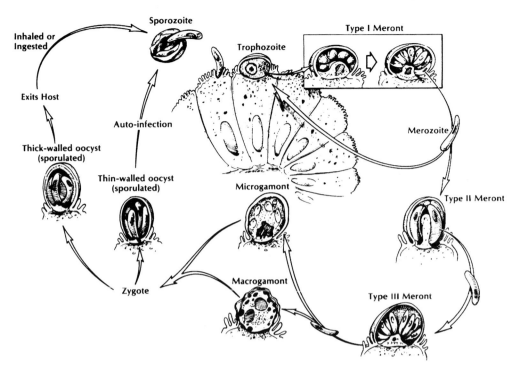

34.7. Proposed life cycle of *Cryptosporidium baileyi* as it occurs in the mucosal epithelium of the intestine (bursa of Fabricius and cloaca) and the respiratory tract of broiler chickens.

INCIDENCE AND DISTRIBUTION. *Cryptosporidium* spp. appear to be present wherever avian hosts are raised commercially. The reported worldwide distribution of *Cryptosporidium* spp. in avian hosts corresponds to the regions where poultry health specialists have used appropriate diagnostic tools, and will continue to expand as awareness of their importance as primary pathogens increases.

CRYPTOSPORIDIOSIS IN CHICKENS. *Cryptosporidium* (probably *C. baileyi*) was diagnosed in 6.8% of 1000 consecutive histology cases of chickens in Georgia (16). In North Carolina, *Cryptosporidium* spp. oocysts were found in the feces of 9 (27.3%) of 33 broilers, 3 (10%) of 30 broiler breeders and 1 (5.9%) of 17 layers (25). Using an enzyme-linked immunosorbent assay (ELISA), 22% of 454 broiler flocks in Delmarva region were found to have birds that were seropositive for *Cryptosporidium* spp. at the time they were processed (6, 36). The number of positives among different companies sampled ranged from 2.8 to 40%. Serologic data demonstrated less cryptosporidiosis in the best 10 than in the worst 10 broiler flocks (ranked by overall mortality). Such investigations do not distinguish between intestinal and respiratory infections (4) (6). These and other data indicate that *Cryptosporidium* spp. are com-

Table 34.5. Distinguishing features of *Cryptosporidium* spp. infecting poultry

Species	Host(s)	Site of Infection	Measurements of Oocysts (µm)
C. baileyi	Chicken, turkey, duck	Bursa of Fabricius, cloaca, respiratory epithelium	6.2 × 4.6 (mean), 6.3–5.6 × 4.8–4.5 (range)
C. meleagridis	Turkey, chicken	Small intestine	5.2 × 4.6 (mean), 6.0–5.6 × 4.8–4.5 (range)
Cryptosporidium spp.	Quail	Small intestine	Approximately 5

Source: (4, 22, 25)

mon intestinal infections in broiler chickens in the United States and Japan (10, 13, 23, 29, 33).

Although less common, respiratory cryptosporidiosis can be a major cause of morbidity and mortality. The factors responsible for naturally occurring outbreaks of respiratory cryptosporidiosis between 4 and 17 wk of age are not understood. The species believed to be responsible for intestinal (bursa of Fabricius and cloaca) and respiratory cryptosporidiosis in chickens is *C. baileyi* (8). Experimentally induced respiratory and intestinal infections in broiler chickens have established the primary pathogenic potential of this parasite (1, 28).

Pathogenesis and Epizootiology. *C. baileyi* generally invades the epithelium of the cloaca and bursa of Fabricius. Oocysts are picked up from heavy fecal contamination of the litter or cages. Respiratory infections apparently result from inhalation or aspiration of oocysts that are present in the environment. As few as 100 oocysts can result in intestinal infections when given orally, or in respiratory infections when inoculated intratracheally. Oocysts of *C. baileyi* are infective at the time they are passed in the feces and no vectors have been identified. Since *C. baileyi* can infect a variety of avian hosts, it is possible that wild birds may serve as carriers. Although *C. baileyi* is not infective for mammals, it is possible that rodents (mice and rats) or perhaps insects could serve as mechanical carriers. Studies of the potential for carrier or transport hosts to spread cryptosporidiosis are needed.

Mild to heavy intestinal and respiratory infections can be demonstrated as early as 3 days after inoculation of oocysts. Intestinal disease is usually mild. No overt signs of gastrointestinal disease occur in chickens receiving oocysts by gavage into the crop.

Signs of respiratory disease may appear within the 1st wk after intratracheal (IT) inoculation of *C. baileyi* oocysts into 7- or 9-day-old broiler chickens. Severe morbidity and sometimes mortality may result (1, 9, 26). IT inoculation of broilers with 4×10^5 *C. baileyi* oocysts produced severe respiratory disease, while equal numbers of oocysts produced asymptomatic intestinal infections. The experimental disease appeared similar to that reported in several naturally occurring outbreaks (10, 23, 29).

Respiratory signs of sneezing and coughing occur in most IT-inoculated chickens by 6 days post inoculation (PI). By 12 days PI, respiratory signs are more severe and many of the birds extend their heads to facilitate breathing. The more severely affected chickens lie on their sterna and are reluctant to move. Severe signs of respiratory disease are present in most IT inoculated birds for about 3–4 wk PI, after which there may be gradual improvement. Birds with respiratory infection had significantly lower weights than birds with intestinal or no

C. baileyi infection when they were inoculated at 7 days of age and sampled 14, 21, and 28 days later (9). The total mean weights of surviving birds in each group did not differ significantly at the end of the 50-day experiment, suggesting a compensatory weight gain following recovery from respiratory cryptosporidiosis. This apparent compensatory weight gain, however, may have been due in part to death of 14% of the smallest birds in the group of chickens with respiratory cryptosporidiosis. Chickens were more resistant to intratracheal inoculation at 28 than at 7 or 14 days of age (28).

Airsacculitis and pneumonia can occur as early as 6 days, but are more common 12–28 days following IT inoculation of *C. baileyi* oocysts. Early in the disease process, posterior thoracic air sacs are slightly thickened and contain foamy, clear to white or gray fluid. By day 12, air sacs may become very thick and contain white caseous exudate. The lungs of birds with severe airsacculitis are almost always affected and exhibit focal consolidation (10–80%), particularly in the ventral region. Abdominal air sacs may also be affected.

Histopathology of IT-inoculated chicks shows large numbers of parasites throughout the microvillous region of the epithelium lining the trachea and bronchi. Deciliation by replacement with developing parasites becomes apparent by 4 days PI (Fig. 34.8). By 12 days, almost all cilia may be replaced by developing parasites and the mucociliary elevator function ceases in affected trachea and bronchi. Histologic lesions include epithelial cell hyperplasia, thickening of the mucosa by mononuclear cell infiltrates with some heterophils, loss of cilia, and discharge of mucocellular exudate into the airways. There is accumulation of mucus, sloughed epithelial cells, lymphocytes, macrophages, and parasites in the tertiary bronchi and atria of the lungs. Affected lobules are expanded by accumulation of exudate and infiltration of mononuclear cells (Fig. 34.9). Affected air sacs lined with respiratory epithelium also contain large numbers of parasites and suffer similar changes.

Respiratory cryptosporidiosis caused high mortality and morbidity in a flock of 16,000 7-wk-old broiler chickens (10). In addition to increased mortality, the performance of birds with respiratory infections is also adversely affected by lower weight gains and higher feed/gain ratios.

Intestinal (cloaca and bursa of Fabricius) cryptosporidiosis in chickens (produced by *C. baileyi*) may result in histologic lesions but does not result in gross lesions or in overt signs of disease. Several reports suggest, however, that performance of broilers can be adversely affected. An unusually high mortality was associated with *C. baileyi* infection in the bursa of Fabricius, and there were lower pigmentation scores when inoculated birds were compared with noninfected controls (1, 18).

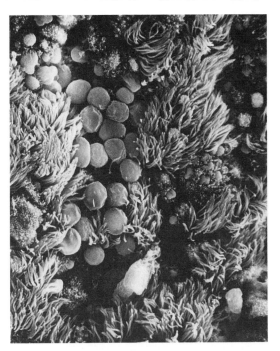

34.8. Scanning electron micrograph of the mucosal surface of the primary bronchi obtained from a broiler chicken 4 days after intratracheal inoculation of *Cryptosporidium baileyi*. Some developmental stages of the parasite can be seen among the cilia of the respiratory surface. At this stage of infection, the mucociliary elevator is probably still functional and the bird would not have overt signs of respiratory distress. On days 10–18 after intratracheal inoculation, developmental stages of the parasite form a virtual monolayer on the respiratory surface. Few or no cilia can be found. (S.L. White, Lilly Research Laboratories)

Interaction of *C. baileyi* and other respiratory pathogens predisposes birds to secondary invasion by *Escherichia coli* because of disruption of the mucociliary elevator (9). Infectious bronchitis virus and *E. coli* also enhance the severity of *C. baileyi*–induced respiratory disease in chickens.

CRYPTOSPORIDIOSIS IN TURKEYS. Two valid species of *Cryptosporidium* found in turkeys are *C. meleagridis* (35) and *C. baileyi*. The intestinal (bursa of Fabricius and cloaca) and respiratory infections produced by *C. baileyi* are similar to those described above for chickens (8, 9, 27).

Slavin reported small intestinal cryptosporidiosis in 1955 (35) due to *C. meleagridis* in a flock of 10- to 14-day-old turkey poults. Illness was associated with diarrhea, unthriftiness, and moderate mortality. More than 30 yr later, several outbreaks of this disease were reported (17, 43).

Turkey poults infected with *C. meleagridis* may develop severe diarrhea. Numerous parasites are present within the brush border of the intestinal mucosa lining the middle and lower small intestine, which becomes pale and distended with cloudy mucoid fluid and gas bubbles. Villi in the affected regions of the intestine become atrophic, the crypts become hypertrophic, and large numbers of lymphocytes, heterophils, and some macrophages and plasma cells accumulate within the lamina propria (17).

There are several case reports of severe respiratory cryptosporidiosis in commercial turkeys caused by *Cryptosporidium* spp. (15, 21, 32, 38). There appear to be two different manifestations of the disease, an upper respiratory involvement that included sinusitis, and a lower respiratory involvement that included colonization of the trachea and bronchi with concomitant airsacculitis and pneumonia. The case reports of upper respiratory tract infections described acute signs of bilateral swelling of infraorbital sinuses, similar to that reported for birds infected with *Mycoplasma* spp., and serous conjunctivitis (15, 21). Case reports of lower respiratory tract infections described signs including rattling, coughing, sneezing, and gasping (32, 38). Microscopic lesions of the infected tissues included deciliation of the epithelium and inflammation.

Inoculation of oocysts of *C. baileyi* isolated from the intestinal tract of broiler chickens into the trachea of turkeys produced respiratory signs the same as those observed in naturally occurring outbreaks (27).

Although there are a number of reports of outbreaks of severe disease, the importance of *Cryptosporidium* spp. as agents of intestinal and respiratory disease in commercially reared turkeys is not clear.

CRYPTOSPORIDIOSIS IN QUAIL. Both respiratory and intestinal cryptosporidiosis have been reported in commercially grown quails, but the species involved has not been adequately described. A case of respiratory cryptosporidiosis was reported in a flock of 4-wk-old quail (*Coturnix coturnix*) in south Australia (39). Clinical signs included depression, sneezing, and respiratory distress; mortality was approximately 10%. Histologic examination revealed parasites in the microvillous region of epithelial cells lining the nasal cavity, trachea, bronchi, salivary glands of the roof of the mouth, esophageal glands, and bursa of Fabricius. Pathologic changes in the respiratory mucosa were similar to those described above for chickens infected experimentally with *C. baileyi*. In five successive hatches of 25,000 young quail (*Colinus virginianus*), there was severe, fatal intestinal cryptosporidiosis (22). Diarrhea developed 4–6 days after hatching and mortality soon exceeded 90%. At necropsy, carcass dehydration was marked. The small intestine had clear, watery contents and

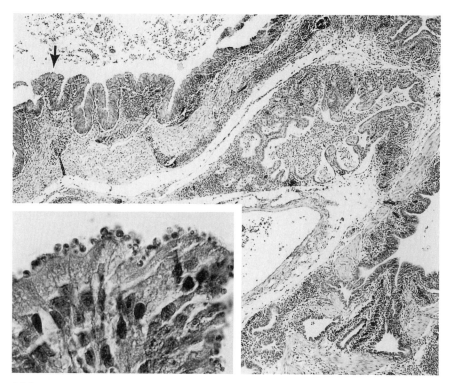

34.9. Histologic section (H & E stained) showing accumulation of lymphoid cells around bronchi in the lungs of a broiler chicken 6 days after intratracheal inoculation of *Cryptosporidium baileyi* oocysts. *Inset*: A higher magnification of the villus (*arrow*) showing the numerous developmental stages of the parasite on the epithelial surface.

the cecum was distended by brown, foamy fluid. Histologic examination of the small intestine revealed shortened villi and enterocytes detached from the tips of villi. Numerous developmental stages of the parasite were observed in the microvillous border of the small intestine, being most numerous in the proximal half. No parasites were observed in the cecum, colon, bursa of Fabricius, respiratory tract, or other tissues. Oocysts measuring approximately 5 µm, which were obtained from the intestines of these infected quail, were not orally infective to day-old broilers.

A similar outbreak was reported from young quail due to a combination of *Cryptosporidium* sp. and a reovirus isolated from intestinal contents (34). Subsequent laboratory studies (19) suggested that the *Cryptosporidium* and not the reovirus was responsible for the intestinal disease.

The organism responsible for this disease in quail appears to be a distinct species of *Cryptosporidium* since its oocysts are smaller than those of *C. baileyi* and since they are not infective to chickens or turkeys.

PREVENTION AND CONTROL.   There are no effective anti-cryptosporidial drugs for prevention or treatment and other approaches to the control are still experimental. Sanitation and immunity may provide some help, but there are no proven programs that can be recommended.

Sanitation.   The oocysts of *Cryptosporidium* spp. infecting poultry are remarkably resistant to chemical agents that readily kill most viral, bacterial, and fungal pathogens. This resistance to chemical agents can be exploited by laboratory researchers trying to separate oocysts from other contaminating microbes; however, destruction of oocysts in commercial production facilities is not considered practical. In the laboratory, oocysts remain viable for months when stored at 4 C in solution of 2.5% potassium dichromate. Oocyst viability is also maintained after a 10–15 min incubation in 25% commercial bleach (sodium hypochlorite), a treatment used to remove other contaminating organic matter. Incubation of *C. baileyi* oocysts for 30 min at room temperature in each of nine commonly used disinfectants mixed with water at the highest concentration recommended by the manufacturers had little or no effect on viability (37). Incubation in

50% ammonia resulted in the greatest reduction in excystation, and 50% commercial bleach destroyed many of the oocysts. Unless a more effective chemical agent is found, large-scale disinfection for cryptosporidiosis in commercial poultry facilities is impractical. The use of a steam cleaner may be a more effective and safer means of disinfecting contaminated cages since exposure to temperatures above 65 C tends to destroy the oocysts.

Immunity. A single intestinal and/or respiratory infection with *C. baileyi* can stimulate an immune response in broiler chickens of sufficient magnitude to clear the parasite from the infected mucosae and to render the host resistant to subsequent intestinal or respiratory challenge with oocysts of the same species (4, 6, 9). Oral or IT inoculation of oocysts into 8- to 14-day-old broilers results in heavy infections of the exposed mucosae for 14–16 days and then a rapid clearance of the parasite. At the time chickens clear primary infections, high titers of circulating antibodies specific to *C. baileyi* can be detected, and the birds exhibit a delayed hypersensitivity reaction to *C. baileyi* oocyst antigens. Data from laboratory studies and from a serologic survey suggest that acquired immunity may protect broilers from cryptosporidiosis during the last several weeks of growout. Studies are needed to identify antigens of *Cryptosporidium* spp. that may be candidates for use as vaccines.

DIAGNOSIS. Active infections in poultry, both respiratory and intestinal, can be diagnosed by identifying oocysts from fluids obtained from the respiratory tract or from the feces. Identification of *Cryptosporidium* spp. oocysts differs somewhat from techniques used for the oocysts of *Eimeria* spp. Techniques include concentration procedures coupled with standard brightfield or with phase contrast microscopy (7), acid-fast staining (14, 31), negative staining (3, 20), and staining with auramine-O for examination under a fluorescence microscope (25). These techniques allow one to readily distinguish *Cryptosporidium* spp. oocysts from yeast cells that are often present in specimens.

Fecal or respiratory specimens can be collected and submitted fresh, in 10% formalin, or in an aqueous solution of 2.5% potassium dichromate. The most effective way of obtaining specimens in the field and in the laboratory is by the use of moist cotton tipped swabs. Vigorous swabbing of the tracheal or cloacal epithelium will remove oocysts from the microvillous border. The swabs are placed in a tube containing 1 mL of water or fixative for transportation to the laboratory. Cryptosporidium infection can also be detected by demonstrating other stages of the life cycle from fresh or stained (24) mucosal scrapings from the microvillous region of the mucosae. These parasites also appear in histologic sections stained with hematoxylin and eosin as 2- to 6-μm basophilic bodies within the brush border of the epithelial cells. The diagnosis can be confirmed by transmission electron microscopy, as this procedure reveals the distinct morphology of developmental stages of *Cryptosporidium* spp. within the mucosal epithelium.

Previous exposure to the parasite can be demonstrated by testing for serum antibodies specific to *Cryptosporidium* sp. (4, 6, 36).

REFERENCES

1. Blagburn, B.L., D.S. Lindsay, J.J. Giambrone, C.A. Sundermann, and F.J. Hoerr. 1987. Experimental cryptosporidiosis in broiler chickens. Poult Sci 66:442–449.

2. Clarke, J.J. 1895. A study of coccidia met with in mice. J Microsc Sci 37:277–302.

3. Current, W.L. 1983. Human cryptosporidiosis. N Engl J Med 309:1326–1327.

4. Current, W.L. 1986. Cryptosporidium sp. in chickens: parasite life cycle and aspects of acquired immunity. In L.R. McDougald, P.L. Long, and L.P. Joyner (eds.). Proceedings of the Georgia Coccidiosis Conference. University of Georgia, Athens, GA, pp. 124–133.

5. Current, W.L. 1989. Cryptosporidium spp. In P.D. Walzer, and R.M. Genta (eds.). Parasitic Infections in the Compromised Host. Marcel Dekker, Inc., New York, pp. 281–341.

6. Current, W.L. and D.B. Snyder. 1988. Development of and serologic evaluation of acquired immunity to Cryptosporidium baileyi by broiler chickens. Poult Sci 67:720–729.

7. Current, W.L., N.C. Reese, J.V. Ernst, W.S. Bailey, M.B. Heyman and W.M. Weinstein. 1983. Human cryptosporidiosis in immunocompetent and immunodeficient persons. Studies of an outbreak and experimental transmission. N Engl J Med 308:1252–1257.

8. Current, W.L., S.J. Upton, and T.B. Haynes. 1986. The life cycle of Cryptosporidium baileyi n. sp. (Apicomplexa, Cryptosporidiidae) infecting chickens. J Protozool 33:289–296.

9. Current, W.L., M.N. Novilla, and D.B. Snyder. 1987. Cryptosporidiosis in poultry: An update (Are Cryptosporidium spp. primary pathogens?). Proceedings of the 22nd National Meeting of the Poultry Health Condemn. Delmarva Poultry Industry, Inc., pp. 17–29

10. Dhillon, A.S., H.L. Thacker, A.V. Dietzel, and R.W. Winterfield. 1981. Respiratory cryptosporidiosis in broiler chickens. Avian Dis 25:747–751.

11. Dubey, J.P., C.A. Speer, and R. Fayer. 1990. Cryptosporidiosis of Man and Animals. CRC Press, Boca Raton, FL.

12. Fayer, R. and B.L.P. Ungar. 1986. Cryptosporidium spp. and cryptosporidiosis. Microbiol Rev 50:458–483.

13. Fletcher, O.J., J.F. Munell, and R.K. Page. 1975. Cryptosporidiosis of the bursa of Fabricius of chickens. Avian Dis 19:630–639.

14. Garcia, L.S., D.A. Bruckner, T.C. Brewer, and R.Y. Shimizu. 1983. Techniques for the recovery and identification of Cryptosporidium oocysts from stool specimens. J Clin Microbiol 18:185–190.

15. Glisson, J.R., T.P. Brown, M. Brugh, R.K. Page, S.H. Kleven, and R.B. Davis. 1984. Sinusitis in turkeys associated with respiratory cryptosporidiosis. Avian Dis 28:783–790.

16. Goodwin M.A. and J. Brown. 1987. Histologic incidence and distribution of Cryptosporidium sp. infection in chickens. J Am Vet Med Assoc 190:1623.

17. Goodwin, M.A., W.L. Steffens, I.D. Russell, and J. Brown. 1988. Diarrhea associated with intestinal cryptosporidiosis in turkeys. Avian Dis 32:63–67.

18. Gorham, S.L., E.T. Mallinson, D.B. Snyder and E.M. Odor. 1987. Cryptosporidiosis in the bursa of Fabricius—a correlation with mortality rates in broiler chickens. Avian Pathol 16:205–211.

19. Guy, J.S., M.G. Levy, D.H. Ley, H.J. Barnes and T.M. Craig. 1987. Experimental reproduction of enteritis in bobwhite quail (Colinus virginianus) with Cryptosporidium and Reovirus. Avian Dis 31:713–722.

20. Heine, J. 1982. Ein einfache Nachweismethode fur Kryptosporidien im Kot. Zentralbl Veterinaermed Reihe B 29:324–327.

21. Hoerr, F.J., F.M. Ranck, Jr., and T.F. Hastings. 1978. Respiratory cryptosporidiosis in turkeys. J Am Vet Med Assoc 173:1591–1593.

22. Hoerr, F.J., W.L. Current, and T.B. Haynes. 1986. Fatal cryptosporidiosis in quail. Avian Dis 30:421–425.

23. Itakura, C., M. Goryo, and T. Unemura. 1984. Cryptosporidial infection in chickens. Avian Pathol 13:487–499.

24. Latimer, K.S., M.A. Goodwin, and M.K. Davis. 1988. Rapid cytologic diagnosis of respiratory cryptosporidiosis in chickens. Avian Dis 32:826–830.

25. Ley, D.H., M.G. Levy, L. Hunter, W. Corbett and H.J. Barnes. 1988. Cryptosporidia-positive rates of avian necropsy accessions determined by examination of auramine o-stained fecal smears. Avian Dis 32:108–113.

26. Lindsay, D.S., and B.L. Blagburn. 1990. Cryptosporidiosis in birds. In j.P. Dubey, C.A. Speer, and R. Fayer, eds., Cryptosporidiosis of Man and Animals, pp. 125–148. CRC Press, Boca Raton, FL.

27. Lindsay, D.S., B.L. Blagburn, and F.J. Hoerr. 1987. Experimentally induced infection in turkeys with Cryptosporidium baileyi isolated from chickens. Am J Vet Res 48:104–108.

28. Lindsay, D.S., B.L. Blagburn, C.A. Sundermann and J.J. Giambrone. 1988. Effect of broiler chicken age on susceptibility to experimentally induced Cryptosporidium baileyi infection. Am J Vet Res 49:1412–1414.

29. Nakamura, K. and F. Abe. 1988. Respiratory (especially pulmonary) and urinary infections of Cryptosporidium in layer chickens. Avian Pathol 17:703–711.

30. O'Donoghue, P.J. 1995. Cryptosporidium and cryptosporidiosis in man and animals. Int J Parasit 25:139–195.

31. Payne, P., L.A. Lancaster, M. Heinzman, and J.A. McCutchan. 1983. Identification of Cryptosporidium in patients with the acquired immunologic syndrome. N Engl J Med 309:613–614.

32. Ranck, F.M., Jr. and F.J. Hoerr. 1986. Cryptosporidia in the respiratory tract of turkeys. Avian Dis 31:389–391.

33. Randall, C.J. 1982. Cryptosporidiosis of the bursa of Fabricius and trachea of broilers. Avian Pathol 11:95–102.

34. Ritter, G.D., D.H. Ley, M. Levy, J. Guy, and H.J. Barnes. 1986. Intestinal cryptosporidiosis and Reovirus isolated from Bobwhite quail (Colinus virginianus) with enteritis. Avian Dis 30:603–608.

35. Slavin, D. 1955. Cryptosporidium meleagridis (sp. nov.) J Comp Pathol 65:262–266.

36. Snyder, D.B., W.L. Current, E. Russek-Cohen, S. Gorham, E.T. Mallison, W.W. Marquardt and P.K. Savage. 1988. Serologic incidence of Cryptosporidium in Delmarva broiler flocks. Poult Sci 67:730–735.

37. Sundermann, C.A., D.S. Lindsay and B.L. Blagburn. 1987. Evaluation of disinfectants for ability to kill avian Cryptosporidium oocysts. Compan Anim Pract 2:36–39.

38. Tarwid, J.N., R.J. Cawthorn, and C. Riddell. 1985. Cryptosporidiosis in the respiratory tract of turkeys in Saskatchewan. Avian Dis 29:528–532.

39. Tham, V.L., S. Kniesberg, and B.R. Dixon. 1982. Cryptosporidiosis in quails. Avian Pathol 11:619–626.

40. Tyzzer, E.E. 1907. A sporozoan found in the peptic glands of the common mouse. Proc Soc Exp Biol Med 5:12–13.

41. Tyzzer, E.E. 1910. An extracellular coccidium, Cryptosporidium muris (gen et sp. nov.) of the gastric glands of the common mouse. J Med Res 23:487–509.

42. Tyzzer, E.E. 1912. Cryptosporidium parvum (sp. nov.), a coccidium found in the small intestine of the common mouse. Arch Protistenkd 26:394–412.

43. Wages, D.P. 1987. Cryptosporidiosis and turkey viral hepatitis in turkey poult. J Am Vet Med Assoc 190:1623.

OTHER PROTOZOAN DISEASES OF THE INTESTINAL TRACT

Larry R. McDougald

HISTOMONIASIS (BLACKHEAD). Histomoniasis is a parasitic disorder of the ceca and liver of many gallinaceous birds. The disease (caused by the protozoan *Histomonas meleagridis*) is characterized by necrotic foci in the liver and ulceration of the ceca, and has also been called infectious enterohepatitis or blackhead. The signs leading to the use of the term *blackhead* are neither pathognomonic nor distinctive since many other diseases may produce a similar appearance (Fig. 34.10A). The roles of the cecal worm *Heterakis gallinarum* and earthworms as accessory hosts of *Histomonas* comprise one of the most intriguing relationships in parasitology.

Although the economic significance of the disease is difficult to ascertain, annual losses from mortality in turkeys has been estimated to exceed two million dollars. Decreased production from morbidity and chemotherapy expense increase cost of the disease. Although histomoniasis is less severe in chickens, losses from morbidity and mortality are estimated to be greater than in turkeys because of the frequency of occurrence and the numbers of birds involved (1). Outbreaks of histomoniasis in leghorn pullets in Georgia caused up to 20% mortality and high morbidity. Chicken houses may become badly contaminated by *Heterakis* worm eggs, causing outbreaks in flock after flock.

History. The disease complex has been re-

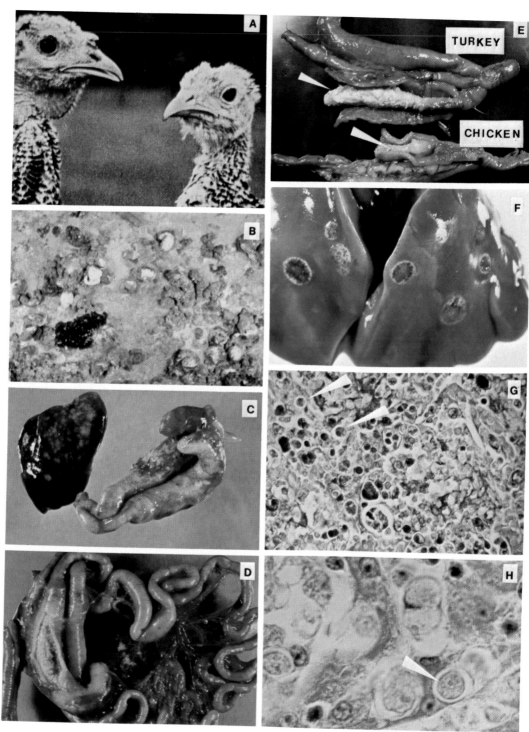

34.10. *A.* (*left*) normal uninfected poult; (*right*) histomonas-infected poult of the same age. Sickly appearance occurs later in course of infection and is not distinctive to histomoniasis. (Hilbrich) *B.* Brilliant yellow material in feces often constitutes the first sign of histomoniasis outbreaks in turkeys. *C.* Liver and cecum from poult 14 days after feeding on *Heterakis gallinarum* ova. Note engorgement of ceca and diffuse nature of liver lesions. (McDougald) *D.* Intestinal tract from experimentally infected turkey showing engorged cecum, core, and inflamed mesenteries. *E.* Chicken and turkey ceca 10 days PI with *Histomonas meleagridis.* Note cecal cores (*arrows*). *F.* Discrete pathognomonic lesions with raised surface from a turkey infected with histomoniasis. *G.* Liver section showing histomonad PAS stain (*arrows*). *H.* Liver sections showing histomonads (*arrows*). H & E. ×1000. (Page).

viewed in depth (16, 17, 22, 27). Histomoniasis in turkeys was first described in 1895. Discovery that a milder form of the disease occurs in chickens that often remained carriers resulted in the first useful recommendation for control. Every poultry producer has learned that turkeys should not be reared with chickens or on range where chickens have been produced during the previous several years. The role of the cecal worm (*Heterakis*) and its eggs and of the earthworm as carriers of the parasite explain this long period of infectivity on uninhabited range.

Although Smith recognized the primary etiologic agent as a protozoan in 1895, Tyzzer was the first to observe that the parasite had flagella as well as pseudopodia (30, 31). The pathogenesis of histomoniasis was elucidated further between 1964 and 1974 by studies showing that certain bacteria are necessary in addition to the histomonads to produce disease. This interesting *Histomonas*-bacteria connection was discovered using germ-free techniques at the Universities of Georgia and Notre Dame.

Incidence and Distribution.
Histomoniasis occurs wherever suitable avian hosts exist. In general, it is more prevalent in areas favoring coexistence of the cecal worm *Heterakis gallinarum* and various earthworm species, but it is regularly reported by diagnostic laboratories in the United States, Canada, and Mexico (1).

Despite improved management and availability of antihistomonal drugs, histomoniasis remains an important, if occasional, disease in chickens, turkeys, and other fowl.

Etiology and Classification.
The causative agent, *Histomonas meleagridis,* was first described under the name *Amoeba meleagridis,* but discovery of flagellate characteristics led Tyzzer to rename the protozoan *H. meleagridis.* A larger (17 µm), nonpathogenic, four-flagellated histomonad found in the cecum was named as a separate species, *H. wenrichi.*

Other agents such as trichomonads and fungi (*Candida albicans*) have been advanced as etiologic agents of blackhead (27). The term *pseudoblackhead* has been popularly applied to cases that did not respond to antihistomonals. Differential diagnosis including demonstration of the organism may be required in such cases.

MORPHOLOGY. *H. meleagridis* in its nonamoeboid state is nearly spherical (3–16 µm in diameter). The amoeboid phase is highly pleomorphic. Pseudopodia may be observed if the slide is warmed during microscopy (see Fig. 34.11). There is a single stout flagellum 6–11 µm in length. There is a large pelta and an axostyle wholly contained within the body of the organism. The parabasal body is V shaped and anterior to the nucleus. The nucleus is spheroid to ellipsoid or ovoid and averages 2.2×1.7 µm.

The tissue forms lack flagella and exist in several different forms: 1) Parasites in the "invasive" stage at the peripheral areas of the lesions (2) are 8–17 µm in size, amoeboid, and appear to form pseudopods. 2) A "vegetative" stage is larger (12–21 µm) and more numerous, and is clustered in vacuoles in degenerating tissue. 3) A third stage present in older lesions is eosinophilic and smaller and may represent a degenerating form.

LIFE CYCLE. The existence of this organism is intimately associated with the cecal nematode *Heterakis gallinarum* and several species of earthworms common to poultry yard soil. Early attempts to find the histomonad in cecal worm eggs were inconclusive until Gibbs (10) demonstrated small bodies seen with the light microscope. Lee (14) observed a small form (3 mm) by electron microscopy and histomonads have been cultured from heterakid eggs in vitro (28).

Histomonads are found in intestinal epithelial cells of very young juveniles or newly hatched worms. The mechanism of egg infection by histomonads has not been determined. Springer et al. (29) found that triturated male worms recently removed from chickens carry viable histomonads. Female worms are less likely to transmit viable histomonads until the heterakid eggs mature. The female worms probably become infected with the histomonads during copulation and incorporate the protozoan into eggs before shell formation.

Earthworms can serve as transport hosts in which heterakid eggs hatch, and the juvenile worms survive in tissues in an infective state. The earthworm thus serves as a means for collection and concentration of heterakid eggs from the poultry yard environment. On range, where climate and soil types favor survival of heterakids and earthworms, the latter must be considered in attempts to control a recurrent histomoniasis problem.

Earthworm transmission of *Histomonas* to the ringnecked pheasant (*Phasianus colchicus torquatus*) has been of documented importance in a partridge-pheasant histomoniasis outbreak at a game-rearing station in central Iowa.

Although direct infection of turkeys by oral ingestion of viable histomonads in fresh droppings is possible, their extremely delicate nature makes this route rather unlikely. Histomonads cannot survive outside the host for more than a few minutes unless protected by the heterakid egg or earthworm.

PATHOGENICITY. Characteristics of the definitive host influence clinical manifestations of infection by *Histomonas meleagridis* more than variations of pathogenicity of the parasite. These characteristics

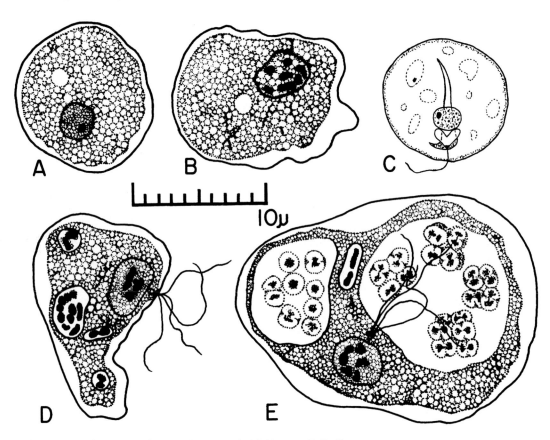

34.11. Examples of *H. meleagridis* (*A, B, C*) compared with *H. wenrichi* (*D, E*)
showing variations for each species associated with environmental conditions. *A.* Tissue type *H. meleagridis* in fresh preparation from liver lesion;
viewed with phase-contrast. *B. H. meleagridis* in transitional stage in lumen of the cecum. Pseudopodia have been formed; distribution of chromatin suggests that binary fission is approaching. However, the flagellum
has not yet appeared. *C.* An organism from culture, with free flagellum
typical of lumen-dwelling forms. (Honigberg and Bennett) *D.* Small *H.
wenrichi,* structurally distinguishable from *H. meleagridis* by presence of
four flagella. *E. H. wenrichi* as viewed in stained smear from cecum in
which packets of *Sarcina* were abundant. Panels *A, B, D,* and *E* are from
camera lucida tracings. Organisms shown in *B* and *D* are from portions of
ceca fixed in Zenker's fluid, sectioned at 6 or 8 μm, and stained with Heidenhain's (*B*) or Wiegert's (*D*) iron hematoxylin. The specimen pictured in
E was fixed in Schaudinn's fluid with 10% glacial acetic acid.

include species, breed, age, and intestinal flora.

Although naturally occurring infections occur in
several species, the turkey is considered the most
susceptible host because most infected turkeys die.
Chickens are easily infected, but often have a
milder form of the disease. Some variation in susceptibility has been found among different breeds
of chickens. Chickens 4–6 wk old and turkeys 3–12
wk old are highly susceptible to infection.

Bacterial flora also plays a role with *H. meleagridis* in development of disease. Lesions of histomoniasis were more severe in turkeys when
Clostridium perfringens was present as a monospe-

cific contaminant than when *Escherichia coli* was
present.

Isolates of *Histomonas* grown in vitro frequently
lose pathogenicity in successive passages. Defined
strains of *H. meleagridis* with varying pathogenicity have not been characterized, with the exception
of *H. wenrichi,* now listed as a separate species.

Pathogenesis and Epizootiology

NATURAL AND EXPERIMENTAL HOSTS. Numerous gallinaceous birds are reported as hosts for *H.
meleagridis.* The turkey, chukar partridge, and

ruffed grouse may be severely affected by histomoniasis, and the chicken, peafowl, guinea fowl, bobwhite quail, and pheasant have a milder form of the disease. Experimentally, the coturnix quail can be infected, but it is a poor host for the parasite.

VECTORS. The role of heterakids as vectors for histomonads is extremely important because they, too, are parasites of gallinaceous birds and protect the histomonad within their egg during transmission from bird to bird. The chicken, by serving as an inapparent host for both heterakids and histomonads, can be an important vector; however, with onset of confinement rearing of chickens and other changes in management of poultry and game bird production, their importance in disseminating *H. meleagridis* was diminished. Wild populations of game fowl, pheasants, and bobwhite quail may serve as vectors. Besides the earthworm, arthropods including flies, grasshoppers, sowbugs, and crickets may serve as mechanical vectors.

INCUBATION PERIOD. Disease is caused when histomonads penetrate the cecal wall, multiply, enter the bloodstream, and eventually parasitize the liver. Overt signs of histomoniasis are apparent from 7 to 12 days and occur most commonly 11 days postinfection (PI). The incubation period is similar following all natural methods of infection, i.e., histomonad-containing heterakid egg, earthworm, and arthropod transmission. Experimentally, lesions develop about 3 days earlier after cloacal inoculation of turkeys with cultured histomonads compared with infection via heterakid eggs.

CLINICAL SIGNS. Early signs of histomoniasis in turkeys include brilliant-yellow feces (Fig. 34.10B), drowsiness, dropping of the wings, walking with a stilted gait, closed eyes, head down close to the body or tucked under a wing, and anorexia. The head may or may not be cyanotic, a sign observed by those who gave the disease the name blackhead. About 12 days PI, turkeys become emaciated. Infections in chickens may be mild and go unnoticed or may be severe and cause high mortality. Sulfur-colored droppings associated with histomoniasis in turkeys are seldom found in chickens, but bloody cecal discharges have been observed. Sometimes gross pathology in chickens may resemble cecal coccidiosis.

CLINICAL PATHOLOGY. Total leukocytes are increased to a maximum count of 70,000/mm³ 10 days PI and return to normal levels 21 days PI. The increase in leukocytes is comprised mainly of heterophils; lymphocyte, basophil, and erythrocyte counts are unchanged.

There is a decline in serum nitrogen, uric acid, and hemoglobin levels during the incubation period, but these return to normal prior to death. Blood sugar levels rise during the cecal phase, decrease during liver lesion development, and drop below normal prior to death. Serum albumin falls very low, but the alpha and beta globulins increase slightly, and the gamma globulins increase greatly during the acute infection in turkeys (20).

Plasma levels of glutamic oxaloacetic transaminase (GOT) and lactic dehydrogenase (LDH) increase as liver lesions develop in turkeys (21), but glutamic pyruvic transaminase (GPT) remains essentially unchanged. There is very little GPT activity in avian liver or other tissues, suggesting that it is not an important enzyme in birds. Appearance of a brilliant yellow urine pigment coincides with depressed liver function and elevated enzyme resulting from tissue damage. In chickens with cecal lesions but without liver lesions, there is an actual decline in plasma levels of GOT, LDH, malic dehydrogenase, and other enzymes, suggesting impaired liver function. Cholinesterase is also depressed, further suggesting depressed liver function, even though gross liver lesions are not apparent. In acutely ill turkeys, the proportion of hemoglobins in the methemoglobin state in the blood is greatly elevated, possibly contributing to cyanosis and the purported blackhead appearance.

MORBIDITY AND MORTALITY. Host response to the infective agent may be variable and is influenced by method and amount of exposure. In naturally occurring infections, mortality usually reaches a peak about the 17th day and then subsides by the end of the 4th wk. Farmer and Stephenson (8) reported that turkeys confined to areas contaminated by chickens have had 89% morbidity and 70% mortality. Experimentally, mortality has reached 100% in turkeys. Although mortality from histomoniasis in chickens is generally low, mortality has exceeded 30% in some naturally occurring infections. Occasionally, a strain of *Histomonas* with high virulence for chickens is found.

GROSS LESIONS. The primary lesions of histomoniasis develop in the ceca and liver (see Fig. 34.10). Lesions are observed initially in the ceca about the 8th day. After tissue invasion by histomonads, cecal walls become thickened and hyperemic. Serous and hemorrhagic exudate from the mucosa fills the lumen of ceca, distends the walls with a caseous or cheesy core, and ulceration of the cecal wall may lead to perforation of the organ and cause generalized peritonitis.

Liver lesions in turkeys are often apparent on the 10th day of infection and are highly variable in appearance. Often the lesion is described as a circular depressed area of necrosis up to 1 cm in diameter and is circumscribed by a raised ring. While these lesions are often seen (Fig. 34.10C,F), they may take on other appearances. In heavy infections lesions may be small, numerous, and mostly subsurface, and they may involve a large part of the liver. In rare cases of recovery, lesions leave purulent scars on the surface of the liver. The liver may be enlarged and discolored green or tan. Lesions in lung, kidney, spleen, and mesenteries are sometimes recognized as white rounded areas of necrosis.

HISTOPATHOLOGY. Initial invasion of the cecal wall results in hyperemia and heterophil leukocyte infiltration, probably a combined response to bacteria, histomonads, and heterakid juveniles (2). Within 5–6 days, numerous histomonads are visible as pale, lightly stained, ovoid bodies within lacunae in the lamina propria and muscularis mucosa. Large numbers of lymphocytes and macrophages have infiltrated tissues by this time, and the heterophil population has also increased. There is a core in the cecal lumen composed of sloughed epithelium, fibrin, erythrocytes, and leukocytes along with trapped cecal ingesta. The core may initially be amorphous and red tinged, but by about 12 days it appears laminated, dry, and yellowish from buildup of successive layers of exudate. By 12–16 days, giant cells appear in the tissues of the cecum. Coagulation necrosis and histomonad invasion extend well into the muscular tunic, extending nearly to the serosa. At about 17–21 days, histomonads are scarce within the tissues, mostly concentrated near the serosal layers. Large numbers of giant cells form and may appear grossly as granulomata bulging upon the serosal aspect of the cecum. Old lesions, after recovery, are characterized by lymphoid centers scattered throughout the cecal tissue. Expulsion of cores and regeneration of epithelium may occur, but the cecum is often abnormally thin and crypts are shallow.

The earliest microscopic lesions are visible in the liver by about 6–7 days PI and consist of small clusters of heterophils, lymphocytes, and monocytes near portal vessels. Histomonads are difficult to locate in these areas. After about 10–14 days, the lesions are enlarged, becoming confluent in some areas. There is extensive lymphocytic and macrophage infiltration, and heterophils are present in moderate numbers. Hepatocytes in centers of the lesions necrose and disintegrate. Many individual or clustered histomonads are visible in lacunae near the periphery of lesions. From 14 to 21 days PI, necrosis becomes increasingly severe, resulting in large areas consisting of little more than reticulum and cellular debris. Histomonads at this stage are present mostly as small bodies in macrophages. If recovery occurs, foci of lymphoid cells remain, along with areas of fibrosis and regenerating hepatocytes.

IMMUNITY

Active. Immunity arising in turkeys that have been naturally or experimentally infected with histomonads is not sufficient to give complete protection against reinfection. Most work with immunity in turkeys has relied on drug-limiting infections, since turkeys usually die from the disease.

Attempts to immunize chickens and turkeys with in vitro attenuated or nonpathogenic histomonads have been only partially successful. Some protection has been demonstrated against cloacal inoculation of pathogenic or attenuated strains of histomonads, but very little against histomonad-containing heterakid eggs (18). Although reports are not in agreement, some protective immunity may be obtained while drug therapy is being administered.

Precipitating antibodies against antigens prepared from infected livers and ceca have been demonstrated in serum of chickens and turkeys 10–12 days PI. Antibodies in turkeys and fowl apparently did not confer resistance to reinfection but were connected with infection of cecal mucosa and persisted in turkeys and fowl for a considerable time (3). Birds recovering from histomoniasis may harbor parasites in the ceca without signs or lesions of the disease (5).

Passive. Attempts to transfer immunity from resistant to susceptible chickens and turkeys by repeated intraperitoneal injections of serum from immune birds have been unsuccessful. When birds receiving immune serum were challenged by cloacal inoculation of infected liver homogenates, turkeys died from histomoniasis and all chickens developed typical cecal lesions (4, 5).

Diagnosis. Most experienced poultry workers make a diagnosis on the basis of gross appearance of lesions, but laboratory confirmation by poultry disease specialists should be sought to rule out concurrent infections with other agents that affect the cecum or liver (coccidiosis, salmonellosis, aspergillosis, upper digestive tract trichomoniasis).

Presence of characteristic lesions is sufficient for presumptive diagnosis. Identification of histomonads requires careful microscopy, preferably with phase-contrast using fresh specimens from birds recently killed in the laboratory and maintained with reasonable warmth during preparation. Histomonads remain active and are more easily identified if the microscope stage is warmed, either with a special stage incubator or small incandescent light bulb.

Histomonads found in the cecal lumen are easily seen and identified, but histomonads found in tissue lesions are nonflagellated and can be differentiated from macrophages and yeast cells only with difficulty.

For routine diagnostic histopathology, any of several stains, including hematoxylin and eosin or periodic acid-Schiff, may be used (13). Excellent cytologic preparations have been made from fresh cultures using Hollande's cupric picroformol and a protein-silver stain.

Where freshly killed birds are available, it is a simple matter to cultivate histomonads in vitro as a diagnostic aid (19), using a modification of Dwyer's (6) medium. If samples are taken from freshly killed birds (before body heat has been lost), the test is over 75% accurate. The medium consists of 85% Medium 199 in Hank's balanced salt solution, 5% chicken embryo extract (CEE50, Gibco), and 10% horse or sheep serum adjusted to pH 7.2. A small amount (10–20 mg) of rice powder (Difco) is added, then tubes are sealed, incubated at 40 C overnight, and observed with an inverted microscope. Cultures obtained in this way can be maintained by subculturing every 2–3 days, but they will become nonpathogenic within 6–8 wk.

Prevention and Control. Since primary means of transmission of histomoniasis occurs through the vehicle of heterakid eggs, successful control measures are directed in large part toward reduction or exclusion of the eggs.

Exclusion of domestic chickens from turkey-raising operations is essential, since chickens may often harbor large numbers of egg-laying cecal worms. Turkey ranges can become severely contaminated with long-lived heterakid eggs, thus creating a situation in which histomoniasis recurs in turkey flocks for many years. Because of the longevity of infectious eggs, range rotation is not practical as a solution. Survival of heterakid eggs may be diminished by providing sunny, well-drained ranges so that lethal effects of solar radiation and dryness can have maximum effect.

Rearing turkeys indoors seems to reduce incidence of blackhead, possibly by eliminating access to earthworms, but this has not helped with chickens. Leghorn pullets often become infected in problem houses where worm eggs have built up in number for several years. In Australia, histomoniasis has been a problem in broilers for many years. In some instances, disinfection may have value in killing worm eggs, but there are little published data.

Management practices alone are rarely adequate to keep the disease at a low level in commercial turkey flocks; therefore, preventive chemotherapy is usually practiced during the high-risk part of the growout. Preventive chemotherapy is not ordinarily practiced with chickens except on problem farms or in localities where there is high incidence of outbreaks.

Five drugs were at one time registered for use in the United States (9), including two arsenicals, two nitroimidazoles, and one nitrofuran (Table 34.6), but recent regulatory action has removed the most useful drugs (nitroimidazoles) from the market. Other drugs are available outside the United States. For preventive use, nitarsone may be effective, but the arsenicals are generally not strong enough for treatment of established infections. The nitroimidazoles (dimetridazole, ipronidazole, or ronidazole) were highly effective for prevention or treatment in chickens or turkeys. These important drugs are still available in many countries. Furazolidone has also been used for treatment of blackhead disease. There is no reported sign of drug resistance in histomonads. For a historical review of older literature on these drugs, see Joyner et al. (12) and Joyner (11).

Table 34.6. Feed additives used in the United States for prevention or treatment of blackhead disease in turkeys[a]

| Drug | Trade name | Supplier | Conditions of Use | | Approval for Chickens |
			Use Level	Withdrawal	
Carbarsone[b]	Carb-O-Sep	Whitmoyer	0.025–0.037%	5	No
Dimetridazole[b]	Emtrymix	Solvay	0.015–0.02%[c] or 0.16–0.08%[d]	5	No
Furazolidone[b]	nf-180	Rhodia/Hess & Clark	0.011%[c]	5	Yes
	Furox	Smith-Kline	0.022%[d]	5	Yes
Ipronidazole[b]	Ipropan	Hoffman-La Roche	0.00625%[c]	4	No
			0.0625%[c]	4	No
Nitarsone	Histostat-50	Solvay	0.01875%	5	Yes

[a]Some products are also available for water treatment.
[b]No longer available in the United States. Information provided for international users.
[c]Preventive level.
[d]Treatment level.

TRICHOMONIASIS. Trichomoniasis in birds, affecting the upper digestive tract, is caused by the flagellated protozoan *Trichomonas gallinae* (Fig. 34.12). In pigeons, it causes a condition known as "canker." Turkeys, chickens, and a wide variety of wild birds are parasitized with varying degrees of pathogenicity (15).

Description. These intestinal flagellates are rapidly moving, pear-shaped protozoa that range in size from 5 to 9 μm in length and from 2 to 9 μm in width (Fig. 34.13). There are typically four free flagella arising from a basal granule at the anterior pole of the organism. A slender axostyle usually extends well beyond the posterior end of the body. An undulating membrane originates at the anterior pole of the body and ends short of the posterior pole, with the enclosed flagellum not trailing free at the posterior end. The flagella and internal structures can only be seen with the aid of phase-contrast microscopy or special stains.

Incidence and Distribution. Squabs usually become infected with their first taste of "pigeon milk" from the crop of adults and usually remain carriers throughout life. With virulent strains, mortality may be as high as 50% before sufficient protective immunity develops. Pigeons are often blamed for transmission of trichomoniasis to turkeys and chickens. The economic impact of the disease in turkeys and chickens is difficult to assess, although infections are occasionally reported. When captive birds of prey such as falcons are allowed to feed on pigeons, infection may result in a condition known as "frounce" among falconers.

Life Cycle. *T. gallinae* reproduces by longitudinal binary fission. Cysts, sexual stages, or vectors are not known. The organism is transferred to squabs by infection of "pigeon milk" from adults. In chicken and turkey flocks, infection is spread by contamination of drinking water and perhaps feed.

Pathogenesis and Pathology. Nearly all pigeons are carriers of this organism. Affected birds may cease to feed and become listless, ruffled in appearance, and emaciated before death. A greenish to yellowish fluid may be seen in the oral cavity and may drip from the beaks of infected birds.

GROSS LESIONS. *T. gallinae* invade the mucosal surface of the buccal cavity, sinuses, pharynx, esophagus, crop, and occasionally the conjunctiva and proventriculus. The liver is frequently invaded, and occasionally other organs—but not the digestive tract below the proventriculus—are involved.

Lesions appear initially as small, circumscribed caseous areas on the surface of the oral mucosa, which may be surrounded by a thin zone of hyperemia. These may enlarge and become confluent. The buildup of caseous material may be sufficient to occlude the lumen of the esophagus partially or completely. These lesions may eventually penetrate tissue and extensively involve other regions of the head and neck, including the nasopharynx, orbits, and cervical soft tissues. In the liver, lesions appear on the surface and extend into the parenchyma as solid, white to yellow circular or spherical masses.

HISTOPATHOLOGY. Pigeons infected with a virulent strain of *T. gallinae* had purulent inflammation with caseation necrosis as the predominant lesion (26). Trichomonads multiplied locally in secretions and on the mucosal surface of the oropharynx. Ulceration of the mucosa with a massive inflammatory response, primarily heterophils, was well established by the 4th day of infection. In the liver, focal necrotic abscesses occurred in all zones of

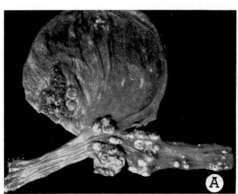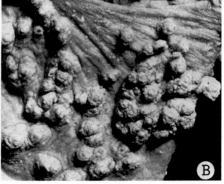

34.12. *A.* Necrotic ulceration of esophagus and crop seen in trichomoniasis. *B.* Close-up of typical pyramidlike necrotic ulcers characteristic of trichomoniasis of upper digestive tract. (Hinshaw and Rosenwald)

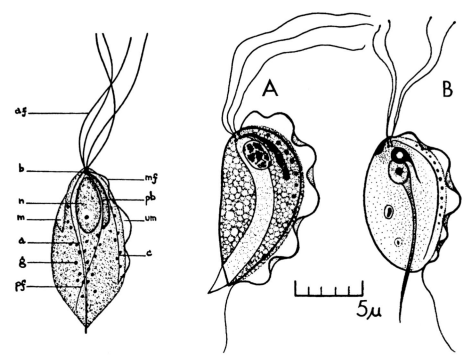

34.13. *Trichomonas gallinae,* semidiagrammatic (*left*): (a) axostyle, (af) anterior flagellum, (b) blepharoplast, (c) costa, (g) cytoplasmic granules, (m) mouth, (mf) marginal filament, (n) nucleus, (pb) parabasal body, (pf) parabasal fibril, (um) undulating membrane (Stabler). Diagrammatic representations of two common trichomonads of lower digestive tract of domestic birds (*right*), as favorable specimens fixed in Schaudinn's fluid and stained with Heidenhain's hematoxylin may appear. A. *Tritrichomonas eberthi.* B. *Trichomonas gallinarum.* (Lund)

lobules, with an inflammatory reaction characterized by mononuclear cells and heterophils. As liver lesions progressed, no intact hepatocytes remained in the center of foci; trichomonads were most numerous at the periphery.

IMMUNITY. The relatively high incidence of infections in otherwise normal pigeons can be attributed to strain variations, acquired immunity, or both. Pigeons are immune to disease from virulent strains of trichomonads after recovery from sublethal trichomoniasis. Plasma from pigeons harboring any of three strains of *T. gallinae* was capable of protecting other pigeons against disease but not infection from a virulent strain.

Antigens of *T. gallinae* have been studied in regard to taxonomy with the conclusion that virulence and antigenic composition were related (7).

Diagnosis. Clinical signs and gross lesions are highly suggestive and may be confirmed by microscopic observation of organisms in direct wet smears from the mouth or crop. Histopathologic ex-

amination or cultivation of organisms in artificial media may help in cases in which the parasites are absent in fresh smears. Trichomoniasis must be differentiated from candidiasis and hypovitaminosis-A, which can produce somewhat similar lesions. History, cultivation for fungi, and histopathologic examination may prove useful in resolving problem diagnoses.

Several other species of flagellates that inhabit the avian gastrointestinal tract are frequently misidentified as *T. gallinae*. These other species of trichomonads and more distantly related flagellates have never been unequivocally demonstrated to be pathogenic for the avian host. Their recognition as harmless commensals will prevent unnecessary expenditures for therapeutic measures.

One trichomonad, *Tetratrichomonas gallinarum* (= *Trichomonas gallinarum*), is a common inhabitant of the cecum of chickens and other gallinaceous birds. This trichomonad or a closely related species has occasionally been isolated from liver and blood. Although lesions have been ascribed to this organism, no confirmation of pathogenicity has come from experimental infection.

Other lower intestinal protozoa such as *Chilomastix gallinarum* (Fig. 34.14), a cyst-forming flagellate with a large cytostomal cleft but no undulating membrane, and *Cochlosoma anatis,* with a ventral sucker covering half the surface of the body, are apparently nonpathogenic. Although additional controlled experiments with flagellates found in the lower intestine are needed, for the present they should not be considered important.

Prevention and Control.   Since *T. gallinae* is transmitted from parent to squab in pigeons, and by contamination of feed and water by oral fluids in the case of domestic fowl, every effort should be made to remove infected birds from a flock. Experimentally, several drugs are active against trichomoniasis in pigeons or turkeys. McLoughlin (24) found dimetridazole useful at a level of 0.05% in drinking water for pigeons. This drug is no longer available in the United States.

HEXAMITIASIS

Etiology and Distribution.   Hexamitiasis, or infectious catarrhal enteritis, of poults is caused by the protozoan *Hexamita meleagridis.* The United States Department of Agriculture (32) estimated that an annual loss of $667,000 occurred from hexamitiasis in turkeys from 1942 to 1951. Only 10 cases, however, were reported in the United States

in 1986 (1). The disease has been reported from several areas of the United States, Canada, Scotland, England, and Germany. The organism has also been found in pheasants, quail, chukar partridge, and peafowl, which may be a source of infection for turkey poults. The eight prominent flagella include four anterior, two anterolateral, and two posterior. The four anterior flagella are recurved along the body (Fig. 34.15). McNeil et al. (25), who named the species, described it as being 6–12.4 × 2–5 µm in size with binucleate large endosomes.

Pathology.   Affected poults do not show specific signs, but a watery diarrhea occurs that may become yellowish later in the course of the disease. The poults at first are nervous and active, but later tend to become listless and huddled. Convulsions and coma may occur as the terminal stage is approached.

Lesions include catarrhal inflammation and atony resulting in distention, especially in the upper small intestine. Intestinal contents are watery, and large numbers of hexamitae may be seen in the crypts upon microscopic examination. A yellowish discoloration of the liver surface was described in an outbreak in Germany.

Diagnosis.   Presence of watery diarrhea and demonstration of hexamitae in fresh smears of duodenal contents are sufficient to establish the diagnosis. Since carrier birds may occur among survivors, presence of *Hexamita* without signs may occur. Hexamitae move very rapidly, with a darting motion, and are quite small compared with other flagellates that may be encountered in the avian digestive tract.

Control and Treatment.   Removal of carrier birds, separation of older stock from poults, and exclusion of other avian host species from the area of the poult flock, along with cleanliness around feeders and waterers should minimize transmission. No effective treatment is known, although butynorate (0.0375%) and chlortetracycline (0.0055%) were approved for use at one time.

MISCELLANEOUS PROTOZOA IN THE DIGESTIVE TRACT.   Several species of the genera *Entamoeba* and *Endolimax* occur naturally in ceca or feces of various domestic fowl or are capable of being established experimentally. Apparently none of these are pathogenic; they exist by feeding on intestinal contents.

The amoebas have irregularly shaped trophozoites and a single nucleus with a more or less prominent endosome and produce cysts that when mature contain one, four, or eight nuclei. These organisms may be difficult to see without using warm smears and phase-contrast microscopy or stained

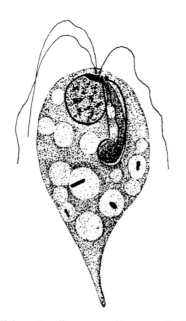

34.14. *Chilomastix gallinarum,* semidiagrammatic, illustrating details of morphology. ×5000. (Boeck and Tanabe)

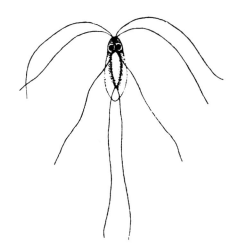

34.15. *Hexamita meleagridis* from intestine of turkey.
×1875. (25)

preparations. Accounts of a number of species have been reported by McDowell (23), Lund (17), and Levine (15).

REFERENCES

1. AAAP Committee on Disease Reporting. 1986. Summary of commercial poultry disease reports. Avian Dis 31:926–987.
2. Clarkson, M.J. 1962. Studies on the immunity to Histomonas meleagridis in the turkey and the fowl. Res Vet Sci 3:443–448.
3. Clarkson, M.J. 1963. Immunity to Histomoniasis (blackhead). Immunology 6:156–168.
4. Clarkson, M.J. 1966. Progressive serum protein changes in turkeys infected with Histomonas meleagridis. J Comp Pathol 76:387–397.
5. Cuckler, A.C. 1970. Coccidiosis and histomoniasis in avian hosts. In G.J. Jackson, R. Herman, and I. Singer (eds.). Immunity to Parasitic Animals. Appleton-Century-Crofts, New York, pp. 371–397.
6. Dwyer, D.M. 1970. An improved method for cultivating Histomonas meleagridis. J Parasitol 56:191–192.
7. Dwyer, D.M. 1974. Analysis of the antigenic relationships among Trichomonas, Histomonas, Dientamoeba, and Entamoeba. J Protozool 21:139–145.
8. Farmer, R.K., and J. Stephenson. 1949. Infectious enetorohepatitis (blackhead) in turkeys: A comparative study of methods of infection. J Comp Pathol 59:119–126.
9. Feed Additive Compendium. 1988. Miller Publishing Company, Minneapolis, MN.
10. Gibbs, B.J. 1962. The occurrence of the protozoan parasite Histomonas meleagridis in the adult and eggs of the cecal worm Heterakis gallinae. J Protozool 59:877–884.
11. Joyner, L.P. 1966. In R.J. Schnitzer and F. Hawking (eds.). Experimental Chemotherapy, vol. 4. Academic Press, New York, pp. 425–428.
12. Joyner, L.P., S.F.M. Davies, and S.D. Kendall. 1963. Chemotherapy of Histomoniasis. In R.J. Schnitzer and F. Hawking (eds.). Experimental Chemotherapy, vol. 1. Academic Press, New York, pp. 333–349.
13. Kemp, R.L., and W.M. Reid. 1966. Staining techniques for differential diagnosis of Histomoniasis and mycosis in domestic poultry. Avian Dis 10:357–363.
14. Lee, D.L. 1969. The structure and development of Histomonas meleagridis (Masticamoebidae: Protozoa) in the female reproductive tract of its host, Heterakis gallinae (Nematoda). Parasitology 59:877–884.
15. Levine, N.D. 1973. Protozoan Parasites of Domestic Animals and of Man, 2nd ed. Burgess, Minneapolis.
16. Lund, E.E. 1969. Histomoniasis. Adv Vet Sci Comp Med 13:355–390.
17. Lund, E.E. 1972. Other protozoan diseases. In M.S. Hofstad, B.W. Calnek, C.F. Hembold, W.M. Reid, and H.W. Yoder Jr. (eds.). Diseases of Poultry, 6th ed. Iowa State University Press, Ames, IA, pp 990–1046.
18. Lund, E.E., P.C. Augustine, and D.J. Ellis. 1966. Earthworm transmission of Heterakis and Histomonas to turkeys and chickens. Exp Parasitol 18:403–407.
19. McDougald, L., and R.B. Galloway. 1973. Blackhead disease in vitro isolation of Histomonas meleagridis as a potentially useful diagnostic aid. Avian Dis 17:847–450.
20. McDougald, L.R., and M.F. Hansen. 1969. Serum protein changes in chickens subsequent to infection with Histomonas meleagridis. Avian Dis 13:673–677.
21. McDougald, L.R., and M.F. Hansen. 1970. Histomonas meleagridis: Effect on plasma enzymes in chickens and turkeys. Exp Parasitol 27:229–235.
22. McDougald, L.R., and W.M. Reid. 1976. Protozoa of Medical and Veterinary Interest, vol. 1. Academic Press, New York, pp. 140–161.
23. McDowell, S., Jr. 1953. A morphological and taxonomic study of the caecal protozoa of the common fowl, Gallus gallus L. J Morphol 92:337–399.
24. McLoughlin, D.K. 1966. Observations on the treatment of Trichomonas gallinae in pigeons. Avian Dis 10:288–290.
25. McNeil, E., W.R. Hinshaw, and C.A. Kofoid. 1941. Hexamita meleagridis sp. nov. from the turkey. Am J Hyg 34:71–82.
26. Perez Mesa, C., R.M. Stabler, and M. Berthrong. 1961. Histopathological changes in the domestic pigeon infected with Trichomonas gallinae (Jones' Barn Strain). Avian Dis 5:48–60.
27. Reid, W.M. 1967. Etiology and dissemination of the blackhead disease syndrome in turkeys and chickens. Exp Parasitol 21:249–275.
28. Ruff, M.D., L.R. McDougald, and M.F. Hansen. 1970. Isolation of Histomonas meleagridis from embryonated eggs of the Heterakis gallinarum. J Protozool 17:10–11.
29. Springer, W.T., J. Johnson, and W.M. Reid. 1969. Transmission of Histomoniasis with male Heterakis gallinarum (Nematoda). Parasitology 59:401–405.
30. Tyzzer, E.E. 1920. The flagellate character of the parasite producing "blackhead" in turkeys Histomonas meleagridis. J Parasitol 6:124–130.
31. Tyzzer, E.E. 1934. Studies on Histomoniasis, or "blackhead" infection, in the chicken and turkey. Proc Am Acad Arts Sci 69:189–264.
32. USDA. 1954. Losses in Agriculture. United States Department Agriculture, ARS, Washington, DC.

OTHER BLOOD AND TISSUE PROTOZOA

Wilfred T. Springer

LEUCOCYTOZOONOSIS. This parasitic disease of birds affects blood and tissue cells of internal organs. Reviews of this and other parasitic diseases have been summarized by Lund (53), Levine (48), and Fallis et al. (21).

Leucocytozoon was assigned to the suborder Haemospororina of the phylum Apicomplexa by a committee of the Society of Protozoologists (51). Levine (48) suggested that similarities in life cycle and ultrastructure of some life stages of *Leucocytozoon*, *Haematroteus*, and *Plasmodium* warrant inclusion of all three genera in a single family, Plasmodiidae.

Criteria for species designation include host range and gametocyte characteristics, such as staining characteristics, size, nature, and extent of distortion of the host cell and altered shape and position of the host cell nucleus (21). Approximately 67 valid species and 34 synonyms have been described. With the exception of a species observed in the teiid lizard in Brazil, all species of *Leucocytozoon* are found in birds (33).

The life cycle includes reproduction by sporogony in insects with schizogony (merogony) in tissue cells, and gametogony in erythrocytes or leukocytes. The disease is prevalent in areas with a suitable ecology and ethology for dipterous invertebrate hosts, simuliid flies and culicoid midges. At least three species of *Leucocytozoon* reported in domestic fowl are known to have caused outbreaks in North America resulting in economic losses in ducks, geese, turkeys and chickens.

LEUCOCYTOZOON SIMONDI MATHIS AND LEGER 1910.

Infection with *L. simondi* has been reported from 27 species of ducks and geese in United States, Canada, Europe, and Vietnam by Hsu et al. (33). They consider *L. anatis* from ducks and *L. anseris* from geese as synonyms of *L. simondi*. Approximately 20% of ducks and geese along the northeastern seaboard of North America each year carry *Leucocytozoon* infections (6). Eighty percent of geese at Seney Wildlife Refuge in Michigan had some parasitemia in 1963 just prior to the egg-laying season, and each year all goslings become infected (32).

ETIOLOGY. Sporogony occurs in the insect vector and may be completed in 3-4 days. Ookinetes develop following fertilization of the macrogametocyte and may be found in the stomach of the insect within 12 hr after a blood meal. Oocysts form from the ookinetes within the stomach of the invertebrate host and produce sporozoites, which migrate to the salivary glands after emerging from the oocyst. Viable sporozoites have been found in vectors up to 18 days after the last blood meal.

Schizogony takes place in such internal organs of the vertebrate host as liver, brain, spleen, and lungs. "Hepatic schizonts" in liver cells measure up to 45 μm when mature. Merozoites and syncytia are released from hepatic schizonts (syncytium refers to cytoplasm bounded by a plasma membrane and containing two or more nuclei). There is some indication that some merozoites may enter parenchymal cells of the liver and initiate another schizogonic cycle, while others enter erythrocytes or erythroblasts to develop into gametocytes. Apparently, syncytia are phagocytized by macrophages or reticuloendothelial cells throughout the body, where they develop into megaloschizonts up to 400 μm in size. Merozoites released from the megaloschizont enter lymphocytes and other leukocytes to form gametocytes.

The gametocytes of *L. simondi* found in the blood average 14.5 × 5.5 μm and usually inhabit elongate spindle-shaped host cells averaging about 48 μm in length. The parasite lies beside the nucleus of the host cell, which is about 30 μm in length. Round gametocytes have been reported also. Elongate gametocytes probably develop exclusively in leukocytes, predominantly lymphocytes and monocytes, while mature round gametocytes are found in erythrocytes. According to Allan and Mahrt (2), each *Leucocytozoon* species has gametogony in only one type of host cell; therefore, the presence of two morphologic types in the same bird indicates a concurrent host infection with two species. Desser et al. (16) observed infections in some areas of northern Michigan that were characterized by presence of both hepatic schizonts and round gametocytes, which he attributed to different strains of *L. simondi*.

Gamonts may be differentiated with a Romanowsky stain based on the dark blue staining cytoplasm of the macrogamete with its red nucleus, and the very pale blue staining cytoplasm of the microgamont with its pale pink nucleus. The microgamonts are more delicate and subject to distortion (48).

PATHOGENESIS AND EPIZOOTIOLOGY. Ducks and geese are suitable hosts for *L. simondi*, but chickens, turkeys, pheasants, and ruffed grouse are not.

Simulium venustum, a bloodsucking fly, was first demonstrated to be the vector among ducks. Other species of this insect shown to be transmitters of

Leucocytozoon are *S. croxtoni, S. euradminiculum* and *S. rugglesi.*

The pathogenicity of *L. simondi* in ducks and geese is well documented. An outbreak of *L. simondi* among ducks in Michigan resulted in 35% mortality. Extensive losses of young goslings attributed to infections of *L. simondi* are observed annually at Seney Wildlife Refuge, with mortality greater than 70% occurring every 4 yr (32).

Clinical signs vary with age and condition of the host. Young ducklings manifest inappetence, weakness, listlessness, dyspnea, and sometimes death within 24 hr. Signs in adults appear less abruptly and consist of listlessness and low mortality. About 60% of fatalities occur 11-19 days postexposure. Some pathologic effects of the disease are anemia, leukocytosis, splenomegaly, and liver degeneration and hypertrophy. Extensive tissue damage was noted in the spleen and heart of ducks carrying megaloschizonts.

Kocan (47) described an anti-erythrocyte factor in sera from acutely infected ducks, which agglutinated and hemolyzed normal untreated duck erythrocytes as well as infected cells. This factor was believed to be a product of the parasite, and its action was intravascular; it may account for the osmotic fragility of erythrocytes and anemia associated with *L. simondi* infections (54).

The greatest number of infections in northern Michigan occur mostly in July, the hottest part of the summer. Gametocytes decrease in number in the blood until midwinter, when they disappear or become scarce and then reappear in the spring.

LEUCOCYTOZOON SMITHI LAVERAN AND LUCET

1905. *L. smithi* was first seen in turkeys in the eastern United States by T. Smith, after whom it is named, and since reported in turkeys in North Dakota, Minnesota, Nebraska, California, Texas, Missouri, France, Germany, the Crimea, and Canada.

In the United States, it is widespread in adult turkeys (73): 289 of 357 turkeys were found infected in Georgia, 60 of 67 in Florida, 4 of 12 in Alabama, and 7 of 9 in South Carolina. The incidence of infection in pen-raised and free-ranging mature wild turkeys in the Cumberland State Forest in Virginia was 100%.

ETIOLOGY. *L. smithi* may be observed in the blood as rounded gametocytes that later become elongate, averaging 20-22 μm in length. They inhabit elongate cells averaging 45×14 μm, with pale cytoplasmic "horns" extending out beyond the enclosed parasite. The host cell forms a long, thin dark band along each side of the parasite; often it is split, forming a band on each side. Gamonts are found only in leukocytes. The staining characteristics of the gamonts with a Romanowsky stain are similar

to those of *L. simondi* (48) (Fig. 34.16A).

Intracellular schizogonous forms are found in the liver. Both schizonts and megaloschizonts were observed and illustrated by Siccardi et al. (65).

Several aspects of the life cycle were described in detail by Newberne and by Wehr (cited by 53); the ultrastructure of gametocytes was defined by Milhous and Solis (58).

PATHOGENESIS AND EPIZOOTIOLOGY. *L. smithi* generally resembles *L. simondi* of Anseriformes, but turkeys are probably not susceptible to the latter. *L. smithi* is not transmissible experimentally to chickens or ducks.

Simulium occidentale, S. aureum, S. meridionale, S. nigroparvum, and *S. slossonae* have been listed as vectors for *L. smithi* (21, 46).

The progress of leucocytozoonosis in susceptible young turkeys may be rapid and fatal. Clinical signs include anorexia, excessive thirst, depression, somnolence, and sometimes muscular incoordination. Death may occur suddenly during the acute stage of the disease.

Heavy infections of *L. smithi*, comparable to those reported for *L. simondi* in ducks, do not seem to occur in mature wild turkeys. Few signs of infection are observed in wild turkeys, possibly because of local factors such as time at which suitable vectors are prevalent and age of birds at first exposure.

Domestic hens infected with *Leucocytozoon* had decreased egg production, egg weight, and hatchability, and higher mortality than uninfected hens (41).

Recovered birds may harbor the parasite in their blood for more than 1 yr (17). There is often loss of vigor, and birds may suffer moist tracheal rales and coughing. Some birds die when subjected to stress. Males showed reduced mating activity (48).

Johnson et al. (39) reported that death results from obstruction of the circulatory system by large numbers of parasites. Congestion of the lungs, small intestine, liver, and spleen, and enlargement of the liver and spleen are frequently observed in affected turkeys. Lund (53) cites descriptive reports of the pathogenesis of the disease.

LEUCOCYTOZOON CAULLERYI MATHIS AND LEGER

1909. *L. caulleryi* is frequently found in chickens in southern and eastern Asia. Infections occur frequently in Japan (60). Reports of leucocytozoonosis in South Carolina, probably caused by *L. caulleryi*, are the only known cases of the disease in chickens in North America. In one survey, 13.6% of domestic yard chickens in South Carolina were infected (63).

ETIOLOGY. *L. andrewsi* and *L. schueffneri* are considered by some protozoologists to be synonymous with *L. caulleryi* (48).

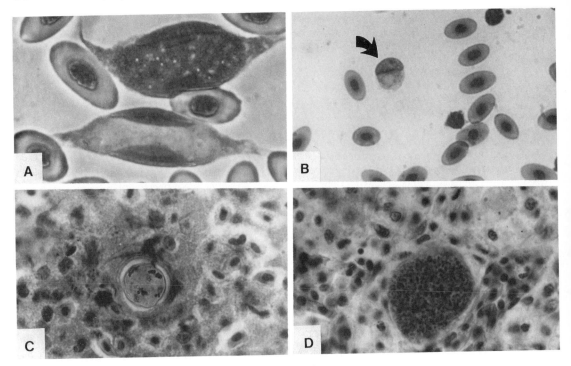

34.16. Photomicrographs of turkey blood containing various stages of *Leucocyto-zoon smithi*. A. Darkly stained macrogametocyte (*upper*) and lightly stained microgametocyte (*lower*). Giemsa stain, ×1250. B. "Round form" often found early in infection (day 16), ×140. C. Megaloschizont in turkey liver; day 9. H & E. ×1000. D. Megaloschizont turkey kidney; day 10. (Dick)

Mature gamonts are round and occupy round host cells, erythrocytes, and leukocytes about 20 μm in diameter. The nucleus of the host cell reportedly disappears after infection, a characteristic that differs from other species with round gametocytes. Others observed that the nucleus was always present in infected cells, leading them to designate the parasite as a new species, *L. andrewsi* (53). Macrogametes (12-15 μm) stain more darkly with Romanowsky stain than microgamonts (10-15 μm), according to Levine (48).

Schizogony occurs in many organs, but more often in lungs, liver, and kidneys. Megaloschizonts and their location in tissues are similar to those of *L. simondi* (21).

PATHOGENESIS AND EPIZOOTIOLOGY. The domestic chicken is the only reported host for this parasite. Insect vectors are *Culicoides arakawa, C. circumscriptus,* and *C. odibilis.* Akiba's discovery that the vector was a species of *Culicoides* and not *Simulium* prompted some to place *L. caulleryi* in a new genus called *Akiba* (21). Leucocytozoonosis epizootics, widespread during summer months in Japan, are serious enough to cause deaths in growing chicks and reduced egg production in hens (60).

Serious outbreaks of *L. caulleryi* in chickens are characterized by hemoptysis and severe renal lesions. Apparently, extensive hemorrhage results in the kidneys when merozoites are released from megaloschizonts. Clopidol has been successfully used in preventive medication, while combinations of pyrimethamine and a sulfonamide have been used in treatment.

***LEUCOCYTOZOON SABREZI* MATHIS AND LEGER 1910.** *L. sabrezi* (*L. schueffneri*, probably a synonym) has been found in domestic chickens in Southeast Asia, causing anemia, thickened oral discharge, and paralysis of the legs. Megaloschizont formation has not been reported for this parasite. Merozoites enter both erythroblasts and leukocytes to form elongate gametocytes within spindle-shaped host cells (6-7 × 4-6 μm), whose nuclei appear as thin bands beside the parasite (21). Macrogametes (22 × 6.5 μm) have a more compact nucleus and stain more darkly with a Romanowsky stain than the microgamonts (20 × 6 μm) (48). The insect vector is unknown.

***LEUCOCYTOZOON SCHOUTEDENI* RODHAM, PONS, VANDENBRANDEN, AND BEQUAERT 1913.** *L.*

schoutedeni, which was found in 50% of chickens in East Africa (21), is unknown elsewhere. Gametocytes are round (11-13 µm) and found in round host cells (18 µm) whose nuclei surround the parasite about one-half of its length. Staining characteristics of the gametocytes have not been reported. The *Simulium* fly serves as the invertebrate host for *L. schoutedeni*.

Diagnosis. *Leucocytozoon* infections are diagnosed by direct microscopic observation and identification of gametocytes in stained blood or schizonts in tissue sections. Solis (69) described the high staining contrast of *Leucocytozoon* in peripheral blood films stained with brilliant cresyl blue.

Treatment and Control. Drug treatment of leucocytozoonosis has had limited success. No effective treatment has been found for *L. simondi*. Pyrimethamine (1 ppm) and sulfadimethoxine (10 ppm) administered simultaneously reportedly will prevent, but not cure, infections of *L. caulleryi*. Clopidol in feed effectively controlled *L. smithi* according to Siccardi et al. (65). This drug (0.0125-0.0250% in feed) has been approved by the Food and Drug Administration for medication of turkeys.

Control requires eliminating the insect vector from the environment of the vertebrate host. A large-scale aerial treatment program using 2% Abate Celatom granules for control of larval *Simulium* substantially reduced adult and larval blackfly populations and reduced the level of *L. smithi* blood parasitemia in turkeys in one study (45).

Repellents sprayed within houses to discourage entrance of the insect vector lowered mortality and incidence of disease, but did not completely prevent infection in the flock (21). Had proper control measures been implemented, an economic disaster might have been avoided when a new turkey enterprise was established in the coastal plain area of South Carolina. It is advisable to grow susceptible birds in areas free of blackflies and midges.

AVIAN MALARIA. Avian malarial infections are caused by parasites of the genus *Plasmodium* and are characterized by the presence of pigment in erythrocytes. Schizogony occurs in blood, and gametocytes are found in mature erythrocytes. Transmission is by mosquitoes. These characteristics distinguish them from other members of the family Plasmodiidae and *Haemoproteus* and *Leucocytozoon* species.

About 65 species of *Plasmodium* from over 1000 different birds have been described, but some 35 or less are considered to be valid (43). The species pathogenic for domestic fowl are found mostly in Asia, Africa, and South America. Malaria outbreaks

in birds on the North American continent are sometimes found in species of the orders Anseriformes, Passeriformes, and Columbiformes.

Etiology. Although many species of *Plasmodium* can be introduced into various domestic fowl, only a few appear to be natural parasites of these birds. *P. gallinaceum* occurs in jungle fowl and domestic hens; *P. juxtanucleare* parasitizes domestic hens and turkeys; *P. durae* and *P. griffithsi* occur in turkeys; *P. lophurae* of the fire-backed pheasant can also parasitize chickens and has been host-adapted to other domestic fowl and ducks; *P. fallax* of guinea fowl has been adapted to various domestic fowl; *P. hermani* will infect domestic and wild turkeys and bobwhite quail (26).

A number of other species that occur primarily in passerine birds can infect domestic fowl or have been experimentally transmitted to them. These include *P. relictum*, *P. elongatum*, *P. cathemerium*, and *P. circumflexum* (43).

Life Cycle. Only a general outline of the malarian life cycle can be given here. Garnham (29) detailed the life cycles extensively and should be consulted for specific information on various species. Greiner et al. (31) presented color plates of 24 species.

Avian plasmodia characteristically develop in culicine mosquitoes of the genera *Culex* and *Aedes*, and rarely in *Anopheles*. Gametocytes from an avian blood meal are taken up by the mosquito, after which gamete formation, oocysts development and sporogony occur. Infective sporozoites entering the avian host from the bite of a mosquito invade cells of the reticuloendothelial system and typically progress through two generations of primary exoerythrocytic schizonts: cryptozoites and metacryptozoites. Merozoites produced by the second generation are released into the bloodstream and invade erythrocytes. An interchange of parasites between blood and reticuloendothelial tissues may occur, resulting in secondary exoerythrocytic schizonts (phanerozoites) in many tissues, especially spleen, kidney, and liver endothelial cells. These may be responsible for subsequent heavy parasitemias.

The initial stage of the merozoite after invasion of the erythrocyte, the trophozoite, is known as the ring form because of its appearance. A vacuole is formed within the parasite surrounded by a band of blue cytoplasm containing a peripheral red-stained nucleus after Romanowsky staining. A characteristic malarial pigment is formed as the parasite consumes and metabolizes the host cell hemoglobin and this is visible in stained smears. Subsequently, nuclear division leads to formation of a mature schizont containing a variable number of nuclei. Merozoites differentiate from the schizont, and the host cell ruptures to release merozoites for infection of other erythrocytes. After several asexual cycles, some merozoites differentiate into gametocytes and await ingestion by a suitable mosquito. The species of avian plasmodia vary in numbers of merozoites formed in exoerythrocytic and erythrocytic stages, in timing of the life cycle, and in morphology of different stages.

Pathology and Pathogenesis. The pathologic effects in avian hosts range from no apparent signs to severe anemia and death. *P. gallinaceum. P. juxtanucleare*, and *P. durae* are the most pathogenic for domestic fowl and may cause 90% mortality. Intense and severe anemia and generalized hypoxia may occur in acute *P. gallinaceum* malaria (43). A similar situation occurs in ducks affected with *P. lophurae*. Severe anemia may also occur in *P. juxtanucleare* infections.

Other pathologic manifestations occur in avian malaria. The exoerythrocytic stages of *P. gallinaceum* may block capillaries in the brain, resulting in death due to central nervous system dysfunction. *P. durae*, which can cause high mortality in turkeys, causes extensive fibrosis in many tissues.

Immunity. Immunologic factors such as antigen–antibody complex and hemagglutinins, and such conditions as splenomegaly, anemia, and nephritis have been studied extensively in *P. gallinaceum* infections (56, 71).

Treatment and Control. The life cycle of the malaria parasite must be broken by eradication of mosquitoes or by isolation of the flock from the vector by suitable housing. Quarantine and import controls diminish the chances of importing malarious fowl into areas such as the United States, which are free from the pathogenic species. Although avian models have been used extensively in chemotherapeutic studies, there are no commercially available medications for treatment of avian malaria. Steck (74) reviewed the literature on malaria chemotherapy.

HAEMOPROTEUS INFECTIONS. *Haemoproteus* infections are characterized by schizogony (merogony) in visceral endothelial cells, gametocyte development in circulating erythrocytes, and presence of pigment in granules in infected erythrocytes. Transmission is by various biting dipterans of the families Hippoboscidae and Ceratopogonidae. Characteristics of *Haemoproteus* are similar enough to *Plasmodium* and *Leucocytozoon* that the genera are placed in the same family, Plasmodiidae. Infections occur throughout tropical and temperate areas of the New and Old Worlds wherever vector species and avian hosts coexist.

Over 120 species of *Haemoproteus* have been reported from birds, mostly in wild waterfowl, raptors, passerines, and some other families of birds (50). Synonymization of many of these species may result as life cycles are defined and cross-transmission studies are conducted. Many of the species designations for avian haemoproteids were evaluated by Bennett and coworkers (5, 77).

Species sometimes found in domestic poultry and pet birds include *Haemoproteus meleagridis*, which has been diagnosed in domestic and wild turkeys (30); *H. columbae* and *H. saccharovi* in pigeons and doves; and *H. nettionis* in waterfowl (53).

Etiology. *H. columbae* of pigeons and doves is the most extensively studied of these parasites. The process of sporogony occurs in two families of flies in which development time differs. Sporogony is completed in 6-7 days in the ceratopogonids or in 7-14 days in the hippoboscids. Schizonts (meronts) of various sizes and numbers of merozoites occur in the pulmonary vascular endothelium in alveolar septa of pigeons. These merozoites invade erythrocytes and mature into gametocytes (1). Further development requires that erythrocytic forms be ingested by a suitable vector in a blood meal.

Vectors include the hippoboscid *Pseudolynchia canariensis* for *H. columbae* and the ceratopogonid *Culicoides* for *H. nettionis* according to Lund (53). Vectors for *H. meleagridis* include *C. edeni, C. hinmani, C. arboricoli, C. knowltoni*, and *C. haemoproteus* (3).

Atkinson (3) studied experimental infections of *H. meleagridis* in turkeys and partially defined the life cycle. He observed developmental stages of ookinetes, oocysts, sporozoites, and megaloschizonts. At least two generations of schizogony occurred. Maturation of the first generation schizonts occurred 5 and 8 days postinfection (PI) and produced elongate merozoites. Second-generation megaloschizonts developed after 8 and 17 days in cardiac and skeletal muscles and yielded spherical merozoites that developed into erythrocytic gametocytes (Fig. 34.17).

Pathogenesis and Pathology. Apparently, most haemoproteid species are well adapted to their host, since few clinical signs have been reported. Signs include severe lameness, diarrhea, severe depression, emaciation, and anorexia in turkeys experimentally infected with *H. meleagridis* (3). There are occasional reports of anemia and enlarged livers attributed to infections. At necropsy, myopathy associated with megaloschizonts was found in wild turkeys infected with *H. meleagridis*. Skeletal muscles contained numerous fusiform cysts oriented in parallel order with muscle fibers (4), and eight pigeons with *H. saccharovi* had enlarged gizzards. *H. nettionis* caused lameness, dyspnea, and sudden death with hemorrhage on the heart as well

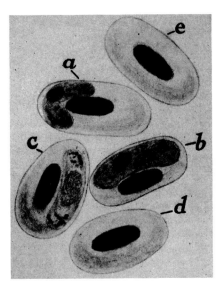

34.17. *Haemoproteus columbae*. Pigeon
blood; (*a,b*) Macrogametocyte in erythrocyte. (*c*) Microgametocyte. (*d,e*)
Normal erythrocyte. (Drake and Jones)

as edematous lungs and swollen firm livers,
spleens, and kidneys in muscovy ducks (*Carina
moschata*); it was nonpathogenic for other species
of ducks (42).

Treatment and Control.   Since life cycles are
incompletely known for most species, specific control measures are difficult to recommend. The control of hippoboscids or ceratopogonids may be of
use in local situations (43). Atebrin and plasmochin
may have marginal effects against *H. columbae*, but
these drugs are not approved for commercial use.

TRYPANOSOMIASIS.   Although trypanosomes have been reported from many species of
wild birds, and some species of domestic birds,
their pathologic significance appears to be minimal
or nil. Even the taxonomic grouping of these organisms is unclear.

Several species have been named, including *Trypanosoma avium*, *T. numidae*, *T. calmetti*, and *T.
gallinarum*. The possibility that the latter three are
synonyms of *T. avium* cannot be ruled out in absence of a rigorous taxonomic study (20).

Observations on *T. avium* and its life cycle were
given by Molyneaux (61), who summarized vector
relationships for all avian trypanosomes and listed
culicine mosquitoes and simuliids as known vectors.

SARCOSPORIDIOSIS.   Sarcosporidiosis is a
parasitic infection caused by apicomplexan protozoa of the genus *Sarcocystis* Lankester 1882. The

disease is recognized by the presence of elongated
cysts (sarcocysts) located in muscles. The nature of
the causative organism was unclear until discovery
that coccidian oocysts appeared when flesh containing sarcocysts was eaten by a suitable final host.
Thus, these parasites are closely related to the
Eimeria and other apicomplexans.

Sarcosporidiosis is not economically important
to the poultry industry, but it occurs extensively in
wild ducks and other birds. Many infected game
birds are discarded annually by hunters for aesthetic
reasons. Sarcosporidiosis does not appear to be a
public health hazard; the parasite is killed by cooking and storage at subfreezing temperatures. Mild
signs were reported, however, by infected human
volunteers given cysts from mammalian sources
(55).

The true biologic nature of *Sarcocystis*, a controversial subject for the past century, and the historic
aspects of sarcosporidiosis were reviewed by
Spindler (72), Levine (48), Long (52), and Melhorn
and Heydorn (57).

Incidence and Distribution.   Avian sarcosporidiosis is found throughout the world in individual birds, but the disease has been reported only
six times in domestic chickens. The incidence is as
high as 40% in ducks and 93% in grackles (22), and
is influenced by species, age, and geographic location of the host. *Sarcocystis* occurs more often in
puddling than diving ducks.

Etiology.   *Sarcocystis horvathi* (*S. gallinarum*,
S. horvathi) is regarded as the etiologic agent for
sarcosporidiosis in chickens (49), and *S. rileyi* (*Bal-
biani rileyi*, *S. anatina*) the cause of sarcosporidiosis in ducks. Based on microscopic differences in
the wall substance of microcysts, however, at least
five different species of *Sarcocystis* are present in
birds (18). Duszynski and Box (19) successfully infected the opossum with tissue cysts from only one
of three species of ducks, suggesting that different
definitive hosts are required to complete the life cycle.

Sarcocystis is classified in the phylum Apicomplexa (49) and the family Sarcocystidae, characterized as having endodyogeny, cysts, or pseudocysts
containing zoites in parenteral cells of the host, and
is a monoxenous parasite of vertebrates (48). The
protozoan classification of *Sarcocystis* is based on
discovery of its coccidial nature with a disporocys-
tid (a tetrazoic isosporan-like oocyst), an obligatory
two-host life cycle, and characteristic ultrastructure
(55, 67). These findings and the lack of evidence of
endodyogeny in its life cycle place the genus *Sarcocystis* within the suborder Eimeriorina.

MORPHOLOGY.   Sarcocysts   (third-generation
meronts) of *S. rileyi*, also called Miescher's tubule,

are elongate, with their long axis parallel to the muscle fibers (Fig. 34.18). They are whitish and smooth walled and appear cylindroid or spindle shaped when removed from the musculature. They are 1.0-6.5 × 0.48-1.0 μm (72). They have double-layered walls, an inner spongy fibrous layer, and an outer dense limiting membrane (48). Sarcocysts are divided into compartments, each of which contains numerous banana-shaped cystozoites (bradyzoites), also called Rainey's corpuscles. Cystozoites are 8-15 μm in length and 2-3 μm in width. Other developmental stages of *S. rileyi* are less well defined. The ultrastructure of *Sarcocystis* was described by Mehlhorn and Heydorn (57).

LIFE CYCLE. Obligatory two-host life cycles have been described from many species of *Sarcocystis* (55). Two vertebrate hosts are required in the life cycle of all these species, usually a carnivorous predator or scavenger and the prey or food animal. Sexual reproduction occurs in the predator (definitive host) and asexual reproduction in the prey (intermediate host). The intermediate host becomes infected by fecal contamination from an infected definitive host.

Studies on transmission of *Sarcocystis* from shoveler ducks (*Anas dypeata*) to the striped skunk

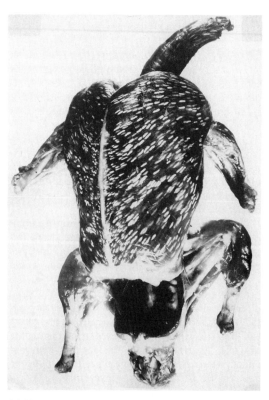

34.18. Severe sarcosporidiosis in wild mallard, naturally occurring infection. (US Dept Interior)

(*Mephitis mephitis*) demonstrated an obligatory two-host life cycle (15, 78). When muscle containing sarcocysts was eaten by skunks, sporocysts (1.4 × 12.4 μm) were shed sporadically from 19 to 63 days PI. Shoveler ducks orally administered sporocysts developed microcysts (80 × 16 μm) in skeletal muscle 85 days later and macrocysts (1-3 × <1 mm) 154 days PI (15). In another study (68), the transmission of *S. falcatula* was demonstrated with the opossum (*Didelphis virginiana*) serving as the definitive host. Although asexual parasites were not found in ducks (*Anas platyrhynchos*) given fecal sporocysts from opossums, the intermediate host spectrum of some avian species of *Sarcocystis* is apparently quite broad (12). Sarcocysts from grackles and cowbirds are also infective to the opossum.

Levine (49) lists the chicken as the intermediate host and the dog as the definitive host for *S. horvathi*. The life cycle for *S. horvathi* is not completely defined.

All species of *Sarcocystis* apparently have similar developmental stages in their life cycle. Sarcocysts in cardiac, smooth, or skeletal muscle tissues are eaten by a definitive host, releasing cystozoites that penetrate the intestinal wall and develop into macrogametocytes and microgametocytes in subepithelial tissues. Oocysts (containing two sporocysts, each with four sporozoites) are produced and are shed in feces as fully sporulated sporocysts. Sporozoites are released when sporocysts are ingested by the intermediate host, and invade the mucosa of the intestine. Schizogony (merogony) occurs in endothelial cells of various organs. After several asexual generations, the merozoites develop into young cyst stages, containing metrocytes and later cystozoites, and mature into the third-generation meronts (sarcocysts) in myocardial, skeletal, and smooth muscle tissues (55, 68).

The life cycles of *Sarcocystis* spp. that infect most species of birds remain incompletely known. More recent findings make earlier postulations of a simple one-host life cycle for any species of *Sarcocystis* less tenable (12, 15).

PATHOGENICITY. The pathogenicity of sarcosporidiosis in most birds is unknown. Box and Duszynski (10) attributed death of 4 of 12 sparrows and morbidity of 3 of 6 canaries to an experimental sarcosporidial infection, but observed no adverse effect from infection in the definitive host (opossum).

Sarcocystin, an endotoxin found in sarcocysts, is toxic for rabbits, mice, and sparrows and may slightly affect other animals. Acting on the central nervous, cardiovascular, and digestive systems, it may cause diarrhea, collapse, and death. There was petechiation of the musculature, anemia, and nephrosis appearing in chickens within 24 hr after subcutaneous (SC) and oral administration of *S. tenella* sarcocysts (70).

Pathogenesis and Epizootiology. Naturally occurring and experimental sarcosporidial infections have been observed in 58 species and 11 orders of birds, including the domestic duck and chicken, but not the turkey (9, 72).

TRANSMISSION, CARRIERS, AND VECTORS. Unsuccessful attempts to transmit *S. rileyi* to young ducks by oral, intramuscular (IM), and intravenous (IV) administration of cystozoites and cohabitation with infected ducks indicate that direct transmission through a one-host cycle does not occur (73).

Sporocyst-contaminated food is the common source of infection for the intermediate host; infection in the carnivorous definitive host results from ingestion of sarcocyst-infected tissues of the intermediate hosts. Cystozoites from sarcocysts in confined migratory ducks were found to be viable at the end of a 3-yr observation period. Thus, intermediate hosts may serve as an available source of infection for prolonged periods over a widespread area. Sarcosporidiosis appears to be most prevalent in hosts that frequently drink from shallow or stagnant water (puddling ducks, cattle, sheep, or swine) (72).

INCUBATION PERIOD. Infections are seldom found in juvenile grackles (22) or in juvenile ducks, which may indicate that the incubation period is long. Cawthorn et al. (15) stated that microcysts and macrocysts were found in ducks 85 and 154 days PI, respectively. Macrocysts were observed in sparrows and canaries 70 days PI (11).

CLINICAL SIGNS. Sarcosporidiosis is usually found in birds that appear normal. Spindler (72) reported that very heavy infections may cause signs of disease, and ducks may fly low and slowly. Adverse signs were not observed in experimentally infected ducks (15); however, Box and Duszynski (10) noted labored breathing and morbidity in canaries and sudden death in sparrows given oocysts.

GROSS LESIONS. Sarcocysts running lengthwise in the musculature of the breast, thigh, neck, or esophagus are the usual lesions associated with avian sarcosporidiosis. Lung consolidation and splenomegaly were observed in infected canaries (10). Lesions have not been seen in definitive hosts with experimental infections.

HISTOPATHOLOGY. Fatty degeneration of muscles, enlargement and rupture of parasitized muscle fibers, and inflammatory responses around sarcocysts in muscles resulting from avian sarcosporidiosis were reported (72).

IMMUNITY. Active and passive immunity have not been demonstrated. Animals have been immunized against sarcocystin by repeated injections of untreated or formalin-treated toxin, and serum from immunized animals gives protection to other animals against the toxin (72).

Diagnosis. Diagnosis is based on identification of sarcocysts or cystozoites in tissues. Large sarcocysts are easily seen in gross specimens; smaller ones and cystozoites can be identified by histologic examination of muscle tissue.

Infections by species of *Sarcocystis* whose life cycles have been defined may be diagnosed in the definitive host by identification of sporocysts in feces and in the intermediate host on the basis of gross lesions or by detecting schizonts in or near endothelial cells of blood vessels in nearly all organs.

SEROLOGY. *Sarcocystis* reacts with cytoplasm-modifying antibody in the Sabin-Feldman dye test but cross-reacts with *Toxoplasma* (72). An indirect fluorescent antibody test in which cystozoites were used as the antigen was successful (75). Munday and Corbould (62) devised a complement-fixation test using an antigen prepared from sarcocysts and found that a titer of 1:10 was indicative of sarcosporidial infections.

Serologic reactions have not been applied in diagnosis of sarcosporidial infections in birds.

Treatment. Chemotherapy of avian sarcosporidiosis has no practical application at this time.

Prevention and Control. The lack of chemotherapeutic or biologic control agents places the burden of control on prevention by breaking the infection cycle. Better knowledge of the parasite life cycles will be necessary for any progress in elimination of these parasites.

TOXOPLASMOSIS. Toxoplasmosis is a parasitic disorder of mammals, birds, and reptiles affecting primarily the central nervous system but sometimes also the reproductive system, skeletal muscles, and visceral organs. The majority of infections are inapparent or latent, with overt toxoplasmosis resulting under favorable ecologic conditions.

Only sporadic outbreaks of toxoplasmosis in chickens have been reported (66). Studies of avian tissues using the mouse inoculation test and histologic examination indicate that a somewhat higher incidence of infection may exist than is apparent. Nevertheless, the disorder is uncommon in chickens and is of little significance to the poultry industry.

Toxoplasmosis is a zoonotic disorder and a human health problem of great concern. Serologic surveys of human populations have shown evidence of infection of 68% in some geographic areas, with an average of 14% throughout the United States (24).

The true nature of *Toxoplasma* as close relatives of *Eimeria* was not known until 1969. The literature presents extensive overviews of history and current knowledge of toxoplasmosis (24, 27, 36, 40, 48).

Etiology. A single species, *Toxoplasma gondii*, is the cause of toxoplasmosis in all hosts. Synonyms for the agent in avian hosts are *T. avium* and *T. paddae*.

T. gondii is a coccidian with sexual stages similar to *Isospora bigemina* (27, 34). Endodyogeny, however, which is not known to occur in *I. bigemina,* is a characteristic of *T. gondii*. Thus current knowledge supports classification close to the coccidian family Eimeriidae. Levine (48) classes *Toxoplasma* in the family Sarcocystidae along with *Sarcocystis*.

Numerous *Toxoplasma* isolates have been designated strains based on varying pathogenicity in different hosts rather than on immunologic variation, although the latter may occur with some strains.

In the free stage, *T. gondii* is crescent shaped (4-6 $\times$ 2-3 µm), with one extremity more rounded than the other and a nucleus near the rounded end. No pseudopods, cilia, or flagella are present. Ultrastructure of developmental stages was reviewed by Levine (48) and Ferguson et al. (25).

LIFE CYCLE. Both schizogonic and gametogenic developmental cycles are known to occur in the intestinal epithelium of some members of the cat family (Felidae). Both an "enteroepithelial" cycle and an "extraintestinal" cycle have been described.

The enteroepithelial cycle occurs only in cats, resulting from infection by encysted organisms (bradyzoites), free or intracellular individual organisms (tachyzoites), or oocysts (23). The prepatent period is 24 days or longer if oocysts are ingested, 5-10 days after ingestion of tachyzoites, and only 3-5 days if bradyzoites are the source of infection. Asexual development may start as early as 12 hr after ingestion, with schizogony occurring in the intestinal epithelium. The number of generations of merozoites that may occur prior to gametogony is undetermined.

The sexual phase of the enteroepithelial cycle occurs also only in intestinal epithelial cells of Felidae. Gametocytes develop throughout the small intestine but more commonly in the ileum. Microgametocytes (7-10 $\times$ 5-8 µm) give rise to 12-32 microgametes (2-5 µm). Following fertilization of the macrogamete (13 µm), oocysts develop and detach unsporulated from the intestinal epithelium. Oocysts are shed for 7-20 days. Sporulation is complete in 1-5 days, depending on environmental temperature and oxygen, and results in develop-

ment of two sporocysts (6-8 $\times$ 5-7 µm), each containing four sporozoites.

The extraintestinal (tissue) cycle apparently constitutes the entire cycle of *T. gondii* in birds and other nonfelines. After oral infection, rapidly multiplying *T. gondii* forms (tachyzoites) reproducing by endodyogeny develop within vacuoles of many cell types. Tachyzoites in the free form spread from cell to cell and may be found in brain, eye, heart, liver, lungs, and nucleated red blood cells of birds. About eight or more organisms tend to accumulate in a host cell, forming pseudocysts (terminal colonies, aggregated), before it disintegrates.

Tachyzoites usually develop into bradyzoites (cells resting or slowly reproducing by endodyogeny with cysts) as chronic toxoplasmosis ensues. Encysted bradyzoites begin to develop intracellularly in the brain, heart, eyes, and skeletal muscles within 1-2 wk as immunity develops. Cysts may persist for the life of the host or, if immunity wanes, bradyzoites may be released and a proliferation of tachyzoites renewed. The tissue cycle may reverse again and cysts form from tachyzoites (27, 37, 40).

Pathogenesis and Epizootiology. Infective oocyts of *T. gondii* are produced only by members of the Felidae (domestic cats, ocelots, pumas, jaguarundi, bobcats, Asian leopards) (40). More than 63 species of birds and 27 species of animals become infected from ingestion of oocysts and develop cysts in tissues without passing oocysts in the feces (66). Naturally occurring infections have been diagnosed in the chickens, turkeys, ducks, and many wild birds (13, 53). Ruiz and Frenkel (64) isolated *T. gondii* from 54% of chickens and 16% of sparrows examined in Costa Rica. *T. gondii* has been reisolated from Japanese quail, bluejays, crows, and chickens after experimental infections (59).

TRANSMISSION, CARRIERS, AND VECTORS. The known modes of transmission of *Toxoplasma* to birds are carnivorism and fecal contamination. Tachyzoites and bradyzoites may be spread by carnivorous ingestion, and sporulated oocysts are spread by cat feces.

The question of congenital infection occurring in chicks from naturally infected parents remains unresolved. Jacobs and Melton (38) found that 12 of 62 pools of reproductive tract tissues from chickens were infected with *T. gondii*, but the parasite could not be isolated from any of 108 eggs from these hens. In another study, 1 of 327 eggs from hens with chronic toxoplasmosis was positive. Iannuzzi and Renieri (35) concluded that toxoplasmas did not survive in unembryonated eggs and was not a factor in transmission. Caballero-Servin (14) reported successful transovarian transmission of the parasite by experimentally infecting hens, which resulted in embryonic mortality and congenital malformation of 18% of the surviving chicks.

Coprophagous arthropods such as flies and cockroaches can serve as transport hosts for the parasite (76). Earthworms ingest toxoplasma oocysts and are a source of infection for chickens (64).

COURSE OF THE DISEASE. The chicken is quite resistant to *T. gondii*, but disease has been observed from both naturally occurring and experimental infections. Variations in the clinical syndrome are attributed to age of host, strain of infective agent, and methods of infection. Clinical signs become apparent in chicks when they are inoculated by the intracerebral (IC) route before 3 wk of age (8) and in chicks inoculated by the intraperitoneal (IP) route before 1 day of age (44). Parasitemia and chronic toxoplasma infections occur in older birds via IV, IP, IM, and SC inoculations.

Clinical signs in chickens include anorexia, emaciation, paleness and shrinking of the comb, drop in egg production, whitish feces, diarrhea, incoordination, ataxia, trembling, opisthotonos, torticollis, and blindness. Clinical signs are apparent 3-12 days after IC inoculation, and all chicks die within 24 hr after onset of clinical signs (7, 8, 44, 53). A rapidly developing outbreak in which most of a flock of chickens were affected and total mortality reached 50% was reported (53). Death occurred in two-thirds of the chicks fed toxoplasma oocysts from cats. Siim et al. (66) noted that infections in turkeys and ducks were mild and suggested that many may be undetected.

GROSS LESIONS. Gross lesions include enlargement of liver and spleen, necrotic hepatitis, pericarditis, myocarditis, ulcerative enteritis, lung congestion, and encephalitis (8, 53).

HISTOPATHOLOGY. In chickens inoculated by IC and IM routes, encysted toxoplasmas were found in the cerebrum, brain stem, optic chiasma, and most frequently, around ventricles and in molecular and Purkinje layers of the cerebellum. Free toxoplasmas were seldom found, and then only in the brain. Toxoplasma cysts were found in the myocardium, pancreas, and testes of chickens infected intramuscularly (8).

Coagulation necrosis and diffuse sinusoidal congestion were observed in the liver. The myocardium, pancreas, and testes were diffusely infiltrated with lymphocytes, plasma cells, and heterophils. In the brain, infection caused lymphocytic lesions and plasma cell-cuffing of blood vessels; lymphocytic infiltration of choroid villi; ependymal proliferation of the lateral ventricle; thickening of leptomeninges; and gliosis of the lateral ventricle and around vessels of the cerebrum, brain stem, and cerebellum.

Diagnosis. *T. gondii* may be isolated and identified by injecting suspensions of infected tissues into various species of laboratory animals, chicken embryos, or cell cultures. Intraperitoneal or IC inoculation of mice with suspensions of brain, liver, lung, or spleen are preferred methods of isolation (28). Mice inoculated with virulent strains die within a few days. When less virulent isolates are suspected, brains should be examined for cyst forms 8-10 wk after mouse inoculation. The isolated organisms should be identified serologically.

Impression smears of peritoneal fluids or tissues stained with Giemsa, or tissue sections of brain, liver, spleen, lung, lymph nodes, and eye often suffice for direct microscopic observation of toxoplasmas.

Toxoplasmas can be grown in the chorioallantoic cavity of 6- to 12-day-old embryonated chicken eggs. Embryos succumb 7-10 days PI with hemorrhage and nodular lesions in skin and viscera. Numerous yellow-white plaques 0.5-3.0 mm in diameter develop on the chorioallantoic and amniotic membranes. Smears of the chorioallantoic membrane and yolk sac stained with Wright's stain reveal numerous free and intracellular toxoplasmas.

SEROLOGY. Present serologic tests for *T. gondii* are not adequate for detecting the presence of the carrier state in most birds. Chickens, Japanese quail, bluejays, and crows did not develop appreciable levels of antibody detectable by the dye test, although *T. gondii* could be isolated from all birds and up to 14 mo PI in chickens (59, 64, 76). With the dye test, low antibody titers (1:16 or less) were measurable in only 3 of 34 infected chickens (44); doves and pigeons, however, develop high antibody levels.

Treatment, Prevention, and Control. Neither prophylactic nor therapeutic chemotherapy has been used to control avian toxoplasmosis.

Prevention of avian toxoplasmosis requires management practices that eliminate the source of infective tachyzoites and oocysts by preventing exposure to rodents, coprophagous arthropods, and cats. Oocysts disseminated throughout the premises are resistant to common laboratory detergents, acids, and alkalis and are, therefore, difficult to destroy. However, they may be destroyed by ammonia, drying, and a temperature of 55 C (48).

REFERENCES
1. Ahmed, F.E., and A.H.H. Mohammed. 1978. Studies of growth and development of gametocytes in Haemoproteus columbae Kruse. J Protozool 25:174–177.
2. Allan, R.A., and J.L. Mahrt. 1987. Populations of Leucocytozoon gametocytes in blue grouse (Dendragapus obscurus) from Hardwicke Island, British Columbia. J Protozool 34:363–366.
3. Atkinson, C.T. 1985. Epizootiology and pathogenicity

of Haemoproteus meleagridis Levine 1961 from Florida turkeys. PhD Dissertation, University of Florida.

4. Atkinson, C.T., and D.J. Forrester. 1987. Myopathy associated with megaloschizonts of Haemoproteus meleagridis in a wild turkey from Florida. J Wildl Dis 23:495–498.

5. Bennett, G.F., and M. Cameron. 1974. Seasonal prevalance of avian hematozoa in passerine birds of Atlantic Canada. Can J Zool 52:1259–1284.

6. Bennett, G.F., and M. Laird. 1973. Collaborative investigation into avian malaria: An international research programme. J Wildl Dis 9:26–28.

7. Biancifiori, F., C. Rondini, V. Grelloni, and T. Frescura. 1986. Avian toxoplasmosis: Experimental infection of chicken and pigeon. Comp Immunol Microbiol Infect Dis 9:337–346.

8. Bickford, A.A., and J.R. Saunders. 1966. Experimental toxoplasmosis in chickens. Am J Vet Res 116:308–318.

9. Borst, G.H., and P. Zwort. 1973. Sarcosporidiosis in Psittaciformes. Z Parasitenkd 42:293–298.

10. Box, E.D., and D. W. Duszynski. 1978. Experimental transmission of Sarcocystis from icterid birds to sparrows and canaries by sporocysts from the opossum. J Parasitol 64:682–688.

11. Box, E.D., and D. W. Duszynski. 1980. Sarcocystis of passerine birds: Sexual stages in the opossum (Didelphis virginiana). J Wildl Dis 16:209–215.

12. Box, E.D., and J.H. Smith. 1982. The intermediate host spectrum in a sarcocystis species of birds. J Parasitol 68:668–673.

13. Burridge, M.J., W.J. Bigler, D.J. Forrester, and J.M. Henneman. 1979. Serologic survey for Toxoplasma gondii in wild animals in Florida. J Am Vet Med Assoc 175:964–967.

14. Caballero-Servin, A. 1974. Congenital malformations in Gallus gallus induced by Toxoplasma gondii. Rev Invest Salud Publica (Mexico) 34:87–94.

15. Cawthorn, R.J., D. Rainnie, and G. Wobeser. 1981. Experimental transmission of Sarcocystis sp. (protozoa: Sarcocystidae) between the Shoveler (Anas clypeata) duck and the striped skunk (Mephitis mephitis). J Wildl Dis 17:389–394.

16. Desser, S.S., J. Stuht, and A.M. Fallis. 1978. Leucocytozoonosis in Canada geese in upper Michigan. 1. Strain differences among geese from different localities. J Wildl Dis 14:124–131.

17. Dick, J. 1978. Leucocytozoon smithi: Persistence of gametocytes in peripheral turkey blood. Avian Dis 22:82–85.

18. Drouin, T.E., and J.L. Mahrt. 1980. The morphology of cysts of Sarcocystis infecting birds in western Canada. Can J Zool 58:1477–1482.

19. Duszynski, D.W., and E.D. Box. 1978. The opossum (Didelphis virginiana) as a host for Sarcocystis debonei from cowbirds (Molothrus ater) and grackles (Cassidiz mexicanus, Quiscalus quiscula). J Parasitol 64:326–329.

20. Fallis, A.M., R.L. Jacobson, and J.N. Raybould. 1973. Haematozoa in domestic chickens and guinea fowl in Tanzania and transmission of Leucocytozoon neavet and Leucocytozoon schouedeni. J Protozool 20:436–437.

21. Fallis, A.M., S.S. Desser, and R.A. Khan. 1974. On species of Leucocytozoon. Adv Parasitol 12:1–67.

22. Fayer, R., and R.M. Kocan. 1971. Prevalence of Sarcocystis in grackles in Maryland. J Protozool 18:547–548.

23. Fayer, R., A.J. Johnson, and P.K. Hildebrandt. 1976. Oral infection of mammals with Sarcocystis fusiformis bradyzoites from cattle and sporocysts from dogs and coyotes. J Parasitol 62:10–14.

24. Feldman, H.A. 1974. Toxoplasmosis: An overview. Bull N Y Acad Med 50:110–127.

25. Ferguson, D.S., W.M. Hutchinson, J.F. Dunachie, and J.C. Siim. 1974. Ultrastructural study of early stages of asexual multiplication and microgametogony of Toxoplasma gondii in the small intestine of the cat. Acta Pathol Microbiol Scand 82:167–181.

26. Forrester, D.J., J.K. Nayar, and M.D. Young. 1987. Natural infection of Plasmodium hermani in the Northern Bobwhite, Colinus virginianus, in Florida. J Parasitol 73:865–866.

27. Frenkel, J.K. 1973. Toxoplasmosis: Parasite life cycle, pathology and immunology. In D.M. Hammond, and P.L. Long (eds.). The Coccidia. Eimeria, Isopora, Toxoplasma, and Related Genera. University Park Press, Baltimore, MD, pp. 343–410.

28. Frenkel, J.K. 1981. False-negative serologic tests for Toxoplasma in birds. J Parasitol 67:952–953.

29. Garnham, P.C.C. 1966. Malaria Parasites and Other Haemosporidia. Blackwell, Oxford, England.

30. Greiner, E.C., and D.J. Forrester. 1980. Haemoproteus meleagridis Levine 1961: Redescription and developmental morphology of the gametocytes in turkeys. J Parasitol 66:652–688.

31. Greiner, E.D., G.F. Bennett, M. Laird, and C.M. Herman. 1975. Avian Hematozoa. I. A color pictorial guide to some species of Haemoproteus, Leucocytozoon, and Trypanosoma. Wildl Dis 68 (WD75-3). [Color fiche].

32. Herman C.M., J.H. Barrows, Jr., and I.B. Tarshis. 1975. Leucocytozoonosis in Canada geese at the Seney National Wildlife Refuge. J Wildl Dis 11:404–411.

33. Hsu, C.-K., G.R. Campbell, and N.D. Levine. 1973. A checklist of the species of the genus Leucocytozoon. J Protozool 20:195–203.

34. Hutchinson, W.M., J.F. Dunachie, K. Work, and J.C. Siim. 1971. The life cycle of the coccidian parasite, Toxoplasma gondii, in the domestic cat. Trans R Soc Trop Med Hyg 65:380–399.

35. Iannuzzi, L., and G. Renieri. 1971. The egg in the epidemiology of Toxoplasmosis. Tests of experimental infections by injection through the shell. Acta Med Vet 17:311–317.

36. Jacobs, L. 1973. New knowledge of Toxoplasma and toxoplasmosis. Adv Parasitol 11:631–669.

37. Jacobs, L. 1973. Toxoplasma gondii: Parasitology and transmission. Bull N Y Acad Med 50:128–145.

38. Jacobs, l., and M.L. Melton. 1966. Toxoplasmosis in chickens. J Parasitol 52:1158–1162.

39. Johnson, E.P., G.W. Underhill, J.A. Cox, and W.L. Threlkeld. 1968. A blood protozoon of turkeys transmitted by Simulium nigroparvum (Twinn). Am J Hyg 27:649–665.

40. Jones, S.R. 1973. Toxoplasmosis: A review. J Am Vet Med Assoc 163:1038–1042.

41. Jones, J.E., B.D. Barnett, and J. Solis. 1972. The effect of Leucocytozoon smithi infection on production, fertility, and hatchability of Broad Breasted White turkey hens. Poult Sci 51:543–545.

42. Julian, R.J., and D.E. Galt. 1980. Mortality in Muscovy ducks (Cairina moschata) caused by Haemoproteus infection. J Wildl Dis 16:39–44.

43. Kemp, R.L. 1978. Haemoproteus. In M.S. Hofstad, B.W. Calnek, C.F. Helmbodt, W.M. Reid, and H.W. Yoder, Jr. (eds.), Diseases of Poultry, 7th ed. Iowa State University Press, Ames, IA, pp. 824–825.

44. Kinjo, T. 1972. Experimental toxoplasmosis in fowls. III. Reactions of chicks at 30–40 days old and one day old. IV. Susceptibility of chick embryos. Sci Bull Coll Agric (Okinawa) 19:407–420.

45. Kissam, J.B., R. Noblet, and G.I. Garris. 1975. Large scale aerial treatment of an endemic area with abate granular larvicide to control black flies (Diptera simuliidae) and suppress Leucocytozoon smithi of turkeys. J Med Entomol 12:359–362.

46. Kiszewski, A.E., and E.W. Cupp. 1986. Transmission of Leucocytozoon smithi (Sporozoa: Leucocytozoidae) by black flies (Diptera simulidae) in New York, USA. J Med Entomol 23:256–262.

47. Kocan, R.M. 1968. Anemia and mechanism of erythrocyte destruction in ducks with acute Leucocytozoon infections. J Protozool 15:455–462.

48. Levine, N.D. 1973. Protozoan Parasites of Domestic

Animals and of Man, 2nd ed. Burgess, Minneapolis, MN.

49. Levine, N.D. 1986. The taxonomy of Sarcocystis (Protozoa: Apicomplexa) species. J Parasitol 72:372–382.

50. Levine, N.D., and G.R. Campbell. 1971. A checklist of the species of the genus Haemoproteus (Apicomplexa, Plasmodiidae). J Protozool 18:475–484.

51. Levine, N.D., J.O. Corliss, F.E.G. Cox, G. Deroux, J. Grain, B.M. Honigberg, G.F. Leedale, A.R. Loeblich III, J. Lom, D. Lynn, E.G. Merinfeld, F.C. Page, G. Poljansky, V. Sprague, J. Vavra, and F.G. Wallace. 1980. A newly revised classification of the protozoa. J Parasitol 27:37–58.

52. Long, P.L. 1982. The Biology of the Coccidia. Univ Park Press, Baltimore, MD.

53. Lund, E.E. 1972. Other protozoan diseases. In M.S. Hofstad, B.W. Calnek, C.F. Helmboldt, W.M. Reid, and H.W. Yoder, Jr. (eds.). Diseases of Poultry, 6th ed. Iowa State University Press, Ames, IA, pp. 990–1046.

54. Maley, G.J.M., and S.S. Desser. 1977. Anemia in Leucocytozoon simondi infections. I. Quantification of anemia, gametocytemia, and osmotic fragility of erythrocytes in naturally infected Pekin ducklings. Can J Zool 55:255–258.

55. Markus, M.B., R. Killick-Kendrick, and P.C.C. Garnham. 1974. The coccidial nature and life-cycle of Sarcocystis. J Trop Med Hyg 77:248–259.

56. McGhee, R. B. 1970. Avian Malaria. In D.J. Jackson, R. Herman, and I. Singer (eds.). Immunity to Parasitic Animals, vol. 2. Appleton-Century-Crofts, New York, pp. 295–329.

57. Melhorn, H., and A.O. Heydorn. 1978. The Sarcosporidia (Protozoa, Sporozoa): Life cycle and fine structure. Adv Parasitol 16:43–91.

58. Milhous, W., and J. Solis. 1973. Turkey leucocytozoon infection. 3. Ultrastructure of Leucocytozoon smithi: Gametocytes. Poult Sci 52:2138–2146.

59. Miller, N.L., J.K. Frenkel, and J.P. Dubey. 1972. Oral infections with Toxoplasma cysts and oocysts in felines, other mammals, and in birds. J Parasitol 58:928–937.

60. Miura, S., K. Ohshima, C. Itakura, and S. Yamogiwa. 1973. A histopathological study on Leucocytozoonosis in young hens. Japan J Vet Sci 35:175–181.

61. Molyneux, D.H. 1977. Vector relationships in the trypanosomatidae. Adv Parasitol 15:1–82.

62. Munday, B.L., and A. Corbould. 1974. The possible role of the dog in the epidemiology of ovine sarcosporidiosis. Br Vet J 130:9–11.

63. Noblet, R., H.S. Moore IV, and G.P. Noblet. 1976. Survey of Leucocytozoon in South Carolina. Poult Sci 55:447–449.

64. Ruiz, A., and J.K. Frenkel. 1980. Intermediate and transport hosts of Toxoplasma gondii in Costa Rica. Am J Trop Med Hyg 29:1161–1166.

65. Siccardi, F.J., H.O. Rutherford, and W.T. Derieux. 1974. Pathology and prevention of Leucocytozoon smithi infection in turkeys. Avian Dis. 18:21–32.

66. Siim, J.C., U. Biering-Sorenson, and T. Moller. 1963. Toxoplasmosis in domestic animals. Adv Vet Sci 8:335–429.

67. Simpson, C.R., and D.J. Forrester. 1973. Electron microscopy of Sarcosystis sp: Cyst wall, micropore, rhoptries, and an unidentified body. Int J Parasitol 3:467–470.

68. Smith, J.H., J.L. Meier, P.J.G. Neill, and E.D. Box. 1987. Pathogenesis of Sarcocystis falcatula in the Budgerigar. II. Pulmonary pathology. Lab Invest 56:72–84.

69. Solis, J. 1973. Nonsusceptibility of some avian species to turkey Leucocytozoon infection. Poult Sci 52:498–500.

70. Sominski, Z.F., D.I. Panasiuk, and R. P. Vilkova. 1971. Pathological-morphological changes during experimental sarcocystis in chickens. Veterinariia 6:68–69.

71. Soni, J.L., and H.W. Cox. 1975. Pathogenesis of acute avian malaria. II. Anemia mediated by a cold-active autohemagglutinin from the blood of chickens with acute Plasmodium gallinaceum infection. Am J Trop Med Hyg 24:206–213.

72. Spindler, L.A. 1972. Sarcosporidiosis. In M.S. Hofstad, B.W. Calnek, C.F. Helmboldt, W.M. Reid, and H.W. Yoder, Jr. (eds.). Diseases of Poultry, 6th ed. Iowa State University Press, Ames, IA, pp. 1046–1054.

73. Springer, W. T. 1984. Other blood and tissue protozoa. In M.S. Hofstad, H. John Barnes, B.W. Calnek, W.M. Reid, and H.W. Yoder, Jr. (eds.). Diseases of Poultry, 8th ed. Iowa State University Press, Ames, IA, pp. 727–740.

74. Steck, E.A. 1971. Chemotherapy of Protozoan Disease, vol. 3. Walter Reed Arm Res Inst (Unnumbered monogr), Sect. 4A, pp. 1–376.

75. Wallace, G.D. 1973. Sarcocystis in mice inoculated with Toxoplasma-like oocysts from cat feces. Science 180:1375–1377.

76. Wallace G.D. 1973. Intermediate and transport hosts in the natural history of Toxoplasma gondii. Am J Trop Med Hyg 22:456–464.

77. White, E.M., and G.F. Bennett. 1979. Avian Haemoproteidae, 12. The hemoproteids of the grouse family Tetraonidae. Can J Zool 57:1465–1472.

78. Wicht, R.J. 1981. Transmission of Sarcocystis rileyi to the striped skunk (Mephitis mephitisy). J Wildl Dis 17:387–388.

35 Developmental, Metabolic, and Other Noninfectious Disorders

C. Riddell

INTRODUCTION. The diseases and conditions discussed in this chapter represent a heterogeneous group; in some cases, the etiology is quite clear, whereas in others it is questionable or unknown. They vary in economic importance and frequency of occurrence. Emphasis has been placed on metabolic diseases of economic importance to the modern poultry industry. Diseases have been classified by body system primarily affected except for the conditions that are discussed under cannibalism or environmental disease.

CANNIBALISM. Many forms of cannibalism occur in domestic fowl and game birds reared in captivity. Weaver and Bird (323) indicated that light breeds of the Mediterranean class are much more prone to these vices than are heavier breeds of the American and Asiatic classes.

Vent Picking. Picking of the vent or region of the abdomen several inches below the vent is the most severe form of cannibalism. This is generally seen in pullet flocks in high production. Predisposing factors are prolapse or tearing of the tissues by passage of an abnormally large egg. Picking of the vent can cause high mortality in turkeys as young as 1 wk of age. Dead poults are anemic and there is generally blood on the tail feathers around the injured vent and on the back of the legs.

Feather Pulling. Feather pulling is most frequently seen in flocks kept in close confinement resulting in lack of sufficient exercise. Nutritional and mineral deficiencies may be contributing factors. Feather picking causes "blueback" in bronze turkeys. Injury to the feather quills allows pigment to escape and tattoo the surrounding area.

Toe Picking. Toe picking is most commonly seen in domestic chicks or young game birds and is often initiated by hunger. Chicks may not find feed because hoppers are too high or too far from the heat source. Feeder space may be inadequate, and the smaller or more timid chicks may be kept from eating by aggressive birds. If the chick cannot find feed, it may pick at its own or a neighbor's toes. It is good practice to put feed on chick box covers or trays and place them under the hover the first few days of brooding.

Head Picking. Head picking usually follows injuries to the comb or wattles caused by freezing or fighting among males. A different form of cannibalism is now being observed in beak-trimmed birds kept in cages. The area about the eyes is black and blue due to subcutaneous hemorrhage, wattles are dark and swollen with extravasated blood, and earlobes are black and necrotic. Even though birds have trimmed beaks and are kept in separate cages, they will reach through the wire and peck at a neighbor or grasp its ear lobes or wattles and shake their heads in much the same fashion as a terrier shaking a rat.

Nose Picking in Quail. Bass (9) reported an unusual form of cannibalism in quail. It is termed "nose picking" since the birds peck at the top of the nose where the fleshy portion merges with the beak. The condition is generally seen in birds 2–7 wk of age kept under crowded conditions. The bird may die as the result of blood loss. If the bird survives, the beak will be permanently deformed and males will be unsatisfactory for breeding stock. This vice occurs only when birds are brooded under artificial conditions. It seldom develops in large pens on the ground in which there is opportunity to pick and scratch. Bass also observed that addition of raw meat to the ration was very effective in preventing and controlling outbreaks.

Etiology. Many causes of cannibalism have been suggested, but often outbreaks of cannibalism occur in one pen, while similar environmental conditions or feeding practices in other pens on the same farm do not cause difficulty. Conditions re-

Grateful acknowledgment is made to Dr. M.C. Peckham, previous author of this chapter, for much of the material on cannibalism and environmental disease, reviews of several conditions, and many of the figures.

ported as predisposing to cannibalism are feeding only pellets or compressed feed, cafeteria system of feeding, excess corn in the ration, insufficient feeder or drinker space, being without feed too long, insufficient nests, nests too light, excessively light pens, high-density rearing systems, too much heat, nutritional and mineral deficiencies, and irritation from external parasites (130, 232). After birds have started picking they will continue their cannibalistic habits without provocation.

Prevention. Cannibalism can best be prevented by providing adequate feed and water space and not permitting birds to go without feed for extended periods. Overcrowding should be avoided; in cages where high-density rearing is practiced, it may be necessary to trim beaks before housing. Careful attention to ventilation and light intensity may preclude an outbreak of cannibalism. In many large-scale commercial operations, beak trimming is necessary to prevent cannibalism. Peckham (243) reviewed old remedies for controlling cannibalism and methods of beak trimming.

ENVIRONMENTAL DISEASE

Heat Prostration. Birds in production are particularly susceptible to high temperatures accompanied by high humidity. Lacking sweat glands, birds' only method of cooling is rapid respiration with mouths open and wings relaxed and hanging loosely at their sides. If body temperatures rise, birds become weak and die due to respiratory, circulatory, or electrolyte imbalances. An attempt to cool the birds can be made by dipping in water or spraying. Every effort should be made to increase circulation of air by running ventilation equipment at full capacity. Cooling the air can be accomplished by using a hose to wet down the floor, walls, ceiling, and outside roof. Adequate drinking water should be available. Preventive measures consist of installation of fans, proper construction of ventilating ducts, insulation of the building, and use of white or aluminum paint on the outside to reflect heat. In southern climates where low production and mortality from heat are constant problems, installation of foggers and sprinklers or evaporative coolers is essential.

Smothering. Smothering is generally caused by birds crowding or piling in a corner. It may occur when birds are moved to new quarters, when they are frightened, or in young birds when they are chilled. The history of the case often indicates that mortality occurs only at night and the flock in general looks healthy. Smothering of baby chicks can occur in chick boxes that are piled too high without an air space between each box, in boxes that do not

have sufficient ventilation holes, or in boxes placed in a closed compartment such as the trunk of a car. Necropsy of chicks that have smothered usually does not reveal enough gross pathology to make a positive diagnosis, but a thorough examination will eliminate other possible causes of death. In broilers and older birds that have smothered, there is congestion of the trachea and lungs, and feathers will be worn off where birds have been trampled. Smothering of chicks in the brooder house can be controlled by putting a circle of corrugated cardboard around the hover for the 1st wk and gradually widening the diameter as chicks get older. This will prevent piling in a corner during the night. When birds are moved to new quarters, the use of a dim light or lantern the first few nights will decrease the possibility of smothering. Birds transferred to new quarters should be checked late in the evening for signs of piling. Frequent observation of the flock is very important the first few days after acquiring a group of new chicks or grown birds.

Dehydration. Dehydration is generally caused by failure of birds to find water, inability to reach the water, or in some cases by a deterring factor in the water. Chicks can survive several days without water but will die beginning on the 4th or 5th day. Mortality will reach its peak during the 5th or 6th day and terminate abruptly if water is provided. Chicks that are not drinking will have succumbed by this period, and survivors are those that have found the water and are drinking. Dehydration can be detected by the chick's inability to "peep" during the later stages, insufficient weight for size and age, and dehydrated and wrinkled skin on the shanks. Other changes are blue discoloration of the beak, dry and dark breast musculature, dark kidneys, accumulation of urates in the ureters, and darkening of the blood. Signs and lesions in older birds are similar to those in chicks, and weight loss is much more noticeable. To prevent dehydration in chicks, water fountains should be placed at the edge of the hover directly on the litter without any platform. When a small drinker is replaced by a large type or automatic drinkers, the old type should be kept for a few days and gradually moved toward the new source of water supply to accustom birds to the change. An electrical charge in the water may be caused by faulty electrical heating devices used to prevent freezing, and birds will not drink.

DISEASES OF THE SKELETON

Crooked Neck. Moorhead and Mohamed (213) reported a crooked-neck syndrome in a flock of 18-wk-old turkeys, with approximately 10% of 8000 birds affected. The principal lesion was an osteodystrophy of the cervical vertebrae. The clinical signs were similar to those of a crooked-neck syndrome attributed to a single recessive gene in brown leghorns. It appears unlikely that the syndrome in turkeys was a genetic defect. The syndrome was common in many turkey flocks in North America circa 1970 and was associated with airsacculitis due to *Mycoplasma meleagridis*. The incidence was reduced by dipping of turkey hatching eggs in tylosin tartrate to control *M. meleagridis* infection (258).

Spondylolisthesis.   Spondylolisthesis is a deformity of the sixth thoracic vertebra causing spinal cord compression and posterior paralysis in broiler chickens. It is commonly called "Kinky Back." Wise (343) and Riddell (262) have written reviews on the condition. A few birds affected with spondylolisthesis are found in most broiler flocks. In some flocks, the incidence of affected birds has reached 2%. The peak incidence occurs at 3–6 wk of age. Affected birds are alert, remain sitting on their hocks with their feet slightly raised off the ground (Fig. 35.1), and use their wings in an attempt to escape when approached. Severely affected birds often become laterally recumbent. Affected birds often die from dehydration if not culled. The posterior paralysis results from rotation of the body of the 6th vertebra along the axis of the spine, with the posterior part of the body moving dorsal and anterior relative to the anterior part. This rotation causes a kyphotic angulation of the floor of the spinal canal between the 6th and 7th thoracic vertebrae, and spinal cord compression (Fig. 35.2). The deformation of the spinal column can be readily recognized by palpating the ventral surface of the spinal column during necropsy. Another form of spondylolisthesis is characterized by steplike defects separating

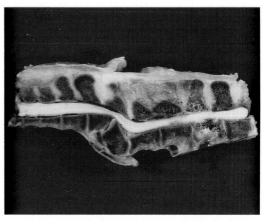

35.2. Midline longitudinal section through thoracic-lumbar region of the spinal column of a broiler chicken with spondylolisthesis, cervical end to right. Rotation of the body of vertebra T6, deformation of T7, and spinal cord compression. (Avian Dis)

the bodies of the 5th, 6th, and 7th thoracic vertebrae. Each vertebral body is displaced ventrally relative to the vertebral body in front, resulting in damage to the spinal cord (72). A diagnosis of spondylolisthesis is best confirmed by removing, decalcifying, and splitting the spinal column along a midline longitudinal plane to allow visualization of the spinal cord compression.

Lordosis and subclinical spondylolisthesis are common in broiler chickens. The lordosis develops after hatching. It can be decreased by slowing the growth rate of the broiler chicken. The incidence of spondylolisthesis can be increased by genetic selection. It is postulated that spondylolisthesis is a development disorder influenced by conformation and growth rate.

Other Abnormalities of the Spine.   Several other spinal deformities occur sporadically at a low incidence in commercial poultry. These deformities include scoliosis and rumplessness and have been reviewed by Riddell (258).

Valgus and Varus Deformation of the Intertarsal Joint.   Deformation of the long bones of the broiler chicken and turkey is a significant cause of economic loss due to culling and death of affected birds. Such deformation includes many different types of twisting or bending of the bones and has been described by terms such as *long bone distortion*, *twisted legs*, or *crooked legs*. The general topic of deformation of the long bones in domestic poultry was reviewed by Riddell (262, 267) and Thorp (307, 308). The most common type of long bone deformation in the broiler chicken is valgus or varus deformation (VVD) of the intertarsal joint

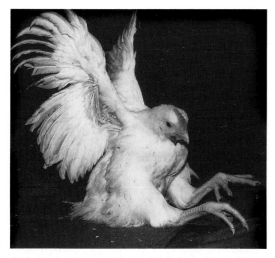

35.1. Broiler chicken with spondylolisthesis. (Avian Dis)

(147, 251, 273). In the turkey, similar deformation of the intertarsal joint is also common but is often associated with varus deformation of the femoral-tibial joint (261). In broiler chickens, the incidence of birds affected with VVD varies from 0.5 to 2.0% in normal broiler flocks, but occasionally affects 5–25% of male broilers in problem flocks (147).

CLINICAL SIGNS AND PATHOLOGY. Broilers may be affected with VVD before 1 wk of age and the incidence increases with birds becoming affected throughout the life of a flock (273). Approximately 70% of affected birds are males (273). The defect may affect both legs but is often unilateral, with the right leg more commonly affected than the left leg (78, 273). Most birds have either valgus or varus deformation, but the occasional bird will have valgus deformation of one leg and varus deformation of the other leg. These birds have been described as "windswept" (65). The major deformity is outward or inward angulation of the distal tibia, with similar but less severe angulation in the proximal metatarsus (Figs. 35.3, 35.4). In some birds, there is an associated outward or internal rotation of the distal tibia. Abnormal rotation of the femur may also be present (78). The degree of angulation varies from mild to very severe. As the severity of the angulation increases, the gastrocnemius tendon becomes displaced and the distal tibial condyles become flattened. In some cases, the angulation progresses to displacement and separation of the tarsal bones from the shaft of the tibia. With severe angulation, birds are forced to walk on the posterior surface of the hock, which becomes bruised and swollen. In some instances, the distal shaft of the tibia will penetrate the skin. Detailed descriptions of the defor-

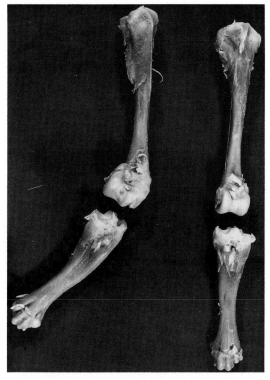

35.4. Tibiotarsal and tarsometatarsal bones from a broiler chicken with unilateral valgus deformation. (Avian Dis)

mity are provided by Randall and Mills (251), Julian (147), and Riddell (263).

PATHOGENESIS AND ETIOLOGY. The pathogenesis of the deformation has not been defined. Similar gross deformation has been reproduced experimentally with several nutritional deficiencies in which there was a generalized disorder of the growth plates of the long bones (262). The classic example of such a deficiency is manganese deficiency, and the syndrome produced was called perosis. Wise (343) proposed the term *chondrodystrophy* to replace *perosis* and this terminology is now widely accepted. No evidence of the microscopic growth plate lesions found in chondrodystrophy has been recognized in VVD (251, 270). The possibility that submicroscopic lesions of the growth plate due to marginal nutritional deficiencies may result in VVD should not be ignored. In the rapidly growing modern broiler chicken, the vascular morphology of the growth plate is irregular, and this may predispose the chicken to VVD (306). Some workers (47, 133, 134) have noted a delay in cortical bone differentiation, which precedes the angulation. Young normal broiler chickens have slight valgus deformation. The angulation is greater in the right leg (77). This

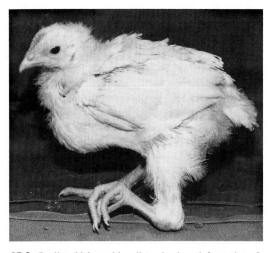

35.3. Broiler chicken with unilateral valgus deformation of the intertarsal joint. (Avian Dis)

small inclination of the growth plate in a rapidly growing chicken may promote deviant growth (251, 274). It has recently been suggested that valgus and varus deformities may each have a different etiologic pathogenesis (179). An association between VVD and dyschondroplasia has been noted (246, 251, 263). Although dyschondroplasia may weaken bones and predispose to deformation, it may be secondary to the deformation (345). In a breeding study, it was observed that VVD was unrelated to dyschondroplasia (259).

The incidence of VVD is influenced by genotype (47) and can be reduced by slowing growth rate (119, 127, 263). A higher incidence of VVD occurs in broiler chickens raised in cages compared with broiler chickens raised in floor pens (119, 255, 263). This may be explained by a lack of exercise in cages (119). Stronger cortical bone in chickens occurs with exercise (278). Different photoperiods will affect the incidence of VVD (37, 269). It is unknown whether this is due to a change in growth rate, amount of exercise, or a hormonal factor. An increased incidence of angular limb deformities has been reported in turkeys subsequent to malabsorption syndrome at an early age (245). A brief review on control of VVD was written by Riddell (266).

Rotated Tibia.   Rotated tibia was reported initially as a significant cause of lameness in turkeys and guinea fowl (262). More recently, it has been reported in broilers (273). Affected birds often have the affected leg extended laterally. Either or both legs may be affected. The defect is restricted to the shaft of the tibia, which is rotated externally often to 90 degrees or greater. There is no angulation of bones, and the hock joint is normal, with no displacement of the gastrocnemius tendon. In some extreme cases, the rotation reaches 180 degrees. In such cases, if both legs are extended ventrally, the two foot pads face in opposite directions (Fig. 35.5). Rotation or torsion of the femur, tibiotarsus, and tarsometatarsus is normal during early development of the chicken. Femurs and tibiotarsi rotate externally, while the tarsometatarsi rotate medially when the axis of the distal articular surface is compared with that of the proximal articular surface (77). Rotated tibia represents excessive and abnormal rotation during development. The cause is unknown, although early rickets has been suggested as a predisposing factor in guinea fowl (11). An increased incidence of rotated tibia has been reported in turkeys subsequent to malabsorption syndrome at an early age (245). Rotated tibia differs from VVD in that no angulation of bones is present, and that in broiler flocks, the peak incidence occurs at 3 wk of age, no sex predisposition is apparent, and the number of birds with either the right leg or left leg affected is approximately equal (273).

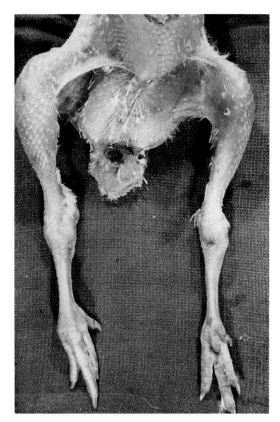

35.5. Turkey with rotated tibia of left leg. Rotation is nearly 180 degrees and the foot pads face in opposite directions.

Crooked Toes.   Crooked toes are a common finding in meat-type chickens and turkeys. The syndrome was reviewed by Riddell (258). An incidence of 4.8–7.7% was reported in broiler chickens in Europe (246), while incidences exceeding 50% were reported in broiler chickens in Australia (215). The deformity, unless very severe, has limited clinical significance. It may interfere with the reproductive performance of breeding cockerels (215). Most digits or a single digit may be bent laterally or medially. Rotation of the phalanges often is present.

The pathogenesis is not understood though it has been proposed that shortening of flexor tendons may cause the deformation. A negative correlation between the presence of twisted legs and slipped tendons and the presence of crooked toes has been reported. The tension in flexor tendons is probably decreased when legs are twisted (246). An increased incidence of crooked toes has been associated with certain types of flooring, infrared brooding, pyridoxine deficiency, and some toxins (258). The syndrome should be differentiated from curly toe paralysis due to riboflavin deficiency.

Dyschondroplasia. Dyschondroplasia is a very common defect associated with the growth plates of meat-type chickens, ducks, and turkeys. It is most commonly recognized in the proximal tibiotarsus, and, hence, the condition is often described as tibial dyschondroplasia. The condition has also been called osteochondrosis by some authors. Osteochondrosis has been used in mammalian pathology to describe a wide range of lesions of growing cartilage, including degenerative and developmental change in both physeal and articular cartilage. The defect that has been called dyschondroplasia in poultry is primarily an abnormal development of physeal cartilage, and dyschondroplasia is the most appropriate name. Reviews on the condition have been written by Wise (344), Riddell (262), Leach and Lilburn (176), Orth and Cook (231), and Thorp (308).

CLINICAL SIGNS AND PATHOLOGY. In many broiler chicken and turkey flocks, up to 30% of birds may have lesions of dyschondroplasia characterized by abnormal masses of cartilage below the growth plate, primarily in the proximal tibiotarsus (Fig. 35.6), but also at other sites. Most birds show no clinical signs. Lesions of tibial dyschondroplasia in broiler chickens have been correlated with anterior bowing of the tibiotarsus and associated lameness (182). If masses of cartilage are very large, signs will include a reluctance to move, a stilted gait, and bilateral swelling of the femoral-tibial joints often associated with bowing of the legs. In a recent survey of leg weakness in broiler chicken flocks processed at 7 wk of age or earlier, few birds were culled because of dyschondroplasia (273). Downgrading of carcasses and trimming of deformed legs at processing have been attributed to dyschondroplasia (29, 273). If broiler chickens are kept to roaster weights, lesions due to dyschondroplasia may be much more severe. In such birds, fractures below the abnormal cartilage in the tibia may cause severe crippling (Fig. 35.7). A high association between leg deformities and tibial dyschondroplasia has been described in turkeys (321). Dyschondroplastic lesions can be recognized on radiographs and with a hand-held lixiscope from 2 wk of age (308).

The abnormal masses of cartilage in the proximal tibia tend to be cone shaped. In mild cases, these cones of abnormal cartilage mainly develop below the posterior medial part of the growth plate, but in severe cases, they develop from the whole growth plate and fill the whole metaphysis. Anterior lateral bowing of the tibia is often associated with larger masses of cartilage. The concave surfaces of such bones have hypertrophied cortices. This is considered an adaptive change (77). Resolution of the abnormal cartilage may start as early as 48 days of age, but sequestra of abnormal cartilage separated from the growth plate and bowing of the tibia may persist to as late as 30 wk of age, even though the proximal growth plate of the tibiotarsus in a chicken closes at 16–17 wk of age. Fractured fibulae have been associated with tibial dyschondroplasia and bowing of the tibia (246). These fractures

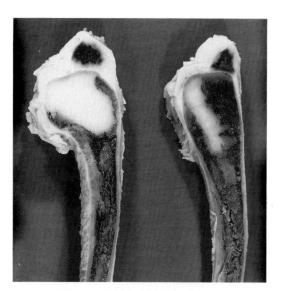

35.6. Medial view of sagittal sections of two proximal tibiotarsal bones from broiler chickens with tibial dyschondroplasia. The abnormal cartilage is only present in the posterior part of the metaphysis (*right*); abnormal cartilage fills the whole metaphysis, and the proximal end of the bone is enlarged (*left*).

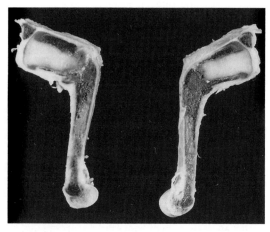

35.7. Sagittal sections of tibiotarsal bones from a roaster chicken with tibial dyschondroplasia. The severe angulation of the bones is due to fractures below the abnormal cartilage.

occur at the *Tuberculum M. iliofibularus*, but are not always associated with abnormal tibiotarsal curvature (63). Dyschondroplasia also occurs, but is less severe, in the proximal and distal femur, the distal tibia, the proximal tarsometatarsus, and the proximal humerus (246). Dyschondroplasia in the femoral head in broiler chickens has been associated with a widened and shortened femoral neck and, in some cases, with fractures of the femoral head (57, 58, 59).

Microscopically, dyschondroplasia is characterized by persistence and accumulation of prehypertrophic cartilage. The separation of the prehypertrophic cartilage from the proliferating cartilage is not sharply demarcated and few vessels penetrate the abnormal cartilage from the metaphysis. Chondrocytes in the abnormal cartilage are small and shrunken and the matrix is more abundant than in normal hypertrophic cartilage. The matrix is not mineralized. It has been suggested that histopathology is essential to differentiate dyschondroplasia from rickets (310). It is possible that in some experimental work, tibial dyschondroplasia has been incorrectly used to describe rachitic lesions.

Ultrastructural studies have demonstrated that the lesion begins in the prehypertrophic zone. The chondrocytes in the abnormal cartilage do not fully hypertrophy, reach only about 40% of their expected size, and then undergo necrosis (109, 120). The abnormal chondrocyte mitochondria retain less calcium and phosphorus as compared to normal chondrocytes. Changes in composition between the abnormal cartilage and normal hypertrophic cartilage that have been reported include lower levels of sulfur, potassium, calmodulin, alkaline phosphatase, and collagen type X (231), and prostaglandin precursors, proteoglycans, and glycosaminoglycans (308). Results have differed between studies. An elevation of alkaline phosphatase was reported in one study. These differences may be the result of examination of different cells or zones of the growth plate (308). Lesion size will influence the metabolic activity of chondrocytes (280). In a recent study of tibial dyschondroplasia in turkeys, reduced activities of alkaline phosphatase and aryl sulfatase were found in dyschondroplastic cartilage, but no major differences were found in protein profiles (253). A 10-fold increase in nonreducible collagen cross-links has been found in the abnormal cartilage in chickens (231). It is not known whether any of these changes in composition are primary. Most may be secondary (231).

PATHOGENESIS AND ETIOLOGY. Detailed discussion of the etiology of tibial dyschondroplasia is provided in the papers written by Leach and Lilburn (176), Orth and Cook (231), Cook et al. (40), and Thorp (308). The pathogenesis of dyschondroplasia

is not well understood. At least three different mechanisms have been suggested. A failure in chondrocyte hypertrophy may result in abnormal cartilage that cannot be invaded by metaphyseal vessels (246). This failure may in part result from rapid bone growth. The presence of the most severe lesions of dyschondroplasia in the proximal tibiotarsus may be due to the growth plate at that site having the most rapid growth. The incidence of tibial dyschondroplasia has been decreased by reducing the growth rate of experimental birds, but there was no direct correlation between growth of individual birds and the development of tibial dyschondroplasia (262). The incidence of tibial dyschondroplasia was reduced by daily fasting (81, 276). This reduction occurred in some experiments without a decrease in body weight, and it was suggested that diurnal rhythms may be important in reducing tibial dyschondroplasia (84). An interrupted- and increasing-light program had no effect on clinical and subclinical tibial dyschondroplasia in roaster chickens (269). An intermittent light program reduced the incidence of tibial dyschondroplasia in one line of broiler chickens, but not in another two lines (350). Occlusion of vascular canals from the epiphysis has been described in the physes of femoral heads with dyschondroplasia. It has been proposed that patent vascular canals from the epiphysis may be necessary for normal chondrocyte hypertrophy (57). Such occlusion of vascular canals is not seen in dyschondroplasia in the proximal tibiotarsus and may be an unrelated lesion. A second possible mechanism is that vascular invasion of the cartilage from the metaphysis may be inadequate. Such inadequacy may be genetically determined or due to trauma in a rapidly growing immature skeleton. Increased weight bearing may increase the incidence of dyschondroplasia (69). A third possible mechanism is defective degradation of cartilage. In *Fusarium*-induced tibial dyschondroplasia a paucity of chondroclasts has been described (121, 322). This change occurred late in the course of the disease and was not considered the primary defect (175). The possibility that dyschondroplasia may be the common endpoint of several different mechanisms cannot be ignored (121).

Recent studies have shown that locally produced peptide growth factors play important autocrine and paracrine roles in development of the growth plate (177). Three important growth factors are insulin-like growth factor-I (IGF-I), basic fibroblast growth factor, and transforming growth factor-ß. A malfunction of one of these factors may be important in the development of tibial dyschondroplasia (308). Fibroblast growth factor-ß, a potent angiogenic factor, is reduced in tibial dyschondroplasia (231). Transforming growth factor-ß expression was reduced in transitional chondrocytes in tibial dyschondroplasia, but its expression was increased where the lesion was being repaired (181). No difference in systemic IGF-I was found between normal chickens and those developing tibial dyschondroplasia, but growth hormone was increased in the abnormal chickens. Systemic as well as local growth factors may be important in the pathogenesis of tibial dyschondroplasia (309, 314). An altered paracrine function of growth plate "macrophages" may result in reduced cartilage degradation and tibial dyschondroplasia (40).

The incidence and severity of tibial dyschondroplasia can be influenced by genetic selection and cation to anion ratio in the ration (262, 349). Though in original reports calcium and phosphorus levels in the ration were considered to have no effect, it has been shown that the incidence and severity of tibial dyschondroplasia in broiler chickens can be increased by feeding high levels of phosphorus relative to the level of calcium (80, 82, 272, 276). Feeding turkeys similar levels of phosphorus and calcium did not result in a high incidence of tibial dyschondroplasia in turkey poults (282). Tibial dyschondroplasia in broiler chickens was not eliminated by feeding a ration containing 1.5% calcium and 0.5% available phosphorus (272). A high level of phosphate affects the cation to anion ratio. Metabolic acidosis may reduce the renal conversion of 25-hydroxycholecalciferol to 1,25-dihydroxycholecalciferol (286). Addition of the latter metabolite of vitamin D to the diet has been shown to decrease the incidence of tibial dyschondroplasia (83, 256, 275, 312). No correlation between the plasma level of 1,25-hydroxycholecalciferol and the incidence of tibial dyschondroplasia was found in one series of experiments, and it was suggested that the ability to utilize the vitamin D metabolite at the receptor level may affect the incidence of tibial dyschondroplasia (84). The incidence of tibial dyschondroplasia was reduced when chicks received ultraviolet radiation or high levels of vitamin D_3 (83). Many of these studies indicate a relationship between rickets and tibial dyschondroplasia. Thorp (308) stated that tibial dyschondroplasia was a form of rickets with a distinct histopathology.

Abnormal cartilage similar to that in tibial dyschondroplasia was produced by feeding a copper-deficient diet to chickens (32), but there are no indications of impaired copper metabolism in chickens with tibial dyschondroplasia, and supplemental copper has failed to prevent tibial dyschondroplasia (176). A high incidence of tibial dyschondroplasia in broiler chickens has been produced with rations contaminated with a fungus, *Fusarium equisete,* with rations containing a fungicide, thiram, or an analog, disulfiram, and with rations containing added cysteine or homocysteine (231). The active compound produced by the fungus has been

characterized and named fusarochromanone. An isolate of *F. oxysporum* has also been shown to induce tibial dyschondroplasia (35). Supplemental copper will prevent the development of tibial dyschondroplasia by all of these compounds (231). None appear to cause a copper deficiency, and copper probably acts by preventing absorption of the compounds from the gut. It has been suggested that thiram and disulfiram may interfere with the hydroxylation of vitamin D, but this has not been supported experimentally. Thiram has been used to produce tibial dyschondroplasia in white leghorn chickens. This was the first time dyschondroplasia had been reported in egg-type chickens (318). More recently, cysteine has been used to produce tibial dyschondroplasia in egg-type chickens (6).

Osteochondrosis. A variety of microscopic degenerate lesions including eosinophilic streaks or scars, occlusion and thrombosis of vascular canals, and necrosis in the growth plate and epiphysis have been described in growing meat-type birds. Though these lesions may be associated with dyschondroplasia, and in some cases, may cause dyschondroplasia (57), in most cases they appear histologically, morphologically, and etiologically dissimilar to dyschondroplasia (201, 274). In this discussion, the term *osteochondrosis* is used for these degenerate lesions. Osteochondrosis has primarily been described in cervical and thoracic vertebrae of broiler chickens (201, 274) and in the femoral head (57, 58, 76, 148, 274) and the antitrochanter (60) of broiler chickens and turkeys.

CLINICAL SIGNS AND PATHOLOGY. Fifty percent of broiler chickens may have osteochondrosis, often without any clinical signs (201, 274). In many studies, osteochondrosis has been described in birds with other skeletal lesions causing lameness, but in two studies, osteochondrosis of the femoral head was the only abnormality detected that could have caused lameness (59, 148).

In affected vertebrae, there is often focal thickening of growth plates associated with eosinophilic streaks following the zone of proliferation or transversing obliquely the growth plate (Fig. 35.8). Many of the streaks enlarge into clefts containing red blood cells and the adjacent cartilage is necrotic (201, 274). The eosinophilic streaks probably represent microscopic tears and the focal thickening of the growth plates appears to be secondary to the tears interfering with endochondral ossification (274).

In affected femoral heads similar eosinophilic streaks are seen in growth plates. Lakes of amorphous eosinophilic material may also be present. In addition, vascular canals in the epiphysis and penetrating the zone of proliferation from the epiphysis

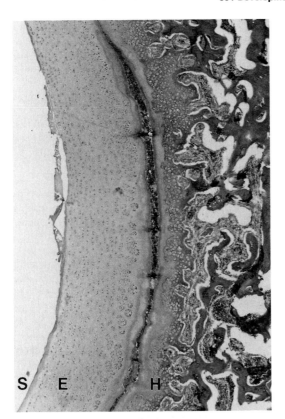

35.8. Osteochondrosis. Midline section of the end of a sixth thoracic vertebral body adjacent to a synovial joint from a broiler chicken. Synovial space (S), epiphysis (E), and top of zone of hypertrophy (H). An eosinophilic streak containing red blood cells follows the zone of proliferation. (Avian Dis)

are occluded with fibrinoid material and contain intact and hemolyzed red blood cells and thrombosed vessels. The growth plate is often thickened and disorganized. Lesions mainly occur on the medial side of the growth plate but also occur laterally. A widened or shortened femoral neck can be associated with these microscopic changes (57). Partial or total femoral head infarction may be associated with the vascular canal occlusion (58). In turkeys, lame because of osteochondrosis, there is often complete separation of the epiphysis and growth plate from the metaphysis. In such birds, the joint capsule may contain brown fluid and necrotic debris (148). In mature chickens, the lesions in the femoral head appear to result in abnormal persistence of growth plate cartilage often with granulation tissue between the cartilage and adjacent trabeculae in the metaphysis. The retained cartilage is disorganized, often necrotic in part and with cystic spaces and fracture lines close to the trabeculae in the metaphysis (59). Such degenerative changes

may result in detachment of the femoral head (74). Similar changes have been reported in the antitrochanter of broiler chickens and turkeys (60) and in the femoral trochanter of broiler chickens (61). Detachment of the proximal femoral epiphysis was observed in broilers that were being downgraded at slaughter as a result of hemorrhage into the thigh musculature. The detachment was probably caused by trauma, and it was suggested that the detachment be described as fracture separation or traumatic epiphysiolysis. It is possible that osteochondrosis may have predisposed to the detachment (76).

Osteochondrosis has been described as a cause of femoral head necrosis in turkeys (148). The term *femoral head necrosis* is nonspecific and has been misused. The use of the term should be discontinued. Necrosis of the femoral head can result from osteochondrosis, dyschondroplasia, or osteomyelitis (148). The term has been applied to the shattering of the femoral head when the femur is osteoporotic, and to the common separation of the proximal femoral epiphysis from the shaft of the femur, which occurs as an artifact when the coxofemoral joint is disarticulated at postmortem. In an experimental study, no evidence was found to support the theory that osteochondrosis might predispose to the separation induced at postmortem (274). A survey of femoral head lesions in commercial broiler chickens indicated that most are due to focal bacterial infection (313).

PATHOGENESIS AND ETIOLOGY. The lesions of osteochondrosis may be due to mechanical forces acting on rapidly growing cartilage (76, 201). The predominance of lesions in the growth plates of vertebrae and the femoral head may be explained by the greater exposure to shear forces of these growth plates than other growth plates (274).

Degenerative Joint Disease. Degenerative changes in joints have been recognized primarily in coxofemoral joints of mature male turkeys (55, 60) and mature meat-type chickens (60, 70), and in the spine of laying hens (351). They have also been reported in the femoral-tibial and intertarsal joints of turkeys (56, 79) and male broiler breeding fowls (70, 74). Duff (55) reviewed early reports of degenerative hip disease in poultry.

CLINICAL SIGNS AND PATHOLOGY. Turkeys with degenerative hip disease assume a stance with abducted pelvic limbs and constantly shift weight from one leg to another and are reluctant to move. The primary gross lesions are found in the articular surface of the antitrochanter. Lesions include areas of surface irregularity, fissures along the dorsocaudal border, and formation of a flap of cartilage that breaks free to give fragments of cartilage within the

joint. Erosions and thinning of the articular cartilage of the trochanter, marginal osteophytes, and
periarticular fibrosis accompany severe lesions
(55). Microscopic changes in the cartilage of the antitrochanter include loss of normal structure, areas
of necrosis, fissures, and massive chondrocyte clusters. Surface fibrillation occurs in the articular cartilage (54).

In the femoral-tibial and intertarsal joints, focal
erosions occur in the articular cartilage with or
without free cartilage bodies in the joint. Flaps of
articular cartilage and osteophytes around the joint
have also been found. Similar microscopic changes
to those described above for lesions in the femoral
head were found associated with evidence of disturbed endochondral ossification in some cases. It
was proposed that the lesion in such cases could be
described as osteochondrosis dissecans (56).

PATHOGENESIS AND ETIOLOGY. The pathogenesis of many of the joint lesions described above is
not clear. Many may result from primary damage to
the articular cartilage, while others may be sequelae
to osteochondrosis (60, 70).

Ligament Failure and Avulsion.
Lesions of
ligaments of the intertarsal joint were first described
as a significant cause of lameness in meat-type
poultry by Craig (42). Lesions have since been reported in the capital femoral ligament in young
adult broiler chickens (62), in the posterior cruciate
and other ligaments of the femoral-tibial joint in
young adult broiler chickens (64, 67, 68, 74) and
turkeys (55, 79), and in the intercondylar and collateral ligaments of the intertarsal joint of turkeys
(79, 146) and broiler chickens (66, 74).

CLINICAL SIGNS AND PATHOLOGY. Lameness
has been attributed to lesions in the capital femoral
ligament. Lesions found include stretching, partial
or total rupture, and avulsion—sometimes with a
piece of cartilage or bone—from the femoral head
insertion. Stretched ligaments sometimes contain
hematomas or are infiltrated with fat. Microscopic
lesions include fraying of collagen bundles, acellu-
larity and hyalinization of the collagen in the tendon, along with necrosis, fissures, and hemorrhage
in cartilage adjacent to the site of insertion (62).
Lameness has also been associated with lesions in
ligaments of the femoral-tibial joint. The posterior
cruciate ligament has been the most commonly affected, but the cranial cruciate, collateral, and caudal meninscofemoral ligaments have also been affected. In the cruciate ligament, total or partial
rupture near the tibial insertion or avulsion from the
tibial insertion occurs. Microscopic lesions are similar to those described for affected femoral capital
ligaments. In addition, multicellular clusters and

mucoid degeneration in the tendons and disorganization of subchondral bone with cysts and granulation at the avulsion site are found (64). Some abnormalities of the menisci of the knee joint have
been associated with ligament disruption (71).
Lameness has also been associated with partial or
total rupture of intercondylar ligament and with
rupture or avulsion of collateral ligaments. Most
microscopic changes in affected ligaments have
been similar to those described for other affected
ligaments (66, 146).

PATHOGENESIS AND ETIOLOGY. Ligament rupture is probably due to trauma. Microscopic lesions
similar to these described in ruptured ligaments
have been described in intact ligaments of broiler-
type chickens, indicating that these changes precede
the rupture (67). In individual male broiler breeding
chickens, tendon or ligament failure is often found
at more than one site, suggesting a predisposition to
ligament and tendon failure in these birds (68). Ligament failure may in part be age related, as the incidence appears to increase with age (74). Ligament
lesions were less severe in turkeys fed a restricted
amount of feed when compared with turkeys fed *ad
libitum* (79). Rupture of ligaments may be secondary to stress induced by limb angulation (66). In
converse, it has been suggested that ligament rupture may result in limb angulation (146, 262).

Cage Layer Osteoporosis/Fatigue.
Cage
layer osteoporosis (fatigue) is the most significant
disease of the skeleton in modern chickens used for
egg production. As the name implies, the major feature of the condition is poor bone structure in laying
chickens kept in cages. In the past, loss of birds in
excess of 3% per month would occur in severely affected flocks. Recent losses have been much
smaller, but poor bone structure in caged laying
hens still causes considerable economic loss due to
bone breakage when birds are processed. A recent
review of welfare problems of laying hens in battery cages stated that poor bone strength due to a
lack of exercise in such cages is probably the greatest single indictment of the battery cage (10). The
early literature relative to the condition was reviewed by Riddell (262).

CLINICAL SIGNS AND PATHOLOGY. Birds initially
are found paralyzed in their cages. They often are
alert, but later become depressed and die from dehydration. Some birds die acutely. The paralysis
gave rise to the term *fatigue*. Paralyzed birds, if removed from their cages and given ready access to
feed and water, will often recover in 4–7 days. On
postmortem examination, paralyzed or dead birds
have bones that are easily broken. Fractures may be
found in leg and wing bones and in the thoracic

spine. Sterna are often deformed, and there is characteristic infolding deformation of the ribs at the junction of the sternal and vertebral components. Parathyroid glands are enlarged. Many birds have regressive ovaries and are dehydrated, while some dead birds have an egg in the oviduct and have died acutely.

On histology, the cortices of bones are thin, with enlarged absorption spaces. Medullary bone is reduced in amount, and largely consists of osteoid. The deformation of the ribs can be seen to be due to small fractures and, often, damage to the spinal cord is associated with the fractures in the thoracic spine.

PATHOGENESIS, ETIOLOGY, AND CONTROL. The paralysis in some birds may be explained by the spinal cord fractures, but these cannot always be found. It is possible that paralysis in some birds, and acute death in others, may be due to hypocalcemia, but this has not been proved. Similar skeletal changes and clinical syndromes have been produced experimentally with low-phosphorus, low-calcium, and vitamin D–deficient diets. Low-calcium and vitamin D–deficient diets produced a severe decrease in egg production, while the low-phosphorus diet only produced a slight decrease. The modern laying hen has a very active calcium metabolism and high egg production may result in a physiologic osteoporosis. Marginal nutritional deficiencies may result in severe osteoporosis and clinical signs. The formation of strong cortical bone and adequate medullary bone prior to egg production may be helpful in reducing cage-layer fatigue. Increased calcium in the ration prior to egg production may be necessary, but it has been suggested that if increased calcium is fed for too long before egg production, the parathyroid gland may be suppressed. Strain of bird and type of housing have been shown to affect the incidence of cage-layer osteoporosis. The clinical condition has been restricted to birds kept in cages. Recent studies have been directed at defining and preventing bone breakage when hens are processed at the end of their production cycle. A greater incidence of freshly broken bones in laying hens after handling at processing time has been described in hens from cages, compared with hens from other housing systems (103). The incidence is influenced by the method of handling (104). Confinement of laying hens in cages has been shown to reduce bone strength significantly (224, 169) and to increase the ease with which bones are broken during handling (169). Perches in cages decreased the severity of osteoporosis (126), but the beneficial effects of perches was relatively minor (342). Treatment of pullets with alendronate—a biphosphonate—just prior to the onset of lay has been shown to decrease

a loss of trabecular bone. Alendronate may have a potential role in preventing osteoporosis in laying hens (311).

DISEASES OF MUSCLES AND TENDONS

Deep Pectoral Myopathy. Deep pectoral myopathy has also been called green muscle disease. Ischemia following exercise in heavily muscled meat-type turkeys and chickens causes the condition. Condemnation of affected muscles has resulted in economic loss in breeder turkeys. The condition was first described in Oregon in breeder turkey hens older than 10 mo of age, with up to 9% of some flocks being affected (53). Several strains of bronze, as well as large, medium, and small white turkeys are affected. Both sexes have the defect (114). The lesion has been recognized in turkeys elsewhere in North America (105) and in the United Kingdom (142). The lesion has also been described in meat-type breeding chickens (115, 143) and in 7-wk-old broiler chickens (257).

CLINICAL SIGNS AND PATHOLOGY. The lesion does not affect the general health of birds and is generally only found at processing. The lesion can be unilateral or bilateral. Chronic lesions result in dimpling or flattening of the breast muscles. These lesions can be detected by palpation (116). Comprehensive descriptions of the pathology of the lesion in turkeys have been provided by Siller and Wight (294), and in broiler breeder chickens by Wight and Siller (338). Lesions in both types of birds are similar. In early lesions, the whole deep pectoral muscle is swollen, pale, and edematous with necrosis in the middle third to three-fifths of the muscle. The overlying fascia is often opaque with edema between the deep and superficial muscles. In older lesions, the edema disappears and the necrotic muscle becomes more prominent and drier with greenish areas. In chronic lesions, the necrotic muscle has shrunk and is uniformly green, dry, and friable and enclosed by a fibrous capsule. It may shrink to a fibrous scar. The muscle posterior to the necrotic muscle becomes atrophied, pale, and sometimes fibrosed. The sternum adjacent to the necrotic muscle is roughened and irregular.

When examined microscopically, the fibers in the green necrotic muscle are swollen and uniformly eosinophilic with discoid necrosis. Nuclei are absent or faint. Blood vessels within the necrotic tissue often contain only nuclei of lysed red blood cells. Surrounding the necrotic tissue, there is an inflammatory reaction with heterophils, macrophages, and giant cells, and in chronic cases, a fibrous capsule. Viable, degenerate, and regenerating muscle fibers are often enveloped by the capsule. Brown pigment and cystlike structures containing yellow material are also found within the capsule. In the muscle posterior to the necrotic tissue, fibers may be atrophied and replaced by fat, and in some instances, fibrosis is present. Vascular lesions consisting of thromboses, intimal proliferation, and aneurysm formation are found in and around the necrotic tissue. Ultrastructural studies on affected muscles have been conducted (142, 338).

PATHOGENESIS AND ETIOLOGY. In an elegant series of experiments Wight (339), Siller (296, 297), and Martindale (185) have demonstrated that deep pectoral myopathy is the result of ischemia secondary to the swelling in a tight fascia of a vigorously exercised muscle. In prior studies, surgical occlusion of arteries to the pectoral muscles in both turkeys and chickens resulted in infarcts similar in appearance to the lesions of deep pectoral myopathy (230, 295). In subsequent studies, temporary occlusion of the subclavian artery combined with electrically induced contractions of the deep pectoral muscle induced necrosis of the muscle in both lightweight and broiler strains of chicken. Similar electrically induced contractions alone produced necrosis of the muscle in the broiler strains, but not in the lightweight chickens (339). Subsequently, it was demonstrated that the necrosis could be produced by voluntary wing movements (296). Surgical incision of the fascia around the deep pectoral muscle prior to exercise, however, would prevent development of the lesion (297). Angiography demonstrated a complete ischemia in the deep pectoral muscle associated with an increase in subfascial pressure following electrical stimulation of the muscle. After 24 hr, the ischemia only persisted in the middle of the muscle (185).

It is possible that the high incidence of deep pectoral myopathy in turkey breeder hens is, in part, the result of the extensive handling these birds receive during artificial insemination. Modification of handling procedures may reduce the incidence (340). Some evidence has been produced for a hereditary predisposition (116). This predisposition may be related to inadequate vasculature in muscles of meat-type birds (339). No specific nutritional factors are known to influence the condition (105, 113), but food restriction may reduce the incidence (338).

Rupture of the Gastrocnemius Tendon.

For many years, lameness due to rupture of the gastrocnemius tendon has been recognized commonly in meat-type chickens and rarely in turkeys. It can cause considerable economic loss in broiler breeder flocks and in broiler chickens raised to roaster weights. The early literature on the condition was reviewed by Peckham (243).

CLINICAL SIGNS AND PATHOLOGY. Up to 20% of a flock may be affected. Most outbreaks have been in broiler breeder chickens older than 12 wk of age, but the condition has been recognized in broiler chickens as early as 7 wk of age. The rupture can be unilateral or bilateral. Onset of lameness is acute. Birds with bilateral rupture have a characteristic posture in which the bird sits on its hocks with its toes flexed (Fig. 35.9). In affected birds, a swelling can be palpated on the posterior surface of the leg just above the hock. With acute lesions, hemorrhage can be seen through the skin. With older lesions, there is green discoloration; with chronic lesions, no discoloration may be apparent, but a very firm mass of abnormal subcutaneous tissue can be palpated. Dissection of acute lesions reveals a blood-filled swelling under the skin on the posterior surface of the leg. Within the hematoma, the free end of the ruptured tendon can be found. The rupture generally occurs as an irregular transverse break just above the hock joint. In older and chronic lesions, the blood is partially or completely reabsorbed and fibrous tissue encloses the end of the ruptured tendon and surrounding tissue. Microscopic lesions are variable. In many acute lesions, there is hemorrhage only. In older lesions, there is fibrous tissue surrounding resolving hematomas and the ruptured tendon. Synovial hyperplasia and infiltration of heterophils and macrophages vary from very little to massive. The infiltration of inflammatory cells occurs within the tendon and in the synovial membranes and cavities, and may be associated with masses of heterophil debris and some bacterial colonies.

PATHOGENESIS AND ETIOLOGY. Duff and Randall (75) reviewed the literature on the causes of rupture of the gastrocnemius tendon. They concluded that tenosynovitis, in particular that due to

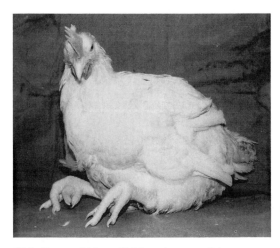

35.9. Roaster chicken with bilateral rupture of the gastrocnemius tendon. Hock-sitting posture with toes directed ventrally is characteristic.

reoviruses, may be implicated in some cases. In other cases, the rupture appears to be spontaneous. In such cases, a frequent concurrent finding is rupture of other pelvic limb tendons or ligaments. In cases associated with tenosynovitis, there was a marked inflammatory response, while in spontaneous rupture, there was a minimal inflammatory response.

The tensile strength of the flexor digitus perforatus and perforans tendon to the third digit is less in meat-type chickens than in egg-type chickens. It has been suggested that this could predispose meat-type birds to tenosynovitis (315). This could also predispose to spontaneous rupture of tendons. Tissue of the gastrocnemius tendon in meat-type birds has a less organized appearance than that in egg-type birds (316). In addition, many meat-type birds have a hypovascular area in the gastrocnemius tendon just above the hock joint. This hypovascular area is associated with thickened chondrocyte plaques, chondrocyte death, and excessive lipid accumulation in the tendon. These changes may predispose to noninfectious tendon rupture (73). Little research has been conducted on the effect of nutrition on tendon strength. In one study, administration of glycine, vitamin C or E, or copper had no effect on tensile strength of tendons (317). In another study, restricted feeding had no effect on tensile strength of tendons, but the ratio of tensile strength to body weight was less in chickens fed *ad libitum* than in those fed a restricted amount of feed (274).

DISEASES OF THE CIRCULATORY SYSTEM

Round Heart Disease in Chickens.
Round heart disease is an acute cardiac failure due to myocardial degeneration in chickens commonly between 4 and 8 mo of age. It used to have a worldwide distribution but has not been reported in commercial poultry flocks for 20 yr. In the past 20 yr, the author has diagnosed a few cases a year in backyard flocks in Saskatchewan but has never diagnosed the condition in large commercial flocks. The literature on the condition was extensively reviewed by Peckham (243). The reader is referred to the review for specific citations. In that review, some papers on round heart disease in turkeys were also discussed. Round heart disease of turkeys is a different syndrome and is discussed under Spontaneous Cardiomyopathy in Turkeys.

CLINICAL SIGNS AND PATHOLOGY.
Morbidity in affected flocks is very low or absent, while mortality may reach 50%. Birds are generally not diagnosed as sick prior to death. The most striking and consistent lesion found at necropsy is an enlarged and yellowish heart. The apex of the heart is blunt

and may be dimpled. Both ventricles are hypertrophied (Fig. 35.10). In some birds, there may be excess gelatinous fluid in the pericardial sac and in a few birds excess fluid is present in the abdominal cavity. Lungs are often edematous and the liver, kidneys, and spleen may be congested. Microscopic lesions consist of vacuolated myocardial fibers with very prominent cell membranes (Fig. 35.11). The vacuolation is due to distension of fibers with fat. Interstitial and perivascular lymphocyte and interstitial heterophil infiltration have been described in some reports, and intranuclear inclusion bodies in other reports.

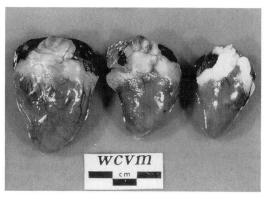

35.10. Round heart disease in chickens. Two enlarged hearts (*left*) in comparison to the normal heart (*right*).

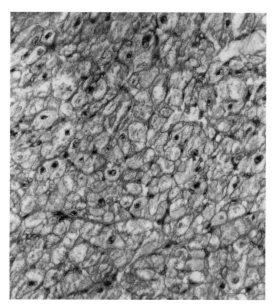

35.11. Histologic section of myocardium from a chicken with round heart disease. The fibers are dilated and vacuolated with prominent membranes. H & E,

PATHOGENESIS AND ETIOLOGY. The etiology is unknown. Numerous attempts to transmit the disease have been unsuccessful. Unspecified toxins, in particular associated with built-up litter, have been suggested as causes. Successful treatment of the syndrome with sodium selenite was reported once, but has not been confirmed. The restriction of the syndrome in Saskatchewan to backyard flocks fed marginal rations supports the concept that round heart disease in chickens may be due to a nutritional deficiency. The microscopic lesions of round heart disease differ from those reported in experimental vitamin E/selenium deficiency in chickens (265).

Spontaneous Cardiomyopathy in Turkeys.

Spontaneous cardiomyopathy has commonly been called round heart disease and less commonly the cardiohepatic syndrome. It is desirable that the term *round heart disease* be discontinued, as the syndrome in turkeys is different in many respects from round heart disease in chickens (183). The early literature on the syndrome has been reviewed by Czarnecki (46) and the reader is referred to this review for more detail and specific citations.

CLINICAL SIGNS AND PATHOLOGY. The highest rate of mortality due to spontaneous cardiomyopathy occurs in young poults, commonly peaking at 2 wk of age and disappearing at 3 wk of age. Recently, the author has observed losses persisting to 14 wk of age. Losses have totaled as high as 22% in some flocks. Affected young turkeys may die suddenly or may have ruffled feathers, drooping wings, and labored gasping breathing prior to death. On postmortem examination, affected young turkeys have greatly enlarged hearts due to dilation of both ventricles. Often, the right ventricle is more dilated. Hydropericardium and ascites may or may not be present. Lungs are generally congested and edematous. Livers may be slightly swollen with rounded edges. In older turkeys from affected flocks, enlarged hearts can still be found, but in these hearts the prominent lesion is an enlargement and hypertrophy of the left ventricle.

Microscopic changes in abnormal hearts are non-specific and include congestion, degeneration of myofibers, focal infiltration of lymphocytes, and in older turkeys, increased fibroelastic tissue under the endocardium of the left ventricle. Vacuolization of hepatic cells, focal necrosis, bile duct hyperplasia, and intracytoplasmic PAS-positive globules in hepatocytes have been described in the swollen livers.

PATHOGENESIS AND ETIOLOGY. The etiology of spontaneous cardiomyopathy is unknown. A genetic influence was demonstrated by breeding trials. Birds with spontaneous cardiomyopathy were selected using electrocardiography, and by mating affected males to affected females, the incidence of the condition was increased in the progeny. Myocardial damage is probably the primary lesion resulting in dilation of ventricles and heart failure. This damage may result from hypoxia in the late embryo or young poult (153). Spontaneous cardiomyopathy has been related to abnormal conditions in incubation (45). Clinical observations indicate that the incidence of spontaneous cardiomyopathy is increased at high altitude and with cold weather (87). Raising turkeys in a hypobaric chamber at an atmospheric pressure of 592 mm Hg (equivalent altitude 2054 m) resulted in a high incidence of spontaneous cardiomyopathy (164). Slowing the growth rate of young poults by dietary manipulation both in a hypobaric chamber at a reduced atmospheric pressure (164) and under commercial conditions (22) reduced the incidence of spontaneous cardiomyopathy. A light program designed to reduce growth rate at an early age also reduced the incidence of spontaneous cardiomyopathy (39). It is probable that an increased oxygen requirement associated with rapid growth and cold may increase the incidence of spontaneous cardiomyopathy (153). Turkey poults kept at a simulated high altitude on a fast-growth diet developed polycythaemia (166). Furazolidone is toxic for turkey poults in concentrations as low as 300 ppm in the feed, and produces a syndrome that is indistinguishable from spontaneous cardiomyopathy. Furazolidone results in changes in enzymes, contractile proteins, and membranes in the myocardium, consistent with a role of tissue hypoxia in the cardiac lesions (209). A suggestion that spontaneous cardiomyopathy might be due to an inherited serum trypsin inhibition has not been confirmed. Further work is needed to determine any relationship between the viral particles seen with the electron microscope in some affected hearts and spontaneous cardiomyopathy. Many factors can cause ascites in poultry (153). A common cause of ascites in commercial poultry is excess sodium in the feed or water. Excess sodium in young broiler chickens causes hypervolemia and right ventricular failure (150). It is probable that with sodium toxicosis, a similar mechanism causes ascites in turkeys.

Ascites and Right Ventricular Failure in Broiler Chickens.

Ascites secondary to right ventricular failure (ARVF) occurs worldwide in growing broiler chickens and is a significant cause of mortality in many flocks. As ARVF is commonly caused by pulmonary hypertension, it has recently been called the pulmonary hypertension syndrome (153). The incidence is increasing. A similar syndrome has been reported in meat-type ducklings (151). The disease was first reported in flocks of broiler chickens reared at high altitudes in Bolivia (106). It has since been described in flocks at high altitudes in Peru (43), Mexico (180), and South

Africa (31, 124). Losses of up to 30% of the birds in some flocks may occur (180). In the past 15 yr it has been reported in flocks at low altitudes in the United Kingdom (3, 305), Canada (159, 264), South Africa (124) and the United States (86). A low incidence of the syndrome has been found in most broiler flocks at processing (264), and mortality may be above 1% in many broiler flocks and occasionally 15–20% in some roaster flocks (160) in Canada.

CLINICAL SIGNS AND PATHOLOGY. The condition may manifest itself as sudden death (159, 305), but often affected birds are smaller than normal and listless with ruffled feathers. Severely affected birds have abdominal distension (Fig 35.12), may be reluctant to move, and are dyspneic and cyanotic (193). Gross lesions include ascites, right-side cardiac enlargement, and variable liver changes. More than 300 mL of straw-colored ascitic fluid with or without fibrin clots explains the abdominal distension (106, 193, 341). Some birds may die before ascites develops (153). The cardiac enlargement includes dilation of the right atrium, sinus venosus, and vena cava as well as the right ventricle (Fig.

35.13) and hypertrophy of both the right ventricle and right muscular atrioventricular valve. Measurement of the ratio of the weight of the right ventricle to the weight of the total ventricles (28) shows a greatly increased ratio in affected birds (124). Nodular thickening of the endocardium, particularly in the region of the right atrioventricular valve, has been described (106). Hydropericardium may be present. The livers in affected birds vary from congested or mottled to shrunken with a grayish capsule and irregular surface. Lungs are congested and edematous (106, 193, 341). Blood from affected birds has increased packed-cell volume, hemoglobin, and red and white blood cell counts. Heterophils and monocytes are increased at the expense of lymphocytes (193).

Microscopic lesions have been described in the heart, liver, lung, and kidney (106, 193, 341). The myocardial fibers are mildly disorganized, with edema and some proliferation of loose connective tissue between fibers, focal hemorrhages, and infiltrations of heterophils. The liver sinusoids may be distended and often the capsule is greatly thickened. Foci of lymphocytes and heterophils in the liver are common. The lungs are often hyperemic with visi-

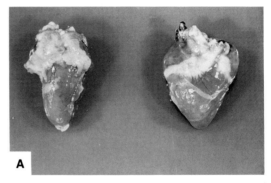
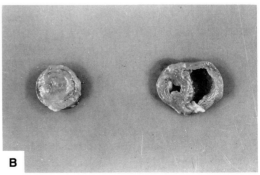

35.13. Right ventricular heart failure in a broiler chicken. *A.* Enlarged heart (*right*) compared with a normal heart (*left*). *B.* Transverse section through the enlarged heart showing dilation and hypertrophy of the right ventricle compared with a transverse section through the normal heart.

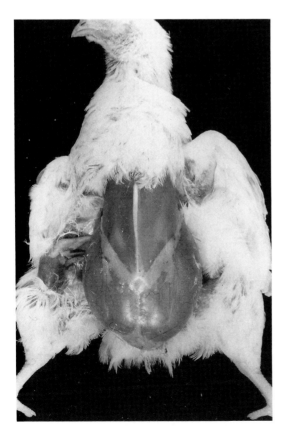

35.12. Broiler chicken with abdomen distended with fluid secondary to right ventricular heart failure.

ble evidence of hemorrhage, edema, and hypertrophy of smooth muscle around the parabronchi, and collapse of the atria and air capillaries. Increased numbers of cartilaginous and osseous nodules have been found in the lungs of birds affected with ascites (189). Kidneys may have congested glomeruli with thickened basement membranes and scattered foci of lymphocytes (193).

Ultrastructural changes in ARVF include myofibril disorganization, mitochondrial abnormalities and hyperplasia in the heart, thickening of alveolar and capillary walls in the lung, and thickened basement membranes and tubular degeneration in the kidney (194, 196, 192). Abnormal calcium deposits have been demonstrated in the mitochondria of cardiac myocytes of birds with ARVF (199). Increased serum troponin T found in live birds with ARVF is another indicator of myocardial damage associated with ARVF (200). An additional ultrastructural observation in some birds with ARVF was the presence of viral particles between muscle fibers in the heart (194). These virus particles were identified as retroviruses (238).

PATHOGENESIS AND ETIOLOGY. Several different mechanisms and a multitude of causes may result in ascites in poultry. The reader is referred to an excellent discussion of this topic by Julian (153) for more detail and references. Ascites can result from obstruction of lymph drainage, decreased plasma osmotic pressure, increased vascular permeability or increased blood pressure. Most of the important syndromes in poultry result from increased blood pressure. Increased blood pressure causing ascites can be split into three categories. In the first category, liver damage interfering with venous return to the liver can result in ascites. Common causes are hepatic toxins in all types of poultry and amyloidosis in ducks. In the second category, primary heart disease affecting valves or the myocardium can cause right ventricular failure and increased venous blood pressure. Spontaneous turkey cardiomyopathy and furazolidone toxicosis are examples in which ascites is probably due to primary heart disease. Other examples include congenital heart defects, endocarditis, monensin and rapeseed oil toxicoses, and viral myocarditis. Ascites in experimental leghorn chickens was attributed to a myocarditis induced by an avian leukosis virus RAV-1 (92). Inoculation of the same virus into meat-type chickens produced myocarditis but no ascites (93). The third and most important category of ascites due to increased blood pressure in poultry is ascites caused by right ventricular hypertrophy and failure secondary to pulmonary hypertension. The syndrome produced by pulmonary hypertension is the subject of the remainder of this section.

Many of the lesions found in ARVF are nonspecific and the result of right ventricular failure. Right ventricular hypertrophy prior to right ventricular failure suggests pulmonary hypertension. The ratio of right ventricle to left ventricle is a measure of pulmonary hypertrophy, until atrophy of the left ventricle in right ventricular failure distorts the ratio (153). The thin right ventricle wall and muscular right atrioventricular flap, instead of valves, in the chicken heart may predispose the chicken to right ventricular failure.

Several factors alone or in combination may cause pulmonary hypertension. A major factor is hypoxemia (291). Hypoxemia results in increased cardiac output, polycythemia, increased hemoglobin, and an increased hematocrit. These changes in the blood produce an increased blood viscosity and larger and more rigid red blood cells, which may have difficulty passing through the capillary bed of the lung, contributing to pulmonary hypertension (207, 198). The resistance to blood flow through the lung may be more important than increased blood flow in the development of pulmonary hypertension in broiler chickens (156).

The high incidence of ARVF at high altitudes can be explained by hypoxia (43); ARVF has been reproduced in hypobaric changes (234, 236, 346, 156). There has been little evidence that reduced environmental oxygen causes ARVF at low altitudes (291, 157). A low-ventilation model with increased CO_2 levels but little decrease in O_2 levels was recently used to reproduce the ARVF. An incidence of 15–35.6% cumulative mortality due to ARVF was reported in two experiments, with an incidence of 4.0% in control birds under normal ventilation in one of the experiments (85, 4, 7). Unfortunately, little information was given on the control birds and normal ventilation. Reduced oxygen concentration from 21 to 19% in one experiment did not affect the blood pressure in experimental broilers susceptible to ascites. This lack of response to low oxygen concentration may have been due to a decreased growth rate (140).

The modern broiler chicken is susceptible to ARVF because its rapid growth causes a high demand for oxygen (160). The incidence of ARVF can be decreased by reducing growth rate (290). The incidence of ARVF is lower in broiler chickens fed mash diets when compared with broiler chickens fed pelleted diets (48, 292). Relative growth of different body organs may be important in the development and control of ARVF. Slower growth of hearts, lungs, and liver relative to whole body growth may increase susceptibility to ascites (141). Feed restriction at an early age decreased ARVF, but also reduced breast muscle growth (1).

Cold temperature is another important factor that causes an increased demand for oxygen and increases the incidence of ARVF (161). Certain feedstuffs may increase the demand for oxygen and the incidence of ARVF (165). In converse, it has been suggested that urease inhibitors in the diet may reduce the incidence of ARVF by decreasing intestinal ammonia and reducing demand for oxygen by the intestinal tract. Supplementing the diet with urease inhibitors caused a decrease in cumulative ascites mortality but also caused a reduction in body weight gains (4, 7).

Features of the modern broiler chicken in addition to rapid growth, which may make it susceptible to developing hypoxemia, include a small lung relative to body size (152, 319), a thicker blood-gas barrier (319), larger and less deformable red blood cells (191, 207), and impaired hemoglobin saturation with oxygen (155, 239). Birds selected for a low feed-conversion ratio may be more susceptible to ARVF (287, 139). Factors that may influence susceptibility include limited thyroid hormone production and a lower capacity for oxygen consumption (288). The ability of these susceptible broiler chickens to maintain growth under adverse environmental conditions may be more important in increasing their susceptibility to ascites than a reduced capacity to use oxygen (139). Addition of 3,3′,5-triiodothyronine to the diet of broiler chickens increased the cumulative mortality linked to ascites. The increase in mortality was greater in an ascites-susceptible line of broiler chickens (49). Abnormal electrocardiographic patterns are found in young chicks that later develop ARVF (225, 226, 237). It is presumed that these abnormal patterns are secondary to early hypoxia in the chicken (237). Lower levels of antioxidants have been reported in the lung and liver of broiler chickens affected with ARVF (85). Though it has been suggested that this may be important in the development of ascites, it is probably a secondary change.

Anemia is a potential factor contributing to hypoxemia but has not been shown to be of major significance under commercial conditions. Right ventricular hypertrophy has been demonstrated in chickens anemic due to infection with *Aegyptionella pullorum* (125). Experimental nitrite toxicosis in broiler chickens produced a transient methemoglobinemia but no ARVF (52). Experimental cobalt toxicosis in broiler chickens produced a polycythemia and ARVF (50). Ascites secondary to right ventricular failure occurring subsequent to phosphorous-deficient rickets has been attributed to hypoxemia resulting from impaired respiration (159).

Hypervolemia may contribute to pulmonary hypertension. Sodium toxicosis resulting in ARVF is the most important cause of hypervolemia in commercial chickens (163). As well as increasing blood volume, excess sodium decreased erythrocyte deformability (210, 208). Furosemide, a diuretic, reduced ARVF mortality in experimental broiler chickens. Though this may be explained on the basis of reduced fluid and electrolyte retention, it may

in part have been due to reduced growth or reduced pulmonary vascular resistance, as furosemide acts as a vasodilator (333).

Increased resistance to blood flow through the lung will contribute to pulmonary hypertension. Clamping of a single pulmonary artery in broiler chickens induced ARVF (327). As discussed above, polycythemia may make it more difficult for the heart to pump blood through the lung. Pulmonary vasoconstriction in mammals occurs with hypoxemia, but there is doubt whether this occurs in chickens (153). Some strains of broiler chickens have thickened muscle coats in their pulmonary arteries (191, 239), and thickened pulmonary arteries have been reported in broiler chickens affected with ARVF (123). Pulmonary vasoconstriction may be mediated by hydrogen ion concentration. The addition of 1% sodium bicarbonate to a broiler ration to cause alkalosis reduced the incidence of ARVF in experimental birds in a hypobaric chamber (235). Supplemental L-arginine reduced the incidence of ARVF mortality in experimental broilers. This was explained on the basis that L-arginine may be required as a substrate for the production of nitric oxide, a powerful endogenous pulmonary vasodilator (334). Ascites secondary to right ventricular failure has been associated with lung damage produced by the drug amiodarone (162), aspergillosis (154), and calcification secondary to excess dietary calcium (19). In Light Sussex chickens, ARVF was associated with feeding a high-calcium diet, but no lung calcification was reported (254). An increase in the number of cartilaginous and osseous nodules was noted in the lungs of birds with ARVF. The possibility that these nodules may contribute to ARVF was discussed, but not proven (197). The nodules may be secondary to hypoxia, but no correlation was found between mean red-cell volume and number of nodules (190).

Acute Death Syndrome in Broiler Chickens.

Acute death syndrome (ADS) describes a condition in which healthy broiler chickens die suddenly for no discernible cause. The syndrome has also been described as sudden death syndrome, heart attack, and flip-over. The latter term has been used because birds dead from the syndrome are commonly found on their backs. The condition was first described as "edema of lungs" in England (122) and subsequently as "died in good condition" in Australia (135). Later, it was reported in Eastern Europe (320), Canada (23, 33), and the United States (27). Birds dead from ADS are found in most broiler flocks. The incidence varies from 0.5 to 4.0% (23, 33, 125, 273, 302). A brief review on ADS was written by Riddell (268).

CLINICAL SIGNS AND PATHOLOGY. Acute death syndrome has been reported to occur from 1 to 8 wk of age, with the greatest losses occurring from 2 to 3 wk of age in most flocks (23, 273, 302). In some broiler flocks, the weekly incidence appears to increase throughout the growing period, suggesting an error in diagnosis or a different syndrome (273). It is possible that birds dying from right heart failure may have been misdiagnosed as ADS (268). Groups of dead birds may be found adjacent to feeder motors or heaters or within feed pans, suggesting the birds may have been startled prior to death (302). In contradiction, no evidence was found in a behavioral study that ADS was precipitated by any environmental event occurring immediately prior to death (222).

Affected chickens show no clinical signs or unusual behavior until less than a minute before death. Birds may squawk during a sudden attack characterized by loss of balance, convulsions, and violent flapping (222). Most birds die on their backs with one or both legs extended or raised, but some may die on their sterna or sides (271, 302). Comparison of blood from birds just after death from ADS with blood from killed healthy birds revealed no consistent differences in serum levels of sodium, potassium, chloride, calcium, phosphorus, magnesium, or glucose. Total lipids were raised in some birds dying from ADS (271).

At necropsy, birds dying from ADS are well fleshed with a full gastrointestinal tract. Livers are enlarged, pale, and friable and, generally, the gall bladder is empty. Kidneys may be pale and the lungs are often congested and edematous (228, 302). The congestion and edema of the lungs may be a postmortem artifact, as it is not found in freshly dead birds (271). The ventricles of the heart are generally contracted and the thyroid, thymus, and spleen may be congested; there may be hemorrhages in the kidney (228). Microscopic lesions reported are nonspecific and consist of congestion, edema, and lymphoid cell infiltration in the lungs; hemorrhages in the kidneys; mild bile duct hyperplasia and periportal lymphoid infiltration in the liver; and mild degeneration and infiltration of lymphoid cells and heterophils in the heart (228). The cellular infiltrations described in the heart of birds dying from ADS have been considered to be normal lymphoid foci and foci of ectopic hemopoiesis (271). Use of an allochrome stain and a hematoxylin-basic fuchsin-picric acid stain did not demonstrate any degenerative changes in hearts of birds dying from ADS (271). In contradiction to these previous studies of the heart in ADS, a more recent study described arteriosclerotic changes and myocardial necrosis mostly in the left ventricle of broiler chickens that had died suddenly without clinical signs (168). The birds studied were 34 to 64 days of age, older than when most ADS mortality occurs and than when birds were examined in one of the prior studies (271). In a study of organ weights, relative liver weights of broilers dead from ADS were significantly greater than the liver weights of control birds, but no significant differences were noted between ADS and control birds in relative weights of lungs, hearts, and intestines (20).

PATHOGENESIS AND ETIOLOGY. The pathogenesis of ADS is not understood. The acute death could be explained by ventricular fibrillation. An increased myocardial irritability in large, fast-growing broiler chickens was found in comparison to slow-growing broiler chickens at 3 wk of age. This increased irritability was no longer present in similar broiler chickens at 6 wk of age (102). Abnormal electrocardiograms have been described in male broiler chickens under stress (99). A suggestion that lactic acid or acid-base balance is involved in ADS was not confirmed (136). It has been suggested that ADS is a metabolic disease and that genetic, nutritional, and environmental factors may affect the incidence (271). Acute death syndrome has primarily been described in broiler-type chickens. White Rock strains are more susceptible than the Light Sussex and New Hampshire crosses used in the early days of intensive broiler chicken production (122). Most modern broiler chicken strains are susceptible (23, 273), but the heritability is low (34). Acute death syndrome was associated with rapid growth in a trial comparing crumble-pellet feeding with all-mash feeding (248). Under field conditions, no correlation was found between growth rate and incidence of ADS (273). A higher incidence of ADS in birds fed a pelleted feed compared with birds fed a mash feed could be due to a factor in the pelleting process, rather than due to the more rapid growth in birds fed the pelleted feed (250). Severe feed restriction eliminated ADS in a small experimental trial (21), but restriction of feed intake for 7 days early in the life of broiler chickens did not significantly reduce the incidence of ADS (277). A lighting program in which birds were exposed to a short photoperiod at an early age decreased early growth rate and also decreased the incidence of ADS (37, 269).

Several nutritional factors have been studied with regard to the incidence of ADS. In a field survey, a higher incidence of ADS was noted in flocks fed wheat-based rations compared with flocks fed corn-based rations. This difference was also noted in some experimental trials (14, 211), but no differences were noted in other nutritional trials (129, 212). It has been suggested that the addition of biotin to broiler rations will reduce the incidence of ADS (128), but this has not been confirmed (129, 303, 324). The content of biotin in liver samples from birds dead from ADS was not significantly different from that in normal flockmates in one study (302), but was lower than that of flockmates dying from other causes in another study (27). Biotin will prevent fatty liver and kidney syndrome (325). A syndrome has been described in which postmortem signs of both fatty liver and kidney syndrome and ADS have been found in dead birds. In particular, affected birds had fatty infiltration in liver, kidney, and heart. It was suggested that an abnormality occurring as a result of fatty liver and kidney syndrome may contribute to the initiation of ADS (324). The total lipid content of livers from birds dead from ADS is increased in a similar amount to that which occurs in livers of birds deficient in biotin, but the alterations in fatty-acid composition that occur in livers of biotin-deficient birds are not found in livers of birds dying of ADS (27). The incidence of ADS has been affected by the type of protein (14) and the level of protein (212). A number of other dietary studies also suggest that an alteration in lipid metabolism may be involved (212, 281, 304). Lipid metabolism may affect cardiac sarcoplasmic reticular transport (36). Increased amounts of calcium, phosphorus, and magnesium (149) or potassium (129) in rations had no effect on the incidence of ADS. Recently, it has been suggested that thiamine may influence the incidence of ADS (38).

In an epizootiologic study of ADS, multiple regression analysis demonstrated negative correlations between the incidence of ADS and flocks with more growing space, larger flocks, flocks raised on hammer-milled straw, and flocks raised in barns with hot-water heating. The authors commented that the correlations did not necessarily indicate causes but suggested areas for future study. No correlations were found with many other management factors including light intensity (273). In an experimental study, it was also shown that light intensity did not affect the incidence of ADS (221), but a field trial suggested that intermittent light may decrease the incidence of ADS (229). Increased light intensity alternating from side to side within pens, when superimposed on a background of low light intensity, had no effect on the incidence of ADS (219, 220). Both acetylsalicylic acid (249) and reserpine (91) have been added to the diet with no effect on the incidence of ADS. A calcium antagonist, verapamil, added to the diet also had no effect on the incidence of ADS (100).

Sudden Death in Turkeys Associated with Perirenal Hemorrhage.

Sudden death in turkeys associated with perirenal hemorrhage (SDPH) has been recognized as a significant cause of mortality in male turkeys between 8 and 14 wk of age in many areas of North America (88, 214, 347). It was first recognized in Israel in 1973 (217). Documented mortality due to SDPH varies from 0.8 to 1.80% (88, 347). Estimates of mortality as high as 6% have been made (214). The syndrome has also been described as hypertensive angiopathy (158, 172).

The dead turkeys are in good condition, with food in their crops and the remainder of the gastrointestinal tract. They have congested and edematous lungs, splenomegaly, congested livers and digestive tracts, and clotted blood surrounding a portion or the whole of the kidneys (90, 173, 214, 347). Perirenal hemorrhage is not a consistent lesion (347). The most significant gross lesion is probably cardiac hypertrophy affecting the left ventricle and intraventricular septum (90, 173). Microscopic lesions include congestion in various organs, with edema in the lungs and hemorrhages in the lungs and kidneys (90, 173). Arterial lesions including internal vacuolation and medial hyperplasia have been found in affected turkeys (90, 158), but have also been recognized in normal control turkeys (214). Hyperplasia of the epithelium and a decrease of colloid in the thyroid glands were noted in the only study in which these glands were examined (173).

The most probable cause of death in SDPH is acute congestive heart failure secondary to cardiac hypertrophy. The renal hemorrhage may result from severe passive congestion, which may be compounded in part by closure of the renal valve in the renal portal circulation (173). The thyroid hyperplasia may contribute to the hypertrophic cardiomyopathy (173). Hypertension is common in young male turkeys (170) and may explain the cardiac hypertrophy and vascular lesions. It has been postulated that poor exercise tolerance in the modern turkey may result in cardiac arrhythmias and SDPH (18). Male turkeys have greater relative left and total ventricular weights than those of females of the same age. This might explain the greater susceptibility of male turkeys to SDPH (17).

Fast weight gain, continuous lighting programs, crowding, and hyperactivity have been suggested as factors that may influence the incidence of SDPH (214). Increased room temperature, toe clipping, step up/step down lighting, and dietary reserpine reduced the incidence of SDPH (89). Dietary aspirin had no effect on the incidence of SDPH (16, 89).

Aortic Rupture in Turkeys.

Aortic rupture or dissecting aneurysm of turkeys is characterized by sudden death in growing turkeys due to internal hemorrhage. The condition has been recognized throughout North America, in Europe, and in Israel. Mortality in the past has been reported to reach 50%, but losses in affected flocks at present usually only reach 1–2%. References to early reports and studies of the syndrome may be found in a review by Peckham (243).

CLINICAL SIGNS AND PATHOLOGY. The condition occurs in birds between 7 and 24 wk of age, with a peak mortality between 12 and 16 wk of age. The incidence is higher in male turkeys. Affected birds die suddenly. Gross and microscopic lesions have been described by McSherry et al. (204) and Pritchard et al. (247). At necropsy, the head, skin, and musculature are anemic. Occasionally, blood will run out of the mouth, or the oral cavity will be bloodstained. Upon internal examination, large clots of blood will be found in the abdominal cavity and beneath the capsule of the kidney. Clotted blood may be present in the pericardial sac, lungs, and leg muscle. Invariably, a longitudinal slit will be present in the aorta between the external iliac and sciatic arteries. In this region, the aorta is dilated; the wall is thin and has lost its elasticity. The tunica intima and media may be thrown into deep folds and partially separated from the tunica adventitia. Fibers of the tunica media may show mild to severe degenerative changes and may be infiltrated with heterophils and macrophages. The media may be thickened due to an increase in ground substance and fibroblastic proliferation. Dissolution or disappearance of the elastic laminae of the media occurs at the site of rupture. Degenerative changes and areas of erosion and cellular infiltration may be present in the adventitia. A marked intimal thickening or a large fibrous intimal plaque often occurs in the region of rupture. Sudan II stains reveal lipid accumulations in the affected intima.

PATHOGENESIS AND ETIOLOGY. Several reports have emphasized the possible role of intimal plaques in the pathogenesis of aortic rupture in turkeys. It has been suggested that these plaques and the absence of an intramural vasa vasorum around the abdominal aorta result in impaired nutrition to, and degeneration of, the media (216). High blood pressure in young male turkeys may also be a precipitating factor, but paradoxically, the administration of diethylstilbestrol decreased blood pressure and increased the incidence of aortic aneurysm (170, 171). Diets containing high levels of protein and fat may increase the incidence of aortic rupture (247). Copper is important in collagen synthesis and it has been suggested that copper deficiency may play a role in aortic rupture. It has been shown that liver levels of copper are low in turkeys dying from aortic aneurysm (98). This was a limited study and further investigation of the possible role of copper in aortic rupture is needed. ß-Aminoproprionitrile, a toxic product that occurs in the sweet pea (*Lathyrus odoratus*), will produce aortic rupture in the turkey but has not been incriminated in the field syndrome (243). Uncontrolled field studies suggest favorable results in treatment of ruptured aorta with reserpine. This has not been confirmed experimentally and such treatment may depress growth rate (243).

DISEASES OF THE RESPIRATORY SYSTEM

Emphysema. Subcutaneous emphysema is caused by an injury or defect in the respiratory tract that permits accumulation of air beneath the skin. This condition has been observed following rough handling and caponizing. After the caponizing operation, the skin incision may heal before the opening in the body wall, with a subsequent accumulation of air beneath the skin. This condition, commonly called a "windpuff," can be alleviated by puncturing the skin with a sharp instrument. In aquatic or flying birds, some of the pneumatic bones such as the humerus, coracoid, and sternum may fracture, allowing air to accumulate beneath the skin. Minor emphysematous bullae are common under the skin ventral to the proximal end of humerus in both turkeys and chickens. It is possible that they may be related to invasion of the humerus by the air sac during the first few weeks of life.

Cartilaginous and Osseous Lung Nodules in Broiler Chickens.
A low incidence of cartilaginous and osseous nodules have been reported in the lungs of birds for several years. Early reports were listed by Maxwell (189). More recent reports from Canada (145, 284) and the United Kingdom (336) indicate that a high incidence of such nodules is common in the modern broiler chicken. The nodules are much less common in egg-type chickens, turkeys, ducks, and geese (284, 336). The incidence of broiler chickens with nodules has been reported to be approximately 60% or greater (189, 284, 336). The incidence is probably 100% as the nodules can only be seen under the microscope and in surveys conducted to date only a limited number of sections of the lungs have been examined. The nodules have been recognized in meat-type chickens from 1 day to 52 wk of age (336). They may be more numerous at 3 wk of age (284), in the left as compared to the right lung (195), and in males (336).

PATHOLOGY. The nodules, though only visible under the microscope, may be as large as 240 μm in diameter (189) and have been classified into hyaline cartilaginous, fibrous cartilaginous, mineralized cartilaginous, and osseous (Fig. 35.14) (189, 284). Hyaline cartilaginous nodules consist of a circular mass of bluish to pink cartilage containing numerous chondrocytes in lacunae. The matrix of fibrous cartilaginous nodules is pink and has a fibrous appearance, lacunae are not apparent and the chondrocytes are pyknotic. Mineralized cartilaginous nodules are similar to fibrous nodules but are in part stained dark blue due to mineralization. The osseous nodules have a variable shape and stain red to purple and contain small cells resembling osteocytes. The nodules are found in the parenchyma of

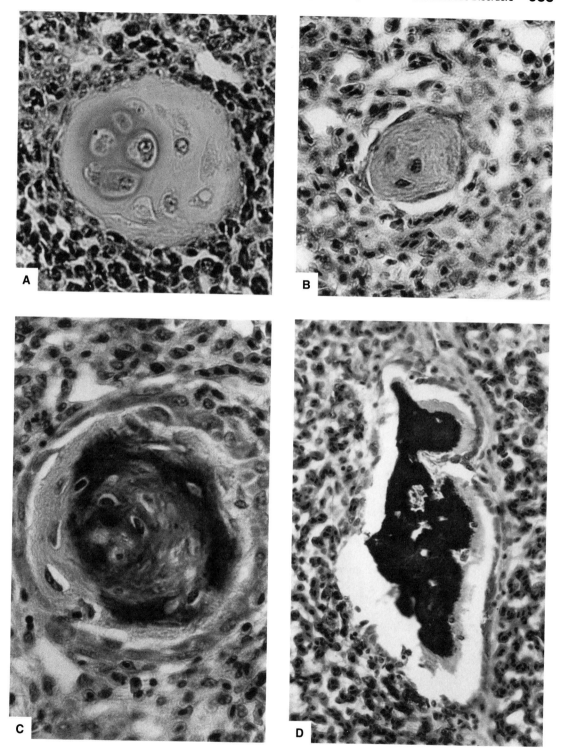

35.14. Cartilaginous and osseous nodules in microscopic sections from the lungs of broiler chickens. *A.* Hyaline cartilaginous nodule. H & E, ×528. *B.* Fibrous cartilaginous nodule. H & E, ×528. *C.* Mineralized cartilaginous nodule. H & E, ×528. *D.* Osseous nodule. Van Kossa stain, ×528. (Avian Dis)

lung lobules. All are located some distance from large airways and blood vessels. No reaction is visible around hyaline cartilaginous nodules, but the other types of nodules may be surrounded by a thin layer of fibrous cells, heterophils, and macrophages. The nodules appear to change with age from hyaline to fibrous to mineralized cartilaginous types, and finally, to an osseous type.

PATHOGENESIS AND ETIOLOGY. The cause and significance of these nodules are unknown. It has been suggested that the nodules may be derived from embolic chondrocytes arising from embryonic cartilage in developing bones (145) or from abnormal growth plates (284). No correlation could be found between incidence of nodules and skeletal deformities (145, 284). It is more probable that the nodules may be derived from chondrocytes displaced from nearby bronchi during early development (336). An increased incidence of nodules has been described in birds suffering from ascites and right heart failure (189, 195, 341). An increase in fibrous tissue in the lungs of such birds may lead to an increase in the number of nodules (189). An increased number of nodules has also been reported in broilers dying from other diseases, but the data could be questioned, as the control birds were kept in separate accommodations (195). The number of nodules is greater in broiler chickens fed *ad libitum* than in broiler chickens fed a restricted amount of food (284). A theory that the nodules may arise from inhaled dietary bonemeal has been disproven by the finding of the nodules in broiler chickens fed rations free of bone meal and animal protein (336).

DISEASES OF THE DIGESTIVE SYSTEM

Miscellaneous Conditions of the Upper Digestive System.
Peckham (243) reviewed four minor conditions of the upper digestive system. These conditions are rarely recognized today and are of limited importance. A stomatitis characterized by diphtheritic patches in the oral cavity of chickens was attributed to *Spirillum pulli*. Beak necrosis, in which the mandible sloughs in chickens, and curled tongue in turkeys were associated with impaction of fine mash feeds in the mouths of affected birds. Crop impaction occurred when large amounts of fibrous material were ingested and formed a ball in the crop.

Pendulous Crop.
Pendulous crop occurs at a low incidence in many chicken and turkey flocks. In some flocks, the incidence may reach 5%. In severely affected birds, the crop is greatly distended and full of feed, particles of bedding, and fluid, which is often foul smelling (Fig. 35.15). The lining of the crop may be ulcerated. Birds continue to eat,

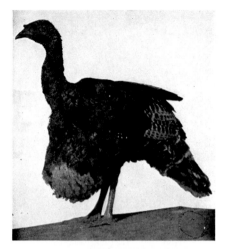

35.15. An 8-mo-old female turkey with pendulous crop of about 5 mo duration. (Peckham)

but digestion is impaired and birds become emaciated. Death may result and carcasses of affected birds are generally condemned at processing. The possible etiologies of pendulous crop were discussed by Peckham (243). A hereditary predisposition has been suggested in turkeys. An increased incidence has been noted in turkeys after increased liquid intake in hot weather. Neither of these factors appear to be important when a high incidence is encountered in modern poultry flocks. The possibility that diet may influence the incidence of pendulous crop is supported by the experimental production of pendulous crops with rations containing cerelose as a substitute for starch. Further research is needed on the etiology of pendulous crop.

Dilation of the Proventriculus in Chickens.
In 4-wk-old chicks fed a purified diet, dilation of the proventriculus was first reported as proventricular hypertrophy by Newberne et al. (218). The abnormality is commonly observed as an incidental finding in broiler chickens. Occasionally, a high incidence in a broiler chicken flock may cause significant carcass contamination when enlarged proventriculi rupture at processing. The enlarged proventriculi have greatly dilated thin walls and are full of feed. The gizzards in affected birds are poorly developed and there is no sharp demarcation between the gizzard and proventriculus (Fig. 35.16). The poor development of the gizzard is generally the result of a finely ground diet lacking in fiber, and the dilation of the proventriculus is secondary (260).

Gizzard Impaction.
Gizzard impaction can cause high mortality during the first 3 wk of life in

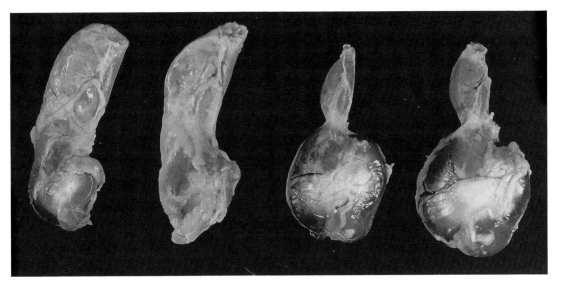

35.16. Gizzards and dilated proventriculi from broiler chickens fed only a commercial broiler starter (*left*) compared with those from broiler chickens fed a broiler starter containing oat hulls (*right*). The former gizzards are small and the proventriculi enlarged. (Avian Dis)

turkey flocks. The condition is rare in chickens. Affected poults are emaciated, with empty intestinal tracts, but gizzards are full of a solid mass of interwoven fibrous material. This fibrous mass often extends into the first part of the duodenum, and in some birds, masses of fibrous material are found lower in the intestine. The impaction results from the birds eating litter that the gizzard is unable to handle. Prevention is aimed at discouraging the eating of litter by young poults.

DISEASES OF THE LIVER

Fatty Liver–Hemorrhagic Syndrome.
This syndrome has been recognized in laying hens in many countries of the world. It occurs primarily in egg-type birds kept in cages, but has also been recognized as a less significant problem in birds kept on litter; outbreaks occur sporadically. Reviews by Butler (30) and Meijering (205) form the basis of the following description.

CLINICAL SIGNS AND PATHOLOGY. In outbreaks of fatty liver–hemorrhagic syndrome (FLHS) there is often a sudden drop in egg production. Hens may be overweight, with large pale combs and wattles covered with dandruff. The first sign of disease is often an increase in mortality, with birds in full production being found dead with pale heads. Mortality usually does not reach 5%. Dead birds have large blood clots in the abdomen, often partially enveloping the liver and arising from the liver (Fig.

35.17). The liver is generally enlarged, pale, and friable; it may have smaller hematomas within the parenchyma. These hematomas may be recent and dark red, or older and green to brown. Similar hematomas may be seen in clinically healthy birds in the same flock if such are examined during or after an outbreak. Large amounts of fat are present in the abdominal cavity and around the viscera. Dead birds are in full production and often have a developing egg in the oviduct.

Microscopic examination of the liver shows hepatocytes distended with fat vacuoles, varying sized hemorrhages and organizing hematomas, and often small irregular masses of uniform eosinophilic material. These masses, which are amyloidlike in appearance, have been identified as a possible derivative of plasma protein and similar to fibrin (337). The fat content of livers generally exceeds 40% dry weight and may reach 70%. The proportion of oleic acid in the lipids is increased. No changes have been found in concentrations of major plasma proteins, the glucose level, or the activities of glutamate-oxalactate transaminase, ß-glucuronidase, and lactate dehydrogenase.

PATHOGENESIS AND ETIOLOGY. The etiology of FLHS was discussed by Squires and Leeson (300) and Hansen and Walzem (107). Excessive consumption of high-energy diets in birds whose exercise is restricted in cages is considered to result in a positive energy balance and excessive fat deposition. This may be compounded by hot weather. Low

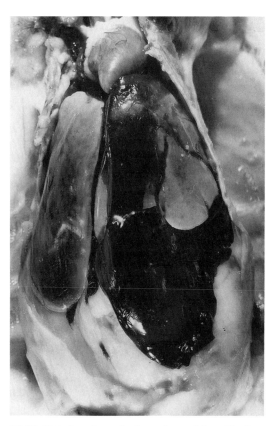

35.17. Fatty liver–hemorrhagic syndrome. A large blood clot is molded over one lobe of the liver. Note excess abdominal fat. (Peckham)

levels of dietary calcium may result in increased feed consumption, liver fat, and liver hemorrhage (279). Laying hens, however, can have high levels of fat in their livers without hemorrhage. The pathogenesis and cause of the hemorrhage has not been defined. Excessive fat may disrupt architecture of the liver and result in weakening of the reticular framework and blood vessels in the liver. A pathogenic relationship between hepatic steatosis and hemorrhage has been suggested (240). Lysis of the reticulin framework of the liver has been reported in FLHS. A strong association of reticulolysis with severity of liver hemorrhage has been described in experimental birds. Rupture of intrahepatic portal veins associated with degenerative changes in the veins was described in the same birds (188). Focal necrosis of hepatocytes leading to vascular injury has been described as another mechanism to explain the hemorrhage (132, 352). It has been postulated that excessive lipid peroxidation of unsaturated fatty acids in the liver may overwhelm cell repair mechanisms and result in tissue damage (300). Quail fed diets designed to induce hepatic steatosis and limit biologic oxidant defenses devel-

oped a syndrome similar to FLHS in chickens. Liver hemorrhage in these quail was reduced by adding vitamin E to the diet, but not by adding glutathione (299). In an attempt to test this postulate in chickens, the diet of a strain of chickens susceptible to FLHS was supplemented with ascorbic acid, tocopherol or L-cysteine. None of these compounds, all of which have a role against oxidation, prevented FLHS (51). The observation of greatly elevated serum calcium and cholesterol in chickens from flocks with FLHS suggests that the syndrome may be due to a hormone imbalance (111, 206). Injection of immature chickens with estradiol has been shown to result in hepatic steatosis and hemorrhage (241). Similar injection of laying hens caused liver enlargement, death from liver hemorrhage, and neurologic disorders (301).

Many papers describing the field treatment of FLHS with specific nutrients, and experiments testing the effect of specific nutrients added to the diet of laying hens on the level of hepatic fat, were reviewed by Butler (30). He concluded that the results were inconsistent and provided no useful conclusions as to the etiology or treatment of FLHS. Stake et al. (301) listed some more recent papers in which the incidence and severity of FLHS were reported to have been reduced by unidentified nutritional factors in alfalfa, dried brewer's grains, soybean mill feed, wheat bran, vitamin E, dried brewer's yeast and torula yeast, fish meal, and fermentation by-products. Increasing the fat content of the diet, especially with fats high in linoleic acid, will decrease liver fat and increase liver content of linoleic acid (205).

In several reports, mortality in laying hens due to liver hemorrhage has been associated with the use of rapeseed meal in the diet (242). As this may occur without the development of fatty livers, it may be a separate syndrome (300). In addition, rapeseed meal has been shown experimentally to increase the extent and severity of liver hemorrhage, but in these experiments, liver hemorrhage also occurred in birds not fed rapeseed meal (188, 242). The possibility of toxins causing FLHS should not be ignored. Aflatoxin has been considered as a possible cause but produces different liver lesions.

DISEASES OF THE URINARY SYSTEM.
An excellent review of renal pathology of the fowl by Siller (293) forms the basis for the following descriptions. These brief descriptions cover only conditions of major importance commonly seen in commercial poultry, and the reader is referred to the above review for more detailed information and descriptions of miscellaneous conditions such as congenital malformations and baby chick nephropathy.

Gout. Gout is a common finding during necropsy of poultry. It is the result of abnormal accumulation of urates and occurs as two distinct syndromes. Articular gout is characterized by tophi, deposits of urates around joints, particularly those of the feet. The joints are enlarged and the feet appear deformed (Fig. 35.18). When these joints are opened, the periarticular tissue is white due to urate deposition, and white semifluid deposits of urates may be found within the joints. Articular gout is a sporadic individual bird problem of little economic importance in poultry. As it has been reproduced by feeding high-protein diets, it is tempting to infer that it results from excess production of uric acid. Studies in a line of chickens bred for susceptibility to articular gout, however, indicate that they may have a defect in tubular secretion of uric acid.

Visceral gout, which has also been called visceral urate deposition, is characterized by precipitation of urates in the kidneys and on serous surfaces of the heart, liver, mesenteries, air sacs, and peritoneum. In severe cases, surfaces of muscles and synovial sheaths of tendons and joints may be involved, and precipitation may occur within the liver and spleen. The deposits on serosal surfaces appear grossly as a white chalky coating, while those within viscera may only be recognized microscopically. Much urate is lost when tissues are processed for histology, but evidence of its presence is often seen as blue or pink amorphous material under the microscope. Feathery crystals or basophilic spherical masses may be seen within tissues under the microscope in some cases.

Visceral urate deposition is generally due to a failure of urinary excretion. This may be due to obstruction of ureters, renal damage, or dehydration. Raised levels of uric acid in the blood have been reported in both renal disease and articular gout in the absence of visceral urate deposition. A change in concentration of some constituent of the intercellular fluid due to renal disease is probably needed to cause precipitation of the urates. Dehydration due to water deprivation is a common cause of visceral

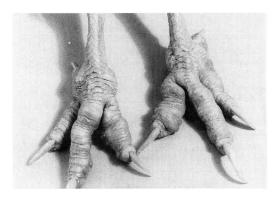

35.18. Gout in a mature chicken causing enlargement and deformity of toes and feet. (Peckham)

gout in domestic poultry. Outbreaks of visceral gout in poultry have also been attributed to vitamin A deficiency, excess dietary calcium, treatment with sodium bicarbonate, and a mycotoxin, oosporein (244). Kidney damage can cause death of birds without visceral gout occurring. Outbreaks of renal gout in which kidneys are enlarged and often distended with urates result when flocks of young chickens are infected with nephrotropic strains of infectious bronchitis virus.

Avian Monocytosis.   The term *avian monocytosis* has been used to describe a variable condition in young laying hens. Prominent features of the condition include cyanosis of the head, diarrhea, monocytosis, hepatic necrosis, and renal gout. The condition was widely reported throughout the world from 1929 to circa 1960. Published reports decreased after 1960, but it was still reported in the American Association of Avian Pathologists' summary of disease reports until 1982 (298). A review of the condition was written by Jungherr and Pomeroy (167). Avian monocytosis is rarely recognized today.

CLINICAL SIGNS AND PATHOLOGY.   In an affected flock, many birds develop inappetence, depression, and diarrhea. Combs and wattles become shrunken and cyanotic. Egg production decreases and up to 50% mortality may occur. Dead birds are often dehydrated and pectoral muscles may have white streaks. The ovaries exhibit regressive changes and free yolk may be present in the abdominal cavity. Catarrhal enteritis and a chalky pancreas have been reported. Livers are often dark in color and may have scattered pinpoint foci of necrosis. The kidneys are generally swollen and contain prominent urate deposits. Microscopic lesions include Zenker's degeneration of breast muscle, focal necrosis in the liver, thickening of basement membranes, dilation of Bowman's space in glomeruli, and degeneration of tubules, with casts and urate crystals associated with heterophils and giant cells in the kidneys. A relative and absolute monocytosis has been reported in the blood of affected birds.

PATHOGENESIS AND ETIOLOGY.   Cumming (44) reviewed the possible etiology of avian monocytosis. He stated that avian monocytosis has never been clearly defined and that the great number of synonyms used exemplifies the confusion regarding the condition. The condition was often called bluecomb. Many different entities may have been included in the bluecomb complex. He noted that a decrease in outbreaks of avian monocytosis in North America in the 1940s coincided with deliberate exposure of young pullets to infectious bronchitis virus. In flocks that were range-reared, many pullets may have reached sexual maturity without exposure to infectious bronchitis. At the same time, soybean meal replaced meat meal in poultry rations. Nephrotropic infectious bronchitis viruses will cause higher mortalities in susceptible chickens if they are fed diets containing meat meal. Other causes of avian monocytosis that have been postulated include water deprivation, nephrotoxic substances in new wheat, overheating, a sodium-potassium imbalance, and other infectious agents (167).

Urolithiasis. In recent years, outbreaks of mortality in laying flocks have been attributed to urolithiasis in both the United Kingdom (15, 252) and the United States (26, 41, 184). Urolithiasis is characterized by severe atrophy of one or both kidneys, distended ureters often containing uroliths, and varying degrees of renal and visceral gout.

CLINICAL SIGNS AND PATHOLOGY. Overall mortality in affected flocks may exceed 2% for several months, and in excess of 50% of this mortality may be due to urolithiasis (15, 184). Renal lesions have been recognized in clinically normal birds in flocks undergoing an outbreak, and 3.2–6.3% of hens in some affected flocks had renal lesions at processing (184). Laying chickens die suddenly and may be in good condition and in full lay (15) or they may have a reduced muscle mass, small pale combs, and white pasting on pericloacal feathers (26). Diffuse visceral urate deposits, atrophied kidneys, and dilated ureters are found in affected birds (15, 26, 184) (Fig. 35.19). The kidney atrophy is often more severe in anterior lobes and is unilateral, but it may be bilateral. The surviving ipsilateral or contralateral lobes may be enlarged. The ureters arising from the atrophied lobes are dilated and full of clear mucus and often contain white irregular concretions or uroliths (26). These uroliths are composed of compact masses of microcrystalline to fine pleomorphic crystals of calcium sodium urate, with random substitution of magnesium and potassium for the calcium and sodium, respectively (227). Microscopic lesions in affected kidneys consist of dilation of ureter branches and tubules, tubular degeneration and loss of tubules, cellular casts, urate crystals, and varying degrees of fibrosis (15, 26). Urolithiasis has been primarily recognized as a disease of laying birds, but reports indicate that lesions and mortality may start during the rearing period (26, 41). In a sequential study of one outbreak, minor focal cortical tubular necrosis was found by microscopic study in grossly normal kidneys of 4-wk-old pullets. In 7-wk-old pullets, the kidneys were grossly swollen with tubular necrosis and casts, eosinophilic globules in glomeruli, and interstitial infiltration of heterophils and lymphocytes. Typical lesions of urolithiasis were found in 14-wk-old birds (26).

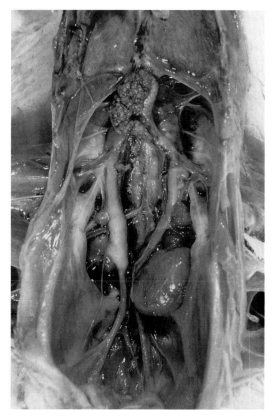

35.19. Urolithiasis in a chicken. Severe atrophy of the right kidney and anterior lobes of the left kidney. The right ureter is distended with white material.

PATHOGENESIS AND ETIOLOGY. Wideman et al. (329) conducted renal function studies on chickens during outbreaks of urolithiasis and concluded that the physiologic impact of the kidney damage was the result of reduced renal mass, rather than of inappropriate renal handling of minerals or electrolytes. A significant reduction in number of glomeruli has also been reported in birds affected by urolithiasis (223). The uroliths may cause sudden death by plugging ureters but probably occur secondary to kidney damage (184). The lesions described in outbreaks of urolithiasis are similar to those described in a long-term study of the pathogenesis of infection of chickens with infectious bronchitis virus (2). In many outbreaks of urolithiasis, it has been difficult to isolate infectious bronchitis virus from affected laying birds (15, 26, 184). This would not be unexpected, as recovery of infectious bronchitis virus was erratic in the long-term study mentioned above. Infectious bronchitis viruses, which have been shown to cause renal damage in experimental chickens, have been isolated in recent outbreaks of urolithiasis (26, 41). In several outbreaks, potential problems in vaccination programs against infectious bronchitis have been identified (15, 41, 184). Excess dietary calcium, in particular if combined with low available dietary phosphorus, fed to growing pullets has caused urolithiasis in experimental trials (94, 289, 330). Exposure of pullets to the Gray strain of infectious bronchitis virus subsequent to feeding a high-calcium laying ration increased the incidence of urolithiasis and gross kidney damage (96). A marked difference in susceptibility to urolithiasis caused by high-calcium diets has been described between two strains of leghorn chickens (178). The more susceptible strain produced more alkaline urine and had a higher proportion of juxtamedullary nephrons (328). Formation of uroliths may be due to high levels of urinary calcium and decreased hydrogen ions in the urine (96). Dietary acidification with ammonium chloride, ammonium sulfate, or methionine has been shown to decrease the incidence of uroliths and gross kidney lesions in urolithiasis induced experimentally with high-calcium diets (95, 178, 326, 331, 332). The use of ammonium chloride was not considered a practical treatment for use in the field because it caused increased water consumption, urine flow, and manure moisture (95). The other compounds did not appear to have this disadvantage (178, 332). Ammonium sulfate was more effective than two forms of methionine in a single trial (178). Water deprivation has been suggested as a cause of urolithiasis on the basis of field observations (144). The fact that some mycotoxins are nephrotoxic led to the suggestion that they should be considered as a potential cause of urolithiasis (184).

DISEASES OF THE EYE

Ammonia Burn.   Ammonia burn describes a keratoconjunctivitis in poultry caused by exposure to ammonia fumes resulting from unsanitary conditions. Peckham (243) reviewed the condition. Affected birds keep their eyelids closed and are reluctant to move. They may rub their head and eyelids against their wings. The cornea has a gray cloudy appearance and may be ulcerated. Edema and hyperemia may be present in the conjunctiva but often may not be very obvious. The condition is generally bilateral and affected birds do not eat and become emaciated. Many birds recover if exposure to ammonia fumes is eliminated. Time of recovery depends on the severity of damage to the cornea and may take 1 mo or longer if lesions are severe. Prevention of the condition is based on proper ventilation and litter management. The ammonia fumes are formed in wet litter.

Blepharoconjunctivitis in Turkeys.   Bierer (12, 13) and Sanger et al. (283) described a disease of breeder turkeys characterized by inflammation of the eyelids, excess lacrimation, and in severe cases, destruction of the eyeball. Mortality was low but morbidity reached 15–40% and resulted in economic loss from poor production performance. White frothy foam at the anterior canthus of the eye was followed by accumulation of caseous exudate and swelling of eyelids, which became encrusted and closed. Ulceration of the cornea resulted in panophthalmitis and destruction of the eyeball. The cause was not determined. Treatment with antibiotics, supplemental vitamin A, and a change to clean warm quarters caused improvement.

Eye-Notch Syndrome.   Eye-notch syndrome refers to a widespread lesion in the eyelid of caged layers (243). The condition appears to start as a small scab or erosion on the lower lid, which develops into a fissure with a tag of flesh attached to one side. The significance and cause of the condition is unknown.

Chorioretinitis and Buphthalmos.   A turkey blindness syndrome due to chorioretinitis and buphthalmos was described in turkeys by Barnett et al. (8). Similar eye abnormalities were previously described in turkeys (285) and in chickens (335).

CLINICAL SIGNS AND PATHOLOGY.   The turkey blindness syndrome occurred in turkey breeder flocks (8). The incidence of eye lesions ranged from 2 to 30%, and egg production was reduced. Blind poults could be recognized by their wandering movement, their tendency to peer at objects in a short-sighted manner, and occasionally by their holding their heads to one side. Blind poults grew normally and were able to locate feed and water. Eyeballs were enlarged by 5–7 wk of age and the corneas flattened. The palpebral fissures became oval. By 16–20 wk of age, many birds had cataracts. Ophthalmoscopic examination of affected eyes revealed pale areas in the retina. On section, severely affected eyes contained an abnormal fluid and some were hard to cut due to bone formation within the eye. Microscopic changes in affected eyes included choroid thickening, degeneration and detachment of the retina, and in severe cases, fibroplasia and islands of ossifying cartilage in the posterior chamber.

PATHOGENESIS AND ETIOLOGY.   Similar lesions to those just described have been induced in experimental turkeys by rearing them on continual artificial light (5, 8). Rearing experimental chickens under continuous light has caused enlargement of eye-balls, decreased corneal curvature, thinning of the retina and an accumulation of fluid in the vitreous body (174). Birds reared on low intensity, but diurnal, light also develop enlarged eyes, but in such eyes the corneas protrude rather than become flattened (118). Eye enlargement in chickens may also be induced by darkness (137).

DISEASES OF THE REPRODUCTIVE SYSTEM

Cystic Right Oviduct. In the female chicken embryo, two Müllerian ducts start to develop into oviducts. The left duct develops into a functional oviduct, while the right duct regresses. If this regression is not complete, partial development will result in a cystic right oviduct. Cystic right oviducts are common incidental findings in postmortem examination of chickens. They vary in size from small, 2-cm diameter, elongated cysts to large fluid-filled sacs up to 10 cm or more in diameter (Fig. 35.20). Small cysts are of little consequence, but large cysts compress the abdominal viscera. The large sacs can result in a bird with a pendulous abdomen and should be differentiated from ascites.

False Layer. The term *false layer* has been used to describe a bird that has the characteristics of a bird in production, visiting the nest regularly but not laying eggs (131). This bird has a normal-appearing ovary and oviduct, but the infundibulum fails to engulf the ovum after it has been ovulated. At necropsy, these birds show excessive amounts of orange-colored fat and have liquid yolk or coagulated yolk in the body cavity. This defect may result

as a sequel to infectious bronchitis at an early age (24, 25).

Internal Layer. In some birds, soft-shelled eggs or fully formed eggs may be found in the peritoneal cavity. This indicates that the yolk progressed normally through the oviduct to a certain point and then reverse peristalsis discharged the egg into the body cavity. A bird with a large accumulation of eggs in the peritoneal cavity may assume a penguinlike posture.

Impacted Oviduct. Occasionally, an oviduct is occluded by masses of yolk, coagulated albumen, shell membranes, and in some instances, fully formed eggs. Large masses of yolklike material may also be found in the oviduct, and upon transection, these masses have the appearance of concentric rings.

Egg-Bound. This term is used to describe a condition in which an egg is lodged in the cloaca but cannot be laid. It may result from inflammation of the oviduct, partial paralysis of the muscles of the oviduct, or production of an egg so large that it is physically impossible for it to be laid. Young pullets laying an unusually large egg are more prone to the problem.

Abnormal Eggs and Depressed Production. Poor egg quality and depressed egg production are common problems that cause great economic loss to the poultry industry. They can be due to a multitude of factors involving nutrition, management, environment, and disease. Reviews related to the topic have been written by Hanson (108), Overfield (233), Wolford and Tanaka (348), and Peckham (243).

DISEASES OF THE INTEGUMENTARY SYSTEM

Contact Dermatitis and Pododermatitis. Erosive lesions affecting the skin on the plantar surface of the feet, the posterior surface of the hocks, or overlying the sternum have been recognized as a significant problem in turkeys in the United Kingdom (186, 344) and in North America (97, 215), and in broiler chickens in the United Kingdom (101, 203), in North America (110), and in Australia (215). Ulcers and erosions of the skin covering the thigh of broiler chickens have been described as scabby hip syndrome in North America (117). A common feature of all of these skin lesions is that they appear to be due to contact irritation and are associated with poor litter conditions.

CLINICAL SIGNS AND PATHOLOGY. The lesions have been described by Martland (186) and Greene

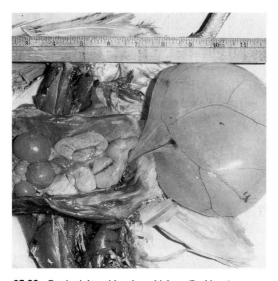

35.20. Cystic right oviduct in a chicken. (Peckham)

et al. (101). Pododermatitis appears as dark black scabs filling ulcers on the ventral metatarsal and digital foot pads. Early changes include enlargement of foot scales, cracks, abrasions, and a superficial scab. These changes proceed to a deep ulcer. Histologic lesions include defective keratin in the *stratum intermedium,* particularly adjacent to the ulcer, and infiltration of heterophils in adjacent epidermis. The center of the lesion is occupied by a necrotic mass of cellular debris, which may enclose plant material and bacteria. The base of the mass is underlain by heterophils and often macrophages and a line of giant cells. Many birds, in addition to the foot lesions, have similar ulcers filled with black scabs on the posterior of the hock and on the breast. In some focal ulcers on the breasts of turkeys, a granulomatous response with giant cells was not noted but connective tissue proliferation occurred below the ulcers (97). Scabby hip syndrome in broiler chickens in North America is characterized by ulcers and erosions covered by scabs on the skin of the thigh of broilers. It differs from other syndromes in that foot and breast lesions were not reported (117). Contact dermatitis has resulted in downgrading of broiler carcasses (203) and experimental studies have demonstrated that severe foot lesions may result in lameness and a depression of body weight (186, 187).

PATHOGENESIS AND ETIOLOGY. Field outbreaks of contact dermatitis have been associated with poor litter conditions (101). In an epidemiologic study, lesions were more frequent with increased stocking density, increased age, and particular feeds, and in male birds in winter (203). In experimental studies, the incidence of dermatitis has been increased by deliberate wetting of litter (112, 186, 187). In an early report of pododermatitis in experimental birds, it was suggested that soybean-based diets may contribute to the condition (138). This has not been confirmed (215). In other early experimental studies, it was also suggested that marginal deficiencies of biotin may cause the condition (110, 112). This appears to be an unlikely cause under modern conditions. Breast blisters involving the formation of a subcutaneous cyst between the skin and the sternum (202) should be distinguished from the ulcerative lesions of contact dermatitis in the skin overlying the sternum. Both may be found in the same flock (187), but the breast blisters are more probably due to prolonged pressure from sitting (202) rather than contact irritation.

Vesicular Dermatitis and Photosensitization.

Vesicular dermatitis characterized by vesicle and scab formation on feet and toes and, occasionally, on unfeathered portions of the head has been described in chickens, turkeys, ducks, and geese. Peckham (243) reviewed the condition and

the reader is referred to his review for specific citations. In outbreaks, up to 20% mortality and severe drops in egg production have occurred. Erythema may proceed vesicle and scab formation. Beak deformation (Fig. 35.21) and scarring of foot webs with upturning of toes (Fig. 35.22) may be sequelae in ducks. The condition in some outbreaks has been shown to be due to photosensitization following ingestion of *Ammi visnaga* and *A. majus* seeds and *Cymopterus watsonii* and *C. longipes* plants and seeds. In some outbreaks of vesicular dermatitis, the photodynamic agent has not been identified. Vesicular dermatitis has been reproduced with *Lolium temulenetum* contaminated with *Cladosporium herboneum* without exposure to sunlight.

Xanthomatosis.
This unusual condition characterized by an accumulation of semifluid yellow-

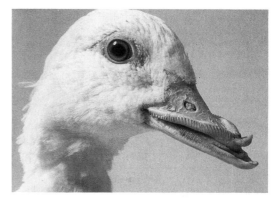

35.21. Chronic lesion of photosensitization in Muscovy duck. Loss of normal epithelium on surface of beak, upturning of edges of beak and foreshortening of upper beak. (Peckham)

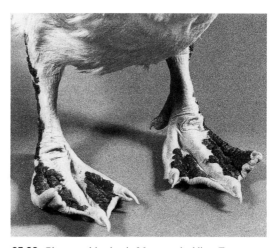

35.22. Photosensitization in Muscovy duckling. Toes upturned and thick brown scabs on footwebs and lateral aspect of legs. (Peckham)

ish material under the skin of chickens was reported as a significant flock problem circa 1960. Peckham (243) reviewed case reports and studies of the condition. White leghorn hens were primarily affected, and the incidence of affected birds in flocks reached 60%. Birds with lesions were bright, active, and in production. Wattles were often swollen. Swellings also occurred on the breast, abdomen, and feathered portions of the legs. The swellings often became nodular and pendulous. Initially, the lesions were soft and fluctuating and contained a honey-colored fluid. Later, they became firm with chalky white areas of cholesterol interspersed through the abnormal thickened subcutaneous tissue. Histopathologic changes included massive infiltration of foamy macrophages (Fig. 35.23), cholesterol clefts (Fig. 35.24), and giant cells. The cause is unknown, but because the xanthomatous tissue contained high levels of hydrocarbons it was postulated that a hydrocarbon in animal feed may have caused the condition.

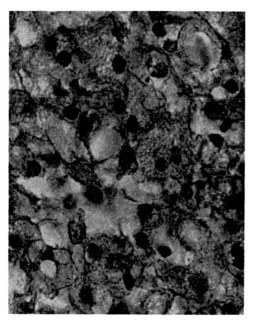

35.23. Histologic section of xanthomatous lesion illustrating vacuolated cytoplasm in foam cells. ×470. (AFIP 54-7256)

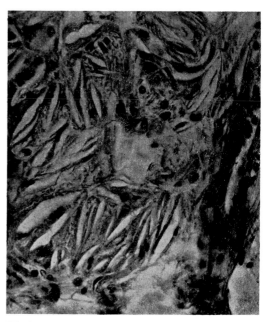

35.24. Histologic section of xanthomatous lesion showing cholesterol clefts. ×470. (AFIP 54-5394)

REFERENCES

1. Acar, N., F.G. Sizemore, G.R. Leach, R.F. Wideman, R.L. Owen, and G.F. Barbato. 1995. Growth of broiler chickens in response to feed restriction regimens to reduce ascites. Poult Sci 74:833–843.

2. Alexander, D.J., R.E. Gough, and M. Pattison. 1978. A long-term study of the pathogenesis of infection of fowls with three strains of avian infectious bronchitis virus. Res Vet Sci 24:228–233.

3. Anonymous. 1985. Upsurge of ascites in broilers. Vet Rec 116:559.

4. Anthony, N.P., J.M. Balog, F.B. Staudinger, C.W. Wall, R.D. Walker, and W.E. Huff. 1994. Effect of a urease inhibitor and ceiling fans on ascites in broilers. I. Environmental variability and incidence of ascites. Poult Sci 73:801–809.

5. Ashton, W.L.G., M. Pattison, and K.C. Barnett. 1973. Light-induced eye abnormalities in turkeys and the turkey blindness syndrome. Res Vet Sci 14:42–46.

6. Bai, Y., and M.E. Cook. 1994. Histological study of tibial dyschondroplasia-like lesion from light-type chicks fed cysteine-supplemental diets. Avian Dis 38:557–562.

7. Balog, J.M., N.B. Anthony, C.W. Wall, R.D. Walker, N.C. Rath, and W.E. Huff. 1994. Effect of a urease inhibitor and ceiling fans on ascites in broilers. 2. Blood variables, ascites scores, and body and organ weights. Poult Sci 73:810–816.

8. Barnett, K.C., W.L.G. Ashton, G. Holford, I. MacPherson, and P.D. Simm. 1971. Chorioretinitis and buphthalmos in turkeys. Vet Rec 88:620–627.

9. Bass, C.C. 1939. Control of "nose-picking" form of cannibalism in young closely confined quail fed raw meat. Proc Soc Exp Biol Med 40:488–489.

10. Baxter, M.R. 1994. The welfare problems of laying hens in battery cages. Vet Rec 134:614–619.

11. Bergmann, V. and M. Pietsch. 1976. Beiträge zur differentialdiagnose der bewegungsstörungen beim junghuhn. 4. Mitt.: Tibiatorsion beim perlhuhn-eine perosisähnliche erkrankung in einem perlhuhnmastbetrieb. Monatsh Veterinaermed 31:581–585.

12. Bierer, B.W. 1956. Keratoconjunctivitis in turkeys: A

preliminary report. Vet Med 51:363–366.

13. Bierer, B.W. 1958. Keratoconjunctivitis in turkeys. II. The relationship of vitamin A, infectious agents and environmental factors to the disease. Vet Med 53:477–483.

14. Blair, R., J.P. Jacob, and E.E. Gardiner. 1990. Effect of dietary protein source and cereal type on the incidence of sudden death syndrome in broiler chickens. Poult Sci 69:1331–1338.

15. Blaxland, J.D., E.D. Borland, W.G. Siller, and L. Martindale. 1980. An investigation of urolithiasis in two flocks of laying fowls. Avian Pathol 9:5–19.

16. Boulianne, M., and D.B. Hunter. 1990. Aspirin: A treatment for sudden death syndrome in turkeys? Proc 39th West Poult Dis Conf, pp. 89–90.

17. Boulianne, M., D.B. Hunter, R.J. Julian, M.R. O'-Grady, and P.W. Physick-Sheard. 1992. Cardiac muscle mass distribution in the domestic turkey and relationship to electrocardiogram. Avian Dis 36:582–589.

18. Boulianne, M., D.B. Hunter, L. Viel, P.W. Physick-Sheard, and R.J. Julian. 1993. Effect of exercise on the cardiovascular and respiratory systems of heavy turkeys and relevance to sudden death syndrome. Avian Dis 37:83–97.

19. Bowes, V.A. 1990. Personal communication.

20. Bowes, V.A., and R.J. Julian. 1988. Organ weights of normal broiler chickens and those dying of sudden death syndrome. Can Vet J 29:153–156.

21. Bowes, V.A., R.J. Julian, S. Leeson, and T. Stirtzinger. 1988. Effect of feed restriction on feed efficiency and incidence of sudden death syndrome in broiler chickens. Poult Sci 67:1102–1104.

22. Breeding, S.W., W.A. McRee, M.D. Ficken, and P.R. Ferket. 1994. Effect of protein restriction during brooding on spontaneous turkey cardiomyopathy. Avian Dis 38:366–370.

23. Brigden, J.L., and C. Riddell. 1975. A survey of mortality in four broiler flocks in western Canada. Can Vet J 16:194–200.

24. Broadfoot, D.I., B.S. Pomeroy, and W.M. Smith, Jr. 1954. Effects of infectious bronchitis on egg production. J Am Vet Med Assoc 124:128–130.

25. Broadfoot, D.I., B.S. Pomeroy, and W.M. Smith Jr. 1956. Effects of infectious bronchitis in baby chicks. Poult Sci 35:757–762.

26. Brown, T.P., J.R. Glisson, G. Rosales, P. Villegas, and R.B. Davis. 1987. Studies of avian urolithiasis associated with an infectious bronchitis virus. Avian Dis 31:629–636.

27. Buenrostro, J.L., and F.H. Kratzer. 1982. A nutritional approach to the "flip-over" syndrome. Proc 31st West Poult Dis Conf, pp. 76–79.

28. Burton, R.R., and A.H. Smith. 1967. Effect of polycythemia and chronic hypoxia on heart mass in the chicken. J Appl Physiol 22:782–785.

29. Burton, R.W., A.K. Sheridan, and C.R. Howlett. 1981. The incidence and importance of tibial dyschondroplasia to the commercial broiler industry in Australia. Br Poult Sci 22:153–160.

30. Butler, E.J. 1976. Fatty liver diseases in the domestic fowl: A review. Avian Pathol 5:1–14.

31. Buys, S.B., and P. Barnes. 1981. Ascites in broilers. Vet Rec 108:266.

32. Carlton, W.W., and W. Henderson. 1964. Skeletal lesions in experimental copper-deficiency in chickens. Avian Dis 8:48–55.

33. Cassidy, D.M., M.A. Gibson, and F.G. Proudfoot. 1975. The histology of cardiac blood clots in chicks exhibiting the "flip-over" syndrome. Poult Sci 54:1882–1886.

34. Chambers, J.R. 1986. Heritability of crippling and acute death syndrome in sire and dam strains of broiler chickens. Poult Sci 65(Suppl 1):23.

35. Chu, Q., W. Weidong, M.E. Cook, and E.B. Smalley. 1995. Induction of tibial dyschondroplasia and suppression of cell-mediated immunity in chickens by Fusarium oxysporum grown on sterile corn. Avian Dis 39:100–107.

36. Chung, H.C., W. Guenter, R.G. Rotter, G.H. Crow, and N.E. Stanger. 1993. Effects of dietary fat source on sudden death syndrome and cardiac sarcoplasmic reticular calcium transport in broiler chickens. Poult Sci 72:310–316.

37. Classen, H.L., and C. Riddell. 1989. Photoperiodic effects on performance and leg abnormalities in broiler chickens. Poult Sci 68:873–879.

38. Classen, H.L., M.R. Bedford, and A.A. Olkowski. 1992. Thiamine nutrition and sudden death syndrome in broiler chickens. Proceedings of the XIXth World's Poultry Congress, vol 1. Amsterdam, pp. 572–574.

39. Classen, H.L., C. Riddell, F.E. Robinson, P.J. Shand, and A.R. McCurdy. 1994. Effect of lighting treatment on the productivity, health, behaviour and sexual maturity of heavy male turkeys. Br Poult Sci 35:215–225.

40. Cook, M.E., Y. Bai, and M.W. Orth. 1994. Factors influencing growth plate cartilage turnover. Poult Sci 73:889–896.

41. Cowen, B.S., R.F. Wideman, H. Rothenbacher, and M.O. Braune. 1987. An outbreak of avian urolithiasis on a large commercial egg farm. Avian Dis 31:392–397.

42. Craig, F. 1967. Traumatic hock disorder in poultry. Proc 16th West Poult Dis Conf, pp. 11–12.

43. Cueva, S., H. Sillau, A. Valenzuela, and H. Ploog. 1974. High altitude induced pulmonary hypertension and right heart failure in broiler chickens. Res Vet Sci 16:370–374.

44. Cumming, R.B. 1969. What has happened to avian monocytosis? World's Poult Sci J 25:218–222.

45. Cummings, T.S. 1988. Hatchery-associated round heart disease in poultry. Proc 125th Annual AVMA Meeting. Portland, Oregon, p. 132.

46. Czarnecki, C.M. 1984. Cardiomyopathy in turkeys. Comp Biochem Physiol 77A:591–598.

47. Dämmrich, K., and G. Rodenhoff. 1970. Skelettveränderungen bei mastküken. Zentralbl Veterinaermed [B] 17:131–146.

48. Da Silva, J.M.L., N. Dale, and J.B. Luchesi. 1988. Effect of pelleted feed on the incidence of ascites in broilers reared at low altitudes. Avian Dis 32:376–378.

49. Decuypere, E., C. Vega, T. Bartha, J. Buyse, J. Zoons, and G.A.A. Albers. 1994. Increased sensitivity to triiodothyronine (T3) of broiler lines with a high susceptibility for ascites. Br Poult Sci 35:287–297.

50. Diaz, G.J., R.J. Julian, and E.J. Squires. 1994. Cobalt-induced polycythaemia causing right ventricular hypertrophy and ascites in meat-type chickens. Avian Pathol 23:91–104.

51. Diaz, G.J., E.J. Squires, and R.J. Julian. 1994. Effect of selected dietary antioxidants on fatty-liver haemorrhagic syndrome in laying hens. Br Poult Sci 35:621–629.

52. Diaz, G.J., R.J. Julian, and E.J. Squires. 1995. Effect of graded levels of dietary nitrite on pulmonary hypertension in broiler chickens and dilatory cardiomyopathy in turkey poults. Avian Pathol 24:109–120.

53. Dickinson, E.M., J.O. Stevens and D.H. Helfer. 1968. A degenerative myopathy in turkeys. Proc 17th West Poult Dis Conf, p. 7.

54. Duff, S.R.I. 1984. The histopathology of degenerative hip disease in male breeding turkeys. J Comp Pathol 94:115–125.

55. Duff, S.R.I. 1984. The morphology of degenerative hip disease in male breeding turkeys. J Comp Pathol 94:127–139.

56. Duff, S.R.I. 1984. Osteochondrosis dissecans in turkeys. J Comp Pathol 94:467–476.

57. Duff, S.R.I. 1984. Dyschondroplasia of the caput femoris in skeletally immature broilers. Res Vet Sci 37:293–302.

58. Duff, S.R.I. 1984. Capital femoral epiphyseal infarction in skeletally immature broilers. Res Vet Sci 37:303–309.

59. Duff, S.R.I. 1984. Consequences of capital femoral dyschondroplasia in young adult and skeletally mature broilers. Res Vet Sci 37:310–319.

60. Duff, S.R.I. 1985. Further studies of degenerative hip

disease; antitrochanteric degeneration in turkeys and broiler type chickens. J Comp Pathol 95:113–122.

61. Duff, S.R.I. 1985. Dyschondroplasia/osteochondrosis of the femoral trochanter in the fowl. J Comp Pathol 95:363–371.

62. Duff, S.R.I. 1985. Hip instability in young adult broiler fowls. J Comp Pathol 95:373–382.

63. Duff, S.R.I. 1985. Fractured fibulae in broiler fowls. J Comp Pathol 95:525–536.

64. Duff, S.R.I. 1985. Cruciate ligament rupture in young adult broiler knee joints. J Comp Pathol 95:537–548.

65. Duff, S.R.I. 1986. Windswept deformities in poultry. J Comp Pathol 96:147–158.

66. Duff, S.R.I. 1986. Rupture of the intercondylar ligament in intertarsal joints of broiler fowls. J Comp Pathol 96:159–169.

67. Duff, S.R.I. 1986. Further studies on cruciate and collateral knee ligaments in adult broiler fowls. Avian Pathol 15:407–420.

68. Duff, S.R.I. 1986. Further studies on knee ligament failure in broiler breeding fowls. J Comp Pathol 96:485–495.

69. Duff, S.R.I. 1986. Effect of unilateral weight-bearing on pelvic limb development in broiler fowls: Morphological and radiological findings. Res Vet Sci 40:393–399.

70. Duff, S.R.I. 1987. Destructive cartilage loss in the joints of adult male broiler breeding fowls. J Comp Pathol 97:237–246.

71. Duff, S.R.I. 1987. Meniscal lesions in the knee joints of broiler fowls. J Comp Pathol 97:451–462.

72. Duff, S.R.I. 1990. Do different forms of spondylolisthesis occur in broiler fowls? Avian Pathol 19:279–294.

73. Duff, S.R.I., and I.A. Anderson. 1986. The gastrocnemius tendon of domestic fowl: Histological findings in different strains. Res Vet Sci 41:402–409.

74. Duff, S.R.I., and P.M. Hocking. 1986. Chronic orthopaedic disease in adult male broiler breeding fowls. Res Vet Sci 41:340–348.

75. Duff, S.R.I., and C.J. Randall. 1986. Tendon lesions in broiler fowls. Res Vet Sci 40:333–338.

76. Duff, S.R.I., and C. J. Randall. 1987. Observations on femoral head abnormalities in broilers. Res Vet Sci 42:17–23.

77. Duff, S.R.I., and B.H. Thorp. 1985. Patterns of physiological bone torsion in the pelvic appendicular skeletons of domestic fowl. Res Vet Sci 39:307–312.

78. Duff, S.R.I., and B.H. Thorp. 1985. Abnormal angulation/torsion of the pelvic appendicular skeleton in broiler fowl: Morphological and radiological findings. Res Vet Sci 39:313–319.

79. Duff, S.R.I., P.M. Hocking, and R.K. Field. 1987. The gross morphology of skeletal disease in adult male breeding turkeys. Avian Pathol 16:635–651.

80. Edwards, H.M., Jr. 1984. Studies on the etiology of tibial dyschondroplasia in chickens. J Nutr 114:1001–1013.

81. Edwards, H.M., Jr., and P. Sorensen. 1987. Effect of short fasts on the development of tibial dyschondroplasia in chickens. J Nutr 117:194–200.

82. Edwards, H.M., Jr., and J.R. Veltmann, Jr. 1983. The role of calcium and phosphorus in the etiology of tibial dyschondroplasia in young chicks. J Nutr 113:1568–1575.

83. Edwards, H.M., Jr., M.A. Elliot, and S. Sooncharernying. 1992. Effects of dietary calcium on tibial dyschondroplasia. Interaction with light, cholecalciferol, 1,25-dihydroxycholecalciferol, protein and synthetic zeolite. Poult Sci 71:2041–2055.

84. Elliot, M.A., and H.M. Edwards, Jr. 1994. Effect of genetic strain, calcium, and feed withdrawal on growth, tibial dyschondroplasia, plasma 1,25 dihydroxycholecalciferol, plasma 25-hydroxycholecalciferol in sixteen-day-old chickens. Poult Sci 73:509–519.

85. Enkvetchakul, B., W. Bottje, N. Anthony, R. Moore, and W. Huff. 1993. Compromised antioxidant status associated with ascites in broilers. Poult Sci 72:2272–2280.

86. Fitz-Coy, S.H. and J.M. Harter-Dennis. 1988. Incidence of ascites in broiler and roaster chickens. Poult Sci 67(Suppl 1):87.

87. Frame, D.D. 1991. Roundheart disease in Utah turkey flocks. Proc 40th West Poult Dis Conf, pp. 95–96.

88. Frank, R.K., J.A. Newman, S.L. Noll, and G.R. Ruth. 1990. The incidence of perirenal hemorrhage syndrome in six flocks of market turkey toms. Avian Dis 34:824–832.

89. Frank, R.K., S.L. Noll, M.E. Halawani, J.A. Newman, D.A. Halvorson, and G.R. Ruth. 1990. Perirenal hemorrhage syndrome in market turkey toms: Effect of management factors. Avian Dis 34:833–843.

90. Frank, R.K., J.A. Newman, and G.R. Ruth. 1991. Lesions of perirenal hemorrhage syndrome in growing turkeys. Avian Dis 35:523–534.

91. Gardiner, E.E., and J.R. Hunt. 1984. Effect of dietary reserpine on the incidence of sudden death syndrome in chickens. Can J Anim Sci 64:1015–1018.

92. Gilka, F., and J.L. Spencer. 1990. Chronic myocarditis and circulatory syndrome in a white leghorn strain induced by an avian leukosis virus: Light and electron microscopic study. Avian Dis 34:174–184.

93. Gilka, F., J.L. Spencer, and J.R. Chambers. 1991. Response of meat-type chickens to infection with RAV-1 avian leukosis virus. Avian Pathol 20:637–647.

94. Glahn, R.P., R.F. Wideman, and B.S. Cowen. 1988. Effect of Gray strain infectious bronchitis virus and high dietary calcium on renal function of Single Comb White Leghorn pullets at 6, 10, and 18 weeks of age. Poult Sci 67:1250–1263.

95. Glahn, R.P., R.F. Wideman, and B.S. Cowen. 1988. Effect of dietary acidification and alkalinization on urolith formation and renal function in Single Comb White Leghorn laying hens. Poult Sci 67:1694–1701.

96. Glahn, R.P., R.F. Wideman, and B.S. Cowen. 1989. Order of exposure to high dietary calcium and Gray strain infectious bronchitis virus alters renal function and incidence of urolithiasis. Poult Sci 68:1193–1204.

97. Gonder, E., and H.J. Barnes. 1987. Focal ulcerative dermatitis ("breast buttons") in marketed turkeys. Avian Dis 31:52–58.

98. Graham, C.L.G. 1977. Copper levels in livers of turkeys with naturally occurring aortic rupture. Avian Dis 21:113–116.

99. Grashorn, M. 1994. Investigations on the aetiology and pathology of sudden death syndrome in meat-type chicken. Arch Geflugelk 58:242–244.

100. Grashorn, M.A., and H.G. Classen. 1993. Use of the calcium antagonist verapamil in experimental investigation of the sudden death syndrome in broilers. Arch Gefluegelkd 57:228–232.

101. Greene, J.A., R.M. McCracken and R.T. Evans. 1985. A contact dermatitis of broilers—clinical and pathological findings. Avian Pathol 14:23–38.

102. Greenlees, K.J., P. Eyre, J.C. Lee, and C.T. Larsen. 1989. Effect of age and growth rate on myocardial irritability in broiler chickens (42861). Proc Soc Exp Biol Med 190:282–285.

103. Gregory, N.G., L.J. Wilkins, S.D. Eleperuma, A.J. Ballantyne, and N.D. Overfield. 1990. Broken bones in domestic fowls: Effect of husbandry system and stunning method in end-of-lay hens. Br Poult Sci 31:59–69.

104. Gregory, N.G., L.J. Wilkins, D.M. Alvey, and S.A. Tucker. 1993. Effect of catching method and lighting intensity on the prevalence of broken bones and on the ease of handling of end-of-lay hens. Vet Rec 132:127–129.

105. Grunder, A.A., K.G. Hollands, and J.S. Gavora. 1979. Incidence of degenerative myopathy among turkeys fed corn or wheat based rations. Poult Sci 58:1321–1324.

106. Hall, S.A., and N. Machicao. 1968. Myocarditis in broiler chickens reared at high altitude. Avian Dis 12:75–84.

107. Hansen, R.J., and R.L. Walzem. 1993. Avian fatty

liver hemorrhagic syndrome: A comparative review. Adv Vet Sci Comp Med 37:451–468.

108. Hanson, B.S. 1968. Disease and egg quality. In T.C. Carter (ed.). Egg Quality. A Study of the Hen's Egg. Br Egg Marketing Board Symp #4. Oliver and Boyd, Edinburgh, Scotland, pp. 171–180.

109. Hargest, T.E., R.M. Leach, and C.V. Gay. 1985. Avian dyschondroplasia. I. Ultrastructure. Am J Pathol 119:175–190.

110. Harms, R.H., and C.F. Simpson. 1975. Biotin deficiency as a possible cause of swelling and ulceration of foot pads. Poult Sci 54:1711–1713.

111. Harms, R.H., and C.F. Simpson. 1979. Serum and body characteristics of laying hens with fatty liver syndrome. Poult Sci 58:1644–1646.

112. Harms, R.H., B.L. Damron, and C.F. Simpson. 1977. Effect of wet litter and supplemental biotin and/or whey on the production of foot pad dermatitis in broilers. Poult Sci 56:291–296.

113. Harper, J.A., and D.H. Helfer. 1972. The effect of vitamin E, methionine and selenium on degenerative myopathy in turkeys. Poult Sci 51:1757–1759.

114. Harper, J.A., P.E. Bernier, J.O. Stevens, and E.M. Dickinson. 1969. Degenerative myopathy in the domestic turkey. Poult Sci 48:1816.

115. Harper, J.A., D.H. Helfer, and E.M. Dickinson. 1971. Hereditary myopathy in turkeys. Proc 20th West Poult Dis Conf, p. 76.

116. Harper, J.A., P.A. Bernier, D.H. Helfer, and J.A. Schmitz. 1975. Degenerative myopathy of the deep pectoral muscle in the turkey. J Hered 66:362–366.

117. Harris, G.C., M. Musbah, J.N. Beasley, and G.S. Nelson. 1978. The development of dermatitis (scabby hip) on the hip and thigh of broiler chickens. Avian Dis 22:122–130.

118. Harrison, P.C., and J. McGinnis. 1967. Light induced exophthalmos in the domestic fowl. Proc Soc Exp Biol Med 126:308–312.

119. Haye, U., and P.C.M. Simons. 1978. Twisted legs in broilers. Br Poult Sci 19:549–557.

120. Haynes, J.S. and M.M. Walser. 1986. Ultrastructure of Fusarium-induced tibial dyschondroplasia in chickens: A sequential study. Vet Pathol 23:499–505.

121. Haynes, J.S., M.M. Walser, and E.M. Lawler. 1985. Morphogenesis of Fusarium sp-induced tibial dyschondroplasia in chickens. Vet Pathol 22:629–636.

122. Hemsley, L.A. 1965. The causes of mortality in fourteen flocks of broiler chickens. Vet Rec 77:467–472.

123. Hernandez, A. 1987. Hypoxic ascites in broilers: A review of several studies done in Columbia. Avian Dis 31:658–661.

124. Huchzermeyer, F.W., and A.M.C. De Ruyck. 1986. Pulmonary hypertension syndrome associated with ascites in broilers. Vet Rec 119:94.

125. Huchzermeyer, F.W., J.A. Cilliers, C.D.D. Lavigne, and R.A. Bartkowiak. 1987. Broiler pulmonary hypertension syndrome. I. Increased right ventricular mass in broilers experimentally infected with Aegyptianella pullorum. Onderstepoort J Vet Res 54:113–114.

126. Hughes, B.O., S. Wilson, M.C. Appleby, and S.F. Smith. 1993. Comparison of bone volume and strength as measures of skeletal integrity in caged laying hens with access to perches. Res Vet Sci 54:202–206.

127. Hulan, H.W., F.G. Proudfoot, D. Ramey, and K.B. McRae. 1980. Influence of genotype and diet on general performance and incidence of leg abnormalities of commercial broilers reared to roaster weight. Poult Sci 59:748–757.

128. Hulan, H.W., F.G. Proudfoot, and K.B. McRae. 1980. Effect of vitamins on the incidence of mortality and acute death syndrome ("flip-over") in broiler chickens. Poult Sci 59:927–931.

129. Hunt, J.R., and E.E. Gardiner. 1982. Effect of various diets on the incidence of acute death syndrome ("flip-over")

of chickens. Poult Sci 61:1481.

130. Huston, T.M., H.L. Fuller, and C.K. Laurent. 1956. A comparison of various methods of debeaking broilers. Poult Sci 35:806–810.

131. Hutt, F.B., K. Goodwin, and W.D. Urban. 1956. Investigations of nonlaying hens. Cornell Vet 46:257–273.

132. Ibrahim, I.K., R.D. Hodges, and R. Hill. 1980. Haemorrhagic liver syndrome in laying fowl fed diets containing rapeseed meal. Res Vet Sci 29:68–76.

133. Itakura, C., and S. Yamagiwa. 1970. Histopathological studies on bone dysplasia of chickens. I. Histopathology of the bone. Jpn J Vet Sci 32:105–117.

134. Itakura, C., and S. Yamagiwa. 1971. Histopathological studies on bone dysplasia of chickens. III. A collective occurence of bowleg (genu varum) among broiler chicks. Jpn J Vet Sci 33:11–16.

135. Jackson, C.A.W., D.J. Kingston, and L.A. Hemsley. 1972. A total mortality survey of nine batches of broiler chickens. Aust Vet J 48:481–487.

136. Jacob, J.P., R. Blair, and E.E. Gardiner. 1990. Effect of dietary lactate and glucose on the incidence of sudden death syndrome in male broiler chickens. Poult Sci 69:1529–1532.

137. Jenkins, R.L., W.D. Ivey, G.R. McDaniel, and R.A. Albert. 1979. A darkness induced eye abnormality in the domestic chicken. Poult Sci 58:55–59.

138. Jensen, L.S., R. Martinson and G. Schumaier. 1970. A foot pad dermatitis in turkey poults associated with soybean meal. Poult Sci 49:76–82.

139. Jones, G.P.D. 1994. Energy and nitrogen metabolism and oxygen use by broilers susceptible to ascites and grown at three environmental temperatures. Br Poult Sci 35:97–105.

140. Jones, G.P.D. 1995. Response of broilers susceptible to ascites when grown in high and low oxygen environments. Br Poult Sci 36:123–133.

141. Jones, G.P.D. 1995. Manipulation of organ growth by early-life food restriction: Its influence on the development of ascites in broiler chickens. Br Poult Sci 36:135–142.

142. Jones, J.M., N.R. King, and M.M. Mulliner. 1974. Degenerative myopathy in turkey breeder hens: A comparative study of normal and affected muscle. Br Poult Sci 15:191–196.

143. Jones, H.G.R., C.J. Randall, and C.P.J. Mills. 1978. A survey of mortality in three adult broiler breeder flocks. Avian Pathol 7:619–628.

144. Julian, R. 1982. Water deprivation as a cause of renal disease in chickens. Avian Pathol 11:615–617.

145. Julian, R. 1983. Foci of cartilage in the lung of broiler chickens. Avian Dis 27:292–295.

146. Julian, R.J. 1984. Tendon avulsion as a cause of lameness in turkeys. Avian Dis 28:244–249.

147. Julian, R.J. 1984. Valgus-varus deformity of the intertarsal joint in broiler chickens. Can Vet J 25:254–258.

148. Julian, R.J. 1985. Osteochondrosis, dyschondroplasia and osteomyelitis causing femoral head necrosis in turkeys. Avian Dis 29:854–866.

149. Julian, R.J. 1986. The effect of increased mineral levels in the feed on leg weakness and sudden death syndrome in broiler chickens. Can Vet J 27:157–160.

150. Julian, R.J. 1987. The effect of increased sodium in the drinking water on right ventricular hypertrophy, right ventricular failure and ascites in broiler chickens. Avian Pathol 16:61–71.

151. Julian, R.J. 1988. Ascites in meat-type ducklings. Avian Pathol 17:11–21.

152. Julian, R.J. 1989. Lung volume of meat-type chickens. Avian Dis 33:174–176.

153. Julian, R.J. 1993. Ascites in poultry. Avian Pathol 22:419–454.

154. Julian, R.J., and M. Goryo. 1990. Pulmonary aspergillosis causing right ventricular failure and ascites in meat-type chickens. Avian Pathol 19:643–654.

155. Julian, R.J., and S.M. Mirsalimi. 1992. Blood oxygen concentration of fast growing and slow growing broiler chickens and chickens with ascites from right ventricular failure. Avian Dis 36:730–732.

156. Julian, R.J., and E.J. Squires. 1994. Haematopoietic and right ventricular response to intermittent hypobaric hypoxia in meat-type chickens. Avian Pathol 23:539–545.

157. Julian, R.J., and B. Wilson. 1992. Pen oxygen concentration and pulmonary hypertension-induced right ventricular failure and ascites in meat-type chickens at low altitude. Avian Dis 36:733–735.

158. Julian, R.J., E.T. Moran, W. Revington, and D.B. Hunter. 1984. Acute hypertensive angiopathy as a cause of sudden death in turkeys. J Am Vet Med Assoc 185:342.

159. Julian, R.J., J. Summers and J.B. Wilson. 1986. Right ventricular failure and ascites in broiler chickens caused by phosphorus-deficient diets. Avian Dis 30:453–459.

160. Julian, R.J., G.W. Friars, H. French, and M. Quinton. 1987. The relationship of right ventricular hypertrophy, right ventricular failure, and ascites to weight gain in broiler and roaster chickens. Avian Dis 31:130–135.

161. Julian, R.J., I. McMillan, and M. Quinton. 1989. The effect of cold and dietary energy on right ventricular hypertrophy, right ventricular failure and ascites in meat-type chickens. Avian Pathol 18:675–684.

162. Julian, R.J., J.A. Frazier, and M. Goryo. 1989. Right ventricular hypertrophy, right ventricular failure and ascites in broiler chickens caused by amiodarone-induced lung pathology. Avian Pathol 18:161–174.

163. Julian, R.J., L.J. Caston, and S. Leeson. 1992. The effect of dietary sodium on right ventricular failure-induced ascites, gain and fat deposition in meat-type chickens. Can J Vet Res 56:214–219.

164. Julian, R.J., S.M. Mirsalimi, L.G. Bagley, and E.J. Squires. 1992. Effect of hypoxia and diet on spontaneous turkey cardiomyopathy (round-heart disease). Avian Dis 36:1043–1047.

165. Julian, R.J., L.J. Caston, S. Mirsalimi, and S. Leeson. 1992. Effect of poultry by-product meal on pulmonary hypertension, right ventricular failure and ascites in broiler chickens. Can Vet J 33:382–385.

166. Julian, R.J., S.M. Mirsalimi, and E.J. Squires. 1993. Effect of hypobaric hypoxia and diet on blood parameters and pulmonary hypertension-induced right ventricular hypertrophy in turkey poults and ducklings. Avian Pathol 22:683–692.

167. Jungherr, E., and B.S. Pomeroy. 1965. Avian monocytosis (so-called pullet disease), infectious nephrosis and bluecomb diseases of turkeys. In H.E. Biester, and L.H. Schwarte (eds.). Diseases of Poultry, 5th ed. Iowa State University Press, Ames, IA, pp. 844–862.

168. Kawada, M., R. Hirosawa, T. Yanai, T. Masegi, and K. Ueda. 1994. Cardiac lesions in broilers which died without clinical signs. Avian Pathol 23:503–511.

169. Knowles, T.G., D.M. Broom, N.G. Gregory, and L.J. Wilkins. 1993. Effect of bone strength on the frequency of broken bones in hens. Res Vet Sci 54:15–19.

170. Krista, L.M., P.E. Waibel, and R.E. Burger. 1965. The influence of dietary alterations, hormones, and blood pressure on the incidence of dissecting aneurysms in the turkey. Poult Sci 44:15–22.

171. Krista, L.M., P.E. Waibel, R.N. Shoffner, and J.A. Sautter. 1967. Natural dissecting aneurysm (aortic rupture) and blood pressure in the turkey. Nature 214:1162–1163.

172. Kumar, M.C. 1986. Hypertensive angiopathy in turkeys: A case report. Proc 35th West Poult Dis Conf, p. 99.

173. Larochelle, R., M. Morin, and G. Bernier. 1992. Sudden death in turkeys with perirenal hemorrhage: Pathological observations and possible pathogenesis of the disease. Avian Dis 36:114–124.

174. Lauber, J.K., J.V. Shutze, and J. McGinnis. 1961. Effects of exposure to continuous light on the eye of the growing chick. Proc Soc Exp Biol Med 106:871–872.

175. Lawler, E.M., J.L. Shivers, and M.M. Walser. 1988. Acid phosphatase activity of chondroclasts from Fusarium-induced tibial dyschondroplastic cartilage. Avian Dis 32:240–245.

176. Leach, R.M., and, M.S. Lilburn. 1992. Current knowledge on the etiology of tibial dyschondroplasia in the avian species. Poult Sci Rev 4:57–65.

177. Leach, R.M., and W.O. Twal. 1994. Autocrine, paracrine and hormonal signals involved in growth plate chondrocyte differentiation. Poult Sci 73:883–888.

178. Lent, A.J., and R.F. Wideman. 1993. Susceptibility of two commercial Single Comb White Leghorn strains to calcium-induced urolithiasis: Efficacy of dietary supplementation with DL-methionine and ammonium sulfate. Br Poult Sci 34:577–587.

179. Leterrier, C., and Y. Nys. 1992. Clinical and anatomical differences in varus and valgus deformities of chick limbs suggest different aetio-pathogenesis. Avian Pathol 21:429–442.

180. Lopez Coello, C., L. Paasch, R. Rosiles, and C. Casas. 1982. Ascites in broilers due to undetermined causes. Proc 31st West Poult Dis Conf, pp. 13–15.

181. Loveridge, N., C. Farquharson, J.E. Heskett, S.B. Jakowlew, C.C. Whitehead, and B.H. Thorp. 1993. The control of chondrocyte differentiation during endochondral bone growth in vivo: Involvement of TGF-ß and the proto-oncogene c-myc. J Cell Sci 105:949–956.

182. Lynch, M., B.H. Thorp, and C.C. Whitehead. 1992. Avian dyschondroplasia as a cause of bone deformity. Avian Pathol 21:275–286.

183. Magwood, S.E., and D.F. Bray. 1962. Disease condition of turkey poults characterized by enlarged and rounded hearts. Can J Comp Med 26:268–272.

184. Mallinson, E.T., H. Rothenbacher, R.F. Wideman, D.B. Snyder, E. Russek, A.I. Zuckerman, and J.P. Davidson. 1984. Epizootiology, pathology and microbiology of an outbreak of urolithiasis in chickens. Avian Dis 28:25–43.

185. Martindale, L., W.G. Siller, and P.A.L Wight. 1979. Effects of subfascial pressure in experimental deep pectoral myopathy of the fowl: An angiographic study. Avian Pathol 8:425–436.

186. Martland, M.F. 1984. Wet litter as a cause of plantar pododermatitis leading to foot ulceration and lameness in fattening turkeys. Avian Pathol 13:241–252.

187. Martland, M.F. 1985. Ulcerative dermatitis in broiler chickens: The effects of wet litter. Avian Pathol 14:353–364.

188. Martland, M.F., E.J. Butler, and G.R. Fenwick. 1984. Rapeseed induced liver haemorrhage, reticulolysis and biochemical changes in laying hens: The effects of feeding high and low glucosinolate meals. Res Vet Sci 36:298–309.

189. Maxwell, M.H. 1988. The histology and ultrastructure of ectopic cartilaginous and osseous nodules in the lungs of young broilers with an ascitic syndrome. Avian Pathol 17:201–219.

190. Maxwell, M.H. 1990. Haematological and histopathological findings in young broilers raised in poorly and well ventilated environments. Res Vet Sci 48:374–376.

191. Maxwell, M.H. 1991. Red cell size and various lung arterial measurements in different strains of domestic fowl. Res Vet Sci 50:233–239.

192. Maxwell, M.H., and H.C.W. Mbugua. 1990. Ultrastructural abnormalities in seven-day-old broilers reared at high altitude. Res Vet Sci 49:182–189.

193. Maxwell, M.H., G.W. Robertson, and S. Spence. 1986. Studies on an ascitic syndrome in young broilers. 1. Haematology and pathology. Avian Pathol 15:511–524.

194. Maxwell, M.H., G.W. Robertson, and S. Spence. 1986. Studies on an ascitic syndrome in young broilers. 2. Ultrastructure. Avian Pathol 15:525–538.

195. Maxwell, M.H., I.A. Anderson, and L.A. Dick. 1988.

The incidence of ectopic cartilaginous and osseous lung nodules in young broiler fowls with ascites and various other diseases. Avian Pathol 17:487–493.

196. Maxwell, M.H., T.T. Dolan, and H.C.W. Mbugua. 1989. An ultrastructural study of an ascitic syndrome in young broilers reared at high altitude. Avian Pathol 18:481–494.

197. Maxwell, M.H., L.A. Dick, I.A. Anderson, and M.A. Mitchell. 1989. Ectopic cartilaginous and osseous lung nodules induced in the young broiler by inadequate ventilation. Avian Pathol 18:113–124.

198. Maxwell, M.H., G.W. Robertson, and C.C. McCorquodale. 1992. Whole blood and plasma viscosity values in normal and ascitic broiler chickens. Bri Poult Sci 33:871–877.

199. Maxwell, M.H., G.W. Robertson, and M.A. Mitchell. 1993. Ultrastructural demonstration of mitochondrial calcium overload in myocardial cells from broiler chickens with ascites and induced hypoxia. Res Vet Sci 54:267–277.

200. Maxwell, M.H., G.W. Robertson, and D. Moseley. 1994. Potential role of serum troponin T in cardiomyocyte injury in broiler ascites syndrome. Br Poult Sci 35:663–667.

201. McCaskey, P.C., G.N. Rowland, R.K. Page, and L.R. Minear. 1982. Focal failures of endochondral ossification in the broiler. Avian Dis 26:701–717.

202. McCune, E.L. and H.-D. Dellmann. 1968. Developmental origin and structural characters of "breast blisters" in chickens. Poult Sci 47:852–858.

203. McIlroy, S.G., E.A. Goodall, and C.H. McMurray. 1987. A contact dermatitis of broilers—epidemiological findings. Avian Pathol 16:93–105.

204. McSherry, B.J., A.E. Ferguson, and J. Ballantyne. 1954. A dissecting aneurism in internal hemorrhage in turkeys. J Am Vet Med Assoc 124:279–283.

205. Meijering, A. 1979. Fatty liver syndrome in laying hens—an attempt to review. World's Poult Sci J 35:79–94.

206. Miles, R.D., and R.H. Harms. 1981. An observation of abnormally high calcium and phosphorus levels in laying hens with fatty liver syndrome. Poult Sci 60:485–486.

207. Mirsalimi, S.M., and R.J. Julian. 1991. Reduced erythrocyte deformability as a possible contributing factor to pulmonary hypertension and ascites in broiler chickens. Avian Dis 35:374–379.

208. Mirsalimi, S.M., and R.J. Julian. 1993. Effect of excess sodium bicarbonate on the blood volume and erythrocyte deformability of broiler chickens. Avian Pathol 22:495–507.

209. Mirsalimi, S.M., F.S. Qureshi, R.J. Julian, and P.J. O'Brien. 1990. Myocardial biochemical changes in furazolidone-induced cardiomyopathy of turkeys. J Comp Pathol 102:139–147.

210. Mirsalimi, S.M., P.J. O'Brien, and R.J. Julian. 1993. Blood volume increase in salt-induced pulmonary hypertension, heart failure and ascites in broiler and White Leghorn chickens. Can J Vet Res 57:110–113.

211. Mollison, B. 1983. Studies of some possible nutritional aspects of sudden death syndrome and abdominal fat pad deposition in broiler chickens. M.S. thesis. University of Winnipeg. Canada.

212. Mollison, B., W. Guenter, and B.R. Boycott. 1984. Abdominal fat deposition and sudden death syndrome in broilers: The effects of restricted intake, early life caloric (fat) restriction and calorie:protein ratio. Poult Sci 63:1190–1200.

213. Moorhead, P.D., and Y.S. Mohamed. 1968. Case report: Pathologic and microbiologic studies of crooked-neck in a turkey flock. Avian Dis 12:476–482.

214. Mutalib, A.A., and J.A. Hanson. 1990. Sudden death in turkeys with perirenal hemorrhage: Field and laboratory findings. Can Vet J 31:637–642.

215. Nairn, M.E., and A.R.A. Watson. 1972. Leg weakness of poultry—a clinical and pathological characterisation. Aust Vet J 48:645–656.

216. Neumann, F., and H. Ungar. 1973. Spontaneous aortic rupture in turkeys and the vascularization of the aortic wall. Can Vet J 14:136–138.

217. Neumann, F., M.S. Dison, U. Klopfer, and T.A. Nobel. 1973. Sporadic renal haemorrhage in turkeys. Refu Vet 30:59–61.

218. Newberne, P.M., M.E. Muhrer, R. Craghead, and B.L. O'Dell. 1956. An abnormality of the proventriculus of the chick. J Am Vet Med Assoc 128:553–555.

219. Newberry, R.C., J.R. Hunt, and E.E. Gardiner. 1985. Effect of alternating lights and strain on roaster chicken performance and mortality due to sudden death syndrome. Can J Anim Sci 65:993–996.

220. Newberry, R.C., J.R. Hunt, and E.E. Gardiner. 1985. Effect of alternating lights and strain on behavior and leg disorders of roaster chickens. Poult Sci 64:1863–1868.

221. Newberry, R.C., J.R. Hunt, and E.E. Gardiner. 1986. Light intensity effects on performance, activity, leg disorders and sudden death syndrome of roaster chickens. Poult Sci 65:2232–2238.

222. Newberry, R.C., E.E. Gardiner, and J.R. Hunt. 1987. Behavior of chickens prior to death from sudden death syndrome. Poult Sci 66:1446–1450.

223. Niznik, R.A., R.F. Wideman, B.S. Cowen, and R.E. Kissell. 1985. Induction of urolithiasis in single comb white leghorn pullets: Effect on glomerular number. Poult Sci 64:1430–1437.

224. Norgaard-Nielson, G. 1990. Bone strength of laying hens kept in an alternative system, compared with hens in cages and on deep litter. Br Poult Sci 31:81–89.

225. Odom, T.W., B.M. Hargis, C.C. Lopez, M.J. Arce, Y. Ono, and G.E. Avila. 1991. Use of electrocardiographic analysis for the investigation of ascites syndrome in broiler chickens. Avian Dis 35:738–744.

226. Odom, T.W., L.M. Rosenbaum, and B.M. Hargis. 1992. Evaluation of vectorelectrocardiographic analysis of young broiler chickens as a predictive index for susceptibility to ascites syndrome. Avian Dis 36:78–83.

227. Oldroyd, N.O., and R.F. Wideman. 1986. Characterization and composition of uroliths from domestic fowl. Poultry Sci 65:1090–1094.

228. Ononiwu, J.C., R.G. Thomson, H.C. Carlson, and R.J. Julian. 1979. Pathological studies of "sudden death syndrome" in broiler chickens. Can Vet J 20:70–73.

229. Ononiwu, J.C., R.G. Thomson, H.C. Carlson, and R.J. Julian. 1979. Studies on effect of lighting on "sudden death syndrome" in broiler chickens. Can Vet J 20:74–77.

230. Orr, J.P., and C. Riddell. 1977. Investigation of the vascular supply of the pectoral muscles of the domestic turkey and comparison of experimentally produced infarcts with naturally occurring deep pectoral myopathy. Am J Vet Res 38:1237–1242.

231. Orth, M.W., and M.E. Cook. 1994. Avian tibial dyschondroplasia: A morphological and biochemical review of the growth plate lesion and its causes. Vet Pathol 31:403–414.

232. Ostrander, C.E. 1957. Control cannabilism in your poultry flock. Cornell Ext Bull 992.

233. Overfield, N.D. 1970. Factors affecting egg quality—field observations. In B.M. Freeman and R.F. Gordon, (eds.). Factors Affecting Egg Grading. Br Egg Marketing Board Symp #6. Oliver and Boyd, Edinburgh, Scotland, pp. 29–52.

234. Owen, R.L., R.F. Wideman, A.L. Hattel, and B.S. Cowen. 1990. Use of a hypobaric chamber as a model system for investigating ascites in broilers. Avian Dis 34:754–758.

235. Owen, R.L., R.F. Wideman, R.M. Leach and B.S. Cowen. 1993. Effect of age at exposure to hypobaric hypoxia and dietary changes on mortality due to ascites. Proc 42nd West Poult Dis Conf, pp. 16–18.

236. Owen, R.L., R.F. Wideman, and B.S. Cowen. 1995. Changes in pulmonary arterial and femoral arterial blood

pressure upon acute exposure to hypobaric hypoxia in broiler chickens. Poult Sci 74:708–715.

237. Owen, R.L., R.F. Wideman, R.M. Leach, B.S. Cowen, P.A. Dunn, and B.C. Ford. 1995. Physiologic and electrocardiographic changes occurring in broilers reared at simulated high altitude. Avian Dis 39:108–115.

238. Payne, L.N., S.R. Brown, N. Bumstead, K. Howes, J.A. Frazier, and M.E. Thouless. 1991. A novel subgroup of exogenous avian leukosis virus in chickens. J Gen Virol 72:801–807.

239. Peacock, A.J., C. Pickett, K. Morris, and J.T. Reeves. 1989. The relationship between rapid growth and pulmonary hemodynamics in the fast-growing broiler chicken. Am Rev Resp Dis 139:1524–1530.

240. Pearson, A.W., and E.J. Butler. 1978. Pathological and biochemical observations on subclinical cases of fatty liver–haemorrhagic syndrome in the fowl. Res Vet Sci 24:65–71.

241. Pearson, A.W., and E.J. Butler. 1978. The oestrogenised chick as an experimental model for fatty liver-haemorrhagic syndrome in the fowl. Res Vet Sci 24:82–86.

242. Pearson, A.W., E.J. Butler, R.F. Curtis, G.R. Fenwick, A. Hobson-Frohock, D.G. Land and S.A. Hall. 1978. Effects of rapeseed meal on laying hens (Gallus domesticus) in relation to fatty liver-haemorrhagic syndrome and egg taint. Res Vet Sci 25:307–313.

243. Peckham, M.C. 1984. Vices and miscellaneous diseases and conditions. In M.S. Hofstad, H.J. Barnes, B.W. Calnek, W.M. Reid, and H.W. Yoder, Jr. (eds.). Diseases of Poultry, 8th ed. Iowa State University Press, Ames, IA, pp. 741–782.

244. Pegram, R.A., and R.D. Wyatt. 1981. Avian gout caused by oosporein, a mycotoxin produced by Chaetomium trilaterale. Poult Sci 60:2429–2440.

245. Perry, R.W., G.N. Rowland, T.L. Foutz, and J.R. Glisson. 1991. Poult malabsorption syndrome. III. Skeletal lesions in market-age turkeys. Avian Dis 35:707–713.

246. Poulos, P.W., Jr., S. Reiland, K. Elwinger, and S.E. Olsson. 1978. Skeletal lesions in the broiler with special reference to dyschondroplasia (osteochondrosis). Acta Radiol Suppl 358:229–275.

247. Pritchard, W.R., W. Henderson, and C.W. Beall. 1958. Experimental production of dissecting aneurysms in turkeys. Am J Vet Res 19:696–705.

248. Proudfoot, F.G., and H.W. Hulan. 1982. Effect of reduced feeding time using all mash or crumble-pellet dietary regimens on chicken broiler performance, including the incidence of acute death syndrome. Poult Sci 61:750–754.

249. Proudfoot, F.G., and H.W. Hulan. 1983. Effects of dietary aspirin (acetylsalicylic acid) on the incidence of sudden death syndrome and the general performance of broiler chickens. Can J Anim Sci 63:469–471.

250. Proudfoot, F.G., H.W. Hulan, and K.B. McRae. 1982. The effect of crumbled and pelleted feed on the incidence of sudden death syndrome among male chicken broilers. Poult Sci 61:1766–1768.

251. Randall, C.J., and C.P.J. Mills. 1981. Observations on leg deformity in broilers with particular reference to the intertarsal joint. Avian Pathol 10:407–431.

252. Randall, C.J., T.B. Blandford, E.D. Borland, N.H. Brooksbank, and S.A. Hall. 1977. A survey of mortality in 51 caged laying flocks. Avian Pathol 6:149–170.

253. Rath, N.C., G.R. Bayyari, J.M. Balog, and W.E. Huff. 1994. Physiological studies of turkey tibial dyschondroplasia. Poult Sci 73:416–424.

254. Reece, R.L. 1991. Ascites syndrome in SPF Light Sussex chickens. J Comp Pathol 105:445–453.

255. Reece, F.N., J.W. Deaton, J.D. May, and K.N. May. 1971. Cage versus floor rearing of broiler chickens. Poult Sci 50:1786–1790.

256. Rennie, J.S., C.C. Whitehead, and B.H. Thorp. 1993. The effect of dietary 1,25-dihydroxycholeciferol in preventing tibial dyschondroplasia in broilers fed on diets imbalanced in calcium and phosphorus. Br J Nutr 69:809–816.

257. Richardson, J.A., J. Burgener, R.W. Winterfield, and A.S. Dhillon. 1980. Deep pectoral myopathy in seven-week-old broiler chickens. Avian Dis 24:1054–1059.

258. Riddell, C. 1975. Pathology of developmental and metabolic disorders of the skeleton of domestic chickens and turkeys. I. Abnormalities of genetic or unknown aetiology. Vet Bull 45:629–640.

259. Riddell, C. 1976. Selection of broiler chickens for a high and low incidence of tibial dyschondroplasia with observation on spondylolisthesis and twisted legs (perosis). Poult Sci 55:145–151.

260. Riddell, C. 1976. The influence of fiber in the diet on dilation (hypertrophy) of the proventriculus in chickens. Avian Dis 20:442–445.

261. Riddell, C. 1980. A survey of skeletal disorders in five turkey flocks in Saskatchewan. Can J Comp Med 44:275–279.

262. Riddell, C. 1981. Skeletal deformities in poultry. Adv Vet Sci Comp Med 25:277–310.

263. Riddell, C. 1983. Pathology of the skeleton and tendons of broiler chickens reared to roaster weights. I. Crippled chickens. Avian Dis 27:950–962.

264. Riddell, C. 1985. Cardiomyopathy and ascites in broiler chickens. Proc 34th West Poult Dis Conf, p. 36.

265. Riddell, C. 1987. Avian Histopathology. American Association of Avian Pathologists, Kennett Square, PA, pp. 32–33

266. Riddell, C. 1990. Effect of management on skeletal problems in poultry. Avian Skeletal Disease Symposium. San Antonio, TX, pp. 59–67.

267. Riddell, C. 1992. Non-infectious skeletal disorders of poultry: An overview. In C.C. Whitehead (ed.). Bone Biology and Skeletal Disorders in Poultry. Carfax Publishing Company, Abingdon, England, pp. 119–141.

268. Riddell, C. 1993. Developmental and metabolic diseases of meat-type poultry. Proc Xth World Vet Poultry Assoc Congr. Sydney, Australia, pp. 79–89.

269. Riddell, C., and H.L. Classen. 1992. Effects of increasing photoperiod length and anticoccidials on performance and health of roaster chickens. Avian Dis 36:491–498.

270. Riddell, C., and J. Howell. 1972. Spondylolisthesis ("Kinky Back") in broiler chickens in western Canada. Avian Dis 16:444–452.

271. Riddell, C., and J.P. Orr. 1980. Chemical studies of the blood, and histological studies of the heart of broiler chickens dying from acute death syndrome. Avian Dis 24:751–757.

272. Riddell, C., and D.A. Pass. 1987. The influence of dietary calcium and phosphorus on tibial dyschondroplasia in broiler chickens. Avian Dis 31:771–775.

273. Riddell, C., and R. Springer. 1985. An epizootiological study of acute death syndrome and leg weakness in broiler chickens in western Canada. Avian Dis 29:90–102.

274. Riddell, C., M.W. King, and K.R. Gunasekera. 1983. Pathology of the skeleton and tendons of broiler chickens reared to roaster weights. II. Normal chickens. Avian Dis 27:980–991.

275. Roberson, K.D., and H.M. Edwards. 1994. Effects of ascorbic acid and 1,25-dihydroxycholecalciferol on alkaline phosphatase and tibial dyschondroplasia in broiler chickens. Br J Poult Sci 35:763–773.

276. Roberson, K.D., C.H. Hill, and P.R. Ferket. 1993. Additive amelioration of tibial dyschondroplasia in broilers by supplemental calcium or feed deprivation. Poult Sci 72:798–805.

277. Robinson, F.E., H.L. Classen, J.A. Hanson, and D.K. Onderka. 1992. Growth performance, feed efficiency and the incidence of skeletal and metabolic disease in full-fed and feed restricted broiler and roaster chickens. J Appl Poult Res 1:33–44.

278. Rodenhoff, G., and K. Dämmrich. 1973. Untersuchungen zur beeinflussung der röhrenknochenstruktur

durch verschiedene haltungssysteme bei masthähnchen. Berl Muench Tieraerztl Wochenschr 86:230–233, 241–244.

279. Roland, D.A., M. Farmer, and D. Marple. 1985. Calcium and its relationship to excess feed consumption, body weight, egg size, fat deposition, shell quality, and fatty liver hemorrhagic syndrome. Poult Sci 64:2341–2350.

280. Rosselot, G., C. Sokol, and R. Leach. 1994. Effect of lesion size on the metabolic activity of tibial dyschondroplastic chondrocytes. Poult Sci 73:452–456.

281. Rotter, B., W. Guenter, and B.R. Boycott. 1985. Sudden death syndrome in broilers: Dietary fat supplementation and its effect on tissue composition. Poult Sci 64:1128–1136.

282. Sanders, A.M., and H.M. Edwards, Jr. 1991. The effects of 1,25-dihydroxycholecalciferol on performance and bone development in the turkey poult. Poult Sci 70:853–866.

283. Sanger, V.L., E.N. Moore, and N.A. Frank. 1960. Blepharoconjunctivitis in turkeys. Poult Sci 39:482–487.

284. Sarango, J.A., and C. Riddell. 1985. A study of cartilaginous nodules in the lungs of domestic poultry. Avian Dis 29:116–127.

285. Saunders, L.Z., and E.N. Moore. 1957. Blindness in turkeys due to granulomatous chorioretinitis. Avian Dis 1:27–36.

286. Sauveur, B., and P. Mongin. 1978. Tibial dyschondroplasia, a cartilage abnormality in poultry. Ann Biol Anim Biochem Biophys 18:87–98.

287. Scheele, C.W., W. DeWit, M.T. Frankenhuis, and P.F.G. Vereijken. 1991. Ascites in broilers. 1. Experimental factors evolving symptoms related to ascites. Poult Sci 70:1069–1083.

288. Scheele, C.W., E. Decuypere, P.F.G. Vereijken, and F.J.G. Schreurs. 1992. Ascites in broilers. 2. Disturbances in the hormonal regulation of metabolic rate and fat metabolism. Poult Sci 71:1971–1984.

289. Shane, S.M., R.J. Young, and L. Krook. 1969. Renal and parathyroid changes produced by high calcium intake in growing pullets. Avian Dis 13:558–567.

290. Shlosberg, A., E. Berman, U. Bendheim, and I. Plavnik. 1991. Controlled early feed restriction as a potential means of reducing the incidence of ascites in broilers. Avian Dis 35:681–684.

291. Shlosberg, A., I. Zadikov, U. Bendheim, V. Handji, and E. Berman. 1992. The effects of poor ventilation, low temperatures, type of feed and sex of bird on the development of ascites in broilers. Physiopathological factors. Avian Pathol 21:369–382.

292. Shlosberg, A., G. Pano, V. Handji, and E. Berman. 1992. Prophylactic and therapeutic treatment of ascites in broiler chickens. Br Poult Sci 33:141–148.

293. Siller, W.G. 1981. Renal pathology of the fowl—a review. Avian Pathol 10:187–262.

294. Siller, W.G., and P.A.L. Wight. 1978. The pathology of deep pectoral myopathy of turkeys. Avian Pathol 7:583–617.

295. Siller, W.G., P.A.L. Wight, L. Martindale, and D.W. Bannister. 1978. Deep pectoral myopathy: An experimental simulation in the fowl. Res Vet Sci 24:267–268.

296. Siller, W.G., P.A.L. Wight, and L. Martindale. 1979. Exercise-induced deep pectoral myopathy in broiler fowls and turkeys. Vet Sci Commun 2:331–336.

297. Siller, W.G., L. Martindale, and P.A.L. Wight. 1979. The prevention of experimental deep pectoral myopathy of the fowl by fasciotomy. Avian Pathol 8:301–307.

298. Springer, W.T. 1984. AAAP 1982 summary of disease reports. Avian Dis 28:816–843.

299. Spurloch, M.E., and J.E. Savage. 1993. Effect of dietary protein and selected antioxidants on fatty liver hemorrhagic syndrome induced in Japanese quail. Poult Sci 72:2095–2105.

300. Squires, E.J., and S. Leeson. 1988. Aetiology of fatty liver syndrome in laying hens. Br Vet J 144:602–609.

301. Stake, P.E., T.N. Fredrickson, and C.A. Bourdeau. 1981. Induction of fatty liver-hemorrhagic syndrome in laying hens by exogenous ß-estradiol. Avian Dis 25:410–422.

302. Steele, P., and J. Edgar. 1982. Importance of acute death syndrome in mortalities in broiler chicken flocks. Aust Vet J 58:63–66.

303. Steele, P., J. Edgar, and G. Doncon. 1982. Effect of biotin supplementation on incidence of acute death syndrome in broiler chickens. Poult Sci 61:909–913.

304. Steele, P., P. O'Malley, and M.C. McGrath. 1983. Personal communication.

305. Swire, P.W. 1980. Ascites in broilers. Vet Rec 107:541.

306. Thorp, B.H. 1988. Pattern of vascular canals in the bone extremities of the pelvic appendicular skeleton in broiler type fowl. Res Vet Sci 44:112–124.

307. Thorp, B.H. 1992. Abnormalities in the growth of leg bones. In C.C. Whitehead (ed.). Bone Biology and Skeletal Disorders in Poultry. Carfax Publishing Company. Abingdon, England, pp. 147–166.

308. Thorp, B.H. 1994. Skeletal disorders in the fowl: A review. Avian Pathol 23:203–236.

309. Thorp, B.H., and C. Goddard. 1994. Plasma concentrations of growth hormone and insulin-like growth factor-I in chickens developing tibial dyschondroplasia. Res Vet Sci 57:100–105.

310. Thorp, B.H., C.C. Whitehead, and J.S. Rennie. 1991. Avian tibial dyschondroplasia: A comparison of the incidence and severity as assessed by gross examination and histopathology. Res Vet Sci 51:48–54.

311. Thorp, B.H., S. Wilson, S. Rennie, and S.E. Solomon. 1993. The effect of a biphosphonate on bone volume and eggshell structure in the hen. Avian Pathol 22:671–682.

312. Thorp, B.H., B. Ducro, C.C. Whitehead, C. Farquharson, and P. Sorensen. 1993. Avian tibial dyschondroplasia: The interaction of genetic selection and dietary 1,25-dihydroxycholecalciferol. Avian Pathol 22:311–324.

313. Thorp, B.H., C.C. Whitehead, L. Dick, J.M. Bradbury, R.C. Jones, and A. Wood. 1993. Proximal femoral degeneration in growing broiler fowl. Avian Pathol 22:325–342.

314. Thorp, B.H., S.B. Jakowlew, and C. Goddard. 1995. Avian dyschondroplasia: Local deficiencies in growth factors are integral to the aetiopathogenesis. Avian Pathol 24:135–148.

315. Van Walsum, J. 1975. Contribution to the aetiology of synovitis in chickens, with special reference to non-infective factors. II. Tijdschr Diergeneeskd 100:76–83.

316. Van Walsum, J. 1977. Contribution to the aetiology of synovitis in chickens, with special reference to non-infective factors. III. Tijdschr Diergeneeskd 102:793–800.

317. Van Walsum, J. 1979. Contribution to the aetiology of synovitis in chickens, with special reference to non-infective factors. IV. Vet Q 1:90–96.

318. Veltmann, J.R., Jr., G.N. Rowland, and S.S. Linton. 1985. Tibial dyschondroplasia in single-comb white leghorn chicks fed tetramethylthiuram disulfide (a fungicide). Avian Dis 29:1269–1272.

319. Vidyadaran, M.K., A.S. King, and H. Kassim. 1990. Quantitative comparisons of lung structure of adult domestic fowl and red jungle fowl with reference to broiler ascites. Avian Pathol 19:51–58.

320. Volk, M., M. Herceg, B. Marzan, M. Kralj, S. Meknic, and V. Tadic. 1974. Investigations of fatal syncope of fowl in broilers. I. Incidence, clinical symptoms, pathomorphological findings and pathogenesis. Vet Arh 44:14–23.

321. Walser, M.M., F.L. Cherms, and H.E. Dziuk. 1982. Osseous development and tibial dyschondroplasia in five lines of turkeys. Avian Dis 26:265–271.

322. Walser, M.M., N.K. Allen, C.J. Mirocha, G.F. Hanlon, and J.A. Newman. 1982. Fusarium-induced osteochondrosis (tibial dyschondroplasia) in chickens. Vet Pathol 19:544–550.

323. Weaver, C.H., and S. Bird. 1934. The nature of cannibalism occurring among adult domestic fowls. J Am Vet Med Assoc 85:623–637.

324. Whitehead, C.C., and C.J. Randall. 1982. Interrelationships between biotin, choline and other B-vitamins and the occurrence of fatty liver and kidney syndrome and sudden death syndrome in broiler chickens. Br J Nutr 48:177–184.

325. Whitehead, C.C., R. Blair, D.W. Bannister, A.J. Evans, and R. Morley Jones. 1976. The involvement of biotin in preventing the fatty liver and kidney syndrome in chicks. Res Vet Sci 20:180–184.

326. Wideman, R.F., and B.S. Cowen. 1987. Effect of dietary acidification on kidney damage induced in immature chickens by excess calcium and infectious bronchitis virus. Poult Sci 66:626–633.

327. Wideman, R.F., and Y.K. Kirby. 1995. A pulmonary artery clamp model for inducing pulmonary hypertension syndrome (ascites) in broilers. Poult Sci 74:805–812.

328. Wideman, R.F., and A.C. Nissley. 1992. Kidney structure and responses of two commercial Single Comb White Leghorn strains to saline in the drinking water. Br Poult Sci 33:489–504.

329. Wideman, R.F., E.T. Mallinson and H. Rothenbacher. 1983. Kidney function of pullets and laying hens during outbreaks of urolithiasis. Poult Sci 62:1954–1970.

330. Wideman, R.F., J.A. Closser, W.B. Roush, and B.S. Cowen. 1985. Urolithiasis in pullets and laying hens: Role of dietary calcium and phosphorus. Poult Sci 64:2300–2307.

331. Wideman, R.F., W.B. Roush, J.L. Satnick, R.P. Glahn, and N.O. Oldroyd. 1989. Methionine hydroxy analog (free acid) reduces avian kidney damage and urolithiasis induced by excess dietary calcium. J Nutr 119:818–828.

332. Wideman, R.F., B.C. Ford, R.M. Leach, D.F.Wise, and W.W.Robey. 1993. Liquid methionine hydroxy analog (free acid) and DL-methionine attenuate calcium induced kidney damage in domestic fowl. Poult Sci 72:1245–1258.

333. Wideman, R.F., M. Ismail, Y.K. Kirby, W.G. Bottje, R.W. Moore, and R.C. Vardeman. 1995. Furosemide reduces the incidence of pulmonary hypertension syndrome (ascites) in broilers exposed to cool environmental temperatures. Poult Sci 74:314–322.

334. Wideman, R.F., Y.K. Kirby, M. Ismail, W.G. Bottje, R.W. Moore, and R.C. Vardeman. 1995. Supplemental L-arginine attenuates pulmonary hypertension syndrome (ascites) in broilers. Poult Sci 74:323–330.

335. Wight, P.A.L. 1965. Histopathology of a chronic endophthalmitis of the domestic fowl. J Comp Pathol 75:353–361.

336. Wight, P.A.L., and S.R.I. Duff. 1985. Ectopic pulmonary cartilage and bone in domestic fowl. Res Vet Sci 39:188–195.

337. Wight, P.A.L., and D.W.F. Shannon. 1977. Plasma protein derivative (amyloid-like substance) in livers of rapeseed-fed fowls. Avian Pathol 6:293–305.

338. Wight, P.A.L., and W.G. Siller. 1980. Pathology of deep pectoral myopathy of broilers. Vet Pathol 17:29–39.

339. Wight, P.A.L., W.G. Siller, L. Martindale, and J.H. Filshie. 1979. The induction by muscle stimulation of a deep pectoral myopathy in the fowl. Avian Pathol 8:115–121.

340. Wight, P.A.L., L. Martindale, and W.G. Siller. 1979. Oregon disease and husbandry. Vet Rec 105:470–471.

341. Wilson, J.B., R.J. Julian, and I.K. Barker. 1988. Lesions of right heart failure and ascites in broiler chickens. Avian Dis 32:246–261.

342. Wilson, S., B.O. Hughes, M.C. Appleby, and S.F. Smith. 1993. Effects of perches on trabecular bone volume in laying hens. Res Vet Sci 54:207–211.

343. Wise, D.R. 1975. Skeletal abnormalities in table poultry—a review. Avian Pathol 4:1–10.

344. Wise, D.R. 1979. Nutrition-disease interactions of leg weakness in poultry. In W. Haresign and D. Lewis (eds.). Recent Advances in Animal Nutrition—1978. Butterworths, London, pp. 41–57.

345. Wise, D.R., and A.R. Jennings. 1972. Dyschondroplasia in domestic poultry. Vet Rec 91:285–286.

346. Witzell, D.A., W.E. Huff, L.F. Kubena, R.B. Harvey, and M.H. Elissalde. 1990. Ascites in growing broilers: A research model. Poult Sci 69:741–745.

347. Wojcinski, H.S.F. 1989. A mortality study of heavy tom turkey flocks in Ontario. D.V.Sc. dissertation, University of Guelph, Guelph, Canada.

348. Wolford, J.H., and K. Tanaka. 1970. Factors influencing egg shell quality—a review. World's Poult Sci J 26:763–780.

349. Wong-Valle, J., G.R. McDaniel, D.L. Kuhlers, and J.E. Bartels. 1993. Correlated responses to selection for high or low incidence of tibial dyschondroplasia in broilers. Poult Sci 72:1621–1629.

350. Wong-Valle, J., G.R. McDaniel, D.L. Kuhlers, and J.E. Bartels. 1993. Effect of lighting program and broiler line on the incidence of tibial dyschondroplasia at four and seven weeks of age. Poult Sci 72:1855–1860.

351. Yamasaki, K., and C. Itakura. 1983. Pathology of degenerative osteoarthritis in laying hens. Jpn J Vet Sci 45:1–8.

352. Yamashiro, S., M.K. Bhatnagar, J.R. Scott and S.J. Slinger. 1975. Fatty haemorrhagic liver syndrome in laying hens on diets supplemented with rapeseed products. Res Vet Sci 19:312–321.

36 Poisons and Toxins

MYCOTOXICOSES

Frederic J. Hoerr

INTRODUCTION. A mycotoxicosis is a disease caused by a toxic fungal metabolite (mycotoxin). Mycotoxins drew attention in the early 1960s when aflatoxin, a mycotoxin produced by *Aspergillus* spp., was discovered to be the cause of disease in poultry and fish. The significance of aflatoxin was accentuated by the disclosure of carcinogenicity. Diseases in humans and animals caused by consumption of moldy food, however, have been recognized since long before the discovery of aflatoxin. Ergotism, moldy corn poisoning of horses, stachybotryotoxicosis, alimentary toxic aleukia, various hemorrhagic syndromes, yellow rice poisoning, and other acute food poisonings are just some of the historically significant mycotoxicoses of humans and animals.

Hundreds of mycotoxins are now recognized (401), but the toxicity, occurrence, and target organs are varied among these naturally occurring toxins. The impact of mycotoxins on poultry production may be measured best indirectly, by improvements in weight gain, feed efficiency, pigmentation, egg production, and reproductive performance that accompany mycotoxin control programs. Overt intoxication is uncommon and diagnostic confirmation even less so, but capabilities are improving and the number of reported confirmations steadily increase.

ERGOTISM

ETIOLOGY AND TOXICOLOGY. Ergotism is a historically important mycotoxicosis characterized by vascular, neurologic, and endocrine disorders (see review 247). Epidemics killed many people in Europe during the Middle Ages. Descriptions of ergotism date back to the Roman Empire and to China of 5000 years ago.

Ergotism is caused by *Claviceps* spp., fungi that attack cereal grains. Rye is especially affected, but also wheat and other leading cereal grains, with regional differences throughout the world. *Claviceps purpurea* is a frequent cause of ergotism because of its wide host range among cereals. The mycotoxins form in the sclerotium, a visible, hard, dark mass of mycelium that displaces grain tissue. In the normal cycle, the sclerotium falls to the ground, germinates, and produces spores that infect the flower of the new crop, and the cycle repeats. Harvest channels the sclerotium into the food chain.

Within the sclerotium are the ergot alkaloids, first described in 1864, which cause ergotism. Lysergic acid is the chemical building block of the 40 or more alkaloids produced by *Claviceps* spp. With individual variation, the alkaloids produce convulsive and sensory neurologic disorders, vasoconstriction and gangrene of extremities, and altered neuroendocrine control of the anterior pituitary gland (276). Some characteristics responsible for toxicity also have pharmacologic benefits.

Ergot has been identified in wheat, barley, oats, rye, rice, and other cereals in Canada, Europe, and Japan (see review 432). Tolerances for ergot in international trade vary, but some countries classify various grains as "ergoty" with sclerotium concentrations of 0.1–0.33%. Rye also has inherent antinutritive factors but ergot, at concentrations that might be encountered naturally (0.33%) has no significant interaction with these factors (268, 269). Weed seed contaminants of grain can also be a source of ergot (313). Pelleting of feeds can increase the toxicity of ergot, perhaps through increased liberation of toxins.

NATURALLY OCCURRING DISEASE. Ergotism occurs as reductions in feed intake and growth; necrosis of the beak, comb, and toes; and diarrhea. Leghorns developed coalescing vesicles and crusts on the comb and wattles, face, and eyelids (vesicular dermatitis, sod disease) (313). Combs and wattles were permanently atrophied and disfigured. Vesicles and ulcers also developed on shanks of the legs and on the toes. In another episode, ergotism spared very young chickens, but those over 6 wk of age failed to grow and had mortality of 25%. Laying hens had reductions in feed consumption and egg production, but no consistent lesions occurred other than those on the skin. Muscovy ducks fed wheat dockage contaminated with 1.17% ergot became listless and lethargic, stopped eating and drinking, and developed diarrhea (384). Most of the ducklings aged 12 wk or younger died but older birds were resistant, in contrast to chickens. Lesions were confined to visceral congestion.

EXPERIMENTAL DISEASE. Wheat ergot causes decreased appetite and growth, and mortality in chickens but the detrimental effects, including mortality, are quite variable (344, 345, 346). Broilers are more sensitive than leghorns. The toxicity is mostly in the alkaloid fraction of the ergot extract, but the predictive value of total alkaloid content is not highly accurate. Ergotamine tartrate, one of the most common alkaloids, causes necrosis of toes and cardiac enlargement in chicks (434). Increased cardiac work load is thought to be due to vasoconstriction and hypertension. Triticale ergot in broiler chicks causes reduction of growth, poor feathering, nervousness, loss of coordination, and inability to stand (33). Intoxication can be fatal.

METABOLISM AND RESIDUES. Ergotamine tartrate accumulates in only trace amounts in broiler chicken tissues when fed at relatively high concentrations (800 mg/kg diet). About 5% of the alkaloid is excreted unchanged and 15–20% is excreted as a complex mixture containing as many as 16 possible metabolites (434).

FUSARIUM MYCOTOXINS. The genus *Fusarium* produces numerous mycotoxins injurious to poultry. Various toxins produced by *Fusarium* produce caustic and radiomimetic injury, cardiac toxicity, and skeletal, digestive, and reproductive disorders.

Trichothecenes

ETIOLOGY AND TOXICOLOGY. Trichothecene mycotoxins are produced by *Fusarium* and its perithecial stages *Calonectria* and *Gibberella,* and the genera *Myrothecium, Stachybotrys, Cephalosporium, Trichoderma, Trichothecium, Cylindrocarpon, Veriticimonosporium,* and *Phomopsis* (see reviews 245, 265, 398). These common soil and plant fungi are found worldwide. In one study, about 20% of investigated isolates were capable of trichothecene production. Of the more than 100 trichothecenes, about half are produced by *Fusarium* (399). The greatest toxin production occurs with high humidity and temperatures of 6–24 C.

Trichothecenes have a tetracyclic sesquiterpene nucleus with a characteristic epoxide ring. Poultry exposure to trichothecenes is likely to be of the non-macrocyclic group, which includes toxins classified as type A (T-2 toxin, neosolanial, diacetoxyscirpenol, and others) and type B (nivalenol, deoxynivalenol, fusarenone-X, and others), reviewed by

Leeson et al. (245). Toxicity resides in the highly stable epoxide ring (265, 398) and is not deteriorated by prolonged storage or normal cooking temperatures (19). As a group but with individual variation, trichothecenes are potent inhibitors of structural lipids (62) and of the synthesis of protein (257) and DNA (398). Many are caustic irritants, a feature used in detection bioassays.

T-2 toxin, diacetoxyscirpenol (DAS), deoxynivalenol (DON, vomitoxin), and nivalenol have been identified in feedstuffs worldwide, including corn, wheat, barley, oats, rice, rye, sorghum, safflower seed, mixed feed, and brewer's grains (see reviews 245, 432). Deoxynivalenol is the most prevalent and is often found with zearalenone, aflatoxin, and other mycotoxins (156, 148, 402). Deoxynivalenol has low toxicity for poultry in contrast to swine in which it causes feed refusal and emesis. For this reason, grains contaminated with deoxynivalenol may be diverted to poultry.

NATURALLY OCCURRING DISEASE. Both historical and recent accounts of trichothecene mycotoxicosis reflect their caustic and radiomimetic effects, expressed as feed refusal, extensive necrosis of oral mucosa and skin in contact with the mold, acute digestive tract disease, and altered bone marrow and immune system function.

Avian fusariotoxicosis occurred in the former Soviet Union during periods when alimentary toxic aleukia was endemic in humans at certain times during the first half of the 20th century. *Fusarium poae* and *F. sporotrichioides* were isolated from grain and green vegetation feedstuffs and were the likely sources of toxins. Chickens with fusariotoxicosis (probable trichothecene mycotoxicosis) had reduced growth, severe depression, and bloody diarrhea (see review 234). Lesions comprised necrosis of oral mucosa, reddening of the gastrointestinal mucosa, mottling of the liver, gallbladder distention, atrophy of the spleen, and visceral hemorrhages. Presumed trichothecene mycotoxicosis caused by *Stachybotrys* spp. occurred in poultry during the 1940s as necrosis of oral and crop mucosa, digestive and neurologic disturbances, blood dyscrasias, and hemorrhagic disease (see review 177).

Broilers. Mycotoxicosis in broilers in the United States was caused by T-2 toxin produced by *Fusarium tricinctum.* Toxin-contaminated feed and litter caused reduced growth, vesicular lesions on the feet and legs, and the oral mucosa was ulcerated and crusted (424). In France, T-2 toxin, neosolaniol, verrucarol, fusarenon-X, and crotocol were trichothecenes identified (1–4 mg/kg) in feed produced from crib-stored corn. Signs and lesions comprised digestive disturbance, reduced growth, rickets, nervous disorders, abnormal feathering, pigmentation defects, and hemorrhages (334). Although infectious bursal disease was a concurrent problem, the situation resolved when unadulterated corn was provided.

Hens. T-2 toxin and HT-2 toxin contamination of feed caused rapid decrease in egg production beginning the day after feed delivery (362). Depression, recumbency, feed refusal, and cyanosis of the comb and wattles also occurred. The ovary and oviduct became atrophied. The situation resolved when nontoxic feed was provided.

Feed contaminated with T-2 toxin (3 mg/kg) caused decreases in feed consumption and egg production, and thin-shelled eggs (166). Yellow crusts and ulcers on the oral mucosa made closing the mouth difficult, and feathers were uneven and poorly formed. Uniformity of oral and feather lesions within cages were noticeably lacking throughout the caged-layer facility. Birds with oral lesions also had yellow-tan, friable livers, swollen kidneys, urate deposits in the ureters, focal ulceration and inflammation of crop mucosa, and thickened, rough lining in the gizzard.

Contamination of grain sorghum with deoxynivalenol (0.3 mg/kg) and zearalenone (1.1 mg/kg) was associated with decreased egg production. Oral ulcers were seen in conjunction with squamous metaplasia of salivary and mucus glands (34). Oral crusts and ulcers in commercial layers, taken as presumptive evidence of thrichothecene exposure, were associated with decreases in egg weight and shell weight (152). The frequency was influenced by strain and was more common in older hens.

Geese and Ducks. Barley contaminated with T-2 toxin (25 mg/kg) caused reduced activity, feed refusal, and increased water consumption in geese and ducks (149, 327). Intoxicated geese died within 2 days and had necrosis and pseudomembranes in the esophagus, proventriculus, and gizzard. Histopathology also revealed degeneration of intestinal epithelium and acute tubular injury in the kidney. Wild geese dying of fowl cholera had concurrent exposure to deoxynivalenol (maximum of 5.0 mg/kg) and zearalenone (maximum of 25 mg/kg) in contaminated corn, postulated to be an immunosuppressive stress (176).

Turkeys. Poults that ate feed contaminated with deoxynivalenol (0.81 mg/kg) and salinomycin (2.2 mg/kg) experienced feed refusal and high mortality (251). In a feeding trial, poults had lower feed consumption and higher mortality, but those fed diets appended with much higher concentrations of deoxynivalenol and salinomycin, alone and in combi-

nation, had no adverse effects. Undetectable toxins were thought to have contributed to the toxicity.

Cranes. Suspected fusariotoxicosis in sandhill cranes (*Grus canadensis*) was associated with trichothecene-producing *Fusarium* isolated from peanuts utilized as a food source in the wild (343). Recurring annual episodes of high mortality were accompanied by clinical signs of loss of motor control to the neck, wings, and legs. Edema was present around the head and neck, but the ulcerative digestive lesions usually attributed to trichothecenes were lacking. Principal lesions were hemorrhages, granulomatous myositis, thrombosis, and vascular degeneration.

EXPERIMENTAL DISEASE. Experimental trichothecene mycotoxicosis in poultry has required several approaches to reproduce fully the disease spectrum observed naturally: purified toxin administered either in solution or in the diet, and toxigenic fungal cultures (see review 207). Collectively, these toxins cause feed refusal, impaired growth and reproductive capability, and whole-body pathology including caustic injury to skin and alimentary mucosa; radiomimetic injury to bone marrow, lymphoid tissues, gastrointestinal tract, and feathers; hepatosis; and thyroid alterations.

Pathology. Many trichothecenes cause erosive and exudative injury to the oral mucosa of poultry fed toxin-appended diets (61, 83, 424, 425). Broiler chickens develop focal, yellow oral plaques that progress to yellow-gray, raised accumulations of exudate with underlying ulcers located near major salivary duct openings on the palate, tongue, and buccal floor. Thick crusts accumulate along the interior margin of the beak (Fig. 36.1A,B). Oral histopathology confirms mucosal necrosis and ulceration, submucosal granulation tissue and inflammatory cells, and crusts of exudate, bacterial colonies, and feed components.

The histopathology of acute lethal oral intoxication by T-2 toxin or diacetoxyscirpenol occurs as necrosis of lymphoid and hematopoietic tissues within 1 hr, rapid cellular depletion, then repletion after 72 hr (182). Discrete foci of hepatocyte necrosis and hemorrhage, and necrosis and inflammation of the gallbladder mucosa are followed by mild proliferation of bile ductules. Necrosis of intestinal epithelium precedes transient shortening of villi and fewer mitotic figures in crypt epithelium. Necrosis also occurs in the mucosa of the proventriculus and gizzard, and in feather epithelium.

Repeated administration of T-2 toxin and diacetoxyscirpenol (183, 184, 426, 429) causes reductions in body weight and skin pigmentation, anemia, and malformed feathers in broilers (Fig. 36.2).

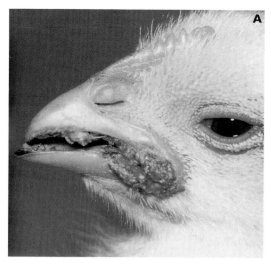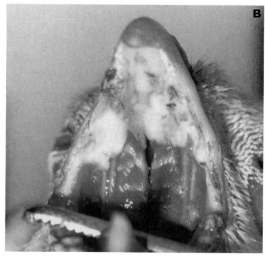

36.1. Fusariotoxicosis. Trichothecene mycotoxins cause chemical irritation of the upper digestive tract mucosa. *A.* Crusts at the beak commissure of a broiler chicken fed diacetoxyscirpenol for 8 days. *B.* Beak and palate ulceration and crusting in a broiler chicken following 14 days consumption of diacetoxyscirpenol (4 mg/kg diet).

Multiple toxins in the scirpenol group cause frayed, misshapen feathers (302). Gross lesions comprise atrophic lymphoid tissues, pale red or yellow bone marrow, and yellowing of the liver (Fig. 36.3). Histopathologic changes include necrosis with cell depletion of lymphoid and hematopoietic tissues, necrosis of hepatocytes, bile ducts, enteric mucosa, and germinal epithelium of feather barbs. Hepato-

cytes have vacuolar change due to lipid accumulation, accompanied by hyperplasia of bile ducts. Thyroid gland follicles are small, contain pale colloid, and have tall epithelial cells.

Trichothecene-producing cultures of *Fusarium* and *Stachybotrys* cause clinical signs and lesions similar to those of the purified toxins (185, 208, 357). Trichothecenes in fungal cultures (a model

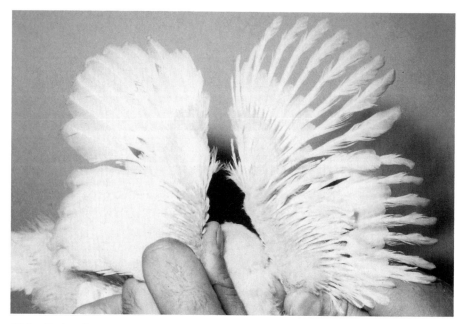

36.2. Feathers from a chicken fed T-2 toxin for 24 days (*right*) are narrow because of radiomimetic injury to the developing barbs; control (*left*).

closer to naturally occurring intoxication) appear more toxic than purified compounds. This suggests that certain trichothecenes, even in low concentrations, may be significant in naturally contaminated feedstuffs.

In mallard ducks, T-2 toxin causes necrosis and caseous plaques throughout the upper alimentary tract, especially in the oropharynx and proventriculus (171, 279). Some develop ulcerative, proliferative esophagitis and proventriculitis. The gizzard lining is thickened, fissured, and ulcerated. Lymphoid tissues are severely atrophied. Muscovy ducks are particularly sensitive to trichothecene injury of oral mucosa, and have been recommended as a bioassay (363).

Acute lethal deoxynivalenol intoxication in broiler chickens occurs as reduced spontaneous activity, dyspnea, diarrhea, visceral gout, and hemorrhages in the subcutis and viscera (198). Broiler and leghorn chicks and turkey poults can tolerate deoxynivalenol at levels likely to be encountered under natural exposure (163, 204, 216, 225). Mild oral plaques and gizzard erosions may occur (249, 272) but only at toxin concentrations much higher than other trichothecenes and greater than those causing feed refusal and emesis in swine.

Egg Production and Reproduction. T-2 toxin, diacetoxyscirpenol, and monoacetoxyscirpenol cause reductions in feed intake, body weight, egg production in leghorn chickens and Nicholas large white turkey hens (8, 9, 63, 378, 429). Decreases in egg production may be abrupt. Hatchability is impaired, although toxins other than trichothecenes may also be involved. Hens recover but are prone to overconsume feed (430). Deoxynivalenol is essentially nontoxic to hens at concentrations likely to be encountered in naturally contaminated grain (24, 163, 164, 216, 227, 228, 249, 273). Adverse effects include minor changes in yolk, white, and shell quality, and embryonic mortality and malformations. Mild changes in dietary intake are likely due to palatability or olfactory responses.

Nutrition. T-2 toxin reduces plasma vitamin E concentrations in broiler chickens (76). The sparing effect of micelle-promoting compounds suggests T-2 toxin impairs lipid metabolism in the intestine.

Hematology. T-2 toxin and diacetoxyscirpenol cause anemia associated with marked hematopoietic depletion in the bone marrow of broiler chickens, although the manner of toxin presentation is important in toxicity (184, 185). T-2 toxin causes leukopenia in leghorn hens (429). Deoxynivalenol fed at prolonged high doses may cause mild anemia and leukopenia (67, 225).

Immunosuppression. Despite the profound effects of many trichothecenes on lymphoid organs and bone marrow (387), measurable immunosuppression has not been documented in chickens or

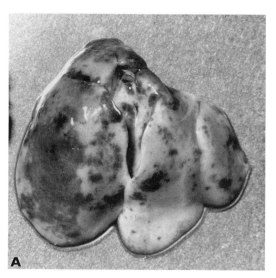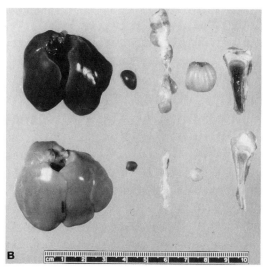

36.3. Experimental trichothecene mycotoxicosis in broiler chickens. *A.* Hemorrhage in the liver occurring 20 hr after consumption of feed mixed with a culture of *Fusarium sporotrichiella* that produced T-2 toxin and neosolaniol. (Avian Pathology) *B.* Fourteen daily oral doses of T-2 toxin causes yellow discoloration of the liver (*top row*) compared with control (*bottom row*). The radiomimetic effects are evidenced by atrophy of the spleen, thymus, and bursa of Fabricius, and yellow discoloration (aplasia) of the bone marrow. (Avian Pathology)

turkeys (30, 335). This may result from using purified toxin-appended diets rather than feeding fungal cultures or oral dosing, which allow greater expression of toxicity by trichothecenes (185).

Coagulation. Broiler chickens fed growth-inhibitory levels of T-2 toxin develop prolonged prothrombin times and have suppressed activity of factor VIII and fibrinogen (95, 98).

Serum Chemistry. Chickens develop changes in serum constituents reflective of lesions in the liver, intestine, muscle, and kidney (63, 64, 65, 306, 429). Serum parameters recover to normal within 10 days after sublethal T-2 intoxication.

Neurotoxicity. Neurotoxicity of T-2 toxin and other trichothecenes is inconsistently reported but occurs as abnormal wing positioning, seizures, and loss of righting response (185, 427). Brain dopamine concentration is increased and norepinepherine is decreased (69).

METABOLISM AND RESIDUES. Liver is the major organ for T-2 toxin metabolism and excretion in the chicken. In broiler chickens, oral T-2 toxin reaches highest concentration in liver at 4 hr, and bile and intestine at 12 hr (66). Eighty-two percent of T-2 toxin and its hydroxylation metabolites are excreted from the body within 48 hr (342). T-2 toxin is the only trichothecene found in liver, but T-2 toxin, HT-2 toxin, neosolaniol, and T-2 tetraol, and others appear in feces (142, 433). Relatively small amounts of T-2 toxin are excreted into the egg (66). Progressively greater amounts of T-2 metabolites are excreted into yolk, but those in egg white peak and remain constant.

Deoxynivalenol fed to broilers at field levels is undetectable in skeletal muscle (117). The concentration in hen plasma reaches only 1% of an oral dose (321), and most is rapidly eliminated in feces. Only low concentrations occur in eggs and diminish when the toxin is withdrawn (321).

Moniliformin

ETIOLOGY AND TOXICOLOGY. Moniliformin is produced by *Fusarium moniliforme* and other *Fusarium* spp. (329) and is cardiotoxic in poultry. *F. moniliforme* causes ear rot, kernel rot, and stalk rot of unharvested corn and may be involved in advanced decay of stored high-moisture shelled corn (see review 47). The fungus also occurs on oats, soybeans, sorghum, barley, and wheat, and corn that visually appears sound. Although moniliformin is quite toxic to poultry, diets made with purified moniliformin are less toxic than toxigenic fungal cultures. *F. moniliforme* also produces fumonisins,

zearalenone and fusariocin A (47), and other toxic fractions (84).

NATURALLY OCCURRING DISEASE. Verification of *F. moniliforme* mycotoxicosis is relatively lacking, although industry reports indicate it is a problem for poultry. Broiler breeders and leghorns fed corn contaminated with *F. moniliforme* had reduced rate of lay and delayed peaks in production (84). Intermittent overconsumption and underconsumption of feed occurred in conjunction with diarrhea, dark fecal droppings with undigested feed, fecal-stained egg shells, and blood smears on egg shells. Contaminated corn was high in moisture, low in protein, and high in crushing strength. The latter causes large particle sizes in the cornmeal leading to digestive disturbance.

EXPERIMENTAL DISEASE. Moniliformin toxicity has been characterized in the chicken, turkey, and duck; lesions are similar in all species. Acute lethal intoxication by purified moniliformin produces mesenteric edema, ascites, and hemorrhages in the digestive tract and skin (78). Subacute toxicity occurs as cyanosis, cardiac enlargement, hydropericardium, and ascites (25, 121). Microscopically, myocardial degeneration occurs as swollen muscle fibers with vacuolation, fragmentation, lysis of myofibrils, and myofiber necrosis. Liver has multifocal vacuolation and swelling of hepatocytes and small foci of hepatocyte necrosis. The cardiac toxicity occurs as bradycardia and changes in the electrocardiogram and is partially alleviated by selenium (277, 436).

Fumonisins

ETIOLOGY AND TOXICOLOGY. *Fusarium moniliforme* also produces the fumonisins, which are the cause of equine leukoencephalomalacia (moldy corn poisoning) (254) and porcine pulmonary edema syndrome (80). Fumonisin B1 is the most common of this group, which is also produced by other species of *Fusarium* (122). The mechanism of fumonisin B1 toxicity is related to disrupted sphingolipid synthesis (409).

EXPERIMENTAL DISEASE. Fumonisin B1 fed as purified toxin or toxigenic culture causes diarrhea, catarrhal enteritis (Fig. 36.4A,B), and impaired weight gain and feed conversion when fed to turkey poults, broiler chicks, and ducklings (26, 40, 122, 243, 410). Poults are more sensitive than chicks, but poultry are quite resistant to fumonisins in comparison to horses and swine. The concentrations that produce toxicity in poultry are higher than those likely to be encountered in naturally contaminated grains (233). *F. moniliforme*, however, produces toxins other than fumonisins that may influence this (411).

Lesions comprise consistent enlargement of the liver, and variable enlargement of kidney, pancreas, and proventriculus and gizzard; atrophy of lymphoid organs; and rickets. Histologically, the liver has multifocal necrosis of hepatocytes, hyperplasia of hepatocytes and bile ductules, and hypertrophy of Kupffer cells. The intestine has villous atrophy and goblet cell hyperplasia. Growth plates are widened in both the zones of proliferating and hypertrophic cartilage. Myocardium and skeletal muscle have mild lesions. Lymphoid tissues are depleted and there is toxicity to macrophages (328).

Fusarochromanone

ETIOLOGY AND TOXICOLOGY. Fusarochromanone is produced by *Fusarium* spp. and causes tibial dyschondroplasia in chickens. Varus and valgus deformities in broiler chicken have been induced by cultures of *Aspergillus niger, A. flavus, F. moniliforme,* and *F. roseum* (358). A strain of *F. roseum* isolated from overwintered barley in Alaska caused a high incidence of tibial dyschondroplasia when fed to broiler chickens (405). Defective chondroclasis was suggested as a possible pathogenesis and chondroclastic activity was found in the water-soluble extract of the culture (244). Of six components identified, one of three fluorescent components (ultraviolet light), TDP-1 (fusarochromanone), induced a 100% incidence of tibial dyschondroplasia when fed to broiler chickens. Tibial dyschondroplasia is a defect in endochondral ossification occur-

ring as a cone of cartilage in the tibiotarsus and other long bones of growing, heavy breeds of chickens, turkeys, and ducks. Lack of vascular penetration of cartilage leads to failure of normal ossification. Rapid growth, genetic predisposition, and various nutritional and management factors also influence the lesion.

EXPERIMENTAL DISEASE. Chicks fed fusarochromanone-producing cultures of *Fusarium* develop lesions in the tibial physis within 4 days (173). The physis becomes thickened and histologically has a thickened transitional zone, especially prominent in the center of the growth plate. Increased dietary copper and zinc have a partial sparing effect (418). The primary site of fusarochromanone action at the cellular and biochemical level is not known. Hypertrophic cartilage has a lower density of chondroclasts (240) and the chondrocytes from the cartilage core have intracellular lipid accumulation, autophagic vacuoles, and necrosis, likely secondary to the increased distance from their vascular source of nutrients (172). Fusarochromanone is only moderately toxic to chondrocytes in vitro (417), and much less so than T-2 toxin. *Fusarium* strains that produce fusarochromanone are also immunosuppressive (418, 419).

Zearalenone

ETIOLOGY AND TOXICOLOGY. Grains infected with the fungus *Gibberella zeae* (*Fusarium graminearum, F. roseum* "Graminearum") are a source of zearalenone (F-2), a mycotoxin with estrogenic ac-

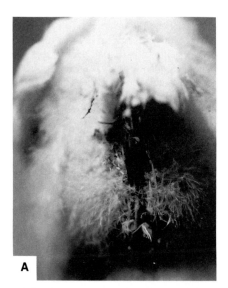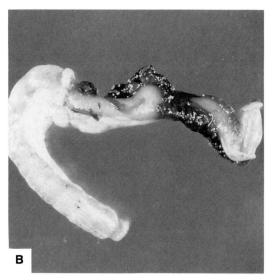

36.4. Diarrhea (*A*) and catarrhal enteritis (*B*) in broiler chickens fed cultures of *Fusarium moniliforme* that produced fumonisin B1.

tivity. Of seven chemical forms, only zearalenone and zearalenol occur naturally. Although zearalenone is the most prevalent and has been closely examined in poultry, zearalenol is three to four times more active estrogenically (266). Zearalenone occurs in corn, sorghum (90), wheat, barley, oats, milo, rye, and other grains (see reviews 364, 432). Toxicity occurs chiefly in swine as reproductive failure. Chickens are more tolerant of zearalenone than are either turkeys or swine, and are an outlet for grains unfit for swine (5, 124). Zearalenone is relatively nontoxic for chickens, but it has potential adverse effects and may be an indicator of other toxins that formed concurrently.

NATURALLY OCCURRING DISEASE. Zearalenone (0.5–5.0 mg/kg) was considered detrimental to broiler breeders that experienced a reduction in egg production although fertility, hatchability, or progeny performance remained normal (29). Affected hens had lowered serum progesterone and ascites in conjunction with cystic inflammation of the oviduct.

EXPERIMENTAL DISEASE. Experimental zearalenone mycotoxicosis has been studied in broiler and leghorn chickens, turkeys, quail, and geese. In general, poultry are tolerant of this mycotoxin. Turkeys are the most sensitive, with reproductive tract and sex hormone–sensitive tissues targeted.

In leghorn chicks, bursa of Fabricius weight increases (377), possibly related to hormone-induced regional swelling in birds. Cysts develop on the peritoneal surface and within the oviduct. Broiler chickens are highly tolerant of zearalenone, with lesions limited to decreased comb and testes weight (7), oviduct enlargement (68), and leukopenia (67). Male turkey poults display precocious strutting behavior and have development of the caruncles and dewlaps, and soft tissue swelling of the vent (6). Japanese quail are resistant (16).

Egg specific gravity, eggshell thickness, and interior egg quality were reduced in leghorns fed corn diets contaminated with *F. roseum.* (377). Serum calcium was decreased and phosphorus was increased (68). Other studies show leghorns highly tolerant of zearalenone (68) and of corn contaminated with *F. roseum* (5, 256). A water-soluble component of *F. roseum* cultures containing neither zearalenone nor trichothecenes caused reduced hatchability (244). In geese, fertility is reduced and spermatogenesis inhibited (298, 299, 300). Eggs produced from turkeys fed *F. roseum* cultures had reduced hatchability, but neither zearalenone nor trichothecenes were the responsible toxins (8).

METABOLISM AND RESIDUES. Zearalenone distributes chiefly to liver and gallbladder (267) and is excreted mainly in feces as zearalenone, and α- and ß-zearalenol (289). In leghorn hens, most is rapidly excreted in feces, but residues may occur in yolk (87).

Other *Fusarium* Toxins. Strains of *F. moniliforme* that produce fusaric acid (73) and fusarocin C (255) are immunosuppressive in chickens. In one study, chicks fed *F. moniliforme* diets developed signs of thiamin deficiency and responded to thiamin therapy (128). Dietary thiamin concentrations were low, possibly due to the thiamin being destroyed or utilization by the mold in the feed. Fumonisin B1 was detected in feed associated with paralysis in quail, but clinical signs could not be reproduced in feeding trials (153).

Aflatoxins

ETIOLOGY AND TOXICOLOGY. Aflatoxins are highly toxic and carcinogenic mycotoxins produced by *Aspergillus flavus, A. parasiticus,* and *Penicillium puberulum* (see review 114). Poultry feeds and ingredients are vulnerable to fungal growth and aflatoxin formation. Aflatoxins are relatively stable in normal food and feed products but are sensitive to oxidizing agents such as hypochlorite (commercial bleach).

The aflatoxins have two fused dihydrofuran rings with various moieties, and members are designated as B1, B2, G1, and G2, after their blue (B) or green (G) color reaction to fluorescent light (365-nm wavelength) and their chromatographic Rf values. Aflatoxin B1 is the most toxic, and hepatotoxicity is the primary effect in nearly all animals. Chronic aflatoxicosis results in neoplasia in many species, usually in the liver, but gallbladder, pancreas, urinary tract, and bone may be involved (see review 297). Although several aflatoxin metabolites are carcinogenic, aflatoxin B1 is most potent. It binds to nuclear and mitochondrial DNA (see review 189) and is a model hepatocarcinogen for mechanisms of tumor initiation in the liver. It may also be active in promotion through oncogene activation, hormone alteration, and dietary interaction.

Aflatoxin-producing fungi and aflatoxin-contaminated animal feedstuffs are recognized worldwide (91, 181, 285, 361, 364, 432), usually with adverse implications for poultry production (209, 214, 250, 274).

NATURALLY OCCURRING DISEASE. Detailed descriptions of the first cases of aflatoxicosis were reviewed in the previous editions (180, 307). What is substantially embedded in the literature as spontaneous aflatoxicosis in now recognized to have significant contributions from cyclopiazonic acid (32) and possibly sterigmatocystin and other toxins.

Lethal aflatoxicosis in ducklings occurred as inappetance, reduced growth (14), abnormal vocalizations, feather picking, purple discoloration of legs and feet, and lameness. Ataxia, convulsions, and opisthotonus preceded death. At necropsy, liver and kidneys were enlarged and pale. With chronicity, ascites and hydropericardium developed, accompanied by a shrunken firm nodular liver, distention of the gallbladder and hemorrhages. Microscopic lesions in the liver were fatty change in hepatocytes, proliferation of bile ductules, and extensive fibrosis, accompanied by vascular and degenerative lesions in pancreas and kidney.

Turkeys developed inappetance, reduced spontaneous activity, unsteady gait, recumbency, anemia, and death (367, 406). At necropsy, the body condition was generally good but there was generalized congestion and edema. The liver and kidney were congested, enlarged, and firm; the gallbladder was full; and the duodenum was distended with catarrhal content. Lethal aflatoxicosis can cause either dark red or yellow discoloration of the liver due to congestion or fat accumulation, respectively (Fig. 36.5). Microscopic lesions in livers consisted of swollen hepatocytes with homogenous, sometimes vacuolated, cytoplasm, karyomegaly, and focal necrosis of centrilobular hepatocytes, followed by hepatocyte regeneration, proliferation of bile ductules and reticuloendothelial cell hyperplasia, and degenerative lesions in the heart, kidney, and intestine.

Aflatoxicosis in chickens closely resembled that in ducks and turkeys (13, 14). The occurrence of skeletal myopathy (134) may have reflected an interaction of selenium and aflatoxicosis (see Experimental Disease).

Aflatoxicosis in poultry is reported from India (71, 320, 331), Malaysia (3), Indonesia (175), Sudan (85), Nigeria (288, 366), Morocco (217), Poland (215), the United Kingdom (235), Australia (42), and the United States (157, 370, 414). The direct and indirect effects of aflatoxicosis include increased mortality from heat stress (broiler breeders) (85); loss of egg production (leghorns) (42); anemia, hemorrhages, liver condemnations (235), paralysis and lameness (288), and impaired performance (214) (broilers); nervous signs (3), impaired performance, and mortality (ducks) (42); impaired

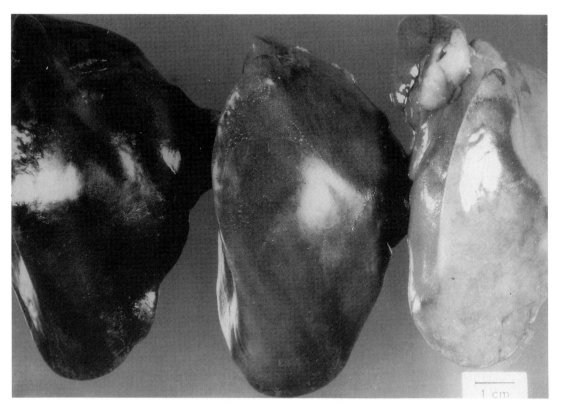

36.5. Lethal aflatoxicosis in turkeys causes liver discoloration from dark red (*left*), due to congestion and necrosis, to yellow (*right*), owing to fat accumulation in hepatocytes. Aflatoxin B1 (200 ppb) was detected in the feed given to these turkeys.

ambulation and paralysis (quail) (414); impaired immunization (turkeys) (174); and increased susceptibility to infectious disease in many species (42, 320). Cases of concurrent aspergillosis and aflatoxicosis confirm that *Aspergillus* spp. are a threat to poultry production in the feed, litter, and environment (331, 366).

EXPERIMENTAL DISEASE. Aflatoxicosis impairs all important production parameters including weight gain, feed intake, feed conversion efficiency, pigmentation, processing yield, egg production, and male and female reproductive performance. Some influences are direct effects of intoxication, while others are indirect, such as from reduced feed intake.

Susceptibility of poultry to aflatoxins varies among species, breeds, and genetic lines. In general, ducklings, turkeys, and pheasants are susceptible, and chickens, bobwhite and Japanese quail, chukar partridge, and guinea fowl are relatively resistant (12, 154, 203, 347, 348). Wide variation exists among breeds, with age and sex also being important (41, 81, 412).

Pathology. The pathology of experimental aflatoxicosis is similar to the naturally occurring disease. Acute intoxication in ducks causes pale, yellow-green discoloration and atrophy of the liver, with the left lobe being more affected (284). Micro-

scopic lesions chiefly involve hepatocytes as cytoplasmic vacuolation (fatty change) and massive necrosis, often accompanied by hemorrhage. Proliferation of bile ductules is evident by the 2nd day and progresses rapidly. Subacute lethal intoxication of ducks, especially those fed cultures of *A. flavus,* causes extensive necrosis and loss of hepatocytes, and explosive proliferation of bile ductules. In nonlethal aflatoxicosis, the liver has principal lesions of fatty change in hepatocytes, karyomegaly, numerous mitotic figures, and proliferation of bile ductules (186). Histologic changes in liver and kidney are illustrated in Figures 36.6 A, B, and C.

Aflatoxicosis in chickens causes yellow, ocher discoloration of the liver, with multifocal hemorrhage and a reticulated pattern on the capsular surface (52). In time, the livers develop white foci as hepatic lipid content increases. Histologic lesions occur as fatty vacuolation of hepatocyte cytoplasm, karyomegaly and prominent nucleoli in hepatocytes, proliferation of bile ducts, and fibrosis. Basophilic, vacuolated, regenerative hepatocytes and inflammation by heterophils and mononuclear cells occur in the portal zones (52, 186). In turkeys, proliferation of bile ductules is prevalent and there are nodules of regenerative, densely eosinophilic hepatocytes that compress adjacent parenchyma (186, 283). Vacuolar change and fibrosis are mild, even in turkeys that die following prolonged toxin ingestion.

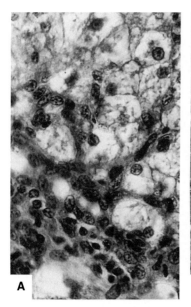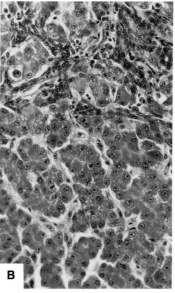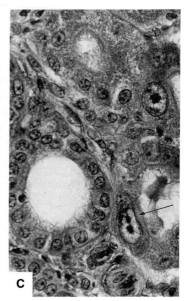

36.6. Aflatoxicosis in ducks fed toxic peanut meal. *A.* Early liver lesion showing degenerative changes in parenchyma and bile duct hyperplasia. H & E, ×1000. *B.* Nodular hyperplasia of liver parenchyma and bile duct hyperplasia are present. H & E, ×398. *C.* Kidney. Proximal tubules are dilated, epithelium is undergoing necrosis, and some nuclei have enlarged bizarre forms with prominent nucleoli (*arrow*). H & E, ×1000.

For the studies above, no aflatoxin-related lesions occurred in either the kidney or major lymphoid tissues. Membranous glomerular lesions and interstitial fibrosis occurred in ducks and goslings of another study (275).

Nutrition and Digestion. Skin pigmentation is a desirable characteristic for broilers in some markets, and carotenoid pigments are fed to produce this effect. Aflatoxin impairs pigmentation in broilers (395) by inhibiting movement and deposition of pigment at several metabolic points (354, 355).

The severity of aflatoxicosis is enhanced by a diet low in fat (160, 339), protein (292, 340), and riboflavin or vitamin D_3 (159, 161), and a diet high in tannic acid (89). Conclusions regarding the need for supplemental vitamin D_3 in aflatoxicosis are equivocal (28, 36); however, aflatoxin influences calcium and phosphorus metabolism by altering the metabolism of vitamin D and parathyroid hormone (145). In broilers, a deficiency of pancreatic amylase and lipase (291) results in steatorrhea, but laying hens are resistant to this effect (337). These variables make it difficult to establish minimum- or no-effect concentrations for aflatoxin in poultry feeds.

Reproduction and Egg Production. Mature leghorn males experience lowered semen volume, testis weight, spermatocrits, and testosterone values caused indirectly by reduced feed intake during aflatoxicosis (359, 360). Lowered testosterone plasma concentration and responsiveness in younger maturing leghorn males are direct effects (75). Reduced body weight and mild anemia occur in broiler breeder males, but semen is unaffected (35, 428).

In broiler breeder hens, hatchability declines before egg production and is the most sensitive parameter of aflatoxicosis (188). Loss of hatchability is due to embryonic death (82). In leghorns, aflatoxin blocks ova maturation and reduces feed efficiency and egg production (205). Like broiler breeders, hatchability is more sensitive than egg production (220). Egg production may be spared despite lesions of hepatotoxicity, although the production decline can be delayed and requires several weeks to return to normal (123, 135). Aflatoxin impairs egg production by reducing synthesis and transport of yolk precursors in the liver. Egg size, yolk weight, and yolk as percent of total egg size are decreased (192). In Japanese quail, impairment of feed conversion, egg production, egg weight, hatchability, and exterior and interior egg quality occur with hepatosis (351). Maturation of both males and females is delayed (97, 295).

Immunosuppression. Spontaneous aflatoxicosis is strongly associated with increased susceptibility to infectious disease (115, 315, 330). Experimental definition of susceptibility through anticipated immunosuppression is less conclusive and lends perspective to the complexity of defining mechanisms of natural toxins. Among the experimental approaches are the use of a single, purified toxin, combinations of purified toxins, crude cultures or culture extracts of a cloned fungal species, and naturally contaminated feeds or grains. Potentially numerous fungal metabolite interactions (and nutritional interactions) likely influence the results and the accuracy of defining an effect at a given concentration.

In chickens, aflatoxin increases susceptibility to, or severity of, cecal coccidiosis, Marek's disease (116), salmonellosis (371, 423), inclusion body hepatitis (350), and infectious bursal disease virus (56, 374). Vaccination failures are emerging as a consequence of aflatoxicosis in chickens (11, 22, 326). Likewise, turkeys experience vaccination failure to *Pasteurella multocida* challenge (316) and increased susceptibility to coccidiosis (416).

Aflatoxin-induced immunosuppression is explained, in part, by atrophy of the bursa of Fabricius, thymus, and spleen (56, 317) regardless of the immune response genetics of the bird (396, 397). Aflatoxin is toxic for B lymphocytes in the late-stage embryo (319). In ducks, lesions in the lymphatic system are accompanied by abnormalities in circulating lymphocytes, suggesting functional disablement (368). There is impaired clearance function of blood phagocytes and the reticuloendothelial system in chickens (53, 54, 263, 270). Serum complement activity is reduced in broilers (381). Cell-mediated immune responses are decreased in both turkeys and chickens (138, 139, 140). Despite the above explanations for aflatoxin-induced immunosuppression, considerable data show no measurable effect on either the histopathology of lymphoid organs or the functional immune response. This has been tested with aflatoxin concentrations far higher than commonly encountered in spontaneously contaminated feedstuffs (113, 138, 139, 140, 186).

Hematology. Aflatoxin causes anemia characterized by reductions in the packed cell volume, erythrocyte count, hemoglobin concentration, and mean corpuscular volume (201, 238, 270). Iron absorption and retention are initially decreased but then compensate (237). Young birds are more susceptible to anemia (238). Total leukocytes are increased, but there is concurrent lymphopenia (238, 393).

Serum Chemistry. Aflatoxin decreases total serum protein, lipoprotein, carotenoid pigment, cholesterol, triglycerides, uric acid, calcium, phosphorus, iron, copper, zinc, and lactate dehydrogenase (100, 125, 201, 332, 394, 400). Serum sorbital dehydrogenase, glutamic dehydrogenase, and potassium are increased (86). Duckling serum protein changes resemble the broiler chicken (282). In selected lines of Japanese quail, the degree of reduction in total protein and albumin and of increase in ß-glucuronidase is correlated with resistance to aflatoxin (312). Blood clotting time and ratio of aspartate aminotransferase to alanine aminotransferase are resistance indicators in ducks (293).

Coagulation. Bruising is a problem during transport and slaughter of poultry, and aflatoxin increases the susceptibility by increasing capillary fragility and reducing shear strength of skeletal muscle (392). It also impairs coagulation in chickens and turkeys by interfering with several coagulation components, notably prothrombin, to affect the extrinsic and common pathways (96, 99, 415). Aflatoxin alters coagulation more than either ochratoxin A or T-2 toxin, but the effects of ochratoxin A last longer (98, 199).

PHARMACOLOGIC INTERFERENCE. Aflatoxicosis can influence drug effectiveness in poultry through alteration of the drug plasma half-life. In broilers, chlortetracycline plasma concentrations are lowered due to decreased drug binding to plasma protein (264). Conclusions differ on aflatoxicosis being either enhanced by the addition of chlortetracycline to feed (239) or diminished (372).

METABOLISM AND RESIDUES. Poultry reared on diets contaminated with aflatoxin constitute a minimal aflatoxin source in the human food chain. Aflatoxins distribute in low concentrations and rapidly clear if nontoxic diets are provided. In broilers, metabolites of aflatoxins B1 and B2 reach highest concentrations in gizzard, liver, and kidney (60) but clear in 4 days. In chickens, aflatoxin B1 is metabolized into conjugated aflatoxins B2a and M1 in the liver (70). Also, NADP-linked cytoplasmic enzymes in duck and chicken livers reduce aflatoxins B1 and B2 to the cyclopentenol, aflatoxicol (304, 305). Aflatoxin B1 is excreted by chickens in the bile, urine, and intestinal content at a ratio of 70:15:15 as six major metabolites including B1, B2, B2a, and M1 (165).

Aflatoxins B1, M1, and aflatoxicol are the metabolites in turkeys, with highest concentrations occurring in liver, kidney, gizzard, and feces (151, 336), and are rapidly cleared when the dietary source is removed. Selenium supplementation is protective in the turkey because it increases the percentage of aflatoxin in the conjugated state (46, 150).

The half-life of aflatoxin B1 in hens is about 67 hr (352). Most is excreted through the bile and intestine, but aflatoxin B1 and aflatoxicol can be identified in ova and eggs for 7 days or longer (206, 391). Aflatoxin B1 accumulates in reproductive organs with transfer to eggs (both yolk and albumen) and hatched progeny (yolk sac and liver) in chickens, turkeys, and ducks (376, 435).

Ochratoxins

ETIOLOGY AND TOXICOLOGY. Ochratoxins are among the most toxic mycotoxins to poultry. These nephrotoxic metabolites are produced chiefly by *Penicillium viridicatum* and *Aspergillus ochraceus* on numerous grains and feedstuffs throughout North America, Europe, and Asia (see review 111). Ochratoxins are isocoumarin compounds linked to L-ß-phenylalanine and are designated A, B, C, and D, and their methyl and ethyl esters. Ochratoxin A is the most common and most toxic, and is relatively stable. Some ochratoxin-producing fungi produce other mycotoxins toxic to poultry, including citrinin.

Ochratoxin is the major determinant in porcine endemic nephropathy, a chronic wasting disease and failure to thrive in bacon pigs in Denmark and Ireland (see review 221).

Ochratoxin A occurs in North America, Europe, and Asia in corn (365, 364), most small grains and in animal feeds (51, 167, 215, 432). Ochratoxin A readily forms in poultry feed under conditions of high temperature and high moisture (17). Ochratoxin A is the predominant toxin in spontaneous disease with ochratoxins B and C occurring only with high concentrations of ochratoxin A (162).

NATURALLY OCCURRING DISEASE. Ochratoxicosis in broilers involving pelleted feed colonized with *A. ochraceus* and *Penicillium* spp. (4) caused mortality and failure to gain weight. Lesions comprised pale discoloration of liver and kidney, and enteritis. Other episodes of ochratoxicosis involving broilers were caused by either contaminated corn or corn gluten meal (162). Growth rate, feed conversion efficiency, and pigmentation were affected, and air sacculitis accompanied the toxin-induced renal disease. Ochratoxin and aflatoxin were causal factors linked to fragile intestines that tore and contaminated carcasses with intestinal content at processing (407). Poultry with enlarged pale kidneys were identified during slaughter inspection (120). Ochratoxin A residues were found in the kidneys, which had atrophy and degeneration of proximal and distal tubules, and interstitial fibrosis.

Turkeys with ochratoxicosis from contaminated corn experienced feed refusal and mortality due to nephrotoxicity and air sacculitis (162). Histopathology confirmed nephrosis as renal edema and necrosis of proximal tubular epithelium. Leghorn hens experienced reductions in egg production and shell quality, and developed nephropathy during two episodes of ochratoxicosis involving contaminated corn (162). Chronic renal disease and diarrhea caused yellow stains on the eggshells, resulting in decreased market value. Experimental feeding of ochratoxin A caused a diarrhea with high urate content and the eggshells had yellow stains (296).

Ochratoxin A occurs in moldy bread and flour (290), which are components of bakery by-product, a poultry feed ingredient. Moldy bread contaminated with ochratoxins A and B caused enteritis in chickens (403).

EXPERIMENTAL DISEASE. Experimental ochratoxin A mycotoxicosis causes primarily renal disease but also influences hepatic, immunologic, and hematopoietic functions, and has significant interactions with other toxins and nutrients.

Pathology. Acute lethal ochratoxin A mycotoxicosis in chickens causes gross lesions of pallor of the liver, pancreas, and kidney, swelling of the kidney, and white urate deposits in the ureter, kidney, heart, pericardium, liver, and spleen (visceral gout) (104, 132, 191, 192, 308). The main histopathologic alteration is acute tubular nephrosis characterized by proteinaceous and urate casts, heterophil inflammation, and focal necrosis of tubular epithelium (308). Some chicks develop cytoplasmic vacuolation and focal necrosis of hepatocytes, followed by foci of fibrosis. Hematopoiesis is suppressed in the bone marrow and lymphocyte depletion occurs in spleen and bursa of Fabricius.

Subacute ochratoxin A mycotoxicosis has been studied in turkeys, ducklings, and chickens and is characterized by increased weight of liver and kidney and decreased weight of lymphoid organs. Of the gamebird species, ringneck pheasants and Japanese quail are most sensitive (347, 348, 349). Gross lesions comprise pallor of the kidney and catarrhal content in the intestine (108). Histologic alterations in kidney include tubular dilatation and cast formation. (49, 108, 193, 253). Hyperplasia of tubular epithelium and interstitial inflammation account for the enlargement seen grossly. Thickening of glomerular basement membranes is dose related.

Lesions in the liver comprise vacuolar change in hepatocytes, associated with increases in glycogen content of liver and skeletal muscle in chickens (112, 196, 408). In ducks, the hepatocyte vacuolation is due to lipid accumulation (49), and in Japanese quail, it is accompanied by proliferation of bile ductules (103). The ultrastructural pathology indicates that the toxicity to kidney and liver originates from sensitivity of mitochondria in the proximal tubules and hepatocytes (38, 49, 108, 388). Severe lymphocytic depletion occurs throughout the immune system. The intestinal lamina propria is expanded by heterophil infiltration, as are the muscular layers (108). Intestinal fragility is associated with apparent decreases in collagen (407), although inflammation may play a role.

Broilers fed ochratoxin A also develop soft bones (108), manifested as increased diameter of the tibia relative to body weight (194) and decreased force required to break the tibia. The histologic changes in bone are generalized skeletal osteopenia with disturbed endochondral and intramembranous bone formation (107). Osteoid formation is defective and osteoporosis develops. Changes in the diaphyseal cortices account for the reduced breaking strength of bones.

Chronic (341 days) ochratoxicosis in hens (222, 383) caused reduced renal function that correlated with mild histologic lesions of ongoing necrosis and regeneration of tubular epithelium.

Nutrition and Digestion. Experimental ochratoxicosis confirmed field observations of feed refusal by turkeys and leghorn hens, but not broilers (44, 45, 325). Ochratoxin A impairs utilization of dietary carotenoids for carcass pigmentation at several metabolic points (200, 353). The toxicity of ochratoxin A is enhanced by vanadium and tannic acid at mycotoxin concentrations likely to occur naturally (223, 224, 226).

Reproduction and Egg Production. Ochratoxicosis in leghorn pullets delays sexual maturity and may block it entirely (72). The reluctance of hens to eat feed contaminated with ochratoxin causes reductions in body weight, egg production, and egg weight (322, 325). Ochratoxin can reduce egg size, interior quality, and shell specific gravity (a measure of shell quality) at concentrations too low to influence the number of eggs produced (389). Japanese quail breeding stock experience reductions of fertility and hatchability due to early embryonic death (323). In chickens, hatchability is reduced by embryonic mortality due to embryonic gout and progeny have reduced growth (72, 286). Ochratoxin A is teratogenic for chicken embryos (141).

Immunosuppression. Immunosuppression by ochratoxin A in poultry (see review 48) stems chiefly from thymic atrophy, although all lymphoid organs are affected (108, 109). Cell-mediated immunity is measurably impaired in broilers and turkeys (110). Humoral immunity occurs secondary to depletion of immunoglobulin-containing cells in lymphoid tissues (109). Phagocytic activity of chicken heterophils is impaired (55), vaccination responses are impaired (119), and the severity of concurrent coccidiosis (190) and salmonellosis is increased (118).

Hematology. Ochratoxin A induces microcytic anemia involving iron metabolism (18, 195) and causes leukopenia (15, 57, 58).

Coagulation. Ochratoxicosis increases the recalcification and prothrombin times (98, 322). Reductions in clotting factors V, VII, and X (99) may occur at ochratoxin concentrations too low to affect growth.

Serum Chemistry. Ochratoxicosis causes serum chemical alterations reflecting damage to the kidney and liver (58, 109, 202, 223, 224, 226, 353), as well as skeletal muscle, pancreas, and bone (118). Renal function is reduced (192, 222, 383).

METABOLISM AND RESIDUES. Dietary ochratoxin A distributes chiefly to the kidney, with lesser concentrations to liver and muscle (129, 133). The biologic half-life in chickens is about 4 hr, and it is rapidly eliminated. Ochratoxin A administered intravenously to Japanese quail distributes to liver, kidney, proventriculus, and ovary and is excreted in bile and in urine (130). Liver and kidney are the tissues of choice to monitor for residues (262), and residues may occur in the absence of renal lesions (222). Residues persist for only 4 days or less when toxic diets are replaced (146, 324). Ochratoxin A distributes to egg yolk and albumin (129), which accounts for reductions in hatchability. Concentrations of ochratoxin A in eggs have low correlation to dose, and several studies found no ochratoxin A in eggs (222, 322).

Citrinin

ETIOLOGY AND TOXICOLOGY. Citrinin is a natural contaminant of corn, rice, and other cereal grains and is produced by many species of *Penicillium* (74) and *Aspergillus* (see review 333). First purified as a yellow crystalline compound from *P. citrinum* in 1931, it received considerable attention because of antibiotic properties against staphylococci and other bacteria before its nephrotoxic properties were discovered. It is a cause of "yellow rice" mycotoxicosis in Japan and has been implicated in porcine endemic nephropathy, which also involves ochratoxin. *A. citrinin* occurs mainly in Canada and northern Europe (see review 432), suggesting toxigenic *Penicillium* may have a competitive advantage in cooler climates.

NATURALLY OCCURRING DISEASE. Spontaneous citrinin mycotoxicosis has not been fully documented. *Penicillium lanosum*, which produced citrinin in culture, was isolated from broiler chicken feed from a house in which the litter was wet and chickens were substantially smaller than expected at slaughter (23, 280). Fungal cultures fed to broiler chicks caused watery fecal droppings and reduced weight gain. At necropsy, kidneys were swollen and the gizzard lining was discolored and fissured. Histopathologic changes in kidney were limited to swelling of tubular epithelial cells and pyknosis.

Mycotic ventriculitis occurred and *P. lanosum* was isolated from the gizzard.

EXPERIMENTAL DISEASE. Citrinin is nephrotoxic to poultry and causes diuresis (155, 253). The diuretic effect is destroyed by heating the toxin (219). It acts directly on the kidney to transiently alter tubular transport processes. Increases in urine flow rates and free water clearance are accompanied by increases in fractional sodium, potassium, and inorganic phosphate excretion (144, 179). Removal of toxin influence causes cessation of the abnormal renal function (143).

Pathology. A single oral lethal dose of citrinin is nephrotoxic to chickens, turkey poults, and Pekin ducklings, with turkeys being the most sensitive. Watery fecal droppings and increased water consumption occur, with epithelial degeneration and necrosis in the proximal and distal tubules (258, 259). The liver may have multifocal necrosis of hepatocytes, hemorrhage, and proliferation of bile ductules. Lymphocyte necrosis and depletion occur in major lymphoid tissues, and is most prominent in ducklings (260, 261). Experimental subacute to chronic dietary toxicity of citrinin in Pekin ducklings results in reduced weight gain and dose-related nephropathy characterized by degeneration, necrosis, mineralization, and regeneration of tubular epithelial cells in cortical and medullary regions, interstitial inflammation and fibrosis (261). Ultrastructural renal pathology of citrinin in leghorn chicks involves proximal tubular epithelium (38).

Egg Production. Laying hens fed citrinin-appended diets developed wet droppings, but egg production and body weight were not affected (10).

Immunity. The histologic evidence of lymphocytic depletion is suggestive of potential immunosuppression; however, citrinin has no effect on humoral or cell-mediated immunity at nephrotoxic doses in broilers (50).

Hematology. *Penicillium citrinum*-contaminated corn containing citrinin caused anemia and leukopenia in leghorn chicks (341).

Serum Chemistry. Hyperkalemia, metabolic acidosis, reduced blood pH, and base excess occur during intoxication (261).

METABOLISM AND RESIDUES. Citrinin fed to broilers is detectable only in the blood and liver (281). Laying hens fed citrinin for 6 wk had distribution of citrinin to skeletal muscle, egg yolk, and egg white (1).

Oosporein

ETIOLOGY AND TOXICOLOGY. Oosporein is a red, toxic, dibenzoquinone metabolite of *Chaetomium* spp. and is capable of causing gout and high mortality in poultry (79, 310). Oosporein was originally extracted from *Oospora colorans* (see review 421). *Chaetomium* spp. have been isolated from numerous feeds and grains, including peanuts, rice, and corn, and cultures are highly toxic in both plant and animal bioassays. *Chaetomium trilaterale* is of particular interest because it produces high concentrations of oosporein on a variety of substrates.

NATURALLY OCCURRING DISEASE. Oosporein mycotoxicosis has occurred in poultry in both North and South America and is characterized by nephrotoxicity, gout, and mortality (421).

EXPERIMENTAL DISEASE. Experimental oosporein mycotoxicosis in young chickens and turkeys occurs as visceral and articular gout related to impaired renal function and elevated plasma concentrations of uric acid (252, 309, 310). Brown et al. (39) found that the renal cortex may show necrosis of the proximal tubules after being fed oosporein for 3 days (Fig. 36.7). Chickens are more sensitive to oosporein than turkeys. Water consumption increases and fecal droppings become fluid. Corn cultures of *Chaetomium*-producing oosporein are more toxic to chickens than the purified organic acid of oosporein. Sodium and potassium salts of oosporein are more toxic than the organic acid and their existence in cultures and naturally contaminated grains explains apparent enhanced toxicity (252).

Pathology. Acute lethal doses of oosporein in chickens and turkeys cause dehydration, swollen pale kidneys, and extensive visceral gout (white uric acid deposits in and on tissues) (310, 311, 431). The liver is mottled and has focal necrosis, and the gallbladder is distended with bile. The proventriculus has an enlarged circumference, the mucosa is covered with exudate, and necrosis may occur at the isthmus. The gizzard lining and intestinal contents are discolored green.

In subacute intoxication, visceral gout is less pro-

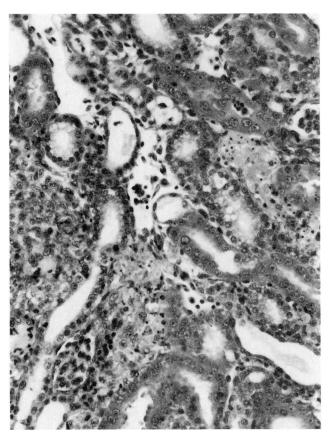

36.7. Kidney from a chicken fed oosporein for 3 days. The renal cortex has necrosis of proximal tubules. ×250. (Brown, Avian Diseases)

nounced or absent, but articular gout (white uric acid deposits in the joints) is common. Histologic lesions in the kidney occur as proximal tubular nephrosis with periodic acid Shiff-positive granules in the macula densa (37). Interstitial granulomas around urate deposits are common. Chicks that survive have interstitial fibrosis, hyperplasia of proximal tubular epithelium, and dilation of centrilobular distal tubules. Glomeruli are atrophic in fibrotic areas and enlarged in normal areas.

Egg Production. Oosporein reduces both feed consumption and egg production at doses capable of inducing nephrotoxicity and gout (431).

Hematology. Oosporein intoxication of broiler chickens has no effect on packed cell volume or hemoglobin concentration (310).

Serum Chemistry. Plasma uric acid concentrations are elevated in chickens and turkeys, and serum chemistry changes are generally reflective of renal toxicity (310, 311, 431).

OTHER MYCOTOXICOSES

Cyclopiazonic Acid. Cyclopiazonic acid is a metabolite of *Aspergillus flavus,* the predominant producer of aflatoxin in feeds and grains. Some features of turkey "X" disease in the United Kingdom in 1959, notably enteritis and opisthotonus, were not fully accountable to aflatoxin and are explained by the presence of cyclopiazonic acid, which has been identified in stored samples from the original episodes (32, 77). The toxin is also produced by *Penicillium* spp. and is a contaminant of meats, outer portions of cheeses (241), peanuts (236), corn, and millet (see reviews 287, 432).

In chickens, cyclopiazonic acid affects weight gain and feed conversion and can be fatal (101). It has additive toxicity with aflatoxin (369) and T-2 toxin (232). Lesions occur in the proventriculus, gizzard, liver, and spleen. The proventriculus is dilated and the mucosa is thickened by hyperplasia and ulceration. Mucosal necrosis occurs in the gizzard. Liver and spleen contain numerous yellow foci of necrosis and inflammation. The reproductive tract of male broiler breeders is impaired (382). Cyclopiazonic acid residues occur in chicken muscle at 14% of a single oral dose, 48 hr after dosing (287). Residues also develop in eggs, in higher concentrations in egg white than yolk (102).

Sterigmatocystin. Sterigmatocystin is a biogenic precursor to aflatoxin B1 and is hepatotoxic and hepatocarcinogenic. It occurs less commonly than aflatoxin and is associated with visibly moldy products (318). Sterigmatocystin is produced on small grains, coffee beans, and cheese by *Aspergil-*

lus versicolor and other *Aspergillus* spp., *Chaetomium* spp., and other cereal fungi. It has been identified in North America, Europe, and Japan (see review 432). Sterigmatocystin is less toxic that aflatoxin, but is produced in higher concentrations (356).

Sterigmatocystin mycotoxicosis occurred in laying hens fed commercial crumbled feed colonized with *A. glaucus* and containing sterigmatocystin (4). Feed intake and egg production was decreased, and brown-shelled eggs were pale. At necropsy, the livers were pale, fatty, and contained hemorrhages. Experimental sterigmatocystin mycotoxicosis in leghorn chicks affects liver, pancreas, lymphoid organs, and kidney (379, 380). Histologically, the liver is congested and has multifocal hemorrhage and necrosis of periacinar hepatocytes accompanied by heterophils. Pancreas has zymogen-granule loading and cytoplasmic vacuolation in exocrine cells. Lymphocyte necrosis and depletion occur in lymphoid organs. Kidney has mild degeneration and necrosis of tubular epithelium. Serum chemistries reflect target organ injury and there is leukopenia. Sterigmatocystin causes reduced embryonic weight, malformations, and mortality in chicken embryos (356). In combination with a low dose of aflatoxin, adverse changes occur in poultry meat and in hematologic parameters (2).

Rubratoxin. Rubratoxins A and B are hepatotoxic mycotoxins produced by *Penicillium rubrum* and *P. purpurogenum* (see review 413). The significance of these fungi for poultry was evident even before aflatoxicosis was defined. In 1958, an investigation of poultry hemorrhagic syndrome yielded these fungi from feed and litter of affected chickens (126). It is noteworthy that *A. flavus* and *P. citrinum,* producers of aflatoxins and citrinin, respectively, were also studied (127). Chicks fed cultures of *P. rubrum* and *P. purpurogenum* developed bloody diarrhea. At necropsy, hemorrhages were in muscles and viscera, and erosions and free blood were in the proventriculus and gizzard. Further studies on purified rubratoxin (20% A, 80% B) have shown relatively low toxicity for chickens (422). Acute lethal intoxication produces congestion and hemorrhages. Dietary rubratoxin causes impaired growth, liver enlargement, and atrophy of the bursa of Fabricius. Hemoglobin, serum protein, and serum cholesterol are reduced, and capillary fragility is increased.

Penicillic Acid. Penicillic acid, discovered in 1913, is a metabolite of numerous species of *Penicillium* and *Aspergillus* (see review 197) and is potentially important to poultry because of high concentrations in corn and poultry feed. Penicillic acid has low toxicity for broiler chickens, and purified toxin has minimal effect when fed solely at concentrations likely to occur naturally (197), but growth and feed conversion are affected when fed with low doses of aflatoxin (2).

Tenuazonic Acid and *Alternaria* Toxins.
Tenuazonic acid is a metabolite of *Alternaria* spp. and has a spectrum of toxicologic and pharmacologic effects (see review 137). Investigations of poultry hemorrhagic syndrome revealed marked toxicity of an isolate of *Alternaria* (127). *Alternaria* spp. are common to corn and agricultural commodities and also produce alternariol, alternariol methyl ether, and altertoxin (see review 432). Tenuazonic acid has moderate toxicity for broiler and leghorn chickens (137). Acute lethal intoxication induces hemorrhages in skeletal muscle, heart, and subcutis. Subacute intoxication also causes hemorrhages, the spleen is pale, and erosions occur in the gizzard lining. Tenuazonic acid-producing cultures of *Alternaria longipes* from tobacco are highly toxic to chicks and cause hemorrhages in the proventriculus and erosion of the gizzard lining (105, 373).

Patulin.
Patulin is a mycotoxin produced by several species of *Aspergillus, Penicillium,* and *Byssochlamys.* Patulin-producing *Penicillium* have been isolated from chick starter feed (74, 248). Patulin has relatively low toxicity for chicks but produces sequential lesions of watery crop content, acute ascites, and hemorrhage in the lumen of the proventriculus, gizzard, and intestine. Growth is suppressed when fed in combination with low doses of aflatoxin (2). Hens fed patulin produce misshapen eggs with reduced calcium content (1).

Other Mycotoxins and Toxigenic Fungi.
Tremorigens, slaframine, and other toxigenic fungi examined for toxicity in poultry, including *Diplodia maydis, Phomopsis leptostromiformis, Helminthosporium maydis Race T,* and uncharacterized metabolites of *Penicillium citrinum,* have been reviewed in a previous edition (180).

DIAGNOSIS.
A definitive diagnosis of mycotoxicosis involves isolation, identification, and quantification of specific toxins. This is usually difficult in the modern poultry production because of the rapid and voluminous use of feed and ingredients. The analytic capability of diagnostic laboratories is also a factor (294). Analyses for aflatoxin and zearalenone are readily available, but analyses for ochratoxins, zearalenol, deoxynivalenol, T-2 toxin, diacetoxyscirpenol, ergot alkaloids, and citrinin are less available. Confirmation of a mycotoxicosis caused by other trichothecenes, cyclopiazonic acid, sterigmatocystin, rubratoxin, or less common mycotoxins is possible in only a few laboratories. Analytic techniques for mycotoxins include chromatography (thin-layer, gas, liquid), mass spectrometry, and monoclonal antibody-based technology. The black light evaluation of grains for *Aspergillus flavus* growth is an acceptable presumptive test for aflatoxin, but does not confirm actual toxin (31). Numerous bioassays are defined for mycotoxin screening tests, but positive test results are presumptive. Laboratory personnel should be consulted before sending samples, as laboratories differ in the capabilities to conduct screening and confirmation tests for mycotoxins. Identification of mycotoxin residues in blood or tissues is possible but not routinely available (178).

If a mycotoxicosis is suspected, a complete diagnostic evaluation is desirable in addition to feed analysis. Other diseases may be occurring in concert with mycotoxins to affect production adversely. A flock rarely experiences a single disease stress. A mycotoxicosis may be suspected but not confirmed by feed analysis, however a complete laboratory evaluation can exclude other significant diseases (187). Birds that have died recently and those obviously sick should be selected for submission.

Moldy feeds may be unpalatable (43), appear unwholesome, and have diminished nutritive value. The energy level fats, vitamins, and amino acids may be affected (21, 20, 271, 338). A fungal presence in feed may reduce performance, but this alone is not definitive evidence of a mycotoxicosis. The presence of fungi in feed does indicate the potential for mycotoxin formation to occur. *Aspergillus, Penicillium,* and *Fusarium* are all mycotoxin-producing fungal genera and are found in most poultry feeds, so the potential is clearly evident (274).

Feed and ingredient samples should be properly collected and promptly submitted to a feed testing laboratory for analysis. Mycotoxin formation may not be uniform in a batch of feed or grain, and multiple samples from different sites increase the likelihood of confirming a mycotoxin formation zone (hot spot). Samples should be collected at all possible sites in the chain of ingredient storage, feed manufacture and transport, feed bins, and feeders within poultry houses. Fungal activity increases as feed is moved from the feed mill to feeder pans (211) and is associated with an increase in fines (small particles of feed) and higher zinc concentrations. Samples of 500 g (1 lb) should be collected and submitted in separate containers. Clean paper bags, properly labeled, are adequate. Sealed plastic or glass containers are appropriate only for short-term storage and transport because grain rapidly deteriorates in airtight containers.

TREATMENT.
Toxic feed should be removed and replaced with unadulterated feed. Poultry generally recover from most mycotoxicoses soon after an uncontaminated diet is available. Treatment of concurrent parasitic or bacterial diseases will alle-

viate additive or synergistic interactions. Substandard management practices are especially detrimental to poultry stressed by mycotoxins and should be corrected. Vitamins, trace minerals (especially selenium), protein, and lipid requirements are increased by some mycotoxins and can be compensated by feed formulation and water-based treatment. Increasing the crude protein and vitamin supplementation can inhibit the effects of aflatoxin (27, 210).

PREVENTION. Prevention of mycotoxicoses centers on acquisition of mycotoxin-free feedstuffs and application of feed manufacturing and management practices that prevent mold growth and mycotoxin formation. This ideally requires access to sufficient laboratory capability to confirm the purchase of ingredients free of mycotoxins, proper storage of ingredients, and feed processing, shipping, and handling procedures to minimize formation. A quality control program can monitor success of these practices (385).

Rapid on-site screening tests for several mycotoxins (aflatoxin, T-2 toxin, ochratoxin, zearalenone) are available in monoclonal antibody-based detection kits. Grain can be screened for potential aflatoxin contamination by examination for green fluorescence under a black (ultraviolet) light to estimate the degree of *A. flavus* contamination. The presence of aflatoxin, however, must be confirmed by a chromatographic procedure (minicolumn technique) or other suitable method.

Mycotoxins form in decayed, crusted, built-up feed in feeders, feed mills, and storage bins (158). Regular inspection of feed bins identifies flow problems like feed separation, central feed-down, and feed bridging (390), which enhance fungal activity and mycotoxin formation. Temperature extremes cause moisture condensation and migration in bins and create high-risk situations for mycotoxin formation (420). Bin inspection and cleaning between flocks to certify absence of feed residue is important. Tandem feed bins allow cleaning between successive feed deliveries. Minimum feed residence time is important, even under cool, dry conditions (147). Adequate ventilation of poultry housing to reduce relative humidity removes moisture available for fungal growth and toxin formation in feeders (214). Selection of feeder equipment that minimizes surface-area contact with feed diminishes mycotoxin formation (212).

Pelleting feed has among its numerous benefits destruction of fungal spores (386) and a decrease in the fungal burden. The combination of pelleting and an antifungal agent has additional effectiveness.

Antifungal agents added to feeds to prevent fungal growth have no affect on toxin already formed but may be cost effective with other feed management practices. As a cautionary note, regulatory approval for use of these various compounds in feeds differs among countries. Organic acids are effective (92, 213), but their effectiveness may be reduced by particle size of feed ingredients (93) and buffering by certain ingredients (94). Organic acids are corrosive and irritating to skin, and some have been modified to counteract this characteristic (303). Other agents showing efficacy in reducing fungal growth or mycotoxin formation include phosphates (tetrasodium pyrophosphate and alkaline sodium polyphosphate) (242), spice oils and extracts (106, 170, 375), and ammonium hydroxide (136). Gentian violet (59, 218) and thiabendazole (131) are effective but no longer approved for use in the United States in most, if not all, animal feeds. Copper sulfate is a poor mold inhibitor for poultry feeds (88). Other prevention strategies include controlled storage atmospheres, irradiation, and fumigation (246).

Detoxification is another approach to utilizing mycotoxin-contaminated feeds while preventing mycotoxicoses. Sorbent compounds can be part of an integrated approach (229). Zeolytes, silica-containing compounds used as anticaking agents and as a shell quality aid, are practical and economical feed additives that can reduce the effects of certain mycotoxins, especially aflatoxin. Hydrated sodium calcium aluminosilicate binds aflatoxin B1 in the digestive tract, possibly by sequestration, and reduces toxicity to chickens (169, 314). This is applicable mainly to aflatoxin, as zeolytes are ineffective against diacetoxyscirpenol and ochratoxin A (203, 231). The adsorbent activity is shown by a number of zeolytic ores (168) and further processing of the silicate-type sorbents may increase their efficacy for protection (230). Bentonite clay also ameliorates aflatoxicosis (404). Other possibilities for preventing mycotoxicoses in the presence of contaminated feeds include specific nutrients involved in forming detoxicants (278). Ammoniation is particularly effective in decontaminating feeds and grains for aflatoxin (301).

REFERENCES

1. Abdelhamid, A.M., and T.M. Dorra. 1990. Study on effects of feeding laying hens on separate mycotoxins (aflatoxins, patulin, or citrinin)-contaminated diets on the egg quality and tissue constituents. Arch Anim Nutr Berlin 4:305–316.

2. Abdelhamid, A.M., and T.M. Dorra. 1993. Effect of feed-borne pollution with some mycotoxin combinations on broiler chickens. Arch Anim Nutr 44:29–40.

3. Abdullah, A.S., and O.B. Lee. 1981. Aflatoxicosis in ducks. Kajian Vet 13:33–36.

4. Abramson, D., J.T. Mills, and B.R. Boycott. 1983. Mycotoxins and mycoflora in animal feedstuffs in western Canada. Can J Comp Med 47:23–26.

5. Adams, R.L., and J. Tuite. 1976. Feeding Gibberella zeae damaged corn to laying hens. Poult Sci 55:1991–1993.

6. Allen, N.K., C.J. Mirocha, S.A. Allen, J.J. Bitgood, G. Weaver, and F. Bates. 1981. Effect of dietary zearalenone on reproduction of chickens. Poult Sci 60:1165–1174.

7. Allen, N.K., C.J. Mirocha, G. Weaver, S. Aakhus-Allen, and F. Bates. 1981. Effects of dietary zearalenone on finishing broiler chickens and young turkey poults. Poult Sci 60:124–131.

8. Allen, N.K., R.L. Jevne, C.J. Mirocha, and Y.W. Lee. 1982. The effect of a Fusarium roseum culture and diacetoxyscirpenol on reproduction of white leghorn females. Poult Sci 61:2172–2175.

9. Allen, N.K., A. Peguri, C.J. Mirocha, and J.A. Newman. 1983. Effects of Fusarium cultures, T-2 toxin and zearalenone on reproduction of turkey females. Poult Sci 62:282–289.

10. Ames, D.D., R.D. Wyatt, H.L. Marks, and K.W. Washburn. 1976. Effect of citrinin, a mycotoxin produced by Penicillium citrinum, on laying hens and young broiler chicks. Poult Sci 55:1294–1301.

11. Anjum, A.D. 1994. Outbreak of infectious bursal disease in vaccinated chickens due to aflatoxicosis. Indian Vet J 71:322–324.

12. Arafa, A.S., R.J. Bloomer, H.R. Wilson, C.F. Simpson, and R.H. Harms. 1981. Susceptibility of various poultry species to dietary aflatoxin. Br Poult Sci 22:431–436.

13. Archibald, R.M., H.J. Smith, and J.D. Smith. 1962. Brazilian groundnut toxicosis in Canadian broiler chickens. Can Vet J 3:322–325.

14. Asplin, F.D., and R.B.A. Carnaghan. 1961. The toxicity of certain groundnut meals for poultry with special reference to their effect on ducklings and chickens. Vet Rec 73:1215–1219.

15. Ayed, I.A.M., R. Dafalla, A.I. Yagi, and S.E.I. Adam. 1991. Effect of ochratoxin A on Lohmann-type chicks. Vet Hum Toxicol 33:557–560.

16. Bacon, C.W., and H.L. Marks. 1976. Growth of broilers and quail fed Fusarium (Gibberella zeae)-infected corn and zearalenone (F-2). Poult Sci 55:1531–1535.

17. Bacon, C.W., J.G. Sweeney, J.D. Robbins, and D. Burdick. 1973. Production of penicillic acid and ochratoxin A on poultry feed by Aspergillus ochraceus: Temperature and moisture requirements. Appl Environ Microbiol 26:155–160.

18. Bailey, C.A., R.M. Gibson, L.F. Kubena, W.E. Huff, and R.B. Harvey. 1989. Ochratoxin A and dietary protein. 2. Effects on hematology, and various clinical chemistry measurements. Poultry Sci 68:1664–1671.

19. Bamburg, J.R., and F.M. Strong. 1971. 12,13-epoxythrichothecenes. In S. Kadis, S.A. Ciegler, and S.J. Ajl (eds.). Microbial Toxins. Academic Press, New York, pp. 207–289.

20. Bartov, I., and N. Paster. 1986. Effect of early stages of fungal development on the nutritional value of diets for broiler chicks. Br Poult Sci 27:415–420.

21. Bartov, I., N. Paster, and N. Lisker. 1982. The nutritional value of moldy grains for broiler chicks. Poult Sci 61:2247–2254.

22. Batra, P., A.K. Pruthi, and J.R. Sandana. 1991. Effect of aflatoxin B1 on the efficacy of turkey herpesvirus vaccine against Marek's disease. Res Vet Sci 51:115–119.

23. Beasley, J.N., L.D. Blalock, T.S. Nelson, and G.E. Templeton. 1980. The effect of feeding corn molded with Penicillium lanosum to broiler chicks. Poult Sci 59:708–713.

24. Bergsjo, B., O. Herstad, and I. Nafstad. 1993. Effects of feeding deoxynivalenol-contaminated oats on reproduction performance of white leghorn hens. Br Poult Sci 34:147–159.

25. Bermudez, A.J., G.E. Rottinghaus, and D.R. Ledoux. 1994. Determination of the no effect level of moniliformin containing Fusarium fujikuroi culture material fed to chickens and turkeys [abst]. Proc Annu Meet Am Vet Med Assoc, p. 127.

26. Bermudez, A.J., D.R. Ledoux, and G.E. Rottinghaus. 1995. Effects of Fusarium moniliforme culture material containing known levels of fumonisin B1 in ducklings. Avian Dis 39:879–886.

27. Beura, C.K., T.S. Johri, V.R. Sadagopan, and B.K.

Panda. 1993. Interaction of dietary protein level on dose response relationship during aflatoxicosis in commercial broilers. I. Physical responses, livability and nutrient retention. Indian J Poult Sci 28:170–178.

28. Bird, F.H. 1978. The effect of aflatoxin B1 on the utilization of cholecalciferol by chicks. Poult Sci 57:1293–1296.

29. Bock, R.R., L.S. Shore, Y. Samberg, and S. Perl. 1986. Death in broiler breeders due to salpingitis: Possible role of zearalenone. Avian Pathol 15:495–502.

30. Boonchuvit, B., P.B. Hamilton, and H.R. Burmeister. 1975. Interaction of T-2 toxin with Salmonella infections of chickens. Poult Sci 54:1693–1696.

31. Bothast, R.J., and C.W. Hesseltine. 1975. Bright greenish-yellow fluorescence and aflatoxin in agricultural commodities. Appl Microbiol 30:337–338.

32. Bradburn, N., R.D. Coker, and G. Blunden. 1994. The aetiology of turkey "x" disease. Phytochem 35:817.

33. Bragg, D.B., H.A. Salem, and T.J. Devlin. 1970. Effect of dietary triticale ergot on the performance and survival of broiler chicks. Can J Anim Sci 50:259–264.

34. Branton, S.L., J.W. Deaton, W.J. Hagler, Jr., W.R. Maslin, and J.M. Hardin. 1989. Decreased egg production in commercial laying hens fed zearalenone- and deoxynivalenol-contaminated grain sorghum. Avian Dis 33:804–808.

35. Briggs, D.M., R.D. Wyatt, and P.B. Hamilton. 1974. The effect of dietary aflatoxin on semen characteristics of mature broiler breeder males. Poult Sci 53:2115–2119.

36. Britton, W.M., and R.D. Wyatt. 1978. Effect of dietary aflatoxin of vitamin D3 metabolism in chicks. Poult Sci 57:163–165.

37. Brown, T.P. 1986. Comparison of renal changes in chickens due to postmortem interval, estrogen, oosporein, citrinin, or ochratoxin A. Diss Abstr B Sci Eng 47:1445–1446.

38. Brown, T.P., R.O. Manning, O.J. Fletcher, and R.D. Wyatt. 1986. The individual and combined effects of citrinin and ochratoxin A on renal ultrastructure in layer chicks. Avian Dis 30:191–198.

39. Brown, T.P., O.J. Fletcher, O. Osuna, and R.D. Wyatt. 1987. Microscopic and ultrastructural renal pathology of oosporein-induced toxicosis in broiler chicks. Avian Dis 31:868–877.

40. Brown, T.P., G.E. Rottinghaus, and M.E. Williams. 1992. Fumonisin mycotoxicosis in broilers: Performance and pathology. Avian Dis 36:450–454.

41. Bryden, W.L., R.B. Cumming, and A.B. Lloyd. 1980. Sex and strain responses to aflatoxin B1 in the chicken. Avian Pathol 9:539–550.

42. Bryden, W.L., A.B. Lloyd, and R.B. Cumming. 1980. Aflatoxin contamination of Australian animal feeds and suspected cases of mycotoxicosis. Aust Vet J 56:176–180.

43. Burditt, S.J., W.M. Hagler, Jr., and P.B. Hamilton. 1983. Survey of molds and mycotoxins for their ability to cause feed refusal in chickens. Poult Sci 62:2187–2191.

44. Burditt, S.J., W.M. Hagler, Jr., J.E. Hutchins, and P.B. Hamilton. 1983. Models of feed refusal syndrome in poultry. Poult Sci 62:2158–2163.

45. Burditt, S.J., W.M. Hagler, Jr., and P.B. Hamilton. 1984. Feed refusal during ochratoxicosis in turkeys. Poult Sci 63:2172–2174.

46. Burguera, J.A., G.T. Edds, and O. Osuna. 1983. Influence of selenium on aflatoxin B1 or crotalaria toxicity in turkey poults. Am J Vet Res 44:1714–1717.

47. Burmeister, H.R., A. Ciegler, and R.F. Vesonder. 1979. Moniliformin, a metabolite of Fusarium moniliforme NRRL 6322: Purification and toxicity. Appl Environ Microbiol 37:11–13.

48. Burns, R.B., and P. Dwivedi. 1986. The natural occurrence of ochratoxin A and its effects in poultry: A review. II. Pathology and immunology. World Poult Sci J 42:48–55.

49. Burns, R.B., and M.H. Maxwell. 1987. Ochratoxicosis

A in young Khaki Campbell ducklings. Res Vet Sci 42:395–403.

50. Campbell, M.L., Jr., J.A Doerr, and R.D. Wyatt. 1981. Immune status in broiler chickens during citrinin toxicosis [abst]. Poult Sci 60:1634.

51. Carlton, W.W., and P. Krogh. 1979. Ochratoxins. In W. Shimoda (ed.). Conference on Mycotoxins in Animal Feeds and Grains Related to Animal Health. Food and Drug Administration Report No. FDA/BVM-79/139, pp. 165–287.

52. Carnaghan, R.B.A., G. Lewis, D.S.P. Patterson, and R. Allcroft. 1966. Biochemical and pathological aspects of groundnut poisoning in chickens. Pathol Vet 3:601–615.

53. Chang, C.F., and P.B. Hamilton. 1979. Impairment of phagocytosis in chicken monocytes during aflatoxicosis. Poult Sci 58:562–566.

54. Chang, C.F., and P.B. Hamilton. 1979. Refractory phagocytosis by chicken thrombocytes during aflatoxicosis. Poult Sci 58:559–561.

55. Chang, C.F., and P.B. Hamilton. 1980. Impairment of phagocytosis by heterophils from chickens during ochratoxicosis. Appl Environ Microbiol 39:572–575.

56. Chang, C.F., and P.B. Hamilton. 1982. Increased severity and new symptoms of infectious bursal disease during aflatoxicosis in broiler chickens. Poult Sci 61:1061–1068.

57. Chang, C.F., W.E. Huff, and P.B. Hamilton. 1979. A leukocytopenia induced in chickens by dietary ochratoxin A. Poult Sci 58:555–558.

58. Chang, C.F., J.A. Doerr, and P.B. Hamilton. 1981. Experimental ochratoxicosis in turkey poults. Poult Sci 60:114–119.

59. Chen, T.C., and E.J. Day. 1974. Gentian violet as a possible fungal inhibitor in poultry feed: Plate assays on its antifungal activity. Poult Sci 53:1791–1795.

60. Chen, C., A.M. Pearson, T.H. Coleman, J.I. Gray, J.J. Peska, and S.K. Aust. 1984. Metabolite deposition and clearance of aflatoxins from broiler chickens fed a contaminated diet. Food Chem Toxicol 22:447–451.

61. Chi, M.S., and C.J. Mirocha. 1978. Necrotic oral lesions in chickens fed diacetoxyscirpenol, T-2 toxin, and crotocin. Poult Sci 57:807–806.

62. Chiba, J., N. Nakano, N. Morooka, S. Nakazawa, and Y. Wanatabe. 1972. Inhibitory effects of fusarenon X, a sesquiterpene mycotoxin, on lipid synthesis and phosphate uptake in Tetrahymena pyriformis. Jpn J Med Sci Biol 25:291–296.

63. Chi, M.S., C.J. Mirocha, H.J. Kurtz, G. Weaver, F. Bates, and W. Shimoda. 1977. Effects of T-2 toxin on reproductive performance and health of laying hens. Poult Sci 56:628–637.

64. Chi, M.S., C.J. Mirocha, H.J. Kurtz, G. Weaver, F. Bates, W. Shimoda, and H.R. Burmeister. 1977. Acute toxicity of T-2 toxin in broiler chicks and laying hens. Poult Sci 56:103–116.

65. Chi, M.S., C.J. Mirocha, H.J. Kurtz, G. Weaver, F. Bates, and W. Shimoda. 1977. Subacute toxicity of T-2 toxin in broiler chicks. Poult Sci 56:306–313.

66. Chi, M.S., T.S. Robison, C.J. Mirocha, S.P. Swanson, and W. Shimoda. 1978. Excretion and tissue distribution of radioactivity from tritium-labeled T-2 toxin in chicks. Toxicol Appl Pharmacol 45:391–402.

67. Chi, M.S., C.J. Mirocha, H.J. Kurtz, G.A. Weaver, F. Bates, T. Robison, and W. Shimoda. 1980. Effect of dietary zearalenone on growing broiler chicks. Poult Sci 59:531–536.

68. Chi, M.S., C.J. Mirocha, G.A. Weaver, and H.J. Kurtz. 1980. Effect of zearalenone on female white leghorn chickens. Appl Environ Microbiol 39:1026–1030.

69. Chi, M.S., M.E. El-Halawani, P.E. Waibel, and C.J. Mirocha. 1981. Effects of T-2 toxin on brain catecholamines and selected blood components in growing chickens. Poult Sci 60:137–141.

70. Chipley, J.R., M.S. Mabee, K.L. Applegate, and M.S. Dreyfuss. 1974. Further characterization of tissue distribution and metabolism of [14C] aflatoxin B1 in chickens. Appl Microbiol 28:1027–1029.

71. Choudary, C., and M.R. Rao. 1982. An outbreak of aflatoxicosis in commercial poultry farms. Poult Advis 16:75–76.

72. Choudhury, H., C.W. Carlson, and G. Semeniuk. 1971. A study of ochratoxin toxicity in hens. Poult Sci 50:1855–1859.

73. Chu, Q.L., W.D. Wu, and E.B. Smalley. 1993. Decreased cell-mediated immunity and lack of skeletal problems in broiler chickens consuming diets amended with fusaric acid. Avian Dis 37:863–867.

74. Ciegler, A., R.F. Vesonder, and L.K. Jackson. 1977. Production and biological activity of patulin and citrinin from Penicillium expansum. Appl Environ Microbiol 33:1004–1006.

75. Clark, R.N., J.A. Doerr, and M.A. Ottinger. 1986. Relative importance of dietary aflatoxin and feed restriction of reproductive changes associated with aflatoxins in the maturing white leghorn male. Poult Sci 65:2239–2245.

76. Coffin, J.L., and G.F. Combs, Jr. 1981. Impaired vitamin E status of chicks fed T-2 toxin. Poult Sci 60:385–392.

77. Cole, R.J. 1986. Etiology of turkey "X" disease in retrospect: A case for the involvement of cyclopiazonic acid. Mycotoxin Res 2:3–7.

78. Cole, R.J., H.G. Cutler, B.L. Doupnik, and J.C. Peckham. 1973. Toxin from Fusarium moniliforme: Effects on plants and animal. Science 179:1324–1326.

79. Cole, R.J., J.W. Kirksey, H.G. Cutler, and E.E. Davis. 1974. Toxic effects of oosporein from Chaetomium trilaterale. J Agric Food Chem 22:517–520.

80. Colvin, B.M., A.J. Cooley, and R.W. Beaver. 1993. Fumonisin toxicosis in swine: Clinical and pathological findings. J Vet Diagn Invest 5:232–241.

81. Colwell, W.M., R.C. Ashley, D.G. Simmons, and P.B. Hamilton. 1973. The relative in vitro sensitivity to aflatoxin B1 of tracheal organ cultures prepared from day-old chickens, ducks, Japanese quail, and turkeys. Avian Dis 17:166–172.

82. Cottier, G.J., C.H. Moore, U.L. Diener, and N.D. Davis. 1969. The effect of feeding four levels of aflatoxin on hatchability and subsequent performance of broilers [abst]. Poult Sci 48:1797.

83. Cristensen, C.M., R.A. Meronuck, G.H. Nelson, and J.C. Behrens. 1972. Effects on turkey poults of rations containing corn invaded by Fusarium tricinctum (cda.) Sny. & Hans. Appl Microbiol 23:177–179.

84. Cunningham, P. 1987. Mycotoxin problems appear to be growing worse. Poult Times 34(24):19.

85. Dafalla, R., Y.M. Hassan, and S.E.I. Adam. 1987. Fatty and hemorrhagic liver and kidney syndrome in breeding hens caused by aflatoxin B1 and heat stress in the Sudan. Vet Human Toxicol 29:252–254.

86. Dafalla, R., A. Yagi, and S.E.I. Adam. 1987. Experimental aflatoxicosis in Hybro-type chicks: Sequential changes in growth and serum constituents and histopathological changes. Vet Human Toxicol 29:222–225.

87. Dailey, R.E., R.E. Reese, and E.A. Brouwer. 1980. Metabolism of [14C]zearalenone in laying hens. J Agric Food Chem 28:286–291.

88. Dale, N. 1987. Copper sulfate as mold inhibitor. Poult Dig 46:311.

89. Dale, N.M., R.D. Wyatt, and H.L. Fuller. 1980. Additive toxicity of aflatoxin and dietary tannins in broiler chicks. Poult Sci 59:2417–2420.

90. D'Andrea, G.H., D.M. Dent, L. Nunley-Bearden, and S.M. Ho. 1987. Zearalenone incidence and toxicosis in Alabama. Auburn Vet 42:4–8.

91. D'Andrea, G.H., L. Nunley-Bearden, D.M. Dent, and S.M. Ho. 1987. Aflatoxin incidence and toxicosis in Alabama. Auburn Vet 42:17–23.

92. Dixon, R.C., and P.B. Hamilton. 1981. Evaluation of

some organic acids as mold inhibitors by measuring CO_2 production from feed and ingredients. Poult Sci 60:2182–188.

93. Dixon, R.C., and P.B. Hamilton. 1981. Effect of feed ingredients on the antifungal activity of propionic acid. Poult Sci 60:2407–2411.

94. Dixon, R.C., and P.B. Hamilton. 1981. Effect of particle sizes of corn meal and a mold inhibitor on mold inhibition. Poult Sci 60:2412–2415.

95. Doerr, J.A. 1979. Mycotoxicosis and avian hemostasis. Diss Abstr B Sci Eng 4127.

96. Doerr, J.A., and P.B. Hamilton. 1981. Aflatoxicosis and intrinsic coagulation function in broiler chickens. Poult Sci 60:1406–1411.

97. Doerr, J.A., and M.A. Ottinger. 1980. Delayed reproductive development resulting from aflatoxicosis in juvenile Japanese quail. Poult Sci 59:1995–2001.

98. Doerr, J.A., W.E. Huff, H.T. Tung, R.D. Wyatt, and P.B. Hamilton. 1974. A survey of T-2 toxin, ochratoxin, and aflatoxin for their effects on the coagulation of blood in young broiler chickens. Poult Sci 53:1728–1734.

99. Doerr, J.A., R.D. Wyatt, and P.B. Hamilton. 1976. Impairment of coagulation function during aflatoxicosis in young chickens. Toxicol Appl Pharmacol 35:437–446.

100. Doerr, J.A., W.E. Huff, C.J. Wabeck, G.W. Chaloupka, J.D. May, and J.W. Merkley. 1983. Effects of low level chronic aflatoxicosis in broiler chickens. Poult Sci 62:1971–1977.

101. Dorner, J.W., R.J. Cole, L.G. Lomax, H.S. Gossar, and U.L. Diener. 1983. Cyclopiazonic acid production by Aspergillus flavus and its effects on broiler chickens. Appl Environ Microbiol 46:698–703.

102. Dorner, J.W., R.J. Cole, D.J. Erlington, S. Suksupath, G.H. McDowell, and W.L. Bryden. 1994. Cyclopiazonic acid residues in milk and eggs. J Agric Food Chem 42:1516–1518.

103. Doster, R.C., G.H. Arscott, and R.O. Sinnhuber. 1973. Comparative toxicity of ochratoxin A and crude Aspergillus ochraceus culture extract in Japanese quail (Coturnix coturnix japonica). Poult Sci 52:2351–2353.

104. Doupnik, B., Jr., and J.C. Peckman. 1970. Mycotoxicity of Aspergillus ochraceus to chicks. Appl Microbiol 19:594–597.

105. Doupnik, B., Jr., and E.K. Sobers. 1968. Mycotoxicosis: Toxicity to chicks of Alternaria longipes isolated from tobacco. Appl Microbiol 16:1596–1597.

106. Dube, S., P.D. Upadhyay, and S.C. Tripathi. 1989. Antifungal, physicochemical, and insect-repelling activity of the essential oil of Ocimum basilicum. Can J Bot 67:2085–2087.

107. Duff, S.R.I., R.B. Burns, and P. Dwivedi. 1987. Skeletal changes in broiler chicks and turkey poults fed diets containing ochratoxin A. Res Vet Sci 43:301–307.

108. Dwivedi, P., and R.B. Burns. 1984. Pathology of ochratoxicosis A in young broiler chicks. Res Vet Sci 36:92–103.

109. Dwivedi, P., and R.B. Burns. 1984. Effect of ochratoxin A on immunoglobulins in broiler chicks. Res Vet Sci 36:117–121.

110. Dwivedi, P., and R.B. Burns. 1985. Immunosuppressive effects of ochratoxin A in young turkeys. Avian Pathol 14:213–225.

111. Dwivedi, P., and R.B. Burns. 1986. The natural occurrence of ochratoxin A and its effects in poultry. A review. Part I. Epidemiology and toxicity. World Poult Sci J 42:32–47.

112. Dwivedi, P., R.B. Burns, and M.H. Maxwell. 1984. Ultrastructural study of the liver and kidney in ochratoxicosis A in young broiler chicks. Res Vet Sci 36:104–116.

113. Dzuik, H.E., G.H. Nelson, G.E. Duke, S.K. Maheswaran, and M.S. Chi. 1978. Acquired resistance in turkey poults to Pasteurella multocida (P-1059 strain) during aflatoxin consumption. Poult Sci 57:1251–1254.

114. Edds, G.T. 1979. Aflatoxins. In W. Shimoda (ed.). Conference on Mycotoxins in Animal Feeds and Grains Related to Animal Health, Food and Drug Administration Report No. FDA/BVM-79/139, pp. 80–164.

115. Edds, G.T., and O. Osuna. 1976. Aflatoxin B1 increases infectious disease losses in food animals. Proc US Anim Health Assoc 80:434–441.

116. Edds, G.T., K.P.C. Nair, and C.F. Simpson. 1973. Effect of aflatoxin B1 on resistance in poultry against cecal coccidiosis and Marek's disease. Am J Vet Res 34:819–826.

117. El-Banna, A.A., R.M.G. Hamilton, P.M. Scott, and H.L. Trenholm. 1983. Nontransmission of deoxynivalenol (vomitoxin) to eggs and meat in chickens fed deoxynivalenol-contaminated diets. J Agric Food Chem 31:1381–1384.

118. Elissalde, M.H., R.L. Ziprin, W.E. Huff, L.F. Kubena, and R.B. Harvey. 1994. Effect of ochratoxin A on Salmonella-challenged broiler chicks. Poult Sci 73:1241–1248.

119. El-Karim, S.A., M.S. Arbid, A.H. Soufy, M. Bastamy, and M.M. Effat. 1991. Influence of metabolite ochratoxin A on chicken immune response. Egypt J Comp Pathol Clin Pathol 4(1):159–172.

120. Elling, F., B. Hald, C. Jacobsen, and P. Krogh. 1975. Spontaneous toxic nephropathy in poultry associated with ochratoxin A. Acta Path Microbiol Scand (A) 83:739–741.

121. Englehardt, J.A., W.W. Carlton, and J.F. Tuite. 1989. Toxicity of Fusarium moniliforme var. subglutinans for chicks, ducklings, and turkey poults. Avian Dis 33:357–360.

122. Espada, Y., R.R. de Gopegui, C. Cuadradas, F.J. Cabanes, and R. Ruiz de Gopegui. 1994. Fumonisin mycotoxicosis in broilers. Weights and serum chemistry modifications. Avian Dis 38:454–460.

123. Exarchos, C.C., and R.F. Gentry. 1982. Effect of aflatoxin B1 on egg production. Avian Dis 26:191–195.

124. Featherston, W.R. 1973. Utilization of Gibberella-infected corn by chicks and rats. Poult Sci 52:2334–2335.

125. Fernandez, A., M.T. Verde, M. Gascon, J. Ramos, J. Gomez, D.F. Luco, and G. Chavez. 1994. Variations of clinical biochemical parameters of laying hens and broiler chickens fed aflatoxin-containing feed. Avian Pathol 23:37–47.

126. Forgacs, J., H. Koch, W.T. Carll, and R.H. White-Stevens. 1958. Additional studies on the relationship of mycotoxicoses to the poultry hemorrhagic syndrome. Am J Vet Res 19:744–753.

127. Forgacs, J., H. Koch, W.T. Carll, and R.H. White-Stevens. 1962. Mycotoxicoses I. Relationship of toxic fungi to moldy-feed toxicosis in poultry. Avian Dis 6:363–381.

128. Fritz, J.C., P.B. Mislivec, G.W. Pla, B.N. Harrison, C.E. Weeks, and J.G. Dantzman. 1973. Toxicogenicity of moldy feed for young chicks. Poult Sci 52:1523–1530.

129. Frye, C.E., and F.S. Chu. 1977. Distribution of ochratoxin A in chicken tissues and eggs. J Food Saf 1:147–159.

130. Fuchs, R., L.E. Applegren, S. Hagelberg, and K. Hult. 1988. Carbon-14-ochratoxin A distribution in the Japanese quail (Coturnix coturnix japonica) monitored by whole body autoradiography. Poult Sci 67:707–714.

131. Gabal, M.A. 1987. Preliminary study on the use of thiabendazole in the control of common toxigenic fungi in grain feed. Vet Human Toxicol 29:217–221.

132. Galtier, P., J. More, and M. Alvinerie. 1976. Acute and short-term toxicity of ochratoxin A in 10-day-old chicks. Food Cosmet Toxicol 14:129–131.

133. Galtier, P., M. Alvinerie, and J.L. Charpenteau. 1981. The pharmacokinetic profiles of ochratoxin A in pigs, rabbits and chickens. Food Cosmet Toxicol 19:735–738.

134. Gardiner, M.R., and B. Oldroyd. 1965. Avian aflatoxicosis. Aust Vet J 41:272–276.

135. Garlich, J.D., H.T. Tung, and R.B. Hamilton. 1973. The effects of short term feeding of aflatoxin on egg production and some plasma constituents of the laying hen. Poult Sci 52:2206–2211.

136. Gazia, N., A.M. Abd-Ellah, and A.N. Dayed. 1991. Chemical treatments of mycotoxin contaminated rations and

possibility of its safety use for chicks. Assiut Vet Med J 25:(49)61–68.

137. Giambrone, J.J., N.D. Davis, and U.L. Diener. 1978. Effect of tenuazonic acid on young chickens. Poult Sci 57:1554–1558.

138. Giambrone, J.J., U.L. Diener, N.D. Davis, V.S. Panangala, and F.J. Hoerr. 1985. Effects of aflatoxin on young turkeys and broiler chickens. Poult Sci 64:1678–1684.

139. Giambrone, J.J., U.L. Diener, N.D. Davis, V.S. Panangala, and F.J. Hoerr. 1985. Effects of purified aflatoxin on broiler chickens. Poult Sci 64:852–858.

140. Giambrone, J.J., U.L. Diener, N.D. Davis, V.S. Panangala, and F.J. Hoerr. 1985. Effect of purified aflatoxin on turkeys. Poult Sci 64:859–865.

141. Gilani, S.H., J. Bancroft, and M. O'Rahily. 1975. The teratogenic effects of ochratoxin A in the chick embryo. Teratology 11:18A.

142. Giroir, L.E., G.W. Ivie, and W.E. Huff. 1991. Comparative fate of the tritiated trichothecene mycotoxin, T-2 toxin, in chickens and ducks. Poult Sci 70:1138–1143.

143. Glahn, R.P. 1993. Mycotoxins and the avian kidney: Assessment of physiological function. World Poult Sci J 49:242–250.

144. Glahn, R.P., and R.F. Wideman, Jr. 1987. Avian diuretic response to renal portal infusions of the mycotoxin citrinin. Poult Sci 66:1316–1325.

145. Glahn, R.P., K.W. Beers, W.G. Bottje, R.F. Wideman, Jr., W.E. Huff, W. Thomas, and W.G. Bottje. 1991. Aflatoxicosis alters avian renal function, calcium, and vitamin D metabolism. J Toxicol Environ Health 34:309–321.

146. Golinnski, P., J Chelkowski, A. Konarkowski, and K. Szebiotko. 1982. Mycotoxins in cereal grain. Part VI. The effect of ochratoxin A on growth and tissue residues of the mycotoxin in broiler chickens. Nahrung 27:251–256.

147. Good, R.E., and P.B. Hamilton. 1981. Beneficial effect of reducing the feed residence time in a field problem of suspected moldy feed. Poult Sci 60:1403–1405.

148. Greenhalgh, R., G.A. Neish, and J.D. Miller. 1983. Deoxynivalenol, acetyl deoxynivalenol, and zearalenone formation by Canadian isolates of Fusarium graminearum on solid substrates. Appl Environ Microbiol 46:625–629.

149. Greenway, J.A., and R. Puls. 1976. Fusariotoxicosis from barley in British Columbia I. Natural occurrence and diagnosis. Can J Comp Med 40:12–15.

150. Gregory, J.F., III, and G.T. Edds. 1984. Effect of dietary selenium on the metabolism of aflatoxin B1 in turkeys. Food Chem Toxicol 22:637–642.

151. Gregory, J.F., III, S.L. Goldstein, and G.T. Edds. 1983. Metabolite distribution and rate of residue clearance in turkeys fed a diet containing aflatoxin B1. Food Chem Toxicol 21:463–467.

152. Grimes, J.L., and W.C. Bridges, Jr. 1992. Relationship of mouth lesions to eggshell quality of commericial laying hens. J Appl Poult Res 1:251–257.

153. Grimes, J.L., T.H. Eleazer, and J.E. Hill. 1993. Paralysis of undetermined origin in bobwhite quail. Avian Dis 37:582–584.

154. Gumbmann, M.R., S.N. Williams, A.N. Booth, P. Vohra, R.A. Earnst, and M. Bethard. 1970. Aflatoxin susceptibility in various breeds of poultry. Proc Soc Exp Biol Med 134:683–688.

155. Gustavson, S.A., J.M. Cockrill, J.N. Beasley, and T.S. Nelson. 1981. Effect of dietary citrinin on urine excretion in broiler chickens. Avian Dis 25:827–830.

156. Hagler, W.M., Jr., K. Tyczkowska, and P.B. Hamilton. 1984. Simultaneous occurrence of deoxynivalenol, zearalenone, and aflatoxin in 1982 scabby wheat from the midwestern United States. Appl Environ Microbiol 47:151–154.

157. Hamilton, P.B. 1971. A natural and extremely severe occurrence of alfatoxicosis in laying hens. Poult Sci 50:1880–1882.

158. Hamilton, P.B. 1975. Proof of mycotoxicoses being a field problem and a simple method for their control. Poult Sci 54:1706–1708.

159. Hamilton, P.B., and J.D. Garlich. 1972. Failure of vitamin supplementation to alter the fatty liver syndrome caused by aflatoxin. Poult Sci 51:688–692.

160. Hamilton, P.B., H.T. Tung, J.R. Harris, J.H. Gainer, and W.E. Donaldson. 1972. The effect of dietary fat on aflatoxicosis in turkeys. Poult Sci 51:165–170.

161. Hamilton, P.B., H.T. Tung, R.D. Wyatt, and W.E. Donaldson. 1974. Interaction of dietary aflatoxin with some vitamin deficiencies. Poult Sci 53:871–877.

162. Hamilton, P.B., W.E. Huff, J.R. Harris, and R.D. Wyatt. 1982. Natural occurrences of ochratoxicosis in poultry. Poult Sci 1:1832–1841.

163. Hamilton, R.M.G., B.K. Thompson, H.L. Trenholm, P.S. Fiser, and R. Greenhalgh. 1985. Effects of feeding white leghorn hens diets that contain deoxynivalenol (vomitoxin)-contaminated wheat. Poult Sci 64:1840–1851.

164. Hamilton, R.M.G., B.K. Thompson, and H.L. Trenholm. 1986. The effects of deoxynivalenol (vomitoxin) on dietary preference of white leghorn hens. Poult Sci 65:288–293.

165. Harland, E.C., and P.T. Cardeilhac. 1975. Excretion of carbon-14-labeled aflatoxin B1 via bile, urine, and intestinal contents of the chicken. Am J Vet Res 36:909–912.

166. Harris, J.R. 1984. Case report on T-2 mycotoxicosis in chickens. Keeping Current (CEVA Laboratories, Inc.) Jan–Feb:2–3.

167. Harvey, R.B., L.F. Kubena, B. Lawhorn, O.J. Fletcher, T.D. Phillips. 1987. Feed refusal in swine fed ochratoxin-contaminated grain sorghum: Evaluation of toxicity in chicks. J Am Vet Med Assoc 190:673–675.

168. Harvey, R.B., L.F. Kubena, M.H. Elissalde, and T.D. Phillips. 1993. Efficacy of zeolitic ore compounds on the toxicity of aflatoxin to growing broiler chickens. Avian Dis 37:67–73.

169. Harvey, R.B., L.F. Kubena, and T.D. Philllips. 1993. Evaluation of aluminosilicate compounds to reduce aflatoxin residues and toxicity to poultry and livestock: A review report. Sci Total Environ SUP-93:1453–1457.

170. Hasan, H.A.H., and A.L.E. Mahmoud. 1993. Inhibitory effect of spice oils on lipase and mycotoxin production. Zentralbl Mikrobiol 148:543–548.

171. Hayes, M.A., and G.A. Wobeser. 1983. Subacute toxic effects of dietary T-2 toxin in young mallard ducks. Can J Comp Med 47:180–187.

172. Haynes, J.S., and M.M. Walser. 1986. Ultrastructure of Fusarium-induced tibial dyschondroplasia in chickens: A sequential study. Vet Pathol 23:499–505.

173. Haynes, J.S., M.M. Walser, and E.M. Lawler. 1985. Morphogenesis of Fusarium sp.-induced tibial dyschondroplasia in chickens. Vet Pathol 22:629–636.

174. Hegazy, S.M., A. Azzam, and M.A. Gabal. 1991. Interaction of naturally occurring aflatoxins in poultry feed and immunization against fowl cholera. Poult Sci 70:2425–2428

175. Hetzel, D.J.S., D. Hoffman, J. van de Ven, and S. Soeripto. 1984. Mortality rate and liver histopathology in four breeds of ducks following long term exposure to low levels of aflatoxins. Singapore Vet J 8:6–14.

176. Higgins, K.F., R.M. Barta, R.D. Neiger, G.E. Rottinghaus, and R.I. Sterry. 1992. Mycotoxin occurrence in waste field corn and ingesta of wild geese in the northern great plains. Prairie Nat 24(1):31–37.

177. Hintikka, E.L. 1978. Stachybotryotoxicosis in poultry. In T.A. Wyllie and L.G. Morehouse (eds.). Mycotoxic Fungi, Mycotoxins, and Mycotoxicoses: An Encyclopaedic Handbook II. Marcel Dekker, New York, pp. 203–208.

178. Hirano, K.Y., Adachi, S. Ishibashi, M. Sueyoshi, A. Bintvihok, and N.H. Kumazawa. 1991. Detection of aflatoxin

B1 in plasma of fowls receiving feed naturally contaminated with aflatoxin B1. J Vet Med Sci 53:1083–1085.

179. Hnatow, L.L., and R.F. Wideman, Jr. 1985. Kidney function of single comb white leghorn pullets following acute renal portal infusion of the mycotoxin citrinin. Poult Sci 64:1553–1561.

180. Hoerr, F.J. 1991. Poisons and Toxins: Mycotoxins. In B.W. Calnek, H.J. Barnes, C.W. Beard, W.M. Reid, and H.W. Yoder (eds). Diseases of Poultry, 9th ed. Iowa State University Press, Ames, IA, pp. 884–915.

181. Hoerr, F.J., and G.H. D'Andrea. 1983. Biological effects of aflatoxin in swine. In U.L. Diener, R.L. Asquith, and J.W. Dickens (eds.). Aflatoxin and Aspergillus flavus in Corn. USDA Southern Cooperative Series Bulletin 279:51–55.

182. Hoerr, F.J., W.W. Carlton, and B. Yagen. 1981. Mycotoxicosis caused by a single dose of T-2 toxin or diacetoxyscirpenol in broiler chickens. Vet Pathol 18:652–664.

183. Hoerr, F.J., W.W. Carlton, B. Yagen, and A.Z. Joffe. 1982. Mycotoxicosis caused by either T-2 toxin or diacetoxyscirpenol in the diet of broiler chickens. Fundam Appl Toxicol 2:121–124.

184. Hoerr, F.J., W.W. Carlton, B. Yagen, and A.Z. Joffe. 1982. Mycotoxicosis produced in broiler chickens by multiple doses of either T-2 toxin or diacetoxyscirpenol. Avian Pathol 11:369–383.

185. Hoerr, F.J., W.W. Carlton, J. Tuite, R.F. Vesonder, W.K. Rohwedder, and G. Szigeti. 1982. Experimental trichothecene mycotoxicosis produced in broiler chickens by Fusarium sporotrichiella var. sporotrichioides. Avian Pathol 11:385–405.

186. Hoerr, F.J., G.H. D'Andrea, J.J. Giambrone, and V.S. Panangala. 1986. Comparative histopathologic changes in aflatoxicosis, In J.L. Richard and J.R. Thruston (eds.). Diagnosis of Mycotoxicoses. Martinus Nijhoff, Dordrecht, The Netherlands, pp. 179–189.

187. Hofacre, C.L., R.K. Page, and O.J. Fletcher. 1985. Suspected mycotoxicosis in laying hens. Avian Dis 29:846–849.

188. Howarth, B., Jr., and R.D. Wyatt. 1976. Effect of dietary aflatoxin on fertility, hatchability, and progeny performance of broiler breeder hens. Appl Environ Microbiol 31:680–684.

189. Hsieh, D.P.H. 1987. Mode of action of mycotoxins. In P. Krogh (ed.). Mycotoxins in Food. Academic Press, San Diego, CA, pp. 149–176.

190. Huff, W.E., and M.D. Ruff. 1982. Eimeria acervulina and Eimeria tenella infections in ochratoxin A-compromised broiler chickens. Poult Sci 61:685–692.

191. Huff, W.E., R.D. Wyatt, T.L. Tucker, and P.B. Hamilton. 1974. Ochratoxicosis in the broiler chicken. Poult Sci 53:1585–1591.

192. Huff, W.E., R.D. Wyatt, and P.B. Hamilton. 1975. Effects of dietary aflatoxin on certain egg yolk parameters. Poult Sci 54:2014–2018.

193. Huff, W.E., R.D. Wyatt, and P.B. Hamilton. 1975. Nephrotoxicity of dietary ochratoxin A in broiler chickens. Appl Microbiol 30:48–51.

194. Huff, W.E., J.A. Doerr, and P.B. Hamilton. 1977. Decreased bone strength during ochratoxicosis and aflatoxicosis. Poult Sci 56:1724.

195. Huff, W.E., C.F. Chang, M.F. Warren, and P.B. Hamilton. 1979. Ochratoxin A-induced iron deficiency anemia. Appl Environ Microbiol 37:601–604.

196. Huff, W.E., J.A. Doerr, and P.B. Hamilton. 1979. Decreased glycogen mobilization during ochratoxicosis in broiler chickens. Appl Environ Microbiol 37:122–126.

197. Huff, W.E., P.B. Hamilton, and A. Ciegler. 1980. Evaluation of penicillic acid for toxicity in broiler chickens. Poult Sci 59:1203–1207.

198. Huff, W.E., J.A. Doerr, P.B. Hamilton, and R.F. Vesonder. 1981. Acute toxicity of vomitoxin (deoxynivalenol) in broiler chickens. Poult Sci 60:1412–1414.

199. Huff, W.E., J.A. Doerr, C.J. Wabeck, G.W. Chaloupka, J.D. May, and J.W. Merkley. 1983. Individual and combined effects of aflatoxin and ochratoxin A on bruising in broiler chickens. Poult Sci 62:1764–1771.

200. Huff, W.E. J.A. Doerr, C.J. Wabeck, G.W. Chaloupka, J.D. May, and J.W. Merkley. 1984. The individual and combined effects of aflatoxin and ochratoxin A on various processing parameters of broiler chickens. Poult Sci 63:2153–2161.

201. Huff, W.E., L.F. Kubena, R.B. Harvey, D.E. Corrier, and H.H. Mollenhauer. 1986. Progression of aflatoxicosis in broiler chickens. Poult Sci 65:1891–1899.

202. Huff, W.E., L.F. Kubena, and R.B. Harvey. 1988. Progression of ochratoxicosis in broiler chickens. Poult Sci 67:1139–1146.

203. Huff, W.E., L.F. Kubena, R.B. Harvey, and T.D. Phillips. 1992. Efficacy of hydrated sodium calcium aluminosilicate to reduce the individual and combined toxicity of aflatoxin and ochratoxin A. Poult Sci 71:64–69.

204. Hulan, H.W., and F.G. Proudfoot. 1982. Effects of feeding vomitoxin contaminated wheat on the performance of broiler chickens. Poult Sci 61:1653–1659.

205. Iqbal, Q.K., P.V. Rao, and S.J. Reddy. 1983. Dose-response relationship of experimentally induced aflatoxicosis in commercial layers. Indian J Anim Sci 53:1277–1280.

206. Jacobson, W.C., and H.G. Wiseman. 1974. The transmission of aflatoxin B1 into eggs. Poult Sci 53:1743–1745.

207. Joffe, A.Z. 1986. Fusarium Species: Their Biology and Toxicology. John Wiley and Sons, New York, pp. 345–384.

208. Joffe, A.Z., and B. Yagen. 1978. Intoxication produced by toxic fungi Fusarium poae and F. sporotrichioides on chicks. Toxicon 16:263–273.

209. Johri, T.S., R. Agarwal, and V.R. Sadagopan. 1986. Surveillance of aflatoxin B1 content of poultry feed stuffs in and around Bareilly district of Uttar Pradesh. Indian J Poult Sci 21:227–230.

210. Johri, T.S., R. Agrawal, and V.R. Sadagopan. 1990. Effect of low dietary levels of aflatoxin on laying quails (Coturnix coturnix japonica) and their response to dietary modifications. Indian J Anim Sci 60:355–359.

211. Jones, F.T., and P.B. Hamilton. 1986. Factors influencing fungal activity in low moisture poultry feeds. Poult Sci 65:1522–1525.

212. Jones, F.T., and P.B. Hamilton. 1987. Research note: Relationship of feed surface area to fungal activity in poultry feeds. Poult Sci 66:1545–1547.

213. Jones, G.M., D.N. Mowat, J.I. Elliot, and E.T. Moran, Jr. 1974. Organic acid preservation of high moisture corn and other grains and the nutritional value: A review. Can J Anim Sci 54:499–517.

214. Jones, F.T., W.H. Hagler, and P.B. Hamilton. 1982. Association of low levels of aflatoxin in feed with productivity losses in commercial broiler operations. Poult Sci 61:861–868.

215. Juszkiewicz, T., and J. Piskorska-Pliszczynska. 1992. Occurrence of mycotoxins in animal feeds. J Environ Pathol Toxicol Oncol 11(3):211–215.

216. Keshavarz, K. 1993. Corn contaminated with deoxynivalenol: Effects on performance of poultry. J Appl Poult Res 2:43–50.

217. Kichou, F., and M.M. Walser. 1993. The natural occurrence of aflatoxin B1 in Moroccan poultry feeds. Vet Hum Toxicol 35:105–108.

218. Kingsland, G.C., and J. Anderson. 1976. A study of the feasibility of the use of gentian violet as a fungistat for poultry feed. Poult Sci 55:852–857.

219. Kirby, L.K., T.S. Nelson, J.T. Halley, and J.N. Beasley. 1987. Citrinin toxicity in young chicks. Poult Sci 66:966–968.

220. Kratzer, F.H., D. Bandy, M. Wiley, and A.N. Booth. 1969. Aflatoxin effects in poultry. Proc Soc Exp Biol Med 131:1281–1284.

221. Krogh, P., and F. Elling. 1977. Mycotoxic nephropathy. Vet Sci Commun 1:51–63.

222. Krogh, P., F. Elling, B. Hald, B. Jylling, V.E. Petersen, E. Skadhauge, and C.K. Svensen. 1976. Changes of renal function and structure induced by ochratoxin A-contaminated feed. Acta Pathol Microbiol Scand 84:215–221.

223. Kubena, L.F., T.D. Phillips, C.R. Creger, D.A. Witzel, and N.D. Heidelbaugh. 1983. Toxicity of ochratoxin A and tannic acid to growing chicks. Poult Sci 62:1786–1792.

224. Kubena, L.F., R.B. Harvey, O.J. Fletcher, T.D. Phillips, H.H. Mollenhauer, D.A. Witzel, and N.D. Heidelbaugh. 1985. Toxicity of ochratoxin A and vanadium to growing chicks. Poult Sci 64:620–628.

225. Kubena, L.F., S.P. Swanson, R.B. Harvey, O.J. Fletcher, L.D. Rowe, and T.D. Phillips. 1985. Effects of feeding deoxynivalenol (vomitoxin)- contaminated wheat to growing chicks. Poult Sci 64:1649–1655.

226. Kubena, L.F., R.B. Harvey, T.D. Phillips, and O.J. Fletcher. 1986. Influence of ochratoxin A and vanadium on various parameters in growing chicks. Poult Sci 65:1671–1678.

227. Kubena, L.F., R.B. Harvey, D.E. Corrier, W.E. Huff, and T.D. Phillips. 1987. Effects of feeding deoxynivalenol (DON, vomitoxin)-contaminated wheat to female white leghorn chickens from day old through egg production. Poult Sci 66:1612–1618.

228. Kubena, L.F., R.B. Harvey, T.D. Phillips, G.M. Holman, and C.R. Creger. 1987. Effects of feeding mature white leghorn hens diets that contain deoxynivalenol (vomitoxin). Poult Sci 66:55–58.

229. Kubena, L.F. R.B. Harvey, T.D. Phillips, and B.A. Clement. 1992. The use of sorbent compounds to modify the toxic expression of mycotoxins in poultry. Proc World Poult Congr 19(1):357–361.

230. Kubena, L.F., R.B. Harvey, W.E. Huff, M.H. Elissalde, A.G. Yersin, T.D. Phillips, and G.E. Rottinghaus. 1993. Efficacy of a hydrated sodium calcium aluminosilicate to reduce the toxicity of aflatoxin and diacetoxyscirpenol. Poult Sci 72:51–59.

231. Kubena, L.F. , R.B. Harvey, T.D. Phillips, and B.A. Clement. 1993. Effect of hydrated sodium calcium aluminosilicates on aflatoxicosis in broiler chicks. Poult Sci 72:651–657.

232. Kubena, L.F., E.E. Smith, A. Gentles, R.B. Harvey, T.S. Edrington, T.D. Phillips, and G.E. Rottinghaus. 1994. Individual and combined toxicity of T-2 toxin and cyclopiazonic acid in broiler chicks. Poult Sci 73:1390–1397.

233. Kubena, L.F., T.S. Edrington, C. Kamps-Holtzapple, R.B. Harvey, M.H. Elissalde, and G.E. Rottinghaus. 1995. Effects of feeding fumonisin B1 in Fusarium moniliforme culture material and aflatoxin singly and in combination to turkey poults. Poult Sci 74:1295–1303.

234. Kurmanov, I.A., and A. Novacky. 1978. Fusariotoxicosis in chickens in the USSR. In T.A. Wyllie and L.G. Morehouse (eds). Mycotoxic Fungi, Mycotoxins, and Mycotoxicoses: An Encyclopaedic Handbook. II. Marcel Dekker, New York, pp. 322–326.

235. Lamont, M.H. 1979. Cases of suspected mycotoxicoses as reported by veterinary investigation centres. Proc Mycotoxins Anim Dis 3:38–39.

236. Lansden, J.A., and J.I. Davidson. 1983. Occurrence of cyclopiazonic acid in peanuts. Appl Environ Microbiol 45:766–769.

237. Lanza, G.M., K.W. Washburn, R.D. Wyatt, and H.M. Edwards, Jr. 1979. Depressed 59Fe absorption due to dietary aflatoxin. Poult Sci 58:1439–1444.

238. Lanza, G.M., K.W. Washburn, and R.D. Wyatt. 1980. Strain variation in hematological response of broilers to dietary aflatoxin. Poult Sci 59:2686–2691.

239. Larsen, C., M. Acha, and M. Ehrich. 1988. Research note: Chlortetracycline and aflatoxin interaction in two lines of chicks. Poult Sci 67:1229–1232.

240. Lawler, E.M., T.F. Fletcher, and M.M. Walser. 1985. Chondroclasts in Fusarium-induced tibial dyschondroplasia. Am J Pathol 120:276–281.

241. Le Bars, J. 1979. Cyclopiazonic acid production by Penicillium camemberti thom and natural occurrence of this mycotoxin in cheese. Appl Environ Microbiol 38:1052–1055.

242. Lebron, C.I., R.A. Molins, H.W. Walker, A.A. Draft, and H.M. Stahr. 1989. Inhibition of mold growth and mycotoxin production in high-moisture corn treated with phosphates. J Food Prot 52:329–336.

243. Ledoux, D.R., T.P. Brown, T.S. Weibking, and G.E. Rottinghaus. 1992. Fumonisin toxicity in broiler chicks. J Vet Diagn Invest 4:330–333.

244. Lee, Y.W., C.J. Mirocha, D.J. Shroeder, and M.M. Walser. 1985. TDP-1, a toxic component causing tibial dyschondroplasia in broiler chickens, and trichothecenes from Fusarium roseum "graminearum." Appl Environ Microbiol 50:102–107.

245. Leeson, S., G. Diaz, and J.D. Summers. 1995. Poultry Metabolic Disorders and Mycotoxins. University Books, Guelph, Canada, pp. 190–326.

246. Leitao, J.G. de Saint Blanquat, J.R. Bailly, and R. Derache. 1990. Preventative measures for microflora and mycotoxin production in foodstuffs. Arch Environ Contam Toxicol 19:437–446.

247. Lorenz, K. 1979. Ergot on cereal grains. Crit Rev Food Sci Nutr 11:311–54.

248. Lovett, J. 1972. Patulin toxicosis in poultry. Poult Sci 51:2097–2098.

249. Lun, A.K., L.G. Young, E.T. Moran, Jr., D.B. Hunter, and J.P. Rodriguez. 1986. Effects of feeding hens a high level of vomitoxin-contaminated corn on performance and tissue residues. Poult Sci 65:1095–1099.

250. Mahipal, S.K., and R.K. Kaushik. 1983. A note on the prevalence of aflatoxicosis in poultry birds in Haryana. Haryana Vet 22:51–52.

251. Manley, R.W., R.M. Hulet, J.B. Meldrum, and C.T. Larsen. 1988. Research note: Turkey poult tolerance to diets containing deoxynivalenol (vomitoxin) and salinomycin. Poult Sci 67:149–152.

252. Manning, R.O., and R.D. Wyatt. 1984. Comparative toxicity of Chaetomium contaminated corn and various chemical forms of oosporein in broiler chicks. Poult Sci 63:251–259.

253. Manning, R.O., T.P. Brown, R.D. Wyatt, and O.J. Fletcher. 1985. The individual and combined effects of citrinin and ochratoxin A in broiler chicks. Avian Dis 29:986–997.

254. Marasas, W.F.O., T.S. Kellerman, and W.C.A. Gelderblom. 1988. Leukoencephalomalacia in a horse induced by fumonisin B1 isolated from Fusarium moniliforme. Onderstepoort J Vet Res 35:197–203.

255. Marijanovic, D.R., P. Holt, W.P. Norred, C.W. Bacon, K.A. Voss, and P.C. Stancel. 1991. Immunosuppressive effects of Fusarium moniliforme corn cultures in chickens. Poult Sci 70:1895–1901.

256. Marks, H.L., and C.W. Bacon. 1976. Influence of Fusarium-infected corn and F-2 on laying hens. Poult Sci 55:1864–1870.

257. McLaughlin, C.S., M.H. Vaughan, I.M. Campbell, C.M. Wei, M.E. Stafford, and B.S. Hansen. 1977. Inhibition of protein synthesis by trichothecenes. In J.V. Rodericks, C.W. Hesseltine, and M.A. Mehleman (eds.). Mycotoxins in Human and Animal Health. Pathotox Publishers, Park Forest South, IL, pp. 263–274.

258. Mehdi, N.A.Q., W.W. Carlton, and J. Tuite. 1981. Citrinin mycotoxicosis in broiler chickens. Food Cosmet Toxicol 19:723–733.

259. Mehdi, N.A.Q., W.W. Carlton, and J. Tuite. 1983.

Acute toxicity of citrinin in turkeys and ducklings. Avian Pathol 12:221–233.

260. Mehdi, N.A.Q., W.W. Carlton, and J. Tuite. 1984. Mycotoxicoses produced in duckings and turkeys by dietary and multiple doses of citrinin. Avian Pathol 13:37–50.

261. Mehdi, N.A.Q., W.W. Carlton, G.D. Boon, and J. Tuite. 1984. Studies on the sequential development and pathogenesis of citrinin mycotoxicosis in turkeys and ducklings. Vet Pathol 21:216–223.

262. Micco, C., M. Miraglia, R. Onori, A. Ioppolo, and A. Mantovani. 1987. Long-term administration of low doses of mycotoxins in poultry. I. Residues of ochratoxin A in broilers and laying hens. Poult Sci 66:47–50.

263. Michael, G.Y., P. Thaxton, and P.B. Hamilton. 1973. Impairment of the reticuloendothelial system of chickens during aflatoxicosis. Poult Sci 52:1206–1207.

264. Miller, B.L., and R.D. Wyatt. 1985. Effect of dietary aflatoxin on the uptake and elimination of chlortetracycline in broiler chicks. Poult Sci 64:1637–1643.

265. Mirocha, C.J. 1979. Trichothecene toxins produced by Fusarium. In W. Shimoda (ed.). Conference on Mycotoxins in Animal Feeds and Grains Related to Animal Health. Food and Drug Administration Report No. FDA/BVM-79/139, pp. 289–373.

266. Mirocha, C.J., B. Schauerhamer, C.M. Christensen, M.L. Niku-Paavola, and M. Nummi. 1979. Incidence of zearalenol (Fusarium mycotoxin) in animal feed. Appl Environ Microbiol 38:749–750.

267. Mirocha, C.J., T.S. Robison, R.J. Pawloski, and N.K. Allen. 1982. Distribution and residue determination of [3H]zearalenone in broilers. Toxicol Appl Pharmacol 66:77–87.

268. Misir, R., and R.R. Marquardt. 1978. Factors affecting rye (Secale cereale L.) utilization in growing chicks. I. The influence of rye level, ergot and penicillin supplementation. Can J Anim Sci 58:691–701.

269. Misir, R., and R.R. Marquardt. 1978. Factors affecting rye (Secale cereale L.) ulitization in growing chicks. III. The influence of milling fractions. Can J Anim Sci 58:717–730.

270. Mohiuddin, S.M., M.V. Reddy, M.M. Reddy, and K. Ramakrishna. 1986. Studies on phagocytic activity and hematological changes in aflatoxicosis in poultry. Indian Vet J 63:442–445.

271. Moran, E.T., Jr., H.C. Carlson, and J.R. Pettit. 1974. Vitamin E-selenium deficiency in the duck aggravated by the use of high-moisture corn and molding prior to preservation. Avian Dis 18:536–543.

272. Moran, E.T., Jr., B. Hunter, P. Ferket, L.G. Young, and L.G. McGirr. 1982. High tolerance of broilers to vomitoxin from corn infected with Fusarium graminearum. Poult Sci 61:1828–1831.

273. Moran, E.T. Jr., P.R. Ferket, and A.K. Lun. 1987. Impact of high dietary vomitoxin on yolk yield and embryonic mortality. Poult Sci 66:977–982.

274. Moreno-Romo, M.A., and G. Suarez-Fernandez. 1986. Aflatoxin-producing potential of Aspergillus flavus strains isolated from Spanish poultry feeds. Mycopathologia 95:129–132.

275. Muller, R.D., C.W. Carlson, G. Semeniuk, and G.S. Harshfield. 1970. The response of chicks, ducklings, goslings, pheasants and poults to graded levels of aflatoxins. Poult Sci 49:1346–1350.

276. Muller, E.E., A.E. Panerai, D. Cocchi, and P. Mantegazza. 1977. Endocrine profile of ergot alkaloids. Life Sci 21:1545–1558.

277. Nagaraj, R.Y., W. Wu, J.A. Will, and R.F. Vesonder. 1996. Acute cardiotoxicity of moniliformin in broiler chickens as measured by electrocardiography. Avian Dis 40:223–227.

278. Nahm, K.H. 1995. Possibilities for preventing mycotoxicosis in domestic fowl. World Poult Sci J 51:177–185.

279. Neiger, R.D., T.J. Johnson, D.J. Hurley, K.F. Higgins, G.E. Rottinghaus, and H. Stahr. 1994. The short-term effect of low concentrations of dietary aflatoxin and T-2 toxin on mallard ducklings. Avian Dis 38:738–743.

280. Nelson, T.S., J.N. Beasley, L.K. Kirby, Z.B. Johnson, and G.C. Ballam. 1980. Isolation and identification of citrinin produced by Penicillium lanosum. Poult Sci 59:2055–2059.

281. Nelson, T.S., J.N. Beasley, L.K. Kriby, Z.B. Johnson, G.C. Ballam, and M.M. Campbell. 1981. Citrinin toxicity in growing chicks. Poult Sci 60:2165–2166.

282. Nemeth, I., and S. Juhasz. 1968. Effect of aflatoxin in serum protein fractions of day-old ducklings. Acta Vet Acad Sci Hung 18:95–105.

283. Newberne, P.M. 1973. Chronic aflatoxicosis. J Am Vet Med Assoc 163:1262–1273.

284. Newberne, P.M., G.N. Wogan, W.W. Carlton, and M.M.A. Kader. 1964. Histopathologic lesions in ducklings caused by Aspergillus flavus cultures, culture extracts, and crystalline aflatoxins. Toxicol Appl Pharmacol 6:542–556.

285. Nichols, T.E. 1983. Economic effects of aflatoxin in corn. In U.L. Diener, R.L. Asquith, and J.W. Dickens (eds.). Aflatoxin and Aspergillus flavus in Corn. USDA Southern Cooperative Series Bulletin 279:67–71.

286. Niemiec, J., W. Borzemska, J. Roszkowski, E. Karpinska, G. Kosowska, and P. Szeleszczuk. 1995. Pathological changes in chick embryos from layers given feed contaminated with ochratoxin A. Med Weter 51(9):538–540.

287. Norred, W.P., R.J. Cole, J.W. Dorner, and J.A. Lansden. 1987. Liquid chromatographic determination of cyclopiazonic acid in poultry meat. J Assoc Off Anal Chem 70:121–123.

288. Okoye, J.O.A., I.U. Asuzu, and J.C. Gugnani. 1988. Paralysis and lameness associated with aflatoxicosis in broilers. Avian Pathol 17:731–734.

289. Olsen, M., C.J. Mirocha, H.K. Abbas, and B. Johansson. 1986. Metabolism of high concentrations of dietary zearalenone by young male turkey poults. Poult Sci 65:1905–1910.

290. Osborne, B.G. 1980. The occurrence of ochratoxin A in mouldy bread and flour. Food Cosmet Toxicol 18:615–617.

291. Osborne, D.J., and P.B. Hamilton. 1981. Decreased pancreatic digestive enzymes during aflatoxicosis. Poult Sci 60:1818–1821.

292. Ostrowski-Meissner, H.T. 1983. Effect of contamination of diets with aflatoxin on growing ducks and chickens. Trop Anim Health Prod 15:161–168.

293. Ostrowski-Meissner, H.T., D.F. Sinclair, I. Komang, and W. Supratman. 1984. Blood analysis in clinical diagnosis of aflatoxicosis in ducks and chickens. Proc World Poult Congr 17:563–565.

294. Ottinger, M.A., and J.A. Doerr. 1980. The early influence of aflatoxin upon sexual maturation in the Japanese quail. Poult Sci 59:1750–1754.

295. Osweiler, G.D. 1986. Mycotoxin diagnosis: A perspective. Proc Am Assoc Vet Lab Diagn 29:221–229.

296. Page, R.K., G. Stewart, R. Wyatt, R. Bush, O.J. Fletcher, and J. Brown. 1980. Influence of low levels of ochratoxin A on egg production, egg-shell stains, and serum uric-acid levels in leghorn-type hens. Avian Dis 24:777–780.

297. Palmgren, M.S., and A.W. Hayes. 1987. Aflatoxins in food. In P. Krogh (ed.). Mycotoxins in Food. Academic Press, San Diego, CA, pp. 56–96.

298. Palyusik, M., and E.K. Kovacs. 1975. Effect on laying geese of feeds containing the fusariotoxins T-2 and F2. Acta Vet Acad Sci Hung 25:363–368.

299. Palyusik, M., K.E. Kovacs, and E. Guzsal. 1971. Effect of Fusarium graminearum on the semen production in geese and turkeys. Magy Allatorv Lapja 26:300–303.

300. Palyusik, M., G. Nagy, and L. Zoldag. 1974. The effect of different Fusarium species on the spermatogenesis in ganders. Magy Allatorv Lapja 8:551–553.

301. Park, D. 1993. Perspectives on mycotoxin decontam-

ination procedures. Food Addit Contam 10:49–60.

302. Parkhurst, C.R., P.B. Hamilton, and A.A. Ademoyero. 1992. Abnormal feathering of chicks caused by scirpenol mycotoxins differing in degree of acetylation. Poult Sci 71:833–837.

303. Paster, N., E. Pinthus, and D. Reichman. 1987. A comparative study of the efficacy of calcium propionate, agrosil and adofeed as mold inhibitors in poultry feed. Poult Sci 66:858–860.

304. Patterson, D.S.P., and B.A. Roberts. 1971. The in vitro reduction of aflatoxins B1 and B2 by soluble avian liver enzymes. Food Cosmet Toxicol 9:829–837.

305. Patterson, D.S.P., and B.A. Roberts. 1972. Aflatoxin metabolism in duck liver homogenates: The relative importance of reversible cyclopentenone reduction and hemiacetal formation. Food Cosmet Toxicol 10:501–512.

306. Pearson, A.W. 1978. Biochemical changes produced by fusarium T-2 toxin in the chicken. Res Vet Sci 24:92–97.

307. Peckham, M.C. 1984. Poisons and toxins. In M.S. Hofstad, H.J. Barnes, B.W. Calnek, W.M. Reid, and H.W. Yoder, Jr. (eds). Diseases of Poultry, 8th ed. Iowa State University Press, Ames, IA, pp. 799–804.

308. Peckham, J.C., B. Doupnik, Jr., and O.H. Jones, Jr. 1971. Acute toxicity of ochratoxins A and B in chicks. Appl Microbiol 21:492–494.

309. Pegram, R.A, and R.D. Wyatt. 1979. Effect of dietary oosporein on broiler chickens. Poult Sci 58:1092.

310. Pegram, R.A, and R.D. Wyatt. 1981. Avian gout caused by oosporein, a mycotoxin produced by Chaetomium trilaterale. Poult Sci 60:2429–2440.

311. Pegram, R.A., Wyatt, R.D., and T.L. Smith. 1982. Oosporein toxicosis in the turkey poult. Avian Dis 26:47–59.

312. Pegram, R.A., Wyatt, R.D., and H.L. Marks. 1986. The relationship of certain blood parameters to aflatoxin resistance in Japanese quail. Poult Sci 65:1652–1658.

313. Perek, M. 1958. Ergot and ergot-like fungi as the cause of vesicular dermatitis (sod disease) in chickens. J Am Vet Med Assoc 132:529–533.

314. Phillips, T.D., L.F. Kubena, R.B. Harvey, D.R. Taylor, and N.D. Heidelbaugh. 1988. Hydrated sodium calcium aluminosilicate: A high affinity sorbent for aflatoxin. Poult Sci 67:243–247.

315. Pier, A.C. 1973. Effects of aflatoxin on immunity. J Am Vet Med Assoc 163:1268–1269.

316. Pier A.C., and K.L. Heddleston. 1970. The effect of aflatoxin on immunity in turkeys. I. Impairment of actively acquired resistance to bacterial challenge. Avian Dis 14:797–809.

317. Pier, A.C., K.L. Heddleston, S.J. Cysewski, and J.M. Patterson. 1972. Effect of aflatoxin on immunity in turkeys. II. Reversal of impaired resistance to bacterial infection by passive transfer of plasma. Avian Dis 16:381–387.

318. Pohland, A.E., and G.E. Wood. 1987. Occurrence of Mycotoxins in foods. In P. Krogh (ed.). Mycotoxins in Food. Academic Press, San Diego, CA, pp. 35–64.

319. Potchinsky, M.B., and S.E. Bloom. 1993. Selective aflatoxin B1-induced sister chromatid exchanges and cytotoxicity in differentiating B and T lymphocytes in vivo. Environ Mol Mutagen 21:87–94.

320. Pramanik, A.K., and H.M. Bhattacharya. 1987. Diseases of poultry in three districts of West Bengal affecting the rural economy. Indian J Vet Med 7:63–65.

321. Prelusky, D.B., H.L. Trenholm, R.M.G. Hamilton, and J.D. Miller. 1987. Transmission of [14C] deoxynivalenol to eggs following oral administration to laying hens. J Agric Food Chem 35:182–186.

322. Prior, M.G., and C.S. Sisodia. 1978. Ochratoxicosis in white leghorn hens. Poult Sci 57:619–623.

323. Prior, M.G., C.S. Sisodia, J.B. O'Neil, and F. Hrudka. 1979. Effect of ochratoxin A on fertility and embryo viability of japanese quail (Coturinx coturnix japonica). Can J Comp Med 59:605–609.

324. Prior, M.G., J.B. O'Neil, and C.S. Sisodia. 1980. Effects of ochratoxin A on growth response and residues in broilers. Poult Sci 59:1254–1257.

325. Prior, M.G., C.S. Sisodia, and J.B. O'Neil. 1981. Effects of ochratoxin A on egg production, body weight and feed intake in white leghorn hens. Poult Sci 60:1145–1148.

326. Pruthi, A.K., P. Batra, and J.R. Sandana. 1992. Comparative studies on cell-mediated immune responses in herpesvirus of turkey vaccinated aflatoxin B1 fed and normally fed chickens. Proc World Poult Congr 19:15–20.

327. Puls, R., and J.A. Greenway. 1976. Fusariotoxicosis from barley in British Columbia II. Analysis and toxicity of suspected barley. Can J Comp Med 40:16–19.

328. Qureshi, M.A., and W.M. Hagler, Jr. 1992. Effect of fumonisin-B1 exposure on chicken macrophage functions in vitro. Poult Sci 71:104–112.

329. Rabie, C.J., W.F.O. Marasas, P.G. Thiel, A. Lubben, and R. Vleggaar. 1982. Moniliformin production and toxicity of different Fusarium species from southern Africa. Appl Environ Microbiol 43:517–521.

330. Rao, V.S. 1987. Persistent Ranikhet disease in a commercial broiler farm—a report. Poult Advis 20:61–65.

331. Rao, A.G., P.K. Dehuri, S.K Chand, S.C. Mishra, P.K. Mishra, and B.C. Das. 1985. Aflatoxicosis in broiler chickens. Indian J Poult Sci 20:240–244.

332. Reddy, D.N., P.V. Rao, V.R. Reddy, and B. Yadgiri. 1984. Effect of selected levels of dietary aflatoxin on the performance of broiler chickens. Indian J Anim Sci 54:68–73.

333. Reiss, J. 1977. Mycotoxins in foodstuffs. X. Production of citrinin by Penicillium chrysogenum in bread. Food Cosmet Toxicol 15:303–307.

334. Renault, L., M. Goujet, A. Monin, G. Boutin, M. Palisse, and A. Alamagny. 1979. Suspected mycotoxicosis due to trichothecenes in broiler fowl. Bull Acad Vet Fr 52:181–188.

335. Richard, J.L., S.J. Cysewski, A.C. Pier, and G.D. Booth. 1978. Comparison of effects of dietary T-2 toxin on growth, immunogenic organs, antibody formation, and pathologic changes in turkeys and chickens. Am J Vet Res 39:1674–1679.

336. Richard, J.L., R.D. Stubblefield, R.D. Lyon, W.L. Peden, J.R. Thurston, and R.B. Rimler. 1986. Distribution and clearance of aflatoxins B1 amd M1 in turkeys fed diets containing 50 or 150 ppb aflatoxin from naturally contaminated corn. Avian Dis 30:788–793.

337. Richardson, K.E., and P.B. Hamilton. 1987. Enhanced production of pancreatic digestive enzymes during aflatoxicosis in egg-type chickens. Poult Sci 66:640–644.

338. Richardson, L.R., S. Wilkes, J. Godwin, and K.R. Pierce. 1962. Effect of moldy diet and moldy soybean meal on the growth of chicks and poults. J Nutr 78:301–306.

339. Richardson, K.E., L.A. Nelson, and P.B. Hamilton. 1987. Effect of dietary fat level on dose response relationships during aflatoxicosis in young chickens. Poult Sci 66:1470–1478.

340. Richardson, K.E., L.A. Nelson, and P.B. Hamilton. 1987. Interaction of dietary protein level on dose response relationships during aflatoxicosis in young chickens. Poult Sci 66:960–976.

341. Roberts, W.T., and E.C. Mora. 1979. Hemorrhagic syndrome of chicks produced by Penicillium citrinum AUA-532 contaminated corn. Poult Sci 58:810–814.

342. Robison, T.S., K.R. Reddy, S.B. Swanson, and M.S. Chi. 1977. Metabolism of T-2 toxin in poultry. University of Minnesota Annual Report to NC 129 (USDA).

343. Roffe, T.J., R.K. Stroud, and R.M. Windingstad. 1989. Suspected fusariomycotoxicosis in sandhill cranes (Grus canadensis): Clinical and pathological findings. Avian Dis 33:451–457.

344. Rotter, R.G., R.R. Marquardt, and J.C. Young. 1985. Effect of ergot from different sources and of fractionated ergot on the performance of growing chicks. Can J Anim Sci 65:953–961.

345. Rotter, R.G., R.R. Marquardt, and G.H. Crow. 1985. A comparison of the effect of increasing dietary concentrations of wheat ergot on the performance of leghorn and

broiler chicks. Can J Anim Sci 65:963–974.

346. Rotter, R.G., R.R. Marquardt, and J.C. Young. 1985. The ability of growing chicks to recover from short-term exposure to dietary wheat ergot and the effect of chemical and physical treatment on ergot toxicity. Can J Anim Sci 65:975–983.

347. Ruff, M.D,. W.E. Huff, and G.C. Wilkins. 1990. Characterization of the toxicity of the mycotoxins aflatoxin, ochratoxin and T-2 toxin in game birds. I. Chukar partridge. Avian Dis 34:717–720.

348. Ruff, M.D,. W.E. Huff, and M.B. Chute. 1992. Characterization of the toxicity of the mycotoxins aflatoxin, ochratoxin and T-2 toxin in game birds. II. Ringneck pheasant. Avian Dis 36:30–33.

349. Ruff, M.D,. W.E. Huff, and G.C. Wilkins. 1992. Characterization of the toxicity of the mycotoxins aflatoxin, ochratoxin and T-2 toxin in game birds. III. Avian Dis 36:34–39.

350. Sandhu, B.S., H. Singh, and B. Singh. 1995. Pathological studies in broiler chicks fed aflatoxin or ochratoxin and inoculated with inclusiion body hepatitis virus singly and in concurrence. Vet Res Commun 19:27–37.

351. Sawhney, D.S., D.V. Vadehra, and R.C. Baker. 1973. Aflatoxicosis in the laying Japanese quail. Poult Sci 52:465–473.

352. Sawhney, D.S., D.V. Vadehra, and R.C. Baker. 1973. The metabolism of [14C] aflatoxins in laying hens. Poult Sci 52:1302–1309.

353. Schaeffer, J.L., J.K. Tyczkowski, and P.B. Hamilton. 1987. Alterations in carotenoid metabolism during ochratoxicosis in young broiler chickens. Poult Sci 66:318–324.

354. Schaeffer, J.L., J.K. Tyczkowski, J.E. Riviere, and P.B. Hamilton. 1988. Aflatoxin-impaired ability to accumulate oxycarotenoid pigments during restoration in young chickens. Poult Sci 67:619–625.

355. Schaeffer, J.L., J.K. Tyczkowski, and P.B. Hamilton. 1988. Depletion of oxycarotenoid pigments in chickens and the failure of aflatoxin to alter it. Poult Sci 67:1080–1088.

356. Schroeder, H.W., and W.H. Kelton. 1975. Production of sterigmatocystin by some species of the genus Aspergillus and its toxicity to chicken embryos. Appl Microbiol 30:589–591.

357. Schumaier, G., H.M. DeVolt, N.C. Laffer, R.D. Creek. 1963. Stachybotryotoxicosis of chicks. Poult Sci 42:70–74.

358. Sharby, T.F., G.E. Templeton, J.N. Beasley, and E.L. Stephenson. 1972. Toxicity resulting from feeding experimentally molded corn to broiler chicks. Poult Sci 52:1007–1014.

359. Sharlin, J.S., B. Howarth, Jr., and R.D. Wyatt. 1980. Effect of dietary aflatoxin on reproductive performance of mature white leghorn males. Poult Sci 59:1311–1315.

360. Sharlin, J.S., B. Howarth, Jr., F.N. Thompson, and R.D. Wyatt. 1981. Decreased reproductive potential and reduced feed consumption in mature white leghorn males fed aflatoxin. Poult Sci 60:2701–2708.

361. Sheridan, J.J. 1980. Some observations on selected mycoses and mycotoxicoses affecting animals in Ireland. Irish Vet J 34:148–154.

362. Shlosberg, A.S., Y. Weisman, V. Handji, B. Yagen, and L. Shore. 1984. A severe reduction in egg laying in a flock of hens associated with trichothecene mycotoxins in the feed. Vet Human Toxicol 26:384–386.

363. Shlosberg, A.S., Y. Klinger, and M. H. Malkinson. 1986. Muscovy ducklings, a particularly sensitive avian bioassay for T-2 toxin and diacetoxyscirpenol. Avian Dis 30:820–824.

364. Shotwell, O.L. 1991. Natural occurrence of mycotoxins in corn. In J.E. Smith and R. Henderson (eds.). Mycotoxins and Animal Foods. CRC Press, Boca Raton, FL, pp. 325–340.

365. Shotwell, O.L., C.W. Hesseltine, and M.L. Goulden. 1969. Ochratoxin A: Occurrence as natural contaminant of a corn sample. Appl Microbiol 17:765–766.

366. Shoyinka, S.V.O., and E.O. Onyekweodiri. 1987. Clinico-pathology of interaction between aflatoxin and aspergillosis in chickens. Bull Anim Health Prod Afr 35:47–51.

367. Siller, W.G., and D.C. Ostler. 1961. The histopathology of an entero-hepatic syndrome of turkey poults. Vet Rec 73:134–138.

368. Slowik, J., S. Graczyk, and J.A. Madej. 1985. The effect of a single dose of aflatoxin B1 on the value of nucleolar index of blood lymphocytes and on the histological changes in the liver, bursa of Fabricius, suprarenal glands and spleen in ducklings. Folia Histochem Cytobiol 13:71–80.

369. Smith, E.E., L.F. Kubena, C.E. Braithwaite, R.B. Harvey, T.D. Phillips, and A.H. Reine. 1992. Toxicological evaluation of aflatoxin and cyclopiazonic acid in broiler chickens. Poult Sci 71:1136–1144.

370. Smith, J.W., and P.B. Hamilton. 1970. Aflatoxicosis in the broiler chicken. Poult Sci 49:207–215.

371. Smith, J.W., W.R. Prince, and P.B. Hamilton. 1969. Relationship of aflatoxicosis to Salmonella gallinarum infections of chickens. Appl Microbiol 18:946–947.

372. Smith, J.W., C.H. Hill, and P.B. Hamilton. 1971. The effect of dietary modifications on aflatoxicosis in the broiler chicken. Poult Sci 50:768–774.

373. Sobers, E.K., and B. Doupnik, Jr. 1972. Relationship of pathogenicity to tobacco leaves and toxicity to chicks of isolates of Alternaria longipes. Appl Microbiol 23:313–315.

374. Somvanshi, R., and G.C. Mohanty. 1991. Pathological studies on aflatoxicosis, infectious bursal disease and their interactions in chickens. Indian J Vet Pathol 15:10–16.

375. Soni, K.B., A. Rajan, and R. Kuttan. 1992. Reversal of aflatoxin induced liver damage by tumeric and curcumin. Cancer Lett 66:115–121.

376. Sova, Z., L. Fukal, D. Trefny, J. Prosek, and A. Slamova. 1986. B1 aflatoxin (AFB1) transfer from reproductive organs of farm birds into their eggs and hatched young. Conf Europeenne d'Aviculture 7:602–603.

377. Speers, G.M., R.A. Meronuck, D.M. Barnes, and C.J. Mirocha. 1971. Effect of feeding Fusarium roseum f. sp. graminearum contaminated corn and the mycotoxin F-2 on the growing chick and laying hen. Poult Sci 50:627–633.

378. Speers, G.M., C.J. Mirocha, C.M. Christensen, and J.C. Behrens. 1977. Effects of laying hens of feeding corn invaded by two species of Fusarium and pure T-2 mycotoxin. Poult Sci 56:98–102.

379. Sreemannarayana, O., R.R. Marquardt, A.A. Frohlich, and F.A. Juck. 1986. Some acute biochemical and pathological changes in chicks after oral administration of sterigmatocystin. J Am Coll Toxicol 5:275–287.

380. Sreemannarayana, O., A.A. Frohlich, and R.R. Marquardt. 1988. Effects of repeated intra-abdominal injections of sterigmatocystin on relative organ weights, concentration of serum and liver constituents, and histopathology of certain organs of the chick. Poult Sci 67:502–509.

381. Stewart, R.G., J.K. Skeeles, R.D. Wyatt, J. Brown, R.K. Page, I.D. Russell, and P.D. Lukert. 1985. The effect of aflatoxin on complement activity in broiler chickens. Poult Sci 64:616–619.

382. Sukspath, S., R.C. Mulley, and W.L. Bryan. 1990. Toxicity of cyclopiazonic acid in mature male chickens. Proc Aust Poult Sci Symp, p. 120.

383. Svendsen, C., and E. Skadhauge. 1976. Renal functions in hens fed graded dietary levels of ochratoxin A. Acta Pharmacol Toxicol 38:186–194.

384. Swarbrick, O., and J.T. Swarbrick. 1968. Suspected ergotism in ducks. Vet Rec 82:76–77.

385. Tabib, Z., F.T. Jones, and P.B. Hamilton. 1981. Microbiological quality of poultry feed and ingredients. Poult Sci 60:1392–1397.

386. Tabib, T., F.T. Jones, and P.B. Hamilton. 1984. Effect of pelleting of poultry feed on the activity of molds and mold inhibitors. Poult Sci 63:70–75.

387. Terao, K., K. Kera, and T. Yazina. 1978. The effects of trichothecene toxins on the bursa of Fabricius in day-old chicks. Virchows Arch B Cell Pathol 27:359–70.

388. Theron, J.J., K.J. van der Merwe, N. Liebenberg, H.J.B. Joubert, and W. Nel. 1966. Acute liver injury in ducklings and rats as a result of ochratoxin poisoning. J Pathol Bacteriol 91:521–29.

389. Tohala, S.H. 1983. A study of ochratoxin toxicity in laying hens. Diss Abstr B Sci Eng 44:655.

390. Toleman, W.J. 1981. Overcoming problems with bulk feed bins. Poult Dig 40:406–408.

391. Trucksess, M.W., L. Stoloff, K. Young, R.D. Wyatt, and B.L. Miller. 1983. Aflatoxicol and aflatoxins B1 and M1 in eggs and tissues of laying hens consuming aflatoxin-contaminated feed. Poult Sci 62:2176–2182.

392. Tung, H.T., J.W. Smith, and P.B. Hamilton. 1971. Aflatoxicosis and bruising in the chicken. Poult Sci 50:795–800.

393. Tung, H.T., F.W. Cook, R.K. Wyatt, and P.B. Hamilton. 1975. The anemia caused by aflatoxin. Poult Sci 54:1962–1969.

394. Tung, H.T., R.D. Wyatt, P. Thaxton, and P.B. Hamilton. 1975. Concentrations of serum proteins during aflatoxicosis. Toxicol Appl Pharmacol 34:320–326.

395. Tyczkowski, J.K., and P.B. Hamilton. 1987. Altered metabolism of carotenoids during aflatoxicosis in young chickens. Poult Sci 66:1184–1188.

396. Ubosi, C.O., P.B. Hamilton, E.A. Dunnington, and P.B. Siegel. 1985. Aflatoxin effects in white leghorn chickens selected for response to sheep erythrocyte antigen. I. Body weight, feed conversion, and temperature responses. Poult Sci 64:1065–1070.

397. Ubosi, C.O., W.B. Gross, P.B. Hamilton, M. Ehrich, and P.B. Siegel. 1985. Aflatoxin effects in white leghorn chickens selected for response to sheep erythrocyte antigen. II. Serological and organ characteristics. Poult Sci 64:1071–1076.

398. Ueno, Y. 1977. Mode of action of trichothecenes. Pure Appl Chem 49:1737–1745.

399. Ueno, Y., K. Ishii, M. Sawano, K. Ohtsubo, Y. Matsuda, T. Tanaka, H. Kurata, and M. Ichinoe. 1977. Toxicological approaches to the metabolites of Fusaria. XI. Trichothecenes and zearalenone from river sediments. Jpn J Exp Med 47:177–184.

400. Umesh, D., V.N. Rao, and H.C. Joshi. 1993. Effect of acute aflatoxin B1 feeding on serum mineral profile in chickens. Indian J Vet Med 13:(2)64–65.

401. Uraguchi, K., and M. Yamazaki. 1978. Toxicology, Biochemistry and Pathology of Mycotoxins. Halsted Press, John Wiley and Sons, New York, pp. 1–106.

402. Vesonder, R.F., A. Ciegler, A.H. Jensen, W.K. Rohwedder, and D. Weisleder. 1976. Co-identity of the refusal and emetic principle from Fusarium-infected corn. Appl Environ Microbiol 31:280–285.

403. Visconti, A., and A. Bottalico. 1983. High levels of ochratoxins A and B in moldy bread responsible for mycotoxicosis in farm animals. J Agric Food Chem 31:1122–1123.

404. Voss, K.A., J.W. Dorner, and R.J. Cole. 1993. Amelioration of aflatoxicosis in rats by Volclay NF-BC, microfine bentonite. J Food Protect 56:595–598.

405. Walser, M.M., N.K. Allen, C.J. Mirocha, G.F. Hanlon, and J.A. Newman. 1982. Fusarium-induced osteochondrosis (tibial dyschondroplasia) in chickens. Vet Pathol 19:544–550.

406. Wannop, C.C. 1961. The histopathology of turkey "x" disease in Great Britain. Avian Dis 5:371–381.

407. Warren, M.F., and P.B. Hamilton. 1980. Intestinal fragility during ochratoxicosis and aflatoxicosis in broiler chickens. Appl Environ Microbiol 40:641–645.

408. Warren, M.F., and P.B. Hamilton. 1981. Glycogen storage disease type X caused by ochratoxin A in broiler chickens. Poult Sci 60:120–123.

409. Weibking, T., D.R. Ledoux, A.J. Bermudez, J.R. Turk, and G.E. Rottinghaus. 1993. Effects of feeding Fusarium moniliforme culture material containing known levels of fumonisin B1 on the young broiler chick. Poult Sci 72:456–466.

410. Weibking, T., D.R. Ledoux, T.P. Brown, and G.E. Rottinghaus. 1993. Fumonisin toxicity in turkey poults. J Vet Diagn Invest 5:75–83.

411. Weibking, T., D.R. Ledoux, A.J. Bermudez, J.R. Turk, and G.E. Rottinghaus. 1995. Effects on turkey poults of feeding Fusarium moniliforme M-1325 culture material grown under different environmental conditions. Avian Dis 39:32–38.

412. Williams, C.M., W.M. Colwell, and L.P. Rose. 1980. Genetic resistance of chickens to aflatoxin assessed with organ-culture techniques. Avian Dis 24:415–422.

413. Wilson, B.J., and R.D. Harbison. 1973. Rubratoxins. J Am Vet Med Assoc 163:1274–1275.

414. Wilson, H.R., C.R. Douglas, R.H. Harms, and G.T. Edds. 1975. Reduction of aflatoxin effects on quail. Poult Sci 54:923–925.

415. Witlock, D.R., and R.D. Wyatt. 1981. Effect of dietary aflatoxin on hemostasis of young turkey poults. Poult Sci 60:528–531.

416. Witlock, D.R., R.D. Wyatt, and W.I. Anderson. 1982. Relationship between Eimeria adenoeides infection and aflatoxicosis in turkey poults. Poult Sci 61:1293–1297.

417. Wright, G.C., Jr., W.F.O. Marasas, and L. Sokoloff. 1987. Effect of fusarochromanone and T-2 toxin on articular chondrocytes in monolayer culture. Fundam Appl Toxicol 9:595–597.

418. Wu, Q.C., M.E. Cook, and E.B. Smalley. 1993. Tibial dyschondroplasia of chickens induced by fusarochromanone, a mycotoxin. Avian Dis 302–309.

419. Wu, Q.C., M.E. Cook, and E.B. Smalley. 1995. Induction of tibial dyschondroplasia and suppression of cell-mediated immunity in chicken by Fusarium oxysporum grown on sterile corn. Avian Dis 39:100–107.

420. Wyatt, R.D. 1986. Mycotoxicosis of poultry—successful prevention and control. Proceedings, Coban Technical Seminar. Elanco, Indianapolis, IN, pp. 1–10.

421. Wyatt, R.D. 1991. Poultry. In J.E. Smith and R. Henderson (eds.). Mycotoxins and Animal Foods. CRC Press, Boca Raton, FL, pp. 553–605.

422. Wyatt, R.D., and P.B. Hamilton. 1972. The effect of rubratoxin in broiler chickens. Poult Sci 51:1383–1387.

423. Wyatt, R.D., and P.B. Hamilton. 1975. Interaction between aflatoxicosis and a natural infection of chickens with Salmonella. Appl Microbiol 30:870–872.

424. Wyatt, R.D., J.R. Harris, P.B. Hamilton, and H.R. Burmeister. 1972. Possible outbreaks of fusariotoxicosis in avians. Avian Dis 16:1123–1130.

425. Wyatt, R.D., B.A. Weeks, P.B. Hamilton, and H.R. Burmeister. 1972. Severe oral lesions in chickens caused by ingestion of dietary fusariotoxin T-2. Appl Microbiol 24:251–257.

426. Wyatt, R.D., P.B. Hamilton, and H.R. Burmeister. 1973. The effects of T-2 toxin in broiler chickens. Poult Sci 52:1853–1859.

427. Wyatt, R.D., W.M. Colwell, P.B. Hamilton, and H.R. Burmeister. 1973. Neural disturbances in chickens caused by dietary T-2 toxin. Appl Microbiol 26:757–761.

428. Wyatt, R.D., D.M. Briggs, and P.B. Hamilton. 1973. The effect of dietary aflatoxin on mature broiler breeder males. Poult Sci 52:1119–1123.

429. Wyatt, R.D., J.A. Doerr, P.B. Hamilton, and H.R. Burmeister. 1975. Egg production, shell thickness, and other physiological parameters of laying hens affected by T-2 toxin. Appl Microbiol 29:641–45.

430. Wyatt, R.D., H.L. Marks, and R.O. Manning. 1978. Recovery of laying hens from T-2 toxicosis [Abstr]. Poult Sci 57 (Suppl 1):1172.

431. Wyatt, R.D., R.O. Manning, R.A Pegram, and H.L. Marks. 1984. Characterization of oosporein toxicosis in mature laying hens [abstr]. Poult Sci 63 (Suppl 1):210.

432. Yoshizawa, T. 1991. Natural occurrence of mycotox-

ins in small grain cereals (wheat, barley, rye, oats, sorghum, millet, rice). In J.E. Smith and R. Henderson (eds.). Mycotoxins and Animal Foods. CRC Press, Boca Raton, FL, pp. 301–324.

433. Yoshizawa, T., S.P. Swanson, and C.J. Mirocha. 1980. T-2 metabolites in the excreta of broiler chickens administered H-labeled T-2 toxin. Appl Environ Microbiol 39:1172–1177.

434. Young, J.C., and R.R. Marquardt. 1982. Effects of er-

gotamine tartrate on growing chickens. Can J Anim Sci 62:1181–1191.

435. Zdenek, Z., Z. Fukal, J. Prosek, A. Slamova, and J. Vopalka. 1986. B1 aflatoxin (AFB1) transfer from reproductive organs of farm birds into their eggs and hatched young [Abstr]. Conf Europeene d'Aviculture 7:618.

436. Zhang, H., and J.L. Li. 1990. Study on toxicological mechanism of moniliformin [Abstr]. J Toxicol Toxin Rev 9:103.

OTHER TOXINS AND POISONS

Richard J. Julian and Thomas P. Brown

INTRODUCTION. Paracelsus recognized 400 yr ago that it is "the dose that makes the poison." Although that may be obvious with known toxic material, it is also true for products such as growth promotants and chemotherapeutic agents usually considered safe. Deliberate overdose may cause illness, and a misplaced decimal in water or feed medication frequently results in toxicity. Sulfaquinoxaline poisoning occurs in meat-type chickens even at recommended doses because of high water intake in warm buildings, particularly in hot weather, or because of poor feed mixing. Disease may also be caused by toxic levels of some nutrients; e.g., excess dietary sodium causes significant losses in chickens and turkeys around the world. High levels of vitamins A and D are toxic. There may be a species or age susceptibility as occurs with the ionophore anticoccidials. Waterfowl are sensitive to some drugs at a dose safe for chickens and turkeys. The immune system seems to be affected by many toxic agents. In addition to disease caused by poisons, the problem of residues in eggs and meat must also be considered. For information on withdrawal times and drug and chemical residues, see Booth (28). It must be remembered that material starts to be deposited in egg yolk 10 days before that egg is laid.

Poisonous substances are widely distributed in nature. Mycotoxins, covered in the previous subchapter, are important to the poultry industry, but toxic agents are also produced by bacteria (botulinum toxin, methylmercury, toxic amines) or occur naturally (selenium, phytotoxins). Pesticides, herbicides, and other synthetic chemicals, metals such as lead, and industrial contaminants add to the list of toxic materials. Many chemicals and human drugs have been given to birds in feed and water to study their toxic effects. These experimental toxicities have not been included except as they may relate to potential naturally occurring poisonings in poultry.

Poisons and toxins are not major causes of production loss or disease in poultry in most countries, although some, such as lead, pesticides, and botulism, are significant in wild birds. In 1985, Terzic

and Curcic (281) reported, however, that 40% of 2065 poisoning cases seen at the Belgrade Veterinary Facility over a 17-yr period were in poultry. Poisoning occurs more frequently in free-range and backyard flocks and in village poultry where birds forage in neighboring gardens and fields or receive household waste and weeds cut from roadsides and fields. Some of these poisonings are malicious. Contaminated litter on the floor and in nest boxes is an added source of toxins in chickens not raised on wire. Since suspected toxicity cases are more likely to be submitted to a diagnostic laboratory than are other sick birds, statistics collected from that source may not be an accurate indication of the incidence of poisoning compared with other disease.

Toxicants covered in this chapter are presented by primary use. Levels of toxic substances that may cause depressed growth in broilers and turkeys or decreased egg production in layers are summarized in Table 36.1.

ANTIMICROBIALS, ANTICOCCIDIALS, AND GROWTH PROMOTANTS. Most reports of poisoning with chemotherapeutic agents involve inappropriate use or overdose of anticoccidials or growth promotants. Toxicity of a variety of chemotherapeutic agents in poultry and pigeons has been reviewed (238, 239).

Sulfonamides. Sulfonamides were used as the primary form of prevention and treatment for coccidiosis in poultry between the early 1940s and late 1950s. Sulfaquinoxaline and sulfamethazine were most widely used. The toxic level of sulfonamides is close to the therapeutic level in poultry, and even the therapeutic level has a detrimental effect on hemopoietic and immune systems. Previous low-level or continuous-preventive medication has a protective effect against subsequent higher doses (88).

Sulfonamides are difficult to mix evenly in feed, which may cause some birds to receive a toxic dose even when a treatment level is used. This is less likely at preventive levels. Both feed and water medication require accurate estimates of feed and

Table 36.1.   Levels in feed (unless otherwise noted) of selected toxins documented to decrease growth rate in broilers and turkeys and reduce egg production in layers.

Toxin	Broilers	Turkeys	Layers
Antimicrobials and Growth Promotants			
Sulfadimethoxine (% in water)	NA[a]	NA	0.05
Sulfaquinoxaline (%)	NA	NA	0.10
Nicabazine (mg/kg)	NA	NA	70
Arsanilic acid (mg/kg)	1000	400	NA
Nitarsone (mg/kg)	300	600	NA
Roxarsone (mg/kg)	90	550	NA
Nutrients and Other Feed- and Water-Related Toxicants			
Aluminum (%)	0.30	0.30	0.15
Arsenic (inorganic pentoxide) (mg/kg)	40	40	40
Boron (mg/kg)	435	435	870
Boric Acid (mg/kg)	2500	2500	5000
Cadmium (mg/kg)	400	400	8-60
Copper (mg/kg)	500–1000	500–1000	1000
Fluoride (mg/kg)	1300	1300	1300
Iodine (mg/kg)	500	500	300
Iron (mg/kg)	200–2000	200–2000	NA
Lead (acetate) (mg/kg)	630	630	630
Mercury (mg/kg)	50	50	5
Molybdenum (mg/kg)	200	200	200
Potassium (%)	0.90	0.90	NA
Selenium (mg/kg)	5	5	80
Sodium (%)	0.80	0.80	0.80
Sodium chloride (%)	2.0	2.0	2.0
Tungsten (mg/kg)	1000	1000	1000
Vanadium (mg/kg)	6	6	20–30
Zinc (mg/kg)	NA	NA	20,000
Other			
Ammonia (ppm)	50	25	75

[a]NA = not available.
Source: (232, 233)

water consumption if each chicken is to receive the correct daily dose. Sulfa poisoning has occurred when no allowance was made for increased water and feed consumption of the modern broiler that eats to its physical capacity rather than to its metabolic need, or, more frequently, for the effect of increased water consumption at high environmental temperature or in hot broiler houses. For broilers, the author recommends one-half of the therapeutic dose, and at temperatures over 27 C (81 F), one-third of the therapeutic dose for water medication. Repeat treatment is hazardous and should not be recommended without a postmortem diagnosis to make sure there is no evidence of sulfa toxicity. Even the newer so-called safe sulfas need to be used with care (53, 239). Under no circumstances should sulfas be given in both feed and water at the same time.

Hemorrhagic syndrome, which occurred frequently when sulfas were in widespread use, is a manifestation of sulfa toxicity and occurs even at therapeutic doses. In addition to blood dyscrasia, bone marrow depression, and thrombocytopenia, sulfonamides depress the lymphoid system and immune function in birds. Focal bacterial granulomas are often found in tissues and organs of chickens dying from sulfa poisoning. Epithelial degeneration in liver, kidney, and other organs may be caused by the direct effect of the drug, but is more likely due to hypoxia secondary to anemia. When determining withdrawal times in layers, the fact that yolk is laid down over a period of 10 days must be considered (26).

Signs.   Chickens and turkeys with sulfa toxicity are depressed, pale, and frequently underweight. In adults, there is a marked decrease in egg production and shell quality; brown eggs may be depigmented (60, 217). Secondary bacterial infections including septicemia and gangrenous dermatitis may follow sulfonamide toxicity (53).

Pathology.   For descriptions of gross and microscopic pathology, see (53, 60, 88).

Hemorrhage in skin, muscles, and internal organs is the most consistent and extensive gross lesion of sulfonamide intoxication. Hemorrhage may be present in comb, eyelids, face, wattles, anterior chamber of the eye, and musculature of breast and thighs. Normal dark-red bone marrow in growing birds changes to pink in mild cases and yellow in severe cases. The entire length of the intestinal tract may be spotted with petechial and ecchymotic hemorrhages, and the cecal lumen may contain blood. Hemorrhage may be present in the proventriculus and beneath the gizzard lining. There may be ulcers at the proventricular–gizzard junction. The liver is swollen, pale red or icteric, and may be studded with petechiae or focal necrosis. The spleen is commonly enlarged, has hemorrhagic infarcts, and contains gray nodular areas. "Paintbrush" hemorrhages occur in the myocardium. Thymus and bursa of Fabricius are small.

Microscopically, areas of caseation necrosis surrounded by a mantle of giant cells occur in liver, spleen, lungs, and kidneys. Lymphocytic and heterophilic infiltration is present at the periphery of necrotic foci. Lymphoid hypoplasia around splenic adenoid sheaths, edema and fibroplasia of the capsule, and macrophages containing hemosiderin are common. Early changes in the liver are periportal mononuclear infiltration associated with bile duct hyperplasia. Hemosiderin deposits are present in necrotic areas, and thrombosis of portal vessels is present. An early change in kidneys is interstitial lymphocytic infiltration. Degeneration and necrosis of tubular epithelium are associated with albuminous casts. Glomeruli are hyperplastic and Bowman's capsule is dilated with albuminous casts. Lungs are congested with interlobular and interstitial edema. Interstitial tissues contain mononuclear foci. There is degeneration and necrosis of lymphocytes and depletion of bursal follicles.

In femoral bone marrow, there is decreased intrasinusoidal erythropoiesis with thrombocytopenia and agranulocytosis, focal increase in extrasinusoidal lymphopoiesis, and, in some instances, myelopoiesis. There are also focal areas of hyalinization, necrosis, and fibroplasia. Hemosiderin deposits and extrasinusoidal edema are present.

Nitrofurans. Nitrofuran use is no longer permitted in some countries. Prominent signs of nitrofurazone (NFZ) toxicity in chicks include depression, incoordination, ruffled feathers, and growth retardation (217). Poor growth may be partially related to feed aversion, since feed consumption drops as the level of NFZ increases. Ducklings on toxic levels of NFZ die suddenly without clinical signs. Nervous signs and hyperexcitability have been described in acute toxicity in chicks and poults. Loud vocalization, opisthotonos, aimless running and flying, and convulsions may be seen.

Furazolidone (FZ) toxicity mainly affects the heart in turkeys, ducks, and chickens (50, 188). Marked individual and age susceptibility to FZ occurs. Some poults, chicks, and ducklings grow well without cardiac damage when fed 400-700 mg FZ/kg feed, whereas others fail to grow, develop ascites, and signs associated with heart failure. Frequency and severity of clinical signs are dose related. Recovery occurred in affected ducklings (294). There also is clinical evidence that FZ may cause nervous signs in chicks and poults and infertility in male breeders (238).

FZ causes dose-related biventricular cardiomyopathy with prominent dilation of ventricles and thinning of either the right or left ventricular wall. Secondary heart failure results in passive congestion with lung edema, or marked congestion of liver and other organs, and ascites depending on whether heart failure is mainly left- or right-sided. Right-sided heart failure with marked cardiac enlargement is usually more common up to 3 wk of age (145).

In turkeys, FZ-induced cardiomyopathy cannot be distinguished from spontaneous turkey cardiomyopathy (STC). The cause of STC is not known, but clinically it is associated with rapid growth, low serum protein, and stressors such as low incubator oxygen, poor ventilation, and fumes from brooders, which might induce ischemic cardiomyopathy. Why high doses of FZ cause dilatory cardiomyopathy is not known (112).

Most microscopic lesions result from heart failure. Cardiac lesions include edema, thinning of myocardial muscle fibers, and multifocal myocytolysis with increased connective tissue. Epicardial fibrosis and endocardial fibroelastosis may also occur. Ultrastructural changes include myofibrillar lysis, clumps of Z-band material, and increased glycogen in myocardial fibers. Changes in heart muscle enzyme levels accompany tissue alterations.

Antibiotics. After subcutaneous injection, gentamicin (an aminogylcoside) causes depression in turkey poults, edema and hemorrhages at the injection site, and large, pale, and degenerated kidneys (21, 243). Aminoglycosides and various other antibiotics used for egg inoculation have caused embryo mortality. Streptomycin and dihydrostreptomycin sulfate injected intramuscularly for sinusitis in turkey poults causes respiratory distress, paresis, and mild convulsions (238, 239).

Ionophores. Ionophores (ion carriers) facilitate movement of some monovalent cations, such as sodium and potassium, and divalent cations such as calcium and magnesium across cell membranes. They can have both anticoccidial and antibacterial activity, and the group is extensively used in poultry and ruminant feeds. Ionophores are coccidiocidal because of their ability to preferentially move ions, usually Na+, into various stages of the parasite.

Toxic levels of ionophores cause potassium to leave and calcium to enter cells, particularly my-

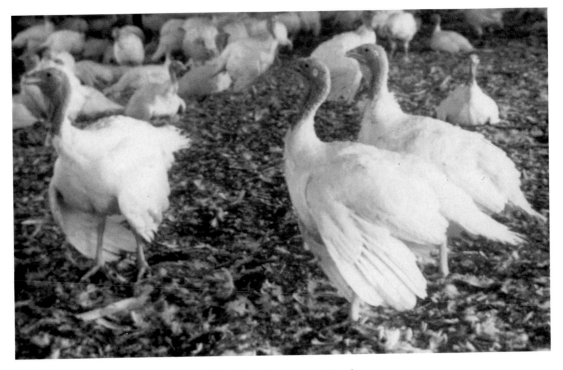

36.8.   Acute ionophore toxicity. Dyspnea and drooping wings are suggestive of
heat stress. (Barnes)

ocytes, resulting in cell death. Signs of toxicity are
related to high extracellular potassium and high intracellular (intramitochondrial) calcium. For more
specific information on metabolism and toxicity of
monensin see (28, 73, 209). Ionophore toxicity
varies with species and age; equidae are very susceptible, and adult poultry, particularly turkeys, are
more susceptible than broilers (115). There is a synergistic effect with antibiotics in the same family of
drugs (283) and increased toxicity with nonrelated
antibiotics, other drugs (30, 36, 72, 162, 220, 226,
238), and low-protein rations (239). Dehydration
because of diarrhea or periods of water and/or feed
deprivation can precipitate toxic events (40, 110).
Monensin, lasalocid, salinomycin, and narasin have
been associated with toxicity in poultry, guinea
fowl, quail, and other species (56, 110, 116, 180,
228, 253, 295).

Signs.   Signs vary from anorexia with depression,
weakness, and reluctance to move to complete
paralysis in which birds lie in sternal recumbency
with neck and legs extended. Less severely affected
birds may show posterior paralysis with legs extended. Dyspnea has occurred in affected adult
turkeys (Fig. 36.8). Signs are associated with muscle damage. Death may follow respiratory failure or
be secondary to dehydration. Mortality is variable

but may exceed 70% (93). In some cases of suspected ionophore toxicity in turkeys, morbidity may
be low with only a few poults paralyzed. The term
knockdown syndrome has been used for this condition (40). Poults with botulism may show similar
signs. Reduced egg production (295) and fertility
with weak chicks also have occurred (221).

Pathology.   Subchronic monensin toxicity (289)
resulted in opaque fibrin plaques on the epicardium,
hemorrhage in coronary fat, and decreased liver
weight. In acutely affected turkeys, pallor and atrophy of mainly type I fibers of legs and back have
been observed associated with monensin use (22,
224, 288). Clinical signs and gross lesions are often
absent in breeders ingesting high levels of monensin (93).
   Microscopic changes in heart and skeletal muscle
consist of scattered areas of hyalinization with muscle necrosis and myofiber degeneration and necrosis. Birds with respiratory signs often have lesions
in tracheal muscles. Type I fibers appear to be selectively affected (116). Heterophils, macrophages,
and occasionally lymphocytes may be present. Frequently, when exposed to low doses or interaction
with other drugs occurs, affected areas are very cellular with large numbers of satellite or sarcolemmal
nuclei, indicating regeneration is occurring (Fig.

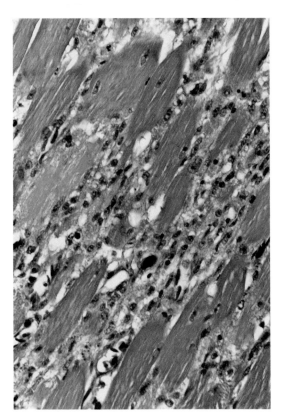

36.9. Muscle from a young turkey with turkey knockdown. Minimal muscle necrosis and inflammation along with increased sarcolemmal or satellite cell nuclei indicating regeneration are characteristic.

36.9). Ultrastructural changes have been described (283). Peripheral neuropathy characterized by edema, demyelination, and axonal degeneration accompanied by marked hypertrophy and hyperplasia of neurilemmal cells may be seen with lasalocid toxicity (110).

Differential Diagnosis. Since there is a marked individual, age, and species variation in susceptibility, and the toxic effect may be potentiated by other drugs, normal levels of ionophore should not be dismissed if clinical signs and histologic changes indicate ionophore toxicity. High serum or plasma levels of muscle enzymes may be useful in differentiating ionophore toxicity from botulism (198). Ionophore toxicity also must be distinguished from vitamin E/selenium deficiency and *Cassia* ingestion, which may produce similar signs and lesions.

Other Anticoccidials. 3,5-dinitro-*o*-toluamide (dinitrotolumide, dinitolmide, DNOT, Zoalene, Zoamix) can cause ataxia, torticollis, incoor-

dination, and reduced growth (143, 217, 238). Nicarbazin (Nicarb) can make broiler chicks listless, dull, and ataxic; in older birds there can be reduced egg production, shell depigmentation, yolk mottling, and reduced hatchability (16, 142, 168). Nicarbazin depresses growth rate at 150 mg/kg feed. Even when used at recommended levels, nicarbazin increases metabolic rate and heat production (18, 238, 301). This makes older broilers more susceptible to heat stress and pulmonary hypertension syndrome. Generally, there are no gross lesions, but there may be hepatic and renal epithelial degeneration (217, 239). Nitrophenide (Megasul) has caused nervous signs but with rapid recovery(217). Ducks and geese may have depressed growth from halofuginone (Stenorol) (19) and reduced skin strength has been found in chickens (109, 184). Use of *t*-butylaminoethanol may result in reduced growth due to choline deficiency.

Antiprotozoals. Organic arsenicals such as dimetridazole (Nitrazol, Emtryl), used for histomoniasis, have caused growth depression, drops in egg production, nervous signs (ataxia, incoordination, tremors), convulsions, and death in geese, ducks, pigeons, and turkeys (238, 239, 242). Waterfowl may be poisoned by doses safe for other poultry. Quinacrine HCl (Atabrine), used for *Haemoproteus* infections in pigeons, was fatal at a dose of approximately 50 mg/kg.

Organic Arsenical Feed Additives. Phenylarsonic acids such as arsanilic acid (*p*-amino-benzene arsanilate) and sodium arsanate, roxarsone (3-nitro-4-hydroxyphenylarsonic acid), and nitarsone (4-nitrophenylarsonic acid, Histostat-50) are used to improve feed efficiency in livestock. *p*-Ureidobenzenearsonic acid (Carb-o-sep, Carbarsone) and dimetridazole (1,2-dimethyl-5-nitroimidazole (Nitrazol, Emtryl) are used for prevention and control of histomoniasis. Toxicity occurs with accidental or deliberate overdose or in dehydrated animals or birds (209). Peripheral neuropathy causing lameness in turkeys developed after they were given twice the recommended level of 3-nitro-4-hydroxyphenylarsonic acid (308). Toxicity, with liver lesions suggestive of inorganic trivalent arsenite, occurred in broilers receiving 10 times the recommended dose of this same growth promotant. Lesions may have resulted from degradation and reduction of the organic product to the trivalent state or, more likely, from biliary excretion of inorganic arsenic present as a contaminant (257). Cysteine exacerbates toxicity, perhaps by reducing the arsenical to the more toxic trivalent state.

Signs. Ataxia and incoordination are usually seen, but stunting and depression also may be prominent signs. Lameness may be evident in turkey poults.

Pathology. Gross changes may be absent, although affected birds are usually small with an empty digestive tract. Microscopically, peripheral nerves may show loss of myelin, fragmentation of axons, and proliferation of neurilemmal cells (239, 243). Ulcerative cholecystitis occurred in turkey poults (35).

ANTHELMINTICS. All anthelmintics are probably toxic if a sufficient overdose is given, but generally birds are more resistant than mammals to anthelmintics.

Benzimidazoles. Cambendazole, mebendazole, and fenbendazole are well tolerated by birds (245).

Imidazothiazoles. Levamisole and tetramisole are not quite as safe as benzimidazoles. The lethal dose-50% (LD_{50}) of tetramisole for chickens is 2.75 g/kg. Geese and captive birds are more susceptible (245); 300 mg/kg is toxic for geese and as little as 66 mg/kg of levamisole is toxic for some wild birds. Anthelmintic activity of *dl*-tetramisole resides in the *l*-isomer (levamisole), so the effective dose of levamisole is half that of tetramisole. This doubles the safety margin. Tetramisole is no longer available in most countries. Levamisole poisoning has occurred in geese being treated for *Amidostomum* infection (313). Levamisole was toxic for ducks parenterally at 40 and 80 mg/kg (114).

Organophosphates. Organophosphorus compounds have caused poisoning in birds eating treated feed intended for horses (135, 177). The resin pellet form of dichlorvos (DDVP) is toxic because it is retained in the gizzard. Colored breeds of chickens are more susceptible than white breeds to coumaphos, and naphthaphos has a narrow safety range for chickens, with 50 mg/kg being fatal (245).

Ivermectin. Ivermectin has a wide safety margin in birds. An oral or injectable dose of 0.1 mg/kg has been suggested (245). Ivermectin is effective against a wide range of parasites. Zeman (314) tried 1.8 mg/kg for *Dermanyssus gallinae*. This dose was more effective in chickens weighing over 450 g. The toxic dose for chickens is 5.4 mg/kg, which causes 4-hr somnolence; 16.2 mg/kg, which causes 24-hr listlessness and ataxia; 48.6 mg/kg resulted in death 5 hr postinjection. Canaries given 20-60 µg/bird IM showed temporary immobility.

Other Anthelmintics. Phenothiazine is relatively nontoxic for birds, and hygromycin B is safe at 8 g/900 kg feed (245).

NUTRIENTS AND OTHER FEED- AND WATER-RELATED TOXICANTS

Amino Acids. Interaction among some amino acids relate to growth, but only methionine is toxic to poultry. Methionine toxicity affects chickens and quail (151, 256) and has caused depressed growth and cervical paralysis in turkey poults (113). Mortality can occur at levels of 1.8% in feed. Methionine attenuates calcium-induced kidney damage (300). Ethinone (a methionine antagonist) toxicity in chicks can be relieved by methionine.

ANTINUTRIENTS. A variety of feed stuffs and potential feed stuffs are poorly digestible, contain factors that inhibit digestion (protein inhibitors), depress growth, cause pasting, or increase skeletal disorders. Antinutritional factors in some of these products (e.g., soybean and some other beans) can be destroyed by heat. The nutritional value of some feedstuffs (e.g., wheat, barley, rye) can be improved by enzymes (31, 103, 133, 141). Antinutrients that can be found in plants include proteases, tannins, saponins, antivitamins, lectins, ß-glucans, pentosans, polysaccharides, concanavalin A, hemagglutinins, vicine, convicine, alkaloids, and sinapines. Feedstuffs known to contain antinutrient factors are alfalfa (144, 282), amaranth (4), jackbeans (69, 171, 205), fababeans (208, 249), lima beans (206), narbon beans (79), soybeans (144, 173), jojoba (12), lupins (32, 222, 247), peas (33), vetch (248), barley, rye, wheat (17, 31, 185), and sorghum (279).

Protein Supplements

FISH AND MEAT MEALS. Gizzerosine, histamine, histidine, and other biogenic amines cause digestive disturbances, stunting, and osteoporosis (132, 276). Biogenic amines result from heating or bacterial spoilage of fish and animal byproducts. Toxic products get into poultry feed through fish or meat meal. Excess acid secretion in the proventriculus is stimulated by gizzerosine, causing gizzard erosion and hemorrhage (131, 191, 254). Broiler chickens may die from hypovolemic shock. Black ingesta and blood may run from the mouth (vomito negro) and contents of the digestive tract are often melanic. Other biogenic amines reduce broiler feed efficiency (154).

Minerals. For information on trace mineral deficiency and toxicity (tissue levels, signs, etc.), see (232, 233). Information on poultry in these references is included for the following minerals: aluminum, arsenic, cadmium, calcium, chloride, chromium, cobalt, copper, fluoride, iodine, iron, lead, magnesium, manganese, mercury, molybdenum, nickel, phosphorus, potassium, selenium, sodium, tungsten, vanadium, and zinc.

ALUMINUM. Aluminum depressed growth rate in chicks, due to decreased feed intake, and egg production in adults when 0.3% was added to the feed (27, 310). Aluminum also may interfere with phosphorus retention (77, 84, 137).

CALCIUM. Excess absorbed calcium is excreted through kidneys; high levels cause ureter and kidney impaction, resulting in nephrosis. Very young birds are most susceptible. High mortality from hyperuricemia with visceral urate deposits may result from kidney damage because of high dietary calcium. Lung pathology with damage to parenchyma from calcium deposits may also occur in young chicks. It is possible that nephrosis and visceral urate deposits in young and dead-in-shell chicks may result from kidney obstruction by calcium. Excess unabsorbed calcium remaining in the intestine increases fecal water content of pullets and hens on high calcium rations. If the source of calcium is dicalcium phosphate, the alkaline solution formed in the upper digestive tract may result in epithelial necrosis (214, 217, 292), particularly if the mineral has been "top-dressed" on feed and birds eat undiluted material.

Urolithiasis in pullet and layer flocks may be caused by high calcium and low phosphorus in pullet rations. The incidence may also be affected by infectious bronchitis virus infection (107).

COBALT. Moderate levels (125 ppm) stimulate polycythemia and induce pulmonary hypertension. Higher levels (500 ppm) cause marked tibial dyschondroplasia and necrosis and fibrosis in pancreas, liver, and skeletal, smooth, and cardiac muscle. All levels reduce feed intake and growth (65).

COPPER. Copper sulfate is added to water for treatment of enteritis or yeast infection, or to clean algae or scum from water lines and drinkers. Addition to feed is another method for treating enteritis and candidiasis. It also may be sprayed on litter to control aspergillus or used as an antifungal preparation on wood. Birds are occasionally poisoned by eating copper sulfate crystals. Diets low in calcium may increase susceptibility to copper toxicity (166). Mortality in turkeys offered water containing copper sulfate may have resulted from dehydration caused by water refusal, rather than from copper poisoning. Toxicity signs are depression and weakness with convulsions and coma terminally (217) or anemia (123, 209, 243). Gross lesions include necrosis of proventriculus and gizzard epithelium with sloughing of koilin lining (127).

FLUORINE. Growth, production, and egg quality were reduced by 700 and 1000 mg sodium fluo-ride/kg feed (111). Leg deformity has also been described.

IODINE. Reduced egg production and weight and increased embryonic mortality in the first wk and at pipping occurred when 350 ppm of iodine was added to the ration of turkey breeder hens (45).

MAGNESIUM. Excess magnesium causes bone abnormalities by replacing calcium and affecting phosphorus utilization (167).

PHOSPHORUS. Excess phosphorus affects growth plate development of bones and increases tibial dyschondroplasia and leg deformities. Phosphate may also be caustic to moist oral and epithelial surfaces.

POTASSIUM. Potassium in the form of fertilizer or potassium permanganate is toxic. The latter causes epithelial necrosis of the digestive tract (217).

SODIUM (SODIUM CHLORIDE, SODIUM BICARBONATE). Excess ionic sodium, usually from sodium chloride in feed or water, causes significant economic losses in poultry in many countries. Most toxicity results from consuming saline water; not water deprivation. Sodium in feed can be toxic for young chicks and poults with or without water deprivation. In some cases of toxicity at apparently low salt levels, analysis may have been for chloride, with salt level calculated from chloride level. When Na^+ toxicity is suspected, both feed and water should be analyzed for Na^+; not estimated from chloride content. There may be sources of Na^+ in feed or water other than sodium chloride. Levels of Na^+ in feed and water are additive.

Young birds are much more sensitive to Na^+ toxicity than are adults, probably because their kidneys are not yet fully developed (186). Water with Na^+ greater than 0.4% (4000 ppm) is quite toxic and will cause high mortality within a few days. Lower levels may be toxic as well, depending on the amount of Na^+ in feed. Levels of Na^+ greater than 0.12% (1200 ppm) are toxic for some chicks and poults and produce heart failure with edema and ascites. Feed with Na^+ greater than 0.85% is toxic for some chicks and poults. Much lower levels will cause heart failure and ascites even when water is available freely. Since steroids increase Na^+ and water retention (255), resulting in hypervolemia, hypertension, right ventricular failure, and ascites, stress may also contribute to Na^+ susceptibility. Birds have poor renal concentrating ability and difficulty reducing plasma osmolality by excretion of salt in excess of water. Some waterfowl have nasal salt glands, which allows them to excrete Na^+ if an excess is ingested.

Two forms of disease result from Na^+ toxicity in

young birds. At high levels, birds develop acute, severe diarrhea and dehydration, lose weight, and die. There is often acute kidney damage, particularly with sodium bicarbonate (187), which may be ischemic because of increased red blood cell rigidity. Potassium may have a protective effect (267). At lower levels, loose droppings also occur, but birds gain weight, at least for 1-2 days, because of associated water retention. Depending on Na+ level, they may subsequently eat less and grow poorly, or continue to eat and grow well. Water retention, with hypervolemia and reduced red blood cell deformability (189), can lead to functional cardiac overload, causing marked right ventricular hypertrophy and dilation, valvular insufficiency, edema, and ascites in chicks (146, 147, 190). At intermediate levels of excess sodium, a variety of clinical signs and pathologic changes are seen, depending partly on how long birds survive with hypertension before heart failure occurs and how long they survive afterward. Many lesions described for Na+ can be attributed to heart failure.

Signs. At low levels of excess Na+, only watery droppings are seen until ascites occurs. At this stage, chicks and poults are dyspneic, depressed, and have a swollen abdomen. At high Na+ levels, birds are obviously sick and depressed within a few hours, with thirst and diarrhea. They may have rough, dirty, wet feathers or down. Nervous signs may be present and some birds may be prostrate. At intermediate levels, stunting of some birds may be prominent. Excess Na+ may cause reduced egg production and increased mortality in adults (57).

Pathology. Chicks with ascites and edema frequently have excess fluid in lungs and hydropericardium. Young males may have cystic dilation of seminiferous tubules (243). There is cardiac hypertrophy, which in chickens is mainly right-sided. Poults have biventricular hypertrophy with dilatory cardiomyopathy. At levels of Na+ causing dehydration, the following also may be seen: cyanosis, myocardial hemorrhage, nephrosis, and enteritis.

Microscopic lesions are frequently secondary to heart failure or dehydration. For a detailed description of histologic lesions, see (192). Glomerulosclerosis (255, 267) may be ischemic in origin. Ultrastructural changes in heart muscle (207) include glycogen accumulation, myofibrillar disarray, Z-band streaming, and disruption of intercalated discs.

SULFATE. The toxic concentration of sulfate is affected by age of the birds, source (water or feed), other salts, etc., and is not clearly defined. Magnesium sulfate may be more toxic than sodium sulfate (285). Diarrhea, reduced growth, and depressed egg production can occur.

SELENIUM. Some plants accumulate selenium (306). Decreased growth and feed intake resulted when there was 4-8 ppm selenium in drinking water (39). Selenium can accumulate in the food chain of aquatic birds causing emaciation, hepatitis, and ascites. Embryo deformity may also occur (203).

ZINC. Toxic levels of zinc (>500 ppm) cause anorexia, depressed growth, reduced egg production, and gizzard and pancreatic lesions (58, 62, 152, 178, 302). Individual birds may be poisoned by ingesting metallic zinc, such as coins or other objects, or galvanized wire from caging in the case of pet birds (240).

Metals and Metalloids

ARSENIC. Inorganic, aliphatic, and trivalent organic arsenicals are used as pesticides, weed and brush killers, and defoliants. Toxic effects include diarrhea, nervous signs, and cyanosis. There is inflammation of the digestive tract including crop, proventriculus, and gizzard, hepatosis, and nephrosis (209, 257). Most reports of arsenic toxicity in birds are experimental, except those associated with grasshopper bait (217). For information on organic arsenicals, see the section on antimicrobials and growth promotants.

CADMIUM. Toxic levels of cadmium found in industrial waste and sewage sludge cause decreased feed intake, decreased growth, and kidney lesions (134, 230, 232, 233, 299). Experimental cadmium toxicity in chicks, poults, and ducklings, and free radical–induced lesions by cadmium, silver, and other minerals have been reported (52, 284).

CHROMIUM AND POTASSIUM DICHROMATE. Chromium from industrial waste or coated metal objects may cause depression, anorexia, and paralysis (134, 232, 233).

LEAD. All species of birds are susceptible to lead poisoning. Lead is the only metallic poison causing significant disease in birds, and most toxicity occurs in wild species, especially waterfowl. Chickens are more resistant than waterfowl (232, 233). Birds as a group are at risk from metallic lead because the material is retained in the gizzard, ground down, and absorbed slowly. Experimental poisoning trials with chickens show an interaction with some nutrients (80, 164) and inhibition of avian bone healing (174).

Lead is widespread in the environment, and there are many possible sources for ingested lead when toxicity occurs. Wild water birds are at greatest risk from ingesting lead shot, which is the main hazard in North America (252) and elsewhere (122). Lead weights from fishing lines are the most important source in England. Pigeons may also ingest lead shot (61). Birds that eat carrion may be poisoned by lead shot ingested with tissues. Backyard and free-range poultry may pick up lead from paint chips, lead batteries, or other lead objects. Chicks have been poisoned by eating contaminated grit (217). Cage birds may be poisoned from the same environmental sources as children and dogs—mainly paint chips, leaded windows, toys, and lead objects (312).

Signs. Most lead poisoning in birds is chronic. Clinical disease is usually seen as wasting, ataxia, lameness or paralysis, and anemia. In acute cases, anorexia, weakness, prostration, and anemia may be prominent. Green diarrhea may result from anorexia, or it may be a direct effect of lead on digestive and nervous systems.

Hematology. Basophilic stippling and abnormal erythrocytes may occur in lead poisoned birds but are not present in all affected birds (Fig. 36.10) (217). Finding anemia with mitosis of erythrocytes and large numbers of immature cells may be more significant.

Pathology. Most lesions probably result from anorexia and debility. Emaciation may be prominent, but many ducks and geese that die from lead poisoning are in good body condition. The carcass may be pale with watery blood. Erosion and ulceration of the gizzard lining can be extensive (Fig 36.11). Impaction of proventriculus is frequently seen and is likely secondary to vagus nerve damage (Fig. 36.12).

Microscopically, the most diagnostic lesions are demyelination of peripheral nerves and focal areas of vascular damage in the cerebellum (136), and acid-fast, intranuclear inclusion bodies in the kidney (Fig. 36.13), liver, and spleen (175, 217, 243). Inclusions are composed of protein-bound lead and can be demonstrated by special staining or electron microscopy (Fig. 36.14) (202). Nephrosis with degeneration and necrosis of tubular epithelial cells containing brown pigment have been described. Hemosiderosis is prominent in the spleen and other organs. Scattered myocardial necrosis associated with hyaline or fibrinoid necrosis of blood vessels (149), arrested mitotic activity in proventricular epithelial cells, and degenerative changes in testes also may be found (182).

Diagnosis. The final diagnosis of lead poisoning is based on blood and tissue levels. In chickens, a blood lead level greater than 4 ppm, a liver lead level greater than 18 ppm wet weight, or a 20 ppm wet weight in kidney would be considered diagnostic (232, 233). Lead levels in bone can also be determined. Acid-fast inclusions in kidney epithelial cells suggest lead poisoning but may be found in birds that could have ingested lead but died from some other cause. Peripheral nerve lesions, in conjunction with fibrinoid necrosis of blood vessels, which may be found throughout the body, not just in brain and heart, are useful in diagnosis, but similar changes are seen in methylmercury poisoning (243). In lead poisoning, however, lesions in the central nervous system are related only to vascular damage.

MERCURY. Organic mercury, used previously as a seed protectant, is discussed below with fungicides. Most organic mercury in the environment today results from methylation by aquatic organisms and action of methogenic bacterial enzymes on elemental mercury from nature (decaying trees) or industry. Tons of mercury as bivalent inorganic mercury, elemental mercury, and phenyl mercury have been discharged into waterways around the world.

Methylmercury, a direct product of biotransformation, gets into small water organisms and enters the food chain when fish eat contaminated plants, insects, or animals (bioconcentration). Fish-eating birds, particularly ducks, may become poisoned from mercury in the food they eat (209). Mercury contamination of pheasants also has occurred. Experimental feeding of low levels of methylmercury resulted in decreased egg production, increased shell-less eggs, and reduced hatchability (209).

Residues in chickens given subclinical amounts of methylmercury were highest in liver, least in muscle, and intermediate in kidney. Eggs had four times as much mercury in albumin compared with yolk (209).

Inorganic mercury of medicinal or industrial waste origin may induce anorexia, enteritis, and nephrosis (209, 232, 233).

TIN. Tin from medicinal sources can cause depression, hunching up, and yellow diarrhea (264).

URANIUM (URANYL NITRATE). Industrial uranium causes depression, anorexia, and nephrosis with severe lesions in collecting tubules, followed by hyperuricemia and visceral urate deposits in birds that survive (161).

VANADIUM. Reduced egg quality, growth, and hatchability all have been attributed to vanadium toxicity (160, 232, 233). Also, there are many reports in the literature of experimental vanadium toxicity.

Vitamins

VITAMIN A. Excess vitamin A reduces egg production (157) and growth rate, and causes osteodystrophy and osteoporosis (278, 286).

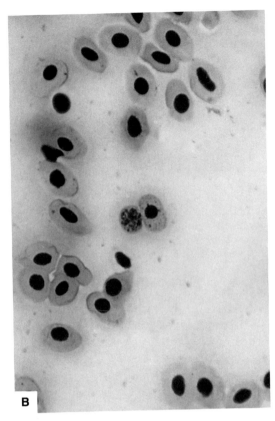

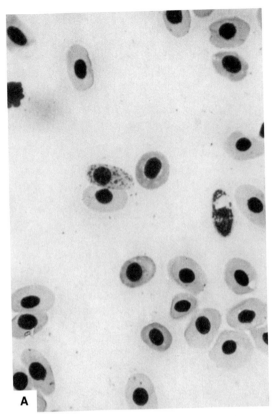

36.10. Duck with lead poisoning. *A*. Immature erythrocytes and two cells showing basophilic stippling. (Barnes) *B*. Basophilic stippling in an erythrocyte adjacent to an immature erythrocyte undergoing mitosis. (Barnes)

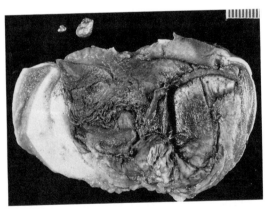

36.11. Gizzard from duck with lead poisoning. Severe erosion, ulceration, and bile staining of koilin lining. Note two lead pellets retrieved from the gizzard. (Barnes)

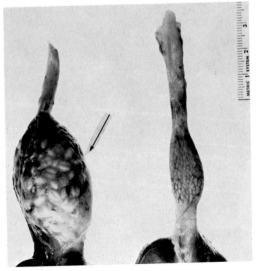

36.12. Lead poisoning, showing distended proventriculus (*arrow*); there were 15 lead shot in gizzard.

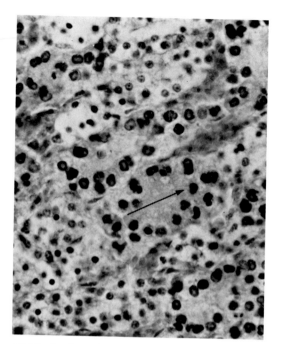

36.13. Lead poisoning. Acid-fast intranuclear inclusion bodies (*arrow*) in kidney of mallard duck. ×480. (Locke)

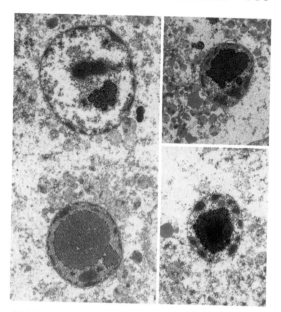

36.14. Proximal renal epithelium from a bird with lead poisoning. Nuclei contain irregular, variable electron-dense inclusion bodies typical of lead accumulation in kidney. Similar inclusions may be present in the liver. (Shivaprasad)

VITAMIN D₃ (CHOLECALCIFEROL). Four percent mortality due to kidney failure occurred in chicks when feed was top dressed with vitamin D₃ powder. Nephrosis with focal mineralization was present throughout the kidneys. Mineralization was also present in walls of arteries, particularly in the proventriculus. Excess vitamin D₃ has also been shown to increase leg abnormalities in broilers (49). Experimentally induced toxicity indicated 25-hydroxycholecalciferol was 100 times as toxic as cholecalciferol (237). A variety of lesions were seen, but renal damage was most significant (194). Poultry, pigeons, and wild birds may also be poisoned by rodenticides in which the toxic agent is 25-hydroxycholecalciferol.

VITAMIN B₆ (PYRIDOXINE). Pyridoxine is toxic for pigeons at levels safe for poultry (90-100 mg/bird, i.e., approximately 200 mg/kg body weight given by injection) (218).

Other

ETHOXYQUIN. Ethoxyquin (1,2-dihydro-6-ethoxy-2,2,4-trimethylquinolone) is a commonly used antioxidant that may be toxic at high levels (6500-12,500 mg/kg feed). Mortality is increased; affected birds have pale, swollen kidneys, dark-brown enlarged livers, and urates in joints. Proximal tubular necrosis in the kidney and accumulations of dark-brown pigment—interpreted to be ethoxyquin—in hepatocytes, bile ducts, and pulmonary blood capillaries are seen microscopically (172).

LIGNOSOL. Calcium lignosulfonate, a pellet binder, may produce black, sticky cecal contents that adhere to the skin of processed broilers, causing increased condemnation from contamination. It has no effect on body weight or feed conversion (231).

NITRATE AND NITRITE. Nitrate is converted to nitrite by bacteria in the digestive tract and is much less toxic than nitrite. High levels of nitrate cause diarrhea, dyspnea, and death. Lower levels affect growth and egg production. Blood hemoglobin is changed to methemoglobin. The effect is greater in young birds, as it is in young mammals, with fetal hemoglobin (66). Most reports of toxicity are experimental, although there are some reports of toxic nitrate levels in leaves and stems of plants (304).

PEN- AND LITTER-RELATED TOXICANTS.

Pen and litter-related toxicants include products accidentally or intentionally incorporated into litter or applied to the pen that result in illness. Some are disinfectants and fumigants discussed below. Except for boric acid, insecticides mixed into the litter (e.g., fire ant control products) or applied to walls, floor, or ceiling are covered later in this chapter. Copper sulfate, often used as a fungicide in litter, has been discussed with food- and water-related toxicants above. Toxic mixtures such as copper–chrome–arsenic formulations are used as preservatives in the timber industry (200). Occasionally, part of the building structure is toxic; geese have been poisoned from eating urea-formaldehyde foam insulation picked from the wall.

BORIC AND ORTHOBORIC ACID. Boric acid is used in litter to control darkling beetles and may be consumed by broilers, which results in reduced growth and abnormal feathering (74, 246).

IRON. Ferrous sulfate hepatahydrate added to litter to reduce ammonia formation was toxic to broilers (291). Affected chicks were depressed and lethargic. Those that died had severe gizzard ulceration and liver degeneration. The LD_{50} of ferrous sulfate is 7010 mg/kg body weight for a single dose. When added to the diet, 3% caused reduced growth and feed intake, while 1.5% had no effect (223).

PENTACHLOROPHENOL. Pentachlorophenol has been used as a pesticide in industry and agriculture, but its primary use is as a wood preservative. Logs may be treated before they leave the forest, or wood may be treated after cutting. Sawdust and shavings from treated wood have frequently been used as poultry litter; chickens can become contaminated from contact with these shavings. Because the product is used for many other purposes, pentachlorophenol may also contaminate broilers or table eggs in other ways.

Illness associated with pentachlorophenol has been caused by toxic impurities such as dioxins (see below). Pure pentachlorophenol can reduce growth, cause kidney hypertrophy, and decrease humoral immune responses (229, 272). It has also been associated with musty taint in eggs and broiler meat. Chlorophenols in litter are metabolized by bacteria and fungi to chloroanisoles. Anisoles have a musty or earthy odor even at very low concentrations, and they are responsible for the taint in eggs and meat from chickens in contact with contaminated litter (101). Reduced hatchability has also been associated with pentachlorophenol contamination (104).

SULFUR. Elemental sulfur may be sprinkled on dirt floors and vaporized by adding water and heating the building before litter is put down. High mortality, ulcerative dermatitis mainly affecting moist areas of the body, irritation of respiratory mucous membranes, and conjunctivitis occurred in chicks placed in treated buildings (225). Lesions probably resulted from sulfur dioxide (from residual sulfur that had not vaporized) dissolving in moisture on the chick's body to form sulfurous acid (H_2SO_3).

DISINFECTANTS AND FUMIGANTS. Fumigants are products producing toxic gases used to control rodents, insects, fungi, and bacteria. They can cause toxicity when inhaled or ingested. Phenolic disinfectants can be toxic when inhaled or absorbed through skin.

Phenolic Compounds and Coal-Tar Derivatives. Phenol, cresol, creolin, carbolineum, and creosote products cause damage to vascular endothelium, epithelia of respiratory and digestive tracts, and parenchymal organs, such as liver and kidney (217). Thymus and bursa of Fabricius are small, but this may result from stunting rather than being a direct effect on the immune system. Hydropericardium is prominent, but ascites and subcutaneous edema are also frequently present if contact is severe. Mortality may be high. Diagnosis is based on a history of contact and by elimination of other causes of ascites and edema. Odor may also provide a useful clue. Cases of creolin toxicity still appear in the literature (170). Coal tar poisoning has been induced in ducks by feeding clay pigeons (42).

Quaternary Ammonium (Cationic Detergents). Use of sanitizers to clean poultry drinkers or treat water has resulted in reduced growth or production and, occasionally, in severe lesions and death in young chicks. High levels of quaternary ammonia cause epithelial irritation of the mouth, pharynx, and upper respiratory tract, resulting in oral, ocular, and nasal discharges. Necrosis of epithelium leads to pseudomembranes in the mouth and epithelial thickening in the esophagus, crop, and proventriculus, with ulcers at the gizzard–proventricular junction (64, 217). Similar lesions have been reported in poults (181).

Chlorine. Low levels (37.5–150 mg/kg) may have a beneficial effect, but high levels (300–1200 mg/kg) result in reduced growth and increased mortality (55).

Formaldehyde. Formaldehyde gas and formalin (a 37% solution of the gas in water, which is then 100% formalin) have been widely used for many years as antibacterial and antiviral agents in the poultry industry. Photophobia and respiratory signs from contact with high levels of formaldehyde are seen occasionally in newly hatched or recently delivered baby chicks and poults. Prolonged exposure to high levels of formaldehyde (which dissolves in liquids on mucous membranes to produce formalin) in the hatcher impairs cilial function and causes tracheal epithelial degeneration and sloughing (251). Air quality during subsequent growout, however, has a greater effect on productivity than does early formaldehyde exposure (250). Epithelial necrosis of eyes, mouth, and trachea with pseudomembranous plaques in the mouth and trachea also may be found. Edematous swellings under the lower beak (105), subcutaneous edema (24) during the acute phase, and ascites or edema occurred later in exposed poults.

Other Fumigants. It must be assumed that most or all chemicals used as fumigants are toxic to poultry (209). A few reports of deliberate or accidental poisoning of poultry by other fumigants appear in the literature (263, 298).

FUNGICIDES. Fungicides are used as seed dressings (protectants), wood preservatives, in paint and plastic, and on cereal crops, fruits, vegetables, and flowers. Previously, poisoning in poultry has usually resulted from incorporation of treated seed into poultry feed.

Organic Mercurials. Mercurial fungicides, frequently ethyl or methyl mercuric chloride, that cause poisoning with central and peripheral nervous lesions in poultry, wild birds, animals, and humans consuming treated seed are no longer in use (125, 126, 243, 270). Signs of organic mercury poisoning may be nonspecific or affected birds may show progressive paralysis or other neurologic signs. Specific gross lesions may be lacking, but microscopically, Wallerian degeneration of peripheral nerves and spinal cord, and neuronal damage in the brain may be present. Vasculitis may also be obvious in some vessels, particularly in the brain.

Thiram. Arasan (active ingredient thiram, a dithiocarbamate) has caused poisoning in poultry, producing lameness and leg deformity in chicks and poults and soft-shelled eggs in layers (217). It is also teratogenic (211). Thiram increases the incidence and severity of tibial dyschondroplasia (81). The LD_{50} is 485–932 mg/kg body weight in pheasants and 2800 mg/kg body weight in mallard ducks (54).

Captan. Captan is an organic seed protectant. It is less toxic than Arasan. It depresses feed consumption, slows growth, and reduces egg production (217).

For descriptions of other organic synthetic fungicides, see (209); pentachlorophenol, a widely used wood preservative, and copper sulfate, a litter treatment, have been covered previously in this chapter.

HERBICIDES

Chlorates. Sodium and potassium chlorates used as herbicides and defoliants are moderately toxic for poultry. They act by converting hemoglobin to methemoglobin. The lethal dose for chickens is 5 g/kg (209).

Organic Synthetic Herbicides. Amitrate (3-amino 1,2,4-triazole) causes hypothyroidism and reduces weight gain in chickens (309). Phenoxyherbicides such as 2,4-D cause kidney enlargement. Some herbicides are toxic for embryos (76). See (209) for additional information.

Dipyridyl Herbicides (Diquat and Paraquat). Paraquat toxicity results from free radical–induced membrane damage caused by inhibition of the glutathione peroxidase system. Selenium is protective. Experimental oral paraquat poisoning in turkeys produced diarrhea, listlessness, and anorexia with terminal convulsions. Gastroenteritis was present at necropsy (269). Turkeys are more resistant than are mammals (123, 209).

INSECTICIDES. Insecticides may be referred to by either their common or registered name. The common name is not capitalized, e.g., carbaryl, while the trade name is, e.g., Sevin® (209). Organic insecticides—organophosphates, organochlorides, and carbamates—have been widely used, some on animals and birds as systemic larvicides and anthelmintics, as well as on buildings and pens. Wild birds have been poisoned by feeding on treated animals (29, 118). Many insecticides are quite toxic for animals as well as insects, arthropods, and helminths. Some more toxic products are used on crops, wood, trees, as soil insecticides, and as seed dressings. Extensive tables presenting general information on insecticides can be found in (209).

Organochloride Insecticides. The mode of action of organochloride (chlorinated hydrocarbon) insecticide toxicity is unknown. Generally, they act to diffusely stimulate or depress the nervous system. Organochloride insecticides often remain longer in the environment than other insecticides. Some more persistent ones have been taken off the market or have restricted use. Because they are fat soluble, organochlorides tend to build up in the food chain and be present in yolks of eggs. There is considerable literature available on insecticide toxicity in wild birds, with emphasis on organochlorides (193).

Signs. Nervous signs varying from excitement with vocalization to tremors, ataxia, and convulsions are prominent. Prostration and death may occur without other signs. Other signs include salivation, vomiting, diarrhea, and depression. Lameness and leg deformity may also occur. There may be decreased egg production, a drop in hatchability, embryo mortality, loss of pigment on pigmented eggs, a change in shell texture (chalky), and eggshell thinning. Administration of atropine to acutely affected birds will not alleviate or modify signs of toxicity.

Pathology. Specific lesions do not occur in organochloride toxicity. Nonspecific changes such as congestion and hemorrhage may be present. Excess cerebrospinal fluid may be noted when brains of affected birds are examined.

CHLORDANE. Chicks develop ataxia and hyperexcitability; hens have reduced body weight, decreased egg production, atrophy and cyanosis of the comb and wattles, and hydropericardium (217).

DDT AND DDE. Hens develop tremors, production drop, and weight loss, and there is eggshell thinning (217).

DIELDRIN. Pigeons, gulls, and other birds may show nervous signs (9, 217).

HEPTACHLOR. This may cause ataxia, salivation, prostration, and death (216, 290).

LINDANE. Diarrhea, vomiting, anorexia, depression, convulsions, and sudden death have been associated with lindane poisoning (25, 217).

MIREX. This has caused embryo mortality (3).

TOXAPHENE. Lameness, thin shells, and osteomalacia may occur (213, 217).

Organophosphorus and Carbamate Insecticides.
These products inhibit acetylcholinesterase, causing acetylcholine to accumulate, which results in overstimulation of parasympathetic nerves and muscles (89). Atropine given to effect often will dramatically reverse clinical signs, but efficacy depends on the type of organophosphorus compound and the duration of the intoxication. Repeated treatments may be necessary. Some organophosphates and carbamates have delayed neurotoxic effects (see below). Chickens and other birds are more susceptible than mammals to this type of toxicity.

Signs. Chicks and poults may die quickly, showing few signs except dyspnea and paralysis, or they may exhibit lacrimation, salivation, diarrhea, tremors, depression, dullness, lethargy, cyanosis,

ataxia, incoordination, and convulsions prior to death. Because of respiratory signs and salivation in early stages, respiratory infection may be suspected initially.

Pathology. Few gross lesions occur. There may be congestion with dark blood, and hemorrhages may be present in heart muscle, on serosal surfaces, and on mucosa of intestines. No specific microscopic changes have been identified.

DIAZINON. Diazinon is used to control fire ants and darkling beetles, but in birds, diazinon can cause incoordination, paralysis, respiratory signs, and death (130). It is also used to control pests in soil and grass, causing death in Canada geese (102, 271).

DICHLORVOS (DDVP). Dichlorvos induces staggering, frothing from the mouth, paralysis, and convulsions (82).

DIMETHOATE. Toxic effects include reduced growth and egg production (259, 260).

FAMPHUR. Mortality in raptors has resulted from famphur toxicity (128).

MALATHION. Malathion causes dullness, salivation, loose droppings, cyanosis, paralysis, and death; lesions include injected subcutaneous vessels and dark congested heart (34, 217). In geese, there may be flaccid paralysis.

MONOCROTOPHOS. Monocrotophos toxicity has been associated with salivation, mortality in quail, and weight loss and embryo abnormalities in chickens (265).

PARATHION. Parathion induces lacrimation, salivation, dyspnea, tremors, and convulsions (217).

CARBAMATES. Various carbamates such as carbaryl, carbofuran, and others are toxic for pheasants, pigeons, turkey poults, chickens, and ducks (13, 83, 235). Signs include reduced growth, lameness, weakness, ataxia, and death. There may be tibial dyschondroplasia, retarded testicular development because of degeneration of seminiferous epithelium, nerve fiber degeneration, and congestion of organs and tissues.

Delayed Organophosphorus Neurotoxicity.
Delayed neurotoxicity occurs several days to weeks after exposure, causing progressive degeneration of peripheral nerves and spinal cord, which leads to weakness and paralysis. Acetylcholinesterase is not affected. Delayed neurotoxicity may result from ingestion or absorption of a va-

riety of triaryl phosphates; chemicals found in phenylphosphorothioate insecticides such as leptophos, cyanofenphos, and their analogues; as well as a variety of industrial chemicals, including fire retardants and lubricants. Malathion and dimethoate may also cause delayed neurotoxicity. Mature chickens, pheasants, and mallard ducklings are highly susceptible (209). Chicks hatched after in ovo exposure also show clinical signs (90). There are many reports of delayed neurotoxicity in chickens from these products. Most describe experimentally induced lesions (1, 2, 78, 163, 176). The author has seen turkeys in Ontario, Canada, with typical clinical signs of ataxia and paralysis and histologic lesions of delayed organophosphorus neurotoxicity in spinal cord and peripheral nerves. Clinical cases occurred in Europe after chickens ate scraps of synthetic leather containing tri-ortho-cresyl-phosphate (TOCP) (217).

Signs. Ataxia, falling sideways, inability to rise, lack of leg reflexes and prostration may be evident. Birds appear bright and eat and drink if given access to food and water for several days.

Pathology. There are no gross lesions. Degeneration of axons and myelin in peripheral nerves and long tracts of the spinal cord are diagnostic. Axons may be swollen, and spheroids may be present in axon spaces. Digestion chambers containing macrophages and debris may be present in subacute cases.

Other Insecticides

PYRETHRUM AND SYNTHETIC PYRETHROIDS. These products are not very toxic to animals or birds and there are no reports of illness (46).

ROTENONE. Rotenone (derris powder) is prepared from roots of *Derris* spp. Mature chickens are resistant (lethal dose 1000-3000 mg/kg); young birds are more susceptible (209). Fish are very susceptible to rotenone.

NICOTINE. Nicotine sulfate (Black Leaf 40®) has been used to paint chicken roosts to control insects and arthropods, particularly northern fowl mite. It has also been used for internal parasites. In low doses, nicotine stimulates the nervous system through an acetylcholinelike activity. At toxic levels, neural transmission is blocked causing death from respiratory paralysis (209).

Signs. Sudden death, occasionally preceded by depression and coma, is seen in affected birds.

Pathology. Since death is from respiratory failure, cyanosis and congestion may be marked. Hemor-

rhages may be present on the heart and in other tissues.

RODENTICIDES, AVICIDES, AND MOLLUSCACIDES

Rodenticides. Information on cholecalciferol and arsenic is presented in the section on Nutrients and Feed- and Water-related Toxicants. (For use of rodenticides, see Chapter 32).

ALPHA-NAPHTHYL THIOUREA (ANTU). ANTU causes depression, anorexia, weakness, prostration, and death. Lesions include pulmonary edema, hydropericardium, fatty change in liver, and myocardial degeneration.

SODIUM MONOFLUOROACETATE (COMPOUND 1080). Signs are reluctance to move, edema of wattles, dyspnea, cyanosis, and nervous signs. Lesions include dark, unclotted blood, pulmonary hemorrhage and edema, clotted blood in the trachea and air sacs, petechiation, enteritis, and hydropericardium (123, 209).

STRYCHNINE. Toxic effects are tonic spasms and respiratory failure (209, 217, 311).

WARFARIN, BRODIFACOUM, AND DIPHACINONE. These anticoagulant rodenticides are sold under a variety of trade names and may be combined with sulfaquinoxaline to interfere with vitamin K synthesis. They inhibit epoxide reductase, which converts vitamin K to its active form. Toxicity causes anemia with fluttering, gasping, and hemorrhages in eyes, mouth, and other tissues (14, 123, 209, 261). Onset may be rapid, and death occurs within 72 hr of ingestion (196). With the long-acting anticoagulants, there is a cumulative effect and if a small amount of anticoagulant is consumed repeatedly, there may be little or no product found in the digestive tract.

PHOSPHOROUS. Elemental yellow, red, and white phosphorus can induce depression, anorexia, diarrhea, ataxia, gastroenteritis, and death (209, 217).

ZINC PHOSPHIDE. Weakness, diarrhea, opisthotonos, and convulsions occur. There is enteritis, ascites, and hydropericardium (119, 261).

For birds, the toxic doses of several rodenticides (α-chloralase, crimidine, pyriminil, phosphorus, α-chlorohydrim) are given in *Clinical and Diagnostic Veterinary Toxicology* (209).

Avicides

AVITROL (4-AMINOPYRIDINE OR 4-AP). Avitrol

causes disorientation and vocalization (distress calls). Affected pigeons may be molested by normal pigeons. Generalized congestion is present at necropsy, and the characteristic small pellets can usually be found in the ventriculus (100, 197).

2-CHLORO-4-ACETOTOLUIDINE (CAT) AND 3-CHLORO-P-TOLUIDINE (CPT). No clinical signs have been described, but kidney necrosis (from CAT) and liver and kidney necrosis (from CPT) occur (106).

Molluscacides

METALDEHYDE. Nervous signs were prominent in ducklings following ingestion of metaldehyde (10).

TOXIC GASES

AMMONIA. Ammonia levels should be less than 25 ppm, but in poorly ventilated litter-type houses, ammonia may exceed 100 ppm (148). High levels of ammonia (50–75 ppm) reduce food consumption and growth rate (59). Egg production is also reduced. Ammonia dissolves in the liquid on mucous membranes and eyes to produce ammonium hydroxide, an irritating alkali causing keratoconjunctivitis. If levels greater than 100 ppm persist, corneal ulceration and blindness can occur. The condition is painful, and photophobia and stunting are marked. At levels of 75–100 ppm, changes in respiratory epithelium include loss of cilia (210) and increased numbers of mucus-secreting cells (8). Heart rate and breathing may be affected and there may be hemorrhages in trachea and bronchi. For a review, see (41).

CARBON MONOXIDE. Carbon monoxide (CO) poisoning may occur in buildings where defective or unventilated gas-catalytic or open-flame brooders or furnaces are in use, or where poultry are exposed to internal combustion-engine exhaust fumes. Affected chicks or poults show drowsiness, labored breathing, and incoordination. Spasms and convulsions may occur prior to death. At postmortem, blood is bright red. Sublethal levels cause stunting (217, 273). In suspected cases, CO should be measured at several locations in the pen with the ventilation system shut off. Carboxyhemoglobin can be measured in blood of affected birds. The author found levels of 70 ppm CO in pens where a repeated high incidence of ascites due to pulmonary hypertension and right ventricular failure occurred. Toxic levels of CO for chickens are: 600 ppm for 30 min causes distress; 2000–3600 ppm is lethal in 1.5–2 hr (209).

AERIAL ENDOTOXIN. Breakdown of bacteria in the litter and environment results in endotoxin in the air in broiler pens. Endotoxin from inhaled air can be found in the blood of people who work in broiler pens (71). The effect of inhaled endotoxin on poultry is not known.

POLYTETRAFLUOROETHYLENE. Fluorinated gases are released when this material, used as a nonstick coating (Teflon) on cookware and ovens, is overheated. Pet birds that inhale the fumes die from lung edema. Histologic examination reveals epithelial necrosis in parabronchi and vascular damage in blood capillaries (274, 296).

Other Toxic Gases. Levels of methane, carbon dioxide, hydrogen sulfide, methyl mercaptan, dimethyl sulfide, and dimethyl disulfide were found to be low in poultry and other livestock buildings in Finland (148), but toxic fumes from liquid manure pits in pig barns have killed humans and pigs in North America, and nitrogen dioxide formed in freshly filled silos has also killed humans and animals in Canada and the United States. Toxic gases associated with livestock production, including poultry, have been reviewed (209). The effect of sulfur dioxide in chickens has been described (91).

HOUSEHOLD AND COMMERCIAL PRODUCTS

ALCOHOL. Ethyl alcohol may be used to dissolve experimental chemicals or drugs given to poultry in feed or water. Clinical signs of intoxication include ataxia and reduced feed consumption. Fatty change in the liver and heart lesions may occur (7, 51). Wild birds are frequently intoxicated from ingesting fermented fruit (94). Pet birds may obtain alcohol inadvertently or it maybe given by the owner.

ANTIFREEZE (ETHYLENE GLYCOL). Ethylene glycol is toxic when ingested because it breaks down to oxalic acid, which combines with calcium to form calcium oxalate. Calcium oxalate crystals block renal tubules and cause tubular epithelial necrosis leading to hyperuricemia and urate nephrosis with visceral urate deposits. Diagnosis is usually based on finding typical crystals and tubular changes on microscopic examination of kidney (243, 244, 275). Liver necrosis is found in pigeons. Other forms of toxicity may occur in other species (209). Coccidia oocysts treated with ethylene oxide were toxic to chicks and caused kidney lesions similar to ethylene glycol (297).

CARBON TETRACHLORIDE. Carbon tetrachloride has been used previously as a household solvent and cleaner. It has also been used to treat tapeworms in chickens (245). It is toxic to animals and birds, interfering with fat metabolism and causing liver and kidney damage. Chickens are more resistant than rats, but low levels cause decreased growth.

FERTILIZER. Lawn, garden, and farm fertilizers contain nitrogen, phosphorus, and potassium. The contents in that order are usually given by numbers representing each element as a percentage of the total. These elements have been discussed above. Fertilizer may be attractive to birds because it is frequently in the form of small hard pellets. Some phosphate fertilizers contain very low levels of radioactive material.

NAPHTHALENE. Mothballs are frequently recommended to keep pets and other animals away from gardens or out of attics. They have also been used in chicken nests for ectoparasite control. Mothballs are toxic and can cause poisoning in poultry and pet birds (158).

UREA. Urea is relatively nontoxic for birds. Because it is used in feed preparations for ruminants, the pellets are occasionally found in poultry feed.

INDUSTRY-RELATED TOXICANTS

Toxic Fat Syndrome, Chick Edema Disease, and Dioxin Toxicity.
Over 30 yr ago, the most toxic dioxin, 2,3,7,8-tetrachlorodibenzodioxin (TCDD), and other dioxins in the same polychlorinated dibenzodioxin group were found as contaminants in industrial fat (tallow from cattle hides) added to poultry feed. This material, which could be distilled from fat, was called "chick edema factor" until it was identified. It caused widespread disease in the broiler industry and in other poultry for several years. Occasional cases of dioxin toxicity (chick edema disease) occurred until about 1970. More recently, TCDD toxicity followed environmental contamination in Italy where adult fowl died with lesions of chick edema disease (227). Dioxin was probably the material causing lesions in toxicity caused by paint containing chlorinated hydrocarbon (183).

Chickens are more susceptible than some mammals to toxic effects of TCDD (209). In chickens, dioxin damages vascular endothelium causing vascular leakage and extensive movement of fluid into body cavities and subcutaneous tissue. The epithelium of some parenchymal organs is damaged and there is degeneration of heart and skeletal muscle.

Since right ventricular hypertrophy and dilation have been described (6) and many lesions in dioxin toxicity are similar to right-sided heart failure from other causes, the possibility of dioxin contributing to right ventricular failure should be considered.

Depending on the level of TCDD in feed, variable numbers of broilers in a flock will show severe signs of stunting, respiratory distress, weakness,

ataxia, and edema. Mortality can occasionally be very high. For a description and review of the syndrome, see (217).

TCDD may be present as a contaminant in herbicides. It and other dioxins are produced by incineration (209) and by industry (85).

Polybrominated Biphenyl (PBB) and Polychlorinated Biphenyl (PCB).
PBBs or PCBs may be accidentally added to feed, get into feed as contaminants (as in oil or grease from equipment), or be present in the environment from industrial contamination and deliberate dumping. Both PBBs and PCBs are toxic to birds. At low levels they affect production, reproduction, hatchability, and offspring viability. Hepatocyte damage and bursal depletion also occur with low-level PBB toxicity (63). Residues may be found in eggs and meat from birds without clinical signs. PBBs are concentrated in eggs at 1.5 times the dietary level (209).

At high levels, lesions of PCB toxicity are similar to dioxin toxicity. It is likely that in some cases, PCBs were contaminated with TCDD.

Crude Petroleum and Oils.
Most information on toxicity of oil to birds deals with environmental contamination and effect of oil spills on waterfowl. Ingested oil causes anorexia, weight loss, incoordination, tremors, and anemia. Lesions include lipid pneumonia, enteritis, hepatosis with fatty infiltration, and nephrosis and degeneration of pancreas, spleen, and bursa (201). Immune responses are impaired. In herring gulls and puffins, lesions suggested a primary toxic hemolytic disease (169) with lymphoid depletion being secondary and stress related.

Oil applied to chicken eggs caused embryo mortality and lesions in organs (48).

Oils and oil products on the feathers and skin can be removed with detergents.

BIOTOXINS.
Biotoxins are poisonous substances produced by living organisms including bacterial toxins such as botulinus toxin, which in birds is frequently associated with toxin-contaminated maggots, bacterial food poisoning, diseases such as necrotic and ulcerative enteritis, gangrenous dermatitis, and mycotoxins. Perhaps, even methylmercury produced by bacteria should be classed as a biotoxin. Insect and snake venoms (165) are also biotoxins. Most of these conditions are of little importance or are discussed in other parts of the text. Botulism is being seen with increasing frequency in housed turkeys and broilers. Birds are very susceptible to botulinus toxin and may show clinical signs following ingestion of very small amounts. The toxin apparently develops in dead birds left in the litter. Birds may pick up toxin from eating decaying tissue or contaminated fly lar-

vae, darkling beetles or litter. An enzyme-linked immunosorbent assay (ELISA), which may be as sensitive as the mouse-inoculation test, has been developed to identify botulinus toxin (see also Chapter 12). Only algae poisoning and rose chafer toxicity are mentioned here.

Algae. Several species of blue-green algae produce a toxin that, when concentrated by rapid algal growth (bloom) in warm bodies of fresh water and a constant light wind blowing the toxic material to the side of the lake, may poison animals and birds consuming it. Toxicity varies directly with concentration (138). Affected chickens may show nervous signs and paralysis before death. Ducks and turkeys have also been poisoned (134). Cyanosis, congestion, and a dilated, distended heart may be seen at necropsy (217). The liver is swollen with necrosis of hepatocytes. Diagnosis is based on identifying toxin in the water (209).

Rose Chafers. Rose chafers (*Macrodactylus subspinosus*) are insects appearing in spring and early summer in eastern and central North America. Young chicks may be poisoned by 15–30 insects (217). Clinical signs include drowsiness, weakness, prostration, and convulsions (217).

PHYTOTOXINS. All or parts of some plants are toxic, or if fed at low levels may only reduce growth rate. Antinutrients are discussed in the section on Nutrients and Other Feed- and Water-Related Toxicants. For additional information on plants that are toxic to poultry and pet birds, see (11, 70, 68, 75, 98, 153, 266, 306).

AVOCADO (*PERSEA AMERICANA*)

Part of Plant. Fruit.

Signs and Lesions. Muscle degeneration, hydropericardium, and subcutaneous edema (37, 120).

BLACK LOCUST (*ROBINIA PSEUDOACACIA*)

Part of Plant. Leaf.

Signs and Lesions. Depression and paralysis; hemorrhagic enteritis.

BLADDER POD (*SESBANIA [GLOTTIDIUM] VESICARIA*)

Part of Plant. Seed.

Signs and Lesions. Diarrhea, cyanosis, prostra-

tion; necrotic enteritis, gizzard ulceration (87).

CACAO (*THEOBROMA CACAO*—THEOBROMINE TOXICITY)

Part of Plant. Bean waste.

Signs and Lesions. Acute cases—nervous signs followed by convulsions and death; cyanosis, cloacal prolapse, and mottled kidneys. Chronic cases—anorexia and diarrhea (217).

CASSAVA (*MANIHOT* SPP.—CYANIDE, POLYPHENOLS)

Part of Plant. Root (tuber).

Signs and Lesions. Sudden death. Depressed growth (86, 215).

CASTOR BEAN (*RICINUS COMMUNIS*)

Part of Plant. Bean.

Signs and Lesions. Progressive paralysis with prostration (like botulism); diarrhea, emaciation, swollen pale mottled liver, hemorrhagic catarrhal enteritis, petechiae, degeneration of lymphoid tissue and parenchymal cells of liver and kidney, bile duct proliferation (140, 204, 217).

COFFEE SENNA, SICKLE POD (*CASSIA OCCIDENTALIS, C. OBTUSIFOLIA*)

Part of Plant. Seed.

Signs and Lesions. Weakness, ataxia, paralysis, decreased egg production, diarrhea; toxic myopathy, pectoralis and semitendinous muscles pale and edematous, muscle degeneration, and necrosis (96, 212, 217, 268, 287).

CORN COCKLE (*AGROSTEMMA GITHAGO*—GITHAGENIN TOXICITY)

Part of Plant. Seed.

Signs and Lesions. Depression, rough feathers, decreased respiratory and heart rate, diarrhea, depressed growth; hydropericardium; caseous necrosis of crop, pharyngeal mucosa, and mouth (129, 217).

COTTON SEED MEAL (GOSSYPOL TOXICITY)

Signs and Lesions. Cyanosis, inappetence, emaciation, reduced egg production and quality; enteritis, degeneration of liver and kidney (217).

COYOTILLO (*KARWINSKIA HUMBOLDTIANA*)

Part of Plant. Fruit and seed.

Signs and Lesions. Depressed growth, cyanosis, and paralysis.

CROTALARIA SPP. (PYRROLIZIDINE ALKALOIDS, MONOCROTALINE TOXICITY)

Part of Plant. Seed, leaf, and stem.

Signs and Lesion. Dull, inactive, reduced feed consumption, stunting, bright yellow-green urates; subcutaneous edema, ascites, hydropericardium, lung edema, hepatitis, bile duct hyperplasia (5, 43, 67, 217, 305).

DAUBENTONIA (*DAUBENTONIA LONGIFOLIA, SESBANIA DRUMMONDII, S. MACROCARPA*)

Part of Plant. Seed.

Signs and Lesions. Weakness, depression, stunting, diarrhea, emaciation; proventriculitis with ulceration and enteritis; liver and kidney degeneration (95, 97, 179, 258).

DEATH CAMAS (*ZYGADENUS* SPP.)

Part of Plant. Leaf, stem, and root.

Signs and Lesions. Weakness, salivation, diarrhea, and prostration (199).

EUCALYPTUS CLADOCALYX (CYANIDE OR PRUSSIC ACID)

Part of Plant. Leaf.

Signs and Lesions. Acute death without premonitory signs.

HEMLOCK (*CONIUM MACULATUM*—CONIINE TOXICITY)

Part of Plant. Seed.

Signs and Lesions. Salivation, weakness, nervous signs, paralysis, diarrhea, reduced growth; hepatic congestion, enteritis (99).

JIMSONWEED (*DATURA STRAMONIUM, D. FEROX*—SCOPOLAMINE, HYOSCYAMINE)

Part of Plant. Seed.

Signs and Lesions. Reduced growth (159).

LEUCAENA LEUCOCEPHALA (MIMOSINE TOXICITY)

Part of Plant. Leaf.

Signs and Lesions. Depressed growth (124).

LILY OF THE VALLEY (*CONVALLARIA MAJALIS*)

MILKWEED (*ASCLEPIAS* SPP.—ASCLEPIDIN TOXICITY)

Signs and Lesions. Weakness and incoordination, convulsions, prostration, leading to death or recovery (217).

NIGHTSHADE (*SOLANUM NIGRUM*—BELLADONNA TOXICITY)

Part of Plant. Immature fruit.

Signs and Lesions. Dilated pupils, incoordination, prostration (117).

NITRATE (NUMEROUS PLANT SPECIES). See section on nitrates and nitrites above.

OAK (*QUERCUS* SPP.—TANNIN TOXICITY)

Part of Plant. Leaf.

Signs and Lesions. There is severe diarrhea, anorexia, and increased water consumption; enteritis, swollen kidneys, and visceral gout; diffuse necrosis of proximal renal tubules. (156).

OLEANDER (*NERIUM OLEANDER*—GLYCOSIDES)

Part of Plant. All parts.

Signs and Lesions. Depression, weakness, diarrhea; gastroenteritis, liver degeneration, death (217, 277).

OXALATE (NUMEROUS PLANT SPECIES—OXALIC ACID)

Part of Plant. Leaf and stem.

Signs and Lesions. Oxalate nephrosis (304). See also section on ethylene glycol above.

PARSLEY, *AMMI MAJUS*, OTHERS (PHOTOSENSITIZATION)

Part of Plant. All parts.

Signs and Lesions. Dermatitis (unfeathered areas); hepatitis (219, 262).

POKEBERRY (*PHYTOLACCA AMERICANA*)

Part of Plant. Fruit.

Signs and Lesions. Ataxia, leg deformity, ascites (15).

POTATO (*SOLANUM TUBEROSUM*—SOLANINE TOXICITY)

Part of Plant. Green or spoiled tubers, peelings, and sprouts.

Signs and Lesions. Incoordination, prostration (teratogenic) (117, 280).

RAGWORT (*SENECIO JACOBEA*—PYRROLIZIDINE ALKALOID)

Part of Plant. All parts.

Signs and Lesions. Focal hepatic necrosis and portal fibrosis (43).

RAPESEED MEAL (ERUCIC ACID/GLUCOSINOLATE TOXICITY; ANTINUTRIENTS—SINAPINE, TANNIN, PHYTIC ACID); CANOLA—LOW GLUCOSINOLATE LEVELS.

Part of Plant. Seed.

Signs and Lesions. Egg taint, hypothyroidism, depressed growth, anemia, sudden death, ruptured liver, hepatitis, ascites, hydropericardium; periacinar hepatic necrosis, fatty change in skeletal and heart muscle (20, 23, 38, 47, 92, 108, 150, 236, 303).

SWEET PEA (*LATHYRUS* SPP.— LATHYRISM)

Part of Plant. Seed (pea).

Signs and Lesions. Skeletal deformity, osteolathyrism (*L. odoratus*); or neurologic disease, neurolathyrism (*L. sativus*) (44, 195, 234).

TANNINS (NUMEROUS PLANT SPECIES). Tannins are antinutrients that occur in a variety of plants. It may be important to determine tannin levels in some feedstuffs such as sorghum (139, 279, 293).

TOBACCO (*NICOTIANA TABACUM*—NICOTINE SULFATE TOXICITY)

Part of Plant. Leaf and stem.

Signs and Lesions. Stunting, reduced production (teratogenic) (217).

VELVETWEED (MALVACEAE FAMILY—CYCLOPENOID FATTY ACIDS)

Part of Plant. Seed.

Signs and Lesions. Pasty, rubbery yolk in eggs (155).

VETCH (*VICIA* SPP.—CYANOGENIC GLYCOSIDE)

Part of Plant. Seed (pea).

Signs and Lesions. Excitability, respiratory distress, convulsions (121, 241).

YELLOW JESSAMINE (*GELSEMIUM SEMPERVIRENS*)

Part of Plant. Whole plant.

Signs and Lesions. Depressed growth (217, 307).

YEW (*TAXUS* SPP.—TAXINE TOXICITY)

Part of Plant. All parts.

Signs and Lesions. Labored breathing, incoordination, collapse; cyanosis.

REFERENCES

1. Abou-Donia, M.B., and A.A. Komeil. 1979. Delayed neurotoxicity of o-ethyl o-4-cyanophenyl phenylphosphonothioate (cyanofenphos) in hens. Toxicol Lett 4:455–459.
2. Abou-Donia, M.B., D.G. Graham, M.A. Ashry, and P.R. Timmons. 1980. Delayed neurotoxicity of leptophos and related compounds: Differential effects of subchronic oral administration of pure technical grade and degradation products on the hen. Toxicol App Pharmacol 53:150–163.
3. Abuelgasim, A., R. Ringer, and V. Sanger. 1982. Toxicosis of mirex for chick embryos and chickens hatched from eggs inoculated with mirex. Avian Dis 26:34–39.
4. Acar, N., P. Vohra, R. Becker, G.D. Hanners, and R.M. Saunders. 1988. Nutritional evaluation of grain amaranth for growing chickens. Poult Sci 67:1166–1173.
5. Alfonso, H.A., L.M. Sanchez, M. de los Angeles-Figeurdo, and B.C. Gomez. 1993. Intoxication due to Crotalaria retusa and C. spectabilis in chickens and geese. Vet Human Toxicol 35:539.
6. Allen, J.R. 1964. The role of "toxic fat" in the production of hydropericardium and ascites in chickens. Am J Vet Res 25:1210–1219.
7. Allen, N.K., S.R. Aakhus-Allen, and M.M. Walser.

1981. Toxic effects of repeated ethanol intubations to chicks. Poult Sci 60:941–943.

8. Al-Mashhadani, E.H., and M.M. Beck. 1985. Effect of atmospheric ammonia on the surface ultrastructure of the lung and trachea of broiler chicks. Poult Sci 64:2056–2061.

9. Amure, J., and J.C. Stuart. 1978. Dieldrin toxicity in poultry associated with wood shavings. Vet Rec 102:387.

10. Andreasen, J.R., Jr. 1993. Metaldehyde toxicosis in ducklings. J Vet Diagn Invest 5:500–501.

11. Arai, M., E. Stauber, and C.M. Shropshire. 1992. Evaluation of selected plants for their toxic effects in canaries. J Am Vet Med Assoc 200:1329–1331.

12. Arnouts, S., J. Buyse, M. M. Cokelaere, and E. Decuypere. 1993. Jojoba meal (Simmondsia chinensis) in the diet of broiler breeder pullets: Physiological and endocrinological effects. Poult Sci 72:1714–1721.

13. Bahl, A.K., and B.S. Pomeroy. 1978. Acute toxicity in poults associated with carbaryl insecticide. Avian Dis 22:526–528.

14. Bai, K.M., and M.K. Krishnakumari. 1986. Acute oral toxicity of Warfarin to poultry, Gallus domesticus: a non-target species. Bull Environ Contam Toxicol 37:544–549.

15. Barnett, B.D. 1975. Toxicity of pokeberries (fruit of Phytolacca americana Large) for turkey poults. Poult Sci 54:1215–1217.

16. Bartov, L. 1989. Lack of effect of dietary factors on nicarbazin toxicity in broiler chicks. Poult Sci 68:145–152.

17. Bedford, M. R., and H. L. Classen. 1993. An in vitro assay for prediction of broiler intestinal viscosity and growth when fed rye-based diets in the presence of exogenous enzymes. Poult Sci 72:137–143.

18. Beers, K. W., T. J. Raup, W. G. Bottje, and T.W. Odom. 1989. Physiological responses of heat-stressed broilers fed nicarbazin. Poult Sci 68:428–434.

19. Behr, K-.P., H. Lüders, and C. Plate. 1986. Safety of halofuginone (Stenorol®) in geese (Anser anser f. dom.), Muscovy ducks (Cairina moschata f. dom.) and pekin ducks (Anas platyrhynchos f. dom.). Dtsch Tieraerztl Wochenschr 93:4–8.

20. Bell, J.M. 1993. Factors affecting the nutritional value of canola meal: A review. Can J Anim Sci 73:679–697.

21. Bennett, W.M. 1989. Mechanism of aminoglycoside nephrotoxicity. Clin Exp Pharm Physiol 16:1–6.

22. Bergmann, V., G. Baumann, and B. Kahle. 1989. Zur Pathologie der akuten Monensin-Vergiftung bei Broilern und Lämmern. Monatsh Vet 44:460–463.

23. Bhatnagar, M.K., S. Yamashiro, and L.L. David. 1980. Ultrastructural study of liver fibrosis in turkeys fed diets containing rapeseed meal. Res Vet Sci 29:260–265.

24. Bierer, B.W. 1958. The ill effects of excessive formaldehyde fumigation on turkey poults. J Am Vet Med Assoc 132:174–176.

25. Blakley, B.R. 1982. Lindane toxicity in pigeons. Can Vet J 23:267–268.

26. Blom, L. 1975. Residues of drugs in eggs after medication of laying hens for eight days. Acta Vet Scand 16:396–404.

27. Bokori, J., S. Fekete, I. Kádar, F. Vetési, and M. Albert. 1993. Complex study of the physiological role of aluminum. II. Aluminum tolerance test in broiler chickens. Acta Vet Hung 41:235–264.

28. Booth, N.H. 1988. Drugs and Chemical Residues in the Edible Tissue of Animals. Chap. 66. In N.H. Booth, and L.E. McDonald (eds.). Veterinary Pharmacology and Therapeutics, 6th ed. Iowa State University Press, Ames, IA, pp. 1149–1205.

29. Bowes, V., and R. Puls. 1992. Fenthion toxicity in bald eagles. Can Vet J 33:678.

30. Braunius, W.W. 1986. Monensin/sulfachloropyrazine intoxicatie bij kalkoenen. Tijdschr Diergeneeskd 111:676–678.

31. Brenes, A., M. Smith, W. Guenter, and R. R. Marquardt. 1993. Effect of enzyme supplementation on the performance and digestive tract size of broiler chickens fed wheat- and barley-based diets. Poult Sci 72:1731–1739.

32. Brenes, A., R.R. Marquardt, W. Guenter, and B.A. Rotter. 1993. Effect of enzyme supplementation on the nutritional value of raw, autoclaved, and dehulled lupins (Lupinus albus) in chicken diets. Poult Sci 72:2281–2293.

33. Brenes, A., B.A. Rotter, R.R. Marquardt, and W. Guenter. 1993. The nutritional value of raw, autoclaved, and dehulled peas (Pisum satirum L.) in chicken diets as affected by enzyme supplementation. Can J Anim Sci 73:605–614.

34. Brown, C., W.B. Gross, and M. Ehrich. 1986. Effects of social stress on the toxicity of malathion in young chickens. Avian Dis 30:679–682.

35. Brown, T.P., C.T. Larsen, D.L. Boyd, and B.M. Allen. 1991. Ulcerative cholecystitis produced by 3-nitro-4-hydroxy-phenylarsonic acid toxicosis in turkey poults. Avian Dis 35:241–243.

36. Broz, J., and M. Frigg. 1987. Incompatibility between lasalocid and chloramphenicol in broiler chicks after a long-term simultaneous administration. Vet Res Commun 11:159–172.

37. Burger, W.P., T. W. Naude, I.B.J. Van Rensburg, C.J. Botha, and A.C.E. Pienaar. 1994. Cardiomyopathy in ostriches (Struthio-camelus) due to Avocado (Persea americana var. guatemalensis) intoxication. J S Afr Vet Assoc 65:113–118.

38. Campbell, L.D. 1987. Effects of different intact glucosinolates on liver hemorrhage in laying hens and the influence of vitamin K. Nutr Rep Int 35:1221–1227.

39. Cantor, A.H., D.M. Nash, and T.H. Johnson. 1984. Toxicity of selenium in drinking water of poultry. Nutr Rep Int 29:683–688.

40. Cardona, C. J., F.D. Galey, A.A. Bickford, B.R. Charlton, and G.L. Cooper. 1993. Skeletal myopathy produced with experimental dosing of turkeys with monensin. Avian Dis 37:107–117.

41. Carlile, F.S. 1984. Ammonia in poultry houses: a literature review. World's Poult Sci J 40:99–113.

42. Carlton, W.W. 1966. Experimental coal tar poisoning in the White Pekin duck. Avian Dis 10:484–502.

43. Cheeke, P.R. 1988. Toxicity and metabolism of pyrrolizidine alkaloids. J Anim Sci 66:2343–2350.

44. Chowdhury, S.D. 1988. Lathyrism in poultry—a review. World's Poult Sci J 44:7–16.

45. Christensen, V.L., and J.F. Ort. 1991. Iodine toxicity in large white turkey breeder hens. Poult Sci 70:2402–2410.

46. Coats, J.R. 1990. Mechanisms of toxic action and structure-activity relationships for organochlorine and synthetic pyrethroid insecticides. Environ Health Perspect 87:255–262.

47. Corner, A.H., H.W. Hulan, D.M. Nash, and F.G. Proudfoot. 1985. Pathological changes associated with the feeding of soybean oil or oil extracted from different rapeseed cultivars to single comb white leghorn cockerels. Poult Sci 64:1438–1450.

48. Couillard, C.M., and F.A. Leighton. 1990. The toxicopathology of Prudhoe Bay crude oil in chicken embryos. Fund Appl Toxicol 14:30–39.

49. Cruickshank, J.J., and J.S. Sim. 1987. Effects of excess vitamin D_3 and cage density on the incidence of leg abnormalities in broiler chickens. Avian Dis 31:332–338.

50. Czarnecki, C.M. 1986. Quantitative morphological alterations during the development of furazolidone-induced cardiomyopathy in turkeys. J Comp Pathol 96:63–75.

51. Czarnecki, C.M., and H.A. Badreldin. 1987. Graded ethanol consumption in young turkey poults: effect on body weight, feed intake and development of cardiomegaly. Res Commun Subst Abuse 8:93–96.

52. Czarnecki, G.L., and D.H. Baker. 1982. Tolerance of

the chick to excess dietary cadmium as influenced by dietary cysteine and by experimental infection with Eimeria acervulina. J Anim Sci 54:983–988.

53. Daft, B.M., A.A. Bickford, and M.A. Hammarlund. 1989. Experimental and field sulfaquinoxaline toxicosis in leghorn chickens. Avian Dis 33:30–34

54. Dalvi, R.R. 1988. Toxicology of thiram: A review. Vet Hum Toxicol 30:480–484.

55. Damron, B.L., and L.K. Flunker. 1993. Broiler chick and laying hen tolerance to sodium hypochlorite in drinking water. Poult Sci 72:1650–1655.

56. Davis, C. 1983. Narasin toxicity in turkeys. Vet Rec 113:627.

57. Davison, S., and R.F. Wideman. 1992. Excess sodium bicarbonate in the diet and its effect on leghorn chickens. Br Poult Sci 33:859–870.

58. Dean, C.E., B.M. Hargis, and P.S. Hargis. 1991. Effects of zinc toxicity on thyroid function and histology in broiler chicks. Toxicol Lett 57:309–318.

59. Deaton, J.W., F.N. Reece, and F.D. Thornberry. 1986. Atmospheric ammonia and incidence of blood spots in eggs. Poult Sci 65:1427–1428.

60. Delaplane, J.P., and J.H. Milliff. 1948. The gross and micropathology of sulfaquinoxaline poisoning in chickens. Am J Vet Res 9:92–96.

61. De Ment, S.H., J.J. Chisolm, M.A. Eckhaus, and J.D. Strandberg. 1987. Toxic lead exposure in the urban rock dove. J Wildl Dis 3:273–278

62. Dewar, W.A., P.A.L. Wight, R.A. Pearson, and M.J. Gentle. 1983. Toxic effects of high concentrations of zinc oxide in the diet of the chick and laying hen. Br Poult Sci 24:397–404.

63. Dharma, D.N., S.D. Sleight, R.K. Ringer, and S.D. Aust. 1982. Pathologic effects of 2,2′,4,4′, 5,5′- and 2,3′,4,4′, 5,5′-hexabromobiphenyl in white leghorn cockerels. Avian Dis 26:542–552.

64. Dhillon, A.S., R.W. Winterfield, and H.L. Thacker. 1982. Quaternary ammonium compound toxicity in chickens. Avian Dis 26:928–931.

65. Diaz, G.J., R.J. Julian, and E.J. Squires. 1994. Lesions in broiler chickens following experimental intoxication with cobalt. Avian Dis 38:308–316.

66. Diaz, G.J., R.J. Julian, and E.J. Squires. 1995. Effect of graded levels of dietary nitrite on pulmonary hypertension in broiler chickens and dilatory cardiomyopathy in turkey poults. Avian Pathol 24:109–120.

67. Dickinson, J.O., and R.C. Braun. 1987. Effect of 2(3)-tertbutyl-4-hydroxyanisole (BHA) and 2-chloroethanol against pyrole production and chronic toxicity of monocrotaline in chickens. Vet Hum Toxicol 29:11–15.

68. DiTomaso, J.M. 1994. Plants reported to be poisonous to animals in the United States. Vet Hum Toxicol 36:49–52.

69. D'Mello, J.P.F., and A.G. Walker. 1991. Detoxification of jackbeans (Canavalia ensiformis): Studies with young chicks. Anim Fed Sci Tech 33:117–127.

70. D'Mello, J.P.F., C.M. Duffus, and J.H. Duffus (eds.). 1991. Toxic Substances in Crop Plants. Royal Society of Chemists, Cambridge, United Kingdom.

71. Donham, K.J. 1991. Air quality relationships to occupational health in the poultry industry. Proc 42nd North Central Avian Disease Conference, Des Moines, IA, pp. 43–47.

72. Dorn, P., R. Weber, J. Weikel, and E. Wessling. 1983. Intoxikation durch gleichzeitige verabreichung von chloramphenicol und monensin bei puten. Prakt Tierarzt 64:240–243.

73. Dowling, L. 1992. Ionophore toxicity in chickens: A review of pathology and diagnosis. Avian Pathol 21:355–368.

74. Dufour, L., J.E. Sander, R.D. Wyatt, G.N. Rowland, and R.K. Page. 1992. Experimental exposure of broiler chickens to boric acid to assess clinical signs and lesions of toxicosis. Avian Dis 36:1007–1011.

75. Dumonceaux, G., and G.J. Harrison. 1994. Toxins. In B.W. Ritchie, G.J. Harrison, and L.R. Harrison (eds.). Avian Medicine: Principles and Application, Wingers Publ. Inc., Lakeworth, FL, pp. 1030–1049.

76. Dunachie, J.F., and W.W. Fletcher. 1970. The toxicity of certain herbicides to hens' eggs assessed by the egg injection technique. Ann Appl Biol 66:515–520.

77. Dunn, M.A., N.E. Johnson, M.Y.B. Liew, and E. Ross. 1993. Dietary aluminum chloride reduces the amount of intestinal calbindin D-28K in chicks fed low calcium or low phosphorus diets. J Nutr 123:1786–1793.

78. Durham, H.D., and D.J. Ecobichon. 1986. An assessment of the neurotoxic potential of fenitrothion in the hen. Toxicology 41:319–332.

79. Eason, P.J., R.J. Johnson, and G.H. Castleman. 1990. The effects of dietary inclusion of narbon beans (Vicia narbonensis) on the growth of broiler chickens. Aust J Agric Res 41:565–571.

80. Edelstein, S., C.S Fullmer, and R.H. Wasserman. 1984. Gastrointestinal absorption of lead in chicks: involvement of the cholecalciferol endocrine system. J Nutr 114:692–700.

81. Edwards, H.M., Jr. 1987. Effects of thiuram disulfiram and a trace element mixture on the incidence of tibial dyschondroplasia in chickens. J Nutr 117:964–969.

82. Egyed, M.N., and U. Bendheim. 1977. Mass poisoning in chickens caused by consumption of organo-phosphorus (dichlorvos) contaminated drinking water. Refu Vet 34:107–110.

83. Ehrich, M., L. Correll, J. Strait, W. McCain, and J. Wilcke. 1992. Toxicity and toxicokinetics of carbaryl in chickens and rats: A comparative study. J Toxicol Environ Health 36:411–423.

84. Elliot, M.A., and H.M. Edwards, Jr. 1991. Some effects of dietary aluminum and silicon on broiler chickens. Poult Sci 70:1390–1402.

85. Elliott, J.E., R.W. Butler, R.J. Norstrom, and P.E. Whitehead. 1988. Levels of Polychlorinated Dibenzodioxins and Polychlorinated Dibenzofurans in Eggs of Great Blue Herons (Ardea herodias) in British Columbia, 1983–87: Possible Impact on Reproductive Success. Progress Notes No. 176. Canadian Wildlife Service, Ottawa.

86. Elzubeir, E.A., and R.H. Davis. 1988. Sodium nitroprusside, a convenient source of dietary cyanide for the study of chronic cyanide toxicity. Br Poult Sci 29:779–783.

87. Emmel, M.W. 1935. The toxicity of Glottidium vesicarium (Jacq) Harper seeds for the fowl. J Am Vet Med Assoc 87:13–21.

88. Faddoul, G.P., S.V. Amato, M. Sevoian, and G.W. Fellows. 1967. Studies on intolerance to sulfaquinoxaline in chickens. Avian Dis 11:226–240.

89. Farage-Elawar, M. 1989. Enzyme and behavioral changes in young chickens as a result of carbaryl treatment. J Toxicol Environ Health 26:119–131.

90. Farage-Elawar, M., and M. Francis. 1988. Effects of fenthion, fenitrothion and desbromoleptophos on gait, acetylcholine and neurotoxic esterase in young chicks after in ovo exposure. Toxicology 49:253–261.

91. Fedde, M.R., and W.D. Kuhlmann. 1979. Cardiopulmonary responses to inhaled sulfur dioxide in the chicken. Poult Sci 58:1584–1591.

92. Fenwick, G.R., C.L. Curl, E.J. Butler, N.M. Greenwood, and A.W. Pearson. 1984. Rapeseed meal and egg taint: Effects of low glucosinolate Brassica napus meal, dehulled meal and hulls, and of neomycin. J Sci Food Agric 35:749–756

93. Ficken, M.D., D.P. Wages, and E. Gonder. 1989. Monensin toxicity in turkey breeder hens. Avian Dis 33:186–190.

94. Fitzgerald, S.D., J.M. Sullivan, and R.J. Everson. 1990. Suspected ethanol toxicosis in two wild cedar waxwings. Avian Dis 34:488–490.

95. Flory, W., and C.D. Hebert. 1984. Determination of the oral toxicity of Sesbania drummondii seeds in chickens. Am J Vet Res 45:955–958.

96. Flunker, L.K., B.L. Damron, and S.F. Sundlof. 1989. Response of White Leghorn hens to various dietary levels of Cassia obtusifolia and nutrient fortification as a means of alleviating depressed performance. Poult Sci 68:909–913.

97. Flunker, L.K., B.L. Damron, and S.F. Sundlof. 1990. Tolerance to ground Sesbania macrocarpa seed by broiler chicks and White Leghorn hens. Poult Sci 69:669–672.

98. Fowler, M.E. 1986. Plant poisoning in pet birds and reptiles. In R.W. Kirk (ed.). Current Veterinary Therapy. IX. W.B. Saunders Co., Philadelphia, PA, pp. 737-743.

99. Frank, A.A., and W.M. Reed. 1990. Comparative toxicity of coniine, an alkaloid of Conium maculatum (poison hemlock), in chickens, quails, and turkeys. Avian Dis 34:433–437.

100. Frank, R., G.J. Sirons, and D. Wilson. 1981. Residues of 4-aminopyridine in poisoned birds. Bull Environ Contam Toxicol 26:389–392.

101. Frank, R., N. Fish, G.J. Sirons, J. Walker, H.L. Orr, and S. Leeson. 1983. Residues of polychlorinated phenols and anisoles in broilers raised on contaminated wood shaving litter. Poult Sci 62:1559–1565.

102. Frank, R., P. Mineau, H.E. Braun, I.K. Barker, S.W. Kennedy, and S. Trudeau. 1991. Deaths of Canada geese following spraying of turf with diazinon. Bull Environ Contam Tox 46:852–858.

103. Friesen, O.D., W. Guenter, R.R. Marquardt, and B.A. Rotter. 1992. The effect of enzyme supplementation on the apparent metabolizable energy and nutrient digestibilities of wheat, barley, oats, and rye for the young broiler chick. Poult Sci 71:1710–1721.

104. Galt, D.E. 1988. Reduced hatchability of eggs associated with pentachlorophenol contaminated shavings. Can Vet J 29:65–67.

105. Gilead, M., and U. Bendheim. 1986. Formalin poisoning in turkeys. Israel J Vet Med 42:193–194.

106. Giri, S.N., A.A. Bickford, and A.E. Barger. 1979. Effects of 2-chloro-4-acetotoluidine (CAT) toxicity on biochemical and morphological alterations in quail. Avian Dis 23:794–811.

107. Glahn, R.P., R.F. Wideman, Jr., and B.S. Cowen. 1989. Order of exposure to high dietary calcium and Gray strain infections bronchitis virus alters renal function and the incidence of urolithiasis. Poult Sci 68:1193–1204.

108. Gough, A.W., and L.J. Weber. 1978. Massive liver hemorrhage in Ontario broiler chickens. Avian Dis 22:205–210.

109. Granot, I., I. Bartov, I. Plavnik, E. Wax, S. Hurwitz, and M. Pines. 1991. Increased skin tearing in broilers and reduced collagen synthesis in skin in vivo and in vitro in response to the coccidiostat halofuginone. Poult Sci 70:1559–1563.

110. Gregory, D.G., S.L. Vanhooser, and E.L. Stair. 1995. Light and electron microscopic lesions in peripheral nerves of broiler chickens due to roxarsone and lasalocid toxicoses. Avian Dis 39:408–416.

111. Guenter, W., and P.H.B. Hahn. 1986. Fluorine toxicity and laying hen performance. Poult Sci 65:769–778.

112. Gwathmey, J.K. 1991. Morphological changes associated with furazolidone-induced cardiomyopathy: Effects of digoxin and propranolol. J Comp Pathol 104:33–45.

113. Hafez, Y.S.M., E. Chavez, P. Vohra, and F.H. Kratzer. 1978. Methionine toxicity in chicks and poults. Poult Sci 57:699–703.

114. Haigh, J.C. 1979. Levamisole in waterfowl: Trials on effect and toxicity. J Zoo Anim Med 10:103–105.

115. Halvorson, D.A., C. Van Dijk, and P. Brown. 1982. Ionophore toxicity in turkey breeders. Avian Dis 26:634–639.

116. Hanrahan, L.A., D.E. Corrier, and S.A. Naqi. 1981. Monensin toxicosis in broiler chickens. Vet Pathol 18:665–671.

117. Hansen, A.A. 1927. Stock poisoning by plants in the nightshade family. J Am Vet Med Assoc 71:221–227.

118. Hanson, J., and J. Howell. 1981. Possible fenthion toxicity in magpies (Pica pica). Can Vet J 22:18–19.

119. Hare, T., and A.B. Orr. 1945. Poultry poisoned by zinc phosphide. Vet Rec 57:17.

120. Hargis, A.M., E. Stauber, S. Casteel, and D. Eitner. 1989. Avocado (Persea americana) intoxication in caged birds. J Am Vet Med Assoc 194:64–66.

121. Harper, J.A., and G.H. Arscott. 1962. Toxicity of common and hairy vetch seed for poults and chicks. Poult Sci 41:1968–1974.

122. Harper, M.J., and M. Hindmarsh. 1990. Lead poisoning in magpie geese Anseranas semipalmata from ingested lead pellet at Bool Lagoon Game Reserve (South Australia). Aust Wildl Res 17:141–145.

123. Hatch, R.C. 1988. Veterinary Toxicology. Section 17. In N.H. Booth, and L.E. McDonald (eds.). Veterinary Pharmacology and Therapeutics, 6th ed. Iowa State University Press, Ames, IA, pp. 1001–1148.

124. Hathcock, J.N., M.M. Labadan, and J.P. Mateo. 1975. Effects of dietary protein level on toxicity of Leucaena leucocephala to chicks. Nutr Rep Int 11:55–62.

125. Heinz, G.H. 1979. Methylmercury:reproductive and behavioral effects on three generations of mallard ducks. J Wildl Manage 43:394–401.

126. Heinz, G.H., and L.N. Locke. 1976. Brain lesions in mallard ducklings from parents fed methylmercury. Avian Dis 20:9–17.

127. Henderson, B.M., and R.W. Winterfield. 1975. Acute copper toxicosis in the Canada goose. Avian Dis 19:385–387.

128. Henny, C.J., E.J. Kolbe, E.F. Hill, and L.J. Blus. 1987. Case histories of bald eagles and other raptors killed by organophosphorus insecticides topically applied to livestock. J Wildl Dis 23:292–295.

129. Heuser, G.F., and A.E. Schumacher. 1942. The feeding of corn cockle to chickens. Poult Sci 2:86–93.

130. Hill, D.L., C.I. Hall, J.E. Sander, O.J. Fletcher, R.K. Page, and S.W. Davis. 1994. Diazinon toxicity in broilers. Avian Dis 38:393–396.

131. Hino, T., T. Noguchi, and H. Naito. 1987. Effect of gizzerosine on acid secretion by isolated mucosal cells of chicken proventriculus. Poult Sci 66:548–551.

132. Horikawa, H., T. Masumura, S. Hirano, E. Watanabe, and T. Ishibashi. 1992. Optimum dietary level of gizzerosine for maximum calcium content in the femur of chicks. Jpn Poult Sci 29:361–367.

133. Huisman, J. 1991. Antinutritional factors in poultry feeds and their management. Proc 8th Eur Symp Poult Nutr, Venezia-Mestre, Italy, World Poult Sci Assoc, pp. 42-61.

134. Humphreys, D.J. 1979. Poisoning in poultry. World's Poult Sci J 35:161–176.

135. Humphreys, D.J., J.B.J. Stodulski, R.R. Fysh, and N.M. Howie. 1980. Haloxon poisoning in geese. Vet Rec 107:541.

136. Hunter, B., and G. Wobeser. 1980. Encephalopathy and peripheral neuropathy in lead-poisoned mallard ducks. Avian Dis 24:169–178.

137. Hussein, A.S., A.H. Cantor, A.J. Pescatore, and T.H. Johnson. 1993. Effect of dietary aluminum and vitamin D interaction on growth and calcium and phosphorus metabolism of broiler chicks. Poult Sci 72:306–309.

138. Jackson, A.R.B., M.T.C. Runnegar, R.B. Cumming, and J.F. Brunner. 1986. Experimental acute intoxication of young layer and broiler chickens with the cyanobacterium (blue-green alga) Microcystis aeruginosa. Avian Pathol 15:741–748.

139. Jansman, A.J.M. 1993. Tannins in feedstuffs for simple-stomached animals. Nutr Res Reviews 6:209–236.

140. Jensen, W.I., and J.P. Allen. 1981. Naturally occurring and experimentally induced castor bean (Ricinus communis) poisoning in ducks. Avian Dis 25:184–194.

141. Jeroch, H., E. Helander, H.J. Schlöffel, K.H. Engerer, H. Pingel, and G. Gebhardt. 1991. Investigation of effectiveness of beta-glucanase containing enzyme preparation "Avizyme®" supplemented to broilers fattening diet based on barley. Arch Geflügelk 55:22–25.

142. Jones, J.E., J. Solis, B.L. Hughes, D.J. Castaldo, and J.E. Toler. 1990. Reproduction responses of broiler-breeders to anticoccidial agents. Poult Sci 69:27–36.

143. Jordan, F.T.W., J.M. Howell, J. Howorth, and J.K. Rayton. 1976. Clinical and pathological observations on field and experimental zoalene poisoning in broiler chicks and the effect of the drug on laying hens. Avian Pathol 5:175–185.

144. Julian, R.J. 1991. Poisons and toxins. In B.W. Calnek, H.J. Barnes, C.W. Beard, W.M. Reed, and H.W. Yoder (eds.). Diseases of Poultry, 9th ed. Iowa State University Press, Ames, IA, pp. 863–884.

145. Julian, R.J. 1993. Ascites in poultry. Avian Pathol 22:419–454.

146. Julian, R.J., G.W. Friars, H. French, and M. Quinton. 1987. The relationship of right ventricular hypertrophy, right ventricular failure, and ascites to weight gain in broiler and roaster chickens. Avian Dis 31:130–135.

147. Julian, R.J., L.J. Caston, and S. Leeson. 1992. The effect of dietary sodium on right ventricular failure-induced ascites, gain and fat deposition in meat-type chickens. Can J Vet Res 56:214–219.

148. Kangas, J., K. Louhelainen, and K. Husman. 1987. Gaseous health hazards in livestock confinement building. J Agric Sci (Finl) 59:57–62.

149. Karstad, L. 1971. Angiopathy and cardiopathy in wild waterfowl from ingestion of lead shot. Connecticut Med 35:355–360.

150. Karunajeewa, H., E.G. Ijagbuji, and R.L. Reece. 1990. Effect of dietary levels of rapeseed meal and polyethylene glycol on the performance of male broiler chickens. Br Poult Sci 31:545–555.

151. Katz, R.S., and D.H. Baker. 1975. Methionine toxicity in the chick: Nutritional and metabolic implications. J Nutr 105:1168–1175.

152. Kazacos, E.A., and J.F. Van Vleet. 1989. Sequential ultrastructural changes of the pancreas in zinc toxicosis in ducklings. Am J Pathol 134:581–595.

153. Keeler, R.F. 1991. Toxicology of Plant and Fungal Compounds. Handbook of Natural Toxins, vol. 6. Marcel Dekker, New York.

154. Keirs, R.W., and L. Bennett. 1993. Broiler performance loss associated with biogenic amines. Proc Md Nutr Conf for Feed Manufacturers, Baltimore, MD, pp. 31–34.

155. Keshavarz, K. 1993. Effect of corn contaminated with velvetweed seeds on eggs. J Appl Poult Res 2:232–238.

156. Kinde, H. 1988. A fatal case of oak poisoning in double-wattled cassowary (Casuarius casuarius). Avian Dis 32:849–851.

157. Kinde, H., H.L. Shivaprasad, F.D. Galey, G. Cutler, and D. Hamar. 1992. Sudden drop in egg production associated with vitamin A toxicity in chickens. Proc Western Poultry Disease Conference, Sacramento, CA, p. 5.

158. Klein, P.N. 1989. The effects of naphthalene and p-dichloro-benzene (mothball chemicals) in canaries and finches fed cumulative amounts in contaminated feed. Proc West Poult Dis Conf, Tempe, AR, p. 164.

159. Kovatsis, A., V.P. Kotsaki-Kovatsi, E. Nikolaidis, J. Flaskos, S. Tzika, and G. Tzotzas. 1994. The influence of Datura ferox alkaloids on egg-laying hens. Vet Hum Toxicol 36:89–91.

160. Kubena, L.F., and T.D. Phillips. 1983. Toxicity of vanadium in female leghorn chickens. Poult Sci 62:47–50.

161. Kupsh, C.C., R.J. Julian, V.E.O. Valli, and G.A. Robinson. 1991. Renal damage induced by uranyl nitrate and oestradiol-17ß in Japanese quail and Wistar rats. Avian Pathol

20:25–34.

162. Laczay, P., F. Simon, Z. Mora, and J. Lehel. 1990. Comparative studies on the toxic interactions of the ionophore anticoccidials with tiamulin in broiler chicks. Arch Gefluegelkd 54:129–132.

163. Larsen, C., B.S. Jortner, and M. Ehrich. 1986. Effect of neurotoxic organophosphorus compounds in turkeys. J Toxicol Environ Health 17:365–374.

164. Latta, D.M., and W.E. Donaldson. 1986. Lead toxicity in chicks: Interactions with dietary methionine and choline. J Nutr 116:1561–1568.

165. Lawal, S., P.A. Abdu, G.B.D. Jonathan, and O.J. Hambolu. 1992. Snakebites in poultry. Vet Hum Toxicol 34:528–530.

166. Leach, R.M., Jr., C.I. Rosenblum, M.J. Amman, and J. Burdette. 1990. Broiler chicks fed low-calcium diets. 2. Increased sensitivity to copper toxicity. Poult Sci 69:1905–1910.

167. Lee, S.R., W.M. Britton, and G.N. Rowland. 1980. Magnesium toxicity: Bone lesions. Poult Sci 59:2403–2411.

168. Leeson, S., L.J. Caston, and J.D. Summers. 1989. The effect of graded levels of nicarbazin on reproductive performance of laying hens. Can J Anim Sci 69:757–764.

169. Leighton, F.A. 1986. Clinical, gross and histological findings in herring gulls and Atlantic puffins that ingested Prudhoe Bay crude oil. Vet Pathol 23:254–263.

170. Lekkas, S., P. Iordanidis, and E. Artopios. 1986. Intoxication by creolin in broilers. Israel J Vet Med 42:114–119.

171. Leon, A.M., J.P. Caffin, M. Plassart, and M.L. Picard. 1991. Effect of concanavalin A from jackbean seeds on short-term food intake regulation in chicks and laying hens. Anim Feed Sci Tech 32:297–311.

172. Leong, V.Y-M., and T. Brown. 1992. Toxicosis in broiler chicks due to excess dietary ethoxyquin. Avian Dis 36:1102–1106.

173. Leske, K.L., C.J. Jevne, and C.N. Coon. 1993. Extraction methods for removing soybean alpha-galactosides and improving true metabolizable energy for poultry. Anim Feed Sci Tech 41:73–78.

174. Lessler, M.A., and D.A. Ray. 1986. Dietary lead inhibits avian bone fracture healing. J Physiol 371:223P.

175. Locke, L.N., G.E. Bagley, and H.D. Irby. 1966. Acid-fast intranuclear inclusion bodies in the kidneys of mallards fed lead shot. Bull Wildl Dis Assoc 2:127–131.

176. Lotti, M. 1992. The pathogenesis of organophosphate polyneuropathy. Crit Rev Toxicol 21:465–487.

177. Ludke, J.L., and L.N. Locke. 1976. Duck deaths from accidental ingestion of anthelmintic. Avian Dis 20:607–608.

178. Lu, J., G.F. Coombs, Jr., and J.C. Fleet. 1990. Time-course studies of pancreatic exocrine damage induced by excess dietary zinc in the chick. J Nutr 120:389–397.

179. Marceau-Day, M.L. 1989. A study on the toxicity of Sesbania drummondii in chickens and rats. Diss Abstr Int B 49:3045.

180. Mathis, G.F. 1993. Toxicity and acquisition of immunity to coccidia in turkeys medicated with anticoccidials. J Appl Poult Res 2:239–244.

181. Mayeda, B. 1968. The toxic effects in turkey poults of a quaternary ammonium compound in drinking water at 150 and 200 ppm. Avian Dis 12:67–71.

182. Mazliah, J., S. Barron, E. Bental, and I. Reznik. 1989. The effect of chronic lead intoxication in mature chickens. Avian Dis 33:566–570.

183. McCune, E.L., J.E. Savage, and B.L. O'Dell. 1962. Hydropericardium and ascites in chicks fed a chlorinated hydrocarbon. Poult Sci 41:295–299.

184. McDougald, L.R. 1990. Coccidiostat toxicities. Proc 25th Natl Meet Poult Health Condemn, Ocean City, MD, pp. 88–93.

185. McNab, J.M., and R.R. Smithard. 1992. Barley ß-glucan: An antinutritional factor in poultry feeding. Nutr Res Rev 5:45–60.

186. Mirsalimi, S.M., and R.J. Julian. 1993. Saline drink-

ing water in broiler and Leghorn chicks and the effect in broilers of increasing levels and age at time of exposure. Can Vet J 34:413–417.

187. Mirsalimi, S.M., and R.J. Julian. 1993. Effect of excess sodium bicarbonate on the blood volume and erythrocyte deformability of broiler chickens. Avian Pathol 22:495–507.

188. Mirsalimi, S.M., F.S. Qureshi, R.J. Julian, and P.J. O'Brien. 1990. Myocardial biochemical changes in furazolidone-induced cardiomyopathy of turkeys. J Comp Pathol 102:139–147.

189. Mirsalimi, S.M., P.J. O'Brien, and R.J. Julian. 1992. Changes in erythrocyte deformability in NaCl-induced right-sided cardiac failure in broiler chickens. Am J Vet Res 53:2359–2363.

190. Mirsalimi, S.M., P.J. O'Brien, and R.J. Julian. 1993. Blood volume increase in salt-induced pulmonary hypertension, heart failure and ascites in broiler and White Leghorn chickens. Can J Vet Res 57:110–113.

191. Miyazaki, S., and Y. Umemura. 1987. Effects of histamine antagonists, an anticholinergic agent and antacid, on gizzard erosions in broiler chicks. Br Poult Sci 28:39–45.

192. Mohanty, G.C., and J.L. West. 1969. Pathologic features of experimental sodium chloride poisoning in chicks. Avian Dis 13:762–773.

193. Mora, M.A., D.W. Anderson, and M.E. Mount. 1987. Seasonal variation of body condition and organochlorines in wild ducks from California and Mexico. J Wildl Manage 51:132–141.

194. Morrissey, R.L., R.M. Cohn, R.N. Empson, H.L. Greene, O.D. Taunton, and Z.Z. Ziporin. 1977. Relative toxicity and metabolic effects of cholecalciferol and 25-hydroxycholecalciferol in chicks. J Nutr 107:1027–1034.

195. Moslehuddin, A.B.M., Y.D. Hang, and G.S. Stoewsand. 1987. Evaluation of the toxicity of processed Lathyrus sativus seeds in chicks. Nutr Rep Int 36:851–855.

196. Munger, L.L., J.J. Su, and H.J. Barnes. 1993. Coumafuryl (Fumarin®) toxicity in chicks. Avian Dis 37:622–624.

197. Nelson, H.A., R.A. Decker, and D.L. Osheim. 1976. Poisoning in zoo animals with 4-aminopyridine. Vet Toxicol 18:125–126.

198. Neufeld, J. 1992. Salinomycin toxicosis of turkeys: Serum chemistry as an aid to early diagnosis. Can Vet J 33:677.

199. Niemann, K.W. 1928. Report of an outbreak of poisoning in the domesticated fowl, due to death camas. J Am Vet Med Assoc 73:627–630.

200. Norton, J., M. Evans, and J. Connor. 1987. Timber treatment and poultry litter. Queensl Agric J 113:105–107.

201. Nwokolo, E., and L.O.C. Ohale. 1986. Growth and anatomical characteristics of pullet chicks fed diets contaminated with crude petroleum. Bull Environ Contam Toxicol 37:441–447.

202. Ochiai, K., K. Jin, C. Itakura, M. Goryo, K. Yamashita, N. Mizuno, T. Fujinaga, and T. Tsuzuki. 1992. Pathological study of lead poisoning in whooper swans (Cygnus cygnus) in Japan. Avian Dis 36:313–323.

203. Ohlendorf, H.M., A.W. Kilness, J.L. Simmons, R.K. Stroud, D.J. Hoffman, and J.F. Moore. 1988. Selenium toxicosis in wild aquatic birds. J Toxicol Environ Health 24:67–92.

204. Okoye, J.O.A., C.A. Enunwaonye, A.U. Okorie, and F.O.I. Anugwa. 1987. Pathological effects of feeding roasted castor bean meal (Ricinus communis) to chicks. Avian Pathol 16:283–290.

205. Ologhobo, A.D., D.F. Apata, A. Oyejide, and O. Akinpelu. 1993. Toxicity of raw lima beans (Phaseolus lunatus L.) and lima bean fractions for growing chicks. Br Poult Sci 34:505–522.

206. Ologhobo, A.D., D.F. Apata, and A. Oyejide. 1993. Utilisation of raw jackbean (Canavalia ensiformis) and jackbean fractions in diets for broiler chicks. Br Poult Sci 34:323–337.

207. Onderka, D.K., and R. Bhatnagar. 1982. Ultrastruc-

tural changes of sodium chloride-induced cardiomyopathy in turkey poults. Avian Dis 26:835–841.

208. Ortiz, L.T., C. Centeno, and J. Trevino. 1993. Tannins in fababean seeds: Effects on the digestion of protein and amino acids in growing chicks. Anim Feed Sci Tech 41:271–278.

209. Osweiler, G.D., T.L. Carson, W.B. Buck, and G.A. Van Gelder (eds.). 1985. Clinical and Diagnostic Veterinary Toxicology. Kendall/Hunt Publishing Co., Dubuque, IA.

210. Oyetunde, O.O.F., R.G. Thomson, and H.C. Carlson. 1978. Aerosol exposure of ammonia, dust and Escherichia coli in broiler chickens. Can Vet J 19:187–193.

211. Page, R.K. 1975. Teratogenic activity of arasan fed to broiler breeder hens. Avian Dis 19:463–72.

212. Page, R.K., S. Vezey, O.W. Charles, and T. Hollifield. 1977. Effects on feed consumption and egg production of coffee bean seed (Cassia obtusifolia) fed to White Leghorn hens. Avian Dis 21:90–96.

213. Page, R.K., O.J. Fletcher, S. Vezey, P. Bush, and N. Booth. 1978. Effects of continuous feeding of toxaphene to white leghorn layers. Avian Pathol 7:289–294.

214. Page, R.K., O.J. Fletcher, and P. Bush. 1979. Calcium toxicosis in broiler chicks. Avian Dis 23:1055–1059.

215. Panigrahi, S., J. Rickard, G.M. O'Brien, and C. Gay. 1992. Effects of different rates of drying cassava root on its toxicity to broiler chicks. Br Poult Sci 33:1025–1042.

216. Panigrahy, B., L.C. Grumbles, and C.F. Hall. 1979. Insecticide poisoning in peafowls and lead poisoning in a cockatoo. Avian Dis 23:760–762.

217. Peckham, M.C. 1982. Poisons and Toxins. Chapt. 34. In M.S. Hofstad, H.J. Barnes, B.W. Calnek, W.M. Reid, and H.W. Yoder, Jr. (eds.). Diseases of Poultry, 8th ed. Iowa State University Press, Ames, IA, pp. 738–818.

218. Peeters, N., N. Viaene, and L. Devriese. 1977. Poisoning in pigeons after administration of vitamin B6 (pyridoxine) [abst no. 700]. Poult Abstr 4:108.

219. Perelman, B., and E.S. Kuttin. 1988. Parsley-induced photosensitivity in ostriches and ducks. Avian Pathol 17:183–192.

220. Perelman, B., J.M. Abarbanel, A. Gur-Lavie, Y. Meller, and T. Elad. 1986. Clinical and pathological changes caused by the interaction of lasalocid and chloramphenicol in broiler chickens. Avian Pathol 15:279–288.

221. Perelman, B., M. Pirak, and B. Smith. 1993. Effects of the accidental feeding of lasalocid sodium to broiler-breeder chickens. Vet Rec 132:271–273.

222. Perez, L., I. Fernandez-Figares, R. Nieto, J.F. Aguilera, and C. Prieto. 1993. Amino acid ileal digestibility of some grain legume seeds in growing chickens. Anim Prod 56:261–267.

223. Pescatore, A.J., and J.M. Harter-Dennis. 1989. Effects of ferrous sulfate consumption on the performance of broiler chicks. Poult Sci 68:1063–1067.

224. Philbey, A.W. 1991. Skeletal myopathy induced by monensin in adult turkeys. Aust Vet J 68:250–251.

225. Phillips, R.A., F.S. Van Sambeek, and R.K. Page. 1995. Acute sulfur toxicity in broiler chicks. Proc 44th West Poult Dis Conf, Sacramento, CA, p. 1.

226. Pietsch, W., and E. Ruffle. 1986. Zur toxizität des monensins und zu problemen seines einsatzes im broilerfutter. Monatsh Vet 41:851–854.

227. Poli, A., and G. Renzoni. 1983. Chick oedema disease in fowls naturally contaminated with 2,3,7,8-tetrachlorodibenzyl-p-dioxin (TCDD) [abst no. 2234]. Poult Abstr 10:273.

228. Potter, L.M., J.P. Blake, M.E. Blair, B.A. Bliss, and D.M. Denbow. 1986. Salinomycin toxicity in turkeys. Poult Sci 65:1955–1959.

229. Prescott, C.A., B.N. Wilkie, B. Hunter, and R.J. Julian. 1982. Influence of a purified grade of pentachlorophenol on the immune response of chickens. Am J Vet Res 43:481–487.

230. Pritzl, M.C., Y.H. Lie, E.W. Kienholz, and C.E.

Whiteman. 1974. The effect of dietary cadmium on development of young chickens. Poult Sci 53:2026–2029.

231. Proudfoot, F.G., and W.F. DeWitt. 1976. The effect of the pellet binder "Lignosol FG" on the chickens digestive system and general performance. Poult Sci 55:629–631.

232. Puls, R. 1994. Mineral Levels in Animal Health: Diagnostic Data, 2nd ed. Sherpa International, Clearbrook, British Columbia, Canada.

233. Puls, R. 1994. Mineral Levels in Animal Health: Bibliographies, 2nd ed. Sherpa International, Clearbrook, British Columbia, Canada.

234. Raharjo, Y.C., P.R. Checke, and G.H. Arscott. 1988. Effects of dietary butylated hydroxyanisole and cysteine on toxicity of Lathyrus odoratus to broiler and Japanese quail chicks. Poult Sci 67:153–155.

235. Rasul, A.R., and J.McM. Howell. 1974. The toxicity of some dithiocarbamate compounds in young and adult domestic fowl. Toxicol Appl Pharmicol 30:63–78.

236. Ratanasethkul, C., C. Riddell, R.E. Salmon, and J.B. O'Niel. 1976. Pathological changes in chickens, ducks and turkeys fed high levels of rapeseed oil. Can J Comp Med 40:360–369.

237. Ratzkowski, C., N. Fine, and S. Edelstein. 1982. Metabolism of cholecalciferol in vitamin D intoxicated chicks. Isr J Med Sci 18:695–700.

238. Reece, R.L. 1988. Review of adverse effects of chemotherapeutic agents in poultry. World Poult Sci J 44:193–216.

239. Reece, R.L., D.A. Barr, W.M. Forsyth, and P.C. Scott. 1985. Investigations of toxicity episodes involving chemotherapeutic agents in Victorian poultry and pigeons. Avian Dis 29:1239–1251.

240. Reece, R.L., D.B. Dickson, and P.J. Burrowes. 1986. Zinc toxicity (new wire disease) in aviary birds. Aust Vet J 63:199.

241. Ressler, C. 1962. Isolation and identification from common vetch of the neurotoxin B-cyano-l-alanine, a possible factor in neurolathyrism. J Biol Chem 237:733–735.

242. Riddell, C. 1984. Toxicity of dimetridazole in waterfowl. Avian Dis 28:974–977.

243. Riddell, C. 1987. Avian Histopathology. American Association of Avian Pathologists, Kennett Square, PA.

244. Riddell, C., S.W. Nielsen, and E.J. Kersting. 1967. Ethylene glycol poisoning in poultry. J Am Vet Med Assoc 150:1531–1535.

245. Roberson, E.L. 1988. Antinematodal Drugs, Chapt. 55. Anticestodal and Antitrematodal Drugs, Chapt. 56. In Booth, N.H. and L.E. McDonald (eds.). Veterinary Pharmacology and Therapeutics. 6th ed. Iowa State University Press, Ames, IA, pp. 882–999.

246. Rossi, A.F., R.D. Miles, B.L. Damron, and L.K. Flunker. 1993. Effects of dietary boron supplementation on broilers. Poult Sci 72:2124–2130.

247. Rothmaier, D.A., and M. Kirchgessner. 1994. White lupins (Lupinus albus, L.)as a replacement for soybean meal in diets for fattening chickens. Arch Gefluegelkd 58:111–114.

248. Rotter, R.G., R.R. Marquardt, and C.G. Campbell. 1991. The nutritional value of low lathyrogenic lathyrus (Lathyrus sativus) for growing chicks. Br Poult Sci 32:1055–1067.

249. Rubio, L.A., A. Brenes, and M. Castano. 1990. The utilization of raw and autoclaved fababeans (Vicia faba L., var. minor) and fababean fractions in diets for growing broiler chickens. Br J Nutr 63:419–430.

250. Sander, J.E., J.L. Wilson, and G.L. Van Wicklen. 1995. Effect of formaldehyde exposure in the hatcher and of ventilation in confinement facilities on broiler performance. Avian Dis 39:420–424.

251. Sander, J.E., J.L. Wilson, G.N. Rowland, and P.J. Middendorf. 1995. Formaldehyde vaporization in the hatcher and the effect on tracheal epithelium of the chick. Avian Dis 39:152–157.

252. Sanderson, G.C., and F.C. Bellrose. 1986. A review of the problem of lead poisoning in waterfowl. Illinois Natural History Survey, 2nd ed., Champaign, IL.

253. Sawant, S.G., P.S. Terse, and R.R. Dalvi. 1990. Toxicity of dietary monensin in quail. Avian Dis 34:571–574.

254. Scott, M.L. 1985. Gizzard erosion. Anim Health Nutr Large Anim Vet (Sept):22–29.

255. Selye, H., and H. Stone. 1943. Role of sodium chloride in production of nephrosclerosis by steroids. Proc Soc Exp Biol Med 52:190–193.

256. Serafin, J.A. 1981. Factors influencing methionine toxicity in young bobwhite quail. Poult Sci 60:204–214.

257. Shapiro, J.L., R.J. Julian, R.J. Hampson, R.G. Trenton, and I.H. Yo. 1988. An unusual necrotizing cholangiohepatitis in broiler chickens. Can Vet J 29:636–639.

258. Shealy, A.L., and E.F. Thomas. 1928. Daubentonia seed poisoning of poultry. Univ Fla Agr Exp Stn Bull 196.

259. Sherman, M., E. Ross, F.F. Sanchez, and M.T.Y. Chang. 1963. Chronic toxicity of dimethoate to hens. J Econ Entomol 56:10–15.

260. Sherman, M., E. Ross, and M.T.Y. Chang. 1964. Acute and subacute toxicity of several organophosphorus insecticides to chicks. Toxicol Appl Pharmacol 6:147–153.

261. Shivaprasad, H.L., and F. Galey. 1995. Diphacinone and zinc phosphide toxicity in a flock of peafowl. Proc 44th West Poult Dis Conf, Sacramento, CA, pp. 116–117.

262. Shlosberg, A., M.N. Egyed, and A. Eilat. 1974. The comparative photosensitizing properties of Ammi majus and Ammi visnaga in goslings. Avian Dis 18:544–550.

263. Shlosberg, A., D. Hadash, S. Tromperl, and M. Meroz. 1976. Poisoning in a flock of chickens after exposure to vapours of methyl bromide and chloropicrin. Refu Vet 33:135–137.

264. Shlosberg, A., S. Held, and R. Bircz. 1978. Poisoning of palm doves with dibutyltin dilaurate. J Am Vet Med Assoc 173:1183–1184.

265. Shlosberg, A., M.N. Egyed, and V. Hanji. 1980. Monocrotophos poisoning in geese caused by drift from crop spraying. Refu Vet 37:42–44.

266. Shropshire, C.M., E. Stauber, and M. Arai. 1992. Evaluation of selected plants for acute toxicosis in budgerigars. J Am Vet Med Assoc 200:936–939.

267. Siller, W.G. 1981. Renal pathology of the fowl—a review. Avian Pathol 10:187–262.

268. Simpson, C.F., B.L. Damron, and R.H. Harms. 1971. Toxic myopathy of chicks fed Cassia occidentalis seeds. Avian Dis 15:284–290.

269. Smalley, H.E. 1973. Toxicity and hazard of the herbicide, paraquat, in turkeys. Poult Sci 52:1625–1628.

270. Snelgrove-Hobson, S.M., P.V.V.P. Rao, and M.K. Bhatnagar. 1988. Ultrastructural alterations in the kidneys of pekin ducks fed methylmercury. Can J Vet Res 52:89–98.

271. Spinato, M.T. 1991. Diazinon toxicity in Canada geese. Can Vet J 32:627.

272. Stedman, T.M., N.H. Booth, P.B. Bush, R.K. Page, and D.D. Goetsch. 1980. Toxicity and bioaccumulation of pentachlorophenol in broiler chickens. Poult Sci 59:1018–1026.

273. Stiles, G.W. 1940. Carbon monoxide poisoning of chicks and poults in poorly ventilated brooders. Poult Sci 19:111–115.

274. Stoltz, J.H., F. Galey, and B. Johnson. 1992. Sudden death in ten psittacine birds associated with the operation of a self-cleaning oven. Vet Hum Toxicol 34:420–421.

275. Stowe, C.M., D.M. Barnes, and T.D. Arendt. 1981. Ethylene glycol intoxication in ducks. Avian Dis 25:538–541.

276. Sugahara, M., T. Hattori, and T. Nakajima. 1992. Effect of dietary gizzerosine from fish meal on mortality and growth of broiler chicks. Anim Sci Tech (Jpn) 63:1234–1239.

277. Tacal, J.V., Jr., B. Daft, and J. McClaine. 1989. Case report: Oleander (Nerium oleander) poisoning in two geese. Proc West Poult Dis Conf, Tempe, AR, p. 167–168.

278. Tang, K.N., G.N. Rowland, and J.R. Veltmann. 1985. Vitamin A toxicity: Comparative changes in bone of the

broiler and Leghorn chicks. Avian Dis 29:416–429.

279. Teeter, R.G., S. Sarani, M.O. Smith, and C.A. Hibberd. 1986. Detoxification of high tannin sorghum grains. Poult Sci 65:67–71.

280. Temperton, H. 1944. Effect of green and sprouted potatoes on laying pullets. Vet Med 39:13–14.

281. Terzic, L., and M. Curcic. 1985. Toxic chemicals and poisoning of farm animals: Survey of cases examined toxicologically and chemically. Vet Glasnik 39:965–973.

282. Ueda, H., and M. Ohshima. 1987. Effects of alfalfa saponin on chick performance and plasma cholesterol level. Jpn J Zool Sci 58:583–590.

283. Umemura, T., H. Nakamura, M. Goryo, and C. Itakura. 1984. Ultrastructural changes of monensin-oleandomycin myopathy in broiler chicks. Avian Pathol 13:743–751.

284. Van Vleet, J.F., G.D. Boon, and V.J. Ferrans. 1981. Induction of lesions of selenium-vitamin E deficiency in ducklings fed silver, copper, cobalt, tellurium, cadmium or zinc: Protection by selenium or vitamin E supplements. Am J Vet Res 42:1206–1217.

285. Veenhuizen, M.F., and G.C. Shurson. 1992. Effects of sulfate in drinking water for livestock. J Am Vet Med Assoc 201:487–492.

286. Veltmann, J.R., Jr., and L.S. Jensen. 1986. Vitamin A toxicosis in the chick and turkey poults. Poult Sci 65:538–545.

287. Venugopalan, C.S., W. Flory, C.D. Hebert, and T. Tucker. 1984. Assessment of smooth muscle toxicity in Cassia occidentalis toxicosis. Vet Hum Toxicol 26:300–2.

288. Wages, D.P., and M.D. Ficken. 1988. Skeletal muscle lesions in turkeys associated with the feeding of monensin. Avian Dis 32:583–586.

289. Wagner, D.D., R.D. Furrow, and B.D. Bradley. 1983. Subchronic toxicity of monensin in broiler chickens. Vet Pathol 20:353–359.

290. Wagstaff, D.J., J.R. McDowell, and H.J. Paulin. 1980. Heptachlor residue accumulation and depletion in broiler chickens. Am J Vet Res 41:765–768.

291. Wallner-Pendleton, E., D.P. Froman, and O. Hedstrom. 1986. Identification of ferrous sulfate toxicity in a commercial broiler flock. Avian Dis 30:430–432.

292. Wallner-Pendleton, E.A., O. Hedstrom, T. Savage, and H. Nakaue. 1989. Toxicity of dicalcium phosphate in the diet of turkey poults. Avian Dis 33:375–376.

293. Waniska, R.D., L.F. Hugo, and L.W. Rooney. 1992. Practical methods to determine the presence of tannins in sorghum. J Appl Poult Res 1:122–128.

294. Webb, D.M., and J.F. Van Vleet. 1991. Early clinical and morphologic alterations in the pathogenesis of furazolidone-induced toxicosis in ducklings. Am J Vet Res 52:1531–1536.

295. Weisman, Y., E. Wax, and I. Bartov. 1994. Monensin toxicity in two breeds of laying hens. Avian Pathol 23:575–578.

296. Wells, R.E., and R.F. Slocombe. 1982. Acute toxicosis of budgerigars (Melopsittacus undulatus) caused by pyrolysis products from heated polytetrafluoroethylene: Microscopic study. Am J Vet Res 43:1243–1248.

297. Wescott, R.B., and H.C. McDougle. 1967. Ethylene oxide toxicosis in chickens. J Am Vet Med Assoc 151:935–938.

298. Westlake, G.E., P.J. Bunyan, P.I. Stanley, and C.H. Walker. 1981. A study on the toxicity and the biochemical effects of ethylene dibromide in the Japanese quail. Br Poult Sci 22:355–364.

299. Whitehead, C.J., D.N. Prashad, and R.O. Blackburn. 1988. Cadmium-induced changes in avian renal morphology. Experientia 44:193–198.

300. Wideman, R.F., B.C. Ford, R.M. Leach, D.F. Wise, and W. Robey. 1993. Liquid methionine hydroxy analog (free acid) and DL methionine attenuate calcium-induced kidney damage in domestic fowl. Poult Sci 72:1245–1258.

301. Wiernusz, C.J., and R.G. Teeter. 1991. Research note: Maxiban™ effects on heat-distressed broiler growth rate and feed efficiency. Poult Sci 70:2207–2209.

302. Wight, P.A.L., W.A. Dewar, and C.L. Saunderson. 1986. Zinc toxicity in the fowl: Ultrastructural pathology and relationship to selenium, lead and copper. Avian Pathol 15:23–38.

303. Wight, P.A.L., R.K. Scougall, D.W.F. Shannon, and J.W. Wells. 1987. Role of glucosinolates in the causation of liver haemorrhages in laying hens fed water-extracted or heat-treated rapeseed cakes. Res Vet Sci 43:313–319.

304. Williams, M.C. 1979. Toxicological investigations on Galenia pubescens. Weed Sci 27:506–508.

305. Williams, M.C., and R.J. Molyneux. 1987. Occurrence, concentration and toxicity of pyrrolizidine alkaloids in Crotalaria seeds. Weed Sci 35:476–481.

306. Williams, M.C., and J.D. Olsen. 1992. Toxicity to chicks of combinations of miserotoxin, nitrate, selenium, and soluble oxalate. In L.F. James, R.F. Keeler, E.M. Bailey, P.R. Cheeke, and M.P.J. Hegarty (eds.). Poisonous Plants: Proceedings of the Third International Symposium. Iowa State University Press, Ames, IA, pp. 143–147.

307. Williamson, J.H., F.R. Craig, C.W. Barber, and F.W. Cook. 1964. Some effects of feeding Gelsemium sempervirens (yellow jessamine) to young chickens and turkeys. Avian Dis 8:183–190.

308. Wise, D.R., W.J. Hartley, and N.G. Fowler. 1974. The pathology of 3-nitro-4-hydroxy-phenylarsonic acid toxicity in turkeys. Res Vet Sci 16:336–340.

309. Wishe, H.I. 1976. The effect of aminotriazole on the thyroid gland and development of the white leghorn chick. Dis Abstr Int 37B:1066–67.

310. Wisser, L.A., B.S. Heinrichs, and R.M. Leach. 1990. Effect of aluminum on performance and mineral metabolism in young chicks and laying hens. J Nutr 120:493–498.

311. Wobeser, G., and B.R. Blakley. 1987. Strychnine poisoning of aquatic birds. J Wildl Dis 23:341–343.

312. Woerpel, R.W., and W.J. Rosskopf. 1982. Heavy-metal intoxication in caged birds. Compend Cont Ed 4: part 1, 729–740; part 2, 801–808.

313. Zajicek, J., O. Kypetova, and P. Matejka. 1985. Levamisole toxicity in breeding geese [abst no. 298]. Poult Abstr 1986 12:35.

314. Zeman, P. 1987. Systemic efficacy of ivermectin against Dermanyssus gallinae (De Geer, 1778) in fowls. Vet Parasitol 23:141–146.

37 Emerging Diseases and Diseases of Complex or Unknown Etiology

INTRODUCTION
Y. M. Saif

The emergence of new diseases and the reemergence of recognized diseases are familiar events in the annals of poultry medicine. Some of these emerging diseases could have been present earlier but were not recognized because of low prevalence, mild signs and lesions, or lack of diagnostic techniques. In other situations, genetic changes in the microorganisms could have rendered them more virulent or pathogenic. Similarly, genetic changes in the bird could have altered its susceptibility and resistance to disease. In addition, changes in environmental conditions or management could result in conditions that are favorable for a microbe to express pathogenic properties. Because of the global activities of the poultry industry resulting in the continual movement of live birds, eggs, and poultry products across political borders, it is difficult to contain an emerging or reemerging disease to a country or a continent. Hence, it is necessary to maintain a vigilant attitude toward poultry health and to sustain capable diagnostic facilities.

There are disease conditions that have multifactorial etiologies including combinations of microbes and, at times, microbes plus nutritional or environmental factors. Examples abound of seemingly harmless microbes that do not cause disease in healthy individuals but can become pathogenic following an insult, although it might be mild, to the host. *Escherichia coli* is a prime example of such a microbe earning it a designation as a universal secondary infection in poultry. In the commercial poultry environment, viruses and bacteria, including some that have the potential of causing disease, are common. Live vaccine viruses, some of which are very mild pathogens, may also be present.

In addition, flocks that are immunocompromised because of infectious or noninfectious agents could present unusual disease syndromes, increased susceptibility to disease, or lack of responsiveness to vaccination. The combinations of etiologies of disease could result in additive or synergistic effects. The pathogenesis of the multiple etiologies is not completely understood, but some mechanisms have been suggested or shown to occur.

The upper respiratory tract and the gastrointestinal tract are continually bombarded by a variety of microbes; yet, disease is not necessarily a common event. Natural and acquired defense mechanisms function efficiently to eliminate infections, inhibit replication, or prevent colonization of tissues by microbes. The mucociliary apparatus of the respiratory tract is a highly efficient system for elimination of microbes and particulate matter. Some viral infections result in deciliation of parts of the respiratory tract and lysis of infected cells, resulting in accumulation of cellular products and debris creating an environment favorable for bacterial multiplication and attachment to cells, which are important events in the pathogenesis of bacterial infections. In the gastrointestinal tract, similar events initiated by viruses have been described, including villous atrophy and consequent increased bacterial replication and adherence to cells. It is a common finding in respiratory and enteric diseases of poultry to encounter a variety of infectious agents. Because of the possible complex etiology of respiratory and enteric disease, it is important to understand the role of the different agents in the disease process. Such understanding should be helpful in designing logical control or prevention strategies.

In this chapter, information is presented on the complexity of respiratory and enteric diseases. In addition, the newly recognized diseases are described.

MULTICAUSAL RESPIRATORY DISEASE

S. H. Kleven and J. R. Glisson

Although much is known about the individual agents responsible for respiratory diseases in poultry, uncomplicated infections with single agents are the exception. Under commercial conditions, complicated infections involving multiple etiologies with viruses, mycoplasmas and other bacteria, immunosuppressive agents, and unfavorable environmental conditions are more commonly observed than simple infections. In addition, respiratory reactions induced by routine vaccination programs may themselves play a major role in the development of respiratory disease.

INTERACTIONS AMONG RESPIRATORY PATHOGENS. Perhaps the best understood examples of multiple respiratory infections are those involving mycoplasmas; this subject has been reviewed previously (8, 25). Although uncomplicated *Mycoplasma gallisepticum* infections in turkeys ordinarily result in respiratory signs, sinusitis, and airsacculitis, simple infection with *M. gallisepticum* or *M. synoviae* in chickens often results in mild or even subclinical disease. Interactions with Newcastle disease (ND) virus or infectious bronchitis virus (IBV) are known to increase the severity of *M. gallisepticum* infection (1, 11, 13, 41, 46, 51, 57). Similar interactions also occur with *M. synoviae* (22, 23, 27, 29, 50, 54).

The virulence of respiratory viruses may influence the severity of mycoplasma infections. With *M. synoviae,* concurrent challenge with high-passage field and vaccine strains of IBV resulted in milder respiratory disease than did exposure to field strains (22), and chicken-passaged vaccine virus resulted in more severe airsacculitis than did the original vaccine when birds were concurrently challenged with *M. synoviae* (23).

The timing of exposure to infectious agents is important in the pathogenesis of complicated infections. Generally, respiratory virus and mycoplasma infection must occur concurrently or within a short period of time for synergism to occur (23, 29), but mycoplasma-free chickens had a milder clinical response to IBV challenge than did chickens that were chronically infected with *M. gallisepticum* (51).

Other infectious agents are also known to interact with *M. gallisepticum.* Synergistic effects between *Haemophilus paragallinarum* and *M. gallisepticum* are well known (2, 26, 32, 38); control of *M. gallisepticum* results in milder respiratory disease due to infectious coryza. Interactions are also known between *M. gallisepticum* and adenovirus (3), re-

ovirus (24), and laryngotracheitis (7).

Three-way interactions between vaccine virus [Newcastle disease virus (NDV) and/or IBV], mycoplasma (*M. gallisepticum* or *M. synoviae*), and *Escherichia coli* resulted in more severe respiratory disease than any two alone. Combinations of any two of the agents resulted in milder disease than the three-way combination, and challenge with only one of the individual agents resulted in very mild or no disease (37, 50). Chickens exposed to infectious bronchitis and *M. gallisepticum* did not become susceptible to *E. coli* until 8 days postchallenge (19).

Interactions with various agents have also been described for *M. meleagridis* in turkeys. Enhanced airsacculitis was observed when germ-free poults were challenged with *M. meleagridis* and *E. coli* (47). An interaction between *M. meleagridis* and *M. synoviae* has been noted for turkey sinusitis (43) but not for airsacculitis (44). Combination infections with *M. meleagridis* and *M. iowae* caused more severe airsacculitis than either agent alone (44). *M. gallinarum,* ordinarily considered to be nonpathogenic, induced airsacculitis in broilers when given in combination with ND/infectious bronchitis vaccine virus (30).

Interactions between *E. coli* and other respiratory agents often occur in the absence of mycoplasma infection. Exposure to *E. coli* or IBV alone resulted in little or no clinical signs or mortality, but challenge with various strains of IBV along with *E. coli* resulted in significantly increased clinical signs and mortality (48, 60). Such a combination challenge with *E. coli* provided a means of evaluating the protection induced by infectious bronchitis vaccine strains against various challenge strains (10). Turkeys exposed to the LaSota strain of NDV had a decreased tracheal mucus transport rate and reduced tracheal clearance of *E. coli* (16). Studies on interactions between *E. coli* and *Bordetella avium* in turkeys have shown that *B. avium*–infected turkeys had higher numbers of *E. coli* in the tracheas and less ability to clear *E. coli* from the tracheas and lungs than did birds free of *B. avium* (52, 53). *B. avium* also adversely affected vaccinal immunity of turkeys to *Pasteurella multocida* (45).

EFFECTS OF IMMUNOSUPPRESSIVE AGENTS. Immunosuppressive agents, especially infectious bursal disease in chickens and hemorrhagic enteritis virus in turkeys, are well known to affect adversely susceptibility to respiratory infections. Challenge of chickens with infectious bursal disease virus has been shown to affect adversely antibody response and resistance to ND (15, 17, 18, 21), infectious bronchitis (18, 42, 58), *M. synoviae*, (18), and *Aspergillus flavus* (40). "Intermediate" vaccine strains of infectious bursal disease virus were highly variable in their interference with development of ND antibodies following ND vaccination (34).

Specific-pathogen–free chickens infected with infectious bursal disease virus and *E. coli* and then challenged with various adenovirus strains developed respiratory signs and lesions, while those infected with infectious bursal disease virus and *E. coli* without adenovirus did not (12).

Control of infectious bursal disease in the field is an essential factor in controlling respiratory disease in broilers.

Association between signs and mortality of colibacillosis in turkeys and presence of hemorrhagic enteritis lesions and viruses in the spleen led to the hypothesis that hemorrhagic enteritis infection often exacerbates colibacillosis (49). This association was subsequently proved in laboratory challenge studies (33). Inclusion of hemorrhagic enteritis virus along with *E. coli* challenge has been useful for induction of colibacillosis in laboratory studies (39). Control of hemorrhagic enteritis is considered to be an essential factor in controlling colibacillosis in turkeys.

Although Marek's disease herpesvirus is well known as an immunosuppressive agent, its role in respiratory disease has not been extensively studied. Chickens infected with Marek's disease virus, however, did not respond as well serologically to *M. synoviae* as chickens that were not challenged (28).

ROLE OF ENVIRONMENTAL FACTORS.

It is evident that environmental factors play a significant role in interacting with infectious agents in the production of respiratory disease in poultry, but there are relatively few published studies of such interactions. Environmental factors that have been studied include atmospheric ammonia, dust, and temperature. Chickens and turkeys continuously exposed to 20 ppm of ammonia showed gross or histologic signs of damage after 6 wk of exposure, and exposed chickens were more sensitive to infection with NDV (5). Turkeys exposed to 10 or 40 ppm of ammonia had deterioration of their normal mucociliary apparatus, excessive mucus production, matted cilia, and deciliation in tracheal tissue (35) and exhibited impaired clearance of *E. coli* from air sac, liver, and lung (36). Chickens exposed to 70 or 100 ppm of ammonia for 4 days exhibited increased thickness of atrial walls and shrinking air capillaries in their lungs (4). Ammonia levels of 25 or 50 ppm resulted in reduced body weights, feed efficiency, larger lung size, and increased airsac-

culitis in chickens challenged with IBV (31).

Atmospheric dust has also been shown to have a detrimental effect on the response to respiratory infections. Atmospheric dust significantly increased the severity and incidence of air sac lesions in turkeys with high or low rates of infection with *M. meleagridis* (6). In a broiler house study, losses from colisepticemia generally peaked 1 wk after coliform numbers peaked in dust samplings (9).

Respiratory disease and airsacculitis condemnations are well known to increase during the winter months, but there have been few studies on the effects of temperature on susceptibility to respiratory disease. Chickens challenged with *M. synoviae* and IBV had more extensive air sac lesions when housed at temperatures of 7–10 C than when housed at 29–24 C or 31–32 C (59).

VACCINATION REACTIONS.

Protection of chickens and turkeys against viral respiratory diseases is dependent upon the widespread use of live respiratory virus vaccines. The live respiratory virus vaccines that have been most widely used are ND vaccines and infectious bronchitis vaccines. Among the live ND vaccines, there are naturally occurring apathogenic strains such as VG/GA, Ulster, and QV4, naturally occurring mild respirotropic lentogenic strains such as B_1 and LaSota, and very limited use of mesogenic strains. Live infectious bronchitis vaccines are typically chicken embryo–passaged field IBV isolates. Chicken-embryo passage is utilized to attenuate the virulence of virulent field IBV isolates. A single IBV isolate, for example Massachusetts 41, may be available as a live vaccine at several different embryo passage levels (virulence attenuation levels).

All of the live respiratory viral vaccines replicate in the bird and cause some degree of cell damage. The clinical manifestation of this viral replication and its resultant pathology is called the "vaccination reaction." The live respiratory virus vaccines are intended to induce an immune response while inducing only minimal pathology, or a minimal vaccination reaction in a healthy bird in a good environment. A normal vaccination reaction for IBV or NDV should become clinically apparent 3–5 days after vaccination and should persist for an additional 3–5 days. If the vaccination reaction appears clinically to be unusually severe or prolonged, it is often referred to as a "rolling" vaccination reaction or, more simply, as a severe vaccination reaction.

Severe or prolonged vaccination reactions following the use of live ND or infectious bronchitis vaccines are a very common occurrence in the commercial poultry industry. Most typically, flocks that undergo a severe vaccination reaction develop respiratory colibacillosis. The pathogenesis of this complex disease interaction follows the same pattern described for the interaction of virulent wild respiratory viruses with *E. coli* (48, 60). Most poultry health specialists agree that respiratory disease that results from the interaction of viral respiratory vaccine viruses with *E. coli* is the most common respiratory disease of commercial poultry.

There are several different sets of circumstances that can culminate in a severe respiratory vaccination reaction, although regardless of the inciting factors, severe respiratory reactions typically culminate in the development of respiratory colibacillosis. Immunosuppression has been demonstrated to enhance the ability of pathogens to induce disease (15, 18). Likewise, immunosuppression can impede a bird's ability to limit replication of a respiratory virus vaccine, allowing a severe vaccination reaction.

Vaccinating birds with respiratory virus vaccines whose respiratory tracts are contaminated with other pathogens can produce a severe vaccination reaction. The most noted examples are *M. gallisepticum* and *M. synoviae* (8). Birds contaminated with *B. avium* or *E. coli,* however, fit a similar pattern. Newly hatched chicks that have hatched in an environment heavily contaminated with *E. coli* may develop severe respiratory reactions when vaccinated at a young age with live ND or infectious bronchitis vaccines.

Some live ND, infectious bronchitis, and infectious laryngotracheitis vaccines may become more virulent if allowed to spread from bird to bird (14, 20, 23). This vaccine "back-passage" can occur in commercial poultry houses if only a portion of the birds are provided with an immunizing dose of the vaccine and the remaining birds in the house become infected by spread of vaccine virus. This type of vaccine reaction appears to be both prolonged in duration and of increased intensity.

Environmental factors can influence the intensity of a vaccination reaction. As discussed earlier, ammonia and dust can interact with respiratory pathogens to enhance the severity of disease (31). This interaction is similar with respiratory vaccine viruses. Improper application of viral respiratory vaccines can enhance the severity of vaccination reactions. Spray application with a very fine spray can allow access of vaccine virus to the deep respiratory tissues and result in excessive viral replication in lungs and air sacs in addition to eliciting a stronger immune response (55). Aerosol vaccination also resulted in more severe airsacculitis after challenge with *M. synoviae* (56). Improper application of vaccines in the drinking water can prevent all birds in a house from receiving an immunizing dose of vaccine, thus providing an opportunity for spread of vaccine virus with a concomitant increase in virulence of the virus.

Since respiratory vaccine viruses of various virulence levels are available, it is important to use the proper vaccine for specific conditions. Typically, very young birds are vaccinated with highly attenuated vaccine viruses and less attenuated vaccine viruses are used in older birds and in birds that have been previously immunized. Severe vaccination reactions can occur, for example, if chicks are vaccinated at the hatchery with a live ND or infectious bronchitis vaccine intended for use in older birds.

REFERENCES

1. Adler, H.E. 1960. Mycoplasma, the cause of chronic respiratory disease. Ann N Y Acad Sci 79:703–712.
2. Adler, H.E., and R. Yamamoto. 1956. Studies on chronic coryza (Nelson) in the domestic fowl. Cornell Vet 46:337–343.
3. Aghakhan, S.M., M. Pattison, and M. Butler. 1976. Infection of the chicken with an avian adenovirus and Mycoplasma gallisepticum. J Comp Pathol 86:1–9.
4. Al-Mashhadani, E.H., and M.M. Beck. 1985. Effect of atmospheric ammonia on the surface ultrastructure of the lung and trachea of broiler chickens. Poult Sci 64:2056–2061.
5. Anderson, D.P., C.W. Beard, and R.P. Hanson. 1964. The adverse effects of ammonia on chickens including resistance to infection with Newcastle disease virus. Avian Dis 8:369–379.
6. Anderson, D.P., R.R. Wolfe, F.L. Cherms, and W.E. Roper. 1968. Influence of dust and ammonia on the development of air sac lesions in turkeys. Am J Vet Res 29:1049–1058.
7. Besrukava, I.Y. 1965. Influence of infectious laryngotracheitis virus on the course of mycoplasmosis in fowls. Veterinariya (Kiev) 5:109–114.
8. Bradbury, J.M. 1984. Avian mycoplasma infections: prototype of mixed infections with mycoplasmas, bacteria and viruses. Ann Microbiol (Inst Pasteur) 135 A: 83–89.
9. Carlson, H.C., and G.R. Whenham. 1968. Coliform bacteria in chicken broiler house dust and their possible relationship to coli-septicemia. Avian Dis 12:297–302.
10. Cook, J.K.A., H.W. Smith, and M.B. Huggins. 1986. Infectious bronchitis immunity: Its study in chickens experimentally infected with mixtures of infectious bronchitis virus and Escherichia coli. J Gen Virol 67:1427–1434.
11. Corstvet, R.E., and W.W. Sadler. 1966. A comparative study of single and multiple respiratory infections in the chicken: Multiple infections (with Mycoplasma gallisepticum, Newcastle disease virus, and infectious bronchitis virus). Am J Vet Res 27:1703–1720.
12. Dhillon, A. 1986. Pathology of avian adenovirus serotypes in the presence of Escherichia coli in infectious-bursal-disease-virus infected specific pathogen-free chickens. Avian Dis 30:81–86.
13. Dunlop, W.R., G. Parke, R.G. Strout, and S.C. Smith. 1964. The effect of sequence of infection on complex respiratory disease. Avian Dis 8:321–327.
14. Eidson, C.S., J.J. Giambrone, B.O. Barger, and S.H. Kleven. 1977. Comparison of the efficacy and transmissibility of conventional NDV vaccines and vaccines prepared after back-passage through chickens. Poult Sci 56:19–25.
15. Farrager, J.T., W.H. Allan, and P.J. Wyeth. 1974. Immunosuppressive effect of infectious bursal agent on vaccination against Newcastle disease. Vet Rec 95:385–388.
16. Ficken, M.D., J.F. Edwards, J.C. Lay, and D.E. Tveter. 1987. Tracheal mucus transport rate and bacterial clearance in turkeys exposed by aerosol to LaSota strain of Newcastle disease virus. Avian Dis 31:241–248.
17. Giambrone, J.J., C.S. Eidson, R.K. Page, O.J. Fletcher, B.O. Barger, and S.H. Kleven. 1976. Effect of infectious bursal agent on the response of chickens to Newcastle disease and Marek's disease vaccination. Avian Dis 20:534–544.

18. Giambrone, J.J., C.S. Eidson, and S.H. Kleven. 1977. Effect of infectious bursal disease on the response of chickens to Mycoplasma synoviae, Newcastle disease virus, and infectious bronchitis virus. Am J Vet Res 38:251–253.

19. Gross, W. 1990. Factors affecting the development of respiratory disease complex in chickens. Avian Dis 34:607–610.

20. Guy, J.S., H.J. Barnes, and L. Smith. 1991. Increased virulence of modified-live infectious laryngotracheitis vaccine virus following bird-to-bird passage. Avian Dis 35:348–355.

21. Hirai, K., S. Shimakura, E. Kawamoto, F. Taguchi, S.T. Kim, and C.N. Chang. 1974. The immunodepressive effect of infectious bursal disease virus in chickens. Avian Dis 18:50–57.

22. Hopkins, S.R., and H.W. Yoder. 1982. Influence of infectious bronchitis strains and vaccines on the incidence of Mycoplasma synoviae airsacculitis. Avian Dis 26:741–752.

23. Hopkins, S.R., and H.W. Yoder. 1984. Increased incidence of airsacculitis in broilers infected with Mycoplasma synoviae and chicken passaged infectious bronchitis vaccine virus. Avian Dis 28:386–396.

24. Johnson, E.P., and C.H. Domermuth. 1956. Some factors in the etiology and control of so-called avian air-sac disease. Cornell Vet 46:409–418.

25. Jordan, F. 1975. Avian Mycoplasma and pathogenicity—A review. Avian Pathol 4:165–174.

26. Kato, K. 1965. Influence of M. gallisepticum infection of chickens infected with H. gallinarum. Natl Inst Anim Health Q 5:183–189.

27. King, D.D., S.H. Kleven, D.M. Wenger, and D.P. Anderson. 1973. Field studies with Mycoplasma synoviae. Avian Dis 17:722–726.

28. Kleven, S.H., C.S. Eidson, D.P. Anderson, and O.J. Fletcher. 1972. Decrease of antibody response to Mycoplasma synoviae in chickens infected with Marek's disease herpesvirus. Am J Vet Res 33:2037–2042.

29. Kleven, S.H., D.D. King, and D.P. Anderson. 1972. Airsacculitis in broilers from Mycoplasma synoviae: effect on air-sac lesions of vaccinating with infectious bronchitis and Newcastle virus. Avian Dis 16:915–924.

30. Kleven, S.H., C.S. Eidson, and O.J. Fletcher. 1978. Airsacculitis induced in broilers with a combination of Mycoplasma gallinarum and respiratory viruses. Avian Dis 22:708.

31. Kling, H.F., and C.L. Quarles. 1974. Effect of atmospheric ammonia and the stress of infectious bronchitis vaccination on Leghorn males. Poult Sci 53:1161–1167.

32. Kuniyasu, C., K. Matsui, S. Sato, and K. Ando. 1967. Serological and bacteriological observation of chickens intranasally inoculated with Mycoplasma gallisepticum. Natl Inst Anim Health Q 7:202–207.

33. Larsen, C.T., C.T. Domermuth, D.P. Sponenberg, and W.B. Gross. 1985. Colibacillosis of turkeys exacerbated by haemorrhagic enteritis virus: Laboratory studies. Avian Dis 29:729–732.

34. Mazariegos, L.A., P.D. Lukert, and J. Brown. 1990. Pathogenicity and immunosuppressive properties of infectious bursal disease "intermediate" strains. Avian Dis 34:203–208.

35. Nagaraja, K.V., D.A. Emery, K.A. Jordan, J.A. Newman, and B.S. Pomeroy. 1983. Scanning electron microscopic studies of adverse effects of ammonia on tracheal tissues of turkeys. Am J Vet Res 44:1530–1536.

36. Nagaraja, K.V., D.A. Emery, K.A. Jordan, V. Sivanandan, J.A. Newman, and B.S. Pomeroy. 1984. Effect of ammonia on the quantitative clearance of Escherichia coli from lungs, air sacs, and livers of turkeys aerosol vaccinated against Escherichia coli. Am J Vet Res 45:392–395.

37. Nakamura, K., H. Ueda, T. Tanimura, and K. Noguchi. 1994. Effect of mixed live vaccine (Newcastle disease and in-

fectious bronchitis) and Mycoplasma gallisepticum on the chicken respiratory tract and on Escherichia coli infection. J Comp Pathol 111:33–42.

38. Nelson, J.B. 1938. Studies on an uncomplicated coryza of the domestic fowl. IX. The cooperative action of Haemophilus gallinarum and the coccobacilliform bodies in the coryza of rapid onset and long duration. J Exp Med 6:847–855.

39. Newberry, L., J. Skeeles, and D. Kreider. 1993. Use of virulent hemorrhagic enteritis virus for the induction of colibacillosis in turkeys. Avian Dis 37:1–5.

40. Okoye, J.O.A., C.N. Okeke, and F.K.O. Ezeobele. 1991. Effect of infectious bursal disease virus infection on the severity of Aspergillus flavus aspergillosis of chickens. Avian Pathol 20:167–171.

41. Omuro, M., K. Suzuki, H. Kawamura, and K. Munakata. 1971. Interaction of Mycoplasma gallisepticum, mild strains of Newcastle disease virus and infectious bronchitis virus of chickens. Natl Inst Anim Health Q 11:83–93.

42. Pejkovski, C., F.G. Develaar, and B. Kouwenhoven. 1979. Immunosuppressive effect of infectious bursal disease virus on vaccination against infectious bronchitis. Avian Pathol 8:95–106.

43. Rhoades, K.R. 1977. Turkey sinusitis: synergism between Mycoplasma synoviae and Mycoplasma meleagridis. Avian Dis 21:670–674.

44. Rhoades, K.R. 1981. Turkey airsacculitis: effect of mixed mycoplasmal infections. Avian Dis 25:131–135.

45. Rimler, R., and K. Rhoades. 1986. Fowl cholera: Influence of Bordetella avium on vaccinal immunity of turkeys to Pasteurella multocida. Avian Dis 30:838–839.

46. Rodriguez, R., and S.H. Kleven. 1980. Pathogenicity of two strains of Mycoplasma gallisepticum in broiler chickens. Avian Dis 24:800–807.

47. Saif, Y.M., P.D. Moorhead, and E.H. Bohl. 1970. Mycoplasma meleagridis and E. coli infections in germ free and specific pathogen free turkey poults: production of complicated airsacculitis. Am J Vet Res 31:1637–1643.

48. Smith, H., J. Cook, and Z. Parsell. 1985. The experimental infection of chickens with mixtures of infectious bronchitis virus and Escherichia coli. J Gen Virol 66:777–786.

49. Sponenberg, D., C. Domermuth, and C. Larsen. 1985. Field outbreaks of colibacillosis of turkeys associated with hemorrhagic enteritis virus. Avian Dis 29:838–842.

50. Springer, W., C. Luskus, and S. Pourciau. 1974. Infectious bronchitis and mixed infections of Mycoplasma synoviae and Escherichia coli in gnotobiotic chickens. I. Synergistic role in the airsacculitis syndrome. Infect Immun 10:578—589.

51. Timms, L.M. 1972. The effects of infectious bronchitis superimposed on latent Mycoplasma gallisepticum infection in adult chickens. Vet Rec 91:185–190.

52. Van Alstine, W., and L. Arp. 1987. Effects of Bordetella avium infection on the pulmonary clearance of Escherichia coli in turkeys. Am J Vet Res 48:922–926.

53. Van Alstine, W., and L. Arp. 1987. Influence of Bordetella avium infection on association of Escherichia coli with turkey trachea. Am J Vet Res 48:1574–1576.

54. Vardaman, T.H., F.N. Reece, and J.W. Deaton. 1973. Effect of Mycoplasma synoviae on broiler performance. Poult Sci 52:1909–1912.

55. Villegas, P., and S.H. Kleven. 1976. Aerosol vaccination against Newcastle disease. I. Studies on particle size. Avian Dis 20:179–190.

56. Villegas, P., S.H. Kleven, and D.P. Anderson. 1976. Effect of route of Newcastle disease vaccination on the incidence of airsacculitis in chickens infected with Mycoplasma synoviae. Avian Dis 20:395–400.

57. Weinack, O., G. Snoeyenbos, C. Smyser, and A. Soerjadi-Liem. 1984. Influence of Mycoplasma gallisepticum, in-

fectious bronchitis, and cyclophosphamide on chickens protected by native intestinal microflora against Salmonella typhimurium or Escherichia coli. Avian Dis 28:416–425.

58. Winterfield, R.W., F.J. Hoerr, and A.M. Fadly. 1978. Vaccination against infectious bronchitis and the immunosuppressive effects of infectious bursal disease. Poult Sci 57:386–391.

59. Yoder, H.W., L.N. Drury, and S.R. Hopkins. 1977. In-fluence of environment on airsacculitis: Effects of relative humidity and air temperature on broilers infected with Mycoplasma synoviae and infectious bronchitis. Avian Dis 21:195–208.

60. Yoder, H.W., Jr., C.W. Beard, and B.W. Mitchell. 1989. Pathogenicity of Escherichia coli in aerosols for young chickens. Avian Dis 33:676–683.

ORNITHOBACTERIUM RHINOTRACHEALE INFECTION

R. P. Chin and R. Droual

INTRODUCTION. *Ornithobacterium rhinotracheale* is a newly named bacterium associated with respiratory disease, decreased growth, and mortality in chickens and turkeys. Infection is characterized by unilateral or bilateral pneumonia, pleuritis, and airsacculitis. Severe lesions are primarily seen in older birds, especially breeders. Economic loss can be considerable when breeders are involved. Presently, there is no known public health significance.

HISTORY. Because *O. rhinotracheale* is difficult to isolate and identify, the organism was not described until 1994 (12). *O. rhinotracheale* may have been present in poultry flocks for many years but was dismissed as a secondary, opportunistic bacterium. The first known isolation of *O. rhinotracheale* was made in Germany in 1981 from 5-wk-old turkeys with respiratory tract infection (9). *O. rhinotracheale*, called *Pasteurella*-like organism, was subsequently isolated in 1986 in the United Kingdom from the trachea of turkeys with mild coughing and tracheitis and from birds in flocks with increased mortality that had unilateral pneumonia suggestive of fowl cholera. In contrast to fowl cholera, the disease did not spread from pen to pen, neither mortality nor morbidity was high, and birds responded satisfactorily to tetracyclines (17). *O. rhinotracheale* also was isolated in Israel from turkeys of various ages with acute exudative pneumonia and airsacculitis in 1986 (1). Since then, approximately 500 isolations from turkeys in Israel have been made. In 1994, *O. rhinotracheale* was reported as the cause of fowl cholera–like lesions in 23-wk-old turkeys in Germany (9). A similar disease was identified in 27- to 42-wk-old breeder turkeys in the United States in 1995 (4).

In 1993, an unidentified, pleomorphic, gram-negative, rod-shaped bacterium was associated with avian respiratory disease in the United States (2). The organism was subsequently identified as *O. rhinotracheale* (16).

O. rhinotracheale has been isolated from birds in Europe (5, 7, 8, 9, 11, 12), Israel (1), South Africa (8, 11, 12), and the United States (2, 4), but is probably distributed worldwide.

ETIOLOGY. *O. rhinotracheale* was previously described as a *Pasteurella*-like organism, *Kingella* sp., Taxon 28, or just a pleomorphic, gram-negative, rod-shaped bacterium (9). *O. rhinotracheale*, in the rRNA superfamily V, was proposed in 1994 based on investigation of 21 isolates (12). The phylogenetic position and various genotypic, chemotaxonomic, and classic phenotypic characteristics of *O. rhinotracheale* have been described (12).

O. rhinotracheale is a gram-negative, highly pleomorphic, nonmotile, nonsporulating bacterium. It appears as short, plump rods 0.2–0.9 µm × 1–3 µm (Fig. 37.1) and has a chemoorganotrophic, mesophilic metabolism (12).

While most *O. rhinotracheale* strains will grow aerobically, microaerobically, or anaerobically, best growth occurs in air enriched with 7.5–10% CO_2. Growth can occur from 30 to 42 C. *O. rhinotracheale* readily grows on 5% sheep blood agar or chocolate agar. At 24 hr, pinpoint colonies (<1 mm in diameter) are observed on sheep blood agar or chocolate agar plates. By 48 hr, colonies are approximately 1–2 mm in diameter, circular, opaque to gray, and convex with an entire edge. Because colonies are very small, especially at 24 hr, they can be masked or overgrown by large numbers of other more robust bacteria, such as *Escherichia coli*.

No growth occurs on MacConkey agar, Endo

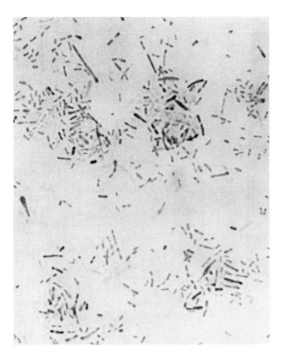

37.1. *Ornithobacterium rhinotracheale* showing highly pleomorphic nature. Gram stain of bacteria from a

agar, Gassner agar, Drigalski agar, or Simmon's citrate medium. It grows poorly on TSI slants with no change in the butt or slant portions of the tube. Isolated organisms are catalase-negative and oxidase-positive. Urease production is variable as determined with both Christensen urea agar slants and urea broths. Occasionally, for positive reactions to be detected, prolonged incubation up to 7 days is required. Indole production is not detected in sulfur-indole-motility media or PPLO media. All isolates are positive for ß-D-galactosidase in *o*-nitrophenyl-ß-D-galactopyranoside broth. Isolates do not hydrolyze gelatin; however, they all produce hyaluronidase. Ability to ferment carbohydrates should be examined using 1% carbohydrate phenol-red broth supplemented with 2% chicken serum. Glucose, galactose, lactose, maltose, and fructose are fermented by a majority of isolates, though this may be variable. Inositol, raffinose, sorbitol, trehalose, and xylose are not fermented.

Because most isolates do not react with standard biochemical tests, they can be further examined using two commercial systems (api-NFT and api-ZYM, bioMérieux, France). Most isolates give positive reactions for urease and all isolates are positive for ß-D-galactosidase (PNPG) in the api-NFT system. Using the api-ZYM system, isolates are positive for alkaline phosphatase, esterase, esterase lipase, leucine aminopeptidase, valine

aminopeptidase, cystine aminopeptidase, trypsin, chymotrypsin, acid phosphatase, phosphohydrolase, α-galactosidase, ß-galactosidase, α-glucosidase, and *N*-acetyl-ß-glucosaminodase. Predominant fatty acids are 15:0 iso, 16:0, 15:0 iso 3OH, 17:0 iso, 16:0 3OH, 17:0 iso 3OH, and unknown peaks with equivalent chain lengths of 13.566 and 16.580.

Using the agar gel immunodiffusion test (AGID), seven distinct serotypes (A, B, C, D, E, F, G) have been identified (14).

PATHOGENESIS AND EPIZOOTIOLOGY.

O. rhinotracheale infections occur naturally in chickens and turkeys. There are also reports of *O. rhinotracheale* being isolated from rooks, and a partridge, chukar, pheasant, and pigeon (2, 12). Mortality rates usually range from 2 to 11% in chickens and turkeys (6, 8).

Although *O. rhinotracheale* infections occur in 3- to 4-wk-old chickens, they are most common in broiler breeders between 24 and 52 wk of age, especially during peak egg production (8). Mortality is slightly increased, feed intake decreased, mild respiratory signs are present, and there may be decreased egg production, poor eggshell quality, and decreased egg size. Mild respiratory signs beginning around 3–4 wk of age, slightly increased mortality, and higher condemnation rates at processing are typical of the infection in young chickens (8).

In turkeys, infections have been seen in 2-wk-old birds, but most severe lesions are seen in older birds (>14 wk) and breeders (8). Infection with *O. rhinotracheale* at 2 wk of age causes respiratory signs and nasal discharge, followed by facial edema and swelling of infraorbital sinuses (8). Birds appear depressed, with ruffled feathers, and have decreased feed and water consumption, which is followed by increased mortality. In older birds, there may only be a sudden increase in mortality. Slight depression and gasping, marked dyspnea, and expectoration of blood-stained mucus can be seen just prior to death. In breeder flocks, there can be a slight (2–5%) decrease in egg production (6).

Experimental infection of 4-wk-old chickens and turkeys via intra–air sac route resulted in decreased growth but no airsacculitis (15). The challenge strain was not reisolated from the air sacs but was incidentally isolated from the brain and joints. Experimental inoculation via aerosol in 14-day-old turkeys produced airsacculitis. In addition, using turkey rhinotracheitis virus as a primer, along with aerosol inoculation, it was possible to produce severe airsacculitis and significant growth depression. Inoculation of 32-wk-old turkeys via intravenous, intramuscular, and intra–air sac routes did not produce any lesions, and the challenge bacterium was not reisolated (3).

Clinical cases in both chickens and turkeys reveal unilateral or bilateral lung consolidation with fibrinous exudate on the pleura (Fig. 37.2). Lesions are similar to those seen in fowl cholera in turkeys but to a lesser extent. In addition, there may be a mild tracheitis and fibrinoheterophilic airsacculitis, pericarditis, and peritonitis.

In clinical cases, microscopic lesions are most common in the lungs, pleura, and air sacs. Lungs (Fig. 37.3) are congested and diffusely affected with large collections of fibrin admixed with macrophages and heterophils in the lumen of air capillaries and parabronchi and pronounced interstitial infiltrates of macrophages and occasional heterophils. There are widespread, coalescing foci of necrosis often centered around the lumen of parabronchi and extending into adjacent parenchyma. Necrotic foci are typically filled with dense aggregates of necrotic, heterophilic infiltrate or exudate in which scattered, small clusters of intralesional bacteria can be found. These bacteria may not be *O. rhinotracheale*. Blood capillaries frequently are distended and contain fibrin thrombi. Pleura and air sacs can be markedly expanded and edematous with interstitial fibrin deposits, diffuse heterophilic infiltrate, scattered small foci of necrotic heterophilic infiltrate, and fibrosis.

DIAGNOSIS.   Trachea, lungs, and air sacs are the best tissues from which to isolate *O. rhinotracheale*. Infraorbital sinus and nasal cavity are also suitable sites for culture, but *O. rhinotracheale* can be easily masked by overgrowth of other bacteria. *O. rhinotracheale* can be isolated on common, nonselective blood or chocolate agar as described

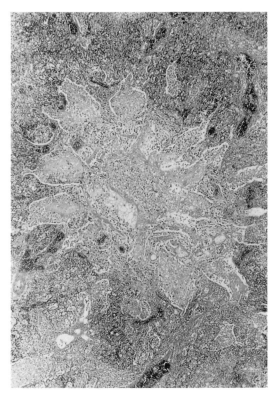

37.3.   Severe fibrinoheterophilic inflammation of lung associated with *Ornithobacterium rhinotracheale* infection in 31-wk-old turkey. H & E, ×15. (De Rosa)

above (see Etiology). Gram stain will reveal characteristic pleomorphic, gram-negative bacteria. Colonies are catalase-negative and oxidase-positive. Additional characterization can be done using biochemical tests (2, 12).

Currently, no commercial antigen or testing kit is available. An indirect ELISA has been developed (8) and used to monitor poultry flocks in Germany. Antibodies to *O. rhinotracheale* were detected in 22.2% (2/9) broiler flocks, 77.3% (17/22) broiler breeder flocks, and 69.2% (27/39) commercial turkey flocks with current or previous respiratory diseases. An ELISA using boiled-extract antigens of three serotypes (A, B, C) has been used for screening purposes and was able to detect maternal antibodies in day-old chickens and turkeys (13).

The major differential diagnosis is fowl cholera. In addition, bacteria causing serositis, such as *E. coli, Reimerella (Pasteurella) anatipestifer,* and *Chlamydia psittaci* must be ruled out. Additional biochemical tests are needed to differentiate *O. rhinotracheale* from *Flavobacterium* spp., *Cytophaga* spp., *Capnocytophaga* spp., and *Pasteurella haemolytica*-like bacteria. Note that the

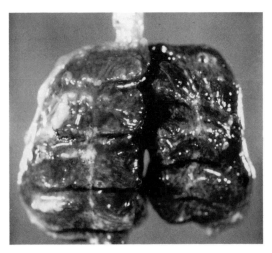

37.2.   Pneumonia and pleuritis associated with *Ornithobacterium rhinotracheale* infection in 31-wk-old turkey. (Shivaprasad)

api-NFT will misidentify this organism as *P. haemolytica* if the urea is negative and, thus, is not recommended for use alone in identifying *O. rhinotracheale*.

TREATMENT. Isolates in Europe have been found to be resistant to gentamicin, ampicillin, apramycin, neomycin, and trimethoprim-sulfonamide in vitro (8). When *O. rhinotracheale* strains isolated from gallinaceous birds were compared with isolates from rooks using the agar dilution method (5), the minimal inhibitory concentrations (MIC) for penicillin-cephalosporin antibiotics were 5 to 20 times higher. These findings suggested that MICs of rook isolates represented the natural sensitivity levels of the species and that all strains from gallinaceous birds tested had acquired resistance. Acquired resistance was also seen with lincosamide, macrolide, quinolone, and tetracycline antibiotics.

In California, all *O. rhinotracheale* isolates have been susceptible to erythromycin, spectinomycin, and streptomycin in vitro. Outbreaks have been treated with one or a combination of oxytetracyclines in the water, chlortetracycline in the feed, or spectinomycin, ceftiofur, and penicillin by injection (4).

Isolates in Virginia were found to be resistant to tetracyclines and apramycin in vitro, but sensitive to almost all other antibiotics tested (10). Penicillin at 10,000 IU/lb was found to be the most cost-effective treatment but is currently losing its efficacy. Chlortetracycline in water (25 mg/lb) or LA-200 (200 mg), ceftiofur (1 mg/lb), and tilmicosin (30 mg/kg) have also been used with some success.

In Germany, water medication with chloramphenicol (500 ppm) and/or amoxicillin (250 ppm for 3–7 days) gave satisfactory results (8).

In the United Kingdom, outbreaks are being treated with tetracyclines in the water with satisfactory results (17).

Currently, there is no commercially available vaccine. Severely affected turkey flocks in Israel, however, have been vaccinated with an autogenous, inactivated, oil-emulsion vaccine for several years with good results (1). In the Netherlands, prelimi-nary trials with an inactivated vaccine in broilers and turkeys have shown promising results (13).

REFERENCES
1. Bock, R.R. 1995. Personal communication.
2. Charlton, B.R., S.E. Channing-Santiago, A.A. Bickford, C.J. Cardona, R.P. Chin, G.L. Cooper, R. Droual, J.S. Jeffrey, C.U. Meteyer, H.L. Shivaprasad, and R.L. Walker. 1993. Preliminary characterization of a pleomorphic gram-negative rod associated with avian respiratory disease. J Vet Diagn Invest 5:47–51.
3. De Rosa, M. 1996. Personal communication.
4. De Rosa, M., R. Droual, R.P. Chin, H.L. Shivaprasad, and R.L. Walker. 1996. Ornithobacterium rhinotracheale infection in turkey breeders. Avian Dis (in press).
5. Devriese, L.A., J. Hommez, P. Vandamme, K. Kersters, and F. Haesebrouck. 1995. In vitro antibiotic sensitivity of Ornithobacterium rhinotracheale strains from poultry and wild birds. Vet Rec 137:435–436.
6. Ghazikhanian, G.Y. 1995. Personal communication.
7. Hafez, H.M. 1994. Respiratory disease conditions in meat turkeys caused by Ornithobacterium rhinotracheale: Clinical signs, diagnostics and therapy. Proc 43rd West Poultry Dis Conf, Sacramento, CA, pp. 113–114.
8. Hafez, H.M. 1996. Current status on the role of Ornithobacterium rhinotracheale (ORT) in respiratory disease complexes in poultry. Arch Geflügelkunde (submitted for publication).
9. Hinz, K.-H., C. Blome, and M. Ryll. 1994. Acute exudative pneumonia and airsacculitis associated with Ornithobacterium rhinotracheale in turkeys. Vet Rec 135:233–234.
10. Opengart, K., F.W. Peirson, G. Blackwell, and G. Meza. 1995. Cholera-like disease in commercial and breeder turkeys of unclear etiology. Proc 132nd Am Vet Med Assoc Meet, Pittsburgh, PA, p. 126.
11. van Beek, P.N.G.M., P.C.M. van Empel, G. Van Den Bosch, P.K. Storm, J.H. Bongers, and J.H. du Preez. 1994. Ademhalingsproblemen, groeivertraging en gewrichtsontsteking bij kalkoenen en vleeskuikens door een Pasteurella-achtige bacterie: Ornithobacterium rhinotracheale or "Taxon 28." Tijdschr Diergeneeskd 110:99–101.
12. Vandamme P., P. Segers, M. Vancanneyt, K. van Hove, R. Mutters, J. Hommez, F. Dewhirst, B. Paster, K. Kersters, E. Falsen, L.A. Devriese, M. Bisgaard, K.-H. Hinz, and W. Mannheim. 1994. Ornithobacterium rhinotracheale gen. nov., sp. nov., isolated from the avian respiratory tract. Int J Syst Bacteriol 44:24–37.
13. van Empel, P. 1995. Personal communication.
14. van Empel, P. 1996. Personal communication.
15. van Empel, P., H. van den Bosch, D. Goovaarts, and P. Storm. 1996. Experimental infection in turkeys and chickens with Ornithobacterium rhinotracheale. Avian Dis (in press).
16. Walker, R.L. 1995. Personal communication.
17. Wilding, P. 1995. Personal communication.

ENTERIC DISEASE COMPLEX

D. L. Reynolds

There are a number of enteric disease conditions affecting young poultry that go undiagnosed with respect to identifying a definitive etiologic agent. Many times, the inability to identify the specific causative organism results from a lack of, or unavailability of, specific assays (reagents), inopportune timing of sample collection, improper handling of appropriate samples and/or other factors that may contribute to a failure to diagnose the causative agent. There have been enteric disease cases, however, involving young poultry where extensive diagnostic procedures were conducted with great care, yet no definitive diagnosis could be made.

A disease (or diseases) of undetermined etiology affecting young poultry has been commonly referred to as "viral enteritis," but a variety of names have been used depending primarily on the avian species involved. Viral enteritis of chickens has been reported from many countries by several different names, including "malabsorption syndrome," "infectious stunting syndrome," "broiler runting syndrome," "pale bird syndrome," and "helicopter disease" (3, 4, 5, 14, 19, 25, 27, 40). More recent reports have indicated that high mortality (spiking mortality) may be associated with this disease syndrome (9). Viral enteritis in turkeys has been frequently termed *turkey viral enteritis, poult enteritis, malabsorption syndrome,* or *maldigestion syndrome* (28, 33, 37). Since the last edition of this text, a number of additional terms such as *stunting syndrome, poult enteritis complex,* and *spiking mortality* (2, 16, 33) have been used to describe similar enteric disease conditions of unknown etiology.

The clinical features of these disease syndromes have common features in turkeys and chickens (4, 28, 33, 37). Typically, birds are affected within the first 2 wk of life and usually display clinical signs of diarrhea, nervousness, growth retardation (stunting), litter eating, and excessive drinking (3, 4, 5, 14, 19, 25, 27, 37, 40). Experimental findings in turkeys have documented that poor feed utilization, depressed weight gains, decreased feed consumption, maldigestion (due to decreased disaccharidase activity), and malabsorption are manifestations of a stunting/malabsorption syndrome (2, 28). Sequelae following the initial clinical signs include poor feather development involving the primary wing feathers, resulting in the "helicopter" chick or poult (4) and development of a rachitic condition (19, 29), which appears to occur more frequently in affected poults than chicks (4). Malabsorption syndrome of poults induces an early osteoporotic lesion associated with hypocalcemia, which

progresses into a rachitic lesion associated with vitamin D depletion and hypophosphatemia (29). Poults that recover from malabsorption have an increased incidence of angular limb deformities (30). In chickens, hypoglycemia occurs, which is directly related to increased mortality (9).

Postmortem findings in affected chickens include enlargement of the proventriculus (25), proventriculitis (19), pancreatic changes (4, 31, 35), thymic involvement (27, 32), bone abnormalities (4, 19, 20), loss of pigmentation of the legs (25), catarrhal enteritis (19), and pale intestines with orange mucus (9). Postmortem findings in affected turkeys typically include distention of the gastrointestinal tract with gas and fluid, loss of tone of the intestinal tract, and dilated ceca with frothy contents (28, 33). Increased mortality has been observed in both chickens and turkeys (especially in spiking mortality cases). In those cases where mortality has been low, morbidity resulting in decreased growth (stunting) and flock unevenness is of greatest concern. Generally, there is little compensatory growth in stunted birds following the course of the disease; therefore, birds remain stunted throughout the grow-out period to market age.

Reported observations and experimental findings have provided strong evidence that this is an infectious disease (2, 19, 38), although the involvement of noninfectious agents has not been completely ruled out (4). Because no recognized enteropathogen(s) has been consistently incriminated as the etiologic agent for this disease, investigators have been searching for viruses and other agents that are associated with this condition. This has led to the discovery and/or identification of numerous viral agents. Those viruses that have been reported to cause viral enteric infections or have been associated with enteric disease of poultry are summarized in Table 37-1. Some of these viruses are discussed further in other chapters or subchapters of this book. Reports on the other enteric viruses are briefly described below.

Several viruses have been either observed or isolated from the intestinal tract of chickens experiencing viral enteritis. Viral particles resembling caliciviruses were demonstrated by electron microscopy (EM) from the intestinal tracts of 4-wk-old chickens with clinical signs of infectious stunting syndrome (41). Similarly, viral particles appearing as small coronaviruses, termed *coronaviruslike particles,* were demonstrated by EM from the intestinal tract of chickens experiencing pale bird syndrome (15). A virus isolated in avian

Table 37.1.   Enteric Viral Infections

Virus Type	Avian Species from Which Identified	Associated Disease/Condition
Adenovirus (group II)	Turkey	Hemorrhagic enteritis
Astrovirus	Turkey	Turkey viral enteritis
Calicivirus	Chicken	Infectious stunting syndrome
Coronavirus	Turkey	Coronaviral enteritis (Bluecomb Disease)
Coronaviruslike particles	Chicken	Malabsorption syndrome
Enterovirus	Turkey	Diarrhea and enteritis
Enteroviruslike virus (particles)	Chicken	Infectious stunting syndrome
FEW virus	Chicken	Infectious stunting syndrome
Fringed membranous particles (FMPs)	Turkeys, chickens, guinea fowl	Poult enteritis complex, diarrhea and enteritis
Herpesvirus	Ducks, geese, swans	Duck plague (duck virus enteritis)
Orthoreovirus	Turkey	Turkey viral enteritis
Parvovirus	Goose	Derzsy's disease
Parvovirus	Chicken	Infectious stunting syndrome
Parvoviruslike virus	Turkey	Enteropathy, stunting, diarrhea
Picornalike virus (Pseudopicornavirus)	Turkey	Enteric and respiratory disease
Reovirus	Chicken	Malabsorption syndrome
Reovirus	Turkey	Infectious enteritis
Rod-shaped viruslike particles (RSVLPs)	Pheasants, chicken, guinea fowl, Japanese quail	Diarrhea and enteritis
Rotavirus	Chicken, duck, guinea fowl, pheasant, turkey	Diarrhea and enteritis
Togaviruslike agent	Chickens, guinea fowl	Infectious stunting syndrome, severe enteric disease

cell culture from intestinal homogenates of 4-day-old chickens showing signs of infectious stunting syndrome has been named the FEW virus (12). Parvoviruses have been identified by EM from the intestinal contents of 10-day-old chickens afflicted with a stunting syndrome (18). There have been conflicting reports on the ability of parvoviruses to cause enteric disease (infectious stunting syndrome) in chickens (10, 17). A togaviruslike agent was isolated and described from pancreatic ducts of chickens having infectious stunting syndrome (13). More recently, a togaviruslike agent was found in guinea fowl with severe enteric disease (6).

The situation in turkeys parallels that of chickens, whereby numerous viruses have been either identified or isolated from poults experiencing enteric disease (33, 34, 36). An enteropathy causing stunting, increased mortality, and diarrhea in young turkeys in which parvoviruses were identified was reported (39). In this disease, parvoviruses were identified by EM from thin sections of the ileal epithelium, which also contained inclusion bodies. Pi-

cornalike viruses (pseudopicornaviruses) have been reported in turkeys displaying signs of enteric and respiratory disease (1).

Although many viral agents have been reported to occur in young chickens and turkeys experiencing enteric disease, a number of points need to be made. First, it is possible (and most probable) that some of the viruses mentioned above are not in themselves the sole etiologic agent for an enteric disease. The ability to detect a viral agent from a diseased host does not in itself constitute a cause and effect relationship for that disease. This point is illustrated by the fact that the most frequently identified viruses from the intestinal tract and/or intestinal contents of chickens and turkeys were bacteriophages (23). Care must be taken not to overinterpret initial findings. For example, fringed membranous particles (FMPs) have been identified by electron microscopy (EM) from the intestinal tracts of chickens, turkeys, and other avian species (16, 26). Fringed membranous particles have been found in birds experiencing enteric disease as well as clinically normal healthy birds. These particles have been described as paramyxolike particles (26) and have often been associated with enteric disease cases in which other enveloped viruses have been identified (16). Fragments of cell membranes can also resemble enveloped viruses (11) and, thus, could account for some FMPs. The identification of FMPs also illustrates the limitations of diagnosing enteric viral diseases by direct EM. Further studies are needed in order to classify many of these viruses correctly into appropriate viral taxons and/or distinguish them from artifacts. Presently, the relationships among morphologically similar viruses are largely unknown.

The second point pertains to the role of each virus and the complexity of enteric disease. The intestinal tract is a highly complex system that has many functions. While providing a means by which the body can derive nutrition from its environment, it also furnishes protective mechanisms to safeguard the host. The intestinal tract itself serves as an environment for other living organisms. The pathogenesis of a viral enteric disease also is a complex entity; likewise, the etiology of an enteric disease may be equally complicated. Combinations of, and interactions among, different viruses and other infectious and noninfectious agents may be necessary to elicit an enteric viral disease or increase/decrease its severity. This point is illustrated by a recent study in which marble spleen disease virus, a group 2 avian adenovirus used as a vaccinating agent against hemorrhagic enteritis in turkeys, was administered concurrently with *Eimeria meleagrimitis* (24). This combination of agents resulted in an exacerbation of the pathogenic effect attributed to the vaccine virus. Paradoxically, results from the same study revealed that when *E. meleagrimitis* was administered concurrently with virulent hemorrhagic enteritis virus (HEV), the pathogenic effect attributed to the virulent HEV was diminished. Another example of the complexity of enteric disease is the observation that broiler chickens vaccinated at 1 day of age with Marek's disease vaccine were less severely affected when an oral inoculum, used to induce malabsorption syndrome, was administered to them at 18 days of age. The protective effect provided by Marek's disease vaccination was attributed to nonspecific stimulation of natural killer cells, since it was postulated that Marek's disease virus was not directly involved as the pathogenic agent (21). The need to delineate and establish what role each virus plays in the etiology and pathogenesis of enteric disease is essential.

A third point is the potential for discovering new enteric viruses. Although many viruses have been identified and associated with enteric disease, the potential for discovering new viruses that play a major role in enteric disease should not be discounted. For example, there has been a report of viruslike particles identified from the intestinal contents of young pheasants experiencing enteric disease (7). These particles are unlike other animal viruses, bacteriophages, or mycoviruses previously reported. These particles do have similarities to plant viruses. Similar rod-shaped viruslike particles have also been observed in enteric samples from chickens (8), guinea fowl, and Japanese quail (22). Whether or not these particles are animal viruses that constitute a new taxon with pathogenic potential for poultry or other animals is yet to be determined.

The poultry industry is a dynamic industry that has in the past made rapid changes in management practices, nutritional programs, and even the bird itself. Such changes could provide an opportunity for new pathogenic enteric viruses to emerge.

REFERENCES

1. Andral, B., and D. Toquin. 1984. Observations et isolements de pseudopicornavirus a partir de dindonneaux malades. Avian Pathol 13:377–388.

2. Angel, C.R., J.L. Sell, and D.W. Trampel. 1990. Stunting syndrome in turkeys: Physical and physiological changes. Poult Sci 69:1931–1942.

3. Bracewell,C.D. 1982. Broiler stunting syndrome: Report of a seminar. World's Poult Sci J 38:222.

4. Bracewell, C.D., and C.J. Randall. 1984. The infectious stunting syndrome. World's Poult Sci J 40:31–37.

5. Bracewell, C. D., and P. Wyeth. 1981. Infectious stunting of chickens. Vet Rec 109:64.

6. Brahem, A., N. Demarquez, M. Beyrie, A. Vuillaume, and H.J.A. Fleury. 1992. A highly virulent togavirus-like agent associated with the fulminating disease of guinea fowl. Avian Dis. 36:143–148.

7. Collins, M.S., R.E. Gough, and B.E. Preece. 1988. Unusual virus-like particles in pheasant small intestines. Vet Rec 123:186.

8. Collins, M.S., R.E. Gough, D.J. Alexander, and D.G. Parsons. 1989. Virus-like particles associated with a "wet litter" problem in chickens. Vet Rec 124:641.

9. Davis, J.F., A.E. Castro, J.C. de la Torre, C.G. Scanes, S.V. Radecki, R. Vasillatos-Younken, J.T. Doman, and M. Teng. 1995. Hypoglycemia, enteritis, and spiking mortality in Georgia broiler chickens: Experimental reproduction in broiler breeder chicks. Avian Dis 39:162–174.

10. Decaesstecker, M., G. Charlier, and G. Meulemans. 1986. Significance of parvoviruses, entero-like viruses and reoviruses in the aetiology of the chicken malabsorption syndrome. Avian Pathol 15:769–782.

11. Doane, F.W., and N. Anderson. 1987. Bacteriophages, non-viral structures and artifacts. In Electron Microscopy in Diagnostic Virology—A Practical Guide and Atlas. Cambridge University Press, New York, NY, pp. 163–175.

12. Farmer, A.M., and J. Taylor. 1985. Infectious stunting syndrome: The isolation of a novel virus. Vet Rec 116:111.

13. Frazier, J.A., H. Farmer, and M.F. Martland. 1986. A togavirus-like agent in the pancreatic duct of chickens with infectious stunting syndrome. Vet Rec 119:208–209.

14. Good, R.E. 1982. The pale bird syndrome. Poult Dig 41:278.

15. Goodwin, M.A., J. Brown, E.C. Player, W.L. Steffens, D. Hermes, and M.A. Dekich. 1995. Fringed membranous particles and viruses in faeces from healthy turkey poults and from poults with putative poult enteritis complex/spiking mortality. Avian Pathol 24:497–505.

16. Goodwin, M.A., M.A. Dekich, K.S. Latimer, and O.J. Fletcher. 1985. Quantitation of intestinal D-xylose absorption

in normal broilers and in broilers with pale-bird syndrome. Avian Dis 29:630–639.

17. Kisary, J. 1985. Experimental infection of chicken embryos and day old chickens with parvovirus of chicken origin. Avian Pathol 14:1–7.

18. Kisary, J., B. Nagy, and Z. Bitay. 1984. Presence of parvoviruses in the intestine of chickens showing stunting syndrome. Avian Pathol 13:339–343.

19. Kouwenhoven, B., F.G. Davelaar, and J. Walsum. 1978. Infectious proventriculitis causing runting in broilers. Avian Pathol 7:183–187.

20. Kouwenhoven, B., M. Vertommen, and J.H.H. van Eck. 1978. Runting and leg weakness in broilers: Involvement of infectious factors. Vet Sci Commun 2:253–259.

21. Kouwenhoven, B., R.M. Dwars, and J.F.M. Smeets. 1992. Wet litter and high feed conversions, a new problem in broilers. In M.S. McNulty and J.B. McFerran (eds.). New and Evolving Virus Diseases of Poultry. Commission of the European Communities, Brussels, Belgium, pp. 243–251.

22. Lavazza, A., S. Pascucci, and D. Gelmetti. 1990. Rod-shaped virus-like particles in intestinal contents of three avian species. Vet Rec 125:581.

23. McNulty, M.S., W.L. Curran, D. Todd, and J.B. McFerran. 1979. Detection of viruses in avian faeces by direct electron microscopy. Avian Pathol 8:239–247.

24. Norton, R.A., J.K. Skeeles, and L.A. Newberry. 1995. The effect of concurrent infections of haemorrhagic enteritis virus or marble spleen disease virus and *Eimeria meleagrimitis* in turkeys. Avian Pathol 24:285–292.

25. Page, R.K., O.J. Fletcher, G.N. Rowland, D. Gaudry, and P. Villegas. 1982. Malabsorption syndrome in broiler chickens. Avian Dis 26:618–624.

26. Pascucci, S., and A. Lavazza. 1992. A survey of enteric viruses in commercial avian species: Experimental studies of transmissible enteritis of guinea fowl. In M.S. McNulty and J.B. McFerran (eds.). New and Evolving Virus Diseases of Poultry. Commission of the European Communities, Brussels, Belgium, pp. 225–241.

27. Pass, D.A., M.D. Robertson, and G.E. Wilcox. 1982. Runting syndrome in broiler chickens in Australia. Vet Rec 110:386–387.

28. Perry, R.W., G.N. Rowland, and J.R. Glisson. 1991. Poult malabsorption syndrome. I. Malabsorption in poult enteritis. Avian Dis 35:685–693.

29. Perry, R.W., G.N. Rowland, and J.R. Glisson. 1991. Poult malabsorption syndrome. II. Pathogenesis of skeletal lesions. Avian Dis 35:694–706.

30. Perry, R.W., G.N. Rowland, and J.R. Glisson. 1991. Poult malabsorption syndrome. III. Skeletal lesions in market-age turkeys. Avian Dis 35:707–713.

31. Randall, C.J., P.J. Wyeth, and R.J. Higgins. 1981. Pancreatic lesions in stunted broilers. Vet Rec 109:125–126.

32. Reese, R.L., P.T. Hopper, S.H. Tate, V.D. Beddome, W.M. Forsythe, P.C. Scott, and D.A. Barr. 1984. Field, clinical and pathological observations of a runting and stunting syndrome in broilers. Vet Rec 115:483–485.

33. Reynolds, D. 1992. Enteric viral infections of young poultry. Poult Sci Rev 4:197–212.

34. Reynolds, D.L., Y.M. Saif, and K.W. Theil. 1987. A survey of enteric viruses in turkey poults. Avian Dis 31:89–98.

35. Riddell, C., and D. Derow. 1984. Infectious stunting and pancreatic fibrosis in broiler chickens in Saskatchewan. Avian Dis 29:107–115.

36. Saif, L.J., Y.M. Saif, and K.W. Theil. 1985. Enteric viruses in diarrheic turkey poults. Avian Dis 29:798–811.

37. Saif, Y.M., D.L. Reynolds, L.J. Saif, and K.W. Theil. 1985. Diarrhea, enteritis, malabsorption, maldigestion, and viruses. Proc 34th West Poult Dis Conf, pp. 61–62.

38. Sell, J.L., D.L. Reynolds, and M. Jeffrey. 1992. Evidence that bacteria are not causative agents of stunting syndrome in poults. Poult Sci 71:1480–1485.

39. Trampel, D.W., D.A. Kinden, R.F. Solorzano, and P.L. Stogsdill. 1983. Parvovirus-like enteropathy in Missouri turkeys. Avian Dis 27:49–54.

40. van der Heide, L. 1982. Malabsorption syndrome in broilers. Clin Vet 105:3.

41. Wyeth, P.J., N.J. Chettle, and J. Labram. 1981. Avian caliciviruses. Vet Rec 109:477.

HYDROPERICARDIUM–HEPATITIS SYNDROME (ANGARA DISEASE)

Simon M. Shane and M. S. Jaffery

INTRODUCTION AND HISTORY. Hydropericardium–hepatitis syndrome (HHS) is an acute, infectious disease of chickens characterized by high morbidity and mortality, excess pericardial fluid, and multifocal hepatic necrosis. Although the specific etiology of HHS has yet to be defined, available evidence suggests the condition is caused by a pathogenic group I adenovirus (15). Other agents may serve as potentiators and increase the severity of the disease under field conditions. Possible contributions of intercurrent immunosuppressive diseases such as infectious bursal disease, Marek's disease, and chicken infectious anemia have not been defined but are believed to be significant. The economic impact of HHS is difficult to determine because the condition occurs concurrently with other diseases of chickens including velogenic Newcastle disease, mycoplasmosis, salmonellosis, Marek's disease, and avian influenza, which are endemic in the broiler industries where HHS occurs (8). Prevalence and severity of HHS outbreaks are related to the density of the poultry population in an area.

Hydropericardium–hepatitis syndrome was first recognized in flocks in Angara Goth near Karachi, Pakistan, in late 1987. Because the disease emerged in this specific geographic area, HHS was initially referred to as "Angara Disease." Within 12 mo, the disease spread rapidly, affecting flocks in most of the intensive broiler growing areas located near urban centers in Pakistan (11).

Outbreaks of HHS were recorded in Mexico in 1989 in the high-density poultry-producing state of Queretaro and became widespread in the broiler-growing areas of five other states by 1990 (12). During 1994, HHS appeared in the high-density poultry areas in the vicinity of Delhi in India; HHS also has been diagnosed in Chile, Iraq (1), and Peru.

Although 3- to 5-wk-old broilers are typically affected, the condition has been identified in immature broiler breeders and commercial layers (2).

ETIOLOGY. Originally, HHS in Pakistan was attributed to a toxicity or nutritional deficiency. An infectious agent was suggested as a possible cause when it was discovered that the disease could be reproduced by inoculating young broilers with bacteria-free liver homogenates from affected birds (10, 13).

Following identification of basophilic intranuclear inclusion bodies in hepatocytes, attempts were made to isolate a viral agent. By late 1988, it was determined that an adenovirus could be the cause of HHS (21). Characteristic hexagonal virions in EM preparations of liver homogenates were subsequently found. Liver and lung extracts from affected birds were positive by agar gel precipitation when tested against group-specific adenovirus antiserum. Filtered homogenates of liver tissue from affected cases inoculated into the chorioallantoic membrane and yolk sac of specific-pathogen–free (SPF) eggs on the 8th day of incubation caused death of embryos within 4–7 days (2).

Studies during 1991 showed that treatment of liver suspensions with ether or chloroform, which normally does not inactivate an adenovirus, eliminated infectivity. Similarly, a suspension of liver from affected birds was infectious after exposure to 60 C for 30 min, which would normally inactivate an adenovirus, although thermostability varies considerably among adenoviruses (see Chapter 23). When liver homogenates were centrifuged at 45,000 rpm for 90 min, the resuspended pellet was infectious, but the supernatant was not. Addition of an inclusion body hepatitis-producing adenovirus to the supernatant restored infectivity, suggesting the presence of an additional viral agent other than the primary adenovirus (3).

Subsequent studies conducted in Mexico in 1994 implicated an RNA virus as an additional agent based on lack of inhibition by 5-bromodeoxyuridine. This agent produced small syncytia in both chick kidney and liver cell preparations (20). A further complication in defining the etiology is the presence of highly pathogenic infectious bursal disease and chicken infectious anemia viruses in areas where HHS occurs. Viruses responsible for these diseases were recovered from liver homogenates derived from infected flocks in Pakistan in addition to group I adenoviruses of serotypes 4 and 11 (24).

More recently, HHS has been reproduced experimentally in Pakistan and Mexico with serotype 4 (strain PARC-1) and serotype 8 (strain DCV-94) avian adenovirus isolates, respectively. Both inclusion body hepatitis and hydropericardium occurred in susceptible chickens following infection (16, 22). The serotype 4 adenovirus also had a predilection for lymphoid tissues, which resulted in immunosuppression (22).

The conflict between the single- and two-virus hypotheses will be resolved following more detailed epidemiologic and laboratory studies (see Chapter 23 for additional information on adenoviral classification, morphology, structure, and laboratory host systems).

PATHOGENESIS AND EPIZOOTIOLOGY

Natural and Experimental Hosts. Immature chickens are the natural hosts; HHS occurs most commonly in 3- to 5-wk-old broilers and immature broiler breeder replacements. A condition resembling HHS has been described in pigeons in Pakistan (6).

Transmission. Because evidence suggests that group I adenoviruses are involved in the etiology of HHS, it is presumed that HHS can be transmitted both vertically and horizontally. Adenoviruses may remain latent in breeding stock until onset of maturity and then be shed following immunosuppression or stress. After 3 wk of age, progeny of infected parent stock may excrete virus for up to 14 wk (19). Horizontal dissemination of virus by carriers may be a significant method of transmission among flocks on multiage farms or in operations without adequate biosecurity (7).

Viral replication in the intestinal tract suggests that fecal contamination of clothing, footwear, and equipment, including transport crates and vehicles, may spread infection under commercial conditions. In the context of poultry farms in Pakistan, lack of biosecurity, close proximity of multiage farms, and live-bird trading promote transmission of viral agents.

Contaminated vaccine prepared in embryos derived from infected flocks may also be a potential source of infection. In a study of risk factors associated with HHS in broiler flocks in Pakistan, it was demonstrated that visits to farms by vaccination crews often predisposed to outbreaks of HHS (9) and subcutaneous or intramuscular injection resulted in infection rates more typical of those seen naturally compared to exposure by aerosol or via contaminated water or litter (5).

Signs, Morbidity, and Mortality. A prevalence rate of 46% was determined in 131 flocks reared on 135 broiler units in the vicinity of Islamabad, Pakistan (9). Nonvaccinated broiler and immature breeder flocks can have mortality as high as 80% if they also are exposed to viscerotropic velogenic Newcastle disease, highly pathogenic infectious bursal disease, and erosive infections such as mycoplasmosis. Duration of infection usually ranges from 9 to 14 days with morbidity of 10–30% and daily mortality of 3–5% (8).

Under experimental conditions, mortality occurs within 2–4 days following inoculation with liver homogenate from an affected flock. Mortality ranges from 30 to 70% depending on the preparation and titer of the homogenate and route of administration (3, 5).

Flocks with HHS show no specific clinical signs; abrupt onset of mortality, lethargy, huddling with ruffled feathers, and yellow, mucoid droppings are characteristic. Affected birds have decreased hemoglobin, packed cell volume, erythrocytes, and total leukocytes. Relative increases in heterophils and decreases in lymphocytes are consistent with stress and viral infections. Decreased albumin production because of liver damage is considered to be responsible for the hypoproteinemia in affected birds, which probably contributes to development of hydropericardium (23). Severe anemia in affected birds might be attributed to coinfection with chicken infectious anemia virus or virulent infectious bursal disease. Lactic dehydrogenase, alkaline phosphatase, and alanine transaminase are elevated in affected birds, which is consistent with hepatic and renal damage (25).

The most striking postmortem lesion is the presence of up to 10 mL of clear transudate in the pericardial sac (Fig 37.4). Generalized congestion and pulmonary edema are evident and the liver and kidneys are usually enlarged, pale, and friable. Under experimental conditions, affected birds may show myocardial and hepatic necrosis. Petechial hemorrhages may be present on the pericardium and beneath the capsule of the liver (11).

Histologic lesions in the heart consist of myocardial edema, degeneration, and necrosis with mild, mononuclear cell infiltration and extravasation of erythrocytes. Multifocal coagulative necrosis with mononuclear cell infiltration and basophilic intranuclear inclusion bodies in hepatocytes is present in the liver. There also may be extensive areas of necrosis in renal epithelium (8, 13).

DIAGNOSIS. Hydropericardium coupled with histologic demonstration of basophilic intranuclear inclusions in hepatocytes is considered highly suggestive of HHS. To confirm the diagnosis, adenovirus can be isolated by infecting embryonic chick liver cells. This procedure is more sensitive than in-

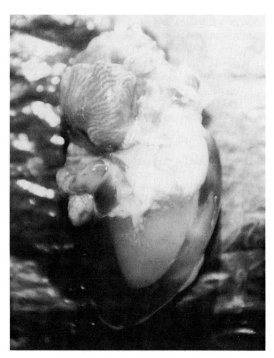

37.4. Heart from chicken with hydropericardium–hepatitis syndrome showing marked distention of pericardial sac by clear fluid.

oculation of 8-day-old embryonated eggs using the yolk sac route (19). The presence of adenovirus in tissue culture is indicated by characteristic cytopathology. Adenoviruses can be demonstrated by negative-stain electron microscopy and identified by a serum neutralization test (18).

TREATMENT. There is no specific treatment for HHS; however, use of an iodophor in the drinking water of affected flocks (0.07–0.1% of a 2.5% solution) reduced mortality and severity of the disease (1).

PREVENTION AND CONTROL. Under conditions prevailing in Pakistan, India, and Mexico, it is neither practical nor economically feasible to maintain strict levels of biosecurity to ensure exclusion of adenovirus from broiler units. The realities of production include multiage placement, sale of live birds, delivery of feed in bags, and employment of workers who maintain domestic poultry. Breeder flocks must be protected from infection by applying an acceptable biosecurity program. Measures include locating farms at least 2 km from commercial units, operating an all-in, all-out placement program with thorough decontamination of houses between successive flocks. Feed should be delivered in bulk and all personnel should be decontaminated before entry to a breeding farm. Live vaccines administered to breeders and their progeny should be manufactured according to accepted international standards and be free of pathogens including adenoviruses and chicken infectious anemia virus.

In areas where HHS is endemic, it is necessary to protect flocks against the primary adenovirus responsible for the condition. A formaldehyde-inactivated vaccine prepared from liver homogenate protected broilers under field conditions in Pakistan (14). A more sophisticated vaccine was prepared by sonicating liver homogenate of SPF chicks followed by inactivation with 0.1% formaldehyde (4). The efficacy of this preparation was demonstrated in a field trial involving 28 flocks comprising 100,000 broilers. Losses due to HHS in the vaccinated group subjected to natural field challenge reached 1.2% in contrast to 20% mortality in non-vaccinated broilers. Mortality in approximately one million broilers in the Rawalpindi area was reduced to 4% compared with 31% in unvaccinated flocks.

A formalin-inactivated oil-emulsion preparation provided 100% protection against challenge as indicated by survival and absence of histologic lesions in an experimental evaluation of five commercial vaccines in Mexico (17). Four other inactivated vaccines provided protection ranging from 0% to 45% against challenge with strain DCV-94, which typically produces 80% mortality in non-vaccinated chicks. Immunofluorescence inhibition demonstrated antibodies in all vaccinated chicks. Survival following challenge was positively correlated with the serologic response stimulated by vaccination.

REFERENCES

1. Abdul-Aziz, T.A., and M.A. Al-Attar. 1991. New syndrome in Iraqi chicks. Vet Rec 129:272.

2. Afzal, M., R. Muneer, and G. Stein. 1991. Studies on aetiology of hydropericardium syndrome (Angara disease) in broilers. Vet Rec 128:591–593.

3. Afzal, M., R. Muneer, G. Stein, Jr., and B.S. Cowen. 1990. Aetiology and control of hydropericardium syndrome (Angara disease) in broilers of Pakistan. Proc 3rd Int Congr Pakistan Vet Med Assoc, pp. 218–228.

4. Ahmad, I., M.I. Malek, K. Iqbal, K. Ahmed, and S. Naz. 1990. Efficacy of formalized liver-organ-vaccine against Angara disease in broilers. Vet Arh 60:131–138.

5. Ahmad, K., I. Ahmad, M.A. Muneer, and M. Ajmal. 1992. Experimental transmission of Angara disease in broiler fowls. Stud Res Vet Med 1:53–55.

6. Akhtar, S. 1994. Hydropericardium syndrome in broiler chickens in Pakistan. World Poult Sci J 50:177–182.

7. Akhtar, S. 1995. Lateral spread of the aetiologic agents of hydropericardium syndrome in broiler chickens. Vet Rec 136:118–120.

8. Akhtar, S., and M. Afzal. 1995. Sindrome de hydropericardio en pollos de engorda en Pakistan: Etiologia, di-

agnostico y control. Proc 20th Annu ANECA Conf, pp. 405–415.

9. Akhtar, S., S. Zahid, and M.I. Khan. 1992. Risk factors associated with hydropericardium in broiler flocks. Vet Rec 131:481–484.

10. Anjum, A.D. 1990. Experimental transmission of hydropericardium syndrome and protection against it in commercial broiler chickens. Avian Pathol 19:655–660.

11. Anjum, M.A., M.A. Sabri, and Z. Iqbal. 1989. Hydropericarditis syndrome in broiler chickens in Pakistan. Vet Rec 124:247–248.

12. Borrego, J.L., and E. Soto. 1995. Reporte de campo de une brote de hepatitis con cuerpos de inclusion (HCI) en reproductoras pesadas a edad temprana. Proc 20th Annu ANECA Conf, pp. 1–4.

13. Cheema, A.H., J. Ahmad, and M. Afzal. 1989. An adenovirus infection of poultry in Pakistan. Rev Sci Tech Off Int Epizoot 8:789–795.

14. Chishti, M., M. Afzal, and A.H. Cheema. 1989. Preliminary studies on the development of vaccine against the hydropericardium syndrome of poultry. Rev Sci Tech Off Int Epizoot 8:797–801.

15. Cowen, B.S. 1992. Inclusion body hepatitis-anaemia and hydropericardium syndromes: Aetiology and control. World Poult Sci J 48:247–254.

16. Gay, G.M., R.A. Retana, M.M.E. Aranda, and A.D. Vasquez. 1995. Implementacion de las pruebas de precipitacion en agar, immunofluorescencia e inhibicion de focos fluorescentes para el diagnostico de la hepatitis con cuerpos de inclusion. Proc 7th Avi-Mex Conference, Mexico, pp. 34–37.

17. Gay, G.M., R.A. Retana, and P.E. Soto. 1995. Valoracion comparativa de una vacuana emulsionada experimental contra la hepatitis con cuerpos de inclusion. Proc 20th Annu ANECA Conf, pp. 118–123.

18. McCracken, R.M., and B.M. Adair. 1993. Avian Adenoviruses. In J.B. McFerran, and M.S. McNulty (eds.). Virus Infections of Birds, vol. 4. Elsevier Science Publishers B.V., Amsterdam, pp. 123–144.

19. McFerran, J.B. 1989. Adenoviruses. In H.G. Purchase, L.H. Arp, C.H. Domermuth, and J.F. Pearson (eds.). A Laboratory Manual for the Isolation and Identification of Avian Pathogens, 3rd ed. American Association of Avian Pathologists, Kennett Square, PA, pp. 77–81.

20. Morales, G.A., V.V. Valle, and D.E. Lucio. 1995. Identifacion de los agentes etiologicos del syndrome del hydropericardio. Proc 20th Annu ANECA Conf, pp. 225–227.

21. Muneer, M.A., M. Ajmal, M. Arshad, M.D. Ahmad, Z.I. Chaudhry and T.M. Khan. 1989. Preliminary studies on hydropericardium syndrome in broilers in Pakistan. Zootech Int (May):46–48.

22. Naeem, K., T. Niazi, S.A. Malik, and A.H. Cheema. 1995. Immunosuppressive potential and pathogenicity of an avian adenovirus isolate involved in hydropericardium syndrome in broilers. Avian Dis 39:723–728.

23. Niazi, A.K., M.Z. Khan, and M. Siddique. 1989. Haematological studies on naturally occurring hydropericardium syndrome in broiler chicks. Vet Rec 125:400.

24. Vos, M., and G. Monreal. 1995. Aislamiento e identificacion de adenovirus de lasaves, con atencion especial en el sindrome del hidropericardio. Proc 20th Annu ANECA Conf, pp. 417–423.

25. Zaman, T., and M.Z. Khan. 1991. Serum profiles in hydropericardium affected broiler chicks. Pakistan Vet J 11:50–52.

HYPOGLYCEMIA–SPIKING MORTALITY SYNDROME OF BROILER CHICKENS

James F. Davis

INTRODUCTION AND HISTORY. Hypoglycemia–spiking mortality syndrome (HSMS) is a disease of uncertain, but probable, infectious etiology, characterized by low morbidity and abrupt onset of high mortality (>0.5%) for at least 3 consecutive days with concurrent hypoglycemia in clinically affected birds. Seven- to 14-day-old broiler chicks are usually affected (1); however, recently the disease has been identified in commercial broilers as old as 42 days (3). Clinical signs include fine head tremors, apparent blindness, ataxia, and coma. Recovery often occurs spontaneously, but rickets, runting/stunting, and airsacculitis frequently develop in survivors.

Hypoglycemia–spiking mortality syndrome was first recognized in broiler flocks on the Delmarva Peninsula in the United States, in 1986 (2). The disease was subsequently described in 1991 (1) from 41 flocks with naturally occurring disease and three flocks with experimental disease. Occurrence of the disease has declined in the Delmarva area but has subsequently increased in the southeastern United States.

Because the etiology is unknown and there is no specific identifying characteristic of the disease (which makes only a clinical definition possible) and because young broilers experience infections with a variety of agents, the relationships among various outbreaks of HSMS remain uncertain. Two clinical forms of the disease have been identified. Type A, which was initially described, is more severe but of shorter duration than Type B, a milder form occurring over a longer period, which was identified later (2). This suggests that either HSMS is one disease caused by a specific etiologic agent that occurs in different forms (possibly because of additional modifying factors) or that similar clinical diseases result from different causative agents.

INCIDENCE AND DISTRIBUTION. Hypoglycemia–spiking mortality syndrome has been reported in Canada, Europe, Malaysia, South Africa, and the United States. Although broiler chicks are most commonly affected, broiler breeder replacements and leghorns are also susceptible.

ETIOLOGY. The etiologic agent(s) of HSMS has not been identified. A serotype-12 avian adenovirus isolated from affected flocks was pathogenic for embryos and chicks but did not cause HSMS (12). Inclusion body hepatitis caused by an adenovirus was identified in a broiler flock with excess mortality and hypoglycemia (9). Evidence for adenovirus infection in other flocks (1) has not been found.

Recently, oral inoculations of unprocessed fecal-intestinal-saline homogenates, fecal-saline homogenates passed through 0.45-μm filters, or crude brain-phosphate buffered saline homogenates from affected chicks have been used to reproduce the disease in susceptible chicks (5, 7). Hypoglycemia–spiking mortality syndrome has also been reproduced using 1) viruslike particles extracted from intestines of affected chicks and banded in a discontinuous Renograffin® gradient, or 2) filtered (0.22-μm porosity filter) homogenate from dead specific-pathogen–free (SPF) embryos inoculated via the yolk sac with banded particles 72 hr earlier (7).

These findings indicate that at least one type of HSMS appears to be caused by an infectious, filterable agent. The agent has yet to be isolated and identified. Arkansas strain of infectious bronchitis virus and avian encephalomyelitis virus have been identified in some of the inocula used to reproduce HSMS experimentally (3, 7). The significance of these two common viral agents of chickens in the disease is currently unknown. Because particles consistent with arenaviruses have been found by direct EM in droppings from affected chicks, immunohistochemistry (IHC) using both monoclonal and polyclonal antibodies to New World arenaviruses has been used to examine formalin-fixed tissues from naturally and experimentally infected chicks. Positive staining was found in the cytoplasm of pancreatic islet and acinar cells, Purkinje cells, neurons, hepatocytes, Kupffer cells, macrophages, histiocytes, and fibroblasts of infected birds, but not in these cells of uninfected, matched controls (5, 7). SPF embryos inoculated via the yolk sac with Renograffin®-banded viruslike particles 72 hr previously were also IHC-positive. Specificity of the IHC reaction in these HSMS-infected embryos and chicks still needs to be determined. It is possible that the antibodies are cross-reacting to an epitope that is present on both arenaviruses and another unidentified agent(s).

To reproduce HSMS, 1- to 2.5-day-old chicks are inoculated orally. Approximately 2 wk later, chicks are fasted for 2–6 hr and, in some cases, sprayed with a cool (25 C) water mist to cause mild stress. Clinical signs of HSMS begin 1.5 to 4 hr after fasting and stressing. Plasma glucose levels are severely depressed in affected chicks; occasionally as low as 17 mg/dL. Unexposed controls remain unaffected by fasting and stressing, and plasma glucose levels remain greater than 150 mg/dL (5, 7).

Hypoglycemia–spiking mortality syndrome also resulted when birds were fed darkling beetles (*Alphitobius diaperinus*) collected from built-up litter on farms where the disease had occurred repeatedly. Whether beetles or other similar insects may serve as mechanical or true vectors of the agent(s) causing HSMS is still unknown (7).

Other factors believed to contribute to HSMS are certain diets, especially ones with high amounts of animal by-products labile to oxidation. An all-vegetable diet resulted in the highest mortality and a marked increase in susceptibility to *Escherichia coli* septicemia (2). Management errors that would lead to birds being without feed or cause them to experience other stressful events will precipitate HSMS in infected birds. Although mycotoxins or other toxic substances might be suspected in the disease because of its abrupt onset and high mortality, these substances have not been identified (2). Feeding cockleburs (*Xanthium* spp.) to chicks did not cause clinical disease or hypoglycemia (8).

PATHOGENESIS AND EPIZOOTIOLOGY.
Clinical signs include huddling, trembling, blindness, loud chirping, litter eating, ataxia, prostration with outstretched legs, and coma. Rapidly growing males in good condition are often most affected (2). Chicks may or may not have diarrhea, but orange mucoid droppings are commonly found. Lameness often occurs after acute clinical signs have subsided.

Gross lesions are nonspecific. Occasionally, hemorrhage and necrosis are evident in the liver. Thymus is markedly atrophied, with other lymphoid organs variably affected. Dehydration is frequently seen along with accumulation of urates in ureters. Also, there are changes consistent with mild enteritis, especially excess fluid accumulation in the lower intestines and ceca. Similarly, microscopic changes are nonspecific and consistent with those expected from the gross lesions. Chicks with gross liver lesions have necrotic hepatocytes secondary to fibrinoid necrosis of hepatic arteries (1, 5, 7). Rarely, similar vascular changes also can be seen in the intestines and gut-associated lymphoid tissue. Rickets and severe lymphoid depletion/necrosis of the bursa of Fabricius have also been observed in affected chicks (1), although these lesions have been inconsistent in more recent cases (5, 7).

Experimentally, the disease seems to have a 10- to 12-day incubation period. At this time, chicks begin passing wet droppings containing undigested feed and huddle together. If chicks are not fasted or stressed, this digestive disorder and the runting-stunting sequelae associated with it may be the only clinical signs seen. Surviving chicks often remain permanently stunted (5). Plasma from stunted or hypoglycemic chicks is often colorless or pale yellow compared with the deep yellow color of plasma from unaffected controls (7). Insulinlike growth factor-1 (IGF-1), a growth-related hormone (13, 14), is significantly depressed in affected chicks (5).

Acutely hypoglycemic chicks, both from the field (4) and from experimental trials (3), have significantly depressed pancreatic glucagon levels. Pancreas from these chicks is histologically normal with no evidence of cell necrosis.

Stress and acute fasting trigger the glucagon–glycogen pathway (glycogenolysis) to maintain adequate blood glucose levels (10, 11). If chicks are deficient in glucagon and/or glycogen, they can rapidly become hypoglycemic. Chicks with HSMS are deficient in both glucagon (4) and glycogen (7), which makes them extremely susceptible to development of hypoglycemia when acutely fasted and/or stressed.

DIAGNOSIS.
A high spike in a mortality curve at 7–14 days of age is suggestive but not diagnostic for HSMS. Varying numbers of chicks may be affected or a high mortality spike may be caused by some other condition. Diagnosis of HSMS is based on the typical clinical findings and demonstrating hypoglycemia in affected chicks. Plasma and/or whole blood can be used for glucose determinations; plasma levels determined with a chemical analyzer are considered to be most accurate. Severely affected chicks typically have blood or plasma glucose levels between 20 and 80 mg/dL. Fasting alone will not result in hypoglycemia (blood glucose <150 mg/dL) in uninfected chicks.

TREATMENT, PREVENTION, AND CONTROL.
There is no specific treatment for the disease. Supportive care based on minimizing stress due to excessive heat, cold, ammonia, poor ventilation, noise, or feed and/or water deprivation is the most important factor (3). Chicks should be left alone and allowed to rest as much as possible in good environmental conditions with continuous availability of feed and water. Multiple vitamins, electrolytes, and liquid vitamin E have been used successfully to reduce mortality (2).

Controlled light–dark exposure programs prevent HSMS, both in the field and experimentally (7). The physiologic basis for this is attributed to melatonin release and a shift from glycogenolysis to gluconeogenesis by the birds exposed to darkness. Control of darkling beetles is important in preventing carryover of HSMS from one flock to the next (see Chapter 32). Vaccination of broiler breeder hens with an experimental formalin-inactivated autogenous vaccine produced from SPF embryos inoculated with the fourth egg passage of Renograffin®-banded viruslike particles (designated "The Oakwood Agent") failed to provide protection against experimental challenge of progeny from the hens (6, 7). Experimental trials with "live" vaccines have not yet been attempted.

REFERENCES

1. Brown, T.P., P.Y. Brunet, E.M. Odor, D.W. Murphy, and E.T. Mallinson. 1991. Microscopic lesions of naturally occurring and experimental "spiking mortality" in young broiler chickens. Avian Dis 35:481–486.
2. Craig, F.R. 1991. Delmarva Mortality Task Force summary. Proc 26th Natl Meet Poult Health Condemn, Ocean City, MD, pp. 12–28.
3. Davis, J.F. 1996. Unpublished observations.
4. Davis, J.F., and R. Vasilatos-Younken. 1995. Markedly reduced pancreatic glucagon levels in broiler chickens with spiking mortality syndrome. Avian Dis 39:417–419.
5. Davis, J.F., J.C. de la Torre, M. Teng, A.E. Castro, J.T. Doman, T.L. Noble, and S. Yuen. 1995. Spiking mortality syndrome in chickens. Vet Rec 136:204.
6. Davis, J.F., A.E. Castro, J.C. de la Torre, C.G. Scanes, R. Vasilatos-Younken, J.T. Doman, S.V. Radecki, and M. Teng. 1995. Hypoglycemia and spiking mortality in Georgia chickens:experimental reproduction in broiler breeder chicks. Avian Dis 39:162–174.
7. Davis, J.F., A.E. Castro, J.C. de la Torre, H.J. Barnes, J.T. Doman, M. Metz, H. Lu, S. Yuen, and P.A. Dunn. 1996. Experimental reproduction of severe hypoglycemia and spiking mortality syndrome using embryo-passaged and field-derived preparations. Avian Dis 40:158–172.
8. Goodwin, M.A., E.T. Mallinson, J. Brown, E.C. Player, K.S. Latimer, N. Dale, W.V. Shaff, and T.G. Dickson. 1992. Toxicological pathology of cockleburs (Xanthium spp.) for broiler chickens. Avian Dis 36:444–446.
9. Goodwin, M.A., D.L. Hill, M.A. Dekich, and M.R. Putnam. 1993. Multisystemic adenovirus infection in broiler chicks with hypoglycemia and spiking mortality. Avian Dis 37:625–627.
10. Guyton, A.C. 1976. Insulin, glucagon, and diabetes mellitus. In A.C. Guyton (ed.). Textbook of Medical Physiology, 5th ed. W.B. Saunders Co., Philadelphia, PA, pp. 1044–1045.
11. Hazelwood, R.L. 1976. Carbohydrate metabolism. In P.D. Sturkie, (ed.). Avian Physiology. Springer-Verlag, New York, pp. 210–232.
12. Mendelson, C., H.B. Nothelfer, and G. Monreal. 1995. Identification and characterization of an avian adenovirus isolated from a "spiking mortality syndrome" field outbreak in broilers on the Delmarva Peninsula, USA. Avian Pathol 24:693–706.
13. Scanes, C.G., E.A. Dunnington, F.C. Buonomo, D.J. Donoghue, and P.B. Siegel. 1989. Plasma concentrations of insulin like growth factors (IGF-)I and IGF-II in dwarf and normal chickens of high and low weight selected lines. Growth Dev Aging 53:151–157.
14. Vasilatos-Younken, R., and C.G. Scanes. 1991. Growth hormone and insulin-like growth factors in poultry growth: required, optimal, or ineffective. Poult Sci 70:1764–1780.

POULT ENTERITIS–MORTALITY SYNDROME ("SPIKING MORTALITY") OF TURKEYS

H. John Barnes and James S. Guy

INTRODUCTION. Poult enteritis–mortality syndrome (PEMS) is an infectious, transmissible disease typically affecting young turkeys between 7 and 28 days of age. The disease is characterized by diarrhea, dehydration, weight loss, anorexia, immunosuppression, growth depression (40% or greater), and mortality (more than 2% between 7 and 28 days). Presently, the etiology is unknown, but enteropathogenic viruses complicated by secondary agents, especially bacteria, appear to be the most likely cause. The relationship of PEMS to other enteric diseases of turkeys is unknown at this time (see previous section on Enteric Disease Complex); some evidence suggests it may be a form of turkey coronaviral enteritis (see also Chapter 27). There is no indication that PEMS may be of public health significance.

Two clinical forms of PEMS have been recognized. Initially, an acute form was observed with a high death loss and a mortality pattern similar to a disease in chickens called "Spiking Mortality" (see previous section). This observation led to the most severe form of PEMS being named "Spiking Mortality of Turkeys" (SMT). Mortality in flocks with SMT is equal to or greater than 9% between 7 and 28 days of age, including at least 3 consecutive days with mortality equal to or greater than 1%. Losses

This disease has emerged so recently and is of such economic importance to the turkey industry that much of the information presented in this section is summarized from clinical and experimental studies conducted in our laboratories and those of Drs. T.P. Brown, F.W. Edens, and M. Qureshi and has yet to appear in published form. It represents our best understanding of PEMS at this time but still should be regarded as preliminary information.

in excess of 50% have occurred, which has often led to depopulation of the remainder of the flock. More recently, a less severe form of PEMS has been recognized, which has been referred to as Excess Mortality of Turkeys (EMT). Mortality in flocks with EMT exceeds 2% during the 7- to 28-day period but does not equal or exceed 1% for 3 consecutive days. Clinical evidence suggests mild or even inapparent infections probably occur; if a flock is first infected at an older age, clinical signs generally are seen and weight loss can still be considerable, but there is little or no mortality. As new knowledge further defines this disease, it is anticipated that a more definitive name for the disease will replace PEMS.

The SMT form of PEMS has a definite seasonal pattern occurring when temperatures and humidity levels are high; i.e., from late spring to early fall. Its geographic distribution is uncertain but appears to be limited to turkey-producing areas of the southeastern United States. Even within this area, it is common to have clusters of outbreaks only in specific localities, apparently related to density of farms and production within affected areas. Economic losses because of mortality, but more especially from reduced weight gain and uneven growth, have been substantial; those for PEMS during 1995 have been estimated at 34 million dollars.

HISTORY, INCIDENCE, AND DISTRIBUTION.

Poult enteritis–mortality syndrome was first recognized as the SMT form in a restricted geographic area along the western North Carolina/South Carolina border in late summer or early fall of 1991. While it is believed that this represents the emergence of a new disease in turkeys, it is also possible that PEMS either occurred previously in a milder form or was so sporadic that it did not attract attention. A similar disease, which has subsequently been identified as turkey coronaviral enteritis, also affected turkey flocks in central Indiana about this same time; its relationship to the North Carolina outbreak is uncertain. In North Carolina, PEMS remained localized until 1994 when flocks throughout the state were affected. The disease has now appeared in additional states and continues to affect most areas of North Carolina, although the severity of the disease still remains greatest in the area where it first occurred.

Epidemiologic studies of the 1994 outbreak in eastern North Carolina identified a close correlation between SMT and EMT on the same farms, suggesting they were different forms of the same disease. Subsequent sentinel studies have corroborated this finding.

ETIOLOGY.

The etiology of PEMS is unknown. Initially, a toxin in the feed, water, or environment was suspected because of the abrupt onset of high mortality. Attempts to incriminate a poison by direct assays and feeding studies were unsuccessful. The infectious nature of the disease was first discovered by Brown (1) at the University of Georgia by exposing normal poults to 1) litter or darkling beetle (*Alphitobius diaperinus*) larvae from affected flocks in western North Carolina, or 2) intestinal homogenates from affected birds. Infectivity of an agent was also apparent in subsequent observations when the disease occurred in sentinels 30 hr after having been placed overnight in an affected flock in eastern North Carolina. In some instances, infective droppings failed to reproduce the disease in susceptible birds after the droppings had been frozen. Ten percent dimethylsulfoxide acts as an effective cryoprotectant. The likely role of darkling beetle larvae in transmission of PEMS has been confirmed experimentally (3).

A variety of enteropathogenic viruses have been identified in affected flocks, but none has been found capable of reproducing the disease or has been consistently associated with the disease. Early findings suggesting that alphaviruses (see Arbovirus Infections, Chapter 31) may have been the cause of PEMS (4) were not confirmed in subsequent studies. A coronavirus or a yet undiscovered virus are presently considered to be the most likely initiating, or "essential," etiologic agent. Coronavirus identified by direct electron microscopy, appeared to be significantly associated with diarrheal diseases in poults including the SMT form of PEMS (5). As a result of changes induced by a putative viral infection in the poults, bacteria, possibly including certain strains of *Escherichia coli*, *Salmonella*, or *Campylobacter*, become important contributors to the disease. Evidence suggests that a virus is primarily responsible for the initial enteric disease, growth depression, and increased susceptibility to bacterial infection, while bacteria are primarily responsible for the mortality. Crop mycosis (see Chapter 16) and heavy intestinal infections with protozoa (trichomonads, *Cochlosoma*, cryptosporidia) (see Chapter 34) are commonly found in affected birds. They are considered to increase the severity of the disease. Nutritional, environmental, and host factors all seem to be important in modulating how severe an outbreak will be.

PATHOGENESIS AND EPIZOOTIOLOGY.

Poult enteritis–mortality syndrome only occurs in turkeys. In the field, hen flocks are often more severely affected than tom flocks. This may, however, be related more to differences in management of the two types of farms because there are no differences based on sex that are apparent after experimental infection. Similarly, all commercial breeds appear to be equally susceptible to the disease. Poults from young breeders are more severely affected and, conversely, poults from recycled hens are more resistant than poults from hens in midproduction.

There is evidence that chickens and cattle may experience inapparent infections with the essential agent. The latter may also serve as a biologic reservoir and maintain the organisms on a farm for an extended period (2). Chickens develop antibodies to the putative essential agent following exposure to infective droppings from affected poults. Cross-transmission studies between chickens and turkeys with their respective spiking mortality syndromes have been unsuccessful, indicating the two diseases are distinct from each other even though they have similar clinical presentations. In addition, hypoglycemia is not a feature of SMT, in contrast to hypoglycemia-spiking mortality syndrome of chickens.

Transmission of the disease is by the fecal–oral route. Attempts to reproduce PEMS experimentally in normal poults using blood or extraintestinal tissue pools have been unsuccessful. Following contact exposure to infected poults, clinical signs develop within 24–36 hr. Using droppings collected at this time for inocula will eliminate cryptosporidia if they are present. Epidemiologic and clinical findings suggest that vertical transmission does not occur. Nor does it appear that there are long-term carriers; sentinels placed in a breeder flock during production that had been affected previously did not contract the disease. It does appear likely that individual poults vary in susceptibility to PEMS, but the responsible factors have yet to be determined.

Clinically there is an initial, brief period of hyperactivity and excess vocalization accompanied by increased water consumption, decreased feed consumption, picking at feed, and eating feathers and litter. Subsequently, the birds become increasingly inactive, somnolent, and anorexic; they huddle together and seek heat sources. Droppings are increased, watery, and pale brown with a fine flocculent appearance. They may drip from the vent of severely affected birds when they are held vertically. Feathers around the vent extending down on the abdomen are wet from contact with liquid feces. Litter conditions in the brooding house deteriorate rapidly following onset of diarrhea. The excess litter moisture likely increases bacterial contamination of the environment and exposure of the poults. Within 3 days, the growth rate markedly decreases, but birds generally continue to gain some weight. By 7 days, growth in many birds will have ceased, with some birds actually losing weight. Mortality is uncommon before 4 days postexposure, peaking on days 5, 6, and 7. A lower secondary peak of mortality often occurs a few days later. Birds that either lose weight or gain the least weight are most likely to die. Lost weight is not regained; recovered tom turkeys can weigh as much as 2–4 kg less than the breed standard when marketed at 20 wk of age. Recovered flocks are more susceptible to other infectious diseases such as colibacillosis and fowl cholera.

Gross Lesions. There are no specific gross lesions that will help to identify PEMS. The overall appearance of an affected bird at necropsy is typical of one with an acute, severe diarrheal disease. Affected poults typically show dehydration, emaciation, and marked muscle atrophy, and occasional birds have osteoporosis (brittle bones) or, less commonly, rickets. Additional findings include enlarged gallbladder; prominent adrenal glands; lack of food in the gastrointestinal tract; litter, often in large amounts, in the gizzard; crop mycosis; thin-walled, dilated intestine containing fluid and gas; ceca distended with watery brown liquid and gas; cloaca and distal rectum distended with feces and urates; extreme thymic and mild to moderate bursal and splenic atrophy; mild to moderate renal swelling; and excess urates visible in ureters. Caseous exudate that accumulates in the bursa of Fabricius to form a bursal core occurs in approximately 10–20% of affected birds later in the disease (Fig. 37.5). Bursal cores may be a characteristic lesion of the disease, but this needs to be confirmed. In one study, bursal cores were still present 5 wk postexposure. Survivors have poor feathering and are stunted.

Histopathology. Typical microscopic lesions of PEMS are found in the intestinal (especially from midjejunum distally) and bursal mucosae. Intestinal and bursal epithelial cells are apparently the

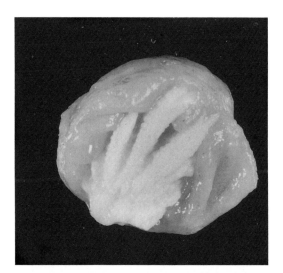

37.5. Caseous exudate has accumulated in the bursa of Fabricius of a turkey poult with poult enteritis–mortality syndrome (PEMS). Such bursal cores can be found in about 10% of infected birds and may represent a characteristic gross lesion of the disease.

target cells for viral infection as determined by light and electron microscopy and immunofluorescence. In the intestinal tract, there is acute enterotyphlitis with villous atrophy; crypt epithelial hyperplasia; a reduction in epithelial cell height, especially on the distal third of affected villi; occasional sloughing of epithelial cells from villous tips; mixed cellular infiltration of the lamina propria, often containing necrotic macrophages; emigration of heterophils into the lumen; and exudation of proteinaceous fluid. Cryptosporidia, intestinal flagellates, and/or increased luminal bacteria, occasionally including long-segmented filamentous bacteria, are frequently present.

In the bursa, epithelial cells undergo degeneration characterized by swelling and pallor. These slough and are accompanied by exudation of proteinaceous fluid and heterophilic inflammation. The normal tall pseudostratified epithelium of the bursa changes to a transitional or, less commonly, a stratified squamous epithelium (Fig. 37.6A). Apoptosis is increased in the bursal follicles, which leads to lymphoid depletion (Fig. 37.6B). In a few birds, luminal exudate in the bursa supports bacterial growth, which intensifies heterophilic exudation leading to production of bursal cores. Other lesions include crop mycosis, which is often severe; moderate to marked lymphoid depletion of spleen and thymus; and organ changes resulting from emaciation and dehydration.

By electron microscopy, viral particles in cytoplasmic vesicles are often numerous in intestinal and bursal epithelial cells, particularly those undergoing degeneration or sloughing into the lumen (Fig. 37.7).

Immunity. Poult enteritis–mortality syndrome causes immunosuppression, probably as a result of damage to lymphoid organs. Because the thymus is most affected, impairment of cell-mediated immunity would be expected to be greater than impairment of humoral immunity. Ability to clear bacteria from the circulation is also impaired (6), which likely provides the basis for increased susceptibility of recovered flocks to subsequent bacterial diseases.

Little is known concerning immunity to the disease itself. A reduction in growth rate, but not mortality, occurred in approximately 20% of recovered birds when they were experimentally reexposed 4 wk after the initial exposure, suggesting that immunity may not be very important in host resistance. Mortality was substantially lower, however, in experimentally infected poults from recovered breeder hens as compared with similar poults from a flock that had not previously experienced the disease. This finding suggests that maternal antibodies may provide some early protection.

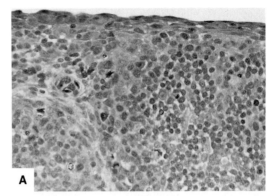

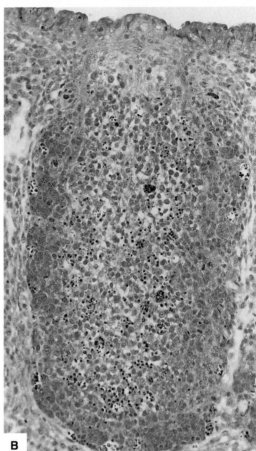

37.6. Bursa of Fabricius from turkey poults with poult enteritis–mortality syndrome (PEMS). *A.* Typical pseudostratified epithelium has been replaced by a squamous epithelium because of sloughing of infected cells. ×70. *B.* Increased apoptosis is occurring in this follicle, which will result in lymphoid depletion. ×70.

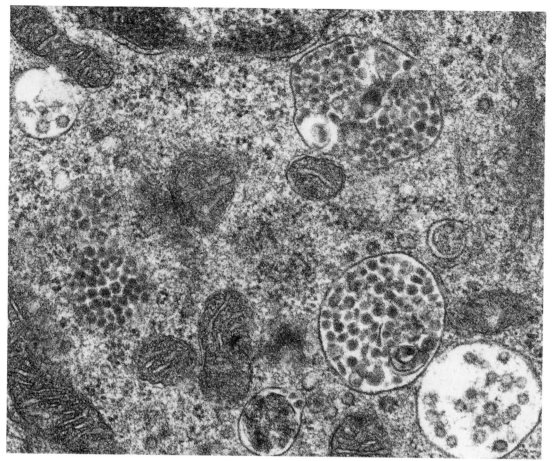

37.7. Bursal epithelium 4 days after exposure to poult enteritis–mortality syndrome (PEMS). Numerous viral particles in cytoplasmic vesicles are characteristic of PEMS. The identity of these particles is not presently known, but they are considered to be the likely cause of the disease. ×58,800.

DIAGNOSIS. Currently, intense efforts are under way to identify the essential agent necessary for PEMS to occur and to develop appropriate diagnostic tests for both antigen and antibody. Until these are available and validated, a tentative diagnosis of PEMS can be made if mortality, due to unknown causes, exceeds 2% in young turkeys between 7 and 28 days of age. This definition should be used for developing control and monitoring programs. Confirmation of PEMS can be made by experimental reproduction of the disease in susceptible poults by inoculation of feces or intestinal homogenates from clinically affected birds, or by placement of sentinels in flocks or environments. The latter approach can be used to detect inapparent infections, carriers, or contaminated premises. Poults that are 1–2 wk of age make good sentinels. At least two blind passages of feces or intestinal homogenates should be made at weekly intervals to amplify any agents

from the inoculum or picked up by the sentinels before calling a flock negative. Mortality of at least 30% and growth depression of at least 40% have been established as criteria for PEMS in experimental studies.

Episodes of acute diarrheal disease are very common in commercial turkey flocks. While they all cause some loss of production and perhaps even a slight increase in mortality, the vast majority are not PEMS, certainly not the SMT form. These common occurrences of enteric disease are lumped together as Poult Enteritis Complex (PEC). When the condition does not fit the criteria of PEMS because of insufficient mortality, this diagnosis should be given rather than one of "mild" SMT or PEMS. Another enteric disease that is intermediate in severity between PEC and PEMS has been variously termed "Stunting Syndrome" or "Feed Refusal Syndrome" (see previous section on Enteric Disease Complex).

This condition is clinically similar to the EMT form of PEMS. The relationship between these two clinical entities is unknown and needs to be resolved. Flocks with suspected PEMS also need to be examined for turkey coronavirus infection. Both antigen- and antibody-detection systems for turkey coronavirus infection are available. Optimum samples are sections of lower jejunum and ileum taken from experimentally exposed poults 4 days postexposure. These should be snap-frozen in a small container or plastic bag submerged in a dry ice/alcohol bath or liquid nitrogen. Direct electron microscopy has not proven very useful for coronaviral diagnosis. Virions often are not numerous enough to detect; furthermore, they are difficult to distinguish from debris, and they frequently lose their characteristic petallike surface projections when being prepared. A possible relationship of turkey coronaviral enteritis to PEMS is suspected but presently uncertain. In any case, the occurrence of any coronavirus infection in turkeys needs to be determined, as it is very likely to be significant (see also Chapter 27).

TREATMENT, PREVENTION, AND CONTROL.

Antibiotics (bacitracin, lincomycin, penicillin) and intestinal astringents (arsenicals, copper) have been used with varying success to control the mortality that occurs with PEMS. Sarafloxacin, a fluoroquinolone recently approved for use in poultry in the United States, is highly effective when used according to manufacturer's directions.

Differences in occurrence and severity of PEMS in flocks of different companies in the same geographic area strongly suggest that nutritional and management factors can have a significant influence on the severity of the disease. One important factor in reducing losses is to stimulate eating during periods of inappetence. Rations for young poults must be carefully formulated with high-quality ingredients. Adding fat to produce a total of 7.5–8% will reduce both mortality and morbidity in affected flocks. Additional carbohydrate and/or fiber may also be helpful, but this has not been confirmed. Feed consistency is extremely important. Mash feeds or poor-quality crumbles containing a high percentage of fines are associated with higher mortality. Adding attractants to the feed such as powdered milk, whole grains, milk replacers, rolled oats, "sweet" (molasses coated) feed, and confectionery sprinkles are helpful. Dumping and recycling feed lines, cycling feeders on and off, and keeping the birds up and moving will stimulate feeding activity. Addition of vitamins and electrolytes to drinking water may provide some nutritional support as well. Milk replacers in the water are useful, but their use has to be closely monitored to prevent blocking of lines and buildup of bacterial contamination.

Affected flocks must be aggressively managed. Ventilation has to be increased to help remove moisture from the litter and house. Heat also will need to be increased to prevent birds from piling and aid in controlling total house moisture. Heavily soiled litter around drinkers and feeders should be removed frequently. Less contaminated areas can be managed by covering them with fresh, dry litter.

Prevention is based on principles of biosecurity (see Chapter 1). Unfortunately, seemingly excellent biosecurity has not proved to prevent occurrence of the disease on new farms, high-security breeding farms, or farms that have been depopulated, thoroughly cleaned and disinfected, and left vacant for periods up to 18 mo. In endemic areas, traditional multiage production is rapidly being replaced by all-in/all-out production and off-site brooding. In the latter production method, brood-only farms supply poults at approximately 5 wk of age to several finishing farms. In this way, both the volume of multiage production and biosecurity of all-in/all-out production can be achieved. It is too early to know what impact these changes may have on PEMS.

Use of formaldehyde to disinfect facilities between flocks is currently considered the best procedure but still does not guarantee that PEMS will not occur. It is important that dead poults be picked up promptly and disposed of in a manner to prevent flies from contacting the carcasses. Control of both beetles and flies is important as they are known, or strongly suspected, vectors of the disease. Arthropod transmission could explain the seasonal and geographic patterns of the disease and why the disease is so difficult to eliminate from affected premises. Limited sentinel studies have shown that recovered flocks can remain a source of the causative agent(s) for 6–8 wk after recovery, but they apparently do not remain persistent carriers. Cattle and other poultry should not be maintained on turkey farms. If present on a farm with affected flocks, cattle may need to be removed to effect control of the disease, as current information suggests they are likely reservoirs.

Procedures that have been tried and judged to be ineffective for controlling PEMS include use of autogenous and approved biologics that could potentially provide cross-protection including use of bursal disease vaccine in day-old poults, heating the house to approximately 90 C (104 F) for at least 3 hr between broods, water acidification, and administration of disinfectants to poults through water.

REFERENCES

1. Brown, T.P. 1995. Personal communication.
2. Brown, T.P., W.H. Emory, and D. Howell, Jr. 1995. Acute enteritis in turkey poults: chickens and cattle as subclinical carriers. Proc 132nd AVMA Meet, Pittsburgh, PA, p. 115.
3. Despins, J.L., R.C. Axtell, D.V. Rives, J.S. Guy, and

M.D. Ficken. 1994. Transmission of enteric pathogens of turkeys by darkling beetle larva Alphitobius diaperinus. J Appl Poult Res 3:61–65.

4. Ficken, M.D., D.P. Wages, J.S. Guy, J.A. Quinn, and W.H. Emory. 1993. High mortality of domestic turkeys associated with highlands J virus and eastern equine encephalitis virus infections. Avian Dis 37:585–590.

5. Goodwin, M.A., J. Brown, E.C. Player, W.L. Steffens, D. Hermes, and M.A. Dekich. 1995. Fringed membranous particles and viruses in faeces from healthy turkey poults and from poults with putative poult enteritis complex/spiking mortality. Avian Pathol 24:497–505.

6. Miles, A.M., and H.J. Barnes. 1995. Factors affecting E. coli clearance in turkeys. Proc 132nd AVMA Meet, Pittsburgh, PA, p. 116

FULMINATING DISEASE OF GUINEA FOWL

H. John Barnes

INTRODUCTION AND HISTORY. Fulminating disease (*maladie foudroyante de la pintade*) of guinea fowl is an infectious, transmissible, acute, viral enteritis of commercial guinea fowl up to 12 wk of age, characterized by severe diarrhea and mortality approaching 100% in young birds (1, 4). Although the cause of the disease remains uncertain, it has been reproduced with a togaviruslike agent (1). Fulminating disease is distinct from a milder, transmissible enteritis, possibly caused by an enteroviruslike virus that occurs frequently and is widespread in guinea fowl (5).

Fulminating disease was first identified in commercial guinea fowl flocks in 1978 and became epidemic in southern France in late 1985 and in 1986 (4). Subsequently, outbreaks have diminished; the disease was no longer affecting flocks by 1991. Why the disease behaved in this fashion is unknown, but it has been speculated that the low density of flocks in the epidemic area may have been partly responsible (1). In spite of its disappearance, the disease remains a potential threat to commercial guinea fowl production because of the high economic losses it can cause and the lack of knowledge about how it can be controlled (1).

INCIDENCE AND DISTRIBUTION. Occurrence of fulminating disease in other areas or avian species is unknown.

ETIOLOGY. The cause of fulminating disease has not been definitively established. *Campylobacter jejuni*, *Chlamydia psittaci*, and protozoa initially associated with the disease have been eliminated as potential causes. A virus is suspected to cause the disease, as it can be reproduced with filtered (0.45 μm) intestinal homogenates from naturally infected guinea fowl. A number of viruses have been associated with the disease including an enteroviruslike virus, a virus isolated in embryos considered to be either a reovirus or herpesvirus that produced diarrhea and weight loss, but not mortality, in experimentally inoculated birds (3), and an agent with a morphology suggestive of a virus in either the *Paramyxoviridae* or *Orthomyxoviridae* family (2). The latter agent was also observed in abnormal droppings from chickens, Muscovy ducks, and turkeys with diarrhea in the same geographic area where fulminating disease of guinea fowl was occurring.

An enveloped virus with characteristics suggesting it may be in the *Togaviridae* family has been identified, purified, and used to reproduce the disease experimentally (1). Buoyant density of the togaviruslike virus concentrated in a sucrose gradient from an intestinal homogenate of guinea fowls orally inoculated 3 days earlier was 1.18 g/mL. The agent hemagglutinated goose erythrocytes (optimum conditions pH 6.3–6.4 at 22 C for 30 min). Spherical particles averaging 85 nm with 6–10 nm surface projections were seen in the purified preparation by electron microscopy. Following ether treatment, particles appeared hexagonal and were approximately 40 nm in diameter. They were distinct from interfering enveloped particles (fringed membranous particles) ranging in size from 50 to 500 nm with 20-nm rectangular surface projections that were found in the intestinal contents of both infected and control birds. Inability to grow this virus in culture has hampered further characterization of the agent (1).

PATHOGENESIS AND EPIZOOTIOLOGY.

Horizontal transmission occurs readily and quickly, most likely by the fecal–oral route. There is no evidence of vertical transmission. High virus titers are present in the intestines of birds 3 days postexposure (1).

Clinical signs include anorexia, lethargy, ruffled feathers, diarrhea, prostration, and emaciation. They are not specific and are typical of any acute, severe, diarrheal disease of birds. Birds die 2–6 days postinfection. At necropsy, intestines are pale, lack tone, and are distended with fluid; gallbladders are prominent because of distension; kidneys are swollen; and multiple, pale foci consistent with necrosis are present in the pancreas. Microscopically, there is mild atrophy of villi, immature enterocytes lacking a brush border on villous tips, and slight infiltration of the lamina propria and submucosa with lymphocytes in the intestines. Acinar cell degeneration and multifocal necrosis are present in the pancreas (1, 4).

DIAGNOSIS.

Diagnosis is based on typical clinical signs in commercial guinea fowl. If the disease is suspected, demonstration of togaviruslike particles in filtrates should be attempted. Serology is not available. Fulminating disease needs to be differentiated from other viral, bacterial, and protozoal diarrheal diseases that may affect guinea fowl (4).

TREATMENT, PREVENTION, AND CONTROL.

There is no specific treatment or prevention method currently available for fulminating disease of guinea fowl. Spread of the disease can be minimized by good biosecurity practices (see Chapter 1). Thorough cleaning and disinfection coupled with all-in, all-out production are useful in controlling the disease on a farm. Affected flocks need to be managed to encourage eating and drinking (flashing lights have been used). Vitamins and minerals, especially vitamin E and selenium, in the water are useful. No vaccine is available (4).

REFERENCES

1. Brahem, A., N. Demarquez, M. Beyrie, A. Vuillaume, and H.J.A. Fleury. 1992. A highly virulent togavirus-like agent associated with the fulminating disease of guinea fowl. Avian Dis 36:143–148.

2. Fleury, H.J.A., G. Morere, N. Demarquez, and A. Vuillaume. 1988. Unidentified viral particles could be associated with enteritis of various commercial bird species. Ann Inst Pasteur 139:449–453.

3. Kles, V., M. Morin, G. Plassiart, M. Guittet, and G. Bennejean. 1992. Isolement d'un virus responsable d'un cas de maladie foudroyante de la pintade. Point Vet 24:283–288.

4. Lecoz, J. 1992. Pathologie de la pintade. In J. Brugere-Picoux and A. Silim (eds.). Manuel de Pathologie Aviaire. Imprimerie du Cercle des Elèves de l'Ecole Nationale Vétérinaire d'Alfort. Maisons-Alfort, France, pp. 281–287.

5. Pascucci, S., and A. Lavazza. 1994. A survey of enteric viruses in commercial avian species: Experimental studies of transmissible enteritis of guinea fowl. In M.S. McNulty and J.B. McFerran (eds.). New and Evolving Virus Diseases of Poultry. Commission of the European Communities, Brussels, pp. 225–241.

MUSCOVY DUCK PARVOVIRUS

H. John Barnes

Muscovy duck disease is an acute, systemic parvoviral infection of young Muscovy ducklings characterized by high mortality; enteric, locomotor, and nervous signs; abnormal feather development; and stunting. The disease is similar to Derszy's disease, a parvoviral infection of geese (see Chapter 31).

The disease emerged in Muscovy ducks being produced in concentrated duck-rearing areas of Brittany in western France in the fall of 1989 (5). Mortality rates as high as 80% occurred in some flocks. Ducks in this region are vaccinated for goose parvovirus (GPV) because that virus is endemic and can cause serious losses in Muscovy ducks (see Chapter 31). Apparent vaccine failures led to the isolation and characterization of a new virus that was found to be related to, but distinct from, goose parvovirus. This virus is provisionally being called duck parvovirus (DPV).

Muscovy duck disease is not known to occur outside of the area where it emerged, although GPV infections have been identified in other countries in Europe and, recently, in Japan (7).

Biologic properties of DPV are similar to those of GPV. It has a density of 1.39–1.42 g/cm^3 and 1.38 g/cm^3 for complete and empty virions, respectively; a diameter of 22–23 nm; three major proteins of 58, 78, and 91 kD; and single-stranded DNA composed of 5600 bases with palindromic ("hairpin") terminal sequences (3).

Duck parvovirus can be differentiated from GPV by cross-neutralization tests (2, 5). Ducklings with high antibody titers to GPV are susceptible to infection with DPV.

Only Muscovy ducks are susceptible to DPV; geese and other types of ducks are resistant (2). Both Muscovy ducks and a variety of types of geese are susceptible to GPV; however, other breeds and types of ducks are resistant. Disease is more severe in younger ducklings than in older ducklings (>5 wk), although the latter are susceptible and respond immunologically when infected.

Duck parvovirus is transmitted horizontally; it is also transmitted vertically when susceptible hens become infected during lay or there is reactivation of latency. Severe disease with high mortality occurs when virus spread occurs among ducklings in the hatcher.

Clinical signs, gross lesions, and histopathology are similar to those of GPV infection (see Chapter 31). Duck parvovirus infection can be differentiated from reovirus infection by the absence of exudative pericarditis, tenosynovitis, or splenic lymphoid hyperplasia (1).

Enzyme-linked immunosorbent assays have been developed to determine antibody titers. Titers in ducklings correspond well with protection against challenge for at least 7 days (2, 6).

Duck parvovirus can be isolated and identified by the same procedures that are useful for isolation of GPV (see Chapter 31). Muscovy duck embryos and cell cultures are preferable for DPV isolation (2). Differentiation of DPV from GPV by serologic and/or molecular methods or cross-neutralization tests may be required to confirm identity of the virus, since Muscovy ducks are susceptible to both GPV and DPV infection.

A chemiluminescent dot blot assay using a nonradioactive digoxigenin-labeled DPV DNA probe will detect DPV antigen in tissues. The method is highly sensitive and specific, but some GPV strains also can be detected with the probe, especially when they are in high concentration. Mammalian parvoviruses and nonviral DNA are not detected (4).

Prevention through good biosecurity practices (see Chapter 1) is important in minimizing spread and introduction of Muscovy duck disease to susceptible flocks.

Control of DPV is based on 1) immunization of breeders to prevent vertical transmission and to provide maternal immunity during the initial period of greatest susceptibility, and 2) day-old vaccination of ducklings to provide active immunity following decline of maternal antibodies. Two inoculations with bivalent, oil-emulsion vaccine containing DPV and GPV have been used in breeders (2, 6). In some flocks, however, maternal antibody levels in ducklings are insufficient to provide protection, especially late in the production cycle (6). Ducklings have been given an inactivated, aqueous DPV vaccine in combination with a live, attenuated GPV vaccine (2).

REFERENCES

1. Dalibard, V., G. Plassiart, Y. Cherel, M. Hurtel, and M. Wyers. 1993. Caractérisation des lésions histologiques de la parvovirose spontanée du canarde barbarie (Cairina moschata). Diagnostic histopathologique différential avec la réovirose. Recl Med Vet 169:763–772.

2. Fournier, D., and D. Gaudry. 1994. Recent discoveries on waterfowl pathology: a new parvovirus of Muscovy ducks in France—field vaccination trials. In M.S. McNulty and J.B. McFerran (eds.). New and Evolving Virus Diseases of Poultry. Commission of the European Communities, Brussels, pp. 183–194.

3. Gall-Recule, G., and V. Jestin. 1994. Muscovy duck parvovirus: Biochemical and genomic characterization. In M.S. McNulty and J.B. McFerran (eds.). New and Evolving Virus Diseases of Poultry. Commission of the European Communities, Brussels, pp. 123–133.

4. Gall-Recule, G., and V. Jestin. 1994. A digoxigenin-labeled probe for the detection of Muscovy duck parvovirus. In M.S. McNulty and J.B. McFerran (eds.). New and Evolving Virus Diseases of Poultry. Commission of the European Communities, Brussels, pp. 157–166.

5. Jestin, V., M-O. Le Bras, M. Cherbonnel, G. Le Gall, and G. Bennejean. 1991. Mise en évidence de parvovirus (virus de la maladie de Derzsy) trés pathogènes dans les élevages de canards de Barbarie. Recl Med Vet 167:849–857.

6. Jestin, V., M-O. Le Bras, and M. Cherbonnel. 1994. Control of Muscovy duck parvoviruses by vaccination. In M.S. McNulty and J.B. McFerran (eds.). New and Evolving Virus Diseases of Poultry. Commission of the European Communities, Brussels, pp. 167–181.

7. Takehara, K., K. Hyakutake, T. Imamura, K-i. Mutoh, and M. Yoshimura. 1994. Isolation, identification, and plaque titration of parvovirus from Muscovy ducks in Japan. Avian Dis 38:810–815.

TRANSMISSIBLE VIRAL PROVENTRICULITIS

Mark A. Goodwin and Scott Hafner

INTRODUCTION

Definition and Synonyms. Transmissible viral proventriculitis (TVP) is defined as transmissible proventricular inflammation in which virus can be found within the lesions (9, 10). Although chicks with proventricular enlargement are commonly said to have proventriculitis, it should be stressed that the lesion diagnosis "proventriculitis" can only be used correctly when there is microscopic evidence of inflammation in the the organ. Additionally, it must be appreciated that etiologic agents other than viruses can cause inflammation in the proventriculus (9).

Economic Significance. Chickens with TVP are more costly to produce than those without the disease (7); it has been estimated that 10 points of feed conversion are lost when chicks in one of the largest broiler-producing companies in the United States suffer outbreaks of viral proventriculitis.

HISTORY. Although broiler chickens throughout the world are commonly plagued by outbreaks of disease characterized at least in part by proventricular enlargement (14, 16), lesions consistent with TVP have only been described in detail in the United States (9, 10), Holland (13, 14, 15), and Australia (22). Other features of illness commonly include whole-body pallor, stunted growth, poor feed conversion ratios, and the passage of undigested or poorly digested feed in the feces (so-called feed passage) (5, 9, 15, 17, 22).

INCIDENCE AND DISTRIBUTION. Definitive prevalence data regarding the global incidence and distribution of TVP are lacking. In one 5-yr study, however, deep nonpurulent necrotizing proventriculitis accompanied by adenoepithelial hypertrophy and hyperplasia constituted 49.5% of the microscopic diagnoses in proventriculi of broiler chickens (9). Intranuclear inclusion bodies were not seen. Unexpectedly, intralesional intranuclear virus was found in proventriculi from each of five cases that were examined with a transmission electron microscope (TEM) (9). Intranuclear virus has not been seen in normal proventriculi.

In a follow-up study, intralesional virus was found in proventriculi from chickens in Texas, Arkansas, Mississippi, and the Delmarva peninsula (7). Light microscopic proventricular lesions in chicks in Holland (13, 14, 15) and Australia (22) were identical to proventricular lesions in U.S. chicks with TVP (9).

ETIOLOGY

Classification. The taxonomic classification of the transmissible virus seen in proventricular lesions has not been determined.

Morphology. In thin sections, intranuclear arrays of distinctly hexagonal virus (average particle size, 68.9 nm) are found. In cells with lysed nuclei, virus is associated with unbound condensed chromatin and is found within vacuolated spaces in the cytoplasm (average particle size, 62.3 nm) (9).

Laboratory Host Systems. Filtered or nonfiltered proventriculus homogenates can be used to transmit virus from infected chicks to specific-pathogen–free (SPF) chicks and commercial broiler chicks.

PATHOGENESIS AND EPIZOOTIOLOGY

Natural and Experimental Hosts. Naturally occurring TVP has only been reported in commercially raised broilers; however, the disease is transmissible to both broilers and SPF leghorns (10). Although the vast majority of chickens diagnosed with TVP are young, this may be a reflection of the age group most commonly presented for diagnosis. Microscopic lesions consistent with a diagnosis of TVP have been seen in chickens as old as 23 wk (7).

Transmission. The routes of natural infection are not known; however, chicks can be experimentally infected by oral and intracoelomic inoculation.

Signs. The predominant signs in chicks with TVP include stunted growth, pallor, unthriftiness, and passage of undigested or poorly digested feed in their feces (9). Naturally occurring cases are associated with poor flock production performance data (8).

Gross Lesions. Naturally or experimentally infected chicks may be significantly smaller than their uninfected counterparts (10). At necropsy, proventriculi are enlarged and mottled with a gray–white–yellow coloration (Fig. 37.8) (9). In formalin-fixed specimens, the proventriculus may

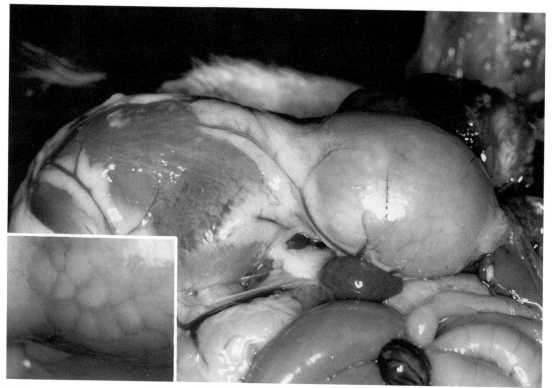

37.8. Proventriculus from a virus-infected broiler chick is enlarged and mottled gray–white–yellow. On close examination, multiple individual glands that are pale can be seen from the serosal surface (*inset*). (Avian Pathology)

have a checkered appearance characterized by subserosal disseminated gray–white polygonal foci that represent individual affected glands. On cut section, the proventricular wall usually is thickened, and the gray-white foci are seen to represent individual glands. Some glands are distended and viscous white material can be expressed from these glands if one uses gentle digital pressure. When viewing the lumenal surface, the mucosa may appear thick and rugose, and papillary orifices may be indistinct (Fig. 37.9).

Microscopic Lesions

LIGHT MICROSCOPY. There is patchy, locally extensive, or diffuse moderate to marked hypercellularity characterized by increased numbers of lymphocytes and macrophages, and fewer plasma cells that infiltrate the connective tissue stroma (tunica propria) (Fig. 37.10A). Inflammatory infiltrates are accompanied by necrosis of the alveolar (oxynticopeptic) pepsinogen- and hydrochloric acid–secreting cells (Fig. 37.10B). These cells have amorphous, granular, or vacuolated cytoplasm and nuclear condensation, fragmentation, or lysis. Fewer attached or sloughed cells have swollen nu-

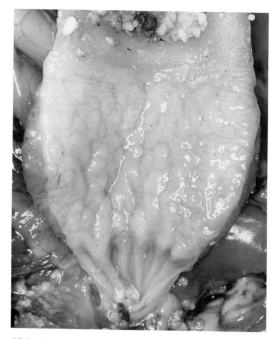

37.9. The proventricular mucosa from a virus-infected chick appears thickened and rugose. Papillary orifices are not distinct. (Avian Pathology)

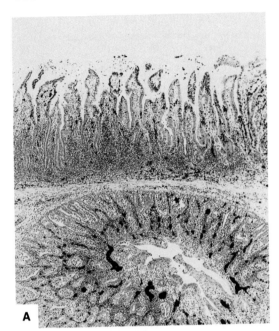

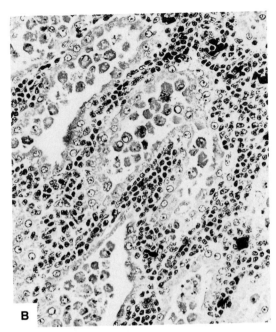

A   **B**

37.10. Microscopic lesions in the proventriculus of a virus-infected chick. *A.* Marked inflammation, adenoepithelial cell hypertrophy and hyperplasia, and early adenoectasia. H & E, ×40. *B.* At higher magnification, marked nonpurulent inflammation is accompanied by degeneration and necrosis of proventricular gland (alveolar) epithelial cells. Some of these alveolar cells have an enlarged nucleus with marginated chromatin and a clear center. H & E, ×397. (Avian Pathology)

clei with marginated chromatin and clear centers. Distinct hyaline or basophilic inclusion bodies are not present. Proliferating (hyperplastic) hypertrophic columnar to low cuboidal cells line primary, secondary, and tertiary gland ducts except where microulcers occur. Cuboidal or low columnar pale basophilic distinctly vacuolated ductlike epithelium appears to replace the destroyed alveolar secretory cells.

Gross and microscopic lesions in chicks with TVP change during the course of infection as follows: During the early stage of infection, i.e., between 5 and 9 days postinfection (DPI), gross lesions consist of multiple focal coalescing subserosal white–gray–yellow foci, and microscopic lesions include hypertrophy of the gut-associated lymphoid tissue (GALT), hyperplasia and piecemeal necrosis of GALT lymphocytes, multifocal, deep necrotizing nonpurulent proventriculitis, necrosis of the alveolar pepsinogen- and hydrochloric acid–secreting (oxynticopeptic) cells giving rise to microulcers, and alveolar cell nuclei have marginated chromatin and clear centers. During the transitional stage of infection (14 DPI), in addition to the above lesions, there is regeneration of the alveolar epithelium and multifocal adenoepithelial hypertrophy and hyperplasia. At the late stage of in-

fection (35 DPI), gross lesions include proventricular enlargement accompanied by prominent widening of the proventriculus–gizzard isthmus, and microscopic lesions consist of GALT hypertrophy, multifocal superficial nonpurulent proventriculitis, multifocal deep necrotizing nonpurulent proventriculitis, hypertrophy and hyperplasia of alveolar and duct epithelium, patchy or diffuse hypercellularity characterized by increased numbers of lymphocytes within the tunica propria, and multifocal adenoepithelial hypertrophy and hyperplasia.

In naturally occurring and experimental disease, virus infection is accompanied by destruction of up to 80% of the pepsinogen- and hydrochloric acid–secreting proventricular alveolar cells (9). The practical implications of such severe lesions are obvious and might explain why whole-body pallor, poor growth, and poor feed conversion are associated with TVP.

TRANSMISSION ELECTRON MICROSCOPY. Degenerating alveolar epithelial cells have either an intact nucleus or no intact nucleus with puddles of electron-dense material interpreted to represent condensed chromatin (Fig. 37.11). Hexagonal virus particles accompany vacuolation and fragmentation of organelles (Fig. 37.12). The size of intralesional virus particles varies from case to case (average size range, 62.3–68.9 nm). Virus particles in intact nuclei tend to be larger than those found in the cytoplasm of cells whose nuclei have lysed (9). Although it is possible that more than one virus might be present in chicks with TVP, it is more likely that harsh chemical treatments (fixation in formalin, exposure to organic solvents during processing, and staining) have adverse effects on virus size, i.e., apparent variations in virus size likely are artifacts; this has been described for chicken infectious anemia virus (18) (see Chapter 30).

Immunity.   Nothing is known about immunity and TVP.

DIAGNOSIS

Isolation and Identification of Agent.   The agent of TVP has not been isolated or identified beyond its TEM appearance in thin sections of fixed and processed proventriculus. A tentative diagnosis of TVP can be made upon finding gross and light microscopic lesions described above. A definitive diagnosis of TVP is made when intralesional hexagonal 62- to 69-nm virus is found.

Attempts to locate intralesional adenovirus or

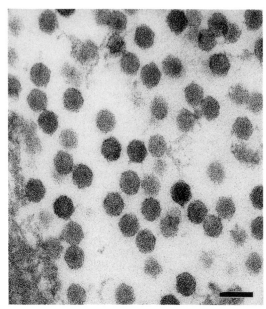

37.12.   Intranuclear virus particles have a hexagonal profile and average 65 nm in diameter. Formalin fixation, uranyl acetate, lead citrate, and osmium tetroxide.

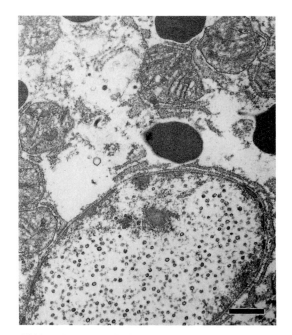

37.11.   Ultrastructurally, hexagonal virus particles are found in an intact nucleus. Notice the prominent large dark secretory granules that are characteristic of proventricular oxynticopeptic cells. Formalin fixation, uranyl acetate, lead citrate, and osmium tetroxide. Bar = 500 nm (Avian Pathology)

polyomavirus nucleic acid have not been successful; however, those findings do not exclude the possibility of adenovirus or polyomavirus infection (9). Intranuclear or intracytoplasmic virus has not been reported in proventriculi from normal or healthy chickens.

Serology.   There is no serologic test for TVP.

Differential Diagnosis.   Several agents or factors other than TVP-virus have been associated with proventricular enlargement and proventriculitis. They include low-fiber diets (23), dietary biogenic amines and mycotoxins (2, 3, 25), reovirus (2, 20), adenovirus (13), tumor-inducing viruses (1, 12, 19, 21, 26), *Cryptosporidium* sp. (6), and idiopathic proliferations of cells interpreted to represent histiocytes (11). Intralesional virus has not been described in any of these reports.

Although some proventriculi from reovirus-infected chicks might appear to be enlarged (2, 20), reovirus-infected chicks usually do not have proventricular enlargement, nor do they have proventriculitis. In fact, there are no data that establish that reoviruses are capable of causing proventriculitis in chickens (4, 24).

TREATMENT.   There is no specific treatment for TVP.

PREVENTION AND CONTROL. There are no specific prevention or control measures for TVP.

REFERENCES

1. Bagust, T.J., T.M. Grimes, and D.P. Dennett. 1979. Infection studies on a reticuloendotheliosis virus contaminant of a commercial Marek's disease vaccine. Aust Vet J 55:153–157.
2. Brugh, M., and R.L. Wilson. 1986. Effect of dietary histamine on broiler chickens infected with avian reovirus S1133. Avian Dis 30:199–203.
3. Dorner, J.W., R.J. Cole, L.G. Lomax, H.S. Gosser, and U.L. Diener. 1983. Cyclopiazonic acid production by Aspergillus flavus and its effects on broiler chickens. Appl Environ Microbiol 46:698–703.
4. Fletcher, O.J., Jr. 1988. Emerging animal diseases. In Poultry Diseases. Proc Second/Asian Pacific Poult Health Conf, Surfers Paradise, Australia, pp. 177–219.
5. Goodwin, M.A. 1993. Runting, stunting, enteritis, and failure to thrive. Proc Symp on Newly-Emerging and Reemerging Avian Diseases: Applied Research and Practical Applications for Diagnosis and Control, Minneapolis, MN, pp. 18–29.
6. Goodwin, M.A. 1995. Esophageal and proventricular cryptosporidiosis in a chicken. Avian Dis 39:643–645.
7. Goodwin, M.A. 1996. Unpublished observations.
8. Goodwin, M.A., K.S. Latimer, E.C. Player, F.D. Niagro, and R.P. Campagoli. 1995. Viral proventriculitis in chickens. Proc 132nd Annu Meet Am Vet Med Assoc, Pittsburgh, PA, pp. 140.
9. Goodwin, M.A., S. Hafner, D.I. Bounous, K.S. Latimer, E.C. Player, F.D. Niagro, R.P. Campagnoli, and J. Brown. 1996. Viral proventriculitis in chickens. Avian Pathol 25:369–379.
10. Goodwin, M.A., S. Hafner, D.I. Bounous, K.S Latimer, E.C. Player, F.D. Niagro, R.P. Campagnoli, and J. Brown. 1997. Transmissible viral proventriculitis in broiler chickens. Avian Pathol 26:(in press).
11. Hafner, S., M.A. Goodwin, E.J. Smith, D.I. Bounous, M. Puette, L.C. Kelley, and K.A. Langheinrich. 1996. Multicentric histiocytosis in young chickens. Gross and light microscopic pathology. Avian Dis 40:202–209.
12. Jackson, C.A.W., S.E. Dunn, D.I. Smith, P.T. Gilchrist, and P.A. MacQueen. 1977. Proventriculitis, "Nakanuke," and reticuloendotheliosis in chickens following vaccination with herpesvirus of turkeys (HVT). Aust Vet J 53:457–458.
13. Kouwenhoven, B., F.G. Davelaar, and J. Van Walsum. 1978. Infectious proventriculitis causing runting in broilers. Avian Pathol 7:183–187.
14. Kouwenhoven, B., M.H. Vertommen, and E. Goren. 1986. Runting in broilers. In J.B. McFerran and M.S. McNulty (eds.). Acute Virus Infections of Poultry. Martinus Nijhoff, Dordrecht, The Netherlands, pp. 165–178.
15. Kouwenhoven, B., R.M. Dewars, and J.F.M. Smeets. 1992. Proc 19th World's Poult Sci Congr, Amsterdam, The Netherlands, pp. 558–561.
16. Martland, M.F. 1989. Advances in runting stunting syndrome research. In R. Pandy (ed.). Progress in Veterinary Microbiology and Immunology, vol. 5. Non-oncogenic Avian Viruses. Karger, Basel, Switzerland, pp. 109–133.
17. McNulty, M.S. 1991. Runting stunting syndrome in broiler chickens. Proc 26th Natl Meet Poult Health Condemn, Ocean City, MD, pp. 115–124.
18. McNulty, M.S. 1991. Chicken anemia agent: A review. Avian Pathol 20:187–203.
19. Mussman, H.C. M.J. Twiehaus. 1971. Pathogenesis of reticuloendothelial virus disease in chicks—an acute runting syndrome. Avian Dis 15:483–502.
20. Page, R.K., O.J. Fletcher, G.N. Rowland, D. Gaudry, and P. Villegas. 1982. Malabsorption syndrome in broiler chickens. Avian Dis 26:618–624.
21. Payne, L.N., and H.G. Purchase. 1991. Leukosis/sarcoma group. In B.W. Calnek, H.J. Barnes, C.W. Beard, W.M. Reid, and H.W. Yoder, Jr. (eds.). Diseases of Poultry, 9th ed. Iowa State University Press, Ames IA, pp. 387–439.
22. Reece, R.L. 1996. Personal communication.
23. Riddell, C. 1987. Alimentary system. In Avian Histopathology. American Association of Avian Pathologists, Kennett Square, PA, p. 49.
24. Robertson, M.D., and G.E. Wilcox. 1986. Avian reovirus. Vet Bull 56:155–174.
25. Stewart, B.P., R.J. Cole, E.R. Waller, and V.E. Vesonder. 1986. Proventricular hyperplasia (malabsorption syndrome) in broiler chickens. J Exp Pathol Toxicol 6-3/4:369–386.
26. Witter, R.L. 1991. Reticuloendotheliosis. In B.W. Calnek, H.J. Barnes, C.W. Beard, W.M. Reid, and H.W. Yoder, Jr. (eds.). Diseases of Poultry, 9th ed. Iowa State University Press, Ames, IA, pp. 439–456.

BIG LIVER AND SPLEEN DISEASE

H. John Barnes

INTRODUCTION AND HISTORY. Big liver and spleen disease (BLS) is an infectious, transmissible disease of uncertain, but probable viral, etiology. It is characterized by decreased egg production, increased mortality, and enlargement of the liver and spleen of mature chickens, especially broiler breeders and, less commonly, egg layers. Infection with the BLS agent has been associated with a condition known as "primary feather drop syndrome" in the United States (8). For recent reviews, see (7, 11).

First recognized in Australia in 1980 (5), BLS is considered the most economically significant disease of broiler breeders in that country (5). Annual losses have been estimated at eight eggs/breeder in 50% of broiler breeder flocks for a value of $2.8 million (8).

INCIDENCE AND DISTRIBUTION. Besides Australia, serologic evidence indicates the BLS agent also infects flocks in the United Kingdom and the United States (7, 8, 10). Further serologic surveys are needed to determine the occurrence, distribution, and significance of the agent and BLS.

ETIOLOGY.

The cause of BLS is considered to be a virus; however, in spite of intensive efforts, it has not been possible to isolate or identify the agent (1, 7). The agent can be propagated in chicken embryos using intravenous inoculation but not by conventional routes of exposure (1, 9). Although BLS can be transmitted to susceptible birds by inoculation with buffy coat cells or suspensions of liver or spleen from affected birds, no agent has been visualized in affected tissues (3, 7). However, antigen in tissue can be detected by immunohistochemistry (1, 6). A BLS-specific, soluble, basic protein antigen with a molecular weight of 18,000 has been isolated from liver of affected birds (6).

Escherichia coli usually can be recovered from birds that develop yolk peritonitis as a consequence of BLS (2, 9), but it is not involved in causing the disease.

PATHOGENESIS AND EPIZOOTIOLOGY

Hosts.

Evidence of naturally occurring infection has only been found in chickens older than 24 wk. Chickens of all ages, including embryos, however, are susceptible to experimental infections. Persistent antigenemia occurred in chickens that hatched following intravenous inoculation as embryos with BLS antigen partially purified from liver homogenates of affected birds. Susceptible chickens placed in contact with these birds became infected for as long as 11 mo after hatching. Antigenemia was greatest in chickens that had been inoculated at 11 days of embryonation (9).

Horizontal transmission occurs among flocks on a farm and when there is contact among birds, but spread within an affected flock may be relatively slow (2). How horizontal transmission occurs has not been determined (1), although the fecal–oral route is suspected (1, 3). Experimental aerosol transmission was unsuccessful (3). The possibility of vertical transmission during clinical infection of the hens, with latency in progeny until onset of production, has been suggested (2).

Clinical Signs.

Morbidity and mortality are low. Affected flocks usually appear normal. Close inspection of potential resting and hiding places may reveal a few sick birds showing lethargy, anemia, and dirty feathers around the vent (5).

Clinical signs vary considerably from inapparent infection, general poor performance, delayed maturity, premature molting, and failure to attain peak production to definite egg drops that may reach 20% accompanied by increased mortality up to 1%/wk for 3–4 wk (2, 5, 8). Small eggs with thin, poorly pigmented shells are produced during the period the flock is affected and often for several wk after apparent recovery. Internal quality, fertility, and hatchability of settable eggs are unaffected. In Europe and the United States, affected flocks tend to have mild or inapparent infections compared with affected flocks in Australia (7).

Hematologic changes include normal packed-cell volumes early, with decreased values later; abnormally small or damaged erythrocytes; enlarged, vacuolated thrombocytes; occasional large blast-type cells; and a leukocytosis due mainly to increased lymphocytes initially followed by increasing monocytes as the disease progresses. Heterophilia is variable. Clotting of blood from affected birds is often delayed (5, 7).

Gross and Microscopic Lesions.

At necropsy, dead birds are in good condition but have empty crops. The most frequently found lesion is an enlarged spleen (2–3 times that of normal). Multiple pale foci on splenic capsular and cut surfaces may be present, especially later in the disease. Usually, the liver is also enlarged and may have variable numbers of small subcapsular hemorrhages. When the liver is involved, there is often evidence of icterus. Occurrence of other lesions is variable but includes pulmonary congestion and edema; enteritis, especially of the duodenum; ovarian regression that may be accompanied by yolk peritonitis; swollen kidneys; and pale plaques and hemorrhages in the pancreas. Splenomegaly is often found when apparently normal birds in an affected flock are examined (2, 3, 5, 7).

Microscopically, five stages can be recognized: 1) lymphoproliferative, 2) pycnotic destructive, 3) macrophage responsive, 4) late responsive, and 5) recovered. There is proliferation of lymphoid tissue in spleen and liver initially. Splenomegaly results from a uniform increase in periellipsoid lymphoblastic regions and variable increases in periarteriolar small lymphocytes. Germinal centers are active. In liver, lymphoid follicles and perivascular lymphoid tissue are increased. These changes precede onset of clinical signs. When signs develop, there is widespread necrosis of lymphoid tissue in the spleen and tissues where lymphoid hyperplasia had occurred earlier. Later, macrophages increase, presumably to remove cell debris and exudate, and scattered heterophils may be found. Reticuloendothelial zones in the spleen become increasingly prominent. Spleens remain enlarged because of increased reticuloendothelial tissue, variable fibrosis, persisting necrotic tissue, and amorphous foci occasionally surrounded by giant cells. Areas of lymphoblastic activity, small lymphocytes, and plasma cells are present. Eventually, there is a return to more normal tissue, although residual lesions and little follicular development can be found (5). At least some aspects of lesion development are suspected to be immune mediated (3).

Immunity. Infection of 1-day-old chicks resulted in presence of antigen in the circulation, but antibody production was delayed in some birds for up to 6 mo. Antibody production did not occur until sexual maturity following oral infection of chickens at 6 wk of age. In mature birds, antigen can be detected prior to antibody, which develops along with splenomegaly and hepatomegaly. Antigen and antibody were detected 2–4 and 3–6 wk, respectively, following intravenous or oral inoculation of susceptible 34- to 36-wk-old broiler breeder hens. Recovered birds apparently remain seropositive for life (3, 7), and a low level of persistent antigenemia occurs (2, 5). Liver contains the highest concentration of BLS antigen (3). Double staining of cells by immunohistochemistry using conjugates to detect antigen and antibody suggests that antigen–antibody complexes commonly occur in affected birds (1, 7).

DIAGNOSIS. Typical clinical signs in mature chickens with enlarged livers and spleens (spleen:body weight ratios greater than 0.001) are sufficient for a presumptive diagnosis (7). Detection of antigen and/or antibody will confirm the diagnosis. Antigen usually precedes or occurs concurrently with antibody (9). Increasing titers and numbers of seropositive birds at 3- to 4-wk intervals compared with those during the acute phase of infection should be demonstrated (2).

Initially, agar gel immunodiffusion tests were developed using extracts from affected tissues and convalescent serum to detect antigen and antibody (5); these are less sensitive than enzyme-linked immunosorbent assays (ELISA) (8, 10). Currently, detection of BLS antibodies and antigen is possible with ELISA tests using purified antigen extracted from spleen and liver of affected birds, or monoclonal/polyclonal antibodies, respectively (4, 8, 10). Immunofluorescence can be used for identifying antigen in frozen tissue sections (6).

Big liver and spleen disease needs to be differentiated from other diseases that produce splenomegaly including group II avian adenovirus infection, Marek's disease, retroviral infections (reticuloendotheliosis and avian leukosis), multi-

centric histiocytosis, systemic protozoal infections, and septicemic diseases including colibacillosis, pasteurellosis, staphylococcosis, and spirochetosis. Other causes of egg-production drops, especially EDS 76 and mycoplasmosis, need to be excluded.

TREATMENT, PREVENTION, AND CONTROL. There is no specific treatment or prevention method currently available for BLS. Thorough cleaning and disinfection of premises after removal of an affected flock can prevent infection of the subsequent flock placed on the farm. Evidence suggests that people can serve as mechanical carriers of the agent and introduce it into susceptible flocks. Practicing good biosecurity is essential for reducing spread of BLS (7) (see Chapter 1).

REFERENCES

1. Clarke, J.K., G.M. Allan, D.G. Bryson, W. Williams, D. Todd, D.P. Mackie, and J.B. McFerran. 1990. Big liver and spleen disease of broiler breeders. Avian Pathol 19:41–50.
2. Crerar, S.K., and G.M. Cross. 1994. Epidemiological and clinical investigations into big liver and spleen disease of broiler breeder hens. Aust Vet J 71:410–413.
3. Crerar, S.K., and G.M. Cross. 1994. The experimental production of big liver and spleen disease in broiler breeder hens. Aust Vet J 71:414–417.
4. Ellis, T.M., C.J. Payne, S.L. Plant, and A.R. Gregory. 1995. An antigen detection immunoassay for big liver and spleen disease agent. Vet Microbiol 46:315–326.
5. Handlinger, J.H., and W. Williams. 1988. An egg drop associated with splenomegaly in broiler breeders. Avian Dis 32:773–778.
6. McAlinden, V.A., A.J. Douglas, F. McNeilly, and D. Todd. 1995. The identification of an 18,000-molecular-weight antigen specific to big liver and spleen disease. Avian Dis 39:788–795.
7. McFerran, J.B. 1994. Big liver and spleen disease. In M.S. McNulty and J.B. McFerran (eds.). New and Evolving Virus Diseases of Poultry. Commission of the European Communities, Brussels, pp. 299–304.
8. Payne, C.J., M.E. Cook, T.M. Ellis, and R.E. Harms. 1991. ELISA testing of US breeders and layers for big liver and spleen disease (BLS). Proc 40th West Poult Dis Conf, pp. 216–218.
9. Payne, C.J., S.L. Plant, T.M. Ellis, P.W. Hillier, and W. Hopkinson. 1993. The detection of big liver and spleen agent in infected tissues via intravenous chick embryo inoculation. Avian Pathol 22:245–256.
10. Todd, D., K.A. Mawhinney, V.A. McAlinden, and A.J. Douglas. 1993. Development of an enzyme-linked immunosorbent assay for the serological diagnosis of big liver and spleen disease. Avian Dis 37:811–816.
11. Williams, W., P. Curtin, J. Handlinger, and J.B. McFerran. 1993. A new disease of broiler breeders—big liver and spleen disease. In J.B. McFerran and M.S. McNulty (eds.). Virus Infections of Birds. Elsevier Science Publishers B.V., Amsterdam, pp. 563–568.

HEPATITIS-SPLENOMEGALY SYNDROME

C. Riddell

INTRODUCTION AND HISTORY. Hepatitis-splenomegaly syndrome is characterized by above-normal mortality in laying hens 30–72 wk of age, with the highest incidence occurring between 40 and 50 wk of age. Weekly mortality increases to approximately 0.3% for several wk during the middle of the production period and may sometimes exceed 1.0% (4, 5, 7). Dead birds have red fluid in their abdomens, and enlarged livers and spleens.

Although first described as hepatitis-splenomegaly syndrome, the disease has also been called necrotic hemorrhage hepatitis-splenomegaly syndrome (4), chronic fulminating cholangiohepatitis (2), necrotic hemorrhagic hepatomegalic hepatitis (7), and hepatitis-liver hemorrhage syndrome (1).

INCIDENCE AND DISTRIBUTION. The syndrome was first reported in western Canada in 1991 (5) and has since been recognized in eastern Canada (7), California (4), and the midwestern United States (2). Caged leghorn hens are typically affected and the disease frequently reoccurs on specific farms (4, 5). Recently, the disease also has been recognized in broiler breeder hens (6) and there is evidence that it may cause sporadic mortality in dual-purpose hens and in small flocks kept on litter (1).

ETIOLOGY. Bacteria have not been routinely isolated from affected livers (4, 5, 7); however, *Campylobacter* spp. were associated with the syndrome in one outbreak (2). Attempts to isolate viruses and identify toxins have been negative (4). The amyloid and hepatic vasculitis are consistent with an immune-mediated disease (1). Similar liver lesions in two young layer flocks in Italy were associated with repeated use of oil-emulsion bacterins (3) but oil-based bacterins have not been used in some of the affected flocks in Canada (7).

PATHOGENESIS AND EPIZOOTIOLOGY. No clinical signs have been recognized in birds prior to death (4, 5, 7). In some outbreaks, there has been an associated drop in egg production of up to 20% (4, 5), but in other outbreaks egg production has not been affected (7).

Dead birds usually are in good condition, with pale combs and wattles (7), but birds in poor condition have been reported (5). Red fluid consistent with unclotted blood is found in the abdomen (4, 5,

7). Livers are enlarged, friable, mottled and stippled with red, yellow, and/or tan foci, and may have subcapsular hematomas and attached blood clots on the surface (4). Splenomegaly has also been reported (5, 7). Affected birds generally have regressive ovaries (4, 5), but active ovaries also have been found (7).

Microscopically, liver lesions varied from multifocal hemorrhage and small pools of amorphous eosinophilic material to extensive areas of necrosis and hemorrhage, infiltration of heterophils and mononuclear cells around portal triads, and separation of hepatocytes by eosinophilic material. In severe cases, discrete granulomas and infiltration of portal veins with mononuclear cells associated with possible thrombosis were recognized. Lesions in spleens consisted of lymphoid depletion and accumulation of eosinophilic material. Eosinophilic material in both livers and spleens was identified as amyloid using Congo red stain (4, 7).

DIAGNOSIS. Diagnosis is based on the typical signs and pathology.

TREATMENT, PREVENTION, AND CONTROL. There is no known treatment. In one outbreak, forced molting of the flock resulted in reduced mortality (4).

REFERENCES

1. Julian, R.J. 1995. Hepatitis-liver hemorrhage syndrome in laying hens. Proc 67th NE Conf Avian Dis, Mystic, CT, p. 17.
2. Kerr, K.M., D.E. Swayne, and G.A. Marsh. 1993. Chronic fulminating cholangiohepatitis associated with Campylobacter species in mature laying chickens. Proc 130th Meet AVMA, Minneapolis, MN, p. 150.
3. Rampin, T., G. Sironi, and D. Gallazi. 1989. Episodes of amyloidosis in young hens after repeated use of antibacterial and emulsion vaccines. Deutsch Tierarztl Wochenschr 96:168–172.
4. Read, D.H., B.M. Daft, J.T. Barton, P.R. Woolcock, G. Cutler, and F. Galey. 1993. Necrotic hemorrhagic hepatitis-splenomegaly syndrome: An unsolved sudden death syndrome in layer leghorn chickens. Proc 36th Ann Meet Am Assoc Vet Lab Diag, Las Vegas, Nevada, pp. 8–9.
5. Ritchie, S.J., and C. Riddell. 1991. "Hepatitis-splenomegaly" syndrome in commercial egg laying hens. Can Vet J 32:500–501.
6. Shivaprasad, H.L., and P.R. Woolcock. 1995. Necrohemorrhagic hepatitis in broiler breeders. Proc West Poult Dis Conf, Sacramento, CA, p. 6.
7. Tablante, N. L., J-P. Vaillancourt, and R.J. Julian. 1994. Necrotic, haemorrhagic, hepatomegalic hepatitis associated with vasculitis and amyloidosis in commercial laying hens. Avian Pathol 23:725–732.

HEPATIC LIPIDOSIS OF TURKEYS

H. John Barnes

Hepatic lipidosis of turkeys is a disease of uncertain, but probable nutritional, etiology. It most frequently affects turkey breeder hen replacements between 12 and 24 wk of age. It is characterized by an abrupt increase in mortality that may approach 5% during a 1- to 2-wk period and by extreme fatty degeneration and massive necrosis of the liver (2). The disease has also been referred to as acute hepatic necrosis.

Sporadic cases of the disease have been seen for the past several years, but only two cases have apparently been described in the literature (2). Flocks in Canada and the United States have been affected.

The cause of hepatic lipidosis is unknown, although nutritional, environmental, and management factors are considered to be involved. Affected flocks are typically on low-protein diets to control growth and development. These diets also may be low in lipotropic factors, especially methionine and cysteine, while still having high energy levels. These amino acids are required for production of apolipoproteins. High peroxide values also have been associated with the disease. High environmental temperatures and/or changes in lighting programs cause the birds to alter eating habits, leading to hepatic deposition of lipid and, eventually, to liver failure. Terminally, lipid peroxidation is considered to contribute to vascular damage, which re-

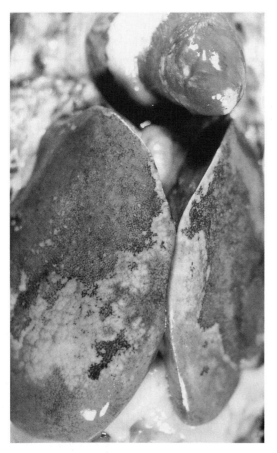

37.13. A 23-wk-old turkey breeder hen with hepatic lipidosis. There is a striking mottled, patchwork pattern apparent in the swollen liver and there are abundant fat deposits around the base of heart and in the abdominal fat pad.

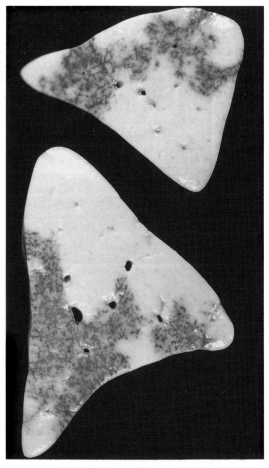

37.14. Cross-section of liver in Fig. 37.13 showing sharp demarcation between pale and dark areas.

sults in lung edema and liver necrosis and hemorrhage (2).

Avian encephalomyelitis (AE) virus and low numbers of *Escherichia coli* have been isolated from affected organs. These are believed to be incidental because turkey breeder hens in this age range are typically vaccinated for AE using live viruses, and it would not be unusual to recover bacteria from livers of seriously affected birds. Inoculation of turkeys with an AE virus isolated from affected hens did not result in disease (1). It is possible that AE virus may interact with noninfectious factors associated with the disease to produce clinical illness.

For a brief period prior to death, affected hens may become inactive and show dyspnea and cyanosis; most often, birds are just found dead. At necropsy, carcasses are in good condition with obvious fat deposits especially in the body cavity. Liver lesions are often striking, consisting of enlargement and a variable number of sharply contrasting pale yellow and dark red areas (Figs. 37.13, 37.14). Other findings include petechial or ecchy-

motic hemorrhages in fat and on organ surfaces, pulmonary congestion and edema, and blood that fails to clot.

Microscopically, virtually all hepatocytes contain single or multiple lipid-filled vacuoles that displace the nucleus. Necrosis and hemorrhage associated with vascular damage are also present. Large confluent areas of fatty degeneration represent pale areas seen grossly, while areas of necrosis and hemorrhage are responsible for dark red areas (2). Occasional nuclei contain prominent condensed nucleoli, probably as a result of cell degeneration, which could be mistaken for viral inclusion bodies (Figs. 37.15 and 37.16).

Diagnosis is based on a history of being on a low-protein, high-energy ration; demonstration of low methionine and/or high peroxides in feed; presence of appropriate environmental and management factors; characteristic gross and microscopic lesions; and failure to isolate significant pathogens (other than AE virus). Hepatic lipidosis needs to be differentiated from acute toxic and infectious diseases that damage the liver.

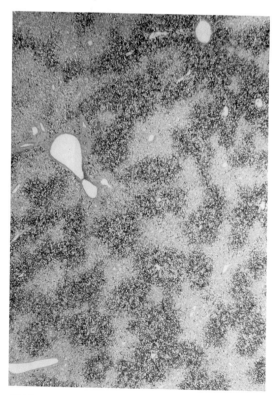

37.15. Liver from turkey breeder hen with hepatic lipidosis. Pale areas consist of hepatocytes that have undergone marked fatty degeneration; necrosis and congested sinusoids and veins are seen in dark areas. ×18.

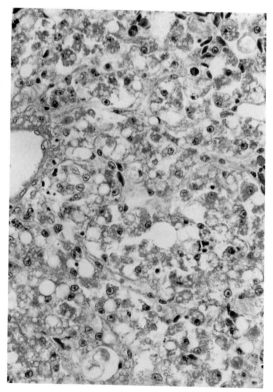

37.16. High-power magnification of Figure 37.15. Vacuoles in hepatocytes replace most of the cytoplasm and displace the nucleus. Some nuclei show margination of chromatin and accentuated nucleolus suggestive of a viral inclusion. ×350.

Administration of vitamin E to affected flocks (25 IU/hen) via water for 7 days reduced mortality (2). Hepatic lipidosis is prevented by having adequate methionine (0.2%) and methionine plus cysteine (0.4%) in the ration (3). Addition of 1 kg 60% choline Cl, 1 kg methionine, and 20 g vitamin B_{12} per ton of feed has been used (2). In some areas, apparent successful prevention of the disease has followed use of a protocol in which the initial AE vaccine is given via water followed by booster inoculation in the wing-web instead of giving two wing-web inoculations.

REFERENCES.

1. Ficken, M. 1996. Personal communication.
2. Gazdzinski, P., E.J. Squires, and R.J. Julian. 1994. Hepatic lipidosis in turkeys. Avian Dis 38:379–384.
3. National Research Council. 1994. Nutrient Requirements of Poultry, 9th ed. National Academy Press, Washington, DC, pp. 35–39.

DERMAL SQUAMOUS CELL CARCINOMA

Scott Hafner and Mark A. Goodwin

INTRODUCTION AND HISTORY. There have been sporadic reports of squamous cell carcinomas in the skin, tongue, pharynx, and esophagus of aged chickens worldwide since the 1800s. Squamous cell carcinomas in older chickens are rarely metastatic (1) but often are locally invasive (3, 7, 8, 13, 16, 21). In contrast, *dermal squamous cell carcinoma* (DSCC) is a term used for lesions usually found in the skin of young broiler chicken carcasses at slaughter. This condition predominantly affects only the dermis and there are no reports of metastasis (5, 6, 11, 12, 17, 22, 23). Some authors accept DSCC as an appropriate name for the lesions in young broiler chickens (5, 6, 14, 22), while others prefer avian keratoacanthoma or keratoacanthoma (11, 12, 17). Keratoacanthomas are regressing tumors of humans that resemble squamous cell carcinomas both grossly and microscopically (2, 15). Naturally occurring DSCC examined in live broiler chickens also regressed (11).

INCIDENCE AND DISTRIBUTION. These ulcerative lesions are most common in broiler chicken carcasses, but similar tumors are also present in the carcasses of older chickens (11). In broilers, the prevalence of carcasses with multiple lesions averages from 0.01% to 0.05%, but may be 0.09% or higher in individual flocks (12, 14, 22, 23). Flocks of chickens slaughtered at less than 48 days of age had an increased prevalence in one study (12), and in some investigations, tumor prevalence was cyclic, lowest in summer months (12, 23). In some surveys, high condemnation rates were associated with dusty houses, with birds placed in new houses, or with certain producers (10).

ETIOLOGY, EPIZOOTIOLOGY, AND PATHOGENESIS. The etiology of the naturally occurring condition is unknown. Experimentally, DSCC developed in two young chickens injected with strains of avian leukosis virus, but other similarly treated chickens did not develop these lesions (4). Repeated topical applications of methylcholanthrene produced regressing lesions originally diagnosed as squamous cell carcinomas (19), then as squamous cell carcinomatoid tumors (20), and finally as keratoacanthomas (18). Applications of methylcholanthrene to chickens chronically infected with fowl pox resulted in papillomas and squamous cell carcinomas. These tumors regressed or resolved to cutaneous horns after applications of the carcinogen ceased. A few metastatic squamous cell carcinomas originated from residual lesions after several years (9).

Gross Lesions. Gross lesions in carcasses are most commonly crater-shaped ulcers with raised margins that occur in feather tracts (Fig. 37.17). Smaller ulcers average 5 mm in diameter and are circular, but large, irregular coalescing ulcers are present on some carcasses (12). Ulcers may be aggregated within feather tracts or scattered throughout tracts. In one study (12), lesions occurred most frequently in dorsopelvic, femoral, and pectoral tracts, but some surveys found no site predilection (22). In live birds, these ulcers are filled with keratin and cell debris (Fig. 37.18). Small (average, 3 mm) nodular lesions often accompany ulcers and appear grossly as enlarged feather follicles (Fig. 37.19). In live young broiler chickens, these nodular lesions progressed to ulcers and all lesions eventually regressed (11).

Histopathology. Nodular lesions appear microscopically as proliferative outgrowths of feather follicle epithelium (Fig. 37.20), cysts originating from feather follicle epithelium, or hyperplastic feather follicles containing hyperkeratotic feathers. Ulcers are composed of a central cup-shaped cavity

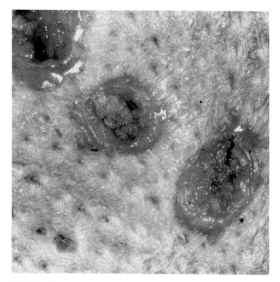

37.17. Typical carcass lesions are craterous ulcers within feather tracts.

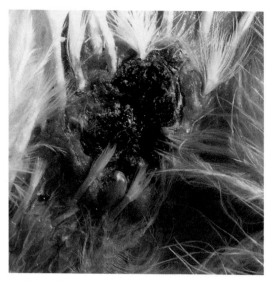

37.18. In live chickens, ulcers contain central masses that are mixtures of keratin, cell debris, and bacteria.

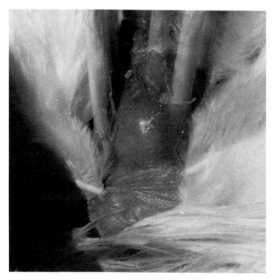

37.19. Early lesions in the skin of live chickens are nodules in the base of feather follicles.

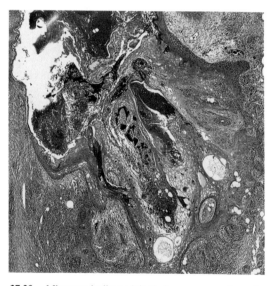

37.20. Microscopically, nodular lesions are expansions of

lined by epithelium and filled with keratin, bacteria, sloughed epithelial cells, and inflammatory cells. Epithelial lips overhang the central keratin mass. The lining epithelium keratinizes toward the central cavity and extends thin strands of keratinocytes into the surrounding dermal fibroplasia (Fig. 37.21). The peripheral fibroplasia contains isolated keratinocytes, heterophils, scattered macrophages, and perivascular lymphocyte aggregates. Carcass lesions are often extensively altered by defeathering, with loss of the central keratin core and much of the lining epithelium.

Ultrastructurally, desmosomes interconnect keratinocytes and these cells contain tonofibrils or keratohyalin granules, but virus particles have not been seen (5, 11).

Pathogenesis. The complete pathogenesis of DSCC is unknown; however, lesions appear to begin at the margin of hyperplastic feather follicles. The peripheral follicular epithelium infiltrates adjacent dermis or expands into small cysts with irregular peripheral margins of invading keratinocytes. There is marked peripheral fibroplasia that contains

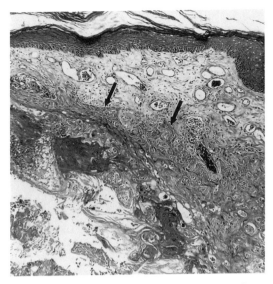

37.21. A section through the epithelial lip of an ulcer from a live bird shows the centrally keratinizing and peripherally invasive lining epithelium (*arrows*) adja-

numerous inflammatory cells. These cysts superficially ulcerate as lesions enlarge. There are overlying epithelial lips that restrain the central mass of keratin and bacteria. After loss of the central keratin core, there is rapid regression to a dermal scar overlaid by reepithelialization.

DIAGNOSIS.　Grossly and microscopically, the differential diagnosis is primarily an ulcerative dermatitis. Adequate examination of microscopic sections confirms the diagnosis.

PREVENTION AND CONTROL.　There are no known methods of prevention and control.

REFERENCES

1. Abels, H. 1929. Die Geschwulste der Vogelhaut. Z Krebsforsch 29:207–210.
2. Ackerman, A.B., and A. Ragaz. 1984. The lives of lesions. Chronology in Dermatopathology. Masson Publishing, New York, NY.
3. Anderson, W.I. and H. Steinberg. 1989. Primary glossal squamous-cell carcinoma in a Spanish Cochin hen. Avian Dis 33:827–828.
4. Beard, J.W. 1980. Biology of avian oncornaviruses. In G. Klein (ed.). Viral Oncology. Raven Press, New York, p. 81.
5. Bergmann, V., A. Valentin, and J. Scheer. 1986.

Hartzkarzinomatose bei Broilern. Monatsh Veterinaermed 41:815–817.
6. Blandford, T.B., A.S. Bremner, and C.J. Randall. 1979. Squamous cell carcinomas in broilers [letter]. Vet Rec 105:334–335.
7. Cardona, C.J., A.A. Bickford, and K. Emanuelson. 1992. Squamous-cell carcinoma on the legs of an Aracauna chicken. Avian Dis 36:474–479.
8. Chin, R.P., and B.C. Barr. 1990. Squamous-cell carcinoma of the pharyngeal cavity in a Jersey black giant rooster. Avian Dis 34:775–778.
9. Duran-Reynals, F. 1952. Studies on the combined effects of fowl pox virus and methylcholanthrene in chickens. Ann NY Acad Sci 54:977–991.
10. Good, R.E. 1991. The importance of squamous cell carcinoma in broilers. In Proc Avian Tumor Virus Symp. American Association of Avian Pathologists, Kennett Square, PA, pp. 56–57.
11. Hafner, S., B.G. Harmon, G.N. Rowland, R.G. Stewart, and J.R. Glisson. 1991. Spontaneous regression of "dermal squamous cell carcinoma" in young chickens. Avian Dis 35:321–327.
12. Hafner, S., B.G. Harmon, R.G. Stewart, and G.N. Rowland. 1993. Avian keratoacanthoma (dermal squamous cell carcinoma) in broiler chicken carcasses. Vet Pathol 30:265–270.
13. James, C. 1968. Neoplasms of the chicken. Ceylon Vet J 16:59–61.
14. Langheinrich, K.A. 1991. Pathology of squamous cell carcinomas in broiler. In Proc Avian Tumor Virus Symp. American Association of Avian Pathologists, Kennett Square, PA, pp. 58–62.
15. Murphy, G.F., and D.E. Elder. 1991. Epidermal (Keratinocytic) Neoplasms. In J. Rosai and L.H. Sobin (eds.). Non-Melanocytic Tumors of the Skin. Atlas of Tumor Pathology. Armed Forces Institute of Pathology, Washington, DC, pp. 11–60.
16. Priester, W.A. 1975. Esophageal cancer in North China; high rates in human and poultry populations in the same areas. Avian Dis 19:213–215.
17. Riddell, C., and P.T. Shettigara. 1980. Dermal squamous cell carcinoma in broiler chickens in Saskatchewan. Can Vet J 21:287–289.
18. Rigdon, R.H. 1959. Keratoacanthoma experimentally induced with methylcholanthrene in the chicken. AMA Arch Derm 79:139–147.
19. Rigdon, R.H., and D. Brashear. 1954. Experimental production of squamous-cell carcinomas in the skin of chickens. Cancer Res 14:629–631.
20. Rigdon, R.H., and M.D. Hooks. 1956. A consideration of the mechanism by which squamous-cell carcinomatoid tumors in the chicken spontaneously regress. Cancer Res 16:246–253.
21. Sugiyama, M., M.H. Yamashina, T. Kanbara, H. Kajigaya, K. Konagaya, M. Umeda, M. Isoda, and T. Sakai. 1987. Dermal squamous cell carcinoma in a laying hen. Jpn J Vet Sci 49:1129–1130.
22. Turnquest, R.U. 1979. Dermal squamous cell carcinoma in young chickens. Am J Vet Res 40:1628–1633.
23. Weinstock, D., M.T. Correa, D.V. Rives, and D.P. Wages. 1995. Histopathology and epidemiology of condemnations due to squamous cell carcinoma in broiler chickens in North Carolina. Avian Dis 39:676–686.

MULTICENTRIC HISTIOCYTOSIS

Scott Hafner and Mark A. Goodwin

INTRODUCTION.   Multicentric histiocytosis is a recently described condition that is grossly characterized by splenomegaly and hepatomegaly accompanied by myriad small white nodules in spleens, livers, and kidneys of young broiler chickens (4). Synonyms for this disease include "big spleen Marek's disease" and "reticuloendotheliosis-like syndrome." It has been hypothesized that lesions of chickens with multicentric histiocytosis are either neoplasms or represent a marked hyperplastic reaction (1, 3, 4, 5).

ETIOLOGY.   No etiologic agent has been identified. Specific-pathogen–free chickens injected with tissues from field cases have developed characteristic gross and microscopic lesions (2). The DNA extracted from lesions of naturally diseased broiler chickens did not contain sequences specific for reticuloendotheliosis viruses, Marek's disease virus, or exogenous leukosis-sarcoma viruses (4, 7). Serum samples from diseased flocks have not implicated Marek's herpesvirus, infectious bursal disease virus, or reoviruses (6).

GROSS LESIONS.   Spleens are enlarged two to four times normal and livers are enlarged twice normal size. Miliary (0.5–2 mm) white-to-yellow nodules are present throughout the spleen and liver. Similar 1- to 5-mm nodules are often visible in the kidney, but gross changes are rare in the pancreas and duodenum. Some diseased birds are pale and are smaller than their flockmates (1, 3, 4, 5).

HISTOPATHOLOGY.   In the spleen, circular nodules of spindle-shaped cells diffusely expand periarteriolar lymphoid sheaths (Fig. 37.22). These histiocytic cells (denoting cells with abundant eosinophilic cytoplasm) contain elongated oval, fusiform, or more bizarrely configured nuclei (Fig. 37.23). Mitotic figures and individual necrotic cells are common in these nodules. The exact lineage of these cells has not been identified by specific markers. Multinucleated cells are not present. A few plasma cells, small lymphocytes, scattered lymphoblasts, and germinal centers are often present within nodules. Similar, but often more heterogenous, nodules diffusely stipple the liver, primarily replacing periportal hepatocytes and bulging into portal veins. Nodules also partially replace the kidneys, pancreas, proventricular glands, and lung. There are diffuse accumulations of histiocytic cells under the mucosal epithelium of the proventriculus and in the duodenal lamina propria. In the duodenum, these cells fill the lamina propria and extend deep into the muscularis. Occasionally, perivascular aggregates of lymphoblasts are present in the musculature of the ventriculus and in cardiac and skeletal muscle (4).

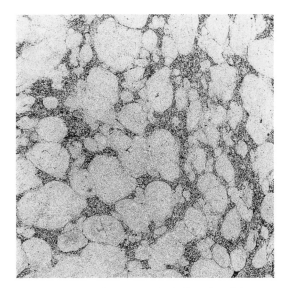

37.22.   Nodules diffusely expand splenic periarteriolar lymphoid sheaths. ×20.

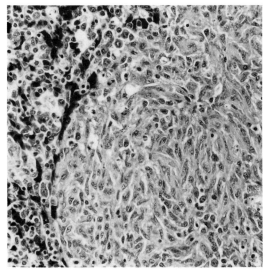

37.23.   Histiocytic spindle-shaped cells contain elongated and pleomorphic nuclei. ×200.

DIAGNOSIS. Histopathology is currently the only method of diagnosis. Nodules are characteristic and are consistently found within specific locations in certain organs (4).

REFERENCES
1. Goodwin, M.A., and S. Hafner. 1994. Multicentric histiocytosis mimicking reticuloendotheliosis in broilers. Proc 29th Natl Meet Poult Health Condemn, Ocean City, MD, p. 56.
2. Hafner, S. 1996. Unpublished observations.
3. Hafner, S., M.A. Goodwin, L. Kelley, M. Puette, D. Bounous, W.L. Steffens, K.A. Langheinrich, and J. Brown. 1994. Multicentric histiocytosis mimicking reticuloendotheliosis in broiler chickens. Proc 66th NE Conf Avian Dis, p. 26.
4. Hafner, S., M.A. Goodwin, E.J. Smith, D.I. Bounous, M. Puette, L.C. Kelley, K.A. Langheinrich, and A.M. Fadly. 1996. Multicentric histiocytosis in young chickens. Gross and light microscopic pathology. Avian Dis 40:202–209.
5. Hall, S.M., M.D. Counts, and M.B. Callaham. 1995. The gross and histological findings in young chickens with a neoplastic condition resembling both reticuloendotheliosis and Marek's disease. Proc 44th West Poult Dis Conf, pp. 68–69.
6. Singbeil, B., J.K. Skeeles, L.A. Newberry, J.K. Dash, J. Beasley, P.S. Wakenell, S.P. Taylor, and A. Mutalib. 1995. Severe acute thymus atrophy in broilers and broiler breeders. 46th North Cent Avian Dis Conf, pp. 121–122.
7. Witter R.L. 1994. Reticuloendotheliosis: Issues and nonissues. Proc 29th Natl Meet Poult Health Condemn, Ocean City, MD, pp. 118–122.

GANGLIOSIDOSIS IN EMUS

A. J. Bermudez

Gangliosidosis is a common inherited neuronal storage disease in mammals that is caused by deficient activity in one of the two enzymes necessary for ganglioside catabolism. Specifically, an inherited defect in ß-galactosidase is associated with GM1 gangliosidosis and an inherited defect in ß-hexosaminidase, or its activator protein, causes GM2 gangliosidosis. Gangliosidoses have been reported in humans (Tay-Sachs and Sandhoff's diseases), cats, dogs, Friesian cattle, Suffolk sheep, and swine. Recently, a similar condition has been reported in emus (*Dromaius novaehollandiae*) (1). The specific metabolic defect in ganglioside metabolism in emus has yet to be characterized.

INCIDENCE AND DISTRIBUTION. With the development of a North American emu industry in the 1990s, emu breeder farms have become a widespread form of alternative agriculture. The distribution of gangliosidosis seems to have paralleled the growth of this industry, with cases reported in Florida, Kentucky, Illinois, Missouri, Oklahoma, Texas, and California.

SIGNS AND PATHOLOGY. Emus with gangliosidosis typically are affected between 3 and 8 mo of age. Two clinical presentations occur. Affected emus may die acutely with no premonitory signs. In these emus, the immediate cause of death is hemorrhage into the body cavity. The source of hemorrhage in these birds may be the liver or may be difficult to locate. The aorta should be examined carefully to rule out a simple case of aortic rupture. The second presentation of emus with gangliosido-

sis is that of a progressive neurologic disease. Affected emus progress from mild to severe ataxia over a period of a month or more. Emus that progress to the neurologic form of the disease will eventually be unable to stand, and these birds are often euthanized because of self-induced trauma resulting from their struggles. Emus with gangliosidosis have a concurrent coagulopathy, which may be demonstrated antemortem by collection of a blood sample into a serum tube. Blood of affected emus often has a prolonged clotting time, typically greater than 2 hr, or may fail to clot altogether. The packed cell volume of blood from affected emus may also be extremely low due to internal hemorrhage.

Gross lesions observed in emus with gangliosidosis are variable. Hemorrhage is the most consistent gross lesion. Hemorrhage is commonly observed in the body cavity or muscles of the leg. Emus affected with prolonged neurologic disease continue to eat, but body condition deteriorates, so at the terminal phase of the disease the affected emu will be thin. Affected emus will also be stunted in comparison to normal hatchmates. The central nervous system of emus with gangliosidosis is unremarkable on gross examination.

Histopathologic changes observed in emus with gangliosidosis are consistent regardless of gross lesions or clinical signs observed in the individual case. The most consistent and diagnostic lesions are observed in the central nervous system and liver. H & E–stained sections of the central nervous system reveal distended neurons containing nonstaining 1- to 2-µm vacuoles (1). These vacuoles are most numerous in the neurons of the cerebrum, pontine nuclei, medulla oblongata, and brain stem. Nissl substance is dispersed by the vacuoles. Toluidine blue staining of sections of paraffin-embedded tissues accentuates the vacuolated appearance of the affected neurons (1) (Fig. 37.24A). Nonstaining, 1- to 2-μm vacuoles are also present in neurons or ganglion cells of the spinal cord gray matter, spinal ganglia, autonomic ganglia, myenteric plexus, and ganglion cell layer of the retina. Ultrastructural evaluation of affected neurons reveals membranous cytoplasmic bodies typical of those seen in mammals with gangliosidosis (1) (Fig. 37.24B). In sections of liver, aggregates of foamy macrophages are consistently present in hepatic sinusoids.

PATHOGENESIS AND EPIZOOTIOLOGY.
The biochemical defect that causes gangliosidosis in emus has not been fully characterized. Analysis of brain gangliosides of an affected 7-mo-old emu revealed 14- and 25-fold increases of GM1 and GM3 gangliosides, respectively, compared with similar tests from control emus (1). Total brain gan-

glioside sialic acids were, on a wet weight basis, 519 μg/g (control A), 658 μg/g (control B), and 1800 μg/g (affected emu). Levels of GD1a and the polysialogangliosides (containing 3 or more sialic molecules) were also twice that of the controls. Gangliosidosis in emus is not caused by any of the enzyme defects that cause this disease in mammals. Furthermore, the disease in emus produces increases in several brain gangliosides. This is unlike the brain ganglioside pattern seen in affected mammals in which, typically, only a single ganglioside is elevated.

Gangliosidosis in emus appears to be inherited in an autosomal recessive fashion with 25% of the progeny being affected. Carrier breeder pairs will produce affected emus in successive years on the same farms with emu breeder pairs that produce normal progeny. A common emu industry practice is to separate breeder pairs that produce affected progeny and match these carrier breeders with emus that do not carry this lethal gene. The progeny of these new pairings do not develop gangliosidosis.

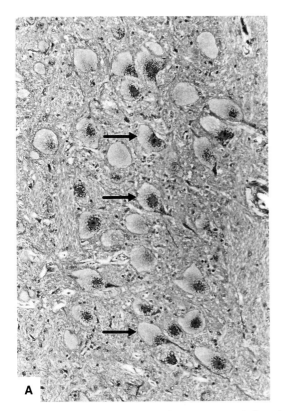
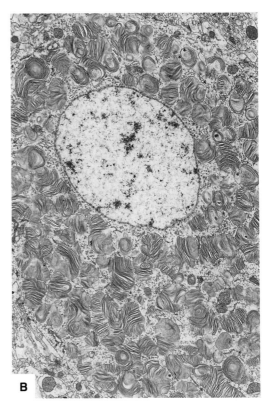

37.24. *A.* Brain stem ganglion with neurons (*arrows*) distended by numerous clear vacuoles. Nissl substance is dispersed by vacuoles. Toluidine blue, ×400. *B.* Transmission electron micrograph of a neuron in the cerebrum with a severe accumulation of membranous cytoplasmic bodies. ×6300. (Avian Dis)

PREVENTION AND CONTROL. The only means of preventing gangliosidosis in emus is by removing all emus that carry this lethal recessive gene from the breeder gene pool. Carrier emus are clinically normal and are appropriate for the slaughter market. Currently, the only means of identifying carriers is by the diagnosis of gangliosidosis in their progeny. Once a pair of carriers have been identified, these emus and all their progeny should be directed to the slaughter market and should not be used as breeders. The practice of splitting up carrier pairs and breeding them to noncarriers should be strongly discouraged because this will only increase the incidence of this lethal gene in the North American emu gene pool.

With further research, the specific enzyme and gene defect that results in gangliosidosis may be characterized. With this information, it may be possible to analyze blood samples of emu breeders for a specific enzyme or gene defect and to eliminate breeders that carry this lethal gene.

REFERENCES
1. Bermudez, A.J., G.C. Johnson, M.T. Vanier, M. Schröder, K. Suzuki, P.L. Stogsdill, G.S. Johnson, D. O'Brien, C.P. Moore, and W.W. Fry. 1995. Gangliosidosis in emus (Dromaius novaehollandiae). Avian Dis 39:292–303.

PIGEON CIRCOVIRUS INFECTION

L. W. Woods and H. L. Shivaprasad

INTRODUCTION. Pigeon circovirus infection (PCI) is a contagious disease affecting primarily young pigeons (3, 4, 9, 10, 11, 13, 14). Mortality is variable but can approach 100%. Clinical signs and mortality are primarily due to an apparent virus-induced immunosuppression with subsequent infection with various secondary viral, bacterial, fungal, and parasitic agents. The virus has yet to be isolated and characterized.

Circovirus infection of pigeons was first reported in California in 1993 (9, 13). Circoviruslike particles were seen in negatively stained preparations of feces from pigeons in South Africa during the same year (1). Suspicious circoviruslike inclusions were noted prior to this (4); a retrospective study of tissues from pigeons examined in Canada in 1986 and several in Australia in 1989 demonstrated circovirus inclusions (14). Circovirus was reported in Australian doves in 1994 (8) and in racing pigeons from Northern Ireland and England in 1995 and 1996, respectively (3, 11). The latter reports suggest PCI is widespread in European pigeons.

ETIOLOGY. Circoviridae is a newly recognized virus family that was previously called circodnaviridae and, prior to that, diminuviridae. Circoviruses are nonenveloped and composed of single-stranded, circular DNA. Particles in negatively stained preparations are typically 14–19 nm, the smallest known animal viruses.

Included in this virus family are porcine circovirus, psittacine beak and feather disease (PBFD) virus, and chicken infectious anemia virus (CIAV) (12). Pigeon circovirus will likely be included in

this group once it is fully characterized. Similar viruses also have been identified in doves (8), canaries (2), and finches (6). Pigeon circovirus is antigenically distinct from PBFD virus but does share some homologous DNA sequences (14). A polymerase chain reaction technique used for PBFD virus (7) does not detect pigeon or passerine circoviruses. Other possible relationships among avian circoviruses are unknown. There have been no reported attempts to infect other avian species with pigeon circovirus.

Limited work has been done to propagate pigeon circovirus. Attempts to grow it in embryonating chicken eggs or in chicken kidney or chicken fibroblast cells have been unsuccessful.

PATHOGENESIS AND EPIZOOTIOLOGY. Pigeon circovirus infection primarily affects young pigeons 2 mo to 1 yr of age, similar to the situation in psittacines infected with PBFD virus (5). Spread appears to be mainly horizontal; occurrence and possible significance of vertical transmission are unknown. Mixing of pigeons during racing is believed to be a common means of virus spread.

A broad range of clinical signs has been reported in pigeons with circovirus infection including lethargy, anorexia, poor racing performance, weight loss, respiratory distress, and diarrhea. Concurrent infections of circovirus-infected pigeons by other agents are common and likely result from immunosuppression associated with the viral infection. In fact, clinical signs are often associated with the secondary infections with agents such as paramyxovirus-1 (PMV-1), poxvirus, adenovirus, herpesvirus, *Escherichia coli, Salmonella ty-phimurium, Mycoplasma* spp., *Pasteurella* spp., *Pseudomonas aeruginosa, Chlamydia psittaci, Candida* spp., *Aspergillus* spp., *Trichomonas* spp., *Haemoproteus* spp., and *Tetrameres* spp. Pigeon circovirus infection appears to also depress vaccinal immunity. Feather loss, a consistent finding of PBFD in psittacine birds, has not been a feature of pigeon circovirus infection outbreaks in California (9, 10, 13, 14); however, loss of wing, tail, and body feathers was observed in circovirus-infected Australian doves (8).

Mortality is variable, ranging from 0 to 100% in young pigeons. It is likely influenced by many factors including virulence of the virus, age of bird when initially infected, and secondary infections (3, 10, 11, 13, 14). Secondary infections are often the immediate cause of death.

Bursal atrophy is sometimes apparent in infected birds (13, 14), but usually gross pathologic lesions are related to secondary infection(s). Microscopically, changes in primary and secondary lymphoid tissues range from lymphofollicular hyperplasia to lymphoid depletion (10, 11, 14). Lymphofollicular hyperplasia is sometimes seen in the spleen, with variable degrees of discrete lymphocellular necrosis. Severe depletion of lymphocytes with diffuse histiocytosis can also be seen. Basophilic, botryoid, crystalline inclusions are evident within the cytoplasm of splenic macrophages (13, 14). In the bursa, changes range from minimal lymphoid de-pletion or, rarely, lymphofollicular hyperplasia (14) with mild, discrete lymphocellular necrosis to cystic bursal atrophy with severe lymphoid depletion (10, 11, 14). Cytoplasmic inclusions have been reported in bursal epithelial cells and sometimes in macrophages (11, 14). In some pigeons, both cytoplasmic and nuclear inclusions can be seen in cells of bursal follicles (Fig. 37.25) (10). Cytoplasmic inclusions are also seen in gut- and bronchial-associated lymphoid tissues (14). Bone marrow hypoplasia involving both erythroid and myeloid cells can occur (10). Lymphocytic infiltrates are variably present in liver, pancreas, kidneys, adrenal glands, thyroid glands, testis, crop, and myocardium (14).

Ultrastructurally, inclusions in macrophages and bursal epithelial cells are large, electron-dense areas containing nonenveloped, icosahedral viral particles, 14–17 nm in diameter, which are often arranged in loose or tight paracrystalline or semicircular arrays (Fig. 37.26).

Knowledge concerning the pathogenesis of infection is limited; however, it is clear that there are similarities among PCI, PBFD, and CIAV infection. Age of the bird when infected or stage of bursal development may determine the effect of the virus on the immune system. Retrospective studies of naturally occurring outbreaks in pigeons suggest depressed vaccinal immunity may occur in some infected birds (14). Presence of numerous concurrent infections that would normally be controlled by humoral or cell-mediated immunity are consistent

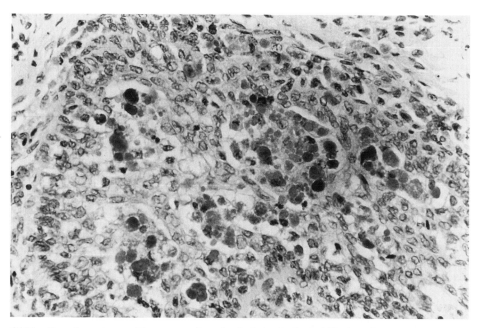

37.25. Bursa from pigeon with numerous circovirus inclusion bodies in follicular cells. H & E, ×300.

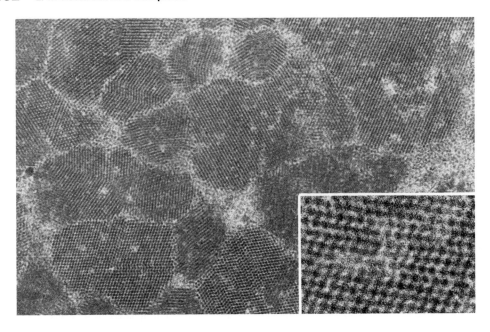

37.26. Paracrystalline viral array in a circovirus inclusion. ×47,520. *Inset*: Icosahedral morphology of virus. ×162,000.

with immune suppression in pigeons with PCI. Immunosuppression may result from bursal atrophy in some birds, while in others viral infection of the monocyte–macrophage system may interfere with microbicidal activity or antigen processing as is believed to occur in psittacine birds with PBFD (5).

DIAGNOSIS. Circovirus infection should be suspected as a possible primary agent in young pigeons with multiple concurrent bacterial, viral, fungal, or protozoal infections. A definitive diagnosis of pigeon circovirus infection is based on histopathology and electron microscopy findings. Characteristic "botryoid" inclusion bodies in mononuclear cells of primary and secondary lymphoid tissue and in follicular cells of the bursa of Fabricius associated with lymphoid depletion should help toward making a definitive diagnosis. Electron microscopy of these inclusions typically reveals nonenveloped, icosahedral viral particles, 14–17 nm in diameter, either loosely arranged or in tight paracrystalline or semicircular arrays. Diagnosis of pigeon circovirus infection by virus isolation or serology is not possible at the present time. A circovirus-specific DNA probe has been developed for the diagnosis of PCI but is not yet available commercially.

TREATMENT, PREVENTION, AND CONTROL. Contact with other pigeons should be minimized and spread of the disease prevented through use of biosecurity practices. Treatment of

the secondary infections that are usually the immediate cause of death in circovirus-infected pigeons may help limit mortality in young pigeons during an outbreak. Because circovirus may interfere with vaccinal immunity, pigeons should not be vaccinated during an outbreak. Pigeons that are vaccinated with PMV-1 should have postvaccinal serum antibody titers evaluated to determine immune response and efficacy of vaccination.

REFERENCES
1. Gerdes, G.H. 1993. Two very small viruses — a presumptive identification [Abstr]. J S Afr Vet Assoc 64:2.
2. Goldsmith, T.L. 1995. Documentation of passerine circoviral infection [Abstr]. Proc Annu Conf Assoc Avian Vet, Philadelphia, PA, pp. 349–350.
3. Gough, R.E., and S.E.N. Drury. 1996. Circovirus-like particles in the bursae of young racing pigeons. Vet Rec 138:167.
4. Graham, D.L. 1990. Feather and beak disease: Its biology, management and an experiment in its eradication from a breeding aviary [Abstr]. Proc Annu Conf Assoc Avian Vet, Phoenix, AZ, pp. 8–11.
5. Latimer, K.S., P.M. Rakich, F.D. Niagro, B.W. Ritchie, W.L. Steffens, R.P. Campagnoli, and D.A. Pesti. 1991. An updated review of psittacine beak and feather disease. J Assoc Avian Vet 5:211–220.
6. Mysore, J., D. Read, and B. Daft. 1995. Circovirus-like particles in finches [Abstr]. Proc Annu Conf Am Assoc Vet Lab Diagn, Histopathology Section, Reno, NV.
7. Niagro, F.D., B.W. Ritchie, K.S. Latimer, P.D. Lukert, W.L. Steffens, and D.A. Pesti. 1990. Polymerase chain reaction detection of PBFD and BFD virus in suspect birds [Abstr]. Proc Annu Conf Assoc Avian Vet, Phoenix, AZ, pp. 25–37.
8. Pass, D.A., S.L. Plant, and N. Sexton. 1994. A laughing dove (Streptopelia senegalensis) with the virus of

psittacine beak and feather disease. Aust Vet J 71:307–308.

9. Shivaprasad, H.L., R.P. Chin, J.S. Jeffrey, R.W. Nordhausen, K.S. Latimer, F.D. Niagro, and R.P. Campagnoli. 1993. A new viral disease of pigeons? Particles resembling circovirus in the bursa of Fabricius [Abstr]. Proc West Poult Dis Conf, Sacramento, CA, pp. 99.

10. Shivaprasad, H.L., R.P.Chin, J.S.Jeffrey, K.S. Latimer, R.W. Nordhausen, F.D. Niagro, and R.P. Campagnoli, R.P. 1994. Particles resembling circovirus in the bursa of Fabricius of pigeons. Avian Dis 38:635–641.

11. Smyth, J.A., and B.P. Carroll. 1995. Circovirus infection in European racing pigeons. Vet Rec 136:173–174.

12. Todd, D., F.D. Niagro, B.W. Ritchie, W. Curran, G.M. Allan, P.D. Lukert, K.S. Latimer, W.L. Steffens, and M.S. McNulty. 1991. Comparison of three animal viruses with circular single-stranded DNA genomes. Arch Virol 117:129–135.

13. Woods, L.W., K.S. Latimer, B.C. Barr, K.S. Niagro, J.D. Campagnoli, R.W. Nordhausen, and A. Castro. 1993. Circovirus-like infection in a pigeon. J Vet Diagn Invest 5:609–612.

14. Woods, L.W., K.S. Latimer, F.D. Niagro, C.R. Riddell, A.M. Crowley, M.L. Anderson, B.M. Daft, J.D. Moore, R.P.Campagnoli, and R.W. Nordhausen. 1994. A retrospective study of circovirus infection in pigeons: Nine cases (1986–1993). J Vet Diagn Invest 6:156–164.

Index

human infection, 82, 85
immunity, 89
  protein intake and, 75
prevention and control
  immunization, 93-94
  management procedures, 82, 83, 91-93
  treatment, 91
Francisella tularensis, 290
Fringed membranous particles (FMPs), 1017-18
Frounce, 896
Fulminating disease of guinea fowl, 1031-32
Fumigated grain, 788
Fumigation, of hatching eggs, 20, 26, 39-40
  E. coli and, 139
  Salmonella and, 85
  Streptococcus and, 301
  toxicity of fumigants, 990-91
Fumonisins, 956-57, 958
Fungal infections, 351-65. *See also* Aspergillosis; Mycotoxicoses
  cryptococcosis, 364
  histoplasmosis, 363-64
  necropsy smears, 36
  rare infections, 365
  thrush, 361-63
Fungicides. *See* Antifungal agents
Furazolidone
  for fowl typhoid, 91
  for histomoniasis, 895
  for pullorum disease, 91
  toxicity, 926, 928, 981
Furosemide, in right ventricular failure, 929
Fusarenone-X, 952
Fusaric acid, 958
Fusariocin A, 956
Fusarium mycotoxins
  fumonisins, 956-57, 958
  fusaric acid, 958
  fusarochromanone, 920, 957
  fusarocin C, 958
  moniliformin, 956
  tibial dyschondroplasia due to, 919
  trichothecenes, 952-56
  zearalenol, 958
  zearalenone, 952, 953, 956, 957-58
  testing for, 967, 968
Fusarochromanone, 920, 957
Fusarocin C, 958

GAL viruses, 607
Gangliosidosis in emus, 1048-50
Gangrenous dermatitis, 265-67
  concurrent infections
    hemorrhagic syndrome, 744
    infectious bursal disease, 730
    reticuloendotheliosis, 265, 468, 475
    Staphylococcus aureus in, 249, 265, 266
  sulfonamide toxicity and, 980
Gapeworm. *See Syngamus trachea*
Gas edema disease. *See* Gangrenous dermatitis
Gases, toxic, 994. *See also* Ammonia

fumes
Gastrocnemius tendon rupture, 924-25
  reoviruses and, 711, 713-14, 715, 925
Gastrointestinal infections. *See* Enteritis
Gastrointestinal tumors, of unknown etiology, 498-99
Gentamicin, toxicity of, 981
Geotrichum candidum, 365
Gibberella, 952, 957-58
Gizzard
  copper excess and, 66
  erosions
    adenoviruses and, 615
    protein supplements and, 984
    thrush and, 362
  impaction, 934-35
  poorly developed, 934
  in vitamin E and selenium deficiency, 55, 68
Gliomas, 416
Gliotoxin, 353
Glutathione peroxidase, 54, 68
  paraquat toxicity and, 991
Going light, in pigeons, 882
Goiters, 504
Gongylonema ingluvicola, 819-20
Goose enteritis. *See* Goose parvovirus infection
Goose hepatitis. *See* Goose parvovirus infection
Goose influenza. *See* Goose parvovirus infection; *Riemerella anatipestifer* infection
Goose parvovirus infection, 777-81
  causative virus, 777-79
  clinical characteristics, 779-80
  diagnosis, 780-81
  epizootiology
    hosts, 779
    incidence and distribution, 777
    transmission, 779
  history, 777
  prevention and control, 781
    bivalent vaccine, 1033
  treatment, 781
Goose venereal disease, 293-94
Gossypol, 996-97
Gout, 936-37
  oosporein and, 937, 965-66
  protein excess and, 48
  vitamin A deficiency and, 50, 937
Government regulation
  chlamydiosis and, 346
  of emergency eradication programs, 599
  of feed additives, 28, 968
  Newcastle disease and, 558-59, 560
  reportable diseases, 27-28
Grain fumigants, 788
Granulomatous disorders, 294, 298
  coligranuloma, 131, 136, 138
Granulosa cell tumors, of ovary, 415, 443
Granulosa-theca cell tumors, 492-93, 494
Gray eye, 369, 382, 384, 395
Gray virus, 721
Green livers, in turkeys, 247, 250, 294

Green muscle disease, 923-24
Grounds, sanitation and cleanup, 17
Grouse disease, 822
Growth rate
  acute death syndrome and, 930
  dyschondroplasia and, 919
  reoviruses and, 712
  right ventricular failure and, 928
  toxic substances and, 979
Guinea fowl, fulminating disease of, 1031-32
Guinea worm, 843
Gynandroblastomas, 494

Haemophilus avium, 180, 181
Haemophilus gallinarum, 179
Haemophilus paragallinarum. See Infectious coryza
Haemoproteus infections, 904-5
  insect vectors, 796, 800, 904, 905
  in intracellular duck infection, 294
  quinacrine treatment, 983
Halofuginone, 875, 876, 877
  toxicity, 983
  in turkeys, 881
Haloxon, 845
Hatchery sanitation, 19-21, 25-26, 139
Hatching eggs
  antibiotic treatment
    for mycoplasmas, 23, 202, 215-16
    for *Salmonella arizonae,* 126
  clean hatchery management, 19-21, 25-26, 139
  fumigation, 20, 26, 39-40
    E. coli and, 139
    Salmonella and, 85
    Streptococcus and, 301
    toxicity, 990-91
  hatchability
    in aflatoxicosis, 961
    in ochratoxicosis, 963
    vitamin D and, 52
  heating to destroy mycoplasmas, 23, 202, 215
  sources of, 20
  storage, 26-27
  warming to prevent sweating, 26
  washing and liquid sterilization, 26, 41
Head picking, 913
Heart attack. *See* Acute death syndrome; Cardiovascular disorders
Heart puncture, 30
Heat prostration, 914
Heavy metal poisoning, 986-87
Helicobacter pamatensis, 290
Helicobacter pullorum, 290
Helicopter disease, 1016
Helminthosporium maydis, 967
Hemangiomas
  clinical characteristics, 440-42
  differential diagnosis, 455
  incidence, 416
  in laboratory host systems, 424
  in nephromas, 443
  viral strains causing, 426, 427
Hemangiopericytomas, 504-5
Hemangiosarcomas, 416

ISBN 0-8138-0427-2

90000>